THE
MERCK
MANUAL

FOURTEENTH EDITION

1st Edition – 1899
2nd Edition – 1901
3rd Edition – 1905
4th Edition – 1911
5th Edition – 1923
6th Edition – 1934
7th Edition – 1940

8th Edition – 1950
9th Edition – 1956
10th Edition – 1961
11th Edition – 1966
12th Edition – 1972
13th Edition – 1977
14th Edition – 1982

VOLUME I

GENERAL MEDICINE

FOURTEENTH EDITION

THE

MERCK
MANUAL

OF

DIAGNOSIS AND THERAPY

VOLUME I

GENERAL MEDICINE

Robert Berkow, M.D., *Editor-in-Chief*

Editorial Board

Donald C. Bondy, M.D.
Philip K. Bondy, M.D.
Alvan R. Feinstein, M.D.
Alfred P. Fishman, M.D.
Robert A. Hoekelman, M.D.

John W. Ormsby, M.D.
Robert G. Petersdorf, M.D.
G. Victor Rossi, Ph.D.
George E. Schreiner, M.D.
John H. Talbott, M.D.

Published by
MERCK SHARP & DOHME RESEARCH LABORATORIES

Division of
MERCK & CO., INC.
Rahway, N.J.

1982

MERCK & CO., INC.
Rahway, N.J.
U.S.A.

MERCK SHARP & DOHME
West Point, Pa.

MERCK SHARP & DOHME INTERNATIONAL
Rahway, N.J.

MERCK SHARP & DOHME RESEARCH LABORATORIES
Rahway, N.J.   *West Point, Pa.*

MSD AGVET DIVISION
Rahway, N.J.

HUBBARD FARMS, INC.
Walpole, N.H.

MERCK CHEMICAL MANUFACTURING DIVISION
Rahway, N.J.

MERCK CHEMICAL DIVISION
Rahway, N.J.

ALGINATE INDUSTRIES LIMITED
London, England

BALTIMORE AIRCOIL COMPANY, INC.
Baltimore, Md.

CALGON CORPORATION
Pittsburgh, Pa.

KELCO DIVISION
San Diego, Calif.

Library of Congress Catalog Card Number 1–31760
ISBN Number 911910–04–2
ISSN Number 0076–6526

First Printing—June 1982
Second Printing—March 1983
Third Printing—April 1984

Printed in the U. S. A.

FOREWORD TO VOLUMES I AND II

These two volumes together contain all of the 14th Edition of THE MERCK MANUAL, with the text rearranged to solve a problem most often encountered by medical students and house officers, to whom these volumes are specifically dedicated. THE MANUAL—probably the most widely used medical text in the world—has steadily grown in size and become too large to be carried conveniently in a jacket pocket or small medical bag. Dividing the book into two smaller volumes provides greater portability for those users who are constantly confronted with a variety of complex problems and need instant access to a pocket-sized reference text.

The objectives of THE MERCK MANUAL have always been ambitious. It covers not only disorders of interest to general internists, but also clinical pharmacology, psychiatry, ophthalmology, otorhinolaryngology, dermatology, dental disorders, special subjects (e.g., clinical procedures, laboratory medicine, radiation reactions and injuries, dental emergencies, and biostatistics), obstetrics, gynecology, and pediatrics. Since the book is used worldwide, more subjects are covered than would be required for a purely domestic text. Furthermore, disease discussions include relevant data about incidence, epidemiology, etiology, pathophysiology, symptoms and signs, and laboratory data, as well as differential diagnosis and treatment. Review of the physical examination, the analysis of symptoms and signs, and the approach to patients with various types of disorders, as well as basic information about major technologic advances, are also discussed in detail. Despite this extraordinary coverage, the size of the book has been well controlled, but achieving pocket-size required a new approach.

Rather than sacrifice coverage, we are offering our readers more choices. The 14th Edition is available in a single volume with a hard cover, as in the past. Additionally, the book has been divided into these two smaller volumes: Volume I covers General Medicine and related subspecialty subjects, while Volume II is limited mainly to Gynecology, Obstetrics, Pediatrics, and Genetics. Some subjects (e.g., poisoning, tables of laboratory values, weights and measures, and certain disease discussions) are reproduced in *both* volumes, for the convenience of the user.

Abbreviations and symbols, used liberally as essential space savers, are listed on pp. xl and xli.

The basic quality of the text, which relates to the excellence of our Editorial Board and distinguished authors, as well as to extensive review procedures, remains the same in the two smaller volumes as that in the single, larger text. We hope you will find these smaller volumes to be of value.

Robert Berkow, M.D.

NOTICE

The authors, reviewers, editors, and publisher of these books have made extensive efforts to ensure that treatments, drugs, and dosage regimens are accurate and conform to the standards accepted at the time of publication. However, constant changes in information resulting from continuing research and clinical experience, reasonable differences in opinions among authorities, unique aspects of individual clinical situations, and the possibility of human error in preparing such an extensive text require that the reader exercise individual judgment when making a clinical decision and, if necessary, consult and compare information from other sources. In particular, the reader is advised to check the product information included in each package of a drug product before prescribing or administering it, especially if the drug is unfamiliar or is used infrequently.

FOREWORD TO EDITION 14

THE MERCK MANUAL first appeared in 1899 as a slender 262-page text titled MERCK'S MANUAL OF THE MATERIA MEDICA. It was expressly designed to meet the needs of general practitioners in selecting medications, noting that "memory is treacherous" and even the most thoroughly informed physician needs a reminder "to make him at once master of the situation and enable him to prescribe exactly what his judgment tells him is needed for the occasion." It was well received and, by the 6th Edition (1934), THE MERCK MANUAL had become highly valued by medical students and house staff also; by the end of World War II the pocket-sized manual was an established favorite ready-reference. Today THE MANUAL is the most widely used medical text in the world. While the book has grown to about 2500 pages, its primary purpose remains the same—to provide useful information to practicing physicians, medical students, interns, residents, and other health professionals.

Fewer physicians now attempt to manage the whole range of medical disorders that can occur in infants, children, and adults, but those who do must have available a broad spectrum of current and accurate information. The specialist requires precise information about subjects outside his area of expertise. All physicians need more and more information for study and examination purposes as well as for patient care. THE MERCK MANUAL continues to try to meet these needs, excluding only details of surgical procedures.

Precisely how do we attempt to meet these needs? First, from a disease orientation, THE MANUAL covers all but the most obscure disorders of mankind, not only those that a general internist might expect to encounter, but also problems of pregnancy and delivery, the more common and serious disorders of neonates, infants, and children, and many special situations. Disorders are mainly organized according to the organ systems primarily affected, on the basis of their etiology (as with most of the infectious diseases and disorders due to physical agents), or on the basis of disciplines (e.g., gynecology, obstetrics, pediatrics, genetics, psychiatry). In addition, THE MANUAL contains information for special circumstances, such as radiation reactions and injuries, problems encountered in deep-sea diving, or dental emergencies. New subjects continue to be added, such as discussions of the principles of clinical biostatistics, Legionnaires' disease, toxic shock syndrome, and geriatric disorders. In fact, this edition has about 400 pages (approximately 20%) more text than the preceding edition. We therefore urge you to check the Index whenever you require information, even on unusual subjects or those not commonly found in other texts.

A completely disease-oriented compendium, however, would have serious limitations. Since patients usually present with complaints or concerns that must be meticulously described, sorted, and deciphered, many chapters are devoted to discussions of symptoms and signs and how to elicit the historical and physical data required for diagnosis. Common clinical procedures and laboratory tests used as diagnostic and management aids are described and are supplemented with information on proper specimen collection and handling. As new and sophisticated laboratory and technologic procedures come forth (e.g., computerized tomography, isotope scanning, ultrasound, mediastinoscopy), they are also described, with comments on their uses, interpretations, and limitations.

Current therapy is presented for each disorder and supplemented with a separate section on clinical pharmacology that describes general principles, new advances (e.g., the role of drug receptors, plasma concentration monitoring), details of pharmacologic groups and specific agents, and even suggestions for prescription writing and the use of placebos. When complex equipment (e.g., respirators, dialyzers) is involved, it is also described. Prophylaxis is emphasized wherever possible. Finally, reference guides are provided for checking normal values, calculating dosages, and converting weights, measures, and volumes to metric equivalents.

Can so many subjects be covered adequately in a single book? You, the reader, must make the ultimate judgment, but we believe the answer is in the affirmative. This edition required a concerted effort by many people, beginning with an internal analysis and critique of the previous edition, even though it enjoyed highly favorable reviews and outstanding reader acceptance. Almost every section of that book was then sent to outside experts, who had had nothing to do with its preparation, to solicit their most candid criticism. Published reviews and letters received from readers were analyzed. Next, the Editorial Board met to compare reviews and critiques and to plan this 14th Edition. Distinguished special consultants were enlisted to provide additional expertise. Then, 272 authors with outstanding qualifications, experience, and knowledge were engaged. Their manuscripts were edited repeatedly in-house to retain every valuable morsel of knowledge while eliminating sometimes elegant, but unneeded, words. Each manuscript was then reviewed by a member of the Editorial Board or a consultant. In many cases, additional special reviewers were invited to comment. Every mention of a drug and its dosage was reviewed by a separate outside consultant. The objectives of all these reviews were to ensure adequate and relevant coverage of each subject, accuracy, and simple and clean exposition. The authors then reworked, modified, and polished their manuscripts. Almost all of the manuscripts were revised at least 6 times; 15 to 20 revisions were not uncommon. We believe that no other medical text undergoes as many reviews and revisions as THE MERCK MANUAL.

The foregoing is a simplified review of the complex, arduous, and rewarding 4½-year enterprise that culminates in the presentation of this 14th Edition of THE MERCK MANUAL. The members of the Editorial Board, special consultants, contributing authors, and in-house editorial staff and their affiliations are listed on the pages that follow. They deserve a degree of gratitude that cannot be adequately expressed here, but we know they will feel sufficiently rewarded if their efforts serve your needs.

We hope this edition of THE MERCK MANUAL will be a welcome aid to you, our readers—compatible with your needs and worthy of frequent use. Suggestions for improvements will be warmly welcomed and carefully considered.

Robert Berkow, M.D., *Editor-in-Chief*
MERCK SHARP & DOHME RESEARCH LABORATORIES
West Point, Pa. 19486

CONTENTS

Volume I

GENERAL MEDICINE

(For Contents of Volume II, see page xxxiii)

§1. INFECTIOUS AND PARASITIC DISEASES *(Cont'd)*

§1. INFECTIOUS AND PARASITIC DISEASES *(Cont'd)*

§2. IMMUNOLOGY; ALLERGIC DISORDERS

§3.   CARDIOVASCULAR DISORDERS *(Cont'd)*

§4.   PULMONARY DISORDERS

§4. PULMONARY DISORDERS *(Cont'd)*

§5. GASTROINTESTINAL DISORDERS

§5.   GASTROINTESTINAL DISORDERS *(Cont'd)*

§6.   HEPATIC AND BILIARY DISORDERS

§8. ENDOCRINE DISORDERS *(Cont'd)*

§11. NEUROLOGIC DISORDERS

§13.   RENAL AND UROLOGIC DISORDERS *(Cont'd)*

§17. DERMATOLOGIC DISORDERS (Cont'd)

§21. CLINICAL PHARMACOLOGY *(Cont'd)*

CONTENTS

Volume II
GYNECOLOGY
OBSTETRICS
PEDIATRICS
GENETICS

(For Contents of Volume I, see page ix)

§3. PEDIATRICS *(Cont'd)*

ABBREVIATIONS AND SYMBOLS

ACTH	adrenocorticotropic hormone	HLA	human leukocyte group A
ADH	antidiuretic hormone	Hz	hertz (cycles/second)
ADP	adenosine diphosphate	ICF	intracellular fluid
ASO	antistreptolysin O (titer)	IgA, etc.	immunoglobulin A, etc.
ATP	adenosine triphosphate	IM	intramuscular(ly)
BCG	Bacillus Calmette-Guerin (vaccine)	IPPB	inspiratory positive pressure breathing
b.i.d.	2 times a day	IU	international unit
BMR	basal metabolic rate	IV	intravenous(ly)
BP	blood pressure	IVP	intravenous pyelogram
BSA	body surface area	K	potassium
BSP	sulfobromophthalein	kcal	kilocalorie (food calorie)
BUN	blood urea nitrogen	kg	kilogram
C	Celsius; centigrade; complement	17-KGS	17-ketogenic steroids
		17-KS	17-ketosteroids
Ca	Calcium	L	liter
CBC	complete blood count	lb	pound
CF	complement fixation, fixating	LDH	lactic dehydrogenase
Ch.	chapter	LE	lupus erythematosus
Ci	curie	m	meter
Cl	chloride; chlorine	M	molar
cm	centimeter	mCi	millicurie
CNS	central nervous system	MCH	mean corpuscular hemoglobin
CO	carbon monoxide; cardiac output	MCHC	mean corpuscular hemoglobin concentration
CO_2	carbon dioxide	MCV	mean corpuscular volume
CPK	creatine phosphokinase	mEq	milliequivalent
CPR	cardiopulmonary resuscitation	mg	milligram
CSF	cerebrospinal fluid	Mg	magnesium
CT	computed tomography	MIC	minimum inhibitory concentration
cu	cubic	min	minute
cu mm	cubic millimeter	mIU	milli-international unit
D & C	dilation and curettage	ml	milliliter
dl	deciliter ($=100$ ml)	MLD	minimum lethal dose
DNA	deoxyribonucleic acid	mm	millimeter
DTP	diphtheria-tetanus-pertussis (toxoids/vaccine)	mM	millimole
		mo	month
D/W	dextrose in water	mol wt	molecular weight
ECF	extracellular fluid	mOsm	milliosmole
ECG	electrocardiogram	MRC	Medical Research Council (units)
EEG	electroencephalogram		
ENT	ear, nose, and throat	N	nitrogen; normal (strength of solution)
ESR	erythrocyte sedimentation rate		
F	Fahrenheit	Na	sodium
FDA	U.S. Food and Drug Administration	ng	nanogram ($=$millimicrogram)
		nm	nanometer ($=$millimicron)
ft	foot; feet (measure)	17-OHCS	17-hydroxycorticosteroids
FUO	fever of unknown origin	OTC	over-the-counter (pharmaceuticals)
GFR	glomerular filtration rate		
GI	gastrointestinal	oz	ounce
gm	gram	P	phosphorus; pressure
G6PD	glucose-6-phosphate dehydrogenase	P_{CO_2}	carbon dioxide pressure (or tension)
GU	genitourinary	P_{O_2}	oxygen pressure (or tension)
h	hour	Pa_{CO_2}	arterial carbon dioxide pressure
HA	hemagglutination, hemagglutinating	Pa_{O_2}	arterial oxygen pressure
		PA_{O_2}	alveolar oxygen pressure
Hb	hemoglobin	pg	picogram ($=$micromicrogram)
HCl	hydrochloric acid; hydrochloride	pH	hydrogen-ion concentration
		p o	orally
HCO_3	bicarbonate	PPD	Purified Protein Derivative (tuberculin)
Hct	hematocrit		
Hg	mercury	ppm	parts per million
HI	hemagglutination-inhibition, inhibiting	p.r.n.	as needed

psi	pounds per square inch	tsp	teaspoon
PSP	phenolsulfonphthalein	u.	unit
q	every	URI	upper respiratory infection
q 4 h, etc.	every 4 hours, etc.	USPHS	United States Public Health
q.i.d.	4 times a day		Service
R, r	roentgen	UTI	urinary tract infection
RA	rheumatoid arthritis	WBC	white blood cell
RBC	red blood cell	WHO	World Health Organization
RF	rheumatic fever; rheumatoid	wk	week
	factor	wt	weight
RNA	ribonucleic acid	yr	year
Sa_{O_2}	arterial oxygen saturation	μ	micro-
SBE	subacute bacterial endocarditis	μm	micrometer; micron
s.c.	subcutaneous(ly)	$m\mu$	millimicron ($=$nanometer)
SGOT	serum glutamic oxaloacetic	μCi	microcurie
	transaminase	μg	microgram
SGPT	serum glutamic pyruvic	μmol	micromole
	transaminase	μOsm	micro-osmole
SLE	systemic lupus erythematosus	/	per
sp gr	specific gravity	$<$	less than
sq	square	$>$	more than
sq m	square meter	$\leq$	equal to or less than
STS	serologic test(s) for syphilis	$\geq$	equal to or more than
TB	tuberculosis	$\cong$	approximately equal to
tbsp	tablespoon	$\pm$	plus or minus
t.i.d.	3 times a day	§	section

EDITOR-IN-CHIEF

CONSULTANTS

J. Julian Chisolm, Jr., M.D.
Associate Professor of Pediatrics, Johns Hopkins University; Program Director, Lead Poisoning Division, The John F. Kennedy Institute for Handicapped Children

Lead Poisoning

John J. Condemi, M.D.
Professor of Medicine and Director of Clinical Immunology, University of Rochester

Immunology; Allergic Disorders

Ralph E. Cutler, M.D.
Professor of Medicine, Loma Linda University

Renal and Urologic Disorders

George E. Downs, Pharm.D.
Associate Professor of Clinical Pharmacy, Philadelphia College of Pharmacy and Science

Pharmaceutical Preparations and Dosages

Eugene P. Frenkel, M.D.
Professor of Internal Medicine and Radiology; Chief, Division of Hematology-Oncology, University of Texas Health Science Center at Dallas

Hematologic Disorders

G. Peter Halberg, M.D.
Clinical Professor of Ophthalmology, New York Medical College; Chief, Glaucoma Service, St. Vincent's Hospital and Medical Center of New York

Glaucoma; Contact Lenses

Charles S. Houston, M.D.
Professor of Environmental Health and Professor of Medicine (Emeritus), University of Vermont

Disorders Due to Physical Agents

Louis Lasagna, M.D.
Professor of Pharmacology and Toxicology and of Medicine, University of Rochester

Clinical Pharmacology

Harold I. Lief, M.D.
Professor of Psychiatry, University of Pennsylvania

Sexually Related Disorders

Fred Plum, M.D.
Anne Parrish Titzell Professor of Neurology, Cornell University; Neurologist-in-Chief, New York Hospital

Neurologic Disorders

Hal B. Richerson, M.D.
Professor of Internal Medicine and Director of Allergy/Immunology Division, University of Iowa

Immunology; Allergic Disorders

John Romano, M.D., D.Sc. (Hon.)
Distinguished University Professor of Psychiatry (Emeritus), University of Rochester

Psychiatric Disorders

Ruth W. Schwartz, M.D.
Clinical Associate Professor of Obstetrics and Gynecology, University of Rochester

Gynecology and Obstetrics

EDITORIAL STAFF

CONTRIBUTORS
Volume I

Hagop S. Akiskal, M.D.
Professor of Psychiatry, Associate Professor of Pharmacology, and Director of Mood Clinic and Affective Disorders Program, University of Tennessee, and Sleep Disorders Center, Baptist Memorial Hospital

Affective Disorders

James K. Alexander, M.D.
Professor of Medicine, Baylor College of Medicine; Chief of Cardiology, Ben Taub General Hospital

Thromboembolism and Infarction

Richard F. Bakemeier, M.D.
Professor of Oncology in Medicine and Associate Director (Educational Programs), Cancer Center, University of Rochester

Tumor Immunology

Joseph A. Baldone, M.D.
Associate Professor of Ophthalmology and Director, Contact Lens Service, Louisiana State University

Eye Disorders

Charlotte F. Baum, B.S., M.A.
Associate Director, School of Physiotherapy, Chaim Sheba Medical Center, Tel-Hashomer, Israel

Special Procedures—Pulmonary

Gerald L. Baum, M.D.
Professor of Medicine, Tel-Aviv University; Director, Pulmonary Division, Chaim Sheba Medical Center, Tel-Hashomer, Israel

Special Procedures—Pulmonary

Laurence H. Beck, M.D.
Associate Professor of Medicine and Associate Chairman, Department of Medicine, University of Pennsylvania

Diuretics

Robert Berkow, M.D.
Editor-in-Chief, THE MERCK MANUAL; Clinical Professor of Medicine and of Psychiatry, Hahnemann Medical College

Toxic Shock Syndrome; Psychiatry in Medicine

Richard W. Besdine, M.D.
Assistant Professor of Medicine, Harvard University; Director of Geriatric Education, Hebrew Rehabilitation Center for Aged

Geriatric Medicine

Don C. Bienfang, M.D.
Assistant Professor of Ophthalmology, Harvard University

Nystagmus; Extraocular Muscle Palsies; Optic Nerve and Visual Pathways

Walter D. Birnbaum, M.D.
Clinical Professor (Emeritus), University of California, San Francisco

Neoplasms of the Bowel; Anorectal Disorders

F. William Blaisdell, M.D.
Professor and Chairman, Department of Surgery, University of California, Davis

Acute Respiratory Distress Syndrome

Harvey Blank, M.D.
Professor and Chairman, Department of Dermatology, University of Miami

Dermatologic Disorders; Reactions to Sunlight

M. Donald Blaufox, M.D., Ph.D.
Professor of Radiology (Nuclear Medicine) and Professor of Medicine; Director, Divisions of Nuclear Medicine, Albert Einstein College of Medicine

Radiation Reactions and Injuries; Diagnostic Use of Radioisotopes

Rodney Bluestone, M.B., F.R.C.P.
Clinical Professor of Medicine, University of California, Los Angeles

Vasculitis; Polyarteritis

Donald C. Bondy, M.D.
Professor of Medicine, University of Western Ontario, London, Canada

Gastrointestinal Disorders—Introduction

William K. Bottomley, D.D.S., M.S.
Professor and Chairman, Department of Oral Diagnosis, Georgetown University

Teeth and Dental Structures; Common Disorders of the Lips and Mouth; Stomatitis; Dental Caries and Its Complications; Periodontal Disease; Preneoplastic and Neoplastic Lesions

Bernard B. Brody, M.D.
Director of Clinical Laboratories, The Genesee Hospital

Laboratory Medicine

F. E. Bruckner, M.B., F.R.C.P.
Director, Department of Rheumatology, St. George's Hospital; Senior Lecturer, University of London, London, England

Neurogenic Arthropathy

Roger J. Bulger, M.D.
President, University of Texas Health Science Center at Houston; Professor of Medicine, University of Texas, Houston

Rat-Bite Fever

George E. Burch, M.D.
Henderson Professor of Medicine (Emeritus),
Tulane University

Myocardial Disease

Benjamin Burrows, M.D.
Professor of Internal Medicine and Director, Division of Respiratory Sciences, University of Arizona

Acute Bronchitis; Chronic Obstructive Pulmonary Disease

Eric D. Caine, M.D.
Assistant Professor of Psychiatry and Neurology, University of Rochester

Neuropsychiatric Syndromes in Organic Cerebral Disease

Burton V. Caldwell, M.D., Ph.D.
Assistant Professor of Medicine and Obstetrics and Gynecology, Yale University

Hypothalamic–Pituitary Relationships; Pituitary

Duncan Catterall, M.D., F.R.C.P.E., F.R.C.P.
Director, James Pringle House, Middlesex Hospital; Medical Teacher, University of London, London, England

Sexually Transmitted Disease

Lawrence N. Chessin, M.D.
Clinical Associate Professor of Medicine, University of Rochester; Head, Infectious Disease Unit, Genesee Hospital

Osteomyelitis

Alan S. Cohen, M.D.
Chief of Medicine and Director, Thorndike Memorial Laboratory, Boston City Hospital; Conrad Wesselhoeft Professor of Medicine, Boston University

Amyloidosis

Sidney Cohen, M.D.
T. Grier Miller Professor of Medicine and Chief, Gastrointestinal Service, University of Pennsylvania

Disorders of the Esophagus

Bentley P. Colcock, M.D., F.R.C.S.I. (H)
Senior Surgeon Emeritus, Lahey Clinic; Associate Clinical Professor of Surgery, Boston University

Diverticular Disease

John J. Condemi, M.D.
Professor of Medicine and Director of Clinical Immunology, University of Rochester

Immunology and Allergic Disorders—Introduction; Biology of the Immune System; Hypersensitivity Reactions

Alastair M. Connell, M.D.
Professor of Internal Medicine and Dean, College of Medicine, University of Nebraska

Bowel Obstruction; Appendicitis; Meckel's Diverticulum; Peritonitis

Lawrence Corey, M.D.
Assistant Professor, Laboratory Medicine, Microbiology and Immunology; Adjunct Assistant Professor of Medicine and Pediatrics, University of Washington

Antimicrobial Chemoprophylaxis

Russell L. Corio, D.D.S., M.S.D.
Chairman, Department of Oral Pathology, Armed Forces Institute of Pathology

Oral Preneoplastic and Neoplastic Lesions

A. Benedict Cosimi, M.D.
Associate Professor of Surgery, Harvard University; Chief, Clinical Transplant Surgery and Associate Visiting Surgeon, Massachusetts General Hospital

Transplantation

Ralph E. Cutler, M.D.
Professor of Medicine, Loma Linda University

Renal Structure and Function; Clinical Evaluation of Genitourinary Disorders; Renal Failure; The Glomerular Diseases; Tubulointerstitial Disease; Acute and Chronic Bacterial Pyelonephritis; Vascular Disease; Cystic Disorders; Hereditary Chronic Nephropathies

David C. Dale, M.D.
Professor of Medicine, University of Washington

Infections in the Compromised Host

W. Howard Davis, D.D.S.
Clinical Professor of Oral Surgery, University of Southern California; Consultant, Long Beach VA Hospital, Long Beach Naval Hospital, and Loma Linda University

Dental Emergencies

Norman L. Dean, M.D.
Associate Clinical Professor of Medicine, Yale University; Director, Pulmonary Medicine, Griffin Hospital

Near-Drowning

Ronald Dee, M.D.
Assistant Clinical Professor of Surgery, Albert Einstein College of Medicine; Visiting Surgeon, Bronx Municipal Hospital Center, and Attending Surgeon, United Hospital

Varicose Veins

Roger M. Des Prez, M.D.
Professor of Medicine, Vanderbilt University; Chief, Medical Service, VA Hospital, Nashville

Tuberculosis; Other Mycobacterial Infections Resembling Tuberculosis

Victor G. deWolfe, M.D.
Senior Physician, Department of Peripheral Vascular Disease; Director, Vascular Laboratory, Cleveland Clinic Foundation

Peripheral Vascular Disorders

Eugene P. DiMagno, M.D.
Professor of Medicine, Mayo Medical School; Consultant in Gastroenterology and Internal Medicine, Mayo Clinic

Cancer of the Pancreas

Gerald S. Dowdy, Jr., M.D.
Baylor College of Medicine

Extrahepatic Biliary Disorders

Eugenie F. Doyle, M.D.
Professor of Pediatrics; Director of Pediatric Cardiology, New York University

Valvular Heart Disease

Douglas Drossman, M.D.
Assistant Professor of Medicine and Psychiatry, University of North Carolina

Functional Dyspepsia and Other Nonspecific Gastrointestinal Complaints

Edward M. Druy, M.D.
Associate Professor of Radiology and Head, Vascular Radiology and Special Procedures, George Washington University

Computerized Transverse Tomography

Edmund L. Dubois, M.D.
Clinical Professor of Medicine, University of Southern California

Discoid Lupus Erythematosus; Systemic Lupus Erythematosus

Robert B. Duthie, M.A., Ch.M., F.R.C.S. (Ed.), F.R.C.S. (Eng.)
Nuffield Professor of Orthopaedic Surgery, University of Oxford; Consultant Advisor in Orthopaedic Surgery, Department of Health and Social Security, England

Bursitis; Tendinitis and Tenosynovitis; Fibromyositis; Spasmodic Torticollis; Neck, Shoulder, and Upper Limb Pain; Low Back Pain and Sciatica

Elliot F. Ellis, M.D.
Professor and Chairman, Department of Pediatrics, State University of New York at Buffalo

Bronchial Asthma

Kent Ellis, M.D.
Professor of Radiology, Columbia University

Radiology

Karl Engelman, M.D.
Associate Professor of Medicine and Pharmacology; Chief, Hypertension and Clinical Pharmacology Section; Director, Clinical Research Center, University of Pennsylvania

Syncope; Orthostatic Hypotension

Carl D. Enna, M.D.
Associate Clinical Professor, Department of Anatomy, Louisiana State University; Senior Member, Clinical Branch and Chief of Surgery, USPHS Hospital (National Leprosarium)

Leprosy

Richard J. Falk, M.D.
Associate Professor and Head, Division of Reproductive Endocrinology and Infertility, Georgetown University; Head, Infertility Clinic, Columbia Hospital for Women

Hypothalamic–Pituitary Relationships; Pituitary

Harvey Feigenbaum, M.D.
Distinguished Professor of Medicine, Indiana University

Ultrasound

Alvan R. Feinstein, M.D.
Professor of Medicine and Epidemiology, Yale University

Streptococcal Infections; Biostatistics for Clinicians

Robert Fekety, M.D.
Professor of Internal Medicine and Physician-in-Charge, Section of Infectious Disease, University of Michigan

Staphylococcal Infections

Stuart C. Finch, M.D.
Professor of Medicine, Rutgers Medical School, Camden; Chief of Medicine, Cooper Medical Center

Leukopenia

Gerald Finerman, M.D.
Professor of Surgery (Orthopaedics), University of California, Los Angeles

Osteitis Deformans

Maxwell Finland, M.D.
Distinguished Physician, VA; George Richards Minot Professor of Medicine (Emeritus), Harvard University; Epidemiology Consultant, Boston City Hospital

Pneumococcal Infections; Pneumonia; Mycoplasmal Pneumonia

Murray M. Fisher, M.D., Ph.D.
Associate Professor of Medicine and Pathology, University of Toronto; Head, Division of Gastroenterology, Sunnybrook Medical Centre, Toronto, Ontario, Canada

Laboratory Evaluation of the Liver and Biliary System; Fatty Liver; Fibrosis and Cirrhosis; Liver Disease Due to Alcohol; Vascular Lesions of the Liver

Alfred P. Fishman, M.D.
William Maul Measey Professor of Medicine, Director of Cardiovascular–Pulmonary Division of Department of Medicine, University of Pennsylvania; Attending Physician, Hospital of the University of Pennsylvania

Approach to the Pulmonary Patient

Lawrence Fleckenstein, Pharm.D.
Department of Pharmacology, Division of Experimental Therapeutics, Walter Reed Army Institute of Research

Drug Absorption and Bioavailability; Drug Distribution; Antiemetics

Noble O. Fowler, M.D.
Professor of Medicine and Director, Division of Cardiology, University of Cincinnati

Pericardial Disease

Irwin N. Frank, M.D.
Professor of Urology, University of Rochester

Renal and Urologic Disorders—Neoplasms; Lower Urinary Tract and Male Genital Tract Infections; Obstructive Uropathies; Myoneurogenic Disorders; Urinary Incontinence; Male Genital Lesions; Genitourinary Trauma

Emil Frei, III, M.D.
Professor of Medicine, Harvard University; Director and Physician-in-Chief, Sidney Farber Cancer Institute

Lymphoma

Eugene P. Frenkel, M.D.
Professor of Internal Medicine and Radiology and Chief, Division of Hematology–Oncology, University of Texas Health Science Center at Dallas

Anemias

Gerald Friedman, M.D., Ph.D.
Assistant Clinical Professor of Medicine, Mt. Sinai School of Medicine

The Irritable Bowel Syndrome

Peter L. Frommer, M.D.
Deputy Director, National Heart, Lung, and Blood Institute

Sudden Cardiac Death

William A. Frosch, M.D.
Professor and Vice Chairman, Department of Psychiatry, Cornell University; Medical Director, Payne Whitney Clinic of The New York Hospital

Psychiatric Emergencies

Timothy S. Gee, M.D.
Associate Professor, Cornell University; Associate Attending Physician, Memorial Hospital; Associate, Memorial Sloan-Kettering Cancer Center

Leukemia

Michael C. Gelfand, M.D.
Associate Professor of Clinical Medicine and Co-Director, Hemodialysis, Hemoperfusion, and Transplantation Service, Georgetown University

Immunologically Mediated Renal Disease

Ray W. Gifford, Jr., M.D.
Head, Department of Hypertension and Nephrology, Cleveland Clinic Foundation

Hypertension

Martin Goldberg, M.D.
Taylor Professor of Medicine and Chairman, Department of Internal Medicine, University of Cincinnati

Diuretics

Peggy L. Goldman, M.D.
Instructor, University of Washington

Manifestations of Infection

Bruce N. Goldreyer, M.D.
Associate Clinical Professor of Medicine, University of Southern California; Director of Diagnostic Cardiology, San Pedro Peninsula Hospital

Cardiac Arrhythmias

M. Jay Goodkind, M.D.
Clinical Associate Professor of Medicine, University of Pennsylvania

Syphilis of the Cardiovascular System; Cardiac Tumors

Robert A. Goodwin, M.D.
Professor of Medicine (Emeritus), Vanderbilt University; formerly Chief, Pulmonary Disease Section, VA Hospital, Nashville

Tuberculosis; Other Mycobacterial Infections Resembling Tuberculosis

G. Peter Halberg, M.D.
Clinical Professor of Ophthalmology, New York Medical College; Chief, Glaucoma Service, St. Vincent's Hospital and Medical Center of New York

Glaucoma; Contact Lenses

Robert W. Hamilton, M.D.
Associate Professor of Medicine/Nephrology and Medical Director, Artificial Kidney Clinic, Bowman Gray School of Medicine

Dialysis; Hemoperfusion, Hemofiltration, and Hemodiafiltration

William J. Harrington, M.D.
Distinguished University Professor, Department of Medicine, University of Miami

Anticoagulants

Donald H. Harter, M.D.
Charles L. Mix Professor of Neurology and Chairman, Department of Neurology, Northwestern University; Chairman, Department of Neurology, Northwestern Memorial Hospital

Slow Virus Infections

Herbert B. Hechtman, M.D.
Senior Associate Professor of Surgery, Harvard University

Venous Cutdown and Cannulation; Measurement of Central Venous Pressure; Pulmonary Artery Catheterization; Pericardial Disease

Stephen E. Hedberg, M.D.
Assistant Clinical Professor in Surgery, Harvard University; Associate Visiting Surgeon and Senior Endoscopist in Gastrointestinal Surgery, Massachusetts General Hospital

Gastrointestinal Bleeding

Paul Henkind, M.D., Ph.D.
Dejur Professor and Chairman, Department of Ophthalmology, Albert Einstein College of Medicine; Director, Department of Ophthalmology, Montefiore Hospital and Medical Center

Retina

Elly P. Hershko, M.D.
Associate Director, Pulmonary Division, Chaim Sheba Medical Center, Tel-Hashomer, Israel

Special Procedures—Pulmonary

John Hetherington, Jr., M.D.
Clinical Professor of Ophthalmology, University of California, San Francisco

Eye Disorders

J. V. Hirschmann, M.D.
Assistant Professor of Medicine, University of Washington; Assistant Chief of Medicine, Seattle VA Medical Center

Superficial Infections; Abscesses

Roland G. Hiss, M.D.
Professor of Postgraduate Medicine and Health Professions Education and Associate Professor of Internal Medicine, University of Michigan

Hemorrhagic Disorders

Paul E. Hodgson, M.D.
Professor of Surgery and Chairman, Department of Surgery, University of Nebraska

Bowel Obstruction; Appendicitis; Meckel's Diverticulum; Peritonitis

Paul D. Hoeprich, M.D.
Professor of Medicine and Chief, Section of Infectious and Immunologic Diseases, University of California, Davis

Erysipeloid; Listeriosis

James W. Holcroft, M.D.
Associate Professor of Surgery, University of California, Davis

Acute Respiratory Distress Syndrome

Joseph H. Holmes, M.D. *(Deceased)*
Professor of Radiology and Medicine (Emeritus), University of Colorado

Diagnostic Ultrasonography

Richard B. Hornick, M.D.
Dewey Professor of Medicine and Chairman, Department of Medicine, University of Rochester

Salmonella Infections; Shigellosis; Tularemia; Leptospirosis

Charles S. Houston, M.D.
Professor of Environmental Health and Professor of Medicine (Emeritus), University of Vermont

Heat Disorders; Cold Injury; High-Altitude Illness

Kenneth A. Hubel, M.D.
Professor of Internal Medicine, University of Iowa

Pancreatitis

Douglas W. Huestis, M.D.
Professor of Pathology, University of Arizona

Blood Transfusion

Daniel A. Hussar, Ph.D.
Remington Professor of Pharmacy and Dean of Faculty, Philadelphia College of Pharmacy and Science

Modification of Drug Response

Harold L. Israel, M.D.
Professor of Medicine, Thomas Jefferson University

Sarcoidosis

George Gee Jackson, M.D.
Robert Wood Keeton Professor of Medicine; Chief, Section of Infectious Diseases, University of Illinois

Respiratory Viral Diseases

I Contributors

Harry S. Jacob, M.D.
Professor of Medicine and Chief, Section of Hematology, University of Minnesota

The Spleen

Ralph F. Jacox, M.D.
Professor of Medicine, University of Rochester; Head, Rheumatology Unit, Strong Memorial Hospital

Wegener's Granulomatosis

Pieter H. Joubert, M.B., B.Ch., F.C.P. (S.A.), D.M.
Professor and Chairman, Department of Pharmacology, Medical University of Southern Africa, Pretoria, South Africa

Modification of Drug Response

Robert J. Joynt, M.D., Ph.D.
Edward A. and Alma Vollertsen Rykenboer Professor of Neurophysiology and Chairman, Department of Neurology, University of Rochester; Neurologist-in-Chief, Strong Memorial Hospital

The Neurologic Examination; Neurologic Disorders—Diagnostic Procedures

Karl D. Kappus, Ph.D.
Center for Infectious Diseases, Centers for Disease Control, USPHS

Rabies

Fred E. Karch, M.D.
Clinical Assistant Professor of Pharmacology and Toxicology and of Medicine, University of Rochester

Topical Antiseptics; Antiviral Drugs; Antihistamines

Nathan G. Kase, M.D.
Professor of Obstetrics and Gynecology, Yale University

Hypothalamic–Pituitary Relationships; Pituitary

Stephen I. Katz, M.D., Ph.D.
Chief, Dermatology Branch, National Cancer Institute

Dermatologic Disorders; Reactions to Sunlight

Thomas Killip, M.D.
Professor of Clinical Medicine, University of Michigan; Chairman, Department of Medicine, Henry Ford Hospital

Congestive Heart Failure; Myocardial Ischemic Disorders

Barbara D. Kirby, M.D.
Assistant Professor of Medicine, University of Washington

Legionnaires' Disease

Lewis Landsberg, M.D.
Associate Professor of Medicine, Harvard University

Multiple Endocrine Neoplasia Syndromes

Edward H. Lanphier, M.D.
Senior Scientist, Department of Preventive Medicine; Assistant Director for Research, The Biotron, University of Wisconsin

Medical Aspects of Diving and Working in Compressed Air

Louis Lasagna, M.D.
Professor of Pharmacology and Toxicology and of Medicine, University of Rochester

Placebos

Daniel M. Laskin, D.D.S.
Professor and Head, Department of Oral and Maxillofacial Surgery, University of Illinois

Temporomandibular Joint Disorders

James B. Lee, M.D.
Professor of Medicine, State University of New York at Buffalo

Prostaglandins

Harvey Lemont, D.P.M.
Professor of Podiatric Medicine and Director, Laboratory of Podiatric Pathology, Pennsylvania College of Podiatric Medicine

Common Foot Disorders

Gerald S. Levey, M.D.
Professor and Chairman, Department of Medicine, University of Pittsburgh

Thyroid

Daniel Levinson, M.D.
Associate Professor, Department of Family and Community Medicine, University of Arizona

Medical Aspects of Air Travel

Michael D. Levitt, M.D.
Associate Chief of Staff for Research, VA Hospital, Minneapolis

Functional Bowel Disease—Gas

Robert I. Levy, M.D.
Director, National Heart, Lung, and Blood Institute

Anomalies in Lipid Metabolism

Pauline Lieberman, M.D.
Director, Intensive Care Unit, Chaim Sheba Medical Center; Instructor in Anesthesia and Intensive Care, Tel-Aviv University, Ramat-Aviv, Israel

Special Procedures—Pulmonary

Yair Lieberman, M.D.
Director, Thoracic Surgery Unit, Tel-Aviv University, Tel-Hashomer, Israel

Special Procedures—Pulmonary

Harold I. Lief, M.D.
Professor of Psychiatry, University of Pennsylvania

Psychosexual Disorders; The Medical Examination of the Rape Victim

Henry S. Loeb, M.D.
Professor of Medicine, Loyola University; Program Director in Cardiology, VA Hospital, Hines

Shock

Mortimer Lorber, D.M.D., M.D.
Associate Professor of Physiology and Biophysics, Georgetown University

Dentistry in Medicine; Approach to the Dental Patient

Stephen E. Malawista, M.D.
Professor of Medicine and Chief, Section of Rheumatology, Yale University

Lyme Disease

Richard G. Masson, M.D.
Chief, Pulmonary Medicine, Framingham Union Hospital; Assistant Professor of Medicine, Boston University

Pulmonary Function Tests

John H. McClement, M.D.
Professor of Medicine, New York University; Director, Chest Service, Bellevue Hospital Center

Bronchiectasis; Atelectasis

Donald S. McLaren, M.D., Ph.D., M.R.C.P.
Reader in Clinical Nutrition, Department of Medicine, The Royal Infirmary, Edinburgh, Scotland

Nutrition—General Considerations; Undernutrition; Vitamin Deficiency, Toxicity, and Dependency; Element Deficiency and Toxicity

Lewis A. Miller, B.A., M.S.
President, Miller Communications, Inc., Norwalk, Connecticut

Office Clinical Records

John A. Moncrief, M.D. *(Deceased)*
Professor of Surgery, University of Texas, San Antonio

Burns

John P. Morgan, M.D.
Medical Professor and Director of Pharmacology Program, Center for Biomedical Education, City University of New York; Associate Professor of Pharmacology and Medicine, Mt. Sinai School of Medicine

Drug Dependence; Prescription Writing; Antidepressants; General Central Nervous System Stimulants and Anorexiants; Sedatives and Hypnotics

W. K. C. Morgan, M.D., F.R.C.P. (Ed.), F.R.C.P. (C)
Professor of Medicine, University of Western Ontario; Director, Chest Diseases Service, University Hospital, London, Ontario, Canada

Occupational Lung Diseases

Roland W. Moskowitz, M.D.
Professor of Medicine, Case Western Reserve University; Director, Division of Rheumatic Diseases, University Hospitals

Osteoarthritis

Don H. Nelson, M.D.
Professor of Medicine and Head, Division of Endocrinology and Metabolism, University of Utah

Adrenal Hypofunction; Adrenal Cortical Hyperfunction; Nonfunctional Adrenal Masses; Corticotropin and Corticosteroids

John C. Nemiah, M.D.
Professor of Psychiatry, Harvard University; Psychiatrist-in-Chief, Beth Israel Hospital

The Neuroses

G. Richard O'Connor, M.D.
Professor of Ophthalmology; Director, Francis I. Proctor Foundation for Research in Ophthalmology, University of California, San Francisco

Uveal Tract

Stephen E. Oshrin, Ph.D.
Associate Professor of Audiology, University of Southern Mississippi

Hearing Aids

Carl M. Pearson, M.D.
Professor of Medicine and Director, Division of Rheumatology, University of California, Los Angeles; Co-Director, Jerry Lewis Neuromuscular Research Center

Ankylosing Spondylitis

Lawrence L. Pelletier, Jr., M.D.
Chief, Medical Service, American Lake VA Medical Center, Tacoma; Associate Professor of Medicine, University of Washington

Bacteroides and Mixed Anaerobic Infections

John A. Penner, M.D.
Professor of Internal Medicine and Director, Division of Hematology–Oncology, Michigan State University

Hemorrhagic Disorders

Peter L. Perine, M.D.
Medical Officer, International Health Programs Office, Centers for Disease Control, USPHS

Endemic Treponematoses; Relapsing Fever

Joseph K. Perloff, M.D.
Professor of Medicine and Pediatrics; Division of Cardiology, University of California, Los Angeles

An Approach to the Cardiac Patient

Robert G. Petersdorf, M.D.
Dean, School of Medicine, and Vice-Chancellor for Health Sciences, University of California, San Diego

Manifestations of Infection; Bacteremia and Septic Shock; Enterobacteriaceae Infections; Familial Mediterranean Fever

Hart deC. Peterson, M.D.
Clinical Associate Professor of Neurology and Pediatrics, New York Hospital–Cornell Medical Center

CNS Infections; Muscular Atrophies and Related Disorders

Marjorie C. Pfaudler, R.N., B.S., M.A., Nursing Education
Associate Professor of Nursing and of Preventive, Family, and Rehabilitation Medicine, University of Rochester

Gastrointestinal and Genitourinary Procedures; Aids for the Disabled Patient; Prevention of Infection—Barriers

Sidney F. Phillips, M.D.
Professor of Medicine, Mayo Medical School; Director, Gastroenterology Unit and Consultant in Gastroenterology, Mayo Clinic

Diarrhea; Constipation; Gastroenteritis: Infective and Toxic

Nathaniel F. Pierce, M.D.
Professor of Medicine, Johns Hopkins University

Cholera

James J. Plorde, M.D.
Professor of Medicine and Laboratory Medicine, University of Washington; Chief, Infectious Diseases and Clinical Microbiology, VA Hospital, Seattle

Bartonellosis; Parasitic Infections

Fred Plum, M.D.
Anne Parrish Titzell Professor of Neurology, Cornell University; Neurologist-in-Chief, New York Hospital

Common Neurologic Manifestations; Seizure Disorders; Sleep Disorders; Cerebrovascular Disease; Trauma of the Head and Spine

Douglas J. Pritchard, M.D.
Assistant Professor of Orthopedic Surgery, Mayo Medical School

Neoplasms of Bones and Joints

C. George Ray, M.D.
Professor of Pathology and Pediatrics, University of Arizona

Viral Diseases—General; Exanthematous Viral Diseases; Herpes Simplex

Stanley E. Read, M.D., Ph.D.
Associate Professor of Pediatrics, University of Toronto, Toronto, Ontario; Adjunct Associate Professor, The Rockefeller University

CNS Infections

Nathaniel Reichek, M.D.
Associate Professor of Medicine and Director, Non-invasive Laboratories, University of Pennsylvania

Phonocardiography

John D. Reid, M.D., F.R.A.C.P.
Professor of Pathology, Northeastern Ohio Universities College of Medicine; Pathology Department, Robinson Memorial Hospital

Carcinoid Syndrome

Eric Reiss, M.D.
Professor of Medicine, University of Miami

Vitamin D Deficiency and Dependency; Parathyroid Disorders

Hal B. Richerson, M.D.
Professor of Internal Medicine and Director of Allergy/Immunology Division, University of Iowa

Hypersensitivity Diseases of the Lungs

Safa M. Rifka, M.D.
Assistant Professor, Reproductive Endocrinology Division, Department of Obstetrics and Gynecology, Georgetown University and Columbia Hospital for Women

Hypothalamic–Pituitary Relationships; Pituitary

B. Lawrence Riggs, M.D.
Professor of Medicine, Mayo Medical School; Chairman, Division of Endocrinology and Metabolism, Mayo Clinic

Osteoporosis

Leonor Rivera-Calimlim, M.D.
Associate Professor, Department of Pharmacology and Toxicology; Assistant Professor, Department of Medicine, University of Rochester

Tranquilizers

William O. Robertson, M.D.
Acting Chairman, Department of Pediatrics, University of Washington; Director, Poison Control Center, Children's Orthopedic Hospital and Medical Center

Poisoning

Gerald P. Rodnan, M.D.
Professor of Medicine and Chief, Division of Rheumatology and Clinical Immunology, University of Pittsburgh

Progressive Systemic Sclerosis; Polymyositis and Dermatomyositis

Robert M. Rogers, M.D.
Professor of Medicine and Anesthesiology and Chief, Pulmonary Medicine, University of Pittsburgh

Cardiac Arrest and Cardiopulmonary Resuscitation; Pulmonary Alveolar Proteinosis

John Romano, M.D., D.Sc. (Hon.)
Distinguished University Professor of Psychiatry (Emeritus), University of Rochester

Psychiatric Disorders—Introduction; Schizophrenic Disorders; Paranoid Disorders

Norman Rosenberg, M.D.
Professor of Surgery, Rutgers Medical School; College of Medicine and Dentistry of New Jersey; Chief, Section of Vascular Surgery, Middlesex General Hospital

Varicose Veins

Harold P. Roth, M.D.
Associate Director for Digestive Diseases and Nutrition, National Institute of Arthritis, Metabolism, and Digestive Diseases

Gastritis; Peptic Ulcer; Malignant Neoplasms of the Stomach

Findlay E. Russell, M.D., Ph.D.
Research Professor, Department of Pharmacology and Toxicology, College of Pharmacy, University of Arizona

Venomous Bites and Stings

Paul S. Russell, M.D.
John Homans Professor of Surgery, Harvard University; Chief, Transplantation Unit, Massachusetts General Hospital

Transplantation

Edwin A. Rutsky, M.D.
Professor of Medicine, University of Alabama in Birmingham

Disturbances in Water, Electrolyte, Mineral, and Acid-Base Metabolism

David B. Sachar, M.D.
Associate Director, Division of Gastroenterology, Mt. Sinai Hospital; Associate Professor of Medicine, Mt. Sinai School of Medicine

Chronic Inflammatory Diseases of the Bowel; Pseudomembranous Enterocolitis

Jay P. Sanford, M.D.
Professor of Medicine and Dean, Uniformed Services University of the Health Sciences

Plague; Melioidosis; Chlamydial Diseases; Arbovirus and Arenavirus Diseases; Cat-Scratch Disease

Dennis R. Schaberg, M.D.
Assistant Professor of Medicine, University of Michigan

Pseudomonas Infections; Campylobacter fetus and Vibrio Infections

Kurt Schapira, M.D., F.R.C.P., F.R.C. Psych.
Department of Psychological Medicine, The Royal Victoria Infirmary, Newcastle upon Tyne, England

Suicidal Behavior

F. D. Schoenknecht, M.D.
Professor, Laboratory Medicine, Microbiology, and Immunology, University of Washington

Use of the Clinical Microbiology Laboratory

George E. Schreiner, M.D.
Professor of Medicine and Director, Division of Nephrology, Georgetown University

Nephrotic Syndrome; Nephrotoxic Disorders

H. Ralph Schumacher, M.D.
Professor of Medicine, University of Pennsylvania; Director, Rheumatology–Immunology Center, VAMC, Philadelphia

Approach to the Patient with Joint Disease; Rheumatoid Arthritis

Robert H. Schwartz, M.D.
Professor of Pediatrics, University of Rochester; Strong Memorial Hospital

Immunodeficiency Diseases

Seymour I. Schwartz, M.D.
Professor of Surgery, University of Rochester

Abdominal Pain

William R. Shapiro, M.D.
Professor of Neurology, Cornell University; Head, Laboratory of Neurological Oncology, Memorial Sloan-Kettering Cancer Center

CNS Neoplasms; Demyelinating Diseases

Gordon C. Sharp, M.D.
Professor of Medicine and Director, Division of Immunology–Rheumatology, University of Missouri, Columbia

Mixed Connective Tissue Disease

Martin A. Shearn, M.D.
Clinical Professor of Medicine, University of California, San Francisco; Director of Medical Education, Kaiser Permanente Medical Center, Oakland

Sjögren's Syndrome

James C. Shelburne, M.D.
Director, Cardiology Department, American Hospital in Paris, Neuilly-sur-Seine, France

Cardiac Catheterization; Angiography

Roger C. Sider, M.D.
Associate Professor of Psychiatry and Director, Adult Ambulatory Services, University of Rochester

The Psychiatric Interview

Fiorindo A. Simeone, M.D., Sc.D. (Hon.)
Professor of Medical Science (Emeritus), Brown University; Surgeon-in-Chief (Emeritus), Miriam Hospital

Arteriosclerosis and Atherosclerosis; Diseases of the Aorta and Its Branches

Jerome B. Simon, M.D., F.R.C.P. (C)
Associate Professor of Medicine, Queen's University, Kingston, Ontario; Head, Division of Gastroenterology, Kingston General Hospital

Hepatic and Biliary Disorders—Introduction; Clinical Features of Liver Disease; Morphologic Evaluation of Liver Disease; Hepatitis; Drugs and the Liver; Postoperative Liver Disease; Hepatic Neoplasms

David P. Simpson, M.D.
Professor of Medicine and Head, Nephrology Section, University of Wisconsin

Renal Disease Associated with Systemic and Metabolic Syndromes

Arthur T. Skarin, M.D.
Associate Professor of Medicine, Harvard University; Associate Physician, Sidney Farber Cancer Institute

Lymphoma

Charles B. Smith, M.D.
Professor of Medicine, University of Utah, and Chief of Medicine, VA Hospital, Salt Lake City

Infectious Arthritis; Reiter's Syndrome; Behçet's Syndrome

Lloyd H. Smith, Jr., M.D.
Professor of Medicine and Chairman, Department of Medicine, University of California, San Francisco

Urinary Calculi

Celia A. Snavely, M.S.W., A.C.S.W.
Nephrology Social Worker and Instructor, Bowman Gray School of Medicine

Psychosocial Aspects of Chronic Dialysis

Gordon L. Snider, M.D.
Professor of Medicine and Chief, Pulmonary Medicine Section, Boston University; Chief, Pulmonary Medicine Section, VA Hospital, Boston

Pleural Disorders; Pneumothorax

James B. Snow, Jr., M.D.
Professor and Chairman, Department of Otorhinolaryngology and Human Communication, University of Pennsylvania

Clinical Evaluation of Complaints Referable to the Ears; External Ear; Tympanic Membrane and Middle Ear; Inner Ear; Nose and Paranasal Sinuses; Nasopharynx; Oropharynx; Larynx; Motion Sickness

Selma E. Snyderman, M.D.
Professor of Pediatrics, New York University

Anomalies in Amino Acid Metabolism

Gabriel Spergel, M.D.
Clinical Associate Professor of Medicine, State University of New York, Downstate Medical Center; Senior Staff Endocrinologist, Brookdale Hospital Medical Center; Chief of Endocrinology, Greenpoint Hospital

Pheochromocytoma

Wesley W. Spink, M.D.
Regent's Professor of Medicine and Comparative Medicine (Emeritus), University of Minnesota

Brucellosis

Walter E. Stamm, M.D.
Assistant Professor, Department of Medicine and Division of Infectious Disease, Harborview Medical Center, University of Washington

Prevention of Infection—Barriers; Neisseria; Hemophilus Infections

Nigel N. Stanley, M.D., M.R.C.P.
Consultant Physician, The Lister Hospital, Stevenage, Hertfordshire, England

Cigarette Smoking

Allen C. Steere, M.D.
Assistant Professor of Medicine, Yale University

Lyme Disease

Marvin J. Stone, M.D.
Chief of Oncology, Baylor University Medical Center; Clinical Professor of Internal Medicine, University of Texas, Dallas

Plasma Cell Dyscrasias

Albert J. Stunkard, M.D.
Professor of Psychiatry, University of Pennsylvania

Obesity

Pavur R. Sundaresan, M.D., Ph.D.
Instructor in Clinical Pharmacology, University of Rochester

Autonomic Drugs; Respiratory Drugs

Richard D. Sweet, M.D.
White Plains, New York

Extrapyramidal and Cerebellar Disorders; Craniocervical Abnormalities; Spinal Cord Disorders; Peripheral Nerve Disorders

Jan P. Szidon, M.D.
Associate Professor of Medicine, University of Chicago; Director, Pulmonary Medicine Division, Michael Reese Hospital and Medical Center

Cor Pulmonale; Goodpasture's Syndrome; Idiopathic Infiltrative Diseases of the Lung

John H. Talbott, M.D.
Clinical Professor of Medicine, University of Miami; Attending Physician, Jackson Memorial Hospital and VA Hospital, Miami

Musculoskeletal and Connective Tissue Disorders—Introduction, Psoriatic Arthritis, Gout, Chondrocalcinosis, Eosinophilic Fasciitis, Polymyalgia Rheumatica

Raymond C. Terhune, D.M.D., M.S.D.
Kailua, Hawaii

Dental Caries and Its Complications

Richard A. Thoft, M.D.
Associate Professor of Ophthalmology, Harvard University; Associate Chief of Ophthalmology, Massachusetts Eye and Ear Infirmary

Ophthalmologic Disorders—Clinical Examination, Ocular Symptoms and Signs, Injuries, Orbit, Lacrimal Apparatus, Eyelids, Conjunctiva, Cornea, and Cataract

George F. Thornton, M.D.
Clinical Professor of Medicine, Yale University; Clinical Professor of Medicine, University of Connecticut; Director, Division of Medicine, Waterbury Hospital Health Center

Streptococcal Infections

Thomas N. Tozer, Pharm.D., Ph.D.
Professor of Pharmacy and Pharmaceutical Chemistry, University of California, San Francisco

Pharmacokinetics and Drug Administration; Drug Elimination; Plasma Concentration Monitoring

Donald P. Tschudy, M.D.
Senior Investigator, Metabolism Branch, National Cancer Institute

Anomalies in Pigment Metabolism

Marvin Turck, M.D.
Professor of Medicine, University of Washington

Bacterial Endocarditis; Antimicrobial Chemotherapy

Gerard M. Turino, M.D.
Professor of Medicine, Columbia University

Pulmonary Insufficiency and Respiratory Failure

John P. Utz, M.D.
Professor of Medicine, Georgetown University

Nocardiosis; Actinomycosis; Systemic Fungal Diseases

George E. Vaillant, M.D.
Professor of Psychiatry, Harvard University

Personality Disorders

Paul P. VanArsdel, Jr., M.D.
Professor of Medicine, and Head, Allergy Section, University of Washington

Disorders Due to Hypersensitivity

Ralph O. Wallerstein, M.D.
Clinical Professor of Medicine, University of California, San Francisco

Polycythemia

William M. Wardell, M.D., Ph.D.
Department of Pharmacology and Toxicology, University of Rochester

Drug Toxicity—Preclinical and Clinical Evaluation, Adverse Drug Reactions, Carcinogenesis, Benefit-to-Risk Ratio

William C. Watson, M.D., Ph.D.
Professor of Medicine, University of Western Ontario; Director of Gastroenterology, Victoria Hospital, London, Ontario, Canada

Malabsorption Syndromes

Michael Weintraub, M.D.
Associate Professor of Pharmacology and Toxicology and of Medicine, University of Rochester

Mechanism of Drug Action; Patient Compliance; Narcotics and Narcotic Antagonists; Nonnarcotic Analgesics, Antipyretics, and Nonsteroidal Anti-inflammatory Drugs

William Weiss, M.D.
Professor of Medicine and Director, Division of Occupational Medicine, Hahnemann Medical University and Hospital of Philadelphia

Lung Abscess

Thomas H. Weller, M.D.
Richard Pearson Strong Professor of Tropical Public Health and Chairman, Department of Tropical Public Health, Harvard School of Public Health

Cytomegalovirus Infection

lvi Contributors

Nanette K. Wenger, M.D.
Professor of Medicine (Cardiology), Emory University; Director, Cardiac Clinics, Grady Memorial Hospital

Exercise and the Heart

Francis C. Wood, Jr., M.D.
Associate Professor of Medicine, University of Washington; Director of Physician Education, Providence Medical Center

Diabetes Mellitus; Hypoglycemia; Glucagon

Walter S. Wood, M.D.
Professor and Chairman, Department of Community and Family Medicine, Loyola University

Anthrax Clostridial Infections

Theodore E. Woodward, M.D.
Professor and Chairman, Department of Medicine, University of Maryland; Physician-in-Chief, University of Maryland Hospital

Rickettsial Diseases

Morton M. Ziskind, M.D. *(Deceased)*
Professor of Medicine; Director, Pulmonary Diseases Section, Tulane University

Tumors of the Lung

C. Gordon Zubrod, M.D.
Professor and Chairman, Department of Oncology, University of Miami; Director, Comprehensive Cancer Care Center of Florida

Cancer Chemotherapy

§1. INFECTIOUS AND PARASITIC DISEASES

1. MANIFESTATIONS OF INFECTION

A healthy individual lives in harmony with his normal body flora, but this balance may be disturbed by disease. **Host defenses** are an important factor in determining whether or not infection will occur. These include anatomic barriers, such as intact skin and the ciliated respiratory mucosa; physiologic barriers, such as gastric acid; immune factors, such as specific antibodies; and phagocytic cells, such as polymorphonuclear neutrophils and macrophages of the reticuloendothelial system. Unknown factors presumably are also involved.

The **microbes that cause disease** are sometimes members of the normal flora. For example, *Streptococcus pneumoniae* and the β-hemolytic *S. pyogenes*, which cause pneumococcal pneumonia and streptococcal pharyngitis, respectively, can exist as part of the normal throat flora. Disease can also be caused by microorganisms that are usually harmless or even beneficial members of the normal flora. An example of this is *Streptococcus viridans* endocarditis in a patient with a heart valve damaged by acute rheumatic fever.

Disease may be caused by a microorganism with a particular virulence for man. Most highly virulent pathogens (e.g., *Yersinia [Pasteurella] pestis*, the causative organism of plague, and *Rickettsia rickettsii*, the causative organism of Rocky Mountain spotted fever) are not part of the normal body flora and predictably will cause disease in man.

Some of the more likely causative pathogens of some common bacterial infections are shown in TABLE 1–1.

TABLE 1–1. CAUSATIVE PATHOGENS IN SOME COMMON BACTERIAL INFECTIONS

	Bronchitis, Acute	Cellulitis	Cystitis	Endocarditis	Furuncles & Carbuncles	Impetigo	Meningitis	Osteomyelitis	Otitis Media	Pneumonia	Prostatitis	Pyelonephritis	Septicemia	Sinusitis	Tonsillitis & Pharyngitis
Enterobacter spp.....			X								√	X	X		
Enterococcus			√	√							√	√			
Escherichia coli......			X				√			√	X	X	X		
Hemophilus influenzae........	X						X		X	√				√	√
Klebsiella spp........			X							√	√	X	X		
Meningococcus......							X						X		
Pneumococcus	X						X		X	X			X	X	
Proteus spp.........			X							√	X	X	X		
Pseudomonas aeruginosa........			√									√	√		
Staphylococcus aureus..........	X			X	X	X	√	X	√	√	√		X	X	
Staph. epidermidis (albus)..........		√		√	√	√						√	√	√	
α-Hemolytic streptococcus				X											
β-Hemolytic streptococcus		X		√		X	√	√	√	√			√	√	X

X = Commonly encountered pathogens;   √ = Less commonly encountered pathogens.

Many **manifestations of infections** are not due to a direct action of the infecting organism and its products but reflect the response of the infected host, and may not appear in patients with impaired host defense mechanisms. They include inflammation at the site of the infection (absent in patients who lack polymorphonuclear leukocytes) and systemic manifestations such as malaise, fever, and chills. Breakdown of local defense barriers around a local inflammatory process may permit dissemination of infection or absorption of toxic material sufficient to cause constitutional symptoms. This occurs when infection spreads from a local focus, either (1) along the lymphatics to the lymph nodes and through the thoracic duct into the bloodstream, or (2) from entry into the bloodstream directly from an extravascular focus. Bacteria, viruses, rickettsias, parasites, and fungi can cause disseminated infection. Individuals with disseminated or generalized infections nearly always present with systemic symptoms if host responses are intact.

Manifestations of infectious diseases are protean because infective agents differ widely and may involve any organ system of the body. Furthermore, many manifestations result from nonspecific host responses rather than from direct actions of infecting organisms.

Infectious illnesses often begin with generalized symptoms: malaise, listlessness, inability to concentrate, and weakness. Myalgias, arthralgias, headache, and anorexia are common nonspecific complaints. Patients may develop more serious symptoms, e.g., hypotension, confusion, and dehydration. A catabolic response occurs at the onset of clinical illness, and weight loss may become prominent in protracted disease.

FEVER

Body temperature > 37.8 C (100 F) orally or 38.2 C (100.8 F) rectally is the cardinal finding in infectious diseases. Fever, exaggerating the normal diurnal variation in body temperature, usually is highest in the late afternoon and early evening. The febrile response is maximal in childhood and diminishes with age. **Hyperthermia,** *a temperature > 41.2 C (106 F)* rectally or orally, is rarely caused by infection. Exceptions include bacterial meningitis and viral encephalitis.

A thermoregulatory center in the hypothalamus controls the temperature by altering skin circulation, sweating, and involuntary muscle activity (shivering). Fever associated with bacterial infection is due to direct action on that thermoregulatory center by endogenous pyrogen, a low molecular weight protein released by leukocytes and other cells after contact with bacteria, their endotoxins, viruses, parasites, other infectious agents, and immune complexes.

Chills raise the temperature to a new level set by the hypothalamus. A single chill typically precedes fever in pneumococcal pneumonia, streptococcal infection, osteomyelitis, tularemia, plague, leptospirosis, typhus, and influenza. However, a chill is not diagnostic of infection and may occur with use of antipyretics or with fever due to allergic reactions, transfusion reactions, or malignancies. Repeated chills are common with aspirin administration and with bacteremias associated with acute pyelonephritis, biliary tract obstruction, endocarditis, and abscesses. **Sweats** usually connote defervescence and commonly occur when the temperature drops to its low diurnal point in the early morning **(night sweats).**

Fever occurs in many noninfectious diseases, including thyrotoxicosis, dehydration in infants and the elderly, ichthyosis and other generalized skin disorders, congenital absence of sweat glands, trauma, myocardial infarction, cerebral thrombosis or hemorrhage, peripheral arterial occlusion, malignant neoplasms, conditions causing intravascular hemolysis, serum sickness, periarteritis nodosa, rheumatic fever, rheumatoid arthritis, and erythema nodosum. Fever may be the sole adverse reaction to drugs; the elevated temperature characteristically remains at a relatively constant level. Many other patterns of fever occur and, although some are associated with particular etiologic agents, the fever curve is usually of little diagnostic aid in the individual patient.

Diagnosis of fever of unknown origin (FUO): Designation as an FUO requires *documentation of fever of at least 38.3 C (101 F) rectally persisting for at least 3 wk without discovery of the cause despite extensive investigation for at least 1 wk.* The differential diagnosis of FUO presents special problems because characteristic or localizing symptoms or signs of a number of febrile diseases may be minimal or lacking at various ages. Causes of fever and their diagnosis in **infants and children** are discussed in Vol. II, Ch. 24. In **adults,** many conditions cause FUO, but infections, collagen-vascular disorders, or occult neoplastic processes (particularly leukemia, lymphoma, and hypernephroma) are commonly found. The history often gives important clues (e.g., a history of drinking contaminated water suggests typhoid; of employment in meat-packing plants, brucellosis; of proximity to rats, typhus or leptospirosis; of being bitten by a rat, rat-bite fever). Usually the diagnosis requires frequent physical examinations, appropriate x-ray studies, blood cultures, and specific antibody titers; at times it requires biopsy of involved lymph nodes, subcutaneous nodules, chronic skin lesions, tender muscles, or liver, as indicated. Blood cultures should be taken 1 to 3 times daily for several days, but seldom is a total of > 6 blood cultures indicated. Serologic tests should be repeated if typhoid, brucellosis, certain virus diseases, or a rickettsial disease is suspected, since a rise in titer as the disease progresses is more significant than a single titer. Malarial parasites must be sought. Liver-spleen scan should be performed in most patients; ultrasonography, arteriography, lymphography, and CT scans are of value in selected patients. Gallium scans are seldom helpful. With a thoughtful, individualized approach to FUO, the cause can be identified in 90% of patients.

Treatment of fever must be directed to its cause. In serious infections, antibiotic therapy must often be instituted before results of cultures and sensitivity studies are known. In general, antipyretic therapy is only appropriate when the diagnosis is clear, but it should be considered when fever is debilitating, causes major symptoms, or affects CNS function. The average oral adult doses of antipyretics are aspirin 0.3 to 1.0 gm q 4 h or acetaminophen 0.3 to 0.6 gm q 4 h. Antipyretics should be given around-the-clock to mitigate acute swings in temperature; however, in some patients with high fever, antipyretics may cause a sudden fall in temperature associated with circulatory collapse. Safer ways to decrease temperature include cold compresses or sponging and use of cooling blankets. The oral temperature should not be reduced to < 38.3 C (101 F). Antipyretic drugs are ineffective in **neurogenic hyperpyrexia** caused by damage to the hypothalamus (e.g., following a CVA or head trauma), but barbiturates may be useful. Sodium pentothal 100 to 200 mg orally or slowly IV, or sodium phenobarbital 75 to 100 mg orally or IM may affect the overactive heat-conserving center. **Heatstroke** is discussed in Ch. 216. Maintaining fluid and electrolyte balance is important, and supplementary sodium chloride may be required. Nutrition should be provided by high-vitamin, high-protein diets in small, frequent feedings; a few patients with prolonged, debilitating fever may require parenteral hyperalimentation.

OTHER MANIFESTATIONS OF INFECTION

Hematologic Manifestations of Infection

Leukocytosis, *an increase in the number of leukocytes in the blood*, characterizes many infectious diseases. Not every kind of white blood cell is increased with every kind of infection; with most bacterial infections, leukocytosis is reflected primarily as neutrophilia. The demand for neutrophils in the tissues is first supplied by increased margination of mature, segmented polymorphonuclear leukocytes **(PMNs)** on the walls of capillaries. As the bone marrow storage pool of mature, segmented neutrophils is exhausted, the proportion of less mature band forms in the peripheral blood increases, and as band forms become depleted, metamyelocytes become the predominant form of neutrophil. Severe infections are sometimes accompanied by a "**leukemoid blood picture**" in which immature, mitotically active leukocytes, including myelocytes, promyelocytes, and myeloblasts, are released into the circulation; careful study is sometimes required to differentiate leukemoid reactions from true leukemias.

In severe infections, the neutrophil stores and productive capacity of bone marrow may be incapable of keeping up with cellular utilization, and **neutropenia** (< 3,000 PMN/cu mm) ensues. This is often an ominous prognostic finding. Diminished ability to mobilize white cells may contribute to the leukopenia found in chronic alcoholics and patients with diabetes mellitus or terminal shock. Neutropenia is frequent in salmonellosis, brucellosis, pertussis, and some rickettsial and viral infections. Abnormalities in neutrophils (e.g., toxic granulations, vacuolization of the cytoplasm, and Döhle bodies) may be signs of severe inflammation.

Antigen-antibody complexes appear to attract eosinophils. Therefore, **eosinophilia** (> 700 eosinophils/cu mm) is common in allergic diseases and helminthic infections, and may be found during the recovery phase in many bacterial infections. **Basophilia** generally is not a response to infectious processes. **Monocytosis** may be present in tuberculosis, brucellosis, syphilis, some rickettsial and protozoal infections, and neutropenia, or during recovery from acute infections. **Lymphocytosis** (> 4,000 lymphocytes/cu mm) is typical in pertussis, is seen in various chronic illnesses, and is prominent during convalescence from acute infections.

Anemia that develops acutely in the course of an infectious disease results from bleeding or from direct destruction of RBCs. The alpha-lecithinase of *Clostridium perfringens* has been associated with hemolysis in vivo; and intraerythrocytic parasitization destroys red cells in malaria and bartonellosis. Cold agglutinins associated with *Mycoplasma pneumoniae*, infectious mononucleosis, or chlamydia infections may cause hemolysis. Chronic infections cause an anemia characterized by an inflammatory block in which there are normal or increased stores of iron in the reticuloendothelial system and decreases in plasma iron and total iron-binding capacity. Saturation of transferrin may be decreased. Cure of the infection is essential to correction of the anemia.

The **erythrocyte sedimentation rate (ESR)** is increased in almost all infectious diseases. Although the test has great sensitivity in indicating active disease, it lacks specificity; any disease that engenders an inflammatory response may be associated with an increased ESR.

Disseminated intravascular coagulation (DIC) (see Ch. 95) is most common in gram-negative infections, but may occur as part of severe gram-positive or viral infections.

Cardiovascular Manifestations of Infection

When there is fever, the pulse is usually increased about 10 beats/min/degree F. With some infections the rate is characteristically slower than would be predicted (e.g., with salmonelloses including typhoid fever, tularemia, brucellosis, bacterial meningitides complicated by increased intracranial pressure, *Mycoplasma pneumoniae*, rickettsialpox, ornithoses, mumps, infectious hepatitis, Colorado tick fever, dengue, and factitious fever). Hypotension with or without shock can occur with severe infections, especially in patients with serious underlying diseases or with the administration of antipyretics. **Septic shock** is discussed separately in Ch. 5.

Renal Manifestations of Infection

Febrile proteinuria—mild, transient proteinuria occurring with fever of any cause—most likely results from nonspecific increased permeability that lets more protein pass through the glomerular membrane. Some infections, such as poststreptococcal glomerulonephritis and the nephritis of chronic endocarditis or parasitic infections, cause structural and functional changes in the kidney, probably as a consequence of immune complex deposition (see Ch. 147). Characteristic changes of immune-complex nephritis involve hematuria or proteinuria, which may become permanent. There may be a transient failure of tubular reabsorption of glucose, which is usually mild in the nondiabetic. With many infections, prerenal azotemia occurs, with an increase in the blood urea nitrogen (BUN) and with normal creatinine. Hypotension may lead to oliguria and, if progressive, to shock. The resultant decrease in renal blood flow causes severe azotemia and a rise in serum creatinine.

Hepatic Manifestations of Infection

Some hepatic dysfunction occurs in many infectious diseases, even without localization of the infectious agent in the liver. Jaundice associated with bacteremia generally indicates a poor prognosis. Intrahepatic cholestasis secondary to hepatocellular dysfunction is the usual finding. Jaundice may also accompany infections that cause massive hemolysis (malaria, bartonellosis, and gas gangrene). Other infectious agents damage hepatic cells (infectious hepatitis, serum hepatitis, infectious mononucleosis, cytomegalovirus, and yellow fever) or create space-occupying lesions (granulomas of TB, brucellosis, schistosomiasis, syphilitic gummas, amebic abscesses, and echinococcal cysts).

Central Nervous System Manifestations of Infection

Nonspecific manifestations of infection (e.g., anxiety, confusion, delirium, stupor, convulsions, or coma) may occur without the presence of the infectious agent in brain tissue. These manifestations of cerebral malfunction usually are proportional to the severity of the infection. More focal findings will usually accompany actual invasion of the brain by infectious agents (see Ch. 124).

---

2. USE OF THE CLINICAL MICROBIOLOGY LABORATORY

The diagnostic or clinical microbiology laboratory assists the physician in diagnosing and managing infections and assists the hospital in controlling hospital-acquired or nosocomial infections. The quality of assistance from the laboratory depends greatly not only on the care with which specimens are collected and transported but also on the relevant clinical information accompanying them. Almost all laboratories can culture, isolate, and identify most microorganisms, and many can also demonstrate antibody responses by serologic technics, including fluorescent antibody procedures, if appropriately collected, paired (acute and convalescent) serum samples are submitted. (City, state, and federal laboratories are usually well equipped to do serologic work and serve as referral centers.) Immunologic technics—e.g., precipitin and immunodiffusion tests, counterimmunoelectrophoresis (CIE), and enzyme-linked immunoadsorbent assays (ELISA)—are being used increasingly for antigen detection in CSF and other body fluids. Some of these technics can demonstrate even minute amounts of antigen in clinical material. Finally, the laboratory guides chemotherapy by testing microorganisms for susceptibility to antibiotics, by periodically tabulating pathogenic organisms and their susceptibility to antibiotics to assess prevailing antibiotic-resistance patterns of key pathogens in a particular institution, and by drug level determinations (assays) in serum or other body fluids.

The most important contribution of the laboratory is its culturing, isolation, and identification work, combined with direct staining procedures.

STAINING PROCEDURES

THE GRAM STAIN

The Gram stain differentiates microorganisms into gram-positive or gram-negative bacilli or cocci; visualizes many fungi, especially yeasts; detects RBCs, WBCs, and many other cellular elements, and provides semiquantitative assessment. Primary Gram stains help control the quality of culturing efforts, e.g., by pointing out organisms that failed to grow, or by suggesting contamination if growth occurs that differs from what has been seen on the smear. Gram staining is important for assessing the etiology of the infectious disease initially and starting at least tentative chemotherapy. Practically all specimens, except blood cultures and perhaps routine throat swabs, should be examined in this way.

Preparing the Smear

With a loop or swab, spread some material onto a clean, labeled slide. The film should be thin, with the material distributed evenly on a defined area of the slide that has been marked with a diamond or grease pencil. Air-dry and then heat-fix by passing the slide, smear side up, through a flame several times. Let cool.

Comments: (1) Swabs with material containing cellular elements should be rolled onto the slide, rather than stirred, in order to preserve cellular details. (2) Overheating destroys cellular detail. It should still be possible to touch the slides, smear side up, to the back of the hand. (3) Heat fixation kills most bacteria, but not spores. (4) Large numbers of RBCs can obscure the bacteria and should be lysed by adding a few drops of distilled sterile water following the heat fixation. After waiting for 3 min, rinse and resume the routine staining procedure. (5) Fluids containing very few cells or bacteria (clear urine or CSF) should not be spread; they should be left as a drop to dry on the slide. With CSF, it is preferable to spin down the specimen and use the sediment to prepare the smear. (6) The tip of a swab may have the most important portion of the clinical material and should be touched to the slide. (7) It is possible to prepare a smear and streak a culture plate with only one swab. If this is necessary, first touch part of the swab to a heat-sterilized *and cooled* slide and then streak the culture plate.

Primary Stain (Crystal Violet)

Flood the smear with crystal violet solution and let stand for 10 to 30 seconds (not critical). Rinse with tap water.

Comments: (1) Crystal violet solution has been reported to contain yeast cells in rare instances. (2) Since some bacteria do not retain their gram-positive characteristics in the acid environment of many clinical specimens, some authorities recommend adding 2 to 3 drops of sodium bicarbonate solution to the crystal violet on the slide. In this instance, mixing should be insured by agitating or tilting the slide back and forth. Let the mixture stand for 30 to 60 seconds before rinsing with tap water.

Iodine Mordant

Flood with Gram's iodine solution for 10 to 30 seconds (not critical). Rinse with tap water.

Decolorization

Decolorize with a 1:1 (v/v) mixture of 95% ethanol and acetone (critical). Decolorize the tilted slide until no more blue dye comes off the thin section of the smear; this will take only a few seconds. Rinse with tap water.

Comments: (1) Overly decolorizing the thinner portion of the smear is probably the most common error. (2) The thinner portions are usually the useful areas for microscopic examinations. (3) Pure acetone alone should be used only by those who are experienced because of the rapidity of decolorization. Most people feel that using ethanol alone is too slow.

Counterstain

Flood the smear with safranin for 10 to 30 seconds (not critical). Rinse with tap water, wipe the back of the slide clean, and let the smear dry.

Comments: (1) Some authorities recommend very gently blotting the smear with absorbent paper to speed the drying. (2) Some gram-negative bacteria, e.g., *Legionella pneumophila*, stain only faintly with this procedure. Prolonged counterstaining with safranin for 2 to 3 min or using carbolfuchsin (for acid-fast bacteria) for 30 seconds is said to give better results.

Interpretation

In a well-stained smear, most gram-positive microorganisms will stain dark purple and most gram-negative bacteria, red. Cellular elements, particularly WBCs, should stain various shades of red in the thin portion of the smear. Many fungi, especially *Candida*, will stain purple. Correct interpretation of many smears requires considerable experience; a laboratory worker familiar with microscopic examination of gram-stained material should be consulted at the slightest doubt and with all critical specimens.

Quality Control

Known cultures of *Escherichia coli* and *Staphylococcus aureus* should be used at regular intervals and with new batches of reagents to insure adequacy of the stain and its differentiating ability. Placing a drop of a suspension of these organisms right and left of the clinical material to be stained serves also as a valid quality control of the staining procedure in critical situations or cases of doubt. In the absence of such cultures, a drop of saliva may be used, since it usually contains numerous gram-positive and gram-negative organisms.

OTHER STAINING PROCEDURES

Other useful staining procedures are special stains for demonstrating acid-fast bacteria, rickettsia, and parasites. Fluorescent antibody procedures for many organisms are available in some laboratories. Unstained or wet-mounts are used for rapid demonstration of live parasites and fungi and motility of microorganisms. Permanently stained preparations are also used for stool and blood parasites. Contrast and visibility in unstained preparations may be enhanced by darkfield, phase contrast, or Nomarski-type differential interference contrast microscopy.

The following discussions in this chapter recommend proven conditions for isolating pathogens and interpreting results correctly.

LABORATORY DIAGNOSIS OF BACTERIAL INFECTIONS

(See TABLE 2–1)

TABLE 2-1. COLLECTING AND HANDLING SPECIMENS FOR LABORATORY DIAGNOSIS OF BACTERIAL INFECTIONS, INCLUDING ACID-FAST BACTERIA AND ANAEROBES

Specimen Type	Patient Preparation	Optimal Specimen and Volume	Container	Collection Technic	Useful Clinical Information	Comments
Anaerobic Cultures						
Actinomycosis	Examine gauze dressing for sulfur granules Skin decontamination (e.g., povidone iodine)	1 ml or more of aspirated material	Special TM; gassed-out tube or syringe with needle in place & covered with plastic sleeve or rubber stopper	Aspirate with syringe from sinus tract or swollen abscess areas Granules may be recovered from secretion in dressing & examined microscopically	History of "lumpy jaw" Chronic infection	Fistulous chronic infections, often in neck, jaw, & upper chest, & sometimes abdominal lesions
Body fluids or secretions	Skin decontamination	1 ml or more	As for actinomycosis	Aspirate into syringe without air; the smaller the volume, the more critical the speed of transport & anaerobic conditions	Foul-smelling discharge Abdominal surgery Septic abortion	For smaller volumes, use smaller syringe For fluids likely to clot, prerinse syringe with heparin solution Instead of needle, sterile plastic catheter may be attached to syringe
Respiratory tract	Coughed-up sputum (contaminated with saliva) not recommended	1 ml or more of transtracheal aspirate, pleural fluid, or pus	As for actinomycosis	Transtracheal aspiration Surgically obtained direct abscess aspiration	Foul-smelling sputum History of aspiration	Regular sputum, nasotracheal, & bronchoscopy aspirates are considered unacceptable specimens by many authorities
Swabs (specially prepared for anaerobic collection & maintained in sterile, gassed-out tube)		As much material or fluid as swab will hold	Special container with prereduced, anaerobically sterilized TM	Sample infected site rapidly Transport to laboratory as soon as possible	Foul-smelling sputum History of aspiration	Do not use ordinary unprepared swabs

Specimen	Precautions	Quantity	Container	How Obtained	Clinical Indications	Remarks
Tissue biopsy (pea-sized or smaller)	As for surgery biopsy	The smaller the specimen, the more vulnerable	Into gassed-out tube, replacing lid immediately	Hold upright to retain CO_2, which is heavier than air	As for body fluids; Gas gangrene	Do not add any fluid, etc.
Tissue biopsy (too large for tube)	As for surgery biopsy	1 cu cm or more	Sterile container (jar, Petri dish)	Usually obtained surgically	As for smaller tissue biopsy	Larger specimens maintain their own anaerobic condition; Do not add fluid
Autopsy Material						
Blood	Best collected before body is handled too much or opened. Decontaminate skin or sear surface of heart or other organ before inserting needle or cutting out tissue block	10 ml right-heart blood	Sterile tube or vacutainer with anticoagulant (heparin or SPS)	From right heart through skin & chest wall or through unopened heart from right ventricle after removal of sternum	Clinical diagnosis; Postmortem interval; Prosector's impression; Previous positive cultures; Suspected infection	Autopsy cultures are often contaminated with bacteria from sinks & water faucets & with enteric bacteria
Tissue		5–10 cu cm cube with 1 serosal or other surface	Sterile jar or screw-capped tube	Cut block, including some normal tissue, from suspicious area		Block of spleen tissue may be submitted in lieu of a blood culture (NOTE: Coccidioidomycosis & TB are frequently discovered only at autopsy)

(Continued)

Abbreviations: SPS, sodium polyanethol sulfonate; TM, transport medium.
Modified from "Collection and Processing of Microbiological Specimens," in *Cumulative Techniques and Procedures in Clinical Microbiology (CUMITECH)*, Vol. 9, 1979. Copyright 1979 by The American Society for Microbiology. Used with permission.

TABLE 2-1.   COLLECTING AND HANDLING SPECIMENS FOR LABORATORY DIAGNOSIS OF BACTERIAL INFECTIONS, INCLUDING ACID-FAST BACTERIA AND ANAEROBES *(Cont'd)*

Specimen Type	Patient Preparation	Optimal Specimen and Volume	Container	Collection Technic	Useful Clinical Information	Comments
Blood						
Peripheral	Skin decontamination with 70% alcohol followed by 2% tincture of iodine or povidone iodine	10 ml (adults & older children), 1–2 ml (infants)	Sterile screw-capped tube or vacutainer with SPS as anticoagulant, or culture bottle for direct inoculation	Sterile venipuncture Specimen drawn through catheter or cannula is less satisfactory	Clinical diagnosis, chemotherapy, antibiotics, immune status Surgery	Recommended number of specimens: For SBE, 2–3 within 24 h; for FUO, 4–6 within 48 h Send to laboratory immediately
Bone marrow	Skin decontamination as for peripheral blood	1 ml or more	As for peripheral blood	Sterile percutaneous aspiration	As for peripheral blood, plus acid-fast bacilli or fungal infection	Smears should be made Recommended by many authorities for diagnosis of systemic histoplasmosis, fungal infections, or miliary TB
Blood bank		Whole unit or leftover from transfusion	Original bottle or container		Recipient & donor histories	May contain few organisms/unit Consider salmonella & malaria & psychrophilic organisms
Body Fluids (other than blood, urine, CSF)			If anaerobes are suspected, use anaerobic technic & container			

Specimen	Preparation	Amount	Container	Collection method	History	Comments
Bile	Surgery	Several ml (first ml from postoperative drain site often contains contaminants)	Sterile tube or jar	Aspiration with syringe during surgery, or from postoperative drainage site, or via nasogastric tube from duodenum	History of salmonella or clostridia infection	Sample may contain gallstones that should be examined also. Duodenal aspirates are sometimes submitted for special tests (Giardia, bacterial overgrowth with coliforms or bacteroides)
Breast milk	Skin decontamination	Several ml	Sterile tube or jar	Gentle manual expression	Abscess	Often yields Staphylococcus aureus &/or Streptococcus pyogenes
Hematomas	Skin decontamination	Several ml	Sterile tube or vacutainer	Sterile aspiration with syringe	Abscess	May clot. When in doubt, use anticoagulant
Joint fluids	Skin decontamination	Several ml	Sterile tube or vacutainer	Sterile aspiration with syringe	History of trauma, previous surgery or infection (gonorrhea)	Often proteinaceous, may clot. Do not add acetic acid or other fluid that may precipitate protein & make cell evaluation impossible. Use distilled sterile water
Pericardial fluid	Skin decontamination	Several ml	As for peripheral blood	Sterile aspiration with syringe	History of TB or previous surgery	Usually a surgical procedure
Peritoneal fluid (including peritoneal dialysis fluid)	Skin decontamination	Several ml or more	Sterile tube or jar	Sterile aspiration, may be quite proteinaceous or clot	History of TB, surgery, cancer	As for joint fluid. Consider also gonorrhea and peritoneal dialysis
Catheter (Tips) Foley catheter		Not recommended				Foley catheters or tips should not be cultured—except unused, as sterility check

(Continued)

TABLE 2-1. COLLECTING AND HANDLING SPECIMENS FOR LABORATORY DIAGNOSIS OF BACTERIAL INFECTIONS, INCLUDING ACID-FAST BACTERIA AND ANAEROBES (Cont'd)

Specimen Type	Patient Preparation	Optimal Specimen and Volume	Container	Collection Technic	Useful Clinical Information	Comments
Catheter (Tips) (Cont'd) Female (Cont'd) Vascular cannulae Central venous pressure lines, umbilical or IV catheters	Skin decontamination	Tip is more relevant; may have infected clot	Sterile jar	Cut off tip with sterile scissors or submit entire catheter	History of infection	Occasionally removed because of sepsis or fever continuing due to colonized catheter tip (yeast is most frequently isolated from hyperalimentation lines)
Central Nervous System						
Brain biopsy	Surgical	Tissue	As for anaerobe cultures	As for anaerobe cultures	History of abscess or cryptococcosis	Needs coordination with pathology and virus laboratory (herpes)
Cerebrospinal fluid	Skin decontamination (usually of lumbar area)	1–5 ml (more if fungi or AFB are suspected)	Sterile, clean screw-capped glass tubes For AFB cultures, use acid-washed glassware	Sterile lumbar puncture Ventricular or sub-occipital tap	Tentative clinical diagnosis &/or suspicion	Since cultures yield more from a larger inoculating volume, an alternate method pools all 3 tubes (after cell counts) to be worked up in microbiology laboratory Supernatant goes to chemistry & serology if required
Meningomyelocele	Skin decontamination	Often only 1 specimen submitted	As for CSF	Sterile aspiration through skin	Infection	Often contaminated or infected with skin flora
Shunt fluid	Skin & catheter decontamination	Often only 1 tube	As for CSF	Sterile aspiration through shunt	Infection	As for meningomyelocele

Ear					
Internal (middle)	Cleanse external canal with mild antiseptic	Usually swabs; if volume allows, submit fluid	Sterile, clean tube TM for swabs	Use sterile funnel if collecting specimen from eardrum or beyond	History of acute or chronic otitis or perforation	If eardrum is perforated, specimen should be collected by otolaryngologist
External	Cleanse external canal with mild detergent	Swab, scrapings, or aspirate fluid	Sterile tube TM for swabs	Obtain specimen from active margin, preferably including fresh secretion from deeper areas	Clinical suspicion	Surface swabbing might miss streptococcal cellulitis or erysipelas
Eye					
Internal	As for surgical specimen	Volume of specimen usually suboptimal	Sterile tube	Surgical technic. Label carefully for left eye & right eye	Trauma. Postoperative infection. Foreign body	Since specimen is usually small & obtained under great difficulty, speed in transport & care in handling are very important
External	Cleanse skin around eye with mild antiseptic. Gently remove makeup, ointment, etc. with sterile cotton & saline	Moistened swabs are used for most cases. For diagnosis of viral or chlamydial infections & for cytology, conjunctival &/or corneal scrapings are necessary. Make 2 slides/lesion	Moist sterile swabs in sterile tubes with small amount of nutrient broth. Alcohol-cleaned glass slides for scrapings to be cultured (AFB, fungi)	Swabbing: Pass moistened swab 2 times over lower conjunctiva; avoid eyelid border lashes (culture these separately in similar fashion if indicated). Scrapings: Use local anesthetic & a platinum spatula; rub spatula with scrapings gently over small area on slide; if too dry, use small amount of water	History & suspected problem, e.g., bacterial, fungal, AFB, inclusion bodies (viral or chlamydial), gonococci only, allergic (vernal) conjunctivitis, chemotherapy	Handle very carefully. Transport to laboratory immediately. Often only few microorganisms present. Scrapings should be done by ophthalmologist. Giemsa and Gram stains are most helpful. (NOTE: OD = right eye, OS = left eye)

(Continued)

TABLE 2-1. COLLECTING AND HANDLING SPECIMENS FOR LABORATORY DIAGNOSIS OF BACTERIAL INFECTIONS, INCLUDING ACID–FAST BACTERIA AND ANAEROBES *(Cont'd)*

Specimen Type	Patient Preparation	Optimal Specimen and Volume	Container	Collection Technic	Useful Clinical Information	Comments
Food		For *food poisoning*, secure remaining food & original container & possibly stomach contents	If possible, sterile container	Material to be sampled for cultures (*Staphylococcus, Salmonella, Vibrio parahaemolyticus*) & for toxin (botulism)	Without history, no workup possible	Hospital laboratories may be asked to work up specimens or to assist with collecting & initial handling. Contact local public health or city laboratory
		For *food check*, secure food samples ready for consumption	If possible, sterile container	Rinse with sterile saline (lettuce, vegetables) or homogenize		
GI Tract Duodenal aspirate	Through tube	Several ml	Sterile tube	Aspiration	History of travel, diarrhea	Examine for bacterial overgrowth, *G. lamblia,* & other parasites
Feces		Several cu cm on 3 consecutive days	Waxed cardboard container with tight-fitting lid	Directly into any clean container	History of travel, diarrhea, suspected food	Avoid contamination with urine, soap, etc. Transport to laboratory immediately or use a buffered glycerol TM
Gastric aspirate In infants	Through tube	Any amount sufficient for smear & culture	Sterile container	To be done by physician During first few days, infant's stomach fluid is not acid	Premature rupture of membranes	May isolate causative agent of septicemia before blood cultures are positive
In adults						(See under AFB and fungal cultures)

Rectal swab	If indicated: proctoscopy, sigmoidoscopy	On 3 consecutive days		Insert swab beyond anal sphincter (1″) & rotate once	As for feces	Inferior to fresh stool
Genital Tract **Female**						
Amniotic fluid		Uncontaminated fluid	Sterile tube	Aspirate with syringe	Premature rupture of membrane	Treat as any other normally sterile body fluid May contain gonococci
Cervix	Wipe cervix clean of vaginal secretion & mucus Use speculum—no disinfectants or lubricants Speculum may be rinsed with warm sterile water	Endocervical secretion uncontaminated Take 2 swabs if smears are to be made as well	As for wound cultures Gonococci survive best if seeded promptly onto chocolate agar either in plates or (better) in bottles for transport	Under direct vision, gently compress cervix with blades of speculum & use a wringing motion with swab; obtain exudate from endocervical glands	Venereal disease Postpartum inspection	Use of ordinary transport medium (Amies or modified Stuart) as a holding medium for > 2 h results in loss of gonococcal viability
Cul de sac	Surgical procedure	Fluid, secretion	Sterile tube (see under anaerobes)	Aspiration through posterior vaginal vault	Venereal disease	Pelvic inflammatory disease
Endometrium	As for cervix	Curettings or aspirates Provide for making smears	Sterile container Anaerobic conditions	If swabs are to be used, collection through a sterile tube sheath will avoid contamination	Postpartum fever Venereal disease	
Intrauterine devices	Surgical	Entire device + secretion, pus, etc.	Sterile container Anaerobic conditions	Surgical removal	History Bleeding	Unusual organisms may be expected, e.g., Actinomyces or Torulopsis or other yeasts
Products of conception (fetus, placenta, membranes)	Surgical	Tissue or aspirates	Sterile container	Select relevant or suspicious areas of tissue; if contaminated, use sampling techniques	History	Occasionally this type of specimen is expelled into toilet & grossly contaminated

(Continued)

TABLE 2-1. COLLECTING AND HANDLING SPECIMENS FOR LABORATORY DIAGNOSIS OF BACTERIAL INFECTIONS, INCLUDING ACID-FAST BACTERIA AND ANAEROBES *(Cont'd)*

Specimen Type	Patient Preparation	Optimal Specimen and Volume	Container	Collection Technic	Useful Clinical Information	Comments
Genital Tract *(Cont'd)* Female *(Cont'd)* Urethra (for gonococci)	Wipe clean with sterile gauze or swab	Swab with urethral secretion or free discharge	Chocolate agar transport bottle	1 h or more after urination; if discharge cannot be obtained by "milking" the urethra, use thin wire swabs to collect material from about 2 cm inside urethra	History of discharge or painful urination	Discharge may be stimulated by stripping & massaging the urethra against the pubic symphysis through the vagina
Uterus, tubes, ovaries	Usually surgical specimen	Tissue, aspirates, or swabs	Sterile container	If surgical specimen, representative samples should be cut & submitted	History Clinical diagnosis	Venereal disease & fungal, anaerobic, & AFB infections have to be kept in mind
Vagina	Speculum use is preferred (see Cervix)	Aspirate or swab for Gram stain, wet mount, & cultures	Sterile container, chocolate agar transport bottle	Simple aspiration or swabbing For *Trichomonas*, aspirates are required	History of discharge	Ulcerations should be checked for soft chancre, syphilis, or genital herpes Yeast & *Trichomonas vaginalis* are common (use wet mount) Role of "clue cells" and *Hemophilus vaginalis* controversial
Vulva (including labia & Bartholin's gland	Do not use alcohol for mucous membranes Skin preparation for regular skin sites	Swab or aspirate (Bartholin's gland abscess)	Sterile container	Collect with swab or aspirate with syringe & needle	History	As for Vagina

Site	Preparation of patient	Specimen	Container	Method of collection	Information needed	Comments
Female & Male						
Darkfield (for Treponema pallidum)	1- to 2-h soak with sterile saline & gauze	Several slide preparations or (better) aspirate into capillary tube	Slide & coverslip or capillary tube	Scrape base of lesion, express fluid, avoid bleeding; Touch slide to fluid & cover with cover glass; or squeeze lesion & collect secretion into capillary tube	Date of questionable intercourse	Transport to laboratory immediately; Motility is seen only in warm material; Seal coverslip or capillary tube with vaseline to protect against drying & O_2
Lymph nodes (inguinal)	Skin decontamination	Biopsy or needle aspiration	Sterile container	Aspiration of lymph node with syringe & needle; If biopsy is done, pathologist has to be involved	History; Venereal disease	Requires arrangements with special laboratory for lymphogranuloma venereum (**LGV**) cultures
Male						
Penis	Do not use alcohol for mucous membranes; Skin preparation for regular skin sites	Swab or aspirate	Sterile container	Vesicles must be opened & secretion submitted as aspirate, on slide or swab for culture & microscopic examinations	Duration of lesion, pain, & discomfort	Viral collection media needed to identify herpes Type 2; Darkfield preparation for syphilis diagnosis; For soft chancre diagnosis, consult with laboratory
Prostate		Secretion for smear & culture	Sterile tube or swab	Digital massage through rectum	History of chronic UTI	Not recommended for gonococcal cultures, but helpful in some chronic UTIs
Urethra	Wipe clean with sterile gauze or swab	Swab with urethral secretion or free discharge	Secretion, slide, &/or swab	Same as for female (above); Thin urethrogenital calcium alginate swabs are preferred	History & duration of painful discharge	In males, diagnosis of gonorrhea can often be made by microscopic examination of a gram-stained smear

(Continued)

TABLE 2-1.   COLLECTING AND HANDLING SPECIMENS FOR LABORATORY DIAGNOSIS OF BACTERIAL INFECTIONS, INCLUDING ACID–FAST BACTERIA AND ANAEROBES *(Cont'd)*

Specimen Type	Patient Preparation	Optimal Specimen and Volume	Container	Collection Technic	Useful Clinical Information	Comments
Lymph Nodes	As for surgery	Tissue or aspirate	Sterile container or syringe	Aspiration, biopsy, or excision	Clinical suspicion Location	Make imprint from cut surface on sterile slide Consider unusual organisms, e.g., LGV, viruses, AFB, actinomycosis, *Yersinia*
Oral Cavity Mucosal surface of gums, tongue, etc.	Rinse mouth	Scrapings or swabs	Swab, tongue blade, slide in sterile container	Scraping, swab	Clinical suspicion Duration	Not submitted for bacterial cultures, but smears for diagnosis of Vincent's angina or yeast infections are valid
Dental abscess, root abscess	Rinse mouth, prepare with dry sterile gauze	Fluid, pus	Sterile, as for anaerobic specimen	Needle & syringe aspiration	Clinical suspicion Duration	Anaerobic bacteria, including *Actinomyces*; certain viridans, streptococci
Pus (abscesses) (See Anaerobic Cultures above & Skin below)						
Respiratory Tract Bronchotracheal secretions or material	Surgical	Secretions, bronchial brushings, tissue	Sterile tube	By incubation or transcutaneous aspiration	Clinical impression	
Epiglottis	Tongue blade, good light source	Swab, etc.	Swab in TM		Age History	Do not swab throat or use tongue blade in cases of acute epiglottitis unless prepared for tracheostomy
Lung	Surgical	Tissue or aspirated fluid	Sterile tube or container (see Anaerobic Cultures)	Percutaneous (under fluoroscopy) or open surgery	Clinical impression	Consider TB, tumor, Legionnaires' disease, anaerobic abscess

Nasopharynx	Swab	Thin wire swab in TM	Swab is passed gently through nostril into nasopharynx Stay near septum & floor of nose Rotate & remove	Suspected agent (e.g., Hemophilus influenzae, Bordetella pertussis)	Send to laboratory immediately
Nose	Swab, etc.	Swab in TM	Rotate swab		Used routinely for Staphylococcus aureus carriers only
Sputum	Careful instruction of patient	Morning specimen, no saliva	Sterile container	Expectoration—if necessary, assisted by saline nebulization, postural drainage, etc.	Clinical impression	Respiratory therapist may be contacted to assist
Throat	Use tongue blade & good light source	One swab	TM	Dislocate membranes & pus, swab inflamed areas	Suspected pathogen (e.g., rule out Group A streptococci & diphtheria or Neisseria gonorrheae)	Do not touch oral mucosa or tongue with swab Routine culture practical only for group A streptococci Many viruses may be detected using 3 swabs for virus cultures
Tracheal aspirate		Sputum without saliva	Sterile container	Through nose or mouth, using sterile tube	Clinical impression	Often done in patient who cannot expectorate sputum
Skin					
Superficial	To clean skin, use 70% alcohol only	Needle aspirate or biopsy	Syringe or sterile container	Open vesicle, aspiration or swab	History Location Trauma	Consider herpes or other viruses if vesicles are present Make multiple smears

(Continued)

TABLE 2–1.　COLLECTING AND HANDLING SPECIMENS FOR LABORATORY DIAGNOSIS OF BACTERIAL INFECTIONS. INCLUDING ACID–FAST BACTERIA AND ANAEROBES *(Cont'd)*

Specimen Type	Patient Preparation	Optimal Specimen and Volume	Container	Collection Technic	Useful Clinical Information	Comments
Skin *(Cont'd)*						
Deep	As for blood culture	Needle aspirate or biopsy	Syringe or sterile container	Aspiration or biopsy	History Location Trauma	If cellulitis is suspected, scarify & obtain specimen from advancing edge. For burn wound, punch biopsy recommended
Tissue	Surgery	At least 1 cu cm unless needle biopsy	Sterile container (see Anaerobic Culture)	Open surgery or needle biopsy	Suspected pathogen Antibiotic therapy	Keep leftover material frozen (−70° C if possible) for further (viral) studies Consult with pathologist
Urine						
Clean voided urine	Careful instruction &/or assistance Follow standard protocol	First AM urine; several ml	Sterile wide-mouthed jar with lid	Clean voided midstream technic	Antibiotic therapy	May be refrigerated If at room temperature for 30 min, specimen is useless for quantitative studies
Catheter urine (indwelling catheter)		First AM urine; several ml	Sterile container	Iodine preparation of aspiration site on catheter	Clinical history	
Bladder urine	Surgical	First AM urine, several ml	Sterile container	Suprapubic aspiration	History	
Acid-Fast Bacteria						
Cerebrospinal fluid	As for other bacteria	5–10 ml or more	Acid-washed or plastic containers approved for AFB work	Aseptically	Previous history, skin test results	

Gastric washings	Patient should be fasting for 12 h before collection in AM	10 ml or more; may have to be repeated	Acid-washed or plastic containers approved for AFB work	Use chilled sterile rubber tube	Alert laboratory to previous history, exposure, & possible chemotherapy	Send to laboratory immediately or neutralize specimen
Respiratory tract	Instruction & assistance to cough up sputum rather than to produce saliva	3–5 early AM samples, 5–10 ml each	Widemouthed acid-washed jars or plastic containers for AFB work	Expectoration. Raising foot of bed during night may produce better specimen next AM	As for gastric washings	In case sputum cannot be raised by expectoration, the following technics may be used: aerosol inhalation, nasotracheal suction, or transtracheal aspiration (see special texts)
Urinary tract	Instruction &/or assistance. Follow standard protocol	Entire midstream specimen	Widemouthed acid-washed or plastic jars approved for AFB work	Clean-voided midstream technic	History, age, & sex are important	24-h urine collection for a pooled specimen is definitely discouraged
Wound tissue	As for other bacterial cultures	As for other cultures	As for urinary tract	Aseptic	History of chemotherapy	If specimen cannot be transported immediately, it should be frozen

The best clinical material for isolating microorganisms is the original material, fluid, pus, or tissue from the infectious process in which the pathogen is suspected. Gross observations such as "bloody," "mucoid," "foul-smelling," or "cloudy" are important and should be communicated. A syringe with aspirated pus, joint fluid, or pleural fluid, etc. is one of the best improvised collection and transport devices. It serves particularly well for fastidious anaerobes as long as no air is drawn in with the fluid and the needle is protected or capped with a sterile cap or stopper. The material should be delivered to the laboratory as soon as possible—at the latest, within 20 to 30 min. Tissue, if it is $\cong$ 1 cu cm or more in volume, keeps organisms alive for at least the same time without special precautions. Any sterile container with a lid, or even a sterile petri dish, is sufficient for **transport** within the hospital. Smaller fragments or biopsies need special protection against drying out and, if anaerobes are suspected, against O_2; special commercially available transport vials with a buffered transport fluid should be used.

Swabs are the least desirable means of specimen collection, since their cotton or fiber tips may be toxic for some microorganisms and the dry fiber surface always adversely affects fastidious organisms in small numbers. Swabs may be used, however, for the throat and skin when only staphylococci or streptococci in large numbers are suspected. In most other instances, the tips should be immersed in the semisolid fluid of transport vials. Date and time of collection should always be noted on the request slip so that the laboratory can detect any unusual delay in transport. Any chemotherapy given at the time of collection, the patient's clinical condition or diagnosis, and any precautions if the specimen is particularly hazardous (e.g., blood or serum from a patient with serum hepatitis) should be written on the request slip.

For many specimens, e.g., sputum and clean-voided, midstream urine specimens, it is essential to insure the patient's cooperation by either personal or written instructions for specimen collection.

If there is any doubt about the best way to collect or transport a specimen, contact the laboratory ahead of time. Many patients, especially those in large institutions, are considerably compromised in their host defenses and immune status and may become "infected" with various unusual microorganisms from their indigenous flora or the environment. Some of the newer agents— e.g., *Legionella pneumophila*, Pittsburgh pneumonia agent—illustrate the problem and demonstrate the need for close cooperation between clinician and laboratory.

LABORATORY DIAGNOSIS OF VIRAL, RICKETTSIAL, AND CHLAMYDIAL DISEASES

(See TABLE 2-2)

In the past, such diagnoses were made mainly on clinical grounds and sometimes confirmed by serologic testing in larger reference centers or public health laboratories. Since the tests require paired serum samples several weeks apart, test results often were not available soon enough to be of value in a particular case. To overcome this problem, many hospitals and medical centers now maintain laboratories for more rapid diagnosis—using, in addition to serology, isolation of the agent by culture technics, direct demonstration by electron microscopy, or use of fluorescent antibody and other immunologic technics for antigen detection, or indirectly by demonstration of giant cells, intracellular inclusions, etc.

It is essential that the physician who is trying to establish a diagnosis of viral, rickettsial, or chlamydial disease consider laboratory diagnosis early (not as an afterthought when all other tests have failed) and communicate with the virologist in charge about specimen collection and the particulars of the case. Most competent laboratories reject specimens submitted "for viral studies" without such communication and detailed clinical information.

Rickettsia, for the most part, are obligate intracellular parasites. Their isolation is very hazardous and done only in a few large reference centers; however, cultural isolation or serologic confirmation should be attempted in selected cases, and the material can be shipped to the reference center. Chlamydia (formerly Bedsonia) are also obligate intracellular parasites, much closer to bacteria than previously thought; again, a large reference center should be contacted for availability of services and shipping details.

LABORATORY DIAGNOSIS OF FUNGAL INFECTIONS

(See TABLE 2-3)

Patients may have superficial fungal infections involving the skin and its appendages or systemic fungal infections involving internal organs and tissues. Superficial infections are usually caused by

TABLE 2–2. COLLECTING AND HANDLING SPECIMENS FOR LABORATORY DIAGNOSIS OF VIRAL, RICKETTSIAL, AND CHLAMYDIAL DISEASES

NOTE: Direct inoculation of clinical material into tissue culture tubes at the bedside is most desirable, particularly if swabs are used for collection. Alternatively, agitate and extricate swab in viral transport medium (**VTM**) in screw-capped vials. If immediate inoculation is not possible, keep specimen or transport vial as close as possible to 4 C (39.2 F) (domestic refrigerator temperature). Only adeno-, entero-, and variola viruses are relatively stable at room temperature or tolerate freezing.

Viral Syndrome or Affected Organ System	*Serology*	*Optimal Specimen*	*Collection Details*	*Comments*
Blood for Culture		Heparinized blood	At least 3 ml (green-topped vacutainer)	Rarely done
Blood for Serology		Clotted whole blood taken during acute phase (within 5 days of onset)	At least 5 ml (red-topped vacutainer) (CAUTION: *Any blood may contain live hepatitis B virus*)	Should be stored frozen at −20 C (−4 F) or lower, for future reference; 2nd sample to be drawn at least 2 wk later
Congenital Syndrome				
Cytomegalovirus	CF	Throat swab	Posterior pharynx as for bacteriology	
		Urine		Fresh AM urine (10 ml or more), preferably repeated 2 or 3 times
Herpes simplex	CF	Throat swab Vesicle fluid	Posterior pharynx See under skin infections	
Enterovirus		Throat swab Feces	Posterior pharynx	
Rubella	HI	Blood for serology		
Eye Syndrome				
Herpes simplex	CF	Conjunctival swab or scraping	Use nasopharyngeal (thin wire) swab to obtain secretion from conjunctiva of eyelid Conjunctival scrapings: wash off in VTM for culture; make smear on clean, dry glass slide for chlamydiae	Eye scraping should be obtained by an ophthalmologist
Adenovirus	CF			
Varicella-zoster	CF			
Vaccinia	CF			

Abbreviations: CF, complement fixation; HI, hemagglutination-inhibition; N, none.

(*Continued*)

TABLE 2–2. COLLECTING AND HANDLING SPECIMENS FOR LABORATORY DIAGNOSIS OF VIRAL, RICKETTSIAL, AND CHLAMYDIAL DISEASES *(Cont'd)*

Viral Syndrome or Affected Organ System	Serology	Optimal Specimen	Collection Details	Comments
Gastrointestinal				
Adenovirus	CF	Feces or rectal swab Throat swab	Fresh feces (at least pea-sized) preferred	For mailing, make 20% suspension in 1 mol/L magnesium chloride & send supernatant
Enterovirus		Feces or rectal swab Throat swab		
Rotavirus		Feces		Electron microscopy or (better) ELISA (enzyme-linked immunosorbent assay) is used in some institutions to demonstrate Rotavirus in stool
Meningoencephalitis				
Arbovirus	HI, CF	Not cultured		
Enterovirus		CSF Throat swab Feces	CSF: Collect at least 1 ml into sterile screw-capped vial without VTM	CSF fluid should be inoculated directly at bedside if possible
Herpesvirus	CF	Throat swab Vesicle fluid		
Mumps virus	CF	Throat swab Urine		
Myocarditis, Pericarditis, Pleurodynia				
Coxsackie B virus	CF	Feces Throat swab (Pericardial fluid)		
Respiratory Syndrome				
Adenovirus	CF or N	Throat swab	Swab posterior pharynx or any visible lesion with dry, sterile cotton swab on wooden applicator; break off in screw-capped vial with VTM	Some wood may be impregnated with toxic preservatives; if this is a problem, extricate swab in VTM without breaking it off in VTM vial

Organism	Method	Specimen	Comments
Cytomegalovirus	CF	Throat swab Urine	
Enterovirus		Throat swab Feces	
Herpes simplex	CF	Throat swab	
Influenza virus	CF or HI	Throat swab	
Mumps virus	CF	Throat swab Urine	
Parainfluenza virus	CF or HI	Throat swab	
Respiratory syncytial virus	CF or N	Nasopharyngeal swab	Use thin wire swab or obtain nasal wash with bulb syringe & 5 ml buffered saline; do not add VTM; transport to laboratory immediately	Inoculation at bedside increases isolation rates
Rhinovirus		Throat swab	
Skin Infections			
Coxsackie A virus		Skin scraping with swab or culturette, also throat swabs	Vesicles or blebs should be ruptured with swab & the base scraped; a slide may be obtained by rolling the swab onto 2 dime-sized areas of a glass slide for fluorescent antibody staining; prepare & air-dry 2 slides	Pox virus may be identified in vesicle fluid by electron microscopy; if Coxsackie A virus is suspected, include feces or rectal swab; with maculo-papular rashes (adeno-, entero-, parainfluenza, respiratory syncytial viruses) only throat swabs are submitted, plus feces for entero- & adenoviruses
Herpes simplex virus	HI		
Varicella-zoster virus	CF		
Vaccinia virus			
Tissue, Biopsies		In sterile container	At least 1 cu cm	Specimen will have to be minced in the laboratory Very small biopsies should be submitted in VTM

(Continued)

TABLE 2–2. COLLECTING AND HANDLING SPECIMENS FOR LABORATORY DIAGNOSIS OF VIRAL, RICKETTSIAL, AND CHLAMYDIAL DISEASES *(Cont'd)*

Viral Syndrome or Affected Organ System	Serology	Optimal Specimen	Collection Details	Comments
Rickettsial Infections		Culture: Whole blood or aseptically obtained tissue	Flash freeze; maintain at −70 C (−94 F) during shipment	Culturing is hazardous & available only in some large reference centers
	CF	Serology: Collect & handle as for virus serology	Paired sera	CF satisfactory for all rickettsial infections except scrub typhus; Weil-Felix agglutination reactions most helpful for epidemic, murine, & scrub typhus & for Rocky Mountain & other tick-borne spotted fevers
Chlamydial Infections	CF	Serology: Collect & handle as for virus serology	Paired sera	Useful for all chlamydial infections
Psittacosis		Culture: Lung tissue	Notify laboratory in advance & obtain special instructions	Possible for psittacosis but quite hazardous
Lymphogranuloma venereum (LGV)		Lymph node aspiration		Possible for LGV but requires special laboratory
Trachoma & Inclusion conjunctivitis		Thin swabs or corneal scrapings	Notify laboratory in advance & obtain special instructions	Quite sensitive & increasingly used for trachoma & inclusion conjunctivitis (TRIC agents)
Nongonococcal urethritis		Thin swabs		

TABLE 2–3. COLLECTING AND HANDLING SPECIMENS FOR LABORATORY DIAGNOSIS OF FUNGAL INFECTIONS

Affected Organ System	Fungus	Optimal Specimen	Collection Details and Comments
Abscess	E.g., Candida, Blastomyces, Cryptococcus	Saline aspirate of abscess contents sent in syringe or transferred to sterile container	Abscess walls & base yield more positive results than pus; specimens should be cultured as soon as possible
Blood	E.g., Candida, Torulopsis, Histoplasma, Cryptococcus	5–10 ml anticoagulated (SPS*) blood; or collect specimen directly into diphasic culture media (Castaneda media)	Specimens should be processed in laboratory on the day collected May encounter other unusual fungi in immuno-suppressed patients
Bone marrow	Histoplasma Candida Cryptococcus Aspergillus Blastomyces	As much as is available, heparinized, in syringe or sterile tube	Specimens should be processed in laboratory on day collected (NOTE: Bone-marrow specimen worked up for systemic mycoses may yield M. tuberculosis)
Body Fluids	Any fungus	Send the anticoagulated fluid in appropriate sterile container	Process as soon as possible
Central Nervous System	Cryptococcus Candida Blastomyces Coccidioides Opportunistic fungi Zygomycetes	As much as is available—i.e., 2–3 ml in sterile screw-capped tubes	Aseptically pool all separate tubes of CSF & centrifuge 10–15 min at ≅2500 rpm; use the sediment for smears & culture Brain lesions may turn out to be Nocardia (not a fungus)
Ear (Otitis externa)	Aspergillus	Scrapings preferred or 1 swab in sterile test tube with enough saline to keep swab moist	If mycelia are grossly visible, send scrapings in petri dish or sterile test tube For specimen from middle or inner ear, use sterile funnel
Eye (Corneal ulcer)	E.g., Fusarium spp., Aspergillus, Zygomycetes, Candida, many others	Inoculate scrapings directly to culture media or send smears to laboratory	Use clean, smooth spatulum to procure scrapings (done by physician) Inner-eye infection (endogenous oculomycosis) most often caused by Candida albicans

* SPS, sodium polyanethol sulfonate.

(Continued)

TABLE 2-3. COLLECTING AND HANDLING SPECIMENS FOR LABORATORY DIAGNOSIS OF FUNGAL INFECTIONS *(Cont'd)*

Affected Organ System	Fungus	Optimal Specimen	Collection Details and Comments
Oral Cavity Mouth (thrush) Tongue	Candida	Tongue depressor scrapings, swab in sterile tube, or smears on glass slide	Split tongue depressor along longitudinal axis & use new edge to scrape lesion; send tongue depressor, with scrapings, in petri dish or sterile tube *Note which end has the specimen*
Respiratory Tract Sputum Transtracheal aspirate	Any fungus *Nocardia* & *Actinomycetes* (not fungi) may be encountered	Expectorated or aspirated specimen from lungs, in sterile container; also tracheal aspirates, broncheal washings, & lung tissue	Early-AM. before-breakfast specimen preferred Patient should either brush teeth & rinse mouth well with water, or a good water- or mouthwash-rinse should just precede collecting specimen; specimen should be processed as soon as possible
Nose Nasopharynx	*Aspergillus* *Allescheria* *Acremonium* *Histoplasma duboisii*	Swab in sterile test tube with saline; nasal scrapings between 2 slides or in petri dish or sterile tube	
Skin System** Fingernail	Dermatophytes, *Candida*	Nail clippings & scrapings in sterile petri dish, between 2 glass microscope slides, or in clean pill envelope	Disinfect infected area with 70% alcohol & use sterile blade to scrape through infected area Do not collect material from under nail Culture within 48 h
Skin	Dermatophytes, *Candida*, *Blastomyces*, *Coccidioides*, Sporotrichosis (deeper with lymph node involvement)	Skin scrapings in sterile petri dish, between 2 glass microscope slides, or in clean pill envelope	Disinfect infected area with 70% alcohol & allow alcohol to dry Scrape from periphery of one or more lesions Be sure to include scrapings from the apparently healthy skin adjoining the lesion *Corynebacterium erythrasmae* causes similar lesions

Hair	Dermatophytes	Pluck several infected hairs & place in sterile petri dish, between 2 glass microscope slides, or in clean pill envelope	Use Wood's light to fluoresce infected hairs, & pluck them for processing; otherwise, pick dull, brittle hairs & follicles from infected areas (Only short hair stubs from broken hair may be available)
Vesicles	Dermatophytes	Snip off tips of several vesicles & submit them in petri dish or test tube	Disinfect vesicular area with 70% alcohol, dry, & snip off tips of vesicles. Vesicular fluids are usually devoid of fungi
Tissue Lymph nodes Liver biopsy	Any fungus	Send biopsy in sterile container. Avoid allowing specimen to dry (use sterile broth)	Try to include walls & central areas of biopsied tissue (liver excepted). Specimens should be cultured as soon as possible
Ulcers	Sporothrix Cryptococcus Blastomyces Histoplasma Coccidioides Dematiaceous fungi Aerobic Actinomycetes	Saline aspirates from the ulcer base & wall in sterile screw-capped tube. If biopsied, include aspirates, ulcer base & wall	Syringe with 25-gauge needle is convenient for collecting aspirates. Specimens should be cultured as soon as possible
Urogenital System Urine	Candida Torulopsis Cryptococcus Blastomyces	50–100 ml in clean sterile container	Midstream specimens collected first thing in AM preferred; should be examined in laboratory on day collected
Prostatic secretions, cervix, vagina	Candida Torulopsis	Moisten swab or secretions in either sterile tube or small amount of sterile saline in a test tube (swabs only)	Specimens should be processed in laboratory on day collected

** Avoid using any topical ointment or antifungal creams or powders for at least 1 wk before specimen is collected. If possible, do not use cotton balls to apply disinfectant; use sponges, etc.

dermatophytes that invade only the epidermis, hair, and nails. However, *Candida albicans* frequently causes superficial infections as well (see Chs. 9 and 191), and *Corynebacterium erythrasmae*, a diphtheroid gram-positive bacterium, may cause similar skin lesions. Therapy is quite different for each of these infections, and the etiology should be established. KOH mount and Gram stain can be very helpful and are easily and quickly done.

The increased number of immunosuppressed patients and the aggressive treatment of leukemia and similar conditions account for the ever-increasing numbers of systemic fungal infections as well as other infections. In some situations, (e.g., IV hyperalimentation) fungi are among the most frequently isolated pathogens. It is essential to forewarn laboratories about the possibility of fungi in the specimen, since the work-up requires additional media and time for incubation. Serologic tests for fungal diseases are only starting to become as helpful as for other microbial diseases. In vitro susceptibility tests for antifungal agents and their assay in serum and other body fluids should be done in large, specialized laboratories.

LABORATORY DIAGNOSIS OF PARASITIC INFECTIONS

(See TABLE 2–4)

Detecting an intestinal parasite is contingent on many factors, among which are quality and number of specimens; for instance, many protozoa, unlike helminths, are shed in sporadic numbers, and repeated examinations may almost double the yield.

For intestinal ova or parasites, 3 stool specimens should, preferably, be collected consecutively every other day. Alternatively, the series may be shortened to 3 consecutive days. Duodenal aspirates or string test specimens may be required. Posttreatment follow-up examinations should be started 2 wk after completion of therapy for helminthic, 4 wk for protozoan, and 6 wk for *Taenia* infections.

Except for a few specific tests, usually no special preparations are required before collecting a stool other than to ensure against contamination with urine, water, dirt, or disinfectants. However, antibiotics, contrast material purgatives, and antacids will adversely affect detection of parasites or decrease to below detectable levels the number of parasites passed; it may be several weeks before such stools become suitable for examination, depending on how soon the interfering compounds are cleared from the GI tract.

Freshly passed stools should be sent to the examining laboratory within 15 min, particularly if they are unformed or diarrheal (i.e., likely to contain motile trophozoites). Do not attempt to keep specimens warm while they are in transit to the laboratory. Formed stools should be refrigerated (*not* frozen) if the examination cannot be effected immediately. If facilities exist, portions of fresh specimen may be emulsified (1 part feces to 3 parts fixative) in polyvinyl alcohol **(PVA)** or 5 to 10% aqueous formalin. Thin fecal smears fixed in Schaudinn's fixative are also useful. Such preserved specimens are suitable for mailing.

If a purgative is attempted, only saline cathartics are recommended. Purged specimens should be examined immediately or preserved. Although the yield of parasites, particularly trophozoites, may be enhanced by catharsis, the process itself disrupts the normal flow of parasites and it may be as long as 1 wk before any parasites can be visualized again.

Anal swabs are useful for detecting pinworms and tapeworms but are unsatisfactory specimens for parasitologic examination.

Specimens collected by sigmoidoscopy should be considered, particularly from patients with a history of amebiasis but a negative series of routine stool examinations. The sigmoidoscopic material should be examined immediately. The specimen is collected with a curette or Volkman's spoon; cotton swabs are unsatisfactory. Sigmoidoscopic specimens and rectal and bladder biopsies should be examined immediately.

For patients with a negative series of stools, one may elect to do the string test for *Giardia* and *Strongyloides*. After overnight fasting, have the patient, in a sitting position, moisten his throat with a sip of water and swallow the string-capsule. The loose end of the string is taped to the patient's neck. The patient should swallow a glass of water at 1 h and at 2 h, but avoid eating anything solid while the string-capsule is in place. After 4 to 6 h, the patient should raise his chin and open his mouth while the physician quickly, but gently, retrieves the string. The string, which dries quickly, should be placed in a sterile container and sent immediately to the laboratory. The patient may swallow more water to remove any bitter aftertaste. As with all critical procedures, advance consultation with the laboratory is essential.

TABLE 2-4. COLLECTING AND HANDLING SPECIMENS FOR LABORATORY DIAGNOSIS OF PARASITIC INFECTIONS

Affected Organ System	Parasite	Optimal Specimen	Collection Details	Comments
Blood	Plasmodium spp.	Thick & thin smears from capillary blood (i.e., finger or earlobe, using disposable lancet) or 5–10 ml fresh anticoagulated blood Thin smears are made same as hematology differential slides; for thick smears, place drop of blood on meticulously clean glass slide & mix into area about 5/8" in diameter Place slide on flat surface; allow blood to dry gently & dust-free before sending slide to laboratory	Collect every 6 h for 3 days Best time to collect specimen is 12 h after a chill Be certain all alcohol disinfectant has evaporated before collecting blood specimen Smears may be made from the tube or anticoagulated blood up to 1 h after collected Slowly dry in covered dish	Wright's or Giemsa stain Glass slides must be very clean If there is any doubt about ability to prepare good slides, collect anticoagulated blood in a tube & send to laboratory for preparation of slides & staining
	Trypanosoma spp.	Place & coverslip drop of capillary blood from a fingerstick onto clean glass slide Alternatively, send 5–6 ml of anticoagulated blood to laboratory		Wright's or Giemsa stain
	Microfilariae	Send 5–10 ml of anticoagulated blood If first specimen is negative, collect one or more to be concentrated For African onchocerciasis, "skin snips" from thigh, buttocks, iliac crest For American onchocerciasis, "skin snips" from scalp, buttocks, face	Wuchereria bancrofti & Brugia malayi: collect between 10 PM & 2 AM Loa loa, Acanthocheilonema perstans, & Mansonella ozzardi: collect between 10 AM & 6 PM For "skin snips," see below under Skin	Wright's or Giemsa stain

(Continued)

TABLE 2-4. COLLECTING AND HANDLING SPECIMENS FOR LABORATORY DIAGNOSIS OF PARASITIC INFECTIONS (Cont'd)

Affected Organ System	Parasite	Optimal Specimen	Collection Details	Comments
Bone Marrow	Leishmania spp	Bone marrow aspirates or thin air-dried smears	Centrifuge 5–10 ml of anticoagulated blood & make buffy coat smears	Wright's or Giemsa stain
Central Nervous System	Naegleria Hartmannella Acanthameba group	Fresh spinal fluid	Aseptic collection Keep specimen temperature	If immediate examination by light of phase microscopy is not possible, fix slides in PVA, Schaudinn's fixative, or 5–10% formalin
Intestinal System Biopsies Jejunal Duodenal	Giardia lamblia Strongyloides	Collected & placed in sterile jar or tube with a little saline, or placed on coverslipped glass microscope slide	Examine immediately	
Rectal	Entamoeba histolytica Schistosoma mansoni Schistosoma japonicum	For schistosomes: biopsy from level of dorsal fold (Houston valve), about 9 cm from anus		
Feces	Entamoeba histolytica Other amebas Trichomonas spp.	3 freshly passed stools collected in AM every other day	If unformed or diarrheal, specimen should be examined within 15 min Formed stools may be refrigerated until examined (see also accompanying text)	Schaudinn's fixative, PVA, or 5–10% formalin
	Giardia lamblia	3 freshly passed stools collected in AM every other day	If initial series of 3 specimens is negative, examine 3 more, 1/wk Duodenal aspirates (string test) may be necessary (see accompanying text)	

	Balantidium coli, Trichuris trichiura, Ascaris lumbricoides, Hookworm, Strongyloides, Tapeworms, Flukes	Up to 3 stools collected daily	Not critical to examine immediately. May be refrigerated
	Enterobius vermicularis	Cellophane tape or anal swab	Collect from area around anus; patient should be resting & quiet for several hours before collecting specimen—usually in AM before bowel movement or bath
Sigmoidoscopy (Proctoscopy)	Entamoeba histolytica	Fresh scrapings collected with a curette or Volkmann's spoon; or with a surgical instrument snip off a piece of mucosa; or aspirate lesion with a 1-ml serologic pipette with a rubber bulb. Cotton-tipped swabs are not satisfactory	If patient has not had a bowel movement shortly before sigmoidoscopy is begun, he should be purged and the procedure not started for 2–3 h. Specimen must be examined immediately or fixed for later examination
Respiratory Tract Sputum	Paragonimus westermani	Fresh sputum	Instruct patient carefully
Aspirates (tracheal, broncheal)	Entamoeba histolytica, Strongyloides, Stercorous Echinococcus granulosus, Hookworm, Ascaris	Any aspirated material; also drainage material	If amebiasis is suspected, specimen should be examined as soon as possible or preserved for later examination
Lung biopsy	All listed above under Respiratory Tract + Pneumocystis carinii	Open lung biopsy. Percutaneous biopsy under fluoroscopy	Collect into sterile container. If needle biopsy, add sterile saline. For Pneumocystis carinii, lung biopsy is best

(Continued)

TABLE 2–4. COLLECTING AND HANDLING SPECIMENS FOR LABORATORY DIAGNOSIS OF PARASITIC INFECTIONS (Cont'd)

Affected Organ System	Parasite	Optimal Specimen	Collection Details	Comments
Skin	Onchocerca volvulus	African cases, "skin snips" from thigh, buttocks, iliac crest For American cases, "skin snips" from face, scapula, buttocks	For "skin snips," disinfect skin with alcohol, insert 25-gauge needle just under epidermis, raise it, & slice off small piece of tissue with a scalpel or razor blade; bleeding should not occur	
	Leishmania spp. Entamoeba histolytica	Ulcer bed	In amebiasis or leishmaniasis, parasites typically are found in the lesion/ulcer wall rather than in the pus	
	Taenia solium Echinococcus granulosus	Regular biopsy technic		
Urogenital System Vagina Urethra Prostatic secretions	Trichomonas spp	1 sterile swab in a tube with small amount of sterile saline	Females should not douche for 3–4 days before collecting specimen Send to laboratory as soon as possible, before trichomonads stop moving	
Bladder	Schistosoma haematobium	Biopsy from area around the trigone		

3. SUPERFICIAL INFECTIONS

CELLULITIS

A diffuse, spreading, acute inflammation within solid (nonhollow) tissues, characterized by hyperemia, leukocytic infiltration, and edema without cellular necrosis or suppuration. It is most commonly evident in the skin and subcutaneous structures but may involve deeper areas.

Etiology

Streptococcus pyogenes (Group A β-hemolytic streptococcus) is the most common cause of superficial cellulitis; diffuse spread of infection occurs because streptokinase, DNAse, and hyaluronidase—enzymes produced by the organism—break down cellular components that otherwise would contain and localize the inflammatory process. *Staphylococcus aureus* occasionally causes a superficial cellulitis typically less extensive than that of streptococcal origin and usually only in association with an open wound or cutaneous abscess. Superficial cellulitis caused by other organisms occurs rarely and generally only with impaired host defenses such as granulocytopenia or tissue ischemia, which prevent localization of infection.

Symptoms and Signs

The lower extremities are the most common sites of infection. A cutaneous abnormality, such as skin trauma, ulceration, tinea pedis, or dermatitis, often precedes the infection; areas of lymphedema or other edema seem especially susceptible. Frequently, however, no predisposing condition or site of entry is evident. The major findings are local erythema and tenderness, frequently with lymphangitis and regional lymphadenopathy. The skin is hot, red, and edematous, with an infiltrated surface resembling the skin of an orange (*peau d'orange*). The borders are usually indistinct, but in **erysipelas,** a type of cellulitis, the raised margins are sharply demarcated. Petechiae are common; large areas of ecchymosis, rare. Vesicles and bullae may develop and rupture, occasionally with necrosis of the involved skin. Systemic manifestations (fever, chills, tachycardia, headache, hypotension, and delirium) sometimes occur, but many patients do not appear ill. Leukocytosis is common, but not constant.

Diagnosis

The diagnosis usually depends on the clinical findings. The responsible organism is difficult to isolate, even with aspiration of the infected area, unless pus has formed or there is an open wound. Blood cultures are only occasionally positive. Serologic tests, especially measurement of anti-DNAse B, will confirm a streptococcal etiology, but are usually unnecessary.

Although cellulitis and deep vein thrombosis are easily differentiated clinically, many physicians confuse the two entities when edema occurs in the lower extremities. The major differences are (1) skin temperature: hot in cellulitis, normal or cool with deep venous thrombosis; (2) skin color: red in cellulitis, normal or cyanotic with deep venous thrombosis; and (3) skin surface: a *peau d'orange* appearance in cellulitis, smooth in deep venous thrombosis. Lymphangitis and regional lymphadenopathy, frequent in cellulitis, do not occur with deep venous thrombosis.

Course and Prognosis

Local abscesses form occasionally and require incision and drainage. Serious but rare complications include development of severe necrotizing subcutaneous infection (streptococcal gangrene or necrotizing fasciitis) and bacteremia with metastatic foci of infection. Even in the preantibiotic era, however, most cases of superficial cellulitis resolved spontaneously. Recurrences in the same area were common, sometimes causing serious damage to the lymphatics, chronic lymphatic obstruction, marked edema, and, rarely, elephantiasis. With antibiotic therapy, such complications are uncommon. Symptoms and signs of superficial cellulitis usually resolve after a few days of antibiotics, but often the clinical manifestations worsen initially, presumably from the abrupt death of organisms and release of their enzymes.

Treatment

Penicillin is the drug of choice. For mild, outpatient cases, penicillin V 250 mg q.i.d., or a single dose of benzathine penicillin 1.2 million u. IM, is adequate. For severe infections requiring hospitalization, aqueous penicillin G 400,000 u. IV q 6 h is indicated. For penicillin-allergic patients, erythromycin 250 mg orally q.i.d. is an effective alternative for mild infections, and parenteral clindamycin or vancomycin can be used for severe cases. When pus or an open wound is present, results of a Gram stain should dictate antibiotic choice. Immobilizing and elevating the affected area help reduce edema; cool, wet dressings may help relieve local discomfort.

LYMPHADENITIS

Inflammation of lymph nodes.

Etiology

Any pathogen—bacterial, viral, protozoal, rickettsial, or fungal—can cause lymphadenitis. The lymph node involvement may be generalized, with systemic infections, or confined to regional lymph nodes draining a local area of infection. **Infections with prominent regional lymphadenopathy include** streptococcal disease, TB or nontuberculous mycobacterial disease, tularemia, plague, cat-scratch disease, primary syphilis, lymphogranuloma venereum, chancroid, and genital herpes simplex. **Generalized lymph node enlargement is frequent in** infectious mononucleosis, cytomegalovirus infection, toxoplasmosis, brucellosis, secondary syphilis, and disseminated histoplasmosis.

Symptoms and Signs

Lymph node enlargement from edema and leukocytic cellular infiltration, the major sign of lymphadenitis, may be asymptomatic or may cause pain and tenderness. With some infections the overlying skin is inflamed, occasionally with cellulitis; abscess formation may occur, and penetration to the skin will produce draining sinuses.

Diagnosis

Lymphadenitis and its cause are usually apparent. Occasionally, however, lymph node aspiration and culture or excisional biopsy may be necessary.

Treatment and Course

Treatment depends on the underlying cause. With resolution of the primary process, lymph node enlargement usually resolves, but sometimes firm, nontender lymphadenopathy persists. Hot, wet applications may help relieve symptoms of acutely painful lymph nodes. Abscesses require surgical drainage (see Ch. 4).

ACUTE LYMPHANGITIS

Acute inflammation of the subcutaneous lymphatic channels, usually caused by Streptococcus pyogenes.

Symptoms and Signs

Streptococci most commonly enter the lymphatic channels from an abrasion, wound, or infection, usually cellulitis, on an extremity. Red, irregular, warm, and tender streaks develop and extend proximally. Regional lymph nodes are typically enlarged and tender. Systemic manifestations such as fever, shaking chills, tachycardia, and headache are common, often are more severe than the cutaneous findings would suggest, and occasionally precede any evidence of significant local infection. Leukocytosis, sometimes marked, is usual.

Diagnosis

Red, irregular linear streaks extending toward regional lymph nodes from a peripheral lesion on an extremity indicate lymphangitis. As in cellulitis, culture of the responsible organism is uncommon unless there is pus, an open wound, or bacteremia.

Course and Treatment

Bacteremia with metastatic foci of infection may occur, often with startling rapidity. Rarely, cellulitis with suppuration, necrosis, and ulceration may develop along the course of the involved lymph channels. Most cases respond rapidly to antibiotic therapy, as discussed under Cᴇʟʟᴜʟɪᴛɪs, above.

CUTANEOUS ABSCESSES

Localized collections of pus causing fluctuant soft-tissue swelling surrounded by erythema. Local cellulitis, lymphangitis, regional lymphadenopathy, fever, and leukocytosis are variable accompanying features. These abscesses usually follow minor skin trauma.

Organisms isolated from cutaneous abscesses are typically the bacteria indigenous to the skin of the involved area. Abscesses in the perineal region (inguinal, vaginal, buttock, and perirectal) contain organisms found in the stool, commonly anaerobes alone or a combination of aerobes and anaerobes. *Peptococcus, Peptostreptococcus, Lactobacillus, Bacteroides,* and *Fusobacterium* species are the predominant anaerobic isolates; α- and nonhemolytic streptococci are the most frequent aerobes. For abscesses on the trunk, extremities, axillae, or head and neck, aerobes alone or a mixture of aerobic and anaerobic flora is usual. The most frequent anaerobic species are *Peptococcus* and *Proprionibacterium*; the most common aerobic organisms are *Staphylococcus aureus* and *epidermidis. Staphylococcus aureus*, found in less than half of cutaneous abscesses in any location, typically occurs in pure culture.

The **treatment** of cutaneous abscesses is incision of the fluctuant area, thorough evacuation of pus from the abscess cavity with careful probing to remove loculations, irrigation with normal saline, and loose packing with a gauze wick that is removed 24 to 48 h later. Local heat and elevation of the affected area, if possible, may hasten resolution of the tissue inflammation. Gram stain, culture, and antibiotic therapy are unnecessary, unless the patient has signs of systemic infection, compromised host defenses, or facial abscesses in the area drained by the cavernous sinus.

NECROTIZING SUBCUTANEOUS INFECTIONS

(Necrotizing Fasciitis; Synergistic Necrotizing Cellulitis)

Severe infections, typically due to a mixture of aerobic and anaerobic organisms, that cause necrosis of subcutaneous tissue, usually including the fascia. When the male genitalia are involved, this infection is called **Fournier's disease.**

Etiology, Pathogenesis, and Pathology

While *Streptococcus pyogenes* (Group A streptococcus) alone may occasionally cause these infections, usually they are caused by a mixture of aerobic and anaerobic bacteria, the most common isolates being aerobic streptococci other than Group A, aerobic gram-negative bacilli, anaerobic gram-positive cocci, and *Bacteroides* species.

These organisms reach the subcutaneous tissue by extension from a contiguous infection or trauma to the area. The trauma, often minor, may be thermal, chemical, or mechanical, including surgical procedures. Involvement of the extremities, the most common site, may occur from infected cutaneous ulcers or infectious complications of previous trauma. Involvement of the perineum, the second most common site, is usually a complication of preceding surgery, perirectal abscesses, perfurethral gland infection, or retroperitoneal infections from perforated abdominal viscera.

The major gross pathologic findings are edema and necrosis of the subcutaneous tissues, including the adjacent fascia; widespread undermining of the surrounding tissue; occlusion of small subcutaneous vessels, leading to dermal gangrene; and absent or minimal muscle involvement. Microscopic abnormalities include intense leukocytic infiltration, microabscess formation, and necrosis in the subcutaneous tissue and adjacent fascia. There is often complete occlusion of the subcutaneous arterioles and venules.

The combination of ischemia, edema, and inflammation in the subcutaneous tissue results in decreased P_{O_2}, permitting growth of obligate anaerobes like *Bacteroides* and promoting anaerobic metabolism by facultative organisms like *E. coli*. This anaerobic metabolism often produces hydrogen and nitrogen, relatively insoluble gases, that may accumulate in subcutaneous tissues and cause crepitus or roentgenographically detectable gas.

Patients with diabetes mellitus seem predisposed to these infections. Possible explanations include (1) small vessel disease, causing tissue hypoxia and therefore promoting anaerobic bacterial metabolism; (2) defective leukocyte function; and (3) elevated tissue glucose, providing abundant nutrients for bacterial growth.

Symptoms and Signs

The skin overlying the infection is tender, red, hot, and swollen; with progression, violaceous discoloration, bullae, crepitus, and dermal gangrene may develop. Fever, nearly always present, typically is accompanied by systemic toxicity, including tachycardia and altered mental status ranging from confusion to obtundation. Evidence of intravascular volume depletion, including hypotension, is frequent.

Laboratory Findings

Polymorphonuclear leukocytosis is usual. With diabetics, the blood glucose is elevated and ketoacidosis may occur. Decreased intravascular volume causes concentrated urine and increased serum creatinine and BUN. Radiographs of the affected area often demonstrate soft-tissue gas.

Diagnosis

Red, hot, tender, and markedly edematous skin suggests an underlying necrotizing subcutaneous infection. Rapid progression or the development of bullae, ecchymoses, dermal gangrene, fluctuance, crepitus, or roentgenographically visible soft-tissue gas confirms the necessity for surgical exploration. Blood cultures should be obtained. Pus aspirated into a syringe percutaneously or during surgery provides the best material for Gram stain and aerobic and anaerobic cultures.

Prognosis

The mortality rate is about 30%. Factors associated with a poor prognosis include old age, the presence of other medical problems, delayed diagnosis and therapy, and insufficiently extensive surgery.

Treatment

Gram stain of pus should determine antibiotic choice. Since both aerobes and anaerobes are usually present, gentamicin and clindamycin, or chloramphenicol alone, will usually be appropriate pending culture results. Large quantities of IV fluids are needed to replace losses into the tissues.

The major element of therapy is extensive incision and debridement. The area involved is typically greater than anticipated by the overlying skin abnormalities, and the incision should be extended until an instrument or finger can no longer separate the skin and subcutaneous tissue from the deep fascia. The most common error is insufficient surgical exposure, and repeating the operation 1 to 2 days later is usually prudent to insure adequate incision and debridement of all affected areas. Amputation of an extremity may be necessary.

4.   ABSCESSES

Collections of pus, usually caused by bacterial infection, in tissues, organs, or confined spaces.

This chapter covers the basic elements of abscess formation; the clinical characteristics of common and important abscesses, based on their location in the body; and the principles of treatment. Specific organisms involved vary greatly and are also discussed elsewhere in the text under appropriate headings. In particular, the frequency, importance, and complexities of mixed anaerobic infections are receiving increasing attention; they are discussed in Ch. 8.

Pathogenesis

Organisms causing an abscess may enter the tissue by (1) direct implantation (e.g., penetrating trauma with an unsterile object); (2) spread from an established, contiguous infection; (3) dissemination via lymphatic or hematogenous routes from a distant site; or (4) migration from a location where they are resident flora into an adjacent, normally sterile area because of disruption of natural barriers (e.g., perforation of an abdominal viscus causing an intra-abdominal abscess).

Predisposing factors to abscess formation include impaired host defense mechanisms (e.g., abnormal leukocyte function); the presence of foreign bodies; obstruction to normal drainage of the urinary, biliary, or respiratory tracts; tissue ischemia or necrosis; hematoma or excessive fluid accumulation in tissue; and trauma.

Abscesses begin as **cellulitis** (see Ch. 3). The separation of cellular elements by fluid or by the space created by cellular necrosis from another cause provides an area where leukocytes can accumulate and form the abscess. The abscess may expand by progressive dissection by pus or by necrosis of surrounding cells. Highly vascularized connective tissue may then invade and surround the necrotic tissue, leukocytes, and debris to limit further spread.

Symptoms, Signs, and Complications

The symptoms and signs of cutaneous or subcutaneous abscesses are heat; swelling; tenderness; redness over the affected site; and, possibly, fever, especially when surrounding cellulitis is present. For deep-seated abscesses the major findings are local pain and tenderness and systemic symptoms, especially fever, but also such nonspecific complaints as anorexia, weight loss, and fatigue. In some locations the predominant manifestation is abnormal organ function, e.g., hemiplegia with a brain abscess.

Complications of abscesses include bacteremia, with spread of infection to distant sites; rupture into adjacent tissue; bleeding from vessels eroded by inflammation; impaired function of a vital organ; and inanition from the systemic effects of anorexia and tissue catabolism.

Treatment

Healing of an abscess usually requires removal of its contents, since these can provoke further inflammation. Drainage may occur spontaneously by rupture of the abscess into adjacent tissue or to the outside surface of the body, sometimes with formation of chronic draining sinuses. Without spontaneous or surgical drainage, an abscess occasionally resolves slowly after proteolytic digestion of the pus results in thin, sterile fluid that is resorbed into the bloodstream. Incomplete resorption leaves a cystic loculation within a fibrous wall, where calcium salts sometimes accumulate to form a calcified mass.

The major elements of adequate drainage are thorough removal of pus, necrotic tissue, and debris (often necessitating blunt dissection to disrupt the fibrous walls surrounding loculated suppuration), and elimination of dead space, which provides a locus for further accumulation of organisms, leukocytes, and debris (often accomplished by packing with gauze—capillary action draws up liquified contents and keeps the wound clean and dry—or by using various types of drains). Predisposing conditions, e.g., obstruction or the presence of a foreign body, require correction if possible.

Systemic antimicrobial agents active against the responsible organisms are indicated for deep-seated infections, but are rarely effective without concurrent surgical drainage. Gram stains, cultures, and sensitivity studies of purulent material removed by aspiration or drainage of the abscess provide an indispensable guide to antibiotic choice by identifying the infecting organisms and their antimicrobial susceptibility.

INTRA-ABDOMINAL ABSCESSES

The 3 types of intra-abdominal abscesses are (1) **intraperitoneal,** (2) **retroperitoneal,** and (3) **visceral.** Though the clinical features vary, most of these abscesses cause fever, leukocytosis, and an increased ESR. Pain, if present, usually occurs near the abscess. Paralytic ileus, either generalized or localized near the infection, may develop, and nonspecific GI symptoms, such as anorexia, nausea, vomiting, and diarrhea or constipation, are common.

Many intra-abdominal abscesses develop from disruption of the GI tract by perforation or inflammation; the infecting organisms, a complex mixture of anaerobic and aerobic bacteria, are part of the normal bowel flora. The most important isolates from these abscesses are aerobic gram-negative rods, e.g., *E. coli* and *Klebsiella*, and anaerobes, especially *Bacteroides fragilis*; effective antimicrobial therapy requires agents active against these organisms. For patients with normal renal function, giving a combination of an aminoglycoside, such as gentamicin 1.5 mg/kg q 8 h, and clindamycin 600 mg q 6 h is effective. Chloramphenicol alone, 500 mg q 6 h, is a reasonable alternative.

INTRAPERITONEAL ABSCESSES

The 3 types of abscesses in this group, **subphrenic, midabdominal,** and **pelvic,** develop from generalized peritonitis due to causes such as trauma, perforated abdominal viscera, or localized peritonitis resulting from infection in a contiguous site. With generalized peritonitis, the effects of gravity and intra-abdominal pressure favor localization to the subphrenic spaces, pelvis, and paracolic gutters lateral to the ascending and descending colon.

SUBPHRENIC ABSCESSES

The subphrenic space, arbitrarily defined as lying below the diaphragm and above the transverse colon, consists of 4 subdivisions. On the right side are the suprahepatic and subhepatic spaces. On the left side, the subhepatic and suprahepatic spaces freely communicate and constitute a single combined subphrenic space. The other left-sided space, lying behind the stomach and anterior to the pancreas, is the lesser sac. About 55% of subphrenic abscesses are right-sided, 25% left-sided, and 20% multiple.

Etiology and Pathogenesis

Most subphrenic abscesses arise from direct contamination of the area following local disease, injury, or, most frequently, surgery. They develop from peritonitis secondary to another cause, such as perforated viscus; extension from an abscess in an adjacent organ; or, most commonly, as a postoperative complication of abdominal surgery, especially on the biliary tract, duodenum, or stomach. The peritoneum may be contaminated during surgery or afterwards from such events as anastomotic leaks. Some develop following spread of infection through the peritoneal cavity from a distant site of contamination (e.g., appendicitis). Factors favoring movement of fluid into subphrenic spaces include the negative pressure in the area generated during the diaphragmatic movement of respiration, and greater intra-abdominal pressure in the lower abdomen, promoting fluid movement superiorly. In a few patients, no predisposing cause is evident (primary subphrenic abscess); presumably, a subclinical peritonitis occurred.

Symptoms and Signs

Clinical manifestations of subphrenic abscesses usually begin subtly, within 3 to 6 wk following surgery, but occasionally do not appear for several months. Fever, nearly always present, may be the only evidence of the abscess. Nonspecific constitutional symptoms such as anorexia and weight loss are common. The most frequent findings relate to the thorax and abdomen. Nonproductive cough, chest pain, dyspnea, and shoulder pain may occur from the effects of the infection on the adjacent diaphragm. Rales, rhonchi, or a friction rub may be audible. Dullness to percussion and decreased breath sounds are present when basilar atelectasis, pneumonia, or pleural effusion occurs.

Abdominal pain, the most common abdominal complaint, is often accompanied by localized tenderness. A mass, wound drainage, or sinus tracts at the previous abdominal incision site are sometimes present. Abdominal distention and hypoactive bowel sounds from paralytic ileus are common.

Diagnosis

Leukocytosis occurs in most patients, and anemia is frequent. Blood cultures are occasionally positive.

Chest x-rays are usually abnormal. The common findings are ipsilateral pleural effusion, elevated or immobile hemidiaphragm, pneumonitis, and atelectasis. Plain abdominal films may reveal extraintestinal gas in the abscess, displacement of adjacent organs, or a soft-tissue density representing the abscess.

A simultaneous liver-lung radionuclide scan may show increased distance between the 2 organs. The value of this test is variable; false positives and negatives occur frequently.

Ultrasonic examination is especially helpful in right-sided subphrenic abscesses. The left-sided subphrenic area is more difficult to examine because of the gas-filled stomach, splenic flexure, aerated lung, and ribs. Moreover, because the spleen varies in shape and size and may contain few echoes, it can resemble an abscess.

Computed tomography (**CT**) generally detects intra-abdominal abscesses, but the subdiaphragmatic area may be difficult to assess, and it may be especially difficult to ascertain whether an abnormality lies just above or below the diaphragm. CT probably should be used when plain films and ultrasound are negative but clinical suspicion of an abscess persists.

Complications, Prognosis, and Treatment

Subdiaphragmatic abscesses may extend into the thoracic cavity, causing an empyema, a lung abscess, or pneumonia. Intra-abdominal complications include incisional breakdown and fistula formation. Occasionally, the abscess may compress the inferior vena cava, causing lower extremity edema.

The mortality of subphrenic abscesses is 25 to 40%, with deaths occurring from uncontrolled infection, malnutrition, and complications of prolonged hospitalization such as pulmonary emboli and nosocomial infections.

The **treatment** is surgical drainage. Antibiotics are adjuncts but not satisfactory substitutes. Adequate nutrition is critical during the often prolonged hospital course.

MIDABDOMINAL ABSCESSES

Midabdominal abscesses, lying between the transverse colon and the pelvis, include **right and left lower-quadrant** and **interloop abscesses.**

Right lower-quadrant abscesses develop most commonly as complications of acute appendicitis and less frequently from colonic diverticulitis, regional enteritis, or a perforated duodenal ulcer with drainage down the right paracolic gutter. Typically, fever, right lower-quadrant tenderness, and a mass develop following symptoms suggesting acute appendicitis. The mass may cause partial or complete small-bowel obstruction. Leukocytosis is usual. **Treatment** includes antibiotics plus surgical drainage. Occasionally, an abscess will resolve on antibiotic therapy alone.

Left lower-quadrant abscesses usually occur from perforation of a diverticulum in the descending or sigmoid colon, less commonly from a perforated colonic carcinoma. The symptoms are those of acute diverticulitis: left lower-quadrant pain, anorexia, and mild nausea followed by fever, leukocytosis, and development of a palpable mass. **Treatment** consists of antibiotic therapy plus surgery. Some surgeons drain the abscess and perform a diverting colostomy, resect the diseased bowel in a 2nd operation, and close the colostomy in a 3rd. Others resect the diseased bowel and bring out the proximal colon as an end colostomy and the distal bowel as a mucous fistula. At a 2nd operation 2 to 3 mo later, they perform an end-to-end anastomosis.

Interloop abscesses, loculations of pus between the folded surfaces of the small and large intestines and their mesenteries, are complications of bowel perforation, anastomotic disruption, or Crohn's disease. The manifestations may be very subtle. Fever and leukocytosis are often the only features; abdominal tenderness, signs of paralytic ileus, or a palpable mass sometimes occur. Plain abdominal films occasionally suggest the diagnosis by the presence of bowel wall edema, separation of bowel loops, localized ileus, and air-fluid levels on upright films. **Treatment** is surgical drainage and appropriate antibiotics.

PELVIC ABSCESSES

Pelvic abscesses usually are complications of acute appendicitis, pelvic inflammatory disease, or colonic diverticulitis. The major symptoms are fever and lower abdominal pain. Abscesses in the Douglas' cul-de-sac, adjacent to the colon, may cause diarrhea; contiguity to the bladder may result in urinary urgency and frequency. Abdominal tenderness is common, and the abscess is usually palpable on vaginal or rectal examination. Leukocytosis is typically present.

Treatment is drainage through the vagina or rectum and appropriate antibiotics, clindamycin and an aminoglycoside (tobramycin or gentamicin) being a good initial choice pending culture results. With abscesses due to pelvic inflammatory disease, some gynecologists treat the patient with fluids, bed rest, and antibiotics, reserving surgery for failure to respond after several days, presence or suspicion of a ruptured abscess, an abscess amenable to drainage via culdotomy or another extraperitoneal route, or uncertain diagnosis.

RETROPERITONEAL ABSCESSES

ANTERIOR RETROPERITONEAL ABSCESSES

These abscesses are complications of acute appendicitis, colonic perforation from diverticulitis or tumor, gastric or duodenal perforation, regional enteritis, or pancreatitis. The major symptoms are fever, abdominal or flank pain, nausea and vomiting, weight loss, and pain in the hip, leg, or knee from psoas muscle involvement. The major findings on examination are fever, abdominal or flank tenderness, and a palpable mass. Pain on extension of the hip is frequent. Leukocytosis is usual. Abnormalities on plain film examination include extraintestinal gas in the abscess, displacement of adjacent organs (such as kidney or colon), and loss of the psoas muscle shadow. Chest films may show ipsilateral diaphragmatic elevation, with or without pleural effusion. Abnormalities shown by excretory urogram include renal or ureteral displacement or hydronephrosis from ureteral obstruction. Barium studies of the intestinal tract may show displacement of adjacent viscera. Computed tomography often defines retroperitoneal abscesses when other studies are negative or equivocal. **Treatment** is drainage and antibiotics. Complications of untreated infection include extension along fascial planes to involve the anterior abdominal wall, thigh, hip, psoas muscle, subphrenic spaces, mediastinum, and pleural cavities. Sometimes intraperitoneal rupture occurs, causing acute bacterial peritonitis.

PERINEPHRIC ABSCESSES

Perinephric abscess nearly always occurs from rupture of a renal parenchymal abscess into the perinephric space between the kidney and its surrounding fascia (Gerota's capsule). Some of these abscesses are staphylococcal and follow hematogenous spread of infection to the kidney from another site, usually cutaneous, with symptoms classically developing 1 to 3 wk after the skin lesions. More commonly, however, perinephric abscesses arise from pyelonephritis, often associated with renal calculous disease, the usual infecting organisms being *E. coli*, *Proteus*, or other aerobic gram-negative rods. Patients are often diabetic.

Symptoms and Signs

The major symptoms are fever, chills, and unilateral flank or abdominal pain, frequently with dysuria. Most patients are febrile and have unilateral flank or abdominal tenderness, often with a palpable mass. Nausea, vomiting, and hematuria occur occasionally. In some patients fever is the only manifestation.

Diagnosis

Leukocytosis and pyuria are common, but not universal. A majority of patients have positive urine cultures; blood cultures are positive in 20 to 40%. Perinephric abscess usually differs clinically from acute pyelonephritis by longer duration of symptoms before hospitalization and by fever following the start of antibiotic therapy; both are usually > 5 days with perinephric abscess and less with acute pyelonephritis.

Chest x-rays are abnormal in about half the patients, revealing ipsilateral pneumonia, atelectasis, pleural effusion, or an elevated hemidiaphragm. In about half the patients, plain abdominal films are also abnormal, showing a mass, calculi, loss of the psoas shadow, or extraintestinal gas in the perinephric area from infection with gas-forming organisms. Findings on excretory urogram, abnormal in about 80% of cases, may include nonvisualizing or poorly visualizing kidney, distorted calyces, anterior renal displacement, and unilateral renal fixation, best demonstrated by fluoroscopy or inspiration-expiration films. Ultrasound and CT are helpful in detecting perinephric abscesses if the other studies are negative or equivocal.

Prognosis and Treatment

The overall mortality rate is about 40%, but prompt diagnosis and therapy usually portend an excellent outcome, especially if the patient has no serious underlying diseases. Treatment is surgical drainage, sometimes requiring nephrectomy if the kidney is extensively involved by infection or stones, and systemic antimicrobial therapy. A reasonable initial choice, pending results of blood, urine, and abscess cultures, is gentamicin.

VISCERAL ABSCESSES

SPLENIC ABSCESSES

Etiology

Most splenic abscesses occur from uncontrolled infection elsewhere and are small, multiple, and clinically silent abnormalities found incidentally at autopsy. Clinically evident splenic abscesses are usually solitary and arise from (1) systemic bacteremia originating in another site, such as endocarditis or salmonellosis, causing infection in a previously normal spleen; (2) infection, presumably of hematogenous origin, in a spleen damaged by blunt or penetrating trauma (with superinfection of a hematoma), bland infarction (such as occurs in hemoglobinopathies, especially sickle trait or hemoglobin SC disease), or other diseases (malaria, hydatid cysts); or (3) extension from a contiguous infection, such as a subphrenic abscess. The most common infecting organisms are staphylococci, streptococci, anaerobes, and aerobic gram-negative rods, including salmonella.

Symptoms, Signs, and Diagnosis

The major symptoms are subacute onset of fever and left-sided pain, often pleuritic, in the flank, upper abdomen, or lower chest that may radiate to the left shoulder. The left upper-quadrant is commonly tender to palpation, and splenomegaly is typical. Rarely, a splenic friction rub is audible. Leukocytosis is usual, and blood cultures sometimes grow the infecting organisms.

Radiographic findings may include a left upper-quadrant mass; extraintestinal gas in the abscess from gas-forming organisms; displacement of other organs, including kidney, colon, and stomach; elevated left hemidiaphragm; and left pleural effusion.

A liver-spleen radionuclide scan and ultrasonic scanning should demonstrate intrasplenic defects with abscesses larger than 2 to 3 cm. A combined lung-spleen radionuclide scan may show an associated left subphrenic abscess. Arteriography, typically showing an avascular mass and mycotic aneurysms, or CT may be helpful when other tests fail to demonstrate a suspected abscess.

Complications and Treatment

Complications of untreated abscesses include hemorrhage into the abscess cavity or rupture into the peritoneum, bowel, bronchus, or pleural space. Splenic abscess is a rare cause of sustained bacteremia in endocarditis despite appropriate chemotherapy. Treatment is systemic antibiotics and splenectomy.

PANCREATIC ABSCESSES

Etiology

Pancreatic abscesses typically develop in a site of pancreatic necrosis, including pseudocysts, following an attack of acute pancreatitis. The usual organisms are bowel flora—aerobic gram-negative rods and anaerobes, but how they reach the pancreas is uncertain.

Symptoms and Signs

In most cases the patient improves after an attack of pancreatitis, but one to several weeks later fever, abdominal pain and tenderness, nausea, vomiting, and, sometimes, paralytic ileus occur. Less commonly, the abscess develops shortly after the attack begins. In those cases the fever, leukocytosis, and abdominal findings so common in acute pancreatitis fail to resolve as quickly as usual; persistence of these features for longer than about 7 days should suggest an abscess. An abdominal mass is palpable in about half the cases.

Diagnosis

The serum amylase may be elevated, but often is normal. Leukocytosis, however, is usually present. The serum alkaline phosphatase may be increased and the albumin decreased. Blood cultures occasionally grow the responsible organism, and sometimes ascitic fluid may be positive when cultured.

Chest x-rays often demonstrate left-sided abnormalities, such as a pleural effusion, basilar atelectasis, pneumonia, or an elevated hemidiaphragm. Plain abdominal films or barium studies of the GI tract may reveal extraintestinal gas in the pancreatic area or displacement of adjacent structures. Ultrasound may show a fluid-filled pancreatic mass, whose contents may have multiple echoes from debris or loculations within the abscess. CT may show a low-density mass within the pancreas that may contain gas and that fails to enhance following intravenously administered contrast material.

Complications, Prognosis, and Treatment

Complications of undrained abscesses include perforation into contiguous structures; erosion into adjacent vessels, such as the left gastric, splenic, and gastroduodenal arteries with exsanguination; and further abscess formation, a frequent occurrence that necessitates reoperation. Even with appropriate surgical and antimicrobial therapy, the mortality rate is about 40%.

Treatment includes surgical drainage and systemic antibiotic therapy. A reasonable choice until culture results are available is chloramphenicol alone or a combination of clindamycin and an aminoglycoside like tobramycin or gentamicin.

HEPATIC ABSCESSES

Etiology and Pathogenesis

Hepatic abscesses are usually amebic or bacterial (pyogenic). Bacterial abscesses occur from (1) ascending cholangitis in a biliary tract partially or completely obstructed by stone, tumor, or stricture; (2) portal bacteremia from an intra-abdominal site, such as diverticulitis or appendicitis; (3) systemic bacteremia originating from a distant location, with organisms reaching the liver via the hepatic artery; (4) direct extension from an adjacent infection outside the biliary tract; and (5) trauma, either penetrating, with direct implantation of bacteria into the liver, or blunt, causing a hematoma that subsequently becomes secondarily infected. A cause is typically obvious, but sometimes the abscess is unexplained. Most abscesses are single, but multiple (usually microscopic) abscesses are common with systemic bacteremia or complete biliary tract obstruction.

Streptococci or staphylococci are the most common bacteria when the infection results from systemic bacteremia. Abscesses originating from a biliary tract infection usually contain aerobic gram-negative rods—e.g., *E. coli* and *Klebsiella*, while those secondary to portal bacteremia from an intra-abdominal infection typically contain both aerobic gram-negative bacilli and anaerobic bacteria.

Symptoms and Signs

With multiple abscesses from systemic bacteremia or biliary tract infection, the onset is usually acute and the principal clinical features of the predisposing disease predominate. With single abscesses, a subacute onset of symptoms occurs over several weeks. Fever is a major, and sometimes the sole, complaint, but most patients also have such symptoms as anorexia, nausea, weight loss, and weakness. Right upper-quadrant pain or tenderness and hepatomegaly occur in about half the cases; right pleuritic chest pain, occasionally. Jaundice is usually apparent only with biliary tract obstruction.

Diagnosis

Common blood test abnormalities include anemia, leukocytosis, elevated ESR, increased alkaline phosphatase, decreased albumin, and mildly elevated bilirubin. Blood cultures are positive in a substantial minority of patients. About half the patients have chest x-rays demonstrating right-sided basilar atelectasis, pleural effusion, pneumonia, or elevated hemidiaphragm.

An abscess larger than 2 cm can usually be detected on radionuclide liver scan or ultrasound examination, which can usually differentiate fluid-filled masses from solid ones and thus help to distinguish liver abscesses from neoplasms. CT and hepatic angiography may also demonstrate the abscess but are usually unnecessary.

In the patient with symptoms of liver abscess and a defect on radionuclide, ultrasound, or CT scans, the most important clinical distinction is between a pyogenic and an amebic abscess. The latter responds well to chemotherapy alone—metronidazole, chloroquine, or emetine, usually without requiring surgical drainage. Features suggesting an amebic etiology are age < 50; single, rather than multiple, defects; a history of diarrhea, especially if bloody; *Entamoeba histolytica* in the stool; and absence of a condition predisposing to bacterial abscesses. Most importantly, nearly all patients with amebic liver abscesses have positive serology for *E. histolytica*.

Complications, Prognosis, and Treatment

Complications of hepatic abscesses include subphrenic abscess formation, bleeding into the abscess cavity, and rupture into the lung, pleural cavity, or peritoneum. With correct diagnosis and appropriate therapy, the mortality rate is 20 to 40%; those with multiple abscesses have a higher mortality rate than those with a single abscess.

Treatment is surgical drainage, including relief of biliary tract obstruction when present, and antimicrobial agents. When the bacteriology is unknown, chloramphenicol alone or a combination of clindamycin and an aminoglycoside like tobramycin or gentamicin should provide adequate coverage until the infecting organisms are identified. To help prevent relapses, antibiotic therapy is usually continued for several weeks following drainage.

URINARY TRACT ABSCESSES

PROSTATIC ABSCESSES

Prostatic abscesses presumably develop as complications of urinary tract infections, especially acute prostatitis, urethritis, and epididymitis. The usual patient is 40 to 60 yr and has frequency, dysuria, or urinary retention. Perineal pain, evidence of acute epididymitis, hematuria, and a purulent urethral discharge are less common signs. Fever is present in only a minority. Rectal examination may show prostatic tenderness and fluctuance, but often prostatic enlargement is the only abnormality, and sometimes the gland feels normal.

Leukocytosis is common. Although pyuria and bacteriuria are frequent, the urine may be completely normal. Blood cultures are positive in a small minority of patients.

Prostatic fluctuance, a purulent urethral discharge, continued or recurrent urinary infections despite antimicrobial therapy, and persistent perineal pain should suggest a prostatic abscess. Many of these abscesses, however, are discovered unexpectedly during prostatic surgery or endoscopy; bulging of a lateral lobe into the prostatic urethra or rupture during instrumentation reveals the abscess.

Treatment is drainage by transurethral evacuation or perineal incision plus appropriate antibiotics. The usual infecting organisms are aerobic gram-negative bacilli or, less frequently, *Staphylococcus aureus*.

HEAD AND NECK ABSCESSES

(See also BRAIN ABSCESS in Ch. 124)

RETROPHARYNGEAL ABSCESSES (See RETROPHARYNGEAL ABSCESS in Vol. II, Ch. 24)

SUBMANDIBULAR SPACE INFECTION (Ludwig's Angina)

A rapidly spreading, bilateral, indurated cellulitis occurring in both the sublingual and submaxillary spaces without abscess formation or lymphatic involvement. Ludwig's angina usually develops from dental or peridontal infection, especially of the 2nd and 3rd mandibular molars. It may occur in association with problems caused by poor dental hygiene (e.g., gingivitis and dental sepsis), tooth extractions, or trauma (e.g., fractures of the mandible, lacerations of the floor of the mouth, peritonsillar abscess). Although not a true abscess, Ludwig's angina resembles one clinically and is treated similarly.

The major manifestations are pain in the area of the involved tooth; severe, tender induration of the submandibular region; trismus; dysphonia; drooling and inability to swallow; and dyspnea and stridor from laryngeal edema and tongue elevation. Fever and systemic toxicity are usual. X-rays of the head and neck are useful to assess the degree of soft-tissue swelling and airway obstruction. **Complications** can include asphyxiation, aspiration pneumonia, lung abscess, and metastatic sepsis.

Treatment includes establishment of an adequate airway, which may require tracheostomy (NOTE: *Obstruction of the airway can progress within hours, and the patency of the airway must be assessed frequently*); penicillin in high doses to treat the oral anaerobes that cause the infection; and incision to drain whatever fluid is present and to relieve the pressure of the swollen, infected tissues. If the patient is allergic to penicillin, chloramphenicol, clindamycin, or a cephalosporin may be used.

PHARYNGOMAXILLARY ABSCESSES

The pharyngomaxillary (lateral pharyngeal, parapharyngeal, or pterygomaxillary) space is a cone-shaped compartment lateral to the pharynx, extending from the sphenoid bone at the base of the skull to the hyoid bone. The styloid bone divides this space into an anterior compartment, closely related to the tonsillar fossa medially and the internal pterygoid muscle laterally, and a posterior compartment containing the carotid sheath and the cranial nerves emerging from their foramina in the base of the skull.

Pharyngomaxillary abscesses usually arise from infections in the pharynx, including the nasopharynx, adenoids, and tonsils. Less common sources are dental infections, parotitis, and mastoiditis. Fever, sore throat, and malaise are usually present. With infections limited to the anterior compartment, trismus, induration along the angle of the jaw, and medial bulging of the tonsil and lateral pharyngeal wall occur. With posterior compartment infection, swelling of the posterior pharyngeal wall and parotid space develops. Trismus is minimal or absent. Involvement of the internal jugular vein within the carotid sheath causes shaking chills, high fever, and bacteremia. Erosion of the internal, external, or common carotid arteries causes profuse hemorrhage. Inferior spread of infection results in neck swelling that obliterates the space beneath the angle of the mandible. **Treatment** is surgical drainage and high-dose penicillin, which is effective against *Streptococcus pyogenes* and the oral anaerobes usually responsible for the infection.

PERITONSILLAR ABSCESSES (See PERITONSILLAR CELLULITIS AND ABSCESS in Ch. 170)

SUPPURATIVE PAROTITIS

Suppurative parotitis, an infection ascending from the mouth, is usually due to *Staphylococcus aureus*, which normally colonizes the opening to Stensen's duct. This infection typically occurs in the elderly or chronically ill patient with a dry mouth from decreased oral intake, from medications with atropine-like effects such as antihistamines or phenothiazines, or following general anesthesia. Fever, chills, and unilateral pain and swelling mark the sudden onset. The gland is firm and tender, with erythema and edema of the overlying skin. Frank pus, expressed from Stensen's duct on compressing the gland, typically shows gram-positive cocci in clumps.

Treatment is a penicillinase-resistant penicillin when *Staphylococcus aureus* is responsible; the antibiotic choice is determined by Gram stain and culture if another organism causes the infection. Improved hydration and oral hygiene are important. Sialagogues (e.g., lemon drops) and massage of the gland help promote drainage through the duct. Surgery is rarely necessary, unless the patient fails to improve after several days of medical management.

MUSCULOSKELETAL ABSCESSES

PYOMYOSITIS

Abscess formation deep within large striated muscles. Muscle abscesses are uncommon. They may develop by spread from a contiguous bone or soft-tissue infection or from a hematogenous route. The latter is thought to be the mechanism of pyomyositis. Presumably, asymptomatic bacteremia occurs with localization of organisms in a muscle damaged by previous, often unrecognized, trauma. Pyomyositis is rare in the USA, but may occur in compromised hosts. It is common in many tropical areas and affects both children and adults, especially the malnourished. The most frequent sites are the quadriceps, gluteus, shoulder, and upper arm muscles, with multiple areas of involvement in about 40% of patients. The initial symptoms are cramping pain followed by edema, worsening discomfort, and mild fever. The muscle may feel indurated at this time. Later, edema and tenderness increase, with obvious fluctuance developing in about half the patients. Leukocytosis is common. In the early indurated stage, needle aspiration may be negative; later it yields thick, yellow pus, nearly always growing *Staphylococcus aureus*. Occasional cases are due to *Streptococcus pyogenes* or *E. coli*. **Treatment** is antibiotic therapy with a penicillinase-resistant penicillin. In the nonsuppurative phase, antibiotics alone suffice; with pus, incision and drainage are mandatory. The extent of involvement at surgery is frequently much greater than anticipated on clinical evaluation.

HAND ABSCESSES

PARONYCHIA (See PARONYCHIAL INFECTIONS in Ch. 190)

FELON

A felon, an infection of the pulp space of the finger pad, nearly always follows minor finger injury (e.g., a splinter or needle prick). Severe local pain, heat, and redness occur, often with lymphangitis and lymphadenopathy. Leukocytosis is common. The abscess rapidly enlarges to involve multiple septae in the distal pulp compartment. Osteitis is a frequent, and osteomyelitis an occasional, complication. **Treatment** is prompt incision, with division of the fibrous septae, to insure adequate drainage.

PURULENT TENOSYNOVITIS

Purulent tenosynovitis occurs from penetrating injury to the flexion creases of the fingers, most commonly the index, middle, and ring fingers. Infection within the tendon sheaths causes rapid tissue destruction and impairment of the gliding mechanisms, leading to loss of finger motion. The major signs are generalized swelling and inflammation of the finger, tenderness over the flexor tendon sheaths, careful maintenance of a flexed finger position, and exquisite pain on active or passive finger extension. Fever, lymphangitis, lymphadenitis, and leukocytosis are usual. **Treatment** is surgical drainage plus antibiotics. Gram stain of the pus should dictate antibiotic choice; streptococci and staphylococci are the usual pathogens.

---

5. BACTEREMIA AND SEPTIC SHOCK

Bacteremia connotes *invasion of the circulation by bacteria.* The term **septicemia** is reserved for *situations in which bacteremia is associated with clinical manifestations of infection.* Bacteremia commonly, and usually transiently, accompanies various surgical manipulations (e.g., incision of an abscess); or it may result from colonization of indwelling intravenous devices and urethral catheters. (For infants, see also NEONATAL SEPSIS AND NEONATAL MENINGITIS under NEONATAL INFECTIONS in Vol. II, Ch. 21.) Bacteremia may be intermittent or sustained, and may cause severe consequences. In patients who abuse intravenous narcotics, gram-positive bacteremia is common and may lead to right-sided bacterial endocarditis even in the absence of cardiac murmurs. The bacteremia of left-sided bacterial endocarditis is usually sustained and may be prolonged. Gram-negative bacteremia is usually intermittent and generally follows primary infection in the GU tract, biliary tree, GI tract, lungs, or, less commonly, skin, bones, or joints. In many patients with chronic diseases no primary focus of infection is apparent.

Symptoms and Signs

Few clinical manifestations are unique to bacteremia. Although variable, fever is almost always present and may be intermittent, with wide diurnal variations (septic, or "spiking"). Chills are common at the onset. Skin eruptions are also common, and may be petechial, purpuric, papular, pustular, or vesicular. Usually gram-negative bacteremia begins abruptly with chills, fever, nausea, vomiting, diarrhea, and prostration.

Diagnosis

The presence of bacteremia is established by blood cultures, which should be performed for both aerobic and anaerobic organisms. A single negative culture does not exclude bacteremia; moreover, in some patients, especially those with prior antibiotic therapy, blood cultures never do become positive.

Complications

Secondary infection of the meninges or of serous cavities, such as the pericardium or larger joints, may occur. Endocarditis (see also BACTERIAL ENDOCARDITIS in Ch. 25) may be the sequel of bacteremia if the pathogen is a streptococcus or staphylococcus; it almost never occurs as a result of gram-negative bacteremias. **Metastatic abscesses** may occur almost anywhere and, when extensive, produce symptoms and signs characteristic of infection in the organ affected. Multiple abscess formation is particularly common with staphylococcal bacteremia. Bacteremia may result in **septic shock,** which is discussed separately, below.

Prognosis

Transient bacteremias associated with surgical procedures, labor and delivery, indwelling intravenous catheters, or urinary catheters are often undetected and probably do not require therapy. However, persistent bacteremia is dangerous; the prognosis depends on the ability to eliminate the source of infection with surgery or antibiotics, and on the status of the underlying disease. When multiple organisms are consistently recovered, polymicrobial bacteremia may be present, auguring a poor outcome. Bacteremia unresponsive to treatment, due to inadequate antibiotic therapy, poor host resistance, or delay in diagnosis, is often fatal.

Treatment of bacteremia is discussed below with septic shock.

SEPTIC SHOCK

When bacteremia is associated with inadequate tissue perfusion, especially with gram-negative organisms or meningococci, **septic shock** with hypotension, vascular collapse, renal failure, and death may ensue. Septic shock usually occurs when bacteremia is due to gram-negative organisms and generally in hospitalized patients with underlying diseases that render them more susceptible. Predisposing factors include diabetes mellitus; cirrhosis; leukemia; lymphoma; disseminated carcinoma; childbirth; surgical procedures; antecedent infection in the urinary, biliary, or GI tracts; indwelling intravenous catheters; treatment with antibiotics, steroids, cytotoxic agents, or inhalation equipment. Septic shock occurs more often in the elderly and in the newborn.

The pathogenesis of septic shock depends upon vasoconstriction of the small arteries and veins, which leads to increased peripheral vascular resistance, pooling of blood in the microcirculation, and decreased cardiac output. With poor perfusion there is tissue anoxia and the decreased blood volume results in hypotension and oliguria. These vasoactive phenomena are related largely to release of endotoxin, the lipopolysaccharide moiety of gram-negative bacillary cell walls, into the circulation.

Symptoms and Signs

Manifestations of bacteremia (see above) usually appear first. When septic shock develops, there are, in addition, tachycardia; tachypnea; hypotension; cool, pale extremities (often with peripheral cyanosis); mental obtundation; and oliguria. Occasionally the findings are subtle, especially in elderly, debilitated patients or infants. Unexplained hypotension, increasing confusion and disorientation, hyperpnea, or oliguria due to decreased renal blood flow may be the only early clues to gram-negative shock. As shock progresses, inadequate renal perfusion may lead to acute tubular necrosis. Heart failure, respiratory insufficiency, and coma may progress to death.

Different hemodynamic patterns are characteristic of endotoxin-related shock. Some patients have normal blood volume, venous pressure, circulation time, and cardiac output, but have decreased peripheral resistance. These patients have warm, dry skin; often they also have cirrhosis. The prognosis in this type of **"warm shock" (hyperdynamic syndrome)** is good unless local acidosis, a consequence of ineffective tissue perfusion and impaired oxygen utilization, eventuates in metabolic acidosis. In other patients, peripheral vascular resistance is increased and there is a decrease in blood volume, central venous pressure, and cardiac output, with hypotension and oliguria. This hemodynamic pattern may be present initially or may follow a period of warm shock.

Most patients with septic shock have deficiencies in several clotting factors, probably due to their consumption in the process of disseminated intravascular coagulation (see Ch. 95). Respiratory failure characterized by decreased pulmonary compliance and irreversible hypoxia, called "**shock lung**" (see Ch. 33), may ensue even after hemodynamic abnormalities have been corrected.

Laboratory Findings

Laboratory data in bacteremia and septic shock vary greatly and depend in many instances on the cause and stage of hemodynamic decompensation. Usually, leukocytosis of between 15,000 and 30,000 WBC/cu mm with a left shift is present. However, relative or absolute leukopenia may be present in severe cases. The platelet count is usually decreased. Urinalysis reveals no specific abnormality. Initially the urine sp gr is increased. However, if oliguria persists, isosthenuria may develop. The BUN and creatinine are increased, and the creatinine clearance declines. Electrolytes vary considerably, with a trend toward hyponatremia and hypochloremia. Potassium may be low or high, depending upon the ability of the kidney to excrete this ion.

Respiratory alkalosis, with a low P_{CO2} and increased arterial pH, is present early and compensates for lactic acidemia. Serum bicarbonate is usually low, while blood lactate is increased. As shock progresses, metabolic acidosis supervenes. Anoxemia with $P_{O2} < 70$ mm Hg is common. Hemodynamic measurements vary as described above. The ECG shows depressed ST segments with T wave inversions and various arrhythmias.

The overall mortality in septic shock ranges from 50 to 90%. If mild to moderate lactic acidemia is present, the prognosis is good. Poor results often follow, due to failure to institute therapy soon enough. Once severe lactic acidemia and decompensated metabolic acidosis become established, shock is often irreversible despite therapy. Because most patients likely to develop septic shock are in the hospital before the symptoms and signs of shock appear, this grave complication of infection is often avoidable by vigilant care.

Treatment

Where available, patients with septic shock should be treated in intensive care units. Pulmonary artery and systemic pressures, arterial and venous pH, arterial blood gases, blood lactate, renal function, and electrolytes should be monitored frequently. Cutaneous vasoconstriction provides a clue to peripheral vascular resistance, but does not accurately reflect blood flow to kidney, brain, or gut. Therefore, hourly urine output should be used to monitor splanchnic blood flow and visceral perfusion. Indwelling urinary catheters are usually required.

Fluid therapy: The central venous pressure **(CVP)** or pulmonary artery pressure should be measured in every patient, and fluid replacement given until the CVP reaches 10 to 12 cm of water or until the pulmonary wedge pressure reaches 12 to 15 mm Hg. Blood volume should be replaced with blood if anemia is present; otherwise, plasma, dextran, human serum albumin, or appropriate electrolyte solutions (usually dextrose-saline with bicarbonate, which is preferable to lactate) are used. Oliguria in the presence of hypotension is not a contraindication to continuing vigorous fluid therapy. The quantity of fluid required often far exceeds the normal blood volume and may amount to 8 to 12 L in a few hours.

Respiration should be supported with nasal oxygen, tracheal intubation, or tracheostomy as necessary. The pulmonary artery pressure may be the best guide for anticipating incipient pulmonary edema. Treatment of shock lung is described in Ch. 33.

Parenteral, bactericidal antibiotics should be administered after cultures of blood and appropriate sites have been taken. Usually at the onset of bacteremia or septic shock, while awaiting cultures and sensitivities, an etiologic diagnosis entails an educated guess based on previous cultures from a primary focus or on the setting in which infection occurs. Pus must be drained and foreign bodies and necrotic tissue must be removed. Failure to do so often results in a poor outcome despite antibiotic therapy. Specific therapy is the same as for the primary infection, but more intense. Since *early* administration of antibiotics may be critical to save the patient's life, an effective regimen for bacteremia of unknown etiology before antimicrobial sensitivities are known is gentamicin 3 to 5 mg/kg/day IM or IV plus either methicillin 6 to 12 gm/day IV or cephalothin or cefazolin 6 to 8 gm/day IV. Carbenicillin 30 gm/day IV may be added if *Pseudomonas* is suspected. As soon as cultures have revealed the putative pathogen, unnecessary agents are stopped. Antibiotics should be continued for several days after shock has resolved and the primary focus of infection has healed adequately.

Vasoactive drugs, particularly alpha-receptor blocking agents (e.g., phenoxybenzamine) or beta-receptor stimulators (e.g., isoproterenol) have been of value in septic shock. Dopamine is now the preferred agent because it enhances renal perfusion. The response to therapy is determined clinically, and return of perfusion to normal is the best guide to stopping vasopressors.

Adrenal corticosteroids in large doses support peripheral resistance and mitigate the cellular injury evoked by endotoxin. While some consider their use controversial, most clinicians will give 30 mg/kg methylprednisolone as a bolus and repeat it at 6- to 12-h intervals for 24 to 48 h.

Control of hemorrhage, with fresh frozen plasma when it is a consequence of clotting factor deficiency or with platelets when due to thrombocytopenia, is important.

Surgical intervention to drain abscesses or excise infected tissues—e.g., infarcted bowel, inflamed gallbladder, infected uterus, or pyonephrosis—should be performed. The patient's condition, although grave, may continue to deteriorate unless the septic focus is removed or drained.

Other therapeutic modalities are indicated, depending on the patient's clinical status, and include mannitol or ethacrynic acid to induce diuresis in patients with oliguria, a rapidly acting digitalis preparation in patients with heart failure, and heparin in patients with disseminated intravascular coagulation.

---

6. INFECTIONS IN THE COMPROMISED HOST

Infections ranging from minor to fatal, caused by normally nonpathogenic organisms in patients whose host defense mechanisms have been compromised. Mainly, the problems presented take place in the hospital setting and are the price of medical advances that have enabled us to deal more effectively with previously unmanageable disorders. Nosocomial infection in the newborn is discussed under NEONATAL INFECTIONS in Vol. II, Ch. 21.

Etiology

Host defense mechanisms—physiologic, anatomic, or immunologic—may be altered or breached by disease or trauma, or by procedures or agents used for diagnosis or therapy. Thus, opportunistic infection may occur if antimicrobial therapy alters the normal relationship between host and microbe, or if the host defense mechanisms have been altered by burns, anemia, neoplasms, metabolic disorders, irradiation, foreign bodies, immunosuppressive or cytotoxic drugs, corticosteroids, or diagnostic or therapeutic instrumentation.

The underlying alteration predisposes the patient to infections from his usually nonpathogenic endogenous microflora or from ordinarily harmless, saprophytic organisms acquired by contact with other patients, hospital personnel, or equipment. The organisms that opportunistically take advantage of the compromised host commonly are resistant to antibiotics, further complicating problems of management. These organisms may be bacteria, fungi, viruses, or other parasites, and the precise character of the host's altered defenses determines which organisms are more likely to be involved.

1. Antibiotic resistance and impaired anatomic host defense mechanisms: Antimicrobial treatment alters the normal microflora of the skin, mucous membranes, and GI tract and may result in **superinfection** (invasion by endogenous or environmental organisms resistant to the antibiotic being given), which is demonstrable microbiologically or clinically. Factors predisposing to superinfection include extremes of age, chronic infection or other debilitating disease, excessive doses of a single antimicrobial, and use of broad-spectrum antibiotics either singly or in combination. The wider the antimicrobial spectrum, the greater the danger of opportunistic infection. Superinfections usually appear on the 4th or 5th day of chemotherapy and may convert a benign, self-limited disease into a serious, prolonged, or even fatal one. They are most often caused by endogenous gram-negative enteric bacilli, fungi, and resistant staphylococci. The diagnosis of superinfection by a normally commensal organism is certain only when the organism is recovered from blood, CSF, or body cavity fluid.

Nosocomial (hospital-acquired) infections are usually acquired from the hospital environment or personnel, the patient's own microflora, or inadequately sterilized equipment, and are commonly due to *Enterobacter, Klebsiella, Serratia, Pseudomonas, Proteus,* or *Candida.* They may replace strains of *Escherichia coli* and many gram-positive organisms, especially when a susceptible patient is given a broad-spectrum antibiotic or massive doses of any antibiotic.

Patients with extensive **burns** or those undergoing diagnostic or therapeutic **procedures** that breach normal anatomic barriers to infection (e.g., tracheostomy, inhalation therapy, urinary tract instrumentation, indwelling urethral or IV catheters, surgery, and surgical prostheses) are vulnerable to infection by endogenous or environmental antibiotic-resistant organisms. Gram-negative bacteria, particularly *Pseudomonas* and *Serratia,* alone or in combination with staphylococci, cause bacteremia in severely burned patients. Significant bacteriuria develops in patients with indwelling urethral catheters, thus increasing the risk of cystitis, pyelonephritis, and gram-negative rod bacteremia. Polyethylene IV catheters may cause sepsis, especially when thrombophlebitis from irritating IV solutions is present. Sepsis due to gram-negative organisms alone or in combination with staphylococci and *Candida* may arise in current or prior IV infusion sites and range from local suppuration to systemic infection and death. Patients with endotracheal tubes or tracheostomies and others who require repeated tracheal suctioning or inhalation therapy with equipment containing a reservoir of nebulization fluid may develop bronchopulmonary infection with nosocomial gram-negative organisms or staphylococci.

2. Impaired cellular or humoral host defense mechanisms: Such **neoplastic** and **immunodeficiency diseases** as leukemia, aplastic anemia, Hodgkin's disease, and myeloma are characterized by selective defects in host resistance. Patients with hypogammaglobulinemia, myeloma, macroglobulinemia, or chronic lymphatic leukemia tend to have deficient humoral immune mechanisms and to develop pneumococcal and staphylococcal pneumonia and gram-negative GU infections. Patients with Hodgkin's disease or acute leukemia, and those receiving intensive **immunosuppressive** or **irradiation therapy** frequently develop gram-negative septicemia secondary to pneumonia. Since these patients also tend to have depressed cellular immune mechanisms, serious infection with *Aspergillus, Candida, Cryptococcus, Histoplasma, Mucor, Nocardia,* or *Staphylococcus* is frequent; herpes zoster, cytomegalovirus, *Pneumocystis,* and *Toxoplasma* infections also occur.

Cytotoxic drugs enhance the susceptibility of tissues to infection by direct cytotoxic action, resulting in severe leukopenia and thrombocytopenia; depression of the primary immune response, including antibody production and cell-mediated immunity; and an altered inflammatory response. Most opportunistic infections in these patients result from the severe leukopenia.

Corticosteroids alter many aspects of host defenses; one of the most important is inhibition of the movement of leukocytes into the inflammatory exudate. Corticosteroids may reactivate healed pulmonary TB, histoplasmosis, coccidioidomycosis, and blastomycosis. Patients receiving corticosteroid treatment (especially those on high dosages) for RA, ulcerative colitis, asthma, sarcoidosis, SLE, and pemphigus, and patients with **Cushing's syndrome** have an increased susceptibility to infection from usual and unusual bacteria; they also tend to develop infections with *Aspergillus, Candida, Cryptococcus, Mucor,* and *Nocardia.*

Prophylaxis

Awareness of the patterns of infections that occur in the compromised host helps greatly in early recognition of infections and initiation of appropriate therapy. It is important to be aware of the specific site of breached defense, the type of defense system that has been weakened or lost, and the characteristics of organisms prevalent in a particular institution, based on continuous epidemiologic hospital surveillance.

Use of broad-spectrum antibiotics, massive doses of any antibiotic, or prophylactic use of systemic antibiotics may ultimately result in infection with resistant bacteria and should be avoided whenever possible. Patients receiving antimicrobial therapy should be watched for signs of superinfection.

Severe hypogammaglobulinemia may require maintenance with immune serum globulin. Tuberculin sensitivity should be determined before a patient is treated with immunosuppressive or corticosteroid agents, and isoniazid **(INH)** treatment should be considered in tuberculin-positive patients. Prophylactic use of trimethoprim **(TMP)**–sulfamethoxazole **(SMZ)** (TMP 5 mg/kg/day and SMZ 20 mg/kg/day) is beneficial to prevent bacterial and *Pneumocystis* infections in patients with leukemia who are undergoing intensive chemotherapy.

The use of **barriers to control and prevent infection** is discussed in detail in Ch. 7. Strict **asepsis** should be maintained in diagnostic and therapeutic manipulative procedures. **Urethral catheters** must be connected to closed sterile drainage bags and the system kept closed. Attendants should wear sterile gloves during **endotracheal** or **tracheostomy suctioning,** and suction catheters should be sterile, disposable, and used only once. Optimally, the masks, tubing, nebulizer jars, and other components of respiratory therapy equipment that connect directly to a patient's airway should be sterilized by steam or gas prior to use and should be changed daily. When steam or gas sterilization is not possible, the equipment should be disinfected with a 2% glutaraldehyde or 2% acetic acid wash followed by thorough rinsing and drying. Alternatively, nebulization of 0.25% acetic acid through the equipment, followed by careful rinsing, is usually satisfactory for daily cleaning of a respirator after it has been assigned to a patient. Special care should be taken to be sure the gas jets have been completely cleaned.

When possible, **IV therapy** should be given through metal or scalp vein needles. IV catheters should be inserted securely, covered with a sterile protective dressing, and removed after 48 h or at the first sign of phlebitis. An ointment of neomycin, polymyxin B, and bacitracin or an iodine ointment—e.g., povidone-iodine—should be applied daily to the cannulation site and the emerging catheter. Thrombophlebitis usually responds to catheter withdrawal and local application of hot compresses.

Treatment

The organisms of opportunistic infection tend to be resistant to most commonly used antibiotics and are difficult to treat once established. Therapy may be merely suppressive unless the underlying condition can be corrected (e.g., removal of urethral or IV catheters, or tracheostomy closure). Cultures, and possibly tissue biopsy (e.g., for *Pneumocystis* infections—see in Ch. 38), should be obtained before starting or altering antibacterial treatment, but at times, while awaiting laboratory results, one may have to begin therapy on the basis of clinical-bacteriologic diagnosis and presumptive sensitivity. When possible, corticosteroid dosage should be reduced while treating an opportunistic infection—except in patients with *Pneumocystis* pneumonia. Severely granulocytic patients with documented infection can be benefited by granulocyte transfusions.

Further details of treatment are given elsewhere in the book, in discussions of specific underlying disorders or procedures and specific organisms.

7. PREVENTION OF INFECTION

IMMUNIZATION PROCEDURES

(See Vol. II, Ch. 23)

BARRIERS

To prevent transmission of infectious diseases within hospitals, special isolation procedures are used for patients who have or are suspected of having certain infections. (For infants, see also NOSOCOMIAL INFECTION IN THE NEWBORN under NEONATAL INFECTIONS in Vol. II, Ch. 21.) In deciding which diseases to isolate and choosing specific isolation procedures, the epidemiology of each infectious disease in the hospital setting must be considered. The usual source of the microorganism in question, its common mode of transmission, and the susceptibility of adjacent patients must all be considered. Not all infections spread readily from patient to patient, and hence not all infections require isolation. In the hospital, most microorganisms are spread by direct or indirect contact (including droplet-spread of microorganisms), airborne transmission, or a contaminated vehicle such as food, water, or drugs. Based on epidemiology, diseases can be sorted into categories of isolation.

Strict isolation prevents the spread of communicable diseases that can be readily transmitted by both contact and airborne routes. It requires a private room with the door kept closed and with an independent air supply; gowns, masks, and gloves worn by all persons entering the room; handwashing in disinfectant material by all persons entering and leaving the room; and special handling of all articles leaving the room to insure their disinfection. **Respiratory isolation** prevents transmission of microorganisms through direct contact or droplets that are spread into the immediate environment by coughing, sneezing, or breathing. It requires a private room with the door kept closed and with an independent air supply; gowns and gloves are not necessary for visitors unless they plan to touch the patient, but they must wear masks; hands must be washed in a disinfectant on entering and leaving the room; and articles directly contaminated with secretions must be disinfected upon leaving the room. **Enteric precautions** prevent spread of diseases that occur through direct or indirect contact with infected feces or heavily contaminated articles. Transmission depends upon ingesting infected material. A private room is not required, although it may be desirable in some cases, particularly for children or uncooperative patients. Persons directly contacting the patient must wear gowns, but masks are not necessary. Gloves are necessary only for persons having direct contact with the patient or with articles contaminated with fecal material; hands must be vigorously washed upon entering and leaving the room; and all articles contaminated with urine or feces must be disinfected or discarded. **Wound and skin precautions** prevent infection from spreading through direct contact with wounds or heavily contaminated dressings. Patients should have private rooms, if possible; gowns must be worn by all persons directly contacting the patients, but masks and gloves are unnecessary except for persons touching infected areas or changing dressings; hands must be washed upon entering and leaving the room; and articles such as instruments, dressings, and linen must be disinfected or discarded. **Discharge precautions** prevent becoming infected through direct contact with wounds or secretion-contaminated articles. The likelihood of cross-infection with diseases in this category is slight. Private rooms are not needed, but the "no touch" dressing technic must be used, careful handwashing should be observed before and after patient care, and potentially infected oral secretions should be disposed of appropriately. **Blood precautions**, procedures that avoid contact with blood or items contaminated with infected blood, are particularly important in patients who have diseases associated with circulation of the etiologic agent in the blood; however, these simple precautions should be observed in all hospitalized patients.

Rooms or areas used for isolation should have handwashing facilities and special containers for soiled linens and for waste disposal. Visiting should be restricted, and *all* visitors (professional or social) must wash their hands upon entering and leaving the isolation area. If required, a mask should be worn over the nose and mouth and should be discarded and replaced as soon as it becomes moist. Masks and gowns are discarded into appropriate receptacles when the visitor leaves the isolation area. Whenever possible, disposable needles, syringes, eating utensils, dishes, and other items are used. Nondisposable items such as thermometers, stethoscopes, sphygmomanometer, and other instruments should be left in the patient's room for the duration of the isolation. Disposal of contaminated materials is important. Used gowns and soiled linens should be bagged immediately and labeled for sterilization by the hospital laundry. Disposable items should be placed in plastic bags and incinerated. Nondisposable items such as instruments or glassware should be rinsed in cold water, double-bagged, and labeled for decontamination. As indicated for each specific disease, items such as body discharges, blood, sputum, vomitus, excreta, soiled dressings, and uneaten food should be flushed down toilets or removed in labeled bags and incinerated. The room and furnishings should be disinfected when the period of isolation is over. Details pertaining to each type of isolation are listed in TABLE 7–1.

Protective isolation (or **reverse isolation**) differs from other isolation procedures in that it attempts to protect the infection-prone patient from contact with potentially harmful microorganisms. It is useful for leukopenic or immunosuppressed patients, cancer patients, and others at high risk of infection. In most hospitals protective isolation consists of a private room with closed door; gowns, masks, and gloves worn by all persons entering the patient's room; handwashing with a disinfectant upon entering and leaving the patient's room; and special disinfection of all items placed in the patient's room. More elaborate forms of protective isolation, used in centers treating many immunosuppressed patients, include special laminar air-flow rooms, serving sterilized food, and giving prophylactic, nonabsorbable oral antibiotics to reduce the patient's intestinal microorganisms. These measures, though effective, are expensive, time-consuming, and not available in most hospitals.

In all forms of isolation, patients experience loneliness, guilt, and anxiety. The necessity for isolation, the procedures to be used, and the anticipated period of isolation should be carefully explained to the patient, with reassurance that the illness, not the person, is being temporarily isolated.

ANTIMICROBIAL CHEMOPROPHYLAXIS

About $1/3$ of all antimicrobial drugs used in hospitals are aimed at preventing, rather than at treating, infection. Prophylaxis is applied most frequently to (1) prevent acquisition of exogenous organisms (as in antimalarial prophylaxis), (2) prevent organisms usually present in one area of the body from gaining access to a normally sterile site (e.g., resident fecal or vaginal flora causing urinary tract infections), or (3) prevent a dormant pathogenic organism from causing disease.

Single-drug prophylaxis directed at a single pathogen has been successful in numerous clinical situations—e.g., in preventing, with benzathine penicillin, recurrent episodes of rheumatic fever secondary to group A streptococcal disease; malaria, with chloroquine; and influenza A, with amantadine.

Short-term antimicrobial prophylaxis is used frequently; the rationale is that brief, low-dose exposure to an antimicrobial—before bacterial multiplication establishes an infection—will abort or ameliorate clinical disease. Examples include penicillin, ampicillin and/or an aminoglycoside preparation such as streptomycin or gentamicin given prior to dental manipulation or other procedures leading to bacteremia, to prevent SBE; and trimethaprim-sulfamethoxazole, mandelamine, or nitrofurantoin given to prevent recurrent urinary tract infections in females. Antibiotics may also prevent disease in close contacts of patients with *Neisseria meningitidis* infection (sulfonamides in sensitive strains; rifampin and/or minocycline in other strains) or with *Corynebacterium diphtheriae* (erythromycin, clindamycin, or penicillin), and in young children who are household or day-care contacts of proven cases of *Hemophilus influenza* type B infection (rifampin or trimethoprim-sulfamethoxazole). Studies indicate that antimicrobial prophylaxis with penicillin or silver nitrate may prevent ophthalmia neonatorum due to *Neisseria gonorrheae* infection, while *Chlamydia trachomatis* conjunctivitis can be prevented with erythromycin or tetracycline ointment. (Tetracycline, although highly effective in the prophylaxis of genital infection with *Neisseria gonorrheae* and *Chlamydia trachomatis*, is not routinely recommended because *N. gonorrheae* resistant to tetracycline may emerge.) Benzathine penicillin injections are routinely used in the prophylaxis of congenital or incubating syphilis.

TABLE 7-1. HOSPITAL ISOLATION RECOMMENDATIONS*

NOTE: Careful handwashing before and after every patient contact is *mandatory*.

Disease	Type of Isolation	Private Room	Mask	Gown	Gloves	Maximum Room Cleaning	Tray Precautions	Excreta & Soiled Articles	Blood	Secreta & Soiled Articles	Duration of Communicability	Comments
Actinomycosis												
1. Draining lesions	SeP									X	Duration of drainage	
2. Other	N											
Agranulocytosis, leukopenia, other compromised hosts	PI	X	X	X	X						Duration of susceptibility	Isolate from patients with any suspected communicable disease (see also Prophylaxis in Ch. 6)
Burns												
1. Extensive	SI	X	X	X	X	X				X	Duration of skin lesions	Acutely ill patients may require protective isolation as well
2. Minor	WSP	D	(X)	(X)	(X)					X		Use careful dressing technic
Chickenpox (varicella)	SI	X	X	X	X	X	X	X	X	X	For 7 days after first vesicles appear; for duration of illness in compromised host	Isolate from highly susceptible patients (e.g., with eczema, burns, leukemia: pregnant women (late 3rd trimester) should not care for the patient; children should be admitted to a nonpediatric unit

(Continued)

* Abbreviations: BP, blood precautions; EnP, enteric precautions; ExP, excretion precautions; N, no isolation or precautions; PI, protective isolation; RI, respiratory isolation; SeP, secretion precautions; SI, strict isolation; WSP, wound and skin precautions; (X), with direct contact; X, all circumstances; D, desirable but optional. (Isolation criteria set by The Center for Disease Control.)

TABLE 7-1. HOSPITAL ISOLATION RECOMMENDATIONS* (Cont'd)

Disease	Type of Isolation	Private Room	Mask	Gown	Gloves	Maximum Room Cleaning	Tray Precautions	Excreta & Soiled Articles	Blood	Secreta & Secreta-Soiled Articles	Duration of Communicability	Comments
Conjunctivitis												
1. Acute infectious of newborn	SeP			(X)	(X)					X	Until discharges from infectious mucous membranes have ceased	
2. Neonatal inclusion blenorrhea	SeP			(X)	(X)							
Cryptococcosis with draining wounds	SeP									X	Until drainage ceases	No isolation for other forms of cryptococcus
CSF rhinorrhea	PI											Isolate from patients with infections
Diarrheal diseases												
1. Amebiasis	EnP				(X)			X				
2. Unknown etiology	EnP				(X)			X				Culture stools of obstetric patients with diarrhea; isolate patient until diagnosis is definite
3. Enterobiasis	EnP	D			(X)	X		X				
4. Gastroenteritis (in patients < 2 yr)	EnP	X		(X)	(X)	X	X	X			48 h after patient is asymptomatic or 1 negative stool culture	Babies should be isolated in suspect nursery
(in patients > 2 yr)	EnP							X				Same as for diarrheal diseases of unknown etiology

Disease	Category								Period of isolation	Comments
5. Nonbacterial gastroenteritis	EnP	X			(X)	X			48 h after patient is asymptomatic	
6. Salmonellosis & shigellosis (bacillary dysentery)	EnP	X		(X)	X	X	X		Until 3 stool cultures, taken 24 h apart & beginning 72 h after cessation of antibiotic therapy, are negative	Clean floors, soiled walls, & equipment, using a phenolic compound
7. Trichuriasis	EnP	D		(X)			X			
8. *Yersinia enterocolitica*	EnP	X		(X)	X		X			
Diphtheria	SI	X	X	X	X	X	X	X	Until 2 cultures, taken from nose & throat at least 24 h after cessation of antibiotic therapy, are negative	Carrier state usually lasts 2–4 wk, may last 6 mo
Encephalitis										
1. Suspect arboviral	N									Isolation unnecessary
2. Mumps	RI	X	X	X	X			X	12–21 days after exposure & until swelling or other signs have cleared	Masks not required for personnel who have had mumps; personnel who have *not* had mumps should *not* care for patient. Susceptible personnel should be vaccinated
3. Herpes simplex	N									Isolation unnecessary in absence of skin lesions
Gas gangrene	WSP	X	X	(X)	(X)			X	Duration of illness	Wear gloves during wound contact; greatest danger is transmission to pre- and postoperative patients
Gastroenteritis										See Diarrheal diseases

(Continued)

TABLE 7-1. HOSPITAL ISOLATION RECOMMENDATIONS* (Cont'd)

Disease	Type of Isolation	Private Room	Mask	Gown	Gloves	Maximum Room Cleaning	Tray Precautions	Excreta & Excreta-Soiled Articles	Blood	Secreta & Secreta-Soiled Articles	Duration of Communicability	Comments
Head lice	SI	X		(X)	(X)	X	X				Until head lice and nits are gone	Caps to be worn by hospital personnel
Hepatitis 1. Asymptomatic HBsAg positive	EnP & BP	D		(X)	(X)		X	X	X	X	Until patient is negative for HBsAg	Transmitted through blood & fecal/oral route; discard needles with extra care to avoid accidental pricking; label all specimens *Bio-hazard;* γ-globulin for hospital personnel only if percutaneous prick occurs
2. Viral, all types	EnP & BP	X		(X)	(X)		X	X	X	X	Duration of illness	
Herpes simplex	SeP	D		(X)	(X)					X	Duration of vesicle, pustule, or scab	
Herpes zoster 1. Disseminated	SI	X	X	X	X	X		X	X	X	Until all lesions are crusted & *dry*	Avoid contact with highly susceptible patients (those on steroids & immunosuppressive therapy, hemodialysis, etc.); see Chickenpox
2. Local	WSP	D		(X)	(X)					X		

Condition	Code								Duration	Comments
Infections or colonization with multiple antibiotic-resistant gram-negative organisms										
1. Wounds, drains, (biliary, chest, etc.)	WSP	D	(X)	X				X	Until resistant organisms are no longer recovered	Gram-negative bacilli resistant to gentamicin; clean floors, soiled walls, & equipment, using a phenolic compound
2. Pulmonary	SeP	X	X	(X)	(X)	X		X		
3. Excreta (urine & stool)	EnP	D		(X)	(X)	X	X			
Malaria	BP					X			Duration of hospital stay	
Measles (rubeola)	RI	X	X	(X)	(X)			X	Isolation for 8–21 days after exposure & for 7 days after rash appears	Susceptible personnel should not care for patient
Meningococcemia	RI	X	X	(X)				X	Until 24 h after start of effective therapy	Chemotherapy for hospital personnel after intimate contact (e.g., mouth-to-mouth resuscitation)
Meningitis										
1. Meningococcal	RI	X	X	(X)				X	Until 24 h after start of effective therapy	Chemotherapy for hospital personnel after intimate contact (e.g., mouth-to-mouth resuscitation)
2. Fungal	N									RI if associated with pulmonary disease; ExP for urinary tract infection
3. Tuberculosis	RI	X	X	(X)				X	Until pulmonary disease has been ruled out	
4. Viral	ExP	D	X	(X)	(X)	X	X	X	Duration of hospital stay	
Mumps	RI	X	X					X		Susceptible personnel should be vaccinated; masks required for young children

(Continued)

TABLE 7-1. HOSPITAL ISOLATION RECOMMENDATIONS* (Cont'd)

Disease	Type of Isolation	Private Room	Mask	Gown	Gloves	Maximum Room Cleaning	Tray Precautions	Excreta & Soiled Articles	Blood	Secreta & Soiled Articles	Duration of Communicability	Comments
Nocardiosis, draining lesions	SeP									X	Until drainage ceases	
Pertussis (whooping cough)	RI	X	X	(X)	(X)					X	Duration of hospital stay	
Pneumocystis carinii	N											Isolate from immunosuppressed patients
Pneumonia (bacterial, unlisted elsewhere)	SeP									X	Duration of illness	See also Streptococcal & Staphylococcal infections & Infections with antibiotic-resistant organisms
Psittacosis (ornithosis)	SeP	X	X							X	Duration of illness	Patient should wear mask when anyone else is in room
Rabies	SI	X	X	X	X	X	X	X		X	Duration of illness	
Respiratory disease 1. Croup, bronchiolitis, pneumonia	SeP	X	X							X	Duration of illness	
2. Febrile undifferentiated exanthem or disease	SeP	X	X	X	(X)			X		X	Duration of illness	
3. Influenza	SeP	X	X							X	Duration of illness	RI desirable if diagnosis made early
Roseola	N											No contact with patients < 4 yr of age

Disease	Category								Duration of hospital stay	Comments
Rubella, congenital syndrome	SI	X	(X)	(X)	(X)		X	X X		Infants with congenital rubella may excrete virus for 2 yr after birth
Rubella (German measles)	RI	X	(X)	(X)	(X)		X		12–21 days after exposure & for 5 days after onset of rash	Pregnant women (at risk during first 5 mo if antibody-negative or unknown) should *not* take care of patient; label all specimens *Bio-hazard*
Salmonellosis & shigellosis										See Diarrheal diseases
Staphylococcal diseases (coagulase-positive) 1. Abscesses, draining wounds, skin lesions a. Minor	WSP	D		(X)	(X)		(X)	X	Until drainage ceases	Mere colonization does not necessarily require isolation
b. Extensive	SI	X	X	X	X	X	X	X		
2. Enterocolitis	EnP	D		(X)	(X)	X	(X)	X	Duration of illness	
3. Pneumonia; draining abscess; tracheobronchitis	SI	X	X	X	X		X	X	Until organism is no longer recovered	Clean floors, soiled walls, & equipment, using a phenolic compound
Streptococcal diseases, Group A 1. Pneumonia	SI	X	X	X	X		X	X	Until 24 h after adequate antibiotic treatment	
2. Skin lesions a. Minor	WSP	D		(X)	(X)		(X)	X		
b. Extensive	SI	X	X	X	X		X	X		
Syphilis, mucocutaneous	SeP	X			(X)		(X)	X	Until 24 h after start of effective therapy	

(Continued)

TABLE 7-1. HOSPITAL ISOLATION RECOMMENDATIONS* (Cont'd)

Disease	Type of Isolation	Private Room	Mask	Gown	Gloves	Maximum Room Cleaning	Tray Precautions	Excreta & Excreta-Soiled Articles	Blood	Secreta & Secreta-Soiled Articles	Duration of Communicability	Comments
Tuberculosis 1. Pulmonary (sputum-proven or suspected)	RI	X	X	(X)	(X)	X	X			X	Until 2 wk after start of therapy; in minimal disease a shorter duration of isolation may be acceptable	Patient must wear mask when in contact with others; during transport in hospital, patient must wear mask & carry tissue & wax-paper bag; label all specimens *Bio-hazard*; use sputum bottles if possible
2. Extrapulmonary (open)	SeP							X		X		
Typhoid fever	EnP	D		(X)	(X)	X	X	X		X	Until 3 consecutive negative stool cultures, taken at least 24 h apart with patient off antibiotics for 72 h, are obtained	
Vaccinia 1. Local vaccination site	N	X		(X)	(X)	X				X		Isolate from highly susceptible patients (e.g., with eczema, burns, leukemia)
2. Eczema vaccination & other generalized complications	SI	X	X	X	X	X	X			X	Duration of skin lesions	

Recent investigations suggest that tetracycline prophylaxis decreases the risk of developing toxigenic *Escherichia coli* ("turista"). Prophylaxis may prove useful in adults—except pregnant women—traveling for > 1 mo in areas with high risk of diarrhea from enterotoxigenic strains that are sensitive to tetracycline. Neomycin or kanamycin have been used to control anaerobic pathogenic *E. coli* diarrhea; ampicillin and neomycin have sometimes been effective in the prophylaxis of shigellosis.

Clinical situations where prophylactic antibiotics are beneficial for **extended periods** (weeks or longer) include use of (1) penicillin and sulfonamides to prevent group A streptococcal disease in persons at high risk of developing rheumatic fever, (2) amantadine for the prophylaxis of influenza A infection in persons at high risk of developing complications of influenza, (3) chloroquine and/or primaquine or pyramethamine and sulfadoxine to prevent malaria in those traveling to endemic areas, (4) isoniazid for contacts of patients with mycobacterium tuberculosis, and (5) trimethoprim-sulfamethoxazole to prevent *Pneumocystis carinii* in cancer patients receiving cytotoxic agents.

Adverse effects are more likely with **multiple drugs** in **high dosages** for **longer periods** than with short-term antimicrobial prophylaxis with a single drug and include superinfection with an organism that has developed resistance to the antibiotics and increased incidence of toxic or allergic reactions. Other disadvantages of such regimens are higher cost and possibly a false assumption that an infection is not the cause of a clinical disease.

Antibiotic prophylaxis is *not* indicated in many bacterial complications of viral respiratory illness (e.g., influenza, complicating secondary bacterial infection of viral exanthems, and acute exacerbations of asthma), and antimicrobials are not useful in preventing colonization of pathogenic organisms in patients in intensive care units. Thus, routine antimicrobial use is not recommended to prevent pneumonia in comatose patients, infections in persons with congestive heart failure, or urinary tract infections in persons with prolonged urethral catheterization; nor is it recommended for patients on high-dose steroid therapy.

In Immunosuppressed Patients

Prophylactic antibiotics and other measures are used to prevent infections in patients with acute leukemia, particularly during the granulocytopenic phase of chemotherapy. Prophylaxis includes barrier isolation, laminar flow rooms, diets low in microbes, and chemoprophylaxis with topical or orofacial antiseptics and nonabsorbable oral antibiotics such as gentamicin, vancomycin, and nystatin, and systemic oral antibiotics such as trimethoprim-sulfamethoxazole. Definitive recommendations on the use of prophylactic antibiotics cannot yet be made because the problem is complex and because various institutions differ in local flora, colonization rates of various pathogens, barrier isolation technics, and diet. In general, total barrier isolation plus use of nonabsorbable oral antibiotics reduces the incidence of infection in patients with acute leukemia who are undergoing chemotherapy. (These measures, however, may not affect the number of remissions or long-term survival.) Whether nonabsorbable oral antibiotics combined with conventional ward care reduce infection rates is not yet clear. Recently, prophylactic use of trimethoprim-sulfamethoxazole has been shown to reduce risk of subsequent bacterial infections. Because infection rates differ, depending on the age of the patient, the type of underlying disease and its severity, and the type of chemotherapy, further studies of routine antimicrobial prophylaxis for immunosuppressed patients are needed.

In Surgery

General guidelines for using prophylactic antibiotics in surgery are described below. Chapters on individual diseases should be consulted for detailed prophylactic regimens.

Use of prophylactic antibiotics must be based on the type of operation. This is especially important when antimicrobials are used to reduce postoperative wound infections; in this situation, antimicrobial use varies, depending on whether the operative procedure is classified as clean, clean-contaminated, contaminated, or dirty. In general, clean operations have an expected wound infection rate of < 5%; clean-contaminated, ≅ 10%; contaminated, ≅ 20%; and dirty, > 30%. Overall use and cost of antimicrobial agents in clean surgery generally exceed the benefits—except when an infection is likely to be catastrophic (e.g., with insertion of prostheses such as cardiac valves, vascular graphs, or artificial joints). For prophylactic antibiotics to be useful in surgery, timing and duration of antimicrobial administration are critical: The antibiotic should be present at the time of potential contamination, and, in general, prophylactic antibiotics should not be continued for > 72 h after a surgical procedure. To date, when directly compared, single-dose antimicrobial prophylaxis has been as effective as multiple-dose prophylaxis for vaginal hysterectomy and for cardiac and biliary tract surgery. When possible, prophylaxis should be carried out with a single dose that is effective against the most frequent postoperative pathogens.

In obstetric and gynecologic surgery, prophylactic antibiotics have reduced febrile morbidity and the duration of hospitalization in those undergoing vaginal hysterectomy, and they may decrease the incidence of endometritis in women undergoing cesarean section after prolonged rupture of the membrane. Most surgeons feel prophylaxis with mechanical bowel preparation and oral or systemic antibiotics is warranted in colorectal surgery. The value of antibiotic prophylaxis in gastroduodenal and biliary tract surgery is more controversial; current data suggest that patients who have impairments of mechanisms that restrict bacterial growth (e.g., those with reduced gastric motility or acidity) or whose biliary tracts are infected preoperatively probably should be given prophylactic antibiotics. Surgical procedures involving foreign bodies (e.g., joint replacement and prostheses) or where infection may lead to severe complications (e.g., cardiac valve surgery) generally warrant short preoperative antimicrobial prophylaxis.

In many areas of surgery where contaminated wounds or procedures are uncommon, such as craniotomies, pulmonary resections, coronary bypass surgery, neurologic surgery, and urologic surgery in those who have sterile preoperative urine cultures, antibiotic prophylaxis is presently of uncertain value.

8. BACTERIAL DISEASES

CAUSED BY GRAM-POSITIVE COCCI

STAPHYLOCOCCAL INFECTIONS

Epidemiology

Pathogenic staphylococci are ubiquitous. They are *normally* carried in the anterior nares of about 30%, and on the skin of about 20%, of healthy adults; hospital patients or personnel have slightly higher rates of carriage. Penicillin-resistant strains are common, especially in hospitals. Certain patients are predisposed to staphylococcal infections: newborns, nursing mothers, and patients with influenza, chronic bronchopulmonary disorders (e.g., cystic fibrosis, pulmonary emphysema), leukemia, neoplasms, renal transplants, tracheostomies, burns, chronic skin disorders, surgical incisions, diabetes mellitus, and indwelling intravascular plastic catheters. Patients receiving adrenal steroids, irradiation, immunosuppressives, or antitumor chemotherapy are also at an increased risk. Predisposed patients may acquire antibiotic-resistant staphylococci from other colonized areas of their own bodies or from infected hospital personnel who may be asymptomatic carriers. Patient-to-patient transmission via the hands of personnel is the most important means of spread.

Unlike other staphylococcal diseases, **staphylococcal food poisoning** (see STAPHYLOCOCCAL FOOD POISONING in Ch. 55) is caused by ingestion of a preformed enterotoxin produced by staphylococci in contaminated food, not by infection with the organism itself. Victims of staphylococcal food poisoning usually are healthy otherwise.

Symptoms, Signs, and Diagnosis

The site of the staphylococcal infection determines its clinical picture. Common presentations include furuncles, carbuncles, abscesses, pneumonia, bacteremia, endocarditis, osteomyelitis, enterocolitis, and gastroenteritis. These are discussed in further detail in other appropriate sections of THE MANUAL, as listed in the Index.

Staphylococcal abscesses and toxic epidermal necrolysis, the "scalded skin syndrome" (for the latter, see Ch. 190 and NEONATAL INFECTIONS in Vol. II, Ch. 21): **Neonatal infections** usually appear within 6 wk after birth. Most commonly seen are pustular or bullous skin lesions, generally located in the axillary, inguinal, or neck skin folds; but multiple subcutaneous abscesses, exfoliation, bacteremia, meningitis, or pneumonia may also occur. Microscopic examination of the pus discloses polymorphonuclear neutrophils and staphylococci, often within the leukocytes.

Nursing mothers who develop breast abscesses or mastitis 1 to 4 wk postpartum should be considered as having penicillin-resistant staphylococcal infections, most probably derived from the nursery via the infant.

Postoperative infections ranging from "stitch abscesses" to extensive wound involvement commonly are due to staphylococci. Such infections may appear within a few days or not until several weeks after an operation; they are particularly likely if the patient received antibiotics at the time of surgery.

Furuncles and **carbuncles** are discussed in Ch. 190.

Staphylococcal pneumonia (see in Ch. 38) should be suspected in patients with influenza who develop dyspnea, cyanosis, or persistent or recurrent fever, and in patients hospitalized with chronic bronchopulmonary disease or other high-risk diseases who develop low-grade fever, tachypnea, cough, cyanosis, and leukocytosis. In neonates, staphylococcal pneumonia is characterized by abscess formation, rapid development of pneumatoceles, and, often, complicating empyema. Microscopic examination of patients' sputum discloses numerous large gram-positive cocci, occasionally within neutrophils.

Staphylococcal bacteremia may occur with any localized staphylococcal abscess and is a common cause of death in severely burned patients, generally 2 to 4 wk after injury. Symptoms and signs are discussed in Ch. 5. Persistent fever is usual and may be associated with shock. Bacterial endocarditis may develop. Diagnosis is established by positive blood cultures.

Staphylococcal osteomyelitis (see also Ch. 113): Acute hematogenous osteomyelitis occurs predominantly in children, causing chills, fever, and pain over the involved bone. Redness and swelling subsequently appear. Periarticular infection frequently results in effusion, suggesting septic arthritis rather than osteomyelitis. The WBC count is usually > 15,000 and blood cultures are often positive. X-ray changes are not apparent for 10 to 14 days; it may be longer before bone rarefaction and periosteal reaction are detected. Acute rheumatic fever is the most common misdiagnosis, but the differential diagnosis is usually not difficult if the delayed development of x-ray abnormalities is appreciated.

Staphylococcal enterocolitis is suggested when hospitalized patients develop fever, ileus, abdominal distention, hypotension, or diarrhea—especially if they have had recent abdominal surgery, broad-spectrum antibiotics, or antibiotics for preoperative bowel preparation. If microscopic examination of the stools discloses clumps of staphylococci, the diagnosis is likely. It is important to rule out infection with toxigenic *Clostridium difficile*, which also can cause colitis (see Ch. 58).

Prophylaxis

Aseptic precautions (e.g., thorough hand washing between patient examinations, sterilization of equipment) are important. Infected patients and their bedding should be isolated from other vulnerable patients. Hospital personnel with active staphylococcal infections, even of a local nature (e.g., boils), should not be allowed in contact with patients or equipment until their infections have been cured. Asymptomatic nasal carriers need not be excluded from patient contact unless the strains are particularly dangerous and the individual is the suspected source of an outbreak.

Treatment

Management includes abscess drainage, antibacterial therapy (parenterally, in a seriously ill patient), and general supportive measures. Cultures should be obtained before instituting or altering antibacterial regimens. Hospital-acquired staphylococci and most community-acquired strains usually are resistant to penicillin G, ampicillin, carbenicillin, streptomycin, and the tetracyclines. These antibiotics should not be used unless the organisms have been proved to be susceptible.

Virtually all strains are susceptible to penicillinase-resistant penicillins (methicillin, oxacillin, nafcillin, cloxacillin, dicloxacillin), cephalosporins (cephalothin, cefazolin, cephalexin, cephradine, cefamandole, cefoxitin), gentamicin, vancomycin, lincomycin, and clindamycin. One of the penicillins is usually the agent of choice, although the cephalosporins and vancomycin are equally effective. Many staphylococcal strains are also sensitive to erythromycin, kanamycin, bacitracin, and chloramphenicol. Chloramphenicol and bacitracin, however, are seldom indicated because they are potentially toxic and alternative agents are available. The choice and dosage of an antibiotic agent depend on the site of the infection, the severity of the illness, and the sensitivity of the organism. In staphylococcal enterocolitis, a nonabsorbed antistaphylococcal agent such as vancomycin 250 to 500 mg q 6 h is given orally, in combination with systemic therapy.

STREPTOCOCCAL INFECTIONS

Classification

Streptococcal infections can be classified **microbially** according to characteristics of the streptococcus and **clinically** according to the type of infection.

When grown on sheep-blood agar, β-hemolytic streptococci produce zones of clear hemolysis around each colony; α-streptococci (commonly called *Streptococcus viridans*) are surrounded by green discoloration due to incomplete hemolysis; and γ-streptococci are nonhemolytic. An additional classification, based on carbohydrates present in the cell wall, divides streptococci into the Lancefield Groups A to O. The members of Group D include enterococcal (*Streptococcus faecalis*, *S. durans*, *S. faecium*) and nonenterococcal (*S. bovis*, *S. equinus*) species. Extracellular Group A streptococcal antigens evoking antibody responses play important roles in the diagnostic tests to be described later.

Clinically, streptococcal infections can be divided into 3 broad groups: (1) the **carrier state**, in which the patient harbors streptococci without apparent infection; (2) **acute illnesses**, often suppurative, caused by streptococcal invasion of tissues; and (3) **delayed, nonsuppurative complications**. The nonsuppurative complications are the inflammatory states of acute rheumatic fever, chorea (discussed in Vol. II, Ch. 24), and glomerulonephritis (in Ch. 148). They occur most commonly about 2 wk after a clinically overt streptococcal infection, but the infection may be asymptomatic and the interval may be under or over 2 wk.

Clinical Manifestations

The symptoms and signs of acute invasive streptococcal infections depend on the affected tissue, the organism, the state of the host, and the host's response.

A **carrier state** exists when streptococci can be identified in material taken from a site that shows no evidence of inflammation. Group D streptococci are normally found in the gut, γ-streptococci in the throat and respiratory tract. β-Hemolytic streptococci of Groups A, B, C, and G—the groups generally regarded as pathogenic for man—can be cultured regularly from normal-looking throats of asymptomatic patients, and the term "carrier state" is usually reserved for such pharyngeal discoveries. The carrier state has importance as a cause of misdiagnosis in many pharyngeal or respiratory illnesses, since bacteriologic demonstration does not prove that a streptococcus is responsible for the associated clinical manifestations.

Acute streptococcal infections can be *primary*, invading normal tissue, or *secondary*, invading tissue compromised by trauma or other disease. The organism in primary invasions is usually the Group A β-hemolytic streptococcus and the site is usually the pharynx. Secondary invasions can be caused by γ-hemolytic streptococci, by Group D streptococci, or by Group A organisms. Group A erysipelas can occur in previously normal skin, or a streptococcal cellulitis can be imposed on traumatized skin or in subcutaneous tissue predisposed by venous insufficiency. A viral pneumonia or degenerative lung disease may be followed by a streptococcal pneumonia; *S. viridans* or Group D streptococci may create bacterial endocarditis; Group D streptococci are frequently found in urinary infections; and the endometritis of a postpartum uterus is often due to enterococci or Group A organisms. Group D streptococci have been recognized recently as common causes of nosocomial wound infections. The eyes, ears, joints, bone, and gut are other sites of secondary streptococcal invasion. Infections with Group B β-hemolytic streptococci *(Streptococcus agalactiae)* are important causes of neonatal sepsis and are reviewed in Vol. II, Ch. 21. In adults, sporadic cases of bacteremia, endocarditis, urinary tract infections, pneumonia, and meningitis have been observed. In addition, Group B β-hemolytic streptococci have been recovered frequently from elderly diabetic patients with cellulitis complicating severe peripheral vascular disease.

Primary or secondary infections can spread through the affected tissues and along lymphatic channels to regional lymph nodes, and can also produce bacteremia. The development of suppuration depends on the severity of infection and the susceptibility of tissue.

The most common type of streptococcal disease is **primary pharyngeal infection with the Group A β-hemolytic organism.** In its typical form, the infection is manifested by sore throat, fever, a beefy red pharynx, and tonsillar exudate. This form occurs in about 20% of patients with Group A infections; the remainder are asymptomatic, have fever or sore throat alone, or have nonspecific symptoms such as headache, malaise, nausea, vomiting, tachycardia. Convulsions may occur in children. The cervical and submaxillary nodes may enlarge and become tender. In children under 4, rhinorrhea is frequent and sometimes the sole manifestation. None of these symptoms (including sore throat) and none of the signs (including pharyngeal exudate or occasional palatal petechiae) are specific for streptococcal infection, and any or all of these clinical features can occur in viral infections, particularly with the adenoviruses and in infectious mononucleosis. The only sign or symptom statistically associated with serologically confirmed streptococcal disease is cervical adenitis. Cough, laryngitis, and stuffy nose are uncharacteristic of streptococcal infection, and their presence suggests that other etiologic agents coexist or have exclusive responsibility for the clinical ailment. Definitive diagnosis rests on the laboratory technics described later.

Though formerly a common ailment, **scarlet fever** is uncommon today, probably because antibiotic therapy prevents the opportunity for the streptococcus to progress in individual patients or to create massive epidemics. Scarlet fever is associated with Group A streptococcal strains that produce an erythrogenic toxin, leading to a diffuse pink-red cutaneous flush that blanches on pressure. The rash, an additional feature of an illness that otherwise resembles streptococcal pharyngitis, is seen best on the abdomen, on the lateral chest, and in cutaneous folds. Among the characteristic manifestations of the rash are **circumoral pallor** surrounded by a flushed face, a "**strawberry tongue**" (inflamed beefy red papillae protruding through a white coating), and **Pastia's lines** (dark red lines in the creases of skin folds). The upper layer of the previously reddened skin often desquamates after the fever subsides. The course and management of scarlet fever are the same as for other clinically evident Group A infections.

Streptococcal pyoderma (impetigo) is covered in Vol. II, Ch. 24.

Laboratory Diagnostic Tests

Acute streptococcal inflammation is regularly associated with an elevation both in ESR (usually > 50 in the Westergren test or uncorrected Wintrobe value) and in WBC count (about 12,000 to 20,000), with 75 to 90% neutrophils, many of which are young forms. The urine commonly shows no specific changes except those attributable to fever (e.g., proteinuria).

The presence of streptococci can be established directly and promptly in material taken from the inflammatory site and examined by bacteriologic technics: overnight incubation on a sheep-blood agar plate or, for Group A organisms, immediate staining with fluorescent antibodies. The fluorescent method obviates the need, when organisms are grown in culture, for serologic testing to differentiate Group A organisms from other β-hemolytic streptococci, but the fluorescence may often produce false-positive reactions with hemolytic staphylococci.

These direct tests can show that streptococci are *present* but *proof of infection* is obtained indirectly from streptococcal antibodies in the serum. The ASO titer rises in only 75 to 80% of infections, and, for completeness, streptococcal antihyaluronidase, antideoxyribonuclease B, antidiphosphopyridine nucleotidase, and antistreptokinase can also be used. Penicillin given early (within the first 5 days) for symptomatic streptococcal pharyngitis may delay the appearance and decrease the magnitude of the antibody response to streptolysin O. Patients with streptococcal pyoderma usually do not have a significant ASO response.

A single value of one antibody titer is only a crude index of recent streptococcal infection. Confirmation requires comparison of sequential specimens for recent *changes* in titer, since a single value may be high as a result of slow "decay" of antibodies from a long antecedent infection. Conversely, a single value lower than the laboratory's upper limit of normal may represent an elevation for an individual patient. Sera need not be taken more often than every 2 wk and may be as far apart as 2 mo. A significant rise (or fall) in titer should span at least 2 tube dilutions, since a 1-tube increment may be due to laboratory variation. For greatest accuracy, the sera under comparison should be saved and tested on the same day, with the same reagents, by the same technician.

Streptozyme, an inexpensive, easily performed test for antibodies to streptolysin O, hyaluronidase, deoxyribonuclease B, and other streptococcal antigens, correlates best with an elevated ASO titer. False-positive results are seen in 3 to 5% of cases. However, 25 to 50% of patients with borderline serologic responses to specific streptococcal extracellular antigens will have false-negative agglutination with the streptozyme test.

Because of the time interval between serial specimens, serologic testing is not useful in managing acute invasive streptococcal infections, where diagnosis depends on clinical manifestations and results of bacteriologic tests. The "serial run" antibody tests are particularly useful, however, in the diagnosis of poststreptococcal inflammatory states. Evidence of a recent Group A streptococcal infection is critical for the diagnosis of rheumatic fever, which can generally be ruled out if no change in titer is demonstrated in a properly performed "serial run" with measurement of other appropriate antibodies besides ASO.

Course and Treatment

The secondarily invasive streptococcal infections can be life-threatening, particularly for a debilitated patient. Septicemias, puerperal sepsis, endocarditis, and pneumonias due to streptococci were frequent causes of death in the preantibiotic era, and remain serious, especially if the infecting organism is an enterococcus. Though Group A streptococci and *S. viridans* are almost always sensitive to penicillin, enterococci are relatively resistant and require treatment with an aminoglycoside in addition to penicillin.

The primary pharyngeal infections, including scarlet fever, ordinarily have a finite course; the fever will drop after several days and recovery is complete within 2 wk. Antibiotics have little effect on the symptoms of streptococcal pharyngitis. Their value is primarily to prevent local suppurative events such as peritonsillar abscess (quinsy), otitis media, sinusitis, and mastoiditis. Most important, they are used to thwart the nonsuppurative complications that may follow untreated Group A infections.

Penicillin is the best therapeutic agent for an established Group A streptococcal infection. A single injection of benzathine penicillin G, at a dose of 600,000 to 900,000 u. IM for small children and 1.2 million u. IM for adolescents or adults, will usually suffice. Since the injection is often painful, oral therapy may be preferred if the patient can be trusted to maintain the regimen. The minor differences of absorption among the diverse oral preparations of penicillin do not seem as important as an adequately high dosage and duration of the regimen. At least 200,000 u. (and perhaps 400,000 u.) of penicillin G or 125 mg (to 250 mg) of penicillin V should be taken q.i.d. for at least 10 days to achieve the effect of a single injection of benzathine penicillin G. The 10-day course *must be completed* even though the patient has become asymptomatic. An alternative plan for patients considered unreliable or unable to take oral medication is to give 3 injections of procaine penicillin (each usually less painful than the one large benzathine dose): 600,000 u. IM is given on the 1st, 4th, and 7th days.

When penicillin is contraindicated, erythromycin 0.5 gm or clindamycin 0.3 gm may be given orally twice daily for 10 days. Sulfadiazine, which is bacteriostatic, should not be used to treat an established infection, though it is highly useful in preventing streptococcal infections. Tetracycline is undesirable because a significant number of Group A streptococci are resistant to it; moreover, in the young it may discolor growing teeth.

Antistreptococcal therapy can often be withheld for 1 or 2 days, until bacteriologic verification has been obtained, without significantly increasing the risk of suppurative or nonsuppurative complications of streptococcal pharyngitis. An effective plan is to begin oral penicillin when infection is suspected and specimens for laboratory tests have been obtained. The treatment is then stopped if laboratory tests fail to confirm the presence of streptococci. Otherwise, oral treatment is continued or replaced by an injectable agent.

Other symptoms of streptococcal infection can be treated with agents such as aspirin for sore throat, headache, or fever. Bed rest is unnecessary unless the patient wants it. Isolation technics are no longer warranted. Among the infected patient's close associates in family or friends, those who are symptomatic or have a history of poststreptococcal complications should be examined for streptococci, then appropriately treated with antibiotics.

RHEUMATIC FEVER (See Vol. II, Ch. 24)

SYDENHAM'S CHOREA (See Vol. II, Ch. 24)

PNEUMOCOCCAL INFECTIONS

Bacteriology

The pneumococcus (formerly called *Diplococcus pneumoniae* and now designated *Streptococcus pneumoniae*) is a gram-positive encapsulated diplococcus, the adjacent surfaces of the cocci being rounded and the ends pointed to give a lancet shape. It sometimes appears as short chains; in old cultures or in purulent exudates, some of the organisms may appear pink. The capsule, visible in ordinary smears stained with methylene blue, consists of a complex polysaccharide that determines serologic specificity and contributes to the virulence and pathogenicity. Some of the 85 or more specific types show cross-reactivity. In the **Neufeld quellung reaction,** the best method for determining type specificity, the capsule swells in the presence of type-specific rabbit antiserum; since this swelling does not occur with other bacteria and does not occur clearly with pneumococci of other types, this method establishes both the species and type of organism. For clinical diagnosis, multivalent antiserum against some groups of specific types is available commercially or from the Center for Disease Control of the USPHS, and a serum against all types is available from the Danish Serum Institute in Copenhagen. Typing may also be carried out by specific agglutination or by immunoelectrophoresis against specific antisera. The specific type of pneumococcal antibody in serum or other body fluids may be determined by counterimmunoelectrophoresis against type-specific polysaccharides.

Distribution of specific serotypes of pneumococci varies among isolates from different clinical types of infections, in carriers, at different times, and in different locations; the commonest types in recent serious infections have been types 1, 3, 4, 7, 8, and 12 in adults and types 6, 14, 19, and 23 in infants and children. The capsular polysaccharides are antigenic in humans and produce type-specific serologic and protective antibody against the whole organism; a polyvalent vaccine containing polysaccharides of 14 types that account for > 80% of pneumococcal infections is available (see Prophylaxis below).

Recovery from pneumococcal infection is usually associated with development of circulating type-specific antibodies.

Epidemiology

Pneumococci commonly inhabit the human respiratory tract, particularly in winter and early spring, when they may be cultured from up to half of the population at any given time. The organisms spread from person to person in droplets, but true epidemics of pneumococcal pneumonia or other infections are rare. Isolation of patients for pneumococcal infections is therefore not generally required.

The patients most susceptible to serious and invasive pneumococcal infections are those with lymphoma, Hodgkin's disease, multiple myeloma, splenectomy, other serious debilitating diseases or immunologic deficiencies, and sickle cell disease. Damage to the respiratory epithelium by chronic bronchitis or common respiratory viruses, notably influenza virus, may predispose to pneumococcal invasion of the pulmonary parenchyma and pneumonia. Pneumococcal pneumonias are highly prevalent among gold and diamond miners in South Africa and New Guinea.

Diseases Caused by Pneumococcus

Pneumonia: Pneumonia, the most frequent serious infection caused by the pneumococcus, is usually lobar pneumonia, but may be bronchopneumonia, or tracheobronchitis without clearly defined parenchymal involvement (see PNEUMOCOCCAL PNEUMONIA in Ch. 38).

Acute purulent empyema of the pleura: Pneumococcus, the most common cause, accounts for about 15% of all empyemas, but < 3% of cases of pneumococcal pneumonia are complicated by empyema (in contrast to sterile pleural effusions, which are more common). The exudate may resolve spontaneously or during therapy of the pneumonia; or it may become thick and fibrinopurulent, sometimes loculated, and require surgical drainage. (See Treatment below and also in Chs. 38 and 45.)

Acute otitis media: The pneumococcus causes about ½ of all cases of acute otitis media in infants (after the newborn period) and children. About ⅓ of all children in most populations will have an attack of acute pneumococcal otitis media in the first 2 yr of life, and recurrent otitis due to pneumococcus is common. Mastoiditis, meningitis, and lateral sinus thrombosis, fairly common complications of otitis media in the preantibiotic days, are rarely seen. (See TABLE 1-1 in Ch. 1 and also ACUTE OTITIS MEDIA in Vol. II, Ch. 24.)

Acute sinusitis: The pneumococcus may cause infections of the paranasal sinuses. Infection of the ethmoidal or sphenoidal sinus may extend into the meninges and produce bacterial meningitis. Sinusitis may become chronic and mixed with other bacteria. (See TABLE 1-1 in Ch. 1 and also SINUSITIS in Ch. 168.)

Acute bacterial meningitis: Except for *H. influenzae* meningitis in children and epidemic meningococcal meningitis, the pneumococcus is one of the most frequent etiologic agents of acute bacterial (purulent) meningitis in all age groups. Pneumococcal meningitis may be secondary to (1) bacteremia from other foci (notably pneumonia), (2) an infection of the ear, mastoid process, or paranasal sinuses (notably the ethmoidal or sphenoidal sinuses), or (3) basilar fracture of the skull involving one of these sites or the cribriform plate. (For the clinical aspects see ACUTE BACTERIAL MENINGITIS in Ch. 124.)

Pneumococcal bacteremia: Bacteremia may accompany the acute phase of pneumococcal pneumonia or meningitis and, of course, is a major manifestation of pneumococcal endocarditis. Pneumococcal bacteremia may also be an apparently primary infection (i.e., without another focus) in susceptible patients (see Epidemiology above) or may occur in an otherwise normal patient during the course of a simple, febrile, viral URI (common cold). In some such cases the pneumococcus is first discovered at autopsy in an infected paranasal sinus, internal ear, or mastoid.

Pneumococcal endocarditis: Pneumococcal endocarditis may complicate the bacteremia accompanying pneumonia or meningitis, or it may occur in patients who have no clinically apparent focus that accounts for the bacteremia. It may occur in patients with or without prior history or evidence of valvular heart disease and rarely may even be fatal without changing murmurs, petechiae, or embolic phenomena. Pneumococcal endocarditis may produce a corrosive valvular lesion, with sudden rupture or fenestration leading to rapidly progressive congestive heart failure; prompt removal and replacement of the diseased valve may be life-saving. It may be possible to visualize the valvular lesion and vegetations by echocardiography or nuclear scanning methods. (See also BACTERIAL ENDOCARDITIS in Ch. 25.)

Pneumococcal peritonitis: Peritonitis caused by pneumococcus, once a common complication of lipoid nephrosis but now seen only rarely, occurs most often in young girls, presumably as an ascending infection from the vagina through the fallopian tubes. The symptoms are similar to those of other causes of acute bacterial peritonitis; the infection responds rapidly to treatment with penicillin. (See also PERITONITIS in Ch. 53.)

Pneumococcal arthritis: The pneumococcus, an uncommon cause of acute purulent (septic) arthritis, can usually be demonstrated by direct smear and by culture of the aspirated purulent synovial fluid. It is usually a complication of pneumococcemia from another focus, especially meningitis or endocarditis. The clinical picture and therapy are similar to those of septic arthritis caused by other gram-positive cocci. (See INFECTIOUS ARTHRITIS in Ch. 103.)

Prophylaxis

A polyvalent pneumococcal polysaccharide vaccine, commercially available, is directed against the 14 types that account for $> 80\%$ of serious pneumococcal infections. It produces specific antibodies against nearly all of these types in most children > 2 yr of age and most adults, reducing pneumonia and other bacteremic infections by about 80% and mortality from such infections by 40%. Its antigenicity and protective effects in infants and young children have not been clearly demonstrated. In the recommended dose of 50 μg of each type in physiologic saline, it is relatively free of side reactions. Protection may last for several years, but in the highly susceptible, especially children, revaccination after 3 yr or more is desirable.

The vaccine is indicated for persons with chronic cardiac disease, chronic bronchitis and bronchiectasis, diabetes, and metabolic disorders, and for elderly and debilitated persons in chronic care facilities. Preliminary data suggest that the vaccine may prevent pneumonia and bacteremia in most but not all patients with sickle cell anemia and in splenectomized patients > 2 yr. Continuous prophylaxis with penicillin has been advocated for splenectomized patients and (to prevent recurrent streptococcal infections) patients with rheumatic heart disease or a history of rheumatic fever. The vaccine may not be effective in preventing pneumococcal meningitis complicating basilar fracture of the skull, and is currently not recommended for pregnant females, children < 2 yr, splenectomized patients with Hodgkin's disease, or anyone hypersensitive to the components. Penicillin V 250 mg b.i.d. to q.i.d. for 5 days at the onset of a common cold may prevent recurrences of pneumococcal pneumonia in patients with chronic bronchitis; however, tetracycline or ampicillin is preferred in patients whose sputum may also contain Hemophilus influenzae.

Treatment

The major therapy for all pneumococcal infections is penicillin G, to which pneumococci of all serotypes have been highly susceptible. (For treatment of pneumococcal pneumonia and of pleural empyema, see PNEUMOCOCCAL PNEUMONIA in Ch. 38.) Generally, doses of procaine penicillin G 600,000 u. IM q 4 or 6 h or penicillin V 250 to 500 mg orally q 3 or 4 h are given for 3 to 5 days for acute pneumococcal otitis media, sinusitis, or arthritis; in arthritis, however, treatment should be kept up for an additional week. Pneumococcal meningitis or endocarditis require much larger doses of penicillin G potassium for injection— 24 million u./day given by intermittent (q 2 h) or continuous IV infusion and maintained for 10 days to 2 wk after the patient is afebrile and cultures of blood and CSF have remained sterile.

Antibiotic resistance: Where strains of pneumococci with marked resistance to penicillin and other antibiotics have been reported (e.g., the USA, Great Britain, South Africa, New Guinea), it is necessary to test for susceptibility to antibiotics.

For patients with pneumococcal pneumonia, meningitis, or endocarditis who are allergic to penicillin, see PNEUMOCOCCAL PNEUMONIA in Ch. 38 and BACTERIAL ENDOCARDITIS in Ch. 25. Patients with endocarditis should be followed closely for evidence of changing murmurs or sudden or progressive heart failure; the latter requires prompt surgical intervention.

CAUSED BY GRAM–NEGATIVE, AEROBIC COCCI

NEISSERIA

Organisms of the genus *Neisseria* include *N. meningitidis*, important cause of meningitis, bacteremia, and other serious infections in both children and adults; *N. gonorrhoeae*, a major cause of sexually transmitted diseases, including urethritis, cervicitis, proctitis, pharyngitis, salpingitis, and epididymitis; and numerous saprophytic *Neisseria* species that commonly inhabit the oropharynx, vagina, or colon but rarely cause human disease. Morphologically, organisms of the genus *Neisseria* can be recognized by their characteristic colonial morphology (small, translucent colonies with umbilicated centers and crenated margins), by Gram stain (small gram-negative cocci, often in chains or pairs), and by their positive oxidase reactions. *N. meningitidis* and *N. gonorrhoeae* can be distinguished from one another and from saprophytic strains on the basis of sugar fermentation reactions. *Neisseria* grow well on solid media containing blood or serum and thrive in a reduced O_2 atmosphere with 5 to 10% CO_2 at 35 to 37 C. Chocolate agar incubated in a candle jar provides a suitable environment.

Since each of the medically important *Neisseria* species is principally responsible for infections of a particular site, gonorrhea infections are discussed in Chs. 151, 162, and 178, and in Vol. II, Ch. 5. Meningococcal infections are discussed under Acute Bacterial Meningitis in Ch. 124.

CAUSED BY GRAM–POSITIVE BACILLI

ERYSIPELOID

An acute, but slowly evolving, skin infection caused by Erysipelothrix rhusiopathiae.

Etiology

Erysipelothrix rhusiopathiae (insidiosa), a gram-positive, noncapsulated, nonsporulating, nonmotile, microaerophilic bacillus with worldwide distribution, is primarily an animal pathogen, especially for swine. Infection in man is chiefly occupational and typically follows a penetrating hand wound in persons who handle fish or animal tissues (e.g., butchers).

Symptoms, Signs, and Diagnosis

Within a week of injury a characteristic raised, purplish-red, nonvesiculated, indurated maculopapule appears, accompanied by itching and burning. Local swelling, though sharply demarcated, may inhibit use of the hand. The border of the lesion may slowly extend outward. Regional lymphatic involvement is absent. The disease is usually self-limiting; discomfort and disability may persist for 2 to 3 wk. Bacteremia is rare but may result in septic arthritis or infective endocarditis (without known valvular heart disease in half the patients).

The characteristic lesion and its course are diagnostic. Culture of a needle aspirate or biopsy specimen taken from the advancing edge of a lesion may yield *Erysipelothrix rhusiopathiae*.

Treatment

Benzathine penicillin G 1.2 million u. IM (600,000 u. in each buttock), or erythromycin 0.5 gm q.i.d. orally for 7 days, is curative.

ANTHRAX (Malignant Pustule; Woolsorter's Disease)

A highly infectious disease of animals, especially ruminants, that is transmitted to man by contact with the animals or their products. Anthrax is an important animal disease. Disease in man is becoming less common, mainly occurring in countries without public health regulations that prevent industrial exposure to infected goats, cattle, sheep, and horses, or to their products. A vaccine, composed of a culture filtrate, is available for those at high risk (veterinarians, laboratory technicians, employees of textile mills processing imported goat hair).

Etiology and Epidemiology

The causative organism, *Bacillus anthracis*, is a large, gram-positive, facultatively anaerobic, encapsulated rod. The spores resist destruction and remain viable in soil and animal products for decades. Human infection is usually through the skin but has followed ingestion of contaminated meat. Inhaling spores under adverse conditions (e.g., the presence of an acute respiratory infection) may result in pulmonary anthrax **(woolsorter's disease),** which is often fatal.

Diagnosis

The occupational history is most important. The organism may be demonstrated in cultures or in gram-stained smears from cutaneous lesions and, in the pulmonary form, from throat swabs and sputum. Mouse inoculation may permit isolation of the organism when primary cultures are unsuccessful.

Symptoms, Signs, and Treatment

The incubation period varies from 12 h to 5 days (generally, 3 to 5 days). The **cutaneous form** begins as a red-brown papule that enlarges with considerable peripheral erythema, vesiculation, and induration. Central ulceration follows, with serosanguineous exudation and formation of a black eschar. Local lymphadenopathy may be present, occasionally with malaise, myalgia, headache, fever, nausea, and vomiting. **Treatment** with procaine penicillin G 600,000 u. IM b.i.d. prevents systemic spread and induces gradual resolution of the pustule. Tetracycline 2 gm/day orally is also effective.

Pulmonary anthrax follows rapid multiplication of spores in the mediastinal lymph nodes. Severe hemorrhagic necrotizing lymphadenitis develops and spreads to the adjacent mediastinal structures. Serosanguineous transudation, pulmonary edema, and pleural effusion occur. Initial symptoms are insidious and resemble influenza. Fever increases; within a few days, severe respiratory distress develops, followed by cyanosis, shock, and coma. Hemorrhagic meningoencephalitis may develop. Lung x-ray may show diffuse patchy infiltration; the mediastinum is widened because of enlarged hemorrhagic lymph nodes. Death is common. Antibiotic therapy is of little value when given at the toxic stage, but early and continuous IV **therapy** with penicillin G 10 million u./day may be lifesaving. Corticosteroids may be of value, but have not been adequately evaluated.

DIPHTHERIA (See Vol. II, Ch. 24)

NOCARDIOSIS

An acute or chronic, often disseminated, granulomatous-suppurative infection caused by the aerobic gram-positive microorganism Nocardia asteroides, *a soil saprophyte.*

Etiology and Epidemiology

The organism usually enters the body via the lung; rarely, via the GI tract or skin. This uncommon disease occurs worldwide at all ages, but incidence is greatest in older adults and more frequent in men than in women. Those who are debilitated or receiving immunosuppressive therapy are most susceptible, but approximately half the patients have no preexisting disease.

Symptoms and Signs

Most cases of disseminated nocardiosis begin as pulmonary infections. Pulmonary nocardiosis may resemble actinomycosis, but *N. asteroides* is more likely to disseminate hematogenously with abscess formation in the brain or, less frequently, in the kidney or in multiple organs. **Skin or subcutaneous abscesses** occur in 1/3 of cases. With **lung lesions,** the most frequent symptoms—including cough, fever, chills, chest pain, weakness, anorexia, and weight loss—resemble those of TB or suppurative pneumonia. In the **metastatic brain abscesses** that occur in 1/3 of cases, the symptoms are severe headache and focal and motor disturbances.

Diagnosis, Prognosis, and Treatment

Diagnosis is by identification of the microorganism in tissue or culture. Though closely related to *Actinomyces israelii, N. asteroides* is not clubbed and becomes arranged in loose clusters of interlacing, slender, branching filaments rather than in the true "sulfur granule" form.

Without treatment, the disease is usually fatal. In those receiving appropriate therapy, the prognosis is poorest in the presence of immunosuppressive therapy, better in CNS infection, and best (> 50% survival) in instances where the lesions occur only in the lungs. *Nocardia* organisms are usually resistant to penicillin in vivo. Sulfonamide **treatment** (e.g., with sulfadiazine 4 to 6 gm/day orally) must be continued for several months, since most cases respond slowly.

ACTINOMYCOSIS (Lumpy Jaw)

A chronic infectious disease characterized by multiple draining sinuses and caused by the anaerobic gram-positive microorganism Actinomyces israelii, *often present as a commensal on the gums, tonsils, and teeth.*

Incidence and Pathology

The disease is seen most often in adult males. In the cervicofacial form, the most common portal of entry is decayed teeth; pulmonary disease results from aspiration of oral secretions; abdominal disease, from a break in the mucosa of a diverticulum or the appendix.

The characteristic lesion is an indurated area of multiple, small, communicating abscesses surrounded by granulation tissue. Disease spreads to contiguous tissue and, rarely, hematogenously. Other anaerobic bacteria are usually also present.

Symptoms and Signs

There are 4 clinical forms of actinomycosis. (1) The **abdominal form** affects the intestines (usually the cecum and appendix) and the peritoneum. Pain, fever, vomiting, diarrhea or constipation, and emaciation are characteristically present. An abdominal mass with signs of partial intestinal obstruction appears, and draining sinuses and fistulas may develop in the abdominal wall. (2) The **cervicofacial form** usually begins as a small, flat, hard swelling, with or without pain, under the oral mucosa or the skin on the neck, or as a subperiosteal swelling of the jaw. Subsequently, areas of softening appear and develop into sinuses and fistulas with a discharge that contains the characteristic "sulfur granules" (rounded or spherical, usually yellowish, granules up to 1 mm in diameter). The cheek, tongue, pharynx, salivary glands, cranial bones, meninges, or brain may be affected, usually by direct extension. (3) In the **thoracic form,** involvement of the lungs resembles TB. Extensive invasion may occur before chest pain, fever, and productive cough appear. Perforation of the chest wall, with chronic draining sinuses, may result. (4) In the **generalized form,** hematogenous spread occurs to the skin, vertebral bodies, brain, liver, kidney, ureter, and (in women) the pelvic organs.

Diagnosis

This is based on clinical symptoms, x-ray findings, and demonstration of A. *israelii* in sputum, pus, or biopsy specimen. (See also TABLE 2–1 in Ch. 2.) In pus or tissue, the microorganism appears as tangled masses of branched and unbranched wavy filaments, or as the distinctive "sulfur granules." These consist of a central mass of tangled filaments, pus cells, and debris, with a midzone of inter-lacing filaments surrounded by an outer zone of radiating, club-shaped, hyaline and refractive fila-ments that take the eosin stain in tissue.

Lung lesions must be distinguished from those of TB and neoplasms. Lesions in the abdomen occur most frequently in the ileocecal region and are difficult to diagnose, except at laparotomy or when draining sinuses appear in the abdominal wall. Aspiration liver biopsy should be avoided be-cause of the danger of inducing a persistent sinus. A tender, palpable mass suggests appendiceal abscess or regional enteritis. Nodules in any location may simulate malignant growths.

Prognosis and Treatment

The disease is slowly progressive. Prognosis relates directly to early diagnosis, is most favorable in the cervicofacial form, and is progressively worse in the pulmonary, abdominal, and generalized forms.

Most cases will respond to medical treatment but, owing to the extensive induration and relatively avascular fibrosis, response is slow and treatment must be continued for at least 8 wk and occasion-ally for > 1 yr. Extensive and repeated surgical procedures may be required. Aspiration is indicated for small abscesses and drainage for large ones. (See TABLE 7–1 under BARRIERS in Ch. 7.) Penicillin G, at least 12 million u./day IV, should be given initially; penicillin V 1 gm orally q.i.d. may be substi-tuted after about 2 wk. Tetracycline 500 mg orally q 6 h may be given instead of penicillin. Treatment must be continued for several weeks after apparent clinical cure.

CAUSED BY GRAM–NEGATIVE, FACULTATIVELY ANAEROBIC BACILLI

ENTEROBACTERIACEAE INFECTIONS

The Enterobacteriaceae comprise *Salmonella, Arizona, Citrobacter, Escherichia, Klebsiella, En-terobacter, Hafnia, Serratia, Proteus,* and *Providencia.* These organisms are readily cultured on ordi-nary media; they ferment glucose, reduce nitrates to nitrites, and are oxidase-negative and catalase-positive. Only the clinically important organisms that are not discussed in other chapters are covered here.

Escherichia coli normally inhabits the GI tract. If normal anatomic barriers are disrupted, the organism may spread to adjacent structures or invade the bloodstream. The site most often infected by E. *coli* is the urinary tract, which is colonized from without; but hepatobiliary, peritoneal, cutane-ous, and pulmonary infections are not uncommon. E. *coli* is an important cause of bacteremia, which often occurs without an overt portal of entry. This organism is also an "opportunistic invader," causing disease in patients who have defects in host resistance due to disease (e.g., cancer, diabe-tes, cirrhosis) or treatment with steroids, x-ray therapy, antineoplastic drugs, or antibiotics.

E. *coli* bacteremia is common in neonates, particularly premature infants (see ACUTE INFECTIOUS NEONATAL DIARRHEA under NEONATAL INFECTIONS in Vol. II, Ch. 21), and certain strains (enteropatho-genic E. *coli*) cause diarrhea in infants and traveler's diarrhea in adults.

When the **diagnosis** of E. *coli* infection is suspected on clinical grounds, it must be confirmed by culture and appropriate biochemical tests; Gram stain does not differentiate E. *coli* from other gram-negative bacteria.

Treatment may be started empirically, and then should be modified on the basis of antibiotic sensitivity studies. Most strains are sensitive to the tetracyclines, chloramphenicol, ampicillin, car-benicillin, the cephalosporins, the aminoglycosides, and trimethoprim-sulfa. In many instances, ther-apy also requires surgery to drain pus, excise necrotic lesions, or remove foreign bodies.

***Klebsiella-Enterobacter-Serratia* infections** are usually acquired in the hospital, mainly by patients with diminished host resistance. In general, these organisms are more resistant to antimicrobials than E. *coli.* As a rule, *Klebsiella, Enterobacter,* and *Serratia* cause infections in the same sites as does E. *coli* and they are also an important cause of bacteremia. They tend to respond to carbenicil-lin and the aminoglycosides; however, many isolates are resistant to multiple antibiotics and sensitiv-ity studies are essential. The sensitivity of *Klebsiella* to the cephalosporins differentiates them from *Enterobacter,* which are generally resistant to these drugs.

Klebsiella pneumonia (see in Ch. 38), a rare pulmonary infection characterized by severe pneumonia (sometimes with expectoration of dark brown or red-currant-jelly sputum), lung abscess formation, and empyema, is most common in diabetics and in patients with alcoholism. If treated early enough, it responds to cephalosporins and aminoglycosides.

Proteus species encompass gram-negative organisms that do not ferment lactose and are characterized by their spreading trait. There are 4 species, *P. mirabilis*, *P. vulgaris*, *P. morganii*, and *P. rettgeri*. *P. mirabilis* causes most human infections and is distinguished from the others by its failure to form indole. These organisms are normally found in soil, water, and the flora of normal feces. They are often cultured from superficial wounds, draining ears, and sputum, particularly in patients whose normal flora has been eradicated by antibiotic therapy. They may also cause deep-seated infections (particularly in the ears and mastoid sinuses, peritoneal cavities, and urinary tracts of patients with chronic urinary tract infections or with renal or bladder stones) and bacteremia.

P. mirabilis is sensitive to ampicillin, carbenicillin, the cephalosporins, and the aminoglycosides. The other 3 species tend to be more resistant, but are sensitive to carbenicillin and the aminoglycosides.

SALMONELLA INFECTIONS

The 1400-odd salmonellas have always been classified according to their antigenic composition; however, there is an attempt to simplify classification by basing it on the clinical presentations caused by the organisms. Three groups are suggested: (1) enteric fever, caused by *Salmonella typhi*; (2) localized disease, *Salmonella choleraesuis*; and (3) gastroenteritis, into which all of the other many salmonellas belong. In this 3rd group the designation will be *Salmonella enteritidis*, with either a biotype or serotype following and the name of the organism, e.g., *S. enteritidis* ser Typhimurium.

Several of the salmonellas are naturally pathogenic only for man (e.g., *Salmonella typhi*), but most are also pathogenic for (and therefore transmissible by) animals. *Salmonella* infection may occur as an asymptomatic carrier state, or as acute gastroenteritis, enteric fever, or a focal disease with or without associated septicemia. An endotoxin is produced, but its role in the varied symptomatology of salmonella infections is undefined. Except for typhoid fever, salmonella infections (especially gastroenteritis) are an increasing public health problem.

TYPHOID FEVER

A generalized infection caused by S. typhi (typhosa), *with involvement of the lymphatic tissues, and characterized by fever, bradycardia, rose-colored eruption, abdominal signs, and splenomegaly.* It is the prototype of the severe enteric salmonella infections.

Epidemiology and Pathology

The source of infection is the feces of asymptomatic carriers or the stool or urine of patients with active disease. Family contacts may be transient carriers. About 2 to 5% of patients become chronic carriers, women 3 times more often than men, and patients with preexisting cholecystitis and cholelithiasis in particular. In communities with poor sanitation, transmission is most frequently by water; next most often by food, especially milk. Transmission in modern urban areas is chiefly through food contaminated by food handlers who are healthy carriers. Flies may spread the organism from feces to food. Infection by direct contact probably does not occur.

The organism enters the body via the GI tract and invades the bloodstream via the lymphatic channels. Peyer's patches, especially in the ileum and cecum, are hyperplastic and, in untreated patients, may develop ulcers. The ulcers heal without scarring. The kidneys and liver usually show cloudy swelling; the latter may show patchy necrosis. The spleen is enlarged and soft. Pulmonary infection is rare.

Symptoms and Signs

The incubation period (3 to 25 days) relates indirectly to the number of organisms ingested. Onset is usually gradual, with chilly sensations (occasionally chills), malaise, headache, anorexia, epistaxis, backache, and constipation. Abdominal pain and tenderness to palpation dominate the clinical picture. Respiratory symptoms other than sore throat are uncommon; in untreated patients, typhoid pneumonia or a secondary pneumonitis may develop.

Without therapy, the temperature rises daily by steps for 7 to 10 days, maintains a peak for another 7 to 10 days, and then falls by lysis by the end of the 4th wk. Relative bradycardia and usually a dicrotic pulse are present. Discrete, rounded, rose-colored spots that blanch on pressure (the diagnostic "**rose spots**") emerge in crops, most commonly on the abdomen and chest, between the 7th and 10th days in about 10% of patients, persist for 2 to 5 days, and then fade. Splenomegaly is usual by the end of the 1st wk. Florid diarrhea occurs late in the disease when intestinal lesions are most manifest. Delirium and stupor are common. Leukopenia and anemia are characteristic and are most marked by the end of the 3rd wk. Leukocytosis, except in children, usually indicates a complication. Albuminuria and casts are frequent.

Atypical clinical manifestations are common. Symptoms may be predominantly pharyngeal (sore throat), abdominal (nausea, vomiting, pain, rigidity), respiratory (bronchitis, pneumonia), renal (nephritis), or neural (meningismus, psychosis). In **ambulatory ("walking") typhoid**, patients are asymptomatic but have typhoid bacillemia.

Complications

Complications occur mainly in untreated patients or when treatment is delayed.

Intestinal hemorrhage may be occult, occasionally progressing to massive hemorrhage. Significant bleeding occurs during the 3rd wk and is indicated by a sudden fall in temperature or an abrupt rise in pulse rate, and by pallor, sweating, hypotension, and, rarely, abdominal pain. The mortality rate of symptomatic hemorrhaging patients is 25%, but this is an unusual complication and blood transfusions prevent death.

Intestinal perforation, the most frequently fatal complication, is most common during the 3rd wk and in adult males, especially those with pronounced abdominal signs. Sharp abdominal pain occurs suddenly, usually in the right lower quadrant, with nausea, vomiting, a fall in temperature, rapid pulse, and muscle spasms; leukocytosis is present. An upright abdominal x-ray showing free air may be helpful in diagnosis.

Relapses: Antibiotic therapy has *increased* the incidence of febrile relapses to 15% from a prior 8%. Fever occurs about 2 wk after cessation of treatment and may only last for several days. If antibiotic therapy is reinstituted, the fever abates rapidly, unlike the slow defervescence seen during the primary illness. Occasionally a second relapse occurs.

Diagnosis

This depends on demonstration of typhoid bacilli in the blood, urine, or feces, or development of a positive Widal reaction. Typhoid bacilli may be cultured from the blood during the first 2 wk; later cultures are less frequently positive. Stool cultures will be positive early in the disease but may be intermittently negative for typhoid bacilli while antibiotic treatment is administered. Afterward, stool cultures may again yield the organism for several weeks to several months. Cultures from bone marrow, rose spots, and liver biopsies have proved to be good sources of typhoid bacilli. The Widal agglutination test becomes positive during the 2nd wk; a progressive rise in agglutination titer is significant. Typhoid bacilli contain both H and O antigens that stimulate corresponding antibodies. Both H and O agglutination titers should be determined, though the O titer is of greater significance because the H agglutinins may remain elevated for years after typhoid immunization, whereas the O titer usually disappears within a year. The Widal test has several deficiencies. Many nontyphoidal strains have cross-reacting O and H antigens that cause significant serum antibody levels, and cirrhosis of the liver is associated with antibody production that can cross-react in the Widal test.

Differential diagnosis should include other salmonella-induced enteric fevers, the major rickettsioses, leptospirosis, miliary TB, malaria, brucellosis, tularemia, infectious hepatitis, and abdominal Hodgkin's disease.

Prognosis

Mortality is < 1% with prompt antibiotic therapy, but may be as high as 30% without specific treatment. Paradoxically, specific chemotherapy has increased the incidence of relapse to about 15%. Convalescence may be slow despite antibiotic therapy because of the loss of body mass due to negative nitrogen balance.

Prophylaxis

Purification of drinking water, pasteurization of milk, preventing chronic carriers from handling food, and complete patient isolation technics are the most successful prophylactic measures. Compulsory surveillance and case-finding in an exposed population is essential for effective control of an epidemic.

Protection induced by typhoid vaccine is incomplete; therefore, recommendations vary. During an epidemic, only exposed persons need be vaccinated; widespread immunization is not indicated. Monovalent acetone-killed typhoid bacilli is the best available vaccine; two 0.5-ml doses s.c. 1 mo apart are recommended; in infants > 6 mo or children < 10 yr, two doses of 0.25 ml of vaccine should be given s.c. 1 mo apart. This vaccine, which has replaced the heat-killed, formalin-preserved typhoid-paratyphoid vaccine, should not be given intradermally, since it may cause severe local reactions when given by this route. Vaccination is not required for travel to endemic areas, but it is advisable for travelers to epidemic areas. Care in selecting restaurants and avoidance of unsafe water, ice in beverages, and contaminated foods are more effective. Unless drinking water is known to be safe, it should be boiled or 2 to 4 drops of 4 to 6% chlorine bleach/L should be added 1/2 h before drinking. Raw leafy vegetables and foods that are kept or served at room temperature should be avoided. Recently prepared foods served hot or chilled, bottled carbonated beverages, and raw foods peeled by the consumer are generally safe.

Treatment

Specific: Chloramphenicol was the drug of choice in all cases until a number of chloramphenicol-resistant strains were isolated during epidemics in Mexico and Southeast Asia. Patients acquiring typhoid fever in these areas should receive ampicillin 100 mg/kg/day IV in 4 equal doses for 14 days; penicillin-allergic patients can be given trimethoprim 8 mg/kg/day with sulfamethoxazole 40 mg/kg/day in 3 divided doses/day for 14 days. Chloramphenicol is effective against strains acquired in other areas. It is given for 14 days—50 mg/kg/day in divided doses q 8 h until the temperature is normal; then 30 mg/kg/day for the remainder of the 2 wk.

Supportive: Despite antibiotics, skilled nursing care remains most important. Stool isolation precautions must be performed carefully. Compulsory hand washing and proper stool disposal are mandatory to prevent spread of the organism. Strict bed rest is not required but is suggested during the antibiotic therapy. Nutrition should be maintained with frequent feedings that are relatively high in calories. Blood replacement may be needed. Cathartics and laxatives should be **avoided**; persistent constipation or distention can be corrected by appropriate fluid and electrolyte therapy. Diarrhea is occasionally distressing, but may be controlled by a clear liquid diet and, if necessary, parenteral nutrition. Adequate fluid replacement is important with high fever. In severely ill patients, corticosteroids may reduce the severity of subjective complaints, delirium, and fever. Prednisone 20 to 40 mg/day orally (or equivalent), given for only the first 3 days of treatment, is sufficient. Management of perforation must be individualized but includes increasing antibiotic coverage, e.g., addition of an aminoglycoside antibiotic such as gentamycin 3.0 to 5.0 mg/kg/day, divided q 8 h or q 6 h. Surgical resection can be dangerous because of friable tissue and poor anesthesia risk. Occasionally patients will develop acute renal failure following the administration of steroids or aspirin because of a sudden significant drop in temperature to hypothermic readings.

Patients with febrile **relapses** should receive chloramphenicol 50 mg/kg/day in divided doses q 8 h for 5 days. If the strain is chloramphenicol-resistant, ampicillin or trimethoprim with sulfamethoxazole (in doses as for the primary disease) should be given for 5 days.

Convalescence

Prolonged bed rest is unnecessary in afebrile patients. Stool cultures should be repeated until they are permanently negative; typhoid bacilli may be isolated for as long as 3 mo after the acute illness.

Carriers

Persistent carriers (persons with positive stool cultures for 1 yr) must be reported to the local health department and prohibited from handling food.

Antibiotic therapy rarely eliminates the carrier state and then only when the biliary tract is normal. If gallstones are present, cholecystectomy with pre- and postoperative antibiotic therapy are necessary; ampicillin 6 gm/day IV for 6 wk is the optimal therapeutic agent.

OTHER SALMONELLA INFECTIONS

The epidemiology of other salmonelloses is similar to that of typhoid, though more complicated, since disease may also occur in man by direct or indirect contact with numerous species of infected animals, their derived foodstuffs, and their excreta. The enormous reservoir of contaminated food products, especially poultry products, has caused a steady increase in the incidence of salmonellosis. Pet turtles have become an important source of infection in recent years. The most common salmonellas involved in the USA are *S. typhimurium, S. heidelberg, S. enteritidis, S. newport, S. infantis, S. agona,* and *S. montevideo.*

Certain types of *Salmonella* cause similar syndromes, including acute gastroenteric, typhoidal (enteric), or focal (with or without septicemia) syndromes, and a carrier state that may persist for weeks or months. The syndromes can occur in any patient singly, in combination, or in sequence. Patients with sickle cell disease or subtotal gastrectomies are prone to develop salmonella infections.

Acute gastroenteritis usually appears 12 to 48 h after ingestion of contaminated food. It may occur as only mild abdominal discomfort with minimal diarrhea lasting less than a day, or, rarely, may be protracted and cholera-like in severity. Fever may occur and persist for 24 h. The stools are usually loose and paste-like, but rarely contain blood or mucus. Diagnosis is confirmed by isolating a *Salmonella* strain from stool cultures. In all cases of suspected bacterial diarrheal illness, attention must be paid to the task of seeking the etiologic agent from the culture. A fresh specimen, delivered promptly to the laboratory, helps to assure good results. The laboratory should be told what organism is suspected or the circumstances associated with the onset of illness, to aid in selection of proper media for isolation. If a transport medium is available, it should be used. A rectal swab may be used to obtain a specimen to look for a carrier state, especially following *Salmonella* infections. The true incidence of septicemia in patients with acute salmonella gastroenteritis is unknown. It does occur and is manifested by low-grade fever and mild abdominal pain; some patients develop localized infections in various body organs.

Focal manifestations of salmonellosis may occur as part of a septicemia or as isolated abscesses. The GI tract, including the appendix and the gallbladder, is frequently involved. Salmonellas tend to migrate to abnormal tissues (e.g., tumors), but can localize and cause necrosis in any part of the body (e.g., lungs, GU tract, soft tissues, CNS, respiratory tract, joints, bones, heart valves).

Paratyphoid: A few strains of salmonella other than *S. typhi* can cause enteric fever, which mimics typhoid fever. Formerly called paratyphoid A and B, newer classifications identify these strains as *S. enteritidis* bioser *paratyphi-A* or ser *paratyphi-B*. The disease and its treatment are identical to that described above for typhoid fever.

Localized abscess caused by *S. cholerae-suis* is a form of salmonella infection that is rare in the USA. As the name implies, it is most often acquired from contaminated pork.

Prophylaxis

Case-reporting is imperative. Methods of controlling animal and human contamination of food-stuffs range from the careful preparation of bone-meal fertilizer to the proper cooking of poultry and poultry products, including eggs and foodstuffs containing dried eggs. Efforts to detect and control other infected animals (e.g., pet turtles) are also important in controlling the disease at its source. Human carriers are not major contributors to the large outbreaks of gastroenteritis. Stool cultures are valuable in detecting Salmonella carriers among hospital personnel.

Treatment

The routine use of antibiotics in uncomplicated acute salmonella gastroenteritis is unwarranted and will prolong the excretion of the organism in the stool. Symptomatic treatment with fluids and a bland diet usually suffices (see SHIGELLOSIS, below, and General Principles of Treatment in Ch. 55). Avoid antispasmodic drugs or paregoric; these agents will prolong the diarrhea and are rarely needed for relief of painful intestinal contractions. Patients with systemic or focal disease should be treated with antibiotics—either ampicillin or chloramphenicol in doses as for typhoid fever, or amoxicillin 50 to 100 mg/kg/day orally in 3 divided doses; the therapeutic response in paratyphoid infection may be somewhat slower than in typhoid fever. Focal abscesses may require surgery.

Carriers should only be given prolonged ampicillin treatment (6 gm/day IV for 6 wk) if they shed organisms for 1 yr. A diseased gallbladder will promote and perpetuate the carrier state; cholecystectomy plus ampicillin (6 gm/day IV for 6 wk) is probably curative.

SHIGELLOSIS (Bacillary Dysentery)

An acute infection of the bowel, caused by Shigella *organisms.*

Etiology and Epidemiology

The genus *Shigella* is divided into 4 major subgroups (A, B, C, and D), which are subdivided into serologically determined types. The genus is worldwide in distribution, but *Shigella flexneri* (B) and *S. sonnei* (D) are found more widely than *S. boydii* (C) and the particularly virulent *S. dysenteriae* (A). *S. sonnei* is the commonest isolate found in the USA.

The source of infection is the excreta of infected individuals or convalescent carriers. Direct spread is by the fecal-oral route; indirect spread, by contaminated food and inanimate objects. Waterborne disease is unusual. Flies serve as mechanical vectors. Epidemics occur most frequently in overcrowded populations with inadequate sanitation. Bacillary dysentery is particularly common in younger children living in endemic areas; adults are relatively resistant to infection and usually have less severe disease.

Convalescents and subclinical carriers are significant infection hazards, but true long-term carriers are rare. Infection imparts little or no immunity, since reinfection with the same strain is possible.

Pathology and Pathophysiology

Shigella organisms penetrate the mucosa of the lower intestine and cause mucus secretion, hyperemia, leukocytic infiltration, edema, and often superficial mucosal ulcerations. This pathological picture describes *Shigella* dysentery, a syndrome frequently preceded by a nonspecific, watery diarrhea. In many patients, dysentery does not occur after the diarrheal phase. The entire colon and often the lower ileum are involved in severe cases. The subacute form, seen almost exclusively in adults, is limited to the lower half of the colon.

Symptoms, Signs, and Course

The incubation period is 1 to 4 days. In younger **children**, onset is sudden, with fever, irritability or drowsiness, anorexia, nausea or vomiting, diarrhea, abdominal pain and distention, and tenesmus. Within 3 days, blood, pus, and mucus appear in the stools. The number of stools generally increases rapidly to 20 or more/day, and weight loss and dehydration become severe. The untreated child may die in the first 12 days; if not, acute symptoms subside by the 2nd wk.

Most **adults** are afebrile, with nonbloody and nonmucous diarrhea and little or no tenesmus. However, onset may be characterized by episodes of griping abdominal pain, urgency to defecate, and passage of formed feces, initially, which temporarily relieves the pain. These episodes recur with increasing severity and frequency. Diarrhea becomes marked, with soft or liquid stools containing mucus, pus, and often blood. Rectal prolapse and consequent fecal incontinence may result from severe tenesmus. The disease usually resolves spontaneously in adults: mild cases in 4 to 8 days, severe cases in 3 to 6 wk. Significant dehydration and electrolyte loss with circulatory collapse and death is largely limited to infants under age 2 yr and to debilitated adults.

In the rare **choleriform type** of bacillary dysentery, onset is sudden, with rice-water or serous (occasionally bloody) stools. The patient may vomit and become rapidly dehydrated.

S. dysenteriae causes a rare form with delirium, convulsions, and coma, but little or no diarrhea; it may be fatal in 12 to 24 h.

Secondary bacterial infections may occur, especially in debilitated and dehydrated patients. Severe mucosal ulcerations may cause significant acute blood loss. Other complications are uncommon, but include toxic neuritis, arthritis, myocarditis, and, rarely, intestinal perforation. Bacillary dysentery does not become chronic and is not an etiologic factor in ulcerative colitis. However, patients with the HLA-B27 genotype have a significant association of Reiter's syndrome following shigella infection.

Laboratory Findings

The bacillus is found in the stools, but bacillemia and bacilluria are rare. Though the WBC count is often reduced at onset, it averages 13,000. Hemoconcentration is common. Plasma CO_2 is usually low, reflecting the diarrhea-induced metabolic acidosis.

Diagnosis

This is facilitated by a high index of suspicion during outbreaks and in endemic areas. Frequently, bacillary dysentery cannot be distinguished from salmonella gastroenteritis except by identification of the offending agent. Ulcerative colitis, diarrhea of nonspecific or viral origin, celiac sprue, cholera, amebiasis, intestinal parasites, and infantile *Escherichia coli* diarrhea should be considered in the differential diagnosis.

Diagnosis is confirmed by isolation of *Shigella* from the stools. Proctoscopic examination is helpful, since specific ulcers can be recognized and adequate culture material obtained. Swabs from ulcers or fresh stool specimens should be taken to the laboratory immediately. Smears of the stools should be examined for blood, pus, and parasites. Agglutinins develop too irregularly to be of diagnostic value.

Prophylaxis

To prevent spread by contaminated food, water, and flies requires good sanitation, with the following precautions: thorough handwashing before handling food; immersion of soiled garments and bedding of dysentery patients in covered buckets of soap and water until they can be boiled; use of screens on houses; use of mosquito netting. Patients and carriers should be managed by proper isolation technics (especially stool isolation). A live oral vaccine is being developed, and field trials in endemic areas seem successful.

Treatment

Fluid therapy: See Ch. 81. Dysentery usually causes isotonic dehydration (equal salt and water loss), with metabolic acidosis and significant potassium loss. Thirst from dehydration can lead to a proportionately excessive water intake, causing hypotonicity.

In infants, especially in hot climates, the fluid lost through sweat and respiration, added to the severe diarrhea, may cause hypertonic serum (see Vol. II, Ch. 22). Premature administration of high-solute fluids (milk, tube feedings, "homemade" electrolyte mixtures) may cause damaging hypertonicity, including convulsions.

Infant feedings: See treatment of Acute Infectious Gastroenteritis in Vol. II, Ch. 24.

Antibiotics: The decision to use antibiotics requires consideration of several factors, including the severity of the disease, age of the patient (for children, see treatment under Acute Infectious Gastroenteritis in Vol. II, Ch. 24), adequacy of sanitation, the likelihood of further transmission, and the possibility of engendering antibiotic-resistant organisms. With proper fluid replacement, antibiotics are often unnecessary, and resistance to them is now widespread, varying with the species. *S. sonnei* isolates are likely to be resistant to ampicillin and tetracycline, but oxolinic acid 20 mg/kg/day in 2 doses at 12-h intervals (for adults) given for 5 days is effective. Despite resistance to tetracycline, successful therapy has been achieved by administering it in a bolus of 3 gm over a half-hour period (in adults). Trimethoprim with sulfamethoxazole (as for typhoid fever) will eradicate organisms quickly from the intestine. Ampicillin 3 gm/day for 5 days will cure most *S. flexneri* infections.

Other treatment: A hot-water bottle helps relieve abdominal discomfort. Absorbent and demulcent methylcellulose preparations do little to alleviate diarrhea and tenesmus. Anticholinergics and paregoric should be avoided in patients with shigellosis. Opiates will induce intestinal stasis, prolong the febrile state, and permit continued organism excretion in the stool. However, individualized use of opiates may be necessary if pain, discomfort, and anxiety are pronounced. Do not maintain continuous use of opiates.

The patient's progress should be followed until the stools are consistently free of *Shigella*.

CHOLERA (Asiatic or Epidemic Cholera)

An acute infection involving the entire small bowel, characterized by profuse watery diarrhea, vomiting, muscular cramps, dehydration, oliguria, and collapse.

Etiology, Epidemiology, and Pathophysiology

The causative organism is *Vibrio cholerae*, serogroup 01, a short, curved, motile, aerobic rod. Susceptibility varies among individuals. Since the vibrio is sensitive to gastric acid, hypo- and achlorhydria are predisposing factors. Persons living in endemic areas gradually acquire a natural immunity.

Cholera is spread by ingestion of water, seafoods, and other foods contaminated by the excrement of persons with symptomatic or asymptomatic infection. Outbreaks of the disease may be explosive and brief or may be protracted. Cholera is endemic in portions of Asia, the Middle East, and Africa. Cases imported into Europe, Japan, and Australia have caused localized outbreaks; an outbreak has also occurred on the Gulf coast of the USA. In endemic areas, outbreaks usually occur during warm months and the incidence is highest in children; in newly infected areas, epidemics may occur during any season and all ages are equally susceptible. Both the El Tor and classic biotypes of *V. cholerae* can cause severe disease; however, mild or asymptomatic infection is much more common with the El Tor biotype. A similar mild form of gastroenteritis caused by non-cholera vibrios is discussed in this chapter under Campylobacter Fetus and Vibrio Infections.

The manifestations of cholera result from the loss of isotonic, watery stools rich in sodium, chloride, bicarbonate, and potassium. *V. cholerae* produces a protein enterotoxin, the enzymes mucinase and neuraminidase, and other less clearly defined substances. The enterotoxin induces hypersecretion of an isotonic electrolyte solution by an intact small-bowel mucosa. The roles of mucinase and neuraminidase in pathogenesis are unclear. Mucinase may be important in reducing a protective effect of intestinal mucin, while neuraminidase may alter the structure of gangliosides in mucosal cell membranes, increasing the content of the specific ganglioside (GM_1) that binds the enterotoxin.

Clinical Course and Prognosis

The incubation period is 1 to 3 days. Cholera can be subclinical; a mild, uncomplicated episode of diarrhea; or a fulminant, rapidly lethal disease. Abrupt, painless, watery diarrhea with vomiting is usually the initial finding; stool loss may exceed 1 L/h but is usually much less. The resultant severe water and electrolyte depletion leads to intense thirst, oliguria, muscle cramps, weakness, and marked loss of tissue turgor, with sunken eyes and wrinkled skin. Hypovolemia, hemoconcentration, anuria, and serious metabolic acidosis with potassium depletion (but with normal serum sodium concentration) occur, and if untreated, result in circulatory collapse, cyanosis, and stupor. Prolonged hypovolemia can cause renal tubular necrosis.

Uncomplicated cholera is self-limited; recovery is within 3 to 6 days. The fatality rate exceeds 50% in untreated severe cases, but is reduced to < 1% with prompt and adequate fluid and electrolyte therapy. Most patients are free of *V. cholerae* within 2 wk, but a few patients become chronic biliary carriers.

Diagnosis

The diagnosis is confirmed by the isolation of *V. cholerae,* serogroup 01, in cultures from direct rectal swabs or fresh stools and its subsequent identification through agglutination by specific antiserum. Cholera must be distinguished from clinically similar disease caused by enterotoxin-producing strains of *Escherichia coli* and from the watery diarrhea with dehydration produced occasionally by salmonella and shigella infections.

Prophylaxis

Proper disposal of human excrement and purification of water supplies are essential in controlling cholera. Precautions also include using boiled water and avoiding uncooked vegetables. Cholera vaccine gives partial protection in endemic areas, but booster injections are required every 6 mo. Prompt prophylaxis with tetracycline 500 mg orally q 6 h in adults is useful in preventing secondary cases among household contacts of cholera patients.

Treatment

Rapid correction of hypovolemia and metabolic acidosis, and prevention of hypokalemia are the objectives. IV infusion should be started promptly with either (a) Ringer's lactate solution; (b) a solution of 8 gm glucose, 4 gm sodium chloride, 6.5 gm sodium acetate, and 1.0 gm potassium chloride per liter; or (c) a 2:1 mixture of normal saline and 0.17 M ($\frac{1}{6}$ M) sodium lactate. Patients in shock require 100 ml/kg; milder cases require only 50 to 80 ml/kg. The infusion should be given very rapidly until BP is normal and pulse is strong. The remainder is then given over a period of 2 h in adults; over 4 to 6 h in children. Water should also be given freely by mouth. Children given either normal saline-sodium lactate or Ringer's lactate solution require additional potassium, which can be supplied by adding potassium chloride 0.7 to 1 gm/L to the IV solution or by giving potassium bicarbonate l ml/kg of a 100 gm/L solution orally q.i.d.

Amounts for replacement of continuing losses should equal measured stool volume. Adequacy of hydration is confirmed by frequent clinical evaluation (pulse rate and strength, skin turgor, and urine output).

Plasma, plasma volume expanders, and vasopressors do not correct the water and electrolyte loss and *should not be used.*

Initial IV rehydration followed by oral or nasogastric administration of a glucose- or sucrose-electrolyte solution is effective in replacing stool losses and is particularly useful in epidemic areas where supplies of parenteral fluids may be limited. Patients with mild disease who are able to drink may be given the oral solution immediately, thus eliminating the need for IV infusion. A solution of 20 gm glucose or 40 gm sucrose, 3.5 gm sodium chloride, 2.5 gm sodium bicarbonate, and 1.5 gm potassium chloride per liter of drinking water should be warmed to 25 to 37 C (77 to 99 F) and given ad libitum in amounts at least equal to stool and vomitus losses. Solid food should be withheld only until vomiting stops and appetite returns.

Early treatment with tetracycline (adults: 500 mg orally q 6 h for 48 h; children: 50 mg/kg/day in 4 divided doses, for 48 h) eradicates vibrios, reduces stool volume by 50%, and terminates diarrhea within 48 h. Furazolidone (adults: 100 mg orally q 6 h for 48 to 72 h; children: 5 mg/kg/day in 4 divided doses, for 48 to 72 h) can be used for tetracycline-resistant strains.

TULAREMIA (Rabbit or Deer-fly Fever)

An acute infectious disease, usually characterized by a primary local ulcerative lesion, profound systemic symptoms, a typhoidlike state, bacteremia, and, not infrequently, atypical pneumonia.

Etiology and Epidemiology

The causative organism, *Francisella tularensis*, is a small, pleomorphic, nonmotile, nonsporulating, aerobic bacillus that enters the body by ingestion, inoculation, or contamination. It can penetrate unbroken skin. Of the 2 major species of *F. tularensis*, Types A and B, Type A is more virulent for man. It is found in rabbits. Type B, usually a mild ulceroglandular infection, comes from rodents. Transmission among animals is by blood-sucking arthropods and by cannibalism.

Hunters, butchers, farmers, fur-handlers, and laboratory workers are most commonly infected. Most cases result from contact with (especially in skinning) infected wild rabbits; others follow handling of other infected animals or birds, contact with infected ticks or other arthropods, and, rarely, eating undercooked infected meat or drinking contaminated water. Man-to-man transmission has not been reported.

Pathology

In disseminated cases, characteristic focal necrotic lesions in various stages of evolution are scattered throughout the body. They are minute (1 mm) to large (8 cm), whitish-yellow, and commonly found in lymph nodes, spleen, liver, kidney, and lung. In most cases, however, necrotic foci are seen externally as the primary lesions found on the finger, eye, or mouth; in pneumonia, foci of necrosis occur in the lung. Microscopically, the focal necrosis is surrounded by monocytes and young fibroblasts, in turn surrounded by large collections of lymphocytes. There may be severe systemic toxicity, but no toxins have been demonstrated.

Symptoms and Signs

The 4 clinical types of tularemia are **ulceroglandular,** 87% of cases, with primary lesions on the hands or fingers; **oculoglandular,** 3%, with inflammation of ipsilateral lymph nodes, probably caused by inoculation of the eye from an infected finger or hand; **glandular,** 2%, with regional lymphadenitis but no primary lesion, is usually cervical and suggests oral ingestion of the bacteria; and **typhoidal,** 8%, a systemic illness with abdominal pain and fever. Tularemic pneumonia may be primary or may be associated with the ulceroglandular manifestations of tularemia.

Onset occurs suddenly, 1 to 10 (usually 2 to 4) days after contact, with headache, chills, nausea, vomiting, fever of 39.5 or 40 C (103 or 104 F), and severe prostration. Extreme weakness, recurring chills, and drenching sweats develop. Within 24 to 48 h an inflamed papule appears at the infection site (finger, arm, eye, or roof of the mouth), except in glandular or typhoidal tularemia. The papule rapidly becomes pustular and ulcerates, producing a clean ulcer crater with a scanty, thin, colorless exudate. The ulcers are usually single on the extremities, but multiple in the mouth or eye. Usually, only one eye is affected. Regional lymph nodes enlarge and may suppurate and drain profusely. A typhoidlike state frequently develops by the 5th day, and the patient may show signs of an atypical pneumonia, in which symptoms are those of other pneumonias (see Ch. 38). A nonspecific roseola-like rash may appear at any stage of the disease. The spleen is often enlarged and perisplenitis may occur. Leukocytosis is common, but the WBC count may be normal with only an increased proportion of polymorphonuclears. In untreated cases, temperature remains elevated for 3 to 4 wk and falls by lysis. Mediastinitis, lung abscess, and meningitis are rare complications.

One attack confers immunity. Mortality is almost nil in treated cases and about 6% in untreated cases. Death is usually from overwhelming infection, pneumonia, meningitis, or peritonitis. Relapses are uncommon, but occur in inadequately treated cases.

Delirium may accompany **tularemic pneumonia** and lead to an initial neurologic diagnosis. Signs of consolidation are frequently present, but suppression of breath sounds and occasional rales may be the only signs in lobular tularemic pneumonia.

Diagnosis

A history of even slight contact with a wild rodent or of exposure to arthropod vectors, the sudden onset of symptoms, and the characteristic primary lesion are usually diagnostic. Laboratory infections are frequently typhoidal or pneumonic, with no demonstrable primary lesion, and are difficult to diagnose. Recovery of the organism from the lesion, lymph nodes, or sputum is diagnostic. *This organism is so highly infectious that the laboratory must have appropriate protective hoods before attempting isolation. Extreme caution is required in handling infected tissues or culture media.* Agglutination tests usually become positive after the 10th day and almost never before the 8th day. A rising titer supports the diagnosis. The serum of brucellosis patients may also react positively to tularemic antigens, but usually in much lower titers.

Prophylaxis

Wild rabbits and other rodents should be handled with great caution, especially in endemic areas. The organisms may be present in the animal and in tick feces on the animal's fur. Protective clothing should be worn and all ticks removed at once. Wild birds and game must be thoroughly cooked before eating; any water that may be contaminated must be disinfected before use.

Treatment

The agent of choice is streptomycin, 0.5 gm IM q 12 h until the temperature is normal; thereafter, 0.5 gm/day for 5 days. Gentamicin 3 to 5 mg/kg/day in 3 divided doses is also effective. Chloramphenicol or tetracycline 500 mg orally q 6 h may be given until the temperature is normal, and then 250 mg q.i.d. for 5 to 7 days; relapses occasionally occur with these 2 drugs, however, and they may not prevent node suppuration. Supportive therapy for pneumonia is the same as for pneumococcal pneumonia (see Ch. 38).

Continuous wet saline dressings are beneficial for primary skin lesions and may diminish the severity of the lymphangitis and lymphadenitis. Large abscesses may be drained, but this is rarely necessary unless therapy is delayed. In ocular tularemia, application of warm saline compresses and use of dark glasses give some relief; 1% homatropine 4 drops q 4 h may be instilled in severe cases. Intense headache usually responds to codeine 15 to 60 mg orally or s.c. q 3 to 4 h.

PLAGUE (Bubonic Plague; Pestis; Black Death)

An acute, severe infection appearing in a bubonic or pneumonic form, caused by the bacillus Yersinia pestis.

Etiology, Epidemiology, and Transmission

The causative organism, *Y. pestis* (*Pasteurella pestis*), is a short bacillus that often shows bipolar staining, especially with Giemsa stain, and may resemble "safety pins."

Plague occurs primarily in wild rodents (e.g., rats, mice, squirrels, prairie dogs), in whom it may be acute, subacute, or chronic, and murine or sylvatic, depending on whether urban or rural rodents are infected. Massive human epidemics have occurred (e.g., the "Black Death" of the Middle Ages); more recently, infection has occurred sporadically or in limited outbreaks.

Plague is transmitted from rodent to man by the bite of an infected flea vector. Man-to-man transmission occurs from inhalation of droplet nuclei spread by coughing patients with bubonic or septicemic plague who have developed pulmonary lesions; primary pneumonic plague is the result. Asymptomatic pharyngeal carriers of *Y. pestis* have been recognized in bubonic plague, but their epidemiologic significance is unknown.

Clinical Features

Bubonic plague is the most common form. The incubation period varies from a few hours to 12 days, but is usually 2 to 5 days. Onset is abrupt and often associated with chills; the temperature rises to 39.5 to 41 C (103 to 106 F). The pulse may be rapid and thready; hypotension may occur. Enlarged lymph nodes **(buboes)** appear with or shortly before the fever. The femoral or inguinal lymph nodes are most commonly involved (50%), followed by axillary (22%), cervical (10%), or multiple (14%) node involvement. The nodes are usually tender, firm, and fixed. The overlying skin is smooth and reddened but usually is not hot. Occasionally a primary cutaneous lesion, varying from a small vesicle with slight local lymphangitis to an eschar, appears at the bite. The patient may be restless, delirious, confused, and incoordinated. The liver and spleen may be palpable. The WBC count is usually 20,000 to 25,000, with neutrophilia. The nodes may suppurate in the 2nd wk. The mortality in untreated patients is about 60%, most deaths occurring from sepsis in 3 to 5 days.

Primary pneumonic plague has a 2- to 3-day incubation period, followed by abrupt onset of high fever, chills, tachycardia, and headache, often severe. Cough, not prominent initially, develops within 20 to 24 h; sputum is mucoid at first, rapidly shows blood specks, and then becomes uniformly pink or bright red (resembling raspberry syrup) and foamy. Tachypnea and dyspnea are present, but not pleurisy. Signs of consolidation are rare and rales may be absent. Chest x-rays show a rapidly progressing pneumonia. Most untreated patients die within 48 h after onset of symptoms.

Other forms of plague: Septicemic plague usually occurs with the bubonic form as an acute, fulminant illness. It may be fatal before bubonic or pulmonary manifestations predominate. **Pharyngeal plague** and **plague meningitis** are less common forms. **Pestis minor**, a benign form of bubonic plague, usually occurs only in endemic areas. Lymphadenitis, fever, headache, and prostration subside within a week.

Diagnosis

This is based on recovery of the organism, which may be cultured from blood, sputum, or lymph node aspirate. Needle aspiration of a bubo is preferable, since surgical drainage may disseminate the organisms. *Y. pestis* can be grown on ordinary culture media or isolated by animal (especially guinea pig) inoculation. Serologic tests include CF, passive hemagglutination, and immunofluorescent staining of a node, secretions, or tissues. A vaccination history does not exclude plague in the differential diagnosis, since clinical illness may occur in vaccinated persons.

Prophylaxis and Treatment

Prevention is based on rodent control and the use of repellents to minimize bites by fleas. Immunization with standard killed plague vaccine gives protection and is recommended for travelers to Southeast Asia.

Treatment should be immediate upon suspicion of plague; prompt treatment reduces mortality to below 5%. In septicemic or pneumonic plague, treatment must begin within 24 h. Streptomycin 30 mg/kg/day IM in 4 equal doses at 6-h intervals for 7 to 10 days is the regimen of choice. Many authorities give higher initial dosages, up to 0.5 gm IM q 3 h for 48 h. Alternative agents include tetracycline 30 mg/kg IV or orally in divided doses. For persons with plague meningitis, chloramphenicol is the drug of choice: a loading dose of 25 mg/kg IV, followed by 50 mg/kg/day in divided doses IV or orally.

Routine aseptic precautions are adequate for patients with bubonic plague. Primary or secondary pneumonic plague requires strict isolation of the patient. All pneumonic plague contacts should be kept under medical surveillance; their temperatures should be taken q 4 h for 6 days. If this is not possible, chemoprophylaxis with tetracycline 1 gm/day orally for 6 days is an alternative, but is not ideal, because of the potential danger of producing drug-resistant strains.

PSEUDOMONAS INFECTIONS

Pseudomonas aeruginosa, a gram-negative, oxidase-positive, motile rod, frequently grows on agar in yellow-green iridescent colonies because two pigments, pyocyanin and fluorescin, are diffused into the medium.

Epidemiology

Pseudomonas can be found occasionally in the axilla and anogenital areas of normal skin, but rarely in stools of adults unless antibiotics are being given. The organism is commonly a contaminant of lesions populated with more virulent organisms, but occasionally it causes infection in tissues that are exposed to the external environment. The most serious infections occur in debilitated patients with diminished resistance due to other disease and/or therapy. *Pseudomonas* infections occur most often in hospitals, where the organism is frequently found in moist areas such as sinks, antiseptic solutions, and urine receptacles. Cross-infection from patient to patient on hands of personnel may occur in outbreaks of urinary tract infection, on burn wards, and in premature-infant nurseries.

Pseudomonas infections can develop in many anatomic locations, including skin, subcutaneous tissue, bone, ears, eyes, urinary tract, and heart valves. The site varies with the portal of entry and the patient's particular vulnerability. In burns, the region below the eschar can become heavily infiltrated with organisms serving as a focus for subsequent bacteremia—an often lethal complication of burns. Bacteremia without a detectable urinary focus, especially if due to *Pseudomonas* species other than *aeruginosa*, should raise the possibility of contaminated IV fluids, medication, or antiseptics used in placing the IV.

Symptoms and Signs

Clinical presentation depends upon the site involved. Otitis externa with purulent drainage, commonly seen in tropical climates, is the commonest form of *Pseudomonas* infection involving the ear. Ocular involvement with *Pseudomonas* generally presents as corneal ulceration, most often following trauma, but contamination of contact lenses or lens fluid has been implicated as causing infection in some cases. *Pseudomonas* osteomyelitis is unusual, although the organism may be found in draining sinuses, especially following trauma or deep puncture wounds.

Pseudomonas is a common cause of urinary infection and usually is seen in patients who have had urologic manipulation or have obstructive uropathy. After *Pseudomonas* has joined with other gram-negative rods in colonizing the oropharynx in hospitalized patients, pulmonary infection can occur in association with endotracheal intubation, tracheostomy, or IPPB treatment. *Pseudomonas* bronchiolitis is common late in the course of cystic fibrosis; isolates have a characteristic mucoid colonial morphology.

Blood isolates of *Pseudomonas* are common in burns and patients with underlying malignancy. The clinical presentation is that of gram-negative sepsis, sometimes with the addition of **ecthyma gangrenosum**, which is a helpful clinical clue. This characteristic skin lesion consists of purple-black areas about 1 cm in diameter with an ulcerated center and surrounding erythema; it is found most often in the axillary or anogenital areas. Rarely, *Pseudomonas* causes endocarditis, usually after open-heart surgery on prosthetic valves or in IV drug abusers. Usually the infected valve must be removed to cure the infection.

Treatment

When infection is localized and external, treatment with 1% acetic acid irrigations or topical agents such as polymyxin B or colistin is effective. Necrotic tissue must be debrided and abscesses must be drained. When parenteral therapy is required, 5 mg/kg/day in divided doses of the aminoglycoside antibiotic tobramycin or gentamicin inhibits most *Pseudomonas.* With clinical response, dosage can be reduced to 3 mg/kg/day to minimize adverse side effects. Dosage must be reduced in renal insufficiency. Amikacin, an aminoglycoside, should be used in treating *Pseudomonas* that has enzyme-mediated resistance to tobramycin and gentamicin. Ticarcillin and carbenicillin are also active against this organism and are used in doses of 24 to 30 gm/day for carbenicillin and 16 to 20 gm/day for ticarcillin. In life-threatening infections or in granulocytopenic patients, an aminoglycoside active against *Pseudomonas* is frequently combined with ticarcillin or carbenicillin. Infections confined to the urinary tract can often be treated with indanyl carbenicillin, an oral preparation useful for urinary infections.

CAUSED BY ANAEROBIC BACILLI

Increased clinical awareness and therapeutic efficacy have followed improved technics for isolating and delineating anaerobic bacteria. The anaerobes can be divided into spore formers (i.e., the clostridia) and an extending taxonomy of other strict and facultative saprophytic gram-negative and gram-positive anaerobes that in the appropriate environment can destroy tissue.

CLOSTRIDIAL INFECTIONS

Clostridia are anaerobic, spore-forming, gram-positive bacilli that exist widely in nature, being found in dust, soil, vegetation, and the GI tracts of humans and animals. Though nearly 100 *Clostridium* species have been identified, relatively few cause disease in humans or animals (see TABLE 8–1). The pathogenic species, in the vegetative form, produce various tissue-destructive and neural exotoxins that have been biochemically and serologically delineated.

The most frequent clostridial infections in humans are benign, self-limited food poisoning (see *Clostridium perfringens* FOOD POISONING in Ch. 55) and incidental wound contamination, which occurs in 10 to 30% of wounds. Lethal clostridial diseases, including gas gangrene (myonecrosis), tetanus, and botulism, are relatively rare but can follow trauma, injection of "street" drugs by addicts, and errors in food canning.

NEUROTOXIC CLOSTRIDIAL DISEASE

Botulism (See in Ch. 55)

Tetanus (Lockjaw)

An acute infectious disease characterized by convulsions and intermittent tonic spasm of voluntary muscles. Spasm of the masseters accounts for the name "lockjaw."

Etiology and Pathogenesis

Tetanus is caused by an exotoxin (tetanospasmin) elaborated by *Clostridium tetani*, a slender, motile, gram-positive, anaerobic, sporulating bacillus. The spores remain viable for years and can be found in soil and in animal feces. Tetanus may follow trivial as well as overtly contaminated wounds, depending on a suitably reduced oxidation-reduction potential of the injured tissue. Drug addicts particularly are prone to develop tetanus, as are patients with burns or surgical wounds. Infection may also develop in the postpartum uterus and a newborn's umbilicus **(tetanus neonatorum).** Clinical disease does not confer immunity.

The toxin enters the CNS along the peripheral motor nerves, or it may be blood-borne to the nervous tissue. The tetanospasmin binds to the ganglioside membranes of nerve synapses and blocks release of the inhibitory transmitter from the nerve terminals, thereby causing a generalized tonic spasticity upon which intermittent tonic convulsions are usually superimposed. Once fixed, the toxin cannot be neutralized.

Symptoms and Signs

The incubation period ranges from 2 to 50 (usually 5 to 10) days. The most frequent symptom is **stiffness of the jaw,** which must always be considered to be caused by tetanus until proved other-

TABLE 8–1. CLOSTRIDIAL DISEASES

Disease	Agent	Major Types in Man	Exotoxin
Tetanus	C. tetani		Tetanospasmin
Botulism	C. botulinum	A, B, E	Neurotoxin (acetylcholine blocks)
Food poisoning	C. perfringens	A (variants?)	Enterotoxin
Pseudomembranous colitis	C. difficile		Cytotoxin
Necrotizing enteritis	C. perfringens	C (?)	
Histotoxic infections: local, uterine, wound infections (myositis, myonecrosis, anaerobic cellulitis)	C. perfringens, C. novyi, C. septicum	A–E A–D A	Lecithinase, protease, collagenase, fibrinolysin, hyaluronidase, deoxyribonuclease, leukocidin

wise. Other symptoms include difficulty in swallowing; restlessness; irritability; stiff neck, arms, or legs; headache; fever; sore throat; chilliness; and convulsions. Later, the patient has difficulty opening his jaws **(trismus)**; spasm of the facial muscles produces a characteristic expression with a fixed smile and elevated eyebrows **(risus sardonicus).** Rigidity or spasm of abdominal, neck, and back muscles—even opisthotonos—may be present. Sphincteral spasm causes urinary retention or constipation. Dysphagia may interfere with nutrition. Painful convulsions with profuse sweating are characteristic and are precipitated by minor disturbances such as a draft or noise, or by jarring the bed. The patient's sensorium usually is clear, but coma may follow repeated convulsions. During convulsions, chest wall rigidity or glottal spasm interferes with respiration, causing cyanosis or fatal asphyxia; since the patient is unable to speak, the immediate cause of death may not be apparent.

The patient's temperature is only moderately elevated except when a complicating infection, such as pneumonia, is present. Respiratory and pulse rates are increased. Reflexes are often exaggerated. Moderate leukocytosis is usual.

Localized tetanus can occur, with spasticity of a group of muscles near the wound but without trismus. The spasticity may persist for weeks.

Diagnosis

A history of a wound in a patient with muscle stiffness or spasm is suggestive. A slight wound may have been overlooked. Tetanus can be confused with meningoencephalitis of other bacterial or viral origin, but the combination of an intact sensorium, normal CSF, and muscle spasms suggests tetanus. Trismus must be distinguished from local causes such as a peritonsillar or retropharyngeal abscess or another local infection. The phenothiazines can induce a tetanus-like rigidity, but other signs of basal ganglia dysfunction are usually evident.

C. tetani sometimes can be cultured from the wound, but its absence does not negate the diagnosis.

Prognosis

The prognosis is poorer if the incubation period is short and symptoms progress rapidly, or if treatment is delayed. Mortality is highest in young and old patients and in drug addicts. The course tends to be milder when there is no demonstrable focus of infection.

Prophylaxis

Immunization: Primary immunization against tetanus with either the fluid or adsorbed toxoid is superior to giving antitoxin at the time of injury. For routine DTP immunization and booster recommendations, see IMMUNIZATION PROCEDURES in Vol. II, Ch. 23.

At the **time of injury,** 0.5 ml of toxoid elicits a protective antibody level in a *previously immunized patient*; this booster dose is not necessary if it is known beyond doubt that the patient has received a booster within the past 5 yr, or within the past 12 mo if the wound is severe and conducive to anaerobic infection. An *inadequately immunized patient* should be given tetanus immune globulin (human) 250 to 500 u. IM, depending on the wound potential and not on age or body wt. At the same time, the first of three 0.5-ml doses of adsorbed tetanus toxoid should be given s.c. or IM at another injection site. The 2nd and 3rd doses of toxoid are given at monthly intervals. Tetanus antitoxin 3000 to 5000 u. IM (CAUTION: *Made from horse or bovine serum; see SERUM SICKNESS in Ch. 19*) should be used *only* if tetanus immune globulin (human) is not available.

Wound care: Prompt, careful wound debridement, especially of deep puncture wounds, is essential, since dirt and dead tissue promote multiplication of *C. tetani.* Penicillin and the tetracyclines are effective against *C. tetani* but are not substitutes for adequate debridement.

Treatment

Therapy involves maintaining an adequate airway; early and adequate use of human immune serum globulin; neutralizing nonfixed toxin; preventing further toxin production; sedation; controlling muscle spasm, hypertonicity, fluid balance, and intercurrent infection; and continuous nursing care.

General principles: The patient should be kept in a quiet room. The patient should be intubated and an adequate airway should be maintained in moderate or severe cases. Tracheostomy should be done when intubation is expected to be prolonged—i.e., about 10 days. Mechanical ventilation may be necessary and obviously so when controlled respirations have been instigated by neuromuscular blockade (see Management of Muscle Spasms, below). O₂ should be humidified. An indwelling IV catheter is preferable to repeated IV administration of fluids and medication. Gastric intubation facilitates feeding; however, IV hyperalimentation avoids the hazard of aspiration secondary to feeding by gastric tube. Since constipation is usual, an initial cleansing enema is helpful; a rectal tube helps to control distention. Catheterization is required if urinary retention occurs. Respiratory toilet, frequent turning, and forced coughing are essential to inhibit hypostatic pneumonia. Hypothermic measures help to reduce high fever. Codeine is useful for pain. Patients with protracted tetanus may manifest a very labile sympathetic nervous system, including periods of hypertension, tachycardia, and myocardial irritability. Ongoing monitoring is indicated, and use of α- or β-blockers may be indicated.

Antitoxin: The benefit of antiserum depends primarily on how much tetanospasmin is already bound to the synaptic membranes. A single IM injection of 3000 u. of tetanus immune globulin (human) should be given. Antitoxin of animal origin is far less preferable, since the patient's serum antitoxin level is not as well maintained and there is considerable risk of serum sickness. If horse serum must be used, however, the usual dose is 50,000 u. IM or 50,000 u. IV (CAUTION: *see* SERUM SICKNESS *in Ch. 19 for necessary precautions*). Human immune globulin or animal antitoxin can be injected directly into the wound, but this is not as essential as proper wound excision and debridement.

Management of muscle spasms: Diazepam is the drug of choice to counter muscle rigidity and induce sedation. The most severe cases may require 10 to 20 mg q 3 h by IV push. Less severe cases can be controlled with 5 to 10 mg q 2 to 4 h orally. Diazepam may not preclude reflex spasms, and effective respiration may require neuromuscular blockade with *d*-tubocurarine or pancuronium bromide. *d*-Tubocurarine (in contrast to pancuronium bromide) may manifest histamine release with unwanted hypotension.

Antibiotics: Although the role of antibiotic therapy is minor in contrast to wound debridement, either penicillin G 2 million u. IV q 6 h or tetracycline 500 mg IV q 6 h should be given. It is not likely to prevent secondary infections (e.g., pneumonia). If pneumonia develops, cultures of the sputum or trachea should be taken, sensitivity tests performed, and an appropriate antibiotic given if necessary. If the patient has an indwelling urethral catheter, the urine should be cultured frequently and antimicrobial therapy given if indicated (see also URINARY CATHETERIZATION in Ch. 228).

Immunization: Since immunity does not follow clinical tetanus, the patient should receive a full immunizing course of toxoid after he leaves the hospital.

HISTOTOXIC CLOSTRIDIAL DISEASE

Etiology and Pathogenesis

The ubiquitous and saprophytic clostridia become pathogenic when the tissues show a reduced oxidation-reduction potential, a high lactate concentration, and a low pH. Such an abnormal anaerobic environment may develop with primary arterial insufficiency or after severe penetrating or crushing injuries. The deeper and more severe the wound, the more prone is the patient to anaerobic infection, especially if there has been even minimal foreign-particle contamination. Clostridial lesions tend to be self-perpetuating once the clostridia have assumed the vegetative form and are producing toxins.

Severe clostridial sepsis may complicate intestinal perforation and obstruction. *C. perfringens* infection may, rarely, complicate simple appendicitis. Clostridia (usually *C. perfringens* Type A) have been implicated in cholecystitis, peritonitis, ruptured appendix, meningitis, lung abscess, brain abscess, endocarditis, pyelonephritis, and osteomyelitis. Clostridial infections may complicate initially aerobic local tissue or organ infections that have become anaerobic by extensive necrosis. Tumors, tissues devitalized by radiation, and even parenteral injection sites can also be susceptible to clostridial infection. Debilitated patients with neoplastic disease or leukemia and patients with diabetes mellitus (because of associated occlusive vascular disease) are at a high risk of developing clostridial infections. The anaerobic environment of intestinal lymphoma and carcinoma permits endogenous *C. perfringens* invasion and replication, resulting in severe local or, rarely, septicemic clostridial disease.

Clinical Types

Uterine Clostridial Infection

This may be a fatal complication of septic abortion; rarely, it also can follow relatively uncomplicated pelvic surgery or childbirth. The patient is toxic and febrile, the lochia is foul-smelling, and the uterus is tender. Gas sometimes escapes through the cervix. Hemolytic anemia may develop as a result of clostridial septicemia and the effect of the toxin lecithinase on the RBC membrane. With severe hemolysis and coexistent toxicity, acute renal failure is to be expected. The mortality rate is then about 50%.

Early **diagnosis** requires a high index of suspicion. Early and repeated Gram stains and cultures of the lochia and blood are indicated, though it should be remembered that *C. perfringens* occasionally can be isolated from the healthy vagina and lochia. X-rays may show local gas production.

Treatment consists of debridement by curettage, and administration of penicillin G 10 million u./day for at least 1 wk. Hysterectomy may be necessary and lifesaving if debridement by curettage is insufficient. Early renal dialysis is needed if acute tubular necrosis develops.

Clostridial Wound Infections

These may occur as local cellulitis, local or spreading myositis, or, most seriously, progressive myonecrosis **(gas gangrene)**. Infection develops hours or days after injury occurs, usually in an extremity after severe crushing or penetrating trauma that results in much devitalized tissue. Similar spreading myositis or myonecrosis may occur in operative wounds, particularly in patients with underlying occlusive vascular disease.

Clostridial cellulitis (anaerobic cellulitis) occurs as a localized infection in a superficial wound, usually 3 or more days after initial injury. Infection may spread extensively along fascial planes, but toxicity is much less severe than in patients with extensive myonecrosis. The exudate is foul-smelling, serous, and brown, with evident crepitation and abundant bubbling of gas. Discoloration and gross edema of the extremity are rare. In clostridial infections associated with primary vascular occlusion of an extremity, extension beyond the line of demarcation and progression to severe toxic myonecrosis are rare.

An initially localized deep **clostridial myositis** rapidly spreads by toxin production in an anaerobic environment, causing edema, gas production, and subsequent myonecrosis. In **myonecrosis**, the exudate is serous and brown, but not necessarily foul-smelling. Pain, tenderness, and edema are usually severe, with dramatic progression over a period of hours. Late in the course, gas crepitation can be felt in about 80% of cases. The wound site may be pale initially, but it becomes red or bronze and finally turns blackish-green. The affected muscle is a lusterless pink, then deep red, and finally gray-green or mottled purple. The patient becomes progressively toxic, though often alert until the terminal stage. In contrast to uterine clostridial infection, septicemia and overt hemolysis are rare with gas gangrene of the extremities, even in terminally ill patients.

Though localized cellulitis, myositis, and spreading myonecrosis may be sufficiently distinctive to permit clinical differentiation and appropriate treatment, precise **diagnosis** often requires thorough surgical wound exploration and visual evaluation of tissue involvement. X-rays may show local gas production. Appropriate anaerobic and aerobic cultures of wound exudate should be taken, to identify the organism. Smears show gram-positive clostridial rods. Typically, there are few polymorphonuclear leukocytes in the exudate. Free fat globules may be demonstrated using Sudan stain. Many wounds, particularly if open, are contaminated with both pathogenic and nonpathogenic clostridia without evident invasive disease. The significance of this must be determined clinically.

Other anaerobic and aerobic bacteria, including members of the family Enterobacteriaceae and *Bacteroides*, *Streptococcus*, and *Staphylococcus* species, alone or mixed, frequently cause clostridia-like severe cellulitis, extensive fasciitis, or gas gangrene in traumatic and postoperative wounds. If polymorphonuclear leukocytes are abundant and the smear shows many chains of cocci, an anaerobic streptococcal or staphylococcal infection should be suspected. An abundance of gram-negative rods may indicate infection with one of the Enterobacteriaceae or a *Bacteroides* species. (See also BACTEROIDES AND MIXED ANAEROBIC INFECTIONS in Ch. 8.)

Anaerobic wound infections, particularly those due to Clostridium *species, can progress from initial injury through the stages of cellulitis to myositis to myonecrosis with shock, toxic delirium, and finally death within one to several days.* Early suspicion and intervention are essential. Anaerobic cellulitis uniformly responds to treatment; however, established and progressive myositis with an associated systemic toxemia carries a mortality rate of 20% or more.

Treatment requires thorough wound debridement, including removal of foreign material and all devitalized tissue. Amputation of an extremity may even be necessary. Penicillin G 10 to 20 million u./day IV should be given as soon as clostridial disease is clinically suspected. Cephalothin 6 to 8 gm/day IV or tetracycline 2 gm/day IV may be substituted in penicillin-allergic patients.

Detection of specific antigenic toxins in the wound or blood is useful only in the rare instance of botulism acquired through a wound portal. For **wound botulism**, early administration of specific or polyvalent antitoxin (see BOTULISM in Ch. 55) is valuable. Polyvalent heterologous antiserum is available for gas gangrene, but its value is questionable compared to that of thorough wound debridement and use of penicillin. Hyperbaric O_2 is helpful in extensive myonecrosis (particularly in extremities) as a supplement to antibiotics and surgery. However, few chambers large enough for surgical and nursing care are available.

Necrotizing Enteritis

In addition to *C. perfringens* food poisoning, clostridia occasionally cause acute inflammatory, sometimes necrotizing, disease in the small and large bowels. A similar process may occur in patients being treated for leukemia. Such clostridial enterotoxemias can occur as isolated cases or as outbreaks and some appear due, at least in part, to contaminated meat. Pig-bel, for example, which occurs in New Guinea, presumably results from eating pork contaminated by *C. perfringens* Type C; it varies from mild diarrhea to fulminant toxemia with dehydration, causing shock and sometimes death.

Clostridia toxins may be responsible for antibiotic-associated pseudomembranous colitis (see Ch. 58) following antibiotics, particularly oral clindamycin therapy. *C. difficile* is the suspected cytotoxic strain.

BACTEROIDES AND MIXED ANAEROBIC INFECTIONS

Etiology and Pathogenesis

Anaerobic bacteria may infect any part of the body, but they often produce disease adjacent to skin or mucous membranes, where numerous anaerobic species coexist with aerobic bacteria as normal human flora. Such infections are usually produced not by a single species but by multiple interacting anaerobic and aerobic species that rely on each other for virulence. Anaerobic flora outnumber aerobic bacteria 1000:1 within the colon, and 10:1 on the skin or within the oropharynx and vagina. When normal tissue barriers and resistance to infection are disrupted, anaerobic bacteria may produce foul-smelling infections characterized by necrosis and abscess formation (see also

Ch. 4). Converting a stable anaerobic commensal existence to progressive host tissue invasion requires an impaired proximate vascular supply. As in all infectious processes, **obstruction** is the *sine qua non* of infection, whether involving the flow of air, blood, lymph, CSF, body excretions, or secretions. Any significant impediment to flow, whether by tumor, trauma, aspiration, stone, or tissue necrosis, can cause stagnation, anoxia, reduced O_2, local lactic acidosis, reduced redox potential, and conversion to bacterial infection or, more commonly, polymicrobial disease.

Many species of endogenous anaerobes appear to be nonvirulent, even in mixed infections. The principal disease-producing anaerobic organisms are gram-positive cocci—peptococci, peptostreptococci, microaerophilic cocci and streptococci; gram-negative bacilli—*Bacteroides* and *Fusobacterium* spp.; gram-positive spore-forming bacilli—*Clostridium* sp.; and gram-positive non-spore-forming bacilli—*Actinomyces, Arachnia, Eubacterium* spp., and *Bifidobacterium eriksoni. Bacteroides fragilis* and anaerobic streptococci are the species most frequently isolated from local lesions and blood cultures.

Superficial mixed-anaerobic infections tend to produce local necrosis and form pseudomembranes on mucosal surfaces; they may cause spreading edema, crepitance, and gangrene in skin and subcutaneous tissues. Anaerobes produce collagenases and proteinases, which form abscesses that frequently complicate deep infections. *Bacteroides* species produce a heparinase that probably contributes to septic phlebitis; they also cause septic pulmonary emboli that may complicate local infections. Foul-smelling, short-chain fatty acids and volatile amines elaborated by anaerobic organisms produce a characteristic fecal odor. Many infections remain localized, but direct extension to other sites, bacteremia, and remote abscess formation in the joints, brain, lung, liver, or other organs may occur.

Symptoms and Signs

Any local or systemic infection can be associated with anaerobic organisms, with or without associated aerobes. Since symptoms and signs vary according to the site involved and predisposing conditions, individual infections caused by mixed-anaerobic organisms are covered in other sections of this book. Clinical syndromes frequently caused by mixed-anaerobic bacteria include dental abscesses, mandibular osteomyelitis, periodontitis, necrotizing gingivitis, necrotizing ulcerative mucositis (cancrum oris), gangrenous pharyngitis (Vincent's angina), chronic sinusitis and otitis media, Ludwig's angina, brain abscess, aspiration pneumonia, putrid lung abscess, pleural empyema, peritonitis, intra-abdominal abscess, liver abscess, endometritis, parametrial abscess, pelvic peritonitis, nongonococcal tubo-ovarian abscess, anaerobic cellulitis, human bite infections, decubitus ulcer and ischemic ulcer infections, and septic thrombophlebitis. Although anaerobes are relatively rare in osteomyelitis and in infective endocarditis, they always should be considered. Anaerobic bacteremia due to organisms such as *Bacteroides fragilis* can induce endotoxemia with disseminated intravascular coagulation and shock indistinguishable from that due to an *Enterobacteriaceae*.

Clinical clues to anaerobic infection include infection adjacent to mucosal surfaces bearing anaerobic flora; pseudomembrane formation on mucosal surfaces; predisposing shock, ischemia, neoplasm, penetrating trauma, foreign body, or perforated viscus; spreading gangrene involving skin, subcutaneous tissue, fascia, and muscle; feculent odor in pus or infected tissues; abscess formation; gas in tissues; septic thrombophlebitis; and failure to respond to antibiotics, particularly whenever the aminoglycosides have been used empirically.

Bacteremia complicating mixed-anaerobic infections may result in fever, rigors, and a critically ill patient. Shock and disseminated intravascular coagulation may occur. Aerobic gram-negative bacilli, *Fusobacterium* sp., *Bacteroides* sp. (most commonly *B. fragilis*), or anaerobic cocci may be isolated from blood cultures.

Diagnosis

When anaerobic infection is suspected, special technics of specimen collection, transport, and culture are necessary to isolate and identify pathogenic anaerobes. Even brief exposure of culture material to air may kill anaerobes; delays in transit to the laboratory may lead to overgrowth of aerobic bacteria and failure to identify anaerobes. If care is not taken to obtain cultures free of contamination by normal flora, contaminants may be mistaken for pathogens. The following specimens are free of contamination and may be cultured for anaerobes: blood; pleural fluid; transtracheal aspirates; pus obtained by direct aspiration, culdocentesis, and suprapubic aspirates; and biopsies of normally sterile tissues. When liquid specimens are obtained by needle and syringe, air should be expelled from the syringe and the needle inserted into a sterile rubber stopper. Transit time to the laboratory should be < 15 min. If delays up to an hour are anticipated, the specimen should be injected into an oxygen-free carrying vial.

Anaerobic culture results usually are not available for 3 to 5 days, and often the clinician must institute therapy before the results are available. In the laboratory, anaerobic cultures should be plated on special media and incubated anaerobically 48 to 72 h before examination. Aerobic cultures and Gram stains should be performed on all specimens. Some anaerobes have characteristic morphology that may be identified on Gram stain. Susceptibility data may not be available for 1 wk or more after initial culture and may not be reliable in many laboratories. If the species of bacteria is known, in most instances its susceptibility can be predicted; therefore, many laboratories do not routinely perform anaerobic susceptibility studies. (See also Ch. 2.)

Prevention

Effective measures to prevent mixed-anaerobic infections include early treatment of localized infection to prevent bacteremia and metastatic disease; debridement, cleansing, removal of foreign bodies, reestablishment of circulation, and early antimicrobial treatment in traumatic wounds; early exploration, drainage, closure of bowel perforation, and antimicrobial treatment in penetrating abdominal wounds; prophylactic antibiotics (penicillin G 300,000 u. IV q 4 h) when amputating ischemic extremities; and neomycin-erythromycin bowel preparation for colon surgery.

Prognosis

Morbidity and mortality from anaerobic and mixed bacterial sepsis tend to be greater than from single aerobic bacteria, and there is more deep-seated tissue necrosis, frequently indifferent to antimicrobial therapy. Bacteremic shock complicating such infections as severe intra-abdominal sepsis or pneumonia has an expected mortality $> 30\%$.

Treatment

Surgical debridement of necrotic tissue, decompression of tissues, and drainage of abscesses often are more important than antimicrobial therapy. Abscesses must be drained adequately, bowel or other organ perforations closed or drained, and devitalized tissue or foreign bodies removed. Closed-space infections, such as empyemas, must be drained. Impaired blood supply should be reestablished; fasciotomies may be required to relieve tissue compression. Septic thrombophlebitis may require vein ligation.

Antimicrobial agents help to check spread of infection and to control bacteremia. Generally, anaerobic infections originating from oral-pharyngeal flora are susceptible to penicillin G. However, if Bacteroides fragilis is isolated, treatment with clindamycin, chloramphenicol, or cefoxitin is indicated. B. fragilis produces a betalactamase and is resistant to penicillin G.

Intra-abdominal or pelvic mixed-anaerobic infections frequently are caused by B. fragilis and aerobic gram-negative bacilli as well as penicillin-susceptible anaerobic and aerobic flora. Due to the multiplicity of organisms with differing susceptibilities, combination antimicrobial therapy usually is indicated. Suitable regimens for adults with mixed-anaerobic intra-abdominal peritonitis or abscess caused by bowel or vaginal flora include (1) penicillin G 4 million u. IV q 4 h, clindamycin 600 mg IV q 6 h, plus gentamicin 1.5 to 1.7 mg/kg IV q 8 h; or (2) penicillin G 4 million u. in the same dosage plus chloramphenicol 1.0 gm IV q 6 h. Gentamicin dosage should be reduced in the presence of renal insufficiency and monitored with peak and nadir serum levels to assure therapeutic nontoxic dosage. Treatment with antibiotics should be continued until the infection in controlled and systemic symptoms have abated. Although the incidence of fatal bone marrow aplasia due to chloramphenicol is low, the drug should be reserved for serious infections. When Pseudomonas aeruginosa or another resistant gram-negative aerobe is present, carbenicillin (24 to 30 gm/day IV in adults) and gentamicin may be substituted for penicillin G, clindamicin, and gentamicin. In patients with penicillin allergy other than anaphylaxis, cefoxitin 2 gm IV q 4 h with gentamicin may be substituted for penicillin G, clindamicin, and gentamicin. In areas where gentamicin resistance is common among aerobic gram-negative bacilli, amikacin may be substituted for gentamicin; however, amikacin should be used as rarely as possible, to minimize development of resistance in susceptible species. Aminoglycosides used in these combinations are not active against anaerobes and are included in combination to control aerobic gram-negative bacilli that often produce gram-negative bacteremia.

Failure to respond to surgical and antimicrobial therapy should prompt reevaluation, looking for undrained sites of infection, persistent drainage from organ perforation, or superinfection by resistant bacteria or fungi (Candida sp., Torulopsis sp.). Sensitivity studies are helpful and should include other antibiotics; e.g., erythromycin and tetracycline. Enteral or parenteral hyperalimentation is important adjunctive therapy, since caloric requirements are high and, commonly, prolonged courses of infection lead to significant protein-calorie malnutrition. Patients with severe mixed-anaerobic intra-abdominal infections who develop acute renal failure have a poor prognosis.

Campylobacter fetus AND VIBRIO INFECTIONS

Campylobacter fetus INFECTIONS

Campylobacter fetus is a motile, curved, microaerophilic, gram-negative rod associated with septic thrombophlebitis, bacteremia, endocarditis, and diarrhea.

Epidemiology

There are 3 subspecies of C. fetus. C. fetus fetus causes venereally transmitted infectious abortion in cattle but is rarely a human pathogen. Subspecies intestinalis and jejuni are human pathogens; intestinalis is primarily associated with bacteremia in adults, often with underlying predisposing disease such as diabetes or malignancy, and jejuni is implicated as a cause of meningitis in infants and of diarrheal disease. The latter 2 subspecies are differentiated by the ability of jejuni to grow at 43 C and its resistance to cephalothin. Although contact with infected animals and ingestion of contaminated food or water have occasionally been implicated, the source of organisms frequently is obscure.

Symptoms and Signs

Bacteremia without localized infection is the most common presentation, although diarrheal disease due to *Campylobacter* is being recognized with increasing frequency. Fever of 38 to 40 C (100 to 104 F) that follows a relapsing or intermittent course is the only constant feature of systemic campylobacter infection, although abdominal pain and hepatosplenomegaly are frequent findings. This infection can also present as classic SBE, septic arthritis, meningitis, or an indolent FUO. Enteritis resembling salmonellosis or shigellosis affects all ages, but peak incidence appears to be in the 1- to 5-yr age group. The diarrhea is watery and often becomes bloody; white blood cells are seen in stained smears of stool.

Diagnosis

Diagnosis, particularly to differentiate from ulcerative colitis (see Ch. 57), requires microbiologic evaluation. *C. fetus* can be recovered from blood and various body fluids, using standard culture media. Isolation from stool in cases of suspected campylobacterial diarrhea requires selective media. Skirrow's medium using 7% lysed horse-blood agar with added vancomycin, polymyxin B, and trimethoprim has been used successfully.

Treatment

Various antibiotics alone and in combination have been used. Tetracycline or chloramphenicol in a dosage of 2 gm/day orally for 10 to 14 days should eradicate the organisms in most instances. Erythromycin 1 to 2 gm/day in 4 divided doses has been effective in treating campylobacterial diarrhea.

NONCHOLERIC VIBRIO INFECTIONS

These vibrios are biochemically or serologically distinct from *V. cholerae* and produce wound infections, enteric sepsis, or diarrhea, depending on the species involved.

Etiology and Epidemiology

The vibrios of importance (other than cholera, which is discussed above under BACTERIAL DISEASES CAUSED BY GRAM-NEGATIVE, FACULTATIVELY ANAEROBIC BACILLI) are *V. parahemolyticus*, *V. alginolyticus*, an as yet unnamed lactose-fermenting (L+) vibrio, and the so-called "nonagglutinable" (NAG) vibrios. *V. parahemolyticus* is a halophilic organism incriminated in food-borne (in inadequately cooked seafood, usually shrimp) outbreaks of diarrhea in Japan and in coastal areas of the USA.

Symptoms, Signs, and Diagnosis

After a 15- to 24-h incubation period, the illness, which usually begins acutely with cramping abdominal pain, watery diarrhea (stools may be bloody and contain polymorphonuclear leukocytes), tenesmus, weakness, and sometimes low-grade fever, subsides spontaneously in 24 to 48 h. The organism neither produces enterotoxin nor invades the bloodstream, but it does damage the gut mucosa. NAG vibrios may cause a cholera-like illness, and they have been isolated from wounds and blood. Neither *V. alginolyticus* nor the L+ vibrio causes enteritis, but both can cause marine wound infection. The L+ vibrio, after oral ingestion by a compromised host, crosses the gut mucosa *without* enteritis and produces septicemia with a high mortality rate.

Wound and bloodstream infections are readily diagnosed with routine cultures. When enteric infection is suspected, vibrio organisms can be cultured from stool on thiosulfate-citrate-bile-sucrose (TCBS) medium; contaminated seafood also yields positive cultures.

Treatment

Noncholeric vibrio infections have been treated with a wide range of antibiotics. Limited experience suggests that 2 gm/day orally of tetracycline or chloramphenicol should be effective. Close attention to repleting volume and electrolyte losses is often needed in the diarrheal disease due to these organisms.

CAUSED BY AEROBIC BACILLI

HEMOPHILUS INFECTIONS

The nonmotile, small gram-negative rods or coccobacilli comprising the genus *Hemophilus* require specific factors (X and/or V) for growth. Most *Hemophilus* species grow well on chocolate agar incubated at 37 C in air. Many *Hemophilus* species are normally found in the upper respiratory passages of both children and adults and rarely cause disease.

H. influenza, the species most important in causing human disease, is one of the leading causes of meningitis, bacteremia, septic arthritis, pneumonia, tracheobronchitis, otitis media, conjunctivitis, sinusitis, and acute epiglottitis in young children. These infections, as well as endocarditis, may occur in adults, but do so uncommonly. They are discussed in Ch. 38 and under ACUTE EPIGLOTTITIS in Vol. II, Ch. 24, MENINGITIS in Ch. 124, and INFECTIOUS ARTHRITIS in Ch. 103. Most *H. influenza* strains that cause serious infections in children or adults are encapsulated, Type B strains. Other *Hemophilus* strains may cause respiratory infections as well. *H. ducreyi* causes the venereal disease chancroid (see Vol. II, Ch. 5).

BRUCELLOSIS (Undulant, Malta, Mediterranean, or Gibraltar Fever)

An infectious disease characterized by an acute febrile stage with few or no localizing signs and a chronic stage with relapses of fever, weakness, sweats, and vague aches and pains.

Etiology and Epidemiology

The causative microorganisms of human brucellosis are *Brucella abortus* (cattle), *B. suis* (hogs), *B. melitensis* (sheep and goats), and *B. rangiferi* (*B. suis* biotype 4; Alaskan and Siberian caribou); *B. canis* (dogs) has caused sporadic infections. Brucellosis is acquired by direct contact with secretions and excretions of infected animals, and by ingesting cow, sheep, or goat milk or milk products (e.g., butter and cheese) containing viable *Brucella* organisms. It is rarely transmitted from person to person. Most prevalent in rural areas, brucellosis is an occupational disease of meat-packers, veterinarians, farmers, and livestock producers; children are less susceptible. Distribution is worldwide.

Clinical Course

The incubation period varies from 5 days to several months (average, 2 wk). Symptoms vary, especially in the early stages. Onset may be sudden and acute, with chills and fever, severe headache, pains, malaise, and occasionally diarrhea; or insidious, with mild prodromal malaise, muscular pain, headache, and pain in the back of the neck, followed by a rise in evening temperature. The total WBC count usually is normal or reduced, with a relative or absolute lymphocytosis. As the disease progresses, the temperature increases to 40 or 41 C (104 or 105 F), subsiding gradually to normal or near-normal in the morning, when profuse sweating occurs. Complications are rare but include SBE, meningitis, encephalitis, neuritis, orchitis, cholecystitis, hepatic suppuration, and bone lesions.

The intermittent fever persists for 1 to 5 wk, followed by a 2-to 14-day remission, when symptoms are greatly diminished or absent; the febrile phase then recurs. Sometimes this pattern occurs only once; occasionally, however, subacute or chronic brucellosis ensues, with repeated febrile waves (undulations) and remissions recurring over months or years. Constipation usually is pronounced; anorexia, weight loss, abdominal pain, joint pain, headache, backache, weakness, irritability, insomnia, mental depression, and emotional instability occur. Splenomegaly appears, and lymph nodes may be slightly or moderately enlarged.

Patients with acute, uncomplicated brucellosis usually recover in 2 to 3 wk. It is unusual for chronic disease to result in prolonged ill health. The disease is rarely fatal.

Diagnosis

Recovery of the organism from the blood, CSF, urine, or tissues is diagnostic, but bacteriologic identification of the disease is not always possible. Agglutination titers of 1:100 or higher are significant; lower titers are highly significant if the agglutinins are IgG immunoglobulins. When the agglutination test is positive but a *Brucella* species cannot be isolated, diagnosis is based on a history of exposure to infected animals or animal products (e.g., ingestion of unpasteurized milk), epidemiologic data, and the characteristic clinical findings and course. Intradermal tests with *Brucella* antigens are of little value in diagnosing active brucellosis.

Prophylaxis

Pasteurization of milk and eating only aged cheese are the most important prophylactic measures. Persons handling animals or carcasses that are likely to be infected should wear rubber gloves and protect skin breaks from bacterial invasion. Every effort should be made to detect the infection in animals and control it at its source.

Treatment

Tetracycline 0.5 gm is given orally q.i.d. for 21 days and should be repeated if relapses occur. Seriously ill patients are also given streptomycin 1 gm IM q 12 h for 1 wk, then 0.5 gm IM q 12 h or 1 gm IM daily for an additional 7 to 14 days. Prednisone 20 mg orally t.i.d. is given for 2 or 3 days if toxemia is present. Severe body pains, especially over the spine, may require codeine 15 to 60 mg orally or s.c. q 4 to 6 h.

Activity should be restricted in acute cases, with bed rest recommended during febrile periods.

MELIOIDOSIS

A glanderslike infection of man and animals, endemic in Southeast Asia, caused by Pseudomonas pseudomallei. This bacillus can be isolated from soil and water. Man may contract melioidosis by contamination of skin abrasions or burns, by ingestion, or by inhalation, but not directly from infected animals or patients.

Clinical Manifestations

Illness may be asymptomatic or occur in various forms. Clinically inapparent infection may be latent for years. Mortality is < 10%, except in acute septicemic melioidosis.

Acute pulmonary infection, the most common form, varies from mild to an overwhelming necrotizing pneumonia. Onset may be abrupt or gradual, with headache, anorexia, pleuritic or dull aching chest pain, and generalized myalgia. Fever is usually over 39 C (102 F). Cough, tachypnea, and rales are characteristic; sputum may be blood-tinged. Chest x-rays usually show upper-lobe consolidation, frequently cavitating and resembling TB. Nodular lesions, thin-walled cysts, and pleural effusion may also be present. The WBC count ranges from normal to 20,000.

Acute septicemic infection: Onset may be abrupt, with disorientation, extreme dyspnea, severe headache, pharyngitis, upper abdominal colic, diarrhea, and pustular skin lesions. High fever, tachypnea, a bright erythematous flush, and cyanosis are present. Muscle tenderness may be striking. There may be signs of arthritis or meningitis. Pulmonary signs may be absent, or rales, rhonchi, and pleural rubs may be present. Chest x-rays usually show irregular nodular (4 to 10 mm) densities. The liver and spleen may be palpable. Liver function tests, SGOT, and bilirubin often are abnormal. The WBC count is normal or slightly increased.

Chronic suppurative infection: Secondary abscesses may develop in the skin, lymph nodes, or any organ. Osteomyelitis is a relatively common presentation. Patients may be afebrile. An acute suppurative form is uncommon.

Diagnosis

Culture of *P. pseudomallei* (which grows on most laboratory media in 48 to 72 h) and HA, agglutination, and CF tests on paired sera aid in diagnosis.

Treatment

Inapparent infection needs no treatment. Antibiotics—usually tetracyclines, chloramphenicol, kanamycin, and sulfonamides—are chosen by susceptibility studies. Mildly ill patients are given either tetracycline or chloramphenicol 40 mg/kg/day orally, or trimethoprim (20 mg)-sulfamethoxazole (100 mg)/kg/day (e.g., 4 tablets, each containing 80 mg of trimethoprim and 400 mg of sulfamethoxazole, orally q.i.d. in 70-kg adult), for a minimum of 30 days. Moderately ill patients are given 2 antimicrobials (e.g., tetracycline plus kanamycin or trimethoprim-sulfamethoxazole) for 30 days, then tetracycline alone or trimethoprim-sulfamethoxazole alone for 30 to 60 days. Patients with severe acute melioidosis are given a triple combination of tetracycline and chloramphenicol, 80 mg/kg/day of each orally or IV, and either sulfisoxazole 140 mg/kg/day orally or IV, kanamycin 30 mg/kg/day IM, or novobiocin 60 mg/kg/day orally. This regimen should be continued until the patient responds clinically (preferably, being afebrile for 48 h) but should not be continued for > 1 wk.

BARTONELLOSIS (*Bartonella bacilliformis* Infection; Carrion's Disease)

A bacterial infection, caused by Bartonella bacilliformis *and seen only in South America, that can be characterized by an acute febrile anemia (Oroya fever) or a chronic cutaneous eruption (Verruga peruana).*

Etiology, Epidemiology, and Pathogenesis

The organism, a small, motile, aerobic, gram-negative bacillus that can be cultured on enriched media, is passed from human to human by the phlebotomine sandfly. Sporadic cases and epidemics occur only at certain altitudes of the Andes in Colombia, Ecuador, and Peru where the vector is found. In nonimmune individuals, the bartonella invade the bloodstream, attach to the surface of erythrocytes, and initiate anemia. They also invade capillary endothelial cells and produce vascular occlusion. This stage of disease is frequently complicated by superimposed bacteremia caused by salmonella or other coliform organisms. As immunity develops, the numbers of bacteria in the blood and in endothelial cells sharply decrease. After a latent period they reappear in the skin and subcutaneous tissue, where they apparently cause hemangioid lesions.

Symptoms and Signs

Oroya fever is characterized by sudden fever, weakness, pallor, muscle and joint pain, severe headache, and, in many cases, delirium and coma. Mortality rates may exceed 50% in untreated patients. **Verruga peruana** may occur in patients with or without previous symptoms of Oroya fever. The skin lesions, ranging from 0.2 to 4 cm in diameter, may be nodular or eroding in nature. They occur in series of crops, usually on the limbs and face, that may persist for from months to years and may be accompanied by pain and fever.

Diagnosis

During the acute phase, the organisms may involve 90% of the erythrocytes and can be easily seen on a stained smear of peripheral blood. During the cutaneous stage, the organisms can be demonstrated in the lesions. Although the peripheral blood smear is usually negative at this stage, bartonella may be recovered from the blood by culture. Salmonellosis, malaria, and amebiasis are important intercurrent infections.

Prophylaxis and Treatment

The sandfly vector can be controlled with insect repellents and residual insecticides. Antimicrobial therapy rapidly terminates the acute febrile illness and hastens involution of cutaneous lesions. The frequency of superimposed salmonella bacteremia makes chloramphenicol (2 gm/day for 7 days) the drug of choice. Transfusions may be required when the anemia is severe.

LISTERIOSIS (See also Neonatal Listeriosis under Neonatal Infections in Vol. II, Ch. 21)

Infection caused by Listeria monocytogenes *and having manifestations that vary according to pathogenesis, site, and age of the patient.*

Etiology, Incidence, and Epidemiology

L. monocytogenes is a gram-positive, non-acid-fast, noncapsulated, nonsporulating, motile, microaerophilic bacillus that is found worldwide and afflicts mammals, birds, arachnids, and crustaceans. Of the 7 major serotypes, Types 4b, 1b, and 1a account for most human listerioses in the USA. Incidence, highest in neonates and in persons over 40, peaks in July and August. It may be significant that 25% of listeriosis patients have a preexisting disease (e.g., cirrhosis, lymphomas, solid tumors). The only proven transmission occurs antepartum and intrapartum, from mother to child, but a human carrier state exists and may be epidemiologically important.

Clinical Forms

Antepartum infection occurs transplacentally. Abortion, premature birth, or stillbirth frequently results. Focal abscesses or granulomas are present in the fetal liver and may be found in any other organ. Listerias may be present in the meconium of live infants, and their presence may be a specific finding in some neonates with cardiorespiratory distress, nausea and vomiting, hypothermia, hepatosplenomegaly, and granulomas of the oropharynx and skin. **Intrapartum infection** usually results in meningitis following a 1-to 4-wk incubation period.

In adults, **meningitis** is the most common form of listeriosis. **Endocarditis** is a rare form, as is **typhoidal listeriosis** with bacteremia and high fever and without localizing symptoms and signs. **Oculoglandular** infection, with ophthalmitis and regional lymph node involvement, follows conjunctival inoculation and, if untreated, may progress to bacteremia and meningitis.

Diagnosis

Listerial infections cannot be identified clinically; isolation of *L. monocytogenes* is necessary for diagnosis. The laboratory must be informed of the possibility of listeriosis when specimens are sent for culture. In neonatal listeriosis, specimens should be taken from cord blood, the infant's CSF and meconium, the mother's lochia and cervical and vaginal exudates, and grossly diseased parts of the placenta. In all listerial infections, IgG agglutinin titers peak 2 to 4 wk after onset.

Treatment

For neonatal listeriosis, penicillin G should be given IV for 2 to 3 wk: 80,000 u./kg q 12 h for infants < 1 wk old; and 110,000 u./kg q 8 h for those 1 to 4 wk old.

For meningitis in the adult, erythromycin and penicillin G are the most active antibiotics and are preferable to tetracycline, which was formerly used most often. For meningitis, penicillin G 240,000 u./kg/day is given IV and continued for 1 wk after defervescence. For endocarditis and typhoidal listeriosis, both penicillin G 240,000 u./kg/day IV and erythromycin 60 to 75 mg/kg/day orally in divided doses q 6 h are given until 4 wk after defervescence. Oculoglandular listeriosis should respond to oral erythromycin or tetracycline 25 to 30 mg/kg/day orally as 4 equal doses q 6 h, continued until 1 wk following defervescence.

CAUSED BY MYCOBACTERIA

TUBERCULOSIS (See also Perinatal Tuberculosis under Neonatal Infections in Vol. II, Ch. 21)

An acute or chronic infection caused by Mycobacterium tuberculosis *and, rarely in the USA, by* M. bovis. TB is characterized clinically by a lifelong balance between the host and the infection, in which pulmonary or extrapulmonary foci may reactivate at any time, often after long periods of latency; TB is characterized pathologically by the formation of tubercles made up of giant cells and epithelioid cells, by a tendency for fibrosis to occur, and by caseation, a unique form of nonliquefying necrosis.

Etiology

M. tuberculosis is an acid-fast, nonmotile rod. The organisms characteristically are sensitive to isoniazid **(INH)** and produce niacin and the enzyme catalase. INH-resistant mutants generally lose their ability to produce catalase, but remain niacin-positive. *M. bovis* is also sensitive to INH, but does not produce niacin. All other mycobacteria are highly INH-resistant, catalase-positive, and niacin-negative. (See Table 8–2.)

Table 8–2. CHARACTERISTICS OF MYCOBACTERIA

Organism	Produce Catalase	Produce Niacin	INH-Sensitive
M. tuberculosis	Yes	Yes	Yes
INH-resistant M. tuberculosis	No (generally)	Yes	No
M. bovis	Yes	No	Yes
Other mycobacteria (excluding M. leprae)	Yes	No	No

Epidemiology

Infection occurs primarily by inhalation. Infectious droplets, which are aerosolized by coughing and dry while suspended in air, may contaminate the air in closed spaces for long periods. In areas where bovine TB has not been eliminated, transmission may occur by ingestion of contaminated milk. Direct inoculation occasionally occurs in laboratory workers.

In 1977, 30,000 cases of TB were reported in the USA; 3000 were fatal, and almost 15% of the cases involved extrapulmonary sites. Case rates vary markedly with such factors as age, race, socio-economic status, and geography. In the USA, most active disease occurs in older individuals (particularly nonwhite males), in contacts of active cases, and in persons known to have had clinical TB in the past who were never adequately treated with drugs; TB is more prevalent and more often resistant to INH or streptomycin (SM) in Mexican and Oriental immigrants than in other Americans. Relapse in adequately treated cases is uncommon.

Pathogenesis

A nonsensitized host has no specific immunologic defense against TB. Infection usually begins in the lower or middle lung fields. With little host reaction and no symptoms, the bacilli spread readily to the draining lymph nodes and, via the bloodstream, can reach any other organ. With the development of tuberculin hypersensitivity 4 to 10 wk later, a small area of pneumonitis develops, multiplication of intracellular bacilli is inhibited at both the initial and metastatic foci, and the infection is usually quickly *arrested*.

In up to 10% or more of new infections, depending on the patient's age and the intensity of the exposure, active disease evolves within 1 to 2 yr. In the remainder, foci of infection remain dormant but viable, with risk of reactivation, for the life of the host. Factors favoring reactivation include waning immunity (due to immunosuppressive therapy, old age, malnutrition, alcoholism, or intercurrent illness—e.g., uncontrolled diabetes or malignancy of the lymphatic or hematologic systems), local injury (destructive pulmonary processes such as lung abscess, cancer, surgery, or local joint or back injury), and some poorly understood intercurrent processes (silicosis, gastric resection).

Prophylaxis

Vaccination with BCG (an attenuated strain of *M. tuberculosis*), still useful in certain parts of the world and in certain groups where the prevalence of TB is high ($>$ 20% of secondary school children positive to tuberculin), is now rarely used in the USA.

Chemoprophylaxis usually consists of **INH** alone, 300 mg daily in adults, 6 to 10 mg/kg in children, for 12 to 18 mo, given as a single dose in the morning. Treatment of **tuberculin-negative** individuals is sometimes appropriate; e.g., when brief exposure of an infant to a known infectious risk (e.g., the mother) cannot be avoided, or when an exposed person has a reduced immune response for any reason. Chemoprophylaxis is indicated in certain **tuberculin-positive** individuals without overt disease: children under age 20; recent tuberculin converters, regardless of age; individuals with pulmonary infiltrates of unknown etiology; persons receiving prolonged corticosteroid therapy; the postgastrectomy patient with x-ray evidence of a quiescent or inactive focus of pulmonary TB; and all patients with silicosis.

Hospitalizing or isolating a patient under treatment is not necessary to prevent spread. The major risk of contagion is before diagnosis; in 10 to 14 days, patients on adequate treatment become noninfectious, despite continued positive sputum by laboratory tests.

PULMONARY TUBERCULOSIS

Childhood Type

Hilar lymphadenopathy is the hallmark of childhood pulmonary TB. Mediastinal nodes draining the initial area of pneumonitis become massively enlarged, usually unilaterally, causing bronchial compression resulting in a brassy, nonproductive cough or, particularly in very young children with flaccid small bronchi, atelectasis distal to bronchial compression. **Serofibrinous pleurisy** with effusion (see PLEURAL TUBERCULOSIS, below) occasionally occurs soon after infection. **Progressive primary TB** is uncommon, but caseation and, very rarely, cavity formation may result. **Hypersensitivity syndromes** include phlyctenular keratoconjunctivitis (a brisk ocular inflammatory reaction to locally deposited tubercle bacilli) and erythema nodosum. Both are rare, probably occur in association with development of tuberculin hypersensitivity, usually are self-limited, and respond to corticosteroids.

Treatment is the same as for adults (see Treatment, in ADULT TYPE, below), except that the dose of INH (10 mg/kg, up to 300 mg) is larger, since children are more resistant to INH induction of pyridoxine deficiency and resulting peripheral neuritis. Corticosteroids may be helpful when bronchial compression by enlarged nodes produces symptoms.

Adult Type

Most pulmonary TB in adults is seen initially in the apical areas of the lung, which have been seeded by bloodstream-spread from an often undetectable primary focus in the lower lung. Progression of the metastatic apical focus takes place while the initial focus is healing. It may occur after a long period of latency, but usually occurs within 2 yr of initial infection. Caseous necrosis, liquefaction, and cavity formation in the apical areas permit spread of infection via the bronchi, typically forming new cavities in the apical and subapical areas on that side and later in the opposite lung. Prior to drug therapy, 50% of cases with cavitary TB were fatal; healing of cavities is now the rule with appropriate drug treatment.

Lower- or middle-lobe progressive TB in adults is being observed more frequently than in the past. The former may represent progressive primary infection and usually occurs in individuals with diminished resistance; the latter is usually due to erosion of the middle lobe bronchus by a calcified hilar node with distal endobronchial spread of infectious material. Other late consequences of calcified hilar nodes include midesophageal traction diverticula and, rarely, bronchoesophageal fistulas.

Symptoms and Signs

Pulmonary TB is asymptomatic at first; signs usually become apparent when the lesion is large enough to be visible on x-ray. Systemic symptoms of fever, malaise, and weight loss are often so gradual as to be unnoticed.

Cough is due to irritative secretions draining into the bronchi from sloughing areas of lung tissue. It is most frequently associated with cavitation and at first occurs only in the morning, as a result of material accumulated in the bronchi overnight. **Sputum,** scanty at first, increases with progressive pulmonary excavation. In a caseous liquefying lesion, it is green and purulent. In chronic disease, with less excavation, the sputum becomes yellowish and mucoid. **Hemoptysis,** occasionally the first symptom, may be due to endobronchial involvement with granulation tissue or to erosion of an artery by an enlarging cavity. It may vary from slight bloody streaking of the sputum to massive, though seldom fatal, hemorrhage. **Pleural** or **chest wall pain** occurs with pleural involvement. **Dyspnea** is common during acute febrile periods. Acute dyspnea may result from a spontaneous pneumothorax or rapidly developing pleural effusion. Rarely, endobronchial spread of infectious secretions causes oral ulcers, painful laryngeal involvement with hoarseness, or gastrointestinal TB that may first call attention to the pulmonary disease.

The pace of the illness varies widely. Particularly in Eskimos, American Indians, and some blacks, the entire upper lobe may be involved together with systemic symptoms, suggesting lobar pneumonia. In others, symptoms may be minimal or absent despite extensive cavity formation and marked fibrosis. Undiagnosed and highly infectious patients may remain in relatively good health for prolonged periods.

Extensive pulmonary TB compromises pulmonary function, and some patients may succumb to respiratory failure or to pulmonary hypertension and cor pulmonale. **Extrapulmonary TB** is discussed below.

Diagnosis

Pulmonary TB is often first suspected on the basis of chest x-ray findings. An apical lesion is most common; a small mottled density is characteristic of early reinfection. Rarefaction may indicate beginning liquefaction and cavitation. Laminagrams help to visualize cavities.

Microscopic identification of acid-fast rods on direct examination of sputum is good presumptive evidence, but it does not exclude other mycobacterial diseases. Histologic evidence of tubercle formation in pulmonary or other tissue is strong but also presumptive evidence for the same reason. Fiberoptic transbronchial lung biopsy often facilitates provisional diagnosis when sputum is negative; however, negative biopsy results do not exclude the diagnosis.

Definitive diagnosis requires cultural identification of M. tuberculosis or M. bovis. Since the growth rate of M. tuberculosis is slow, culture is time-consuming and results may not be available for 3 to 6 wk. An early morning sputum collection is the best source. Alternatively, sputum swallowed during the night may be obtained by aspirating gastric contents immediately after the patient awakens and prior to his leaving the bed. The specimen should also be plated on media containing various concentrations of INH, streptomycin, and, if possible, other antituberculous drugs for initial drug sensitivity studies. A high degree of INH resistance, with the ability to form catalase, is often the first evidence that the infection is due to another mycobacterial species.

The **tuberculin test** is an important adjunct to diagnosis. The standard test material is purified protein derivative **(PPD),** which is stabilized by including a polysorbate detergent in the diluent. First strength tuberculin (1 tuberculin unit or **TU)** is useful in individuals in whom a high degree of hypersensitivity might be anticipated, such as young children. Most epidemiologic data are based on 5 TU (intermediate strength). Second strength PPD is 250 TU. Antigen can be applied by the scratch (Pirquet's) test and by multiple-puncture tine and Heaf tests, but the most satisfactory method is careful intradermal administration (Mantoux test). Palpable induration (not erythema) of over 10 mm 48 h after administration of 5 TU by the Mantoux technic is diagnostic of tuberculous infection, though not necessarily of active TB. A smaller reaction (5 to 9 mm of induration) is labeled doubtful and may be due to infection with other mycobacteria. Many patients with active TB do not react to 5 TU; such patients should be tested with 250 TU. Some patients seriously ill with proven TB do not initially react to even this larger dosage, but usually revert to positive with clinical improvement. Accordingly, a negative tuberculin test does not exclude a diagnosis of TB.

Treatment

Principles of drug therapy: (1) At least 2 drugs are required for pulmonary TB; in extensive disease, 3 drugs are desirable. (2) Response to drug therapy and prognosis as to potential relapse can be predicted by the rapidity of sputum conversion from positive to negative. When this occurs within 3 mo, successful outcome without additional drugs is usual. When sputum conversion is delayed past 4 or 5 mo, the probability of an emerging drug-resistant population is greater and 2 new drugs to which the infection is known to be sensitive should be added. (3) Since most treatment failures are based on lack of patient compliance, the least inconvenient and disagreeable drug regimen is preferred. (4) INH should be part of all treatment regimens except in the unusual circumstance of unacceptable drug toxicity, and probably when rifampin **(RMP)** is being given for retreatment of INH-resistant TB. (5) Therapy with drug regimens other than those containing both INH and RMP should be continued at least 18 to 24 mo after sputum has become negative for tubercule bacilli. Regimens containing both INH and RMP can be as short as 9 mo. (6) INH + RMP has been widely accepted as initial therapy for all patients, administered for 9 mo, with SM or EMB added during the first 2 to 3 mo in advanced cases or where there is suspicion of drug resistance. This regimen carries some risk of increased hepatotoxicity and no better final outcome than INH + EMB in moderate disease or INH + EMB + SM (2 mo) in advanced disease, given for 18 to 24 mo. There is concern that noncompliant patients who take drugs irregularly may develop resistance to both major agents in regimens containing both INH and RMP. (7) In renal failure, drugs largely excreted by the kidneys (EMB, INH, aminoglycosides) are best avoided or administered at reduced dosage with control of serum levels; RMP can be administered without dosage alteration.

Initial treatment regimens: (See TABLE 8–3.) In generally well individuals with moderately advanced disease, the INH + EMB regimen is simple, nontoxic, and effective. In extensive disease and in patients with markedly compromised general health, INH + EMB + SM (SM for 2 mo) and INH + RMP or INH + RMP + EMB (EMB for 2 mo) are equally effective, differing only in that the last 2 regimens can be discontinued after 9 mo. In the 1st and 3rd regimens, when bacteriologic response is favorable and the infection is known to be drug sensitive, the SM or EMB is usually given only during the initial 2 or 3 mo.

Retreatment regimens: (See TABLE 8–3.) Principles of the therapy of treatment failures are complex. In general, if rifampin **(RMP)** has not been given previously, it is the keystone of retreatment, in combination with at least 1 and preferably 2 other drugs also not previously given.

Specific antimicrobial drugs: Isoniazid (INH) is bactericidal and the least toxic, least expensive, and most easily administered antituberculous agent (see TABLE 8–3 for dosages). Concentrations in the CSF are approximately 20% of those in the serum; with meningeal inflammation, the concentration approaches that in the serum. Penetration into other tissues is also excellent.

Toxic reactions: Transient minor **elevations of serum transaminase** occur in as many as 10% of patients; **jaundice** is seen in about 1%; fatalities due to severe liver injury, histologically resembling chronic active hepatitis, occur in about 0.1% of some treatment groups. *The risk increases progressively with age, and is further increased in daily users of alcohol.* Minor transaminase elevations ($<$ 5 $\times$ normal) usually subside without stopping the drug but must be closely followed. Jaundice, usually associated with symptoms of hepatitis, requires *stopping the drug and not giving it again to avoid fatality.*

INH-induced **pyridoxine deficiency,** which may cause peripheral neuritis, is dose-related, occurring in about 2% of patients taking the usual 300-mg daily dose but in $>$ 10% of those taking INH in increased dosages. Routine administration of pyridoxine, 50 to 100 mg/day, is necessary in those receiving increased INH dosage and in patients, especially alcoholics, in whom baseline pyridoxine deficiency might be expected. Many administer it in the same dosage in all cases, although the need for this has not been established. If pyridoxine-deficiency peripheral neuritis does develop, INH should be temporarily discontinued and pyridoxine 300 mg/day administered until symptoms disappear. INH can then be resumed together with a reduced pyridoxine dosage. **INH hypersensitivity** may be manifested by fever, skin rash, and, rarely, agranulocytosis. **Drug interactions:** INH interferes with phenytoin metabolism; phenytoin blood levels should be monitored to avoid toxicity.

Rifampin (RMP) is at least as potent as INH; some authorities recommend its use routinely with INH in all initial treatment cases, but others do not. Hepatotoxicity, as with INH, is possible. Other untoward effects are assumed to be immunologic in origin, since anti-RMP antibodies inevitably appear; these effects include serum-sickness-like syndromes, thrombocytopenia, and, rarely, acute renal failure. These effects are uncommon when dosage is given daily, but occur more frequently with dosage intervals $>$ 72 h and especially with doses $>$ 600 mg given on a less-than-daily basis. Dosage is given orally on an empty stomach (see TABLE 8–3 for dosages). It is always administered with at least one other drug to which the infecting microbial population is sensitive, since resistance can develop promptly and when it does all drug effect is lost. **Drug interactions** occur with many drugs; RMP has been reported to accelerate the metabolism of coumarin anticoagulants, oral contraceptives, corticosteroids, digitoxin, oral hypoglycemic agents, and methadone.

TABLE 8-3. SUGGESTED SCHEME OF TREATMENT FOR TUBERCULOSIS

	Recommended Regimen*
Initial Treatment, Pulmonary	
Chemoprophylaxis†	INH for 12–18 mo
Minimal disease	INH + EMB for 18 mo
Moderately advanced or far advanced disease	INH + EMB for 18–24 mo INH + EMB + SM (SM for 2 mo; INH + EMB for 18–24 mo) INH + RMP for 9 mo INH + RMP + EMB (EMB for 2 mo, INH + RMP for 9 mo)
Re-treatment, Pulmonary	
Drug-sensitive	As above
INH-resistant‡	RMP + 2 other effective§ drugs
INH- + EMB- + SM- + RMP-resistant	3 effective§ drugs; preference, in order: capreomycin, pyrazinamide, ethionamide, cycloserine, kanamycin, amikacin
Intermittent Supervised Initial Treatment	
	INH + EMB + SM daily for 2 mo followed by twice weekly INH 15 mg/kg + either EMB 50 mg/kg or SM 25–28 mg/kg INH + RMP (with or without SM for 2 mo) daily followed by twice weekly INH 15 mg/kg + RMP 600 mg or 10 mg/kg (the usual dose)
Extrapulmonary (life-threatening)	
Miliary, meningeal, renal, spinal, pericardial	INH + SM or INH + RMP (with or without SM)
Extrapulmonary (other)	
Lymphatic, bone & joint, excluding spinal; pleural; peritoneal; GU, excluding renal; upper airways (laryngeal, oral, middle ear) in the absence of concomitant pulmonary disease (rare); GI in the absence of pulmonary disease (uncommon)	INH + EMB or INH + RMP

* INH = isoniazid 300 mg/day (single dose in the morning) in adolescents and adults, 10 to 30 mg/kg (single dose) in infants and small children. For chemoprophylaxis in children, 6 to 10 mg/kg (single dose in the morning).

EMB = ethambutol 25 mg/kg/day for 2 mo or until sputum becomes negative or while under close observation; reduced to 15 mg/kg/day for prolonged or relatively unsupervised use (single dose in adults; divided dose in older children; not used in younger children).

SM = streptomycin 1 gm/day (single dose) in adults; 20 mg/kg (single dose) in children. Usually discontinued after 8 to 16 wk when sputum conversion has occurred promptly in regimens initially containing 3 drugs.

RMP = rifampin 600 mg/day (single dose) in adults; 15 to 20 mg/kg (single dose) in children.

† Instances in which progressive infection has not been established (see chemoprophylaxis above).

‡ With exception of RMP-containing regimens, INH included in spite of in vitro resistance.

§ Effective here means that the infecting microbial population is sensitive to that drug.

Streptomycin (SM), the 3rd major antituberculous agent, is given IM in a dosage of 1 gm/day for adults; after the initial response to treatment has been established, the dosage may be reduced to 1 gm 3 times/wk. (See also TABLE 8-3 for dosages.) Compromised renal function is a relative contraindication to its use; when SM is required despite the presence of azotemia, the dosage must be reduced and serum drug concentrations should be monitored. The minimal inhibitory serum concentration for sensitive strains of M. tuberculosis is 0.2 µg/ml, 20 to 50 times less than the peak serum concentration after a 1-gm dose. CSF penetration is poor. Intrathecal SM is **not recommended**.

SM causes selective toxicity for the 8th cranial nerve, particularly the vestibular apparatus, and the vestibular injury tends to be permanent. Since patients over age 50 may become permanently ataxic, they should not be given SM if possible. Caloric testing of vestibular function and audiologic examination are recommended before and during treatment. SM may also cause allergic reactions, including drug fever, agranulocytosis, and a serum-sickness-like illness. Flushing, itching, and fullness of the head immediately after injection are bothersome histamine-like reactions not necessarily associated with the more serious allergic and toxic signs.

Ethambutol (EMB) is the most desirable companion drug to INH (except when INH and RMP are used together) and is well absorbed by mouth. The recommended dosages are given in TABLE 8-3. Some authorities do not give EMB to children, especially young children; other authorities prescribe it for older children if clinical testing for optic neuritis is carried out. Optic neuritis with visual field constriction and loss of ability to distinguish the color green, a dose-related side effect, is completely reversible when detected early. EMB should be avoided in uremia; when this is impossible it should be administered at a decreased dosage, 8 to 10 mg/kg.

Capreomycin, pyrazinamide, ethionamide, cycloserine, kanamycin, and **amikacin** are effective and useful in special situations (see TABLE 8-3), but their use is limited by toxicity.

Other modes of therapy: Bed rest and **hospitalization** are indicated by the patient's general condition. Since patients receiving chemotherapy become noninfectious rapidly, most can quickly return to work and other normal activity. **Surgical resection** has limited usefulness. If sputum conversion is delayed, drug resistance emerges, or thick-walled cavities or dense confluent disease persists after 5 to 9 mo of effective chemotherapy, resection may be performed provided that the remaining pulmonary tissue will be adequate. When resection is performed because of drug resistance, 2 drugs not previously given are administered together with the drugs previously given.

Adjunctive corticosteroid therapy may be advantageous in patients with extensive disease and profound hypoxemia and toxicity (as in extensive miliary TB or extensive bronchogenic spread); those who remain toxic, anemic, catabolic, and febrile for many weeks despite effective chemotherapy; and those with tuberculous meningitis. For patients who remain toxic and catabolic, prednisone 30 to 40 mg/day is sufficient. In patients in whom the inflammatory response is life-threatening, an initial larger dose (60 mg/day) is advisable. Guided by whether or not the symptoms reappear, the dosage is progressively decreased after 2 or 3 wk, and then discontinued. Using corticosteroids in tuberculous pleurisy and pericarditis is controversial. Corticosteroids are also used for replacement (rather than pharmacologic) therapy in patients with coexistent Addison's disease.

EXTRAPULMONARY TUBERCULOSIS

Extrapulmonary TB represents an increasing proportion of cases. It may result from lymphohematogenous spread; dissemination of contaminated pulmonary secretions via the bronchi to the upper air passages, mouth, and GI tract (intracanalicular spread); or direct extension to contiguous tissue. Sites seeded by lymphohematogenous spread prior to the development of tuberculin hypersensitivity may be undetectable for some time and then appear as an isolated clinical syndrome or syndromes without evidence of recent or remote pulmonary TB. Extrapulmonary lesions produced by intracanalicular spread respond promptly to drug therapy for the pulmonary disease and rarely achieve clinical prominence.

Treatment differs from that of cavitary pulmonary TB (see TABLE 8-3 and the preceding discussions of specific drugs for dosages and other details of drug regimens). The drug regimen is determined by urgency rather than by the possibility of emerging resistance. Prompt treatment with a multiple-drug regimen may be required when the anatomic location carries special risk, as in tuberculous meningitis, pericarditis, or spondylitis (Pott's disease). Initial treatment with INH + EMB is adequate when there is no immediate threat of loss of vital function, as in tuberculous lymphadenitis, peritonitis, or peripheral arthritis.

Miliary Tuberculosis (Generalized Hematogenous or Lymphohematogenous Tuberculosis)

When metastatic foci are located near blood vessel lumina, development of hypersensitivity and its attendant necrosis may result in secondary reseeding of the bloodstream, causing **early postprimary tuberculous septicemia (hyperacute miliary TB).** High fever and general toxicity are usually present. Tuberculous meningitis is a common complication, particularly in young children. Early in the course, the chest x-ray may be negative because the inflammatory foci are small; the tuberculin test may also be negative. Choroidal tubercles are usually present and are important in diagnosis. Cultures of sputum or gastric contents are often positive; urine cultures are occasionally positive even without demonstrable GU involvement. Examination and culture of the bone marrow or liver may provide the only evidence of tuberculous infection; fiberoptic transbronchial lung biopsy is more often productive than either bone marrow or liver biopsy. **Maximally effective drug therapy** is indicated, usually with INH + SM or INH + RMP.

Late hematogenous dissemination or chronic hematogenous TB follows breakdown of a long-standing, previously quiescent and undetected, usually extrapulmonary focus of TB. Multiple, widely spaced episodes of bacteremic seeding may occur from these foci. This may produce a serious febrile illness much like that occurring soon after initial infection, but may produce a less acute process with low grade or absent fever, anemia, and wasting. In some, the usual cellular components of the inflammatory process may be lacking, a process termed **nonreactive TB**, in which myriads of tubercle bacilli exist in the tissues with only a sparse nonspecific cellular response. The clinical manifestations may be extremely subtle, consisting simply of loss of appetite and weight, and failure to thrive. Fever may be absent. Marrow involvement occasionally produces syndromes resembling primary hematologic diseases such as refractory anemia, thrombocytopenia, and leukemoid reaction. There is often no evidence of pulmonary disease, and the tuberculin test often is negative.

Diagnosis may be established by culture of any body fluid or tissue. Bone marrow and liver biopsies are important, and fiberoptic transbronchial lung biopsy more important. *The key to diagnosis is keeping the syndrome in mind*, and, in the absence of contraindications, it may be appropriate to assess results of a therapeutic trial of INH + EMB. Response is prompt; abrupt improvement in health, nutrition, and vigor generally supports the diagnosis. When the diagnosis is established on histologic or cultural grounds rather than by response to therapeutic trial, double drug **therapy** with INH + SM or INH + RMP is usually recommended.

Central Nervous System Tuberculosis

Tuberculous meningitis develops following rupture of a metastatic subependymal focus of TB into the subarachnoid space (not via bloodstream contamination of the CSF). It usually develops several weeks after the initial manifestations of the miliary process. Incidence is highest in children aged 1 to 5 yr, but the disease may occur at any age. Symptoms may be acute and resemble bacterial meningitis, or may be chronic with emphasis on headache and perhaps behavioral changes. Usually, however, there are alterations in consciousness, ranging from drowsiness to stupor or coma; various cranial nerve or long-tract signs may be present. Permanent sequelae include convulsive disorders, communicating hydrocephalus, subarachnoid block, mental retardation, and focal neurologic abnormalities.

Diagnosis is suspected in the presence of active TB or a history of TB or of exposure to it. The tuberculin test is usually positive, but confirmation is by CSF examination. When 4 serial spun sediment specimens are examined, the result is positive in > 75%. In most cases, the cell count is between 100 and 600/cu mm and is principally mononuclear. However, polymorphonuclear cells may predominate, especially early in the course of the illness. CSF protein concentration is usually elevated, and the CSF glucose content is typically less than half that in a simultaneously obtained blood sample. A low CSF glucose content and mononuclear pleocytosis are characteristic, but may also accompany fungal meningitis, meningeal involvement with carcinoma or lymphoma, and, rarely, partially treated bacterial meningitis. CSF culture is usually positive (even when cells are scant), but therapy must begin before these long-delayed results are available.

Treatment consists of maximum chemotherapy, usually with INH + SM or INH + RMP. Adjunctive therapy with corticosteroids (e.g., prednisone 60 mg/day orally in 4 divided doses) is recommended for inflammatory complications. The symptoms of meningeal inflammation are an excellent guide to the duration of corticosteroid therapy and the rapidity of dosage tapering. Usually, initial dosage is given for about 2 wk and discontinued by 4 to 6 wk.

Tuberculomas produce symptoms of mass brain lesions, usually without signs of infection, and are most often discovered at craniotomy for intracranial mass. Removal carries a risk of spread of infection and, accordingly, **chemotherapy** (INH + RMP for 18 mo) is always administered after resection.

Pleural Tuberculosis

Pleural TB occurs in at least 2 forms differing in pathogenesis and clinical import. **Primary serofibrinous pleurisy with effusion** may occur without discernible pulmonary parenchymal disease. It most often occurs soon after initial infection but may be seen any time during the course of pulmonary TB. The necrotizing effect of hypersensitivity causes a subpleural focus to rupture suddenly into the pleural space and produce an allergic effusion of mononuclear cells, protein, and pleural fluid enzyme (LDH) concentrations characteristic of exudates. Systemic symptoms may be marked or entirely lacking. A high degree of reactivity to tuberculin is commonly present. Pleural effusions with a mononuclear pleocytosis in a tuberculin-positive individual should be considered tuberculous unless proved otherwise. Tubercle bacilli are rarely seen on direct examination of the fluid; culture is positive in about 1/3 of the cases. Thoracoscopy or thoracotomy reveals many small tubercles studding the pleural surfaces. Pleural needle biopsy should be performed; histologic evidence of TB is present in most patients and culture of the biopsy specimen is often positive. **Treatment** is usually with INH alone. Although the pleural involvement is usually self-limited and resolves with no visible residua, or, rarely, with some pleural fibrosis, most untreated patients develop progressive TB in the lung or elsewhere within 5 yr.

Tuberculous empyema is usually a chronic and generally progressive complication of an established focus of chronic pulmonary TB. The pleural fluid is frankly purulent and loculation is common. Bronchopleural fistula may be the initial cause or a complication of the empyema, and surgical drainage is usually required for resolution. When spontaneous pneumothorax is followed by a tuberculous empyema or bronchopleural fistula, surgical drainage is usually required in addition to chemotherapy as for established pulmonary TB.

Tuberculous Pericarditis

Tuberculous pericarditis is usually due to direct extension from involved mediastinal nodes, or, rarely, to hematogenous dissemination. It may begin acutely, with systemic symptoms and rapid development of compromised cardiac function, or it may be indolent, sometimes becoming apparent only as constrictive pericarditis. There may be no evidence of coexistent TB in the lungs or elsewhere, but the tuberculin test is usually positive.

The presence of a pericardial effusion or constrictive pericarditis can be readily established, but it is extremely difficult to prove the tuberculous etiology of the effusion. The risk of morbidity is considerable, and some mortality is associated with pericardiocentesis; the fluid obtained rarely provides prompt evidence of TB, since culture reports not only are delayed but also are positive in less than half the cases. Pericardial biopsy considerably improves diagnostic accuracy by providing tissue for histologic study and culture, but even then the reports may be false-negative.

Therapy requires a maximal chemotherapeutic regimen, usually INH + SM or INH + RMP. There is uncertainty concerning the proper use of corticosteroids and surgery in treatment; corticosteroid treatment combined with antimycobacterials may prevent chronic scarring and constriction in some cases, although this is not certain and is risky when etiologic diagnosis is in doubt. Pericardiocentesis may be necessary to relieve or prevent cardiac tamponade but is not without risk and should be performed in controlled situations, preferably a cardiac catheterization laboratory. Pericardiectomy is indicated for chronic constrictive or restrictive pericarditis or if pericardial effusion is associated with considerable hemodynamic compromise. It is often the best and most definitive measure to establish the diagnosis. Pericardiectomy is technically simpler done early in the course, since later dense and visceral-pericardial adhesions may create a difficult surgical situation.

Genitourinary Tuberculosis

Tuberculous pyelonephritis begins as a small cortical focus, seeded hematogenously, and progresses after the infection reaches the medulla. Local symptoms may be subtle or absent (though fever and weight loss may be present) and the patient often appears to be in surprisingly good health. Renal cavities may be seen on IVP as calyceal deformities with areas of reflux of the dye from the pelvis to the interstitial area. When the process is longstanding, renal calcification and pyelographic evidence of pyelonephritis may be the only signs. Symptoms of lower urinary tract involvement due to intracanalicular spread from the kidneys to the ureters, bladder, seminal vesicles, and even prostate are variable. Cystitis with pyuria but no culturable bacterial pathogens suggests tuberculous infection. Once the infection reaches the pelvis, inflammation of other genitourinary organs develops. Indolent, draining, perineal fistulas or an unexplained epididymal mass may be the first evidence of genitourinary TB.

Treatment consists of multiple-drug therapy, usually INH + SM, or possibly, in older or uremic individuals, INH + EMB. Frequent pyelograms are indicated during the course of treatment to detect possible ureteral constriction. Nephrectomy is seldom indicated. Treatment with INH alone is satisfactory for TB localized to the epididymis, testes, or perineum.

Tuberculous salpingo-oophoritis is probably acquired hematogenously. It may remain clinically silent or may present as acute or chronic pelvic inflammatory disease and may cause sterility. Laparotomy may be required for diagnosis. Culture of uterine scrapings or culture and biopsy of cervical lesions is occasionally diagnostic. Response to **chemotherapy** (INH + EMB) is usually prompt; surgery is unnecessary in most cases.

Tuberculosis of the Gastrointestinal Tract

TB may occur anywhere in the GI tract as superficial mucosal ulcerations caused by continuous surface contamination, or as hyperplastic involvement of a viscus wall presenting as an obstructing lesion. The latter may occur without obvious active pulmonary TB and is almost always discovered during surgery for a suspected carcinoma. Where bovine TB is common, contaminated milk may produce primary lesions in the GI tract, most frequently in the oropharynx. Superficial mucosal involvement of the **small and large intestine** may result in profound malabsorption, and TB of the **cecum,** probably the most frequent form of intestinal TB, may cause obstruction or bleeding with diarrhea.

Treatment of gastrointestinal TB is with INH + EMB.

Tuberculous Peritonitis

Tuberculous peritonitis may be due to spread from adjacent lymph nodes, a GI focus, or tuberculous salpingo-oophoritis. Clinically, it ranges from an indolent illness with a doughy-feeling abdomen, local tenderness, and systemic signs of infection, to a process resembling acute bacterial peritonitis. The peritoneal exudate is usually mononuclear.

The main consideration in differential diagnosis is peritoneal carcinomatosis. Peritoneoscopy with biopsy under direct vision or a limited laparotomy are the best ways to make a diagnosis. Prompt response to antituberculous **chemotherapy** (INH + EMB) is expected.

Tuberculosis of the Adrenals

TB of the adrenals occurs occasionally as a result of hematogenous dissemination. The glands may be totally destroyed, causing adrenal cortical insufficiency (Addison's disease). **Treatment** with INH alone is adequate, but corticosteroid replacement therapy is also necessary.

Tuberculosis of the Liver

TB of the liver is frequent in patients with both pulmonary and extrapulmonary TB, but it is seldom of clinical importance. Granulomas usually heal without scarring; only with miliary TB do signs such as jaundice and hepatomegaly appear. **Diagnosis** is made by liver biopsy, and a portion of the tissue obtained should be cultured. The serum alkaline phosphatase and 5'-nucleotidase tend to be elevated. **Treatment** is that of hematogenous TB; no specific treatment of the liver is indicated. Tuberculoma, tuberculous cholangitis, and tuberculous pyelophlebitis are all extremely rare.

Tuberculosis of Bones and Joints

TB of a peripheral joint is usually monarticular and involves the hip, knee, elbow, or wrist, producing a purulent arthritis from which organisms are easily recovered. Rarely, cystic areas of osteomyelitis due to TB are found in the long bones or digits. Response to **chemotherapy** (INH alone) is usually prompt. Immobilization and avoidance of weight bearing may be required to relieve pain.

Tuberculous spondylitis (Pott's disease) is a serious form of TB; neurologic damage frequently occurs. Symptoms are variable. Nagging local back pain may be present and may be referred to the anterior abdominal wall and mistaken for appendicitis or another abdominal disorder. A tender, prominent spinal process may develop because of anterior wedging of 2 vertebral bodies. A paraspinal abscess may extend and present as a mass in the groin or the supraclavicular space; symptoms may develop because tissue is dissected by the abscess. A paraspinal abscess that compresses the spinal cord or granulation tissue that intrudes on the anterior aspects of the cord causes symptoms ranging from minor loss of bowel and urinary sphincter control to abrupt and irreversible paraplegia.

X-rays reveal anterior destruction of 2 or more adjacent vertebral bodies, loss of the intervertebral disk, anterior wedging of the vertebrae, and presence of a paraspinal abscess. Spondylitis due to staphylococci, gram-negative enterobacteria, and, less commonly, fungus infections such as blastomycosis may produce similar clinical and x-ray evidence. If active TB is or has been present elsewhere in the body, a strong presumptive **diagnosis** of tuberculous spondylitis can be made. However, surgical exploration of the lateral aspects of the vertebral column is often necessary to provide tissue for culture and histologic study.

Treatment with chemotherapy, usually INH + SM, and bed rest is usually satisfactory in neurologically uncomplicated disease. Posterior spinal fusion is safe and probably contributes to the firmness of healing (if instability of the spine is likely), but morbidity following prolonged immobilization is substantial. A major conflict surrounds the usual orthopedic recommendation that the spinal column be explored and debrided extensively along its anterior aspect. Serious worsening of the neurologic status of the patient has occurred and the procedure should be *avoided* if possible, except when mandated by progressive paralysis of legs or sphincters.

Tuberculous Lymphadenitis

Before the control of bovine TB, most tuberculous lymphadenitis occurred as **scrofula**, cervical lymphadenitis due to primary infection in the oropharyngeal lymphatic tissue. Scrofula, now rare in this context, is common in other mycobacterial infections. Currently, TB of the lymph nodes represents lymphohematogenous spread from a primary pulmonary focus. The process may be disseminated or localized. Diagnosis is usually made by excisional biopsy. Response to INH alone is usually prompt and complete.

Tuberculosis of the Mouth, Middle Ear, Larynx, and Bronchial Tree

TB of the mouth is almost always associated with a pulmonary cavity, but an oral ulcer or a tooth socket that does not heal after dental extraction may suggest an otherwise silent pulmonary cavitary lesion. **Tuberculous otitis media**, presumably extended via the eustachian tube, is characterized by persistent drainage and multiple perforations of the tympanic membrane. Profound conductive hearing loss and intracranial complications may occur. **Tuberculous involvement of the larynx** is rare and usually due to infectious bronchial secretions, or, occasionally, to hematogenous spread. Severe pain may occur on swallowing and hoarseness is common. Laryngeal carcinoma must be excluded. **Bronchial TB** invariably accompanies cavitary pulmonary TB. The draining bronchi are superficially infected, granulation tissue forms, and, rarely, cicatrization and obstruction occur. Hemoptysis in pulmonary TB often originates from inflamed bronchial mucosa. Considerable bronchial distortion is almost always present following extensive pulmonary TB. Response of these types of TB to any INH-containing drug regimen is prompt and excellent.

OTHER MYCOBACTERIAL INFECTIONS RESEMBLING TUBERCULOSIS

Mycobacteria other than the tubercle and lepra bacillus cause disease in man pathologically and clinically similar to TB. They include *M. kansasii* and *M. marinum* (Group I), *M. scrofulaceum* (Group II), *M. intracellulare* and *M. avium* (Group III), and *M. fortuitum* (Group IV). *M. chelonei* subsp. *abscessus* is generally not included in this Runyon grouping. The organisms are INH-resistant, catalase-positive, and niacin-negative. They may cause chronic pulmonary disease and, rarely, (usually in immunologically compromised patients) disseminated disease in adults, cutaneous abscesses and granulomas, and, particularly in children, bone and joint involvement, lymphadenitis, and disseminated disease including meningitis. Person-to-person transmission has not been proved; the organisms presumably exist in the environment.

Pulmonary disease: *M. intracellulare* and *M. kansasii* are the usual etiologic agents. Most cases occur in white men over age 40. Systemic symptoms are frequently absent, but progressive pulmonary insufficiency occurs. Chemotherapy with 2 effective drugs or 3 or more partially effective drugs is based on demonstrating drug sensitivities of the organism. In the absence of drug sensitivity testing, RMP, EMB, and SM may be an effective combination, particularly in *M. kansasii* infection, though not in *M. intracellulare* infection. Resection of cavities may be helpful in *M. intracellulare* infections, but is seldom necessary in *M. kansasii* infections. Coexistent chronic lung disease and the anatomic extent of infection often make this impossible.

Cutaneous disease: "Swimming pool" granuloma is a protracted but self-limited superficial granulomatous ulcerating infection caused by *M. marinum* contracted from contaminated swimming pools and occasionally from home aquariums. The infection is pathologically similar to TB. Healing occurs spontaneously, though RMP may hasten healing. *M. abscessus* causes a deeper and more persistent cutaneous granulomatous abscess on the exposed parts of the body. Its epidemiology is unknown and the response to drug treatment is virtually nil.

Bone and joint involvement: Widespread lytic bone disease may rarely occur in children. Joint involvement, and, more rarely, cutaneous fistula formation may occur as complications. The infections are usually drug-resistant, but RMP, EMB, and SM may be tried.

Lymphadenitis: In the USA, these organisms probably cause infectious granulomatous lymphadenitis more frequently than does the tubercle bacillus. The portal of entry is probably the eye, pharynx, GI tract, or abraded skin. Many cases are due to local spread from the site of primary infection. Response to drug therapy varies; surgical excision is recommended when the process persists.

Disseminated disease is rare, occurring particularly in children and in immunologically compromised older individuals. It may resemble malignant reticuloendotheliosis, except that the causative organisms are readily recovered. Meningitis may also occur, and, rarely, extensive miliary-like pulmonary involvement. Treatment with maximum chemotherapy (INH, SM, RMP, or another combination based on sensitivity testing) is usually tried, almost always with disappointing results.

LEPROSY (Hansen's Disease)

A chronic infectious disease caused by Mycobacterium leprae, *an organism with high infectivity but low pathogenicity and with a predilection for cooler regions—skin, mucous membranes, and peripheral nerves.*

Etiology and Distribution

M. leprae, an acid-fast bacillus, is the etiologic agent. Leprosy has incubation periods from 1 to 30 yr and progresses slowly. Transmission, most often via infected nasal discharges, possibly occurs also by fomites and arthropods. Only about 5% of contacts acquire the disease; others appear to be immune. Leprosy is found mainly within a broad equatorial band that includes Southeast Asia, Africa, and South America. Of the estimated 12 to 20 million cases, about 2000 are in the continental USA. Endemic foci exist in Texas, Louisiana, and Hawaii. The disease is also seen in California, Florida, and New York City, primarily among immigrants.

Types and Clinical Course

In all types, lesions of the skin and peripheral nerves dominate early clinical findings. Leprosy is classified on a spectrum reflecting degrees of host immunity.

Indeterminate leprosy is difficult to diagnose. The earliest skin lesion, usually a poorly defined, hypopigmented or erythematous macule 1 or 2 cm in diameter, generally shows nonspecific inflammation involving blood vessels, sweat and sebaceous glands, hair follicles, and cutaneous nerves. Organisms are few and may not be detected, but a presumptive diagnosis can be made if the cutaneous nerves are inflamed. The lesions tend to heal spontaneously, but may progress to any of the 3 more distinct types.

Tuberculoid leprosy is characterized by skin lesions that are localized initially to the skin or peripheral nerves. Lesions of the skin tend to be large, well-defined, single or few in number, anesthetic, and asymmetric. The inflammatory response is intense, with epithelioid and Langhans' cells resembling a tubercle surrounded by many lymphocytes. Bacilli are few and difficult to find. Characteristically, caseation necrosis destroys nerve bundles, and often one or more extremities become paralyzed. Resistance to the infection is high, and spontaneous recovery may occur; however, peripheral nerves can be destroyed.

Lepromatous leprosy is a generalized infection involving skin, oral, nasal, and upper respiratory mucous membrane, the anterior aspect of the eye, cutaneous and peripheral nerve trunks, the reticuloendothelial system, adrenal glands, and testes. The entire body surface may be involved so diffusely that no distinct lesion is identifiable. The numerous small skin lesions have poorly defined margins. Macules are most common; papules, nodules, or plaques also occur. Numerous bacilli are easily found in tissue specimens. Patient resistance to M. leprae is low, and untreated disease is progressive.

Dimorphous (borderline) leprosy has clinical and pathologic features of both tuberculoid and lepromatous "polar" types in various combinations, and subclassification, from dimorphous-tuberculoid to dimorphous-lepromatous, depends on the relative numbers of epithelioid cells and macrophages. M. leprae usually are numerous. Dimorphous leprosy is unstable and may regress ("reversal reaction") toward the tuberculoid form or progress ("downgrading reaction") toward the lepromatous form, depending on the effects of treatment and shifts in the patient's immunologic status.

Nerve lesions: In all stages of all forms of leprosy, M. leprae invades peripheral nerves, particularly the terminal cutaneous branches (producing anesthesia of a skin lesion) or the nerve trunk (producing anesthesia along its cutaneous innervation). Advanced disease results in "glove" and "stocking" anesthesia. Paralysis and deformity follow sensory loss. Facial paralysis usually is limited to lagophthalmos, which may end in blindness from trauma and infection involving the insensitive cornea. Claw-hand, foot-drop, and claw-toe deformities are common and may be accompanied by ulcers and secondary infection. Insensitivity leads to neglected injuries (e.g., destruction of the fingers, resulting in a "mitten hand"); about 25% of patients have some disfigurement and disabling deformity.

In lepromatous disease, peripheral nerves may be enlarged, yet the patient may show little clinical change or deformity. Sensory loss may be widespread, but motor impairment develops insidiously over several years. Reflexes are not affected. Impairment of touch and temperature sensation occurs early, whereas deep-pain perception and proprioception are lost later. In tuberculoid leprosy, caseation necrosis destroys segments or entire fascicles of the nerve, producing more sudden paralysis. Painful neuritides usually are associated with "acute reaction" episodes.

Acute reactions: Reversal reactions, seen in all but pure lepromatous leprosy, apparently result from spontaneous increases in patients' cell-mediated immunity to M. leprae. In a reversal, e.g., from dimorphous toward tuberculoid, the lesions become erythematous and edematous and may progress to necrosis and ulceration. Erythema nodosum leprosum (ENL) reactions, by contrast, probably are mediated by humoral factors and resemble the Arthus phenomenon (see Type III Hypersensitivity Reactions in Ch. 18). ENL occurs in lepromatous patients and in some dimorphous cases with dominant lepromatous features. Multiple painful erythematous nodules develop that may form pustules or progress to ulceration and necrosis. ENL often is accompanied by fever and sometimes by neuritis, lymphadenopathy, arthritis, iridocyclitis, orchitis, proteinuria, and leukocytosis.

Other manifestations (mainly in progressive dimorphous and lepromatous types): Nasal stuffiness and epistaxis occur early; later, ulceration and necrosis destroy supporting cartilages, causing nasal deformity and collapse. Earlobe enlargement and loss of eyebrows are common. Isolated lesions of the lip, tongue, and palate must be differentiated from malignancy.

Leprosy affects the eyes in several ways: by direct infection, acute reaction, or damage of the zygomatic branch of the facial nerve, which leads to paralysis of the orbicularis oculi muscle. Conjunctivitis, keratitis, corneal ulceration, iridocyclitis, anterior choroiditis, and glaucoma may occur and, if untreated, may lead to blindness.

Orchitis, often leading to atrophy, and gynecomastia occur in advanced lepromatous leprosy. Peripheral lymph nodes enlarge and may develop abscesses. In advanced lepromatous disease, the spleen, bone marrow, liver, and kidney are involved and amyloidosis occasionally develops; death is due to renal failure.

Diagnosis

Leprosy may mimic other diseases involving the skin and peripheral nerves. The diagnosis is established by biopsy. Skin smears indicate the extent and progress of the disease. The lepromin test (intradermal injection of autoclaved bacilli from human lepromas) usually is positive in tubercu-

loid and negative in lepromatous polar types. An early positive lepromin reaction in tuberculin-negative *children* (it is positive in nearly all normal adults) is diagnostic. The lymphocyte transformation
test and the leukocyte migration inhibition test provide in vitro evidence of cell-mediated immunologic responsiveness to the bacillus.

Prophylaxis and Treatment

Control requires active case-finding and early treatment. A patient controlled by therapy poses no
public health problem. Results of prophylaxis with BCG vaccine or dapsone in highly endemic areas
have been inconclusive. In the USA, contacts without disease should be examined every 6 to 12 mo.
Cure by immediate active therapy can be expected if a lesion is found early.

Sulfones are the drugs of choice, but sulfone-resistant organisms are becoming prevalent and
combined therapy is recommended for multibacillary forms. Though paucibacillary cases may heal
spontaneously, every active case should be treated and cure can then be expected. In most early
cases of multibacillary forms, the disease may be cured or arrested. Medication must be taken regularly and in adequate dosages, since small dosages or interrupted therapy may produce sulfone-
resistant bacilli, with exacerbation or relapse of the disease, even after several years of inactivity.

Dapsone (4,4'-diaminodiphenyl sulfone, **DDS**) 50 mg/day (or to 10 mg/kg/wk) orally is recommended for **indeterminate** and **tuberculoid types.** It is given without interruption, even during reactions, until 2 yr after the disease becomes inactive. For **dimorphous** and **lepromatous leprosy,**
intensive combined therapy is given initially. Recommended regimens include (a) rifampin 600
mg/day for a minimum of 2 wk plus dapsone 100 mg/day indefinitely; (b) rifampin 1500 mg in a
single dose on the first day of treatment plus dapsone 100 mg/day indefinitely; or (c) clofazimine 100
mg/day for 2 mo, then 100 mg 3 times/wk for 4 mo, plus dapsone 100 mg/day indefinitely. Rifampin
is bactericidal for *M. leprae,* whereas the other drugs are bacteriostatic. However, resistance to
rifampin may occur. Clofazimine combines bacteriostatic with anti-inflammatory properties and is
considered the best second-line drug and the drug of choice for severe longstanding multibacillary
cases, especially those associated with acute reaction. Skin pigmentation limits its usefulness. As
with rifampin, "bacterial persisters" can be isolated after many years of continuous clofazimine
treatment. Rifampin is available commercially; clofazimine, from the USPHS Hospital in Carville, La.

Primary **dapsone resistance** has been reported in all types of leprosy and in contacts of cases of
secondary resistance; secondary dapsone resistance, however, has been reported only in multibacillary disease. Drug resistance should be suspected if the disease progresses or relapses, if bacilli are
found in new lesions, or if there is no response to dapsone therapy in 3 to 6 mo. Concern about drug
resistance should be confirmed with mouse-footpad drug sensitivity studies before therapy is
changed. Recommended regimens for treating dapsone-resistant patients include (a) rifampin 600
mg/day for 1 mo plus clofazimine 100 mg/day for 6 mo, then 100 mg 3 times/wk indefinitely; (b)
rifampin 600 mg/day for 1 mo plus ethionamide 375 mg/day indefinitely; (c) ethionamide 375
mg/day for 3 mo plus clofazimine 100 mg/day for 6 mo, then 100 mg 3 times/wk indefinitely; or (d)
clofazimine 100 mg/day for 6 mo plus ethionamide 375 mg/day indefinitely.

Side effects from dapsone 100 mg/day or less are infrequent. Mild anemia is a common finding.
Patients with G6PD deficiency, however, may experience more severe hemolysis; therefore, they
should be given antileprosy drugs not related to the sulfones. Agranulocytosis is a potentially serious
but rare complication. (Peripheral neuropathy, reported in other diseases, is attributed to considerably larger doses of dapsone than those used in leprosy.)

Sulfoxone is given if there is gastric intolerance to DDS; 330 mg are equivalent to about 50 to 100
mg of DDS. Solasulfone and acedapsone (4,4'-diacetyldiaminodiphenyl sulfone, DADDS) are experimental drugs in the USA.

Mild **reactional states** are treated with bed rest, analgesics, and sedatives. More severe reactions
may be managed with bed rest and corticosteroids, thalidomide, or clofazimine.

Prednisone 30 to 60 mg/day is given when a serious complication, such as paralysis, necessitates
immediate treatment. After the desired response, the dosage is cut gradually. If therapy is required
for more than several months, prednisone should be replaced by thalidomide or clofazimine.

Thalidomide, an experimental drug in the USA but available through the USPHS Hospital, Carville,
La., currently is the treatment of choice for ENL reactions. The initial dose of 300 mg/day may be
continued for several months. Because of teratogenicity, it is **contraindicated** in women of childbearing age. The drug does not affect the underlying disease.

Clofazimine is slow-acting and seldom given initially to control acute reaction. Usually it supplements antileprosy drugs prescribed for patients with chronic recurring ENL. The initial dosage, 300
mg/day, may be decreased to a minimum of 100 mg 3 times/wk in case of severe GI complaints.
Treatment becomes less effective when doses are given at intervals of a week or more. Clofazamine
may be the only alternative to prolonged high-dose corticosteroid therapy for severe reactions.

Moderate reactions are sometimes treated with other drugs, including potassium antimony tartrate
(tartar emetic), stibophen, and chloroquine.

DDS or other specific therapy for the disease must be continued during episodes of acute reaction, or the disease deteriorates and becomes chronic; therapy is discontinued only if thalidomide or
clofazimine fails to control the acute reaction or the patient experiences serious steroid side effects.

Immediate recognition and treatment of **eye problems** are essential. ENL iridocyclitis is an emergency. The pupil is dilated, using atropine eyedrops or ointment 1% q 6 h for 3 days and then once

daily until the reaction subsides. Hydrocortisone drops or ointment 1% is also applied q 4 h for the first 3 days, then b.i.d. until the inflammation subsides. These drugs are given in addition to the treatment for the ENL reaction. Lagophthalmos is another serious complication, especially when associated with corneal anesthesia. Corneal dryness is treated with commercial artificial teardrops or ophthalmic mucin substitutes. Physiotherapeutic measures are instituted to strengthen weakened eyelid muscles; if no improvement follows, surgery is indicated. Glaucoma and cataracts may follow iridocyclitis. In general, the patient should be referred to an ophthalmologist for management of these problems.

Supportive care is important to protect insensitive eyes, hands, and feet from repeated infections and injuries that lead to blindness and mutilation. Deformities may be corrected surgically to improve function. Shoes can be built to conform to residual deformity and bear weight evenly. The patient must understand his problems and their potential dangers and observe early changes. Physicians at the USPHS Hospital in Carville, La., are always available to the medical profession for consultation on leprosy-related matters.

CAUSED BY SPIROCHETES

SYPHILIS (See Ch. 162)

ENDEMIC TREPONEMATOSES (Endemic Syphilis, Yaws, and Pinta)

Chronic nonvenereal spirochetal infections, spread by body contact. Treponema pallidum II (**endemic syphilis**), *T. pertenue* (**yaws**), *and T. carateum* (**pinta**) *are morphologically and serologically indistinguishable from T. pallidum* (**syphilis**).

Endemic syphilis is mainly found in Arab countries of the eastern Mediterranean and North Africa; yaws, in humid equatorial countries; and pinta, among the Indians of Mexico, Central America, and northern South America.

Clinical Course

Endemic syphilis (nonvenereal syphilis, Bejel) begins in childhood as a mucous patch, usually on the buccal mucosa, followed by papulosquamous and erosive papular lesions of the trunk and extremities. Periostitis of the bones of the legs is common. Gummatous lesions of the nose and soft palate develop in later stages.

Yaws (frambesia) begins as a granulomatous or macular lesion at the inoculation site, usually on the legs, after an incubation period of several weeks. The lesion heals but is followed by a generalized eruption of soft granulomas of the face, extremities, and buttocks, often at mucocutaneous junctions. These granulomas heal slowly and may relapse. Keratotic lesions may develop on the soles and cause painful ulcerations ("crab" yaws). Destructive lesions may develop years later, including periostitis (particularly of the tibia), proliferative exostoses of the nasal portion of the maxillary bone (**goundou**), juxta-articular nodules, gummatous skin lesions, and, ultimately, mutilating facial ulcers, particularly around the nose (**gangosa**).

Pinta begins at the inoculation site as small papules that progress to erythematous plaques in several months. Erythematous, squamous patches develop later, mainly on the extremities, face, and neck. After several years, slate-blue patches develop, usually symmetrically and generally on the face and extremities and over bony prominences; these later become depigmented, resembling vitiligo. Hyperkeratosis may occur on the soles and palms.

Diagnosis and Treatment

Diagnosis is made from the typical appearance of lesions in persons from endemic areas. The VDRL and FTA-ABS tests are positive but do not distinguish these diseases from venereal syphilis. Early lesions are often darkfield-positive for spirochetes indistinguishable from *T. pallidum*.

In each disease, one IM injection of 2.4 million u. of benzathine penicillin G produces healing, with rapid disappearance of the spirochetes. Children < 100 lb should receive 1.2 million u. Destructive lesions leave a scar. Public health control of each disease is based on active case finding and the prophylactic treatment of family and childhood contacts with benzathine penicillin.

RELAPSING FEVER (Tick, Recurrent, or Famine Fever)

An acute infectious disease caused by several species of spirochetes, transmitted by lice and ticks, and characterized by recurrent febrile paroxysms lasting 3 to 5 days, separated by intervals of apparent recovery.

Etiology and Epidemiology

Relapsing fever is the term applied to recurrent fevers, clinically similar but etiologically distinct, caused by different *Borrelia* spirochetes. The insect vector may be the soft ticks of the genus *Ornithodoros* or the head and body louse, depending on geographic location. The louse-borne relapsing fevers are endemic only in parts of Africa; the tick-borne, in the Americas, Africa, Asia, and Europe. In the USA, the disease is generally confined to the western states.

The various species of *Borrelia* are morphologically similar. They are delicate, threadlike organisms 8 to 30 μ long, with pointed ends and 4 to 10 large, irregular coils. They appear in the blood during a paroxysm, and can be found in internal organs, especially the spleen and brain.

The louse is infected by feeding on a patient during the febrile stage. The spirochetes are not transmitted directly to man, but are released and enter abraded skin or bites when the louse is crushed. Ticks acquire the spirochetes from rodents acting as reservoirs, and infect man when spirochetes in the tick's saliva or coxal fluid (excreta) enter the skin as the tick bites.

Symptoms, Signs, and Prognosis

After an incubation period of about 7 days, sudden chills usher in the disease, followed by high fever, tachycardia, severe headache, vomiting, muscle and joint pain, and often delirium. An erythematous macular or purpuric rash may appear early over the trunk and extremities; subcutaneous or submucous hemorrhages may be present. Mild polymorphonuclear leukocytosis may occur. Late in the course of the fever, jaundice, hepatomegaly, splenomegaly, myocarditis, and cardiac failure may appear, especially in cases of louse-borne disease. Fever remains high for 3 to 5 days, then clears abruptly by crisis.

The patient is usually asymptomatic for several days to a week or more; relapse, related to the cyclic development of the parasites, then occurs with all the former symptoms and signs. Jaundice is more common during relapse. The illness clears as before, but from 2 to 10 similar paroxysms may follow at intervals of 1 to 2 wk. The paroxysms become progressively less severe, and recovery eventually occurs as the patient develops immunity.

The mortality rate is generally low (0 to 5%) but may be considerably higher in very young, old, malnourished, or debilitated persons, or during epidemics of louse-borne fever.

Diagnosis

Relapsing fevers may be confused with malaria, dengue, yellow fever, leptospirosis, typhus, influenza, and the enteric fevers. The diagnosis is suggested by the recurrent fever and confirmed by the appearance of spirochetes in the blood during a paroxysm. Darkfield examination or thick and thin Wright- or Giemsa-stained blood smears will disclose the spirochetes. In tick-borne infection, intraperitoneal injection of the patient's blood into a mouse or rat produces large numbers of spirochetes in the animal's tail blood within 3 to 5 days.

Prophylaxis

Dusting the undergarments and inner surfaces of clothing with DDT, malathion, or lindane powders will protect against relapsing fever resulting from infestations of body or head lice. Tick-borne infections are more difficult to prevent because of the inadequacy of insect control measures (see ROCKY MOUNTAIN SPOTTED FEVER in Ch. 10).

Treatment

Therapy should be started early in the paroxysm or during the afebrile stage, but should be avoided near the end of a paroxysm because of the danger of a Herxheimer reaction, which is regularly seen and occasionally fatal in louse-borne infection. The severity of the Herxheimer reaction and the transient hypotension that follows it may be lessened by giving acetaminophen 0.65 gm orally 2 h before and 2 h after the first dose of tetracycline or erythromycin. In tick-borne fever, a tetracycline or erythromycin 0.5 gm orally q 6 h is given for 5 to 10 days; a single 0.5-gm oral dose of either drug cures louse-borne fever. The dose should be proportionately reduced in children. When vomiting or severe disease precludes oral administration, tetracycline 500 mg in 100 or 500 ml of saline may be given IV once or twice/day.

Dehydration and electrolyte imbalance should be corrected with parenteral fluids. Codeine 30 to 60 mg orally q 4 to 6 h may be used to relieve severe headache. Nausea and vomiting should be treated with dimenhydrinate 50 to 100 mg orally or rectally (or 50 mg IM) q 4 h, or with prochlorperazine 5 to 10 mg orally or IM 1 to 4 times/day. If heart failure occurs, specific therapy is indicated (see Ch. 25).

LEPTOSPIROSIS (Weil's Disease or Syndrome; Infectious [Spirochetal] Jaundice; Canicola Fever)

An inclusive term for all infections due to an organism of the genus Leptospira, *regardless of serotype.* About 130 serotypes have been identified. A single serotype may cause various clinical features, or a single syndrome (e.g., aseptic meningitis) may be caused by multiple serotypes.

Epidemiology

Leptospirosis, a zoonosis, occurs in several domestic and wild animal hosts and varies from inapparent illness to fatal disease. A carrier state exists in which animals shed leptospires in their urine for months. Human infections occur by direct contact with an infected animal's urine or tissue, or indirectly by contact with contaminated water or soil. Abraded skin and exposed mucous membranes (conjunctival, nasal, oral) are the usual portals of entry in man. Infection occurs at any age. At least 75% of those infected are males. Leptospirosis can be an occupational disease (e.g., of farmers or sewer and abattoir workers), but most patients are exposed incidentally during recreational activities. Dogs, immersion (e.g., swimming) in contaminated water, and rats are the most common probable sources. The 40 to 140 cases reported annually in the USA occur mainly in late summer and early autumn.

Clinical Features

The incubation period ranges from 2 to 20 (usually 7 to 13) days. The disease is characteristically biphasic. The **leptospiremic phase** is abrupt in onset, with headache, severe muscular aches, chills, and fever. Conjunctival suffusion is characteristic, usually appearing on the 3rd or 4th day. Spleno- and hepatomegaly are uncommon. This phase lasts 4 to 9 days, with recurrent chills and fever that often spikes to $>$ 39 C (102 F). Defervescence follows; then, on the 6th to 12th day of illness, the **second** or "**immune**" **phase** occurs, correlating with appearance of antibodies in the serum. Fever and earlier symptoms recur and meningismus may develop. CSF examination after the 7th day discloses pleocytosis in at least 50% of the patients. Iridocyclitis, optic neuritis, and peripheral neuropathy occur infrequently. If acquired during pregnancy, leptospirosis may cause abortion even during the convalescent period.

Weil's syndrome is a form of severe leptospirosis with jaundice and, usually, azotemia, hemorrhages, anemia, disturbances in consciousness, and continued fever. Onset is similar to that of the less severe forms; the signs of hepatocellular and renal dysfunction appear from the 3rd to 6th day. Renal abnormalities include proteinuria, pyuria, hematuria, and azotemia. Hemorrhagic manifestations are due to capillary injury. Thrombocytopenia may occur. The hepatic damage is minimal, and complete healing occurs.

Aseptic meningitis may occur with any serotype. The CSF cell count is between 10 and 1000/cu mm (usually $<$ 500), with predominantly mononuclear cells. CSF sugar is normal; protein is $<$ 100 mg/100 ml.

Mortality is nil in anicteric patients. With occurrence of jaundice, mortality is about 15%; in patients over 60, the rate is doubled.

Laboratory Findings

The WBC count is normal or slightly elevated in most cases but may reach 50,000 in severely ill, icteric patients. Leukocytosis $>$ l5,000 suggests liver involvement. There are usually $>$ 70% neutrophils, a finding that may help to differentiate leptospirosis from viral illnesses. In jaundiced patients, intravascular hemolysis may cause marked anemia. Serum bilirubin, usually $<$ 20 mg/100 ml, may reach 40 mg/100 ml in severe infection; BUN is usually $<$ 100 mg/100 ml. These findings indicate liver and renal involvement. Most patients with aseptic meningitis do not manifest significant disease of liver and kidney.

Investigations include the search, toward the end of the 1st wk, for spirochetes in the blood and assay for antibodies. Blood is drawn for staining, darkfield examination for spirochetes, culture, guinea pig inoculation, and acute phase serologic antibodies. After the 1st wk, *Leptospira* may be found in the urine and guinea pig inoculation may be positive.

Diagnosis

Meningitis or meningoencephalitis, influenza, hepatitis, acute cholecystitis, and renal failure must be included in the differential diagnosis. With the enteroviruses, which commonly cause aseptic meningitis, there is usually no history suggesting biphasic illness. Such a history favors leptospirosis or perhaps cytomegalovirus infections.

Leptospires may be isolated from the blood, urine, or CSF during the first phase by inoculation onto Fletcher's medium. Serologic technics, including slide and microscopic agglutination tests and an indirect fluorescent antibody method, may be used during the second phase.

Treatment

Antibiotics such as penicillin, streptomycin, the tetracyclines, chloramphenicol, and erythromycin are effective in experimental infections, but their value in man is uncertain. They are not beneficial if given later than 4 days after onset of the disease. In severe illness, penicillin G 6 to 12 million u./day IM or IV or tetracycline 2 gm/day orally or IV is often recommended. Fluid and electrolyte therapy are necessary for azotemia or jaundice. Isolation is not required, but care is needed in disposing of urine.

RAT-BITE FEVER

Rat-bite fever represents 2 clinically similar but etiologically distinct diseases that may follow a rodent bite. **Streptobacillary rat-bite fever,** caused by the pleomorphic gram-negative bacillus *Streptobacillus moniliformis,* is more common in the USA than **spirillary rat-bite fever,** caused by *Spirillum minus.* Rat-bite fever follows up to 10% of rat bites. It is mainly a disease of ghetto dwellers and the socially deprived, and it is also a hazard to biomedical laboratory personnel. It may be mistaken for a viral infection.

Streptobacillary Rat-bite Fever

S. moniliformis is present in the oropharynx of healthy rats. Epidemics have been associated with ingestion of unpasteurized, contaminated milk **(Haverhill fever),** but infection is usually a consequence of a bite by a wild rat or mouse.

The primary wound usually heals promptly, but after an incubation period of 1 to 22 (usually < 10) days, the patient abruptly develops a viral-like syndrome with chills, fever, vomiting, headache, and back and joint pains. The WBC count ranges between 6,000 and 30,000. A morbilliform, petechial rash appears in about 3 days on the hands and feet of most patients. Polyarthralgia or arthritis, usually affecting the large joints asymmetrically, develops in many patients within a week and may persist for several days or for months if untreated. SBE and abscesses in the brain or other tissues are rare but serious complications.

Streptobacillary rat-bite fever usually can be differentiated on clinical grounds from spirillary rat-bite fever, but can be confused with Rocky Mountain spotted fever, infection with Coxsackie B virus, and meningococcemia. **Diagnosis** is confirmed by culturing the organism from blood or joint fluid. Agglutinins develop during the 2nd or 3rd wk and are diagnostically important if the titer increases.

Treatment consists of either procaine penicillin G 1.2 million u./day IM or penicillin V 2 gm/day orally for 7 to 10 days. Erythromycin 2 gm/day orally may be an alternative in cases of penicillin hypersensitivity.

Spirillary Rat-bite Fever (Sodoku)

Spirillum minus infection is acquired through a rat or, occasionally, a mouse bite. The wound usually heals promptly, but inflammation recurs at the site after an incubation period of 4 to 28 (usually > 10) days, accompanied by a relapsing fever and regional lymphadenitis. The WBC count ranges between 5,000 and 30,000. VDRL tests are false-positive in half the patients. A roseolar-urticarial rash sometimes develops, but is less prominent than the streptobacillary rash. Systemic symptoms commonly accompany the fever. Arthritis is rare. In untreated patients, 2- to 4-day cycles of fever usually recur for 4 to 8 wk but, rarely, febrile episodes recur for > 1 yr.

Diagnosis is made by demonstration of the spirillum in blood smears or tissue from the lesions or lymph nodes, or by Giemsa stain or darkfield examination of blood from inoculated mice. If the physician is unaware of previous rat bite in cases with long incubation periods, he may easily confuse the disease with malaria, meningococcemia, or *Borrelia recurrentis* infection, all of which are characterized by relapsing fever.

Treatment: Procaine penicillin G 1.2 million u./day IM or, for patients allergic to penicillin, tetracycline 2 gm/day orally is given for 7 days.

---

9.   SYSTEMIC FUNGAL DISEASES

(Systemic Mycoses)

The important systemic mycoses are discussed in this chapter. Dermatophytoses and other skin infections can be found in Ch. 191; pulmonary disorders caused by hypersensitivity to fungi are discussed in Ch. 41; fungal diseases affecting the GU system can be found in Ch. 151.

General Diagnostic Principles

Several considerations are important in the diagnosis of the deep mycoses.

1. Many of the causative fungi are "opportunists," not usually pathogenic unless they enter a compromised host. (See also Ch. 6.) Opportunistic fungus infections are particularly apt to occur and should be anticipated in patients after ionizing (x-) irradiation and during therapy with corticosteroids, immunosuppressives, or antimetabolites; they also tend to occur in patients with azotemia, diabetes mellitus, bronchiectasis, emphysema, TB, Hodgkin's disease or other lymphoma, leukemia, or burns. Candidosis, aspergillosis, phycomycosis, nocardiosis, and cryptococcosis are typical opportunistic infections.

2. Fungal diseases occurring as primary infections may have a typical geographic distribution. For example, in the USA, coccidioidomycosis is virtually confined to the southwest, while histoplasmosis occurs in the East and Midwest, especially in the Ohio and Mississippi River valleys. Blastomycosis is restricted to North America and Africa; paracoccidioidomycosis, often called South American blastomycosis, is confined to that continent. However, travelers can develop a symptomatic infection some time after returning from such endemic areas.

3. The major clinical characteristic of virtually every deep mycosis is its chronic course. Septicemia or an acute pneumonia is rare. Lung lesions develop slowly. Months or years may elapse before medical attention is sought or a diagnosis is made.

4. Symptoms are rarely intense; fever, chills, night sweats, anorexia, weight loss, malaise, and depression may all be present.

5. When a fungus disseminates from a primary focus in the lung, the manifestations may be characteristic. Thus, cryptococcosis usually appears as meningitis, progressive disseminated histoplasmosis as hepatic disease, and blastomycosis as a skin lesion.

6. Delayed cutaneous hypersensitivity tests and serologic tests are available for only 3 or 4 of the infections discussed in this chapter. Even in these, the tests become positive either so late (e.g., coccidioidomycosis) or so infrequently (e.g., blastomycosis) that they are of no diagnostic value for the acutely ill patient.

7. The diagnosis is usually confirmed by isolation of the causative fungus from sputum, bone marrow, urine, blood, or CSF, or from lymph node, liver, or lung biopsy. When the fungus is a commensal of man or is prevalent in his environment (e.g., *Candida, Aspergillus*), it is difficult to interpret its isolation from such specimens as sputum, and confirmatory evidence of tissue invasion is necessary to attribute an etiologic role to it.

8. In contrast to viral and bacterial diseases, fungal infections can be diagnosed histopathologic- ally with a high degree of reliability. It is the distinctive fungal morphology, not the tissue reaction to the fungus, that permits specific etiologic identification.

9. Even when the microorganism has been demonstrated histopathologically in tissues, the ac- tivity of the disease must be established before treatment is begun. Culture of the causative microor- ganism or such clinical and laboratory findings as fever, leukocytosis, elevated ESR, abnormal liver function, worsening of chest film findings, or elevated serum globulins are helpful as indications for therapy.

General Therapeutic Principles

General medical care, surgery, and chemotherapy constitute modes of treatment for systemic fungus infections. **Ketoconazole**, a new antifungal imidazole derivative, appears to have major ad- vantages: oral dosage, broad antifungal activity, and minimal adverse effects; but testosterone syn- thesis may be blocked, usually transiently, and serious idiosyncratic hepatotoxicity may occur. Current usage is 200 to 400 mg orally once a day with a meal. It may be given for prolonged periods to establish and maintain clinical remission or to prevent reinfection. Because **amphotericin B** is used in many systemic mycoses, it is covered in detail here. Indications and directions for other therapeutic measures are given below in the discussions of specific mycoses.

Amphotericin B, a fungicidal and fungistatic antibiotic, has reversed the prognosis of many fungal infections. An initial IV dose of 0.1 mg/kg/day is increased by 0.05 to 0.10 mg/kg every day until 1.0 mg/kg (but not exceeding 50 mg/dose) is given daily or every other day. The antibiotic is dissolved in 5% D/W (optimal concentration, 0.1 mg/ml). (CAUTION: *Saline solution precipitates the drug and should not be used. Follow the manufacturer's instructions in preparing and storing solutions.*)

The drug should be given over a 2- to 6-h period. Reactions are usually mild, but some patients may experience chills, fever, headache, anorexia, nausea, and, occasionally, vomiting, particularly with the initial injections. The severity of reactions may be reduced by giving aspirin or an antihista- mine (e.g., diphenhydramine 50 mg) before, after 3 h, and at the end of treatment. If this therapy is ineffective, hydrocortisone 25 to 50 mg IV may be given at the beginning of the amphotericin B infusion.

Chemical thrombophlebitis may occur; adding heparin to the infusion (or into the tubing just prior to starting the injection) may lessen the incidence.

The BUN or serum creatinine should be determined before and periodically during treatment. A slight increase can be ignored. A moderate rise may be reversed by giving the drug on alternate days, but if not, treatment should be discontinued until the levels approach normal. If this requires only a few days, treatment can be resumed with the previous dose, but if a longer period is neces- sary, therapy should be restarted with a smaller dose. Serum potassium should be determined regu- larly, since hypokalemia is common and occasionally is dramatic and dangerous. Oral liquid supplements are usually sufficient; rarely, potassium IV (not added to the amphotericin B infusion) may be necessary (see DISTURBANCES IN POTASSIUM METABOLISM, in Ch. 81).

Intrathecal injection may be indicated in meningitis, but great care must be taken to ensure proper dose and volume: 50 mg of amphotericin B should be painstakingly dissolved in 10 ml of sterile water. The total volume should then be diluted in a 250-ml bottle of 5% D/W from which 10 ml has been removed. From 0.5 ml (0.1 mg) to 5.0 ml (1.0 mg) should then be drawn into a 10-ml syringe, further diluted to 10 ml with CSF, and injected *slowly* (over at least 2 min). A lumbar, cisternal, or ventricular (by an Ommaya reservoir) site may be used.

HISTOPLASMOSIS

An infectious disease caused by Histoplasma capsulatum, *characterized by a primary pulmonary lesion and occasional hematogenous dissemination, with ulcerations of the oropharynx and GI tract, hepatomegaly, splenomegaly, lymphadenopathy, and adrenal necrosis.*

Etiology and Incidence

H. capsulatum in tissue is an oval budding cell 1 to 5 μ in diameter. Infection follows inhalation of dust that contains the spores. Severe disease is more frequent in men.

Chest x-ray surveys in certain geographic areas have demonstrated many residents with symptom- less, nontuberculous, occasionally calcified pulmonary lesions; delayed cutaneous hypersensitivity reactions to histoplasmin suggest widespread but subclinical infection. The highest incidence of such hypersensitivity is in the Ohio and Mississippi River valleys.

Symptoms and Signs

There are 3 recognized forms of the disease. The **primary acute form** causes symptoms (fever, cough, malaise) indistinguishable in endemic areas (except by culture) from otherwise undifferenti- ated URI or grippe-like disease. The **progressive disseminated form** follows hematogenous spread from the lungs and is characterized by hepatomegaly, lymphadenopathy, splenomegaly, and, less frequently, oral or GI ulceration. Addison's disease is an uncommon but serious manifestation. The lesions in the liver are granulomatous, show the intracellular fungus, and may lead to hepatic calcification. Addison's disease of other etiology, lymphoma, Hodgkin's disease, leukemia, and sarcoidosis must be differentiated. The **chronic cavitary form** produces pulmonary lesions indistinguishable, except by culture, from cavitary TB. The principal manifestations are cough, increasing dyspnea, and eventually disabling respiratory embarrassment. That histoplasmosis is a cause of uveitis has been postulated but not proved.

Diagnosis

Demonstration of *H. capsulatum* by culture is diagnostic. Specimens for culture may be obtained from sputum, lymph nodes, bone marrow, liver biopsy, blood, urine, or oral ulcerations. Tissues may also be examined microscopically after staining (Gomori's methenamine silver, periodic acid-Schiff, or Gridley). Delayed cutaneous hypersensitivity and CF tests are of no diagnostic value, since they are usually negative early in the disease.

Prognosis and Treatment

The acute primary form is usually benign; it is fatal only in those rare cases with massive infection. The progressive disseminated form has a high mortality. In the chronic cavitary form, death results from severe respiratory insufficiency.

Primary acute disease rarely requires chemotherapy (see amphotericin B and also ketoconazole in General Therapeutic Principles, above). The disseminated form responds to amphotericin B; in the chronic cavitary form, the fungi disappear with therapy, but fibrotic lesions show little change.

COCCIDIOIDOMYCOSIS

(San Joaquin or Valley Fever)

An infectious disease, caused by the fungus Coccidioides immitis, *occurring in a* **primary form** *as an acute, benign, self-limiting respiratory disease, or in a* **progressive form** *as a chronic, often fatal, infection of the skin, lymph glands, spleen, liver, bones, kidneys, meninges, and brain.*

Etiology, Incidence, and Pathology

The disease is endemic in the southwestern USA and occurs most frequently in men aged 25 to 55. Infection is acquired by inhalation of spore-laden dust. Individuals contracting the disease while traveling through endemic areas may not develop manifestations until later, after leaving the area.

The basic pathologic change is an acute, subacute, or chronic granulomatous process with varying degrees of fibrosis. Lesions may show central necrosis; the organisms are surrounded by lymphoctyes and by plasma, epithelioid, and giant cells. Cavitation or granuloma ("coin lesion") formation may occur in chronic lung infection.

Symptoms and Signs

Primary pulmonary coccidioidomycosis, the more common form, may occur asymptomatically, as a mild URI, as acute bronchitis, occasionally with pleural effusion, or as pneumonia. Symptoms, in descending order of frequency, include fever, cough, chest pain, chills, sputum production, sore throat, and hemoptysis. Physical signs may be absent, or occasional scattered rales and areas of dullness to percussion may be present. Leukocytosis is present and the eosinophil count may be high. Some patients develop **"desert rheumatism,"** a more recognizable form with conjunctivitis, arthritis, and erythema nodosum.

Progressive coccidioidomycosis develops from the primary form; evidence of dissemination may appear a few weeks, months, or, occasionally, years after primary infection or long residence in an endemic area. Symptoms include continuous low-grade fever, severe anorexia, and loss of weight and strength. Progressive cyanosis, dyspnea, and mucopurulent or bloody sputum are present in the pulmonary type. The bones, joints, skin, viscera, brain, and meninges may be involved as the disease spreads.

Diagnosis

Coccidioidomycosis should be suspected in a patient with an obscure illness who has been or is in an endemic area. Diagnosis is established by finding the characteristic spherules of *C. immitis* in sputum, gastric washings, pleural fluid, CSF, pus from abscesses, biopsy specimens, or exudate from skin lesions by direct examination or culture. In the tissues, the fungus appears as thick-walled, nonbudding spherules 20 to 80 μ in diameter.

A delayed cutaneous hypersensitivity reaction to coccidioidin or spherulin usually appears 10 to 21 days after infection, but is characteristically absent in progressive disease. Precipitating and CF antibodies are present regularly and persistently in the progressive form but only transiently in acute primary cases.

Prognosis and Treatment

For primary pulmonary coccidioidomycosis, treatment is not needed and the outlook is excellent. The progressive type, however, is fatal in 55 to 60% of cases. Amphotericin B (see amphotericin B and also ketoconazole in General Therapeutic Principles, above) is indicated in all patients with the progressive form. Results are less satisfactory than in blastomycosis or histoplasmosis. Meningitis requires prolonged intrathecal administration, usually for years. Untreated meningitis is fatal.

CRYPTOCOCCOSIS

(Torulosis)

An infectious disease due to the fungus Filobasidiella neoformans *(formerly known as* Cryptococcus neoformans *or* Torula histolytica), *with a primary focus in the lung and characteristic spread to the meninges and occasionally to the kidneys, bone, and skin.*

Incidence and Pathology

Distribution is worldwide. In the USA, more cases occur in the Southeast, in adults aged 40 to 60, and in men more often than in women. Individuals with Hodgkin's disease are particularly susceptible.

CNS lesions include diffuse meningitis, meningeal granulomas, endarteritis, infarcts, areas of softening, increase in neuroglia, or extensive tissue destruction. Cutaneous lesions appear as acneiform pustules or granulating ulcers. Subcutaneous and visceral lesions are deep nodules or tumorlike masses filled with gelatinous material. Acute inflammation is minimal or absent, but infiltration with lymphocytes and fibroblasts, and with plasma, "foam," and giant cells, is seen occasionally.

Symptoms and Signs

Meningitis with headache is the most common form. The patient seeks medical care because of blurred vision or is brought to the physician because of such mental disturbances as confusion, depression, agitation, or inappropriate speech or dress. CSF examination shows elevated protein and cell count (mostly lymphocytes) in about 90% of patients, and decreased glucose in 50%; *F. neoformans* can be seen on India ink examination in 60%.

Though the infection is acquired via the respiratory route with a primary focus in the lung, it has only recently been recognized that a benign, rarely progressive, pulmonary form occurs, often as a complication of other lung disease. Cough or other symptoms of the underlying pathologic changes in the lung are usually present.

The kidney is the next most common organ involved. *F. neoformans* can be cultured from the urine in about 30% of patients with cryptococcal meningitis. Although renal infection is usually asymptomatic, pyelonephritis with renal papillary necrosis has been reported.

Skin lesions (pustules or ulcers) and bone lesions (osteomyelitis) are seen less frequently.

Diagnosis

This is strongly suggested by finding, with an India ink preparation, the budding yeast surrounded by a clear capsular area in sputum, pus, other exudates, or CSF. Similar encapsulated yeast forms, seen on proper staining of fixed tissues, are also almost diagnostic. Isolation in culture and identification of the causative fungus confirm the diagnosis.

Prognosis and Treatment

Treatment with amphotericin B (see General Therapeutic Principles, above) has reduced the fatality rate of the meningeal form to about 15%. Though daily and total dosages are not firmly established, a 2- to 3-gm total dose seems reasonable. Patients with nonprogressive pulmonary disease may need no treatment. Skin, bone, and renal infections require therapy, though these forms are intermediate in severity.

Alternatively, once sensitivity has been demonstrated, flucytosine 50 to 150 mg/kg/day orally at 6-h intervals may be given for nonmeningitic forms. Each dose is preferably taken over a 15-min period, and dosage is continued for at least 6 wk. Flucytosine is not metabolized significantly when taken orally; it is excreted primarily by the kidney. Renal and hematologic status should be determined before therapy and the drug must be given with extreme caution to patients with impaired renal function or bone marrow depression. The lower dose is given initially if the BUN or serum creatinine is elevated or if there is renal impairment. Frequent monitoring of renal, hematologic, and hepatic function is essential throughout therapy.

Adverse reactions include GI disturbances; rash; anemia; leukopenia; thrombocytopenia; occasionally, elevation of hepatic enzymes, BUN, and creatinine; and, infrequently, confusion, hallucination, or headache. Leukopenia, thrombocytopenia, and, occasionally, elevated SGOT have occurred, which can be due to the drug, to underlying disease, to the infection, or to a combination of all three.

BLASTOMYCOSIS

(North American Blastomycosis; Gilchrist's Disease)

An infectious disease caused by the fungus Blastomyces dermatitidis, *primarily involving the lungs and occasionally spreading hematogenously, characteristically to the skin.*

Etiology and Incidence

B. dermatitidis is a fungus of unknown natural source. Most reported cases are from the USA, chiefly in the southeastern states and the Mississippi River valley, and occur in men aged 20 to 40. A sufficient number of cases from widely scattered sites in Africa now precludes geographic limitation of the disease name.

Symptoms and Signs

Pulmonary form: Primary pulmonary blastomycosis frequently forms patches of bronchopneumonia that appear, on chest film, to fan out from the hilum like a neoplastic growth. Onset is usually insidious. A dry hacking or productive cough, chest pain, fever, chills, drenching sweats, and dyspnea are initial symptoms.

Systemic form: Sites of hematogenous spread include skin, prostate, epididymis, testis, bone, subcutaneous tissue, and, rarely, oral or nasal mucosa. The vertebrae, tibia, and femur are more commonly involved than other bones; swelling, heat, and tenderness are present over the lesion. Genital tract lesions are characterized by painful swelling.

Skin lesions begin as papules or papulopustules on exposed surfaces and spread slowly. Painless miliary abscesses, varying from pinpoint to 1 mm in diameter, develop on the advancing borders. Irregular, wartlike papillae form on the surfaces. As the lesions enlarge, the center heals with a typical atrophic scar. A fully developed individual lesion appears as an elevated verrucous patch measuring 2 cm or larger with an abruptly sloping, purplish-red, abscess-studded border. Ulceration may occur if bacteria are present.

Diagnosis

Isolation in culture and identification of *B. dermatitidis* is diagnostic. Diagnosis is almost as certain if thick-walled budding yeasts, about 15 μ in diameter and without a capsule, are seen on direct examination of pus, sputum, or exudate, or after appropriate tissue fixation and staining. Skin and serologic tests are of no value.

Pulmonary disease must be distinguished from TB, other fungus infections, and bronchogenic carcinoma. Skin lesions resemble sporotrichosis, TB, iodism, or, especially, basal cell carcinoma. Genital involvement mimics TB.

Prognosis and Treatment

In most untreated patients, the disease is slowly and fatally progressive. Amphotericin B (see General Therapeutic Principles, above) is highly effective. Improvement begins within a week, with a rapid disappearance of organisms.

Hydroxystilbamidine isethionate is occasionally useful for this infection (e.g., in patients with a renal disorder or with nonprogressive blastomycosis limited to the skin). However, storage and administration are difficult, and the manufacturer's instructions for use of the drug must be carefully followed. Dosage is begun with 25 mg/day IV and increased in increments of 25 mg/day until 225 mg/day is reached; this dose is continued until a total of 8 gm has been given. Alleviation of symptoms usually begins after 14 days, but little improvement in the lesions is noted before 30 days. Improvement usually continues for 3 to 6 mo after the last dose. Occasionally, the course of treatment must be repeated. Rarely, facial numbness in the sensory distribution of the 5th cranial nerve occurs. Fever occurring near the end of the first week of therapy suggests a Herxheimer-like reaction.

PARACOCCIDIOIDOMYCOSIS

(South American Blastomycosis)

An infectious disease of the skin, mucous membranes, lymph nodes, and internal organs, caused by the fungus Paracoccidioides brasiliensis (*formerly* Blastomyces brasiliensis). *The disease occurs only in South and Central America, most frequently in men aged 20 to 50, and especially in the coffee-growers of Brazil.*

Symptoms and Signs

There are 4 clinical forms. (1) The **cutaneous form** occurs most often on the face, frequently at the nasal and oral mucocutaneous borders. The typical lesion is a slowly expanding ulcer with a granular base and numerous pinpoint yellowish-white areas in which the fungus is abundant. Regional lymph nodes enlarge, become necrotic, and discharge through the skin. (2) In the **lymphatic form,** there is massive painless enlargement of the cervical, supraclavicular, or axillary lymph nodes. (3) In the **visceral form,** the liver, spleen, and abdominal lymph nodes enlarge. Abdominal pain may be the first symptom. (4) In the **mixed type,** cutaneous, lymphatic, and visceral lesions are present simultaneously.

Diagnosis and Treatment

Identification of *P. brasiliensis* in pus, biopsy, or culture is diagnostic. Treatment with amphotericin B (see General Therapeutic Principles, above) is effective sulfonamides are suppressive but not curative. Ketoconazole (see General Therapeutic Principles, above), a new agent under investigation, shows promise in this disorder.

SYSTEMIC CANDIDOSIS
(Candidiasis; Moniliasis)

Invasive disease caused by Candida *spp., especially* C. albicans, *and manifested by septicemia, endocarditis, meningitis, or, rarely, osteomyelitis.* Topical *Candidal* spp. infections are discussed in other appropriate sections of THE MANUAL.

Etiology and Incidence
The infections are usually caused by *C. albicans.* Superficial candidosis is universal, but patients with leukemia, or with organ transplants, or receiving immunosuppressive or antibacterial therapy are especially prone to *C.* spp. septicemia. *C.* spp. (frequently *C. parapsilosis*) endocarditis is related to intravascular trauma such as cardiac catheterization, surgery, or indwelling venous catheters.

Symptoms and Signs
C. spp. **endocarditis** resembles bacterial disease, with fever, heart murmur, splenomegaly, and anemia; large vegetations and emboli to major vessels are frequently present and are differential features. Renal involvement is usually found on laboratory and autopsy examination. *C.* spp. **septicemia** usually resembles gram-negative bacterial sepsis in frequency of fever, shock, azotemia, oliguria, renal shutdown, and fulminant course. *C.* spp. **meningitis** is chronic, like cryptococcal meningitis, but lacks the latter's usually fatal outcome when untreated. *C.* spp. **pyelonephritis** and pulmonary disease are less well characterized. **Osteomyelitis** is rarely encountered; it resembles that due to other microorganisms.

Diagnosis
Because *C.* spp. are commensals of man, their culture from sputum, mouth, vagina, urine, stool, or skin must be interpreted cautiously. To confirm the diagnosis, the culture must be complemented by a characteristic clinical lesion, exclusion of other etiology, and histologic evidence of tissue invasion. Isolation from blood or CSF, however, establishes the presence of *C.* spp. infection and supports the appropriate clinical impression: septicemia, endocarditis, or meningitis.

Treatment
Such predisposing conditions as diabetic acidosis must first be controlled. In systemic candidosis, amphotericin B IV is preferable therapy (see General Therapeutic Principles, above). As an alternative, flucytosine may be given as for cryptococcosis (see above) if the isolate is sensitive to it. Ketoconazole (see General Therapeutic Principles, above) appears promising in investigational studies in this disorder.

ASPERGILLOSIS

An infectious disease of the lung, with occasional hematogenous spread, caused by various Aspergillus *spp., especially* A. fumigatus. A noninvasive pulmonary disorder may also occur as an allergic reaction to *A. fumigatus* (see ALLERGIC BRONCHOPULMONARY ASPERGILLOSIS in Ch. 41).

Etiology, Symptoms, and Signs
The fungus, an "opportunist," appears after antibacterial or antifungal therapy (to which it is usually resistant) in bronchi damaged by bronchitis, bronchiectasis, or tuberculosis. The "fungus ball" (aspergilloma), a characteristic form of the disease, appears on the chest film as a dense round ball, capped by a slim meniscus of air, in a cavity; it is composed of a tangled mass of hyphae, fibrin, exudate, and a few inflammatory cells. Aspergillomas usually occur in old cavitary disease (e.g., tuberculosis) or, rarely, in patients with rheumatoid spondylitis. Symptoms (cough, productive sputum, dyspnea) and findings on physical examination or chest film are usually those of the underlying disease. However, hemoptysis has been a disturbing and even occasionally fatal complication. In the presence of leukemia, organ transplantation, or corticosteroid or immunosuppressive therapy, dissemination to the brain and kidneys may occur. The clinical picture in this form is a typical septicemia: fever, chills, hypotension, prostration, and delirium.

Diagnosis and Treatment
Because it is a commensal of man, culture of *A.* spp. from sputum, mouth, or bowel must not be considered diagnostic unless a clinically compatible illness is present, other causes have been eliminated, and tissue invasion has been demonstrated. In disseminated and pulmonary disease, amphotericin B should be given IV (see General Therapeutic Principles, above), although tolerated doses are usually ineffective, since most strains are resistant.

PHYCOMYCOSIS
(Mucormycosis)

A term that includes numerous clinical conditions associated with the presence of broad, nonseptate hyphae. In most cases, the fungus has been visualized in tissues only microscopically. When cultured, it has been either a *Rhizopus, Absidia,* or *Basidiobolus* spp. One form of the disease, subcutaneous phycomycosis, occurs in southeast Asia and Africa as a self-limited, multiple, grotesque, subcutaneous swelling of the neck and chest. **Rhinocerebral phycomycosis,** more familiar in the USA, is a fulminant and usually fatal primary infection of the nose, sinus, or orbit seen in patients with diabetic acidosis or immunosuppressive disorders or drugs. Severe pain, fever, orbital cellulitis, proptosis, purulent nasal drainage, and gangrenous and necrotic destruction of septum, palate, or orbital or sinus bones are usually present. Early invasion of vessels and spread to the brain causes convulsions, aphasia, and hemiplegia. The clinical appearance is diagnostic, but bacterial abscesses, histoplasmosis or TB of the oral cavity, or lethal midline granuloma occasionally mimic rhinocerebral phycomycosis. It has been difficult to culture the fungi clearly present in tissues at biopsy or autopsy. **Treatment** includes control of the underlying acidosis and amphotericin B therapy, given empirically, since the causative fungus has not usually been available for sensitivity studies.

MADUROMYCOSIS

(Madura Foot; Mycetoma)

A fungus infection of the feet (and occasionally the upper extremity), characterized by chronicity, tumefaction, and multiple sinus formation, and progressing until ended by excision, amputation, or death.

About half the cases are caused by *Nocardia* spp., the remainder by some 20 different fungi and bacteria. The disease is most prevalent in the tropics and southern USA and is usually contracted between ages 21 and 40.

Symptoms, Signs, and Diagnosis

The first lesion may be a small papule, a deep-seated fixed nodule, a vesicle with an indurated base, or an abscess that ruptures and produces a fistula. Early lesions are granulomatous but are later surrounded by a dense fibrous capsule and intersected by fibrous trabeculae. Lesions are usually nontender unless secondary infection is present. The disease progresses slowly; 6 to 8 papules or abscesses may form in succession and then disappear. Months or years may pass before muscles, tendons, fascia, and bone are destroyed.

In advanced cases, the foot characteristically appears as a grotesque, swollen, club-shaped mass of cystlike areas with multiple draining and intercommunicating sinuses and fistulas that discharge an "oily" or serosanguineous fluid. Characteristic fungus granules in the discharge measure 0.5 to 2 mm, are irregularly shaped, and vary in color. The patient is able to walk until deformity or muscle wasting intervenes. Systemic symptoms are rare. The course may be prolonged for 10 yr or longer, the patient eventually dying from sepsis or intercurrent disease, unless the infecting organism is sensitive to an antimicrobial agent. Diagnosis is made from the clinical course, appearance, and demonstration of the characteristic colored granules in the exudate.

Treatment

Cases caused by *Actinomyces* spp. should be treated with penicillin or a tetracycline (see ACTINO-MYCOSIS in Ch. 8); those caused by *Nocardia* spp. with a soluble sulfonamide (see NOCARDIOSIS in Ch. 8). No specific treatment is known for other types. Amputation of the limb may be required to prevent fatal spread of secondary bacterial infection.

SPOROTRICHOSIS

An infectious disease caused by the plant saprophyte Sporothrix, *and characterized by the formation of nodules, ulcers, and abscesses, usually confined to the skin and superficial lymph channels but occasionally affecting the lung or other tissues (synovial membranes). Farm laborers and horticulturists, especially those handling barberry bushes, are most often infected.*

Symptoms and Signs

The most common form, cutaneous-lymphatic, occurs characteristically on the arm and hand. The primary lesion, usually on the finger, begins as a small, movable, nontender, subcutaneous nodule that slowly enlarges, adheres to the skin, becomes pink and later necrotic, and finally ulcerates. In a few days or weeks, similar discolored subcutaneous nodules appear along the course of the lymphatics draining the area. Local pain, heat, and general symptoms (fever, chills, malaise, or anorexia) are notably absent.

Inhalation of the microorganism apparently can cause pneumonia, localized infiltrates, or cavities (sometimes bilateral). Symptoms are relatively mild, and the course is chronic.

Though *S. schenckii* has only rarely been cultured from the blood, it seems reasonable to explain other extracutaneous disease as hematogenous dissemination either from a subclinical cutaneous lesion or, perhaps more likely, from a pulmonary focus. Bone, periosteum, or synovium is involved in 80% of such cases; muscle and eye, in others. Involvement of the spleen, liver, kidney, genitalia, or CNS is rare.

Diagnosis

Isolation and identification of *S. schenckii* in culture is diagnostic. Unlike other pathogenic fungi, *S. schenckii* can rarely be seen in fixed tissue, even with special stains.

Prognosis and Treatment

The cutaneous-lymphatic form is chronic, indolent, and rarely fatal. It responds readily to potassium iodide saturated solution initially 1 ml orally t.i.d., increased by 1 ml/day to an optimal dose of 3 to 4 ml t.i.d. The solution may be diluted in water or other beverage and should be taken after meals. Therapy must be continued and may be well tolerated for prolonged periods. However, iodism may appear at any time as an irritative phenomena of the skin and mucous membranes (e.g., rashes, coryza, conjunctivitis, stomatitis, laryngitis, bronchitis). When symptoms develop, the dose should be decreased or the drug temporarily stopped. After a 1- to 2-wk interruption, the drug may be cautiously resumed at a lower dosage. It may be considered essential to continue iodide medication despite iodism; in such cases, iodide sensitivity may lessen or disappear despite continued therapy.

In disseminated disease, IV amphotericin B (see General Therapeutic Principles, above) is necessary, since about 30% of patients have died, in some instances despite extensive treatment with iodides.

CHROMOMYCOSIS

(Chromoblastomycosis; Verrucous Dermatitis)

An infectious disease caused by Hormodendrum pedrosoi, H. compactum, *or* Phialophora verrucosa, *and characterized by warty cutaneous nodules which slowly develop into large papillomatous vegetations that tend to ulcerate.* Incidence is worldwide, but highest in the tropics. The disease is prevalent from age 30 to 50, primarily in men.

Symptoms, Signs, and Diagnosis

The infection, usually unilateral, begins on the foot and leg, or sometimes on other exposed parts, especially where the skin is broken. The early lesion is a small, itching, enlarging papule resembling ringworm. The patch is dull red or violaceous in color, is sharply demarcated, and has an indurated base. New crops projecting 1 or 2 mm above the skin may appear several weeks or months later along the paths of lymphatic drainage. Hard, dull red or grayish cauliflower-like nodules may develop in the center of the patch and gradually cover the infected extremities. Lymphatics may be blocked, itching may be present, and secondary infection may lead to ulceration. From 4 to 15 yr may elapse before the entire extremity is involved.

In late cases, the diagnosis is made from the clinical appearance. Early lesions may be mistaken for dermatophytoses and must be differentiated by finding the characteristic dark brown septate bodies in pus or biopsy specimens.

Prognosis and Treatment

The disease is rarely fatal but complete surgical excision is the treatment of choice. A few reports suggest that amphotericin B, instilled into the lesion, may be effective even in advanced cases. More recently flucytosine has been the recommended chemotherapy.

RHINOSPORIDIOSIS

A probably infectious disease caused by Rhinosporidium seeberi, *characterized by large, friable, sessile or pedunculated polyps on the mucous membranes of the nose, eyes, larynx, and vagina, and occasionally on the skin of the ears or penis.* The disease, apparently contracted by swimming in stagnant water, occurs most often in boys and young men in India and Ceylon. The diagnosis is established by identifying the ovoid spores (measuring 7 to 9 μ) in smears, or by demonstrating the characteristic spore-filled sporangia (200 to 300 μ) in biopsy material.

Prognosis and Treatment

The disease is rarely fatal, but the patient may die of secondary infection. Complete excision of the early lesions is curative.

GEOTRICHOSIS

A variety of conditions, none yet characterized or studied, existing in a patient from whom Geotrichum candidum *has been cultured.* Since the microorganism is a commensal of man, its isolation from the mouth and bowel is etiologically meaningless. No clinical condition has been consistently associated with *Geotrichum*, although there have been rare reported cases of fungemia.

PENICILLIOSIS

A term used to include the rarely encountered, disparate instances when a species of apparently multiplying Penicillium *has been recovered from deep tissues* (e.g., the brain, orbit, or kidney). Like *Candida* and *Geotrichum*, *Penicillium* is a commensal in the bowel and is found in stool.

10.   RICKETTSIAL DISEASES

A variety of illnesses manifested by sudden onset, a course of fever of one to several weeks, headache, malaise, prostration, peripheral vasculitis, and, in most cases, a characteristic rash. Most rickettsias are maintained in nature by a cycle involving an animal reservoir and an insect vector (usually an arthropod) that infects humans.

Most of the members of the order Rickettsiales are obligate intracellular organisms that resemble viruses and bacteria. Like bacteria, they possess metabolic enzymes, have cell walls, utilize O_2, and are susceptible to antibiotics; like viruses, they require living cells for growth. Most are pleomorphic coccobacilli that stain purple with Giemsa, pink to red with Castaneda, and bright red with Giménez stains. During convalescence they usually induce serum agglutinins against specific *Proteus* strains **(Weil-Felix reaction)** and various types of antibodies to specific rickettsial antigens. Since many of the rickettsias are localized to geographic areas, knowing where the patient lives or has recently traveled often helps in diagnosis.

In some rickettsioses, rickettsias multiply at the site of an arthropod attachment and produce a local lesion (eschar). They penetrate the skin or mucous membranes and multiply in the endothelial cells of small blood vessels, causing a vasculitis consisting of endothelial proliferation, perivascular infiltration, and thrombosis. The endovasculitis is responsible for the rash, encephalitic signs, and gangrene of skin and tissues.

Rickettsioses comprise 4 groups: (1) **typhus**—epidemic typhus, Brill-Zinsser disease, murine (endemic) typhus, and scrub typhus; (2) **spotted fever**—Rocky Mountain spotted fever, Eastern tick-borne rickettsioses, and rickettsialpox; (3) **Q fever**; and (4) **trench fever.**

EPIDEMIC TYPHUS

(European, Classic, or Louse-Borne Typhus; Jail Fever)

An acute, severe, febrile disease characterized by prolonged high fever, intractable headache, and a maculopapular rash. The agent, Rickettsia prowazekii, *is transmitted by lice.*

Etiology and Epidemiology

Rickettsia prowazekii is prevalent worldwide and transmitted to man in feces of the human body louse, *Pediculus humanus*, when a puncture wound is contaminated by scratching. Dried louse feces may also infect the mucous membranes of the eyes or oral cavity. Lice become infected on febrile patients and transmit illness to susceptible humans. Man is the natural reservoir of infection. A human form of epidemic typhus fever has been identified in the USA that is occasionally contracted after contact with squirrels or their ectoparasites; the illness is generally milder than classic typhus and is identified by serologic methods.

Symptoms and Signs

Following the 7- to 14-day incubation, fever, headache, and prostration begin suddenly. Temperature reaches 40 C (104 F) in several days and remains at a high level, with slight morning remission, for about 2 wk. Headache is generalized and intense. Small pink macules appear on the 4th to 6th day, usually in the axillae and on the upper trunk; they rapidly cover the body, usually sparing the face, soles, and palms. Later the lesions become dark and maculopapular; in severe cases, the rash becomes petechial and hemorrhagic. Splenomegaly occurs in some cases. Hypotension occurs in most seriously ill patients, and vascular collapse, renal insufficiency, encephalitic signs, ecchymosis with gangrene, and pneumonia are poor prognostic signs. Fatalities are rare in children < 10 yr, but mortality increases with age and may reach 60% in those > 50.

Prophylaxis

Immunization and louse control are highly effective. Live and killed vaccines are available. Lice may be eliminated by dusting infested persons with DDT, malathion, or lindane.

For **diagnosis** and **treatment**, see Differential Diagnosis of Rickettsial Diseases and Therapy of Rickettsial Diseases, below.

BRILL–ZINSSER DISEASE

Recrudescence of epidemic typhus, occurring years after an initial attack.

Etiology and Epidemiology

Patients who develop Brill-Zinsser disease either acquired epidemic typhus earlier in life or lived in an endemic area. *R. prowazekii* persist as viable organisms long after recovery. Apparently when host defenses falter, rickettsia are activated, causing recurrent typhus. Lice that feed on patients may acquire infection and transmit the agent. Also, *R. prowazekii* may be isolated from the blood of such patients by animal inoculation.

The disease is sporadic, occurring at any season and in the absence of infected lice. A history of epidemic typhus or residence in an endemic area is helpful.

Symptoms and Signs

The illness, almost always mild, resembles epidemic typhus in the character of the rash, circulatory disturbances, and hepatic, renal, and nervous system changes. The remittent febrile course lasts about 7 to 10 days; the rash is often evanescent or absent. Mortality is nil.

For **diagnosis** and **treatment,** see Differential Diagnosis of Rickettsial Diseases and Therapy of Rickettsial Diseases, below.

MURINE (ENDEMIC) TYPHUS

(Rat-Flea Typhus; Urban Typhus of Malaya)

An acute febrile disease clinically similar to, but milder than, epidemic typhus, caused by Rickettsia mooseri *and transmitted to humans by rat fleas.*

Etiology and Epidemiology

The causative agent, *R. typhi (mooseri),* resembles other rickettsias morphologically, in staining characteristics, and in intracellular parasitism. The animal reservoir is wild rats, mice, and other rodents; the agent is transmitted to man by rat fleas (*Xenopsylla cheopis*). This illness, sporadic and worldwide in distribution, is more prevalent in congested areas where rats abound, but the incidence is low.

Symptoms and Signs

Following an incubation of 6 to 18 days (mean 10), a shaking chill develops, associated with headache and fever. The fever lasts about 12 days and terminates by lysis. The rash and other manifestations are similar to those of epidemic typhus but are much less severe. The early exanthem is sparse and discrete. Although mortality is low, fatalities may occur in elderly patients.

Prophylaxis

Incidence of murine typhus has been decreased by reducing rat and rat-flea populations through securing foundations of food depots and granaries and by dusting rat runs, burrows, and harborages with DDT or another residual insecticide. There is no effective vaccine.

For **diagnosis** and **treatment,** see Differential Diagnosis of Rickettsial Diseases and Therapy of Rickettsial Diseases, below.

SCRUB TYPHUS

(Tsutsugamushi Disease; Mite-Borne Typhus; Tropical Typhus)

A mite-borne infectious disease caused by Rickettsia tsutsugamushi *and characterized by fever, a primary lesion, a macular rash, and lymphadenopathy.*

Etiology and Epidemiology

This disease occurs in the Asiatic-Pacific area bounded by Japan, India, and Australia; *R. tsutsugamushi* is transmitted in nature by trombiculid mites (usually *Leptotrombidium akamushi* and *L. deliensis*) transovarially and by feeding on forest and rural rodents, including rats, voles, and field mice. Human infection follows a chigger (mite larva) bite.

Symptoms and Signs

After an incubation period of 6 to 21 days (average 10 to 12 days), onset is sudden, with fever, chilliness, headache, and generalized lymphadenopathy. At onset of fever, a local lesion (eschar) often develops at the site of the chigger bite. The lesion is common in Caucasians but rare in Asians. It begins as a red, indurated lesion about 1 cm in diameter and eventually vesiculates, ruptures, and becomes covered with a black scab; regional lymph node enlargement occurs. Fever rises during the 1st wk, often to 40 to 40.5 C (104 to 105 F). Headache is severe and commonly present, as is conjunctival injection. A macular rash develops on the trunk during the 5th to 8th day of fever and often extends to the arms and legs. It may disappear rapidly or become maculopapular and intensely colored. Cough is present during the 1st wk of fever, and pneumonitis may develop during the 2nd wk. In severe cases, pulse rate increases, blood pressure decreases, and delirium, stupor, and muscular twitching develop. Splenomegaly may be present, and interstitial myocarditis is more common than in other rickettsioses. In untreated patients, high fever may persist for 2 wk or more, then fall by lysis over several days. With specific therapy, defervescence usually begins within 36 h and recovery is prompt and uneventful.

Prophylaxis

Clearing brush and spraying infested areas with residual insecticides eliminate or decrease mite populations. Mite repellents, e.g., dimethyl phthalate or benzyl benzoate, should be used by individuals likely to be exposed.

For **diagnosis** and **treatment,** see Differential Diagnosis of Rickettsial Diseases and Therapy of Rickettsial Diseases, below.

ROCKY MOUNTAIN SPOTTED FEVER

(Spotted Fever; Tick Fever; Tick Typhus)

An acute febrile disease caused by Rickettsia rickettsii *and transmitted by ixodid ticks.*

Etiology, Epidemiology, and Pathology

R. rickettsii is limited to the Western Hemisphere. Initially recognized in the Rocky Mountain states, it occurs in practically all states (except Vermont) in the USA, especially on the Atlantic seaboard. Hard-shelled ticks (family Ixodidae) harbor *R. rickettsii*, and infected females transmit the agent transovarially to their progeny. Ticks are the natural reservoir, and animals provide blood nourishment. *Dermacentor andersoni* (the wood-tick) is the principal vector in the western USA; *D. variabilis* (dog tick) and *Ambloyomma americanum* (lone-star tick) are common vectors in the eastern and southern USA. The organism is also maintained in rabbits and other small mammals. The disease occurs mainly from May to September, when adult ticks are active and persons are most apt to be in areas infested by ticks. In southern states, cases occur throughout the year. The incidence is high in children under age 15 and in others who frequent tick-infested areas for work or recreation. Recent studies suggest that the disease may, rarely, be transmitted directly from person to person via infectious aerosol produced by the cough of a patient with respiratory-tract involvement; this is an important mechanism of transmission.

Small blood vessels are the sites of the characteristic pathologic lesion. Rickettsia propagate within damaged endothelial cells, and vessels may be blocked by thrombi. The major sites of vasculitis are the skin, subcutaneous tissues, CNS, lungs, heart, kidneys, liver, and spleen.

Symptoms and Signs

A history of tick bite is elicited in about 70% of patients. The incubation period averages 7 days but varies from 3 to 12 days; the shorter the incubation period, the more severe the infection. Onset is abrupt, with severe headache, chills, prostration, and muscular pains. Fever reaches 39.5 or 40 C (103 or 104 F) within several days and remains high (for 15 to 20 days in severe cases), though morning remissions may occur. An unproductive, harassing cough develops. On about the 4th day of fever, a rash appears on the wrists, ankles, palms, soles, and forearms; it rapidly extends to the neck, face, axilla, buttocks, and trunk. Often a warm water or alcohol compress will bring out the rash. Initially macular and pink, it becomes maculopapular and darker. In about 4 days, the lesions become petechial and may coalesce to form large, hemorrhagic areas that later ulcerate. Neurologic symptoms include headache, restlessness, insomnia, delirium, and coma, all indicative of an encephalitis. Hypotension develops in severe cases. Hepatomegaly may be present, but jaundice is infrequent. Localized pneumonitis may occur. Untreated patients may develop such complications as pneumonia, tissue necrosis, and circulatory failure, with such sequelae as brain and heart damage. Cardiac arrest with sudden death occasionally occurs in fulminant cases.

Prognosis

Starting antibiotic therapy early has significantly reduced mortality, formerly about 20% and much higher in localized areas and in adults over age 50. No serious sequelae result if therapy is instituted early.

Prophylaxis

A tissue-culture–derived, inactivated vaccine is under development and will be recommended for persons who frequently encounter ticks during work or recreation. Tick repellents such as dimethyl phthalate should be used by all who live or work in tick-infested areas. Good personal hygiene should be practiced, with frequent searches for ticks, particularly in children. Engorged ticks should be removed with care and not crushed between the fingers because of danger of transmission. Gradual traction of the head part with a small forceps will dislodge the tick. The point of attachment should be swabbed with alcohol. Although no practical means exist to rid entire areas of ticks, tick populations may be reduced in endemic areas by controlling small-animal populations; spraying the area with DDT, dieldrin, or chlordane is also helpful.

For **diagnosis** and **treatment**, see DIFFERENTIAL DIAGNOSIS OF RICKETTSIAL DISEASES and THERAPY OF RICKETTSIAL DISEASES, below.

TICK-BORNE RICKETTSIOSES OF THE EASTERN HEMISPHERE

(North Asian Tick-Borne Rickettsiosis; Queensland Tick Typhus;
African Tick Typhus [Fièvre Boutonneuse])

Mild to moderately severe febrile diseases, transmitted by ixodid ticks and characterized by an initial lesion, satellite adenopathy, and an erythematous maculopapular rash.

Etiology and Epidemiology

The etiologic agents of the 3 diseases in this category (listed above) belong to the spotted fever group of rickettsia and, with *R. rickettsii* and *R. akari*, possess common group antigens that are demonstrated by agglutination, complement fixation, rickettsiae microagglutination, and indirect fluorescent antibody reactions. North Asian tick-borne rickettsiosis, caused by *R. sibirica*, is found in Armenia, Central Asia, Siberia, and Mongolia; Queensland tick typhus, caused by *R. australis*, in

Australia. Fièvre boutonneuse, the prototype of the 3, caused by *R. conorii*, occurs throughout the African continent, in India, and in areas of Europe and the Mideast adjacent to the Mediterranean, Black, and Caspian Seas. It often is known by the area in which it occurs (e.g., Indian tick typhus, Marseilles fever).

The epidemiology of these tick-borne rickettsioses resembles that of spotted fever in the Western Hemisphere. Ixodid ticks and wild animals maintain the rickettsias in nature; if humans intrude accidentally into the cycle, they break the transmission chain. In certain areas, the cycle of fièvre boutonneuse involves domiciliary environments, with the brown dog tick, *Rhipcephalus sanguineus*, as the dominant vector. Transovarial transmission of rickettsias occurs in various ticks.

Symptoms, Signs, and Prognosis

The 3 tick-borne rickettsioses of the Eastern Hemisphere resemble one another closely; they are milder than spotted fever. After a 5-to 7-day incubation period, fever, malaise, headache, and conjunctival injection develop. With the onset of fever a local lesion appears (termed **eschar**, or, in fièvre boutonneuse, **tache noire**), a small buttonlike ulcer 2 to 5 mm in diameter with a black center. Usually the regional or satellite lymph nodes are enlarged. About the 4th day of fever, a red maculopapular rash appears on the forearms and extends to most of the body, including the palms and soles. Fever lasts into the 2nd wk of illness. Complications are rare. Death is rare except among aged or debilitated patients.

For **diagnosis** and **treatment**, see Differential Diagnosis of Rickettsial Diseases and Therapy of Rickettsial Diseases, below.

RICKETTSIALPOX
(Vesicular Rickettsiosis)

A mild, self-limited, febrile disease with an initial local lesion and a generalized papulovesicular rash, caused by Rickettsia akari *and transmitted from its murine host by mites.*

First observed in New York City, rickettsialpox has also occurred in other US areas and in Russia, Korea, and Africa. The vector, a small, colorless mite, *Allodermanyssus sanguineus*, is widely distributed. It infects the house mouse (*Mus musculus*) and some species of wild mice, and can transmit *R. akari* transovarially. Humans may be infected by either chigger or adult mite bites.

Symptoms and Signs

An eschar resembling the tache noire of fièvre boutonneuse appears about 1 wk before onset of fever. Initially a small papule 1 to 1.5 cm in diameter, it develops into a small ulcer with a dark crust that heals leaving a scar; regional lymphadenopathy is present. The fever is intermittent and lasts about a week, with chills, profuse sweating, headache, photophobia, and muscle pains. Early in the febrile course, a generalized maculopapular rash with intraepidermal vesicles appears, sparing palms and soles. The disease is mild; no deaths have been reported.

Prophylaxis

Mouse harborages must be destroyed and the vector controlled by residual insecticides.

For **diagnosis** and **treatment**, see Differential Diagnosis of Rickettsial Diseases and Therapy of Rickettsial Diseases, below. Treatment is usually not indicated because the disease is so mild.

Q FEVER

An acute disease characterized by sudden onset of fever, headache, malaise, and interstitial pneumonitis, caused by Coxiella burnetii (Rickettsia burnetii). *In contrast to other rickettsial diseases, the illness is not associated with a cutaneous exanthem or agglutinins for* Proteus *strains (Weil-Felix reaction).*

Etiology and Epidemiology

The route of infection is usually inhalation of infected aerosols. Worldwide in its distribution, Q fever is maintained as an inapparent infection in domestic animals; sheep, cattle, and goats are the principal reservoirs for human infections. *C. burnetii* persists in feces, urine, milk, and tissues (especially the placenta), so that fomites and infective aerosols form easily. Cases occur among workers whose occupations bring them in close contact with domestic animals or their products. The disease can also be contracted by ingesting infective raw milk.

C. burnetii is also maintained in nature through an animal-tick cycle. In the USA, Q fever was first recognized in persons bitten by *Dermacentor andersoni*. Various arthropods, rodents, other mammals, and birds are naturally infected and may play a role in human infection.

Symptoms and Signs

The incubation period varies from 9 to 28 days (average 18 to 21 days). Onset is abrupt, with fever, severe headache, chilliness, severe malaise, myalgia, and, often, chest pains. Fever may rise to 40 C (104 F) and persist for 1 to > 3 wk. Rash is absent. A nonproductive cough with x-ray evidence of pneumonitis often develops during the 2nd wk of illness. Mortality is < 1% in untreated patients, and even lower with antibiotic therapy.

In fatal Q fever, lobar consolidation usually occurs and the gross appearance of the lungs may resemble that of bacterial pneumonia. However, histologic changes in Q fever pneumonia are similar to those of psittacosis and some viral pneumonias. An intense interstitial infiltrate about the bronchioles and blood vessels extends into the adjacent alveolar walls. Plasma cells are numerous. The bronchiolar lumina may contain polymorphonuclear leukocytes. The alveolar lining cells are swollen, and the alveoli contain desquamated lining cells and large mononuclear cells.

Hepatitis occurs in about 1/3 of patients with the protracted form. In this type there is fever, malaise, hepatomegaly with right upper abdominal pain, and possibly jaundice. Headache or respiratory signs are frequently absent. Liver biopsy specimens show diffuse granulomatous changes, and *C. burnetii* may be identified by immunofluorescence. Lobar pneumonia may be particularly severe in aged or debilitated patients. There are several forms of chronic Q fever, such as chronic hepatitis and endocarditis. Chronic Q fever hepatitis must be differentiated from other liver granulomas, e.g., tuberculosis, sarcoidosis, histoplasmosis, brucellosis, tularemia, and syphilis. Endocarditis caused by *C. burnetii* is serious but uncommon. Clinically, it simulates SBE, with aortic valve involvement more common. Routine blood cultures are persistently negative.

Diagnosis

Diagnosis is made by clinical suspicion and by demonstration of phase I type antibodies in the patient's serum. Clinically, during early stages Q fever simulates many infectious diseases, such as influenza, other viral infections, salmonellosis, malaria, hepatitis, brucellosis, and, later on, many forms of bacterial, viral, and mycoplasmal pneumonias. Contact with animals, animal products, or ticks is an important clue.

C. burnetii may be isolated from the blood. The Weil-Felix reaction is negative. Specific CF and agglutinating antibodies appear during convalescence. Agglutination tests are more sensitive than CF tests; fluorescent antibody tests are helpful. *C. burnetii* exists in two phases, I and II; antibodies against Phase I organisms are rarely produced in infected human serum, but when present indicate chronic Q fever.

Prophylaxis

Animal-to-man transmission must be prevented: milk should be pasteurized; dust control in pertinent industries is essential; and animal placentas, feces, and urine should be incinerated. The sputum and urine of Q fever patients should be autoclaved and the patient isolated. Vaccines made from Phase I rickettsias are effective and should be used to protect slaughterhouse and dairy workers, rending plant workers, herders, woolsorters, farmers, and others at risk. These vaccines are not available commercially, but may be obtained from special laboratory groups—e.g., the US Army Medical Research Institute of Infectious Diseases in Frederick, Maryland.

Treatment (See also THERAPY OF RICKETTSIAL DISEASES, below)

Tetracycline and chloramphenicol are effective. In acute disease, treatment should be continued until the patient has been afebrile for about 5 days. The course of illness may be shortened by giving tetracycline 250 mg orally q 4 or 6 h. Chloramphenicol may be used in young children.

In endocarditis, treatment is prolonged and tetracycline is preferred. Some cures without surgical intervention have been reported, but when antibiotic treatment is only partially effective, it is necessary to replace damaged valves. Clear-cut regimens for chronic hepatitis have not been determined.

TRENCH FEVER

(Wolhynian Fever; Skin-Bone Fever; Quintan Fever)

A rare louse-borne febrile disease observed mainly in military populations during World Wars I and II.

Etiology and Epidemiology

The causative organism, *Rochalimaea (Rickettsia) quintana*, grows extracellularly, unlike other rickettsias, and multiplies in the gut lumen of the body louse. One strain has been cultivated in blood agar. *R. quintana* is transmitted to man by the rubbing of infected louse feces into abraded skin or into the conjunctiva. Humans are the reservoir, since *R. quintana* persists in the blood for months after clinical recovery. The disease is endemic in Mexico, Tunisia, Eritrea, Poland, and the USSR.

Symptoms and Signs

Following a 14- to 30-day incubation period, onset is sudden, with fever, weakness, dizziness, headache, and severe back and leg pains. Fever may reach 40.5 C (105 F) and persist for 5 to 6 days. In about half the cases, fever recurs 1 to 8 times at 5- to 6-day intervals. A transient macular or papular rash and, occasionally, hepatomegaly and splenomegaly are present. Although recovery is usually complete in 1 to 2 mo and mortality is negligible, the illness may be prolonged and debilitating.

The disease is marked by persistent rickettsiemia present during the initial attack, during relapses (which are common), and throughout the symptomatic periods between relapses. Rickettsiemia may persist for long periods, and clinical relapse has been reported 10 yr after the original attack.

Diagnosis

The disease may be suspected in persons living where louse infestation is heavy. Leptospirosis, typhus fever, relapsing fever, and malaria must be ruled out. The organism may be identified by xenodiagnosis: normal body lice excrete *R. quintana* about 1 wk after ingestion of the patient's blood. Antibodies can be demonstrated by fluorescence or CF tests during convalescence.

Prophylaxis and Treatment

Body lice must be controlled (see EPIDEMIC TYPHUS, above). *R. quintana* is highly sensitive to in vitro chloramphenicols and the tetracyclines, but there are no reliable data regarding clinical efficacy. Aspirin and codeine are indicated for control of discomfort.

DIFFERENTIAL DIAGNOSIS OF RICKETTSIAL DISEASES

Differentiation of the rickettsioses from other acute infectious diseases is difficult during the first several days before the rash. History of lousiness, flea infestation, or tick bite in known endemic areas of typhus, Rocky Mountain spotted fever **(RMSF)**, or other tick-borne rickettsial diseases are helpful clues.

The rash of **meningococcemia**, which may be pink, macular, maculopapular, or petechial in the subacute form, and petechial confluent, or ecchymotic in the fulminant type, resembles RMSF or epidemic typhus. The meningococcal rash develops rapidly in the acute type and when ecchymotic is usually tender to palpation; the rickettsial rash usually appears on about the 4th febrile day and gradually, over several days, becomes petechial.

RMSF is often confused with measles. In **rubeola**, the rash begins on the face, spreads to the trunk and arms, and soon becomes confluent; the rash of **rubella** usually remains discrete. Postauricular lymph nodes and lack of toxicity favor rubella.

In murine typhus, the illness is milder than RMSF or epidemic typhus, the rash is nonpurpuric, nonconfluent, and less extensive; renal and vascular complications are uncommon. Differentiation of RMSF from murine typhus may be difficult and require the results of specific serologic reactions. (Treatment cannot be delayed until this distinction is made.) Epidemic louse-borne typhus fever causes all of the profound physiologic and pathologic abnormalities of RMSF, including peripheral vascular collapse, shock, cyanosis, ecchymotic skin necrosis, gangrene of digits, azotemia, renal failure, delirium, and coma. The rash of epidemic typhus usually appears first over the axillary folds and trunk; later it spreads peripherally, rarely involving the palms, soles, and face. Local eschars occur in patients with scrub typhus, rickettsialpox, and, occasionally, spotted fever. The epidemiologic history often helps in differentiation. The rash in rickettsialpox is vesicular, whereas in tick-borne typhus it is often obviously maculopapular. **Tularemia** is associated with an eschar and there is no exanthem.

Rickettsialpox, a member of the spotted fever group, is mild; there is usually an initial eschar at the point of the mite attachment, and the rash, in the form of vesicles with surrounding erythema, is sparse. **Varicella** must be ruled out, since similar oral lesions occur in both diseases.

A rash in Q fever is unusual and in trench fever is sparse.

Patients with scrub typhus have all of the clinical and pathologic manifestations of RMSF and epidemic typhus. Scrub typhus occurs in different geographic areas; there is frequently an eschar with satellite adenopathy.

Several types of confirmatory **laboratory tests** aid diagnosis: serologic tests, isolation and identification of *R. rickettsii* from blood or tissues, or identification of the agent in skin or other tissues by immunofluorescence technics.

Serologic tests, to be useful, require 3 serum samples during the 1st, 2nd, and 4th to 6th wk of illness.

Weil-Felix reaction: Strains of *Proteus* OX-19 are agglutinated by sera of patients with epidemic murine fever and RMSF; however, they provide no specificity for these diseases. In RMSF and other tick-borne rickettsioses, agglutinins for *Proteus* OX-19 and OX-2 appear; *Proteus* OX-K agglutinins occur in scrub typhus. The Weil-Felix reaction is not significantly reactive in patients with rickettsialpox, Brill-Zinsser disease, Q fever, or trench fever.

A single convalescent serum titer of $1/160$ to $1/320$ is usually diagnostic, but a demonstrated rise in titer is of greater value. *Proteus* agglutinins may appear as early as the 5th day and are generally present by the 12th febrile day. A maximum titer is generally reached in early convalescence and declines rapidly to nondiagnostic levels in several months. In approximately 10% of cases, *Proteus* agglutinins fail to appear. When antibiotics are given during the first few days of illness, the titer may be delayed, but it usually reaches the same level.

Complement-fixation reaction: The various rickettsial diseases can be differentiated by using group-specific, soluble rickettsial antigens. Using specific rickettsial antigens, the serologic patterns of RMSF and typhus are distinctive. In the USA, louse-borne typhus does not occur except as Brill-Zinsser disease (recurrent epidemic typhus fever). Spotted fever and typhus group rickettsiae possess 2 types of CF antigens; the soluble fraction is common to all members of the group, while purified fractions are more specific for individual rickettsiae. Various member-diseases of the spotted fever group, such as Rocky Mountain spotted fever, rickettsialpox, fièvre boutonneuse, north Asian tick-borne rickettsiosis and Queensland tick typhus, may be distinguished by use of type-specific washed rickettsial-body antigen. Antibodies during response to a primary infection of RMSF and typhus are usually 19S globulins. CF antibodies appear during the 2nd and 3rd wk of these illnesses and later in those treated with antibiotics within the first 3 to 5 days of illness. Under these circumstances, a later convalescent specimen should be taken at 4 to 6 wk. In Brill-Zinsser disease, antibodies appear rapidly after several days of illness and are 19S type. Q fever antigens are specifically diagnostic. In acute infections, antibodies to phase II antigens appear; phase I antibodies indicate chronic infection such as hepatitis or endocarditis.

Other serologic tests: Using purer antigens, other serologic procedures for rickettsioses not only distinguish between specific rickettsial infections but also help determine the type of immunoglobulin in acute (IgM) and late or recurrent (IgG) illnesses such as Brill-Zinsser disease (recurrent typhus fever). The Weil-Felix and CF tests are useful for routine diagnosis; microscopic agglutination (MA), immune fluorescence antibody (IFA), and hemaglutination (HA) reactions are valuable for identification and are becoming standard procedures. IFA and CF tests help confirm trench fever. *R. akari* shares a common antigen with other members of the spotted fever group but can be differentiated from them by demonstrating a rising titer of specific CF antibodies. *R. conori*, *R. sibirica*, and *R. australis* share a common antigen with *R. rickettsii* and *R. akari*, but are differentiated by CF and mouse toxin neutralization tests and by cross-immunity tests in guinea pigs.

Isolating and identifying rickettsia: If isolation is attempted, blood should be obtained, prior to antibiotic treatment, from febrile patients with spotted or typhus fever (see TABLE 2–2, p. 24). Male guinea pigs are inoculated intraperitoneally with 2 to 4 ml of defibrinated blood or emulsified clot. Details of how to establish infection may be found in standard laboratory texts.

Identification of *R. rickettsii* in tissues: Immunofluorescence technics have been used to detect *R. rickettsii* and *R. prowazekii* in tissues of chick embryos, guinea pigs, and vector ticks. Identifiable rickettsiae have been visualized in skin lesions of patients with RMSF as early as the 4th day of illness or as late as the 10th day. Rickettsia may be stained by IFA technic in formalized tissues.

THERAPY OF RICKETTSIAL DISEASES

Those principles necessary for treating all rickettsioses are (1) specific chemotherapy and (2) supportive care. Measures advisable for all rickettsioses are described here; variations are described in specific subsections.

Prompt alleviation of signs and symptoms occurs if therapy begins early, when the rash first appears. *Since untreated patients with RMSF may become moribund or die before definitive serologic data are available, treatment should begin as soon as a presumptive diagnosis is made.*

Chloramphenicol and the tetracyclines are specifically effective; they are rickettsiostatic, not rickettsiocidal. Optimal antibiotic regimens are (1) chloramphenicol, an initial oral dose of 50 mg/kg or (2) tetracycline, 25 mg/kg. The same dosage is given subsequently in daily doses divided equally and given at 6- to 8-h intervals until the patient improves and has been afebrile for about 24 h. IV preparations are used for the loading dose and subsequent doses in patients too ill to take oral medication. In critically ill patients who are first observed late in the course of severe illness, large doses of adrenocortical steroids, given for about 3 days in combination with specific antibiotics, are recommended. All patients with rickettsioses respond promptly to antibiotic treatment when it is initiated early in illness, before serious tissue changes have occurred. Obvious clinical improvement is usually noted within 36 to 48 h, with defervescence in 2 to 3 days. In scrub typhus the response is even more dramatic. In those patients first treated during the later stages, clinical improvement is slower and fever extends over longer periods. Patients seriously ill with the typhus spotted fever group often have circulatory collapse, oliguria, anuria, azotemia, anemia, hyponatremia, hypochloremia, edema, and coma that must be managed. In mildly and moderately ill patients these alterations are absent, making management less complicated.

Proper mouth care, swabbing the oral cavity and using mouthwashes, may help prevent gingivitis and parotitis. Turning the patient frequently will help avert pressure sores over bony prominences and prevent aspiration pneumonia. Negative nitrogen balance can be avoided by generous protein supplements with frequent feedings. Protein intake of 3 to 5 gm protein/kg of normal body weight, with adequate carbohydrate and fat to make the diet palatable, is usually well tolerated. In uncooperative patients when there is no abdominal distention, IV alimentation or hourly liquid protein feedings by gastric tube are helpful.

In critically ill patients, attention is given to parenteral alimentation with glucose and amino acid supplements. Small whole blood transfusions are indicated when anemia is present. Judicious use of serum albumin may improve the circulation. With oliguria, anuria, and azotemia, the circulation should not be overloaded; results of laboratory tests and clinical judgment guide therapy. Dialysis is indicated if there is clear-cut evidence of acute tubular necrosis.

11. CHLAMYDIAL DISEASES

The organisms responsible for psittacosis, lymphogranuloma venereum **(LGV)**, trachoma, and and inclusion conjunctivitis, are now classified in the genus *Chlamydia* (*Bedsonia, Miyagawanella*), which is divided into 2 species: *C. psittaci*, which causes psittacosis, and *C. trachomatis*, which consists of several strains, often referred to as the "TRIC agents," that cause LGV, trachoma, and inclusion conjunctivitis. Recently *C. trachomatis* has also been shown to cause a number of sexually transmitted diseases, including nongonococcal urethritis and epididymitis in the male, cervicitis, urethritis, and pelvic inflammatory disease in women, Reiter's syndrome in HLA-B27 haplotype individuals, and neonatal conjunctivitis and pneumonia transmitted from an infected mother to her newborn.

The chlamydias are nonmotile, obligate intracellular parasites. Although originally considered viruses because they multiply in the cytoplasm of host cells, the chlamydias are more closely related to bacteria, since they contain both DNA and RNA, have a cell wall that is chemically similar to that of gram-negative bacteria, possess ribosomes, grow well in the yolk-sacs of embryonated eggs, and are susceptible to the tetracyclines and erythromycin. Chlamydia can be isolated from infected secretions or tissues in appropriate tissue cultures (see TABLE 2–2, p. 24).

PSITTACOSIS is discussed in Ch. 38. Sexually transmitted urethritis is in Ch. 162 and LGV is in Vol. II, Ch. 5. Epididymitis is in Ch. 151; REITER'S SYNDROME is in Ch. 103; NEONATAL PNEUMONIA is in Vol. II, Ch. 21; and the ophthalmic disorders TRACHOMA and INCLUSION CONJUNCTIVITIS are in Ch. 178. CAT-SCRATCH DISEASE, not yet established as a chlamydial disease, is discussed under PRESUMPTIVE VIRAL DISEASES in Ch. 12.

12. VIRAL DISEASES

GENERAL

Viruses: *The smallest of parasites; intracellular molecular particles, in some instances crystallizable, with a central core of nucleic acid and an outer cover of protein; wholly dependent on cells (bacterial, plant, or animal) for reproduction.* The nucleic acid core (RNA or DNA) represents the basic infectious material, being able in many cases to penetrate susceptible cells and initiate infection alone.

Though most viruses are invisible in the light microscope (size variation, about 0.02 to 0.3 μ), they can be seen by electron microscopy and measured by various biophysical and biochemical methods. Like most other parasites, animal viruses stimulate host antibody production.

Several hundred different viruses may infect man. Many have been recognized only recently, so their clinical effects or even relationships are not fully delineated. Many viruses usually produce inapparent infections and only occasionally overt disease; nevertheless, because of their wide (sometimes universal) prevalence and their numerous distinct serotypes, they create important medical and public health problems.

The viruses occurring primarily in man are spread chiefly by man himself, mainly via respiratory and enteric excretions. Such viruses (see TABLE 12–1) are found in all parts of the world, their spread being limited by inborn resistance, prior immunizing infections or vaccines, sanitary and other public health control measures, and, in a few instances, by chemoprophylactic agents.

Many viruses pursue their biologic cycle chiefly in animals, man being only a secondary or accidental host. The zoonotic viruses (see TABLE 12–2), in contrast to the specifically human agents, are limited to those geographic areas and environments able to support their extrahuman natural cycles of infection (vertebrates or arthropods, or both).

Two properties of certain viruses are noteworthy because of their implications: (1) oncogenicity and (2) a prolonged incubation period. (1) Oncogenic properties of some animal viruses are well known (e.g., Rous sarcoma of chickens, Shope rabbit papilloma, murine leukemia viruses), but as yet no virus has been identified as the primary cause of human malignancy. However, some human viruses (e.g., adenovirus Type 12) can induce tumors in hamsters, particles resembling viruses have been observed by electron microscopy in certain human malignant cells, and Epstein-Barr virus has been found in association with some lymphoid tissue malignancies, such as Burkitt's lymphoma. (2) Kuru, a rare disease confined to natives of New Guinea and characterized by chronic degeneration of the CNS, has been transmitted and passed in primates. Symptoms appear after a prolonged incubation period of about 18 mo; hence the agent has been termed a **"slow" virus.** Slow viruses have also been found in sheep and other animals. The implications for man are clear: some of the

TABLE 12–1. HUMAN VIRAL DISEASES: NATURAL CYCLE CHIEFLY IN MAN; PERSON-TO-PERSON SPREAD*

Virus Groups & Categories	No. Known Sero-types	Most Important Syndromes	Serotypes	Prevalence, Distribution	Diagnostic Leads	Specific Therapy	Specific Prophylaxis
Respiratory Influenza A, B, & C	3	Influenza; AFRD; acute bronchitis & pneumonia; croup	A (with many possible subtypes), B, C	Epidemic, occasionally pandemic (A, B); endemic (C)	Clinical & epidemiologic features; serologic; virus isolation	None	Vaccine (moderately effective) Amantadine (A)
Parainfluenza 1–4	4	AFRI (children); acute bronchitis & pneumonia; croup	1 (Sendai, HA-2) 2 (CA, SV-5) 3 (HA-1, SF-4)	1: Local epidemic; 1 & 3: widely in children	Clinical not defined; serologic; virus isolation	None	Vaccines under study
Mumps	1	Parotitis, orchitis, meningoencephalitis	1	Global: most children; some adults	Clinical features; serologic; virus isolation	None	Vaccine
Adenoviruses	33	AFRD (children); ARD (adults); APCF; EKC; viral pneumonia; acute follicular conjunctivitis	1–10, 14, 21	1–3, 5–7: Children 4, 7, 14, 21: Adults 8: Local EKC	APCF, EKC: Clinical features Most: Serologic & virus isolation	None	Vaccine (4,7) for military epidemic situations
Reoviruses	3	Mild RI	(?)	Widely in children; may be same as in animals	Serologic; virus isolation	None	None
Respiratory syncytial	1 (3 sub-types)	U & L RI (infants); mild URI (adults)	1 (?)	Pediatric clinics & hospital wards	Serologic & isolation & identification of viruses	None	None
Infectious mononucleosis	1	Infectious mononucleosis	Epstein-Barr virus	Widespread; apparent chiefly in young adults	Heterophil agglut.; diff. WBC count; fluorescent antibody	None	None

					Clinical features		
Rhinoviruses	(?)	Common cold; acute coryza with or without fever	>95; probably 100's	Universal: especially in cold months		None	None
Enteric Polioviruses	3	Poliomyelitis (paralytic); aseptic meningitis; AFRD (children)	1, 2, & 3	Almost universal; + in warm months; + at younger ages	Paralysis typical; serologic; virus isolation	None	Vaccines: Live (oral) Killed (injected)
Coxsackieviruses	30 (A's: 24; B's: 6)	Herpangina: epidemic pleurodynia; aseptic meningitis; myocarditis; pericarditis; AFRD (children); paralytic disease; fever & exanthem	A's: 2, 4–10, 16, 21, 23 B's: 1–6	Varies with types; most persons infected; + in warm months; + in children	Virus isolation; serologic difficult, due to so many serotypes	None	None
Echoviruses	31**	Aseptic meningitis; fever & exanthem; meningoencephalitis with rash; diarrhea neonatorum; paralytic disease; myocarditis; pericarditis; ARD	4, 6, 8, 11, 14, 16, 18, 20, 30	As for coxsackieviruses	As for coxsackieviruses	None	None
Epidemic gastroenteritis	3 (?)	Epidemic nausea & vomiting	Rotaviruses; astro-viruses, "adenolike;" "parvo/picorna-like"	Local epidemics (children); + in colder months; + in neonates	Clinical & epidemiologic features, electron microscopy of diarrheal stools	None	None

(Continued)

* Developments are so rapid that no summary can be fully up to date. Main abbreviations: **AFRD**, acute febrile respiratory disease: **AFRI**, acute febrile respiratory illness; **APCF**, acute pharyngoconjunctival fever; **ARD**, acute respiratory disease; **CA**, croup-associated; **EKC**, epidemic keratoconjunctivitis; **HA**, hemadsorption; **LRI**, lower respiratory illness; **SF-4**, shipping fever; **SV-5**, a simian myxovirus; **URI**, upper respiratory illness.
** Types 9, 10, and 28 have been reclassified: these numbers are no longer used.

TABLE 12–1. HUMAN VIRAL DISEASES: NATURAL CYCLE CHIEFLY IN MAN; PERSON-TO-PERSON SPREAD *(Cont'd)*

Virus Groups & Categories	No. Known Sero- types	Most Important		Prevalence, Distribution	Diagnostic Leads	Specific	
		Syndromes	Serotypes			Therapy	Prophylaxis
Exanthems Rubeola	1	Measles; encephalomyelitis	1 known	Almost universal; monkeys also infected; CNS involvement rare	Clinical features; serologic; virus isolation	None	Vaccines
Rubella	1	German measles	1 (?)	Universal; birth defects from infection during 1st trimester of pregnancy	Clinical & epidemiologic features; serologic	None	Vaccines
Varicella-zoster	1	Chickenpox	1 known	Almost universal (children); occasionally in adults	Clinical features; serologic; virus isolation	None	γ-Globulin
	Same	Herpes zoster	Same	Common in adults; reactivation or reinfection	Same	None	None
Herpes simplex	2	Herpes labialis; herpetic gingivo-stomatitis; eczema; keratoconjunctivitis; encephalitis; vulvovaginitis	2 established	Recurrent labial, almost universal; gingivo-stomatitis frequent in infants & children; others rare	Clinical features; serologic; virus isolation	Idoxuri-dine (IDU) Adenine arabin-oside (Ara-A)	None
Roseola infantum	1 (?)	Rose rash, infants (Exanthem subitum)	Not isolated	Widespread: early childhood	Clinical features	None	None

Variola	1	Smallpox	1 known	Formerly epidemic & endemic (unless vaccinated)	Clinical features	None	None
Erythema infectiosum	2 (?)	"Fifth" disease; rash, malaise	Not isolated	Sporadic outbreaks	Atypical exanthems	None	None
Persistent (Latent) Cytomegaloviruses (salivary gland)	1	Congenital defects (cytomegalic inclusion disease); hepatitis (CMV mononucleosis)	1 established	Virus widespread; recognized disease uncommon	Clinical features; serologic; virus isolation	None	None
Hepatitis 1. Type A	1	Hepatitis A	1 established	Widespread; often epidemic	Clinical & epidemiologic features	None	γ-Globulin; vaccine under study
2. Type B	1	Hepatitis B	1 established	Widespread; may follow use of whole blood & derivatives or contaminated equipment	Clinical features; serologic	None	Strict aseptic precautions; screening for hepatitis B surface antigen; vaccine; γ-globulin
3. Non-A, Non-B	?	? Hepatitis C	?	Similar to Type B	Clinical features; serologic exclusion of Types A & B	None	None
Papovavirus	1	Warts (Verrucae)	Not definitely established	Universal; common; often recurrent	Clinical examination & biopsy	None	None
Molluscum contagiosum	1	Molluscum contagiosum tumors	1 established	Infrequent	Clinical examination & biopsy	None	None

TABLE 12-2. VIRUSES TRANSMITTED FROM NATURE TO MAN (ZOONOSES)

Virus Groups & Categories	No. Known Serotypes	Most Important Syndromes	Serotypes	Prevalence, Distribution	Diagnostic Leads	Specific Therapy	Specific Prophylaxis
Arboviruses* Group A	>250	1. Western equine encephalitis (WEE) 2. Eastern equine encephalitis (EEE) 3. Venezuelan equine encephalitis (VEE) 4. Chikungunya encephalitis 5. Mayaro disease	Same designations as clinical syndromes	1. N. & S. America 2. N. & S. America 3. Gulf states to S. America 4. Africa, S.E. Asia, India 5. S. America, Trinidad	Serologic; pathologic; virus isolation	None	Effective vaccines can be made; except for yellow fever, none in general use
Group B		1. Yellow fever 2. Dengue 1–4 3. Japanese encephalitis 4. Murray Valley encephalitis 5. St. Louis encephalitis 6. Russian spring-summer encephalitis 7. Omsk hemorrhagic fever 8. Kyasanur Forest disease 9. Powassan		1. Africa, Cen. & S. America 2. Tropics & subtropics worldwide 3. Asia, Australia, New Zealand 4. Australia, New Guinea 5. N. & S. America 6. USSR, E. Central Europe, Malaya 7. USSR 8. India 9. N. America			
Group C (Bunyamwera supergroup)		1. Bunyamwera and 13 others 2. Marituba and 12 others 3. California encephalitis and 8 related types		1. Africa, S. America, Finland, USA 2. S. America, Central America 3. Probably worldwide; common in midwest USA			

Group	No.	Clinical diseases	Serotypes known	Geographic distribution	Diagnosis		Prevention
Phlebotomus fever group		1. Naples, Sicilian fevers 2. Punta Toro, Chagres fevers 3. Candiru fever		1. Italy, India, Egypt 2. Panama 3. Brazil			
Ungrouped		1. Rift Valley fever 2. Crimean-Congo hemorrhagic fever		1. E. Africa, Egypt 2. USSR, Central Africa, W. Pakistan			
Diplornavirus (Reovirus-like)	1	Colorado tick fever	1 known	Western USA	Serologic; virus isolation	None	None
Rabies	1	Rabies (Hydrophobia)	1 known	Worldwide; domestic & wild animals; infrequent in man	Hist'y, clin. & path. findings; virus isolation	None	Effective vaccines available
Herpesvirus simiae (B virus)	1	Encephalomyelitis	1 known	Chiefly lab. workers exposed to monkeys, simian tissue cultures	Virus isolation	None	None
Arenaviruses*	≥11	1. Lassa fever 2. Machupo (Bolivian hemorrhagic fever) 3. Junin (Argentinian hemorrhagic fever) 4. Lymphocytic choriomeningitis	Same designations as clinical syndromes	1. Africa 2. S. America 3. S. America 4. Worldwide; chief reservoir: rodents	Virus isolation, serology	None	None
Unclassified viruses	2	1. Marburg virus (hemorrhagic fever) 2. Ebola virus (hemorrhagic fever)		1. Africa 2. Africa	Virus isolation, serology	None	None

*See also Table 12–5 in ARBOVIRUS AND ARENAVIRUS DISEASES, below. Arthropod vectors of most arboviruses are one or more genera and species of mosquito, ticks (Russian spring-summer encephalitis, Crimean hemorrhagic fever), and sandflies (Phlebotomus fever). Arbovirus Groups A and B are now reclassified as Togaviruses.

chronic degenerative diseases, previously with no known etiology, now appear to be due to slow virus infections. Besides kuru, these include subacute sclerosing panencephalitis, progressive multifocal leukoencephalopathy, Creutzfeldt-Jakob disease, and progressive rubella encephalitis. Probably in the future other human diseases will also be linked to slow viruses. (See SLOW VIRUS INFECTIONS below.)

Diagnosis of Viral Infections
In theory, most viral infections can, by some means, be recognized; in practice, diagnosis often remains difficult. A few viral diseases can be diagnosed accurately on clinical and epidemiologic grounds (e.g., several well-known exanthems), but many diagnoses depend on retrospective tests (e.g., serologic examination of acute and convalescent sera), unless an adequately equipped diagnostic virology laboratory is available in the community for more rapid diagnosis by such procedures as culture or immunofluorescence microscopy. During large epidemics (e.g., of influenza), laboratory diagnosis of early cases may aid in recognizing and managing those cases occurring subsequently. Many state health laboratories and the National Center for Disease Control can also offer diagnostic assistance.

Viruses of man and animals are isolated from secretions, excretions, and tissues by inoculating susceptible animals, chick embryos, and cultures of living cells (see TABLE 2–2, beginning on p. 21). Presence of the virus usually is indicated by disease and antibody responses in the animals or by cytopathogenic effects and antigen production in tissue cultures. Specific details of diagnosing viral diseases are discussed in THE MANUAL in relation to the discussion of each disease.

Prophylaxis and Treatment
Viral diseases are not susceptible to antibiotics. In certain viral illnesses, particularly those liable to superinfection with bacterial pathogens, antibiotics have been used to prevent complications. The efficacy of such treatment is debatable; moreover, indiscriminate use of antibiotics in viral infections (e.g., measles) may be harmful.

Results from the laboratory and from clinical trials hold out hope that the barriers—chiefly intracellular multiplication—to effective use of chemotherapeutic or chemoprophylactic drugs against viruses and viral diseases may soon be breached, if not broken. Examples are idoxuridine (IDU) and its derivatives for herpes simplex keratitis, methisazone for smallpox, amantadine for influenza A, adenine arabinoside for herpes simplex encephalitis, and exogenous or endogenous interferon, a protein of low molecular weight that is produced by certain cells when stimulated by a variety of substances (e.g., bacteria, some viruses, nucleic acids) and that nonspecifically inhibits replication of a wide range of viruses in the cells of the host producing it. (See also ANTIVIRAL DRUGS in Ch. 246.)

In many common, undifferentiated illnesses—the most frequent manifestations of prevalent viruses—decisions concerning the use of chemotherapeutic agents or antibiotics are often complicated by the difficulties of making a definitive diagnosis. In such instances, the best guides are the severity and course of the illness, blood and x-ray findings, and clinical judgment. Because antibiotics cannot be expected to influence most viral illnesses favorably, lack of response should suggest the need for stopping them and seeking a more specific therapy, if such exists.

Effective prophylactic virus vaccines available for general use to provide active immunity include those for influenza, measles, mumps, poliomyelitis, rabies, rubella (German measles), smallpox, and yellow fever. An adenovirus vaccine is available and effective, but should be used only in population groups subject to high risk, such as military recruits. Vaccines are also available for passive immune prophylaxis (see IMMUNIZATION PROCEDURES in Vol. II, Ch. 23). Other vaccines are being developed.

EXANTHEMATOUS VIRAL DISEASES
(See MEASLES; RUBELLA; ROSEOLA INFANTUM; ERYTHEMA INFECTIOSUM; CHICKENPOX; and SMALLPOX in Vol. II, Ch. 24)

HERPES ZOSTER (Shingles; Zona; Acute Posterior Ganglionitis)
An acute CNS infection involving primarily the dorsal root ganglia and characterized by vesicular eruption and neuralgic pain in the cutaneous areas supplied by peripheral sensory nerves arising in the affected root ganglia.

Etiology, Incidence, and Pathology
Herpes zoster is caused by the varicella-zoster virus, the same virus that causes chickenpox. It may be activated by local lesions involving the posterior root ganglia, by systemic disease, particularly Hodgkin's disease, or by immunosuppressive therapy. It may occur at any age but is most common after age 50. Inflammatory changes occur in the sensory root ganglia, the posterior horn of the gray matter, the meninges, and the dorsal and ventral roots.

Symptoms and Signs
Prodromal symptoms of chills and fever, malaise, and GI disturbances may be present for 3 or 4 days before distinctive features of the disease develop, with or without pain along the site of the future eruption. On about the 4th or 5th day, characteristic crops of vesicles on an erythematous base appear, following the cutaneous distribution of one or more posterior root ganglia. The in-

volved zone is usually hyperesthetic, and the associated pain may be severe. The eruptions occur most often in the thoracic region and spread unilaterally. They begin to dry and scab about the 5th day after their appearance. Zoster may become generalized. If dissemination occurs or the lesions persist beyond 2 wk, an underlying malignancy or immunologic defect becomes more suspect.

One attack of herpes zoster usually confers immunity. Most patients recover without residua, except for occasional scarring of the skin. However, postherpetic neuralgia may persist for months or years, most frequently in the elderly.

Geniculate zoster (Ramsay Hunt syndrome) results from involvement of the geniculate ganglion. There is pain in the ear and facial paralysis (rarely permanent) on the involved side. Vesicular eruptions are present in the external auditory canal and on the auricle, the soft palate, and the anterior pillar of the fauces. (See also HERPES ZOSTER OTICUS in Ch. 167.)

Ophthalmic herpes zoster (see also in Ch. 179) follows involvement of the gasserian ganglion. There is pain and a vesicular eruption in the distribution of the ophthalmic division of the 5th nerve. A 3rd nerve palsy may be present. Vesicles on the tip of the nose indicate the nasociliary branch of the 5th nerve and the cornea are involved, with possible development of corneal ulcerations and opacities.

Diagnosis

Though difficult in the preeruption stage, diagnosis is made readily after the vesicles appear in characteristic distribution. Pleurisy, trigeminal neuralgia, Bell's palsy, and, in children, chickenpox must be differentiated. The pain may resemble that of appendicitis, renal colic, cholelithiasis, or colitis, depending on the location of the involved nerve. Herpes simplex virus may produce nearly identical zosteriform lesions. Herpes simplex tends to recur, but herpes zoster rarely ever does. The viruses can be differentiated serologically and by culture.

Treatment

There is no specific therapy. However, a corticosteroid, if given early, may relieve pain in severe cases. The initial dose should be relatively large (e.g., prednisone 50 mg/day orally for an adult), and duration should not exceed 3 wk; all the precautions associated with prescribing corticosteroids should be observed. Locally applied wet compresses are soothing. Aspirin 600 mg, alone or with codeine 15 to 60 mg, orally q 4 to 6 h, may relieve pain. Recent trials suggest that immunosuppressed patients with herpes zoster may benefit from treatment with adenine arabinoside or exogenous human interferon if begun before dissemination develops; however, both agents are still considered experimental for this purpose.

For ophthalmic herpes zoster, see Ch. 179. (CAUTION: *Before using corticosteroids one must be certain that the disease is not acute ocular herpes simplex, in which corticosteroids are* **contraindicated;** *close supervision and follow-up of the patient are required*)

RESPIRATORY VIRAL DISEASES

Viral infections of the respiratory tract usually are acute illnesses with variable local and systemic manifestations. Coryza (common cold), pharyngitis, laryngitis (including croup), and bronchitis are common respiratory syndromes. Infectious asthma can resemble allergic causes. Nonpneumonic respiratory distress is frequently caused by viral infection; viral pneumonia is often unrecognized. Febrile syndromes without respiratory symptoms can mimic bacterial infections. In infants, such illnesses probably are caused more often by viruses than by bacterial sepsis. In adults, acute febrile "flu" can be produced by one of many viruses and is not distinguishable clinically from the specific infections described below under influenza.

THE COMMON COLD (Upper Respiratory Infection, URI; Acute Coryza)

An acute, usually afebrile, catarrhal respiratory tract infection, with major involvement in any or all airways, including the nose, paranasal passages, throat, larynx, and often the trachea and bronchi.

Etiology

Many viruses cause the common cold, including rhino-, influenza, parainfluenza, respiratory syncytial, corona, adeno-, certain echo-, and coxsackieviruses. More than 100 sero-specific rhinovirus types have been established and many viruses are still untyped. Pinpointing the specific etiology of each illness by virus isolation or serologic tests is rarely necessary in practice. The common cold has a striking seasonal relation. Spring, summer, and fall colds are more often picornavirus infections; late fall and winter colds are most frequently paramyxo- or myxovirus infections.

Predisposing factors have not been clearly identified. Chilling of the body surface will not by itself induce colds, and susceptibility is not affected either by the person's health and nutrition or by upper respiratory tract abnormalities (e.g., enlarged tonsils or adenoids). Infection may be facilitated by excessive fatigue, emotional distress, or allergic nasopharyngeal disorders and during the midphase of the menstrual cycle.

Pathogenic bacteria that inhabit the nasopharynx are the cause of infrequent purulent complications such as otitis media and sinusitis. Bronchitis may be of viral etiology, but secondary bacterial infection is common.

Symptoms and Signs

Onset is abrupt after a short (1 to 3 days) incubation period. Illness generally begins with throat discomfort, followed by sneezing, rhinorrhea, and malaise. Characteristically it is an afebrile illness, but fever of 38 to 39 C (100 to 102 F) can occur in infants and children. Pharyngitis, laryngitis, and tracheitis with substernal tightness and burning discomfort are variable symptoms related to the individual patient and the etiologic agent. Secretions thicken in the course of uncomplicated infection. Hacking cough often lasts into the 2nd wk. Severe tracheobronchial involvement with purulent sputum suggests primary or secondary bacterial invasion. Purulent sinusitis or otitis media are other bacterial complications. In the absence of complications, symptoms normally resolve in 4 to 10 days.

Diagnosis

Clinical symptoms and signs are nonspecific. Bacterial infections, allergic rhinorrhea, and other disorders also cause catarrhal upper respiratory tract symptoms and at their onset may be confused with primary coryza. Differentiation depends on the course of the symptoms. The presence of fever and more severe symptoms usually differentiates influenza. Leukocytosis indicates a disorder other than an uncomplicated common cold.

If exudate is present, a smear for microscopic examination is recommended, with attention given to the number of polymorphonuclear cells and the character of the bacteria. Eosinophilia in secretions suggests an allergic etiology. In the early phase of an epidemic of viral respiratory infections, nasopharyngeal washings or garglings should be sent to local public health or academic laboratories for specific virus identification and an acute phase serum specimen collected for serologic confirmation.

Prophylaxis

Immunity is type-specific. Effective experimental vaccines have been prepared for single types of rhinoviruses or myxoviruses, but the large number of types and strains of causative viruses has precluded production of a useful vaccine. Many other measures to prevent acquisition and spread of common colds have been tried, including polyvalent bacterial vaccines, alkalis, citrus fruits, vitamins, ultraviolet light, and glycol aerosols, but none has been unequivocally effective. In controlled trials, large (as much as 2 gm/day) prophylactic oral doses of vitamin C have not altered the frequency of acquisition of common rhinovirus colds or the amount of virus shedding, but some studies have shown a reduced duration of disability among persons who took as much as 8 gm/day on the first day of disease. Such persons might act as carriers, since the person's sense of well-being is enhanced but virus shedding is not reduced.

Large doses of exogenous human interferon and prophylactic administration of a chemical interferon inducer, N,N-dioctadecyl-N′N′-bis(2-hydroxyethyl) propanediamine, have shown protective and beneficial effects; however, biologic and logistic limitations prevent their practical use.

Treatment

A warm, comfortable environment and measures to avoid direct spread of infection are recommended for all persons. Rest at home is indicated for children, preadolescents, and all febrile patients. Though antipyretics and analgesics are commonly used, their benefit, except on fever, is doubtful. Under some conditions, aspirin can increase virus shedding while producing only slight symptomatic improvement and is therefore not recommended unless symptoms are severe enough to keep the patient at home in relative isolation.

To dry the nasal mucosa, atropine 0.25 mg orally t.i.d. or belladonna tincture 0.3 to 1 ml orally t.i.d. are sometimes useful. Oral phenylpropanolamine 15 to 50 mg, 0.5% phenylephrine or ephedrine nose drops or spray, or a nasal inhaler (not more often than q 3 or 4 h) can provide temporary nasal decongestion. Steam inhalations will relieve chest tightness. If necessary, cough syrups (especially those containing codeine; e.g., terpin hydrate and codeine 5 to 10 ml orally q 3 to 4 h) can be used to control coughing; an expectorant (e.g., iodinated glycerol 60 mg orally q.i.d. or potassium iodide saturated solution 300 to 600 mg [0.3 to 0.6 ml] orally q 2 h) may help. In persons with nasal allergy, antihistamines may reduce rhinorrhea, but they are of no use in other people. Ascorbic acid or high doses of citrus juices are popular, mostly on lay recommendation; no adequate scientific data confirm any benefit. Antibiotics do not affect viruses and are *not recommended* unless a specific bacterial complication develops.

RESPIRATORY SYNCYTIAL VIRUS (RSV) (See Vol. II, Ch. 24)

INFLUENZA (Grippe; Grip; "Flu")

A specific acute viral respiratory disease characterized by fever, coryza, cough, headache, malaise, and inflamed respiratory mucous membranes. It usually occurs as an epidemic in the winter. Prostration, hemorrhagic bronchitis, pneumonia, and sometimes death occur in severe cases.

Etiology

Influenza is caused by myxoviruses. These are RNA viruses 80 to 120 nm in size with a core of helical nucleic acid and a soluble nucleoprotein (NP or S) antigen. On the basis of the reaction of this antigen with specific antibody in a CF test, influenza viruses are classified into Types A, B, and C. The virion has a limiting membrane and is enveloped in a coat composed principally of 2 glycoproteins, one having hemagglutinating activity (HA) and one having enzymatic activity as a neuramini-dase (NA), which are the strain-specific antigens. Myxoviruses require a specific glycoprotein receptor site on the cell surface for attachment by the hemagglutinin. The virus is then engulfed, its envelope fuses with the vacuolar membrane, and the viral genetic material enters the cell. After intracellular replication of the viral components, the virus is assembled at the cell surface and is released from the cell by a budding process in which the viral NA participates.

Different serotypes of influenza A viruses are numbered H_0N_1, H_1N_1, H_2N_2, and H_3N_2 according to the major surface antigens of strains that have caused epidemics of disease in humans since the virus was first isolated in 1933. Currently both H_3N_2 and H_1N_1 types are causing prevalent disease. Usually only the most recent serotype causes epidemics, but strains can recycle after several years of absence, probably by genetic reconstitution of infectious viruses, rather than reemergence from a reservoir. Influenza B viruses show strain-specific variations, but the cross-relationship among strains is much greater than with influenza A. Specific numbers are not assigned to the Type B surface antigens. Influenza C is not a prevalent virus, and serotypes, if they occur, are not defined.

Epidemiology

Influenza A virus is the most frequent single cause of clinical influenza, which is also caused by influenza B, paramyxo-, and sometimes rhino- or echoviruses. Spread is by person-to-person con-tact and airborne droplet spray contaminates articles with viruses and may infect people. Infection produces sporadic respiratory illness every year. Acute epidemics occur about every 3 yr, generally nationwide during late fall or early winter. A major shift in the prevalent antigenic type of influenza A virus has occurred about once in a decade, resulting in an acute pandemic. Persons of all ages are afflicted, but prevalence is highest in school children, and severity is greatest in the very young, aged, or infirm. Persons at high risk of developing severe disease are those with chronic pulmonary diseases; those with valvular heart disease with or without congestive heart failure, or other heart disease with pulmonary edema; pregnant women in the 3rd trimester; and persons who are aged, very young, or confined to bed. Influenza B, but not influenza C, has infrequently caused equally severe disease.

Epidemics often occur in 2 waves—the first in students and active family members, the second mostly in shut-ins and persons in semi-closed institutions. Influenza B causes epidemics about every 5 yr and is much less often associated with pandemics. Influenza C is an endemic virus that sporadi-cally causes mild respiratory disease.

Symptoms and Signs

During the 48-h incubation period, transient asymptomatic viremia may occur before infection localizes in the respiratory tract. Influenza A or B is sudden in onset, with chilliness and fever up to 39 to 39.5 C (102 to 103 F) developing over 24 h. Prostration and generalized aches and pains (most pronounced in the back and legs) appear early. Headache is prominent, often with photophobia and retrobulbar aching. Respiratory tract symptoms may be mild at first, with sore throat, substernal burning, nonproductive cough, and sometimes coryza; later the respiratory disease becomes domi-nant. Cough can be severe and productive. The skin, especially on the face, is warm and flushed. The soft palate, posterior hard palate, tonsillar pillars, and posterior pharyngeal wall may be red-dened, but there is no exudate. The eyes water easily and the conjunctiva may be mildly inflamed. Usually, after 2 to 3 days acute symptoms subside rapidly and fever ends, though fever lasting up to 5 days may occur without complications. Abnormal bronchociliary clearance and altered bronchiolar air flow are regularly present. Weakness, sweating, and fatigue may persist for several days or occa-sionally for weeks.

In severe cases, hemorrhagic bronchitis and pneumonia are frequent and can develop within hours. Fulminant fatal viral pneumonia occasionally occurs; dyspnea, cyanosis, hemoptysis, pulmo-nary edema, and death may proceed as soon as 48 h after onset of the influenza. Such severe disease is most likely to occur during a pandemic caused by a new influenza A serotype and in persons at high risk.

Complications

Secondary bacterial infection of the bronchi and sometimes pneumonia are suggested by persis-tence of fever, cough, and other respiratory symptoms for more than 5 days. Pneumonia should be suspected if dyspnea, cyanosis, hemoptysis, rales, a secondary rise in temperature, or a relapse develops. With pneumonia, cough increases and purulent or bloody sputum is produced. Crepitant or subcrepitant rales can be detected over the involved pulmonary segments. The bacterial etiology of this secondary pneumonia is related to age and environment. Pneumococci, streptococci, and Hemophilus influenzae are common causes, especially in ambulatory nonhospitalized or young pa-tients. Pneumococci, staphylococci, and Klebsiella pneumoniae are the most common causes in older, infirm, or hospitalized patients. (See also Ch. 38.)

Encephalitis, myocarditis, and myoglobinuria may also occur as complications of influenza, usu-ally during convalescence. The virus is rarely recovered from affected organs and the specific rela-tionship and pathogenesis of these diseases cannot be positively established. However, an increase in such diseases regularly follows influenza A pandemics. Reye's syndrome (see also Vol. II, Ch. 24), characterized by encephalitis, hepatitis, and lipidemia, has been prominently associated with epi-demics of influenza B.

Diagnosis

Clinical influenza is an experience of people universally and a frequently made lay diagnosis. The specific disease cannot be diagnosed clinically except during epidemics. In the early stages of infection or in uncomplicated cases, chest examination is usually normal. In mild cases, the symptoms are those of a febrile or afebrile common cold. Pulmonary symptoms may be those of bronchitis or atypical pneumonia, especially during epidemics. In distinguishing influenza from other respiratory tract infections, one should consider the season and whether an influenza epidemic is in progress; the mode of onset and severity of symptoms; and the presence or absence of a tonsillar or pharyngeal exudate, other signs of localized infection, or evidence of suppurative disease. The leukocyte count is normal in uncomplicated cases; sometimes a leukopenia with a relative lymphocytosis may be present. Fever and severe constitutional symptoms differentiate influenza from the common cold. An exudate is often present over the tonsils and pharyngeal wall in hemolytic streptococcal tonsillitis and sometimes with adenoviral infection, but not in influenza. Petechiae or ulcers on the palate might signify infectious mononucleosis or a herpes or coxsackie viral infection.

A **specific diagnosis** of influenza can be made by virus isolation or serologic tests. During the first several days, the virus can be recovered from respiratory secretions. The specimen can be collected as sputum, but more often throat washings are obtained by gargling a buffered saline solution, usually with a small amount of protein such as albumin or gelatin; if necessary, diluted skim milk can be used. The recently prevalent strains of influenza virus have not been difficult to isolate either in tissue cultures or embryonated eggs. During epidemics, it is important to isolate and identify influenza viruses early. For this purpose, State Health Laboratories and, through them, the National Center for Disease Control and International Influenza Reference Centers assist in strain identification.

Serologic tests used are predominantly CF and HI tests. Serial serum specimens are best, the first collected at the onset of illness and another a week or more later. The 2 specimens are tested simultaneously to demonstrate a rise in the specific antibody titer. If only a single serum specimen is available after the disease is already well developed, a high CF antibody titer may indicate recent infection; the HI titer may reflect previous infection or vaccination.

Leukocytosis, with young granulocytes in the blood smear, is a valuable diagnostic sign of complicating bacterial pneumonia. Purulent sputum should be smeared, gram-stained, and examined for leukocytes and bacteria. Appropriate sputum and blood cultures and other examinations should be made to identify the specific bacterial species and to determine the extent of secondary infection.

Prognosis

Recovery is the rule in uncomplicated influenza. However, viral pneumonia and other virus-related complications may cause death in some patients, especially those identified above as being at high risk. Chemotherapy decreases the fatality rate of severe secondary bacterial pneumonia.

Prophylaxis

Vaccines that include the prevalent strains of influenza viruses effectively reduce the incidence of infection among vaccinees for 1 or 2 yr after vaccination. The immunity is less when appreciable antigenic drift occurs in the virus, and when a major antigenic mutation occurs no significant protection is afforded unless the new strain is incorporated into the vaccine. Vaccine is prepared as inactivated whole virus or as subunits of the virus, either semi-purified viral hemagglutinin or disrupted virion components. Both types of vaccine are equally protective. Under development are new attenuated live virus vaccines given intranasally. They have the advantage of eliciting specific secretory antibody at the portal of virus entry.

Vaccination is especially important for the aged and for patients with cardiac, pulmonary, or other chronic diseases. Pregnant women expected to deliver during the winter months should be vaccinated also. Immunization, preferably in the fall, usually consists of 1 dose of vaccine, but when new strains arise primary immunization should consist of 2 injections of vaccine containing the new strains, given 1 mo apart. About 2 wk is required for immunity to develop after vaccination. Because immunity from vaccination lasts only 1 or 2 yr, an annual booster dose early in the fall is required for optimal protection. Primary or booster doses are 0.5 to 1 ml s.c. or IM. With the presently available purified vaccines, local or constitutional reactions are uncommon or minor, except sometimes in children.

Amantadine 100 mg orally b.i.d. (for adults) can be used prophylactically against influenza A. It is ineffective against influenza B. During influenza A epidemics, it should be given to family members and other close contacts of patients and to persons at high risk. Persons at high risk of infection who have not been vaccinated previously should receive vaccine during the period of administration of amantadine. Amantadine may be discontinued in 3 wk, or, if vaccine cannot be given, amantadine must be continued for the duration of the epidemic, usually 6 or 8 wk. In some persons amantidine causes nervousness or insomnia.

Influenza renders the patient temporarily immune to reinfection with the same virus serotype and incompletely immune to variants from antigenic drift; it has no effect on other strains of influenza virus.

Treatment

Amantadine has a beneficial effect on fever and respiratory symptoms if given early in uncomplicated influenza A. It has no clinical benefit when used for pneumonia, but might improve the recovery of pulmonary function. The basic treatment otherwise is symptomatic. The patient should remain in bed or rest adequately and avoid exertion during the acute stage and for 24 to 48 h after the temperature becomes normal. If constitutional symptoms of acute uncomplicated influenza are severe, antipyretics and analgesics (e.g., aspirin 600 mg, alone or with codeine 15 to 30 mg, orally q 4 h) are helpful. To relieve nasal obstruction, 1 or 2 drops of 0.25% phenylephrine may be instilled into the nose periodically. Gargles of warm isotonic saline are useful for sore throat. Steam inhalation may alleviate respiratory symptoms somewhat and also prevent drying of secretions. Treatment of respiratory symptoms may be unnecessary in less severe cases. A codeine cough mixture (e.g., terpin hydrate and codeine 5 to 10 ml orally q 3 to 4 h) may be indicated during some stages of the disease. Complicating bacterial infections require appropriate antibiotics.

PARAINFLUENZA VIRUSES

A group of viruses causing a number of respiratory illnesses varying from the common cold to influenza-like pneumonia, with febrile croup as their most common manifestation.

Etiology

The parainfluenza viruses are RNA paramyxoviruses and consist of 4 serologically distinct agents categorized as Types 1, 2, 3, and 4. Early human isolates of parainfluenza Types 1 and 3 were called "hemadsorption (HA) viruses." The initial Type 2 isolates were designated "croup-associated (CA) viruses." Though the 4 types tend to cause diseases of different severity, they share common antigens, as evidenced by cross-reactive antibody responses, and are similar structurally and biologically. Type 4 has antigenic cross-reactivity with mumps. Though each type of parainfluenza virus has a corresponding serotype that causes specific diseases in animals, cross-infection of animals to man or vice versa either does not occur or the transfer is very inefficient. The corresponding strains of animal origin for Types 1, 2, and 3 are Sendai virus (mice), Simian virus 5 (SV-5), and shipping fever virus of cattle (SF-4).

Epidemiology

Infections with Types 1 and 3 are common in early childhood; sharp localized outbreaks occur in nurseries, schools, pediatric wards, and orphanages. Widespread community epidemics are prevented by almost universal immunity in adults. Infection with each type produces different epidemiologic patterns. Parainfluenza infections occur in all seasons, but epidemic disease in the fall is more likely to be due to Type 1, which comprises ½ of the isolates. The epidemic types, 1 and 2, tend to recur reciprocally every other year. Type 3 disease is endemic, highly contagious, occurs in all seasons, and causes ⅓ of the infections. The incubation period is usually 24 to 48 h with Type 3, and 4 to 5 days with Type 1. Type 2 is more sporadic and causes modest epidemics of infantile croup (acute laryngotracheobronchitis). The parainfluenza viruses are a chief cause of this condition. Type 4 causes mild respiratory illness, but only rarely.

Second and even third infections with the same strains of virus, particularly with Types 1 and 3, are not uncommon, though the partial immunity developed during previous episodes may reduce the spread and severity of subsequent infections.

Symptoms and Signs

The most common illness produced in children is an acute febrile respiratory infection that is clinically indistinguishable from influenza or other respiratory virus infection occurring in the same age group. Onset is marked by fever and moderate coryza. The degree of malaise is directly related to the height of the fever. In many cases, the temperature does not exceed 38 or 39 C (101 or 102 F); in others, it may peak several times to 40 C (104 F). Moderate sore throat and a dry cough usually develop early in the disease. Hoarseness and croup are prominent symptoms in many cases; this **acute laryngotracheobronchitis** (see Croup in Vol. II, Ch. 24) is the most severe and dangerous manifestation of parainfluenza virus infections in children.

Fever may subside promptly or continue for 2 or 3 days. In some patients, particularly those who develop lower respiratory tract involvement, fever lasting a week or more may recur one or more times.

Bronchitis and "walking" pneumonia often develop during or after the initial acute episode in children and sometimes adults infected with Type 3. Pneumonia is detected by auscultation that reveals moist rales in one or more lung areas, or by chest x-ray. Bacterial complications are not common.

Diagnosis

A specific diagnosis of parainfluenza infection cannot be made clinically. Virus isolation and identification require tissue culture inoculation. CF, HI, and hemadsorption-neutralization tests with acute and convalescent sera will confirm a parainfluenza infection but serologic cross-reactions can make it difficult to identify the specific parainfluenza virus without a viral isolate.

Prognosis

Except for infantile croup, illnesses due to the parainfluenza viruses, although frequent, are usually mild, self-limited, and of brief duration. The bronchitis and pneumonia associated with Type 3 infections seldom cause serious disability and are rarely, if ever, fatal.

Prophylaxis and Treatment

No effective vaccine is available and there is no specific therapy. Rest and a comfortable environment are the best remedies. Aspirin is not recommended unless the fever is high or the symptoms prevent sleep. If necessary, antitussives (e.g., codeine 1 to 1.5 mg/kg/day orally in 6 divided doses) will suppress cough. For treatment of croup, see that discussion in Vol. II, Ch. 24.

ADENOVIRUSES

A group of viruses causing a variety of acute febrile disorders characterized by inflammation of the respiratory and ocular mucous membranes and hyperplasia of submucous and regional lymphoid tissue.

Etiology

Adenoviruses are DNA viruses 60 to 90 nm in size. The virion is shaped like an icosahedron. Three major antigens can be directly related to the capsid structures. Most important is the hexon, a 6-sided capsomere comprising 240 of the 252 capsomeres. It reacts with specific antisera in a non-type-specific CF reaction and thus serves as a group antigen to identify all types of adenoviruses. However, virus-neutralizing antibody is type-specific. The 2nd major antigen is associated with a penton, a 5-sided capsomere located at the 12 common vertices of the 20 triangles that form the icosahedron. It is a type-specific antigen that can be differentiated in neutralization or HI tests. The 3rd antigen is a fiber antigen related to the threadlike structure extending from the apices of the virion. Not infrequently, adenoviruses have another smaller DNA virus associated with them, called **adenoassociated virus (AAV).** It is a defective virus that requires complementation by adenovirus in order to replicate. The importance of AAV in adenovirus infections is not known.

Epidemiology

About 4 to 5% of clinically recognized respiratory illnesses in civilian populations are caused by adenoviruses. Of the 33 known serotypes, only a few have been adequately observed in relation to human disease to determine their prevalence and ability to produce illness (see Table 12–3). **Different serotypes have quite different epidemiologies:** Types 1, 2, and 5 cause sharp, limited outbreaks of respiratory or enteric illness during the first few months or years of life. Type 2 has been relatively more common in some of these episodes. In older children and adults, Type 3 causes a characteristic syndrome of acute pharyngoconjunctival fever **(APC),** especially among patrons of summer camps and swimming pools. Acute respiratory disease **(ARD)** occurs in military camps and is caused by Types 4, 7, 14, and 21. In some countries, ARD epidemics have also been apparent among civilian populations, but not in the USA. Epidemic keratoconjunctivitis **(EKC)** is caused by one of several types and is seen largely in industrial plants and eye clinics.

Adenoviruses also infect the intestinal tract, usually without causing symptoms, although enteritis, mesenteric adenitis, and intussusception can occur. Following infection with Types 1, 2, and 5, the virus may remain latent in the tonsils and adenoids; about 80% of excised tonsils yield such virus.

The ratio of manifest disease to infection rates varies with the different syndromes and serotypes and according to the season when infected. In winter, infection of military recruits with adenovirus Types 4 or 7 causes recognizable illness in most cases and about 25% require hospitalization for fever and lower respiratory tract disease. APC occurs in a high proportion of Type 3 infections in the summer. The ratio of illness to infection is lower with Types 1, 2, 5, and some of the less studied, higher numbered adenoviruses.

Pathology

Adenoviral infections are rarely fatal and have few, if any, recognizable long-term pathologic effects. Some deaths have occurred with giant-cell pneumonia associated with adenovirus Types 3, 4, or 7. Autopsies have disclosed microscopically an extensive and unique inclusion body pneumonia, the intranuclear inclusions appearing to be similar to those considered characteristic of adenoviral cellular invasions in tissue cultures. Biopsies of superficial lesions produced by adenoviruses in conjunctival and pharyngeal mucosa show capillary dilation, occasional submucous hemorrhage, and mononuclear leukocyte infiltration, but no intranuclear inclusions. The conjunctivitis caused by the common respiratory types of adenoviruses is benign, but keratoconjunctivitis caused by Type 8 can produce corneal opacities and impaired vision.

Symptoms and Signs

Acute febrile respiratory disease is the usual manifestation of known adenoviral infection in children. Adenoviruses Types 1, 2, 3, 5, and 6 have been isolated most commonly, though infection with these types is often not directly associated with any specific illness. Infection is airborne or waterborne (by swimming), or acquired by direct contact. The incubation period is 2 to 5 days. In a typical outbreak confined to a household or nursery, some affected children have fever only, without localizing signs; others have fever and pharyngitis; others have fever with pharyngitis, tracheitis, and bronchitis, a moderately persistent nonproductive cough, and, rarely, pneumonia. Cough with adenoviral pneumonia has been confused with pertussis in children. Pharyngeal lymphoid hypertrophy sometimes persists and leads to eustachian tube obstruction and possibly otitis media. Regional lymph nodes are frequently enlarged and sometimes tender, but they never suppurate. Laboratory findings are generally within normal limits, though some children may show a lymphocytosis.

TABLE 12-3. SYNDROMES CAUSED BY ADENOVIRUSES

Disease	Serotypes Implicated		Comments
	Common	Less Common	
Respiratory only: Acute febrile respiratory disease of children	1, 2, 3, 5, 6	Other types	Probably the most frequent manifestation of adenoviruses; Types 1, 2, & 5 endemic; Type 3 occasionally epidemic; more prevalent during cold months
Acute respiratory disease (ARD)	4, 7	14, 21	Epidemic in military recruits; sporadic in adult civilians; Types 4 & 7 infections rare in children
Viral pneumonia: Infants	7	1, 3	Rare; occurs in hospital nurseries; may be fatal; similar to Goodpasture's inclusion body pneumonitis
Adults	4, 7	3	Predominantly associated with acute respiratory disease; cold agglutinins not developed
Ocular only: Acute follicular conjunctivitis	3, 7	2, 6, 9, 10, 21	Sporadic; adults chiefly affected; in children, usually associated with respiratory & systemic effects
Epidemic kerato-conjunctivitis (EKC)	8 (classic)	3, 7 (mild)	Epidemic; adults mainly affected; widespread in Japan, rare in USA
Combined respiratory & ocular: Acute pharyngo-conjunctival fever (APC)	3, 7	1, 2, 5, 6, 14, 21	Epidemic in children; sporadic in adults; summer epidemics frequently associated with swimming in pools or lakes

A disease syndrome designated **ARD (acute respiratory disease)** is observed in military recruits during periods of mobilization. Adenovirus Types 4 and 7 have been reported in most outbreaks in the USA, but Types 14 and 21 have also been incriminated. ARD is marked by malaise, fever, chills, and headache. Respiratory manifestations include nasopharyngitis, hoarseness, and dry cough. The disease may resemble streptococcal pharyngitis with exudate on the faucial pillars and posterior pharyngeal wall. Cervical adenopathy is present, but the nodes are not as tender as in streptococcal pharyngitis. Viremia and viruria may occur and there may be a fine erythematous macular rash on the body, but the viruria occurring with these respiratory strains of adenoviruses does not produce symptoms like those of the epidemic hemorrhagic cystitis that occurs as a primary disease with Type 11. Physical signs are minimal except in about 10% of patients, who develop rales and x-ray evidence of pneumonia. Fever usually subsides within 2 to 4 days; convalescence, while uneventful, may require another 10 to 14 days.

Viral pneumonia of infants, due chiefly to Type 7, is a rare but specific clinicopathologic entity. Small outbreaks have occurred in France, the USA, and Japan, with fatalities due to extensive pneumonia. Onset is sudden, affecting infants in the first few days or weeks of life, with high fever and rapid upper and lower respiratory tract involvement. The pneumonia is lobular but may be so extensive as to suggest lobar pneumonia. Several fatal cases developed a maculopapular rash and encephalitis, with focal necrosis apparent in the brain, skin, and lungs.

Acute pharyngoconjunctival fever (APC) produces the clinical triad of fever, pharyngitis, and conjunctivitis. Infection is sometimes waterborne. The incubation period is 5 to 8 days. Adenovirus Types 3 and 7 have been reported in nearly all outbreaks. In a typical outbreak, 50% or more of the patients have all 3 components, while others may have only 1 or 2. The conjunctivitis is initially unilateral and sometimes painful. Involvement of the lower respiratory tract may occur in addition to pharyngitis. The illness usually subsides within a week, but follicular conjunctivitis may persist for another week.

Conjunctivitis without constitutional symptoms appears to be a rather common manifestation of infection with several different adenovirus serotypes. It occurs most often in young adults, chiefly parents of children with APC, and is self-limited and benign. Onset is sudden and usually unilateral. Symptoms and signs include a foreign-body sensation in the eye, lacrimation, and focal erythema of the palpebral and bulbar conjunctiva. The discharge is mucoid but not purulent. The other eye is subsequently involved in about half the patients, usually less severely. Persistent follicular enlargement of submucous lymphoid tissue under the palpebral conjunctiva, even resembling early trachoma, may be seen about 2 to 4 days after onset. Preauricular and posterior cervical lymphadenopathy, more prominent on the same side as the more involved eye, is usual. A mild sore throat occasionally develops, often on the same side as the affected eye. The course is usually mild, though focal conjunctival hemorrhages and extensive periorbital edema occasionally occur.

Epidemic keratoconjunctivitis (EKC) is a specific, sometimes severe, epidemic disease caused by adenovirus, especially Type 8. Observed for many years in Japan, it became epidemic in the USA during World War II, chiefly among shipyard workers on both coasts. It has occurred only sporadically in this country since then, but widespread epidemics have occurred in Europe and Asia. Onset is sudden, one eye showing redness and chemosis followed by periorbital swelling, preauricular lymphadenopathy, and superficial corneal opacities. Unlike herpetic keratitis, it does not result in corneal ulceration; local pain like that from foreign-body irritation is usual, however. The other eye may become involved within a week. Systemic symptoms and signs are mild or absent. The illness usually lasts 3 to 4 wk, though opacities may persist much longer and vision has sometimes been permanently impaired.

Mild, transient corneal involvement has been observed in eye infections (e.g., APC) with other adenoviruses (Types 3 and 7), but the opacities are seldom noticeable except to an ophthalmologist.

Diagnosis

Clinical identification of adenoviral infection is only presumptive, except in typical APC, EKC, and ARD in military recruits; in these conditions the clinical or epidemiologic characteristics, or both, are unique. During the acute stages of adenoviral illnesses, the virus can be isolated from respiratory and ocular secretions, and frequently from feces and urine. Several serologic procedures (CF, HI, and neutralization tests) can be performed on acute and convalescent sera. A 4-fold rise in the serum antibody titer indicates recent adenoviral infection. The CF test is group-specific for any adenovirus serotype. HI and neutralization tests are type-specific. Commercial antigen is available for the CF test but not for the latter 2 tests.

Prognosis

Adenoviral infections are generally benign and of relatively short duration. Except for rare cases of fulminating primary pneumonia in young infants, even severe adenoviral pneumonia is not fatal.

Prophylaxis

Live Type 4 and 7 adenovirus vaccine, given orally in an enteric-coated capsule, has caused a marked reduction in ARD in military populations. Spread of the vaccine virus to family members can occur, but it is of no importance under the conditions of military use. The live oral vaccine is neither recommended nor available for civilian use. Vaccines for other serotypes have not been developed.

Treatment

Treatment is symptomatic and supportive. Bed rest at home or infirmary care may be required during the acute febrile period. Aspirin is not recommended unless headache and malaise are distressing; analgesics such as codeine are rarely necessary. Severe pneumonia in infants and EKC require early hospitalization and close supervision to prevent death in the former and permanently impaired vision in the latter. Topical corticosteroids relieve symptoms and shorten the course of EKC and adenoviral conjunctivitis. Such therapy is dangerous in ulcerative corneal conditions, however, and should always be supervised by an ophthalmologist.

HERPES VIRUSES

HERPES SIMPLEX (Fever Blister; Cold Sore)

A recurrent viral infection characterized by the appearance on the skin or mucous membranes of single or multiple clusters of small vesicles, filled with clear fluid, on slightly raised inflammatory bases.

Etiology

The infecting agent is the relatively large herpes simplex virus (herpesvirus hominis, **HVH**). There are 2 HVH strains. Type 1 commonly causes herpes labialis and keratitis; Type 2 is usually genital and is transmitted primarily by direct contact with lesions, most often venereally. The time of initial HVH infection is usually obscure, except in the primary systemic infection that is occasionally seen in infants (see NEONATAL HERPES SIMPLEX VIRUS INFECTION under NEONATAL INFECTIONS in Vol. II, Ch. 21) and is characterized by generalized or localized cutaneous and mucosal lesions accompanied by severe constitutional symptoms. Localized infections ordinarily occur more frequently in childhood, but may be delayed until adult life. Presumably, the virus remains dormant in the skin or nerve ganglia, and recurrent herpetic eruptions can be precipitated by overexposure to sunlight, febrile illnesses, physical or emotional stress, or certain foods and drugs. The trigger mechanism is often unknown.

Symptoms and Signs

The lesions may appear anywhere on the skin or mucosa, but are most frequent about the mouth, on the lips, on the conjunctiva and cornea, and on the genitalia. Following a short prodromal period of tingling discomfort or itching, small tense vesicles appear on an erythematous base. Single clusters vary in size from 0.5 to 1.5 cm, but several groups may coalesce. Herpes simplex on skin tensely attached to underlying structures (e.g., the nose, ears, or fingers) may be painful. The vesicles persist for a few days, then begin to dry, forming a thin yellowish crust. Healing usually begins 7 to 10 days after onset and is complete by 21 days. Healing may be slower, with secondary inflammation, in moist body areas. Individual herpetic lesions usually heal completely, but recurrent lesions at the same site may cause atrophy and scarring.

Variations and Complications

Genital herpes is discussed in Vol. II, Ch. 5, herpes simplex keratitis in Ch. 179, and primary and recurrent herpetic stomatitis and herpes labialis in ORAL HERPETIC MANIFESTATIONS in Ch. 208. Gingivostomatitis and vulvovaginitis may occur as a result of herpes infection in infants or young children. Symptoms include irritability, anorexia, fever, gingival inflammation, and painful ulcers of the mouth and occasionally of the vulva and vagina. In infants and sometimes in older children, primary infections may cause extensive organ involvement and fatal viremia. Women with Type 2 HVH infection late in pregnancy may transmit the infection to the fetus, with the development of severe viremia (see in NEONATAL INFECTIONS in Vol. II, Ch. 21). Herpes simplex is an occasional cause of severe encephalitis. Type 2 HVH has been associated with usually self-limited aseptic meningitis or lumbosacral myeloradiculitis syndromes. **Kaposi's varicelliform eruption (eczema herpeticum)** is a potentially fatal complication of infantile or adult atopic eczema; patients with extensive atopic dermatitis should **avoid** exposure to persons with active herpes simplex. Herpes simplex may be followed by typical erythema multiforme, but the relationship is uncertain because a variety of other infectious agents and drugs can induce an identical syndrome.

Diagnosis

Herpes simplex may be confused with herpes zoster, but the latter rarely recurs and usually causes more severe pain and larger groups of lesions that are distributed along the course of a sensory nerve. Differential diagnosis also includes varicella, genital ulcers or gingivostomatitis due to other causes, and vesicular dermatoses, particularly dermatitis herpetiformis and drug eruptions. When herpes simplex is suspected, cultures for the virus, a progressive increase in serum antibodies (in primary infections), and biopsy findings confirm the diagnosis.

Prophylaxis

Smallpox vaccinations may be dangerous and should not be done. Patients who find sunlight a precipitating factor should avoid overexposure and apply a topical sunscreen preparation (e.g., 3.5% digalloyl trioleate or 10% sulisobenzone lotion).

Treatment

No local or systemic chemotherapeutic agent is effective, with the possible exception of topical idoxuridine (**IDU**) in superficial herpetic keratitis. Reports on this compound in cutaneous herpes are conflicting. Topical treatment with acyclovir has also shown promise in experimental studies.

Gentle cleansing with soap and water is recommended, but keeping lesions moist may aggravate the inflammation and delay healing. Drying lotions or liquids (e.g., camphor spirit or 70% alcohol) may be applied to oozing skin lesions. In secondary infections, topical antibiotics (e.g., neomycin-bacitracin ointment) or, if severe, appropriate systemic antibiotics, are indicated. Topical treatment with neutral red dye and phototherapy (photoinactivation), and with topical ether or alcohol, has been suggested, but their efficacy appears to be nil. (CAUTION: *Corticosteroids, either topical or systemic, should not be used in ocular herpes simplex because the lesions may progress to hypopyon or corneal perforation.*)

In herpes simplex with systemic manifestations, vigorous supportive therapy (control of electrolyte balance, parenteral fluid, blood transfusions, and systemic antibiotics) may be necessary. Systemic treatment with vidarabine (adenine arabinoside) has been attempted in serious infections such as encephalitis or disseminated neonatal disease. Such therapy has been shown to be of benefit in herpes simplex encephalitis, if begun before the patient becomes comatose. Acyclovir, a new antiviral agent, has shown promise for the therapy of severe herpes infections, but is still undergoing investigational studies.

INFECTIOUS MONONUCLEOSIS (See Vol. II, Ch. 27)

CYTOMEGALOVIRUS (CMV) INFECTION (Cytomegalic Inclusion Disease) (See also CONGENITAL AND PERINATAL CYTOMEGALOVIRUS INFECTION under NEONATAL INFECTIONS in Vol. II, Ch. 21)

A virus infection occurring congenitally, postnatally, or at any age, and ranging in severity from a silent infection without consequences, through disease manifested by fever, hepatitis, and (in neo-

nates) severe brain damage, to stillbirth or perinatal death. The restrictive appellation "cytomegalic inclusion disease" refers to the intranuclear inclusions found in enlarged infected cells.

Etiology and Epidemiology

The human cytomegaloviruses ("salivary gland viruses") are a subgroup of agents closely related to the herpes group of viruses, which have the propensity for remaining latent in man. Cytomegaloviruses are highly host-specific and cannot be propagated in laboratory animals or in most nonhuman cell cultures.

The cytomegaloviruses are ubiquitous. Infected individuals may excrete virus in the urine or saliva for months; virus may be demonstrable in human cervical secretions, semen, feces, and milk; fresh blood from asymptomatic infected donors may produce disease in susceptible recipients. Infection may be acquired transplacentally, during birth, or by contact with infected secretions or excretions at any time thereafter. High infection rates may occur at early ages in closed populations such as orphanages. The incidence of infection gradually increases with age; 60 to 90% of adults have experienced infection. CMV disease in an immunologically impaired adult may be a newly acquired infection or an activation of a latent process.

Symptoms and Signs

Congenital infection: The extent of the pathologic process is highly variable. Most commonly, infection is manifested only by cytomegaloviruria in an otherwise apparently normal infant. At the other extreme, CMV infection may cause abortion, stillbirth, or postnatal death from hemorrhage, anemia, or extensive hepatic or CNS damage. Infants born with severe nonfatal disease typically have a low birth weight and develop fever, hepatitis with jaundice, and hemorrhagic manifestations such as purpura. Hepatosplenomegaly, thrombocytopenia, chorioretinitis, microcephaly, and periventricular cerebral calcification may be present. The prognosis must be guarded in overt cases because psychomotor retardation, spastic diplegia, blindness, deafness, or seizures may develop. Infants with inapparent infections may later manifest hearing defects.

Acquired infection: Infections acquired postnatally or later in life are often asymptomatic. An acute febrile illness, termed **cytomegalovirus mononucleosis** or **cytomegalovirus hepatitis**, may result from iatrogenic or spontaneous contact with CMV. **Postperfusion syndrome** develops 2 to 4 wk after transfusion with fresh blood containing CMV and is characterized by fever lasting 2 to 3 wk, hepatitis of variable degree with or without jaundice, a characteristic atypical lymphocytosis resembling that of infectious mononucleosis, and occasionally a rash. CMV infection in patients with malignancy or receiving immunosuppressive therapy may cause pulmonary, GI, or renal involvement. This complication is of major import, with a 50% attack rate and high associated mortality in some reported transplantation series.

Diagnosis

CMV may be isolated from urine or other body fluids by inoculation of human fibroblastic cell cultures. However, CMV may be excreted for months or years after infection and cytomegaloviruria must be interpreted accordingly. The appearance of specific CF antibodies during illness provides supportive evidence. Morphologic demonstration of infected cells in urine is of limited value.

Congenital infection must be differentiated from bacterial, viral (e.g., rubella), and protozoan (e.g., toxoplasmosis) infections. Acquired infection must be differentiated from viral hepatitis and infectious mononucleosis. The absence of pharyngitis or lymphadenopathy, and a negative heterophil antibody test, are helpful in ruling out infectious mononucleosis.

Treatment

There is no specific therapy. Trials of drugs that interfere with viral DNA synthesis (floxuridine, cytarabine, and others) have not yielded clear-cut results.

ENTEROVIRAL DISEASES

(See Vol. II, Ch. 24)

CENTRAL NERVOUS SYSTEM VIRAL DISEASES

(See also Ch. 124)

POLIOMYELITIS (See Vol. II, Ch. 24)

MUMPS (See Vol. II, Ch. 24)

RABIES (Hydrophobia)

An acute infectious disease of mammals, especially carnivores, characterized by CNS irritation followed by paralysis and death.

Etiology and Epidemiology

The etiologic agent is a neurotropic virus often present in the saliva of rabid animals. The use of monoclonal antibodies has recently revealed that rabies virus, previously thought to be stable, is as unstable in tissue culture as is the influenza virus. Several serotypes have been defined in the laboratory and from street isolates collected from different parts of the world. These serologic differences may account for occasional vaccine failures. The ability to identify distinct virus serotypes is expected to provide new information of value in epidemiology and vaccine production.

Rabid animals transmit the infection by biting animals or humans. Rabies may also be acquired by exposure of a mucous membrane or fresh skin abrasion to infected saliva. Four cases of apparent respiratory infection have been reported, 2 following laboratory exposure and 2 from the atmosphere of a cave infested by millions of guano bats. Worldwide, rabid dogs still present the highest risk to man. In the USA, where vaccination has largely controlled canine rabies, bites of infected wild animals have caused most cases of human rabies since 1960.

Infected dogs may have either **furious rabies**, characterized by agitation and viciousness, followed by paralysis and death; or **dumb rabies**, in which paralytic symptoms predominate. Rabid wild animals may show "furious" behavior, but less obvious changes (diurnal activity of normally nocturnal bats, skunks, and foxes; lack of normal fear of humans) are more likely.

Pathology

The virus has an affinity for nervous tissue. It travels from the site of entry via peripheral nerves to the spinal cord and the brain, where it multiplies; subsequently it continues through efferent nerves to the salivary glands and into the saliva. Postmortem examination shows vessel engorgement and associated punctate hemorrhages in the meninges and brain; microscopic examination shows perivascular collections of lymphocytes but little destruction of nerve cells. The presence of intracytoplasmic inclusion bodies **(Negri bodies)**, usually in the cornu Ammonis, is pathognomonic of rabies, but these are not always found.

Symptoms and Signs

In man, the incubation period varies from 10 days to > 1 yr (average, 30 to 50 days). It is usually shortest in patients with extensive bites or bites about the head or trunk. The disease commonly begins with a short period of mental depression, restlessness, malaise, and fever. Restlessness increases to uncontrollable excitement, with excessive salivation and excruciatingly painful spasms of the laryngeal and pharyngeal muscles. The spasms, which result from reflex irritability of the deglutition and respiration centers, are easily precipitated—e.g., by a slight breeze or an attempt to drink water. As a result, the patient cannot drink, though his thirst is great (hence, "hydrophobia"). Death from asphyxia, exhaustion, or general paralysis formerly occurred within 3 to 10 days, but with modern supportive care patients may survive much longer.

Diagnosis

The fluorescent antibody test and virus isolation have replaced examination of the animal's brain for Negri bodies as the preferred method of diagnosis. An asymptomatic dog or cat that bites a human should, when practicable, be confined and observed by a veterinarian for 10 days. If the animal remains healthy, it can be safely concluded that it was not infectious at the time of the bite. When the biting animal was apparently rabid or was a wild animal (i.e., whenever a biting animal must be proved uninfected to avoid human treatment), it should be killed immediately and the brain submitted to a diagnostic laboratory for fluorescent antibody testing.

In patients, diagnosis is suggested by a history of a compatible animal bite (infrequently absent) and confirmed by viral testing once the characteristic clinical symptoms appear. The diagnosis should be considered in cases with severe, progressive encephalitis or ascending paralysis with encephalitis. Hysteria due to fright may follow a bite and give the impression of rabies, but the symptoms should subside promptly once the patient is assured that he is in no immediate danger and can be protected from rabies.

Control

The prevention and control of rabies require restraint of dogs by their owners and impoundment of stray dogs. Immunizing 70% or more of the canine population has effectively restricted transmission of the disease, even in areas where rabies is endemic among wildlife.

Controlling rabies in wildlife reservoirs is more difficult, especially when the wildlife host population is dense. Locally, rabies becomes self-limiting because it decimates susceptible hosts until epidemic disease can no longer be propagated. Adequate systematic reductions of host species yield the same result and prevent spread; however, these expensive control efforts are best limited to locales where human contact with wildlife is high (e.g., campgrounds).

Prophylaxis

Postexposure: Rabies rarely occurs in man if proper local and systemic prophylaxis is carried out immediately after exposure. **Local wound treatment** may be the most valuable preventive measure. The contaminated area should be cleansed immediately and thoroughly with a 20% solution of medicinal soft soap. Deep puncture wounds should be flushed, using a catheter and soapy water. Cauterizing or suturing the wound is not advised.

Systemic postexposure prophylaxis (see TABLE 12–4) should be started immediately (1) if the animal is rabid or develops rabies during confinement or (2) if a domestic animal that is not available for observation or examination was behaving in an atypical manner or its biting was unprovoked *and* there is rabies in the area. Among wild animals, skunks, raccoons, foxes, and bats are particularly suspect and, unless proved uninfected by examination, their bites generally necessitate rabies treatment. Rabbits and rodents (including squirrels, chipmunks, rats, and mice) are rarely infected and their bites seldom justify rabies treatment. State or local health departments may be consulted on these decisions.

Administration of rabies immune globulin or antirabies serum for **passive immunization** followed by vaccine for **active immunization** gives the best specific postexposure prophylaxis. Both passive and active immunizing products should be used concurrently. The preferred products are human rabies immune globulin **(RIG)** for passive immunization with human diploid cell rabies vaccine **(HDCV)** for active immunization. If these products are unavailable, antirabies serum **(ARS)** of equine origin may be substituted for RIG and duck embryo vaccine **(DEV)** may be substituted for HDCV. For **passive immunization,** RIG is given only once—at the beginning of antirabies prophylaxis. The recommended dose is 20 IU/kg. If possible, up to ½ of the total dose is infiltrated around the wound; the remainder is given IM. If ARS is used, 40 u./kg is given in the same manner.

Active immunization with HDCV or DEV should also begin immediately. HDCV is given in a series of five 1-ml IM injections (e.g., in the deltoid area) beginning on the day of exposure, followed by injections on days 3, 7, 14, and 28. Serum collected 2 to 3 wk after the 5th injection should be tested (through arrangement with the state health department) for antibody response; if the response is inadequate, a 1-ml booster injection should be given. Alternatively, the World Health Organization recommends that a 6th injection be given 90 days after the 1st injection. HDCV has replaced DEV as the vaccine of choice for postexposure prophylaxis because HDCV produces a superior immune response and few adverse reactions; local reactions at the injection site are usually minor, and systemic reactions are rare. Prophylaxis should not be interrupted because of minor adverse reac-

TABLE 12–4. POSTEXPOSURE ANTIRABIES GUIDE

The following guide should be used in conjunction with knowledge of the animal species involved, circumstances of the bite or other exposure, vaccination status of the animal, and presence of rabies in the region. Advice from local or state public health officials may be sought to help determine the need for prophylaxis.

Animal and Its Condition		Treatment of Exposed Human*
Species	Condition at Time of Attack	

Wild
  Skunk, Fox, Coyote,
  Raccoon, Bat, other
  wild carnivore
	Regard as rabid	RIG + HDCV†‡

Domestic Dog, Cat	Healthy (and available for observation)	None§
	Escaped (unknown)	RIG + HDCV†
	Rabid or suspected rabid	RIG + HDCV†

Others
  Including Livestock,
  Rodents, Rabbits
	Consider individually: Bites of rodents seldom require prophylaxis	

RIG = Human rabies immune globulin; HDCV = Human diploid cell vaccine; DEV = Duck embryo vaccine.

  * Clean bites with soap and water. For rabies prophylaxis, give both RIG and HDCV† immediately.
  † If HDCV is unavailable, use DEV.
  ‡ Discontinue vaccine if fluorescent antibody tests of animal killed at time of attack are negative.
  § Begin RIG + HDCV† at first sign of rabies in biting dog or cat during holding period (10 days).

Adapted from USPHS Advisory Committee on Immunization Practices (ACIP) Recommendations, *Morbidity and Mortality Weekly Report* Vol. 29, No. 23, 1980.

tions that can be managed with antihistamines, anti-inflammatory and antipyretic agents; for serious systemic or neuroparalytic reactions, consideration should be given to choosing an alternate vaccine or discontinuing vaccination. Individual assistance in each situation may be sought from the state health department or the Centers for Disease Control, Atlanta, GA 30333.

If HDCV is unavailable, DEV may be given s.c. either in one 1-ml injection/day for 21 days, or in two 1-ml injections/day for 7 days followed by one 1 ml/day for 7 days. The initial series in either regimen should be followed by 2 additional injections 10 and 20 days after the last infection. Serum collected at the time of the final injection should be tested for adequate antibodies and additional vaccine given if needed. Injection sites (preferably the lower abdomen, lower back, and lateral aspects of the thighs) should be rotated to minimize discomfort.

Preexposure: Because of the relative safety of HDCV and DEV, prophylactic vaccination of persons with a high occupational risk of exposure to rabid animals is well justified. HDCV is preferred and is given in the deltoid area in a series of three 1-ml IM injections, with the 2nd injection 7 days after the 1st, and the 3rd one 2 or 3 wk later. If DEV is used, 2 alternative regimens are recommended: either two 1-ml doses of DEV s.c. in the deltoid area 1 mo apart with a 3rd inoculation 6 mo later, or (for more rapid immunization) three 1-ml doses 1 wk apart with a 4th inoculation 3 mo later. Serologic confirmation of antibody response should be obtained 2 to 3 wk after the last injection, and booster doses given, if needed, until antibody is detected. Persons with continuing exposure should have booster doses (1 ml) every 2 to 3 yr unless their antibody titers remain satisfactory. If a previously immunized person (antibody response confirmed) is bitten by a rabid animal, he should receive two 1-ml injections of HDCV immediately and another 3 days later, or 5 daily doses of DEV and a booster dose 20 days after the 5th dose. Passive immunization is not given.

Treatment

If rabies develops, treatment is symptomatic. Vigorous supportive treatment is **recommended** and expert consultation should be sought to assist in clinical management. Although death from rabies was once considered inevitable if symptoms developed, recovery has occurred following aggressive, vigorous, supportive treatment to control respiratory, circulatory, and CNS symptoms.

SLOW VIRUS INFECTIONS

In these slowly developing, progressive diseases, responses to viral infections appear many years after the initial infections. The etiology may be conventional viruses or infectious agents lacking some properties of conventional viruses.

SUBACUTE SCLEROSING PANENCEPHALITIS (SSPE) (See Vol. II, Ch. 24)

PROGRESSIVE MULTIFOCAL LEUKOENCEPHALOPATHY

A rare, rapidly progressive, demyelinating CNS disorder that occurs mainly in patients with underlying depression of cell-mediated immunity.

Etiology and Epidemiology

The disease is caused by the JC virus, a human papovavirus that replicates in human fetal glial cell tissue cultures. It is commonly associated with disorders of the reticuloendothelial system, such as leukemia and lymphoma, but may occur in any disease with concomitant depression of cell-mediated immunity. A few cases have occurred in patients without a detectable immune disorder. The disease affects adults of all ages, men more frequently than women.

Symptoms, Signs, and Diagnosis

Onset may be gradual or insidious, but the course is relentlessly progressive. The duration from onset of symptoms to death is usually 1 to 4 mo. The neurologic findings reflect diffuse asymmetrical involvement of the cerebral hemispheres. Pyramidal tract involvement manifested by hemiparesis is the most commonly encountered finding. Progressive intellectual impairment of varying severity occurs in $\frac{2}{3}$ of patients. Aphasia, dysarthria, and hemianopsia are other frequent findings. Sensory changes and cerebellar and brainstem signs may be present. Occasionally an incomplete or complete transverse myelitis appears. Headaches and convulsive seizures are rare.

CSF studies, skull x-rays, and cerebral angiograms are normal. Abnormalities in radioactive and CT brain scan have been noted. The EEG commonly shows diffuse and focal abnormalities corresponding to the underlying asymmetric pathology, but these findings are not pathognomonic of the disease. Serologic studies do not confirm the diagnosis because $\frac{2}{3}$ of a normal population have antibodies against JC virus and underlying immunologic abnormalities in most patients with progressive multifocal leukoencephalopathy make serologic tests unreliable. Brain tissue confirms the diagnosis by identifying the JC virus, using IFA staining or electron microscopic agglutination.

Treatment

There have been isolated reports of favorable therapeutic responses to cytosine or adenine arabinoside, but a treatment of proven effectiveness is not yet available.

PROGRESSIVE RUBELLA PANENCEPHALITIS (See Vol. II, Ch. 24)

CREUTZFELDT–JAKOB DISEASE (Subacute Spongiform Encephalopathy)

A progressive, inevitably fatal, slow virus disease of the CNS, characterized by progressive demen-tia and myoclonic seizures and affecting adults in mid-life.

Etiology and Epidemiology

The disease occurs throughout the world, but little is known about its mode of transmission. Human-to-human transmission has occurred inadvertently during organ transplantation and by the use of contaminated brain electrodes, and the incidence of neurosurgical procedures is more common in Creutzfeld-Jakob patients than would be expected by chance. The agent has been recovered from the CSF. It occurs primarily in adults, men and women alike, with peak incidence in the late 50s.

The disease can be transmitted to primates and small rodents, and it causes scrapie-like tissue damage in goats. The infectious agent appears similar to the agent that causes scrapie of sheep. It is unusually resistant to inactivation by heat, formalin, or exposure to ultraviolet light or x-rays.

Symptoms and Signs

Dementia, invariably present and often the first manifestation of illness, is commonly evidenced by self-neglect, apathy, or irritability. Some patients complain of easy fatigability, somnolence, or insom-nia or other sleep disorders. Disorientation may be noted and may progress to profound and global intellectual defects. Other abnormalities of higher cortical function—e.g., aphasia, apraxia, dyslexia, dysgraphia, agnosia, left-right disorientation, and unilateral neglect—may occur. Palmomental and snout reflexes are frequently present.

Myoclonus, often provoked by sensory stimuli, usually appears within the first 6 mo of the illness. Cerebellar disturbances also occur. Corticospinal tract involvement is common, as manifested by extensor plantar reflexes, clonus, and hyperreflexia. In certain cases, anterior horn cell involvement is prominent, with muscular atrophy and fasciculations. Signs of basal ganglia involvement, such as hypokinesia, dystonic posturing, cogwheel rigidity, tremor, and choreathetoid movements may de-velop. Cranial nerve palsies may be noted occasionally. Ocular disturbances are frequent and in-clude visual field defects, diplopia, dimness or blurring of vision, and vision agnosia.

The disease ends in death after a 3- to 12-mo illness, commonly with a complicating pneumonia.

Diagnosis

The CSF is normal. A CT brain scan or pneumoencephalography may show cerebral and cerebel-lar atrophy. The EEG often shows a local or generalized disorganization, which progresses to a characteristic pattern of paroxysms of sharp waves and spikes against the slow background or, in some cases, a "burst suppression" pattern of low voltage activity. Creutzfelt-Jakob disease should be considered in a patient with a rapidly progressive dementia appearing in mid-adult life, especially if accompanied by myoclonic seizures. There are no specific tests, but the diagnosis can be con-firmed by finding the typical spongiform vacuolar changes and astrocytic proliferation in brain tissue.

Treatment

To prevent transmission of the disease, *caution must be exercised in handling fluids and other materials from patients suspected to have Creutzfeld-Jakob disease.* The infective agent can be destroyed by autoclaving and other treatments, but many standard methods of sterilization, such as exposure to formalin, may be ineffective in destroying the agent.

Treatment of the disease is nonspecific and symptomatic.

KURU

A progressive neurologic disorder transmitted during cannibalistic rites and occurring only in natives of the New Guinea highlands.

Etiology and Epidemiology

The scrapie-like infectious agent appears to enter the body during cannibalistic practices. The infectious origin of the illness has been confirmed by innoculating brain material into higher primates and other animals.

Symptoms and Signs

Patients exhibit various movement disorders; i.e., cerebellar abnormalities, rigidity of the limbs, and clonus. Occasionally, coarse athetosis and choreiform movements are present and the patient shows an exaggerated startle response. Emotional lability is present, with pathologic bursts of laugh-ter. Dementia may be present in advanced stages. Death usually occurs 3 to 12 mo after onset of the disease. In a terminal state, the patient is generally totally placid, mute, and unresponsive. Death is caused by severe decubitus or hypostatic pneumonia.

Diagnosis

Routine laboratory tests are unrevealing. No serologic changes or responses have been detected. The diagnosis can be made by noting characteristic spongiform changes and astrocytic proliferation in brain tissue.

Treatment

There is no known treatment for the disorder.

ARBOVIRUS AND ARENAVIRUS DISEASES

Arboviruses: *Viruses that are maintained in nature through transmission between vertebrate hosts and hematophagous arthropods; they multiply in both the vertebrates and the arthropods.* **Arenaviruses:** *Lymphocytic choriomeningitis and morphologically related viruses that are transmitted by rodents and can show man-to-man transmission.*

TABLE 12-5. IMPORTANT ARBOVIRUS AND ARENAVIRUS DISEASES IN MAN: CLINICAL AND EPIDEMIOLOGIC FEATURES

Major Clinical Syndrome	Viral Agent	Group Classification	Vector	Major Distribution
Fever, malaise, headaches, myalgia	Venezuelan equine encephalitis (VEE)	Group A	Mosquito	Fla., Tex., La., Mexico, Central America, Northern S. America
	Naples Sicilian	Phlebotomus fever	Sandfly	Italy, India, Egypt, Iran, Pakistan
	Punta Toro Chagres	Phlebotomus fever	Sandfly	Panama
	Candiru	Phlebotomus fever	Sandfly	Brazil
	Colorado tick fever	Ungrouped	Tick	Western USA
	Rift Valley fever	Ungrouped	Mosquito	E. Africa, Egypt
Fever, malaise, headaches, myalgia, arthralgia, rash	Chikungunya	Group A	Mosquito	S. Africa, India, S.E. Asia
	O'nyong-nyong	Group A	Mosquito	E. Africa, Egypt
Fever, malaise, headaches, myalgia, rash, lymphadenopathy	Dengue 1–4	Group B	Mosquito	Worldwide (includes Caribbean, Hawaii)
	West Nile	Group B	Mosquito	S. & W. Africa, Middle East, India, Malaysia
Fever with CNS involvement	Eastern equine encephalitis (EEE)	Group A	Mosquito	Eastern Canada & USA, Caribbean, Eastern S. America
	Western equine encephalitis (WEE)	Group A	Mosquito	Canada, USA, Mexico, Brazil, Argentina
	Japanese encephalitis	Group B	Mosquito	Japan, China, S.E. Asia, Malaysia, Australia, New Zealand
	Kyasanur Forest disease	Group B	Tick	India
	Murray Valley encephalitis	Group B	Mosquito	Australia, New Guinea
	Powassan	Group B	Tick	Canada, USA
	St. Louis encephalitis	Group B	Mosquito	USA, Caribbean, Panama, Brazil, Argentina
	California encephalitis	California Group	Mosquito	USA
	Lymphocytic choriomeningitis	Arenavirus	Rodent	Worldwide (includes USA)

(Continued)

Modified from *Harrison's Principles of Internal Medicine,* edited by M. M. Wintrobe et al, ed. 7. Copyright 1974 by McGraw-Hill, Inc. Used with permission of McGraw-Hill Book Company.

TABLE 12-5. IMPORTANT ARBOVIRUS AND ARENAVIRUS DISEASES IN
MAN: CLINICAL AND EPIDEMIOLOGIC FEATURES *(Cont'd)*

Major Clinical Syndrome	Viral Agent	Group Classification	Vector	Major Distribution
Fever, malaise, headaches, myalgia, hemorrhagic signs	Chikungunya	Group A	Mosquito	S.E. Asia, Malaysia, India
	Dengue 1-4	Group B	Mosquito	S.E. Asia, Caribbean, India, Philippines, Polynesia
	Omsk hemorrhagic fever	Group B	Tick	USSR
	Yellow fever	Group B	Mosquito	Africa, Central & S. America
	Crimean-Congo hemorrhagic fever	Ungrouped	Tick	S. USSR, Central Africa, W. Pakistan, Bulgaria
	Junin (Argentinian hemorrhagic fever)	Arenavirus (Tacaribe group)	Rodent	Argentina
	Machupo (Bolivian hemorrhagic fever)	Arenavirus (Tacaribe group)	Rodent	E. Bolivia
	Lassa	Arenavirus	Rodent Man-to-Man	Central W. Africa
	Far Eastern or Korean hemorrhagic fever or nephropathia epidemica	?Arenavirus	Rodent	E. USSR, Manchuria, China, Korea, Scandinavia

ARBOVIRUS ENCEPHALITIDES

The arboviruses **(ar**thropod-**bo**rne viruses) number > 250; at least 80 immunologically distinct arboviruses cause disease in humans. Arboviruses are transmitted among vertebrates by biting insects, chiefly mosquitoes and ticks. Birds are often important sources of infection for mosquitoes, which then transmit the infection to horses, other domestic animals, and humans. Man is a "dead-end" host (i.e., incidental to the natural cycle and ineffective in virus perpetuation) for most of the agents, but is a definitive host (i.e., part of the natural cycle and necessary for transmitting the infection) in urban yellow fever, phlebotomus fever, chikungunya, mayaro, oropouche, and dengue. The agents are widely distributed throughout the world, depending on the availability of lower vertebrate hosts and appropriate vectors.

The arboviruses are classified by antigenic structure into 24 groups and 1 supergroup with 11 subgroups; there is also an ungrouped category for agents showing no serologic relationships. Many of the important disease-producing agents are in Group A (Eastern, Western, and Venezuelan equine encephalitis viruses) or Group B (the viruses of yellow fever; dengue; West Nile fever; St. Louis, Murray Valley, and Japanese encephalitis; and Kyasanur Forest disease).

In the USA, Western equine encephalitis **(WEE)** occurs throughout the country in all age groups, but a disproportionate number of cases occur in children < 1 yr old. Eastern equine encephalitis **(EEE)** occurs in the eastern USA, mainly in young children and persons > 55 yr, and has a higher mortality rate than WEE. In children < 1 yr old, WEE and EEE tend to be severe, with permanent sequelae. Epidemics of both WEE and EEE are associated with epizootics in horses. Urban and rural outbreaks of St. Louis encephalitis have occurred throughout the USA; morbidity and mortality are greatest in older age groups. The California encephalitis virus group is widely distributed throughout the USA, and mainly affects children in rural or suburban areas.

Symptoms, Signs, and Treatment

Arboviruses may cause CNS syndromes (including aseptic meningitis and encephalitis), minor nonspecific febrile illnesses, and, most commonly, inapparent infection. Except in epidemics, the clinical findings in meningitis and encephalitis rarely permit specific identification. Headache, drowsiness, fever, vomiting, and stiff neck are the usual presenting symptoms. Tremors, mental confusion, convulsions, and coma may develop rapidly. Paralysis of the extremities occasionally occurs. Treatment is supportive, as in other viral encephalitides (see in Ch. 124).

YELLOW FEVER

An acute arbovirus infection of variable severity, characterized by sudden onset, fever, a relatively slow pulse, and headache. Intense albuminuria, jaundice, and hemorrhage, especially hematemesis, are characteristic but occur only in the proportionately few severe cases.

Etiology and Epidemiology

The virus of **urban yellow fever** is transmitted by the bite of an *Aedes aegypti* mosquito infected 2 wk previously by feeding on a viremic patient. **Jungle (sylvatic) yellow fever** is transmitted by *Haemogogus* and other forest canopy mosquitoes which acquire the virus from wild primates. Yellow fever is endemic in central Africa and areas of South and Central America.

Symptoms and Signs

(1) Period of incubation: *3 to 6 days.* Prodromal symptoms are usually absent. **(2) Period of invasion:** *2 to 5 days.* Onset is sudden, with fever of 39 to 40 C (102 to 104 F). The pulse, usually rapid initially, by the 2nd day becomes slow for the degree of fever present **(Faget's sign).** The face is flushed and the eyes are injected; the tongue margins are red and the center is "furred." Nausea, vomiting, constipation, epigastric distress, headache, muscle pains (especially in the neck, back, and legs), severe prostration, restlessness, and irritability are common symptoms. If mild, the illness ends at this stage after 1 to 3 days. **(3) Period of remission:** In moderate or severe illness, the fever falls by crisis 2 to 5 days after onset and a remission of several hours or days ensues. **(4) Period of intoxication:** *3 to 9 days.* The fever recurs but the pulse remains slow. Jaundice, extreme albuminuria, and hematemesis ("black vomit"), the three characteristic clinical features, appear. Oliguria or anuria may occur, and petechiae and mucosal hemorrhages are common. The patient is dull, confused, and apathetic. Delirium, convulsions, and coma occur terminally. **(5) Period of convalescence:** This is usually short except in the most severe cases. There are no known sequelae.

Diagnosis and Laboratory Findings

Albuminuria occurs in 90% of patients, usually on the 3rd day, and may reach 20 gm/L in severe cases. The WBC count is usually low and drops to 1500 to 2500 by the 5th day; leukocytosis may occur terminally. Experimental evidence suggests that disseminated intravascular coagulation may occur. Serum bilirubin is mildly elevated.

The clinical features are nonspecific during the period of invasion, but the diagnosis is suggested by Faget's sign. During the period of intoxication, the characteristic triad of intense albuminuria, jaundice, and hematemesis should suggest the diagnosis. Diagnosis is confirmed by isolation of the virus from the blood, by a rising antibody titer, or at autopsy by the characteristic midzonal liver cell necrosis. Needle biopsy of the liver during illness is **contraindicated** by the risk of hemorrhage.

Prognosis

Up to 10% of clinically diagnosed cases end fatally but overall mortality is actually lower, since many mild or inapparent infections are undiagnosed.

Prophylaxis

Active immunization with the 17D strain of live attenuated yellow fever virus vaccine (0.5 ml s.c. every 10 yr) effectively prevents outbreaks and sporadic cases. In the USA, the vaccine is given only at USPHS-authorized Yellow Fever Vaccination Centers. Countries vary in their vaccination requirements; current information and addresses of vaccination centers can be obtained from state and local health departments.

To prevent further mosquito transmission, patients should be isolated in well-screened rooms sprayed with residual insecticides. Since transmission of infection can occur through laboratory accidents, hospital and laboratory personnel should be careful to avoid self-inoculation with patients' blood.

Eradication of urban yellow fever requires widespread mosquito control and mass immunization. During sylvatic outbreaks, work in the area should be discontinued pending immunization and mosquito control.

Treatment

Management is supportive and directed toward alleviating major symptoms. Complete bed rest and nursing care are important. Correction of fluid and electrolyte imbalance is imperative (see Ch. 81).

Hemorrhagic tendencies should be combated with calcium gluconate 1 gm IV once or twice/day, or with phytonadione (see VITAMIN K DEFICIENCY, Treatment, in Ch. 78). Transfusion may be necessary. Therapy with heparin should be considered if there is evidence of disseminated intravascular coagulation (low fibrinogen levels, prolonged thrombin time, thrombocytopenia, and elevation of fibrin split products in full-blown cases; in less acute forms some of these laboratory findings may not occur). Typical heparin dosage is 50 to 100 u./kg initially, then 10 to 15 u./kg/hour, given by IV infusion.

Nausea and vomiting may be alleviated with dimenhydrinate 50 to 100 mg orally or rectally, or 50 mg IM, q 4 to 6 h; or with prochlorperazine 5 to 10 mg orally, parenterally, or rectally q 4 to 6 h. Fever may be reduced with tepid-water sponge baths. Headaches may require codeine 15 to 60 mg orally or s.c. q 4 to 6 h, or meperidine 50 to 100 mg orally or IM q 4 to 6 h.

DENGUE (Breakbone or Dandy Fever)

An acute febrile disease characterized by sudden onset, with headache, fever, prostration, joint and muscle pain, lymphadenopathy, and a rash that appears simultaneously with a second temperature rise following an afebrile period. A hemorrhagic fever syndrome associated with dengue occurs in children (see below).

Dengue is endemic throughout the tropics and subtropics; outbreaks have occurred in the Caribbean, including Puerto Rico and the US Virgin Islands, since 1969. Cases have also been imported in tourists returning from Tahiti. The causative agent, a Group B arbovirus with 4 distinct serogroups, is transmitted by the bite of *Aedes* mosquitoes.

Clinical Course

Following an incubation period of 3 to 15 (usually 5 to 8) days, onset is abrupt, with chills or chilly sensations, headache, postorbital pain on moving the eyes, lumbar backache, and severe prostration. Extreme aching in the legs and joints occurs during the first hours of illness. The temperature rises rapidly to as high as 40 C (104 F), with a relative bradycardia and hypotension. The bulbar and palpebral conjunctivas are injected, and a transient flushing or pale pink macular rash (particularly of the face) usually appears. The spleen may be soft and slightly enlarged. Cervical, epitrochlear, and inguinal lymph nodes are usually enlarged.

Fever and other symptoms persist for 48 to 96 h, followed by rapid defervescence with profuse sweating. This ushers in an afebrile period, with a sense of well-being, which lasts about 24 h. A second rapid temperature rise follows, usually with a lower peak than the first, producing a "saddleback" temperature curve. A characteristic maculopapular eruption simultaneously appears, usually spreading from the extremities to cover the entire body except the face, or distributed patchily over the trunk and extremities. The palms and soles may be bright red and edematous. The fever, rash, and headache and other pains constitute the **"dengue triad."** Cases have occurred without the second febrile period.

Mortality is nil in typical dengue. Convalescence is often prolonged, lasting several weeks, and accompanied by asthenia. An attack produces immunity for a year or more.

Diagnosis and Laboratory Findings

Leukopenia is present by the 2nd day of fever; by the 4th or 5th day, the WBC count has dropped to 2000 to 4000 with only 20 to 40% granulocytes. Moderate albuminuria and a few casts may be found.

Dengue may be confused with Colorado tick fever, typhus, yellow fever, or other hemorrhagic fevers. Serologic diagnosis may be made by HI and CF tests using paired sera, but is complicated by cross-reactions with other Group B arbovirus antibodies.

Prophylaxis and Treatment

Prevention requires control or eradication of the mosquito vector. To prevent transmission to mosquitoes, patients in endemic areas should be kept under mosquito netting until the second fever has abated. **Treatment** is symptomatic. Complete bed rest is important. Aspirin 600 mg and codeine 15 to 60 mg may be given orally q 4 h for severe headache and myalgia.

DENGUE HEMORRHAGIC FEVER SYNDROME (DHFS; Philippine, Thai, or Southeast Asian Hemorrhagic Fever)

An acute disease occurring in children living where dengue is endemic, and characterized by an abrupt febrile onset followed by hemorrhagic manifestations and circulatory collapse. It is prevalent in Southeast Asia and India, and recently occasional cases have occurred in the Caribbean. Virtually all patients are under age 10.

Symptoms and Signs

Onset is abrupt, with fever, headache, nausea, vomiting, abdominal pain, cough, pharyngitis, and dyspnea. Shock occurs 2 to 6 days after onset, with sudden collapse or prostration, cool clammy extremities (the trunk is often warm), weak thready pulse, and circumoral cyanosis. Bleeding tendencies occur, usually as purpura, petechiae, or ecchymoses at injection sites; sometimes as hematemesis, melena, or epistaxis; and occasionally as subarachnoid hemorrhage.

Hepatomegaly is common, as is bronchopneumonia with or without bilateral pleural effusions. Myocarditis may be present. Mortality ranges from 6 to 30%; most deaths occur in infants < 1 yr old.

Laboratory Findings and Diagnosis

Hemoconcentration (Hct > 50%) is present during shock; the WBC count is elevated in 1/3 of the patients. Thrombocytopenia (< l00,000/cu mm), a positive tourniquet test, and a prolonged prothrombin time are characteristic and indicative of the coagulation abnormalities. Minimal proteinuria may be present. SGOT levels may be moderately increased. Serologic tests usually show high CF antibody titers against Group B arboviruses, suggestive of a secondary immune response.

Presumptive diagnosis is based on abrupt onset of fever followed by sudden shock or collapse 2 or more days later, and bleeding abnormalities, including thrombocytopenia without manifest bleeding.

Treatment

The degree of hemoconcentration, dehydration, and electrolyte imbalance must be evaluated immediately and monitored closely for the first few days, since shock may occur or recur precipitously. Cyanotic patients should be given O_2. Vascular collapse and hemoconcentration require immediate and vigorous fluid replacement, preferably with a crystalloid solution such as Ringer's lactate (overhydration must be avoided). Plasma or human serum albumin should also be given if there is no response in the first hour. Fresh blood or platelet transfusions may control bleeding. Agitated patients may be given paraldehyde, chloral hydrate, or diazepam. Hydrocortisone, pressor amines, α-adrenergic blocking agents, and vitamins C and K are of doubtful value.

LYMPHOCYTIC CHORIOMENINGITIS (LCM)

An acute viral infection caused by an RNA virus now classified as an arenavirus, usually appearing as an influenza-like illness or aseptic meningitis, which may be associated with rash, arthritis, orchitis, or parotitis.

LCM infection is endemic in rodents. Human infection results most commonly from exposure to dust or food contaminated by the gray house mouse or hamsters, which harbor the virus for life and excrete it in urine, feces, semen, and nasal secretions. When transmitted by mice the disease occurs primarily in adults, in the winter.

Clinical Course

An influenza-like illness develops 5 to 10 days after exposure. Fever, usually 38.5 to 40 C (101 to 104 F), with rigors is uniform. Over half the patients may experience malaise, weakness, myalgia (especially in the lumbar area), retro-orbital headache, photophobia, anorexia, nausea, and lightheadedness. Less common symptoms include sore throat and dysesthesia. In the first week of illness, physical findings are few; there may be relative bradycardia and pharyngeal injection without exudate. After 5 days to 3 wk, patients may improve for 1 or 2 days. Many then relapse with recurrent fever, headache, skin rashes, swelling of metacarpophalangeal and proximal interphalangeal joints, meningeal signs, orchitis, parotitis, and alopecia of the scalp. Patients with aseptic meningitis almost always recover without sequelae. With encephalitis, up to 33% of patients have neurologic residua.

Laboratory Findings, Diagnosis, and Treatment

Leukopenia (WBC, 2000 to 3000) and thrombocytopenia (platelets, 50,000 to 100,000) are almost uniform during the first week of illness. Chest radiographs may reveal basilar pneumonitis. In patients with meningeal signs, the CSF usually contains several hundred cells/cu mm, but occasionally > 1000. Lymphocytes predominate (> 80%), even early. Decreased CSF glucose, with concentrations as low as 15 mg/100 ml, has been reported in up to 25% of patients.

The clinical manifestations cannot be differentiated from those of many other viruses.

Therapy is supportive.

LASSA FEVER

A serious systemic arenavirus infection that involves most visceral organs but spares the CNS.

Etiology and Epidemiology

After Lassa fever was first recognized in Lassa, Nigeria in 1969, outbreaks occurred in Nigeria, Liberia, and Sierra Leone. Cases have been imported into the USA and the United Kingdom. *Mastomys natalensis*, a small rat that commonly inhabits houses and is widespread in Africa, is a reservoir of the virus. Most human cases probably result from contamination of food with rodent urine, but human-to-human transmission can occur through contact with urine, feces, saliva, vomitus, or blood. The outbreaks in Nigeria and Liberia were primarily hospital-associated, spreading from an index case to hospital workers or other patients. In Sierra Leone, where most cases were acquired outside of hospitals, 6% of the residents in the endemic area had antibody against Lassa virus, while only 0.2% were recognized as having had clinical disease. About 2/3 of the cases have been women, a predilection that may relate to exposure rather than to differences in susceptibility.

Symptoms and Signs

The incubation period is 1 to 24 days, 10 days being usual. The onset of severe symptoms is gradual; most patients have symptoms for 4 to 5 days before hospitalization. The initial symptoms—sore throat, fever, chilliness, headache, myalgia, and malaise—are followed by anorexia, vomiting, and pains in the chest and epigastrium. The sore throat becomes more severe during the 1st wk; patches of white or yellow exudate may appear on the tonsils and may coalesce into a pseudomembrane. Early in the course, relative bradycardia is common. Generalized nontender lymphadenopathy occurs in some patients. During the 2nd wk, severe lower abdominal pain and intractable vomiting are common. Facial and neck swelling and conjunctival edema are seen in 10 to 30%. Occasionally, patients have tinnitus, epistaxis, bleeding from the gums and venipuncture sites, maculopapular rashes, cough, and dizziness. During the acute stage, systolic BPs of < 90 mm Hg with pulse pressures of < 20 mm Hg occur in 60 to 80% of patients. During the 2nd wk, patients who will recover defervesce, while fatally ill patients often develop shock, clouded mental status, agitation, rales, pleural effusion, and, occasionally, grand mal seizures. The illness lasts from 7 to 31 days (average, 15 days) in those who survive and 7 to 26 days (average, 12 days) in fatal cases.

Laboratory Findings and Diagnosis

Hct values are normal. Early, in $1/3$ of the patients the WBC count drops to < 4000, with relative neutrophilia. Platelet counts remain normal. Urinalyses reveal proteinuria, which is often massive. Chest radiographs may show basilar pneumonitis and pleural effusions. SGOT and SGPT values become elevated (10 × normal), as do levels of creatine phosphokinase (CPK) and lactic dehydrogenase (LDH). The diagnosis may be made quickly by staining conjunctival scrapings with fluorescent-labelled anti-Lassa serum. Confirmation requires growth of the virus in tissue culture or a fourfold rise in antibody with a CF test; however, the latter is rarely positive before the 14th day. Virus may be isolated from blood.

Prognosis

The severity of infection correlates with the level of viremia, elevations in transaminase values, and fever. Mortality rates have varied between 16 and 45%; however, in women who were pregnant or delivered within 1 mo, mortality was 50%. Among survivors, late sequelae include deafness in about 5% and occasional instances of alopecia, iridocyclitis, and transient blindness.

Prophylaxis and Treatment

In Sierra Leone, barrier nursing (surgical masks, gowns, and gloves) has been effective. In the USA, maximum isolation, including use of goggles, high efficiency masks, and a negative pressure room with no air circulation, is recommended. Surveillance of contacts also is recommended.

Management is supportive and directed toward alleviating major symptoms. *Correction of fluid and electrolyte imbalance is imperative.* Infusion of immune plasma from convalescent patients has been used, but the limited experience is equivocal in results. In experimental Lassa fever in monkeys, an antiviral agent, ribavirin, has significantly decreased mortality.

PRESUMPTIVE VIRAL DISEASES

CAT-SCRATCH DISEASE (Nonbacterial Lymphadenitis; Benign Lymphoreticulosis)

A febrile disorder characterized by lymphadenitis, thought to be transmitted by cats.

Etiology

Although no etiologic agent has been isolated, available evidence suggests that the etiologic agent belongs to the genus *Chlamydia*. Several animals have been considered to be carriers, particularly cats, because > 90% of cases follow cat scratches.

Symptoms and Signs

A few days after a minor scratch, a papule or pustule develops at the site. Regional lymphadenopathy develops within 2 wk, usually unilaterally and in relation to the scratch site (i.e., axillary, epitrochlear, submandibular, cervical, or inguinal). The nodes are initially firm and tender, but later become fluctuant and may drain with fistula formation. Pathologic examination of involved nodes shows hyperplasia, a granulomatous response, and then suppurative necrosis and microabscess formation. Fever, malaise, headache, and anorexia accompany the lymphadenopathy. Erythema nodosum, thrombocytopenic purpura, Parinaud's syndrome (conjunctivitis associated with palpable preauricular lymph nodes), and osteolytic lesions occur but are uncommon. Encephalitis is a rare but severe complication, usually occurring one or more weeks after onset.

Diagnosis, Treatment, and Prognosis

Diagnostic criteria include persistent (> 3 wk) regional lymphadenopathy, a history of cat contact, characteristic histopathology, negative studies for other common causes of lymphadenitis, and a positive intradermal skin test with cat-scratch antigen (not commercially available).

Therapy with tetracycline may shorten the course. Spontaneous node regression usually occurs within 4 wk. Surgical excision may be necessary, especially if fistulas drain. Prognosis is excellent.

13. PARASITIC INFECTIONS

(NOTE: Several of the drugs mentioned in this chapter are not available commercially in the USA but may be obtainable as investigational drugs from the Parasitic Diseases Branch of the Center for Disease Control in Atlanta, Georgia.)

PROTOZOAL DISEASES

AMEBIASIS (Entamebiasis)

An infection of the colon caused by Entamoeba histolytica. *It is most commonly asymptomatic, but symptoms ranging from mild diarrhea to dysentery may occur.*

Etiology, Epidemiology, and Incidence

There are 2 forms of *E. histolytica*: the motile trophozoite and the cyst. The trophozoite, the parasitic form, dwells in the bowel lumen, where it feeds on bacteria or tissue. With diarrhea, the fragile trophozoites pass unchanged in the liquid stool and rapidly die. If diarrhea is not present, the organisms usually encyst before leaving the gut. The cyst, the infective form of the organism, resists environmental changes and may be spread either directly from person to person or indirectly via food or water. **Direct spread** appears to be more common in the USA, where it occurs in situations of compromised personal hygiene (e.g., among sexual partners, particularly male homosexuals and institutionalized, mentally retarded individuals). **Indirect spread** is more frequent in poorly sanitized areas of the world, including migrant labor camps and Indian reservations in the USA. Fruits and vegetables may be contaminated when they are fertilized by human feces, washed in polluted water, or prepared by an asymptomatic cysts-passer. Faulty hotel and factory plumbing has resulted in 2 water-borne epidemics; more commonly, amebiasis is sporadic. The infection rate in the USA is about 1 to 5%. The carrier rate may exceed 50% in areas of the world where sanitation is poor.

Pathogenesis

Excystation of ingested cysts occurs in the small intestine. The released trophozoites are carried to the colon, where they grow and multiply in the bowel lumen as commensals. Change in the organism's virulence or the host's resistance may lead to tissue invasion and disease.

The trophozoites penetrate the mucous membrane mainly in regions of fecal stasis—the cecum, appendix, ascending colon, sigmoid colon, and rectum. The earliest lesion is a small abscess, usually in the submucosa; later, ulcers form that tend to be ragged and undermined. The lesions are focal and discrete in mild cases, but may spread and become confluent, with hemorrhage, edema, and sloughing of large areas of mucosa. Although the muscular coat limits penetration by the ameba, it is occasionally destroyed and perforation results; amebas enter the radicles of the portal vein and are carried to the liver. Most of the amebas are probably destroyed, but one or more large hepatic abscesses develop if the survivors are numerous and multiply. Further spread of the disease is usually by direct extension from the liver into the pleura, right lung, and pericardium.

Symptoms and Signs

Because of the infrequency of tissue invasion, most patients, particularly those living in temperate climates, are asymptomatic. Symptoms occur with tissue invasion. These may be so vague as to be recalled only after successful therapy, but more often intermittent diarrhea and constipation, flatulence, and cramping abdominal pain occur. There may be tenderness over the liver and ascending colon, and the stools may contain mucus and blood.

Amebic dysentery, common in the tropics but uncommon in temperate climates, is characterized by episodes of frequent semifluid or fluid stools, often containing blood, flecks of mucus, and hordes of active trophozoites. Slight fever may be present. Between relapses, symptoms diminish to recurrent cramps and loose or very soft stools due to colitis, yet emaciation and anemia increase.

Complications and Sequelae

Hepatic amebiasis: Tender hepatomegaly frequently accompanies amebic colitis. This syndrome, formerly termed "diffuse amebic hepatitis," probably reflects a nonspecific periportal inflammation and not amebic liver infection. **Liver abscess** may develop during or 1 to 3 mo after an attack of dysentery, or may be unassociated with dysentery. Abscesses occur most frequently in adult males. The abscesses are usually single and develop insidiously, but symptoms may begin abruptly. Symptoms include pain or discomfort over the liver, aggravated by movement and occasionally referred to the right shoulder; intermittent fever; sweats; chills; nausea; vomiting; weakness; and weight loss. Jaundice is unusual, except in mild degree. The abscess may perforate into the subphrenic space, right pleural cavity, right lung, and other adjacent organs.

Symptoms of **subacute appendicitis** may occur during clinical or subclinical amebic infection as a result of diffuse amebic invasion of the appendix and cecum. Surgery in such cases often results in

TABLE 13–1. COMMONLY ENCOUNTERED

Condition	Causative Organism (Synonyms or Varieties)	Geographic Distribution	Source of Infection	Portal of Entry (& Stage)
Roundworms				
Ascariasis	*Ascaris lumbricoides* (Giant intestinal roundworm)	Cosmopolitan, more common in warm, moist climates	Fecal contamination of soil (eggs) Contaminated vegetables	Mouth (embryonated eggs)
Hookworm infection	a) *Ancylostoma duodenale* (Old World type) b) *Necator americanus* (Tropical type)	a) Temperate & warm, moist climates b) Warm, moist climates	Fecal contamination of soil (larvae)	Skin, usually feet, possibly mouth (filariform larvae)
Strongyloidiasis	*Strongyloides stercoralis* (Threadworm)	Southern USA, moist tropics	Fecal contamination of soil (larvae)	Skin, usually feet (filariform larvae)
Trichuriasis	*Trichuris trichiura* (Whipworm)	Warm, moist climates Uncommon in USA	Fecal contamination of soil (eggs)	Mouth (embryonated eggs)
Enterobiasis	*Enterobius vermicularis (Oxyuris vermicularis;* pinworm, seatworm)	Cosmopolitan, esp. in children	Eggs from contaminated fomites Anus-finger-mouth	Mouth (embryonated eggs)
Tapeworms				
Dwarf Tapeworm infection	*Hymenolepis nana*	Southern USA, in children Cosmopolitan	Eggs contaminating environment	Mouth (eggs)
Beef Tapeworm infection	*Taenia saginata*	Cosmopolitan	Poorly cooked or raw infected beef	Mouth (cysticercus larvae in infected beef)
Pork Tapeworm infection	*Taenia solium*	Rare in USA; common in Latin America, Asia, USSR, E. Europe	Poorly cooked infected pork	Mouth (cysticercus larvae in infected pork)
Fish Tapeworm infection	*Diphyllobothrium latum*	Northern Minn. & Mich.; Canada Cosmopolitan	Infected fresh-water fish	Mouth (larvae in infected fresh-water fish flesh)

INTESTINAL PARASITIC INFECTIONS

Most Common Symptoms	Diagnostic Findings	Therapeutic Agents	Remarks
Bronchial symptoms, eosinophilia* (larval stage) Colicky pains, "acute abdomen"	Immature eggs in stool Worms evacuated in stool, occasionally vomited	Pyrantel pamoate Mebendazole	May block intestine, biliary or pancreatic duct
Abdominal pain, anemia, cardiac insufficiency, retarded growth	Immature eggs in stool	Pyrantel pamoate Mebendazole	Prophylaxis: Use sanitary latrines, wear shoes, treat infected persons
Radiating pain in pit of stomach, diarrhea	Larvae in stool Larvae in duodenum	Thiabendazole	Prophylaxis: As for hookworm
Diarrhea, abdominal pain, anemia, weight loss	Immature eggs in stool	Mebendazole	May produce dysenteric syndrome or acute appendicitis; rectal prolapse in children
Perianal & perineal pruritus	Eggs in perianal swabs; adult worms per anum	Pyrantel pamoate Mebendazole	Often involves entire family
Diarrhea, abdominal discomfort, in massive infections in children	Eggs in stool	Niclosamide Paromomycin	May be symptomless
Usually asymptomatic, anal passage of proglottids, abdominal distress, "acute appendix"	Proglottids of adult worms in stool; eggs near anus	Niclosamide Paromomycin	May be symptomless Prophylaxis: Thoroughly cook all suspected beef
Similar to *T. saginata*	Eggs and proglottids of adult worms in stool; eggs near anus	Niclosamide Paromomycin	May be symptomless Ingested eggs may produce human cysticercosis Prophylaxis: Thoroughly cook all pork in infected areas
Mild GI symptoms; may cause pernicious anemia	Immature eggs in stool	Niclosamide Paromomycin	May be symptomless Prophylaxis: Thoroughly cook or freeze fresh-water fish

* Note: Eosinophilia often accompanies intestinal helminthiasis.   *(Continued)*

TABLE 13-1. COMMONLY ENCOUNTERED

Condition	Causative Organism (Synonyms or Varieties)	Geographic Distribution	Source of Infection	Portal of Entry (& Stage)
Tapeworms *(Cont'd)* Sparganosis	*Diphyllobothrium mansoni*	Several areas, incl. southern USA Cosmopolitan	a) Drinking water containing infected Cyclops (primary host) b) Direct contact with flesh of intermediate host	a) Usually mouth (larval stages) b) Skin
Echino-coccus	*Echinococcus granulosus*	Sheep-raising areas of the world, Alaska	Canine feces	Mouth (eggs)
Protozoa Amebiasis	*Entamoeba histolytica*	Cosmopolitan; common in warm, moist climates	Feces-contaminated water, food, fomites	Mouth (cyst)
Giardiasis	*Giardia lamblia*	Cosmopolitan	Human feces	Mouth (cyst)
Flukes Intestinal	a) *Fasciolopsis buski* b) *Heterophyes, Metagonimus*	In USA only as rare infections imported from Orient or tropics	a) Vegetation b) Fresh-water fish	Mouth (encysted metacercarial larva)
Hepatic	a) *Fasciola hepatica* (sheep liver fluke) b) *Clonorchis sinensis*	a) Cosmopolitan in sheep-raising countries b) Orient	a) Watercress containing metacercarial cysts b) Fresh-water fish	a) Mouth (encysted metacercarial larva) b) Mouth (encysted larva)
Pulmonary	*Paragonimus westermani* (Oriental lung fluke)	a) Africa b) Orient, extensive foci c) Latin America	Crabs or crayfishes containing metacercarial cysts	Mouth (encysted metacercarial larva)

INTESTINAL PARASITIC INFECTIONS *(Cont'd)*

Most Common Symptoms	Diagnostic Findings	Therapeutic Agents	Remarks
Inflamed subcut. tissue containing sparganum larva	Sparganum larva in subcut. tissues	Surgical excision	Adult worm in intestine of various nonhuman mammals
Abdominal mass, pain, pulmonary "coin lesion," cough, hemoptysis	Compatible history, liver or lung cyst, positive serology	Surgical excision	Patients with small, calcified hepatic cysts & Alaskan variety pulmonary cyst require surgery only if symptomatic

a) Intestinal
  1. Mild
  2. Dysentery
 	
b) Amebic abscess
	Trophozoite stage or cyst in stool	a) 1. Metronidazole, Diiodohydroxyquin, or Diloxanide furoate
		   2. Metronidazole & Diiodohydroxyquin + Emetine or Dehydroemetine
		b) Metronidazole *or* Emetine & Chloroquine phosphate
			Amebiasis may be asyndromic in individuals or populations

Mucous diarrhea, abdominal pain, weight loss	Vegetative stage or cyst in stool	Metronidazole Quinacrine	Prevalent in children in day-care centers and patients with immunoglobulin deficiencies. A cause of "travelers' diarrhea"
Usually asymptomatic abdominal pain, diarrhea, at times intestinal obstruction	Eggs in stool	a) Tetrachloroethylene b) Tetrachloroethylene	Primary intermediate hosts are fresh-water snails
Hepatic colic, cholecystitis	a) Immature eggs in stool or biliary drainage b) Eggs in stool & duodenal contents	a) Bithionol† b) None	a) Sheep infected in USA, but only 1 confirmed human infection b) Infections in USA from imported dried or pickled fish
Peribronchiolar distress, with hemoptysis	Immature eggs in stool or sputum Serology	Bithionol†	Related species in wild mammals and hogs in USA

† Available in USA from Center for Disease Control.   *(Continued)*

TABLE 13-1. COMMONLY ENCOUNTERED

Condition	Causative Organism (Synonyms or Varieties)	Geographic Distribution	Source of Infection	Portal of Entry (& Stage)
Flukes (Cont'd) Blood (Schisto- somiasis)	a) *Schistosoma japonicum* b) *S. mansoni* c) *S. haematobium*	a) Orient b) Africa, Latin America c) Africa, Near East	Infested water containing fork-tailed larvae from snail hosts	Skin (active fork-tailed cercariae)

peritonitis and death. If there is reasonable suspicion that the symptoms are of amebic origin, it is advisable to delay surgery for 48 to 72 h in order to observe the effects of chemotherapy (see Treatment, below).

Penetration of the muscle layers of the colon occasionally results in a vigorous granulomatous reaction, producing tissue masses or ameboma that may obstruct the bowel and be mistaken for carcinoma.

The lungs, brain, and other organs are occasionally infected by **hematogenous spread** from the intestines. Skin lesions, especially around the perineum and buttocks, and, particularly, traumatic and operative wounds are occasionally infected with amebas.

Diagnosis

Intestinal amebiasis, suggested by the clinical picture and epidemiologic setting, is confirmed by demonstration of *E. histolytica* in the stool or tissues. Wet mounts of liquid and semiformed stools should be examined immediately for trophozoites. Bloodstained flecks of mucus in the stool are more likely to contain amebas. Formed stool should be examined, by direct and concentration methods, for cysts. If examination is delayed, a portion of the stool should be placed in a preservative for cysts (5% formalin) and trophozoites (polyvinyl alcohol). Diagnosis may require examination of 3 to 6 stool specimens. Since antibiotics, antacids, antidiarrheal agents, enemas, and intestinal radiocontrast agents may interfere with recovery of the parasite, their administration should be postponed until the stool has been examined.

Proctoscopy often demonstrates mucosal lesions in symptomatic patients. The lesions should be aspirated and the material examined for trophozoites. Biopsy specimens from the lesions may also show trophozoites.

Extraintestinal amebiasis is more difficult to diagnose. Stool examination is usually negative, and recovery of the trophozoite from pus is uncommon. In patients suspected of having an amebic liver abscess, a therapeutic trial of amebicides may be the single most helpful diagnostic tool.

Serologic tests are positive in almost all patients with amebic liver abscess and in more than 80% of those with acute amebic dysentery. However, since antibody titers may persist for months or years, serologic tests are less helpful in endemic areas. The tests are positive in only about 10% of asymptomatic carriers, suggesting that tissue invasion is a prerequisite of antibody formation. The indirect HA test appears to be the most sensitive test available.

Differential Diagnosis

Nondysenteric amebiasis is often misdiagnosed as irritable bowel syndrome, regional enteritis, or diverticulitis. **Amebic dysentery** may be confused with bacillary dysentery, salmonellosis, schistosomiasis, or ulcerative colitis. In contrast to bacillary dysentery, the stools in amebic dysentery are more fecal and less frequent, watery, or purulent. They characteristically contain tenacious mucus and flecks of both fresh and altered blood. Unlike shigellosis, salmonellosis, and ulcerative colitis, they do not contain large numbers of leukocytes.

Hepatic amebiasis and amebic abscess must be differentiated from other hepatic infections, including abscesses due to bacterial infection and infected echinococcus cysts. Fever, local pain and tenderness, and hepatomegaly are significant findings. Serologic tests are usually positive in hepatic amebiasis; amebas are found in the stools in about 1/3 of cases.

When an abscess is present, the liver is usually enlarged and tender, but it may not be palpable. X-rays may show elevation and fixation, or impaired excursion of the right leaf of the diaphragm. Radioisotopic liver scanning may show the extent of the abscess, while ultrasonic scanning may demonstrate it to be fluid-filled. The ESR and alkaline phosphatase may be elevated. The abscesses contain thick, semifluid material ranging from yellow to chocolate brown and composed of cytolyzed remains of tissue. A needle biopsy may show pus, but motile amebas are difficult to find in the abscess material and cysts are not present.

INTESTINAL PARASITIC INFECTIONS *(Cont'd)*

Most Common Symptoms	Diagnostic Findings	Therapeutic Agents	Remarks
Dysentery, fibrosis of intestinal or bladder walls, hepatic fibrosis (a,b), hematuria (c)	Embryonated eggs in stool (a,b), or urine (c)	a) Antimony potassium tartrate, Niridazole† b, c) Niridazole†, Sodium dimercaptosuc-cinate†, Hycanthone‡	Related flukes cause "swimmer's itch" in bathers in USA and elsewhere

† Available in USA from Center for Disease Control.

Prophylaxis

Controlling the spread of *E. histolytica* requires preventing access of human feces to the mouth. The high incidence of asymptomatic carriers complicates the problem.

Treatment

General: This is directed at relieving symptoms, replacing blood, and correcting fluid and electrolyte losses.

Chemotherapy:

Course A (asymptomatic intestinal amebiasis): Metronidazole, diiodohydroxyquin, or diloxanide furoate may be given orally. For adults, metronidazole 750 mg orally t.i.d. for 10 days is recommended; for children, 35 to 50 mg/kg/day orally in 3 divided doses, also for 10 days. The comparable dose of diiodohydroxyquin is 650 mg t.i.d., or 30 to 40 mg/kg/day in 3 divided doses for children. For both, the drug is given for 20 days. Diloxanide furoate is given for 10 days, 500 mg t.i.d. in adults and 20 mg/kg/day in 3 doses for children.

Course B (symptomatic intestinal amebiasis): Metronidazole should be given *in combination* with diiodohydroxyquin. In severe dysentery, emetine 1 mg/kg/day (maximum 65 mg) or dehydroemetine 1 to 1.5 mg/kg/day (maximum 90 mg) given by deep s.c. or IM injection may be added to the above regimen until symptoms are controlled (maximum 5 days). (CAUTION: *Emetine and dehydroemetine are toxic; patients receiving them should be confined to bed and placed on cardiac monitors. Therapy should be stopped promptly if such signs of toxicity as tachycardia, hypotension, muscular weakness, marked GI effects, or dermatoses appear*) Pregnancy and cardiac disease are **contraindications.**

Course C (extraintestinal amebiasis): Metronidazole, given in the dosage mentioned above, is the drug of choice. Alternatively, emetine or dehydroemetine can be given for 5 days in the manner described for severe amebic dysentery. If one of the latter 2 drugs is used, it should be combined with oral chloroquine phosphate to diminish the risk of relapse. The dosage is 1 gm/day orally for 2 days, then 500 mg/day for 3 wk. The dose for children is 10 mg/kg/day (maximum 600 mg/day) for the same duration.

Emetine, dehydroemetine, or chloroquine can be used in a therapeutic trial. A favorable response is so characteristic that it constitutes an important diagnostic aid. A therapeutic trial of metronidazole, however, may lead to an erroneous diagnosis, since it is also effective against many anaerobic bacteria that commonly cause pyogenic liver abscess.

Criteria of cure: Ideally, the patient should not be discharged until 3 stool examinations, performed daily for 3 days after completion of treatment, are negative. One of the specimens should be obtained after catharsis. Since amebiasis tends to relapse, stools should be reexamined with reasonable frequency—if feasible, 1, 3, and 6 mo after treatment. Recurrence of GI symptoms does not require amebicidal drug therapy unless parasitic relapse has been proved by demonstration of *E. histolytica.*

GIARDIASIS

An infection of the small intestine caused by Giardia lamblia. It is commonly asymptomatic, but clinical manifestations ranging from flatulence to malabsorption may occur.

Etiology and Epidemiology

The *G. lamblia* trophozoite attaches itself to the mucosa of the duodenum and jejunum by means of a central sucker and multiplies by binary fission. The organisms are passed in normal stool as cysts. In this resistant form, they spread the disease from host to host by fecal-oral routes, either directly, as between children or sexual partners, or indirectly via food or water. Water-borne epidemics involving remote mountain streams, well water, and chlorinated community systems have all been implicated. Both humans and wild animals may serve as reservoirs.

The infection is found worldwide, especially in areas of poor sanitation and in children; rates > 50% have been noted in day care centers. Infection rates are also high among travelers, male homosexuals, and patients with gastrectomies, decreased gastric acidity, chronic pancreatitis, and immunoglobulin deficiencies. In the USA, about 4% of stools submitted for parasitologic examination contain *G. lamblia* cysts.

Pathogenesis and Symptoms and Signs

Symptoms are commonly absent or mild, but intermittent nausea, eructation, flatulence, epigastric pain, abdominal cramps, and diarrhea may occur. In severe cases, malabsorption can lead to significant weight loss and bulky, malodorous stools. The severity of the malabsorption is related to the degree of infection, but the pathogenesis of these manifestations is unknown. Mechanical blockade of the microvilli, damage to their brush border, altered mobility, and mucosal invasion have all been suggested as possible mechanisms.

Diagnosis

The diagnosis is made by finding the organism in the stool or duodenal secretions. In acute infections the parasite can be readily found in the stool; in chronic cases excretion is irregular, requiring repeated stool examinations. Alternatively, duodenal contents—obtained with a nylon string (Enterotest®) or by aspirations through a gastric tube—can be examined for trophozoites.

Treatment

Of the 3 drugs available in the USA for treatment of giardiasis, the most frequently recommended is quinacrine 100 mg t.i.d. for 5 days. Although it is highly effective (70 to 95% cure rate), it may produce GI disturbances and, rarely, toxic psychosis. Metronidazole 250 mg t.i.d. for 7 days is equally effective and better tolerated, but it is not currently licensed for use in giardiasis and there is concern over its potential carcinogenicity. Furazolidone is less effective than either of these agents but is available as a suspension, making it useful in children. Although the FDA has approved it, it has been shown to induce neoplasia in experimental animals.

Household and sexual contacts should be examined and, if infected, treated. Pregnant women should be treated only if they show significant symptoms.

MALARIA

A protozoan infection characterized by paroxysms of chills, fever, and sweating, and by anemia, splenomegaly, and a chronic relapsing course.

Etiology and Epidemiology

Malarial parasites of 4 types, each with a different biologic pattern, may affect man: *Plasmodium vivax, P. falciparum, P. malariae,* and *P. ovale.* Infection occurs through the bite of an infected anopheles mosquito, transfusion of blood from an infected donor, or use of a common syringe by drug addicts.

Most hyperendemic malarious areas are in the tropics. Chemotherapeutic agents and insecticides have made autochthonous malaria rare in the USA and many other parts of the world, but visitors from malarious areas may introduce the infection; returning armed forces personnel have caused small sporadic epidemics.

Pathogenesis

The life cycle of the malarial parasite begins when a female anopheles mosquito, feeding on a patient with malaria, ingests blood containing gametocytes. These undergo sexual development (sporogony) within the mosquito, to end as sporozoites located in the insect's salivary glands. The mosquito injects the sporozoites into man, and the parasite multiplies asexually in the liver parenchymal cells. Little is known of the pathologic changes accompanying this asymptomatic fixed-tissue (**exoerythrocytic**) phase. After a period of maturation ranging from days to months (average, 2 to 4 wk), merozoites are released and invade the RBCs, initiating the clinical or **erythrocytic** phase of the disease. *P. vivax* and *P. ovale* exoerythrocytic parasites persist in the liver cells, periodically "seeding" the bloodstream with new merozoites to cause a relapse. *P. falciparum* and, presumably, *P. malariae* do not persist in the liver cells; however, in untreated infections erythrocytic parasites may persist from months (*P. falciparum*) to years (*P. malariae*) and produce recrudescent clinical disease.

All 4 parasites multiply asexually within the RBCs (schizogony) to produce a new generation of merozoites. The RBCs rupture and these merozoites are released into the circulating plasma to enter intact RBCs and repeat the erythrocytic cycle. Gametocytes rather than merozoites are formed in some RBCs. These gametocytes cannot self-replicate, and they die unless ingested by the anopheles mosquito for completion of the sexual cycle.

Pathology

After prolonged untreated malarial infection or repeated relapses, persistent hepatosplenomegaly develops. The spleen is usually soft and full of malarial pigment. The sinusoids are filled with numerous parasitized RBCs and the macrophages contain ingested malarial pigment. The Kupffer cells may be distended with parasites and pigment. There are no characteristic changes in other organs except the presence of scattered malarial pigment in macrophages. In fatal falciparum malaria, however, the brain is slate gray and punctate hemorrhages are often scattered throughout the brain substance. The capillaries are choked with parasite-infected RBCs.

Symptoms and Signs

The incubation period is usually 10 to 35 days, often followed by a short (2 to 3 days) prodrome of irregular low-grade fever, malaise, headache, myalgia, and chilly sensations that is frequently misidentified and treated as influenza.

In **vivax** and **ovale malaria,** the primary attack begins abruptly with a shaking chill, followed by fever and sweats with irregularly remittent fever. Within a week the typical paroxysmal pattern of the disease is established. The initial chill may be preceded by a short period of malaise or headache. The fever lasts from 1 to 8 h; after it subsides, the patient feels well until the next rigor. A rigor occurs q 48 h in uncomplicated vivax malaria.

In **falciparum malaria,** there may be a chilly sensation rather than a shaking chill; the temperature rises gradually and falls by lysis. The paroxysm may last 20 to 36 h, there is more prostration than in vivax malaria, and headache is prominent. During intervals between paroxysms, which are exceedingly variable (36 to 72 h), the patient usually feels miserable and has a low-grade fever.

In **malariae malaria,** the disease more frequently begins abruptly with a paroxysm, which then recurs at 72-h intervals.

In falciparum malaria, fever of 40 C (104 F) or severe headache, drowsiness, delirium, confusion, or parasitemia in excess of 100,000 organisms/cu mm may indicate impending **cerebral malaria,** usually a fatal complication. Delirium may accompany high fever in vivax malaria, but cerebral manifestations are uncommon.

In both falciparum and vivax malaria, the periodicity of the chills and fever is influenced by numerous factors, including dual infection (by more than 1 plasmodium species), strain differences, and immunity. The WBC count is usually normal, with an increase in the percentage of lymphocytes and monocytes. Mild jaundice usually develops if the disease persists untreated, and the spleen and liver become enlarged.

Chronic malaria with low-grade parasitemia occurs in partially immune subjects in hyperendemic areas and may be accompanied by malaise, listlessness, periodic headache, anorexia, fatigue, and mild fever. These symptoms may culminate in acute attacks of chills and fever, considerably milder and of shorter duration than in the primary attack.

Blackwater fever, a rare complication, is characterized by intravascular hemolysis and hemoglobinuria. It occurs, perhaps exclusively, in chronic falciparum malaria, especially in patients treated with quinine. Primaquine may cause hemolysis in individuals with G6PD deficiency (see Curative Therapy, below).

Diagnosis

Periodic attacks of chills and fever without apparent cause always suggest malaria, particularly if the individual has been in a malarious area within the year and if the spleen is enlarged. Diagnosis depends on demonstration of the parasite in the stained blood smear; more than one smear may be required, since the intensity of parasitemia often varies. It is important to identify the type of plasmodium, as this will influence therapy and prognosis.

If fever persists after adequate antimalarial therapy in patients with suspected malaria, the original diagnosis was in error.

Prognosis

Untreated vivax malaria subsides spontaneously in 10 to 30 days, but may recur at variable intervals. The prognosis becomes less favorable if intercurrent infection supervenes or if the individual was in poor general health when the attack began. Antimalarial therapy produces excellent results in vivax and falciparum malaria. Untreated falciparum malaria has a high mortality rate.

Prophylaxis and Suppression Therapy

Attempts to induce immunity with vaccines are still in experimental stages. Patients with malaria, however, develop a gradual immunity that considerably modifies the clinical course. This immunity has a degree of strain specificity.

Preventive measures include control of mosquito breeding places and use of residual insecticide sprays in homes and outbuildings, screens (or mosquito netting where screens are not feasible) on doors and windows, and mosquito repellents and sufficient clothing (particularly after sundown, to protect as much of the skin surface as possible against mosquito bites). Contact between malaria patients and mosquitos must be prevented to avoid further spread of infection.

Chloroquine phosphate 500 mg (300-mg base) (children, 5-mg base/kg) orally once/wk protects travelers to malarious areas by suppressing the erythrocytic infection and thus the clinical manifestations of malaria. In Asia and Latin America, where chloroquine-resistant strains of P. falciparum malaria exist, 25 mg of pyrimethamine and 500 mg of sulfadoxine (available in a combination tablet in endemic areas) should also be taken orally each week. These drugs should be started 2 wk before arrival in the area and continued for 6 wk after leaving, since this continued use eradicates P. falciparum and P. malariae. In other types of malaria, primaquine must be given in addition to chloroquine (see Curative Therapy, below).

Treatment

1. Treatment of the acute attack: The drug of choice in all types of malaria except drug-resistant falciparum malaria is chloroquine. The dose is 1 gm of chloroquine phosphate (600-mg base) (children, 10-mg base/kg) orally, followed by 500 mg (300-mg base) (children, 5-mg base/kg) in 6 h, and then 500 mg (300-mg base)/day for 2 days. The total dose for adults is 2.5 gm (1.5-gm base). Patients who are comatose or vomiting may be given chloroquine hydrochloride 250 to 375 mg (200- to 300-mg base) IM q 6 h (children, 5-mg base/kg q 12 h). Oral therapy with chloroquine phosphate should be resumed as soon as possible.

Chloroquine-resistant strains of *P. falciparum* (any case contracted in Central or South America or the Far East may be resistant) should be treated with quinine, pyrimethamine, and a sulfonamide, all given concurrently. Quinine sulfate 600 mg t.i.d. (children, 25 mg/kg/day in 3 doses) is given orally for 10 days. If oral therapy is precluded, 600 mg of quinine dihydrochloride (children, 25 mg/kg/day in 3 doses) may be diluted in 300 ml saline or glucose and given IV over 30 min. The dose may be repeated q 8 h, but oral therapy should be restarted as soon as possible. In cases with renal failure, the dose is limited to 600 mg once/day. Quinine may cause tinnitus and, occasionally, drug fever or allergic purpura. Pyrimethamine 25 mg b.i.d. (children < 10 kg, 6.25 mg/day; 10 to 20 kg, 12.5 mg/day) is given orally for 2 days. It is a folate antagonist and may cause or accentuate anemia. Sulfadiazine 500 mg orally q.i.d. (children, 100 to 200 mg/kg/day in 4 doses, to a maximum of 2 gm/day) is given for 5 days.

2. Curative therapy: Because *P. falciparum* and *P. malariae* parasites do not have a persistent hepatic (exoerythrocytic) phase, the disease is cured once the acute attack is adequately treated as outlined above.

In other types of malaria, the exoerythrocytic and erythrocytic parasites must be eradicated to prevent relapse. Primaquine phosphate 26.3 mg (15-mg base)/day (children, 0.3-mg base/kg/day) orally for 14 days accomplishes this in 80 to 90% of primary infections. It may be given at the same time as chloroquine or afterward. A second course of primaquine may be given if relapse occurs. Primaquine may cause intravascular hemolysis in patients with G6PD deficiency, but this is infrequent and generally benign if the recommended therapeutic doses are given. Abdominal cramps and methemoglobinuria may also occur with primaquine.

3. Gametocidal therapy: Gametocytes usually appear 2 to 3 days after onset of the erythrocytic phase and may persist for long periods, particularly in falciparum malaria. They do not produce symptoms, but indicate preexisting infection and serve as a source of infection for the anopheles mosquito.

P. vivax and *P. malariae* gametocyte development can be prevented by suppression with chloroquine (see Prophylaxis and Suppression Therapy, above), or by adequate and prompt treatment of the acute attack. *P. falciparum* gametocytes, once developed, are resistant to suppressive drugs, but are susceptible to primaquine; 15 mg (base)/day for 3 days or a single 45-mg dose will sterilize the gametocytes.

LEISHMANIASIS

A group of conditions caused by a species of Leishmania *and transmitted by several phlebotomine sandflies.* The manifestations may be visceral, mucocutaneous, or cutaneous, and the strain of the infecting organism and the host's immunologic status apparently can greatly modify the clinical manifestations. The incubation period is weeks to months.

KALA-AZAR (Visceral Leishmaniasis; Dumdum Fever)

Epidemiology, Pathogenesis, and Findings

Kala-azar occurs in India, China, Russia, Africa, the Mediterranean basin, and several South and Central American countries. Children and young adults are particularly susceptible. The protozoa (*L. donovani*) invade the bloodstream and localize in the reticuloendothelial system, causing fever, pronounced splenomegaly, emaciation, and pancytopenia. The fever is seldom sustained and recurs irregularly. The liver and lymph nodes may become enlarged. Hypergammaglobulinemia is present. The parasite may be demonstrated in needle biopsy of the liver, spleen, bone marrow, or lymph nodes, or in cultures from these tissues or from blood. Sensitive serologic tests have been developed but are not generally available. The leishmanin skin test is negative during active disease. The fatality rate is 90% in untreated cases but generally below 10% in treated cases.

Treatment

General: Bed rest, oral hygiene, and good nutrition are important. Transfusions are useful for anemia; antibacterial chemotherapy is indicated for bacterial complications.

Specific: Pentavalent antimony compounds and aromatic diamidines are the drugs of choice. Sodium antimony gluconate (sodium stibogluconate) is given once daily, slowly IV or IM in distilled water. The generally accepted dosage is 0.1 ml (10 mg antimony)/kg/injection (maximum, 600 mg antimony/day; minimum, 200 mg/day) for 6 to 10 days. If toxic effects (nausea, vomiting) appear, the drug should be given on alternate days, its dosage reduced or its administration stopped. Three 10-day courses as above, separated by 10-day intervals, may be given in resistant (African) cases.

Kala-azar encountered in the Sudan is resistant to antimony; pentamidine 4 mg/kg/day IM for up to 15 days must be used instead.

ORIENTAL SORE (Cutaneous Leishmaniasis; Tropical Sore; Delhi or Aleppo Boil)

Epidemiology and Findings

Oriental sore occurs in China, India, the Near East, the Mediterranean basin, and Africa as far south as Nigeria and Angola. It is characterized by single or multiple sharply demarcated, ulcerating, granulomatous, autoinoculable skin lesions. Secondary infection is usual. The only systemic symptoms are those due to secondary infection. *Leishmania tropica* may be demonstrated in smears or cultures of curettings from the sides or base of the ulcer. The leishmanin skin test is positive. Healing occurs spontaneously in 2 to 18 mo, leaving a depressed scar.

Treatment

Excellent results are obtained by infiltrating the indurated edge and base of the ulcer with 6 ml of sodium antimony gluconate 3 or 4 times every other day. CO_2 snow, infrared therapy, and radiotherapy may also be effective. When lesions are numerous, sodium antimony gluconate should be given parenterally as for kala-azar, above. Antibiotics are indicated for secondary infections.

AMERICAN LEISHMANIASIS (Espundia; Forest Yaws; Uta; Chiclero Ulcer)

This disease may manifest itself as localized cutaneous ulcers resembling oriental sore or as metastatic mucocutaneous lesions known as *Espundia*. The localized lesions, caused by *L. mexicana*, usually occur on the face; they are known as chiclero ulcers, since they primarily affect persons who enter forests to gather chicle. Uta, a similar disease found in Peru, is caused by *L. braziliensis peruviana. Espundia*, which causes ulcerative lesions of the nose and pharynx, occurs in southern Mexico and Central and South America. It is caused by *L. braziliensis braziliensis*. Untreated, the disease may persist for years, with death resulting from secondary infection. **Diagnosis** is by demonstrating the parasites in biopsy material or by culture of material from the ulcer edge.

Treatment of the early cutaneous lesions is as recommended above for oriental sore. The extensive lesions of later stages require sodium antimony gluconate or pentamidine as for kala-azar (see above).

DIFFUSE CUTANEOUS LEISHMANIASIS

This form of the disease, characterized by widespread skin lesions resembling those of lepromatous leprosy, presumably results from a specific defect of cell-mediated immunity to the leishmanial organism. In South America, it is caused by *L. mexicana amazonensis*; in Ethiopia, by *L. tropica aethiopica*. The diagnosis is made by demonstrating the organisms in the skin lesions. The disease is resistant to treatment.

TRYPANOSOMIASIS (African Sleeping Sickness; Chagas' Disease)

A chronic disease caused by protozoa of the genus Trypanosoma. *T. brucei* var. *gambiense* and *rhodesiense* produce African sleeping sickness (Gambian and Rhodesian trypanosomiasis); *T. cruzi* causes Chagas' disease (South American trypanosomiasis), seen in South and Central America. The African forms of trypanosomiasis are spread by the bite of the tsetse fly (genus *Glossina*). Chagas' disease is transmitted by contamination of the bite wound of the "assassin" or "kissing" reduviid bugs (*Triatoma* and related Reduviidae) with the infected feces of the insect.

Symptoms, Signs, and Course

African trypanosomiasis is characterized by irregular fever, generalized lymphadenopathy (particularly of the posterior cervical chain), cutaneous eruptions, and areas of painful localized edema. CNS symptoms, such as tremors, headache, apathy, and convulsions, later predominate and progress to coma and death. Rhodesian trypanosomiasis is more severe and more often fatal than Gambian trypanosomiasis.

Acute Chagas' disease occurs predominantly in young children and is characterized in the early stages by fever, lymphadenopathy, hepatosplenomegaly, and facial edema. Rarely, meningoencephalitis or convulsive seizures may occur, sometimes causing permanent mental or physical defects or death. Acute myocarditis is common and may be fatal. Chronic Chagas' disease may be mild or even asymptomatic, or may be accompanied by myocardiopathy, megaesophagus, and megacolon, with fatal outcome. These late manifestations probably result from lymphocyte-mediated destruction of muscle tissue and nerve ganglions during the acute stage of the disease. In Brazil and Argentina the disease is often severe; in Chile, usually mild.

Diagnosis

Recognition of African trypanosomiasis depends on demonstration of the trypanosomes. Early in the disease, they may be found in smears of peripheral blood or in fluid aspirated from an enlarged lymph node. In advanced stages, they may be found only in the CSF.

Chagas' disease is identified by demonstration of trypanosomes in the peripheral blood or leishmanial forms in a lymph node biopsy, or by animal inoculation or culture, xenodiagnosis, or CF tests.

Prophylaxis

Prophylaxis against African trypanosomiasis includes protection against the vector flies, avoidance of endemic areas, or chemoprophylaxis. Pentamidine 4 mg/kg IM every 3 to 6 mo confers a high degree of protection against the Gambian form of disease, but its use in the Rhodesian variety is controversial. Pentamidine may produce cryptic infections and cause diabetes; therefore it should be used only in persons in great danger of being infected.

Reduviid bugs, the vectors of Chagas' disease, inhabit poorly constructed houses and outbuildings. Residual spraying with 5% γ-benzene hexachloride is most effective in controlling the vector.

Treatment

There is no satisfactory treatment for Chagas' disease. Prolonged administration of nifurtimox, a nitrofurazone derivative, may effect parasitologic cure. Chronic organ damage, however, appears irreversible.

Suramin is the drug of choice for both early Rhodesian and Gambian trypanosomiasis. It is given IV as a 10% solution in distilled water; an initial test dose of 100 mg (to exclude hypersensitivity) is followed by 1 gm on the next day and on days 3, 7, I4, and 2I, for a total of 5 gm. (CAUTION: *Renal impairment*)

Melarsoprol, a trivalent arsenical, is more toxic than the above drugs, but is effective in all stages of Gambian and Rhodesian trypanosomiasis. It should be used when the CNS is involved. Patients with minimal to moderate neurologic involvement are given three 3-day courses of 3.6 mg/kg/day IV, each course 2 wk apart. Melarsoprol causes the usual arsenical toxicity: GI, neurologic, and renal.

Patients with severe neurologic involvement may develop a reactive encephalopathy when given melarsoprol. Prior treatment with suramin may help to avert this complication, which is apparently due to release of trypanosomal antigen. Suramin is given in 2 to 4 alternate-day doses of 250 to 500 mg IV. Melarsoprol is then given in 3 daily or alternate-day doses of 1.5, 2.0, and 2.2 mg/kg IV. After a 7-day interval, 3 doses of melarsoprol, 2.5, 3.0, and 3.6 mg/kg/day, are given; after another 7-day interval, a third course of 3.6 mg/kg/day is given for 3 days.

TOXOPLASMOSIS

A generalized or CNS granulomatous disease caused by Toxoplasma gondii. Asymptomatic infections are common; serologic surveys show that 7 to 94% of various populations are infected. The disease occurs worldwide.

Etiology and Pathogenesis

T. gondii is a small intracellular protozoan parasite that can infect any warm-blooded animal. It invades and multiplies asexually within the cytoplasm of nucleated host cells. With the development of host immunity, multiplication slows and tissue cysts are formed. Sexual multiplication occurs in the intestinal cells of cats (and apparently only cats); oocysts form and are shed in the stool. Transmission may occur transplacentally, by ingestion of raw or undercooked meat containing tissue cysts, or, perhaps most importantly, by exposure to oocysts in cat feces.

Symptoms and Signs

Neonatal congenital toxoplasmosis (see also CONGENITAL TOXOPLASMOSIS under NEONATAL INFECTIONS in Vol. II, Ch. 21) is acquired transplacentally, the mother presumably having acquired a primary infection at conception or later during pregnancy. Abortion may ensue if infection occurs early in pregnancy. Infection later in pregnancy may result in miscarriage or stillbirth, or in the birth of a living child with clinical disease. The disease may be severe, fulminating, and rapidly fatal, or there may be no symptoms at all. Symptoms of subacute infection may begin shortly after birth, but more often appear months or several years later. Chronic chorioretinitis; severe jaundice; hepatosplenomegaly; maculopapular rash; thrombocytopenic purpura; intracerebral calcification; convulsions, opisthotonos, psychomotor disturbances, or other CNS symptoms; and hydrocephalus or microcephaly are common. Blindness and severe mental retardation may result. Chronic disease, with relapses, occurs in patients who survive the subacute phase. Visceral lesions, aside from those in the liver, are unusual and heal more readily than CNS lesions.

Acquired toxoplasmosis is seldom symptomatic and is usually recognized serologically. However, symptomatic infection may present in any of 3 ways:

1. The more common **mild lymphatic form** may resemble infectious mononucleosis. It is characterized by cervical and axillary lymphadenopathy, malaise, muscle pain, and irregular low fever. Mild anemia, hypotension, leukopenia, lymphocytosis, and slightly altered liver function may be present. More commonly, it presents as asymptomatic cervical lymphadenopathy.

2. An acute, **fulminating, disseminated infection** occurs primarily in immunologically incompetent patients, often with a rash, high fever, chills, and prostration. Some patients may develop meningoencephalitis, hepatitis, pneumonitis, or myocarditis.

3. **Chronic toxoplasmosis** causes severe retinochoroiditis (posterior uveitis); muscular weakness, weight loss, headache, and diarrhea may be present. Symptoms are vague and indefinite, and diagnosis is difficult. In the USA, uveitis is seldom due to *Toxoplasma* infection.

Diagnosis

The diagnosis is usually established serologically. IgM antibodies, which are detected by the indirect fluorescent antibody procedure (IgM-IFA), appear during the 1st wk of illness, peak within 1 to 2 wk, and revert to normal within 3 wk to several months. IgG antibodies arise more slowly, peak in 1 or 2 mo, and then may remain high and stable for months to years. They are also detected with the indirect fluorescent-antibody **(IgG-IFA)** technic, but may also be measured with the Sabin-Feldman dye, indirect hemagglutination, and the CF tests. A positive IgM-IFA test ($>$ 1:20) or a 2-tube rise in one of the IgG tests usually indicates the presence of acute disease. Acute disease should also be assumed present if the IgG-IFA or dye test titers exceed 1:1000 in the presence of lymphadenopathy in a pregnant woman or encephalitis in an immunocompromised host.

The parasite has been isolated during the acute phase of the disease by injecting mice with biopsy material from lymph nodes, muscle, or other tissues.

Prognosis

The prognosis is poor in congenital toxoplasmosis acquired during the 1st trimester. Affected children die in infancy or suffer chronic destructive CNS lesions. Infections acquired during the 3rd trimester are usually asymptomatic. The prognosis in acquired postnatal toxoplasmosis is good. The general mildness of postnatally acquired infection is indicated by the large number of persons with latent or cured toxoplasmosis, and by the fact that the disease is rarely fatal in adults. Reactivation of toxoplasmosis in immunosuppressed patients usually ends in death.

Treatment

Acute toxoplasmosis of newborns, pregnant women, and immunosuppressed patients should be treated with standard oral doses of trisulfapyrimidines or sulfadiazine plus pyrimethamine 25 mg (1 mg/kg for children) daily for 3 to 4 wk. The hematologic toxicity of pyrimethamine can be minimized with the daily administration of folinic acid (10 mg). Since pyrimethamine is teratogenic in animals, sulfonamides alone should be used in the first trimester of pregnancy. Other patients with active disease do not require specific therapy unless a vital organ (eye, brain, heart) is involved or constitutional symptoms are severe and persistent. Corticosteroids are often useful in these situations to control the inflammatory reaction. Periodic blood counts may be obtained during therapy to monitor the hemotoxicity of pyrimethamine.

BABESIOSIS

A cosmopolitan infection of animals caused by intraerythrocytic parasites of the genus Babesia. Human disease is rare. The organisms are transmitted by hard-bodied ticks and produce a febrile hemolytic anemia. In splenectomized patients the infection has a high mortality rate and closely resembles falciparum malaria, with high fever, hemolytic anemia, hemoglobinuria, jaundice, and renal failure. A patient with an intact spleen has a milder illness that usually resolves spontaneously in weeks or months. Most cases in the USA have been of this milder type and have been acquired on offshore islands of New York and Massachusetts. **Diagnosis** requires demonstration of the parasites, which resemble those of malaria, in Giemsa-stained smears of peripheral blood. In contrast to *Plasmodium* spp., however, neither gametocytes nor malaria pigment can be seen. The presence of tetrads and basket-shaped parasites is also helpful.

Treatment is usually not required in patients with intact spleens. In infections that are life-threatening, clindamycin 300 to 750 mg IV q 6 h and quinine 650 mg orally q 6 h appear to be effective.

DISEASES CAUSED BY WORMS

INTESTINAL NEMATODES

ENTEROBIASIS (See TABLE 13–1 in this chapter and PINWORM INFESTATION in Vol. II, Ch. 24)

TRICHURIASIS (Whipworm Infection; Trichocephaliasis)

An infection caused by Trichuris trichiura *and characterized by abdominal pain and diarrhea.*

Etiology, Pathogenesis, and Epidemiology

Infection results from ingestion of eggs that have incubated in soil for 2 or 3 wk. The larva hatches in the small intestine, migrates to the colon, and embeds its anterior head in the mucosa. Mature females produce about 5000 eggs/day, which are passed in the stool.

This parasite is found principally in the subtropics and tropics, where poor sanitation and a warm, moist climate provide the conditions necessary for incubating the eggs in soil. Clinically significant infections are uncommon in the USA.

Symptoms, Signs, and Diagnosis

Only heavy infection causes symptoms—abdominal pain and diarrhea. Very heavy infections may cause intestinal blood loss, anemia, weight loss, appendicitis, and, in children and parturient women, rectal prolapse.

The characteristic barrel-shaped eggs are usually readily found in the stool.

Prophylaxis and Treatment

Prevention depends upon adequate toilet facilities and good personal hygiene.

Mebendazole 100 mg orally b.i.d. for 3 days has been highly effective and is the drug of choice. The drug should not be used in pregnancy because it is teratogenic in animals. Light infections (those that require stool concentration procedure for their detection) do not require treatment.

ASCARIASIS

An infection caused by Ascaris lumbricoides *and characterized by early pulmonary and later intestinal symptoms.*

Etiology, Epidemiology, and Pathogenesis

The life cycle of the ascarids resembles that of *Trichuris* except for a phase of larval migration through the lungs. Once the larva hatches, it migrates through the wall of the small intestine and is carried by the lymphatics and bloodstream to the lungs. Here it passes into an alveolus, ascends the respiratory tract, and is swallowed. It matures in the jejunum, where it remains as an adult worm. Disease may be caused by both the larval migration through the lung and the presence of the adult worm in the intestine. Malabsorption may result with heavy worm loads; the pathogenesis is not clearly understood.

The disease occurs worldwide but is concentrated in warm, poorly sanitated areas where it is maintained largely by the indiscriminate defecation and ingestion habits of children.

Symptoms, Signs, and Diagnosis

Fever, cough, wheezing, eosinophilic leukocytosis, and migratory pulmonary infiltrates may be present during the phase of larval migration through the lungs. Heavy intestinal infection may cause abdominal cramping and, occasionally, intestinal obstruction. Adult worms may rarely obstruct the appendix, or the biliary or pancreatic ducts.

Infection with the adult worm is usually diagnosed by finding eggs in the stool. Occasionally, adult worms are passed in the stool or vomited. Larvae are occasionally found in the sputum during the pulmonary phase.

Prophylaxis

Prevention requires adequate sanitation. Drug prophylaxis has been successful in endemic areas.

Treatment

Pyrantel pamoate 11 mg/kg (maximum, 1 gm) in a single oral dose, or mebendazole 100 mg b.i.d. for 3 days is also effective. Mebendazole should not be used in pregnancy (see TRICHURIASIS, above).

HOOKWORM DISEASE

A symptomatic infection caused by Ancylostoma duodenale *or* Necator americanus *and characterized by abdominal pain and iron-deficiency anemia.* Asymptomatic hookworm infection is more common than symptomatic disease.

Etiology, Pathogenesis, and Epidemiology

The life cycles of the 2 worms are similar. Eggs are discharged in the stool and hatch in the soil after a 1- to 2-day incubation period, releasing a free, living larva that molts a few days later and becomes infective to humans. The larvae penetrate human skin, reach the lung via the lymphatics and blood, ascend the respiratory tract, are swallowed, and, about a week after skin penetration, reach the intestine. They attach by their mouths to the mucosa of the upper small intestine and suck blood.

About 25% of the world's population is infected with hookworms. Infection is most common in warm, moist areas with poor sanitation. *A. duodenale* is found in the Mediterranean basin, India, China, and Japan. *N. americanus* is found primarily in tropical areas of Africa, Asia, and the Americas; it is the species found in the USA.

Symptoms and Signs

A pruritic maculopapular rash ("ground itch") may develop at the site of larval penetration. Larval pulmonary migration occasionally causes pulmonary symptoms (see ASCARIASIS, above). Adult worms often cause epigastric pain. Whether iron-deficiency anemia and hypoalbuminemia result from intestinal blood loss depends upon whether the gut losses are replaced in the diet; this, in turn, is related to the worm load and to dietary adequacy. Growth retardation, cardiac failure, and anasarca may accompany chronic severe blood loss. In most infections, however, anemia does not develop.

Diagnosis

In symptomatic infections, the typical eggs are usually readily detected in the stool. If the stool is not examined for several hours, the eggs may hatch and release larvae that may be confused with those of *Strongyloides.*

Prophylaxis

Preventing soil pollution and avoiding direct skin contact with the soil are effective but impractical measures in most endemic areas. Periodic mass treatment and dietary iron supplements may be effective.

Treatment

General supportive treatment and correction of anemia take first priority. Anemia usually responds to oral iron therapy, but parenteral iron or blood transfusions may be required in severe cases. Anthelmintic therapy may be given as soon as the patient's condition is stable. Several effective agents are available. Pyrantel pamoate 11 mg/kg (maximum, 1 gm) orally is given in a single dose. Mebendazole 100 mg orally b.i.d. for 3 days is equally effective but should not be used in pregnant women (see TRICHURIASIS, above).

STRONGYLOIDIASIS (Threadworm Infection)

An infection caused by Strongyloides stercoralis *and characterized by eosinophilia and epigastric pain.*

Etiology, Pathogenesis, and Epidemiology

The life cycle closely resembles that of the hookworm, except that the eggs hatch while still in the intestine, and larvae rather than ova are passed in the stool. The larvae generally molt in the soil and develop into the infective filariform stage. Occasionally, the larvae molt in the intestine or on the perianal skin, and the filariform larvae then invade the host directly ("autoinfection" or "hyperinfection") without going through a soil phase. This can result in an extremely heavy worm load.

The disease is endemic in the tropics and is generally found in the same climatic and sanitary conditions favorable to the spread of hookworm. It may also occur in temperate areas in unsanitary, crowded institutions.

Symptoms, Signs, and Diagnosis

Transient bouts of linear urticaria and erythema may accompany autoinfection. Pulmonary manifestations similar to those seen in ascariasis (see above) may occur as a result of larval migration through the lungs. Heavy intestinal infection may cause epigastric pain and tenderness, vomiting, and diarrhea. Potentially fatal massive autoinfection and widespread larval migration may occur in immunodepressed patients, and these often are accompanied by severe enterocolitis and gram-negative bacteremia.

Larvae are found in the stool; several specimens should be examined, since only a few larvae may be present. Examination of duodenal aspirates or jejunal biopsies may also demonstrate the larvae.

Prophylaxis and Treatment

Prevention is generally as above, for hookworm. Thiabendazole 25 mg/kg b.i.d. orally for 2 or 3 days is effective treatment. In disseminated disease, treatment should be continued for 5 days.

TISSUE NEMATODES

TRICHINOSIS (Trichiniasis)

A parasitic disease caused by Trichinella spiralis, *characterized initially by GI symptoms, and later by periorbital edema, muscle pains, fever, and eosinophilia.*

Etiology, Pathogenesis, and Epidemiology

Infection with the roundworm *T. spiralis* results from eating raw or inadequately cooked or processed pork or pork products (rarely, meat of bears and some marine mammals) containing encysted larvae (trichinae). The cyst wall is digested in the stomach or duodenum and the liberated larvae penetrate the duodenal and jejunal mucosa. Within 2 days, the larvae mature sexually and mate, after which the males play no further role in disease causation. The females burrow into the intestinal wall and begin to discharge living larvae by the 7th day. Each female may produce over 1000 larvae. Larviposition continues for about 4 to 6 wk, after which the female worm dies and is digested. The minute (0.1 mm) larvae are carried by the lymphatic and portal circulation to the bloodstream, and from there to various tissues and organs. Only those larvae reaching skeletal muscle survive; they penetrate individual fibers, causing myositis. They grow to 1 mm in length, coil up, encyst, and eventually calcify. Encystment is complete by the end of the 3rd mo. The larvae may remain viable for several years. The diaphragm and tongue, and the pectoral, eye, and intercostal muscles are especially involved. Larvae reaching the myocardium and other nonskeletal muscles are surrounded by a focus of inflammatory reaction and die. In animals, the encysted larvae are the source of infection for the next host.

Trichinosis occurs worldwide but is rare or absent in native populations of the tropics and where swine are fed root vegetables, as in France. In the USA, it has become sporadic and less frequent; outbreaks are usually caused by consumption of ready-to-eat pork sausages.

Symptoms and Signs

The clinical course is markedly irregular, severity varying with the number of invading larvae, the tissues invaded, and the physiologic condition of the patient. Many patients remain asymptomatic. GI symptoms and slight fever may appear within 1 or 2 days after ingestion of infected meat, but manifestations of systemic larval invasion usually do not appear for 7 to 15 days. Edema of the upper eyelids appears suddenly about the 11th day of infection and is one of the earliest and most characteristic signs. This may be followed by subconjunctival and retinal hemorrhage, pain, and photophobia. Muscle soreness and pain, urticaria, subungual hemorrhage, thirst, profuse sweating, fever, chills, weakness, prostration, and a rapidly rising eosinophilia may develop shortly after the ocular signs. Soreness is especially pronounced in the muscles of respiration, speech, mastication, and swallowing. Severe dyspnea, sometimes causing death, may occur. Fever is generally remittent, rising to 39 C (102 F) or higher, remaining elevated for several days, and then falling gradually. Eosinophilia usually begins in the 2nd wk, reaches its height (20 to 40% or more) in the 3rd or 4th wk, then gradually declines. It may be obscured by concomitant bacterial infection. Lymphadenitis, encephalitis, meningitis, visual or auditory disorders, pneumonitis, pleurisy, and myocarditis may develop in the 3rd to 6th wk, as the widely disseminated larvae outside the skeletal muscles are destroyed by inflammatory reaction; if myocardial failure develops, it occurs between the 4th and 8th wk. Most symptoms disappear by about the 3rd mo, although vague muscular pains and fatigue may persist for months.

Diagnosis

During the intestinal stage of infection, symptoms are nonspecific and no diagnostic laboratory procedures are available. Diarrhea, nausea, vomiting, and other GI disturbances may be recalled later by the patient. A history of ingesting ready-to-eat pork sausage or insufficiently cooked pork or bear meat, followed by acute gastroenteritis or acute facial edema (particularly of the upper eyelids) is helpful in diagnosis. Eosinophilic leukocytosis usually appears within 2 wk of infection. Muscle biopsy performed during the 4th wk of infection may demonstrate larvae or cysts. Even when trichinae cannot be demonstrated in the biopsy specimen, a diffuse myositis may indicate active trichinosis. The parasite is rarely found in the infected meat, or in the patient's stool, blood, or CSF.

Commercially available skin test antigens are unreliable at present and their use is discouraged. Available serologic tests include CF, precipitin, indirect fluorescent antibody, and (probably the best) bentonite flocculation. False negative results can occur occasionally with each; therefore, 2 or more tests should be employed routinely. Since these tests may also remain positive for years, they are of most value if they are initially negative and then turn positive.

Skeletal manifestations of trichinosis must be differentiated from acute rheumatic fever, acute arthritis, angioedema, and myositis; **febrile states** from TB, typhoid fever, sepsis, undulant fever; **pulmonary manifestations** from pneumonitis; **neurologic manifestations** from meningitis, encephalitis, and poliomyelitis; and **eosinophilia** from Hodgkin's disease, eosinophilic leukemia, and polyarteritis nodosa.

Prognosis

This is good in most cases. Unfavorable prognostic signs are the absence of an eosinophilic response, or a sudden fall in the eosinophil level to 1% or zero during the acute phase.

Prophylaxis

Trichinosis can be prevented by thoroughly cooking all pork and pork products. Larvae can generally be rendered nonviable by freezing the meat at -15 C for 3 wk or -18 C for 1 day; however, larvae from arctic mammals appear to survive even colder temperatures. Hogs should not be fed raw garbage, since it may contain infected pork wastes.

Treatment

Symptomatic and supportive therapy is aimed at assisting the patient to survive the acute toxemia, which terminates when the larvae become encysted. Muscular pains are usually relieved by bed rest, but may require analgesics such as aspirin or codeine. Corticosteroids are indicated for patients with severe allergic manifestations or myocardial or CNS involvement. Prednisone 20 to 60 mg/day orally in divided doses is given for 3 or 4 days; dosage is then gradually reduced and the drug is discontinued in 10 days.

Thiabendazole, 25 mg/kg b.i.d. orally for 5 to 10 days, is highly effective against the parasite, but the clinical response is variable.

TOXOCARIASIS (Visceral Larva Migrans)

A widely distributed clinical syndrome resulting from invasion of human viscera by nematode larvae (e.g., Toxocara canis *and* cati, *normally intestinal parasites of dogs and cats), with subsequent prolonged migration of the larvae through the body.* It usually occurs as a relatively benign disease in children aged 2 to 4, but may afflict older patients.

Etiology and Pathogenesis

The source of infection is the fully embryonated egg of the parasite found in soil contaminated by feces of infected dogs and cats. Children's sandboxes are attractive defecating sites for cats and are a potential hazard. The eggs may be transferred either directly to the mouth as the child plays in or eats (geophagia) the contaminated soil or indirectly through contaminated food or other objects. The incubation period varies from weeks to several months, depending on the intensity and number of exposures and on the sensitivity of the patient.

The eggs hatch in the intestine after ingestion. Liberated larvae penetrate the intestinal wall and are widely disseminated in the body by the systemic circulation. Almost any tissue may be involved, particularly the CNS, eye, liver, lung, and heart. The larvae may remain alive for many months, causing damage by their wanderings and by tissue sensitization. They produce a focal granulomatous reaction, though the larvae themselves may be difficult to demonstrate in tissue sections. The parasites do not complete their development in the human body.

Symptoms, Signs, and Diagnosis

Clinically, patients present with fever, cough or wheezing, and hepatomegaly. Skin rash, splenomegaly, and recurrent pneumonia occur in some patients. Eye lesions (chorioretinitis), which may be mistaken for retinoblastoma, may be seen in older children and adults, usually in the absence of other clinical manifestations of disease.

High eosinophilia (> 60%), hepatomegaly, pneumonitis, fever, and hyperglobulinemia are suggestive. Liver biopsy and demonstration of a larva or its fragments in the typical granulomatous lesion may be helpful in the diagnosis. Reliable serologic tests have been developed recently. The prognosis is good; the disease is self-limited (6 to 18 mo in the absence of reinfection).

Prophylaxis and Treatment

Infected pet dogs and cats, particularly those under 6 mo of age, should be dewormed regularly (under veterinary direction), and children's sandboxes should be covered when not in use.

No proven treatment is available. Thiabendazole 25 to 50 mg/kg for 7 to 10 days is probably the treatment of choice; or diethylcarbamazine 2 mg/kg t.i.d. orally after meals for 2 to 4 wk may be helpful, although it has no demonstrable activity against ascarids. Prednisone 20 to 40 mg/day orally, with reduced dosage after 3 to 5 days, helps to control symptoms.

FILARIASIS

A group of diseases occurring in tropical and subtropical countries and caused by Filarioidea.

Etiology and Pathogenesis

Wuchereria bancrofti is found only in humans; *Brugia malayi* is often spread to man from animal hosts. The adult filarioidea live in the human lymphatic system. Microfilariae released by gravid females are found in the peripheral blood, usually at night. Infection is spread by many species of mosquitoes; vectors of *W. bancrofti* are *Aedes, Culex,* and *Anopheles;* of *B. malayi, Anopheles* and *Mansonia.* The microfilariae are ingested by the mosquito, undergo development in the insect's thoracic muscles, and, when mature, migrate to its mouthparts. When the infected mosquito bites a new host, the microfilariae penetrate the bite puncture and eventually reach the lymphatics, where they develop to the adult stage.

Pathology

Inflammation and fibrosis occur in the vicinity of the adult worms, producing progressive lymphatic obstruction. The microfilariae probably do not contribute directly to the host reaction.

Symptoms and Signs

The incubation period may be as short as 2 mo. The "prepatent" period (from time of infection to appearance of microfilariae in the blood) is at least 8 mo. Clinical manifestations depend on the severity of the infection; they may include lymphangitis, lymphadenitis, orchitis, funiculitis, epididymitis, lymph varices, and chyluria. Chills, fever, headache, and malaise may also be present. Elephantiasis and other late severe sequelae occur with long-time residence in endemic areas and repeated reinfection. An aberrant form of filariasis (tropical eosinophilia) is characterized by hypereosinophilia, presence of microfilariae in the tissues but not the blood, and high titers of antifilarial antibodies. Clinically, the patient may present with lymphadenosplenomegaly or with cough, bronchospasm, and chest infiltrates.

Diagnosis

Microfilariae may be found in blood or lymph fluid. An intradermal antigen (prepared from *Dirofilaria immitis*) is useful when microfilariae cannot be demonstrated, but is not completely reliable.

Prophylaxis and Treatment

Promising results have been obtained in controlling filariasis by combining mass treatment and mosquito control.

Diethylcarbamazine 2 mg/kg orally t.i.d. after meals for 3 to 4 wk eliminates microfilariae from the bloodstream. In many patients it also kills adult worms or impairs their reproductive capacity, resulting in permanent clearing of the microfilariae. Severe allergic reactions and abscess formation may follow its use, but may be controlled by antihistamines or corticosteroids.

Surgical intervention is indicated only to alleviate certain types of elephantiasis, especially of the scrotum. Elephantiasis of the legs is treated by elevation and elastic bandages.

ONCHOCERCIASIS (River Blindness)

A disease resulting from infection by Onchocerca volvulus *and characterized by fibrous nodules in the skin and subcutaneous tissues.* Ocular findings are common; blindness may result. The disease, spread by the bite of black flies (*Simuliidae*), occurs in southern Mexico, Guatemala, Venezuela, Colombia, Yemen, and central Africa. **Diagnosis** depends on demonstration of microfilariae in skin snips or nodules.

Treatment

Microfilariae, but not adult worms, are destroyed by diethylcarbamazine, given orally after meals. Since an allergic reaction to the dead microfilariae can result in ocular damage if the eye is involved in the infection, initial dosage is limited to 0.1 to 0.2 mg/kg/day. Dosage is gradually increased to 2 to 3 mg/kg t.i.d. and then maintained at this level for 1 wk. An antihistamine and prednisone 20 to 40 mg/day orally may be necessary to prevent the acute allergic inflammation in and around the eye that follows the rapid destruction of numerous microfilariae.

Adult worms are eliminated by surgically removing the nodules; suramin (CAUTION: *Toxicity*) in a test dose of 100 mg IV, followed by 5 weekly injections of 1 gm IV, is also effective.

LOIASIS (Calabar Swellings)

A form of filariasis found in west and central Africa, caused by Loa loa *and transmitted by the bite of flies of the genus* Chrysops. The disease is characterized by localized transient swellings (calabar swellings) caused by migration of adult worms in the subcutaneous tissues. The worms may also migrate across the eye beneath the conjunctiva. Microfilariae are found in the calabar swellings and peripheral blood; eosinophilia is common.

Treatment

Diethylcarbamazine 2 mg/kg orally t.i.d. after meals for 14 days kills both the microfilariae and adult worms. Since allergic reactions are common during the first part of treatment, an antihistamine and prednisone 10 to 30 mg/day orally should be given concurrently during the first 4 days of treatment.

DRACUNCULIASIS (Dracontiasis; "Fiery Serpent"; Guinea Worm)

A disease caused by the presence of the guinea worm (Dracunculus medinensis) *in subcutaneous tissues.* It is endemic in India, Pakistan, the Near East, tropical Africa, certain West Indies islands, and the Guianas. Infection follows ingestion of water containing infected crustacea (*Cyclops*). The larvae penetrate the intestinal wall, mature in the retroperitoneal space, and migrate to the subcutaneous tissue, producing skin ulcers through which the female discharges larvae. Intense local itching and burning may result. **Diagnosis** is possible only after the adult worm reaches its destination under the skin, at which time its head may be seen in the base of the ulcer, or larvae may be demonstrated in the discharge.

Treatment consists of slow extraction of the adult worm by gradual traction on its head over a period of 10 days. Administering thiabendazole 25 mg/kg b.i.d. for 2 days or niridazole 25 mg/kg in 3 divided doses for 3 days leads to rapid symptomatic improvement; it is uncertain whether the worms are killed or just expelled. Surgical removal is not recommended. Septic and foreign-body reactions should be treated appropriately.

DIROFILARIASIS (Heartworm)

Dirofilaria immitis, a large filaria, lives in the right heart of dogs. Microfilariae are released into the peripheral blood, where they are taken up by several species of mosquitoes. If they are subsequently transmitted to man by an infected mosquito (an exceedingly rare event), they find their way to the lung to produce well-defined pulmonary nodules. The patient may experience chest pain, cough, and, occasionally, hemoptysis. **Diagnosis** is made by histologic examination of pulmonary nodules. No treatment is indicated.

TREMATODES

SCHISTOSOMIASIS (Bilharziasis)

A visceral parasitic disease caused by blood flukes of the genus Schistosoma.

Etiology, Pathogenesis, and Epidemiology

The schistosomes that affect man are digenetic trematodes. Fresh-water snails are the intermediate hosts. Human infection follows contact (by bathing, wading, etc.) with the free-swimming cercariae of the parasite that penetrate the skin and are carried to the intrahepatic portal circulation, where they mature in 1 to 3 mo. The adult worms then migrate to the venules of the bladder or intestines. Three species cause clinical disease: *S. haematobium* causes symptoms in the GU system or the lower colon and rectum; *S. mansoni* and *S. japonicum* cause disturbances in the small intestine, colon, and rectum.

The disease is endemic in Africa, the Middle East, and Cyprus (*S. haematobium*); Egypt, areas of northern and southern Africa, certain West Indies islands, and the northern ⅔ of South America (*S. mansoni*); and Japan, central and south China, the Philippines, the Celebes, Thailand, and Laos (*S. japonicum*). *S. mansoni* is frequently encountered in Puerto Ricans residing in the USA.

Several schistosome species do not dwell in man, but are capable of causing dermatitis (**"swimmer's itch"**) and are seen in the USA as well as elsewhere. The definitive hosts are usually migratory birds; both fresh and salt water mollusks serve as intermediate hosts.

Symptoms and Signs

Initially, a pruritic papular dermatitis appears where the cercariae entered the skin. In "swimmer's itch" the disease never progresses beyond this point. In other forms, the adult worm develops in the liver, causing fever, eosinophilia, and often urticaria, hepatosplenomegaly, and lymphadenopathy. When the adults migrate to the viscera, the damage caused by the reaction to their eggs produces symptoms referable to the affected visceral structures (cystitis, chronic diarrhea). Hepatic cirrhosis, portal hypertension and resulting splenomegaly, ascites, and esophageal varices may occur from inflammation and fibrosis around eggs that have been carried back to the liver by the portal blood flow, especially in *S. mansoni* and *S. japonicum* infections. With the establishment of venous collaterals, eggs may be transported to other organs of the body as well. Eggs of *S. haematobium* and *S. mansoni* may cause pulmonary damage; those of *S. japonicum* and *S. mansoni* may cause CNS damage.

Diagnosis

Eggs are found in the stool (*S. japonicum* and *mansoni*) or urine (*S. haematobium*), or in rectal or bladder biopsies. Repeated stool examinations using concentration technics may be necessary. Positive skin and serologic tests are not sufficient basis for therapy, but should lead to a vigorous search for eggs. Only the demonstration of living eggs in a patient warrants initiation of treatment.

Prophylaxis

Control of the disease is difficult and depends upon proper disposal of urine and feces, use of molluscacides, provision of a pure water supply, and treatment with anthelmintics.

Treatment

Since the severity of schistosomiasis depends on the intensity of infection, the aim of therapy is to reduce the worm load. Prolonged or repeated courses of antischistosomal agents in an attempt to effect a cure are unwarranted because of the toxicity of available agents. Niridazole and the trivalent antimony compounds are the preferred therapeutic agents. The former agent in the dose of 25 mg/kg/day orally in 2 divided doses for 5 to 7 days is the drug of choice for *S. mansoni* and *S. haematobium* infections. Cure rates in *S. japonicum* infections are low; nevertheless, niradazole treatment will usually substantially reduce total egg output even in this disease, leading many authorities to recommend this agent for all 3 parasites. Mental confusion, psychosis, and, less commonly, convulsions may occur during treatment but disappear when the drug is discontinued.

Tartar emetic (antimony potassium tartrate) is the most toxic, but most effective, of the trivalent antimonials and is probably the drug of choice in *S. japonicum* infections. It is given slowly IV as a 0.5% solution 2 or 3 h after a light meal. The needle should be wiped with a sterile sponge; extravasation of fluid should be **avoided** since the solution irritates tissues and may cause sloughing. The patient should remain recumbent for at least an hour after treatment. The drug is given on alternate days. The initial dose is 40 mg (8 ml). If tolerated, the dose is increased by 20 mg (4 ml) every other day, to a maximum dose of 140 mg (28 ml). This last dose is continued until a total of 15 injections has been given.

Toxic effects of tartar emetic include coughing immediately upon injection (which is not important), nausea, vomiting, stiff joints and muscles, a sense of constriction of the chest, upper abdominal pain, cardiac arrhythmias, dizziness, and collapse. Hepatitis, nephritis, or hemolytic anemia may occur occasionally. The drug should be stopped at once if critical toxic reactions occur during injection. Following any major toxic effect, subsequent doses should be reduced, or administration of the drug temporarily or permanently discontinued, according to the circumstances. Severe coughing can be controlled or avoided by giving future doses in 2 portions 1 h apart.

Stibocaptate (sodium antimony dimercaptosuccinate), another trivalent antimony, can be used in all 3 infections if the primary drugs mentioned above cannot be used. It is given IM 8 mg/kg once or twice weekly for a total of 5 doses. (CAUTION: *Trivalent antimonials are contraindicated in liver, kidney, and cardiac disease*) Hycanthone, a thioxanthone given as a single IM injection, is also effective against *S. mansoni* and *S. haematobium*, but its mutagenic and hepatotoxic properties limit its usefulness.

Patients should be examined for the presence of living eggs 3 and 6 mo after treatment. Retreatment is indicated if egg excretion has not decreased markedly.

CLONORCHIASIS

An inflammation of the liver resulting from ingesting cysts of the fluke Clonorchis sinensis.

Etiology and Epidemiology

Clonorchis sinensis is an important liver fluke of humans (see SCHISTOSOMIASIS above and TABLE 13-1 for other flukes infesting humans): it lives for 20 to 50 yr in the biliary tree and passes operculated eggs into the feces. The egg, on reaching fresh water, hatches into a free-swimming miracidium that is ingested by the intermediate snail host. After multiplying and further development within the snail, thousands of free-living cercariae are released and must enter 2nd intermediate hosts—e.g., freshwater fish, such as the carp and salmon, where they encyst to form metacercariae. Infections follow ingestion of raw, dried, salted, or pickled fish containing these metacercariae. The larvae are released in the duodenum, enter the common bile duct, and migrate to the 2nd-order bile ducts (or, occasionally, the gallbladder and pancreatic ducts), where they mature in about 1 mo into adult, flat flukes varying from a few mm to several cm in length. Endemic in the Far East (where dogs, cats, pigs, and other animals also serve as reservoirs), the infection is found elsewhere most frequently among immigrants from that area and in fish imported from there.

Symptoms, Signs, and Complications

Light infections are usually asymptomatic. Apparent cases occur mainly in adults, when the worm load accumulates to > 500. Initially the patient may have fever, chills, tender hepatomegaly, mild jaundice, and eosinophilia. The mature worms, feeding on secretions from the biliary duct mucosa and possibly on cellular elements, cause chronic cholangitis with inflammation of the biliary tree, proliferation of the biliary epithelium, and progressive portal fibrosis. In heavy infections (10,000 to 20,000 flukes), portal fibrosis may be associated with portal hypertension and may extend into the liver parenchyma, resulting in liver cell death and fatty change. Jaundice is usually caused by biliary obstruction due to a mass of flukes or to stone formation. Other complications of severe clonorchiasis include cholangiocarcinoma (a metaplastic change in the irritated biliary epithelium), suppurative cholangitis, and chronic pancreatitis.

Diagnosis

Clinical and epidemiologic findings often suggest the diagnosis, which can be confirmed only by finding the eggs in the feces or duodenal contents. The light brown, ovoid eggs measure 29 × 16 μm, have a conspicuous opercular rim and a posterior knob, and are difficult to distinguish from the eggs of the trematodes *Metagonimus*, *Heterophyes*, and *Opisthorchis*. Alkaline phosphatase and bilirubin may be elevated. Eosinophilia is variable. A plain film of the abdomen occasionally demonstrates intrahepatic calcification. In acute symptomatic disease, liver scan is usually negative but may show multiple areas of diminished uptake, and percutaneous transhepatic cholangiography often shows dilatation of peripheral intrahepatic bile ducts. The adult worms (5 × 15 mm in diameter) look like round filling defects.

Prophylaxis and Treatment

Thorough cooking of freshwater fish prevents infection. No treatment is advised for asymptomatic patients. No consistently effective treatment is known; for symptomatic clonorchiasis, chloroquine diphosphate (300 mg base) two 250-mg tablets t.i.d. for 3 to 6 wk is most frequently prescribed. Biliary obstruction may require surgery.

CESTODES

Beef Tapeworm Infection (*Taenia saginata* Infection; Taeniasis Saginata)

A usually asymptomatic infection of the intestinal tract caused by the cestode Taenia saginata.

Etiology, Pathogenesis, and Epidemiology

The adult worm inhabits the human intestinal tract and is composed of a small head (scolex), 1 to 2 mm in diameter, and up to 1000 hermaphroditic proglottids that give the worm its characteristic ribbonlike shape. The worm measures 4.5 to 9 m (15 to 30 ft). Egg-bearing proglottids are passed in the stool and ingested by cattle. The eggs hatch in the cattle, invade the intestinal wall, and are carried by the bloodstream to striated muscle, where they encyst (cysticercus stage). Humans are infected by ingesting the cysticercus in raw or undercooked beef.

The infection is particularly common in Africa, the Middle East, Eastern Europe, Mexico, and South America. Infection in the USA is uncommon, but still occurs in California and New England.

Symptoms, Signs, and Diagnosis

The infection is usually asymptomatic, although epigastric pain, diarrhea, and weight loss may occur. Occasionally, the patient may feel an active proglottid crawling through the anus.

The diagnosis is usually made by finding the characteristic proglottids or, more rarely, the scolex in the stool. The perianal area may also be examined by pressing the sticky side of cellophane tape against the area, placing the tape on a glass slide, and microscopically examining it for eggs deposited by ruptured proglottids.

Prophylaxis

Infection may be prevented by thoroughly cooking beef at a minimum of 56 C (133 F) for 5 min. Meat inspection and adequate toilet facilities also help to control infection.

Treatment

A single dose of 2 gm niclosamide is given as 4 tablets (500 mg each) that are chewed one at a time and swallowed with a small amount of water. The worm is then usually digested by the time it is passed. The stool should be rechecked in 3 mo and 6 mo to make certain a cure has been obtained.

Paromomycin 1 gm taken orally every 15 min for 4 doses is somewhat less effective, but has the advantage of being commercially available.

Pork Tapeworm Infection (*Taenia solium* Infection; Cysticercosis)

An intestinal infection caused by the adult cestode Taenia solium. *Infection with the larvae (cysticerci) causes* cysticercosis, *an occasional occurrence in man.*

Etiology, Pathogenesis, and Epidemiology

The adult *T. solium* measures 2.5 to 3 m (8 to 10 ft) in length, and is composed of a scolex armed with several hooklets and a body composed of 800 to 1000 proglottids. The gravid proglottids have fewer uterine branches than gravid *T. saginata* proglottids have. The life cycle resembles that of *T. saginata* except that hogs rather than cattle serve as the normal intermediate hosts. Humans may also act as intermediate hosts either by ingesting the eggs directly, or by regurgitating gravid proglottids from the intestine to the stomach where the embryos are released, penetrate the intestinal wall, and are carried to the subcutaneous tissue, muscle, viscera, and CNS. Viable cysticerci cause only a mild tissue reaction; dead larvae, however, provoke a vigorous reaction.

T. solium infections are frequent in Asia, Russia, Eastern Europe, and Latin America; infection in the USA is rare.

Symptoms and Signs

Infection with the adult worm is usually asymptomatic. Heavy larval infection (cysticercosis) may cause muscle pains, weakness, fever, or, if the CNS is involved, meningoencephalitis or epilepsy.

Diagnosis

In adult worm infections, eggs may be found in the perianal area or stool. The proglottids or scolex must be recovered from the stool and examined in order to differentiate *T. solium* from *T. saginata*. Cysticercosis should be suspected in any patient who lives in an endemic area and develops neurologic findings. Calcified cysticerci may be seen on x-ray. Encysted larvae may occasionally be recovered in biopsied subcutaneous nodules. A hemagglutination test has been developed, but its usefulness is uncertain.

Prophylaxis and Treatment

Infection may be prevented by thoroughly cooking pork.

The intestinal infection is treated as described above for *T. saginata*. However, since these agents result in proglottid disintegration, with release of eggs, their use could theoretically cause cysticercosis.

Fish Tapeworm Infection (Diphyllobothriasis)

An intestinal infection caused by the adult cestode Diphyllobothrium latum.

Etiology, Pathogenesis, and Epidemiology

The adult worm possesses several thousand proglottids, and measures 4.5 to 9 m (15 to 30 ft) in length. Operculated ova (*D. latum* are the only eggs of the tapeworm group that are operculated) are released from the proglottid in the intestinal lumen and are passed in the stool. The egg, as it hatches in fresh water, releases the embryo, which is eaten by small crustaceans. They may, in turn, be ingested by a fish. Humans are infected by eating raw or undercooked infected fish.

The infection occurs in Europe (particularly Scandinavia), Japan, Africa, South America, Canada, and, in the USA, in Florida and the North Central States. Uncooked "lutefisk" or "gefilte fish" often harbor infection.

Symptoms, Signs, and Diagnosis

Infection is usually asymptomatic, although mild GI symptoms may be noted. Rarely, an anemia that resembles pernicious anemia may develop, presumably because of host-tapeworm competition for vitamin B_{12}.

Operculated eggs are easily found in the stool.

Prophylaxis and Treatment

All fresh-water fish should be thoroughly cooked, or frozen at -10 C (14 F) for 48 h. Treatment requires niclosamide or paromomycin (see Beef Tapeworm Infection, above).

Echinococciasis (*Echinococcus granulosus* Infection)

A tissue infection of humans caused by the larval stage of Echinococcus granulosus.

Etiology, Epidemiology, and Pathogenesis

The adult worm is found in the small intestines of dogs, wolves, and other canines. It measures 5 mm in length and consists of a scolex and 3 proglottids. The terminal or gravid proglottid splits, releasing into the stool eggs that are morphologically identical to those of *T. saginata*. These eggs pass to the external environment and are ingested by an intermediate host, e.g., sheep, moose, or human; the embryos penetrate the intestinal wall and the portal circulation carries them to the liver, or beyond to the lung, brain, kidney, bones, and other tissues. Surviving larvae develop into hydatid cysts that slowly enlarge to produce pressure symptoms. The cyst is fluid-filled and contains scolices, brood capsules, and 2nd-generation (daughter) cysts containing infectious scolices. When the intermediate is eaten by a carnivore the scolices are released into the GI tract, where they develop into adult worms.

The dog is the principal definitive host and the sheep the most common intermediate. (In Alaska and western Canada, wolves act as the definitive host and moose as the intermediate.) Human infection, often acquired in childhood during play with infected dogs, is most common in the sheep-raising areas of the world, including South Africa, Australia, New Zealand, the Middle East, central Europe, and South America. In the USA, autochthonous cases have been reported among southwestern Indian, California Basque, and Utah shepherds.

Symptoms and Signs

The majority of cysts are found in the liver, where, after remaining asymptomatic for decades, they finally produce abdominal pain or a palpable mass. Jaundice may occur if the bile duct is obstructed. Rupture into the bile duct, abdominal cavity, peritoneal cavity, or lung may produce fever, urticaria, or a serious anaphylactoid reaction. The released scolices may produce metastatic infection. Pulmonary cysts are usually discovered on routine chest x-ray. Some rupture, and cough, chest pain, and hemoptysis result.

Diagnosis

Radioisotopic and ultrasonic scanning will reveal the fluid-filled liver cysts. Chest x-ray may demonstrate a round, often irregular, pulmonary mass of uniform density. The skin test is usually positive but lacks both sensitivity and specificity. Serologic tests are positive in approximately 60% of pulmonary and 90% of hepatic lesions.

Prophylaxis and Treatment

Dogs in sheep-raising areas should be wormed repeatedly. The carcasses and offals of sheep should be destroyed to prevent access of dogs to material containing hydatid cysts.

There is no established medical therapy. Surgical excision offers the only hope of cure. Patients with small hepatic cysts or pulmonary lesions acquired in Alaska need surgery only if they are symptomatic or the cysts enlarge with time; all others require surgery.

---

14.   DISEASES OF UNCERTAIN ETIOLOGY

SARCOIDOSIS

A multisystem granulomatous disorder of unknown etiology, characterized histologically by epithelioid tubercles involving various organs or tissues, with symptoms dependent on the site and degree of involvement.

Etiology and Incidence

The cause is unknown. A single provoking agent (e.g., a slow virus) or disordered defense reactions triggered by a variety of insults may be responsible; genetic factors may be important. Sarcoidosis occurs predominantly between ages 20 and 40 and is most common among northern Europeans and American blacks. The incidence in some advanced countries exceeds that of TB.

Pathology

The characteristic histopathologic findings are multiple noncaseating epithelioid granulomas, with little or no necrosis, that may resolve completely or proceed to fibrosis. They occur commonly in mediastinal and peripheral lymph nodes, lungs, liver, eyes, and skin, and less often in the spleen, bones, joints, skeletal muscle, heart, and CNS.

Symptoms and Signs

Symptoms depend on the site of involvement and may be absent, slight, or severe. Function may be impaired by the active granulomatous disease or by secondary fibrosis. Fever, weight loss, and arthralgias may be initial manifestations. Persistent fever is especially common with hepatic involvement. Peripheral lymphadenopathy is common and usually asymptomatic. Even insignificant nodes may contain characteristic tubercles.

Mediastinal adenopathy often is discovered by routine chest x-ray. X-ray findings of bilateral hilar and right paratracheal adenopathy are virtually pathognomonic; adenopathy occasionally is unilateral. **Diffuse pulmonary infiltration** may accompany or follow the adenopathy; this infiltration may have a diffuse fine ground-glass appearance on x-ray, may occur as reticular or miliary lesions, or may be present as confluent infiltrations or large nodules that resemble metastatic tumors. Pulmonary involvement, which may also occur without visible adenopathy, is usually accompanied by cough and dyspnea, but these symptoms may be minimal or absent. Pulmonary fibrosis, cystic changes, and cor pulmonale are end results of longstanding progressive disease.

Skin lesions (plaques, papules, and subcutaneous nodules) frequently are present in patients with severe chronic sarcoidosis. Nasal and conjunctival mucosal granulomas may occur. **Erythema nodosum** with fever and arthralgias is a frequent manifestation in Europe, but less common in the USA.

Hepatic granulomas are found in 70% of patients examined by percutaneous biopsy, even if patients are asymptomatic with normal liver function tests. Hepatomegaly is noted in fewer than 20% of patients; progressive and severe hepatic dysfunction with portal hypertension and esophageal varices is rare.

Granulomatous uveitis occurs in 15% of cases; it is usually bilateral, and may cause severe loss of vision from secondary glaucoma if untreated. Retinal periphlebitis, lacrimal gland enlargement, conjunctival infiltrations, and keratitis sicca occasionally are present. **Myocardial involvement** may cause angina, congestive failure, or fatal conduction abnormalities. Acute **polyarthritis** may be prominent; chronic periarticular swelling and tenderness may be associated with osseous changes in the phalanges. **CNS involvement** is of almost any type, but cranial nerve palsies (especially facial paralysis) are most common. **Diabetes insipidus** may occur. **Hypercalcemia** and **hypercalciuria** may cause renal calculi or nephrocalcinosis with consequent renal failure, but prednisone therapy has reduced the frequency and importance of disordered calcium metabolism.

Laboratory Findings

Leukopenia frequently is present. Hyperglobulinemia is common among blacks. Elevated serum uric acid is not uncommon, but gout is rare. Serum alkaline phosphatase may be elevated as a result of hepatic involvement. Depression of delayed hypersensitivity is characteristic, but a negative second-strength tuberculin reaction reliably excludes a complicating TB.

Pulmonary function tests show restriction, decreased compliance, and impaired diffusing capacity. CO_2 retention is uncommon, since ventilation rarely is obstructed except in patients with endobronchial disease or in late stages with severe pulmonary fibrosis. Serial measurements of pulmonary function are a guide to treatment and to the course of the disease.

Diagnosis

A clinical diagnosis may be made in asymptomatic patients with typical chest x-ray findings, but the diagnosis must be considered in the presence of the symptoms and signs described above even if (as in about 10% of patients) the chest x-ray is normal. Tissue biopsy, with microbiologic as well as histologic examination, is essential if symptoms are present and corticosteroid therapy seems indicated. When superficial or palpable lesions (e.g., in skin, lymph nodes, palpebral conjunctiva) are present, biopsy is positive in 87% of specimens.

When physical examination is negative, transbronchial biopsy by fiberoptic bronchoscope is the best initial procedure for securing histologic evidence of sarcoidosis. This technic has shown granulomas in 60 to 90% of patients, whether the chest x-ray reveals pulmonary infiltration or hilar adenopathy alone.

If this approach is not available or fails to show granulomas, other possible biopsy sites include the mediastinum, which can be approached by mediastinotomy or mediastinoscopy; the lungs, approached by intercostal biopsy; or random biopsies of skeletal muscle and conjunctiva. Liver biopsy shows granulomas in 70% of cases, and can be useful. Scalene fat-pad biopsy is obsolete in view of the higher yields of other methods.

Local sarcoid reactions in a single organ and granulomas due to infection or hypersensitivity must be excluded. In questionable cases, histologic evidence of granulomas should be sought in more than one site. The Kveim reaction, a granulomatous reaction appearing 4 wk after intradermal injection of extracts of sarcoid spleen or lymph node, is positive in 50 to 60% of patients, but reliable antigens are not available in the USA.

Angiotensin converting enzyme **(ACE)** is elevated significantly in sera of patients with sarcoidosis, presumably reflecting macrophage activity. Tissue levels are highest in sarcoid lymph nodes rather than in pulmonary tissues. Elevations greater than 2 standard deviations occur in 60% of patients with sarcoidosis, but these elevations are also seen in 10% of patients with TB or lymphoma; therefore, elevated ACE has limited diagnostic value, but may prove useful in following the course of sarcoidosis.

TB still must be distinguished from sarcoidosis, but aspergillosis and cryptococcosis are now more frequent complications of sarcoidosis. Hodgkin's disease also must be excluded. It is uncertain whether the typical sarcoid granulomas found in 5% of liver biopsies done for staging of Hodgkin's disease indicate 2 concurrent diseases or a sarcoid reaction to the neoplasm.

Course and Prognosis

Evaluating treatment is difficult, since spontaneous improvement or clearing is common. Massive hilar adenopathy and extensive infiltrates may disappear in a few months or years. Mediastinal adenopathy persists without change for many years in about 10% of cases. In 1/3 of the patients, complete clearing of the disease occurs; another 1/3 recover, but with minor residua; in the remaining 1/3, progressive disease requires treatment. Mortality is < 5%. Gradual pulmonary fibrosis, leading to pulmonary insufficiency, pulmonary hypertension, and cor pulmonale, is the leading cause of disability and death; pulmonary hemorrhage from aspergillosis is the second most common cause of death.

Treatment

No available therapeutic agents have been shown to prevent progressive tissue damage and fibrosis of the lungs. Corticosteroids accelerate clearance of symptoms, physiologic disturbances, and roentgenographic changes; but after 5 yr no difference is demonstrable between treated and untreated patients. Asymptomatic hilar or peripheral adenopathy needs no treatment. Corticosteroid therapy should be given to suppress troublesome or disabling symptoms such as dyspnea, severe arthralgia, or fever, and should be started promptly if active ocular disease, respiratory failure, hepatic insufficiency, cardiac arrhythmia, CNS involvement, or hypercalcemia is present. Prednisone therapy is required by 1/3 of white patients and 2/3 of black patients with sarcoidosis.

Prednisone 40 to 60 mg/day orally may be given when a prompt effect is desired, but doses of 10 to 15 mg/day by mouth usually are adequate to control the inflammatory reaction. If doses > 15 mg/day are given, alternate-day schedules should be employed. Treatment may be needed for weeks, for years, or indefinitely. Maintenance doses of 5 to 10 mg/day are surprisingly effective in controlling symptoms and radiologic changes in many chronic cases. Clinical examination, x-rays, and pulmonary function studies should be made at frequent intervals when dosage is being reduced or medication terminated. Serious complications of corticosteroid therapy are infrequent with low-dose therapy in this disease. Concomitant isoniazid therapy, 300 mg/day for a year, is indicated only for the few patients given corticosteroids who have positive tuberculin skin tests.

Methotrexate and chlorambucil occasionally are effective in sarcoidosis, but dramatic improvement with these agents is rare. They deserve a trial only when corticosteroids fail or are contraindicated.

FAMILIAL MEDITERRANEAN FEVER (FMF)

An inherited disorder of unknown etiology, usually characterized by recurrent episodes of fever, peritonitis, and pleuritis and less commonly by arthritis and skin lesions. FMF occurs predominantly in patients of Armenian, Arabic, and Sephardic Jewish ancestry and is rare in individuals of other ethnic backgrounds.

Clinical Course and Complications

Discrete attacks generally begin between ages 5 and 15. They vary greatly in duration and frequency, usually lasting 24 to 48 h but occasionally as long as 7 days, and occurring from twice weekly to as rarely as once a year. They consist of fever; abdominal pain, which may be severe; pleuritic chest pain; and, less commonly, arthritis, involving primarily the large joints, and skin lesions (painful, erythematous areas of swelling) on the lower legs.

The most serious complication of FMF in the USA is drug addiction. Amyloidosis is a major complication in Israel but is rare in North America. Amyloid infiltration usually involves the kidneys, and the patients die of renal failure (see Ch. 83). The prognosis is good if amyloidosis does not occur.

Diagnosis and Treatment

The diagnosis is based on a history of typical acute attacks, an appropriate ethnic background, and, usually, a positive family history. There is no specific laboratory test for the diagnosis. The WBC and the ESR are generally elevated during attacks but are normal between them.

Attacks may be prevented by administering colchicine 0.6 mg orally t.i.d. and may be aborted by giving the drug more frequently (e.g., 0.6 mg orally every hour for 4 h, then q 2 h for 4 h, then orally t.i.d.). The mechanism of action of the drug is unknown. Use of narcotics to treat pain is unwise, and surgery is contraindicated. A few successful renal transplants have been performed to arrest progression of renal failure from amyloidosis.

TOXIC SHOCK SYNDROME (TSS)

A syndrome characterized by high fever, vomiting, diarrhea, confusion, and skin rash that may rapidly progress to severe and intractable shock. This syndrome was first described in children (8 to 17 yr old) in 1978. In 1980, a large number of cases began to be recognized, predominantly in young women (age 13 to 52 yr), almost always associated with menstruation and the use of vaginal tampons. The incidence is not known, but estimates made from small series suggest about 3 cases/100,000 menstruating women. Overall, about 700 cases were reported in the USA in 1980. By 1981, after widespread publicity, as well as withdrawal of some vaginal tampons from the market, the incidence in women was noted to drop precipitously. About 15% of cases occur in men.

Etiology and Pathogenesis

The exact cause of TSS is unknown, but almost all cases have been found to have an infection with pyrogenic exotoxin-producing strains of phage-group I *Staphylococcus aureus*. The organism has been found in mucosal (nasopharynx, vagina, trachea) or sequestered (empyema, abscess) sites. In menstruating women it has been found in the vagina in almost every case and the affected women used vaginal tampons for their menses. During the past few years, tampon manufacturers have been modifying the absorbent material to increase absorbency and more completely obstruct outflow from the vagina. Presumably, women most at risk are those with preexisting *S. aureus* colonization of the vagina who also use tampons on a continuous basis for their menses. Conceivably, mechanical factors related to tampon use result in the bacterial exotoxin being able to enter the bloodstream through a mucosal break or via the uterus to the peritoneal cavity.

Symptoms and Signs

The onset is sudden, with fever of 102 to 105 F (39 to 40.5 C) that remains elevated and is associated with headache, sore throat, nonpurulent conjunctivitis, profound lethargy, intermittent confusion without focal neurologic signs, vomiting, profuse watery diarrhea, and a diffuse, sunburnlike erythroderma. The syndrome may progress rapidly (within 48 h) to hypotension, orthostatic syncope, and shock. Between the 3rd and 7th days after onset, desquamation of the skin occurs and may lead to epidermal sloughing, particularly of the palms and soles.

Other organ systems are usually involved, resulting in mild nonhemolytic anemia, moderate leukocytosis with a predominance of immature granulocytes, and early thrombocytopenia followed by thrombocytosis. Although clinically important bleeding phenomena rarely occur, the prothrombin time and partial thromboplastin time tend to be elevated. Particularly in children, impaired perfusion of the extremities may be associated with profound hypotension. Renal dysfunction, characterized by diminished urine output and increases in BUN and creatinine, is almost universal. Laboratory evidence of hepatocellular dysfunction (hepatitis) and skeletal myolysis are common during the 1st wk of illness. Cardiopulmonary involvement occurs, manifested by peripheral and pulmonary edema (despite abnormally low central venous pressures, suggesting adult respiratory distress syndrome).

Mortality rates range between 8 and 15%, but may not reflect the true incidence, since these figures are probably based on recognition of only more severe cases. Recurrence is common in women who continue to use tampons during the first 4 mo following an episode of TSS, although there is evidence that women treated with antibiotics to eradicate *S. aureus* do not fit this pattern.

Diagnosis

TSS resembles Kawasaki's disease (mucocutaneous lymph node syndrome) (see also under Miscellaneous Infections in Vol. II, Ch. 24), but can usually be differentiated on clinical grounds. Shock usually is not seen in Kawasaki's disease; the skin rash is maculopapular in Kawasaki's, but a diffuse erythema in TSS; azotemia and thrombocytopenia are rarely seen in Kawasaki's disease and are common in TSS. Kawasaki's disease generally occurs in children < 5 yr of age and the staphylococcal exotoxin is different from that in TSS. Other disorders to be considered in differential diagnosis are scarlet fever, Reye's syndrome, the staphylococcal scalded-skin syndrome, meningococcemia, Rocky Mountain spotted fever, leptospirosis, and viral exanthematous diseases. These are ruled out by specific differences in the clinical picture and appropriate cultures and serologic studies.

Treatment

Patients suspected of having TSS should be hospitalized immediately and treated intensively. Immediate consideration must be given to supportive care, particularly adequate fluid and electrolyte replacement to prevent or treat hypovolemia, hypotension, or shock. Since shock may be profound and resistant, large quantities of fluid and electrolyte are sometimes required. Specimens for Gram stain and culture should be obtained from mucosal surfaces and blood. After these specimens have been obtained, it is probably appropriate to treat with a β-lactamase-resistant penicillin or a cephalosporin. While present evidence is unclear whether antibiotics modify the acute course of the illness, eradication of staphylococcal foci does appear to have protective value against recurrences.

In addition to eradicating *S. aureus*, precise recommendations for prevention (primary or secondary) cannot be made with certainty. However, it seems prudent to advise women to avoid constant use of tampons throughout the menstrual period, intermittently using napkins or other hygienic measures. Additionally, it may be advisable to avoid newer designs of tampons promoted for maximum absorbency.

§2. IMMUNOLOGY; ALLERGIC DISORDERS

15. INTRODUCTION

The science of immunology began with an attempt to understand resistance to infection, which was initially thought to be the only function of the immune system. Its relationship to hypersensitivity (allergy) was recognized early in this century and led to elucidation of the general biologic functions of the immune system, including a role in immunity to cancer, prevention of tissue transplantation from one individual to another, and the capability of *causing* diseases by injuring normal tissue.

These functions are accomplished in man by a complex immune system that has emerged through the phylogenetic scale, retaining elements of all the immune responses noted in other vertebrate species. When operating normally, several immunologic processes result in very precise functions: **recognition** and **memory of, specific response to,** and **clearance of, foreign substances** (chemical and cellular antigens) that either penetrate the protective body barriers of skin and mucosal surfaces (microorganisms, transplanted tissue) or arise de novo (malignant transformation). These processes depend on (1) the development of T and B cell lymphocytes; (2) clonal proliferation of immunologically committed T and B lymphocytes; (3) plasma cell differentiation and antibody production; (4) T cell differentiation into memory, activated, helper, and suppressor cells; (5) macrophages, required for processing antigen; (6) phagocytosis by polymorphonuclear leukocytes and by macrophages and other cells of the reticuloendothelial system; and (7) amplification of the immune response by lymphokines, the complement system, lysosomal enzymes, vasoactive amines, and kallikreins. These same protective processes may, under special circumstances, result in injury; the result is a hypersensitivity disorder or an autoimmune disease. When the immune system fails, the result may be an immunodeficiency disease or the growth of malignant cells.

GLOSSARY OF IMMUNOLOGIC TERMS

Activated lymphocyte: A T cell that has become stimulated by contact with antigen and is therefore able to induce a cell-mediated immune reaction.

Afferent phase (limb): The stages of the immune response concerned with the way in which foreign substances come in contact with macrophages and T and B lymphocytes, are recognized, are processed, and stimulate the immune response.

Allergen: An antigen responsible for a hypersensitivity reaction, especially an atopic or IgE-mediated reaction.

Allergy: Synonymous with hypersensitivity, but often restricted to immediate-type IgE-mediated reactions (e.g., atopic diseases).

Alloantibody: See Isoantibody.

Alloantigen: See Isoantigen.

Allogeneic: Denoting tissues that are antigenically distinct, but from the same species (said of tumors and transplants).

Allograft (homograft): Transfer of tissue between members of the same species.

Alternative pathway of complement: See Complement.

Amplification: Originally, the various processes of the immune system that augmented the phylogenetically primitive mechanisms of phagocytosis and the inflammatory response. Now often used to refer to any processes capable of increasing the effects of activated T cells or antibody molecules. *Examples:* The effects of opsonization by antibody, complement activation, mast cell release of vasoactive amines, and the production of lymphokines by activated T cells.

Anamnestic response: See Immune response, secondary.

Anergy: Inability to react to specific antigens; it may be either humoral or cell-mediated, but usually refers to inability to mount delayed-type skin reactions.

Antibody: An immunoglobulin molecule with a specific amino acid sequence and tertiary surface configuration that enable it to react specifically with a matching site on the surface of a homologous antigen. Antibodies are produced by plasma cells in response to stimulation by antigen.

Antigen: A substance capable of combining with antibody and of eliciting a specific immune response, either humoral (antibody production) or cell-mediated. Sometimes used to mean a substance that can combine with an antibody but cannot by itself elicit an immune response, but such a substance is more properly called a **hapten.** (See Hapten; Immunogen.)

Antigenic determinant: The specific configuration on the surface of an antigen that determines its ability to react with a corresponding configuration on an antibody. (*Synonyms*: Epitope, Combining site, Antigenic grouping.) Sometimes used to mean the combining site on the surface of an antibody.

Antiglobulin (anti-immunoglobulin): Antibody directed against an immunoglobulin molecule (i.e., an **anti-antibody**). May be an alloantibody or an autoantibody (e.g., rheumatoid factors). Antibody produced in one individual against an immunoglobulin from another individual, the immunoglobulin here acting as an antigen.

Arthus reaction: The development of an inflammatory lesion due to the action of precipitating antibodies (**precipitins**) with antigen, and characterized by induration, edema, hemorrhage, and necrosis within hours after intradermal injection of antigen to which the individual has been sensitized. It is caused by complement-dependent antigen-antibody complexes, which precipitate in and around blood vessels, especially capillaries and venules, plugging the vessels and causing exudation of fluid rich in polymorphonuclear neutrophils.

Atopy: An inherited tendency to develop asthma, hay fever, and other IgE-mediated hypersensitivity to allergens that provoke no immune reactions in most persons. (*Adjective*: Atopic.)

Autoantigen: An endogenous tissue component that stimulates an immune reaction (e.g., **autoantibody** production) in the person in whom it exists.

Autochthonous tumors: Tumors arising in the same host.

Autograft: Transfer of tissue from one location to another in the same individual.

Autoimmune disease: A clinical disorder resulting from an immune response against an autoantigen. The term does not refer to diseases in which there are autoantibodies of no pathologic significance.

B cell: A lymphocyte, probably derived from bone marrow in man, which is responsible for the production of humoral antibodies. (*Synonyms*: B lymphocyte, Thymus-independent lymphocyte; when used adjectivally, synonymous with Humoral.)

Blastogenic factor (BF): A lymphokine that is capable of inducing other lymphocytes to undergo transformation into lymphoblasts. (*Synonyms*: Lymphocyte transforming factor, Mitogenic factor.)

Blocking antibody: An antibody that can block the combination of an antigen with another antibody (e.g., in IgE-mediated hypersensitivity, antibody that combines with antigen and inhibits the effect of further antigen-antibody reaction); or an antibody that can prevent T cell-antigen reactions (*Synonym*: In tumor immunology, Enhancing antibody. See that term; see also Immunologic enhancement.)

Bradykinin: A basic nonapeptide that is one of the vasoactive plasma kinins. It is detectable in the serum in experimental anaphylaxis and may play a role in IgE-mediated reactions.

Bursa of Fabricius: A gut-associated (juxta-cloacal) lymphoepithelial organ in birds, responsible for B cell formation and subsequent antibody production. The bone marrow is the presumed equivalent in man.

Carcinoembryonic antigen (CEA): A protein-polysaccharide complex found in colon carcinomas, and in normal fetal gut, pancreas, and liver. It may also be detected in the serum of patients with colon carcinoma and inflammatory disease of the small intestine, colon, and liver.

Carrier protein: Protein to which a hapten can become attached, enabling the hapten to induce an immune response (either cell-mediated or humoral).

Cell-mediated (cellular): Pertaining to those aspects of the immune response that are under the control of thymus-dependent (T) cells. (See Immune response, cell-mediated.)

Central phase: The stage of the immune response concerned with the formation of antibody.

Chemotaxis: Enhanced migration of cells in the presence of chemical substances, usually toward the substance. Leukocyte chemotaxis, which occurs in response to substances released during an immune reaction, is a part of the inflammatory response.

Clonal inhibition factor: See Lymphotoxin.

Clonal proliferation: Asexual division of a single cell (first into 2 cells, then into 4 cells, etc.), resulting in a large number of progeny cells (the **clone**) that are genetically identical to the original cell.

Combining site: On an antigen, the antigenic determinant (epitope); on an antibody, the corresponding surface configuration (paratope, antigen-binding site) that controls the specificity of the antibody to link only with a matching (or very similar) antigenic configuration. The antibody configuration and specificity are determined by the amino acid sequence at the combining site.

Committed lymphocyte: Originally, a lymphocyte that was able to respond only to a specific antigen as a result of prior contact with that antigen. Now, a lymphocyte that has been "programmed," by passage through the thymus (T cell) or bone marrow (B cell), to react against a single (or very similar) antigen (i.e., committed even before the first contact) and to develop along a particular line—

i.e., into T or B memory cells, helper or suppressor T cells, or antibody-producing plasma cells. (*Synonyms*: Immunologically competent cell, Small lymphocyte, Immunocyte.)

Complement: A complex series of 18 distinct enzymatic proteins, when one includes inhibitors, acting as 9 functioning **components** designated C1 through C9 (C1 has 3 subunits, C1q, C1r, and C1s), which are activated sequentially in a manner similar to the coagulation factors. **Complement activation** by the **classic pathway** takes place when antibody of the IgM or IgG class combines with antigen and activates C1s, stimulating the full cascade of sequential events. An **alternative pathway** exists whereby properdin activates C3, bypassing the initial components (C1, C4, and C2). As the components are activated **(fixed),** they participate in a variety of immunobiologic activities, including anaphylatoxin production, leukocyte chemotaxis, opsonization, phagocytosis, antibody-mediated cytolysis, and antibody production.

Complement-dependent: Requiring the participation of activated complement components.

Cross-reaction: The reaction between an antibody and an antigen with a nonhomologous but very similar combining site.

Cytotoxic antibodies: Antibodies that cause damage to antigen-bearing cells, especially in the presence of complement. Such antibodies may be cytolytic or may cause damage to the cell membrane without lysis.

Cytotoxic factor: A lymphokine which causes the destruction of human tissue culture cells.

Cytotoxic T cell (killer cell): T lymphocyte subset that lyses target cells when in direct contact with target cells.

Delayed hypersensitivity: A T-cell–mediated hypersensitivity reaction manifested as an inflammatory reaction to the intradermal injection or topical administration of an appropriate antigen, which becomes manifest only after several hours, takes 24 to 48 h to reach maximum, and slowly subsides. Since it is one of the major indicators of **cell-mediated immunity,** it is often used as a synonym for that term.

Derepression: In genetic theory, the inactivation of a repressor substance with the result that normally inactivated genetic material is able to exert an effect; hence, in tumor immunology, the activation (by a carcinogen) of genetic material that is normally suppressed during fetal development.

Efferent phase (limb): The stages of the immune response during which immune reactions are brought about by the interactions of antibodies or T cells with antigen.

Enhancing antibody: In tumor immunology, an antibody that complexes with tumor-specific antigens present on the tumor surface, preventing (blocking) destruction of the tumor by T cells, thus favoring (enhancing) the growth of the tumor. (See Blocking antibody; Immunologic enhancement.)

Epitope: The region on the surface of an antigen that is responsible for its specific interaction with an antibody having a matching (or very similar) site. (*Synonyms*: Antigenic determinant, Combining site. See also Specific.)

Fetoproteins: Proteins found in fetal tissue and in a number of malignant diseases. (*Synonym*: Fetoglobulins.)

Graft rejection: The immunologic reaction between the graft recipient and antigens present in the graft which results in necrotic destruction of the graft. The reaction may be of the immediate (antibody-mediated) type, but is more often a delayed (cell-mediated) reaction (the latter is sometimes called a **host-vs.-graft reaction**).

Graft-vs.-host reaction: Reaction of a graft containing immunologically competent T cells against antigens in the tissues of a graft recipient whose immunologic competence is defective or has been reduced by irradiation or immunosuppressive drugs.

Hapten: A substance that reacts specifically with antibody but is unable to induce antibody formation unless attached to other "carrier" molecules, usually proteins.

Helper cell: A T cell that is able to augment specific antibody production by interaction with an appropriate B cell.

Heterograft: See Xenograft.

Heterotopic: Situated in an abnormal location (said of grafts placed in an abnormal site in the recipient—e.g., a kidney transplant placed in the iliac fossa).

Histiocyte: See Macrophage.

Histocompatibility antigens: Genetically determined isoantigens, carried on the surface of most nucleated cells, which are important in transplantation because they elicit the immune reactions responsible for rejection of the graft when donor and recipient are histoincompatible. (Often used synonymously with Transplantation antigens; HLA antigens.)

HLA (Human Leukocyte Antigen) **system; complex; loci; antigens:** A term referring to a chromosome region having a complex of genetic loci with a multiplicity of alleles which govern a number of human tissue antigens. Originally of greatest importance in transplantation as the major mediators of graft rejection, the HLA antigens have become highly significant of late because of the newly discovered statistical associations between certain HLA alleles and a number of otherwise unrelated disorders. At present, 4 distinct loci are identified, which are designated HLA-A, HLA-B, HLA-C, and HLA-D. HLA-DR is the same as HLA-D.

Homograft: See Allograft.

Homologous: Having matching parts. Said of antigens and antibodies that have matching combining sites and are therefore specific for one another.

Host-vs.-graft reaction: See Graft rejection.

Humoral: Pertaining to bodily fluids (as opposed to cellular elements); hence, those aspects of the immune response that are associated with circulating antibody. (See also Immune response, humoral.)

Hypersensitivity: An immunologically mediated reaction that damages host tissue. The 4 types of hypersensitivity reactions are discussed in Ch. 18. (See also Allergy.)

Immune: Properly, resistant to a disease because of the formation of antibodies or the development of cellular immunity; now often used to refer to any aspect of the immunologic system and its functions.

Immune adherence: A complement-dependent adherence of antigen-antibody complexes or antibody-coated antigens (e.g., bacteria) to particulate material such as RBCs.

Immune complex: A macromolecular complex made up of antigen and antibody **molecules** bound specifically together. May be present in the circulation or deposited in vessel walls or tissues. (See Ch. 18.)

Immune deficiency: Any condition in which a deficiency of humoral or cell-mediated immunity exists.

Immune response (strictly, **Specific immune response**): The changes that occur in the immune system in response to antigen.

Immune response, cell-mediated (or **cellular**): The development, proliferation, and differentiation of T cells after exposure to antigen, and the consequent phenomena of delayed hypersensitivity, graft rejection, and defense against malignant cells and certain viral, fungal, and bacterial infections.

Immune response, humoral: The development, proliferation, and differentiation of B cells after exposure to antigen, resulting in antibody production and consequent immunity or hypersensitivity.

Immune response, nonspecific: The various responses of the immune system that do not depend on the specific recognition of and reaction to antigen.

Immune response, primary: The response of immunologically competent cells on first exposure to an antigen. B cells, after a short lag period, produce a small amount of antibody (chiefly IgM) and differentiate into B memory cells and cells capable of becoming plasma cells. The response in T cells is undetectable, but they differentiate into T memory cells and helper or suppressor cells.

Immune response, secondary: The accelerated response that ensues on subsequent exposure to an antigen by B and T cells that have undergone a primary response to that antigen. B cells rapidly develop into plasma cells that produce large amounts of antibody (chiefly IgG). T cells transform into activated lymphocytes and induce such reactions as delayed hypersensitivity and graft rejection. (*Synonyms*: Anamnestic response, Booster response.)

Immunity: Properly, the state of being highly resistant to a disease, especially an infectious disease, because of the presence of antibodies (or activated T cells). **Active immunity** results from antigenic stimulation (either through natural infection or inoculation), is manifested by the prompt production of antibodies (or delayed skin test) in response to antigenic challenge, and is long-lasting or permanent. **Passive immunity** results from administration of exogenous antibodies (or T cells or transfer factor), does not induce antibody formation because no antigenic stimulation takes place, and therefore is not lasting. (Delayed sensitivity passively transferred with lymphocytes or transfer factor is longer lasting.) (*Verb*: **Immunize**.)

Immunization: The administration of antigen, antibodies, sensitized T cells, or transfer factor in order to induce reactivity, usually protection, to antigenic substances.

Immunocyte: See Committed lymphocyte.

Immunogen: A substance that is capable of inducing an immune response.

Immunoglobulin: A protein produced by plasma cells, usually having antibody activity. Each immunoglobulin is composed of one or more molecules, each molecule being made up of 2 light and 2 heavy polypeptide chains linked by disulfide bonds. The nature of the heavy chains determines whether the immunoglobulin is IgG, IgM, IgA, IgD, or IgE, the **5 major classes** in man. Most myeloma globulins are immunoglobulins in structure but appear to have no antibody activity. (See Antibody.)

Immunologic enhancement: In tumor immunology, the enhancement of tumor growth by substances (enhancing or blocking antibodies) that inhibit the antitumor activity of T cells.

Immunologic tolerance: Failure to respond to a substance that normally induces an immune response. It may result from fetal or postnatal contact with antigen (when the immature immune system is unable to distinguish foreign substances from "self"), or may result from initial contact later in life with very low amounts of antigen **(low-zone tolerance)** or very large amounts **(high-zone tolerance; immunologic paralysis).**

Immunologically competent cell: A cell that is capable of responding to antigen and engaging in an immune response—i.e., a B cell or T cell. Most commonly used in reference to cells that have had prior contact with antigen.

Immunotherapy: Stimulation of the immune system for the purpose of treating disease.

Isoantibody: Antibody against isoantigen. *Example*: anti–B-blood-group antibody).

Isoantigen: An antigen that occurs in different allelic forms in a species; one allelic form induces an immune response in an individual with a different allele. *Examples*: Blood group antigens, histocompatibility antigens. (*Synonym*: Allotypic antigen.)

Isogeneic: See Syngeneic.

Isograft: Transfer of tissue between identical twins.

Killer cell: (See Cytotoxic T cell; T cell.)

Kinins: Peptides having the ability to produce vasodilation and smooth muscle contraction, formed from kininogens in the plasma by the action of esterases known as kallikreins. (See also Bradykinin.)

Lymphocyte transformation: The name given to the change in morphology seen when lymphocytes are cultured in the presence of specific antigen or nonspecific mitogens (phytohemagglutinins). The cells increase in size and resemble blast cells (blastogenesis).

Lymphoid tissue, central (primary): Thymus, bone marrow (and, in birds, bursa of Fabricius); the sites at which stem-cell–derived lymphoid cells take on the properties that later characterize them as T cells and B cells.

Lymphoid tissue, peripheral (secondary): Lymph nodes, spleen, and blood; the sites at which lymphocytes are found in large numbers. T cells are found in **thymus-dependent areas**—around the central arterioles in the white pulp of the spleen and in the paracortical and deep cortical regions of lymph nodes. B cells are found in **thymus-independent areas**—the germinal follicles and perifollicular regions of the spleen, and the germinal centers, far cortical areas, and medullary cortex of lymph nodes. Of the circulating lymphocytes, 30% are B cells and 70% are T cells.

Lymphokines: Soluble factors released by activated T lymphocytes which induce the changes noted in cellular immunity, delayed hypersensitivity, and tissue rejection. (*Synonyms*: T cell mediators, T cell effectors.)

Lymphotoxin (LT): A lymphokine that injures lymphocytes and prevents clonal proliferation of lymphocytes. (*Synonym*: Clonal inhibition factor.)

Lysosome: A cytoplasmic vacuole (present in many cells, an example of which are the granules of WBCs) containing various hydrolytic enzymes important in intracellular digestion.

Macrophage: A cell of the mononuclear phagocytic system characterized by its capacity to phagocytose both foreign and endogenous particulate substances; it may also play a role in making antigens recognizable to lymphocytes. **Macrophages** are present in subcutaneous and connective tissue, lymph nodes, bone marrow, spleen, lung, liver, and brain; those stimulated by inflammation are mobile and highly phagocytic. **Angry (activated) macrophages** are unusually phagocytic; this activity is thought to be an effect of a lymphokine, migration inhibitory factor. **Monocytes** are circulating macrophages; **histiocytes**, tissue macrophages.

Mast cell: A connective tissue cell containing strongly basophilic cytoplasmic granules that release pharmacologically active agents such as heparin, histamine, eosinophilic chemotactic factor, and slow reactive substance—all important mediators of immediate-type hypersensitivity reactions. When antigen reacts with IgE bound to the mast cell surface, stimulation occurs and the cell secretes or releases its active agents.

Memory cell: A T cell or B cell that has encountered a specific antigen and is therefore committed to respond in an enhanced fashion on subsequent encounter with the same antigen.

Migration inhibitory factor (MIF): A lymphokine that causes macrophages to agglutinate and thereby prevents their migration.

Mitogenic factor: See Blastogenic factor.

Monocyte: See Macrophage.

Opsonins: Substances that can adhere to bacteria and other cells, enhancing their phagocytosis. Some are heat-stable antibodies; others are heat-labile components of complement.

Opsonization (opsonification): The facilitation of phagocytosis by opsonins; e.g., the increase in phagocytosis that occurs after the attachment of antibody or complement component, especially C3, to cells.

Orthotopic: Located in the normal anatomic site; said of tissue transferred from a donor to a similar site in a recipient (e.g., a heart transplant).

Paralysis, immune: See Immunologic tolerance.

Paratope: See Combining site.

Phytohemagglutinin (PHA): A hemagglutinin derived from bean plants which is capable of inducing lymphoblast transformation and mitosis of both T and B lymphocytes in man.

PK (Prausnitz-Küstner) reaction: A local passive transfer test for identifying IgE antibodies. Serum from the allergic individual is injected intradermally into a nonallergic individual, and the specific allergen is applied to the site by scratch or intradermally 48 h later. A typical wheal-and-flare reaction occurs in 15 to 20 min at the test site if skin-sensitizing antibody to the test allergen is present.

Plasma cell (plasmacyte): The antibody-producing progeny of the B cell. A mononuclear cell with abundant, strongly basophilic **(pyroninophilic)** cytoplasm, prevalent in the extracellular plasma of lymphoid tissue but relatively uncommon in peripheral blood.

Primary immune response: See Immune response, primary.

Properdin: A globulin with gamma motility that is part of the alternative (properdin) pathway of complement. (See Complement.)

Properdin system: Same as alternative pathway of complement. (See Complement.)

Reaginic antibody: See Skin-sensitizing antibody.

Rosette formation: The clustering of RBCs around lymphocytes seen during in vitro tests using various reagents to detect T or B cells. Most commonly, sheep RBCs are used to detect T cells.

Secondary immune response: See Immune response, secondary.

Sensitized lymphocyte: A lymphocyte that has participated in a primary immune response and can therefore act as an effector of immunologic reactions on another encounter with its homologous antigen.

Skin reactive factor: A lymphokine that causes an inflammatory process in the skin of animals, including an increase in vascular permeability.

Skin-sensitizing antibody: Antibody (usually of the IgE class) capable of producing a PK reaction. Recently, IgG_4 subclass skin-sensitizing antibodies have been described. The skin sensitization depends on combination with receptors on mast cells and release of mediators after combination of the antibody with specific antigen. (*Synonyms for IgE*: Reaginic, atopic, anaphylactic, or PK antibody.)

Slow-reacting substance [of anaphylaxis] **(SRS-A):** A substance released during mast cell degranulation that appears later and persists longer than histamine; it causes slow, prolonged smooth muscle contraction.

Specific: (1) With respect to antibodies (or T cells) and their corresponding antigens—reacting only with one another because of identical combining sites; hence (2) pertaining to those aspects of the immune system having to do with the recognition of, remembrance of, and reaction to, a particular antigen by B cells, T cells, their progeny cells, and their products. The **specificity** of an antibody (and presumably of a T cell), and of a protein antigen, is determined by the amino acid sequence at the combining site; the specificity of a polysaccharide antigen, by its sugar side chains.

Suppressor cell: A T cell, circulating monocyte, or macrophage that can inhibit antibody production by plasma cells.

Syngeneic: Having identical genotypes (said of individuals or tissues—e.g., identical twins or grafts between them). (*Synonym*: Isogeneic.)

T cell: A lymphocyte altered by passage through the thymus, which becomes responsible for the phenomena of cellular immunity. (*Synonyms*: Thymus-dependent lymphocyte; when used adjectivally, synonymous with Cell-mediated, Cellular.) T cell subsets include T_H (helper cells), T_S (suppressor cells), T_D (delayed hypersensitivity effector cells), and T_K (killer cells).

Thymus-dependent (T-cell–dependent): Requiring the participation (in an immune response) or presence (in tissue) of T cells. (See also Lymphoid tissue, peripheral.) Usually refers to B cells that require T helper cells to produce antibody.

Thymus-independent: See B cell; Lymphoid tissue, peripheral.

Tolerance: See Immunologic tolerance.

Transfer factor: An extract derived from the lymphocytes of an individual with delayed hypersensitivity which, when injected into a previously nonreactive individual, will induce delayed hypersensitivity in the recipient. The reaction is specific; i.e., the recipient will show delayed hypersensitivity only to the antigen that originally induced the reaction in the donor.

Transplantation antigens: The genetically determined antigens that stimulate the immunologic response occurring when blood cells or tissues are transplanted from a donor into a non-syngeneic recipient. Included are the histocompatibility antigens and the blood group antigens.

Tumor-associated transplantation antigens: Antigens present on tumor cells which, when injected into normal syngeneic animals, protect the recipient from developing a tumor by causing a graft rejection reaction if cells from the same type of tumor are injected. The antigens may be tumor-specific (present on tumor cells but not on normal cells), or may be normally present but intracellular, released through some effect of the neoplastic process on the cell membrane. (The terms tumor-specific transplantation antigens, TSTA, are used synonomously.)

Unblocking factors: In tumor immunology, substances present in the serum which decrease (unblock) the action of enhancing or blocking antibody. These substances may be antibody, antigen-antibody complexes, or circulating antigen.

Uncommitted lymphocyte: A lymphocyte (either T or B) that has not yet had its initial encounter with antigen. Since progenitors of lymphocytes are now thought to become programmed for (committed to) their specific antigens at the time when they pass through the thymus or bone marrow and develop into T or B cells, the concept of an uncommitted lymphocyte no longer holds true; however, the term is still used in the above sense.

Xenograft (heterograft): A graft between members of different species.

---

16. BIOLOGY OF THE IMMUNE SYSTEM

The **immune response** in humans is divided into humoral (antibody) and cellular or cell-mediated (delayed immunity) components. **Humoral** processes involve the interactions between antigens and antibodies; **cellular** processes involve the interactions between antigens and certain specialized (thymus-influenced) lymphocytes, which act both directly and through the elaboration of substances other than antibody. The humoral and cell-mediated processes are thought of as **specific** for 2 reasons: (1) The lymphocytes and antibodies recognize, remember, and respond to unique pattern configurations on the surfaces of antigens; and (2) each lymphocyte and each antibody responds only to one specific antigenic configuration.

Other mechanisms of the immune system, such as phagocytosis and complement activation, are **nonspecific** since they do not involve such pattern recognition. However, these nonspecific processes often act in concert with antibodies and lymphocytes in reactions against antigenic substances.

Current concepts have evolved from study of animal models and humans and are depicted in FIG. 16-1. A primitive stem cell originates in the yolk sac, migrates through the liver and spleen, and settles in the bone marrow. These stem cells are thought to be multipotential and to develop into precursors of the lymphoid, myeloid, erythroid, and megakaryocytoid series. There is evidence to suggest that the stem-cell–derived lymphoid cells in the bone marrow are already committed to become T and B cells, and are called pro-thymocytes and pro-B cells. The pro-thymocyte migrates to the thymus where it develops the characteristics of a T cell. The pro-B cell becomes a B cell probably in the bone marrow, possibly also in the spleen. The 2 types of cells are identical in appearance at this time in their development and are already programmed for the antigens to which they will respond.

CELLULAR IMMUNE SYSTEM
(Delayed Sensitivity; Cell-Mediated Immunity)

That portion of the immune system mediated by T cells and which is responsible for delayed skin tests, delayed hypersensitivity, graft rejection, and an important defense against malignant cells, viral infection, fungal infection, and some bacteria. The specific type of immune response is mediated by *small* lymphocytes in man, and in most animals is dependent upon the presence of the thymus at birth.

In man, the thymus anlage is differentiated into a compact epithelial structure that can participate in the immune response by the 12th wk of gestation. The pro-thymocyte migrates from the bone marrow to the thymus, where it proliferates and differentiates into thymic lymphoid cells **(T cells)**. Each cell is programmed for the number of antigens to which it will react. These cells leave the thymus to circulate in the blood as "long-lived" small and medium-sized lymphocytes with a life span up to 5 yr. Some settle in lymph nodes and the spleen, specifically the corticomedullary junction of lymph nodes and cuffing the penicilliary arteries in the spleen.

In the blood, T cells comprise 70% of circulating lymphocytes and can be distinguished by 2 surface markers: (1) receptors for normal sheep RBCs **(SRBC),** which can be detected by observing rosette formation (collection of RBCs around lymphocytes) when SRBCs are mixed with lymphocyte

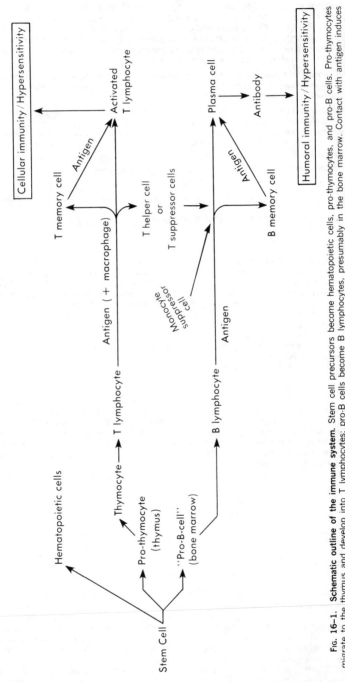

FIG. 16–1. Schematic outline of the immune system. Stem cell precursors become hematopoietic cells, pro-thymocytes, and pro-B cells. Pro-thymocytes migrate to the thymus and develop into T lymphocytes; pro-B cells become B lymphocytes, presumably in the bone marrow. Contact with antigen induces lymphocytic differentiation; for this process, T cells may require macrophage participation and some B cells require T helper (or suppressive) cell participation. Both first and later contacts with antigen result in activated T cells or plasma cells, the mediators, respectively, of cellular and of humoral immunity and hypersensitivity.

preparations; (2) specific T cell antigen, detected by immunofluorescence using antiserum prepared in animals immunized with human thymus cells (thoracic duct cells) and rendered specific for T cells by absorption with B cell lymphocytes derived from patients with chronic lymphatic leukemia. Some antigens, such as proteins from bacteria, viruses, fungi, and protozoa, can induce a cellular immune response directly. Haptens such as nickel, rhus antigen (poison ivy), and paraphenylenediamine (hair dye) are capable of inducing a cellular immune response after combining with tissue proteins (carrier protein).

As discussed later, macrophages are considered to be necessary for processing and presenting all antigens to T cells. On initial contact with antigen, the T cell undergoes clonal proliferation and differentiates into sensitized lymphocytes or **committed** T cells with various functions. Some cells become **activated** and are responsible for mediating cellular immunity or resulting in injury to host tissue (hypersensitivity reactions). Others become T **memory cells,** thereby increasing the number of cells with the ability to react to specific antigen. Still others are presumed to become **helper** or **suppressor cells** and regulate the production of antibody by B cells by concentrating antigen on their surfaces or releasing a local humoral factor responsible for stimulating B cells to produce antibody. These are important because of data suggesting that autoimmune diseases and some immunologic deficiency disorders may be due to defects of suppressor T cells, autoimmune diseases representing a decrease in suppressor activity and immunologic deficiency representing a result of excessive suppressor activity of T cells. If the immunogen is a major histocompatibility antigen, then killer cells that are **cytotoxic T cells** for target cells bearing the antigen are generated.

The activated T lymphocyte mediates cellular immunity by a direct toxic effect, reacting directly with cell-membrane–associated antigens, or by releasing various soluble factors called **lymphokines.** Lymphokines are referred to as the chemical mediators of cellular immunity, and several factors have now been defined: Migration inhibitory factor **(MIF)** causes macrophages to become sticky and agglutinate in the area of delayed sensitivity. It also augments the bactericidal activity of macrophages **(macrophage activation).** Blastogenic factor **(BF,** lymphocyte transforming factor **[LTF],** mitogenic factor) is capable of inducing other lymphocytes to undergo transformation into lymphoblasts. Cytotoxic factor causes the destruction of human tissue culture cells. Lymphotoxin **(LT,** cloning inhibitor factor **[CIF])** prevents clonal proliferation of lymphocytes and damages lymphocytes. Skin reactive factor produces vasodilatation and an inflammatory response in the skin of animals. Interferon has an antiviral effect within the cells.

HUMORAL IMMUNE SYSTEM

That portion of the immune system mediated by antibodies produced by B cells.

In birds, it is quite clear that the bursa of Fabricius (a gut-associated lymphoepithelial organ) is the site at which a pro-B cell becomes a B cell capable of producing immunoglobulins. The bursal equivalent in man has not been established, but the bone marrow is considered the most likely site. Other possible areas include gut-associated lymphoid tissue (such as that found in the appendix, the cecum, and Peyer's patches), the liver, and the spleen. B cell maturation is thought to take place in 2 stages. The pro-B cell is first converted into a B cell capable of producing immunoglobulin of the IgM class. Some of these cells migrate to the blood, spleen, and peripheral lymph nodes and continue to produce IgM. Others differentiate to cells producing IgG, some of which migrate to peripheral tissues while others remain in the bone marrow to later become IgA-producing cells. The sequence of development of IgD- and IgE-producing cells has not been established. The role of IgD on cell surfaces has not been determined. IgD is found on a great majority of all B lymphocytes in adult animals (man included), as well as shortly after birth. Since IgD is found only in very low amounts in serum, it may be that its principal role is as a membrane receptor. What is clear is that the IgM-bearing cell is necessary for the development of IgA, IgG, and IgD plasma cells.

B cells, which comprise 30% of blood lymphocytes, are "short-lived," having a life span of 15 days. Though morphologically indistinguishable from T cells, they can be distinguished by technics that detect surface markers: (1) immunoglobulins of the major classes can be detected on the surface with fluorescein-labeled anti-immunoglobulin (immunofluorescent technic). The largest proportion of cells, however, bear surface IgD and IgM; (2) receptors for the 3rd component of complement (C3 receptors) can be detected by the adherence of complement-coated RBCs to the surface of B cells, forming "rosettes"; (3) receptors for immunoglobulins can be detected by adherence of antigen-antibody complexes or aggregated γ-globulin to B cells. B cells can also be evaluated by histologic examination: in the lymph node they make up the outer cortical area containing germinal centers and medullary cord; in the spleen they compose the germinal follicles and perifollicular areas.

The B cells in peripheral tissues are precommitted to respond to a limited number of antigens. The first interaction between antigen and antibody is known as the **primary immune response,** and the B cells committed to respond to this antigen undergo differentiation and clonal proliferation. Some of these become **memory cells** and others differentiate into mature antibody-synthesizing **plasma cells.** The principal characteristics of the primary immune response are a latent period before the appearance of antibody, the production of only a small amount of antibody, chiefly IgM, and, most importantly, the creation of a large number of memory cells that are capable of responding to the same antigen in the future.

The **secondary (anamnestic** or **booster) immune response** takes place on subsequent encounters with the same antigen. Its principal characteristics are a rapid proliferation of B cells, a rapid differentiation into mature plasma cells, and the prompt production of large quantities of antibody. This antibody, which is chiefly of the IgG class, is released into the blood and other body tissues where it can effectively encounter and react with the antigen.

T and B Cell Interaction

Cooperation between T and B cells appears to be important in the immune response, but the phenomenon leaves much to be elucidated. For example, a secondary (humoral) immune response to a hapten will not occur unless there are T cells present that are capable of interacting with the hapten's carrier protein. In the humoral immune response to antigens, the need for T cell cooperation varies according to the nature of the antigen. Polymeric antigens such as *Salmonella* flagella protein, pneumococcal polysaccharide, *Escherichia coli* lipopolysaccharide, and povidone (polyvinylpyrrolidone) are T-cell–independent antigens, capable of inducing antibody formation (predominantly IgM) in T-cell–deprived animals. Other antigens are T-cell–dependent (e.g., the monomeric form of flagellar *Salmonella* antigen)—they require the presence of T cells to induce production of large amounts of IgM and IgG antibodies, although small amounts of both can be produced without T cells. The need for T cell cooperation also depends on the class of immunoglobulin produced. IgG production seems to be more T-cell–dependent than IgM, while IgA and IgE are still more dependent on the presence of T cells. More recently it has been recognized that T suppressor cells are composed of 2 populations. One population of cells acts nonspecifically and can inhibit immunoglobulin production, while another is antigen-specific and specifically inhibits antibody production. In addition, the impaired immunoglobulin production observed in multiple myeloma has been demonstrated to be due in part to the presence of a monocyte or macrophage that prevents the maturation of normal B cells into immunoglobulin-secreting cells.

Humoral Immunity

Immunity can be active or passive. In **active immunization,** antibody production is stimulated by administration of antigen or by exposure to naturally occurring antigens such as bacteria, viruses, or fungi. In **passive immunization,** pre-formed antibodies actively produced in another person or animal are given to the recipient in the form of serum or γ-globulin. The protection offered by humoral antibody may be direct, such as toxin or viral neutralization by serum IgG or viral neutralization by secretory IgA, or may depend upon activation of the complement system.

ANTIGENS

Antigen Structure and Antigenicity

Antibodies combine with antigens by virtue of matching combining sites on the 2 molecules, which fit together much like the pieces of a jigsaw puzzle. The antigenic combining sites that are recognized by antibody molecules are specific configurations, known as **epitopes** or **antigenic determinants,** which are present on the surfaces of large molecules of high mol wt such as proteins, polysaccharides, and nucleic acids. It is the presence of at least one such epitope that makes a molecule an **antigen.**

In fact, 2 essentials are required for a substance to be antigenic (immunogenic), i.e., capable of both binding to antibody and inducing an immune response: (1) the sum of the antigenic determinants on its surface must make up a configuration that differs from configurations recognized by the immune system as "self"; and (2) the substance must be of sufficient mol wt (about 10,000 as a minimum). Plausibly, the larger the molecule, the more room on its surface for antigenic determinants; and the greater the number of "foreign"-looking antigenic determinants present on its surface, the greater will be its antigenicity.

A **hapten** is a substance of lower mol wt than an antigen, which can *react* specifically with antibody but which is unable to *induce* antibody formation unless attached to another molecule, usually a protein (the **carrier protein**). Examples of haptens are the allergenic substances in penicillin and numerous other drugs; and nickel, rhus antigen (poison ivy), and paraphenylenediamine (hair dye). The former are capable of inducing a humoral immune response, and the latter a cellular immune response, when they combine with carrier protein.

The combining sites of antibody and the antigen to which it is committed fit avidly together, with a strong force of attraction, because the matching areas on the surface of each molecule are relatively large. The same antibody molecule can also combine **(cross-react)** with related antigens if their surface determinants are similar enough to the determinants on the homologous (original) antigen. However, the antigen-antibody binding in such cross-reactions is weaker because smaller surface areas are in close contact, because of the differences in configuration.

The processing of an antigen by initial phagocytosis appears to be important to its antigenicity, although the role of the macrophage in the initial recognition of a substance as antigen is unclear. The lymph nodes and spleen are rich in phagocytic cells as well as in lymphocytes. When antigen first enters the body it is trapped and largely metabolized by these phagocytes. A small proportion of the antigen, localized on the surface of the macrophage, comes into contact with nearby T cells. These T cells will participate in either the production of cellular immunity or the production of humoral antibody by T-dependent B cells. T-cell–independent antigens do not require macrophages to stimulate antibody production. Cytoplasmic bridges between macrophages and lymphocytes have been observed, suggesting that the macrophage transfers genetic information to the lymphocyte by attaching messenger RNA to the antigen, and that the RNA of the antigen-RNA complex genetically "instructs" the lymphocyte to recognize the attached antigen. Or it may be that the RNA or lysosomal enzymes within the macrophage alter the structure of the foreign molecule to produce or enhance its antigenicity. This processing of antigen appears to be most important in the primary immune response. In the secondary immune response, antigen interacts with antibody fixed to the dendritic macrophages of cortical lymphoid follicles before it can be ingested by the macrophage.

IMMUNOGLOBULINS (Antibodies)

The antibodies (immunoglobulins [Ig]) offer humoral protection against viruses and bacterial pathogens such as pneumococci, Hemophilus influenzae, streptococci, and staphylococci. IgM is the predominant antibody in the primary immune response, and IgG in the secondary immune response. Other special biologic properties of the different Ig classes are described below.

Immunoglobulin Structure

Immunoglobulins are a family of serum proteins with antibody activity which are remarkably heterogeneous but which have a number of common properties. The γ-globulin fraction of serum is rich in antibody activity, but other globulin fractions also contain antibody.

The molecular subunits of the immunoglobulins all have a similar structure: each is composed of 4 polypeptide chains—2 identical **heavy chains** and 2 identical **light chains** (so called because of their relative mol wt)—joined into a Y shape by disulfide bonds. There are 5 major types of heavy chains, which give their name to the **5 major Ig classes** in man: IgM, IgG, IgA, IgD, and IgE (see TABLE 16–1). There are 2 types of light chains, called κ and λ; a single molecule has only 1 type of light chain, but molecules of both types are found in all 5 of the major classes. Thus, there are 10 different types of Ig molecules. IgG, IgD, and IgE are each monomers, i.e., made up of I molecule (2 heavy and 2 light chains). IgM is a polymer of 5 molecules (10 heavy chains, 10 light chains), while IgA occurs in 3 forms—as a monomer and as polymers of 2 and 3 molecules.

Additional chains have been identified. Joining (J) chains link the 5 subunits of IgM and the 2 or 3 subunits of IgA; and secretory IgA has an additional polypeptide chain, secretory component (SC, secretory piece, transport piece), which is produced in epithelial cells and added to the IgA molecule.

Antibody Structure and Specificity

The Y-shaped Ig molecule is divided into a **variable region,** located at the distal ends of the Y arms, in which the amino acid sequence differs for the various antibody molecules, and a **constant region,** where the amino acid sequence is relatively constant for each Ig class. Electron microscopy has shown that the variable regions hold the concave **combining sites (antigen-binding sites)** of the antibody molecules. It is the great variety of possible amino acid sequences in the variable regions that confers **specificity** on the antibodies, since each clone of B cells can produce its own specific amino acid sequence, and thus its own antibody configuration that is specific for a particular antigen.

The structure-function relationships of the antibody molecule were originally studied by fragmentation with proteolytic enzymes. Papain splits the molecule into 2 univalent fragments designated **Fab** (antigen-binding), which contain the variable regions and thus the combining sites, and one fragment designated **Fc** (crystallizable), which contains most of the constant region. Pepsin produces a fragment designated **F(ab')$_2$**, which retains divalent antibody activity.

Both B and T cells are capable of recognizing and responding to antigen, but the way in which this occurs is still unclear. B cells (but not T cells) carry small amounts of Ig bound to the cell surface, and it is assumed that this surface Ig serves as a specific recognition antibody in the initiation of an immune response. The T cell recognition site has not been defined. Antibodies of the IgM, IgG, and IgA classes are all capable of responding to the same antigen. One hypothesis to explain this assumes that the B cells derived from a single pro-B cell may differentiate (during the process of B cell maturation described above) into a family of B cells genetically programmed to synthesize antibodies of a single antigenic specificity, while having representative cells committed to the production of each antibody class. The cells undergoing this differentiation from IgM- to IgG- to IgA-producing cells are not yet plasma cells—the development of B cells is independent of antigenic stimulation, but differentiation into plasma cells capable of synthesizing goodly amounts of antibody does require antigenic stimulation.

By use of the ultracentrifuge, sedimentation coefficients can be determined for each Ig protein. IgM has the highest sedimentation coefficient—19S, while IgG is 7S. In addition to these broad classes, it is now recognized that Ig subclasses exist, termed IgG$_{1,2,3,4}$, IgA$_{1,2}$, and IgM$_{1,2}$. These distinctions may be important, since specific biologic functions are beginning to be associated with various subclasses; e.g., IgG$_4$ does not fix complement or bind to monocytes, whereas the other 3 IgG subclasses do; IgG$_3$ has a half-life significantly shorter than the other 3.

TABLE 16–1. CHARACTERISTICS OF THE IMMUNOGLOBULINS

Immuno-globulin Class	Heavy Chains	Light Chains	Addi-tional Chains	No. of Basic Molecules	Sub-classes	Molecular Weight	Sedimen-tation Coefficient	Mean Survival $T^{1/2}$ (days)	Mean Serum Conc. (Adult; mg/100 ml)	Biologic Properties
IgM	μ	κ, λ	J	5	IgM_1 IgM_2	900,000	19S	1	45–150	Appears early in immune response; efficient agglutinator & opsonizer; fixes complement; major antibody for polysaccharides, gram-neg. bacteria
IgG	γ	κ, λ		1	IgG_1 IgG_2 IgG_3 IgG_4	150,000	7S	23	720–1500	Most abundant; found esp. in extravascular fluids; crosses placenta; subclasses 1, 2, & 3 fix complement (1 & 3 > 2); major antibody for antitoxins, viruses, bacteria
IgA	α	κ, λ	J SC	1–3	IgA_1 IgA_2	170,000	7–15S	6	90–325	Major immunoglobulin in seromucous secretions at body surfaces
IgD	δ	κ, λ		1		180,000	7S	3	3	Not yet identified
IgE	ϵ	κ, λ		1		200,000	8S	2	0.03	Found in seromucous secretions; levels increased in parasitic infections; mediator of atopic allergies

J = joining chain; SC = secretory component

Biologic Properties of Antibodies

The amino acid structure in the constant region of the heavy chain in the antibody molecule appears to determine certain biologic properties of the immunoglobulins. Each class of Ig has its own characteristics.

IgG, the most prevalent type of serum Ig, diffuses readily into the extravascular spaces, and is the only Ig that crosses the placenta. As the prime mediator of the secondary immune response, it provides the body's chief serologic defenses against bacteria, viruses, and toxins. Different subclasses of IgG neutralize bacterial toxins, fix complement, and enhance phagocytosis by opsonization. Commercial γ-globulin is almost entirely IgG. IgG can also inhibit other antigen-antibody interactions, and one suggested mechanism for desensitization in atopic allergies is the development of **blocking IgG antibodies,** which prevent IgE-antigen interactions.

IgM (macroglobulin) is largely confined to the bloodstream. It is the earliest globulin to appear after antigenic challenge, but if IgM is the only antibody to respond to the antigen, immunologic memory is not achieved. The large IgM molecules also fix complement and are active opsonizers, agglutinators, and cytolytics that assist the reticuloendothelial system in eliminating many kinds of microorganisms. Most antibodies to gram-negative organisms are IgM globulins.

IgA (secretory antibody) is found in the seromucous secretions of body tracts exposed to the external environment (saliva, tears, respiratory and GI tract secretions, colostrum), where it provides an early antibacterial and antiviral defense. Secretory IgA is synthesized in the subepithelial regions of the GI and respiratory tracts and is present in combination with locally produced secretory component. Few IgA-producing cells are noted in the lymph node and spleen. Most of serum IgA appears to be derived from secretory IgA, and when this is so, both should have the same antibody specificities despite structural differences between the 2 forms, serum IgA not containing secretory component. Serum IgA contains antibodies against brucella, diphtheria, and poliomyelitis.

The biologic activity of **IgD** is not yet known. It is present in serum in extremely small amounts, but is prominent on B lymphocytes. It is speculated that their role may be that of cell-bound antigen receptor involved in triggering of antibody synthesis. **IgE (reaginic, skin-sensitizing,** or **anaphylactic antibody),** like IgA, is secreted chiefly in the respiratory and GI subepithelium. IgE is the mediator of atopic allergies; its beneficial role is not established, though it may be active against parasitic and respiratory infections.

Immunoglobulin serum assays are useful diagnostically and for following the course of therapy. IgG and IgD have a Svedberg sedimentation value of 7S; IgM of 19S; and IgA of 9 to 13S. These immunoglobulins are present in reasonably high concentrations and can therefore also be determined by the size of precipitin rings that form in gels containing specific antibody to each. This is an easier, less cumbersome, and more practical method than ultracentrifugation. Many laboratories are using a **nephelometer** to quantitate specific protein concentrations of many serum proteins, including immunoglobulins. It determines protein concentration, using the principle of molecular light scatter. The technic is based on the concept that antiserum to the protein to be measured will form immune complexes. These scatter an incident beam of light, and the amount of light scatter is proportional to the concentration of the antigen. **Immunoelectrophoresis** qualitatively identifies the immunoglobulins. **Electroimmunodiffusion** is more rapid and more specific, and can be quantitative. IgE is present in serum in minute quantities and may be measured by **radioimmunoassay** (see also Ch. 230). A simplified modification, paper radioimmunosorbent test (PRIST), is used by most laboratories. IgE is elevated in atopic diseases (such as exogenous asthma, hay fever, and atopic dermatitis), parasitic diseases, far-advanced Hodgkin's disease, and E-monoclonal myeloma.

MONOCLONAL ANTIBODIES

The heterogeneous nature of antibodies produced in animals and the contamination of such antibodies with animal serum proteins have until recently handicapped immunologists in their efforts to prepare both diagnostic antibodies and those to be used as probes in research. (For example, the specificity of the antinuclear antibody test depends in part on the antibody to human γ-globulin produced in animals. Since the strength of the diagnostic reagent may vary, titers of positive reactions will differ among laboratories and even among preparations in the same laboratory. Differences also occur in the material these antibodies are detecting.) Since all immunologic tests utilizing antibody, such as radioimmunoassays and nephelometry, depend on antibodies to the target material (e.g., insulin), universal use of antibodies of the same specificity and strength is clearly advantageous.

The **hybridoma** technic (the procedure by which 2 cells are fused [hybrid], one an antibody-producing cell, the other a myeloma cell) now permits preparation of a continuous supply of antibody produced by a single B cell **(monoclonal antibody).** This antibody is produced by immunizing a mouse with an antigen such as a cell preparation from a human thymus. The spleen is removed from the immunized mouse and a suspension of cells prepared. Cell fusion is then carried out with mouse myeloma cells that are in perpetual tissue culture and are not producing antibody. From this suspension of cells, one can then isolate individual plasma cells that are producing monoclonal antibodies. This single cell will then multiply, thereby resulting in a tissue culture preparation producing large amounts of antibody. With this technic portions of the cells can be deep-frozen, protecting against accidental losses.

Applications of the technic are broad. Antibodies to specific T cells such as suppressor and helper cells can now be prepared, and their appearance or disappearance determined in certain diseases. It is expected that monoclonal antibodies will be given to transplant recipients in the future to prevent graft rejection. Differences in the effectiveness of antilymphocyte antibodies in preventing graft rejection are clearly related to their specificity. With pure antibody of known specificity, one may be able to modify, rather than eliminate, response. Specific monoclonal antibodies to tumor antigens such as leukemia, teratoma, neuroblastoma, and sarcoma are now being sought; these antibodies can obviously be used diagnostically, or can be combined with cytotoxic agents to permit delivery of the agent to a specific tumor cell.

Monoclonal antibodies are additionally attractive because they are similar to other chemical reagents with precisely defined characteristics; they will eventually revolutionize diagnostic antibody reagents such as those used in radioimmunoassays. As research reagents, they will permit comparison of different investigative results without the concern that any differences might be due to the antibody preparation used. There is also a financial advantage; maintaining a tissue culture is much less expensive than maintaining an experimental animal.

MEASUREMENT OF CELLULAR AND HUMORAL IMMUNITY

A number of in vivo and in vitro technics are available to evaluate the presence and functional competence of T and B cells. Since these procedures are often used in the evaluation of suspected immunodeficiency disorders, they are discussed in Ch. 17. The cell-mediated phenomenon of delayed hypersensitivity is also discussed under Type IV Hypersensitivity Reactions in Ch. 18.

Delayed sensitivity can be passively transferred from one individual to another with an extract prepared from immune lymphocytes (transfer factor). A successful transfer is demonstrated when the recipient is converted from skin-test–negative to skin-test–positive. The conversion only applies to those antigens to which the donor has a positive delayed skin test.

The complement fixation (CF) test is most commonly used in the diagnosis of viral diseases by detecting the presence of specific antibody to viruses in a patient's serum. The serum is first heated to destroy its complement activity. Subsequently, antigen (such as a virus particle) and a known amount of complement are added to the mixture. The presence of antigen and antibody in the mixture will utilize complement, thus reducing its activity. Any remaining free complement is detected by adding antibody-sensitized RBCs, which will undergo lysis in the presence of free complement. The absence of hemolysis indicates that the antigen-antibody complex has fixed all the available complement.

THE COMPLEMENT SYSTEM

An important process by which antibody production leads to immunity or hypersensitivity occurs when antibody combines with antigen and initiates complement activity. The activation of complement involves over 18 distinct plasma proteins, if one includes inhibitors. They react sequentially and mediate a number of biologically significant consequences. Phenomena that have been described in vitro include immune adherence (adherence of antigen-antibody complexes or antibody-coated bacteria to macrophages or RBCs); production of anaphylatoxin (a protein that causes release of histamine from mast cells or basophils); chemotaxis (causing the migration of cells toward the area where complement activity is present); phagocytosis; lysis of cells (RBCs, nucleated cells, and many bacteria); and modulation of the immune response.

For historic reasons the first 4 components to react are numbered out of order as C1, C4, C2, and C3; but the remaining 5 components are numbered sequentially C5 through C9. The first component of human complement is composed of 3 distinct protein molecules called C1q, C1r, and C1s. The first stage of activation of the classic complement cascade begins when C1q recognizes antibodies and binds to them. This binding leads to activation of C1s, which continues the complement cascade by reacting with C4. In general the activation of the components of the complement system involves enzymatic cleavage of each component into 2 fragments, the larger of which joins the preceding activated component to generate a new enzymatic activity capable of cleaving the next component.

The classic pathway of complement activation (see Fig. 16–2) begins when C1q comes in contact in vivo with antigen-antibody complexes or, in vitro, with aggregated IgG or IgM. If the antigen is a virus, viral neutralization occurs in the course of activation when the first 2 components of complement (C1 and C4) have been activated. This may be an important defense mechanism during the early phases of a viral infection when limited amounts of antibody are present.

In guinea pigs when C2 is activated, a kinin-like factor (distinct from bradykinin) is generated; it is similar to a kinin-like activity noted in patients with hereditary angioedema during the active phase of the disease. In activating C3, C3a and C3b are produced. When the antigen is a cell, C3b attaches to a cell membrane receptor that is separate from the site of attachment of C142, resulting in immune adherence and phagocytosis. The fragment C3a is also called anaphylatoxin and is capable of releasing histamine from mast cells. Recent work in animals and man suggests that complement, up to and including C3, is important in the development of the humoral immune response. Its role and mechanisms of action, however, remain to be defined. C5a, which has anaphylatoxin and chemotactic properties, is generated in binding C5. Subsequently, when C6 and C7 are activated a trimolecu-

$$C1 \xrightarrow{\text{AgAb}} \overline{C1s}$$

$$C4 \xrightarrow{\overline{C1s}} \overline{\begin{array}{c}C1s4b\\C14b\end{array}} \quad \text{Viral neutralization when antibody limited}$$

$$C2 \xrightarrow{\overline{\begin{array}{c}C1s4b\\C14b\end{array}}} \overline{\begin{array}{c}C1s4b2a\\C142\end{array}} \quad \text{C3 convertase—ability to cleave C3 on contact}$$

$$+$$

Fragment with kinin-like activity

$$C3 \xrightarrow{\overline{\begin{array}{c}C1s4b2a\\C142\end{array}}} \overline{\begin{array}{c}C1s4b2a3b\\C1423b\end{array}} \quad \begin{array}{l}\text{Phagocytosis of RBC, bacteria, or}\\ \text{other particles; immune adherence; production of antibody}\end{array}$$

$$+$$

C3a   Anaphylatoxin

$$C5 \xrightarrow{\overline{\begin{array}{c}C1s4b2a3b\\C1423\end{array}}} \overline{C14235b}$$

$$+$$

C5a   Anaphylatoxin; chemotaxis

$$C6 + C7 \xrightarrow{\overline{C1-5b}} \overline{C1-7}$$

$$+$$

$$\overline{C567} \quad \text{Chemotaxis}$$

$$C8 \xrightarrow{\overline{C1-7}} \overline{C1-8} \quad \text{Slow or partial lysis}$$

$$C9 \xrightarrow{\overline{C1-8}} \overline{C1-9} \quad \text{Rapid lysis}$$

FIG. 16-2. **Classic pathway of complement activation.** The initiating antigen (Ag) can be erythrocyte, bacteria, virus, other cell, or any other antigen; the antibody (Ab) can be IgG_1, IgG_3, IgG_2, or IgM. A bar over the component indicates that the component has acquired enzymatic or other biologic activity.

lar complex, C567, is formed; it either fixes on the cell membrane or remains in solution and is chemotactic for leukocytes, macrophages, and probably eosinophils. When RBCs, bacteria, or nucleated target cells in tissue culture have reacted with complement components from 1 through 8, slow or partial lysis occurs. When all 9 components of complement have reacted, rapid lysis of cells occurs.

An alternative pathway (see FIG. 16-3) for the activation of the terminal complement components from C3 to C9 has also been described, in which activation of C3 by certain bacterial polysaccharides and aggregated immunoglobulins is accomplished without prior activation of C1, C4, and C2. Another name for the alternative pathway is the **properdin system.** The diagram is only an outline, since there are many unanswered questions concerning the exact steps in this pathway. An unusual feature, however, is the positive feedback through C3b. The C3b resulting from fluid phase activation of either the classical or alternative pathway is capable of reacting with factor B to form additional C3bBb, also called amplification convertase, which can split native C3, resulting in the generation of additional C3b and C3a.

Inhibition occurs at points in the complement cascade. There is an inhibitor (C1 esterase inhibitor) present for the activated first component, and C3b inactivator and B1H, 2 inhibitors for the C3b fraction of the 3rd component, which also inhibits the alternate pathway. There may also be a C6 inactivator and C1q- + C4-binding proteins.

Activation of this same complement system, which is so important for host defense, can also result in **injury of normal tissue** by several mechanisms: (1) the generation of anaphylatoxins that produce increased vascular permeability, edema, and smooth muscle contraction; (2) the generation of chemotactic factors that result in migration of polymorphonuclear cells into an area of inflammation. When these cells break down they release lysosomal enzymes that are proteolytic and destroy tissue;

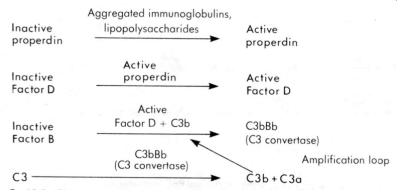

FIG. 16-3.   **Alternative pathway of complement activation.** The initiating substance may be endotoxin, yeast cell wall, bacterial capsules, or IgA.

(3) destruction of RBCs in autoimmune hemolytic anemia; (4) activation of the kinin system, which results in vasodilatation, increased vascular permeability, and pain. The clinical counterparts of these processes involve hypersensitivity reactions Types II and III elaborated by Gell and Coombs (see Ch. 18).

17.   IMMUNODEFICIENCY DISEASES

A diverse group of conditions, characterized chiefly by an increased susceptibility to various infections with consequent severe acute, recurrent, and chronic disease, which result from one or more defects in the specific or nonspecific immune systems.

The **primary immunodeficiencies** are divisible into **specific** and **nonspecific** groups. The former result from failure to manifest efficient humoral (B cell, plasma cell, immunoglobulin [Ig], antibody) responses or cellular (T cell) responses, or from a combined deficiency in both humoral and cellular functions. Complement deficiencies (opsonic defect) and disorders of phagocytosis, chemotaxis, and intracellular bacteriolysis make up the latter, nonspecific, group.

Genetic features distinguish the primary immunodeficiency disorders from **secondary immunodeficiency,** such as (1) hypogammaglobulinemia secondary to hypercatabolism (nephrotic syndrome—which causes renal loss of γ-globulins; protein-losing enteropathy—GI loss); (2) certain lymphopenic states (intestinal lymphangiectasia—GI loss; radiation, cytotoxic drugs—bone marrow and lymphoid tissue suppression); (3) immunodeficiencies associated with malignancy, malnutrition, aging, and debilitation; (4) certain diseases in which cellular immune anergy develops, such as Hodgkin's disease, sarcoidosis, leprosy, and miliary TB; and (5) the impaired phagocytosis that results from the neutropenia or pancytopenia caused by toxic drug reactions, radiation, antimetabolite therapy, and leukemia and other malignancies.

A **perinatal immunodeficiency state** exists (see also IMMUNOLOGIC STATUS OF THE FETUS AND NEWBORN in Vol. II, Ch. 21; and HOST DEFENSES IN THE NEWBORN under NEONATAL INFECTIONS in Vol. II, Ch. 21) because the immune system of the fetus and neonate is still immature. Although it is physiologic, the immunodeficiency puts the fetus and infant at risk of susceptibility to infection. Infection during early gestation can result in multiple congenital anomalies (congenital rubella); infection at or near term can cause multiple organ involvement and persistence of the organism (herpes simplex, cytomegalovirus); while postnatal infection can range in severity from localized oral candidiasis (thrush) to overwhelming gram-negative septicemia and meningitis. The prolonged shedding of contagious virus that occurs in infants after intrauterine infection indicates a complex impairment of both specific and nonspecific immune mechanisms. A **normal physiologic immunodeficiency** also occurs at age 3 to 6 mo, when IgG derived from the mother by active placental transport reaches its nadir. A relative hypogammaglobulinemia exists, and normal infants may experience their first infections during this period. Premature infants may experience more profound hypogammaglobulinemia, since their maternal endowment of IgG is less than that of term infants. Hypogammaglobulinemia soon disappears as serum levels of IgG, IgA, and IgM increase, because of continued immunoglobulin synthesis by the newborn. However, some infants have sluggish synthesis, and IgG and antibody levels may remain low until age 18 to 24 mo. This condition, which may be familial, has been called **transient**

hypogammaglobulinemia of infancy. Recurrent diarrhea, otitis media, and episodes of respiratory infections with wheezing may occur. These children may need to be treated with γ-globulin until endogenous synthetic rates become normal.

PRIMARY SPECIFIC IMMUNODEFICIENCY DISORDERS

These disorders, recognized only since 1952, were formerly classified as either congenital or acquired, based on age at the time of recognition. It is now known that most primary specific immunodeficiency disorders are genetically determined, even though the time of clinical onset is variable, being dependent upon both the nature and severity of the immunologic defect and upon chance exposure to infectious agents.

Although most of these disorders appear to be genetically determined, intrauterine stress (e.g., viral infection such as rubella) may play a necessary role in some cases. Thus, for example, selective IgA deficiency is a complication of congenital rubella, but it is also known to occur familially. No genetic influence is known in DiGeorge syndrome, and the intrauterine events which lead, in this condition, to abnormal development of the 3rd and 4th pharyngeal pouches also remain unexplained.

Advances in immunochemistry and immunobiology have made it possible to distill the basis of classification, from clinical description alone, to functional deficits, to cellular deficiencies, and finally to the molecular and genetic origins of disease (see TABLE 17–1). Therapy has paralleled this understanding. Use of γ-globulin to replace a functional deficit has been supplanted by "engineering" (cellular, molecular, and genetic) to correct some immunodeficiencies more specifically, using histocompatible bone marrow transplants, fetal thymic implants (see Ch. 20), and transfer factor (see Principles of Treatment, below) for "immunoreconstitution."

Pathology

The pathologic changes seen in lymphoid tissue depend on the type of defect. Acellular T-cell–dependent areas in spleen and lymph nodes are found in pure T cell defects (e.g., DiGeorge syndrome); absence of germinal follicles in pure B cell deficiencies (e.g., infantile X-linked agammaglobulinemia); and rudimentary reticular structures in both central and peripheral lymphoid tissue in severe combined (T and B cell) immunodeficiency **(SCID).** In selective IgA deficiency (with or without ataxia telangiectasia), in X-linked immunodeficiency with hyper-IgM, and in some common variable immunodeficiencies, patients possess lymphoid tissue with evident T and B cell areas. They have both T and B cells, but some or all of the latter are unable to differentiate into plasma cells and produce immunoglobulins. It appears that excessive inhibition of B cells by suppressor T cells or the absence of helper T cells underlies the Ig deficiency. In some of the disorders this deficiency is total; in others, only certain immunoglobulins are lacking. At times follicular hyperplasia occurs, which may be clinically expressed as lymphadenopathy, nodular intestinal lymphoid hyperplasia, and splenomegaly.

Clinical Features

The nature and the degree of the specific immunologic defect determine the age of onset, clinical expression, severity, and types of infections to which the patient is susceptible. When considered with genetic data (family history and sex), these clinical clues are diagnostically helpful in pinpointing the specific defect. Patients with severe combined T and B immunodeficiency (SCID) develop viral, bacterial (*Staphylococcus, Escherichia coli, Enterobacter, Klebsiella*), fungal (*Candida*), or protozoal (*Pneumocystis carinii*) infections (severe diarrhea, pneumonia, otitis media) and failure to thrive in early life, most frequently before age 6 mo, and rarely survive beyond age 12 to 18 mo. Patients with pure T cell deficiency have similar infections and early onset of disease. Those with pure B cell defects (especially infantile X-linked agammaglobulinemia) usually become symptomatic at age 6 to 12 mo when placentally transferred IgG antibodies have reached low levels. Infections with extracellular pyogenic bacteria (staphylococci, streptococci, pneumococci, *Pseudomonas, Hemophilus influenzae*, meningococci) are the rule.

Evaluation of Suspected Immunologic Deficiency

Immunodeficiency is suspected when the clinical picture is one of severe acute, acute recurrent, or chronic infection. The following discussion suggests routes to the diagnosis of immunodeficiency and delineation of the immunologic defect. It must be remembered that defects may exist singly or in combinations, and may be partial or complete. Partial deficiencies in T and/or B cell functions also may become more profound with time. This loss of function has been called **abiotrophy.** It occurs with aging and more rapidly in ataxia telangiectasia. It is also the reason that common variable hypogammaglobulinemia may appear to be "acquired."

History: The **time of onset** of infections and the **causative organisms** give important clues. Onset before age 6 mo suggests a cell-mediated defect; onset after age 6 mo, a humoral defect. Recurrent staphylococcal infections with granuloma formation suggest chronic granulomatous disease; recurrent pneumococcal infections suggest splenic disorders (sickle cell [HbS] disease or splenic aplasia); and other gram-positive infections suggest a defect in complement-associated antibodies. Salmonella infections may be a sign of sickle cell disease; pseudomonas infections suggest a deficiency of IgM; and other gram-negative infections, a defect in T cell function. Fungal infections point

TABLE 17-1. PRIMARY SPECIFIC IMMUNODEFICIENCY DISORDERS

Type	Genetics	Cellular Defect	Clinical Features	Therapy‡
Defective humoral immunity				
Selective immunoglobulin (IgA) deficiency (Janeway Type 3 dysgammaglobulinemia)	Autosomal recessive or dominant	B*	Most common disorder. Bronchitis, sinusitis, malabsorption, steatorrhea; or asymptomatic	Avoid gamma globulin and plasma (anaphylaxis)
Immunodeficiency with variable onset and expression (common variable type)	Autosomal recessive or dominant	B† T	2nd most common disorder. Recurrent infection, both viral and bacterial	Gamma globulin; fresh-frozen plasma
Infantile X-linked (Bruton's) agammaglobulinemia	X-linked recessive	B	Recurrent infection with extracellular pyogenic pathogens	Gamma globulin; fresh-frozen plasma
Transient hypogammaglobulinemia of infancy	Familial	B	Recurrent infection with extracellular pyogenic pathogens	Gamma globulin
X-linked immunodeficiency with hyper-IgM (Janeway Type 1 dysgammaglobulinemia)	X-linked recessive	B*	Recurrent infection, thrombocytopenia, aplastic and hemolytic anemia	Immunotherapy under study
Defective cellular immunity				
Thymic hypoplasia (DiGeorge syndrome)	No evidence	T	Usually fatal in infancy; frequent viral, fungal, or pneumocystis infection	Human fetal thymus implantation
Episodic lymphopenia with lymphocytotoxin	Unknown	T	Recurrent viral and bacterial infection; lymphopenia; eczema	Immunotherapy under study
Nucleoside phosphorylase deficiency	Autosomal recessive	T	Recurrent infections	Immunotherapy under study

Combined immunodeficiency diseases

Disease	Inheritance	Cells	Clinical features	Therapy‡
Cellular immunodeficiency with abnormal immunoglobulin synthesis (Nezelof's syndrome)	Unknown	B† T	Recurrent pneumonia	Gamma globulin; transfer factor; thymus implantation
Ataxia telangiectasia	Autosomal recessive	B T	Cerebellar ataxia; telangiectasias (esp. conjunctival); frequent sinopulmonary infection in cases with low IgA	Fresh-frozen plasma (caution in those with IgA deficiency)
Immunodeficiency with thrombocytopenia and eczema (Wiskott-Aldrich syndrome)	X-linked recessive	B T	Frequent infection with viruses, fungi, and pyogens; eczema; bleeding	Transfer factor; fresh-frozen plasma
Immunodeficiency with thymoma	Unknown	B T	Recurrent infections with pyogens, sometimes with viruses, fungi	Thymectomy (thymic transplant usually not indicated)
Immunodeficiency with short-limbed dwarfism	Autosomal recessive ?	B T	Short-limbed dwarfism; lymphopenia	Immunotherapy under study
Severe combined immunodeficiency (SCID) (1) Autosomal recessive—"Swiss type" (a) with ADA** deficiency (b) with normal ADA (2) X-linked (thymic alymphoplasia) (3) Sporadic		B T S B T S B T S B T S	Severe viral, bacterial, fungal infection; diarrhea; failure to thrive	Bone marrow transplantation; fetal thymus implantation; fetal liver transplantation; gamma globulin; irradiated plasma; transfer factor
Immunodeficiency with hematopoietic hypoplasia (reticular dysgenesis)	Unknown	B T S	Rarely survive beyond first few weeks of life	Bone marrow transplantation

B = B cells; T = T cells; S = Stem cells.

* Involves some, but not all, B cells.

† Encountered in some, but not all, patients.

‡ Therapy also includes appropriate antibiotic and antiviral therapy for all conditions.

** Adenosine deaminase.

to a T cell defect. Generalized vaccinia may be the result of a cell-mediated defect or, rarely, a humoral defect; cytomegalovirus, *P. carinii*, and *Giardia lamblia* infections occur with either T cell or B cell defects.

In evaluating recurrent infections in children, it must be remembered that recurrent otitis media, a few bouts of pneumonia, frequent tonsillitis, or sequential viral diseases, are more likely to represent one end of the spectrum of ordinary childhood susceptibility to infection than to be a sign of immunodeficiency. Moreover, respiratory allergies may resemble recurrent URIs and at first be misconstrued. When chronic and recurrent pulmonary disease occurs in children and young adults, not only immunodeficiency disorders but also congenital anomalies, cystic fibrosis, immotile cilia syndrome, and α_1-antitrypsin deficiency should be included in the differential diagnosis.

Family history: Points to be noted include the occurrence of early deaths or failure to thrive, recurrent infections, collagen vascular diseases, and malignancies, as well as the occurrence of specific hereditary disorders such as ataxia telangiectasia or the Wiskott-Aldrich syndrome. If possible, a pedigree chart should be constructed to determine any hereditary patterns.

Physical examination: The size of lymphoid and reticuloendothelial organs should be noted. Lymph nodes, tonsils, and adenoids are enlarged in some humoral defects, especially in some immunodeficiencies with variable onset and expression (*common variable type*) where there is a defect in the conversion of B cells to Ig-secreting plasma cells. They may be small in either cellular (*combined immunodeficiency*) or humoral (*X-linked agammaglobulinemia*) defects. Posteroanterior and lateral chest x-rays should be obtained for neonates, to determine the presence or absence of the thymus; abdominal x-rays and a radioisotope scan may be helpful in visualizing the spleen, or establishing its absence. The spleen is absent in congenital aplasia, may be enlarged or small and fibrotic in sickle cell disease, and is enlarged in some humoral and cellular defects. Since the liver is also a reticuloendothelial organ, it may also become enlarged, presumably as a compensatory phenomenon. Hepatosplenomegaly occurs when B cells are present but cannot mature to plasma cells because of successive T cell suppressor activity.

Eczema is common in the Wiskott-Aldrich and hyperimmunoglobulinemia-E syndromes; a nonspecific dermatitis is often present in chronic granulomatous disease. Certain physical signs are specific: the child's appearance is typical in the DiGeorge syndrome, adenosine deaminase deficiency, and short-limbed dwarfism. Telangiectasias, especially conjunctival, occur in ataxia telangiectasia; neonatal hypocalcemic tetany in the DiGeorge syndrome; and partial albinism in the Chédiak-Higashi syndrome.

Laboratory studies and tests: Laboratory confirmation of immunodeficiency can be quite extensive and can require sophisticated procedures available only at a large hospital or academic laboratory. However, certain laboratory tests are widely available, and some can be performed as office procedures. Persistent or periodic lymphopenia below 1000 or 2000 cells/cu mm suggests a cell-mediated defect; cyclic or persistent neutropenia may accompany either cell-mediated or humoral immunodeficiency. Coombs-positive hemolytic anemia occurs in certain humoral defects; thrombocytopenia, in the Wiskott-Aldrich syndrome. Serum calcium is low in the DiGeorge syndrome.

Tests of humoral immunity: Many laboratories are now able to determine serum Ig levels. Immunoelectrophoresis may be used to identify agammaglobulinemia, a deficiency of IgG, IgM, or IgA, or the presence of immunoglobulins of limited mobility. The technic is not quantitative, however, and in order to obtain specific levels of IgG, IgM, IgA, or IgD, radial immunodiffusion or nephelometry is used; IgE is determined by radioimmunoassay. (These procedures are described under PRINCIPLES OF MEASUREMENTS in Ch. 230.)

The presence of normal serum Ig levels (see TABLE 17–2) does not necessarily mean that antibody synthesis is intact: determining the presence or amount of Ig does not identify its antibody specificity. To determine **antibody content,** the most commonly used technics are gel precipitation (a known antigen is combined with serum in a liquid gel medium; if antibody to that antigen is present in the serum a solid sediment forms) and agglutination (the antigen is a cell or a particulate substance— bacteria, RBCs, latex particles—to which antigen is attached; in the presence of the specific antibody, agglutination occurs).

Specific antibody assays are significant in children who have had or have been immunized against measles, rubella, mumps, influenza A or B, tetanus, diphtheria, or poliomyelitis. A positive Schick test in an immunized person indicates an IgG defect; except in patients of blood group AB, A and B isohemagglutinin titers indicate an IgM defect. If no specific antibodies are found on assay, antibody responsiveness to diphtheria, tetanus, hemophilus B, typhoid, poliomyelitis, mumps, measles, or blood group substances can be tested by vaccine or antigen injection. (CAUTION: *Not with live or attenuated vaccines.*) Antibody stimulation by other antigenic substances (bacterial, viral, carbohydrate) can also be tested.

To determine **local immune function,** the IgA level in saliva, bronchial washings, and nasal secretions may be determined; tissue obtained by biopsy of respiratory or GI mucosa may be examined for immunoglobulins by fluorescent microscopy; or tetanus toxoid may be applied to the nasal mucosa, which is then examined for the presence of toxoid-induced antibody. Positive skin tests for immediate-type (atopic) hypersensitivity indicate the presence of specific IgE in the skin; skin tests for mast-cell–fixed IgE may also be performed with anti-IgE antibody. Circulating allergen-specific IgE can be measured in serum by RAST (radioallergosorbent test) technic.

TABLE 17-2. IMMUNOGLOBULIN LEVELS IN NORMAL CHILDREN
EXPRESSED AS PERCENT OF NORMAL ADULT LEVELS

Immunoglobulin	IgG	IgM	IgA
Adult	1158 ± 305 mg/100 ml	99 ± 27 mg/100 ml	200 ± 61 mg/100 ml
Newborn	89% ± 17%	11% ± 5%	1% ± 2%
1 – 3 mo	37 ± 10	30 ± 11	11 ± 7
4 – 6 mo	37 ± 16	43 ± 17	14 ± 9
7 – 12 mo	58 ± 19	55 ± 23	19 ± 9
13 – 24 mo	66 ± 18	59 ± 23	25 ± 12
25 – 36 mo	77 ± 16	62 ± 19	36 ± 19
3 – 5 yr	80 ± 20	57 ± 18	47 ± 14
6 – 8 yr	80 ± 22	66 ± 25	62 ± 23
9 – 11 yr	97 ± 20	80 ± 33	66 ± 30
12 – 16 yr	82 ± 11	60 ± 20	74 ± 32

Values represent mean ± 1 S.D. *Above **percentages** can be applied when local laboratories determine their own normal adult values.*

Adapted from E.R. Stiehm and H.H. Fudenberg, *Pediatrics* Vol. 37, pp. 715–727, May 1966. Copyright American Academy of Pediatrics, 1966. Used with permission of the Academy and the author.

Since B cells have identifiable surface markers, the number of peripheral **circulating B cells** can be determined. Surface immunoglobulins can be detected with fluorescein-labeled anti-immunoglobulins specific for the Fc components of IgG, IgA, IgM, and IgD (immunofluorescence—see TYPE II REACTIONS in Ch. 18); a B cell receptor for the 3rd component of complement (C3 receptor) can be detected by the adherence of complement-coated RBCs to the B cells, forming rosettes; and a receptor for the Fc portion of the antibody molecule can be detected with antigen-antibody complexes or aggregated γ-globulin. A bone marrow biopsy will detect signs of maturation or arrest of cells in the neutrophil series and will determine the presence or absence of **plasma cells**; architectural changes in a lymph node, determined by biopsies performed before and after local immunization (e.g., DTP in the thigh, with inguinal node biopsy), will enable determination of **B cell and plasma cell function**. Rectal biopsy tissue may also be examined for lymphoid tissue, B cells, and plasma cells.

Tests of cell-mediated immunity: A lymphocyte count above 2000/cu mm suggests that the cell-mediated immune system is normal. However, repeated blood counts may be necessary to detect periodic or progressive lymphopenia, which occurs with partial deficiencies of the cell-mediated immune system.

A number of antigens are now commercially available for specific **delayed-hypersensitivity skin tests** (see TABLE 17-3). These tests are usually performed by injecting 0.1-ml amounts of the antigen into the skin. If T memory cells for the test antigen are present, induration and erythema become apparent at the test site at about 24 h, peak at 48 h, and then resolve over the next day or two. In order to test a patient's ability to *develop* cell-mediated immunity, a test must be performed with an antigen that he has not previously encountered. The antigens most commonly used are dinitrochlorobenzene (DNCB) and dinitrofluorobenzene (DNFB). These are applied to the skin as in a patch test

TABLE 17-3. COMMERCIALLY AVAILABLE ANTIGENS FOR EVALUATING
DELAYED HYPERSENSITIVITY

Antigen*	Concentration	
	Initial	Final
Candida albicans, 500 PNU/ml	1:1,000	1:10
Trichophyton, 500 PNU/ml	1:1,000	1:10
Mumps	1:1	—
Diphtheria-tetanus fluid toxoid	1:10	1:1
Streptokinase-streptodornase	1:1,000	—
PPD (tuberculin)	5 T.U.	250 T.U.
Histoplasmin	1:1	—
1–Chloro–2,4–dinitrobenzene (DNCB)	1% in acetone (Sensitizing dose)	0.1% in acetone (Test dose)

* DNCB 0.25 ml is applied to intact skin as in patch testing (see TYPE IV HYPERSENSITIVITY REACTIONS in Ch. 18); other antigens are given intradermally in 0.1-ml doses.

(see TYPE IV REACTIONS in Ch. 18), but first in a sensitizing dose and then in a test dose. If the patient's T cells are immunologically competent, a contact dermatitis will follow the test dose. These tests are more reliable in children and adults than in neonates: delayed hypersensitivity reactions are more difficult to induce and to elicit in neonates because their immune system is still immature. A positive delayed skin test to *Candida albicans* can usually be elicited in a normal 1-yr-old.

The patient's ability to reject a skin graft from an unrelated (and hence incompatible) donor also indicates his cell-mediated immunologic competence. The procedure is seldom used in humans as a diagnostic test, as there is the potential hazard of inducing a graft-vs.-host reaction (GVH disease).

A number of sophisticated **in vitro tests** can be performed to evaluate cellular immunity and the presence of T memory cells. The occurrence of rosette formation when sheep RBCs (SRBC) are mixed with lymphocyte preparations indicates the presence of T cells but not their functional capacity. For this purpose, a specimen of the patient's lymphocytes may be placed into short-term culture and their response to the addition of antigen observed. T memory cells will proliferate and enlarge **(lymphocyte transformation)**. These large cells can be counted directly. Alternatively, the amount of radioactive **thymidine** incorporated by the lymphocytes (indicating protein synthesis) may be used as a measure of transformation. It is also possible to measure the supernatant for lymphokines after antigen has been added to the lymphocytes; the **MIF** (migration inhibitory factor) **assay** is the one most commonly used and indicates the presence of activated T cells.

Phytohemagglutinin **(PHA)**, an extract from the seeds of a bean plant, stimulates lymphocyte transformation and thymidine incorporation in both T and B memory cells and although it cannot be used as a measure of cellular immunity alone, testing with this mitogen is useful when humoral immunity is known to be normal.

Principles of Treatment

Precautions: Patients with either T or B cell defects should be protected from exposure to infectious disease, and should not be immunized with live virus vaccines. Use of corticosteroids and immunosuppressive drugs is also **contraindicated** in these patients, and they should not be subjected to splenectomy, since these therapeutic measures will compromise the remaining immunologic defenses. In addition, patients with T cell deficiency should not be given fresh blood or plasma transfusions, since these may induce a graft-vs.-host reaction. Irradiated blood and plasma may be used. For those with selective IgA deficiency, γ-globulin, blood, or plasma should be avoided if possible, because production of anti-IgA antibodies may result in an anaphylactic reaction. Surgery should be avoided in patients with thrombocytopenia; and patients with splenomegaly should avoid contact sports and other activities that increase the risk of splenic rupture.

Infections: When a patient with an immunodeficiency disorder develops an infection, it is safest to assume that it is bacterial and to begin antibiotic therapy as soon as specimens have been taken for culture, later changing the therapy as indicated by the culture results. The possibility of viral, fungal, or *P. carinii* superinfection must be borne in mind. The therapy of choice for *P. carinii* infections is trimethoprim-sulfamethoxazole (see PNEUMONIA CAUSED BY *Pneumocystis carinii* in Ch. 38); for cytomegalovirus, idoxuridine **(IDU)**, floxuridine, or cytarabine **(Ara-C)**; for generalized herpes simplex infection, IDU or Ara-C; and for severe *Candida* or *Aspergillus* infection, amphotericin B (see General Therapeutic Principles in Ch. 9). Some patients may need continuous antibiotic in addition to γ-globulin therapy to minimize recurrent infections.

γ-**Globulin** provides mostly IgG, and cannot effectively replace IgA or IgM. However, it is the treatment of choice in panhypogammaglobulinemia. γ-Globulin will not correct cell-mediated, phagocytic, or complement deficiencies. It is **contraindicated** in selective IgA deficiency (because of a tendency to anaphylaxis) and in thrombocytopenic states (risk of bleeding at the injection site). The usual dose is 0.6 ml/kg IM of 16.5% γ-globulin. Initially, a loading dose of 1.8 ml/kg (as 3 separate injections) is given; then 0.6 ml/kg every 3 to 4 wk, to maintain IgG serum levels at 200 mg/100 ml. The maximum tolerable dose is about 20 to 30 ml. It is given only IM; intravascular injection must be avoided. Aged preparations may contain aggregated γ-globulin and should not be used because they may cause local, toxic, or anaphylactic reactions.

Fresh-frozen plasma infusion provides the 3 major immunoglobulins, IgG, IgA, and IgM. If obtained from specifically immunized donors, it provides specific antibodies. It can be used in place of the large initial loading dose of γ-globulin, and is also useful in patients with disorders causing large renal or GI losses of γ-globulin, and in patients with thrombocytopenia. It has been used with some success in certain complement defects, particularly in C5 dysfunction and C1-esterase inhibitor deficiency. Fresh-frozen plasma is **contraindicated** in selective IgA deficiency since, like γ-globulin, it may cause anaphylaxis. In T cell deficiencies, it may cause a graft-vs.-host reaction, but the risk can be reduced by allowing the plasma to age for 2 wk and by irradiation with 3000 R, which eliminates the T cells in the plasma. The usual dose is 15 to 20 ml/kg, given every 3 to 4 wk in hypogammaglobulinemia, and weekly or biweekly in opsonic and complement deficiencies. The plasma should be tested for syphilis and hepatitis before use.

Transfer factor, a nonviable dialyzable extract of activated lymphocytes, given subcutaneously, has shown promise in treatment of the Wiskott-Aldrich syndrome and chronic mucocutaneous candidiasis. When taken from a donor who responds strongly to delayed hypersensitivity skin tests, it has induced conversion of T cell anergy in patients for 6 to 12 mo, though more frequent doses may be necessary. Transfer factor does not induce graft-vs.-host reactions or cause hepatitis, but local and febrile reactions may occur. Nephrotic syndrome, monoclonal gammopathy, hemolytic anemia, and malignancy have occurred in a few cases treated with transfer factor. Whether these rare side effects are due to transfer factor is not yet known.

Lymphocyte infusions are useful in T cell disorders, but donors must be HLA-identical or a graft-vs.-host reaction may occur. Bone marrow transplantation supplies stem cells and has been effective in SCID, but again the donor must be HLA-identical. Fetal (< 8 wk gestation) liver transplants have also been successful in a few cases of SCID. Thymus implantation has been effective in restoring T cell immunity in the DiGeorge syndrome and in some cases of SCID. The success of this procedure may be due to thymic humoral substances such as thymosin, which increases both in vitro and in vivo T cell function. Thymus instruction of T cells may also result in helper function towards B cells and subsequent immunoglobulin production. The thymus from a fetus of < 14 wk gestation is implanted IM, subcutaneously, or intraperitoneally. Although the risk of a graft-vs.-host reaction is minimal, the thymus graft is usually rejected and the procedure may need to be repeated to maintain T cell function. Lymphocyte infusions, bone marrow transplants, thymus implants, and fetal liver transplants are performed only at specialized centers.

SELECTIVE IGA DEFICIENCY

This is the most common Ig deficiency. Occurring in 1:400 to 1:500 persons, it is 10 times more common than panhypogammaglobulinemia. Most of these patients have normal numbers of circulating B cells with IgA surface markers. They have a defect in terminal maturation of B lymphocytes into IgA-secreting plasma cells. This can be due either to the presence of selective IgA suppressor T cells or to an intrinsic defect in IgA B cells. Both autosomal dominant and autosomal recessive modes of inheritance have been described. Some people with IgA deficiency have no problems and are healthy, possibly because they can substitute low-mol-wt IgM for the deficient IgA and are thus able to maintain immunologic defense at the levels of the GI and sinopulmonary epithelium. Other patients have recurrent sinopulmonary infections or severe malabsorption and diarrhea with intestinal nodular hyperplasia. Incidence of selective IgA deficiency rises in patients with respiratory allergy, chronic urticaria, celiac disease (gluten-induced enteropathy), ulcerative colitis, regional enteritis, RA, SLE, and ataxia telangiectasia, and in families of patients with agammaglobulinemia. IgA-deficient children with recurrent viral respiratory disease and chronic serous otitis media have been observed to synthesize IgA spontaneously as their infections become less frequent and their clinical conditions improve. Therefore, their serum IgA levels should be determined yearly. In addition, although prospective studies of individuals with selective IgA deficiency have not been done, the association of this deficiency with other diseases should be kept in mind.

Treatment is symptomatic. IgA cannot be replaced with γ-globulin or plasma, as anaphylactic reactions are likely to occur. Prognosis is good to excellent with symptomatic management, especially if the defect is not accompanied by associated conditions.

IMMUNODEFICIENCY WITH THYMOMA

A combined immunodeficiency disorder associated with thymoma (either benign or malignant) occurring in adulthood and characterized by recurrent infections, chronic diarrhea, stomatitis, aplastic anemia, thrombocytopenia, chronic hepatitis, arthritis, and diabetes mellitus. Myasthenia gravis may coexist. The disorder occurs after age 20 and twice as often in women as in men. There is no known inheritance pattern.

Immunologic studies have shown deficiency of IgG, IgA, and IgM, impaired antibody response to injected antigens, lymphopenia, negative skin tests to delayed hypersensitivity antigens, and lack of lymphocyte transformation on in vitro testing.

Onset of symptoms is gradual. Infections become recurrent, especially affecting the respiratory tract and skin. Both bacterial and viral infections occur. Septicemia may ensue. Chronic diarrhea suggests intestinal Giardia infection. The thymoma (usually spindle-cell) is diagnosed by finding a mass in the anterior mediastinum on x-ray. Tracheal compression by the mass may cause wheezing. The appearance of the thymoma may precede or follow by years the clinical and laboratory signs of immunodeficiency. Therefore, adults with "acquired" immunodeficiency should be examined for this complication.

Prognosis is generally poor, the progressive immunologic deterioration eventually leading to fatal infection. Death is often from cytomegalovirus or P. carinii infection. Treatment consists of γ-globulin and antibiotics to control the recurrent infections; γ-globulin therapy may also control chronic diarrhea in some cases. Excision of the thymoma is indicated, but this does not improve immunologic function.

PRIMARY NONSPECIFIC IMMUNODEFICIENCY DISORDERS

The phagocytic system is impaired in congenital neutropenia or pancytopenia because the number of phagocytic cells is reduced. Primary nonspecific immunodeficiency syndromes involving functional deficits of phagocytic cells may occur as a result of (1) complement deficiencies, which cause impaired chemotaxis and adherence; (2) impaired chemotaxis due to a defect in WBCs; (3) failure to kill phagocytized bacteria because of an intracellular enzyme defect (chronic granulomatous disease); and (4) failure to kill phagocytized bacteria because of a lysosomal defect (Chédiak-Higashi syndrome).

COMPLEMENT DEFICIENCIES

Primary deficiencies of components of the complement system have been described; though case reports are few, they have added to our understanding of the protective role of complement against infection. **Secondary complement deficiency** may be the result of complement consumption, as occurs during serum sickness, the early stages of acute post-streptococcal glomerulonephritis, and acute active SLE. Complement activation and its biologic effects are described in Ch. 16. Patients with **deficient C3** lack the crucial link for activation of both classic and alternative pathways, and clinically resemble those with agammaglobulinemia, with recurrent pyogenic bacterial infections of the sinuses, ears, and lungs. They require treatment with antibiotics. Inherited **C1q, C1r, and C1s deficiencies** have been described in patients with SLE and in their relatives. **C2 and C4 deficiencies** have also been described in collagen vascular diseases such as dermatomyositis and SLE. Recurrent infections may be associated with the disease and its treatment with corticosteroids rather than with the complement deficiency. **C5 deficiency** has been described in a patient with SLE, and **C7** in a family and patient with scleroderma. The former patient had recurrent infections but had been receiving corticosteroid treatment. A small number of patients have been described with **C6 or C8 deficiency.** They have had gonococcal and meningococcal infections (arthritis, septicemia, and meningitis), suggesting that the late components of complement are important in the bodily defense against *Neisseria.*

In addition to the above, **familial dysfunction of C5** has been described. It occurs in infants and is similar to Leiner's disease, with failure to thrive, widespread refractory seborrheic dermatitis, chronic diarrhea, and recurrent sepsis. Total hemolytic complement and immunoquantitation of C5 are normal, but there is a defect in phagocytosis of yeast particles that is corrected by the addition of normal C5. Patients have responded to the infusion of fresh plasma. However, the syndrome resembles the symptoms of combined immunodeficiency, and prior to plasma therapy normal cell-mediated immunity should be demonstrated in order to avoid the risk of graft-vs.-host reactions.

---

18.   HYPERSENSITIVITY REACTIONS

At the present stage of knowledge it is difficult to formulate a classification that adequately categorizes the gamut of diseases in which hypersensitivity phenomena may play a role. These diseases range from hay fever (which results from hypersensitivity to an exogenous antigen, is limited to the respiratory and ocular mucosal surfaces, and lacks systemic morbidity) to SLE (a multisystem disease with significant morbidity, and which is associated with hypersensitivity to autoantigens). There are, moreover, those diseases in which antibodies to host tissues can be demonstrated even though their pathologic significance is unknown; for example, the antibody to heart tissue that appears following heart surgery or myocardial infarction.

Proposed classifications include those based on the time required for the appearance of symptoms or skin test reactions after exposure to antigen (such as immediate and delayed hypersensitivity), on the type of antigen (such as drug reactions), or on the nature of organ involvement. These classifications, however, have not taken into account that more than one type of immune response may be occurring or that more than one type may be necessary to produce immunologic injury. While this is also true of the Gell and Coombs classification of hypersensitivity reactions into 4 types, theirs has proved to be clinically and conceptually helpful and has come to be widely used. It is based on animal experiments in which the 4 types of reaction can be clearly distinguished. Although the processes involved are often more complex in the clinical setting, the Gell and Coombs classification does allow one to plan a diagnostic and therapeutic approach to a clinical problem. It should be emphasized that in order to be classed as a hypersensitivity reaction a pathologic process must be the result of a specific interaction between antigen (exogenous or endogenous) and either humoral antibodies or sensitized lymphocytes. This definition therefore excludes those diseases in which antibodies are demonstrated but have no known pathophysiologic significance, even though their presence may have diagnostic value.

TYPE I REACTIONS

(Immediate-Type, Atopic, Reaginic, Anaphylactic, or IgE-Mediated Hypersensitivity Reactions)

Reactions resulting from the release of pharmacologically active substances such as histamine, slow-reactive substance of anaphylaxis (SRS-A), and eosinophilic chemotactic factor (ECF) from

IgE-sensitized basophils and mast cells after contact with specific antigen. The released substances cause vasodilatation, increased capillary permeability, smooth muscle contraction, and eosinophilia. The consequent clinical manifestations include urticaria, angioedema, hypotension, and spasm of bronchial, GI, or uterine musculature.

The clinical conditions in which Type I reactions play a role include allergic extrinsic asthma, seasonal allergic rhinitis, systemic anaphylaxis, reactions to stinging insects, some reactions to foods and drugs, and some cases of urticaria.

Diagnostic Tests

The most convenient test for the detection of IgE-sensitized mast cells is the **direct skin test.** Solutions for direct skin tests are made from extracts of materials which are inhaled, ingested, or injected, such as wind-borne pollens from certain trees, grasses, and weeds; house dust; animal danders; molds; foods; insect venoms; horse serum; and certain drugs. The tests are performed either by applying the test solutions to scratches or shallow punctures of the skin or by injecting them intradermally. The former is usually safer because less antigen is introduced, and is often done initially to identify materials which may cause a systemic reaction if injected intradermally. Scratches about 1 cm long and 2.5 cm apart are made with a needle on the forearm or back, and a drop of concentrated (1:20) test extract is placed on each scratch. Alternatively, the skin is punctured through a drop of test extract with commercially available scarifiers or a darning needle (prick technic). Control tests are performed simultaneously, using the diluent by prick and intradermally and either histamine (0.01 mg histamine base/ml) or morphine sulfate (0.1 mg/ml), which is a mast cell degranulator, intradermally. The diluent should give a negative test result and the latter 2 substances should produce a wheal measuring 1 cm or less. The histamine and morphine tests determine the reactivity of the capillaries in the skin and the presence of mast cells capable of releasing histamine. The tests are especially important as controls when the patient has been taking drugs, such as antihistamines and hydroxyzine, that are known to inhibit skin tests by blocking the effect of histamine on blood vessels, and drugs such as codeine, meperidine, and morphine, which are mast cell degranulators.

A positive wheal-and-flare reaction is usually obvious by 15 to 20 min after the test extract is applied. If the diameter of the wheal is more than 0.5 cm larger than the diluent control wheal, the test is positive and an intradermal test should not be performed. An intradermal test can be done if the reaction is smaller than this or if the patient has dermatographia so that there is a question whether the wheal and flare are immunologically mediated.

In the intradermal test, a tuberculin syringe and short-bevel No. 26 needle are used to inject 0.02 ml of a 1:500 or 1:1000 concentration of the test extract into the skin. A wheal more than 0.5 cm larger than the diluent control wheal, appearing in 15 min, is a positive reaction. The size of the skin test reaction shows a rough correlation with clinical symptoms, although some patients with large reactions do not have symptoms and some patients with small intradermal skin test reactions do have symptoms. Therefore, most physicians monitor the patient with periodic clinical reevaluations to determine the significance of skin tests.

A **radioallergosorbent test (RAST)** or a **passive transfer test** (the **PK** [Prausnitz-Küstner] reaction) may be performed when, occasionally, direct skin testing is not possible because of generalized dermatitis, extreme dermatographia, or the patient's anxiety. The **RAST** detects the presence of antigen-specific serum IgE. In this test, a known antigen, in the form of an insoluble polymer-antigen conjugate, is mixed with the serum to be tested. Any IgE in the serum that is specific for the antigen will attach to the conjugate. Adding ^{125}I-labeled anti-IgE antibody and measuring the amount of radioactivity taken up by the conjugate determines the quantity of antigen-specific IgE in the patient's circulation.

Many commercial laboratories are now able to perform the RAST, but if a laboratory cannot test for antigens of interest to the physician, a **PK test** may be performed. (Since serum from the patient is injected into another individual in this test, the patient should first be tested for syphilis and hepatitis-associated antigen, and SGOT, SGPT, alkaline phosphatase, and bilirubin levels should be obtained.) Serum from the patient is obtained under sterile precautions or sterilized by filtration, and 0.1-ml amounts are injected intradermally into several sites in a nonallergic subject (usually a relative). After 48 h, these sites are tested with antigen as in the direct skin test. Indirect skin testing is possible because IgE antibody in the patient's serum can adhere to the recipient's mast cells.

Leukocyte histamine release, another in vitro test, detects antigen-specific IgE on sensitized basophils by measuring antigen-induced histamine release from the patient's leukocytes. Though not widely used diagnostically, this test has given valuable insight into the kinetics of histamine release and has been useful in evaluating drugs for their ability to inhibit histamine release.

Provocative challenge is performed when a positive skin test has raised a question concerning the role of the particular antigen in the production of symptoms. The antigen is applied to the eyes, nose, or lungs. **Ophthalmic testing** offers no advantage over skin testing and is rarely positive when skin tests are negative. However, it is sometimes used in testing hypersensitivity to pollens in suspected atopic conjunctivitis. A small amount of antigen (e.g., dried pollen or an aqueous extract of pollen in the same concentration as used for intradermal testing) is applied to the lower conjunctival sac. An appropriate control (e.g., the diluent or dried pine pollen) is used in the other eye. A positive response is characterized by burning, smarting, itching, or redness of the bulbar conjunctiva exceeding that in the control eye. Edema often follows. If a positive reaction occurs, the eye should be irrigated with isotonic saline, then a drop of epinephrine 1:1000 instilled.

Nasal challenge is occasionally performed. There are numerous methods for introducing the antigen—insufflating dried pollen into the nose, spraying aqueous extract from a squeeze bottle or by nebulizer, or inserting a cotton pledget soaked in aqueous extract. Response is positive if itching, sneezing, and rhinorrhea occur, accompanied by a change in the appearance of the mucosa.

Bronchial inhalation challenge has long been used by European allergists to select the antigens to be used for immunotherapy. Although it remains predominantly an investigative tool in this country, some allergists use bronchial challenge when the clinical significance of a positive skin test is unclear.

Total IgE level determination is also used in evaluating patients with Type I reactions using a paper radioimmunosorbent test (PRIST). Serum IgE levels may be elevated in allergic asthma, allergic bronchopulmonary aspergillosis, parasitic infections, and eczema; they are normal in allergic alveolitis. Very high IgE levels are seen in allergic bronchopulmonary aspergillosis and can therefore be used to distinguish this form of allergic lung disease from asthma induced by pollen, dust, and mold and from nonallergic forms of asthma. The normally wide range of IgE levels, however, limits its usefulness in separating allergic from nonallergic asthma.

Provocative food testing may be performed when regularly occurring symptoms are suspected of being food-related and skin tests are of doubtful clinical significance (see also Diagnosis of Gastrointestinal Allergy in Ch. 19). Certain foods are eliminated or incriminated as allergens by their individual and gradual addition to a basic diet composed of relatively nonallergenic foods (see TABLE 18–1). When symptoms are relatively infrequent and food is thought to be the cause, a food diary may be useful. Common food allergens include milk, eggs, fish, shellfish, nuts, wheat, citrus fruits, tomato, and chocolate, and all products containing one or more of these ingredients. Except for acute anaphylactic-type reactions to foods, food intolerances, idiosyncrasies, and vague constitutional symptoms (fatigue, headache, insomnia) have not been demonstrably due to Type I hypersensitivity.

Most of the common allergens and all suspected foods must be eliminated from the starting diet. No foods or fluids may be consumed other than those specified in the starting diet. Eating in restaurants is not advisable, since the patient (and physician) must know the exact composition of all meals. Furthermore, one must always be certain of the purity of products used—for example, ordinary "rye" bread contains some wheat flour.

If no improvement occurs after 2 wk on a given diet, another should be tried. If symptoms are relieved, one new food is added to the diet and eaten regularly for 3 to 7 days or until symptoms recur. Alternatively, small amounts of the food to be tested are eaten in the physician's presence and

TABLE 18–1. ELIMINATION DIETS—ALLOWABLE FOODS

Foodstuff	Diet No. 1* (No beef, pork, fowl, milk, rye, corn)	Diet No. 2* (No beef, lamb, milk, rice)	Diet No. 3* (No lamb, fowl, rye, rice, corn, milk)
Cereal	Rice products	Corn products	
Vegetable	Lettuce, spinach, carrots, beets, artichokes	Corn, tomatoes, peas, asparagus, squash, string beans	Lima beans, beets, potatoes (white and sweet), string beans, tomatoes
Meat	Lamb	Chicken, bacon	Beef, bacon
Flour (bread or biscuits)	Rice	Corn, 100% rye (ordinary "rye" bread contains wheat)	Lima beans, soybeans, potatoes
Fruit	Lemons, pears, grapefruit	Peaches, apricots, prunes, pineapple	Grapefruit, lemons, peaches, apricots
Fat	Cottonseed oil, olive oil	Corn oil, cottonseed oil	Cottonseed oil, olive oil
Beverage	Tea, coffee (black), lemonade		Tea, coffee (black), lemonade, juice from approved fruit
Miscellaneous	Tapioca pudding, gelatin, cane sugar, maple sugar, salt, olives	Cane sugar, gelatin, corn syrup, salt	Tapioca pudding, gelatin, cane sugar, maple sugar, salt, olives

* Diet No. 4: Should symptoms persist when on the above 3 elimination diets, the daily diet may be restricted to whole milk, 2000 to 3000 ml.

the patient's reactions are observed. Aggravation or recrudescence of symptoms following the addition of a new food is the best evidence of allergy to that item. Such evidence should be verified by noting the effect of removing that food from the diet for several days, then restoring it.

Since allergy to one or another ingredient may exist, vitamin supplements should not be added until some therapeutic response to the diet has been obtained. In severely restricted diets, a multivitamin preparation of synthetic origin may be added after the first 3 days.

TYPE II REACTIONS

(Cytotoxic Reactions; Cytolytic Complement-Dependent Cytotoxicity; Cell-Stimulating Reactions)

Reactions that result when antibody reacts with antigenic components of a cell or tissue elements or with an antigen or hapten that has become intimately coupled to cells or tissue. The antigen-antibody reaction may cause opsonic adherence through coating of the cell with antibody; it is then called immune adherence, which occurs by activation of complement components through C3, with consequent phagocytosis of the cell; or activation of the full complement system with consequent cytolysis or tissue damage. In some situations stimulation of secretory organs such as the thyroid may occur.

Clinical examples of cell injury in which antibody reacts with antigenic components of a cell are Coombs-positive hemolytic anemias, antibody-induced thrombocytopenic purpura, leukopenia, pemphigus, pemphigoid, myasthenia gravis, Graves' disease, and pernicious anemia. These reactions occur in patients receiving incompatible transfusions, in hemolytic disease of the newborn, and in neonatal thrombocytopenia. They may also play a part in multisystem hypersensitivity diseases such as SLE. For a discussion of renal effects, see Ch. 147.

The mechanism of injury is best exemplified by the effect on RBCs. In hemolytic anemias the RBCs are destroyed either by intravascular hemolysis or by macrophage phagocytosis, predominantly within the spleen. In vitro studies have demonstrated that in the presence of complement some complement-binding antibodies such as the blood group antibodies anti-A and anti-B cause rapid hemolysis; others such as anti-Le cause a slow lysis of cells; and still others do not damage cells directly but cause their adherence to and phagocytosis by phagocytes. By contrast, Rh antibodies on RBCs do not activate complement, and they destroy cells predominantly by extravascular phagocytosis.

Examples of Type II reactions in which the antigen is a component of tissue include *early acute* (hyperacute) graft rejection of a transplanted kidney, which is due to the presence of antibody to vascular endothelium, and Goodpasture's syndrome, which is due to antibody reacting with glomerular and alveolar basement membrane endothelium. In experimental Goodpasture's syndrome complement is an important mediator of injury, but the role of complement has not been clearly determined in the early acute graft rejection.

Examples of reactions that are due to haptenic coupling with cells or tissue include many of the drug hypersensitivity reactions, such as penicillin-induced hemolytic anemia and purpura.

Antibody-dependent cell-mediated cytotoxicity is a newly described form of Type II immunologic injury that has been observed in mice; its role in human disease has not been defined. In this reaction cells that have been coated with antibody are destroyed by lymphocyte-like cells that do not have T or B cell markers and have been called K (killer) cells. Whether complement plays a role in the reaction is not yet known.

Another effect of antibody is to stimulate cell function, as occurs with an immunoglobulin, the long-acting thyroid stimulator **(LATS)**. LATS is found in the IgG fraction of serum and is considered to be an autoantibody directed against some determinant on the thyroid cell membrane, causing excessive hormone secretion.

Diagnostic Tests

A Type II reaction is tested (1) by detecting the presence of antibody or complement on the cell or on tissue, or (2) by detecting the presence, in serum, of antibody to a cell surface antigen, a tissue antigen, or an exogenous antigen. Although complement is often required for Type II cell injury and may be detected on the cell or in the tissue, total serum hemolytic complement activity is not depressed as it often is in Type III hypersensitivity reactions.

The direct antiglobulin and anti-non-γ-globulin tests detect antibody and complement on RBCs, respectively. These tests use rabbit antisera, one to immunoglobulin and the other to complement. When these reagents are mixed with RBCs coated with immunoglobulin or complement, agglutination occurs. Antibodies eluted from these cells have demonstrated both a specificity for RBC blood group antigens and an ability to fix complement, thus demonstrating that they are true autoantibodies and account for the complement present on the RBCs in the direct non-γ-globulin test.

The indirect antiglobulin test is used to detect the presence of a circulating antibody to RBC antigens. The patient's serum is incubated with RBCs of the same blood group (to preclude false results due to incompatibility) and the antiglobulin test is then performed on these RBCs. Agglutination confirms the presence of antibody to RBC antigens.

In penicillin-induced hemolytic anemia the patient has a positive direct Coombs' test while receiving penicillin but has a negative indirect antiglobulin test. The patient's serum, however, will agglutinate the indirect-test RBCs if they are coated with penicillin.

Fluorescent microscopy is most commonly used to detect the presence of immunoglobulin or complement in tissue (by the direct technic) and can also be used to determine the specificity of a circulating antibody (by the indirect technic). In the **direct immunofluorescent technic,** animal antibody specific for human immunoglobulin or complement is labeled with a fluorescent dye (usually fluorescein) and then layered on tissue. When the tissue is examined under the fluorescent microscope, a typical fluorescent color (green for fluorescein) indicates the presence of human immunoglobulin or complement in the tissue. Direct immunofluorescence can also be used to detect the presence of other serum proteins, tissue components, or exogenous antigen as long as specific animal antibodies to them can be produced. The technic itself does not indicate a Type II reaction unless the antibody can be eluted from the tissue and its specificity for tissue antigens determined.

In Goodpasture's syndrome the immunofluorescent pattern is seen as a linear fluorescence on kidney and lung basement membrane. When antibody is eluted from the kidney of patients with Goodpasture's syndrome and layered on normal kidney or lung, it attaches to the basement membrane and gives the same linear fluorescent pattern when tested with fluorescein-labeled antibody to human γ-globulin **(indirect immunofluorescence).**

In pemphigus the direct immunofluorescent technic reveals antibody to an antigen present in the intercellular cement of the prickle cell layer; in pemphigoid, to an antigen in the basement membrane. In both diseases the antibody is detectable by the indirect immunofluorescence technic. The indirect immunofluorescence technic is used to detect tissue-specific circulating antibodies in many other disorders, e.g., thyroiditis (antithyroid antibodies) and SLE (antinuclear antibodies, anticytoplasmic antibodies).

TYPE III REACTIONS

(Immune Complex or Soluble Complex Hypersensitivity Reactions; Toxic Complex Reactions)

Reactions that result from deposition of soluble circulating antigen-antibody (immune) complexes in vessels or tissue. The antigen-antibody complexes activate complement and thereby initiate a sequence of events that results in polymorphonuclear cell migration and release of lysosomal proteolytic enzymes and permeability factors in tissues, thereby producing an acute inflammatory reaction. The consequences of immune complex formation depend in part on the relative proportions of antigen and antibody in the complex. With an excess of antibody, the complexes rapidly precipitate near the site of the antigen (e.g., within the joints in rheumatoid arthritis) or are phagocytosed by macrophages and are therefore not toxic. With a slight excess of antigen, the complex tends to be more soluble and may cause systemic reactions by being deposited in various tissues.

Examples of clinical conditions in which Type III reactions appear to play some role are serum sickness due to serum, drugs, or viral hepatitis antigen, SLE, RA, polyarteritis, cryoglobulinemia, hypersensitivity pneumonitis, bronchopulmonary aspergillosis, acute glomerulonephritis, chronic membranoproliferative glomerulonephritis, and associated renal disease (see Ch. 147). In bronchopulmonary aspergillosis, drug- or serum-induced serum sickness, and some forms of renal disease, a Type I reaction is thought to precede the Type III reaction.

The classic laboratory examples of Type III reactions are the Arthus reaction and experimental serum sickness.

In the **Arthus reaction,** animals are first hyperimmunized to induce large amounts of circulating IgG antibodies and are then given a small amount of antigen intradermally. The antigen precipitates with the excess IgG and activates complement, so that a highly inflammatory, edematous, painful local lesion rapidly appears, which may progress to a sterile abscess containing many polymorphonuclear cells, and then to gangrene. A necrotizing vasculitis with occluded arteriolar lumens can be seen microscopically. No lag period precedes the reaction because antibody is already present.

In **experimental serum sickness,** a large amount of antigen is injected into a nonimmunized animal. After a lag period, antibody is produced; when this reaches a critical level, antigen-antibody complexes form which are deposited in endothelial vessels (particularly in glomeruli), where they produce widespread vascular injury characterized by the presence of polymorphonuclear leukocytes. During the appearance of the vasculitis a fall in serum complement can be detected, and antigen, antibody, and complement can be found in the areas of vasculitis. The antigen-antibody complexes are not capable of inducing injury by themselves, however, but require the presence of a Type I reaction to enhance vascular deposition.

Diagnostic Tests

Type III reactions can be suspected in human disease when a vasculitis occurs that is similar to the conditions observed in experimentally induced Arthus reaction and serum sickness. In polyarteritis this is the only clinical evidence to support a presumed Type III reaction. Further support to document a Type III reaction may be obtained by direct immunofluorescence tests (as described above for Type II reactions), which may indicate the presence of antigen, immunoglobulin, and complement in the area of vasculitis.

In experimental studies, fluorescent microscopy shows a coarse granular deposit ("lumpy bumps") along the basement membrane when animal glomeruli are stained for the presence of immunoglobulin and complement. A similar distribution can be seen in Type III human renal diseases (see Ch. 147). The electron microscope can also be used to detect electron-dense deposits (similar to those seen in experimental serum sickness), which are felt to be the antigen-antibody complexes. Rarely, the presence of both antigen and antibody can be detected by immunofluorescence in the inflamed tissue—this has been demonstrated in the renal disease of SLE and the vasculitic lesions of hepatitis-antigen–associated serum sickness.

Further evidence in support of a Type III reaction is obtained by demonstrating the presence of circulating antibody to antigens such as horse serum, hepatitis antigen, DNA, RF, and mold spores. In SLE, for example, a rise in antibody to native undenatured, double-stranded DNA and a fall in serum complement occur during exacerbations of renal disease. If the antigen is unknown, levels of total serum complement and of the early components (C1, C4, or C2) can be tested; a depressed level indicates classic complement activation and therefore that a Type III reaction is occurring. The C4 assay is the one most readily available.

In allergic pulmonary aspergillosis an intradermal skin test with aspergillus antigen may produce a Type I wheal-and-flare reaction followed by a Type III (painful edematous) reaction.

Until recently, detection of immune complexes in the serum was by cryoprecipitation (using the property of some complexes to precipitate in the cold). Sophisticated equipment could also detect soluble complexes by analytic ultracentrifugation and sucrose density gradient centrifugation. Several tests detecting circulating immune complexes have now been developed that depend on the ability of complexes to react with complement components (such as C1q-binding assays) and the ability of complexes to inhibit the reaction between monoclonal RF and IgG. Assays such as the Raji cell assay are based on the interaction of immune complexes containing complement components with cellular receptors, e.g., a C3 receptor on the Raji cell. Other assays are available, but the 3 mentioned are the most commonly used.

TYPE IV REACTIONS

(Cellular, Cell-Mediated, Delayed, or Tuberculin-Type Hypersensitivity Reactions)

Reactions caused by sensitized lymphocytes (T cells) after contact with antigen, which result from direct cytotoxicity or from the release of lymphokines, or a combination of both. Delayed hypersensitivity differs from the other immune reactions in that it is mediated by sensitized lymphocytes and not by antibody. Thus, transfer of delayed hypersensitivity from sensitized to normal persons can be demonstrated with peripheral blood leukocytes or with an extract of these cells (transfer factor), but not with serum.

The T lymphocyte that has been sensitized (activated) by contact with antigen may cause immunologic injury by a direct toxic effect or through the release of soluble substances (lymphokines). In tissue culture, activated T lymphocytes have been demonstrated to destroy "target" cells to which they have been sensitized, when they are brought into direct contact with the target cells. The lymphokines released from activated T lymphocytes include several factors affecting the activity of macrophages, skin reactive factor, and a lymphotoxin.

Examples of clinical conditions in which Type IV reactions are felt to be important are contact dermatitis, allograft rejection, granulomas due to intracellular organisms, some forms of drug sensitivity, thyroiditis, and encephalomyelitis following rabies vaccination. The evidence for the last 2 is based on experimental models and, in human disease, on the appearance of lymphocytes in the inflammatory exudate of the thyroid and the brain.

Diagnostic Tests

A Type IV reaction can be suspected when an inflammatory reaction is characterized histologically by perivascular lymphocytes and macrophages. Delayed-hypersensitivity skin tests (see Tests of cell-mediated immunity in Ch. 17) and patch tests are the most readily available methods of testing for delayed hypersensitivity.

Patch tests are performed to identify allergens causing a contact dermatitis. The suspected material (in appropriate concentration) is applied to the skin under a nonabsorbent adhesive patch and left for 48 h. If burning or itching develops earlier, the patch is removed. A positive test consists of erythema with some induration and, occasionally, vesicle formation. Because some reactions do not appear until after the patches are removed, the sites are reinspected at 72 h. Patch testing is done after the patient's contact dermatitis has cleared in order to prevent its exacerbation.

Lymphocyte transformation and **thymidine incorporation** are in vitro tests that can be performed in a patient with a negative skin test, when the antigen is known, to determine whether the defect is an inability of the skin to react to lymphokines or an inability of T cells to produce lymphokines. The best correlate with delayed hypersensitivity, however, is the production of migration inhibitory factor. (For a discussion of these tests, see Ch. 17.)

19. DISORDERS DUE TO HYPERSENSITIVITY

ATOPIC DISEASES
(Allergic Disorders)

Disorders caused by Type I hypersensitivity, resulting from the release of vasoactive substances by mast cells and basophils that have been sensitized by the interaction of antigen primarily with IgE (reaginic or skin-sensitizing antibody). The terms **hypersensitivity** and **allergy** are often used synonymously to mean an exaggerated response to an antigen, leading to various types of tissue damage.

The most common human allergic disorders—hay fever (seasonal allergic rhinitis), asthma (particularly in children), infantile eczema, and some cases of urticaria and GI food reactions—are atopic diseases. Patients with atopic diseases have in common an inherited predisposition to develop hypersensitivity to substances (allergens) in the environment that are harmless to 80% of people. Features similar to atopy have been identified in several mammalian species.

Diagnostic Procedures

History: Review of the symptoms, their relation to the environment and to seasonal and situational variations, and their clinical course should yield sufficient information to classify the disease as atopic. The history and clinical course are more valuable than tests in determining whether a patient is allergic, and it is inappropriate to subject the patient to extensive skin testing unless reasonable clinical evidence exists for atopy. Age of onset may be an important clue (e.g., childhood asthma is much more likely to be atopic than asthma beginning after age 30). Also indicative are symptoms that are seasonal (e.g., correlating with specific pollen seasons), or appear after exposure to animals, hay, or dust, or develop in specific environments (e.g., at home, at work).

It is also helpful, for advising the patient, to investigate the effects of nonspecific contributory factors, such as tobacco smoke and other pollutants, cold air and cold beverages, certain drugs, and life stresses.

Tests: These are used to confirm sensitivity to an antigen when it is suspected that the patient is allergic. For details on direct and passive-transfer skin tests, the radioallergosorbent test (RAST), provocative challenge tests, and leukocyte histamine release, see TYPE I HYPERSENSITIVITY REACTIONS in Ch. 18.

Nonspecific findings: Eosinophilia is associated with some atopic conditions, particularly asthma and eczematous eruptions, but its absence does not rule out allergy. **IgE levels** are of diagnostic significance in eczema, since they are elevated and will rise during exacerbations and fall during remissions. IgE levels are also elevated in atopic asthma but are often normal in allergic rhinitis.

Treatment

Avoidance: Eliminating the allergen is the preferred treatment. This may require a change of diet, occupation, or residence; withdrawal of a drug; or removal of a household pet. Some locales, free of allergens such as ragweed, are havens for afflicted persons. When complete avoidance is impossible, as in the case of house dust, exposure may be reduced by removing dust-collecting furniture, carpets, and draperies, frequent wet-mopping and dusting, and installing a high-efficiency air-filtering system.

Symptomatic therapy: Relief of symptoms with drugs should not be neglected while the patient is being evaluated and specific control or treatment is being developed. The proper use of antihistamines, sympathomimetics, and corticosteroids is outlined for each disease category in the discussions that follow. In general, corticosteroids are appropriate for treatment of potentially disabling conditions that are self-limited and of relatively short duration (seasonal asthma due to pollens; serum sickness; infiltrative lung disease; severe contact dermatitis). In such cases there is little chance that long-term use, with its associated side effects, will be necessary.

Desensitization (hyposensitization, immunotherapy): When it is not feasible to avoid an allergen or to control it sufficiently to relieve symptoms of atopic disease, desensitization can be attempted by injecting an extract of the allergen subcutaneously in gradually increasing doses. Several specific effects can be demonstrated, although there is no test that correlates absolutely with clinical improvement. The titer of blocking (neutralizing) antibody increases proportionately to the dose administered. Sometimes, particularly when high doses of pollen extract can be tolerated, the serum IgE level falls significantly. In addition, peripheral blood basophil histamine release is reduced from pretreatment levels on incubation with antigen (or an increased amount of antigen is required to release 50% of the basophil histamine). This effect may not be specific—the reduced leukocyte hypersensitivity of some patients applies to antigens not used in desensitization and to anti-IgE antibody as well.

Clinical results are most satisfactory when injections are continued year-round. Depending on the degree of sensitivity, the first dose is 0.1 ml of a dilution ranging from 1:100,000 to 1:100,000,000. The dose is increased weekly or biweekly by 75% (or less) until a maximum tolerated concentration has been reached, e.g., 0.3 ml of a 1:50 dilution. For crude pollen extracts, this amounts to about 30 μg of protein nitrogen (3000 protein nitrogen u.). Once the maximum dose has been reached, it can be maintained at monthly intervals year-round. Even in seasonal allergies this **perennial method** is superior to preseasonal or co-seasonal treatment methods.

The major allergens used for desensitization are the inhalants that usually cannot be effectively avoided: pollens, house dust, and molds. Whole-body extracts of stinging insects were used for many years to treat patients who experienced generalized reactions, but should be replaced by venom, which is clearly more effective and is now available for desensitization. Animal dander desensitization should be used only for those who cannot avoid exposure, such as veterinarians or laboratory workers. There is no indication for food desensitization.

Adverse reactions to desensitization: Patients are often extremely sensitive, particularly to pollen allergens, and if an overdose is given, can experience constitutional reactions varying from a mild cough or sneezing to generalized urticaria, severe asthma, and anaphylactic shock. To prevent such reactions, one must (1) check that the proper dilution is used, (2) increase the dose by small increments, (3) repeat the same dose (or even decrease it) if the local reaction from the previous injection is large (2.5 cm in diameter or greater), and (4) reduce the dose when a new extract is used. Reducing the dose of pollen extract during the pollen season is often wise also. Intramuscular and intravascular injection must be *avoided*.

Despite the best precautions, reactions occur occasionally. Since the severe, life-threatening ones develop within 20 min, patients must remain under observation for that time. The first signs of an impending reaction may be sneezing, coughing, and chest tightness, or a generalized flush, tingling sensations, and pruritus. A tourniquet should be applied above the injection site at once, and the site infiltrated with 0.2 ml of epinephrine 1:1000. (The tourniquet should be released in 15 min.) If the reaction is mild, a double dose of an antihistamine can then be given orally (e.g., diphenhydramine 100 mg or chlorpheniramine 8 mg) and 0.3 ml of epinephrine 1:1000 can be given s.c. in the opposite arm. However, if symptoms and signs of shock have developed, IV fluids should be started and epinephrine 1:10,000, 1 to 2.5 ml IV, should be given over about 10 min, and other measures instituted for treatment of anaphylaxis (see below). Corticosteroid therapy will not help during the acute reaction, but may be helpful in preventing the late 4- to 6-h asthmatic or urticarial reaction that may develop after the patient has recovered from the first reaction and gone home.

Occasionally, a generalized reaction such as urticaria may appear 30 min to several hours after an allergen injection. This can be treated with an antihistamine alone. Following any generalized reaction, the next dose of allergen should be reduced by ⅓ or ¼, and later increments kept as small as is practicable (usually 0.03 to 0.05 ml).

ALLERGIC RHINITIS

A symptom complex including hay fever and perennial allergic rhinitis, characterized by seasonal or perennial sneezing, rhinorrhea, nasal congestion, pruritus, and often conjunctivitis and pharyngitis.

HAY FEVER (Pollinosis)

Hay fever, the acute seasonal form of allergic rhinitis, is generally induced by wind-borne pollens. The **spring** type is due to tree pollens (e.g., oak, elm, maple, alder, birch, cottonwood); the **summer** type, to grass pollens (e.g., Bermuda, timothy, sweet vernal, orchard, Johnson) and to weed pollens (e.g., sheep sorrel, English plantain); the **fall** type, to weed pollens (e.g., ragweed). Occasionally, hay fever is due primarily to airborne fungus spores. Important geographic regional differences occur.

Symptoms and Signs

The nose, roof of the mouth, pharynx, and eyes begin to itch gradually or abruptly after onset of the pollen season. Lacrimation, sneezing, and clear, watery nasal discharge accompany or soon follow the pruritus. Frontal headaches, irritability, anorexia, depression, and insomnia may appear. The conjunctiva is injected, and the nasal mucous membranes are swollen and bluish red. Coughing and asthmatic wheezing may develop as the season progresses. Many eosinophils are present in the nasal mucus during the season.

Diagnosis

The nature of the allergic process and even the responsible allergen is often suspected from the history. Diagnosis is confirmed by the above physical findings, skin tests, and the accompanying eosinophilia in blood or secretions.

Treatment

Symptoms may be diminished by avoidance of the allergen (see above). Most patients obtain adequate relief with oral antihistamines (e.g., chlorpheniramine, in sustained-release form, 12 mg q 8 h; triprolidine 2.5 mg q 8 h). If these drugs are too sedating, a different drug should be used (e.g., slow-release brompheniramine 12 mg orally q 8 h). Sympathomimetics are often used in combination with antihistamines. Phenylpropanolamine, phenylephrine, or pseudoephedrine are available in many antihistamine-decongestant preparations. Ephedrine 25 mg orally q 4 h is more effective, but its central-stimulating effects limit its use.

When nasal symptoms are not relieved adequately by antihistaminic treatment, intranasal dexamethasone spray is usually effective. Two metered doses t.i.d. are used initially; each dose is freon-propelled from a container that delivers dexamethasone 0.084 mg/dose. When symptoms have been relieved, dosage is reduced to 1 dose b.i.d. for the remainder of the season. Severe intractable extranasal symptoms may require a short course of systemic corticosteroid treatment (prednisone 10 mg orally b.i.d., with gradual reduction in dose; an alternate-day regimen may also be used).

Cromolyn sodium may help prevent the progression of pollen-induced symptoms if treatment is begun early in the season. It has been available as a 2% solution in England for several years. A 4% solution is undergoing investigational trials now in the USA.

Desensitization treatment (see above) is advised if drug treatment is poorly tolerated, if corticosteroids are needed during the season, or if asthma develops. Treatment should begin soon after the pollen season has ended.

PERENNIAL ALLERGIC RHINITIS

In contrast to hay fever, symptoms of perennial rhinitis vary in severity (often unpredictably) throughout the year. Extranasal symptoms such as conjunctivitis are uncommon, but chronic nasal obstruction is often prominent and may extend to eustachian tube obstruction. The resultant hearing difficulty is particularly common in children. The **diagnosis** of allergic rhinitis is supported by a positive history of atopic disease, the characteristic bluish-red mucosa, numerous eosinophils in the nasal secretions, and positive skin tests (particularly to house dust, feathers, animal danders, or fungi, and occasionally to foods). Some patients have complicating sinus infections and nasal polyps.

Certain patients suffer from chronic rhinitis, sinusitis, and polyps and often have negative skin tests. These patients are not allergic but often have aspirin and indomethacin sensitivity and should be evaluated also for sensitivity to sodium benzoate (a food preservative) and tartrazine (a yellow food coloring) by a trial elimination of these food additives from the diet. Despite the negative skin tests, these patients have numerous eosinophils in their tissues and nasal secretions. A subset suffers only from chronic rhinitis. Some patients with mild but annoying chronic continuous nasal obstruction or rhinorrhea have no demonstrable allergy, polyps, infection, or drug sensitivity, a condition identified as **vasomotor rhinitis** (see Ch. 168).

Treatment

Management is similar to that for hay fever if specific allergens are identified, except that systemic corticosteroids, even though effective, should be avoided because of the need for prolonged use. Surgery (antrotomy and irrigation of sinuses, polypectomy, submucous resection) may be necessary after allergic factors have been controlled or ruled out. The subset of patients with chronic nonspecific rhinitis and eosinophilia mentioned above may respond very well to topical dexamethasone. For many patients the only treatment is reassurance, antihistamine and vasoconstrictor drugs, and advice to avoid topical decongestants, which produce after-congestion and, when used continuously, may aggravate or perpetuate chronic rhinitis **(rhinitis medicamentosa).**

ALLERGIC PULMONARY DISEASE

The lungs can be involved in known or suspected allergic reactions in several ways, depending on the nature of the allergen and its route of entry. Specific disorders are discussed in Ch. 41 and under BRONCHIAL ASTHMA in Ch. 34.

ANAPHYLAXIS

Generalized anaphylaxis is an acute, often explosive, systemic reaction characterized by urticaria, respiratory distress, and vascular collapse and occasionally by vomiting and abdominal cramps. It occurs in a previously sensitized person when he again receives the sensitizing antigen. This Type I reaction occurs when antigen reaches the circulation. Histamine, slow-reactive substance (SRS-A), and other mediators released when the antigen reacts with IgE on basophils and mast cells cause the smooth muscle contraction and vascular dilatation that characterize anaphylaxis. The most common causative antigens are foreign serum and other proteins, certain drugs, desensitizing injections, and insect stings. **Anaphylactoid reactions** are clinically similar to anaphylaxis, but occur after the *first* injection of certain drugs (histamine, polymyxin, pentamidine, morphine, contrast media), and have a dose-related, toxic-idiosyncratic mechanism rather than an immunologically mediated one.

Pathogenesis

The wheezing and GI symptoms are caused by smooth muscle contraction. Vasodilatation and escape of plasma into the tissues causes the urticaria and results in a decrease in effective plasma volume, which is the major cause of shock. Fluid escapes into the lung alveoli and may produce pulmonary edema. Obstructive angioedema of the upper airway may also occur. Rarely, myocarditis develops if the reaction is prolonged.

Symptoms and Signs

Typically, in 1 to 15 min, the patient complains of a sense of uneasiness and becomes agitated and flushed. Palpitation, paresthesias, pruritus, throbbing in the ears, coughing, sneezing, and difficulty in breathing are other typical complaints. Primary cardiovascular collapse can occur in the absence of respiratory symptoms. Nausea and vomiting are less common. The symptoms and signs of shock may develop within another 1 or 2 min, and the patient may become incontinent, convulse, become unresponsive, and die.

Prophylaxis

Patients with the greatest risk of anaphylactic reactions to a drug are those who have reacted previously to that drug. Yet anaphylactic deaths still occur in patients who do not give such a history. The risk of a reaction to horse serum is sufficiently high that routine skin testing before giving the serum is *mandatory* (see under SERUM SICKNESS, below). Routine skin testing before other drug treatment is neither practicable nor reliable, except for penicillin. Tests for penicillin hypersensitivity are discussed under DRUG HYPERSENSITIVITY, Mechanisms, below.

Prophylaxis for the patient who needs antiserum (e.g., for botulism, diphtheria, or snake and black widow spider bites) is described below under SERUM SICKNESS.

Long-term desensitization is effective and appropriate for prevention of insect-sting anaphylaxis but has rarely been attempted in patients with a history of drug or serum anaphylaxis. Instead, if treatment with a drug or serum is essential, rapid desensitization must be carried out under carefully controlled conditions (see DRUG HYPERSENSITIVITY, below; BACTERIAL ENDOCARDITIS in Ch. 25; and SERUM SICKNESS, below).

Treatment

Immediate treatment with epinephrine is imperative. It is a pharmacologic antagonist to the effects of the chemical mediators on smooth muscle, blood vessels, and other tissues.

For mild reactions such as generalized pruritus, urticaria, angioedema, mild wheezing, nausea, and vomiting, 0.3 to 0.5 ml of aqueous epinephrine 1:1000 should be given s.c. If an injected antigen has caused the anaphylaxis, a tourniquet should be applied above the injection site and 0.1 to 0.2 ml of epinephrine 1:1000 also injected into the site, in order to reduce systemic absorption of the antigen. This may suffice for a mild reaction, although a second injection of epinephrine s.c. may be required. Once symptoms have resolved, an oral antihistamine should be given for 24 h.

For more severe reactions, with massive angioedema but without evidence of cardiovascular involvement, patients should be given diphenhydramine 50 to 100 mg IV (for an adult) in addition to the above treatment, to forestall laryngeal edema and to block the effect of further histamine release. When the edema is responding, 0.3 ml of an aqueous suspension of long-acting epinephrine 1:200 s.c. can be given for its 6- to 8-h effect, and an oral antihistamine should be given for the next 24 h, and possibly a corticosteroid to suppress the late phase of a dual reaction.

For severe respiratory reactions that do not respond to epinephrine, IV fluids should be started and aminophylline 6 mg/kg IV should be given over 10 to 20 min, followed by 0.5 mg/kg/h, more or less, to maintain a theophylline blood level of 10 to 20 μg/ml. Endotracheal intubation or tracheostomy may be necessary, with O_2 administration at 4 to 6 L/min.

The most severe reactions usually involve the cardiovascular system, causing severe hypotension and vasomotor collapse. IV fluids should be started and the patient should be recumbent with legs elevated. Epinephrine (1:1000) 0.25 to 0.5 ml added to 10 ml saline can be given slowly IV, repeating the dose in 5 to 10 min if necessary. Side effects include headache, tremulousness, nausea, and arrhythmias. The underlying severe hypotension may be due to vasodilation, hypovolemia from loss of fluid, myocardial insufficiency (rarely), or a combination of these. Each has a specific treatment and often the treatment of one exacerbates the others. The appropriate therapy may be clarified if central venous pressure (CVP) and left atrial pressure can be obtained (see also in Ch. 23). A low CVP and normal left atrial pressure indicate peripheral vasodilation and/or hypovolemia. Vasodilation should respond to the epinephrine (which will also retard the loss of intravascular fluid).

In most cases, hypovolemia is the major cause of the hypotension. The CVP and left atrial pressure are both low, and large volumes of saline must be given, with monitoring of the BP, until the CVP rises to normal. Colloid plasma expanders such as dextran are rarely necessary. Only if fluid replacement does not restore normal BP should one initiate treatment cautiously with adrenergic drugs such as metaraminol.

In the rare instance of myocardial insufficiency, both CVP and left atrial pressure will be elevated. Isoproterenol 1 mg is diluted in 500 ml of 5% dextrose and infused at a rate of 0.5 to 1 ml/min. The patient should be monitored carefully, for the isoproterenol may cause cardiac arrhythmias and hypotension due to peripheral vasodilation.

Cardiac arrest may occur, requiring immediate resuscitation (see CARDIAC ARREST AND CARDIOPULMONARY RESUSCITATION in Ch. 25). Further therapy depends on ECG findings.

When all the above measures have been instituted, diphenhydramine (50 to 75 mg IV slowly over 3 min) and corticosteroids may then be given for treatment of slow-onset urticaria, asthma, laryngeal edema, or hypotension. Hydrocortisone sodium succinate 100 mg (or equivalent) should be given q 1 to 2 h IV until symptoms are controlled, then q 2 to 4 h for 24 h IV, and then discontinued. Complications such as myocardial infarction and cerebral edema should be looked for and treated specifically.

Patients with severe reactions should remain in a hospital under observation for 24 h following recovery to ensure adequate treatment in case of relapse.

Any person who has had an anaphylactic reaction to a stinging insect should be provided with a kit containing a pre-filled syringe of epinephrine and an epinephrine nebulizer to allow prompt self-treatment of any future reaction. Such an individual should also be evaluated for venom immunotherapy (desensitization).

URTICARIA; ANGIOEDEMA

(Hives; Giant Urticaria; Angioneurotic Edema)

Urticaria: Local wheals and erythema in the dermis. Angioedema: A similar eruption, but with larger edematous areas that involve subcutaneous structures as well as the dermis.

Etiology

Acute urticaria and angioedema are essentially anaphylaxis limited to the skin and subcutaneous tissues and can be due to drug allergy, insect stings or bites, desensitization injections, or ingestion of certain foods (particularly eggs, shellfish, nuts, or fruits). Some food reactions occur explosively following ingestion of only minute amounts. Others (such as reactions to strawberries) may occur only after overindulgence, and possibly result from direct (toxic) histamine liberation. Urticaria may accompany or even be the first symptom of several viral infections, including hepatitis, infectious mononucleosis, and rubella. Some acute reactions are unexplained, even when recurrent. If acute angioedema is recurrent, progressive, and never associated with urticaria, a hereditary enzyme deficiency should be suspected (see HEREDITARY ANGIOEDEMA, below).

Chronic urticaria and angioedema lasting more than 3 wk are more difficult to explain, and only in exceptional cases can a specific cause be found. They occur equally in nonatopic and atopic subjects. Occasionally, unsuspected chronic drug or chemical ingestion is responsible, e.g., from penicillin in milk, from the use of nonprescription drugs, or from preservatives, dyes, or other food additives. Chronic underlying disease (SLE, polycythemia vera, lymphoma, or chronic sinus or dental infection) should be ruled out. Though suspected frequently, controllable psychogenic factors are not often identified. Urticaria caused by physical agents is discussed in PHYSICAL ALLERGY, below.

Symptoms and Signs

In **urticaria**, pruritus (generally the first symptom) is followed shortly by the appearance of wheals that may remain small (1 to 5 mm) or may enlarge. The larger ones tend to clear in the center, and may be noticed first as large (more than 20 cm across) rings of erythema and edema. Ordinarily, crops of hives come and go, a lesion remaining in one site for several hours, then disappearing, only to reappear elsewhere. **Angioedema** is a more diffuse swelling of loose subcutaneous tissue: dorsum of hands or feet, eyelids, lips, genitalia, mucous membranes. Edema of the upper airway may produce respiratory distress, and the stridor may be mistaken for asthma.

Diagnosis

The cause of acute urticaria is usually obvious. Even when it is not, a diagnostic workup is seldom required because of the self-limited, nonrecurrent nature of these reactions. In chronic urticaria, an underlying chronic disease should be ruled out by obtaining a CBC, ESR, urinalysis, and a dental and sinus examination. Eosinophilia is uncommon in urticaria. Other tests such as stool examination for ova and parasites, serum complement, and antinuclear antibody are not worthwhile unless there are clinical indications other than urticaria.

Treatment

Acute urticaria is a self-limited condition that generally subsides in 1 to 7 days; hence, treatment is chiefly palliative. If the cause is not obvious, all nonessential medication should be stopped until the reaction has subsided. Symptoms can usually be relieved with an oral antihistamine (e.g., diphenhydramine 50 to 100 mg q 4 h or cyproheptadine 4 to 8 mg q 4 h). Corticosteroids (e.g., prednisone 30 to 40 mg/day orally) may be necessary for the more severe reactions, particularly when associated with angioedema. Topical corticosteroids are of no value. Epinephrine 1:1000, 0.3 ml s.c., should be the first treatment for **acute pharyngeal or laryngeal angioedema**. This may be supplemented with topical treatment, e.g., nebulized epinephrine 1:100, and an intravenous antihistamine (e.g., diphenhydramine 50 to 100 mg). This usually prevents airway obstruction, but one must be prepared to perform a tracheostomy and give O_2.

Although the specific cause of **chronic urticaria** can seldom be identified and removed, spontaneous remissions occur within 2 yr in about half the cases. Control of stressful life situations often helps, and may even effect a permanent remission. Certain drugs (e.g., aspirin) may aggravate symptoms, as will alcoholic beverages, coffee, and tobacco smoking; if so, they should be avoided. When urticaria is produced by aspirin, sensitivity to related compounds (e.g., indomethacin) and to the food- and drug-coloring additive tartrazine should be investigated (see also PERENNIAL ALLERGIC RHINITIS, above). Oral antihistamines with a sedative effect are beneficial in most cases (e.g., cyproheptadine 4 to 8 mg q 4 h or hydroxyzine 25 to 50 mg t.i.d.). All reasonable measures should be used before resorting to corticosteroids, which are frequently effective but, once started, may have to be continued indefinitely. A few patients with intractable urticaria are hyperthyroid.

HEREDITARY ANGIOEDEMA

A form of angioedema transmitted as an autosomal dominant trait and associated with a deficiency of serum inhibitor of the activated first component of complement. In 85% of cases, the deficiency is due to a lack of the C1 esterase inhibitor **(C1 Inh)**; in 15%, to C1 Inh malfunction. A positive family history is the rule, but there are exceptions. The edema is characteristically unifocal, indurated, painful rather than pruritic, and not accompanied by urticaria. Attacks are often precipitated by trauma or viral illness, and are aggravated by emotional stress. The GI tract is often involved, with nausea, vomiting, colic, and even signs of intestinal obstruction. The condition may cause fatal upper airway obstruction. **Diagnosis** may be made by measuring C4, which is low, even between attacks, or more specifically by demonstrating deficiency of C1 Inh by immunodiffusion or bioassay technics.

Treatment

The usual symptomatic treatment used in angioedema is unsuccessful; the edema progresses until complement components have been consumed. Acute attacks that threaten to produce airway obstruction should therefore be treated promptly by establishing an airway. Epinephrine and an antihistamine should be given, as in other forms of angioedema (see above); but there is no proof that these drugs are effective.

For short-term prophylaxis, as before a dental procedure or surgery, ε-aminocaproic acid (an inhibitor of fibrinolysis) 10 to 15 mg should be given. Fresh frozen plasma is also used for the same purpose. Although there is a theoretic concern that a complement substrate in the plasma might provoke an attack, in practice this has not been observed. Recently, a partially purified C1 Inh fraction of pooled plasma has been shown to be safe and effective for prophylaxis.

For long-term prophylaxis, ε-aminocaproic acid 10 mg/day is effective in reducing the number and severity of attacks; but it is still an experimental drug because of side effects. Androgens are also effective. Of these, danazol 200 mg orally t.i.d., oxymethalone 5 mg/day, and methyltestosterone 10 mg/day (buccal tablets) are not only effective but also have been shown to raise the low C1 Inh and C4 toward normal. The first 2 are impeded androgens; i.e., masculinizing effects are low. They still occur, however, and in women particularly, the dose should be reduced to the smallest that is effective.

PHYSICAL ALLERGY

A condition in which allergic symptoms and signs are produced by exposure to cold, sunlight, heat, or mild trauma.

Etiology

The underlying cause is unknown in most cases. Photosensitivity (see Ch. 214 and CONTACT DERMATITIS in Ch. 189) may sometimes be induced by drugs or topical agents, including certain cosmetics. Cold and light sensitivity, in many but not all cases, can be passively transferred with serum that contains a specific IgE antibody, suggesting an immunologic mechanism involving a physically altered skin protein as antigen. The serum of a few patients with cold-induced symptoms contains cryoglobulins or cryofibrinogen; these abnormal proteins may be associated with a serious underlying disorder such as a malignancy, a collagen vascular disease, or chronic infection. Cold may aggravate asthma or vasomotor rhinitis, but cold urticaria is independent of any other known allergic tendencies. Heat sensitivity usually produces cholinergic urticaria, which is also induced in the same patients by exercise, emotional stress, or any stimulus that causes sweating. **Dermatographia (dermographism),** a wheal-and-flare reaction seen after scratching or firmly stroking the skin, is usually idiopathic but occasionally is the first sign of an urticarial drug reaction. The sensitivity of about half the cases studied can be passively transferred by serum and appears to be IgE-mediated. Urticaria has also occurred following a persistent, vibratory stimulus (familial), and even after water exposure ("aquagenic").

Clinical Features

Pruritus and unsightly appearance are the most common complaints. Cold sensitivity is usually manifested by urticaria and angioedema, which develop most typically after exposure to cold is terminated and during or after swimming or bathing. Bronchospasm and even histamine-mediated shock may occur in extreme cases and result in drowning. Sunlight may produce urticaria or a more chronic polymorphous skin eruption.

The skin lesions in cholinergic urticaria are small, highly pruritic, discrete wheals surrounded by a large zone of erythema. Cholinergic urticaria appears to be caused by an unusual sensitivity to acetylcholine, and administration of acetylcholine or methacholine may reproduce the lesions, but in only about 1/3 of cases. The most reliable test is exercise, with occlusive garments to promote sweating.

Prophylaxis and Treatment

The use of drugs or cosmetics should be reviewed with the patient, particularly if photosensitivity is suspected. Protection from the physical stimulus is necessary, but most patients want more help than this when seeking medical attention. Management of photosensitivity is discussed in Ch. 214 and under CONTACT DERMATITIS in Ch. 189.

For relief of itching, an antihistamine with sedative effects should be given orally (diphenhydramine 50 mg q.i.d.; cyproheptadine 4 to 8 mg q.i.d.). Cyproheptadine has been noted to be the most effective in cold urticaria. Hydroxyzine 25 to 50 mg orally q.i.d. is the preferred drug for cholinergic urticaria; anticholinergic drugs are ineffective at tolerable doses. Prednisone 30 to 40 mg/day orally should be given in severe light eruptions other than urticaria to shorten the clinical course; the dose is gradually reduced as treatment becomes effective.

ALLERGIC CONJUNCTIVITIS

(See also VERNAL [ALLERGIC] CONJUNCTIVITIS in Ch. 178)

Atopic conjunctivitis of an acute or chronic catarrhal form is usually part of a larger allergic syndrome such as hay fever, but may occur alone through direct contact with airborne substances such as pollen, fungus spores, various dusts, or animal danders.

Symptoms, Signs, and Diagnosis

Itching is prominent and may be accompanied by excessive lacrimation. The conjunctiva is edematous and hyperemic. The cause is often suggested by the history and may be confirmed by skin testing. If *atopic* conjunctivitis is suspected but skin tests are equivocal, an ophthalmic challenge (see TYPE I HYPERSENSITIVITY REACTIONS in Ch. 18) occasionally will be positive. Since so few antigens can be tested in a reasonable period, ophthalmic challenge has limited application. *It should not be used for diagnosis of contact hypersensitivity.*

Treatment

An identified or suspected causative allergen should be avoided. Frequent use of a bland eyewash (e.g., buffered 0.65% saline) may reduce the irritation. Contact lenses should not be worn. In atopic conjunctivitis, antihistamines given orally usually are helpful. A topical antiseptic is available (0.5% antazoline phosphate), but only in combination with the vasoconstrictor naphazoline 0.05 to 0.1% as an ophthalmic solution. The frequency of contact dermatitis is less than with topical dermatologic antihistamines. However, most patients respond as well if not better to an oral antihistamine plus a topical vasoconstrictor than to the topical combination, so it is not necessary to assume the very small risk of sensitization. One should be aware, though, that the preservative in any topical solution may also sensitize the patient. In severe cases, and in most cases of contact hypersensitivity, more effective relief is provided by a corticosteroid ophthalmic ointment (e.g., hydrocortisone 2.5% or dexamethasone 0.05% applied t.i.d. or q.i.d). *Intraocular pressure should be checked before and regularly during such treatment, and treatment should be terminated as soon as possible.* Cromolyn sodium may be helpful (see HAY FEVER, above). Indications for desensitization are similar to those for hay fever; patients with contact hypersensitivity cannot be desensitized.

OTHER ALLERGIC EYE DISEASES

The **lids** may be involved by angioedema or urticaria, contact dermatitis, or atopic dermatitis. Contact dermatitis of the eyelids, a Type IV hypersensitivity reaction, may be caused by various ophthalmic medications or drugs conveyed by the fingers to the eyes (e.g., antibiotics by drug handlers) or by face powder, nail polish, or hair dye. The **cornea** may become involved by extension of allergic conjunctivitis or by a variant of superficial punctate keratitis, leading rarely to scarring.

Pain, photophobia, and circumcorneal inflammation indicate probable **uveitis.** In most cases the cause is unknown; it may, rarely, be due to a specific environmental allergen, and bacterial hypersensitivity of the cell-mediated type (Type IV hypersensitivity) may be suspected. **Sympathetic ophthalmia** (see in Ch. 181) is felt to be a hypersensitivity reaction to uveal pigment. **Endophthalmitis phacoanaphylactica** is caused by allergy to native lens protein. The reaction, which is severe, occurs typically in the remaining lens after one lens has been removed uneventfully, though it may follow trauma or inflammation involving the lens capsule. Prompt treatment by an ophthalmologist is required in these serious ophthalmic conditions.

GASTROINTESTINAL ALLERGY

An uncommon symptom complex due to ingestion of specific food or drug allergens, manifested by nausea, vomiting, crampy abdominal pain, and diarrhea. GI symptoms from food or drugs more often represent nonspecific intolerance or are secondary to digestive enzyme defects (as in celiac disease and disaccharidase deficiency); hypersensitivity to food allergens is more commonly manifested as urticaria or angioedema.

Symptoms and Signs

The severe (but rare) acute reaction to food is characterized by nausea, vomiting, diarrhea, and violent abdominal pains associated with the other symptoms of anaphylaxis (see above). Less severe reactions—chronic crampy pain, diarrhea, and, often, urticaria—are more common. Most people prone to severe reactions can detect traces of the offending food in their mouths by the rapid onset of mucosal burning or itching.

Occasionally, cheilitis, aphthae, pylorospasm, spastic constipation, irritable colon, pruritus ani, and perianal eczema have been attributed to food allergy, but the association is difficult to prove. **Eosinophilic enteropathy,** which may be related to specific food allergy, is an unusual illness with pain, cramps, and diarrhea that is associated with blood eosinophilia, eosinophilic infiltrates in the gut, protein-losing enteropathy, and other signs of atopic disease. Rarely, dysphagia occurs, indicating esophageal involvement.

Diagnosis

Severe food allergy is usually obvious to the patient. When it is not, diagnosis is difficult and the condition must be differentiated from functional GI problems. Skin tests are of limited value except in young children, in whom low sensitivity tests (e.g., prick tests) correlate well with oral challenge tests. A detailed history, physical examination, and elimination diets assist in establishing a diagnosis. The regular occurrence of symptoms after ingestion of a particular food (see discussion of provocative food testing in Ch. 18, TYPE I HYPERSENSITIVITY REACTIONS) is usually the only practical diagnostic clue, but the association is not specific for allergy.

Treatment

Except for elimination of the offending foods, there is no specific treatment. Elimination diets can be used both for diagnosis and treatment (see Ch. 18, TYPE I HYPERSENSITIVITY REACTIONS) but are often misleading. When only a few foods are involved, abstinence is preferred. Sensitivity to one or more foods may disappear spontaneously. Oral desensitization (by first eliminating the offending food for a time and then giving small, daily increased amounts) has not been proved effective. Heating certain foods (e.g., milk) may reduce their antigenicity by protein denaturation. Antihistamines are of little value except in acute general reactions with urticaria and angioedema. Oral cromolyn sodium has been used with apparent success in other countries, but the oral form has not been approved for use in the USA. Prolonged corticosteroid treatment is not indicated except in eosinophilic enteropathy.

For treatment of the severe, potentially fatal acute attack, see URTICARIA; ANGIOEDEMA, and ANAPHYLAXIS, above.

DRUG HYPERSENSITIVITY

Drug eruptions are discussed in Ch. 196. Discussed here are other hypersensitivity reactions that can follow oral or parenteral drug administration. Contact dermatitis, which is a Type IV hypersensitivity reaction that follows topical use, is discussed in Ch. 189; and drug reactions that result from other than immunologic mechanisms are also discussed in Ch. 242.

Before attributing a given reaction to a drug, one should appreciate that placebos also may cause unwanted effects. Nausea, tachycardia, excessive sweating, epigastric disturbance with diarrhea, dry mouth, headache, easy fatigue, somnolence, and even skin rashes have been reported by persons taking inert substances in double-blind studies. Nevertheless, true reactions due to drugs are important and constitute a major medical problem. The literature on specific drugs should be consulted for the most likely adverse reactions.

With **overdosage of a drug,** toxic effects occur in direct relation to the total amount of drug in the body, and can occur in any patient if the dose is large enough. *Absolute* overdosage results from an error in the amount or frequency of administration of individual doses. *Relative* overdosage may be seen in patients who, because of liver or kidney disease, do not metabolize or excrete the drug normally.

In **drug idiosyncrasy,** the adverse reaction develops on the first use of the drug. It may be the same toxic reaction ordinarily expected at higher doses (also called *intolerance*) or it may be an exaggeration of a common mild side effect, such as antihistaminic sedation, or it may be unique. Reactions due to genetically determined enzyme deficiencies are being identified in steadily increasing numbers. Hemolytic anemia, for example, develops in patients with G6PD deficiency during treatment with any of several drugs. Succinylcholine apnea and isoniazid (INH) peripheral neuropathy are other examples from the field of pharmacogenetics.

Most toxic and idiosyncratic reactions (e.g., hyperergic reactions from anesthetic agents) differ sufficiently from allergic reactions to cause no confusion. There are a few exceptions. Toxic or idiosyncratic reactions from drugs with a direct histamine-releasing action (e.g., radiographic contrast media, opiates, pentamidine, polymyxin) may present as urticaria or even as anaphylactoid reactions. Hemolytic anemia may be allergic (e.g., penicillin, stibophen) or due to enzyme deficiency. Drug fever may be allergic, toxic (e.g., amphetamine, tranylcypromine), or even pharmacologic (e.g., etiocholanolone).

Allergic reactions have the following characteristics: (1) The reaction occurs only after the patient has been exposed to the drug (not necessarily for therapy) one or more times without incident. (2) Once hypersensitivity has developed, the reaction can be produced by doses that are far below therapeutic amounts, and usually below those levels that give idiosyncratic reactions. (3) The clinical features are restricted in their manifestations. Skin rashes (particularly urticaria), serum sickness, unexpected fever, anaphylaxis, and eosinophilic pulmonary infiltrates appearing during drug therapy are almost always due to hypersensitivity; some cases of anemia, thrombocytopenia, or agranulocytosis may be. Rarely, vasculitis develops after repeated exposure to a drug (e.g., sulfonamides, iodides, penicillin), and nephropathy (e.g., penicillin) and liver damage (e.g., halothane) have been reported in circumstances consistent with development of specific hypersensitivity.

Mechanisms of Drug Hypersensitivity

Protein and large polypeptide drugs can stimulate specific antibody production by straightforward immunologic mechanisms. Perhaps the smallest molecule that is potentially antigenic is **glucagon**, with a mol wt of about 3500. Most drug molecules are much smaller than this. By themselves the drugs cannot act as antigens, but as **haptens** some can bind covalently to proteins, and the resulting conjugates will stimulate antibody production specific for each chemical. It is likely that most drug hypersensitivity requires the prior formation of hapten-protein conjugates. The drug, or one of its metabolites, must be chemically reactive with protein, and must form a stable covalent bond. The usual serum-protein binding common to many drugs is much weaker and is of insufficient strength for antigenicity.

The specific immunologic reaction has been determined only for benzylpenicillin. This drug does not bind firmly enough with tissue or serum proteins to form an antigenic complex, but its major degradation product, benzylpenicillenic acid, can combine with tissue proteins to form benzylpenicilloyl **(BPO)**, the **major antigenic determinant** of penicillin. Several **minor antigenic determinants** are formed in relatively small amounts, by mechanisms that are not as well defined. IgE antibodies to the BPO determinant cause the urticaria that follows penicillin administration, while IgE antibodies to minor determinants are usually responsible for anaphylaxis as well as urticaria. In addition, IgG antibodies have been demonstrated to the major but not to the minor determinants. It is felt that these act as "blocking antibodies" to BPO, modifying or even preventing a reaction to BPO, while the lack of blocking IgG antibodies to the *minor* determinants seems to explain the ability of these determinants to induce anaphylaxis.

A BPO-polylysine conjugate (benzylpenicilloyl-polylysine), is commercially available for **skin testing**. Since the minor determinants are not available, penicillin G in dilutions of 1000 u./ml and 10,000 u./ml may be used. Skin testing is first performed by the scratch technic with the more dilute, then with the more concentrated, dilution. Negative scratch tests may be followed by intradermal testing. If skin tests are positive, the patient risks an anaphylactic reaction if treated with penicillin. Negative skin tests minimize but do not exclude the risk of a serious reaction. Moreover, skin tests with penicillin are themselves sensitizing (they stimulate IgE production), so that in most instances a patient should be tested to rule out penicillin allergy only immediately before essential penicillin therapy is begun. Since they detect only Type I (IgE-mediated) reactions, skin tests will not predict the occurrence of morbilliform eruptions or hemolytic anemia.

The semisynthetic penicillins (e.g., ampicillin, carbenicillin, amoxicillin) all cross-react with penicillin, so that penicillin-sensitive patients often (though not always) react to them as well. Cross-reactions also occur with the cephalosporins, but to a lesser degree. Treatment with a cephalosporin should be started with great *caution* if the patient gives a history of a severe reaction, such as anaphylaxis, to penicillin.

Hematologic Type II drug reactions may develop by any of 3 mechanisms, examples of which are as follows: (1) In penicillin-induced anemia, the antibody reacts with the hapten, which is firmly bound to the RBC membrane, producing agglutination and increased destruction of RBCs. (2) In stibophen- and quinidine-induced thrombocytopenia, the drug forms a soluble complex with its specific antibody. The complex then reacts with nearby platelets (the "innocent bystander" target cells) and activates complement, which alone remains on the platelet membrane and induces cell lysis. (3) In other hemolytic anemias, the drug (e.g., methyldopa) appears to alter the RBC surface chemically, thereby uncovering an antigen that induces and then reacts with an autoantibody, usually of Rh specificity. These disorders are discussed in detail in §9, HEMATOLOGIC DISORDERS.

Diagnosis

Toxic-idiosyncratic and **anaphylactic reactions** are sufficiently unique in kind or in time that the offending drug is usually easily identified. **Serum-sickness–type reactions** are most often due to the penicillins or cephalosporins, but occasionally sulfonamides, phenylbutazone, sulfonylureas, or thiazides are responsible. **Photosensitization** is characteristic of sulfonamides, psoralens, tetracyclines, and griseofulvin. All drugs except those deemed absolutely essential should be stopped. When **drug fever** is suspected, the most likely drug is stopped (e.g., penicillin, isoniazid, sulfonamides, barbiturates, quinidine). Reduction in fever within 48 h implicates that drug. If fever is accompanied by granulocytopenia, drug toxicity rather than allergy is a positive cause and is a much more serious matter (see GRANULOCYTOPENIA in Ch. 96).

Allergic pulmonary reactions to drugs are usually infiltrative, with eosinophilia, and can be produced by gold salts, penicillin, and sulfonamides, among others. The most common cause of an acute pulmonary reaction is nitrofurantoin. This is probably allergic but usually not eosinophilic.

Hepatic reactions may be primarily cholestatic (phenothiazines and erythromycin estolate are most frequently involved) or hepatocellular (rifampin, hydantoins, isoniazid, methyldopa, sulfonamides, and many others). The usual **allergic renal reaction** is interstitial nephritis, most commonly due to methicillin; other antimicrobials and furosemide have also been implicated.

A syndrome similar to SLE can be produced by several drugs, most commonly hydralazine and procainamide. The syndrome is associated with a positive test for antinuclear antibody and is relatively benign, sparing the kidneys and CNS.

Allergic reactions in blood transfusion recipients to components in donor blood are discussed under ALLERGIC REACTIONS, in Ch. 93.

Diagnosis of any drug hypersensitivity reaction can be confirmed by challenge, i.e., by readministering the drug; but reproducing most allergic reactions to confirm the relationship may be risky, and is seldom warranted.

Laboratory tests for specific drug hypersensitivity (e.g., RAST, histamine release, basophil or mast cell degranulation, lymphocyte transformation) are either unreliable or remain experimental. Tests for hematologic drug reactions are an exception (see Diagnostic Tests under TYPE II HYPERSENSITIVITY REACTIONS in Ch. 18).

Skin tests for immediate-type (Type I) hypersensitivity help in diagnosis of reactions to penicillin (see under DRUG HYPERSENSITIVITY, Mechanisms, above), xenogeneic serum, and some vaccines and polypeptide hormones, but for most drugs they are unreliable.

Treatment

It is usually necessary to stop treatment with the offending drug if the reaction appears to be allergic, in contrast to toxic and some idiosyncratic reactions, where the dose can often be reduced and still be effective without causing a reaction. Sometimes a drug that may be life-saving must be continued despite allergic manifestations. Treatment of bacterial endocarditis with penicillin, for example, may be continued despite the appearance of a morbilliform eruption, urticaria, or drug fever. Urticaria is treated in the usual manner, including corticosteroids if necessary.

Rapid desensitization to a drug may be necessary if sensitivity has been established by history and positive challenge or (for penicillin) a positive skin test, and if no alternative exists (see BACTERIAL ENDOCARDITIS, in Ch. 25). Expert consultation is advised if this situation arises.

Most reactions clear within a few days after a drug is stopped. Treatment can usually be limited to symptom control. For example, drug fever or a nonpruritic skin rash usually requires no treatment. However, if a patient is acutely ill, with signs of multiple system involvement, or with exfoliative dermatitis, intensive corticosteroid treatment is required (e.g., prednisone 40 to 80 mg/day orally). More information on treatment of specific clinical reactions will be found in the pertinent chapters in this volume.

SERUM SICKNESS

An allergic reaction usually appearing 7 to 12 days after administration of a foreign serum or certain drugs, characterized by fever, arthralgias, skin rash, and lymphadenopathy.

Etiology

The most common cause of serum sickness is not serum, but penicillin and related drugs (see DRUG HYPERSENSITIVITY, above). Reactions from horse serum antitoxins occur in at least 5% of persons given the serum for the first time. Anaphylaxis and serum sickness were frequent medical problems when antisera, usually obtained from horses, were used extensively for passive immunization. Serum reactions have become infrequent with current active-immunization programs and antibiotics, and with the development of human immune sera for tetanus and rabies. However, horse antiserum is still used in managing diphtheria, botulism, and venomous snake and spider bites; and anti-lymphocyte or -thymocyte serum from horses and other species is being used increasingly to suppress immune reactions to transplanted organs.

The injected serum or drug is slowly excreted, so that it remains in the circulation long enough to stimulate the production of specific IgG antibodies that form soluble complexes with the antigen to cause a Type III reaction; IgE antibodies and consequently a Type I reaction may also be produced. (See Ch. 18 for a discussion of the immunologic mechanisms.) Both types of reaction probably contribute to symptoms.

Prophylaxis in Using Animal Serum to Avoid Anaphylaxis

Before giving any animal serum or animal serum product, it is imperative to ascertain whether the patient has ever received serum before and whether he has a history of asthma, hay fever, urticaria, or other allergic symptoms—particularly on exposure to horses. A positive history calls for special caution to avoid acute anaphylactic (Type I) reactions.

Regardless of history, any person about to receive a foreign serum *must be tested first.* Some written instructions still call for an intracutaneous test using 0.1 ml of a 1:10 dilution, but this procedure is unsatisfactory and may be dangerous: it produces many false-positive reactions and is likely to produce a generalized reaction in an allergic patient. A patient who is not atopic and who has not received horse serum previously should first be given a **scratch test** with a 1:10 dilution; if this is negative, 0.02 ml of a 1:10 dilution is injected intracutaneously. A wheal more than 0.5 cm in diameter will develop within 15 min if the patient is sensitive. All patients who may have received serum previously (*whether or not they reacted*) and those with a suspected allergic history should be tested first with a 1:1000 dilution. Negative skin test results make anaphylaxis (Type I reaction) unlikely but do not predict the incidence of subsequent serum sickness (Type III reactions).

If the skin test is positive and serum must be used, serial dilutions should be used for skin testing to determine that dilution to which the patient is skin-test–negative. **Desensitization for Type I (anaphylactic) hypersensitivity** is then carried out using 0.1 ml of the first skin-test–negative dilution injected s.c. or slowly IV; although not the standard method, the IV approach gives the physician control of both concentration and rate of delivery. If no reaction occurs in 15 min, the dose is doubled every 15 min until a dose approximating 1 ml of undiluted serum is reached. This amount of undiluted serum is then injected IM and if no reaction occurs in 15 to 20 min, the full dose can then be given. Oxygen and a syringe of 1:1000 epinephrine should always be on hand to initiate prompt treatment should a reaction occur (see ANAPHYLAXIS, above). If a patient does react, it may still be possible to proceed cautiously by reducing the amount injected after pretreatment with antihistamines and corticosteroids, given as for acute urticaria, and then increasing at small intervals. The treatment dose of antiserum for sensitive patients should be *twice* the usual dose to allow for some inactivation by the patient's antibodies.

Symptoms and Signs of Serum Sickness

Onset is usually several days after injection of the serum or drug but may be much sooner than the usual 7 days if the patient has been exposed previously **(accelerated serum sickness)**. Urticaria is the usual skin manifestation. Less frequently, the rash may be multiform or morbilliform; rarely, it is scarlatiniform or purpuric. Most patients have polyarthritis or periarticular edema. Temporomandibular arthritis may be severe, and has been confused with tetanus. When fever occurs, it is mild and lasts for only 1 or 2 days. Adenopathy develops in the region draining the injection site and may become generalized. Splenomegaly is sometimes present. Occasionally, abdominal pain and diarrhea may accompany other symptoms. Myocarditis may develop but is rare. Peripheral neuritis is the only complication that may cause irreversible injury. Surprisingly, glomerulonephritis, so prominent in experimental serum sickness in animals, is rarely a problem.

Diagnosis

A history of serum or drug administration and the characteristic symptoms and signs usually make diagnosis obvious. A positive immediate (IgE-mediated) skin test supports the diagnosis and predicts an anaphylactic risk, but is of little help in predicting the development of serum sickness, since the patient need not be sensitive at the time of testing.

Treatment

Since the disease is self-limited, treatment is usually restricted to relief of symptoms. Pruritus is treated with an antihistamine as for acute urticaria; arthralgias, with salicylates (aspirin 0.6 to 1.5 gm orally q 4 h). If these are not adequate, prednisone 30 mg/day orally is almost always effective. The corticosteroid dose is gradually reduced to zero after symptoms have been relieved. Early, intensive corticosteroid treatment is necessary if the rare complications of peripheral neuritis or myocarditis develop. Large doses of cyproheptadine (0.7 mg/kg/day) or hydroxyzine (5 mg/kg/day) given soon after the serum have been effective in reducing the incidence of serum sickness.

AUTOIMMUNE DISORDERS

Disorders in which the immune system produces autoantibodies to an endogenous antigen, with consequent injury to tissues.

Considered here are the pathogenetic immunologic mechanisms underlying autoimmune diseases (see also TABLE 19–1). Clinical aspects of the specific disorders are presented elsewhere in this volume.

Development of the Autoimmune Response

Although precise details of the autoimmune response are incompletely understood, there is no need to postulate a special mechanism by which organisms recognize their own antigens as "self" and thereby do not respond to them immunologically. The outcome of antigenic stimulation, whether antibody formation or activated T cells or tolerance, seems to depend on the same factors with autoantigen as with exogenous antigen.

Four possible mechanisms for developing an immune response to autoantigens are recognized:

1. Hidden or sequestered antigens (e.g., intracellular substances) may not be recognized as "self"; if released into the circulation they may induce an immune response. This occurs in sympathetic ophthalmia with the traumatic release of an antigen normally sequestered within the eye. Autoantibody alone may not produce disease because it cannot combine with the sequestered antigen. For example, antibodies to sperm and heart muscle antigens are blocked by the basement membrane of the seminiferous tubules and myocardial cell membrane, respectively. Immunologically active T cells, however, may not have such restrictions and would be more effective in producing injury.

2. The "self" antigens may become immunogenic because of chemical, physical, or biologic alteration. Certain chemicals couple with body proteins and render them immunogenic, as seen in contact dermatitis. Photosensitivity exemplifies physically induced autoallergy: ultraviolet light alters skin protein, to which the patient becomes allergic. Biologically altered antigens are seen in New Zealand mice that develop autoallergic disease resembling SLE when persistently infected with an RNA virus known to combine with host tissues, altering them sufficiently to induce antibody.

TABLE 19-1. AUTOIMMUNE DISORDERS

	Disorder	Mechanism or Evidence
Highly Probable	Hashimoto's thyroiditis	Cell-mediated and humoral thyroid cytotoxicity
	Systemic lupus erythematosus	Circulating immune complexes
	Goodpasture's syndrome	Anti-basement membrane antibody
	Pemphigus	Epidermal acantholytic antibody
	Receptor autoimmunity	
	Graves' disease	TSH receptor antibody (stimulatory)
	Myasthenia gravis	Acetylcholine receptor antibody
	Insulin resistance	Insulin receptor antibody
	Autoimmune hemolytic anemia	Phagocytosis of antibody-sensitized erythrocytes
	Autoimmune thrombocytopenic purpura	Phagocytosis of antibody-sensitized platelets
Probable	Rheumatoid arthritis	Immune complexes in joints
	Progressive systemic sclerosis	Nucleolar and other nuclear antibodies
	Mixed connective tissue disease	Antibody to extractable nuclear antigen (ribonucleoprotein)
	Pernicious anemia	Anti-parietal cell and intrinsic factor antibodies
	Idiopathic Addison's disease	Humoral and (?) cell-mediated adrenal cytotoxicity
	Infertility (some cases)	Antispermatozoal antibodies
	Glomerulonephritis	Glomerular basement membrane antibody, or immune complexes
	Bullous pemphigoid	IgG and complement in basement membrane
	Sjögren's syndrome	Multiple tissue antibodies
	Diabetes mellitus (some)	Cell-mediated and humoral islet cell antibodies
	Adrenergic drug resistance (some asthmatics)	β-adrenergic receptor antibody
Possible	Chronic active hepatitis	Smooth muscle antibody
	Primary biliary cirrhosis	Mitochondrial antibody
	Other endocrine gland failure	Specific tissue antibodies in some cases
	Vitiligo	Melanocyte antibody
	Vasculitis	Some cases: immunoglobulin and complement in vessel walls, low serum complement
	Post-myocardial infarction, cardiotomy syndrome	Myocardial antibody
	Many other inflammatory, granulomatous, degenerative, and atrophic disorders	No reasonable alternative explanation

3. Foreign antigen may induce an immune response that cross-reacts with normal "self" antigen. Examples are the cross-reaction that occurs between streptococcal M protein and human heart muscle or the encephalitis that can follow rabies vaccination in which an autoimmune cross-reaction probably is initiated by animal brain tissue in the vaccine.

4. Autoantibody production may be a result of mutational change in immunocompetent cells. This may explain the monoclonal autoantibodies seen occasionally in patients with lymphoma.

Probably the autoimmune reaction is normally held in check by the action of a population of specific suppressor T cells. Any of the above processes could lead to, or be associated with, a suppressor T cell defect.

The role of other complex mechanisms demonstrable experimentally still needs clarification. For example, adjuvants such as alum or bacterial endotoxin, while not antigenic themselves, enhance the antigenicity of other substances. Freund's adjuvant, an emulsion of antigen in mineral oil with heat-killed mycobacteria, is usually required in order to produce autoimmunity in experimental animals.

Genetic factors play a role in autoimmune disorders. Relatives of patients with autoimmune disorders often show a high incidence of the same type of autoantibodies, and the incidence of autoimmune disease is higher in identical than in fraternal twins. Women are more often affected than men are. The genetic contribution appears to be one of predisposition. In a predisposed population a number of environmental factors could provoke disease; in SLE, for example, these might be latent virus infection, drugs, or tissue injury such as occurs with ultraviolet light exposure. This situation would be analogous to the development of hemolytic anemia as a consequence of environmental factors in persons with G6PD deficiency, a predisposing genetically determined biochemical abnormality.

Pathogenetic Mechanisms

The pathogenetic mechanisms of autoimmune reactions are, in many cases, better understood than the way in which autoimmune antibodies develop. In some autoimmune hemolytic anemias, the RBCs become coated with Type II autoantibody; the complement system responds to these antibody-coated cells just as it does to similarly coated foreign particles, and the interaction of complement with the antibody complexed to the cell surface antigen leads to RBC phagocytosis or cytolysis.

Autoimmune renal injury can occur as the result of either a Type II or Type III reaction. The Type II reaction occurs in Goodpasture's syndrome, in which lung and renal disease is associated with the presence of an anti-basement membrane antibody (see Ch. 42). The best-known example of autoimmune injury associated with soluble antigen-antibody complexes (Type III) is the nephritis associated with SLE (see in Chs. 104 and 147 and below). Another example is a form of membranous glomerulonephritis that is associated with an immune complex containing renal tubular antigen. Although it is possible that post-streptococcal glomerulonephritis could be due in part to streptococcus-induced cross-reacting antibodies, there is as yet no proof of this.

A variety of autoantibodies are produced in SLE and other systemic (as opposed to organ-specific) autoimmune diseases. Antibodies to formed elements in the blood account for autoimmune hemolytic anemia (see in Ch. 92), thrombocytopenia, and possibly leukopenia; anticoagulant antibodies may cause bleeding problems. Antibodies to nuclear material result in the Type III deposition of antigen-antibody complexes, not only in glomeruli, but also in vascular tissues and in skin at the dermal-epidermal junction. Synovial deposition of aggregated IgG-RF-complement complexes occurs in RA. Rheumatoid factor (RF) is usually an IgM globulin (occasionally IgG or IgA) with specificity for a receptor on the constant region of the heavy chain of autologous IgG. The IgG-RF-complement aggregates can also be found within neutrophils, where they cause the release of lysosomal enzymes that contribute to the inflammatory joint reaction. Plasma cells are also present in large numbers within the joint, and may synthesize anti-IgG antibodies. T cells and lymphokines are also found in rheumatoid joints and may contribute to the inflammatory process. The process that sets off the immunologic events is unknown; it could be a bacterial or viral infection. In SLE the low serum complement level reflects the widespread immunologic reactions taking place; in RA, by contrast, serum complement is normal but intrasynovial complement levels are low.

In pernicious anemia, autoantibodies capable of neutralizing intrinsic factor can be found in the GI lumen. Autoantibodies against the microsomal fraction of gastric mucosal cells are even more common. It is postulated that a cell-mediated autoimmune attack against the parietal cells results in the atrophic gastritis that, in turn, reduces the production of intrinsic factor but still allows absorption of sufficient vitamin B_{12} to prevent the megaloblastic anemia. If autoantibodies to intrinsic factor should also develop in the GI lumen, however, B_{12} absorption will cease and pernicious anemia will develop.

Hashimoto's thyroiditis is associated with autoantibodies to thyroglobulin, the microsomes of thyroid epithelial cells, a thyroid cell-surface antigen, and a second colloid antigen. Tissue injury and eventual myxedema may be mediated both by the cytotoxicity of the microsomal antibody and by the activity of specifically committed T cells. Low-titered antibodies are also found in patients with primary myxedema, suggesting that it is the end result of unrecognized autoimmune thyroiditis. An autoimmune reaction is also involved in thyrotoxicosis (Graves' disease), and about 10% of patients eventually develop myxedema spontaneously; many more do so after ablative therapy. Other antibodies, unique to Graves' disease, are called thyroid-stimulating antibodies. They react with TSH receptors in the gland and have the same effect on thyroid cell function that TSH normally has.

20. TRANSPLANTATION

The transfer of living tissues or cells from one individual to another, with the objective of maintaining the functional integrity of the transplanted tissue in the recipient.

GENERAL CONSIDERATIONS

Despite surgical technics making transplantation of almost any tissue feasible, the clinical use of transplantation to remedy disease is still limited for most organ systems. The greatest obstacle is the **rejection reaction,** which generally destroys the tissue shortly after transplantation (except in special circumstances, such as corneal grafts or transplants between identical twins). Nevertheless, with improved understanding of immune mechanisms and methods for preventing rejection, organ transplantation may save many patients with otherwise fatal disease.

Use of cadaver organs in transplantation has become more prevalent. The concept of brain death gradually is gaining acceptance, and the Uniform Anatomical Gift Act of 1973 allows adults to assign their organs for later use as transplants under such circumstances.

Transplants are categorized by the genetic relationship between donor and recipient and by the site of transplantation. An **autograft** is a transfer of tissue from one location to another in the same individual (e.g., bone grafting for fracture stabilization). An **isograft** is a graft between identical twins; an **allograft (homograft)** is one between genetically dissimilar members of the same species. **Xeno-grafts (heterografts)** are transplants between members of different species. A tissue or organ graft is **orthotopic** if it is transferred to an anatomically normal recipient site—as in a heart transplant. If the transplant is to an anatomically abnormal site, it is **heterotopic**—as in the transplantation of a kidney into the iliac fossa of the recipient.

IMMUNOBIOLOGIC PRINCIPLES

Allografts or xenografts may be rejected through either a cell-mediated or a humoral immune reaction of the recipient against antigenic components present on the donor's cell membranes. These **transplantation, or histocompatibility, antigens** are found on all nucleated cells of the body. The strongest antigens are governed by a complex of genetic loci and are termed **HLA** (see below); together with the major blood group **(ABO)** antigens, they are the chief transplantation antigens presently detectable in man. Because transplantation antigens can be identified by their effects in vitro, tissue typing (see TISSUE COMPATIBILITY, below) is possible.

The principal mechanism of rejection is the **acute lymphocyte-mediated immune reaction** against transplantation antigens **(host-vs.-graft reaction)**. A delayed hypersensitivity response similar to the tuberculin reaction, it causes graft destruction days to months after transplantation and is character-ized histologically by a mononuclear cellular infiltration of the allograft, with varying degrees of hemorrhage and edema. Usually, vascular integrity is maintained; thus, cell-mediated rejection may be reversed in many cases by intensifying immunosuppressive therapy. After successful reversal of an acute lymphocyte-mediated rejection episode, histologic examination shows that severely dam-aged elements of the graft have healed by fibrosis, and the remainder of the graft appears to be normal. It is interesting to note that the allograft will then often survive for prolonged periods, even though the immunosuppressive drug dosages have been reduced to very low levels. This process of "graft adaptation" is most likely explained by development in the recipient of donor-specific sup-pression, perhaps mediated by suppressor cells.

Occasionally, **late graft deterioration** occurs in immunosuppressed patients. This chronic type of rejection is often insidious but relentless in progression, despite increased immunosuppressive mea-sures. The pathologic picture differs from that of acute rejection. The vascular endothelium is pri-marily involved, with extensive proliferation that gradually occludes the vessel lumen, resulting in ischemia and fibrosis of the graft.

The role of humoral antibody in graft rejection is obvious when the recipient has been **presensi-tized** (by pregnancy, blood transfusion, or previous transplantation) to HLA antigens present in the graft. Transplantation in these circumstances almost invariably leads to **hyperacute rejection**, caus-ing destruction of the graft within hours or even minutes after revascularization (see TISSUE COMPATI-BILITY, below). This antibody-mediated rejection reaction is characterized by small-vessel thrombosis and graft infarction and cannot be reversed by any known immunosuppressive technics (unlike lymphocyte-mediated rejection). Paradoxically, in some instances blood transfusion appears to be protective, possibly by suppressing the immune response (see TISSUE COMPATIBILITY, below). The role of humoral antibody in more delayed graft destruction is probably also important but is still unclear.

A result similar to antibody-mediated rejection usually occurs if a graft is transplanted in defiance of the blood group barriers normally observed in blood transfusions. Therefore, **pretransplant evalu-ation** must include verifying the ABO compatibility between donor and recipient and the existence of a negative cross-match for tissue antibodies (lack of significant reactivity between donor leukocytes and recipient serum in vitro), as well as tissue typing for HLA compatibility.

Methods are also being explored to measure the host's immune response to the graft after trans-plantation. Such **immunologic monitoring** includes enumeration of lymphocyte subpopulations; measurement of lymphocyte-mediated cytotoxicity (LMC) or complement-dependent cytotoxic (CTC) antibodies directed against donor-specific antigens; or the blastogenic response of recipient lym-phocytes stimulated by mitogens such as phytohemagglutinin. These assays attempt to provide a means of assessing responses to treatment and to diagnose rejection prior to functional deteriora-tion of the allograft. Completely reliable and reproducible methods of monitoring immune responses, however, remain to be established.

THE HLA SYSTEM

A group of tissue antigens governed by a chromosomal region bearing a number of genetic loci, each with multiple alleles, that have relevance to transplantation rejection reactions and are markers of the prevalence of several nonimmunologic disorders.

The immunologic response to this group of genetically linked antigens is the major cause of most graft rejection episodes in organ transplantation. Also, awareness is growing of the statistical associ-

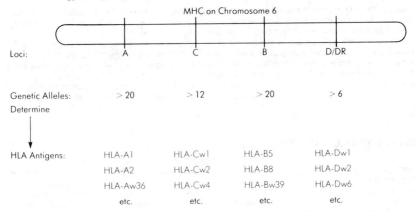

FIG. 20-1.   **Schematic illustration of major histocompatibility complex (MHC) in man.** Allelic genes at each of the four loci determine the cell membrane antigens. A typical example is an individual carrying the specificities: HLA–A1, HLA–A3; HLA–B7, HLA–B8; HLA–Cw1, HLA–Cw2; HLA–Dw2, HLA–Dw3.

ation of certain of these antigens with a variety of diseases. Although some of these disorders may have immunologic features, the pathogenetic meaning of such associations is unknown.

The antigens, termed **HLA** (for **h**uman **l**eukocyte group **A**), are controlled by a complex of genes at several closely linked loci collectively called the major histocompatibility complex **(MHC)**, which is located on the 6th chromosome. Four genetic loci (Loci A, B, C, and D) within the MHC have been identified to date. The genes are allelic—that is, a number of different forms of each gene are found in the population. By mendelian laws, each person has 2 alleles from each locus or, possibly, a pair of identical alleles. (See FIG. 20-1.)

Because the alleles were numbered before their loci were identified, those on Loci A and B are not numbered consecutively. Those alleles that are still provisional are designated with a "w." The difficulties encountered in identifying and sorting out this complex allelic system led to much confusion in original nomenclature. Since 1975, the WHO committee on leukocyte nomenclature has periodically met to assign universally accepted designations to well-recognized individual alleles of each locus (e.g., HLA-A1, HLA-B5, HLA-Cw1, HLA-Dw1). Because of the extensive research into this area, the number of named specificities is rapidly expanding.

The antigens associated with Loci A, B, and C are identified serologically, and are therefore often referred to as **SD** (**s**erologically **d**etermined) antigens. The antigens governed by Locus D are best identified by a **m**ixed **l**ymphocyte **c**ulture **r**eaction, and are often termed **MLR** or **LD** (**l**ymphocyte **d**etermined); these antigens show significant functional differences from the A-, B-, and C-locus antigens, and are probably different structurally.

While any of the HLA antigens may participate in transplantation reactions, there has been a suggestion, as yet incompletely confirmed, that those located on Locus D (including DR or D-related) are of special importance. The antigens having a statistical association with various presumably autoimmune disorders and with lymphoid-cell neoplasms are primarily B- and D-locus antigens. Evidence is now accumulating to suggest that other immunologic disorders, such as atopic allergy, are also associated with a particular HLA genotype. In addition, complement components C2, C4, C8, and properdin factor B have been found to be governed by genes closely linked to the D locus.

Statistical associations between some disorders and HLA antigens are considered to be established: B27 with ankylosing spondylitis, Reiter's syndrome, and psoriatic spondylitis; B13 and Bw17 with psoriasis. Probable associations include Dw1 with chronic active hepatitis, Dw2 with multiple sclerosis, Dw3 with myasthenia gravis, and Dw4 with RA. A great many other associations have been reported, some of them negative. For example, persons with Hodgkin's disease or malignant lymphomas were reported to have a decreased incidence of A11; those with psoriasis, a decreased incidence of B12; and those with rheumatic fever, a decreased incidence of A3. However, because of the difficulties of testing for individual HLA antigens, the reliability of such associations, both negative and positive, depends on accumulating more data.

TISSUE COMPATIBILITY

The degree of similarity of the genetically determined tissue antigens on donor and recipient cells.

Histocompatibility (or tissue) typing of peripheral blood or lymph node lymphocytes is performed prior to transplantation. The goal is to identify serologically the HLA-A, -B, and -C antigens and, by appropriate donor selection, to minimize the antigenic differences between donor and recipient. HLA-D antigens can be determined by mixed lymphocyte culture tests, and the related antigens of the DR series can be determined serologically. Histocompatibility matching of HLA-A and -B antigens has significantly improved functional survival of transplants between related individuals. Results between unrelated individuals also show definite correlations with typing tests for compatibility of HLA-A and -B antigens, although less clearly, since the complex histocompatibility differences in an outbred population introduce many more variables. More recent approaches have evaluated the importance of donor-recipient compatibility for HLA-DR antigens, since they are closely related to the MLR HLA-D gene products. Preliminary studies in renal allograft recipients appear to show a better survival rate in patients sharing one or two HLA-DR antigens with the donor.

A good primary source for HLA tissue-typing antibodies is the serum of multiparous women, who have formed antibodies to fetal transplantation antigens that were inherited from the father but are absent on the mother's cells. Another source is serum from patients who have previously rejected an allograft. In each case, the antisera are multispecific; i.e., they contain antibodies against many or all of the transplantation antigens that were present in the fetus or allograft but absent in the mother or graft recipient. As a result, tissue typing requires large test-cell panels in which the antisera can be grouped to represent a specific antigen identified in common by each group. Newer technics for isolating single transplantation antigens from cell membranes have been developed, and monospecific antisera have been produced by immunization of volunteer donors and use of suitable serum absorption reactions to remove unwanted antibodies. The use of hybridoma technics to produce monoclonal antibodies also promises a ready source of monospecific typing antisera.

Detecting specific presensitization of the recipient against donor antigens is more important than matching for donor-recipient histocompatibility antigens prior to transplantation. Such presensitization most commonly results from prior blood transfusions or pregnancies and is evaluated by a lymphocytotoxic test between recipient serum and donor lymphocytes in the presence of complement. A positive cross-match usually indicates the presence of antibodies in the recipient's serum directed against donor HLA-A, -B, and -C antigens, commonly foreboding hyperacute rejection of the allograft and therefore generally considered to be a contraindication to transplantation. Some antibodies identified in the lymphocytotoxic cross-match are now known to be directed against antigens present on the B lymphocyte subpopulation of peripheral blood (perhaps against HLA-D antigens) but not on T lymphocytes, platelets, or most other nucleated cells. The significance of such a positive B cell cross-match is not clear, since transplantation in its presence does not necessarily result in early failure.

The role of blood transfusions in dialysis and transplantation is controversial. Transfusions have been shunned to avoid sensitization of potential transplant recipients. However, many transplant groups noted better allograft survival in those recipients receiving transfusions, suggesting that transfusion may cause a suppression of the immune response. The dilemma between risking dangerous presensitization vs. achieving a beneficial immunosuppressive effect is presently being dealt with by transfusing potential transplant recipients only with buffy-coat–poor red cell preparations. With the use of frozen washed red cell transfusions, the risk of presensitization is even further reduced, probably because of the absence of viable leukocytes in these preparations.

IMMUNOSUPPRESSION IN TRANSPLANTATION

Immunosuppressive agents are used to control the rejection reaction caused by antigenic differences remaining after tissue typing and donor-recipient matching. Since these drugs suppress all immunologic reactions and also the metabolism of rapidly dividing cells, overwhelming infection is the leading cause of death in transplant recipients. Nevertheless, carefully selected and administered immunosuppressive treatment has been primarily responsible for the present success of clinical transplantation.

Except after isografts, immunosuppressive therapy can rarely be stopped completely after transplantation. However, intensive immunosuppression is usually required only during the first few weeks after transplantation or during rejection crises. Subsequently, the graft often seems to become accommodated and can be maintained with relatively small doses of immunosuppressives and fewer adverse effects.

The antimetabolite **azathioprine**, a key immunosuppressive drug, is given orally or IV, usually beginning at the time of transplantation; doses of 1.5 to 3 mg/kg are usually tolerated indefinitely by the transplant recipient. Its primary toxic effects are bone marrow depression and hepatitis (a reactivation of viral hepatitis may be the underlying factor).

Cyclophosphamide has been substituted in patients who do not tolerate azathioprine; equivalent doses are apparently equal in immunosuppressive activity. This alkylating agent is also used in much larger doses as one of the primary immunosuppressive drugs in bone marrow transplantation, but severe toxicity (hemorrhagic cystitis, alopecia, and infertility) is common.

Prednisone or **methylprednisolone** is usually given in high doses (2 to 30 mg/kg) at the time of transplantation and then reduced gradually to a maintenance dose of 10 to 20 mg/day given indefinitely. It has been suggested that administration of the drug on an alternate-day basis avoids many of the steroid side effects, particularly important in children, where growth is desirable. Many centers utilize this approach, although the risk of rejection is somewhat increased. Should allograft rejection occur, the dose is sharply increased again, risking serious side effects, especially an increased susceptibility to a variety of infections. Because prednisone causes persistent adrenal suppression, supplemental corticosteroids are needed during periods of increased stress such as infections, major trauma, or surgery, but not for a minor stress such as a viral URI. (See also Ch. 251.)

A new agent, the fungal metabolite **cyclosporin A,** has been highly immunosuppressive in some animal models, possibly by promoting a type of suppression specifically directed to donor antigens. Clinical evaluation is limited, but encouraging results have been reported; toxicity, however, including an unusual incidence of lymphomas, remains to be defined.

Presently, **irradiation** for immunosuppression is of limited clinical use in transplantation. The graft and local recipient tissues are sometimes irradiated, either as an adjunctive prophylactic immunosuppressive measure or during treatment for established rejection. The total dose (usually 400 to 600 rads) is below the threshold that might cause serious radiation injury of the graft itself. Extracorporeal irradiation of the recipient's blood or lymph as it traverses a surgically created fistula has been somewhat successful but is too cumbersome for use on a large clinical scale. In treating refractory leukemia, whole-body irradiation in 1000-rad doses combined with chemotherapy destroys the host's immunologic capability (and residual leukemic cells as well). Irradiation is followed by a bone-marrow allograft.

Recently, interest in irradiation therapy has been renewed, stimulated by the observation that treatment directed (by suitable shielding such as that used for Hodgkin's disease) toward all lymphoid centers (total lymphatic irradiation [TLI]) appears to provide a profound but relatively safe suppression of cell-mediated immunity. Application of this technic to transplantation is in its infancy but appears promising.

Attempts have been made to specifically suppress *cellular* immunity with equine or rabbit antiserum against human lymphocytes or thymus cells, leaving the recipient's *humoral* immunologic response intact and preserving his defenses against many bacterial infections. **Antilymphocyte serum (ALS)** or its **globulin fraction (ALG)** may be useful adjuncts, allowing other immunosuppressive measures to be used in lower, less toxic, doses. However, only recently have preparations and regimens for their use become sufficiently standardized to justify the regular use of ALS or ALG in specific circumstances, such as treatment of established rejection. Utilization of the newly available technics of antibody production by **hybridized cells (hybridomas)** should now provide the means for rapid development of therapeutic reagents directed specifically against only selected lymphocyte populations. Such reagents can thus be administered with a minimum of side effects and nonspecific suppression. Possible adverse reactions to heterologous sera include anaphylactic reactions, serum sickness, or antigen–antibody–induced glomerulonephritis, but using highly purified serum fractions, giving them IV, and combining them with other immunosuppressive agents seems to reduce the incidence of these reactions.

Transplant biologists hope to provide specific and selective suppression of the recipient's response only to the foreign antigens on the graft. Such **immunologic tolerance (unresponsiveness)** is best exemplified by the prenatal development of a specific unresponsive state to one's own body constituents. Induction of tolerance to foreign antigens in the adult has been accomplished experimentally by careful selection of conditions, such as antigen dose, route of injection, and short-term use of other immunosuppressive agents; however, the clinical usefulness remains uncertain.

Enhancement is a phenomenon that provides another approach to specific immunologic unresponsiveness. Although the presence of antibodies against donor antigens is usually associated with accelerated rejection, such antibodies, especially when infused passively into the recipient in low dosages, may paradoxically suppress active immune responses and result in prolonged transplant survival. Enhancement of transplant survival may depend especially (but not exclusively) on the presence of anti–HLA-D antibodies. Clinical application of this phenomenon is still investigational.

KIDNEY TRANSPLANTATION

Since long-term success can be expected in 50 to 90% of renal allografts, all patients with terminal renal failure should be considered for transplantation except those at risk from another life-threatening condition. In addition, patient rehabilitation following successful transplantation is generally much more complete than that achieved with hemodialysis, not only because of the freedom from the requirement of prolonged treatments 3 times weekly but also because of the beneficial metabolic functions of the kidney, such as erythropoietic stimulation and calcium homeostasis. Patient survival 1 yr after transplantation from a living related donor is over 95%, with approximately 75 to 80% of the allografts functioning. Subsequently, an annual patient or graft loss of 3 to 5% is observed. The 1-yr patient survival rate following transplantation from a cadaver donor is approximately 90%, and graft survival ranges between 50 to 70% at various centers. In subsequent years, some 5 to 8% of grafts or patients are lost annually. Transplantation in patients over age 55 has been felt by some groups to represent an unacceptable risk to the recipient. However, with the use of more limited immunosuppression and immunologic monitoring, it has been possible to proceed with allografting in selected patients even in their 7th decade, with results quite comparable to those in younger patients.

Pretransplant preparation includes hemodialysis to ensure a relatively normal metabolic state, and provision of a functional, infection-free lower urinary tract. Bladder reconstruction, nephrectomy of infected kidneys, or construction of an ileal conduit for draining the allograft may be required. Prolonged hemodialysis is avoided in pretransplant patients if possible, since the repeated transfusions that are often required may sensitize the patient to transplantation antigens or result in hepatitis. Paradoxically, in those patients who do not develop such sensitization, transfusions may be protective (see TISSUE COMPATIBILITY, above).

Donor Selection and Kidney Preservation

Kidney allografts are obtained from living relatives or cadaver donors, excluding donors with a history of hypertension, diabetes, or malignant disease except possibly those with neoplasms originating in the CNS. Living donors are also carefully evaluated for emotional stability, normal bilateral renal function, freedom from other systemic disease, and histocompatibility. HLA antigens, because of their mode of inheritance, are identical in 25% of siblings. Transplantation between HLA-compatible siblings is successful in over 90% of cases, and less immunosuppression is generally needed. Transplants from other siblings and from parents tend to be less successful, depending on the degree of histoincompatibility between donor and recipient. A living donor gives up reserve renal capacity, may have complex psychologic conflicts, and faces some morbidity from the nephrectomy; yet the significantly improved long-term prognosis for recipients of a well-matched allograft justifies the consideration of the related donor in most instances.

More than half of kidney transplants are nevertheless from cadavers, in many instances from previously healthy persons who have sustained fatal brain damage but maintain stable cardiovascular and renal function. Following brain death or circulatory arrest, the kidneys are removed as quickly as possible and cooled by perfusion. For simple hypothermic storage, special cooling solutions containing large concentrations of poorly permeating substances, such as glucose or mannitol, and electrolyte concentrations approximating intracellular levels (e.g., Collins or Sachs solution) are used to flush the kidney, which is then stored in the iced solution. Kidneys preserved by this method usually function well if transplanted within 24 h. By using the more complex technic of continuous pulsatile hypothermic perfusion with an oxygenated, plasma-based perfusate, kidneys have been successfully transplanted after ex vivo perfusion of up to 72 h.

Transplant Procedure and Immunosuppression

The transplanted kidney is usually placed retroperitoneally in the iliac fossa. Vascular anastomoses are performed to the iliac vessels, and ureteral continuity is established. The role of prophylactic antibiotics for these patients is unclear. Some groups recommend a short course of broad-spectrum coverage to prevent wound infections; others have achieved similar results relying on wound lavage and careful surgical technics. Other measures, such as interferon administration, remain investigational. Pneumococcal vaccine is generally administered only to patients undergoing splenectomy as well. Despite prophylactic immunosuppressive therapy begun just before or at the time of transplantation, most recipients undergo one or more acute rejection episodes in the early post-transplant period. Rejection is suggested by deterioration of renal function, hypertension, weight gain, tenderness and swelling of the graft, fever, and appearance of protein, lymphocytes, and renal tubular cells in the urine sediment. If the diagnosis is unclear, percutaneous needle biopsy is performed to obtain tissue for histopathologic evaluation. Rejection may be reversed by intensified immunosuppression, or may progress until the transplant is no longer functioning. If rejection is not reversed, immunosuppression is tapered, and the patient either is returned to hemodialysis or receives a subsequent transplant.

Most rejection episodes and other complications occur within 3 to 4 mo after transplantation. The majority of patients then return to more normal health and activity, but immunosuppressive medication, usually azathioprine and prednisone (see IMMUNOSUPPRESSION IN TRANSPLANTATION, above), must be maintained unless toxicity or severe infection occurs, since even brief cessation may precipitate rejection.

Late Complications

Some patients suffer irreversible chronic graft rejection, with progressive hypertension and gradual deterioration of renal function that may necessitate nephrectomy and retransplantation. Other late complications include azathioprine toxicity, increasing side effects of prednisone administration, recurrent glomerulonephritis, and acute or chronic infections. In addition, the incidence of malignancy in renal allograft recipients has increased. The risk of epithelial carcinoma is 4 to 5 times higher than normal; of lymphoma, about 30 times. Management of these neoplasms is similar to that for cancer in nonimmunosuppressed patients. Reduction or interruption of immunosuppression is not generally required in treating squamous cell epitheliomas but is recommended for more aggressive tumors and lymphomas.

BONE MARROW TRANSPLANTATION

The clinical use of bone marrow transplantation in patients suffering hematopoietic or lymphoreticular disease is slowly expanding. Common indications have been severe aplastic anemia, refractory leukemia, or congenital immunodeficiency syndromes. However, as success rates have continued to improve, this approach has been extended to patients even earlier in the course of their disease, i.e., to patients with acute leukemia in remission but with a known poor prognosis. With expected continuing advances in knowledge of transplantation biopsy, use of this procedure will undoubtedly increase. The transplantation procedure itself is simple—aspiration of marrow from the donor and IV infusion of the marrow into the recipient—but long-term successful engraftment continues to be difficult to achieve; about 70% of patients with aplastic anemia and even fewer with leukemia survive > 1 yr.

In addition to graft rejection by the host, other factors complicate the procedure. Because of the underlying disease and the vigorous pretransplant immunosuppression, pancytopenia usually occurs before the graft begins to function, seriously predisposing to opportunistic infection or spontaneous hemorrhage. Also, **graft-vs.-host (GVH) disease,** characterized by fever, exfoliative dermatitis, hepatitis, diarrhea or abdominal pain, ileus, vomiting, and weight loss, often develops as a result of the immunologically competent donor cells being administered to a severely depressed host. Despite the use of HLA-identical donors and postgraft immunosuppression, GVH disease occurs in 2/3 of patients and accounts for many deaths after marrow engraftment.

For nonmalignant conditions, immunosuppressive preparation of the marrow recipient is directed solely to reducing immunocompetence, usually by cyclophosphamide 30 to 50 mg/kg/day for several days, or large doses of antilymphocyte globulin **(ALG)** for 7 to 10 days. In leukemia, therapy must also be directed at the malignant cells. Total-body irradiation is commonly used, with the addition of antileukemic drugs for some patients. Methotrexate is usually given after transplantation to suppress GVH disease; established GVH disease has been successfully reversed with ALG. More recently, successful prevention of GVH disease has been achieved by incubation of the donor marrow (with monoclonal antibody to T lymphocytes) prior to transplantation.

If failure of engraftment, sepsis, GVH disease, and recurrence of leukemia are avoided, a long-term stable condition develops in which host and donor marrow cells exist compatibly **(chimerism).** Immunosuppressive therapy may often be stopped after several months of stable chimerism without resultant graft rejection (in contrast to the situation with long-surviving allografts of other tissues) or recurrent GVH reaction.

SKIN TRANSPLANTATION

Skin allografts are valuable for patients with extensive burns or other causes of massive skin loss. Covering the denuded area reduces fluid and protein losses and discourages invasive infection. By alternating strips of autografts and allografts, the entire denuded area can be covered in a patient with insufficient donor sites to permit the use of autografts alone. The allografts are rejected, but these secondarily denuded areas can then be re-covered with autografts taken from healed original donor sites. Allografts are also used as dressings for infected burns or wounds; the wounds rapidly become sterile and develop well-vascularized granulations on which autografts will take readily.

Patients (especially children) with extensive (usually lethal) burns have been treated early with immunosuppression, generally ALG, followed by excision of the burns and wound closure with allografts. The allografts can be maintained for several months while the patient's own skin is repeatedly harvested and used to replace the allografts. Once the burns are completely autografted, immunosuppression is stopped. The benefit of immediate and complete wound closure in these immunosuppressed patients apparently outweighs the risk of increased incidence of infection, since > 50% of patients with burns covering 75 to 90% of the body surface have survived when treated in this fashion.

TRANSPLANTATION OF OTHER ORGANS

Fetal **thymus implants** obtained from stillborn infants may restore immunologic responsiveness to children with thymic aplasia and consequent lack of normal development of the lymphoid system. Because the recipient is immunologically unresponsive, immunosuppression is not required; however, GVH disease may be severe.

Autografts and even, rarely, **allografts of parathyroid tissue** with host immunosuppression have been successfully performed. Parathyroid autotransplantation has been recommended by some groups for treatment of patients with primary or secondary hyperplasia, persistent hyperparathyroidism after surgical exploration, or following total thyroidectomy for cancer. The technic involves removal of all parathyroid tissue from the neck, with placement of a few small slivers of tissue in a muscle pocket in the forearm, where the tissue can later be easily identified if hypercalcemia recurs. Allografts may be undertaken for patients with iatrogenic hypoparathyroidism whose medical management is unsatisfactory. Since immunosuppression is required, this procedure is rarely indicated unless the patient also is receiving a renal allograft, for which suppression will be necessary anyway.

Transplantation of the liver, heart, lung, and pancreas is more experimental, but some recipients have survived as long as 10 yr with a cardiac allograft. Since only cadaver donors can be used and no artificial organs are available to sustain terminal patients awaiting transplantation, the logistic problems are more formidable than with kidney transplantation.

Liver transplantation is still investigational but has shown slowly improving results, with a number of allografted patients having survived > 5 yr. Failure of liver transplantation has often been due to technical complications, particularly of the biliary drainage anastomosis, but newer procedures appear to be overcoming this problem. Because of biliary drainage problems, these patients have an unusually high incidence of bacteremia. Usual indications for liver transplantation include severe chronic hepatic failure, as in cirrhosis or biliary atresia, and primary malignant disease such as hepatoma. Patients with malignancy must be carefully selected, since any nonresected tumor may rapidly disseminate once immunosuppression is begun. Acute liver failure is usually not an indication for transplantation, because prognosis is difficult to assess and also because medical personnel may be infected by viruses.

The allograft may replace the diseased liver orthotopically or be used as an accessory heterotopic organ. A heterotopic transplant is less traumatic but tends to atrophy if excluded from the portal circulation.

Rejection may be suggested by the development of hepatomegaly, light-colored stools, and complaints of anorexia, right flank pain, and fever. Jaundice, elevations in serum enzyme determinations, and reduced uptake of radioisotope on liver scan are corroborative findings. Because of the likelihood of technical problems with the biliary drainage, invasive studies including laparotomy may be required to establish the diagnosis. Liver allografts appear to be less aggressively rejected than kidney or heart tissue. Azathioprine, prednisone, and ALG usually are given initially (see IMMUNOSUPPRESSION IN TRANSPLANTATION, above) in doses similar to those used for renal recipients; maintenance dosage can generally be lower. Some groups recommend substituting cyclophosphamide for azathioprine in the early post-transplant period because of the possible hepatotoxicity of the latter.

Cardiac transplantation was restricted to a few centers but is gradually increasing as long-term survival rate and rehabilitation levels approach those of patients receiving cadaver-donor renal allografts. End-stage coronary artery disease and cardiomyopathy are the common indications for cardiac transplantation. In addition, patients who could not be weaned from temporary cardiac assist devices following myocardial infarction or nontransplant surgery have received transplants successfully.

Immunosuppressive regimens are similar to those for kidney or liver transplantation. The onset of rejection may be heralded by fever, malaise, tachycardia, hypotension, and cardiac failure that is predominantly right-sided. Arrhythmias are common in more severe rejection cases. In milder cases, rejection may be suggested by ECG changes only, and is confirmed by transvenous endomyocardial biopsy. Immunologic monitoring to detect rejection prior to functional deterioration of the graft is becoming increasingly helpful. Because no artificial organ is available to maintain patients, potential recipients often die while awaiting transplantation or during severe rejection. Nevertheless, cardiac transplantation is a realistic endeavor for patients with no practical alternatives.

Lungs are particularly difficult to transplant, primarily because of devastating infection in a transplanted organ continually exposed to nonsterile ambient air and dependent on the cough mechanism, which is disrupted by transplantation. Doubts concerning the functional capacity of a lung immediately after transplantation also have discouraged widespread attempts at lung transplantation.

Pancreatic transplantation offers hope of reestablishing normal carbohydrate homeostasis in diabetes and possibly preventing the development of microangiopathic lesions of the eye, kidney, and other organs. However, transplantation of pancreatico-duodenal grafts has been accompanied by severe morbidity and only short-term success, because of complications arising from the exocrine portion of the gland. More successful results have recently been achieved using segmental transplantation of the tail of the pancreas, with the pancreatic duct either occluded by a polymer solution or left to drain intraperitoneally. Efforts are also being directed toward transplantation of islet cell preparations that can be infused IV—usually into the liver via the portal system. Using this technic, diabetes has been successfully prevented following total pancreatectomy for chronic pancreatitis and autografting of islet tissue. Problems with obtaining sufficient viable donor tissue and controlling the rejection reaction, however, continue to limit islet cell allografting.

Cartilage is unique in that chondrocytes are among the few types of mammalian cells that can be allografted without succumbing to the immune response. In children, cartilage grafts obtained from cadaver donors may be used to replace congenital nasal or ear defects. In adults, autografts (usually from rib cartilage) are more commonly used to treat severe injuries. Utilization of cartilage allografts to resurface articular joints destroyed by arthritis has been attempted, but technical obstacles still make joint replacement with prosthetic devices preferable.

Bone grafting is widely used, but except for autografts only a small portion of transplanted bone survives in the recipient. The allografts at first "take," but the immunologic response destroys the cells a week or so later. However, the remaining dead matrix has a bone-inducing capacity that stimulates host osteoblasts to recolonize the matrix and lay down new bone, thus serving as a scaffolding for bridging and stabilizing defects until new bone is formed. Massive resection of malignant bone tumors and reconstruction by implantation of composite bone and cartilage allografts are possible practical approaches to salvaging extremities that would otherwise be amputated. Cadaver allografts are preserved by freezing to decrease immunogenicity of the bone (which is dead at the time of implantation) and glycerolization to maintain chondrocyte viability. No postimplantation immunosuppression is used. Although these patients develop anti-HLA antibodies, early follow-up reveals no evidence of cartilage degradation.

21. TUMOR IMMUNOLOGY

The demonstration of immune responses in experimental animals to spontaneously occurring tumors, to carcinogen- or viral-induced tumors, and to transplanted tumors has stimulated much interest in seeking similar immune responses in man over the past 3 decades. The availability of syngeneic strains of animals has permitted a distinction to be made between immune reactions directed against tumor-specific (or tumor-associated) transplantation antigens and histocompatibility antigens also present on tumor cells. The absence of such a distinction in man, except in the unusual circumstance of identical twins, has made the study of human anti-tumor immunity more complex. Nevertheless, it seems likely that the presence of immunogenic surface configurations on human neoplastic cells permits their recognition by immunocompetent host cells as well as their interaction with humoral antibodies. The significance of such recognitions and reactions in the pathogenesis of tumors, and the potential for augmenting them in favor of the host, is currently the object of intensive laboratory and clinical investigation. It is fair to state, however, that at the time of this writing a decade of clinical trials with human cancer immunotherapy—most of it involving so-called "nonspecific" immunotherapy—has resulted in major reservations concerning the efficacy of such therapy.

TUMOR-SPECIFIC TRANSPLANTATION ANTIGENS (TSTA)

Most induced or transplanted experimental animal tumors have been shown to immunize syngeneic recipients against subsequent challenge with the same tumor but not against transplantation of normal tissues or other tumors. Such findings indicate the presence of antigens that are associated with the tumor cells but are not apparent on normal cells. These antigens are known as **tumor-specific** or **tumor-associated transplantation antigens (TSTA)**. (The term "tumor-associated" may be more accurate, since such markers may be normally inapparent cell components that become manifest during the neoplastic process, as explained below.)

The findings are particularly well demonstrated by chemical carcinogen-induced tumors, which tend to have individual antigenic specificity that varies from tumor to tumor, even with tumors induced by the same carcinogen; and by virus-induced tumors, which tend to show cross-reactivity between tumors induced by a given virus.

Suggested mechanisms for the origin of such antigens include (1) new genetic information introduced by a virus; (2) alteration of genetic function by carcinogens, possibly through derepression, by which genetic material that is normally inactive, except perhaps during embryonic development, is activated and becomes expressed in the cell phenotype; (3) uncovering of antigens that are normally "buried" in the cell membrane, through the inability of neoplastic cells to synthesize membrane constituents such as sialic acid; (4) release of antigens that are normally sequestered in the cell or its organelles, through the death of neoplastic cells.

Technics to demonstrate TSTA in animal tumors include standard tissue transplantation methods, immunofluorescence, cytotoxicity tests using dye uptake or radioisotope release, prevention of tumor growth in vitro or in vivo by exposing the tumor to lymphoid cells or serum from immunized donors, delayed hypersensitivity skin tests, and lymphocyte transformation in vitro.

Evidence for TSTA in human neoplasms has been demonstrated with several neoplasms, including Burkitt's lymphoma, neuroblastoma, malignant melanoma, osteosarcoma, and some GI carcinomas. Choriocarcinomas in women possess paternally derived histocompatibility antigens that may serve as "tumor-specific" antigens in eliciting an immune response. The complete cure of choriocarcinomas by chemotherapy may be attributable, at least in part, to such an immune response.

HOST RESPONSES TO TUMORS

CELLULAR IMMUNITY

The importance of lymphoid cells in tumor immunity has been repeatedly demonstrated in experimental animal tumor systems. In humans, the growth of tumor nodules has been inhibited in vivo by mixing suspensions of a patient's lymphocytes and tumor cells, suggesting a cell-mediated reaction to the tumor. In vitro studies have demonstrated that lymphoid cells from patients with certain neoplasms show cytotoxicity against corresponding human tumor cells in culture. This has been found with neuroblastoma, malignant melanoma, sarcomas, and carcinomas of the colon, breast, cervix, endometrium, ovary, testis, nasopharynx, and kidney. Similar antitumor cytolytic properties have been demonstrated with lymphocytes from members of the families of neuroblastoma and osteosarcoma patients, suggesting common exposure to a suspected environmental agent. The significance of such reactions in controlling tumor growth is not clear at this time. However, it seems likely that one or more types of lymphocytes, primarily associated with T cell differentiation, are capable of damaging tumor cells in vivo.

HUMORAL IMMUNITY

Humoral antibodies that react with tumor cells in vitro are produced in response to a variety of animal tumors induced by chemical carcinogens or viruses. However, antibody-mediated protection against tumor growth in vivo has only been demonstrable in certain animal leukemias and lymphomas. By contrast, lymphoid-cell–mediated protection in vivo occurs in a broad variety of animal tumor systems.

Anti-tumor antibodies may include the following types. (1) **Cytotoxic antibodies:** These are generally complement-fixing antibodies directed against surface antigens of relatively high density. In general, IgM antibodies are more cytotoxic in transplantation systems than are IgG antibodies. (2) **Enhancing** or **blocking antibodies:** Generally IgG antibodies, possibly complexed with soluble antigen, these *favor* the growth of a tumor rather than inhibit it. The mechanisms for such immunologic enhancement are not understood but may involve (a) binding with TSTA and blocking their immunogenicity (afferent enhancement); (b) reacting with and inhibiting immunologically competent cells (central enhancement); (c) coating of tumor cells and thus preventing their interaction with lymphoid cells (efferent enhancement). The enhancement of human tumors seems likely, since blocking antibodies have been demonstrated in vitro. (3) **Unblocking factors:** These factors are not yet characterized completely, but may be antibodies. They decrease the blocking activity of enhancing antibodies or antigen-antibody complexes. They have been detected in the sera of patients following surgical removal of all clinically apparent tumor tissue. The exact relationship of cytotoxic, blocking, and unblocking, factors is not yet clear; i.e., whether or not the presumed antibodies involved are distinct from each other is not known.

Humoral antibodies directed against *human* tumor cells or their constituents have been demonstrated in vitro in the serum of patients with Burkitt's lymphoma, malignant melanoma, osteosarcoma, neuroblastoma, and digestive system carcinomas. Antibodies to melanoma cells and to carcinoembryonic antigen (see below) are usually found in patients *without* disseminated disease; the reasons are unknown. Perhaps a failure to produce such antibodies permits metastasis; or perhaps antibodies are formed but are promptly absorbed by the large tumor mass.

Interest has also been directed toward "anti-antibodies" in human malignancy. In melanoma patients, antibodies have been demonstrated that appear to interact with the $F(ab')_2$ fragment of anti-melanoma cytoplasm IgG antibodies. This complicated and possibly delicate balance between potentially beneficial and potentially detrimental immune responses requires clarification to assist in planning immunotherapeutic maneuvers. Shifting this balance in favor of the host by removing factors inhibiting humoral antitumor immunity is a relatively unexplored area of human immunotherapy.

ALTERATIONS OF HOST IMMUNE REACTIVITY

Tumors that possess TSTA are able to grow in vivo, which suggests a deficient host response to the TSTA. Possible mechanisms include the following: (1) Specific immunologic tolerance to TSTA (e.g., because of prenatal exposure to the antigen, possibly viral in origin). This may involve suppressor cells in a manner not well understood at present. (2) Suppression of the immune response by chemical or viral carcinogens. (3) Suppression of the immune response by treatment, especially cytotoxic chemotherapy and radiation therapy. Occurrence of > 100 times the expected incidence of tumors in patients undergoing immunosuppressive therapy for renal transplantation suggests an impairment of postulated "immune-surveillance" mechanisms, which are theorized to inhibit growth of newly transformed neoplastic cells, or an impairment of immunity to oncogenic viruses, among possible explanations. Also, tumors have been inadvertently transplanted to immunosuppressed human kidney recipients, and these may regress when immunosuppression is discontinued. (4) Suppression of the immune response by the tumor itself. Deficient cellular immunity can be associated with recurrence and dissemination of tumors. This has been repeatedly demonstrated with a variety of human tumors, most dramatically in Hodgkin's disease, which appears to involve a variable defect in T cell function. An immunoglobulin reacting with the host's lymphocytes appears to be associated with this defect. Deficient humoral immunity occurs in association with neoplasms involving abnormal B cell derivatives, such as multiple myeloma and chronic lymphocytic leukemia. Recent investigation implicates a macrophage-related suppressor cell in the humoral immune deficiency state of myeloma.

IMMUNOTHERAPY OF HUMAN TUMORS

During the 1970s, extensive clinical investigation was conducted on cancer immunotherapy, stimulated by effectiveness of immunologic manipulation in experimental animal tumor systems. A variety of biologic modifiers have been employed, including both "specific" immunization with tumor cells or fractions thereof and "nonspecific" immunization with such materials as bacterial vaccines, thymic extracts, white blood cell fractions, and several chemical immunoadjuvants. These attempts at immunotherapy often have involved patients with far-advanced cancer, having large tumor-cell burdens and impaired immune mechanisms that had little chance of being effectively augmented. Cautious investigation of these therapeutic approaches with patients who have relatively poor prognoses, but at a time when their disease is *limited*, seems justifiable at present, e.g., in a patient whose recurrent malignant melanoma in lymph nodes has been surgically resected. All such immunologic approaches to cancer are at this time experimental and not considered to be standard therapy. The possibility exists of shifting in an *unfavorable* direction the delicate balance between factors stimulating and inhibiting immunologic defenses against a tumor.

Experimental Therapeutic Methods

Large tumor masses are, if possible, reduced by prior surgery, radiotherapy, or chemotherapy to facilitate potential effectiveness of immunologic mechanisms.

1. **Active immunization with tumor cells.** (a) **Autochthonous tumors** (tumors arising in the same host) have been used after irradiation or neuraminidase treatment in kidney carcinoma and malignant melanoma patients, among others. Mixing the tumor cells with a bacterial adjuvant (see below) may enhance the immunogenicity of such vaccines. Clinical improvement associated with such therapy has been seen in a minority of patients so treated, but variables such as dose and timing require additional study. Cell culture and hybridization technics help make available larger numbers of tumor cells for use in vaccines. (b) **Allogeneic tumor cells** (cells from other patients) have been used after their irradiation in acute lymphoblastic leukemia and acute myeloblastic leukemia in conjunction with BCG or other adjuvants (see below) after remission has been induced by intensive chemotherapy and radiotherapy. Prolongation of remissions or improved reinduction rates have been reported in some series but not in others. (c) **Tumor cell extracts** and purified TSTA are being studied. It is possible that the integrity of tumor cell membranes must be maintained to some extent to provide the steric configurations required for immunogenicity. (d) **Activation of autologous lymphocytes in vitro:** Lymphoid cells, separated from peripheral blood or obtained from the thoracic duct, have been incubated with tumor cells in vitro and then reinfused. Autologous blood lymphocytes have also been activated in vitro with lymphocyte mitogens such as phytohemagglutinin and then reinfused.

2. **Passive immunization.** (a) **Antiserum:** Antilymphocyte serum has been used in chronic lymphocytic leukemia, resulting in a temporary decrease in lymphocyte counts. Humoral antibody, both autologous and allogeneic, might be made more effective if association with soluble tumor antigens or immunoglobulin "anti-antibodies" could be reversed or prevented. (b) **Lymphoid cells:** Allogeneic blood leukocytes, from other cancer patients previously grafted with the recipient's tumor, have been transfused ("adoptive" immunotherapy) in studies with malignant melanoma and other tumors. Some remissions have occurred, but graft-vs.-host reactions may result, as with bone marrow transplantation. (c) **Transfer factor:** This dialyzable leukocyte extract, capable of transferring delayed hypersensitivity reactivity from one individual to another, has been studied as a means of transferring antitumor immunity in malignant melanoma, renal carcinoma, lymphomas, and a variety of other human tumors. Responses have been reported, although not as frequently in cancer patients as in patients with cell-mediated immune deficiency disorders and chronic infection.

3. **Nonspecific immunotherapy.** (a) **Interferons** are a series of proteins derived from fibroblasts or WBCs which possess anti-tumor activity that may originate partially from immunologically mediated mechanisms. Current studies with human cancer patients show some promise although slowed by limited availability and purity. (b) **Thymosin,** an extract of bovine thymus, appears to stimulate maturation of several early stages of T cell development and to increase the ability of mature T cells to respond to antigens. Clinical studies suggest that survival of certain cancer patients, including those with small-cell lung carcinoma, may be increased when receiving thymosin in addition to chemotherapy. (c) Skin malignancies have regressed after induction of delayed hypersensitivity to dinitrochlorobenzene and subsequent direct application of **dinitrochlorobenzene** to the tumor. (d) **Bacterial adjuvants,** such as **BCG** (attenuated tubercle bacilli), extracts of BCG such as **MER** (methanol-extracted residue), or killed suspensions of *Corynebacterium parvum* have been used in randomized trials, with or without added tumor antigen, in a broad variety of human cancer patients, usually in association with intensive chemotherapy or radiation therapy. Direct injection of BCG into melanoma nodules almost always leads to regression of the injected nodules, and occasionally of distant, non-injected nodules as well. Recent studies suggest that MER may help prolong chemotherapy-induced remission duration in acute myeloblastic leukemia and that BCG added to combination chemotherapy may increase survival in advanced breast cancer and possibly in non-Hodgkin's lymphoma. BCG injected intrapleurally after resection of localized bronchogenic carcinoma may improve survival, although not when nodal or other metastases are present. Numerous other studies with these immunoadjuvants, however, have shown no beneficial effects. (e) **Chemical immunomodulators** such as levamisole (a veterinary antihelminthic agent) and glucan (a polyglucose) are being examined both in animal systems and in human trials. Suggestive beneficial effects have been reported in some studies, but these await confirmation.

In summary, nonspecific immunotherapy has resulted in very limited therapeutic benefit, if any at all. Better understanding of the mechanisms involved in its action, and its utilization with sources of TSTA whenever possible, seems necessary for satisfactory application in cancer therapy.

TUMOR IMMUNODIAGNOSIS

Many tumors release antigenic substances into the circulation. These antigenic macromolecules may eventually provide sensitive indicators of the presence of a variety of malignancies, yielding a valuable immunologic approach to the early diagnosis of neoplastic disease, particularly if detectable by technics appropriate for mass screening programs. They can also aid in monitoring patients for tumor recurrence after therapy.

Carcinoembryonic antigen (CEA) is a protein-polysaccharide complex found in colon carcinomas and in normal fetal gut, pancreas, and liver. Use of a sensitive radioimmunoassay permits detection of increased levels in the blood of patients with colon carcinoma. However, the specificity of this technic is currently under investigation, since positive tests have also occurred in cirrhosis, in ulcerative colitis, and with other cancers, including those of the breast, pancreas, and bladder. α-**Fetoprotein (AFP)** is an antigen migrating with the α-globulins in electrophoresis, and is found in serum from patients or animals with primary hepatoma and from patients with ovarian or testicular embryonal carcinoma. β-**Subunit of human chorionic gonadotropin (βHCG)** is measured by immunoassay and is a very useful marker in patients with residual testicular choriocarcinoma or embryonal carcinoma.

22. AN APPROACH TO THE CARDIAC PATIENT

Cardiovascular clinical diagnosis depends on a synthesis of information from the history, physical signs, ECG, chest x-rays, and special laboratories. Specialized laboratory studies should not be ordered until the initial clinical assessment has provided a basis for judging the need for other procedures such as echocardiography, exercise testing, radionuclide imaging, cardiac catheterization, and angiographic studies. The sequence used in gathering clinical information can vary with the situation; for example, the physical examination of an infant or a young child best begins during a period of calm. The impressions gained from initial findings usually influence the objectivity with which subsequent findings are appraised. By the end of the clinical assessment, unlikely considerations should have been deemphasized or discarded, and probabilities should have been brought into sharp focus.

THE HISTORY

Knowledge of the natural history of cardiovascular disease helps to establish the diagnosis as well as the prognosis. Considerations may be narrowed to relatively few probabilities based upon the history alone.

Leading questions should be minimized or avoided. Questions are best phrased in a neutral fashion or with reversed implications in order to increase the likelihood of a reliable answer. For example, a patient with chest pain is best asked, "What aggravates or relieves the pain or chest discomfort?" rather than an anticipatory, "Doesn't nitroglycerin abolish the chest pain?" Clarity must be assured; too often patients are embarrassed to say that they do not understand the questions.

Initial questions should be general, serving as a framework and providing an overview. Can ordinary day-to-day activities be performed without limitations? What is the patient's assessment of his/her general state of health? Can a child keep up with playmates, or is special effort needed? Nonspecific complaints are often noncardiac in origin. For example, anxiety causes fatigue more commonly than does heart disease, which is seldom responsible for fatigue alone; breathlessness can be simple hyperventilation; and paroxysmal nocturnal dyspnea may represent the hyperpneic phase of Cheyne-Stokes respiration in an elderly patient given inappropriate sedatives, especially barbiturates.

More pointed, detailed inquiries follow. In a patient with heart failure believed to be cardiomyopathic, an accurate history of excessive alcohol ingestion can be crucial. An exacerbation of cardiac failure may be due to exposure to heat and humidity rather than to deterioration of basic ventricular function. Aggravation of angina may reflect anemia, tachyarrhythmias, or thyrotoxicosis rather than progressive coronary arterial obstruction. Painful fingertips (infective endocarditis) are especially apt to disturb a typist. Tight shoes at the end of the day may indicate the edema of heart failure, but a single tight shoe (asymmetric swelling) is more likely due to varicose edema. Ascites is sometimes recognized by the patient as inappropriate tightness of belt or waistband. The general question of palpitations should be followed by detailed questions that may identify a specific arrhythmia. Imitating the patterns of rate and rhythm by tapping one's chest (or the patient's chest) may allow such identification. A history of allergies is important in advising prophylaxis for infective endocarditis, and a history of bleeding disorders is important to establish before embarking upon cardiac surgery employing rigid prosthetic valves and anticoagulants.

A fundamental difference between pediatric and adult cardiology is the patient's state of health apart from the cardiac or vascular disease. The infant or child with a cardiac or circulatory disorder is usually free or relatively free of other diseases. In the adult, however, cardiac abnormalities are likely to be accompanied by a variety of noncardiac (or even other cardiac) disorders that interact with the primary heart disease to varying degrees. Accordingly, the "noncardiac" history—while always important—is especially so in older patients.

THE PHYSICAL EXAMINATION

The Physical Appearance

Attention should first be directed to the *general* physical appearance, then to *detailed* deviations from normal. For example, the general appearance of chronic illness—catabolic effect of chronic congestive heart failure—usually is readily apparent. Certain general appearances identify diseases associated with predictable types of cardiac or vascular disorders, such as Marfan's syndrome with aortic root/mitral valve abnormalities and Down's syndrome with endocardial cushion defect. Detailed physical examination provides a host of diagnostic insights. Mild pectus excavatum, kyphoscoliosis, or loss of thoracic kyphosis is often associated with mitral valve prolapse, while more pronounced abnormalities of these thoracic configurations can alter the physical examination of the heart and produce signs that mimic organic heart disease. Pretibial and presacral edema are time-honored details of physical appearance that do not always represent congestive heart failure. Varicose veins that are inapparent in the supine position may be obvious when the patient stands. Subungual splinter hemorrhages occur in normal people, but the important white-centered conjunctival petechiae or retinal Roth spots of infective endocarditis are overlooked unless specifically sought. Symmetric cyanosis in an elderly patient with nicotine-stained fingers and barrel chest reflects chronic obstructive lung disease. Cyanosis of the feet but not of the hands is a sign of patent ductus arteriosus with reversed shunt.

The Arterial Pulse

The ancient art of feeling the pulse is helpful in diagnosis. The radial, brachial, carotid, femoral, dorsalis pedis, posterior tibial, and digital (fingertips) pulses are all accessible and, except for the digital pulses, should be palpated routinely to determine their presence and quality. Tactile impression is heightened by using a single finger for palpation, preferably the thumb. To compare 2 pulses, the arteries should be palpated at the same time or in rapid sequence; the alternating method is appropriate for examining the carotids. The brachials and carotids are best for assessing the quality of the pulse since their wave form gives a more accurate impression of the central aortic pulse than either the more distal radial or femoral. However, pulsus alternans amplifies peripherally and therefore may be more apparent in distal pulses such as the radial and femoral.

The examiner should sit or stand comfortably at the patient's right side and should use the right hand to support the patient's elbow, leaving the thumb free to explore the antecubital fossa for the brachial artery. The patient should relax the arm. Once the examining finger or thumb is in place, the patient's forearm can be gently raised or lowered, while the pressure applied to the artery is varied until the maximum pulsation is felt. When the examiner's right thumb palpates the patient's left carotid artery, the contralateral jugular venous pulse can be timed. The examiner can feel digital pulsations by gently gripping the patient's fingertips. Digital pulses can be accurately timed if the examiner palpates the ipsilateral radial artery while using the free hand to support the patient's wrist. The femoral pulse in an infant should be sought only while the leg is voluntarily relaxed.

Palpating the arterial pulsations provides information about (1) the cardiac rate and rhythm, (2) differential pulsations (right-left or upper-lower extremities), (3) arterial thrills, and (4) wave form. An initial impression of rate and rhythm is useful even though this information is also derived from other sources. Comparative palpation of 2 arteries is useful in acquired cardiovascular disease (peripheral obstructive disease) and in congenital cardiac disease such as coarctation of the aorta (upper-lower extremity) or supravalvular aortic stenosis (right-left brachials and carotids). The neck should be examined for arterial thrills by selective palpation over both subclavian and carotid arteries and in the suprasternal notch. Arterial thrills in the neck, although frequently caused by aortic stenosis, may occur in some normal children with innocent supraclavicular systolic murmurs and in some adults with acquired occlusive disease. Analysis of the wave form of an arterial pulse is useful; specific attention should be paid to the ascending limb, the peak, and the descending limb. Each crest should be compared with the next to detect cyclic differences in rate of rise and amplitude characteristic of **pulsus alternans,** a subtle clinical sign of left ventricular failure. Quality and amplitude should be compared during normal expiration and inspiration to detect the inspiratory decline in pulse pressure of **pulsus paradoxus.** However, the most common cause of pulsus paradoxus in a general hospital is not pericardial effusion or constrictive pericarditis, but the inspiratory fall in intrathoracic pressure in pulmonary emphysema with decreased lung compliance, especially when bronchospasm coexists.

The Jugular Veins

The jugular venous pulse should be examined for (1) the venous pressure and wave form, (2) information on conduction defects and arrhythmias, and (3) anatomic/physiologic inferences. The deep (internal) and superficial (external) jugular veins provide a convenient, accurate, and reproducible means of assessing right atrial pressure and wave form. Since it is normal for the jugular veins to distend passively when the patient is supine, the trunk must be elevated to the level at which excursions of the deep jugular vein are maximal, generally about 35 to 45 degrees above the horizontal. The head can then be adjusted upward or to either side by gently moving the chin but must not be tilted too far upward or turned too sharply since these maneuvers tense the sternocleidomastoid muscle and may obliterate the underlying deep jugular vein. An oblique light source should be directed across the area being examined so that the shadows will throw the highlights into relief. It is generally convenient for the examiner to place the right thumb on the patient's left carotid and inspect the venous pulsations on the patient's right side. The free hand can adjust the light source. The superficial jugular vein is readily recognized since it distends when the vessel is compressed gently just above the clavicle. When the compression is released, the crest of the distended column falls to a level approximating the mean right atrial pressure. This procedure is not needed when venous pressure is elevated.

The deep jugular venous pulsations must be distinguished from carotid arterial pulse. Pulsations asynchronous with the carotid cannot be arterial and therefore must be venous. The carotid pulse is palpable, but the venous pulse is not. Carotid pressure remains the same or falls slightly with inspiration, but inspiration may make the jugular venous A wave more prominent because augmented venous return tends to increase the force of right atrial contraction. Venous pulsations cease if the

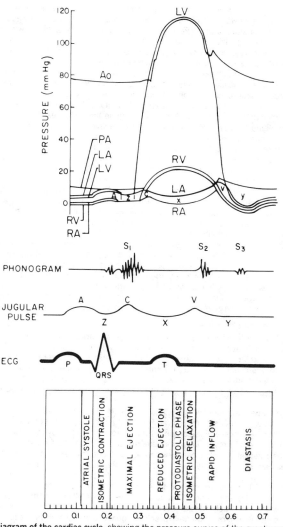

Fig. 22–1.   **Diagram of the cardiac cycle,** showing the pressure curves of the great vessels and cardiac chambers, heart sounds, jugular pulse wave, and the ECG. Ao, aorta; PA, pulmonary artery; LA, left atrium; LV, left ventricle; RA, right atrium; RV, right ventricle. For illustrative purposes, the time intervals between the valvular events have been modified and the z point has been prolonged. (Adapted from *The Heart,* ed. 3, edited by J. W. Hurst et al, copyright 1974 by McGraw-Hill, Inc.; and *A Primer of Cardiology,* ed. 4, by G. E. Burch, copyright 1971 by Lea & Febiger. Used with permission.)

deep jugular vein is compressed at the root of the neck; the pressure required does not affect the carotid pulse. Abdominal compression with the palm of the hand may transiently augment venous, but not arterial, pulsations.

The deep jugular vein pulsates in response to phasic changes in right atrial pressure (see Fig. 22–1). The individual components of the venous pulse should be identified by timing them with simple clinical references, such as the carotid pulse or the heart sounds. It is useful to time the venous pulse first with the carotid so that the physical examination will not be interrupted for auscultatory orientation. During subsequent cardiac auscultation, the venous pulse can be reassessed to confirm or identify specific features that may not have been clear using the carotid reference alone. Two positive venous waves (crests) and 2 descents (troughs) occur in each normal cardiac cycle. The first positive wave is the A wave of atrial contraction, which immediately precedes the carotid pulse. The first trough—the X descent or descending limb of the A wave—is generally interrupted by the carotid arterial pulse with which it seems to coincide. The second positive wave—the V wave of passive atrial filling—follows the carotid pulse by a perceptible interval. The second trough—the Y descent—is clearly diastolic and represents the descending limb of the V wave. The Y descent begins early in diastole as the tricuspid valve opens and the right atrial pressure falls passively.

Timing with heart sound references requires selection of a precordial site where the first and second sounds (S_1, S_2) are heard well. The examiner holds the stethoscope in place with the right hand, and a light source can be adjusted with the left hand. The A wave coincides with or immediately precedes S_1. The Y descent begins just after S_2, when the tricuspid valve opens.

Jugular venous pressure can be determined conveniently and accurately. The vertical levels (crests) of the A wave, V wave, and the superficial jugular vein are determined after the patient's trunk has been elevated above the horizontal to an angle that achieves the maximum excursion of the deep jugular veins. The sternal angle of Louis or the level of the suprasternal notch is the most suitable reference for measuring the crests of the waves. A centimeter rule can be placed vertically at the sternal angle with a tongue blade crossing it perpendicularly at the level of the crest of the wave to be measured. The height can then be read in centimeters above the sternal angle. Although the superficial jugular vein as a rule reliably reflects mean right atrial pressure, occasionally venoconstriction collapses the vessel despite an elevated venous pressure. If the measured heights of the wave forms are normal or borderline, additional information can be gained by observing the response to gradual, sustained abdominal compression for 30 to 60 seconds (**hepato-** or **abdominojugular reflux**). Normally, the pressure rises transiently and no more than 2 cm. With compromised right ventricular function, a greater and more sustained rise occurs.

Conduction defects and arrhythmias can sometimes be diagnosed from the jugular pulse. In sinus rhythm, an A wave precedes each carotid pulse. Prolongation of the A wave to carotid pulse interval reflects prolongation of the P-R interval. The A wave disappears in atrial fibrillation, occurs twice as often as the carotid pulse in 2:1 heart block, and amplifies and becomes synchronous with the carotid in junctional rhythms. Similarly, anatomic/physiologic inferences can be drawn. A giant presystolic A wave means that a hypertrophied right atrium contracts against a resistance (tricuspid stenosis or the thick-walled hypertrophied right ventricle of pulmonary hypertension or isolated pulmonic stenosis). An early, large V wave followed by a brisk Y descent implies tricuspid regurgitation.

Precordial Palpation and Movements

The important precordial movements transmitted by the heart can generally be palpated or seen by the clinician. The information gained includes (1) the systolic movements caused by the ventricles, the great arteries, and the atria; (2) the vibrations or movements caused by heart sounds; and (3) the transmitted vibrations of murmurs; i.e., the thrills. Percussion supplies little additional information, but before beginning methodical palpation, it is useful to percuss briefly to establish the presence of a left thoracic heart, a left stomach, and a right liver to avoid overlooking situs inversus (mirror image dextrocardia).

Palpation should be conducted systematically and should be preceded by inspection of precordial movements, which are sometimes more readily seen than felt. A good source of oblique illumination will highlight the movements, which can be brought into further relief by inking an X on the skin over the site being observed. The visualized movements can be timed by using the carotid pulse or the heart sounds as references. With experience, one can determine not only whether an impulse is systolic or diastolic, but also whether it occurs in mid-diastole, presystole, early systole, or late systole. For both inspection and palpation, each of the following sites should be considered: apex, left and right sternal borders (interspace by interspace from 1st to 5th), subxyphoid, suprasternal notch, right sternoclavicular junction, and ectopic sites, especially above the apex for postinfarction left ventricular aneurysm. Each movement should initially be sought with the flats of the fingers, then with the tips of several fingers, and finally precisely localized with the tip of the first or second finger. Parasternal impulses (right ventricle, pulmonary artery, ascending aorta) can be appreciated better during full exhalation. Precordial movements are best palpated with the undersurface of the fingertips, but thrills may be more readily detected with the heads of the metacarpal bones. The parasternal impulses are best analyzed with the patient supine, and the apical movements are more clearly defined with the patient in a partial left lateral decubitus position.

Systolic movements of the ventricles: Identification, localization, and characterization of the ventricular movements should replace the term "point of maximum impulse"; recognition of left and right ventricular impulses is fundamental. If the **left ventricle** forms the cardiac apex, there is a positive systolic movement with simultaneous medial retraction that identifies the plane of the interventricular septum and confirms that the lateral impulse is left ventricular. Although the quality of the left ventricular impulse is more accurately assessed with the patient in the left lateral decubitus position, ventricular size is best estimated by returning the patient to the supine position while keeping the finger over the site of the systolic ventricular movement. Normally, the left ventricular impulse is a gentle, localized tap; excitement or exercise may increase its prominence but not its duration. The impulse becomes appropriately quick, abrupt, and dynamic as the stroke volume and ejection rate increase (aortic regurgitation), and it becomes slow, steady, and sustained as resistance to ejection increases (aortic stenosis). A prominent left ventricular impulse is usually associated with augmented retraction of the precordium overlying the right ventricle. These asynchronous movements, when exaggerated, impart a rocking motion to the chest.

Right ventricular movement is assessed at the left sternal border (3rd through 5th interspaces) and beneath the xiphoid. The infundibulum underlies the 3rd interspace, and the body of the right ventricle underlies the 4th and 5th interspaces. The right ventricle may impart an impulse to the ends or tips of the fingers if the flat of the hand is placed beneath the xiphoid and directed up toward the diaphragm. A brief, tapping, left sternal edge impulse is occasionally found in children or adults with thin chest walls and narrow anteroposterior dimensions. In some patients with small linear hearts, the left ventricular impulse is felt so close to the sternal edge that it cannot be distinguished from a right ventricle until the patient is turned to a left lateral position. In this position the heart falls away from the midline so that the left ventricle can be identified by detecting medial retraction not apparent when the patient is supine. The right ventricle is normally palpable in the healthy newborn while the left ventricle is not. The normal dominance of the left ventricle develops as the infant grows and the chest begins to retract over the right ventricle.

As the right ventricle enlarges, normal left sternal border retraction is replaced by a positive systolic movement with lateral retraction in the region of the ventricular septum. A pure right ventricular impulse causes a positive movement at the left sternal edge with retraction at the apex. A pure left ventricular impulse causes a positive movement at the apex with medial retraction. With combined ventricular impulses, the positive movements at apex and left sternal edge are separated by an area of retraction near the intervening ventricular septum.

Systolic impulses of the aorta and pulmonary trunk may be seen and palpated. A dilated aortic root causes a distinct impulse in the 2nd or 3rd right interspace (aortic aneurysm), and a right aortic arch may cause a subtle right sternoclavicular impulse. Systolic distention of an enlarged pulmonary trunk (as in atrial septal defect or pulmonary hypertension) may transmit a systolic impulse in the 2nd left interspace.

Systolic expansion of dilated atria, especially in patients with mitral or tricuspid regurgitation, imparts distinctive movements to the chest wall. The left atrium is a posterior chamber, so systolic expansion moves the heart forward, the rigid vertebral column serving as an immobile fulcrum preventing posterior displacement. The movement may be mistaken for an intrinsic right ventricular impulse, but left atrial expansion occurs perceptibly later than the impulses imparted by either ventricle. This subtle difference in timing can be detected by simultaneously identifying S_1. Systolic expansion of an enlarged right atrium may cause an impulse to the right of the sternum in some patients with gross tricuspid regurgitation.

Vibrations and movements caused by heart sounds: Heart sounds may be palpable because of the intensity of their vibrations or because of the discrete precordial movements that they impart. The loud S_1 of mitral stenosis can generally be felt over the left ventricular impulse. Pulmonic ejection sounds are palpated in the 2nd left interspace and may wax with expiration and wane with inspiration. The impact of the pulmonic component of S_2 (pulmonary hypertension) is characteristically felt in the 2nd left interspace, although this sound may be palpated as a tap in some normal children or thin adults. An augmented atrial contribution to ventricular filling can be felt as presystolic distention of either the left or right ventricle and may be more readily detected by palpation than by the auscultatory counterpart (fourth heart sound [S_4]). Rapid ventricular filling may be associated with discrete mid-diastolic distention of the left ventricle corresponding to an abnormal third heart sound (S_3). A physiologic or normal S_3 is rarely palpable or visible.

A palpable murmur is called a thrill. Murmurs that reach or exceed Grade IV/VI commonly transmit their vibrations through the chest wall as thrills. A thrill should be defined in terms of its site of maximum intensity, the direction of its radiation from that site, and its duration. Thrills should be sought at each precordial site as well as in the neck (suprasternal notch, carotids, subclavians). Thrills may be better appreciated with the heads of the metacarpal bones than with the fingertips, although the hand should not be arched when the metacarpals are applied.

Auscultation

Accurate cardiac auscultation requires a quiet room, a comfortable patient, and a stethoscope equipped with bell, diaphragm, and well-fitting earpieces. Auscultation should not only be conducted in the supine, sitting, and left lateral positions, but should also be accompanied by appropriate physical maneuvers. Simple respiration or somewhat exaggerated inspiratory and expiratory excursions are useful in assessing S_2, a right-sided S_3 and S_4, and tricuspid murmurs. Isometric exercise (clenched fists), Valsalva's maneuver, squatting, and prompt standing are important in patients with mitral valve prolapse or hypertrophic obstructive cardiomyopathy.

Orderly auscultatory analysis requires identification of the phases of the cardiac cycle and their related acoustic events (see FIG. 22-2). S_1 and S_2 establish the framework into which murmurs and additional sounds can be placed. If a stethoscope is applied to the chest with the right hand, the thumb of the left hand can palpate the carotid pulse, the onset of which identifies the S_1 complex, even at rapid heart rates. Alternatively, S_1 and S_2 can be identified at the base of the heart (where the cadence and comparative intensities often make recognition easier). The stethoscope is then moved toward the sternal edge and apex in steps so that the auscultatory interpretation gained at the base is not lost. Once the framework of the basic cardiac cycle is established, the auscultatory events should be analyzed in sequence: S_1, systole, S_2, early diastole, mid-diastole, presystole. The sequence with which precordial sites are examined is best related to the normal direction of blood flow;

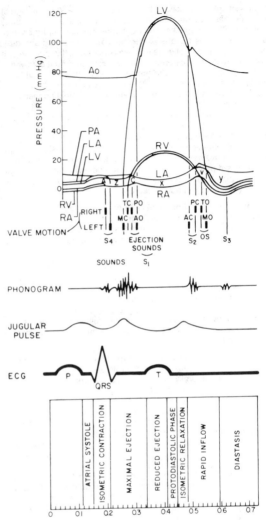

FIG. 22-2. **Diagram of the cardiac cycle,** showing records of valvular events, the pressure curves of the great vessels and cardiac chambers, heart sounds, jugular pulse wave, and the ECG. Valve motion: MC and MO, mitral component and opening; TC and TO, tricuspid component and opening; PC and PO, pulmonary component and opening; AC and AO, aortic component and opening; Ao, aorta; PA, pulmonary artery; LA, left atrium; LV, left ventricle; RA, right atrium; RV, right ventricle; OS, opening snap of atrioventricular valves. (Adapted from *The Heart,* ed. 3, edited by J. W. Hurst et al, copyright 1974 by McGraw-Hill, Inc.; and *A Primer of Cardiology,* ed. 4, by G. E. Burch, copyright 1971 by Lea & Febiger. Used with permission.)

i.e., the inflow valves—apex and lower left sternal edge—followed by the outflow valves—the left and right base. Repetitive use of a consistent sequence minimizes the chance of oversight. Attention should also be directed to nonprecordial sites, including the axilla, back, neck, and abdomen.

There are **4 basic heart sounds.** The S_1 complex is readily identified by timing with the carotid pulse. S_2 should always be assessed at the left base during respiration so that the aortic and pulmonic components can be properly recognized. The terms "A_2" and "P_2" should be applied to the aortic and pulmonic components, respectively, only when both are heard simultaneously, normally during inspiration at the left base. Variations in splitting and intensity of S_2 are important. S_3 and S_4 coincide with the 2 diastolic filling periods of each cardiac cycle—one passive and occurring in mid diastole, and the other initiated by active atrial contraction and occurring in presystole. These sounds may be normal (physiologic) or abnormal (pathologic). Their presence sometimes produces a cadence or **gallop rhythm**. A number of sounds are not found in the normal heart so their presence is immediately suspect; these sounds include opening snaps, ejection sounds, and mid-to-late systolic clicks. Ejection sounds can be either aortic or pulmonic. Opening snaps are almost always mitral, and mid-to-late systolic clicks almost always originate in the mitral apparatus (leaflet/chordal tensing in mitral prolapse).

A cardiovascular **murmur** is a relatively prolonged series of auditory vibrations. Analysis of a murmur should begin with assessing its intensity (loudness), frequency (pitch), configuration (shape), quality, duration, direction of radiation, and timing in the cardiac cycle. Diagnostic conclusions can then be drawn from murmurs that fit given descriptions. According to their timing within the cardiac cycle, there are 3 basic categories of murmurs—systolic, diastolic, and continuous. **Systolic murmurs** are best classified according to their time of onset and termination. A **midsystolic murmur** begins after S_1 and ends before S_2. A **holosystolic murmur** begins with S_1 and occupies all of systole, reaching S_2. **Early systolic murmurs** begin with S_1, diminish in a decrescendo fashion, and end well before S_2. **Late systolic murmurs**—often but not invariably introduced by mid-to-late systolic clicks—begin in mid-to-late systole and rise in a crescendo to S_2. **Diastolic murmurs** are best classified according to their time of onset. An **early diastolic murmur** begins with S_2; a **mid-diastolic murmur** begins at a clear interval after S_2; and a **late diastolic** (presystolic) **murmur** begins immediately before S_1. A **continuous murmur** starts in systole and continues without interruption through S_2 into all or part of diastole. A continuous murmur does not necessarily persist throughout the entire cardiac cycle.

The Chest and Abdomen

Examining the chest and abdomen is an important part of the cardiovascular physical diagnosis. The rales of alveolar edema are important features of pulmonary venous congestion in the adult, and are seldom heard in the infant in whom pulmonary edema is largely, if not exclusively, interstitial. In the latter setting, tachypnea, absent rales, and hepatomegaly identify congestive heart failure. Examination of the abdomen may focus on the splenomegaly of infective endocarditis, the ascites of constrictive pericarditis, or an aortic aneurysm in a hypertensive patient with abdominal pain or tenderness.

---

23. SPECIAL DIAGNOSTIC PROCEDURES

Constant correlation of clinical and laboratory information has advanced the inferences that can be drawn from clinical material alone. Laboratory study should clarify, discriminate, and quantify a relatively select number of diagnostic hypotheses derived from clinical appraisal. Specialized laboratory methods are divided into several general categories. The first includes noninvasive technics that can be applied with little or no special preparation of the patient, are safe and convenient, and cause no discomfort. Phonocardiograms, recordings of precordial displacement (apex- or kinetocardiograms), and especially echocardiograms extend the clinical appraisal and carry no risk. The second group includes stress testing (treadmill or, less commonly, bicycle exercise). The third group includes cardiac catheterization and related technics such as selective angiocardiography and intracardiac electrophysiologic investigations. These methods are not routine extensions of the clinical evaluation but should be reserved for problems that cannot be satisfactorily resolved without them. The selection of patients for such studies depends partly on the confidence with which clinical information from other sources can be assembled and interpreted. These special diagnostic procedures are discussed below.

NONINVASIVE DIAGNOSTIC PROCEDURES

THE ELECTROCARDIOGRAM

Interpretation of the ECG can be approached in either of two ways. The tracing can be used to support and extend impressions already gathered from the history, physical signs, and x-rays, or a clinical evaluation may begin with the ECG and be completed by gathering, interpreting, and relating the history, physical signs, and x-rays to the ECG. Thus, objective ECG impressions can be achieved without compromising the complete synthesis of the clinical information derived from other sources.

Optimum benefit from the interpretation of an ECG requires (1) a technically satisfactory tracing; (2) a descriptive analysis of each component of the tracing; and (3) diagnostic conclusions based upon these descriptive analyses. Electrophysiologic information extends materially the value of the ECG, especially in the interpretation of rhythm and conduction disturbances. The vectorcardiogram can often clarify complex or disputed features in the scalar ECG.

An analysis of the ECG should be conducted in the same sequence each time. The cardiac rhythm should be studied first. Using a relatively long strip of a single lead, generally lead II, will facilitate this analysis. P waves should first be sought, and the regularity or irregularity of the rhythm should be determined. A regular rhythm should be further identified as sinoatrial, junctional, infranodal, or artificially paced. An irregular rhythm may be completely erratic as in atrial fibrillation or may have a recurrent pattern, such as the group beating of simple bigeminy or Wenckebach periods. (See also CARDIAC ARRHYTHMIAS in Ch. 25.)

In analyzing the complexes and intervals, attention should be focused on the P wave, P-R interval, P-R segment, QRS complex, S-T segment, T wave, Q-T interval, and U wave. The electrical axis should be established, especially in the frontal plane. When completed, these descriptive analyses should suggest certain diagnoses, such as left or right atrial abnormality, ventricular hypertrophy, bundle branch block, fascicular block, aberrant ventricular conduction, myocardial ischemia or infarction, pericardial disease, nonspecific alterations in S-T segments or T waves, drug effect (e.g., digitalis), or metabolic fault (e.g., hyper- or hypokalemia, hyper- or hypocalcemia).

PHONOCARDIOGRAPHY

Graphic display of heart sounds and murmurs as recorded from chest wall microphones.

Cardiovascular sounds are recorded simultaneously from multiple sites along with the ECG, respiratory cycle, and one or more external cardiovascular impulses (carotid pulse, jugular venous pulse, apex cardiogram). Sound recordings usually are made from the 2nd and left intercostal spaces, the 4th intercostal space, and the cardiac apex. Filters are used to permit selective recording of high- and low-frequency events.

Phonocardiography and external pulse recordings have three principal uses. First, they provide a permanent objective record of acoustic data. Second, they are invaluable tools in teaching cardiac physical diagnosis. Finally, they permit detailed analysis of the temporal relationships and contours of heart sounds, murmurs, and impulses. Such analysis provides diagnostic and physiologic information that may elude a bedside examiner.

Common issues amenable to phonocardiographic analysis are discussed below. Reference to FIG. 23–1 will help to visualize the phenomena described.

Events around the first heart sound (S_1): S_1 may have as many as four components and an overall duration of up to 120 msec. At the bedside, differentiating a split S_1 from combinations with a fourth heart sound (S_4) or an S_1-ejection sound **(ES)** is often difficult. The phonocardiogram readily identifies an S_4 by the following features: onset before the QRS complex; simultaneous occurrence with the A wave of the apex cardiogram; lower frequency than S_1; apical localization of the left-sided S_4; localization at the lower left sternal edge; and inspiratory augmentation of the right-sided S_4. An aortic ES is identified by its close relationship to the carotid upstroke. Inspiratory diminution in intensity may identify a pulmonic ES.

Sequence and intensity of the components of the second heart sound (S_2): The relative intensity, direction of splitting, and respiratory behavior of the aortic and pulmonic components of S_2 **(S_2A and S_2P)** may be difficult to analyze at the bedside. On the phonocardiogram S_2A is identified by the fact that it always precedes the dicrotic notch of the carotid pulse tracing (usually by 40 msec or less) and comes closer to the Q wave of the ECG during inspiration than during expiration. S_2P has no fixed relationship to the carotid pulse tracing, and the Q-S_2P interval increases during inspiration and shortens during expiration.

Early diastolic sounds: Bedside differentiation of mitral and tricuspid opening snaps **(OS)** from the third heart sound **(S_3)** can be difficult. Phonocardiographically, the OS is higher in frequency than S_3 and occurs at or before the nadir (O point) of the apexcardiogram, 50 to 120 msec after S_2A. In contrast, S_3 is simultaneous with the rapid filling wave of the apexcardiogram and occurs 100 to 200 msec after S_2A.

Murmur timing and contours: Differentiation between early systolic, midsystolic, holosystolic, and late systolic murmurs and recognition of crescendo-decrescendo and plateau configurations are often made more easily by phonocardiography than by auscultation.

Abnormalities of the jugular venous pulse: Excessively large A waves occur when right atrial emptying is impaired by reduced right ventricular compliance or tricuspid valve obstruction. Obliteration of the X descent by a positive systolic wave is an important sign of tricuspid regurgitation. Delay in the Y descent is an important sign of tricuspid stenosis.

Abnormalities of the arterial pulse contour: The slowed upstroke of aortic stenosis and the brisk upstroke of aortic regurgitation and hypertrophic subaortic stenosis are readily demonstrated. The double systolic pulses due to aortic regurgitation, hypertrophic subaortic stenosis, or aortic stenosis and regurgitation can be distinguished from each other or from a prominent anacrotic notch in mild aortic stenosis.

Abnormalities of the apexcardiogram: Increased forcefulness of left atrial systole will, in the absence of mitral obstruction, generate a prominent A wave on the apexcardiogram (more than 17% of the total excursion). Pressure loading of the left ventricle produces an abnormally sustained systolic

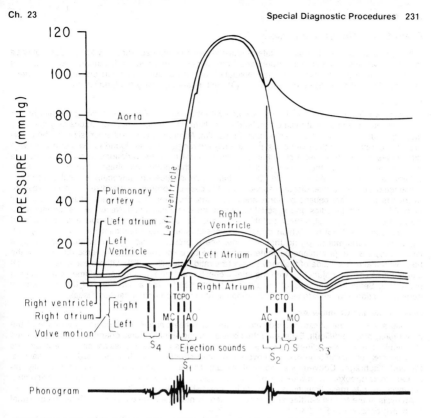

FIG. 23-1. **Schematic representation of the cardiac cycle,** showing pressure recordings from the right atrium and ventricle, pulmonary artery, left atrium and ventricle, and aorta. S₄, 4th heart sound; S₁, 1st heart sound; MC, mitral closure; TC, tricuspid closure; PO, pulmonic valve opening; AO, aortic valve opening; S₂ 2nd heart sound; AC, aortic closure; PC, pulmonic closure; TO, tricuspid opening; MO, mitral opening; OS, opening snap; S₃, 3rd heart sound. Time is on the horizontal axis, and the total duration of the record is one second. (Adapted from *The Heart,* ed. 3, edited by J. W. Hurst et al, copyright 1974 by McGraw-Hill, Inc. Used with permission.)

plateau. Bifid systolic plateaus of various types are seen in hypertrophic subaortic stenosis, mitral valve prolapse, coronary artery disease with segmental dyskinesia or aneurysm, and severe mitral regurgitation. The rapid filling wave is impaired by mitral stenosis, but accentuated by volume overloading of the left ventricle or severe left ventricular dysfunction.

Systolic time intervals: Simultaneous recording of the carotid pulse contour, ECG, and S₂A permits the measurement of total electromechanical systole (Q-S₂A interval), left ventricular ejection time (**LVET** = carotid upstroke to dicrotic notch), and the pre-ejection period (**PEP** = Q-S₂A minus LVET). Rate-corrected LVET tends to reflect alterations in stroke volume if left ventricular outflow obstruction is absent. The normal PEP/LVET ratio, which does not require rate correction, is 0.345 ± 0.036. Since nonvalvular heart disease tends to increase the ratio in proportion to the reduction of stroke volume, measurement of systolic time intervals may be a useful noninvasive index of left ventricular function.

RADIOLOGY

X-ray examination of the heart is essential to the diagnosis and management of many cardiac disorders. The major radiologic technics are (1) **plain chest roentgenography** (ordinarily frontal and lateral chest x-rays; in special cases oblique, inspiration-expiration, decubitus, or other views may be required); (2) **fluoroscopy;** (3) **cardiac ultrasonography;** (4) **angiocardiography** (including coronary arteriography); and (5) **radionuclide imaging** of the heart and evaluation of cardiac function. Plain chest films, fluoroscopy, and ultrasound are discussed here; angiography is discussed below and radionuclide imaging is discussed in Ch. 227.

PLAIN CHEST ROENTGENOGRAPHY

Interpretation of plain frontal and lateral chest x-rays has been advanced by knowledge obtained from observations at the time of surgery and from special roentgenographic studies. Examination of frontal and lateral chest films includes evaluation of the possibility of heart disease from 3 main aspects: (1) heart size, (2) heart shape, and (3) the lungs—especially the lung vasculature.

Heart Size

The conventional frontal chest x-ray is made with the patient close to and facing the film holder and with the x-ray source at least 6 ft behind the patient. This arrangement produces only a slightly magnified (usually < 10%) cardiac outline on the film. Although the overall heart size can be determined accurately from the plain chest film, the normal range has been found to overlap greatly with the ranges of abnormal heart size. Factors that account for wide variations in normal heart size include the heart rate, the phases of the heart cycle, the depth and phase of respiration, blood volume, and body weight and build. Overall heart size is often unequivocally normal despite the presence of severe cardiac disease, especially in the case of coronary artery disease and in pressure overloads such as are caused by aortic stenosis. Thus, precision in determining heart size is mainly helpful in statistical studies and in serial studies of the same individual. Nevertheless, certain judgments are of value, and observation of the plain chest film should permit categorization of the heart size as follows: (1) **normal** (which does not necessarily exclude significant cardiac disease); (2) **significantly abnormal** (implying that heart disease is present); and (3) **borderline** (necessarily a large group). Some physicians estimate cardiac size by comparing the transverse diameter of the heart with that of the inside of the bony thorax (the ratio is usually < 1:2). Others estimate the frontal cardiac area (or, in conjunction with the lateral chest x-ray, the total cardiac volume) when judging heart size. Serial comparisons of the same patient's heart sizes avoid many of the problems of normal variation and provide valuable information about the course of cardiac disease.

Heart Shape and Chamber Analysis

While a view of the chest may indicate an abnormal heart shape, determining the cause of the abnormality may be difficult. Estimating the sizes of the individual cardiac chambers from a plain film is difficult, and precise delineation of the heart chambers is usually impossible since the chambers are intimately clustered together and covered by other structures, such as pericardium, mediastinal fat, and diaphragm. Conventional signs of specific chamber enlargement, often dogmatically described in textbooks, are frequently difficult to apply, and in some cases are frankly misleading. However, despite these limitations, study of the heart shape is worthwhile.

Analysis of the frontal cardiac silhouette is aided by noting 4 segments along the **left mediastinal (or heart) border** (see FIG. 23–2a).

1. The upper or first segment is the convexity made by the lateral profile of the distal aortic arch, which tends to become more prominent as the aorta becomes more tortuous and enlarges with age. This segment is characteristically continuous with the margin of the descending aorta on the chest film.

2. The second segment is related to the main pulmonary artery margin and becomes relatively more prominent when the main pulmonary artery enlarges in response to pulmonary hypertension or the poststenotic dilation of pulmonary valve stenosis.

3. The third segment is a concave margin in most adults. This is the region of the left atrial appendage, and when the left atrium enlarges, this segment tends to become straight or, more significantly, convex.

4. The fourth segment of the left heart border is the ventricular region, a convexity usually produced by the lateral aspects of the left ventricle, though when the right ventricle is very large, it may form this border in the frontal projection.

On the **right mediastinal (or heart) border** (see FIG. 23–2a), 2 major segments should be routinely noted:

1. The upper segment in young people is usually the lateral aspect of the superior vena cava, while in older people this margin is more commonly produced by the ascending aorta.

2. The lower convex segment on the right border is the lateral contour of the right atrium. This segment tends to become more prominent and longer in the presence of right atrial enlargement; it can also be made more prominent by simple displacement of the right atrium due to enlargement of other parts of the heart or because of pericardial effusion. The azygous vein is often seen on the frontal chest film as an ovoid increase in density just lateral to the right main bronchus. This structure may dilate in response to venous and right atrial pressure elevation. The azygous vein also varies greatly in size because of the relative pressure changes produced by respiratory effort. Also, a paratracheal lymph node may not be distinguishable from the azygous vein on a single chest film.

The **lateral chest film** (FIG. 23–2b) is useful in evaluating heart size and configuration since the lateral dimensions of the mediastinum and heart are shown and can be measured and compared. A margin of the intrathoracic inferior vena cava, concave posteriorly, is usually seen just above the right diaphragm. It is typically pushed back by a large right atrium and ventricle, while with left ventricular dilation this region is overlapped progressively by the posterior aspect of the left ventricle. The right ventricle and the main pulmonary artery form the anterior and anterior-superior aspects of the lateral heart silhouette. Increased prominence of these margins, especially extension of

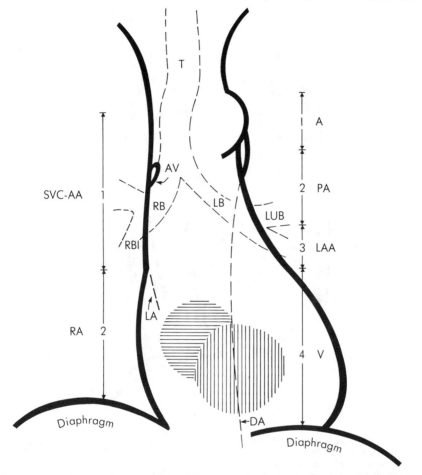

FIG. 23–2a. Diagram of normal adult heart as shown on the frontal chest roentgenogram. The left border of the mediastinum is divided into 4 segments: (1) distal aortic arch segment; (2) main pulmonary artery segment; (3) left atrial appendage segment; (4) ventricular segment. The right border is divided into 2 segments: (1) the superior vena cava or ascending aortic segment; (2) right atrial segment. LA indicates the right margin of the left atrium, often seen in this region in the normal person; T, trachea; AV, azygous vein; RB, right main bronchus; RBI, right intermediate bronchus; LB, left main bronchus; LUB, left upper lobe bronchus; DA, left margin of descending aorta. The horizontally-lined area represents usual position of the aortic valve, while the vertically-lined area represents usual position of the mitral valve. The tracheal and main bronchial outlines are shown. (From *Nomenclature and Criteria for Diagnosis of Diseases of the Heart and Great Vessels*, ed. 8, 1979. Copyright 1979 by the Criteria Committee of the New York Heart Association, Inc. Used with permission.)

the cardiac density superiorly in the retrosternal region, is a sign of right ventricular dilation. Such changes, however, are easily confused with the increased density in the same general region that may be caused by a dilated tortuous ascending aorta. In the lateral view the right and left hilar arteries and major bronchi are often well seen. The posterior upper aspect of the heart silhouette (in the region overlying the spine) is typically produced by the left atrium. Since ordinarily the esophagus courses directly posterior to the left atrium, this margin of the heart may be more precisely observed after opacifying the esophagus by ingestion of barium sulfate. Prominence of this posterior border of the heart and secondary displacement of the esophagus is typical of left atrial dilation.

Meaningful analysis of the cardiac configuration is aided by appreciation of 2 important points:
    1. **The left atrium is of pivotal importance in cardiac chamber analysis,** since the margins of this chamber can usually be appreciated on the frontal chest film. The maximal outline of the left atrium

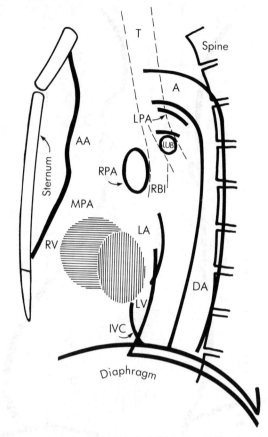

FIG. 23–2b.   **Diagram of normal adult heart in the left lateral projection.** A, aorta; LPA, left pulmonary artery at left hilus arching over LUB, circular image of left upper lobe bronchus; RPA, right pulmonary artery at right hilus; LA, dorsal margin of left atrium; LV, dorsal margin of left ventricle; IVC, dorsal margin of intrathoracic inferior vena cava; RV, ventral margin of right ventricular outflow tract; MPA, ventral margin of main pulmonary artery; AA, ventral margin of ascending aorta; RBI, right intermediate bronchus; DA, descending thoracic aorta; T, trachea. The horizontally-lined area represents usual position of the aortic valve, while the vertically-lined area represents usual position of the mitral valve. (From *Nomenclature and Criteria for Diagnosis of Diseases of the Heart and Great Vessels,* ed. 8, 1979. Copyright 1979 by the Criteria Committee of the New York Heart Association, Inc. Used with permission.)

can be approximated by noting the positions of (1) the right main and intermediate and left main bronchial air shadows; (2) the second (or double) contour produced by the left atrium, usually seen close to the right heart border; (3) the left heart margin in the region of the left atrial appendage (Segment 3); (4) the general increase in heart density in the region of the left atrium when it has a prominent posterior bulge; and (5) mitral valve or valve anulus calcification when present.

The lateral view, especially with barium in the esophagus, is helpful in locating the posterior margins of the left atrium, particularly since slight left atrial enlargement is most impressive along its dorsal margin. A disproportionately enlarged left atrium deforms the cardiac silhouette by producing notable bronchial displacement, a straightening or especially a convexity of the left heart border, or an unusually prominent double contour on the right. In most cases of chronic left ventricular disease, the left atrial enlargement parallels but is not disproportionate to that of the left ventricle. In acute left ventricular dilation, the left atrium typically does not enlarge as much as the ventricle. Atrial fibrillation increases atrial size. The left atrium may be exceptionally small in some disorders; e.g., atrial septal defect.

2. The individual ventricular outlines cannot be clearly discriminated from each other on the basis of the silhouette of the ventricular region of the heart alone. On the frontal chest film the part of the heart per se to the left of the midline and not accounted for by left atrium can be considered the ventricular region. In adults, enlargement of this region is due to left ventricular enlargement in over 90% of cases, but in some cases right ventricular dilation or pericardial effusion can produce precisely the same appearance. Lengthening of the long axis of the ventricular region and its lateral margin toward the left costophrenic angle suggests left ventricular dilation. On the lateral view increased thickness of the heart at the level of the diaphragm also favors left ventricular enlargement. Calcifications in aortic or mitral valves, in coronary arteries, or in old myocardial infarcts, when present, help to identify the outline of the left ventricle.

Since the right ventricle seldom forms a border in the frontal projection, its dilation produces only nonspecific enlargement of the ventricular region. Dilation of the right ventricle does, however, tend to displace its outflow tract and the main pulmonary artery cephalad and to the left, resulting, on the lateral view, in encroachment on the retrosternal clear space from below. The value of this feature is limited in diagnosing right ventricular enlargement since it can be mimicked by a prominent ascending aorta or even a normal thymus gland (especially if the anterior-posterior dimension of the mediastinum is small).

The Lungs and the Pulmonary Vasculature

The pulmonary vasculature provides information concerning many aspects of the circulatory state and, in particular, of left ventricular function. The size of central pulmonary arteries (the main pulmonary artery and its hilar branches) provides an index of the pulmonary artery pressure. The sizes of the more peripheral pulmonary vessels reflect pulmonary blood volume and are also rough indicators of the pulmonary BP and flow. Prominence of the region of the right ventricular outflow tract and especially dilation of the central pulmonary arteries are the most important signs suggesting right ventricular enlargement. Dilation of the main pulmonary arteries (after discounting the effects of aging and normal variations) indicates pulmonary hypertension or poststenotic dilation; right ventricular hypertension is implied, and right ventricular hypertrophy and/or dilation is almost certainly present.

High pulmonary capillary pressure (> 22 mm Hg) secondary to left heart dysfunction produces pulmonary edema. Interstitial edema shows as a linear pattern with increased prominence of the interstitial architecture of the lungs, including the interlobular septa. Alveolar pulmonary edema presents as a more homogeneous lung density, often in a patchy distribution, due to filling of the peripheral air spaces with fluid. Alveolar edema produces the typical clinical picture of pulmonary edema, but in most cases of pulmonary edema both alveolar and interstitial components are present. Edema of either type tends to obliterate the outlines of the peripheral lung vasculature. In left heart failure loss of visibility of the peripheral lung vasculature due to edema occurs first in the lower lungs. Even mild elevation of the pulmonary vascular pressures secondary to left heart failure causes some changes on the chest film. An early change is increased distention of the peripheral vasculature of the upper lungs, where the vessels are normally relatively small because of low intravascular pressure in the erect position. The peripheral vessels in the lower lungs tend to appear smaller with increasing left heart and pulmonary capillary pressures, ultimately becoming invisible because of pulmonary edema. FIG. 23-3 diagrams several characteristic x-ray patterns of the pulmonary vasculature.

CARDIAC FLUOROSCOPY

Cardiac fluoroscopy has limited diagnostic value and gives the patient a relatively large dose of radiation. However, it is often worthwhile in the initial workup of perplexing patients with significant valvular or congenital heart disease and in a number of special diagnostic situations. Fluoroscopy is most worthwhile for detecting cardiac calcifications (valvular, pericardial, myocardial, tumorous, or coronary), unusual pulsations, effects of respiratory motion, and esophageal displacement (by the left atrium, great vessels, etc.), and for noting the position and motion of epicardial fat in relation to the cardiac borders in suspected pericardial effusion.

ULTRASOUND

The principles and technics of ultrasound are discussed further in Ch. 226. The principal use of ultrasound in the diagnosis of cardiovascular disorders is **echocardiography**. This noninvasive diagnostic tool uses pulsed-reflected ultrasound to visualize internal cardiac structures. The ultrasonic transducer is placed over the surface of the chest, usually along the left sternal border, and the ultrasonic beam is directed toward various portions of the heart. Occasionally the transducer will be placed in the subxiphoid area, in the suprasternal notch, or in the supraclavicular area. Every cardiac structure that is roughly perpendicular to the ultrasonic beam will be recorded on the oscilloscope. All 4 cardiac valves can be visualized, and internal dimensions of both ventricles and the left atrium can be measured. If the structure intersected by the ultrasonic beam moves, a wavy line is inscribed on the echocardiogram. A stationary structure like the chest wall is visualized as a straight line. Ultrasound does not traverse air or bone well, and satisfactory echocardiograms are difficult to obtain in patients with emphysema or thick chests.

FIG. 23-4 shows a diagram of an echocardiogram as the ultrasonic beam is directed toward the apex of the heart (position 1) and then is gradually moved toward the base of the heart (position 4).

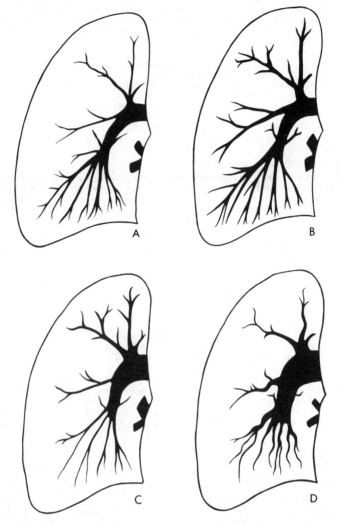

FIG. 23–3. **Diagrams of the pulmonary vasculature** as shown on the frontal chest film in erect adult (right lung).
   A. *Normal pulmonary vasculature.* Note that the larger peripheral vessels are in the lower lung.
   B. *General increase in prominence of pulmonary vasculature.* Typical of large left-to-right shunts in congenital heart disease and high blood volume–high output states; e.g., anemia, pregnancy, overhydration.
   C. *Distended upper lung field vessels and relatively small lower lung field vessels* (which may not be visible in the presence of edema), typical of chronic left heart failure; e.g., severe mitral stenosis.
   D. *Dilated tortuous central pulmonary arteries with relatively small peripheral pulmonary arteries,* typical of acquired chronic severe pulmonary hypertension due to a high peripheral pulmonary resistance. (From *Nomenclature and Criteria for Diagnosis of Diseases of the Heart and Great Vessels,* ed. 8, 1979. Copyright 1979 by the Criteria Committee of the New York Heart Association, Inc. Used with permission.)

Initially, the ultrasonic beam traverses part of the right and left ventricles in the vicinity of the posterior papillary muscle **(PPM).** In this position, one can visualize the chest wall, the anterior right ventricular wall, a small portion of the right ventricular cavity, the interventricular septum, the left ventricular cavity, the PPM, the posterior left ventricular wall, and the lung. As the beam begins to move toward the base of the heart, the PPMs become continuous with structures originating from the mitral valve. One can again see the cavities of the right and left ventricles, together with the interven-

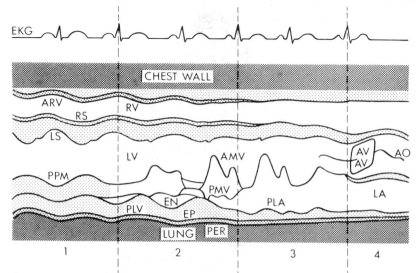

Fig. 23–4. **Diagram of an M-mode scan of the heart** from the apex (1) to the base (4) of the heart. ARV, anterior right ventricular wall; RV, right ventricular cavity; RS, right side of the interventricular septum; LS, left side of the interventricular septum; LV, left ventricular cavity; PPM, posterior papillary muscle; PLV, posterior left ventricular wall; EN, posterior left ventricular endocardium; EP, posterior left ventricular epicardium; PER, pericardium; AMV, anterior mitral valve leaflet; PMV, posterior mitral valve leaflet; PLA, posterior left atrial wall; AV, aortic valve; AO, aorta; LA, cavity of the left atrium. (From H. Feigenbaum: "Clinical Applications of Echocardiography," in *Progr. Cardiovasc. Diseases* 14: 531–558, May 1972. Used by permission of Grune & Stratton, Inc., and the author.)

tricular septum and the posterior left ventricular wall. With further movement of the ultrasonic beam toward the base of the heart, the mitral valve assumes its maximum amplitude and the anterior mitral valve inscribes a characteristic "M" appearance during diastole. The left ventricular wall now becomes the posterior left atrial wall. Moving even further medially and superiorly, the ultrasonic beam traverses the root of the aorta and the body of the left atrium. Within the aortic root, 2 of the aortic valve leaflets produce a box-like configuration during systole. Further changes in the direction of the ultrasonic beam allow echoes from the tricuspid valve and the pulmonic valve to be recorded.

Two-dimensional or cross-sectional echocardiography provides spatially correct images of the heart that are important supplements to the standard M-mode examination. These "real time" images are recorded on videotape or movie film and look much like cineangiograms. Three frames from a two-dimensional echocardiogram are shown in Fig. 23–5.

The Mitral Valve

Mitral stenosis: The first cardiovascular abnormality for which echocardiography was shown to be useful in diagnosis was mitral stenosis. In mitral stenosis normal closure of the anterior leaflet of the mitral valve in early diastole is decreased. Movement of the posterior mitral leaflet is also altered; instead of moving opposite to the anterior leaflet, it moves in the same direction, resulting in marked diminution of the distance between the 2 leaflets during diastole. The echocardiographic appearance of the valve can assess the degree of fibrosis or restriction of motion, thus helping to decide whether a commissurotomy will be successful or whether the valve must be replaced. With two-dimensional echocardiography, the stenotic mitral orifice and the degree of stenosis can be visualized.

Other mitral valve abnormalities: The mitral valve echogram is also useful in diagnosing a prolapsed mitral valve; the echocardiogram shows a posterior or downward displacement of the posterior and frequently the anterior mitral leaflet during systole. Completely disrupted mitral valves also have a characteristic echocardiographic appearance. Torn chordae or flail valves show chaotic motion both during systole and diastole. Valvular vegetations 3 mm or more in diameter frequently produce distinctive echoes on the mitral valve leaflets. With aortic insufficiency, the mitral valve leaflets usually exhibit a very fine fluttering motion during diastole.

Physiologic mitral valve data: The motion of the mitral valve echoes is related to the left ventricular diastolic pressure. When the left ventricular diastolic pressure is elevated in patients with aortic

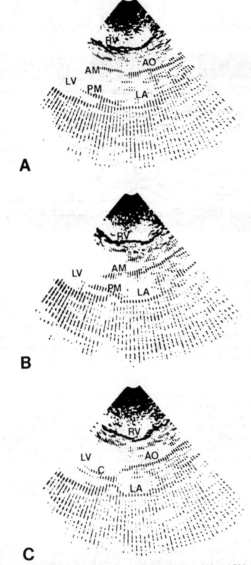

FIG. 23–5.　**Three frames from a two-dimensional echocardiogram.** AM and PM, the anterior and poste-rior mitral leaflets; C, chordae tendineae; LV, left ventricle; LA, left atrium; and AO, aorta in early diastole (A), mid-diastole (B), and systole (C). FIG. 23–5A, taken in early diastole, shows the mitral leaflets fully opened. In FIG. 23–5B, a mid-diastolic frame, the mitral valve is partially closed. The closed mitral valve with chordae tendineae attached is recorded in the systolic frame (FIG. 23–5C).

insufficiency, premature closure of the mitral valve is frequent. In coronary artery disease or left ventricular hypertrophy, the atrial component of the left ventricular pressure is markedly elevated and distorts the closure of the mitral valve characteristically. The onset of closure begins earlier and the completion of closure is delayed. When left ventricular diastolic pressure is elevated throughout diastole, as in congestive heart failure, the rate of opening of the mitral valve is decreased. The separation between the 2 mitral valve leaflets may also give a gross estimation of the amount of blood flowing through this orifice.

Other Cardiac Valves

Less diagnostic information is obtained from the aortic valve echogram than from the mitral valve. With aortic stenosis, the number of echoes from the aortic valve leaflet is increased. Echocardiography can detect a thickened aortic valve but M-mode echocardiography rarely provides information concerning the degree of stenosis. Two-dimensional echocardiography is improving our ability to diagnose congenital aortic stenosis and to quantitate the degree of stenosis. Vegetations on the aortic valve can be detected as a mass of eccentrically placed echoes with no restriction of motion of the leaflets. Information that can be obtained about the tricuspid and pulmonary valves is also limited. The diastolic slope of the tricuspid valve is decreased in the presence of tricuspid stenosis. Ebstein's anomaly produces a characteristic echocardiogram. The pulmonary valve echogram is useful in diagnosing pulmonary hypertension and pulmonary stenosis.

Evaluation of Cardiac Chambers

Echocardiography provides internal dimensions for both ventricles and the left atrium. The left ventricular internal dimensions are between the interventricular septum and the posterior left ventricular wall. The thickness of the posterior left ventricular wall and the interventricular septum can also be measured, and left ventricular dilation can be distinguished from left ventricular hypertrophy. From the dimensions during both systole and diastole, the corresponding ventricular volumes and the vigor with which the ventricle contracts can be estimated, provided that the ventricle contracts uniformly and is not grossly distorted in shape. In patients with segmental heart disease, as occurs with coronary artery disease, echocardiography can be used to assess the contractility of the individual segments of the left ventricular chamber. Cross-sectional echocardiography of the left ventricle can evaluate areas of the chamber not recorded on the M-mode tracing, determine the extent of myocardial damage, and detect ventricular aneurysms. These additional capabilities of ultrasonic examination are particularly useful in patients with coronary artery disease.

The right ventricular dimension obtained by echocardiography is particularly useful in detecting right ventricular dilation with volume overload states such as atrial septal defect. In addition to increasing the distance between the anterior right ventricular wall and the right ventricular interventricular septum, a right ventricular volume overload usually produces paradoxic or flat motion of the interventricular septum. When a pressure overload dilates the right ventricle, the interventricular septum retains its normal motion. Left bundle branch block also produces a characteristically abnormal pattern of septal motion.

The left atrial dimension on echocardiography correlates well with angiographic left atrial size and is considerably more accurate than estimations of left atrial size from plain chest x-rays and fluoroscopy. A dimension for the root of the aorta can also be obtained. Echocardiography may be helpful in detecting dissection of the root of the aorta.

Cardiac Tumors

One of the most dramatic uses of echocardiography is in the detection of atrial tumors, usually left atrial myxomas. These are commonly pedunculated and attached by a long stalk in the left atrium, so they plop in and out of the mitral orifice behind the mitral valve. On the echocardiogram, a mass of echoes is seen just behind the anterior leaflet of the mitral valve during diastole. With ventricular systole, this mass of echoes appears within the body of the left atrium. Right atrial tumors are less common but also can be detected echocardiographically; these tumors appear as a mass of echoes in the vicinity of the tricuspid valve. Ventricular tumors have also been seen echocardiographically.

Hypertrophic Subaortic Stenosis

Echocardiography is exceptionally useful in idiopathic hypertrophic subaortic stenosis. Demonstrable bulging or anterior displacement of the anterior mitral leaflet during systole is quantitatively related to the degree of subvalvular obstruction present. In addition, a midsystolic closure of the aortic valve corresponds to the reduction of aortic valve flow with the obstruction. Thirdly, and possibly most specifically, the hypertrophied interventricular septum can be found. The septal hypertrophy is usually out of proportion to the thickness of the posterior left ventricular wall.

Congenital Heart Disease

Many congenital anomalies can be detected by echocardiography, including atrial septal defect, pulmonary stenosis, discrete subaortic stenosis, supravalvular aortic stenosis, coarctation of the aorta, patent ductus arteriosus, transposition of the great vessels, hypoplastic right and left ventricles, Ebstein's anomaly, atrioventricular canal abnormalities, tetralogy of Fallot, truncus arteriosus, double outlet right ventricle, and a variety of cardiac malpositions. Echocardiography is particularly useful in newborn infants and in deciphering some of the more complicated congenital abnormalities seen in pediatric cardiology.

Pericardial Effusion

Pericardial fluid appears on the echocardiogram as a relatively echo-free space between the posterior left ventricular epicardium and the pericardium. In addition, a similar echo-free space frequently occurs between the chest wall echoes and the anterior right ventricular wall echo. Echocardiographic detection of pericardial effusion is extremely sensitive and reliable and is the diagnostic procedure of choice when available.

Doppler Ultrasound

Doppler ultrasound is also used to diagnose cardiovascular disorders. This modality primarily records the **velocity of moving echoes,** usually moving columns of blood, and is particularly useful in diagnosing peripheral vascular disease. Recently the Doppler technic has been combined with pulsed ultrasound to make recording the velocity of intracardiac blood possible. This development promises to provide significant diagnostic information (see also Ch. 226).

INVASIVE DIAGNOSTIC PROCEDURES

VENOUS CUTDOWN AND CANNULATION

Venous cutdown and cannulation are necessary when it is impossible or hazardous to locate a vein large enough for a needle to enter percutaneously; e.g., when a patient is in shock and all normally accessible veins are collapsed, is obese, or is very young. The procedure is also used when large amounts of fluid must be given rapidly (e.g., in cardiac arrest). Indwelling catheters extending from the cephalic, external or internal jugular, or subclavian vein into the superior vena cava may be used to administer hypertonic solutions and to measure central venous pressure (see below). For brief periods of cannulation, the cephalic vein in the upper arm is often used.

Procedure: For extremities, a tourniquet is applied and the vein is palpated. Using antiseptic precautions and local anesthesia, the skin is incised; strict asepsis must be maintained around the insertion site, because an indwelling venous catheter or cannula may result in nosocomial infection or phlebitis. The vein is exposed and ligated; a second ligature, passed proximal to the first, under the vein, is left untied. The vein is then cut partially through between the 2 ligatures. The tourniquet is released. A saline-filled cannula, catheter, or large-bore needle (at least 16-gauge) is inserted into the vein opening, and the second ligature is tied around it just tightly enough to secure it. To avoid possible obstruction of the catheter or cannula, it is connected immediately to an IV infusion. The wound is closed with interrupted sutures; one suture holds the catheter in place. Sterile dressings are applied and the tubing is securely taped until fluid administration has been completed. The catheter or cannula should be changed if local pain, swelling, and erythema appear or if FUO occurs. The cannula is removed by withdrawing it gently after cutting the holding suture, and a pressure dressing is applied.

MEASUREMENT OF CENTRAL VENOUS PRESSURE

The central venous pressure **(CVP)** reflects right ventricular end-diastolic pressure or preload. It is an extremely poor indicator of left ventricular function. CVP monitoring of cardiac response to blood volume changes requires extreme caution, particularly in treating congestive heart failure. In general, a hypotensive patient with a CVP < 5 mm Hg may be given fluid safely, although the hypotension may not be reversed. Fluid must be given with caution if the CVP is more than 15 mm Hg, since it will not usually reverse the hypotension. Because CVP is an unreliable guide to volume status or to left ventricular function, pulmonary artery catheterization (see below) should be considered if cardiovascular instability persists after trial therapy.

Procedure: The superior vena cava may be reached percutaneously or by venous cutdown (see above) via the cephalic, subclavian, or internal or external jugular vein. Percutaneous subclavian vein catheterization is used most often. The patient's legs are elevated to distend the vein and the skin is prepared with antiseptic. A percutaneous needle-catheter (14-gauge; 17-gauge for infants) attached to a 10-ml syringe is used to enter the vein, usually from below the clavicle. Gentle backpressure is maintained once the needle pierces the skin; dark blood flows into the syringe when the vein is entered. To reduce the risk of air embolism, the patient inhales deeply and then holds his breath (Valsalva's maneuver) while the syringe is quickly removed and the catheter is inserted through the needle into the vein. The syringe is replaced and the return of blood is ensured; the catheter is then connected to an IV infusion with a 3-way valve inserted into the tubing, and the catheter is taped securely to the chest. A chest x-ray will verify the position of the catheter and exclude the possibility of pneumothorax.

To monitor the CVP, a manometer is attached to the 3-way valve and a "zero reference point" (e.g., the midaxillary line) is selected and marked on the patient's skin with tape. CVP is recorded at end exhalation with the patient supine and the base of the manometer at the level of the "zero point." The valve is opened to fill the manometer with fluid, then changed to allow direct communication between the subclavian vein and the manometer. The fluid level in the manometer should fall (to the CVP), then fluctuate slightly with respiration. Once the reading is taken, the 3-way valve is adjusted to allow resumption of the IV infusion.

Precautions: Patients must be warned that sudden movements could dislodge the indwelling catheter. Thrombophlebitis is less likely with subclavian cannulation than with external jugular or cephalic. The risk of sepsis is always present with an indwelling catheter. One form of septic complication results from catheter damage to the tricuspid valve and bacterial endocarditis (especially seen in burn patients). The usual infectious complication relates to a bacteremia originating from platelet-fibrin deposits on the catheter tip, or a local cellulitis originating from the site of skin perforation.

The hazard of pneumothorax should discourage the use of subclavian punctures in patients with chest injury and in those patients with particularly stiff or low-compliant lungs. In addition, placement should not be distal to an injury; e.g., after liver trauma an upper torso placement is proper.

CARDIAC CATHETERIZATION

A primarily diagnostic technic in which a flexible catheter is passed along veins or arteries into the heart in order to explore the heart structure, to measure pressures and blood-gas levels in the heart chambers and associated blood vessels, and to inject radiopaque dyes for angiography (see below).

Indications

Cardiac catheterization provides otherwise unavailable information in many types of heart disease. Its earliest use was to verify the presence of a septal defect or patent ductus arteriosus by passing the catheter through it. Congenital and acquired malformations of the heart can be accurately described from the results of catheterization, and thus corrective surgery can be better planned. Measurements of blood-gas levels at various points may enable localization and quantification of a shunt. BP measurements at various points in the heart and great vessels and calculation of pressure gradients across valves provide useful quantitative information. Calculations of cardiac output and vascular resistance may also be diagnostically useful in some patients.

Patients referred for cardiac catheterization include those in whom noninvasive studies have not provided a diagnosis, those in whom medical treatment is no longer effective and surgery is contemplated, and those for whom more precise definition of the extent and severity of the heart lesion is sought. Also, cardiac catheterization is often the most accurate means of acquiring data needed in clinical research. Infants with congenital heart disease are referred for cardiac catheterization when an exact diagnosis is needed for early surgery; their small size and grave illness call for careful technic in performing the procedure, but many of the same principles of adult catheterization apply.

Emergency cardiac catheterization is rarely indicated in adult cardiology. Rapid cardiac catheterization may be employed in cardiac tamponade since pericardial fluid may be demonstrated by angiography. Pulmonary embolism with hemodynamic deterioration can be rapidly diagnosed by pulmonary angiography. Bypass grafting for coronary artery disease may create new indications for emergency cardiac catheterization; unstable angina (or preinfarction syndrome) and even uncomplicated myocardial infarctions in young patients seen within 2 to 4 h of the onset of symptoms may be indications for emergency catheterization and coronary angiography if bypass grafting is contemplated. Sound medical judgment and common sense are important in reaching a decision.

Contraindications

There is no absolute contraindication to cardiac catheterization. Coexisting medical problems involving other organ systems, such as overwhelming infection and irreversible brain damage, are relative contraindications. Catheterization should be avoided in severe congestive heart failure unless surgery is contemplated to alleviate this condition.

Data

Measurements that are usually made during cardiac catheterization include intracardiac pressures, pressure pulse tracings, and blood-gas saturations. Cardiac output and vascular resistance can be calculated. Various other substances (e.g., pyruvates, lactates, and citrates) can be analyzed in arterial and coronary sinus blood to obtain information on myocardial metabolism.

Imaging with radiopaque dyes is discussed in ANGIOGRAPHY, below, and in Ch. 227.

Pressures: BP can be measured in both atria, both ventricles, the pulmonary arteries, and the peripheral arteries as the catheter is passed through those parts of the heart (see TABLE 23–1 for normal values). The **pulmonary capillary wedge pressure** is often measured during catheterization of the right side of the heart; the catheter is advanced into a pulmonary artery until it will go no further. Blood samples taken in the "wedged" position are as highly oxygenated as peripheral arterial samples, and the pressure tracing (which is lower than the pulmonary artery pressure and rises suddenly when the catheter is withdrawn) reflects that of the left atrium. Changes in the pulmonary capillary wedge pressure are similar to changes in left atrial pressure except in rare instances when there is obstruction of the pulmonary veins.

"Pressure gradients," *differences of pressure across a valve*, are the most accurate means of evaluating valvular function. Normal pressure pulse tracings are shown in FIG. 22–1. The normal atrial pressure curve consists of (1) a small rise caused by atrial contraction (A wave), followed by a fall (X descent); (2) a momentary rise due to valvular closure and early ventricular systole (C wave); (3) a fall with ventricular systole and "descent of the base" (moving the "floor" of the atrium downward); (4) a steady rise as blood flows in from the great veins while ventricular contraction continues (V wave); (5) a sudden fall as the atrioventricular valves open (Y descent); and (6) a second steady rise as blood flows in from the great veins while the atrioventricular valves remain open—"diastasis."

Mitral or tricuspid stenosis causes high atrial pressure, with slow fall in early diastole. In mitral or tricuspid insufficiency, ventricular systole produces a prominent atrial systolic V wave. The slow-rising "anacrotic" aortic pulse in aortic stenosis and the "collapsing" pulse in aortic insufficiency are well shown in arterial pressure tracings. When the heart fails as a pump, one of the earliest indices of myocardial failure may be a rise in the ventricular end-diastolic pressure to > 12 mm Hg in

TABLE 23-1. NORMAL PRESSURES IN HEART AND GREAT VESSELS

Pressures (mm Hg)	Average	Range
Right atrium	2.8	1 – 5
Right ventricle		
Peak-systolic	25	17 – 32
End-diastolic	4	1 – 7
Pulmonary artery		
Mean	15	9 – 19
Peak-systolic	25	17 – 32
End-diastolic	9	4 – 13
Pulmonary artery wedge		
Mean	9	4.5 – 13
Left atrium		
Mean	7.9	2 – 12
A Wave	10.4	4 – 16
V Wave	12.8	6 – 21
Left ventricle		
Peak-systolic	130	90 – 140
End-diastolic	8.7	5 – 12
Brachial artery		
Mean	85	70 – 105
Peak-systolic	130	90 – 140
End-diastolic	70	60 – 90

Modified from N. O. Fowler, *Cardiac Diagnosis and Treatment*, ed. 2. Copyright 1976 by Harper & Row, Publishers, Inc. Used with permission.

the left ventricle or > 5 mm Hg in the right ventricle. With continued high end-diastolic ventricular pressures, cardiac dilation eventually results. When ventricular distensibility is reduced (e.g., in constrictive pericarditis or stiffened endocardium or myocardium), atrial pressure curves exhibit a W form: an early diastolic dip ("snap-open" effect), followed by a sharp dip caused by descent of the base, succeeded in turn by a plateau. With restricted ventricular filling (as may occur in constrictive pericarditis, pericardial tamponade, infiltrative myocardiopathies, and occasionally in biventricular failure), an early diastolic component of ventricular pressure tracings resembles the square root sign; i.e., a sudden dip followed by a plateau.

Normally there is no significant difference between right atrial and right ventricular diastolic pressures, but the right atrial tracing is ventricularized in tricuspid insufficiency. There is normally no gradient between the left ventricle and the aorta during systole; however, there is a clear difference between pressure tracings taken from the aorta and those in the systemic arteries. The distal arteries reflect a higher pulse pressure than the central aorta by 30 to 40%. These changes are usually ascribed to resonance characteristics in the peripheral arteries.

The diastolic pressures of the left ventricle in conjunction with accurate volume data may help to describe the compliance characteristics of that chamber. In the absence of information on left ventricular volume, however, pressure elevations cannot be ascribed solely to decreased compliance.

Blood gases: Normal values are shown in TABLE 23-2. A central circulatory shunt is an abnormal communication between the pulmonary and systemic circulations connecting either of the 2 pairs of cardiac chambers or the great vessels. Blood may be shunted from left to right, from right to left, or in both directions. Determination of O_2 content of blood at different levels within the heart and great vessels aids in determining the presence, direction, and volume of central shunts. Left-to-right shunts under 15% usually cannot be detected by blood-O_2 sampling. Since 1 gm of Hb normally combines at sea level with 1.33 ml of O_2, O_2 content can be calculated from measurement of O_2 saturation and Hb.

The O_2 saturation of blood in the superior vena cava and pulmonary artery is approximately equal; blood in the inferior vena cava usually has a much higher O_2 saturation because of the relatively higher oxygenation of renal venous blood. Blood in the coronary sinus is markedly desaturated. Significant mixing does not occur in the right atrium and possibly not in the right ventricle; therefore, "mixed venous" blood is usually obtained from pulmonary arteries.

A 10% increase in O_2 saturation of the right side of the heart may indicate a left-to-right shunt. The maximal difference in O_2 content between the pulmonary artery and the right ventricle is 0.5 ml/100 ml; between the right ventricle and the right atrium, 0.9 ml/100 ml; and between the right atrium and the superior vena cava, 1.9 ml/100 ml. If the O_2 content of blood in a chamber exceeds that of the more proximal chamber by more than these values, a left-to-right shunt at that level is probably

TABLE 23-2. BLOOD AND BLOOD GASES

Arterial O_2 saturation	$\dfrac{O_2 \text{ Content}}{O_2 \text{ Capacity}} \times 100 = 95\%$
Pulmonary arterial O_2 saturation	$= 75\text{–}80\%$
Whole blood O_2 capacity	17–21 ml of O_2/100 ml of blood
Arterial O_2 content	16.5–20.0 ml/100 ml of blood
Mixed venous O_2 content	10–16 ml/100 ml of blood
pH (arterial plasma)	7.39–7.41
CO_2 combining power (venous plasma)	21–30 mEq/L
Arterial CO_2 content (whole blood)	20–25 mEq/L
Arterial and alveolar CO_2 tension (Pa_{CO_2})	37–41 mm Hg

present. Right-to-left shunts are strongly suspected if the arterial O_2 saturation (Sa_{O_2}) is less than normal (95%) in the absence of lung disease, pulmonary congestion, or alveolar hypoventilation. Arterial unsaturation associated with increased O_2 content of blood samples drawn beyond the site of the shunt suggests the presence of a bidirectional shunt.

Cardiac output (CO) and flow: The volume of blood ejected by the heart each minute is the CO; the normal range in the resting state is 4 to 8 L/min. Usually the CO is expressed in relation to the BSA as the **cardiac index (CI)**—L/min/sq m of BSA. BSA is calculated from the DuBois and DuBois height-weight equation: BSA sq m = (wt in kg)$^{0.425}$ × (ht in cm)$^{0.725}$ × 0.007184. Various nomograms for BSA have been devised based on this equation, although the assumption that the absolute CO varies with the size of the individual is open to question. (See TABLE 23-3 for normal values for CO and related measurements.)

Various methods are used to calculate the CO: the Fick technic and indicator-dilution technics are among those most commonly used. The **Fick technic** is based on the principle that the difference between the O_2 concentrations in arterial and mixed venous blood represents the amount of O_2 taken up by each unit of blood as it passes through the lungs. Thus the CO can be calculated from the subject's O_2 uptake for a given period of time and the O_2 saturations of mixed venous and arterial blood samples. Accurate measurement of CO by this method requires that the heart rate, respiratory rate, O_2 consumption, and respiratory exchange rate be stable for 6 to 8 min.

The **indicator-dilution technic** is based on the principle that the degree of dilution of an indicator injected into the circulation is a measure of the flow. A known amount of the indicator is injected into the venous system and its concentration in a peripheral artery is recorded. The concentration curve is divided into 3 segments: (1) appearance time (from the injection to the first appearance of the indicator in the artery); (2) build-up time (from the first appearance to peak concentration); and (3) disappearance time (from the peak concentration to a minimal value). Changes in these segments are important in detecting shunts and evaluating valvular regurgitation and heart failure.

In a normal subject an increased tissue demand for O_2 is met by both increased CO and increased O_2 extraction. In a normal subject, exercise sufficient to double the resting O_2 consumption increases

TABLE 23-3. NORMAL VALUES FOR CARDIAC OUTPUT AND RELATED MEASUREMENTS

Measurements	Units	± S.D.
O_2 uptake	143 ml/min/sq m	14.3
Arteriovenous O_2 difference	4.1 ml/100 ml	0.6
Cardiac index	3.5 L/min/sq m	0.7
Stroke index	46 ml/beat/sq m	8.1
Total systemic resistance	1130 dynes sec cm^{-5}	178
Total pulmonary resistance	205 dynes sec cm^{-5}	51
Pulmonary arteriolar resistance	67 dynes sec cm^{-5}	23

From B. G. Barratt-Boyes and E. H. Wood, "Cardiac output and related measurements and pressure values in the right heart and associated vessels, together with an analysis of the hemodynamic response to the inhalation of high oxygen mixtures in healthy subjects," *Journal of Laboratory and Clinical Medicine* 51: 72–90, 1958. Used with permission of the C. V. Mosby Co. and the authors.

the A-V O_2 difference by no more than 3 ml/100 ml. The CO normally increases 800 to 1500 ml/min for every 100 ml increase in O_2 consumption with exercise. Patients with heart failure or limited cardiac reserve must meet an increased O_2 demand primarily by increasing tissue extraction, thus increasing the A-V O_2 difference. Low resting CO with an inadequate response to exercise may result from inadequate ventricular filling (as in mitral or tricuspid stenosis or constrictive pericarditis) or inadequate ventricular emptying (as in pulmonary or aortic stenosis or when myocardial contractility is impaired). High CO is encountered in such conditions as anxiety, fever, severe anemia, thyrotoxicosis, beriberi, and various A-V fistulas.

Vascular resistance and valve areas: Vascular resistance is the impedence to blood flow through a segment of the circulation and is frequently expressed as the pressure differential across the vascular bed divided by the flow through that bed. It is difficult to define resistance adequately in terms of cardiac dynamics, and a change in resistance through a given segment of the circulation does not define the cause of the change. Resistance can be given in either absolute units (1 dyne/sq cm at a flow of 1 cu cm/sec, or 1 dyne sec cm^{-5}) or resistance units (a pressure of 1 mm Hg at a flow of 1 L/min). It is sometimes calculated using the CI rather than the CO, and the resulting resistance indices are considered to be more comparable between individuals. (See Table 23–3 for normal resistance values.) Pulmonary arteriolar (or vascular) resistance is an estimation of the resistance between the main pulmonary artery and the pulmonary venous bed. It is calculated from the mean pulmonary artery pressure and the mean pulmonary artery wedge pressure, and is elevated in pulmonary hypertension, cor pulmonale, some cases of mitral stenosis, left ventricular failure, and some left-to-right shunts. The total pulmonary resistance, calculated from the mean pulmonary artery pressure and the left ventricular mean diastolic pressure, includes the pulmonary arteriolar resistance, the pulmonary venous resistance, and the resistance across the mitral valve.

Total systemic resistance is an estimation of the resistance between the systemic arteries and the capillary bed. Since the capillary bed is assumed to have no pressure, total systemic resistance is calculated by dividing the mean arterial pressure by the CO. It is normally < 20 resistance units and is most commonly elevated in systemic hypertension.

An expression of the areas of the mitral and aortic valves can be calculated from the pressure gradients across them and the CO. Normal valve areas are given in Table 23–4. Clinical disability occurs with mitral valve areas of 1 sq cm or less and generally with an aortic valve area of 0.75 sq cm or less (and always when it is 0.5 sq cm or less). Tricuspid and pulmonary valve areas can also be calculated, but this is rarely done clinically. Similar formulas can be used to calculate the size of a patent ductus arteriosus or the size of atrial or ventricular septal defects.

Myocardial energetics: Decreased availability of O_2 for metabolism within the myocardium, or myocardial hypoxia, and the resulting shift to an anaerobic metabolism can be detected by an increased lactate-pyruvate concentration ratio in coronary sinus blood. Myocardial citrate extraction is significantly decreased in coronary artery disease. However, too much emphasis should not be placed on substrate analysis without accurate steady-state measurements of coronary flow.

Catheterization Procedure

Equipment: All fluoroscopy should be done with an image intensifier and television system. Using videotape instant replay recorders, the angiography can be reviewed immediately and the physician can determine whether additional views are needed. A wide variety of catheters are used for the various procedures, and they are constantly being revised. The catheters must be radiopaque, nonthrombogenic, and flexible enough to bend without becoming soft and unmanageable at body temperatures. Flow-directed catheters have a small balloon at the tip that allows venous flow to direct them into the pulmonary artery from peripheral veins. These catheters are frequently used at the bedside in the ICU and are a valuable adjunct in the management of seriously ill patients.

Since blood samples may be drawn at any time during the procedure for analysis of O_2 and CO_2 content, oximetric devices that allow continual rapid determination of O_2 saturation are needed. Electrocardiographic monitoring is essential, and the ECG should be displayed simultaneously with the other information so that arrhythmias may be detected instantly. A sophisticated analysis of atrial, A-V nodal, junctional, His bundle, and ventricular conduction systems is now available and may become part of the catheterization data.

A DC defibrillator in perfect working order should be in the catheterization laboratory at all times in case of refractory ventricular arrhythmias. Wall outlets for O_2, a source of negative pressure for

Table 23–4. VALVE AREAS AND VALVE FLOWS

Measurements	Units
Aortic area	2.6 – 3.5 sq cm
Aortic valve flow	250 ml/SEP/sec
Mitral area	4 – 6 sq cm
Mitral valve flow	150 ml/DFP/sec

SEP, systolic ejection period; DFP, diastolic filling period.

suction, and an emergency tray containing epinephrine, isoproterenol, atropine, lidocaine, morphine, and needles for intrathoracic injection should be immediately available.

Preparation: The patient should be prepared psychologically before catheterization. The procedure, its purpose, and specific details such as the number of needle punctures and their sites should be explained specifically. For children or infants thiopental 9 mg/kg rectally is used for anesthesia.

Right heart catheterization: In adults the femoral or antecubital veins may be used for entering the right side of the heart. A small cutdown is usually used on the arms. A medial arm vein is usually more satisfactory than the lateral vein since the lateral circulation enters the subclavian vein at right angles, and advancing the catheter past this right angle may be difficult. The femoral vein is usually entered via the Seldinger technic, in which a spring wire is inserted into the vein through the needle and the catheter is passed over the spring wire into the vein after the needle is removed. The spring wire is then removed from the catheter. Usually no difficulty is encountered in advancing a catheter from a peripheral vein to the right atrium, through the tricuspid valve to the right ventricle, and across the pulmonary valve into one or both pulmonary arteries. For selective catheterization of the coronary sinus, the catheter should be advanced to the tricuspid valve and turned somewhat posteriorly to enter the sinus.

Left heart catheterization: Methods of obtaining information from the left side of the circulation include (1) retrograde arterial catheterization via an arteriotomy in the right brachial artery or via percutaneous femoral artery puncture and (2) transseptal technics. The catheter can usually cross the aortic valve into the left ventricle without difficulty in the retrograde technic, even when the aortic valve is stenotic. Transseptal catheterization involves passing a catheter from the right femoral vein to the right atrium, through the atrial septum, into the left atrium, and then across the mitral valve into the left ventricle.

Occasionally the left ventricle cannot be entered via retrograde or transseptal technics, and a direct percutaneous puncture is indicated. Pressures should be monitored continuously during this procedure, and the needle should be kept in the chamber as short a time as possible. This procedure is relatively free of complications and is useful despite its dramatic aspects.

Complications

The mortality and complication rates for cardiac catheterization vary with the procedures and the expertise of the catheterization team. No more than 2 deaths should occur per 1000 catheterizations, including those performed for angiography and selective coronary angiography. Although the complications can be serious problems, they are uncommon in centers where at least 200 to 300 cardiac catheterizations are performed each year. The risk of complications is low (under 4%), but it is not negligible.

Arrhythmias—ventricular tachycardia, ventricular fibrillation, and cardiac arrest—are the most serious complications of cardiac catheterization. Isolated premature ventricular contractions, atrial fibrillation, or supraventricular arrhythmias are relatively easily controlled, usually of short duration, and rarely of physiologic significance. Ventricular arrhythmias are most common during selective coronary angiography. Catheter withdrawal and/or DC cardioversion usually restore sinus rhythm and do not preclude completing the procedure. The incidence of ventricular fibrillation during coronary angiography is < 0.4% in men and somewhat higher in women; the reason for this difference is not known.

Most cases of **pericardial tamponade** during catheterization are complications of transseptal technics. Some degree of pericardial tamponade can be expected in about 25% of patients whose cardiac wall is perforated during catheterization.

Arterial trauma includes dissection, thrombosis, A-V fistulas, false aneurysms, and bleeding. It is slightly more common with the Seldinger technic and more frequent in patients with conditions that produce wide pulse pressures, such as A-V fistulas, high-output states, or aortic regurgitation. Removing intra-arterial clots with Fogarty catheters at the time of arterial closure has reduced the incidence of brachial artery thrombosis to between 1 and 4%. If there is no palpable radial pulse at the end of arterial closure, a vascular surgeon should explore the arterial lumen and repair the artery.

Profound **hypotension** is associated usually with an allergic reaction, systemic sepsis, or perforation of a chamber of the heart. Occasionally vagal episodes can produce transient but remarkable hypotension that can be corrected with small amounts of atropine. Allergic reactions are usually related to contrast material or the catheter material. If there is a history of allergy to iodine-containing dyes, precautions should be taken during angiography.

Bacterial endocarditis and **systemic sepsis** rarely follow cardiac catheterization. **Local infections** around the catheter entry into the skin are more common and may occasionally prolong hospitalization.

Systemic and pulmonary emboli can complicate cardiac catheterizations. Systemic emboli usually result from clots that form at the end of a catheter and are flushed into the systemic circulation. Myocardial infarctions, cerebrovascular accidents, and other systemic complications have been reported. Thrombophlebitis, a rare occurrence at the site of venous catheterization, has resulted in pulmonary thromboembolism and pulmonary infarction. Catheters have become knotted and broken. The lumen can become thrombosed, and the catheter will be useless and dangerous if it is left in the vascular system for long without adequate flushing.

Hemorrhage may occur at a site of entry into a vein but is more common at an arterial entry. Heparin, commonly used during cardiac catheterization to prevent clotting, increases the risk of serious bleeding. The nursing and house staff should be made aware of this possibility, and the patient should be observed closely for 24 h after the catheterization.

PULMONARY ARTERY CATHETERIZATION

Passage of a flow-directed catheter from a superficial vein to the pulmonary artery is indicated in acutely ill patients with (1) hypotension resistant to therapy; (2) sudden respiratory failure manifested by dyspnea, tachypnea, and hypoxia; (3) failure of 2 or more organ systems. Catheter passage is > 95% successful.

Procedure

A 4-lumen, No. 7 French catheter is used in adults. The lumena are: (1) **distal**—for measuring pulmonary artery and pulmonary arterial wedge pressure **(PAWP)** and for withdrawing blood; (2) **balloon**—for inflating with 1 ml of air to help advance the catheter and measure PAWP; (3) **proximal**—for measuring right atrial or central venous pressure and for injecting iced dextrose and water; (4) **thermistor**—for measuring cardiac output by using a temperature-sensing device which describes a temperature-time curve after injection of iced dextrose and water.

The catheter is usually inserted via a cutdown on a vein in the medial antecubital fossa; the femoral or external jugular veins are alternative sites. Percutaneous introduction is also common; a 10-gauge needle is used to enter the internal jugular vein. Then the pulmonary artery catheter is inserted and the needle withdrawn. Partial inflation of the balloon permits blood flow to propel the catheter after it is advanced into a major vein such as the axillary or subclavian.

The position of the catheter tip is determined by pressure monitoring using a strain gauge transducer coupled to the distal lumen. The right ventricle has been entered when the systolic pressure suddenly increases to about 30 mm Hg; diastolic pressure is similar to right atrial or vena caval pressure. When the catheter is in the pulmonary artery, the transducer characteristically shows a systolic pressure equivalent to that in the right ventricle and a narrow pulse pressure, so that the diastolic pressure is higher than right ventricular end-diastolic or central venous pressure.

Further movement of the catheter wedges the balloon in a distal pulmonary artery. Since this vascular segment no longer has blood flow, there is no kinetic energy loss or pressure drop across the pulmonary capillary bed. The strain gauge transducer now reflects pressure in the pulmonary veins. This pressure is equivalent to left ventricular end-diastolic pressure **(LVEDP)** except in 3 circumstances: when mitral stenosis is present; when high levels (> 10 cm H_2O) of positive end-expiratory pressure **(PEEP)** are used; and when the pulmonary artery balloon is excessively inflated (deflating the balloon produces the characteristic pulmonary arterial pressure).

A chest x-ray should follow catheter passage to verify proper placement. The patency of the proximal and distal lumena is maintained with a slow infusion (4 ml/h) of dilute heparinized saline (1000 u./L) through a millipore filter.

When measuring cardiac output, the pulmonary artery catheter must not be in the wedge position. To measure the cardiac output, 10 ml of 5% D/W at 0 C (32 F) is rapidly injected into the proximal lumen and a temperature-time curve is constructed using the thermistor located at the end of the catheter. The thermistor signal is usually electronically integrated and a direct measure of flow is obtained in < 1 min.

Precautions

When the catheter enters the right ventricle, *the ECG must be monitored and lidocaine must be available, since the catheter frequently induces ventricular irritability.* Further passage of the catheter into the pulmonary artery usually corrects the arrhythmia, but *severe arrhythmias or persistent minor ones demand termination of the procedure.* Balloon rupture is frequent if > 1 ml of air is used for inflation. Air embolism, though theoretically possible, has not been a problem. Knotting of the catheter has been infrequent. Pulmonary infarction may result if the catheter remains in the wedge position for more than several minutes. Strict asepsis while inserting the catheter, during repositioning and blood withdrawal, cardiac output measurements, and pressure monitoring should prevent phlebitis and septic complications. The catheter should not stay in the pulmonary artery > 3 to 4 days.

Measurements and Their Interpretation

Common causes of peripheral hypotension can be defined (see TABLE 24–1). Hydrostatic and increased permeability pulmonary edema can be differentiated using the PAWP. The composition of mixed venous blood, particularly mixed venous O_2 tension **(P$\bar{v}_{O_2}$)**, can be determined using the catheter. If the P$\bar{v}_{O_2}$ decreases to < 30 mm Hg, the prognosis is poor. Therapy may be evaluated, such as the effects of inotropic drugs, intra-aortic balloon assist, fluid infusions, or respiratory therapy. Since mechanical ventilation may depress cardiac output, particularly when combined with high levels (> 10 cm H_2O) of PEEP, thermodilution measured flow in combination with arterial O_2 content **(C$_a$O$_2$)** measurement may be used to calculate O_2 delivery (cardiac output × C$_a$O$_2$) and thereby determine an optimal PEEP setting. In most critically ill patients, fluid is infused until the cardiac index (cardiac output/BSA) is normal or slightly increased; i.e., exceeds 2.5 L/min/sq m with the

PAWP < 12 mm Hg. When the PAWP is > 12 mm Hg, the cardiac index can be raised by β agonists (e.g., dopamine), and by correction of pH and Hct.

Other derived variables, including pulmonary vascular resistance and right and left ventricular stroke work **(LVSW)**, have clinical and research applications. Starling-type myocardial performance curves have been constructed from measurements of LVSW and PAWP during and after a rapid fluid infusion. These curves yield information regarding cardiac function at different filling pressures. Pulmonary artery end-diastolic pressure may be substituted for the PAWP if pulmonary vascular resistance is normal and if the heart rate is slow. The ratio of the pulmonary artery end-diastolic pressure to PAWP may be used as an index of pulmonary vascular resistance.

ANGIOGRAPHY

Radiographic recording of contrast material injected into arteries, veins, or heart chambers to define anatomy, disease, or direction of blood flow.

Technic

Procedure: Contrast material can be injected (1) through a needle into a peripheral vein; (2) through a catheter into the right heart chamber, across the atrial septum into a left heart chamber, or through the aorta into the left cardiac chambers; or (3) through a needle directly into a major artery. Successful angiography depends on the catheter position, the size of the catheter lumen, the amount of contrast material injected, the rate of injection, and proper positioning of the catheter and the patient. The choice of contrast material depends on its viscosity, lack of toxicity, and the efficiency of opacification; iodinated compounds are usually used. When large chambers are to be opacified, power injection is most suitable; hand injections are used for selective arteriography of individual small vessels such as the coronary arteries.

For suspected cardiac anomalies such as septal defect and narrowed outlets, the contrast material is injected proximal to the lesion or into the chamber with the higher pressure (see also CARDIAC CATHETERIZATION, above). In valvular incompetence the contrast material is injected into the chamber with the higher pressure distal to the valve. If technical difficulties preclude the best positioning of the catheter, the injection should be made in the nearest convenient site and circulation of the contrast material filmed. For example, with a left atrial myxoma, injecting into the left atrium is not advisable because a tumor fragment may be dislodged; therefore, the pulmonary arteries are injected and contrast material is filmed as the left atrium is opacified.

Recording: Most x-rays are taken at 3 to 6 times/second. For studies of anomalies such as congenital heart lesions, cut film provides excellent detail. Biplane angiocardiography (lateral and frontal exposures) gives a 3-dimensional perspective of the cardiac chambers and great vessels. Unlike static films, cinecardiograms can be monitored during the injection, and the injection sequence can be simultaneously recorded on videotape and instantly replayed. The resolution of details on individual cine frames is only ⅓ that of conventional x-rays, but the motion is a more natural expression of the heart, and details are apparent that are not appreciated on still films.

Physiologic Effects and Complications

All contrast media are hypertonic and are excreted by the kidneys. The cardiovascular response includes tachycardia, a slight fall in systemic pressure, and a rise in cardiac output. A transient sense of warmth, especially in the head and face, is universally experienced after injection of contrast media. Nausea, vomiting, and coughing are minor side effects. Major complications such as cardiac arrest, anaphylactoid reactions, shock, convulsions, cyanosis, and renal toxicity are rare. Patients with a high Hct are susceptible to clotting, and the Hct should be $< 65\%$ before the angiogram is performed. Allergic reactions may include urticaria and conjunctivitis, which respond to diphenhydramine. Bronchospasm, edema of the larynx, and dyspnea are potential but rare reactions. Ventricular arrhythmias are common if the catheter tip contacts the ventricular endocardium. Ventricular fibrillation is a potential but rare hazard. ECG monitoring and an emergency tray including necessary drugs, resuscitation equipment, O_2, endotracheal tubes, defibrillator, and transvenous pacing wires should always be available.

Specific Structures

Right ventricle and pulmonary valve: Direct injection of contrast material into the apex of the right ventricle allows an appreciation of tricuspid valve competence and demonstrates the pulmonary valve, the subvalvular region, and the proximal pulmonary arteries. The right ventricular outflow tract is best seen with the patient in a steep lateral position, which also demonstrates the relation of the pulmonary artery to the aorta and occasionally the presence of a ventricular septal defect or communication between the right ventricle and the aorta.

Pulmonary artery: Pulmonary angiography is the most definitive technic for the diagnosis of acute pulmonary embolism; intraluminal filling defects of arterial cutoffs are diagnostic. Contrast material is usually injected into the main pulmonary artery or right ventricular outflow tract, but selective injection into one or both pulmonary arteries may be indicated.

Left atrium: Space-occupying lesions such as myxoma or clots are the usual reasons for opacifying the left atrium. Direct injection into the left atrium may be hazardous in such cases, and the levo phase of a pulmonary angiogram is currently used to visualize it.

Left ventricle: The long axis of the left ventricle can best be seen in a 30- to 45-degree right anterior oblique projection, and ventricular aneurysms or areas of asynergy of the anterior wall are best demonstrated in this view. This projection also permits a "side-on" view of the A-V valves and separates the left atrium from the left ventricle so that any mitral regurgitation can be seen. The left anterior oblique projection is used to define the left ventricular outflow area and subvalvular aortic obstruction as well as the motion of the interventricular septum and left ventricular posterior wall. Cineangiography is valuable in assessing the motion of the left ventricle and evaluating ventricular performance. Ventricular asynergy is the term applied to abnormal ventricular wall motion; localized abnormalities are termed myocardial asynergy and are divided into (1) akinesis (absence of wall motion); (2) dyskinesis (paradoxic systolic expansion); (3) hypokinesis (diminished motion); and (4) asynchrony (disturbed temporal sequence of contraction).

After left ventricular mass and volume are determined from single plane or biplane angiocardiograms, end-systolic and end-diastolic volumes and the ejection fraction can be calculated mathematically. Stroke volume is the difference between end-diastolic and end-systolic volume, and the ejection fraction is the ratio of stroke volume to end-diastolic volume. The normal heart ejects 50 to 60% of its end-diastolic volume with each systole under resting conditions.

Aorta: Aortic regurgitation is best visualized by injecting contrast material into the ascending aorta in a 60-degree left anterior oblique or left lateral projection. Aorto-pulmonary windows, coarctations of the aorta, and patent ductus arteriosus also are commonly diagnosed from aortic angiocardiograms.

Coronary arteries: Indications for coronary arteriography include (1) chest pain refractory to medical management and probably due to coronary artery disease; (2) chest pain of uncertain etiology refractory to medical management; (3) aortic stenosis that might be corrected by aortic valve replacement, especially in patients with a history of angina or syncope; (4) unexplained congestive heart failure possibly due to a left ventricular aneurysm; and (5) medically uncontrolled angina pectoris when a surgical procedure is contemplated for relief of pain.

In 1958 Sones perfected methods of selectively catheterizing the coronary arteries. In the Sones technic the right brachial artery is entered via an arteriotomy, and a tapered catheter with a flexible tip is passed to the coronary orifice. This procedure is safe but requires training and expertise. The Judkins technic involves percutaneous entry into the femoral arteries and the passage of preformed catheters to the coronary ostia. Coronary venography into the coronary sinus is also possible.

There are no absolute contraindications to coronary arteriography, although relative contraindications include a myocardial infarction within the past 3 mo (unless surgical treatment is contemplated) or debilitating disease of some other major organ system. Passing catheters into the heart and injecting contrast media in the coronary arteries is associated with recognizable hazards. Cardiac arrhythmias, ventricular fibrillation, and asystole may occur and should be treated promptly. Temporary transvenous pacemakers are routinely inserted into the right ventricle before any angiographic procedure in patients who have experienced conduction disturbances. Angina may develop and should be treated with sublingual nitroglycerin. Clots from the catheter can produce myocardial infarction or cerebrovascular accidents and the catheter must be kept well flushed and free from thrombi. The mortality rate of coronary angiography should not be $> 1{:}1000$ to $2{:}1000$ (0.15%), and in centers where the procedure is done > 400 times/yr, the mortality is even lower.

PERICARDIOCENTESIS (See PERICARDIAL DISEASE in Ch. 25)

---

24. GENERALIZED CARDIOVASCULAR DISORDERS

ARTERIOSCLEROSIS; ATHEROSCLEROSIS

Arteriosclerosis is a generic term for a number of blood vessel diseases, **atherosclerosis** being the most important. Others include **Mönckeberg's arteriosclerosis**, in which there is focal calcification of the media of small arteries; **arteriolosclerosis**, in which hyalinization of small arteries occurs, usually secondary to hypertension; and **involutional changes**, which accompany increasing age and are characterized by loss of elastic tissue, spotty calcification, and intimal thickening.

Atherosclerosis: *An arterial lesion characterized by intimal thickening due to localized accumulations of lipids, known as atheromas.* The great clinical importance of atherosclerosis is due to its predilection for coronary, cerebral, and renal, as well as peripheral arteries. Its complications are the major causes of death in the USA; death classified as degenerative and arteriosclerotic heart disease represents 33% of all deaths, and cerebral vascular disease is the 3rd most common cause of death in the USA after heart disease and cancer.

Pathology and Pathogenesis

The atherosclerotic plaque, or **atheroma**, is the characteristic lesion and represents the end of a process that begins with the deposition of lipid in the smooth muscle cells of the intima and media of the vessel wall. This initial deposition of lipid appears as a fatty streak in the arterial wall. Since fatty streaks appear in childhood and in both high- and low-risk populations, whether or not they are transformed into plaques is uncertain. However, fatty streaks probably precede plaque formation, since both involve the same anatomic sites. The mechanism of atheroma development remains unclear, and several hypotheses have been developed compatible with the available evidence. The initial lesion probably is at the intimal barrier. Lesions of the intimal barrier may be produced experimentally by various mechanical measures. Factors such as turbulence, hypertension, and hypoxia are considered important. Following such injury, smooth muscle cells proliferate, and some migrate to the intima where they are affected by the blood elements with which they come in contact, especially platelets and lipoproteins. Platelets contain a factor that stimulates smooth muscle cell proliferation and migration. Lipoproteins, especially low-density lipoproteins **(LDL)**, attach to smooth muscle cells and stimulate their growth. The uptake of LDL can convert what ordinarily would be a limited tissue response to injury into atherosclerosis by introducing cholesterol, a major component of the LDL, into the vessel wall. Smooth muscle cells also synthesize collagen, elastin, and other proteins that are present in increased amounts in the atheromatous lesion. The collagen causes accumulation of fibrous tissue, which becomes laden with lipids and cellular debris.

Risk Factors

If one or more of certain biochemical, physiologic, and environmental factors, known as risk factors, is present in an individual, the possibility of his suffering from atherosclerosis and its complications increases. Removal or modification of the risk factors in a population seems to diminish the incidence of the complications of atherosclerosis, such as coronary heart disease. The major risk factors are (1) **hypertension,** (2) **elevated serum lipids,** specifically cholesterol and triglycerides, (3) **cigarette smoking,** (4) **diabetes mellitus,** and (5) **obesity.** Other presumed risk factors include physical inactivity, certain types of behavioral patterns and personality, hardness of the drinking water, and a family history of premature atherosclerosis. The risk of arteriosclerosis also increases with age. The death rate from coronary heart disease among white men aged 25 to 34 is about 10:100,000; at age 55 to 64 it is nearly 1,000:100,000. This relationship to age may be due to the time required for the lesions to develop or to the duration of exposure to risk factors. Male sex is an important risk factor; at ages 35 to 44 the death rate from coronary heart disease among white men is 6.1 times that among women. In nonwhites, for unknown reasons, the sex difference is less apparent. Diabetic arteriosclerotic disease and hyperlipidemia are discussed below; hypertension, smoking, and obesity are discussed elsewhere.

Symptoms, Signs, and Diagnosis

Atherosclerosis is characteristically silent until stenosis, thrombosis, aneurysm, or, rarely, embolus supervenes. Symptoms and signs may develop gradually as the atheroma slowly encroaches upon the vessel lumen. When a major artery is acutely occluded by thrombosis, embolism, dissecting aneurysm, or trauma, the symptoms and signs may be dramatic. Clinical findings (see Ch. 28) occur distal to the obstructive lesion in tissues whose circulation depends upon the affected artery. Specific ischemic disorders related to occlusion are described in Chs. 25, 27, and 122.

Prophylaxis and Treatment

In many societies the incidence of atherosclerosis is much lower than in ours, and attempts to prevent atherosclerosis by focusing on the risk factors seem useful. Diabetes mellitus and obesity should be treated early and adequately. Cigarette smoking should be limited or stopped. Regular exercise may help to prevent clinical coronary disease and may be a useful therapeutic measure. Lowering BP reduces the incidence of stroke and probably congestive heart failure, although it has not been shown to decrease the incidence of myocardial infarction. Hypertensive individuals should be identified and treated early. Treatment of hyperlipidemia has not been proved to prevent atherosclerosis. However, the considerable evidence relating hyperlipidemia to atherosclerosis makes reducing serum lipid levels reasonable, especially when they are elevated. Hyperlipidemia can be treated (1) by treating the population in general, which in Western nations has higher serum lipid levels than are desirable, and (2) by treating patients with clearly defined hyperlipidemia. The main step in preventing hyperlipidemia in the general population is to change Western dietary habits. Fat intake should be reduced, and many saturated fats replaced with polyunsaturated fats. The intake of cholesterol and saturated and short-chain fatty acids, such as occur in meats and dairy products, should be reduced. Such a diet is consumed by many populations in the world and is well tolerated. Weight reduction to normal, or even slightly below current statistical norms, is recommended. The treatment of individuals with hyperlipidemia is more complex and is discussed in Ch. 82.

Treatment of atherosclerosis is directed at its complications, such as angina pectoris, myocardial infarction, arrhythmias, heart failure, kidney failure, stroke, and peripheral arterial occlusion. These subjects are covered under individual subject headings.

DIABETIC ARTERIOSCLEROTIC DISEASE

Three types of vascular disease are seen in diabetes mellitus: (1) **diabetic microangiopathy,** characterized by diffuse thickening of the capillary basement membrane and microaneurysms; (2) **arteriolar disease,** frequently associated with hypertension; and (3) **atherosclerosis,** involving primarily the medium-sized and larger arteries. This discussion is limited to atherosclerosis. Microvascular disease and other aspects are discussed under DIABETES MELLITUS in Ch. 90. No histopathologic difference between diabetic and nondiabetic atherosclerotic lesions can be demonstrated, but the incidence of atherosclerosis is higher in diabetics than in nondiabetics. Peripheral vascular disease has been estimated to occur 11 times more frequently and to develop about 10 yr earlier in diabetics than in nondiabetics. Gangrene is about 50 times more frequent in diabetic men than in nondiabetic men over age 40, and 70 times more frequent in women in this age group. The incidence of coronary artery disease is greater and life expectancy is shorter among diabetic women than among nondiabetic women. In nondiabetic patients, larger vessels such as the aortoiliac or femoropopliteal arteries are most likely to be involved, with relative sparing of the leg arteries. In contrast, involvement of the peroneal, anterior and posterior tibial, and digital arteries of the legs is greater in diabetic patients.

Unexplained geographic differences occur in diabetic vascular disease. Diabetic patients in some groups in Israel, North Africa, and the Middle East have a low incidence of coronary artery disease, and the incidence of atherosclerosis, including peripheral vascular disease, in Japanese diabetics is small.

An abnormal glucose tolerance test has been found in about 37% of men and 42% of women with coronary artery disease who were not known to have diabetes mellitus. The high incidence of atherosclerotic disease in diabetes mellitus is unexplained, and the relationship to blood glucose appears to be independent of coexisting hypercholesterolemia or hypertension. A correlation between hyperglycemia and hypertriglyceridemia has been found in some studies, but other data are contradictory.

Symptoms and Signs

Peripheral arterial disease (arteriosclerosis obliterans) in diabetic patients is usually manifested by the effects of **ischemia**, which are often complicated by **neuropathy** and **infection**. The foot of the diabetic patient is very susceptible to all forms of trauma; the heel is particularly vulnerable. The common response is infection and gangrene. Specific symptoms and signs are similar to those seen in any patient with occlusive arterial disease (see below, and in Ch. 28).

The clinical manifestations of diabetic **neuropathy** that may complicate peripheral vascular disease include sensory disturbances, plantar ulcers, trophic skin lesions and ulcers, autonomic neuropathy (anhidrosis, vasodilation, edema, erythema, atrophy of skin and subcutaneous tissues), and the neuropathic or Charcot joint, a painless degenerative arthropathy involving chiefly the tarsometatarsal and metatarsophalangeal joints. When **infections** occur, pyogenic organisms are frequently associated with a fungal infection. A mycotic infection frequently is the initial process, leading to wet interdigital lesions, cracks, fissures, and ulcerations that favor secondary bacterial invasion. Infections also commonly result from manipulation of an ingrown toenail, plantar corn, or callus. Infections may progress to cellulitis, lymphangitis, and involvement of the deeper soft tissues by abscess formation, osteomyelitis, and gangrene. The neuropathy renders infection and gangrene relatively painless in the diabetic.

HYPERLIPIDEMIA

Serum lipids and lipoproteins participate in the pathogenesis of atherosclerosis, and regimens that decrease serum lipid and lipoprotein levels are important aspects of treatment. The association between hyperlipidemia and the presence of arteriosclerosis is deduced from the following observations: (1) The high lipid content of the atherosclerotic lesions is qualitatively similar to that in the blood. (2) Lesions can be produced in animals by feeding them diets that increase serum lipid levels. (3) Patients with clinical evidence of atherosclerosis, especially those with coronary heart disease and those in younger age groups, tend to have higher serum lipid levels than patients of the same age with no arteriosclerosis. (4) Patients with various forms of hyperlipidemia have an increased incidence of arteriosclerosis. (5) Prospective studies show a correlation between the occurrence of arteriosclerotic disease, especially coronary heart disease, and the serum cholesterol and triglyceride levels. (6) Epidemiologic studies show that the incidence of coronary heart disease is highest in populations with the highest serum lipid levels. Normal levels of serum cholesterol and triglycerides and specific abnormalities and their management are discussed in detail under ANOMALIES IN LIPID METABOLISM in Ch. 82.

HYPERTENSION

ARTERIAL HYPERTENSION

Elevation of systolic and/or diastolic blood pressure, either primary (essential hypertension) or secondary.

Etiology

Primary or essential hypertension is not linked to a single etiology. It may be only a quantitative deviation from average (rather than a qualitative change) and a reflection of polygenic inheritance of BP, with hypertensives occupying the upper quartile of a bell-shaped distribution curve for BP. Heredity predisposes to hypertension, but environmental, neurogenic, humoral, and vascular factors also interact and influence BP to various extents. Most patients with primary hypertension show heightened vascular and cardiac reactions to sympathetic stimuli. Whether this hyperresponsiveness resides in the sympathetic nervous system, its receptors, or the tissues that it innervates is not known, but it may precede the development of sustained hypertension. No measurable abnormality in catecholamine metabolism has been identified consistently in primary hypertension. A "resetting" of the carotid sinus baroreceptors so that this homeostatic mechanism tends to maintain rather than combat increased arterial pressure has been demonstrated in animals and humans, but this is a result rather than the cause of sustained hypertension. Some authorities implicate the kidney in the etiology of primary hypertension, but serial observations suggest instead that functional and structural abnormalities (arteriolar nephrosclerosis) follow the hypertension. Renin secretion may be suppressed, normal, or increased in primary hypertension.

New information indicating that prostaglandins may play an important role in BP regulation and the development of hypertension is discussed in Ch. 252.

The arteriolar walls of hypertensive animals contain more water and sodium than normal. This encroachment on the lumen may increase peripheral resistance, but it is not necessarily the inciting mechanism. There is no evidence that excessive sodium ingestion, emotional stress, or obesity causes hypertension, although each of these factors may aggravate preexisting hypertension or hasten the appearance of hypertension in genetically predisposed individuals.

Secondary hypertension is associated with bilateral renal parenchymal disease (e.g., chronic glomerulonephritis or pyelonephritis, polycystic renal disease, collagen disease of the kidney, or obstructive uropathy) or with such potentially curable disorders as pheochromocytoma, Cushing's syndrome, primary aldosteronism, hyperthyroidism, myxedema, coarctation of the aorta, renal vascular disease, and unilateral renal disease. It may also be associated with use of oral contraceptives. The etiologic mechanisms in secondary hypertension are not as obvious as they might seem. Other mechanisms are also involved when hypertension due to some readily identifiable cause (e.g., catecholamine from pheochromocytoma, renin and angiotensin from renal artery stenosis, or aldosterone from adrenal cortical adenoma) has persisted for some time. The longer the hypertension has existed, the less likely it is that surgery will restore normal BP.

Hypertension associated with chronic renal parenchymal disease is due to various combinations of 2 mechanisms, one apparently renin-dependent and another volume-dependent. In most patients with renal parenchymal disease and hypertension, increased renin activity cannot be demonstrated in peripheral blood, and in these patients meticulous attention to fluid balance readily controls BP. The renal medulla probably elaborates one or more depressor substances (including prostaglandins) that tend to keep BP within normal range; absence of these substances due to renal parenchymal disease or bilateral nephrectomy would permit the BP to rise. Modest hypertension sensitive to sodium and water balance is characteristic of anephric animals and humans (**renoprival hypertension**).

Renovascular hypertension (caused by occlusion of a renal artery or its branches) is discussed separately in this chapter, below, and **malignant hypertension (malignant nephroangiosclerosis)** is discussed in Ch. 152.

Prevalence

It is estimated that there are 35 million hypertensives (BP $\geq$ 160/95 mm Hg) in the USA ($>$ 15% of the adult population). About 25% do not know that they are hypertensive. Hypertension is almost twice as frequent in blacks (nearly 30% of adults) as in whites, and morbidity and mortality are greater in blacks. Before age 50 it is more common in white men than in white women, while after age 50 it is more frequent in women. There is no difference in prevalence between black men and black women. Prevalence increases with age; nearly 25% of whites and almost 50% of blacks over age 65 are hypertensive. Between 85 and 90% of cases are primary; in 5 or 10% hypertension is secondary to bilateral renal parenchymal disease, and only 1 or 2% of cases are due to a potentially curable condition.

Pathology

No pathologic changes occur early in primary hypertension. Ultimately, generalized arteriolar sclerosis develops; it is particularly apparent in the kidney and is characterized by medial hypertrophy and hyalinization. Nephrosclerosis is the hallmark of primary hypertension. Left ventricular hypertrophy and, eventually, dilation develop gradually. Coronary, cerebral, aortic, renal, and peripheral atherosclerosis are more common and more severe in hypertensives since hypertension accelerates atherogenesis. Tiny Charcot-Bouchard aneurysms are frequently found in perforating arteries, especially in the basal ganglia, in hypertensive patients and may be the source of intracerebral hemorrhage.

Malignant hypertension is characterized by widespread necrotizing arteriolitis with fibrinoid changes and proliferative endarteritis, especially in, but not confined to, the kidneys. (See Ch. 152.)

Hemodynamics

Not all patients with primary hypertension have normal cardiac output and increased peripheral resistance. Cardiac output is increased and peripheral resistance is inappropriately normal for the level of cardiac output in the early labile phase of primary hypertension. Peripheral resistance increases and the cardiac output returns to normal after a period of time, probably because of autoregulation. Patients with high, fixed diastolic pressures often have decreased cardiac output. The role of the large veins in the pathophysiology of primary hypertension has largely been ignored, but venoconstriction early in the course of the disease may contribute to the increased cardiac output.

Plasma volume tends to decrease as BP increases, although some patients with primary hypertension have expanded plasma volumes. Plasma renin activity **(PRA)** is usually normal but may be suppressed in some (about 25%) and elevated in others (about 15%). The accelerated (malignant) phase of hypertension is usually accompanied by elevated PRA. Plasma volume and PRA variations are evidence that primary hypertension is more than a single entity or that different mechanisms are involved in different stages of the disorder.

Renal blood flow gradually decreases as the diastolic BP increases and arteriolar sclerosis begins to appear. Coronary, cerebral, and muscle blood flow are maintained unless there is concomitant severe atherosclerosis in these vascular beds. GFR remains normal until late in the disease, and, as a result, the filtration fraction is increased. The hypertensive kidney excretes a sodium load more rapidly than the normal kidney until the GFR begins to decline.

In the absence of cardiac failure, cardiac output is normal or increased, and peripheral resistance is usually high in hypertension associated with pheochromocytoma, primary aldosteronism, renal artery disease, and renal parenchymal disease. Plasma volume tends to be high in hypertension due to primary aldosteronism or renal parenchymal disease and is lower than normal in pheochromocytoma.

Systolic hypertension (with normal diastolic pressure) is not a discrete entity. Often it is the result of increased cardiac output or stroke volume (e.g., labile phase of primary hypertension, thyrotoxicosis, A-V fistula, or aortic regurgitation); in the elderly, with normal or low cardiac output, it usually reflects inelasticity of the aorta and its major branches ("arteriosclerotic hypertension").

Symptoms and Signs

Primary hypertension is asymptomatic until complications develop. Symptoms and signs are nonspecific and arise from complications in target organs; they are not pathognomonic for hypertension since identical symptoms and signs can develop in normotensives. Dizziness, flushed facies, headache, fatigue, epistaxis, and nervousness are not caused by uncomplicated hypertension. Complications include left ventricular failure; atherosclerotic heart disease; retinal hemorrhages, exudates, papilledema, and vascular accidents; cerebrovascular insufficiency; and renal failure. Hypertensive encephalopathy due to severe hypertension and cerebral edema is encountered only in hypertensive patients (see also Ch. 122).

On the basis of retinal changes, Keith, Wagener, and Barker classified hypertension into 4 groups which have important prognostic implications: Group 1—constriction of retinal arterioles only; Group 2—constriction and sclerosis of retinal arterioles; Group 3—hemorrhages and exudates in addition to vascular changes; Group 4 (malignant hypertension)—papilledema.

A fourth heart sound and broad, notched P-wave abnormalities on the ECG are among the earliest signs of hypertensive heart disease. Physical, x-ray, and ECG evidence of left ventricular hypertrophy may appear later. Aortic dissection or leaking aneurysm of the aorta may be the first sign of hypertension or may complicate untreated hypertension. Polyuria, nocturia, diminished renal concentrating ability, proteinuria, microhematuria, cylindruria, and nitrogen retention are late manifestations of arteriolar nephrosclerosis.

Diagnosis

Diagnosis of primary hypertension depends on (1) demonstrating that the systolic and diastolic BP are usually, but not necessarily always, higher than normal and (2) excluding secondary causes. At least 2 BP determinations should be made on 3 separate days before labeling a patient hypertensive. For patients in the low hypertension range and especially for patients with marked labile BP, more than this minimum number of determinations are desirable. The upper limit of normal BP in adults is 140/90 mm Hg; it is much lower for infants and children. A somewhat higher limit, especially for systolic pressure, is acceptable (though probably not normal) for patients over age 60 yr. Sporadic higher levels in patients who have been resting for > 5 min suggest an unusual lability of BP that may precede sustained hypertension.

TABLE 24–1 lists the basic or minimal evaluation recommended for patients with mild hypertension. The more severe the hypertension and the younger the patient, the more extensive the evaluation should be. Rapid sequence IVP, chest x-ray, ECG, screening tests for pheochromocytoma, and renin-sodium profiling are not necessary routinely. Plasma renin activity has not been helpful in diagnosis, prognosis, or drug selection.

Besides elevating BP, **pheochromocytoma** usually produces symptoms (various combinations of headache, palpitations, tachycardia, excessive perspiration, tremor, and pallor) that should alert the physician to this possibility. Diagnosis depends on demonstrating increased urinary or plasma concentrations of catecholamine or increased urinary concentrations of its metabolic products, metanephrines and VMA. (The catecholamines, such as epinephrine and norepinephrine, are eventually metabolized in the body to a common product, 3-methoxy-4-hydroxymandelic acid, which is frequently called vanillylmandelic acid **[VMA].**) For a full discussion of pheochromocytoma, see Ch. 88.

Hypokalemia not due to diuretics should suggest **primary aldosteronism.** Proteinuria, cylindruria, or microhematuria with or without nitrogen retention early in the course of hypertension is strong evidence of underlying **primary renal disease.** Absent or markedly reduced femoral arterial pulsations in a hypertensive patient under age 30 is presumptive evidence of **coarctation of the aorta.**

TABLE 24-1. MINIMAL EVALUATION FOR PATIENTS WITH MILD AND
MODERATE HYPERTENSION (140-180/90-115)

History and physical examination
Complete blood count
Routine urinalysis (with microscopic examination)
Serum levels of importance: BUN and/or creatinine, potassium, cholesterol, uric acid, glucose, HDL cholesterol
Serum triglycerides (for patients less than age 60 yr)

Renovascular hypertension is discussed below. Cushing's syndrome, collagen disease, acute porphyria, hyperthyroidism, myxedema, and some CNS disorders which also must be excluded, as well as aldosteronism, are discussed in detail in this volume. Toxemia of pregnancy can be found in Vol. II.

Prognosis

An untreated hypertensive patient is at great risk of developing disabling or fatal left ventricular failure, myocardial infarction, cerebral hemorrhage or infarction, or renal failure at an early age. Hypertension is the most important risk factor predisposing to coronary and cerebral atherosclerosis. The higher the BP and the more severe the changes in the retina, the worse is the prognosis. Fewer than 5% of patients with Group 4 or malignant hypertension characterized by papilledema survive 1 yr without treatment. Effective medical control of hypertension will prevent or forestall all complications and will prolong life in patients whose diastolic BP is > 90 mm Hg. Coronary disease is the most common cause of death among treated hypertensive patients.

Treatment

There is no cure for primary hypertension, but appropriate therapy can modify its course. It is estimated that approximately 50% of the 35 million hypertensive patients in the USA have their BP adequately controlled. At least 8 million are not aware that they have hypertension. The Federal Government (through the National High Blood Pressure Education Program), the American Heart Association, and other organizations are urging screening programs for hypertension and other risk factors for atherosclerosis and appropriate treatment for those found to be at risk.

General measures: Sedation, extra rest, prolonged vacations, admonitions not to worry, and half-hearted attempts at weight reduction and dietary sodium restriction are poor substitutes for effective antihypertensive drug therapy. Patients with uncomplicated hypertension should live normal lives as long as they keep their BP controlled with medication. Dietary restrictions should be imposed to control diabetes mellitus, obesity, or blood lipid abnormalities. In mild hypertension, weight reduction to ideal levels and modest dietary sodium restriction may make drug therapy unnecessary; if a diuretic is given, a very low-salt diet (< 5 gm/day) usually is not required. Prudent exercise should be encouraged and cigarette smoking discouraged to reduce the risk of atherosclerotic heart disease.

Congestive heart failure, symptomatic coronary atherosclerosis, or cerebrovascular disease and renal failure should be treated in the usual manner and do not contraindicate judicious antihypertensive therapy. Hypertension increases both the maternal hazards of pregnancy and the fetal mortality rate. Close prenatal supervision, dietary sodium restriction, and antihypertensive drugs will decrease maternal but not fetal mortality. When hypertension cannot be controlled or azotemia supervenes, the pregnancy should be terminated.

Specific antihypertensive therapy: All patients with diastolic BP averaging 90 mm Hg or more should receive antihypertensive drugs if weight control and limitations in dietary sodium do not normalize BP. When complications are present or impending or when the diastolic BP is > 105 mm Hg, drug therapy should not be deferred while awaiting the uncertain results of dietary therapy. There are no data on the efficacy of antihypertensive therapy for borderline hypertension or for systolic ("arteriosclerotic") hypertension of the elderly. Except in elderly patients, the goal of therapy should be to reduce BP to normal (i.e., < 140/90 mm Hg) or as nearly normal as the patient and his cardiovascular system can tolerate. The 1980 report of the Joint National Committee on Detection, Evaluation and Treatment of High BP recommended reducing diastolic BP to ≤ 85 mm Hg based on the findings of the Hypertension Detection and Follow-up Program (HDFP). Usually it is advantageous to have the patient measure his own BP at home.

When diastolic pressure is 90 to 115 mm Hg, treatment is usually started with an oral diuretic. All thiazide derivatives and their congeners are equally effective in equivalent doses (see TABLE 24-2). Metolazone and the loop diuretics, furosemide and ethacrynic acid, are no more effective than the thiazides in managing hypertension, but unlike the thiazides, they are effective when renal function is impaired and hence are preferred for hypertension associated with chronic renal failure. The distal tubular diuretics (spironolactone, triamterene, and amiloride) do not cause hypokalemia, hyperuricemia, or hyperglycemia, but they are not as effective as the thiazides in controlling hypertension. Potassium supplementation is not needed with kaliuretic diuretics unless the patient is also receiving digitalis, is going to have an operation, or is symptomatic from hypokalemia. As much as 100 mEq/day of potassium chloride is needed to prevent hypokalemia, and most patients will not ingest this much. Spironolactone 25 mg q.i.d., triamterene 100 mg t.i.d., or amiloride 5 to 10 mg once daily can be added to the regimen instead of potassium supplementation. The antihypertensive action of diuretics seems to be due to a modest reduction in plasma volume and a decrease in vascular reactivity, possibly mediated by shifts in sodium from intra- to extracellular loci.

TABLE 24–2. ORAL DIURETIC DRUGS USEFUL AS ANTIHYPERTENSIVE AGENTS

Diuretic Agents	Trade Name	Usual Daily Dose* (mg)	Side Effects
Benzothiadiazine derivatives			
Chlorothiazide	Diuril	500–1500†	
Hydrochlorothiazide	HydroDIURIL Esidrix Oretic	50–150†	Unpleasant taste
			Dry mouth
			Weakness
Hydroflumethiazide	Saluron	50–150†	Muscle cramps
Bendroflumethiazide	Naturetin	5–15	GI irritation
			Skin rash
Trichlormethiazide	Naqua Metahydrin	4–12	Photosensitivity (except ethacrynic acid)
			Hypokalemia
Methyclothiazide	Enduron	5–15	Hyponatremia
Benzthiazide	Exna Aquatag	100–150†	Hyperuricemia
			Hyperglycemia
Polythiazide	Renese	4–8	Hypercalcemia (except furosemide & ethacrynic acid)
Cyclothiazide	Anhydron	2–4	
Phthalimidine derivative			Nerve deafness (ethacrynic acid & furosemide only when given IV)
Chlorthalidone	Hygroton	25–50	
			Impotence
Quinazoline derivatives			Pancreatitis
Quinethazone	Hydromox	100–150†	Marrow depression
Metolazone	Zaroxolyn Diulo	2.5–10	Purpura
			Azotemia
Anthranilic acid derivative			
Furosemide§	Lasix	40–1000‡	
Phenoxyacetic acid derivative			
Ethacrynic acid§	Edecrin	100–300‡	
Distal tubular diuretics (potassium sparing)			
Spironolactone	Aldactone	50–100‡	GI irritation, gynecomastia, impotence, menstrual irregularities, lethargy, hyperkalemia, hyponatremia, dry mouth, hirsutism
Triamterene	Dyrenium	100–300†	Hyperkalemia, hyponatremia, GI irritation

* Given once daily unless otherwise indicated.
† Usually divided and given twice daily.
‡ Usually divided and given four times daily.
§ Loop diuretics.

If the diuretic does not adequately control the hypertension, a sympathetic depressant drug should be added to the regimen (see TABLES 24-3 and 24-4). A β-blocker is preferred because its side effects are better tolerated. Drugs such as methyldopa, reserpine, and clonidine, which have a central action, are more likely to produce drowsiness, lethargy, and sometimes depression than are the others. Methyldopa and clonidine reduce sympathetic nervous activity by stimulating the α_2-adrenergic receptors in the brainstem. Reserpine depletes the brain of norepinephrine and serotonin and also depletes the peripheral sympathetic nerve ending of norepinephrine. Prazosin is a postsynaptic α_1-adrenergic blocking drug.

A vasodilator (hydralazine) can be added as a third agent (see TABLES 24-3 and 24-5). It is a direct vasodilator that does not act on the autonomic nervous system centrally or peripherally. Minoxidil, more potent than hydralazine, is associated with side effects including sodium and water retention and hirsutism which is poorly tolerated by women. It should be reserved for severe, resistant hypertension.

The fourth step is to add either guanethidine or clonidine to the regimen (see TABLE 24-3). Guanethidine blocks sympathetic transmission at the neuroeffector junction and, like reserpine, depletes tissue stores of norepinephrine. It is usually reserved for patients with severe hypertension, whose BP has not responded optimally to the drugs already mentioned.

In Europe, especially in the United Kingdom and Scandinavia, antihypertensive therapy is initiated with a β-blocking agent. BP frequently is controlled without adding other drugs, but it is often necessary to use enormous doses (up to 1 to 3 gm propranolol daily). Fortunately, the side effects of β-blockers, including bradycardia, are not dose-related once the dose has been increased above 200 or 300 mg of propranolol or metoprolol. Most physicians in the USA do not use monotherapy, but subscribe to the step-care approach outlined in TABLE 24-3.

Pargyline is a nonhydrazine monoamine oxidase inhibitor that inhibits sympathetic transmission at the neuroeffector junction, perhaps by formation of a false neurotransmitter, octopamine. It is as potent a hypotensive as guanethidine and has similar side effects except that it does not produce bradycardia or diarrhea. Its usefulness is limited by the food and drug incompatibilities shared by all monoamine oxidase inhibitors; *dangerous hypertensive crises can be induced if the large stores of norepinephrine that accumulate because monoamine oxidase is inhibited are suddenly released by tyramine, ephedrine, amphetamines, or other indirect sympathomimetic agents.* Some foods (aged cheese, chicken livers, pickled herring) and beverages (Chianti wine) contain enough tyramine to trigger such crises. The antihypertensive dose of pargyline ranges from 10 to 150 mg/day in a single dose. Its use should be restricted to depressed hypertensive patients or those who cannot tolerate guanethidine because of diarrhea.

For moderately severe hypertension (diastolic pressure between 115 and 130 mm Hg), it is usually advisable to start therapy with an oral diuretic and a sympathetic depressant (e.g., β-blocker, methyldopa, clonidine, prazosin, or reserpine) simultaneously. For severe hypertension (diastolic pressure > 130 mm Hg), therapy should be started with an oral diuretic, a β-blocker, and hydralazine simultaneously.

Prompt BP reduction with parenteral agents is indicated for patients with **hypertensive encephalopathy** or other hypertensive emergencies. Diazoxide or sodium nitroprusside is usually employed for this purpose. Both are very potent vasodilators and must be given IV. Because diazoxide is a nondiuretic thiazide derivative that can cause fluid retention if given without a diuretic, furosemide 40 or 80 mg IV is usually given with it. The usual dose of diazoxide is 300 mg given by IV bolus injection which reduces BP to normal within 3 to 5 min, and the effect of one injection may last 12 h. If a more gradual reduction in BP is desired, bolus injections of 100 mg may be given sequentially q 5 to 10 min until the BP has reached the optimal level. Side effects include nausea, vomiting, hyperglycemia, tachycardia, and, only occasionally, hypotension (without shock).

Sodium nitroprusside given by continuous IV infusion in D5W (50 to 100 mg/L) can reliably and promptly reduce BP in a hypertensive crisis, but its evanescent effect and its potency require almost

TABLE 24-3. STEPS IN THE MEDICAL TREATMENT OF HYPERTENSION

Step	Suggested Agent
1. Give an **oral diuretic**	Usually a thiazide or related diuretic; use furosemide if azotemia is present
2. Add a **sympathetic depressant**	β-blocker or methyldopa or clonidine or prazosin* or reserpine
3. Add a **vasodilator**	Hydralazine (minoxidil in resistant hypertension)
4. Add another **sympathetic depressant****	Guanethidine or clonidine

* Prazosin can also be used as an alternative to hydralazine in Step 3.
** When a β-blocker is used in Step 2, there may be merit in using phenoxybenzamine (10 to 20 mg q.i.d.) in Step 4.

TABLE 24–4. ANTIHYPERTENSIVE DRUGS THAT DEPRESS THE SYMPATHETIC NERVOUS SYSTEM

Drug	Trade Name	Dose (mg)	Side Effects
Central and peripheral inhibition			
Reserpine (single alkaloid)	Serpasil	0.1–0.25/day	Lethargy, fatigue, sedation, depression, activation of peptic ulcer, nasal congestion, parkinsonian-like state, impotence, diarrhea, bradycardia
Methyldopa	Aldomet	250–1000 b.i.d.	Lethargy, sedation, dry mouth, impotence or loss of ejaculation, depression, abnormal liver function tests with or without hepatic necrosis, positive direct Coombs' test (hemolytic anemia rare), nasal congestion, drug fever, retroperitoneal fibrosis (rare), myocarditis (rare), skin rash, orthostatic hypotension
Central inhibition			
Clonidine	Catapres	0.1–1.2 b.i.d.	Drowsiness, dry mouth, impotence, constipation, hypertensive overshoot following sudden withdrawal, GI irritation
Neuroeffector blockade			
Guanethidine	Ismelin	10–200/day	Orthostatic hypotension worse after prolonged recumbency, exercise hypotension, nasal congestion, diarrhea, impotence or loss of ejaculation
Pargyline	Eutonyl	10–200/day	Orthostatic hypotension worse after recumbency, exercise hypotension, nasal congestion, bradycardia, impotence or loss of ejaculation; interactions with drugs such as tyramine, ephedrine, & amphetamines & with foods containing tyramine to produce hypertensive crisis
Receptor blockade			
Alpha			
Prazosin	Minipress	1/day*–20 b.i.d.	Orthostatic hypotension (usually with first dose or with increments in dosage), headache, tachycardia, palpitations, fatigue, nausea, weakness, impotence or loss of ejaculation
Beta			
Propranolol	Inderal	40–160 b.i.d.†	Fatigue, listlessness, GI irritation, depression, bradycardia, impotence, bizarre mental aberrations, hyperglycemia, nightmares, insomnia. Precautions: congestive heart failure (impending or actual), 2° or 3° heart block, bronchial asthma, chronic occlusive arterial disease with peripheral ischemia, brittle insulin-dependent diabetes mellitus (may mask the warning symptoms of hypoglycemia)
Metoprolol‡	Lopressor	50–160 b.i.d.	
Nadolol	Corgard	40–320/day	
Pindolol	Visken	5–30 b.i.d.	
Timolol	Blocadren	10–30 b.i.d.	
Atenolol‡	Tenormin	50–100/day	

* Small test dose of 1 mg advisable to minimize risk of "first dose effect" (orthostatic hypotension and syncope).
† Doses up to 3 gm daily have been used in United Kingdom.
‡ Cardioselective β-blockers are less likely to aggravate asthma or peripheral ischemia than nonselective β-blockers. Nevertheless, in large doses selectivity is only relative and precautions must be observed in giving cardioselective β-blockers to asthmatics or patients with occlusive arterial disease.

TABLE 24–5. ANTIHYPERTENSIVE DRUGS THAT ACT DIRECTLY ON
VASCULAR SMOOTH MUSCLE

Drug	Trade Name	Dose Range (mg)	Side Effects
Hydralazine	Apresoline	25–150 b.i.d.	Headache, flushing palpitation, tachycardia, fluid retention, aggravation of angina, GI irritation, lupus-like syndrome, drug fever, skin rash, psychosis
Minoxidil	Loniten	2.5–20 b.i.d.	Headache, flushing palpitation, tachycardia, fluid retention, aggravation of angina, GI irritation, hirsutism

continuous monitoring of BP in an intensive care unit. It produces venodilation as well as arteriolar dilation and therefore reduces both pre- and afterload, making it especially useful for managing hypertensive patients with congestive heart failure. Side effects include nausea, vomiting, agitation, muscular twitching, and cutis anserina if BP is reduced too rapidly. Acute psychosis from thiocyanate intoxication can result from prolonged therapy. The drug should be discontinued if the blood thiocyanate concentration exceeds 12 mg/100 ml.

Reserpine, methyldopa, or trimethaphan may be given parenterally to manage hypertensive encephalopathy, but these agents are usually less desirable than diazoxide or sodium nitroprusside.

Inhibition of angiotensin II is a new concept in the control of hypertension which is actively being investigated. Some angiotensin II analogues have been synthesized which block the angiotensin II receptor. One of these is Sar[1]-ala[8] angiotensin II (Saralasin). These agents must be given IV, thus limiting their usefulness in managing hypertension. At this time they must be considered investigational tools for identifying hypertension that is angiotensin II-dependent.

Another approach to angiotensin II inhibition is inactivation of the enzyme that converts angiotensin I to angiotensin II (converting enzyme). SQ14225 (captopril) is the first orally effective converting enzyme inhibitor, and preliminary trials suggest that it is a potent agent that will control hypertension when other drugs have failed.

Prostaglandins and calcium antagonists may also offer new possibilities in the treatment of hypertension (see in Ch. 252).

RENOVASCULAR HYPERTENSION

Acute or chronic elevation of systemic BP caused by partial or complete occlusion of one or more renal arteries or their branches, often surgically correctable.

Etiology and Pathophysiology

Stenosis or occlusion of one or both main renal arteries or their branches or an accessory renal artery or its branches can cause hypertension by inciting the release of the enzyme renin from the juxtaglomerular cells of the affected kidney. Presumably, the decrease in pulse amplitude rather than the decrease in blood flow stimulates renin secretion. The area of the lumen must be decreased by at least 60% before the occlusion is hemodynamically significant. Renin acts on an α-2-globulin in the plasma (renin substrate) to form a decapeptide (angiotensin I) and ultimately an octapeptide (angiotensin II) that is one of the most potent pressor substances known.

In patients over age 50 yr (usually men), the most frequent cause of renal arterial stenosis is atherosclerosis; in younger patients (usually women), it is one of the fibrous dysplasias. Rarer causes of renal arterial stenosis or obstruction include emboli, trauma, inadvertent ligation during surgery, and extrinsic compression of the renal pedicle by tumors.

Symptoms, Signs, and Diagnosis

Renovascular hypertension should be suspected when hypertension first develops in a patient under age 30 or over age 50 or whenever previously stable hypertension abruptly accelerates. Rapid progression to malignant hypertension within 6 mo of onset is suggestive of renal artery disease.

A systolic-diastolic bruit in the epigastrium, usually transmitted to one or both upper quadrants, is the most important physical finding. Unfortunately, about 50% of patients with renovascular hypertension do not have systolic-diastolic bruits in the abdomen. Trauma to the back or flank or acute pain in this region with or without hematuria should alert the physician to the possibility of renovascular hypertension, but these historic features are rare. Renovascular hypertension is characterized by both high cardiac output and high peripheral resistance.

Both renovascular and primary hypertension are usually asymptomatic, and only a difference in history, the presence of an epigastric bruit, or abnormalities on an IVP will distinguish them clinically. The main justification for diagnostic evaluation is to find a surgically curable lesion.

None of the available tests for renovascular hypertension is ideal. All give false-positive and false-negative results; all are expensive; and some are hazardous. The most widely used test for screening purposes is the rapid sequence IVP, although it has been shown that nearly 20% of patients with renovascular hypertension will have a normal IVP. The renal flow scan may be as useful as urography for screening, but does not give as much anatomic information. A positive excretory urogram is indicated by a differential of > 1.5 cm in vertical axis length of the kidneys (allowing for the fact that the left kidney is normally 0.5 cm longer than the right), and by delay of the ischemic kidney in excreting the contrast media.

Aortography and selective renal arteriography can establish the diagnosis of renovascular disease and are useful in determining operability and planning the best surgical approach. A normal rapid sequence urogram does not contraindicate arteriography if other indications warrant it. However, a lesion found on an arteriogram may not be responsible for the hypertension. Further study is necessary to define the probable significance of lesions and the probable response to surgical therapy (see below).

Prognosis and Treatment

Without surgical or medical treatment, the prognosis in renovascular hypertension is similar to untreated primary hypertension. Most investigators have found that appropriate surgery will relieve hypertension if the renal vein renin activity **(RVRA)** ratio (involved to uninvolved side) is $> 1.5:1$. However, many patients with RVRA ratios less than this have also been cured of hypertension by revascularization or removal of the ischemic kidney. There is evidence that short duration of hypertension (< 5 yr) and appropriate abnormalities on the rapid sequence intravenous urogram, when considered together, are just as reliable in predicting the outcome of surgery as is RVRA ratio. To enhance the reliability of the RVRA ratio, blood should be obtained from the renal veins under conditions of sodium depletion to stimulate the release of renin. This can be accomplished by use of a 0.5-gm sodium diet and oral diuretics for 48 h or by injecting 40 to 80 mg furosemide IV and obtaining blood 30 min later. Bilateral lesions, which occur in 35% of cases, make the rapid sequence urogram and the RVRA ratio less dependable. Peripheral venous renin activity is often normal in renovascular hypertension.

Revascularization of the involved kidney with a saphenous vein bypass graft is recommended for younger patients with fibrous dysplasia of the renal artery. The cure rate is 90% with proper selection, and the surgical mortality rate is $< 1\%$. If disease in the arterial branches precludes adequate revascularization, nephrectomy may be considered but medical treatment is preferable if the BP can be controlled.

Atherosclerotic patients have been found to respond less well to surgery, presumably because they are older and have more extensive vascular disease within the kidneys and throughout the vascular system. Their hypertension may persist and surgical complications occur more commonly. Surgical mortality is higher than for young patients with fibrous dysplasia of the renal artery. Since renovascular hypertension responds to antihypertensive drugs as does primary hypertension (see ARTERIAL HYPERTENSION, above), medical treatment is preferable to surgery unless the BP cannot be controlled or unless bilateral involvement or a lesion in an artery to a solitary kidney threatens renal function. The decision as to surgery must be individualized on the basis of the patient's overall status, age, the type of renal arterial disease, and prior response to medical therapy. When possible, surgery should involve repair and revascularization instead of nephrectomy.

SYNCOPE

(Fainting)

Syncope is usually defined as *the sudden loss of consciousness,* but, in general usage, includes *near-total loss of consciousness or the sensation that such loss is impending.* The altered state of consciousness is usually brief and usually occurs with the subject upright. Recovery usually is spontaneous and is often associated with the subject's falling or assuming a horizontal position. Both cardiovascular and noncardiovascular conditions may cause syncope.

Etiology and Pathophysiology

Both primary cardiovascular disorders and secondary cardiovascular failure due to other than cardiac disease may result in impaired circulation due to decreased effective cardiac output and cerebral perfusion. Upright posture accentuates the ineffective cardiac output. Ventricular tachyarrhythmias (ventricular fibrillation or tachycardia) frequently result in shock and syncope. Less commonly, atrial tachyarrhythmias (atrial fibrillation, flutter, or paroxysmal atrial tachycardia) also result in syncope, especially if there are other coexisting cardiac lesions that already impair cardiac output. Bradyarrhythmias (severe bradycardia, Stokes-Adams) may also produce syncope. Patients with severe valvular and subvalvular aortic stenosis may faint when engaging in activities requiring abrupt increases in cardiac output. Acute myocardial infarction or acute pulmonary embolism (with or without associated arrhythmias) rarely results in syncope unless the patient goes into profound shock.

In syncope not due to primary cardiovascular disease, **vasovagal attacks (vasodepressor syncope)** caused by fright, trauma, or pain are most common. Reflex inhibition of sympathetic activity with augmented vagal activity results in decreased peripheral resistance, decreased cardiac output, peripheral vasodilation, and bradycardia. Subjects frequently note nausea, become pale, and sweat. In patients with severe asthmatic episodes or protracted coughing spells, **prolonged and marked elevation of intrathoracic pressure** may so impair venous return to the heart that BP also falls to levels producing syncope. Similarly, severe straining while having a bowel movement or in attempt ing to void (as occurs commonly in elderly men with prostatic hypertrophy) may result in loss of consciousness. **Orthostatic hypotension** due to any cause (see below) may also be severe enough to cause syncope when the patient is upright. Occasionally, especially in elderly patients, a sensitive carotid sinus mechanism may result in reflex hypotension. This may be induced by pressure caused by a tight collar, manual massage, or even by turning the head in a particular direction.

Noncardiovascular causes of syncope may be further divided into neurologic and metabolic etiologies that alter cerebral function. Syncope rarely occurs after stroke unless there is global involvement, but it may occur during or after seizure activity. The postictal state after grand mal seizures is frequently associated with loss of consciousness, and transient lapses in consciousness are common during petit mal seizures. Loss of consciousness due to profound hypoglycemia or drugs rarely occurs abruptly, but usually evolves over a period of minutes or more. Syncope may also occur as a result of hyperventilation and its metabolic sequela during severe anxiety states.

Symptoms and Signs

The patient usually notes sudden onset of a pervasive sense of weakness, giddiness, distortion and dimming of vision, sweating, nausea, and sometimes vomiting, together with a sensation of impending loss of consciousness. If he can lie down quickly, loss of consciousness may be averted and the other symptoms begin to recede. An injurious fall is rare. The entire episode may last only seconds or up to 30 min. Convulsions, loss of bowel or bladder control, drowsiness, disorientation, or amnesia do not occur. In simple syncope, the patient is strikingly pale and sweating profusely. The pulse may be impalpable or very slow and BP tends to be low. Symptoms and signs remit promptly in the horizontal position.

Diagnosis

Recognizing the cause of loss of consciousness is not usually difficult, especially when the patient can give a complete or even partial history. Stokes-Adams attacks are especially suspect when syncope does not occur in the upright position. Additional clues can be obtained from the reports of witnesses to the event; examination of the pulse, BP, and precordium; evidence of prior seizure activity, etc. Where repetitive attacks have occurred without evident cause, thorough cardiovascular, neurologic, and metabolic evaluation is necessary, especially to rule out recurrent inapparent arrhythmias, seizures, or obscure metabolic factors.

Treatment

Immediate treatment of syncope is frequently unnecessary, since the more common cardiovascular mechanisms of decreased cardiac output are usually remedied by the patient's falling or putting himself into the horizontal position. Well-meaning but ill-informed bystanders sometimes aggravate the situation by propping the subject upright or carrying him in an upright position. Raising the legs of a supine patient is useful in restoring effective cardiac output. Specific therapy is dictated by the precise etiology of the syncopal episode.

ORTHOSTATIC HYPOTENSION

An excessive fall in BP on assuming the erect position. The condition is not a disease entity itself, but a manifestation of abnormalities in normal BP regulation.

Pathophysiology

On arising to the erect position there is normally considerable pooling of blood in the dependent venous capacitance vessels. The subsequent transient decrease in venous return and cardiac output results in a reduction of BP, which is sensed by the baroreceptor mechanisms of the aortic and carotid sinus areas. Activation of autonomic reflexes results in rapid restoration of systolic BP to normal, a slight overshoot in diastolic pressure, and tachycardia. These changes are primarily mediated through increased sympathetic discharge resulting in augmented vasomotor tone of the capacitance veins and an increase in heart rate and myocardial contractile force to enhance cardiac output; peripheral arterial tone is also increased by similar mechanisms. When the afferent, central, or efferent portions of the reflex arc are impaired by a primary disease process or a drug, or in the presence of hypovolemia or impaired myocardial function, these compensatory mechanisms may be inadequate to compensate fully for the reduced pressure. Hence, BP falls to levels that result in markedly decreased tissue perfusion, manifested first by the effects of impaired cerebral blood flow.

Etiology

The most common cause of symptomatic orthostatic hypotension is the use of **drugs that impair autonomic reflexes,** usually excessive doses of antihypertensive drugs such as methyldopa, guanethidine, clonidine, reserpine and rauwolfia alkaloids, and ganglionic blocking drugs (mecamylamine, hexamethonium, pentolinium). Vasodilator therapy for hypertension usually is not associated with a greater BP reduction in the standing position since autonomic reflexes remain intact. The use of diuretics is associated with significant orthostatic hypotension only when volume depletion and dehydration are produced. Orthostatic hypotension is not generally caused by β-adrenergic blocking drugs, but α-adrenergic blockers (phentolamine and phenoxybenzamine), indicated only for treating hypertension due to pheochromocytoma, may be causative. Another α-blocker, prazosin, may cause orthostatic hypotension, especially when initiating therapy.

Several groups of drugs used in nervous and mental disorders reduce BP in the standing position as an important side effect. Monoamine oxidase inhibitors (isocarboxazid, phenelzine, and tranylcypromine) used in depression may also reduce BP with symptoms of orthostatic hypotension. Less commonly the tricyclic antidepressants (nortriptyline, amitriptyline, desipramine, imipramine, and protriptyline) may reduce BP in the standing position, as may the phenothiazine antipsychotic drugs such as chlorpromazine, promazine, and thioridazine. Additional drugs that may occasionally cause orthostatic hypotension include quinidine, L-dopa, barbiturates, and alcohol. The interference with autonomic reflexes due to the drugs cited above is a reversible pharmacologic effect. In contrast, the antineoplastic drug vincristine may produce severe, long-lasting orthostatic hypotension as a result of its neurotoxic side effects.

Acute or semi-acute severe **reductions in intravascular volume** may produce moderate to severe orthostatic hypotension due to the decrease in cardiac output despite intact autonomic reflexes. Acute hemorrhage, severe vomiting or diarrhea, excessive use of diuretics, or protracted sweating or osmotic diuresis (as in uncontrolled diabetes mellitus) all may lead to marked volume contraction, dehydration, and orthostatic hypotension unless there is adequate fluid and electrolyte replacement. Similarly, adrenocortical insufficiency (Addison's disease) may lead to hypovolemic orthostatic hypotension in the absence of adequate salt intake.

Neuropathic disorders may interrupt the sympathetic reflex arc at one of several sites with consequent impairment of the normal adrenergic responses to standing. Diseases commonly associated with orthostatic hypotension are diabetes mellitus, amyloidosis, porphyria, tabes dorsalis, pernicious anemia, uremia, Parkinson's disease, Guillain-Barré syndrome (postinfectious polyneuropathy), and Riley-Day syndrome (familial dysautonomia). Surgical sympathectomy in the treatment of severe hypertension, vasospastic disorders, or peripheral vascular insufficiency also results in reduction of BP in the standing position. Approximately 2/3 of patients with pheochromocytoma and some patients with primary hyperaldosteronism and *severe* hypokalemia may present with hypertension in the supine position and paradoxic orthostatic hypotension.

Two poorly understood and possibly related primary neuropathic disorders frequently associated with severe orthostatic hypotension are the **Shy-Drager syndrome** and the entity known as **idiopathic orthostatic hypotension.** These conditions are characterized by widespread lesions affecting not only the sympathetic nervous system, but also the parasympathetic nervous system, basal ganglia, and spinal tracts. Early manifestations include marked decreases in sympathetic motor tone, especially to the arterial and venous system in the legs. Lesions spread in an ascending fashion with other prominent signs and symptoms; they include loss of hair on the lower extremities, loss of sweating in an ascending order, and, eventually, the development of autonomic denervation of other organs, resulting in atony of the bowel, bladder, and stomach; decreased salivation and tearing; mydriasis; and impaired visual accommodation. Focal neurologic signs may appear, including tremor, rigidity, incoordination, and pyramidal tract signs (compatible with extrapyramidal, cerebellar, and pyramidal degeneration). Cerebellar ataxia or muscular atrophy and fasciculations compatible with anterior horn cell disease may be present. The most severe orthostatic hypotension occurs in these conditions, and as the autonomic denervation progresses, patients lose cardiac sympathetic innervation with resulting bradycardia despite marked reduction in BP when standing. Paradoxically, in these patients BP in the supine position may be somewhat elevated despite severe orthostatic changes because of loss of parasympathetic as well as sympathetic regulation of the cardiovascular system.

Symptoms, Signs, and Diagnosis

Mild to moderate acute reductions in cerebral blood flow may result in a feeling of faintness, lightheadedness, and mental or visual blurring, and more severe reductions produce sudden syncope and even generalized seizures. Many other phenomena may appear in orthostatic hypotension; these usually relate to the specific disorder causing the condition (see above). The diagnosis is made on the basis of symptoms suggestive of hypotension and the demonstration of marked reductions in BP in the standing position. A specific etiologic diagnosis must be based upon each patient's presenting circumstances.

Prognosis and Treatment

The prognosis depends upon the underlying cause. Orthostatic hypotension due to hypovolemia or drug effects is usually reversed by therapy directed at these problems. When the underlying disorder is chronic and unremitting, the orthostatic hypotension may be controlled until the basic disease process progresses and other organs are involved. In these instances therapy can be directed only toward increasing cardiac output or peripheral vasoconstriction, and not toward the underlying disease. Usually, BP may be maintained at an asymptomatic, though somewhat reduced, level in the standing position, but in the advanced stages of the Shy-Drager syndrome or idiopathic orthostatic hypotension, this may be impossible with pharmacologic therapy alone, and some form of counterpressure device may be needed.

In milder cases, the peripherally active adrenergic agent ephedrine (25 to 50 mg orally q 3 to 4 h while awake) may support the BP in a tolerable range. If this proves ineffective, volume expansion, by increasing salt intake or giving salt-retaining hormones, frequently is helpful. Usually, it is sufficient to increase sodium chloride intake by 5 to 10 gm above normal dietary intake by liberal salting of food; patients who find this unpalatable can use sodium chloride tablets. In addition, fludrocortisone

(0.1 to 0.5 mg orally each day) usually produces a weight gain of 3 to 5 lb due to salt retention and extracellular fluid volume expansion and provides better maintenance of the standing BP. This drug requires adequate salt ingestion and is not effective unless there is evidence of weight gain and fluid accumulation. Congestive heart failure in patients with impaired myocardial function is a possible danger of this therapy, but the development of dependent edema in the absence of elevated venous pressure or pulmonary symptoms does not contraindicate continuation of therapy. Due to the potassium-wasting effects of the mineralocorticoid and the high sodium intake, hypokalemia may occur. The serum potassium should be carefully monitored and replacement therapy should be instituted if needed. A recent report suggests that propranolol 40 to 240 mg/day orally may further enhance the beneficial effects of salt and steroid therapy.

Nonsteroidal anti-inflammatory agents result in salt retention and the inhibition of prostaglandin synthesis. One of these agents, indomethacin (25 to 50 mg orally t.i.d.), has been reported to produce beneficial effects in patients with orthostatic hypotension. However, since a dangerous pressor drug reaction has been described in other patients when indomethacin and sympathomimetic drugs (ephedrine, phenylpropanolamine, etc.) were used together, *this combination should be avoided*. Oral administration of monoamine oxidase inhibitors plus amphetamines, tyramine, or other indirectly acting sympathomimetic agents has also been suggested for use in this condition, but the concomitant use of these drugs may be very dangerous with the potential for lethal hypertensive reactions, and is *not recommended*.

Venous pooling in the lower extremities may also be reduced mechanically to enhance cardiac output and BP while standing. In mild cases elastic hose may be useful, but tightly fitted, specially tailored pressure stockings or leotards may be necessary. In the most serious cases, BP may be maintained only with an inflatable aviator-type antigravity suit to produce sufficient lower extremity and abdominal counterpressure.

SHOCK

A state in which blood flow to peripheral tissues is inadequate to sustain life because of insufficient cardiac output or maldistribution of peripheral blood flow, usually associated with diminished peripheral circulation, hypotension, and reduced urine output.

Etiology and Pathophysiology

Shock may be due to inadequate intravascular volume (hypovolemic), to inadequate cardiac function (cardiogenic), to inadequate vasomotor tone (vasodilation), or to combinations of these factors.

Hypovolemic shock: Inadequate intravascular volume (absolute or relative) produces diminished ventricular filling and a reduction in stroke volume which, unless compensated for by increased heart rate, results in a decreased cardiac output. Acute hemorrhage following trauma is a common cause of hypovolemic shock, or hemorrhage may occur in a preexisting (often unrecognized) disease such as peptic ulcer, esophageal varices, or aortic aneurysm. Hemorrhage may be apparent (hematemesis or melena) or concealed (ruptured ectopic pregnancy) and should always be considered in patients presenting with shock. Since shock may develop within minutes (before homeostatic hemodilution) following acute blood loss, the Hb and Hct may be normal, and this finding does not rule out hemorrhage as the cause of shock.

In the absence of hemorrhage, hypovolemic shock may follow increased losses of body fluids. It usually takes several hours to develop and is frequently associated with a rising Hb or Hct. Fluid may be lost from the body surface following thermal or chemical injury or may be sequestered in the peritoneal cavity in response to generalized peritonitis following perforation of the GI tract or pancreatitis. Fluid may also be pooled within or lost from the GI tract due to vomiting or diarrhea from a variety of conditions including small or large bowel obstruction, paralytic ileus, or gastroenteritis. Excessive renal losses of fluid leading to hypovolemic shock may occur in diabetes mellitus or insipidus, adrenal insufficiency, "salt-losing" nephritis, the polyuric phase following acute tubular damage, and after administration of potent diuretic agents. Hypovolemic shock may also develop when intravascular fluid is lost to the extravascular space because of increased capillary permeability secondary to anoxia or cardiac arrest or as the result of acute hypersensitivity reactions.

In addition to excessive fluid loss, hypovolemic shock may be due to inadequate fluid intake, often associated with modest increases in fluid loss. Frequently these patients, because of neurologic or physical disability, cannot respond to thirst by increasing fluid intake. In hospitalized patients, hypovolemia may be compounded when early signs of circulatory insufficiency are incorrectly ascribed to cardiac failure and fluids are withheld for fear of precipitating pulmonary edema.

Cardiogenic shock: Although cardiac output is reduced as in hypovolemic shock, the reduction is secondary to ventricular failure in cardiogenic shock. Blood volume is adequate, and the cardiac output will not be significantly improved by fluid administration. Cardiogenic shock may result from mechanical interference with ventricular filling, as during tension pneumothorax and pericardial tamponade, or from interference with ventricular emptying, as in massive pulmonary embolism. In these conditions proper diagnosis and immediate specific therapy may be lifesaving. Cardiogenic shock also may result from a disturbance of heart rate or rhythm, frequently associated with preexisting cardiac disease. Inadequate myocardial contraction, a third mechanism for cardiogenic shock, is most commonly due to acute myocardial infarction, but may also occur in valvular heart disease, in cardiomyopathies, following administration of drugs that depress myocardial function, or in severe hypoxemia secondary to pulmonary or neurologic disease.

Vasodilation: Hypovolemic shock may be *relative* in that circulating blood volume is normal but insufficient for adequate cardiac filling. A variety of conditions may cause widespread venous and/or arteriolar dilation. If cardiac output does not increase commensurate with reduced vascular resistance, arterial hypotension develops, and if arterial pressure falls below a critical level, vital centers will be inadequately perfused. The degree of hypotension necessary to cause the shock syndrome varies and often is related to the presence of preexisting vascular disease. Thus, a modest degree of hypotension that is tolerated well by a young, relatively healthy individual might result in severe cerebral, cardiac, or renal dysfunction in a patient who has significant arteriosclerosis in vessels supplying these organs. Widespread vasodilation may occur following severe cerebral trauma or hemorrhage **(neurogenic shock),** hepatic failure, or ingestion of certain drugs or poisons. Shock associated with bacterial infection **(bacteremic** or **septic shock)** may be partly due to the effects of endotoxin or other chemical mediators on resistance vessels, resulting in vasodilation and decreased vascular resistance (see Ch. 5). In addition, some patients with acute myocardial infarction and shock appear to have inadequate compensatory vasoconstriction in response to the decreased cardiac output.

Symptoms and Signs

The manifestations associated with shock may be due to the shock state itself or to the underlying disease process. Findings in patients with **hypovolemic** or **cardiogenic shock** are similar. Mentation may be preserved, but lethargy, confusion, and somnolence are common. The hands and feet are cold, moist, and often cyanotic and pale. Capillary filling time is prolonged and, in extreme cases, a bluish reticular pattern may appear over large areas. The pulse is weak and rapid unless there is associated heart block or terminal bradycardia; in some instances only femoral or carotid pulses can be felt. Tachypnea and hyperventilation are present, but apnea may be a terminal event when the respiratory center fails due to inadequate cerebral perfusion. BP taken by cuff tends to be low or unobtainable, but, direct measurement by intra-arterial cannula often gives significantly higher values.

The findings in **septic shock** (see also Ch. 5) may be similar to those in hypovolemic and cardiogenic shock, but with some significant differences. Fever, usually preceded by chills, is generally present. *Elevated* cardiac output is associated with diminished total peripheral resistance, possibly accompanied by hyperventilation and respiratory alkalosis. Thus, early symptoms may include the onset of a shaking chill, rapid rise in temperature, warm flushed skin, a bounding pulse, and falling and rising BP **(hyperdynamic syndrome).** Urinary flow is decreased despite the high cardiac output. Mental status is usually markedly impaired, and mental confusion may even be a premonitory sign preceding hypotension by 24 h or more. However, these findings are variable and may not be apparent even in patients whose markedly increased cardiac output and reduced vascular resistance are confirmed by direct hemodynamic measurement. The presence of fever and hypotension suggest septic shock; in later stages hypothermia is common.

Manifestations of the underlying disease process may be important clues to the diagnosis of shock. Acute blood or fluid loss from a ruptured aorta, spleen, or tubal pregnancy or from peritonitis can be suspected from the physical findings. Signs of generalized dehydration are helpful in recognizing hypovolemia in patients with neurologic, GI, renal, or metabolic disorders. Cardiogenic shock is suggested by engorged neck veins, signs of pulmonary congestion, and a gallop rhythm. A systolic murmur may indicate ventricular septal rupture or mitral insufficiency, either of which may result in shock after acute myocardial infarction. Pericardial tamponade is suggested by muffled heart sounds, a pericardial rub, and a paradoxical pulse. Massive pulmonary embolism is suspected in patients with a parasternal lift, a loud fourth heart sound at the left sternal border, and an accentuated, widely split pulmonary closure sound. Septic shock tends to occur at the extremes of age and is more common in men than in women. The signs of preexisting pulmonary, GI, or urinary tract infection may be present, as may signs of an underlying malignancy or debilitating disease resulting in altered immunity against infection. In women of childbearing age, septic abortion is a common cause of shock.

Diagnosis

The diagnosis of shock requires evidence of insufficient tissue perfusion that is due to either reduced cardiac output or inadequate peripheral vasomotor tone. Within the framework of those conditions known to result in the shock syndrome, most consider shock to be present in any patient who develops a significant fall in arterial pressure, a urine flow of < 30 ml/h, and a progressive increase in the arterial lactic acid concentration associated with reduced arterial P_{CO_2} and bicarbonate levels. The diagnosis of shock would be supported by the presence of signs relating to hypoperfusion of specific organs (obtundation, ECG abnormalities, peripheral cyanosis) or signs relating to compensatory mechanisms (tachycardia, tachypnea, diaphoresis). In the earliest stages of shock, especially septic shock, many of the above signs might be absent or undetected if not specifically sought. Thus, treatment might not be initiated until the shock is irreversible. None of these findings *alone* is specific for the shock syndrome; each must be evaluated in the context of the overall clinical setting. The arterial BP, in particular, may be reduced to levels commonly associated with the shock syndrome in patients who otherwise show no evidence of inadequate tissue perfusion. In such patients, reversal of hypotension with vasopressor agents might do more harm than good.

Hypovolemic shock is diagnosed by demonstrating normal or reduced ventricular filling pressure with a low cardiac output and the shock syndrome. A right ventricular filling pressure or central venous pressure **(CVP)** < 7 cm H_2O (5 mm Hg) suggests hypovolemia; however, the CVP may be above this level when hypovolemic shock occurs with preexisting pulmonary hypertension. A better index to left ventricular filling is obtained by floating a balloon-tipped catheter into the pulmonary artery and measuring pulmonary end-diastolic **(PEDP)** or wedge **(PWP)** pressure, both of which are usually closely related to the actual left ventricular pressure during diastole. A low PEDP or PWP suggests that hypovolemia is causing or contributing to the shock syndrome. When hypovolemia is suspected, a therapeutic trial with volume loading may help confirm the diagnosis. Hypovolemia can be assumed to be present when arterial pressure and urine flow are improved and the clinical manifestations of shock are reduced with small increments in CVP or PWP following rapid infusion (100 ml/10 min) of a colloid such as dextran, plasma, or serum albumin.

Cardiogenic shock is diagnosed by demonstrating reduced cardiac output associated with an increased ventricular filling pressure. Since hypovolemia may occur with acute myocardial infarction or preexisting heart disease, the shock cannot be assumed to be due entirely to myocardial damage. Pericardial tamponade, tension pneumothorax, or massive pulmonary embolism can usually be diagnosed if thought of. When myocardial damage is sufficient to result in shock, the ECG is usually diagnostic of acute infarction; the ECG is also helpful in identifying arrhythmias that may, in themselves, cause shock.

Shock secondary to vasodilation is suspected in patients with cerebral trauma, sepsis, or drug intoxication, but hypovolemia, which is frequently also present, must be excluded. Myocardial dysfunction secondary to release of a myocardial depressant factor or inadequate coronary perfusion may also complicate shock due to vasodilation.

Prognosis

Untreated, shock is usually fatal. Prognosis following development of shock depends on the cause, the presence of preexisting or complicating illness, time between onset and diagnosis, and adequacy of therapy. The mortality in shock due to massive myocardial infarction and in elderly patients with septic shock remains extremely high.

Treatment

First aid: Prior to hospitalization, the usual first aid measures apply. The patient should be kept warm and his feet raised slightly to improve venous return. Hemorrhage should be stopped, airway and ventilation checked, and respiratory assistance given if necessary. Nothing should be given by mouth, and the patient's head should be turned to avoid aspiration if emesis occurs. Narcotics should generally be avoided, but severe pain may be treated with morphine 2.5 to 5.0 mg IV, repeated if necessary. Anxiety may be due to cerebral hypoperfusion, and sedatives or tranquilizers should *not* be given.

Definitive therapy: Vital functions may have to be stabilized before diagnostic procedures can be carried out. Profound hypotension may result in depression of respiratory function, which rapidly leads to hypoventilation, worsening acidosis, hypoxemia, and death. Assisted ventilation with high O_2 concentrations should be instituted promptly. Airway obstruction from secretions or gastric contents must be removed.

If hemorrhage is suspected, a large (16- to 18-gauge) catheter should be inserted into a peripheral vein (femoral or internal jugular) by direct skin puncture for the infusion of blood or other fluids and the administration of medication. Analysis of arterial pH and blood gases may be helpful. Giving sodium bicarbonate IV may help to reverse metabolic acidosis.

Monitoring: Patients in whom shock is not immediately reversed should be considered critically ill and definitive treatment should be continued in a special care area (e.g., ICU, CCU). Careful monitoring should be followed: (1) ECG; (2) arterial BP—preferably by direct intra-arterial cannula; (3) ventricular filling pressure (CVP, or preferably PEDP or PWP); (4) respiratory rate and depth; (5) urine flow (usually by indwelling bladder catheter); (6) arterial blood pH, P_{O2}, and P_{CO2}; (7) body temperature; and (8) clinical status including sensorium, pulse volume, skin temperature, and color. Measuring cardiac output using thermodilution technics is also very helpful in patients requiring extended treatment. A well-designed flowsheet is extremely valuable. Serial measurements of blood volume, plasma oncotic pressure, Hct, and EEG may also be helpful.

Hypovolemic shock is treated by restoring intravascular volume and eliminating the underlying cause. Rapid infusion of fluids to elderly patients may precipitate pulmonary edema; therefore, monitoring of CVP, PEDP, or PWP is helpful during therapy even after the diagnosis of hypovolemia has been established. Generally PEDP or PWP should not be raised above 18 to 20 mm Hg by fluid replacements. The primary measurements to follow are BP, PEDP or PWP, and urine flow. CVP monitoring is helpful when PEDP or PWP measurements are not available. The precise mode and type of fluid to be given are determined by the specific circumstances and are guided by frequent determination of Hct and serum electrolytes. Saline is as good as any other solution, but large quantities may cause pulmonary edema. After approximately 40 to 50% of the calculated blood volume is replaced, whole blood or a colloid solution should be given. Whole blood should be cross-matched, but in an urgent or desperate situation giving 1 to 2 u. of O, Rh-negative blood is an alternative. Colloid solutions include dextran, plasma, or reconstituted 5% human serum albumin, all of which lack RBCs and will dilute the Hct. Serum albumin is the most physiologic and safest, but it is expensive and may not be available. Fresh frozen plasma carries the risk of hepatitis B. Dextran is an excellent osmotic expander, but using > 1 L is not advised because it can alter coagulation and may make cross-matching inaccurate.

Shock that fails to respond to volume replacement may be due to insufficient volume administration while bleeding or fluid loss continues or may be due to complicating factors such as myocardial damage or coexisting septic shock. When hypovolemia is not the probable cause or when BP does not respond promptly to volume administration, a pressor agent (levarterenol given by controlled IV infusion or metaraminol given by IM injection—see TABLE 24-6) may be considered to raise the systolic pressure to between 90 and 100 mm Hg. The use of pressor agents is controversial; they are generally overused and *should be limited to carefully selected situations*. Although they can increase peripheral resistance and elevate the BP by stimulating receptors, the elevated BP may be falsely reassuring since already impaired peripheral and visceral microcirculation is worsened. Vasopressors are used primarily to enhance the force of the heart beat and to increase coronary artery blood flow; e.g., in profound cardiac failure associated with critically reduced coronary perfusion. Inadequate coronary perfusion may be manifested by ischemic chest pain, ECG changes, and arrhythmias. Some authorities recommend simultaneous use of an α-adrenergic blocking agent such as phenoxybenzamine or massive doses of corticosteroids (e.g., hydrocortisone 2 to 10 gm IV) to prevent adverse effects on the peripheral circulation.

Bradycardia and other arrhythmias, if due to hypoxemia, acidosis, or hypotension, often respond to the above measures, but specific antiarrhythmic drugs, cardioversion, or temporary cardiac pacing may be necessary (see CARDIAC ARRHYTHMIAS in Ch. 25).

Cardiogenic shock is treated by improving cardiac performance. Shock following **acute myocardial infarction** should be treated by O_2 inhalation, stabilization of cardiac rate and rhythm, and volume expansion if indicated by normal or low CVP, PEDP, or PWP. Morphine 3 to 5 mg given IV over a 2-min period may relieve severe chest pain and help restore BP; the initial dose can be repeated after 10 min if there is no evidence of respiratory depression. Atropine 1 mg IV is often effective in reversing the bradycardia and hypotension that frequently occur very early after the onset of symptoms, particularly in inferior-posterior infarctions. Atropine will also help prevent the undesired vagal effects of morphine. Levarterenol or dopamine is used to maintain arterial systolic pressure above 90 mm Hg (but not above 110 mm Hg). Because it markedly increases O_2 demand, isoproterenol is *contraindicated* in patients with shock after acute myocardial infarction except temporarily to increase heart rate before transvenous pacing is begun when shock is associated with severe bradycardia. Isoproterenol may also be of value in patients with severe mitral regurgitation. Digitalis is not

TABLE 24–6. INOTROPIC CATECHOLAMINES

Drug	Route of Administration and Dosage	Hemodynamic Actions
Levarterenol (Norepinephrine)	8 mg/500 ml D5W continuous IV infusion at 0.25 ml (0.004 mg) to 1 ml (0.016 mg)/min	α-adrenergic: vasoconstriction β-adrenergic: inotropic and chronotropic*
Metaraminol	5 to 10 mg by IM injection	Same as levarterenol with slower onset and dissipation of effect
Isoproterenol	2 mg/500 ml D5W continuous IV infusion at 0.25 ml (0.001 mg) to 1 ml (0.004 mg)/min	β-adrenergic: vasodilation, inotropic, and chronotropic
Dopamine	500 mg/500 ml D5W continuous IV infusion at 0.25 ml (0.25 mg) to 1 ml (1 mg)/min	α-adrenergic: vasoconstriction† β-adrenergic: inotropic, chronotropic, and vasodilation† Nonadrenergic: renal and splanchnic vasodilation
Dobutamine	500 mg/500 ml D5W continuous IV infusions at 0.25 ml (0.25 mg) to 1 ml (1 mg)/min	β-adrenergic: inotropic‡

* Effect not apparent if arterial pressure elevated too much.
† Effects depend upon dosage given and underlying pathophysiology.
‡ Chronotropic, arrhythmogenic, and direct vascular effects are minimal at lower doses.

routinely used in shock but may be of value in patients with supraventricular tachycardia or signs of pulmonary congestion. In the absence of severe hypotension, dobutamine infusion may be used to improve cardiac output and reduce left ventricular filling pressure somewhat. Tachycardia and arrhythmias may occasionally occur during dobutamine administration, particularly at higher doses. Vasodilators such as nitroprusside and nitroglycerin, which act to increase venous capacitance and/or lower systemic vascular resistance, reduce the workload imposed on the damaged myocardium and may also be of value in patients who do not have severe arterial hypotension. Combination therapy such as dopamine or dobutamine with nitroprusside or nitroglycerine may be particularly useful but requires close monitoring of infusion rates as well as clinical and hemodynamic responses. Since the early use of mechanical circulatory assistance, particularly intra-aortic balloon counterpulsation, appears to be extremely valuable for temporarily reversing shock in patients with acute myocardial infarction, it should be considered whenever the above measures do not result in prompt clinical improvement. Although the mortality is high, emergency coronary and left ventricular cineangiography followed by surgical correction of mechanical defects such as ruptured ventricular septum, mitral regurgitation, or localized aneurysmal dilation and/or by coronary artery bypass may be required for patients who cannot be successfully weaned from the intra-aortic balloon.

Management of **shock due to vasodilation** is primarily supportive while treating the underlying cause. Little can be done when shock follows massive irreversible cerebral damage. Shock due to sepsis should be treated by eliminating hypovolemia as a causative factor and by maintaining an adequate arterial pressure with vasoactive agents (see Ch. 5). Isoproterenol is occasionally of value, but levarterenol may be necessary. Dopamine is an inotropic agent that is less vasoconstrictive than levarterenol and causes less vasodilation than isoproterenol but selectively improves mesenteric and renal blood flow; it may have advantages over other vasopressors in selected patients. Appropriate antibiotics and surgical drainage of abscesses are important and necessary adjuncts in treating septic shock.

Other considerations: Pericardial tamponade requires pericardiocentesis, and in life-threatening situations, pericardial fluid may have to be removed at the bedside. Under less urgent circumstances surgical creation of a pericardial window or pericardectomy may be advisable to avoid recurrence. **Massive pulmonary embolism** resulting in shock is treated by supportive measures (levarterenol, digitalis) to improve cardiac function and with IV heparin to prevent recurrent thrombosis. In patients who cannot be stabilized with these measures, emergency pulmonary angiography and surgical embolectomy should be considered. The use of urokinase or streptokinase to lyse clots already formed remains experimental but may be of value.

Pulmonary complications that often coexist or develop in patients with shock must not be overlooked. Massive doses of corticosteroids (hydrocortisone 2 to 10 gm IV) may reduce cellular damage and have been advocated for patients with shock, especially septic shock. When given with levarterenol and similar agents, steroids may block their adverse effects on peripheral or visceral microcirculation without hampering their inotropic effect on the heart. Mannitol (15 gm in 100 ml H_2O IV) or furosemide (40 to 80 mg IV) may help prevent renal tubular damage resulting from diminished renal perfusion.

SYPHILIS OF THE CARDIOVASCULAR SYSTEM

Etiology and Pathology

Treponema pallidum invades the bloodstream and lymphatics in the first 2 to 3 days of primary acquired syphilis, but cardiovascular symptoms usually occur during the late phase of the disease, 10 to 25 yr after the initial infection. The organisms enter the perivascular lymphatic spaces of the vasa vasorum of large blood vessels, especially the aorta and particularly those adjacent to the mediastinum, after passing through the lungs. The resultant inflammatory response leads to an **obliterative endarteritis of the vasa vasorum** with scarring of the layers of the aorta. Cardiovascular involvement is rare in congenital syphilis, but it may appear in untreated patients 15 to 20 yr after birth; the lesions are identical to those of acquired syphilis.

During the secondary phase of syphilis, **acute myocarditis** may occur, resulting rarely, in the late phase, in **myocardial gummas**, which occur most often in the upper portion of the interventricular septum and sometimes on the free wall of the left ventricle. In the former site they cause varying degrees of atrioventricular conduction disturbances, including complete or incomplete heart block. Gummas of the free wall may result in scarring and aneurysm formation with subsequent rupture and sudden death.

Aortitis occurs in about 70 to 80% of patients with untreated syphilis but is usually asymptomatic and is discovered only at postmortem examination. The most significant involvement follows the densest lymphatic distribution of the ascending aorta in the supravalvular portion, and the least follows the sparest lymphatic supply, that of the descending aorta. **Complications** of aortic insufficiency, aneurysm, and coronary ostial stenosis develop in about 10% of patients with syphilitic aortitis. Aortic insufficiency, the most common complication, results from gradual dilation of the root of the aorta. As scarring involves the commissures of the aortic cusps, rolling the free edges of the valve, the valve cusps retract so that the valve leaflets coapt incompletely. Aortic insufficiency may also be due to syphilitic involvement of the ascending aorta with scarring and aneurysmal dilation of the sinuses of Valsalva. Aortic aneurysms are the second most common lesion. Scarring of the aortic wall, especially in the ascending and transverse arch, results in saccular aneurysms in 10% of patients with aortitis and fusiform dilation of the aorta in 45%. Syphilitic aortitis in the supravalvular region of the aorta may involve the coronary ostia, producing cicatricial narrowing. Stenosis may lead to anginal pain but rarely results in myocardial infarction, since a prolonged time permits the development of collateral myocardial circulation.

Symptoms, Signs, and Diagnosis

A composite of clinical syndromes, signs, and laboratory findings suggests the diagnosis and includes serologic tests, a history of treated or untreated syphilis, x-ray changes, aortic insufficiency, cardiomegaly, and chest pain. The VDRL test (or a similar cardiolipin test) is reactive in about 75% of active cases of syphilitic cardiovascular disease, and CSF serology is reactive in almost 50%. The fluorescent treponemal antibody test is a sensitive indicator of the presence of active or previous syphilitic disease. Serologic tests are discussed further in Ch. 162. Radiologic examination, including chest x-rays, barium swallow, CT, and angiocardiography, may be needed to confirm the diagnosis.

The diagnosis of **syphilitic aortitis** is suggested clinically by widening of the aortic root and a fine pattern of linear calcification on the lateral and anterior walls of the ascending aorta on chest x-ray; increased retrosternal dullness to percussion and a loud, musical tambour quality of the aortic second sound on physical examination; circulatory embarrassment or cardiac failure; chest pain; and paroxysmal nocturnal dyspnea. Syphilitic aortitis is more likely in patients under age 40 yr who have these clinical findings, do not have hypertension or rheumatic heart disease, and have reactive serologic tests.

Since **syphilitic aortic insufficiency** is characterized by the absence of significant aortic stenosis, it may be distinguished from rheumatic heart disease or a congenital bicuspid aortic valve in which significant stenosis may occur. The murmur of syphilitic aortic insufficiency, unlike the murmur of rheumatic aortic insufficiency, is often transmitted to the right of the sternum, where it is best heard in the 3rd or 4th intercostal space of the right sternal border. The symptoms and signs of syphilitic aortic insufficiency are otherwise similar to those of other forms of aortic insufficiency. (See VALVULAR HEART DISEASE in Ch. 25.)

Syphilitic aneurysms may enlarge and produce symptoms by compressing or eroding adjacent structures in the mediastinum and chest wall. Symptom complexes secondary to aneurysm formation include a brassy cough and stridor from pressure on the trachea; bronchial stenosis and subsequent pulmonary collapse or infection; dysphagia secondary to esophageal compression; hoarseness secondary to compression of the recurrent laryngeal nerve; and painful erosion of the sternum and ribs or spine from the repeated pulsations of the dilated aorta. Rarely, an aneurysm may present as a pulsating mass on the chest wall, but more often, since aneurysms tend to bulge anteriorly and laterally, they cause dullness to percussion to the right of the sternum and a loud systolic murmur. An aneurysm may rupture, producing sudden death, but saccular aneurysms are often protected from rupture by laminated clots within their lumens; clots, however, do not prevent the continual enlargement of the aneurysm. Widening of the intracardiac portion of the ascending aorta may be detected by echocardiography or angiography. Aneurysms of the descending aorta are usually asymptomatic and are diagnosed on x-ray. Abdominal aneurysms are usually not due to syphilis.

Patients with **coronary ostial stenosis** complain of angina on effort or emotion, and the pain is frequently very severe at night. Complete coronary occlusion is uncommon, but sudden death may occur. ECGs show S-T segment depression and inverted T waves over the left ventricle, although these changes may only be apparent after exercise.

Prognosis

Uncomplicated syphilitic aortitis may have a prolonged course; asymptomatic patients have a good prognosis, and unless complications develop, they may live a normal life span. The degree of cardiovascular involvement in late syphilis is perhaps the most significant factor in determining the duration of life following the onset of symptoms. Aortic insufficiency, although often asymptomatic for 15 to 20 yr, may cause coronary artery insufficiency or congestive heart failure, and only 30 to 40% of patients live > 10 yr after syphilitic aortic insufficiency is diagnosed. Less than 20% of patients who have congestive heart failure when syphilitic aortic insufficiency is diagnosed survive 5 yr or longer, and < 6% survive 10 yr; the average life span after the onset of congestive heart failure is about 3 yr. Syphilitic aortic aneurysms carry a grave prognosis; the average life span after onset of symptoms is about 6 mo.

Treatment

The treatment of syphilitic aortitis and its complications includes treating the infection itself (see the treatment of latent syphilis in Ch. 162). Congestive heart failure secondary to aortic insufficiency is treated as usual (see CONGESTIVE HEART FAILURE in Ch. 25). Angina pectoris due to coronary ostial stenosis that can be demonstrated on coronary arteriography may be treated by endarterectomy of the coronary ostia to relieve the stenotic segments. Aortic insufficiency associated with aortitis or an aneurysm may be treated by prosthetic replacement of the ascending aorta and aortic valve. Aneurysms of the ascending and transverse arch of the aorta are usually treated by surgical resection and prosthetic replacement of that portion of the aorta.

25. DISEASES OF THE HEART AND PERICARDIUM

CONGESTIVE HEART FAILURE (CHF)

(For CHF in infants, see Vol. I, Ch. 23)

A clinical syndrome in which the heart fails to propel blood forward normally, resulting in congestion in the pulmonary and/or systemic circulation and diminished blood flow to the tissues because of reduced cardiac output. The condition, usually easily recognized at the bedside, is caused by many different kinds of heart disease. Adverse consequences of the series of physiologic events that initially compensate for reduced performance of the heart as a pump lead to the symptoms and signs of clinical CHF.

Physiology

The clinical findings and rational treatment of CHF are best understood by first reviewing normal heart function and the effect of disease. At rest and during exercise, the amount of venous return, cardiac output **(CO)**, and the distribution of blood flow and delivery of O_2 to tissues is delicately balanced by nervous, humoral, and intrinsic factors to meet body needs. Since the energy of cardiac muscle contraction is a function of the length of the muscle fiber prior to stimulation, cardiac stroke work is directly proportional to the length or degree of stretch of the myocardial fiber in the normal heart. Recent work suggests that in the abnormal heart, left ventricular outflow resistance or aortic impedance is important in regulating pump performance. It is useful to describe cardiac function in terms of the **ventricular function curve (the Frank and Starling relationship**—Fig. 25–1**)**. As the figure depicts, the output of the heart, which can be measured in various ways, is dependent upon the diastolic length of cardiac muscle fiber. Fiber length is not easily measured at bedside so that end-diastolic pressure is used as an index of volume or stretch with the assumption that during the period of observation, diastolic compliance, the stiffness of the ventricle, is unchanged during a given set of observations. Often this assumption is not justified, but end-diastolic pressure is easily measured, and it is useful in conceptualizing abnormal cardiac function. The axes of the ventricular function curve can be related to the symptoms of patients with heart disease. Dyspnea, congestion, and edema develop as ventricular filling pressure rises, as depicted on the abscissa. Peripheral hypoperfusion, fatigue, and peripheral cyanosis develop as CO falls, as depicted on the ordinate.

A variety of factors such as catecholamine level, contractility, and energetics are thought to create a family of Frank-Starling curves. Changes in muscle stretch and diastolic volume probably play a minor role in response of the normal heart. When contractility is reduced by disease, however, increased diastolic volume and pressure result in improved CO. It is generally assumed, but difficult to prove, that after a certain point on the curve, cardiac function progressively declines as filling pressures increase creating a descending limb. In myocardial disease contractility usually is reduced, and the function curve is displaced downward so that much greater stretch and higher filling pressures are required to produce a small increment in CO. Stimulation of the sympathetic nervous system or injection of catecholamines increases cardiac contractility and moves the ventricular function curve upward, but this mechanism is probably not very helpful in the presence of advanced cardiac disease. Changes in afterload or outflow resistance may be more important in controlling ventricular function in the diseased myocardium.

Ventricular filling pressure or **preload** is altered by changes in blood volume, venomotor tone, myocardial contractility, and ventricular stiffness or compliance. Thus, systemic or pulmonary venous pressure is determined both by myocardial function and factors affecting the veins directly. In the failing heart, venomotor tone is increased to maintain a high ventricular filling pressure. Systemic venous pressure falls in hypovolemic states and rises in hypervolemia. When the atrioventricular valves open, venous return is propelled and to some degree sucked into the ventricle during diastole. Most filling occurs in the early part of diastole. Atrial contraction adds only a small volume to the ventricle, but this atrial "kick" stretches the well-filled ventricle and creates a small but significant increment in ventricular end-diastolic pressure. This maximizes cardiac performance by providing optimal diastolic stretch but minimizes mean ventricular filling pressure (i.e., minimizes pulmonary venous and systemic venous pressures). In patients with decreased myocardial function, loss of the normal atrial "kick," as in atrial fibrillation, will reduce CO and arterial systolic pressure and increase mean venous pressures.

The stiffness or compliance of the ventricle and its contractility influence the position of the heart on the ventricular function curve. Factors which control compliance are not well understood, but thick, hypertrophied hearts are stiff or noncompliant and hence have high filling pressure (e.g., idiopathic hypertrophic subaortic stenosis, severe aortic stenosis with ventricular hypertrophy).

Increased **afterload** (*the resistance against which the heart contracts*), as in hypertension or aortic stenosis, causes hypertrophy of the myocardium, an increase in cell size. Myocardial capacity for hyperplasia or increase in cell number is negligible, and myocardial hypoxia possibly results from

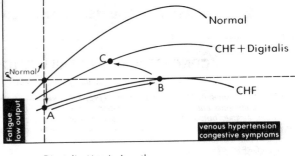

Systolic Pressure
Stroke Volume
Cardiac Output
Stroke Work
Cardiac Work

Diastolic Muscle Length
End-Diastolic Pressure
End-Diastolic Volume

FIG. 25–1. **Frank-Starling relationship.** *Ordinate,* ability of ventricle to function as a pump. *Abscissa,* direct or indirect measurements of length or stretch of myocardial fiber. Dotted lines depict resting normal values; the normal curve includes point of intersection. Note that under normal conditions left ventricular systolic pressure, stroke volume, and work increase rapidly as the myocardial fiber is lengthened at end diastole. There is a family of ventricular function curves depicting cardiac performance under normal and abnormal conditions. During heart failure consequent to myocardial insufficiency, ventricular performance falls sharply (Point A). Reduced stroke volume causes increased end diastolic volume with consequent stretchings of diastolic muscle length. Ventricular function moves to the right on a relatively flat ventricular function curve to achieve relatively normal resting cardiac performance (Point B). Thus, compensation in heart failure to maintain adequate resting cardiac performance results from increased ventricular diastolic volume and pressure. Treatment of the failing ventricle with digitalis improves the ventricular function curve, which, however, remains abnormal. Ventricular function moves to Point C with adequate or improved cardiac performance at rest and reduced but still abnormal muscle length, end diastolic pressure, and volume. In patients with fatigue as the main symptom of heart failure, cardiac output tends to be low while ventricular filling pressures are inordinately high. (Adapted from J. F. Spann, D. T. Mason, R. Zelis: "Recent Advances in the Understanding of Congestive Heart Failure (II)" in *Modern Concepts of Cardiovascular Disease* Vol. 39, pp. 79–84, Feb. 1970. Used by permission of the American Heart Association, Inc., and the author.)

hypertrophy because neovascularization is deficient (multiple areas of fibrosis are commonly present in the hypertrophied ventricle).

Acute changes in myocardial contractility are largely modulated through the sympathetic nervous system. Sympathetic discharge to the heart generally has greater influence than circulating catecholamines. Sympathetic regulation of contractility is markedly reduced in CHF and advanced myocardial disease, because the myocardial concentration of the neurotransmitter norepinephrine is greatly decreased. Giving digitalis is the prime therapeutic maneuver to enhance the contractile state in patients with CHF.

Reduction in afterload, as might occur with standing or vasodilation accompanying exertion, induces more complete ventricular emptying, thus increasing the **ejection fraction** (systolic volume/end-diastolic volume). Acute increase in afterload has the opposite effect. When an individual rises from the sitting or supine position, venous inflow momentarily falls, stroke volume falls, systolic pressure declines somewhat, and the heart rate increases. Generally, CO does not fall despite the stroke volume decrease because the increased heart rate permits a constant volume/minute. Within moments of continued standing, systemic arterial and venous tone increases, venous return or preload rises to the control state, stroke volume increases, and the heart rate slows. The sequence of changes reflects the critical importance of reflex adjustment, largely mediated through baroceptor mechanisms, in maintaining adequate cardiac performance. Therapeutic reduction in afterload has become an important new modality in treating chronic myocardial failure.

In some situations the sequence of ventricular contraction may significantly influence ventricular performance. Ventricular activation is abnormal in bundle branch block. If the myocardium is diseased, ventricular function can be adversely affected. Patchy ventricular dysfunction **(dyskinesia)** is characteristic of coronary artery disease and influences ventricular performance adversely in ways not yet completely understood.

Recently, attention has focused on the important influence of afterload in controlling ventricular function. **Afterload** may be defined as *those factors opposing ventricular emptying when the semilunar valves open at the end of isovolumic contraction.* In patients with poor left ventricular function, an increase in afterload (e.g., a rise in arterial pressure) results in increased ventricular filling pressure and a decline in CO. A reduction in afterload increases myocardial fiber shortening and hence increases stroke volume. In the abnormal ventricle, reduction of afterload may significantly decrease ventricular diastolic pressures. Long-term afterload reduction with drugs is becoming an accepted form of therapy for chronic ventricular failure.

Ultrastructure: The fundamental contractile unit of the heart is the sarcomere, which consists of interdigitating bands of actin and myosin protein connecting through dynamic crosslinks of troponin, tropomyosin, and calcium. The fibers of actin are anchored to the intercalated discs or Z bands. According to current understanding, electrical depolarization mobilizes free calcium ions, stimulating alteration in the crosslinks so that the filaments of actin and myosin slide by each other and the muscle contracts. The performance of the heart as a pump can be described by these ultrastructural relationships. A direct relationship between initial sarcomere length and force of contraction has been demonstrated and Frank-Starling curves can be constructed for individual sarcomeres.

Energetics: The major determinants of myocardial O_2 need are heart rate, contractile state, and afterload or systolic tension. Pressure work is far more costly metabolically than volume work. Thus, patients with aortic stenosis have greater myocardial O_2 requirements than patients with severe aortic regurgitation. A rough index of myocardial O_2 demand under different loads can be calculated by multiplying the heart rate by the systolic pressure.

Because of its obligate oxidative metabolism, the heart depends on coronary blood flow and O_2 delivery for sustained normal function. It extracts more O_2 per unit of flow than any other tissue. Coronary sinus P_{O2} is the lowest of a venous sample from any organ. Any factor that reduces coronary blood flow, such as increased ventricular wall tension, hypotension, tachycardia, or coronary artery obstruction, may compromise ventricular function. Anaerobic metabolism can provide only about 10 to 30% of the energy needed for sustained myocardial contraction. Anaerobiosis results in increased lactate production so that the principal metabolic sign of myocardial hypoxia is increased lactic acid concentration in the coronary sinus.

No effective therapeutic modalities to increase myocardial energy production or substrate utilization are currently available. However, methods of reducing cardiac work by reducing the heart rate, altering contractility, or decreasing systolic afterload can improve the performance of the failing ventricle. When left ventricular function is impaired, reflex arterial vasoconstriction increases impedance to left ventricular ejection and reduces stroke volume. Thus treatment with a vasodilator to reduce impedance may improve ventricular performance by reducing cardiac work to a more tolerable level.

Exercise and cardiac reserve: Cardiac reserve may be defined as *unutilized ability of the resting heart to deliver O_2 to the tissues.* Reserve mechanisms include alterations in heart rate, systolic and diastolic volume, stroke volume, and tissue extraction of O_2. In well-trained young adults during maximal exercise, CO may increase from its resting normal value of 6 L/min to 25 L/min or more; O_2 consumption increases from 250 to 1500 ml/min or more; heart rate may increase from a sedentary 72 to 180 beats/min. The increased demand of the body for O_2 to meet metabolic requirements is met by a marked increase in CO (stroke volume × heart rate) and by greater than normal extraction of O_2 from capillary blood in the tissues. In the normal young adult at rest, arterial blood contains approximately 18 ml O_2/100 ml of blood, and mixed venous or pulmonary artery blood contains about 14 ml/100 ml. The arteriovenous O_2 difference (A-V_{O2}) is thus about 4.0 ± 0.4 ml O_2/100 ml of blood. During exercise the increase in CO, even to maximal levels, is insufficient to meet tissue metabolic needs; hence the tissues extract more O_2, and mixed venous blood O_2 content falls considerably. The A-V_{O2} difference widens to 12 to 14 ml/100 ml.

In heart failure, stroke volume is reduced and relatively fixed so that the major components of cardiac reserve are heart rate and tissue extraction of O_2 as reflected in the A-V_{O2} difference. Measurement of systemic A-V_{O2} difference is one of the most sensitive indices of ventricular performance available. An increase in resting systemic arterial-pulmonary artery O_2 difference greater than normal is irrefutable evidence of compromised ventricular function. With the Swan-Ganz pulmonary artery catheterization technic and bedside measurement of blood gases, this index of cardiac function is readily available, easily interpreted, and provides valuable clinical physiologic information.

Oxyhemoglobin dissociation: Availability of O_2 to the tissues is largely influenced by the oxyhemoglobin dissociation curve (FIG. 25–2). The position of this curve is frequently expressed as P_{50}, the partial pressure of O_2 in blood at 50% oxyhemoglobin saturation; normal P_{50} is 27 ± 2 mm Hg. An increase in P_{50} indicates a rightward shift of the oxyhemoglobin dissociation curve (decreased affinity of Hb for O_2). Alterations in this curve provide another reserve mechanism in heart failure. Shift of the curve to the right, downward displacement, means that for a given P_{O2} less O_2 is combined with Hb and the saturation is lower; at the capillary, more O_2 is released and thus available to the tissues. Increased hydrogen concentration (reduced pH) shifts the oxyhemoglobin dissociation curve to the right (Bohr effect). A major factor influencing the position of the curve is the concentration of 2,3-diphosphoglycerate **(DPG)** in Hb. Increased DPG alters the spatial relationships within the Hb molecule, reducing its affinity for O_2 and shifting the curve to the right. Increased DPG and a favorable rightward shift enhancing O_2 availability at the tissues occurs in anemia, hypoxia, and heart failure.

Etiology and Pathophysiology

The sequence of events leading to the clinical manifestations of heart failure begins when the myocardium cannot contract with sufficient force to maintain a normal stroke volume. Because of

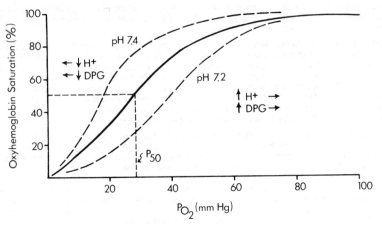

FIG. 25–2. Oxyhemoglobin dissociation curve. Arterial oxyhemoglobin saturation (*ordinate*) is curvilinearly related to partial pressure of O_2 (*abscissa*). P_{O_2}, at 50% saturation, P_{50}, is normally 27 mm Hg. The dissociation curve is shifted to the right by increased H^+ concentration and increased RBC diphosphoglycerate. The curve is shifted to the left by decreased H^+ and lower RBC diphosphoglycerate. Hb characterized by rightward shifting of the curve has a *decreased* affinity for O_2; Hb characterized by a leftward shift of curve has an *increased* affinity for O_2.

incomplete emptying, the ejection fraction (stroke volume/end-diastolic volume), normally over 50%, falls. End-diastolic volume increases, shifting the ventricle to the right on the Frank-Starling curve with a consequent rise in end-diastolic pressure. The increased diastolic stretch induces a more forceful systolic contraction, enabling the ventricle to maintain adequate cardiac work at the expense of greater diastolic volume and tension (FIG. 25–1). As the process proceeds, ventricular filling pressure and hence venous pressure, pulmonary or systemic, gradually increases while CO falls and the A-V_{O_2} difference widens. Systemic arterial pressure is maintained by an increase in peripheral vascular resistance. The resultant rise in left ventricular outflow resistance may further adversely affect myocardial performance.

In most forms of heart disease, either the right or the left ventricle is primarily affected. **Left ventricular failure** is characterized by reduced CO and increased pulmonary venous pressure. The cardinal clinical signs are dyspnea on exertion and fatigue. Elevation of pulmonary venous pressure to the level of plasma protein oncotic pressure (about 24 mm Hg) leads to increased lung water, reduced pulmonary compliance, and a rise in the O_2 cost or work of breathing. Left ventricular failure occurs characteristically in hypertension, aortic valve disease, patent ductus arteriosus, large ventricular septal defect, mitral regurgitation, and coronary artery disease.

Right ventricular failure is most commonly caused by left ventricular failure secondary to pulmonary arterial hypertension induced by pulmonary vascular changes and by elevated pulmonary venous pressure. Right ventricular failure is characterized by systemic venous hypertension and edema; fatigue and low CO are late manifestations. Diseases causing right ventricular failure include any form of left ventricular failure, mitral stenosis, primary pulmonary hypertension, multiple pulmonary embolization, pulmonary stenosis, tricuspid regurgitation, and atrial septal defect. The volume overload and increased systemic venous pressure in conditions such as polycythemia, overtransfusion, acute renal failure with overhydration, and obstruction of the vena cava may cause marked systemic venous hypertension, but myocardial function is usually normal, at least initially.

Although mitral stenosis and left atrial myxoma are characterized by dyspnea and high pulmonary venous pressure, these developments are not due to left ventricular failure, since left ventricular function is usually normal. The concept of left atrial failure in these conditions has been proposed.

Biventricular failure characteristically occurs in the myocardiopathies (alcoholic, viral, and nonspecific) and in chronic constrictive pericarditis, but the presenting symptoms are usually those of right ventricular failure. Both right and left *ventricular* filling pressures are elevated approximately equally, but systemic fluid retention and edema occur more readily with lower *right atrial* pressures than with the left atrial pressures needed to produce pulmonary edema. Therefore, such patients may manifest considerable edema with little or no dyspnea. CO is usually sharply reduced and fatigue is a prominent symptom.

Pulmonary effects: Pulmonary venous hypertension and increased lung water alter pulmonary mechanics and ventilation-perfusion relationships. Dyspnea has been correlated with increased work of breathing and elevated pulmonary venous pressure, although the exact cause of the subjective symptom is still debated. With increased pulmonary venous pressure, fluid escapes from the pulmonary capillary into the interstitial space and alveoli with consequent alveolar collapse and atelectasis. Pleural effusions of CHF characteristically accumulate in the right hemithorax. Lymphatic drainage is greatly enhanced but cannot mobilize the continual increase in lung water. Unoxygenated pulmonary arterial blood is shunted past nonaerated alveoli, decreasing mixed pulmonary capillary P_{O2}. A combination of alveolar hyperventilation due to increased lung stiffness and reduced arterial P_{O2} is characteristic of left ventricular failure. Thus, arterial blood gas analysis reveals an increased pH and a reduced P_{CO2} (respiratory alkalosis) with decreased saturation and P_{O2} (increased intrapulmonary shunting). Increasing the inspired O_2 concentration will increase arterial P_{O2} and improve O_2 delivery to the tissues, but the pulmonary shunting limits the response.

Renal function: Renal blood flow and GFR are reduced in CHF, and blood flow within the kidney is redistributed. The filtration fraction is reduced, and filtered sodium is decreased, but tubular sodium absorption is enhanced. In advanced CHF, hyperaldosteronism develops, further increasing salt and water retention. Other as yet poorly defined extrarenal factors, both reflex and humoral, also seem to influence sodium retention. Antidiuretic hormone (ADH) is not directly involved in the altered fluid balance of CHF. As a result of the renal changes, the blood volume, total body sodium, and water are increased. These alterations are partly compensatory since they enhance myocardial fiber stretch by increasing ventricular volume, but they also lead directly to the congestive clinical manifestations of heart failure.

Hepatic function: Reduced splanchnic blood flow and increased venous pressure characteristic of CHF cause liver engorgement and decreased nutrient hepatic blood flow. Moderate hepatic dysfunction commonly occurs in right heart failure, with approximately equal elevations of conjugated and unconjugated bilirubin, increased prothrombin time, and rise in hepatic enzymes such as alkaline phosphatase, AST (SGOT), and ALT (SGPT). These enzyme elevations are usually modest, but in severely compromised circulatory states with marked reduction of CO and hypotension, hepatic central necrosis and the manifestations of liver failure may be severe enough to suggest hepatitis with acute hepatic failure. In advanced CHF reduced aldosterone breakdown by the liver further contributes to fluid retention.

Other organs: Chronic severe venous hypertension has been associated with the syndrome of protein-losing enteropathy characterized by marked hypoalbuminemia. Bowel infarction, acute and chronic GI hemorrhage, and malabsorption syndromes may complicate low CO states. Peripheral gangrene in the absence of large vessel occlusion has been reported in patients with chronic markedly reduced CO. Chronic irritability and decreased mental performance may reflect severely reduced cerebral blood flow and hypoxia in chronic low-output states.

Symptoms and Signs

CHF may be predominantly left- or right-sided, may develop gradually, or may present suddenly with acute pulmonary edema.

Left ventricular failure may become apparent early with undue tachycardia, fatigue with exertion, dyspnea with mild exercise, and intolerance to cold. Paroxysmal nocturnal dyspnea and cough reflect the movement of excess fluid from the extremities to the lungs that occurs when a patient with borderline left ventricular compensation lies down. These symptoms may be important early clues. Occasionally, pulmonary venous hypertension and increased pulmonary fluid manifest primarily as bronchospasm and wheezing. In advanced CHF severe cough is a prominent symptom. Rusty tinged or brownish sputum due to blood and the presence of heart failure cells are common. Frank hemoptysis presumably due to ruptured pulmonary varices from bronchial veins is not common but may occur, and large amounts of blood may be lost. Physical findings are influenced by the type of heart disease. Signs of left ventricular failure include reduced carotid pulsations, diffuse and laterally-displaced apical impulse, palpable and audible 3rd and 4th heart sounds, accentuated pulmonic 2nd sound, inspiratory basilar rales, and right-sided pleural effusion.

Acute pulmonary edema is a dramatic and life-threatening manifestation of acute left ventricular failure. A sudden rise in left ventricular filling pressure to high levels results in rapid movement of plasma fluid through pulmonary capillaries into the interstitial spaces and alveoli. The patient presents with extreme dyspnea, cyanosis, tachypnea, hyperpnea, restlessness, and anxiety with a sense of suffocation. Pallor and diaphoresis are common. The pulse may be thready, and the BP may be difficult to obtain although direct measurement reveals a normal central aortic pressure. Respirations are grunting and labored with inspiration, and expiration is prolonged. Expiratory rales are widely dispersed over both lung fields anteriorly and posteriorly. In some patients the major manifestation is marked bronchospasm or wheezing, termed **cardiac asthma.** Vigorous, noisy respiratory efforts often prevent careful examination of the cardiovascular system. Hypoxia is severe, and cyanosis is deep. CO_2 retention is a late, ominous manifestation.

Right ventricular failure: The principal symptoms include increasing fatigue, awareness of fullness in the neck, fullness in the abdomen, occasionally an ache in the right upper quadrant of the abdomen, ankle swelling, and (in advanced stages) ascites. Pertinent signs include evidence of venous hypertension, abnormally large A or V waves in the external jugular pulse, an enlarged and tender liver, murmur of tricuspid regurgitation, and pitting edema of the lower extremities. Cyanosis may occur with either left or right ventricular failure. In the former the cause is central, and the cyanosis reflects hypoxia; in the latter, it is due to capillary stasis and the increased A-V$_{O2}$ difference with resultant marked venous oxyhemoglobin unsaturation. Improvement in the color of the nail bed with vigorous massage suggests the presence of peripheral cyanosis. Central cyanosis cannot be altered by locally increasing blood flow.

There are no *specific* ECG findings in CHF. Abnormalities such as ventricular hypertrophy, acute myocardial infarction, or bundle branch block may provide clues to the etiology of the heart disease. Analysis of rhythm is often helpful; determining whether arrhythmias are primary or secondary is important. The recent development of rapid atrial fibrillation, for example, may precipitate acute left ventricular failure and requires prompt treatment. On the other hand, frequent ventricular premature beats may be secondary and may subside when the heart failure is treated.

Chest x-rays are helpful in evaluating the presence and severity of CHF and its cause. Hilar congestion and the "butterfly" or "batwing" configuration of increased vascular markings are characteristic of left ventricular failure. Recognition of edema surrounding bronchioles, peribronchial cuffing, may help establish that CHF is the cause of pulmonary infiltrates. Kerley B lines reflect chronic elevation of left atrial pressure and represent chronic thickening of the intralobular septa from edema. Careful examination of the cardiac silhouette, evaluation of chamber enlargement, and a search for intra- or extracardiac calcifications are important x-ray clues to the etiology of the primary cardiac abnormality.

Treatment

Management of CHF is based on the physiologic concepts, specific etiology, and pathophysiology outlined above. Therapy includes rest, oxygenation, measures to improve myocardial contractility, correction of arrhythmias, diuresis, sodium restriction, and reduction of afterload if possible. Even in the most urgent situation the cause of the CHF must be determined, correctable conditions searched for, and contributing factors eliminated.

Rest: Reduction of heart rate and cardiac work by bed rest and sedation contributes importantly to management. The degree of restriction depends upon the severity of the CHF. Sedation with diazepam 5 to 10 mg orally as needed and flurazepam 15 to 30 mg orally at bedtime is often helpful.

Contributing factors: An important component of management is the recognition and control of factors that may be causing increased cardiac demands or adversely affecting myocardial function, such as hypertension, anemia, excess salt intake, excess alcohol, arrhythmias, thyrotoxicosis, fever, increased ambient temperature, or pulmonary emboli.

Rhythm: Arrhythmias should be evaluated as primary or secondary. Usually, arrhythmias are secondary to CHF and improve with therapy. Frequent ventricular premature or atrial premature beats will usually subside as the congestion improves. However, some arrhythmias may require specific treatment. In rapid atrial fibrillation, for example, control of the ventricular rate or cardioversion may resolve the failure. Persistent "sinus tachycardia" at a rate of 150 may actually be atrial flutter with 2:1 A-V block requiring specific therapy.

Digitalis: Adequate dosage with digitalis has been a major component of therapy in chronic CHF. Digitalis suppresses ventricular arrhythmias, increases venous tone, increases renal blood flow, slows heart rate, prolongs A-V conduction, and in toxic doses or the presence of hypokalemia may induce ventricular extrasystoles. Its primary action is to increase myocardial contractile force, leading to a decreased diastolic ventricular volume, decreased ventricular wall tension, reduced ventricular filling pressure, increased stroke volume, and both reflex and direct slowing of heart rate. The net effect is increased cardiac work at reduced metabolic cost.

Since improved ventricular performance in the patient with CHF may follow reduction in filling pressure (preload) by use of diuretics or reduction in afterload by use of vasodilators, controversy over the role of digitalis in treatment of heart failure has developed. While many clinicians favor its use, effective treatment of CHF is possible with reduced doses or no digitalis.

Digoxin or digitoxin may be given orally, IM, or IV. IM injection is not recommended because the alcohol preparation is extremely painful and irregularly absorbed. Ouabain and deslanoside are given IV only. Physicians should be thoroughly familiar with 2 preparations, one short-acting and one longer-acting. Familiarity with use and properties of digoxin and digitoxin will suffice in most clinical situations. The properties and dosages of digitalis preparations are outlined in TABLE 25–1.

Since digitalis compounds are eliminated from the body in proportion to their concentration, large doses have traditionally been given rapidly (digitalization) for initial full therapeutic effect, followed by lower maintenance doses (see TABLE 25–1). However, digitalis has a narrow toxic-therapeutic ratio, and currently low-dose schedules are being advocated. When a reasonably effective digitalis level has accumulated, increased doses enhance the risk of toxicity with only a small increment in therapeutic effect (see FIG. 25–3). When there is no urgent need, standard maintenance doses of digitalis can be given orally without an initial loading dose. Digitalization will be achieved in this manner in about 5 days with digoxin and in 10 to 14 days with digitoxin. This approach is favored in elderly, ambulatory patients who do not need rapid treatment, who may be seen only intermittently, and who may be confused by changing dosages. Digitalis blood levels may be helpful in evaluating absorption when the drug is given orally and in regulating the dosage in difficult cases. The serum sample should be drawn not less than 6 h after the most recent dose, or falsely high values will be

TABLE 25-1. DIGITALIS PREPARATIONS—ROUTES OF ADMINISTRATION, PHARMACOKINETICS, DOSAGES

	Digoxin	Digitoxin	Deslanoside	Ouabain
Preferred route*	Orally, IV	Orally, IV	IV	IV
Percent GI absorption	85%	100%		
Onset of effect, IV	15–30 min	$1/2$–2 h	10–30 min	5–10 min
Peak effect, IV	4–6 h	6–12 h	1–2 h	$1/2$–2 h
Plasma half-life	30–36 h	5–7 days	30–36 h	18–25 h
Excretion, metabolism	Renal	Hepatic, GI	Renal	Renal, GI

Plasma level
  Therapeutic
  Toxic
	1.0–1.4 ng/ml
	> 2 ng/ml
		20–30 ng/ml
		> 40 ng/ml		

Digitalization schedule†
Oral, 24 h
	0 h: 0.5 mg
	8 h: 0.25 mg
	16 h: 0.25 mg
	24 h: 0.25 mg
	Thereafter, daily
	  maintenance
	  dose‡
		0 h: 0.6 mg
		8 h: 0.3 mg
		16 h: 0.2 mg
		24 h: 0.1 mg
		Thereafter, daily
		  maintenance dose		

Oral, 48 h	0.25 mg
	  q 8 h × 6
	Thereafter, daily
	  maintenance
	  dose‡
		0.2 mg q 8 h × 6
		Thereafter, daily
		  maintenance dose		

Oral, gradual	0.25 mg/day (digitalization achieved in 5–7 days)‡	0.1 mg/day (digitalization achieved in 10–14 days)		

IV, 24 h	0 h: 0.5 mg
	6 h: 0.25 mg
	12 h: 0.125 mg
	18 h: 0.125 mg
	Thereafter, daily
	  maintenance
	  dose‡
		0 h: 0.6 mg
		8 h: 0.3 mg
		16 h: 0.2 mg
		24 h: 0.1 mg
		Thereafter, daily
		  maintenance dose
			0 h: 0.6 mg
			6 h: 0.4 mg
			12 h: 0.2 mg
			18 h: 0.2 mg
			24 h: 0.2 mg
				0 h: 0.3 mg
				4 h: 0.2 mg
				8 h: 0.1 mg
				12 h: 0.1 mg‡

Daily maintenance
  dose, oral
	0.25–0.375
	  mg/day
		0.1 mg 5 times/wk
		to 1.5 mg/day		

* IM injections are *not* recommended because they are painful and absorption is erratic.
† Doses are designed to produce effective but prudent plasma and tissue concentrations (see text for details).
‡ Abnormal renal function prolongs plasma half-life, necessitating *reduction* in suggested dosage.

obtained. Obtaining blood levels at peak effect, 6 to 8 h after dosage, and at the nadir, just before the next dose, is often useful.

Digitalis toxicity may result from overdosage, hypokalemia, advanced degenerative heart disease associated with conduction abnormalities and thus an increased sensitivity to the drug, or a combination of these factors. The maintenance dosage should be carefully planned to avoid excess accumulation. Deliberate digitalis underdosage, combined with sodium restriction and diuresis to produce additional therapeutic effects, is often prudent. Continual alertness to the possibility of potassium loss with diuresis and appropriate replacement with supplementary dietary potassium chloride are important in preventing toxicity. Because digoxin is largely eliminated by the kidneys, digitoxin may be preferable in patients with actual or suspected renal disease; renal function may be considerably compromised although the BUN remains within a normal range. Although digitoxin is largely eliminated by the liver, even advanced liver failure seems to have little effect on blood level.

Systemic toxic effects of digitalis include nausea, vomiting, anorexia, diarrhea, confusion, amblyopia, and xerophthalmia. The most important toxic effects of the drug are life-threatening arrhyth-

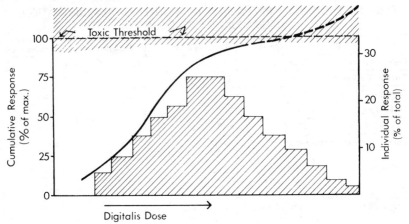

Fig. 25–3. **Theoretical dose–response relationships for digitalis.** The left ordinate indicates the linear curve of the cumulative dose–response curve up to 100% of the maximum therapeutic effect. Note the imprecise location of the toxic threshold. The pharmacologic effect of the drug increases rapidly with increasing digitalis dosage. The maximum therapeutic effect cannot be precisely determined clinically. Furthermore, the toxic threshold may vary according to potassium level, P_{O_2}, metabolism, and as yet undetermined factors. Continued increased dosage assures achievement of toxic effects. The histogram represents the percent of individuals responding to a given dose (right-hand ordinate). Note that some individuals obtain satisfactory therapeutic response at low dosage; others require very high doses. The dose–response curve (on the left) is the integral of distribution of individual responses.

mias due to the drug's direct effect on the A-V node, causing a prolonged P-R time, Wenckebach phenomenon, and ultimately complete heart block. Nonparoxysmal junctional tachycardia developing in the presence of atrial fibrillation is a frequently overlooked but serious sign of digitalis toxicity. Digitalis increases the automaticity of Purkinje fibers and may enhance reentry, resulting in coupled extrasystoles, ventricular tachycardia, or ventricular fibrillation. Bidirectional ventricular tachycardia is a pathognomonic sign of digitalis intoxication. The development of a new arrhythmia or worsening of a previous one while the patient is taking digitalis should always raise the suspicion of digitalis intoxication.

The first step in treating digitalis toxicity is to discontinue the drug. The ECG should be closely monitored throughout all treatment. If the serum potassium is low, 80 mEq of potassium chloride IV should be given in 1 L 5% D/W at a rate of 6 ml/min (0.5 mEq/min). Ventricular arrhythmias are treated with a 50- to 100-mg bolus of lidocaine IV, repeated in 3 to 5 min until a therapeutic effect is obtained, a total of 300 mg is given, or CNS toxicity occurs. When the arrhythmia is controlled, a continuous infusion of 2 to 4 mg/min should be started. Alternatively, phenytoin (diphenylhydantoin) 100 mg q 3 to 5 min can be given slowly up to a total of 1000 mg. Heart block is best treated with a temporary pervenous pacemaker. Isoproterenol is *contraindicated* in digitalis intoxication because of the increased tendency to ventricular arrhythmia. Digitalis cannot be dialyzed since it is either protein-bound or rapidly fixed to tissues. Cholestyramine resin may be useful in digitoxin overdosage since it binds intestinal digitoxin and interrupts the enterohepatic circulation. Suicide attempts due to digitalis overdosage are especially difficult to treat because of the large amount of drug ingested. Hyperkalemia due to displacement of K^+ from cells develops. Drug-specific antibody fragments (FAB) have been evaluated experimentally and are available from special centers in the USA for IV administration for severe cases.

Diuretics: Diuretics and sodium restriction are essential to long-term management of CHF. In both acute and chronic CHF, the importance of reliable daily weights cannot be overemphasized for gauging the effectiveness of therapy and adjusting diuretic dosages. Ambulatory patients can weigh themselves at home at the same time of day under the same conditions and keep a daily log.

Table 25–2 lists details of various diuretics (see also Ch. 255). In mild CHF, thiazide diuretics such as hydrochlorothiazide 50 mg/day or chlorothiazide 500 mg daily or b.i.d. are useful. Increasing the dosage does not significantly increase the diuretic effect. Supplemental potassium chloride is generally needed since chronic diuresis causes hypokalemic alkalosis. Increased daily ingestion of foods with a high potassium content, such as bananas and orange juice, may suffice for adequate replacement, but liquid preparations of 20 to 40 mEq potassium chloride b.i.d. to q.i.d. may be necessary. Potassium salts other than potassium chloride are generally not useful since both potassium and chloride must be replaced. Potassium-sparing diuretics such as triamterene 50 to 100 mg/day may

TABLE 25–2. CLINICAL AND PHARMACOLOGIC PROPERTIES OF DIURETICS

Preparation	Relative Potency	Site of Action	Onset of Action	Advantages	Adverse Effects	Dosage, Route of Administration
Thiazides	Moderate	Excreted into proximal tubule, inhibit Na and Cl absorption in distal segment	1–2 h	Mild, relatively nontoxic, oral administration, antihypertensive	K loss, hyperglycemia, decreases platelets, ineffective when GFR < 20 ml/min	Chlorothiazide 500–2000 mg orally/day Hydrochlorothiazide 50–200 mg orally/day
Ethacrynic acid	High	Inhibition of Cl transport in ascending limb of loop of Henle	**Orally:** 1 h **IV:** 10–20 min	Rapid onset, high potency, independent of acid-base balance, effective even when GFR is reduced	GI symptoms, excessive diuresis, hypovolemia, K loss and hypokalemia, hyperuricemia, transient or irreversible deafness when given in large doses in renal failure or administered IV	**Orally:** 50–400 mg/day **IV:** Initially, 50 mg: may increase dose depending on response
Furosemide	High	Inhibition of Cl transport in ascending limb of loop of Henle	**Orally:** 1 h **IV:** 10–20 min	Rapid onset, high potency, independent of acid-base balance, effective even when GFR is reduced	Excessive diuresis, hypovolemia, K loss and hypokalemia, hyperuricemia, transient or irreversible deafness especially when used with aminoglycoside antibiotic	**Orally:** 40–200 mg, 1, 2, or 3 times/day **IV:** 40 mg initially; may increase dose to 200–400 mg depending on response
Spironolactone	Moderate to low	Aldosterone homolog, competitive inhibition for receptor site in distal tubule Secondary: inhibition of aldosterone biosynthesis	2–3 days for maximum effect	Useful in combination with more proximal-acting diuretic to spare K	Hyperkalemia when K salts are given concomitantly or renal function is reduced markedly	25–50 mg orally b.i.d. to q.i.d.
Triamterene	Moderate	Inhibition of Na resorption in distal tubule	1–2 h	Useful in combination with more proximal-acting diuretic to spare K	Hyperkalemia when K salts are given concomitantly or renal function is reduced markedly	100 mg orally b.i.d. to t.i.d.

be useful, but combinations such as hydrochlorothiazide 25 mg and triamterene 50 mg are usually not effective in more severe cases. Spironolactone 25 to 50 mg t.i.d. may be useful in severe CHF and hypokalemia; however, it is expensive and may induce hyperkalemia. Spironolactone seems to be most effective in hyperaldosterone states, which are unusual except in severe and refractory CHF. The "loop" diuretics such as furosemide or ethacrynic acid are highly effective. Their advantages include rapid onset of action both IV and orally, lack of accumulation, and increasing effectiveness with increasing dose; their disadvantage is their potency. Overdosage may cause hypovolemia, hyponatremia, and profound hypokalemia, and they should be used cautiously. Small initial doses and careful evaluation of response is wise. Oral doses of furosemide should start with 40 mg, increasing to 80 or 160 mg daily or b.i.d. depending on the response; higher dosages may be needed. IV doses of 20 to 40 mg can be given initially and increased as needed. In refractory cases bolus injections are more effective than slow infusion. Nerve deafness due to specific and potentially nonreversible ototoxicity has occurred shortly following IV injection of both "loop" diuretics.

Sodium restriction: Reduction of salt intake is an important but frequently neglected aspect of the management of CHF; neglect of this factor is a major cause of refractoriness to treatment. Habits of salt usage in cooking and at the table vary and should be evaluated for each patient. Many patients may only need to eliminate table salt and avoid salted foods (ham, bacon, peanuts, french fries, etc.). Restriction below 2 gm of sodium (87 mEq), about 5 gm of sodium chloride, may be necessary in severe cases. Advanced CHF may require the combination of potent diuretics and severe restriction of sodium to 0.5 to 1.5 gm/day.

Acute pulmonary edema is a medical emergency demanding prompt and effective treatment. Unless in shock, the patient should sit upright, preferably with legs dangling. High concentrations of O_2 should be given by mask or nasal cannula. Increasing expiratory pressure may be helpful since the raised intrathoracic pressure impedes venous return thus reducing ventricular filling pressure. Morphine sulfate 4 to 6 mg IV or 10 to 15 mg IM reduces agitation, decreases the respiratory rate, and has some effect toward slowing heart rate and lowering BP; these effects reduce the work of breathing and cardiac work. In severe cases rotating tourniquets are effective: BP cuffs are applied to 3 limbs, inflated midway between diastolic and systolic pressures, and deflated q 10 to 20 min. *The BP cuffs should not be applied to the limb into which an IV infusion is running.* Occasionally phlebotomy is necessary, and the rapid removal of 300 to 500 ml of blood may have a dramatic effect. Inhalation of alcohol mist to reduce the surface pressure of the alveolar fluid has been advocated. Effective therapy includes the IV administration of a rapidly acting diuretic; e.g., IV injection of furosemide 40 mg or ethacrynic acid 50 mg to initiate a prompt diuresis in 15 to 20 min, thus decreasing the plasma volume and ventricular filling pressure. Most patients with acute pulmonary edema can be treated successfully without digitalis, although it may be needed later to prevent further episodes. If digitalis is given, low doses are mandated because of the rapidly changing clinical situation, including aggressive diuresis. Not more than 50% of the digitalizing dose should be given initially.

The cause of the pulmonary edema should be diligently sought. In valvular heart disease, sudden onset of a rapid arrhythmia such as atrial flutter or fibrillation may precipitate pulmonary edema that responds to cardioversion. Pulmonary edema due to a hypertensive crisis or significant systolic hypertension may respond to a vasodilator such as apresoline or nitroprusside. Deliberate reduction of afterload with nitroprusside in refractory cases despite lack of hypertension may be useful.

Refractory heart failure: In some patients chronic or acute CHF persists despite appropriate therapy. In such cases an orderly approach is useful. Has the etiology been established? Have mitral stenosis, aortic stenosis, excess alcohol intake, thyrotoxicosis, pulmonary emboli, anemia, or other contributing factors been overlooked? Are drug doses optimal? (Some patients require very large doses of "loop" diuretics for effective diuresis.) Is the oral digitalis being absorbed? (Small bowel disorders and interference by other drugs such as neomycin or antacids containing magnesium trisilicate inhibit absorption of digoxin.) Is the patient adhering to an adequate low-salt diet? Hyponatremia in the presence of an elevated venous pressure and edema must reflect excess water intake rather than low body sodium and is a clue to inadequate fluid and sodium restriction. It must be recognized, of course, that even the best medical efforts may fail in the face of advanced myocardial disease and that with low CO, venous hypertension, and refractory edema, the patient will succumb.

Afterload reduction or vasodilator therapy: A recent important therapeutic advance is the use of vasodilators to reduce afterload in treatment of CHF, usually due to myocardiopathy responding poorly to conventional measures. A variety of drugs have been utilized including nitroglycerin, nitroprusside (see under ANTIHYPERTENSIVE VASODILATORS in Ch. 248), isosorbide dinitrate, hydralazine, prazosin, and minoxidil. Treatment is based on the recognition that in the presence of myocardial failure, compensatory increases in peripheral vascular resistance that maintain BP may adversely influence cardiac function because of the greater ventricular afterload. The aim of therapy is to reduce left ventricular filling pressure (pulmonary wedge pressure) and improve CO without inducing tachycardia or lowering BP. If monitoring facilities and technics for pulmonary artery catheterization (Swan-Ganz) are available, the acute response of the patient to a vasodilator may be tested during cautious infusion of nitroprusside with constant hemodynamic monitoring. If the patient responds favorably, ambulatory treatment with vasodilators, such as isosorbide dinitrate 2.5 to 5 mg sublingually q 3 to 6 h as needed, combined with hydralazine 25 to 75 mg t.i.d., may be useful. A variety of

TABLE 25–3. EFFECTIVE VASODILATORS FOR TREATMENT OF CONGESTIVE HEART FAILURE*

Drug	Route of Administration	Dose	Vasodilator Effect Venous	Arterial	Heart Rate	Duration of Action	Comments
Na nitroprusside	IV	20–300 µg/min	++	+++	↓	3–5 min	Titer response by changing rate of infusion. Nausea, vomiting, sweating, headache with excess vasodilation. Metabolate thiocyanate accumulates with prolonged infusion with weakness, hypoxia, nausea, delirium. Use fresh solutions no more than 4 h old. BP should be monitored continuously.
Hydralazine	PO	50–200 mg/day	0	+++	↑	6–12 h	Increases stroke volume, heart rate, and cardiac output in normals and CHF. Drug-induced lupus occurs at doses > 400 mg/day largely in whites, who are slow acetylators. If reflex tachycardia is severe, it may be counteracted by concomitant use of beta blocker.
Nitroglycerine	SL UNG	0.4–0.6 mg q 2–6 h 2% ointment, 2.5–5 cm q 4–6 h	+++	+	↓	10–20 min	Effect on coronary arteries controversial. Relieves coronary spasm (Prinzmetal). Increases endocardial blood flow. Reflex tachycardia can occur with excess dosage. Peak blood concentration 4 min after sublingual dose. Half-life = 1–3 min.
Isosorbide dinitrate	SL PO	5–30 mg, q 3–6 h 20–80 mg, q 3–6 h	+++	+	↓	1½–3 h	Adjust frequency of dose to desired response. Oral doses required are larger than previously thought, but tolerance may develop. See comments under nitroglycerine.
Prazosin	PO	3–10 mg	++	++	↓	5–10 h	Selective α₁—adrenergic blocker. Half-life = 3 h, but longer in heart failure. First-dose phenomenon of postural hypotension and syncope; start slowly with 1 mg t.i.d.
Minoxidil	PO	10–40 mg/day	0	++	↑	6–12 h	Reflex tachycardia. Fluid retention, spontaneous pericardial effusion, and hypertrichosis may occur.

* Abbreviations: IV = intravenous; PO = per os; SL = sublingual; UNG = unguent

vasodilators have been used clinically (see TABLE 25-3). An adequate dose of the vasodilator must be administered and the patient closely watched for evidence of adverse effects. Long-term studies comparing different drug programs and depicting the safety and efficacy of vasodilators in the management of chronic CHF suggest that some patients are greatly benefited by this form of treatment. Caution and close follow-up are important.

Prazosin (see TABLE 25-3), a quinazoline derivative, is a new oral vasodilator antihypertensive agent that has major peripheral vascular relaxing effects, produced by postsynaptic α_1 blockade. It dilates both venules and arterioles, thus reducing both preload and aortic impedance in a balanced fashion in patients with heart failure. Its effects, then, are similar to those of nitroprusside, with the advantage that it can be given orally. Accordingly, its use is being explored not only in the treatment of acute, severe heart failure but in chronic and less severe heart failure. Attenuation of its effects over time has been reported; however, it appears not to be true tachyphylaxis, but a result of physiologic adaptations that may respond to such measures as increasing the drug dosage, adding spironolactone, increasing other diuretic dosage, or temporary cessation of prazosin usage.

COR PULMONALE (CP)

Enlargement of the right ventricle secondary to malfunction of the lungs that may be due to intrinsic pulmonary disease, an abnormal chest bellows, or a depressed ventilatory drive. The term does not include right ventricular enlargement secondary to left ventricular failure, congenital heart disease, or acquired valvular heart disease. CP is usually chronic but may be acute and reversible.

Etiology

A number of disease processes can lead to CP. The most common cause of **chronic CP** is chronic obstructive pulmonary disease **(COPD)**—chronic bronchitis, emphysema. Other possible causes include extensive loss of lung tissue from surgery or trauma, chronic recurrent pulmonary emboli, primary pulmonary hypertension, pulmonary veno-occlusive disease, scleroderma, diseases leading to diffuse interstitial fibrosis, kyphoscoliosis, obesity with alveolar hypoventilation, neuromuscular diseases involving respiratory muscles, and idiopathic alveolar hypoventilation. **Acute CP** usually results from massive pulmonary embolization, but acute reversible exacerbations of chronic CP often occur in patients with COPD, usually during acute respiratory infections.

Pathogenesis

CP is directly caused by alterations in the pulmonary circulation that lead to pulmonary arterial hypertension and thereby impose an increased mechanical load on right ventricular emptying. **Pulmonary hypertension** can be caused by irreversible reduction in the size of the vascular bed, as in diseases primarily affecting pulmonary blood vessels (e.g., embolization or scleroderma) or as in massive loss of lung tissue (e.g., from emphysema or surgery). However, the most important mechanism leading to pulmonary arterial hypertension is alveolar hypoxia, which results either from localized inadequate ventilation of alveoli that are well perfused or from a generalized decrease in alveolar ventilation. Alveolar hypoxia, whether acute or chronic, is a potent stimulus of pulmonary vasoconstriction, and chronic alveolar hypoxia, in addition, promotes hypertrophy of smooth muscle in the pulmonary arterioles. These hypertrophied vessels then respond vigorously to acute hypoxia. Hypercapnic acidosis acts synergistically with hypoxemia to augment the pulmonary vasoconstriction. During chronic hypoxia, anatomic and vasomotor effects are often intensified, both by increased blood viscosity arising from secondary polycythemia and by increased cardiac output. Even though increased pulmonary capillary pressure does not contribute per se to the pathogenesis of pulmonary arterial hypertension in CP, independent disease of the left ventricle is often aggravated by hypoxemia and acidosis, and respiratory insufficiency in turn is intensified if left ventricular failure induces pulmonary edema.

Symptoms, Signs, and Diagnosis

CP should be suspected in all patients with the disorders mentioned above under Etiology. Signs of right heart enlargement appear early and are readily discernible in acute CP. In chronic CP caused by pulmonary vascular disease, dyspnea may be slight or absent at rest, even when frank right ventricular failure is present. Some patients suffer syncopal attacks on exertion, and substernal anginal pain is common. Physical signs include left parasternal systolic lift and a loud pulmonic 2nd sound (S_2P). Murmurs due to functional tricuspid and pulmonic insufficiency may occur. Chest x-rays show right ventricular and pulmonary arterial enlargement. ECG evidence of right ventricular hypertrophy correlates well with the degree of pulmonary hypertension. Gallop rhythm, distended jugular veins, hepatomegaly, and edema may be seen in patients with right ventricular failure.

In CP due to disease of the pulmonary parenchyma, the clinical manifestations of the primary disease frequently overshadow those of CP. The major symptoms and signs (dyspnea, cough, cyanosis, and wheezing) are also seen in left heart failure, and differentiation may be difficult. Arterial blood gases are helpful in such cases since appreciable hypoxemia, hypercapnia, and acidosis are unusual in left heart failure unless there is also frank pulmonary edema. Because pulmonary hyperinflation and bullae cause a realignment of the heart in these patients, the physical examination, x-rays, and ECG may be relatively insensitive indicators of the right ventricular enlargement.

Treatment

Therapy of the primary pulmonary disorders is discussed in the appropriate chapters in §4. Therapy of right heart failure is discussed in Congestive Heart Failure, above. Phlebotomy during hypoxic CP has been suggested, but the beneficial effects of decreased blood viscosity are not likely to outweigh the effects of reducing the O_2-carrying capacity of the blood; also, substantial polycythemia is uncommon in hypoxic CP. Digitalis is not as effective in hypoxic CP as in other forms of congestive heart failure. Diuretics can improve pulmonary gas exchange in hypoxic CP, presumably by relieving extravascular fluid accumulation in the lungs. Vigorous use of diuretics, however, can lead to metabolic alkalosis, which diminishes the effectiveness of CO_2 as a respiratory stimulus. Potassium and chloride losses must be carefully replaced when diuretics are used. The continuous use of O_2 can reduce pulmonary hypertension and prevent polycythemia in hypoxic patients, but does not reduce overall mortality.

CARDIAC ARRHYTHMIAS

Normal sinus rhythm originates within pacemaker cells of the sinoatrial (S-A, sinus) node (at the junction of the superior vena cava and high right atrium). These cells represent the primary electrical generator (pacemaker) for the normal human heart. Conduction within the sinus node is slow, since it must occur through cells which themselves are automatic and partially depolarized. The sinus node depolarizes at least 80 to 120 msec before the start of the P wave on the ECG. Recent indirect human studies of sinoatrial conduction suggest it to be considerably longer than previously estimated and at least part of this conduction delay is due to specialized perionodal fibers that surround the sinus node. The P wave is inscribed on the ECG as the electrical impulse spreads over first the right and then the left atrium (Fig. 25–4). The total duration of atrial excitation is generally 80 to 100 msec and represents the normal P wave duration. The impulse travels from the S-A node to the atrioventricular (A-V) node preferentially via three specialized tracts within the atria, but may be conducted by ordinary atrial myocardium as well. Conduction velocity within these specialized pathways is more rapid than in ordinary atrial myocardium, and the excitation wave enters the A-V node about 40 msec after the P wave begins.

Conduction through the A-V node is also slow, and A-V nodal refractoriness is generally longer than that of any other cardiac tissue. After the impulse has crossed the A-V node it is still on the atrial side of the anulus fibrosus and it should be remembered that the A-V node is not responsible for A-V conduction but rather for the sequence and rapidity with which impulses are presented to the A-V or His bundle. The bundle of His conducts propagating impulses between the atria and ventricles (Fig. 25–4). It runs along the tricuspid valve ring to the area of the trigone of the tricuspid valve, penetrates the anulus fibrosus, and continues down through the membranous interventricular septum as a discrete fascicle.

At the point where membranous septum becomes muscular septum, the His bundle divides into three major fascicles. The right bundle continues down the right ventricular endocardial surface and does not branch or result in depolarization of myocardium until it reaches the anterior right ventricular papillary muscle and apex of the right ventricle. The main left bundle crosses the summit of the muscular interventricular septum to emerge on the left side of the heart just below the noncoronary cusp of the aortic valve. At this point it divides (at least functionally) into a left posterior division which cascades down the mid and posterior left side of the interventricular septum. Recent studies suggest a portion of this posterior division behaves like an independent conduction fascicle and is responsible for providing input for septal depolarization. The anterior portions of the left bundle divide into a thinner, free-running left anterior division which runs to the anterior papillary muscle of the left ventricle before its terminal branches begin. This anterior superior fascicle of the left bundle controls the appropriate timing of activation of the anterolateral and basilon portions of the left ventricle.

None of this conduction—i.e., within the atrial specialized tracts, A-V node, bundle of His, three fascicles, and terminal His-Purkinje system—has electrical manifestations on the surface ECG, although specialized intracardiac recording technics may record some of these events (Fig. 25–4). The surface ECG depicts only depolarization of atrial (P waves) and ventricular (QRS complexes) myocardium. The relationship between depolarization of these specialized cardiac tissues and the surface ECG is depicted in Fig. 25–4.

The S-A node and these specialized cardiac tissues all contain cells capable of automaticity (spontaneous Phase IV diastolic depolarization) with the probable exception of the A-V node. The intrinsic rhythmicity is highest in the S-A node and the rate of each of the other latent cardiac pacemakers decreases with increasing distance from the S-A node. The rhythm of the heart is therefore normally controlled by the rhythmicity of the S-A node. If the sinus node, either reflexly or due to intrinsic disease, slows sufficiently, one of the other cardiac pacemaking tissues assumes its function.

Most arrhythmias are accompanied by symptoms. Some arrhythmias can be detected and correctly diagnosed by physical examination (from characteristic changes in pulse rate, rhythm, or change in heart sounds, or from the relationship between atrial and ventricular mechanical events), but arrhythmias are actually diagnosed with any degree of accuracy only with the ECG. More recently developed intracardiac recording technics have significantly augmented our knowledge of

A

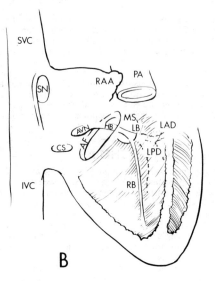

B

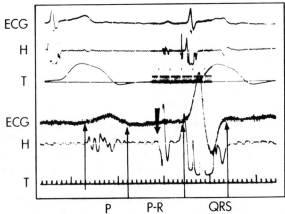

FIG. 25–4.   **Relationship between cardiac conduction system and ECG.**
  A. A schematic diagram of the human heart, labeled as follows: SVC, superior vena cava; IVC, inferior vena cava; SN, sinus node; CS, coronary sinus; RAA, right atrial appendage; PA, pulmonary artery; AF, anulus fibrosus; AVN, atrioventricular node; HB, bundle of His; MS, membranous septum; RB, right bundle; LB, left bundle; LAD, left anterior division; LPD, left posterior division.
  B. Electrical events associated with cardiac excitation. The upper and lower portions (identical except that the lower portion is time-expanded) include an electrocardiogram (ECG), a His bundle electrogram (H), and time marks (T) at 10- and 100-msec intervals. In the upper portion a pressure tracing shows the recording site of the His bundle electrogram to be within the right ventricle. In the lower portion a P wave lasting 90 msec is illustrated between 2 vertical ascending arrows. A QRS of 95 msec is similarly illustrated. During the isoelectric P-R segment of the surface ECG, the depolarization of the His bundle is shown by the heavier descending arrow. Conduction time from the onset of the P wave to His bundle depolarization (A-H interval) is normal at 150 msec. Conduction time within the infranodal structures (H-V interval) is slightly prolonged at 55 msec (normal = 40–50 msec).

both normal and abnormal heart rhythms. A careful history, physical examination, evaluation of physical manifestations, but primarily, an understanding of the basic mechanism of any cardiac arrhythmia, are all necessary to estimate the patient's prognosis.

NORMAL SINUS RHYTHM

The average adult heart generally beats 72 to 78 times/min while at rest. However, from birth to old age the sinus rate progressively decreases. Normal sinus rhythm in the infant, a rate of 110 to 150, is sinus tachycardia in the adult. Also, heart rates below 60 may occur in as many as 33% of hospitalized men and 19% of hospitalized women. In deciding whether the sinus rate is too fast or too slow, the patient's age and the circumstances of the examination are important.

SINUS BRADYCARDIA

A slow sinus rhythm characterized on ECG by an atrial rate < 60 beats/min and by a sequence of atrial depolarization (i.e., P wave morphology) which reflects initiation of the impulse from the area of the high right atrium (Fig. 25-5).

Etiology

Sinus bradycardia is most frequently the result of increased vagal tone, is common in athletes and young persons in vigorous health, and often occurs normally during rest or sleep. It is also common in noncardiac conditions such as myxedema, jaundice, recovery from illness causing sinus tachycardia, and increased vagal tone from GI disturbances, and occasionally results from medicinal intoxication. In organic heart disease, it is commonly the result of digitalis excess or the use of β-blocking agents such as propranolol.

Sinus bradycardia also commonly results from intrinsically depressed automaticity within the S-A node of elderly patients with arteriosclerotic heart disease and is benign in the absence of symptoms. Chronic and inappropriate sinus bradycardia—where sinus rate does not increase appropriately with exercise or emotion—is a recognized form of S-A node dysfunction and may occur in the total absence of other forms of heart disease.

Mechanism

Sinus bradycardia is the result of slowed diastolic depolarization within all the S-A pacemaker cells. This slowed automaticity is often caused by acetylcholine release via vagal efferent fibers, although it may be due to intrinsic cellular membrane abnormalities in the pacemaker cells or a lack of appropriate sympathetic innervation.

Symptoms and Signs

Sinus bradycardia with rates between 40 to 60 is generally without symptoms provided the patient is sedentary or at rest. Since the major augmentation of cardiac output which occurs with exercise, however, is a function of increasing heart rate rather than stroke volume, the patient with a fixed, low, or narrow range of sinus rates, although asymptomatic at rest, may be severely limited in terms of exercise tolerance. Slower sinus rates may result in cardiac outputs which are insufficient even at rest and result in fatigue and decreased exercise tolerance. *Sinus rates < 30 beats/min require emergency treatment.* Sinus bradycardia < 20 beats/min may result in syncope, convulsions, and even death, due to the emergence of other cardiac arrhythmias and severely depressed cardiac output resulting in cerebral anoxia.

Treatment

Asymptomatic patients require no treatment. If chronic sinus bradycardia causes diminished cardiac output and loss of myocardial reserve, vagolytic agents (atropine) or sympathomimetic drugs (isoproterenol) are rarely long-term solutions; a permanent endocardial atrial, ventricular, or A-V sequential pacemaker should be implanted. Pacemakers which are sensitive to increasing demand for cardiac output and which respond with an increasing paced rate are now being developed. Pacemaker therapy is clearly indicated if episodic sinus bradycardia results in near-syncope, vertigo, faintness, or episodic loss of consciousness.

Acute sinus bradycardia < 40 beats/min should be treated first by administration of atropine 0.5 to 1 mg IV, repeated if no effect is seen within 4 min. If atropine is ineffective, as may be the case in patients with the "**sick sinus syndrome**," isoproterenol IV may be life-saving. Very small doses (0.5 μg/min) should be used initially since these patients may be extremely sensitive to IV isoproterenol. The dosage may then be increased in order to raise the sinus rate to the desired level. Emergency percutaneous temporary pacemaker insertion (generally via the right subclavian vein) may prove lifesaving when slow heart rates are incompatible with coronary or cerebral oxygenation. For patients with repeated symptomatic episodes of sinus bradycardia, pacemaker therapy is the only long-term solution.

SINUS TACHYCARDIA

A sinus rhythm > 100 beats/min in an adult (Fig. 25-6).

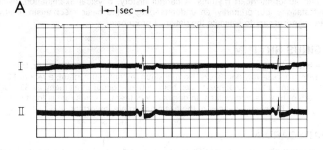

Fig. 25–5. Sinus bradycardia.

A. A marked sinus bradycardia (20 beats/min).

B. ECG leads I, II, III, V_1, and V_6 are shown with an atrial electrogram (A), a His bundle electrogram (H), and time marks at 100- and 1000-msec intervals. The ECG demonstrates sinus bradycardia at a cycle length of 1200 msec. The remainder of the ECG, with the exception of anterolateral T wave abnormalities, is within normal limits.

Etiology

In sinus tachycardia, neural mechanisms affect the rate of automaticity of the sinus node pacemaker cells. Specifically, sinus tachycardia occasionally results from decreased vagal tone with diminished acetylcholine release. More typically, increased sympathetic tone with catecholamine release in the area of the sinus node results in a faster rate of spontaneous diastolic depolarization of intrinsically automatic cells and therefore an increase in heart rate. Emotion, exercise, thyrotoxicosis, hypotension, hypoxia, hyperthermia, anemia, hemorrhage, and infections are frequent noncardiac causes. Heart failure will increase the sinus rate reflexly, and inflammatory diseases of the pericardium, myocardium, or endocardium are frequently accompanied by sinus tachycardia. Sympathomimetic drugs (nicotine, caffeine, marijuana) all increase the heart rate. Habitual use of belladonna alkaloids or propantheline for GI disturbances may cause persistent sinus tachycardia.

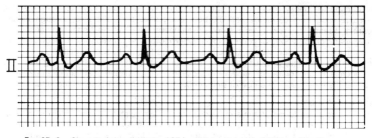

FIG. 25–6. Sinus tachycardia (rate, 107 to 115 beats/min). ECG lead II is shown.

Symptoms and Signs

An increase in sinus rate rarely gives rise to symptoms, but the patient may be aware of both the fast rate and increased forceful contraction of the heart. Sinus tachycardia usually increases cardiac output, and is almost always the result, rather than the cause, of heart failure. Unlike paroxysmal tachycardia, sinus tachycardia does not start and stop suddenly. Rather, an episode begins gradually, with the heart rate increasing over several minutes, and tapers off in the same way when its cause is removed.

Diagnosis

The diagnosis of sinus tachycardia is made electrocardiographically when the rate of P waves is between 100 and 180/min, and atrial depolarization is consistent with origin at the junction of the high right atrium and superior vena cava. Maneuvers that increase vagal tone, such as carotid sinus massage, temporarily slow the heart rate; but it returns to its tachycardic level as soon as carotid sinus pressure is removed.

Prognosis

The prognosis is that of the causative condition. Sinus tachycardia has no intrinsic significance when it is due to anemia, hemorrhage, or hyperthyroidism. It is clinically significant when it results from congestive heart failure, active myocarditis, myocardial infarction, or other primary myocardial disease.

Treatment

Although β-blocking agents such as propranolol may slow the heart rate, therapy should be directed at the cause. In congestive heart failure, digitalis will slow the heart to a normal rate. Propranolol may be useful in the occasional patient with hyperdynamic heart syndrome, where diminution in cardiac rate and contractility will diminish the cardiac palpitations.

SINUS ARRHYTHMIA

A common variant of regular sinus rhythm characterized by cyclic changes in heart rate due to periodic fluctuation in the discharge rate of the sinus node.

Sinus arrhythmia is the result of alternate increases and decreases in vagal and sympathetic tone. In the respiratory variety, the heart rate increases with inspiration and slows with expiration. In the nonrespiratory variety, the same phasic changes occur but are unrelated to respiration. Sinus arrhythmia produces no symptoms.

Diagnosis

The P wave morphology remains identical throughout, but the interval between P waves shows a phasic increase and decrease which generally varies by $<$ 160 msec. A relationship to respiration, if present, is easily identified. Confusion between sinus arrhythmia and atrial premature depolarizations can be avoided by recognizing that sinus arrhythmia is repetitive and cyclical.

Treatment

No treatment is required. In general, the more bradycardic the patient, the greater will be the sinus arrhythmia. Treating sinus bradycardia (e.g., with atropine or other vagolytic agents) diminishes the arrhythmia, but is of no clinical consequence.

SICK SINUS SYNDROME (Sinus Node Dysfunction Syndromes)

A variety of syndromes associated with inadequate sinus node function most commonly resulting in the cerebral manifestations of lightheadedness, dizziness, and near or true syncope.

Etiology

Coronary artery disease is the most common single cause of sinus node dysfunction, and on an acute basis right coronary artery occlusion with subsequent ischemia and vagal influences on sinus node function frequently result in inadequate sinus node function. However, a variety of cardiac diseases ranging from cardiomyopathies, both congestive and infiltrative, through inflammatory myocardial disease may result in sinus node dysfunction. The 2nd most common cause is progressive degeneration of sinoatrial conduction, a sclerotic process analogous to degeneration of the interventricular conduction system; these processes are frequently seen together.

Although abnormalities of sinus node function can be divided into those involving abnormal sinus node pacemaker function (automaticity) and those that are a function of abnormal sinoatrial conduction, by far the most frequent cause of sinus node dysfunction syndromes is the latter.

Symptoms and Signs

The most common forms of sinus node dysfunction are related to **intermittent sinoatrial block.** Here, one sees varying degrees of block ranging from sinoatrial Wenckebach through high-degree sinoatrial block with what has been called "sinus arrest." Most episodes of "sinus arrest" actually represent prolonged periods of high-degree sinoatrial block. The patient basically in sinus rhythm, who has a prolonged period of sinoatrial block, experiences symptoms related to the duration of the asystolic period—weakness, dizziness, pre- or near-syncope, or actual fainting episodes.

The 2nd most common form of sinus node dysfunction syndrome is that of **tachycardia-bradycardia syndrome,** wherein a patient with inadequate sinoatrial conduction experiences paroxysmal atrial arrhythmias. In these patients, episodes of supraventricular tachycardia, atrial flutter, or atrial fibrillation result in a variable period of depression of sinoatrial conduction. Hence, following the termination of any of these arrhythmias, there is a prolonged pause before sinus rhythm resumes. Again, during this asystolic period, its length will determine the patient's symptoms, which may range from near-syncope to actual loss of consciousness. Although it has been assumed that sinoatrial function is depressed by retrograde conduction into the sinus node with abnormal reset of sinus node pacemaker activity, more recent evidence suggests that sinoatrial block following termination of these arrhythmias is responsible for the patient's symptomatic episode.

Occasionally patients have **persistent sinus bradycardia** which is symptomatic. This form of abnormal pacemaker activity may result in lethargy and weakness.

Although occasionally aware of palpitations in the tachycardia-bradycardia syndrome, most patients are unaware of any cardiac irregularities accompanying or preceding their near syncopal or true syncopal episodes. These episodes are usually short-lived and are most frequently described as "grey-outs" rather than a true loss of consciousness. There are no neurologic sequelae provided the patient does not have intrinsic CNS disease. The severity of the symptoms are, of course, related to the duration of the asystolic period.

Diagnosis

The diagnosis of sinus node dysfunction may be suspected in elderly patients with episodes of presyncope or near syncope, particularly if associated with a prior history of palpitations. The diagnosis is made with accuracy, however, only with ECG documentation of episodes of sinoatrial block, atrial tachycardias followed by prolonged periods of high degree sinoatrial block, or paroxysmal complete sinoatrial block. Electrophysiologic stimulating procedures have been used to determine the normal responsiveness of sinus node tissue in patients. Single atrial premature beats are evoked during electrophysiologic testing, or the atria is paced at rates in excess of the sinus node rate. Prolonged sinoatrial recovery times following single premature beats or prolonged sinus node reset times following atrial pacing is highly suggestive of sinus node dysfunction. The incidence of false-negative results with electrophysiologic testing, however, indicates that the best method for documenting sinus node dysfunction is careful ECG monitoring, such as with Holter monitors with or without invasive electrophysiologic testing.

Treatment

Although initially tried in a variety of forms, sympathetic stimulation or parasympathetic inhibition as treatment for intermittent sinus node dysfunction syndromes or sick sinus syndrome has been totally unsuccessful. At the present time, any symptomatic patient with sinus node dysfunction requires the implantation of a permanent demand pacemaker. Several varieties of demand pacemakers are available, but the relative advantages or disadvantages of standard ventricular demand pacing as opposed to AV sequential pacing or dual demand pacing has yet to be elucidated.

PREMATURE DEPOLARIZATION (Premature Beats; Premature Contractions)

Depolarization of the atria or ventricles, or both, that occurs before the next expected sinus beat. Such depolarizations can arise from the S-A node, the atrial specialized conduction system, ordinary atrial myocardium, the His bundle, any of the three interventricular fascicles, or the terminal branches of the His-Purkinje system. The A-V node is *not* a site of impulse formation and hence the term "nodal premature beats" is meaningless, while the term "junctional premature beats" is too broad. Junctional premature beats arise within either the bundle of His or the three fascicles of the interventricular conducting system. Since the significance of premature depolarizations depends on the site of impulse formation, each will be considered separately.

ATRIAL PREMATURE DEPOLARIZATIONS

Although atrial premature beats **(APBs)** may occur in normal hearts. they are more often associated with organic heart disease, especially rheumatic and arteriosclerotic, and with conditions that
tend to increase ventricular filling pressures on either side of the heart. APBs are a common result of
sympathomimetic drugs, tobacco, caffeine, and CNS disturbances.

Mechanism

It is unresolved whether APBs represent the firing of ectopic automatic cells within the atrial myocardium or the atrial conduction pathways, or reflect reentry within localized areas of atrial myocardium. Current information derived from excised human atrial myocardial samples shows that under
diseased conditions ordinary atrial myocardium is capable of automaticity. Portions of both mitral
and tricuspid valves have been shown to exhibit pacemaker activity as well as to participate in re-
entrant arrhythmias. It is likely that both automaticity and re-entry are responsible for specific atrial
premature depolarizations. Clinical differentiation is currently impossible.

Symptoms, Signs, and Diagnosis

Most patients complain of a "skipped beat," flutter, or extra beats in the chest, but generally
disregard them until their frequency causes alarm. Depending on the timing of the premature beat,
heart sounds may be identical to or totally different from normal. Very early APBs may not allow
sufficient ventricular filling to produce a palpable pulse. The diagnosis of an APB is certain if an S_4
gallop sound precedes the premature beat.

On ECG, atrial premature depolarizations, irrespective of their site of origin, interrupt sinus rhythm
in a characteristic manner, producing a premature P wave (FIG. 25–7). If the P wave is conducted to
the ventricles, then the premature P wave is followed by a premature QRS complex. No QRS complex is seen if the APB occurs while the A-V node or subsidiary A-V conducting structures are
refractory. The length of the cycle surrounding the APB is determined by its prematurity and by sinus
node function, but finding a pause equal to, less than, or greater than fully compensatory is not an
aid in diagnosis. In APBs late in the sinus cycle the premature depolarization does not enter the
sinus node. The sinus node discharges on time but atrial myocardium is refractory. The next sinus
impulse is on time and the pause surrounding the APB is fully compensatory. APBs occurring during
the midportion of the sinus cycle retrogradely enter the sinus node discharge and reset its dominant
pacemakers. A pause less than compensatory and generally $\leq$ 130% of the preceding sinus cycle
results. (Very prolonged sinus reset times > 150% of the preceding sinus cycle may be an indication
of sinus node dysfunction.) APBs occurring very early in the sinus cycle may find S-A conduction
pathways refractory and fail to enter and discharge the sinus node. The next S-A impulse is capable
of re-exciting the atrium and an interpolated APB results.

The contour of the premature P wave may suggest the source of the APBs. Origin in the low right
atrium, for example, typically produces inverted P waves in the inferior electrocardiographic leads II,
III, and aVF. Origin in the anterior left atrium may cause inverted anterior precordial P waves. Origin
within the atrium is certain if a P wave is the first event of the premature beat complex since there is
no way for a premature beat originating below the atrial level to result in atrial depolarization prior to
depolarization of ventricular myocardium.

Treatment

The treatment of APBs is directed at the cause. If, for example, ventricular filling pressures are
high, indicating heart failure, the use of **digitalis** may abolish APBs. In the absence of heart disease,
mild sedation, as with phenobarbital or diazepam, may help, and the use of caffeine and nicotine
should be eliminated.

Quinidine or **procainamide** may suppress APBs in organic heart disease. A test dose of quinidine
sulfate 200 mg orally is given to exclude idiosyncrasy. If, within 4 h, no tinnitus, deafness, urticaria,

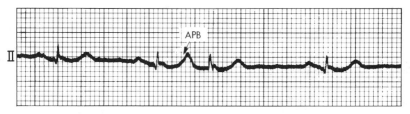

FIG. 25–7. **Atrial premature depolarization (APB).** ECG lead II is shown. Following the 2nd beat of
sinus origin, the T wave is deformed by an APB. Since the APB occurs relatively early during the sinus
cycle, the sinus node pacemaker is reset and a pause less than fully compensatory precedes the next sinus
beat.

diarrhea, or falling BP appears, 300 to 400 mg q 4 to 6 h may be started. Quinidine blood levels continue to rise during the initial 72 h of therapy, so that quinidine should not be considered ineffective after a trial period of only 24 to 48 h. It should be remembered that digitalis blood levels may rise to toxic levels when quinidine is added to a previously well tolerated digoxin dosage regimen. Nausea and vomiting is more likely the result of digitalis excess than quinidine intolerance when these two drugs are used together.

If quinidine cannot be given because of idiosyncrasy or GI intolerance (cramps and diarrhea predominate), procainamide is a useful substitute. It is essentially 100% absorbed and reaches maximum blood levels within 30 min after an oral dose. A dosage of 500 mg to 1 gm orally q 3 to 6 h is given initially; 2 to 4 gm/day are usually needed to control APBs. A lupus-like syndrome with arthralgias, fever, and pleuropericarditis may develop with long-term procainamide therapy.

An ECG should be taken frequently (e.g., after every other dose) during the first 3 days of quinidine or procainamide therapy. Prolongation of the Q-T interval and QRS widening are ECG manifestations of toxicity, and the quinidine or procainamide should either be stopped or used with great caution if QRS widening is 25% or more.

Propranolol 40 to 320 mg/day orally may also be used for the control of APBs. Although generally not as effective as quinidine, in patients where GI intolerance to quinidine has been demonstrated, a trial of propranolol is definitely indicated. When propranolol is used, its β-adrenergic blocking effect and slowing of sinus rate must be considered. Disopyramide phosphate appears to have little if any effect on isolated APBs or atrial arrhythmias in general. Newer, still experimental antiarrhythmic drugs should be reserved for arrhythmias with more clinical significance than simple APBs.

His Bundle and Fascicular Premature Depolarizations

Etiology

His bundle and fascicular premature beats (Fig. 25–8) formerly were called **junctional** or **nodal premature beats.** They may occur in normal hearts during periods of stress or of excess catecholamine production; in organic heart disease, they may be the result of ischemia or digitalis excess. Fascicular premature beats have been shown to be an occasional concomitant of acute myocardial infarction.

Mechanism

The most likely mechanism for His bundle and fascicular premature depolarizations is enhanced automaticity within these structures. Whether due to ischemia or the effects of digitalis, the rate of spontaneous diastolic depolarization within certain cells of the His bundle or the fascicles becomes higher than that of the sinus node and a premature beat occurs.

Diagnosis

Symptoms and signs are identical to those described above for APBs. His bundle premature beats are diagnosed on ECG by the presence of a premature QRS complex morphologically identical to conducted QRS complexes that is *not* preceded by a premature atrial complex. There is generally a retrograde P wave within or just after the QRS complex, although it is often hard to detect.

Fascicular premature beats occur most commonly in acute myocardial infarction, and arise within either the anterior or posterior fascicle of the left bundle branch. The normal rhythm is interrupted by a premature QRS complex whose morphology reflects right bundle branch block plus either left anterior or left posterior hemiblock, depending on the originating fascicle. The more characteristic the bundle branch block pattern, the more likely it is that the premature depolarization originates within one of the fascicles of the left bundle branch.

Given the conduction properties of the A-V node, a premature beat originating below the A-V node cannot result in a P wave prior to a QRS complex. Therefore, if the premature beat complex begins with a P wave, the beat is most likely an atrial premature depolarization. If it begins with a normal QRS complex that is followed by a P wave, its site of origin is most likely within the bundle of His.

Treatment

The treatment of His bundle and fascicular premature depolarizations is as for APBs, except that lidocaine and phenytoin may be useful. Since their incidence is not common, it is difficult to state the aggressiveness with which these premature depolarizations should be treated. In the presence of acute myocardial infarction, however, the fact that the refractoriness of the A-V node does not protect the ventricular myocardium from depolarization during its vulnerable period would suggest that an early His bundle PB could be as ominous as an early VPB in the initiation of more life-threatening ventricular arrhythmias.

Ventricular Premature Depolarizations

Etiology

Ventricular premature depolarizations (Fig. 25–9) may occur in normal or diseased hearts, or as a result of digitalis excess. In normal hearts, any process causing excess catecholamine release may result in ventricular premature beats **(VPBs).** Peri-, epi-, or myocardial inflammatory states may also

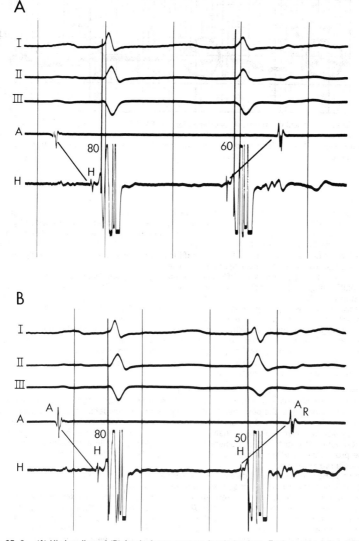

FIG. 25–8.   **(A) His bundle and (B) fascicular premature depolarizations.** Each panel records ECG leads I, II, and III, an atrial electrogram (A), and a His bundle electrogram (H). Heavy vertical lines represent 1-second intervals. In each panel a normal sinus beat is followed by the premature beat originating from high within the ventricular specialized conduction system but below the A-V node. In panel A, the fact that the H-V interval (60 msec) is almost normal and the QRS morphology is normal indicates the origin of this premature beat to be within the His bundle. In panel B the shorter H-V interval and the QRS morphology resembling a right bundle branch block pattern indicate the origin of this premature beat to be within the main left bundle. Note that in each panel the first observable electrical event during the premature beat is depolarization of the His bundle, and each premature beat conducts retrograde across the A-V node to result in atrial excitation.

precipitate VPBs. Myocardial stretching, as in congestive heart failure, or ischemia, as in coronary artery disease, results in a high incidence of VPBs. VPBs occur in > 90% of patients with acute myocardial infarction and under these circumstances may be an ominous precursor of sudden cardiac death.

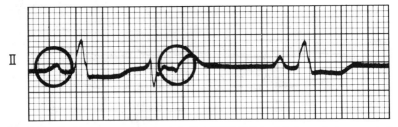

FIG. 25–9. **Ventricular premature depolarization (VPB).** ECG lead II demonstrates normal sinus rhythm with an upright P wave (first circle) followed by premature depolarization of the ventricles. The premature inverted P wave (second circle) following this VPB is the result of ventriculoatrial conduction (VAC). After the VPB, sinus rhythm resumes.

Diagnosis

Symptoms and signs are identical to those described above for APBs. VPBs are diagnosed on ECG when the sinus rhythm is interrupted by a premature QRS complex (not preceded by a premature P wave) whose morphology is distinctly abnormal and unlike the morphology of conducted QRS complexes. The ECG patterns of VPBs originating from the distal His-Purkinje system do not resemble any form of classic bundle branch block, and the more bizarre the QRS complex, the more distal its site of origin within the His-Purkinje system is likely to be.

Depending on their timing, each VPB may be interpolated ("sandwiched") between two normal sinus beats or may cause the next sinus beat to block in the A-V node, giving rise to a fully "compensatory pause." VPBs often cause retrograde conduction to the atria and may or may not reset the sinus node, giving rise to a pause less than compensatory. *The cycle surrounding any premature beat is not helpful in diagnosing its site of origin.* The presence of a premature depolarization of ventricular origin may be made with certainty when a QRS complex initiates the premature beat complex and the sequence of ventricular activation is abnormal. There is no way that a premature depolarization originating above the level of the A-V node could result in ventricular depolarization prior to that of the atrium—and vice versa. Although morphologic diagnostic criteria for VPBs may be helpful, the above criteria are absolute.

Treatment

Frequent VPBs in a patient without heart disease may or may not require therapy. They are frequently more annoying to the physician than to the patient. If no evidence of valvular heart disease is found by echocardiogram and physical examination; and no evidence of ischemic heart disease elicited by history, exercise ECG, or thallium myocardial perfusion studies, a Holter monitor should be performed to determine the characteristics of the VPBs present. In the absence of organic heart disease probably only VPBs occurring early in the cycle (R on T VPBs) in salvos or as ventricular tachycardia require therapy.

Chronic VPBs in organic heart disease are an altogether different problem. It has been recognized that ventricular ectopic activity in the presence of valvular heart disease and, more specifically, in the presence of coronary artery disease represents a physiologic abnormality frequently requiring correction. The key to the urgency with which VPBs must be treated in these patients is based upon their underlying organic heart disease and the malignancy of the ventricular arrhythmias encountered. For example, in patients presenting with VPBs in whom mitral valve prolapse is documented both clinically and echocardiographically to be the etiology of their ventricular ectopic activity, a trial of VPB suppression with standard antiarrhythmic drugs is indicated. There is a small but discrete incidence of sudden death resulting from ventricular ectopic activity—ventricular fibrillation—in these patients and, hence, frequent ventricular premature depolarizations should be suppressed if possible with antiarrhythmic drugs.

In patients with coronary artery disease or myocardiopathies with severely depressed left ventricular function, the aggressiveness with which ventricular ectopic activity should be treated is even greater. In these two classes of patients, an initial assessment of ventricular performance should be made. Exercise ECG with or without thallium myocardial perfusion testing and wall motion studies should be utilized as a means of evaluating the severity of left ventricular dysfunction, since ectopic activity in the presence of depressed left ventricular dysfunction from either cause becomes significantly more clinically important. When possible a Holter monitor (24-h tape recording) should be made in all patients prior to the initiation of antiarrhythmic therapy. This not only allows a baseline in order to determine the severity of the ventricular arrhythmias under consideration but also allows for the subsequent determination of drug efficacy after antiarrhythmic drugs have been instituted.

Once the decision has been made to treat ventricular premature depolarizations present in patients with organic heart disease, standard antiarrhythmic drugs available are basically limited to 5. Although digitalis is occasionally effective in diminishing the frequency of VPBs or abolishing them completely in patients with severe left ventricular dysfunction, in general a specific antiarrhythmic drug should be used. Not necessarily in this order of preference, the following should be considered:

1. Procainamide: Procainamide is a potent antiarrhythmic drug which is rapidly absorbed and has a relatively short clinical half-life. It should be given in dosages of 375 to 500 mg q 4 h, but in refractory cases recent suggestions of much higher dosing regimens, up to 6 to 10 gm/day of oral procainamide, have been suggested. Drug efficacy should be determined with the use of frequent Holter monitors and, when using high levels of this medication, peak and trough procainamide levels are useful. The demonstration of adequate procainamide blood levels without suppression of ventricular ectopic activity would suggest moving to another antiarrhythmic drug.

The most common side effects of procainamide include GI disturbance (primarily upper GI with bleeding and nausea), but significant autoimmune inflammatory lupus-like reactions are not uncommon. These vary from arthralgias to frank arthritis and have included the development of skin rashes and pleural and pericardial effusions.

2. Quinidine sulfate: Although quinidine sulfate in isolated tissue preparations behaves similarly to procainamide and is a Class 1 antiarrhythmic drug which prolongs action potential duration and refractoriness, in clinical situations quinidine has been shown to be effective in cases where procainamide has failed and vice versa. After an initial test dose of quinidine sulfate 200 mg orally, dosage regimens of 200 to 400 mg q 6 h are generally used for suppression of ventricular ectopic activity. Again, careful observation of the patient with ECG and/or Holter monitoring will disclose drug efficacy. Serum quinidine levels are also readily available and should be followed to determine if a lack of efficacy is due to low serum blood levels or a nonresponse of the arrhythmia under consideration.

Quinidine is a moderately well-tolerated drug causing GI symptoms in many patients. GI bloating and diarrhea are its commonest side effects but fever, liver disease, and thrombocytopenia have all been seen. It should be remembered that quinidine may cause a significant *increase* in ventricular ectopic activity and, by prolonging ventricular refractoriness, has even been implicated as a cause of sudden death due to ventricular fibrillation **(quinidine syncope).**

3. Propranolol: Propranolol as an antiarrhythmic affects the ventricular myocardium both directly and reflexly as a β-blocking agent. It prolongs conduction, action potential duration, and refractoriness, having significant effects on A-V nodal conduction as well as the incidence of ventricular ectopic activity. Dosage regimens for propranolol vary widely in the chronic setting; 10 mg q.i.d. up to regimens of 320 mg/day have been used for the control of ventricular premature depolarizations, but since propranolol is a depressant of myocardial function, higher dosage levels may be precluded by the presence of severe left ventricular dysfunction in the patients under consideration. In addition to its depressant effect on left ventricular performance, its β-blocking activity may cause GI disturbance, nightmares, and, in patients with bronchospastic pulmonary disease, a severe exacerbation of airways obstruction.

4. Phenytoin enjoyed a brief vogue as an antiarrhythmic drug for ventricular ectopic activity. Although occasionally effective in the patient with chronic heart disease and ectopic activity, its current use should probably be restricted to those patients with ventricular ectopic activity which is the result of digitalis excess. Its efficacy as a long-term antiarrhythmic drug has not withstood the test of time.

5. Disopyramide phosphate is a more recent antiarrhythmic drug with significant abilities to depress ventricular ectopic activity. Dosage regimens of 100 to 300 mg q.i.d. may be used to suppress ectopic activity, but again, careful observation of the ECG and/or Holter monitor is indicated. Major side effects are a reflex increase in sinus rate, difficulty in visual accommodation, and difficulty with urination. In patients with depressed left ventricular dysfunction, disopyramide phosphate may be a very potent depressant of myocardial contractility resulting in severe exacerbations of chronically existing congestive heart failure.

A variety of new and experimental antiarrhythmic drugs recently available in the USA should probably be reserved for patients with malignant and life-threatening arrhythmias until clinical efficacy and toxicity are clearly established.

As opposed to careful prolonged clinical trials in patients with chronic organic heart disease and VPBs, *VPBs occurring in patients with acute myocardial infarction require more urgent correction.* The effect of an initial bolus of **lidocaine** 50 to 100 mg IV on the sinus rate, BP, and ECG should be noted. An IV infusion of 2 mg/min should also be started immediately. If the VPBs are not controlled by this initial regimen, 50-mg boluses of lidocaine may be repeated q 5 min to a maximum of 325 to 375 mg or until undesirable CNS side effects occur and the infusion rate may be increased gradually to 4 mg/min.

The immediate toxic effects of IV lidocaine consist of transient auditory disturbances and disorientation followed by muscular twitching and finally by overt convulsions. Lidocaine should be discontinued and IV **procainamide** begun if signs of CNS toxicity begin to develop or the VPBs are not controlled. Procainamide 100 mg IV is given q 5 min until either the VPBs are controlled, a maximum dosage of 1000 to 1200 mg has been given, or procainamide toxicity occurs. The QRS and Q-T intervals should be measured before each dose. Procainamide, in addition to its slight myocardial depressing effect, is a potent peripheral vasodilator; the occurrence of hypotension precludes its continued use. If the 5-min doses of procainamide abolish the VPBs, then an IV infusion of procainamide 2 to 6 mg/min should be started immediately. Since a patient with myocardial ischemia is likely to develop primary ventricular fibrillation if the VPBs are not abolished, every possible attempt should be made to control them. Although effective in 98% of myocardial infarction patients, in nonresponders lidocaine and pronistyl may be used simultaneously.

For VPBs resulting from digitalis toxicity, phenytoin 100 mg IV is given q 5 min until CNS toxicity occurs or the VPBs are abolished. Propranolol 1 mg IV q 2 to 3 min to a maximum of 5 to 7 mg also may help to abolish VPBs. *Hypotension should be avoided.* If hypokalemia is present, it should be corrected.

PAROXYSMAL SUPRAVENTRICULAR TACHYCARDIA (Paroxysmal Atrial Tachycardia [PAT]; Paroxysmal Nodal Tachycardia)

A condition in which the heart rate suddenly increases to 100 to 200 beats/min and 1:1 A-V conduction is maintained.

Mechanism

Although it had been assumed for years that paroxysmal atrial and paroxysmal nodal tachycardias were the result of the sudden takeover of cardiac rhythm by an ectopic atrial or junctional focus, intracardiac electrocardiography has now shown that these rhythms are the same and are initiated and maintained by atrial reentry via the A-V node. The arrhythmia develops spontaneously when a single atrial depolarization enters the A-V node during a specific portion of its relative refractory period. Because the impulse is propagating very slowly toward the ventricles, this physiologically slowed conduction through the A-V node allows the impulse to be reflected back to the chamber of its origin and to reenter the atrium. Although the majority of patients utilize the A-V node for both the antegrade and retrograde limbs of the re-entry pathway, recent studies have demonstrated a variety of concealed tracts bypassing the A-V node in a retrograde direction thus suggesting a congenital basis for this electrophysiologic disorder. However conducted retrogradely, once the impulse is in the atrium, if the A-V node is again receptive, the cycle may be repeated continuously. The result is supraventricular tachycardia **(SVT).**

Any mechanism which allows A-V conduction to become significantly slowed will allow reentry within or adjacent to the A-V node and the development of paroxysmal SVT. However, the specific physiologic or anatomic substrate of SVT is still unknown. It characteristically occurs in young persons with no evidence of organic heart disease, but may also occur in older patients with arteriosclerotic cardiovascular disease.

Symptoms and Signs

The patient with spontaneous APBs may or may not be aware of single premature beats, but at the beginning of a paroxysm the sudden, rapid, regular fluttering sensation in the chest is easily noticed. Most patients feel weak and faint, but true syncope is rare. Arterial BP falls and giant atrial waves in the neck cause a feeling of tightness and palpitations. Shortness of breath is not uncommon, and older patients may develop angina during the paroxysm. Polyuria often occurs during or after attacks. Recent studies have shown that the almost simultaneous diastolic filling of atria and ventricles results in hemodynamic derangements far more severe than previously recognized. Paroxysmal SVT is considerably less benign than previously thought.

Diagnosis

The ECG (FIG. 25–10) shows an atrial rate of 150 to 214 beats/min (average, 187) where each atrial impulse is conducted to the ventricles with a normal QRS morphology. When P waves are seen, they are generally inverted in the inferior leads and follow the QRS complex. More frequently, however, P waves occur simultaneously with QRS complexes and are difficult to discern. Paroxysmal atrial tachycardia cannot be differentiated from paroxysmal His bundle or fascicular tachycardia by the ability to discern P waves between QRS complexes since the tachycardias may all have the same rate, the only difference being the degree of A-V nodal conduction delay. The diagnosis is established by observing the onset of the tachycardia on the ECG, since an APB exhibits prolonged A-V conduction and initiates SVT (FIG. 25–11), or by observing its cessation, since the last beat of SVT is followed by a prolonged pause before the sinus rhythm resumes its slower rate (FIG. 25–12).

Treatment

In the **acute attack,** the patient should assume the supine position. Significant hypotension is the rule rather than the exception and whether mediated by a decrease in stroke volume or increased left atrial stretch, hypotension is greatly exaggerated by the upright position.

Since SVT requires A-V nodal conduction for at least one limb of its re-entrant pathway, any maneuver which prolongs or temporarily interrupts conduction via the A-V node must result in a termination of SVT. Valsalva's maneuver should be tried, with ECG monitoring; gagging or vomiting may also increase vagal tone enough to interrupt the tachycardia. Most episodes of paroxysmal SVT can be terminated with **carotid sinus massage** (providing the patient is not markedly hypotensive), and this should be the next therapeutic maneuver. Atropine should always be on hand, and the carotid sinus should be palpated and then gently massaged before firm massage is applied. When carotid sinus massage is effective, the rate of the SVT slows slightly and then there is a long pause, after which sinus rhythm resumes.

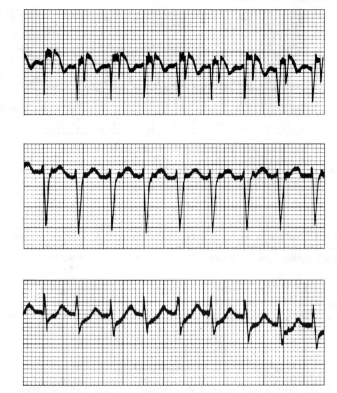

Fig. 25–10.   **Supraventricular tachycardia (SVT).** An atrial electrogram (A) and ECG leads V_1 and V_6 are simultaneously recorded. Although P waves are not readily apparent in the ECG leads, the rapid deflection following the QRS complex in the atrial electrogram represents the P wave. In this arrhythmia each P wave generates the next QRS complex with a P-R interval of 240 msec.

If carotid sinus massage is ineffective, edrophonium IV is given. Again with atropine close at hand, a 1-mg test dose is given. If there is no idiosyncratic reaction, 10 mg IV is then given as a bolus. The anticholinesterase effect of this drug allows acetylcholine to build up at the A-V node and thus terminates many episodes of SVT.

When the patient is hypotensive, vagal maneuvers may not be sufficient to interrupt paroxysmal SVT because of sympathetic nervous system overactivity. Metaraminol as an increasing IV infusion should be given to raise the BP to normal levels and then vagal maneuvers attempted again. If still unsuccessful, the infusion rate of metaraminol may be increased and used to elevate the BP to 160 to 180 mm Hg; by reflex vagal activity, this may terminate the SVT. Propranolol has also been advocated in the emergency therapy of SVT. Its depressant effect on A-V nodal conduction and rapid onset of action when given IV make it an excellent choice. Caution is advised when propranolol is given in the presence of compromised left ventricular function or significant hypotension.

Verapamil is a new slow channel blocking antiarrhythmic drug which has potent effects on A-V nodal conduction. Recent studies suggest it is effective both in patients with standard A-V nodal re-entrant SVT as well as those with concealed bypass tracts. Given intravenously, it has become the treatment of choice for rapid termination of paroxysmal SVT. However, long-term prophylaxis is less effective.

If all these emergency procedures fail, the patient may either be digitalized or cardioverted and should be hospitalized. For the younger patient whose hemodynamic function is not seriously compromised by a sustained rate of 180 beats/min, digitalization is the therapy of choice. Digoxin 0.5 mg IV, followed by 0.25 mg IV q 4 to 6 h usually results in resumption of sinus rhythm. Immediate DC cardioversion is advisable if the patient is older and hemodynamically compromised by the SVT or if ischemic chest pain is present. For cardioversion, anteroposterior paddles are suggested and the amount of electrical energy required may be only 10 to 50 watt-seconds. In all patients with paroxysmal SVT a temporary atrial pacemaker may be used to initiate APBs, which render the A-V node refractory and thereby immediately terminate SVT. The electrical conversion of SVT by programmed

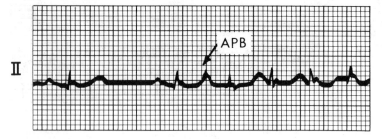

II

FIG. 25–11.   **Onset of supraventricular tachycardia (SVT).** In ECG lead II, 2 normal sinus beats are followed by an atrial premature depolarization (APB), which distorts the T wave of the 2nd sinus beat. This APB shows prolonged A-V conduction and initiates an episode of sustained SVT with a cycle length of 340 msec (rate, 160 beats/min).

atrial stimulation is uniformly successful and essentially without risk. Single atrial premature depolarizations or atrial pacing at rates in excess of SVT are equally effective. Implantable permanent pacemakers with circuits designed to sense and convert episodes of SVT by programmed stimulation have already been used in patients with frequently occurring or refractory SVT.

ATRIAL ECTOPIC TACHYCARDIA

Etiology

These atrial tachycardias are generally nonparoxysmal. They tend to occur in patients with organic heart disease—particularly those with hypokalemia, digitalis excess (PAT with block—see below), or myo- or pericarditis—and following the overconsumption of alcohol.

Mechanism

In contrast to paroxysmal SVTs, atrial ectopic tachycardias (**AET**) *are* the result of a rapidly firing automatic focus located within the atrial myocardium. Premature beats initiating these tachycardias usually occur late in the atrial cycle and arise well outside the refractory period of the A-V node. Their rate is totally unrelated to A-V conduction. For this reason, drugs or maneuvers affecting A-V nodal conduction do not terminate AETs but may produce varying degrees of A-V block.

Symptoms and Signs

Although the atrial rate of AETs is similar to that seen in paroxysmal SVT, the generally present 2:1 A-V block tends to lessen symptoms. Patients with 1:1 A-V conduction experience symptoms identical to those of paroxysmal SVT.

Diagnosis

A rapid, regular atrial rate of 150 to 214 is seen on the ECG. Because depolarization does not originate within the sinus node, the P waves are abnormal in contour. Although occasionally difficult, in general AET may be distinguished from SVT even when 1:1 A-V conduction is present. In AET the rate is not a function of A-V conduction, PR intervals tend to be < 50% of the cycle length (short), and discrete P waves are seen preceding each QRS complex. In SVT atrial and ventricular depolarizations occur almost simultaneously since the PR interval is so long (> 60% of the cycle length) and discrete P waves are rarely seen.

Absolute distinction between SVT and AET is possible utilizing vagal maneuvers. With an ectopic atrial tachycardia, these will produce increasing A-V block, Wenckebach periods, and 2:1 or 3:1 A-V conduction without altering the atrial rate (FIG. 25–13). The tachycardia continues unabated despite A-V block because these arrhythmias are unrelated to A-V nodal conduction.

If the ECG captures the initiating atrial premature depolarization, one can see that it occurs late in the atrial cycle, well past the relative refractory period of the A-V node. The tachycardia then demonstrates the "warm-up" phenomenon characteristic of pacemakers, in that subsequent atrial cycles increase in rapidity until the eventual cycle length of the tachycardia is established.

Treatment

AETs are unresponsive to vagal maneuvers and to therapy designed to increase A-V nodal refractoriness. They are, however, responsive to medications which suppress atrial automaticity. These include quinidine, procainamide, and propranolol (given as for APBs), but not phenytoin or lidocaine. AETs can neither be initiated nor terminated by single stimulated premature beats nor terminated by rapid atrial stimulation such as overdrive suppression. Although cardioversion may temporarily convert the patient's rhythm to sinus, some suppressant medication must be used in order to prevent AET from recurring.

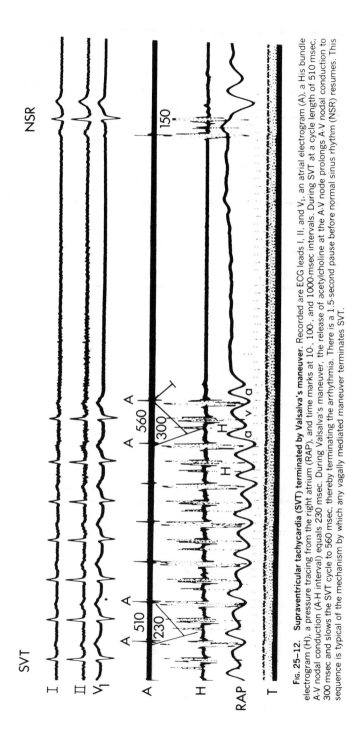

Fig. 25-12. Supraventricular tachycardia (SVT) terminated by Valsalva's maneuver. Recorded are ECG leads I, II, and V_1, an atrial electrogram (A), a His bundle electrogram (H), a pressure tracing from the right atrium (RAP), and time marks at 10-, 100-, and 1000-msec intervals. During SVT at a cycle length of 510 msec, A-V nodal conduction (A-H interval) equals 230 msec. During Valsalva's maneuver, the release of acetylcholine at the A-V node prolongs A-V nodal conduction to 300 msec and slows the SVT cycle to 560 msec, thereby terminating the arrhythmia. There is a 1.5-second pause before normal sinus rhythm (NSR) resumes. This sequence is typical of the mechanism by which any vagally mediated maneuver terminates SVT.

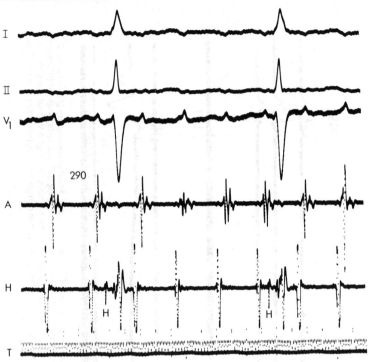

FIG. 25–13.   **Atrial tachycardia with block.** Recorded are ECG leads I, II, and V_1, an atrial electrogram (A), a His bundle electrogram (H), and time marks at 10- and 100-msec intervals. The atrial cycle length is 290 msec (a rate slightly above 200 beats/min). A 4:1 A-V nodal block is present, since depolarization of the His bundle follows only every 4th atrial beat.

ATRIAL ECTOPIC TACHYCARDIA WITH BLOCK (PAT with Block)

All AETs may demonstrate A-V block, but the designation **PAT with block** is generally used when digitalis excess is the cause. Since digitalis acts to prolong A-V conduction, these atrial tachycardias always demonstrate at least 2:1 A-V nodal block (FIG. 25–13). The mechanism and diagnosis is as described above, but **treatment** differs. Since the ventricular response in PAT with block is generally fairly slow, simply waiting for the digitalis level to fall often allows the arrhythmia to end spontaneously. Giving potassium will speed this sequence. Both quinidine and procainamide can be used if discontinuing digitalis does not terminate the tachycardia, but cardioversion is *contraindicated* for PAT with block since *the presence of digitalis excess may result in life-threatening ventricular arrhythmias.*

ATRIAL FLUTTER

An arrhythmia wherein continuous electrical activity within the atrium is organized into regular cyclic waves with a cycle length of about 200 msec, producing an atrial rate between 240 and 400 (approximately 300).

Etiology

Atrial flutter (much less common than atrial fibrillation) may occur in any organic heart disease, but particularly in arteriosclerotic heart disease, myocardial infarction, rheumatic heart disease, and inflammatory diseases of the atrium. In some patients atrial flutter is paroxysmal, and without known cause.

Mechanism and Diagnosis

The mechanism of atrial flutter has long been debated, but recent electrophysiologic evidence from both human and canine studies strongly suggests it is as follows: Atrial flutter is initiated by single APBs which occur during the relative refractory period of the atrial myocardium. As a result, the slow spread of atrial excitation through refractory muscle results in continuous atrial electrical reentry, via ordinary atrial myocardium. Direct recordings from inside the atrium demonstrate regular atrial activity with a fixed periodicity and an isoelectric segment between atrial cycles. Atrial flutter is probably independent of both the S-A and the A-V nodes for its maintenance. Since perpetration of atrial flutter requires re-entry via ordinary atrial myocardium, the atrial excitation waves in flutter must approximate the cycle length of the arrhythmia itself, the ECG appearance is one of a regular saw-tooth base line, particularly in the inferior leads where continuous atrial electrical activity is usually seen. (FIG. 25-14). This, plus determining that an atrial rate between 240 and 400 exists with a regular cycle length, is diagnostic. Since maintenance of the arrhythmia does not depend on A-V nodal conduction, some degree of A-V block is always present (FIG. 25-15). This may be 2:1, 4:1, or less commonly 3:1 or 5:1. Atrial flutter with 1:1 A-V conduction may be a life-threatening arrhythmia since ventricular rates of 300/min are encountered. These extremely rapid ventricular rates are generally the result of some form of A-V nodal bypass tract. Atrial flutter with high degrees of A-V block *in the absence of digitalis* suggests intrinsic A-V nodal pathology, and conduction may not be normal when sinus rhythm is restored.

Since atrial flutter generally occurs at a rate of 300 and the usual degree of block in the undigital-ized patient is 2:1, the ventricular response is 150. If the characteristic saw-tooth does not appear on the ECG, it is difficult to distinguish sinus tachycardia, atrial tachycardia with 1:1 conduction, and atrial flutter with 2:1 conduction. **Carotid sinus massage** can be useful. If the degree of A-V block can be increased from 2:1 to 4:1, diagnostic saw-tooth flutter waves will appear.

Symptoms, signs, and treatment are discussed below under atrial fibrillation.

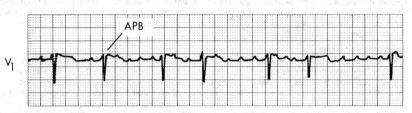

FIG. 25-14.   Onset of atrial flutter. ECG lead V_1 is recorded. Following the 2nd normal sinus beat, an atrial premature depolarization (APB) with a coupling interval of 140 msec initiates a sustained atrial rhythm with a cycle length of 200 msec (rate, 300 beats/min) and variable A-V block.

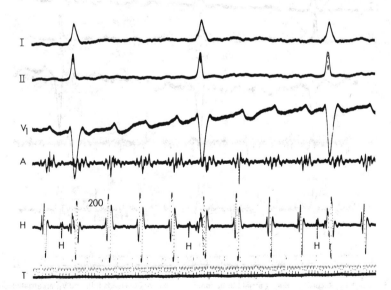

FIG. 25-15.   Recordings during atrial flutter. Recorded are ECG leads I, II, and V_1, an atrial electro-gram (A), a His bundle electrogram (H), and time marks at 10- and 100-msec intervals. Note the broad, notched, but regular atrial depolarizations at a cycle length of 200 msec (rate, 300 beats/min); 4:1 A-V nodal block exists, since depolarization of the His bundle occurs only after every 4th flutter wave.

ATRIAL FIBRILLATION

An arrhythmia which results from the continuous and chaotic reentry of electrical impulses within the atrial myocardium. Since electrical activity is continuous and chaotic, it is difficult to discuss an atrial rate, but recordings from inside the atrium demonstrate rapid activity at cycle lengths between 100 and 200 msec (Fig. 25–16).

Etiology

Atrial fibrillation is much more common than atrial flutter, and occurs in the same diseases. In young patients atrial fibrillation is most commonly idiopathic or the result of rheumatic mitral valvular disease. In older patients, arteriosclerotic heart disease is the major cause. The presence of atrial fibrillation generally indicates disease or stretching of the left atrium. Thus hypertensive heart disease with left atrial enlargement, congestive cardiomyopathy, or particularly mitral stenosis with enlarged and diseased left atrium are common etiologies. Echocardiography to exclude silent mitral valve disease should be undertaken in all patients with paroxysmal atrial flutter or fibrillation.

Mechanism

Atrial fibrillation is generally initiated by a single APB occurring very early during the refractory period of the atrial myocardium (Fig. 25–17). This single impulse then "fragments" due to the variable refractory periods of adjacent atrial myocardium not yet fully repolarized. These partially depolarized cells then result in very slow intra-atrial conduction. Continuous reentrant excitation waves occur within both atria if excitability and refractoriness vary enough from one portion of atrial myocardium to the next. The arrhythmia depends on a disparity between refractoriness and conduction velocity in various parts of the atrium, and, therefore, significant atrial myocardial disease must exist. The mechanism is independent of S-A or A-V nodal reentry and maneuvers or drugs affecting A-V nodal conduction will not change the basic rate of atrial fibrillation although they diminish the ventricular response.

Symptoms and Signs

At the onset of both flutter and fibrillation, symptoms are generally similar to those of paroxysmal tachycardia except that the patient is frequently aware of an irregularly irregular pulse. Palpitations, near-syncope, pallor, nausea, weakness, lightheadedness, and fatigue occur in atrial fibrillation because the ventricular response is rapid and irregular. When cardiac reserve is extremely limited by

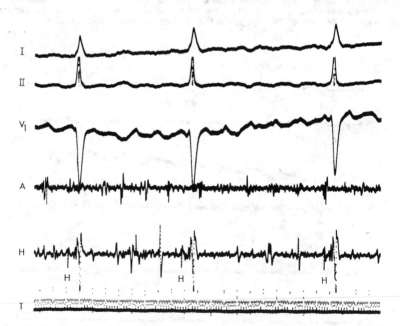

Fig. 25–16.   **Recordings during atrial fibrillation.** Recorded are ECG leads I, II, and V₁, an atrial electrogram (A), a His bundle electrogram (H), and time marks at 10- and 100-msec intervals. Electrical activity within the atrial electrogram shows no regularity. A chaotic continuous series of wave fronts occurs within the atrium, which represents atrial fibrillation. Each QRS complex is preceded by depolarization of the His bundle, indicating the supraventricular origin of each QRS complex.

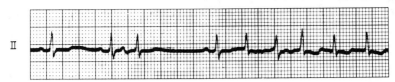
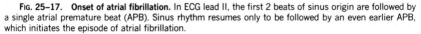

FIG. 25-17. **Onset of atrial fibrillation.** In ECG lead II, the first 2 beats of sinus origin are followed by a single atrial premature beat (APB). Sinus rhythm resumes only to be followed by an even earlier APB, which initiates the episode of atrial fibrillation.

left ventricular disease or in severe mitral stenosis, cardiogenic shock or acute pulmonary edema may occur. The severity of symptoms is directly proportional to the rapidity of the ventricular response and augmented by the degree of underlying left ventricular dysfunction. In mitral stenosis the diastolic filling period is curtailed by the rapid ventricular response, and left atrial and pulmonary capillary wedge pressures rise precipitously.

In atrial flutter, physical examination usually shows a regular radial pulse with a rate of about 150. Flutter waves and regular cannon A waves are frequently seen in the jugular venous pulse. In atrial fibrillation, the pulse is irregularly irregular and although venous pressures are elevated, no discrete A waves are seen. When the ventricular rate is particularly rapid, some beats expel little or no blood into the aorta and fail to cause a discernible pulse at the wrist. The difference between the number of apically heard beats and those felt at the wrist is known as a **pulse deficit.** The more rapid the ventricular response in atrial fibrillation, the greater the pulse deficit is likely to be.

Course and Prognosis

Both atrial flutter and fibrillation tend to occur paroxysmally before becoming constant, regardless of their etiology. Although sustained atrial flutter is extremely uncommon, sustained atrial fibrillation is one of the most common atrial arrhythmias encountered clinically. In the prognosis of atrial fibrillation, cause is a factor, as is the fact that atrial mural thrombi tend to develop with prolonged fibrillation, particularly in patients with mitral stenosis. Arterial emboli are common in fibrillation, extremely rare in flutter.

Diagnosis

In atrial fibrillation the ECG shows irregular, coarse fibrillatory, nonperiodic wave forms in the baseline (reflecting the continuous atrial reentry), most easily identified in lead V_1 (FIG. 25-18). The chaotic electrical activity causes irregularly irregular A-V nodal conduction and therefore conducted QRS complexes on the ECG show no regular periodicity. Intracardiac ECGs reveal the continuous chaotic high-frequency electrical activity with no isoelectric segment (FIG. 25-16).

Treatment

The primary aim of therapy in atrial fibrillation and in atrial flutter is to slow the ventricular response, thereby increasing the cardiac output. If the patient shows evidence of severe cardiac compromise (such as shock or pulmonary edema), it is best to terminate the arrhythmia immediately by DC cardioversion, but if the rapid ventricular response is well tolerated, digitalis therapy is recommended. Digitalis decreases the ventricular response by slowing A-V conduction, and occasionally will convert flutter or fibrillation into regular sinus rhythm. More often, after the patient is fully digitalized and the ventricular response acceptably slowed, quinidine sulfate 400 mg q 6 h or procainamide 1 gm q 6 h is given to convert fibrillation to sinus rhythm; these drugs are effective in 50% of patients. If 3 days of such therapy does not convert the arrhythmia and the fibrillation has not been protracted, digitalis should be withheld for 24 h and DC cardioversion should then be attempted.

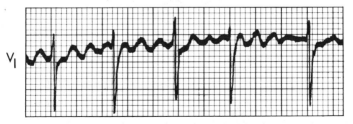

FIG. 25-18. **Atrial fibrillation—ECG characteristics.** These are most easily documented in lead V_1 where irregular waves of varying amplitude and frequency demonstrate the rhythm to be due to atrial fibrillation.

For the occasional patient in whom digitalis does not effectively slow the ventricular response, and if congestive heart failure is not a therapeutic problem, propranolol 0.5 to 1 mg IV every minute for a total dose of 2 mg generally decreases the ventricular response to a rate < 100 and occasionally converts atrial fibrillation to sinus rhythm directly.

Once atrial flutter or fibrillation is terminated, therapy is given to prevent recurrences. Quinidine, procainamide, and propranolol, in that order, are the drugs of choice, and should be continued for as long as the underlying cause of the atrial fibrillation exists. Verapamil may be extremely useful in paroxysmal atrial flutter or fibrillation both because of its effects on atrial myocardium directly and also because its profound slowing of A-V nodal conduction results in a slower ventricular response when fibrillation occurs.

The hazard of releasing arterial emboli during cardioversion for atrial fibrillation is probably not significantly greater than the risk of emboli from the fibrillation itself. Because this hazard exists, however, many believe that 3 wk of anticoagulant therapy should precede cardioversion, especially if the patient has had a prior arterial embolus. The need for cardioversion, and for anticoagulant therapy, must be determined for each patient. A maintained sinus rhythm is less likely to follow cardioversion (1) the longer the atrial fibrillation has lasted, (2) the worse the atrial myocardial disease, (3) the larger the atrial muscle mass, (4) the worse the predisposing coronary artery disease, and (5) in the presence of inflammation or infarction. The hemodynamic advantages of sinus rhythm over atrial fibrillation with a well-controlled ventricular response are generally small, but in patients with atrial fibrillation the best prophylaxis against arterial emboli is conversion to and maintenance of sinus rhythm.

MULTIFOCAL ATRIAL TACHYCARDIA

An arrhythmia which results from multiple areas of enhanced automaticity within ordinary atrial myocardium.

The underlying rhythm is generally sinus or sinus tachycardia. It is interrupted by frequent atrial premature depolarizations **(APBs)**, which occur singly, in pairs, or frequently in salvos of 3 to 15 beats in a row. The P wave morphology varies greatly from beat to beat as does A-V conduction. These salvos of APBs occur without sequence or specific repetitive pattern and result in periods of rapid, irregular heart action.

Etiology

Although multifocal atrial tachycardia may occur with all forms of cardiac disease, it is most commonly seen in patients with severe chronic pulmonary disease, respiratory insufficiency, and/or theophylline excess. An acute exacerbation of underlying respiratory illness is the commonest predisposing factor to the development of multifocal atrial tachycardia.

Mechanism

Atrial irritability is enhanced by pulmonary hypertension with elevated right atrial pressures and right atrial stretch. This, combined with systemic hypoxia, the use of sympathomimetic agents in the treatment of pulmonary disease, and/or elevated theophylline levels, results in multiple areas of enhanced automaticity within ordinary atrial myocardium. These multiple abnormal atrial pacemaker cells fire singly or in salvos, thus producing the characteristic pattern of this arrhythmia.

Symptoms and Signs

Multifocal atrial tachycardia is usually asymptomatic and the symptoms which predominate are those of the underlying pulmonary disease. Sustained rapid heart rates, however, may exacerbate left ventricular dysfunction precipitated by hypoxemia and result in an overall worsening of the cardiopulmonary status.

Diagnosis

Multifocal atrial tachycardia is generally distinguishable from atrial fibrillation by finding discrete if irregular and multiform atrial activity preceding each QRS complex. Irregular rates of 100 to 180 beats/min are common and intracardiac ECGs merely reflect the varying atrial depolarization sequence engendered by various foci of abnormal atrial automaticity. Since patients with multifocal atrial tachycardia generally have a high level of sympathetic nervous system activity (intrinsic or iatrogenic), vagal maneuvers generally do not result in A-V block or a slowing of ventricular response in multifocal atrial tachycardia.

Treatment

The treatment of multifocal atrial tachycardia should be directed at correcting its underlying cause rather than at the rhythm itself. Ventilatory assistance in patients with respiratory insufficiency, hypoxemia, and hypercapnia may be mandatory. If the patient is receiving aminophylline or a similar therapeutic agent, theophylline levels should be measured and carefully observed. Digitalis may be helpful in treating the patient's overall cardiopulmonary state but is of no specific advantage in the therapy of multifocal atrial tachycardia. Similarly, antiarrhythmic agents such as quinidine or procainamide are generally less effective in converting this rhythm than is correction of the patient's underlying pulmonary disease. Propranolol and other β-blocking agents are specifically to be avoided because of their tendency to increase bronchospasm and worsen the patient's respiratory status.

HIS BUNDLE RHYTHMS

An arrhythmia which results from sustained enhanced automaticity within the bundle of His.

Junctional rhythms of various rates from 70 to 150 may arise due to spontaneous Phase IV diastolic depolarization (enhanced automaticity) within the bundle of His or the subsequent branching portions of the interventricular conducting system. These ectopic tachycardias are generally nonparoxysmal and tend to be of relatively short duration. They result in normal impulse propagation through the ventricles and hence a QRS of normal duration and morphology. Generally, 1:1 retrograde conduction across the A-V node is present.

His bundle rhythms and tachycardia may occur in ischemic heart disease, acute myocardial infarction, rheumatic heart disease, or digitalis excess.

Symptoms, Signs, and Diagnosis

The patient may be totally asymptomatic or may be aware of a rapid heart beat. The sensation of palpitation is enhanced when 1:1 ventriculoatrial conduction results in cannon A waves which are sensed in the neck. Carotid sinus massage may transiently slow, but not terminate, these rhythms.

On ECG (Fig. 25–19), His bundle rhythms and tachycardias are diagnosed by the regular QRS complexes of generally normal duration and morphology that are either dissociated from an atrial rhythm (i.e., sinus rhythm, atrial flutter or fibrillation) or are accompanied by 1:1 ventriculoatrial conduction. Under these circumstances, an inverted P wave may be seen early in the S-T segment, during the QRS complexes, or following the QRS in leads II, III, and aVF.

Treatment

Immediate cardioversion is required if His bundle tachycardias are very rapid, have resulted in cardiac compromise, and are not the result of digitalis excess. If the patient's digitalis status is unknown, or the arrhythmia is fairly well tolerated, then antiarrhythmic medications (quinidine, procainamide, propranolol) should be given to treat and to suppress the redevelopment of these tachycardias. Digitalis will only increase the automatic rate of the His bundle focus and should not be used.

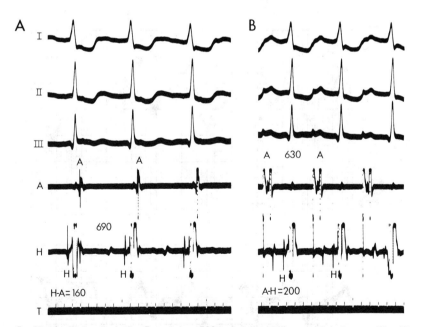

Fig. 25–19. **His bundle rhythm.** Recorded are ECG leads I, II, and III, an atrial electrogram (A), a His bundle electrogram (H), and time marks at 10- and 100-msec intervals.

A. A sustained rhythm with a cycle length of 690 msec is shown to originate within the bundle of His. Each QRS complex is preceded by depolarization of the His bundle and this sustained His bundle rhythm results in 1:1 ventriculoatrial conduction. The retrograde A-V nodal conduction time has an H-A interval of 160 msec.

B. The origin of the rhythm within the His bundle is substantiated since atrial pacing at a cycle length of 630 msec shows antegrade conduction with a normal A-H interval of 200 msec.

VENTRICULAR TACHYCARDIA (VT)

A regular ventricular rhythm with broad QRS complexes and a rate between 100 and 200 beats/min.

Etiology

VT may occasionally be paroxysmal in young patients without other evidence of heart disease, but it occurs most commonly in arteriosclerotic heart disease, coronary artery disease with myocardial ischemia, and digitalis excess. Paroxysmal VT is generally encountered in patients with coronary artery disease complicated by ventricular aneurysm formation. It may also be seen in patients with congestive cardiomyopathies and otherwise healthy patients with mitral valve prolapse. Recently, paroxysmal VT has been found in patients with isolated right ventricular dysplasia.

Mechanism

The mechanism of VT is variable. With digitalis excess it is most likely the result of enhanced automatic activity in the terminal branches of the His-Purkinje system, generally on the left side of the heart. In myocardial ischemia or infarction, it is probably the result of localized reentry within the His-Purkinje system and ventricular myocardium, specifically involving the ischemic or infarcted cells. Recent studies of patients with paroxysmal VT complicating coronary artery disease have shown the arrhythmia to be initiated and sustained by a specific re-entrant circuit utilizing slow conduction within or around an area of ventricular aneurysm formation.

Symptoms and Signs

VT is generally a hemodynamically disastrous rhythm, and critical symptoms at its onset—hypotension, cardiogenic shock, and pulmonary edema—are all common. The patient may or may not be aware of palpitations. The pulse is regular and thready; if A-V dissociation is present, the first heart sound will vary in intensity and cannon A waves may be seen in the neck. The mere fact, however, that a rapid wide QRS tachycardia is hemodynamically well tolerated should not exclude the diagnosis of VT. Some patients with well-preserved ventricular function may be totally asymptomatic although in VT at rates as high as 200/min.

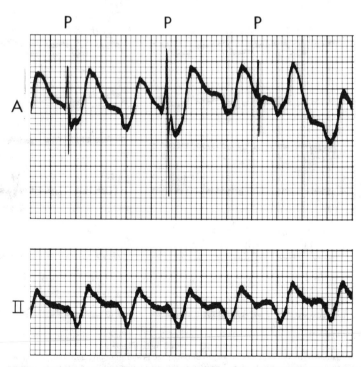

Fig. 25–20. **Ventricular tachycardia—ECG characteristics.** The rapid ventricular response with A-V dissociation establishes the diagnosis. An atrial electrogram (A) and ECG lead II are simultaneously recorded. Although P waves are not apparent in the ECG, the intra-atrial electrogram shows sharp spiking P waves at a regular cycle length considerably slower than those of the QRS complexes, indicating ventricular tachycardia.

Diagnosis

The ECG shows wide, regular QRS complexes whose rate exceeds that of the atrial rhythm (Fig. 25–20). Although ventriculoatrial conduction can occur, most often the atria remain under control of the sinus node and 2/3 of patients in VT demonstrate A-V dissociation. This results in P waves "marching through" the QRS complexes. The ventricular origin is also indicated by the presence of fusion beats (QRS morphology partly resembling the observed tachycardia and the normal) or "capture" (conduction of a dissociated P wave through the A-V node, resulting in both premature and normal ventricular depolarization). Carotid sinus massage has no effect on this tachycardia. Intracardiac electrograms demonstrate that His bundle depolarization does not precede each QRS complex, thereby establishing the more distal ventricular origin of the tachycardia (Fig. 25–21).

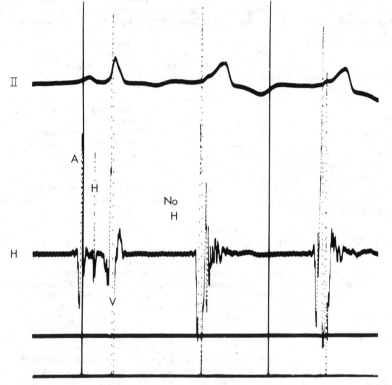

Fig. 25–21.   Ventricular tachycardia. Recorded are ECG lead II and a His bundle electrogram (H). The first beat shows normal A-V conduction with A, H, and V occurring in their usual sequence. This beat is then followed by 2 premature QRS complexes. The His bundle electrogram shows no His bundle depolarization preceding these QRS complexes and thereby demonstrates their origin to be within the distal His-Purkinje system, well below the level of the His bundle.

Treatment

VT is usually a cardiac emergency. In acute myocardial infarction, immediate cardioversion should be undertaken. Lidocaine is the treatment of choice if digitalis excess is a possible cause or if the patient's state of digitalization is unknown. A bolus of lidocaine 50 to 100 mg IV is given over 1 to 2 min. This can be repeated after 3 to 5 min, since its action is so rapid. Additional lidocaine boluses of 50 mg may be given at 5-min intervals until a maximum of 325 to 375 mg is reached or significant CNS side effects are encountered. If lidocaine terminates the tachycardia, a constant infusion of 2 to 4 mg/min is begun. (CAUTION: *Too rapid an IV injection will result in toxic blood levels with auditory aberrations and diffuse muscular twitching, followed by seizures and, possibly, respiratory arrest.*) If the VT is unresponsive to lidocaine, procainamide 100 mg IV should be given q 5 min until either the arrhythmia is suppressed, there is QRS widening, or the patient becomes hypotensive. If procainamide is effective, it should be continued as an IV infusion at 2 to 6 mg/min, then orally, 500 mg to 1 gm q 3 to 6 h.

If the VT is unresponsive to either lidocaine or procainamide, propranolol is given IV 1 mg q 2 to 3 min to a total dose of 3 to 5 mg. Propranolol is *contraindicated* in bronchospastic lung disease, and it frequently causes a further decrease in cardiac output and arterial BP if the VT is not converted.

In VT resulting from digitalis excess, phenytoin 100 mg IV q 5 min is particularly effective. Its efficacy in VT resulting from ischemia or infarction is less clear.

Once the VT has been terminated, further episodes must be prevented by the continued use of a suppressive drug. Lidocaine and procainamide (in that order) are most effective in the presence of acute myocardial infarction; otherwise quinidine or propranolol should be given. Several new classes of antiarrhythmic drugs have recently been advocated for the treatment of paroxysmal VT unresponsive to quinidine, procainamide, or propranolol. Disopyramide phosphate may be effective but its deleterious effect on left ventricular function must be seriously considered. Mexiletine and encainide are currently under investigation.

A totally new slow channel blocking drug, amiodarone, has undergone extensive testing in patients with refractory VT. The agent is given orally and requires 2 to 4 wk before adequate tissue levels are achieved. Its extremely slow elimination allows a once/day dosage regimen and clinical investigations thus far show a drug efficacy far superior to any antiarrhythmic agent previously administered on a long-term basis.

In patients with paroxysmal VT unresponsive to standard or newer antiarrhythmic drugs, serious consideration should be given to electrophysiologic investigation and cardiac surgery to correct their potentially life-threatening arrhythmias. Recent studies have shown that in patients with paroxysmal VT, appropriately timed induced ventricular premature depolarizations will result in the initiation of episodes of VT identical to those occurring spontaneously. Intracardiac electrophysiologic mapping both at the time of cardiac catheterization and heart surgery have shown that most of these patients have a specific re-entrant pathway utilizing ordinary ventricular myocardium and a slow pathway involving the center of periphery of a pre-existent ventricular aneurysm. Thus, as single induced ventricular premature depolarizations may initiate VT, so they may also be used to terminate it. Once the pathway has been mapped, if drug therapy is found to be ineffective, surgical exploration with resection of the ventricular aneurysm and specifically resection of that portion of the endocardial His-Purkinje system involved in the re-entrant pathway responsible for VT will result in complete and permanent abolition of this arrhythmia. It should be noted that blind resection of the area of ventricular aneurysm formation has a < 50% success rate. Thus, careful endo- and epicardial mapping at the time of surgery is essential in order to assure the success of this procedure for the prevention of paroxysmal VT.

VENTRICULAR FIBRILLATION

An irregular and chaotic ventricular arrhythmia with a rapid rate and disorganized spread of impulses throughout the ventricular myocardium. Since electrical activity is chaotic, ventricular systole becomes an uncoordinated event, mechanical activity cannot occur, and cardiac output and BP fall to zero. Heart sounds become inaudible and syncope occurs, followed within minutes by death. **Ventricular fibrillation is a fatal arrhythmia if not immediately terminated** (see also CARDIAC ARREST AND CARDIOPULMONARY RESUSCITATION, below).

Etiology

Acute myocardial infarction is the most common cause. Ventricular fibrillation is likely to occur within minutes and is probably the mechanism in most cases of sudden death. Ventricular fibrillation is occasionally the result of general anesthesia or of overdosage with digitalis, quinidine, or procainamide.

Mechanism

The mechanism of ventricular fibrillation is comparable to that of atrial fibrillation. An initiating ventricular premature beat falling during the refractory period of the ventricular myocardium results in irregular, slow, and chaotic impulse transmission throughout both ventricles. This electrical activity is maintained as multiple reentrant cycles until death supervenes (FIG. 25–22).

Diagnosis

The ECG diagnosis of ventricular fibrillation is easy. All electrical activity is chaotic, and although the QRS complexes may initially be saw-toothed, they diminish in amplitude and increase in frequency until a wandering and erratic baseline is the only evidence of cardiac electrical activity (FIG. 25–22). If ventricular fibrillation is not terminated, electrical activity ceases and the ECG becomes a straight line.

Treatment

Treatment should be primarily directed at prevention, particularly in acute myocardial infarction. Since VPBs herald and initiate this arrhythmia, their suppression will prevent ventricular fibrillation in most patients. Recent studies have clearly demonstrated that the prophylactic use of lidocaine may virtually abolish ventricular fibrillation in acute myocardial infarction. Should ventricular fibrillation develop, *immediate DC defibrillation is the only effective therapy*, and must be followed by an antiarrhythmic regimen designed to prevent further episodes. Lidocaine and procainamide are generally

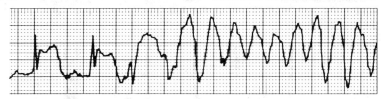

FIG. 25–22. **Ventricular fibrillation.** Two sinus beats in a patient with an acute inferior myocardial infarction are followed by a VPB, which initiates an episode of ventricular fibrillation.

effective. Bretylium tosylate has a mechanism of action unlike other antiarrhythmic drugs and may not only prevent repetitive fibrillation but may, under certain circumstances, chemically defibrillate the patient.

Paroxysmal ventricular fibrillation in the absence of acute myocardial infarction (sudden cardiac death) is now recognized as a specific electrophysiologic entity. Studies where patients have been revived from out-of-hospital sudden cardiac death and ventricular fibrillation show that, although most have coronary artery disease, many have not sustained an acute myocardial infarction. The prognosis of this resuscitated group of patients, however, is extremely poor; the incidence of recurrent sudden cardiac death due to ventricular fibrillation is about 50% within 2 yr. Although not clearly established, it is suggested that all patients resuscitated from out-of-hospital ventricular fibrillation in the absence of myocardial infarction should be placed on some form of antiarrhythmic therapy. Many of these patients demonstrate malignant ventricular ectopic activity on repeated Holter monitoring and, thus, antiarrhythmic drug efficacy can be judged. All patients resuscitated from out-of-hospital sudden cardiac death should undergo extensive investigation of their cardiac anatomy and function; echocardiography, treadmill testing, Holter monitoring, and probably cardiac catheterization with coronary arteriography are indicated. Recent studies again suggest that amiodarone may be the most effective drug thus far used for the prevention of paroxysmal ventricular fibrillation and recurrent sudden cardiac death.

HEART BLOCK

Conditions in which the spread of cardiac electrical excitation is slowed or interrupted in a portion of the normal conduction pathway.

SINOATRIAL (S-A) BLOCK

Impulse transmission is physiologically very slow in S-A node tissues because many cells within the node undergo spontaneous diastolic depolarization, and each successive cell is activated at a low resting membrane potential. Estimates of normal S-A conduction range from 40 to 120 msec. This normally slow conduction may become pathologically slowed even more by disease, and S-A block results.

Impulses originating within pacemaker cells of the S-A node are initiated by normal Phase IV diastolic depolarization, but the impulse is prevented from leaving the area of the sinus node and exciting surrounding atrial myocardium. Thus deprived of their primary pacemaker, the atria and ventricles fail to contract unless a subsidiary pacemaker arises elsewhere within the cardiac conduction system. Subsidiary pacemakers, generally located within the bundle of His or atrial specialized conduction system, have an intrinsically slower rate of impulse generation. Depending on the degree of S-A block, either an escape beat or an escape rhythm results.

Various forms of S-A block may occur.

Sinoatrial Wenckebach periods: During regular sinus rhythm, impulses emerging from the S-A node may demonstrate progressive conduction delay until one is finally blocked. Since depolarization of the S-A node is not recorded by the ECG, this form of S-A block appears as progressive shortening of the P-P interval until finally one P wave is "dropped." 5:4, 4:3, and 3:2 Wenckebach periods may be recognized on ECG.

2:1 Sinoatrial block: The sinus node is firing at a regular rate; suddenly, alternate impulses fail to emerge from the sinus node to excite the atrial myocardium. This results in a sudden slowing of the P wave rate, with a cycle length during the slow rhythm that is exactly twice that of normal sinus rhythm (FIG. 25–23). The P wave morphology must remain the same and sinus arrhythmia is minimal.

Higher degrees of S-A block: Impulses emerging from the sinus node may also be blocked with a 3:1, 4:1, or 5:1 periodicity. This would result in atrial cycles three, four, and five times the length of the basic sinus rhythm.

Complete S-A block (sinus arrest): During normal sinus rhythm, P waves may suddenly stop. This condition, previously known as "sinus arrest," is much more likely to be the result of complete S-A block. Cardiac arrest will follow unless a subsidiary pacemaker (escape rhythm) develops.

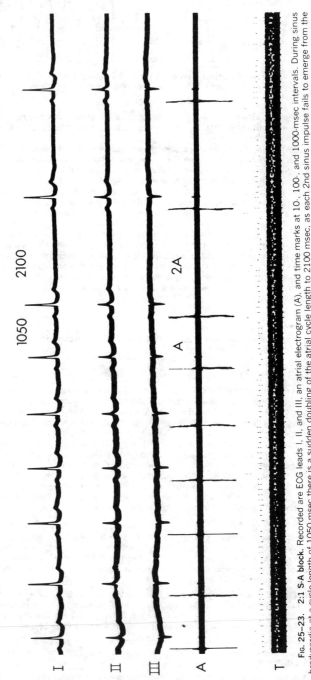

Fig. 25–23. 2:1 S-A block. Recorded are ECG leads I, II, and III, an atrial electrogram (A), and time marks at 10-, 100-, and 1000-msec intervals. During sinus bradycardia at a cycle length of 1050 msec there is a sudden doubling of the atrial cycle length to 2100 msec, as each 2nd sinus impulse fails to emerge from the sinus node.

Etiology

S-A block may occur in arteriosclerotic and chronic rheumatic heart disease, but is most common in patients with coronary artery disease. Sinoatrial Wenckebach periods and 2:1 S-A block are commonly the result of vagotonia or digitalis excess. The combination of digitalis and quinidine frequently gives rise to sinus node dysfunction. Hyperkalemia rarely results in S-A block, but may cause **sinoventricular rhythm**—a progressive diminution of P wave amplitude until the P waves disappear, despite the fact that pacemaker function remains within the sinus node.

Symptoms, Signs, and Diagnosis

S-A block is apt to be an intermittent event in elderly patients. S-A Wenckebach periods and 2:1 S-A block seldom cause symptoms, but higher degrees of S-A block may prolong cardiac asystole enough to diminish cerebral perfusion and cause dizziness, near-syncope, or, rarely, syncope and convulsions. Physical examination may reveal the rhythm change characteristic of each type of block, and the ECG shows the absence of P waves in a characteristic pattern. A normal jugular venous pulse is preserved. Paroxysmal S-A block may be an exasperatingly difficult diagnosis to establish. Most patients are elderly and complain of infrequent paroxysms of lightheadedness or near syncope. Frequently, prolonged in-hospital monitoring or repeated Holter monitors are required before a symptomatic period accompanied by S-A block is demonstrated.

Prognosis and Therapy

The prognosis of S-A block depends on its cause, frequency, and the duration of the asystolic periods. Elderly patients with S-A block tend to have increasingly frequent symptomatic periods. Neither atropine, ephedrine, nor isoproterenol therapy is successful in patients with symptomatic S-A block. Permanent demand pacemaker implantation is the treatment of choice. The site of implantation (atrial, ventricular, or bifocal) depends on the physiologic state in the remainder of the A-V conduction system. If the P-R interval and QRS duration are normal, a permanent atrial pacemaker is the preferred therapy.

INTRA–ATRIAL BLOCK

Slowed conduction of the propagating cardiac impulse through the atrial myocardium. Intra-atrial block is generally the result of atrial myocardial disease, either secondary to rheumatic or coronary artery disease, or the result of infiltrative primary myocardial diseases.

Diagnosis is made by finding broad P waves lasting 120 msec or more on the ECG. They are frequently notched and may be of low amplitude. Intra-atrial block is, in itself, asymptomatic and **therapy** is not required. Patients with intra-atrial block and slowed atrial conduction, however, are frequently prone to the subsequent development of atrial arrhythmias such as flutter and fibrillation.

ATRIOVENTRICULAR (A-V) BLOCK (A-V Nodal Block)

Prolonged or blocked impulse propagation from atrial to ventricular myocardium, resulting from abnormal conduction across the A-V node.

Etiology

A-V nodal block is usually the result of A-V nodal ischemia secondary to acute inferior myocardial infarction, digitalis toxicity, vagal stimulation (e.g., from carotid sinus hypersensitivity or parasympathomimetic drugs), or primary A-V nodal disease. It also may occur in acute rheumatic fever and congenitally.

Mechanism and Diagnosis

A-V nodal block may be incomplete, intermittent, or complete. In **incomplete A-V nodal block** (prolonged A-V nodal conduction), the transmission of impulses across the A-V node is prolonged, but 1:1 conduction is still present (FIG. 25–24a). The conduction delay is seen on ECG as a prolongation of the P-R interval beyond 200 msec. The contours of the P waves and QRS complexes remain normal. As the degree of block increases, A-V conduction time is prolonged until some P waves fail to reach the bundle of His and ventricular myocardium, resulting in intermittent A-V conduction. **Intermittent A-V nodal block** characteristically takes the form of **Wenckebach periodicity**. The P-R interval progressively lengthens until finally one P wave fails to result in a QRS complex. The cycle then repeats. A-V nodal Wenckebach periods are generally 3:2, 4:3, or 5:4 cycles, according to the number of impulses which precede the "dropped" beat. Other forms of intermittent A-V nodal conduction may also occur. Impulses may block within the A-V node in a pattern of 2:1, 3:1, or even 4:1 A-V block (FIG. 25–24b). In these higher degrees of A-V nodal block, the P waves are normal, and every second, third, or fourth wave is followed by a QRS complex of *normal* contour with a constant P-R interval.

As A-V nodal conduction becomes more abnormal, **complete A-V nodal block** may occur. In this condition, none of the P waves seen on the ECG results in QRS complexes. The ventricles are controlled by a subsidiary pacemaker (escape focus), most often from the bundle of His. As a result, the P waves are entirely dissociated from the QRS complexes, and the form of the QRS complexes remains identical to that seen before block occurred. This point is important in differentiating com-

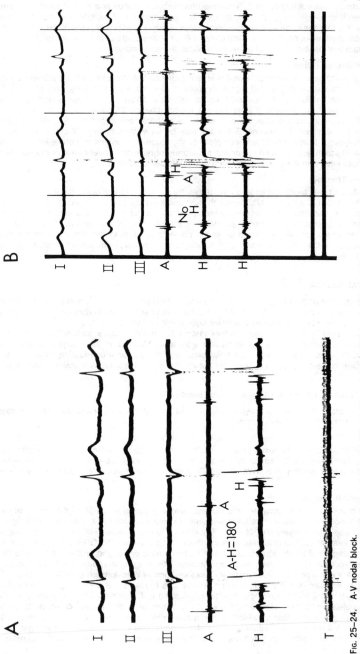

Fig. 25-24. A-V nodal block.

A. Prolonged A-V nodal conduction (first degree A-V block). Recorded are ECG leads I, II, and III, an atrial electrogram (A), a His bundle electrogram (H), and time marks at 10- and 100-msec intervals. The P-R interval is prolonged because conduction from atrium to the His bundle (A-H interval) is abnormally long (180 msec). P-R interval prolongation generally results from A-V nodal conduction delay.

B. 2:1 A-V nodal conduction. Every 2nd atrial depolarization of sinus origin fails to traverse the A-V node and excite the His bundle, resulting in 2:1 A-V block within the A-V node.

plete A-V nodal from infranodal block. The escape focus within the bundle of His generally fires at a rate of 40 to 70 beats/min. Thus, complete A-V nodal block is only moderately symptomatic.

Symptoms and Signs

Incomplete and intermittent A-V nodal blocks usually are without symptoms. The patient may recognize complete A-V nodal block as a slower heart beat accompanied by weakness or fatigue. Syncope is rare, but may occur when the rate of the subsidiary pacemaker is extremely slow. Complete A-V block may be recognized on physical examination by the varying intensity of the first heart sound and the lack of correlation between jugular venous pulsations and carotid pulses. This results in characteristic cannon A waves when a P wave is superimposed upon a QRS complex and atrial and ventricular mechanical systole occur simultaneously.

Therapy

A-V nodal block of any type is rarely permanent. When it is the result of inferior myocardial infarction, it almost always disappears within 72 h after onset. Therapy (atropine, or the implantation of a temporary cardiac pacemaker) is required only if the patient is symptomatic. A-V nodal block resulting from digitalis intoxication is best treated by withholding the drug. Although potassium or phenytoin may decrease the block, these drugs should be avoided in complete A-V nodal block caused by digitalis excess because they may slow the subsidiary pacemakers and thus increase rather than diminish symptoms. However, atropine or isoproterenol, even if they do not reverse the A-V nodal block, will speed the His bundle pacemaker and improve cardiac output. Permanent cardiac pacemakers are almost never required in patients with A-V nodal block, as the condition producing it is generally transient.

INFRANODAL A-V BLOCK

A type of A-V block in which impulses traverse the A-V node normally, but are blocked within the ventricular specialized conduction system; that is, within the bundle of His or all three fascicles of the cardiac conduction system.

Etiology

Infranodal A-V block is the result of either arteriosclerotic coronary artery disease, intrinsic degeneration of the ventricular conduction system, or infiltrative diseases such as amyloid, syphilis, or tumor. The ventricular conduction system may also be damaged by the deposition of calcium in the anulus of the aortic or mitral valves. Acute myocardial infarction with occlusion of the left anterior descending coronary artery proximal to its first septal perforating branch may result in ischemia or infarction of the proximal ventricular specialized conducting system and the development of complete infranodal A-V block.

Mechanism

Impulses traversing a normal A-V node find an infranodal conduction system in which all three fascicles (right bundle, and anterior and posterior divisions of the left bundle branch) are abnormal. During periods of conduction, which is generally 1:1, patients usually demonstrate block in one or more branches of the fascicles; i.e., **bundle branch block (BBB)**. Suddenly, and without apparent cause, conduction fails in all three fascicles (complete infranodal A-V block), either as an isolated event or over a series of successive beats. A subsidiary pacemaker must take over cardiac excitation or cardiac arrest and death will result. Since the impulses are blocked within the fascicles, this pacemaker is distal in the His-Purkinje system and its rate is extremely slow. The inciting cause for the sudden loss of conduction, and its equally sudden resumption, is presently unknown.

Symptoms and Signs

Infranodal A-V block is most common in elderly patients and results in syncope which, when of this etiology, is referred to as a **Stokes–Adams attack**. Episodes are unheralded and short-lived, but tend to increase in frequency. The pulse is usually between 20 and 50 beats/min. Cannon A waves may also be recognized in the jugular venous pulse. Only an ECG can distinguish nodal from infranodal A-V block, but the presence of syncope suggests that it is infranodal.

Diagnosis

The ECG almost always shows intraventricular conduction disturbances during sinus rhythm. During periods of 1:1 conduction, one may find right bundle branch block plus left anterior hemiblock, right bundle branch block plus left posterior hemiblock, or left bundle branch block. Left bundle branch block with a superiorly oriented mean frontal plane axis is a commoner precursor of complete A-V block than previously recognized. The P-R interval is generally normal. During the period of complete infranodal A-V block, P wave morphology is normal (Fig. 25–25). QRS complexes are wide and bizarre, with a rate between 20 and 50 beats/min, and (in contrast to those of complete A-V nodal block) are entirely different from those observed during conducted rhythm. The wide QRS complexes and their very slow rate prove that the block is infranodal. Intracardiac ECGs show that each P wave propagates across the A-V node and activates the bundle of His, but is blocked distally to it (Fig. 25–26).

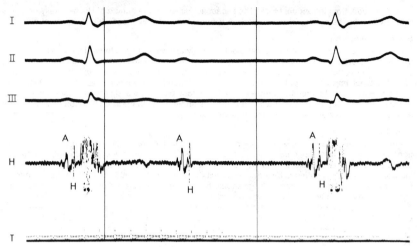

FIG. 25–25.   **2:1 Infranodal A-V block with right bundle branch block (RBBB).** Recorded are ECG leads I, II, and III, a His bundle electrogram (H), and time marks at 10- and 100-msec intervals. The ECG demonstrates RBBB on the conducted beats. Each atrial depolarization (A) is followed by depolarization of the His bundle (H), but alternate His bundle depolarizations fail to excite the ventricular muscle.

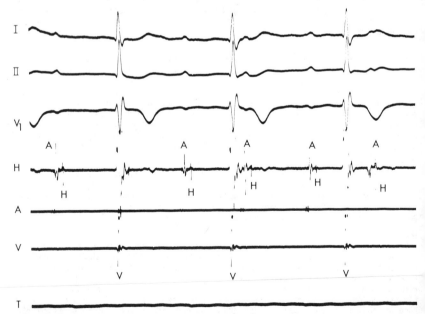

FIG. 25–26.   **Complete infranodal A-V block.** Recorded are ECG leads I, II, and V₁, a His bundle electrogram (H), atrial electrogram (A), ventricular electrogram (V), and time marks (T). Each atrial beat of sinus origin (A) is followed by depolarization of the His bundle but conduction proceeds no further, and QRS complexes are the result of an independent idioventricular pacemaker.

Therapy

Implantation of a permanent right ventricular endocardial demand pacemaker is the only therapy for intermittent complete infranodal A-V block. These have markedly reduced the former mortality rate of almost 50% over 2 yr in patients with true Stokes-Adams seizures. In the emergency situation, if the patient has lost consciousness and has a slow heart rate, the subsidiary focus may be speeded up by isoproterenol 1 to 3 μg/min IV. Atropine is probably ineffective. Even in an emergency, implanting a temporary demand pacemaker is preferable to the use of sympathomimetic drugs. Transvenous percutaneous temporary pacemaker insertion via the subclavian vein is optimal; transthoracic pacemaker insertion has only rarely been effective.

INTRAVENTRICULAR (IV) BLOCK (Intraventricular Conduction Defect; IVCD)

This includes the various bundle branch or fascicular blocks as well as other forms of intraventricular conduction defects (IVCDs).

Bundle Branch Block (BBB)

The cardiac impulse originating in the sinus node follows a normal pathway until it reaches the trifurcation of the common bundle of His. At this juncture, impulse propagation in one or more of the three fascicles is slowed or interrupted, resulting in a characteristic appearance of the QRS complex on the ECG, according to whether the block is **right bundle branch block (RBBB), left bundle branch block (LBBB),** or **left anterior and posterior divisional block.**

Etiology

IVCDs may occur in arteriosclerotic, rheumatic, and, occasionally, congenital heart disease; in all forms of myocarditis; transiently during myocardial infarction; or as a result of primary or metastatic cardiac tumors or any other myocardial infiltrative process. The commonest cause of IVCDs is intrinsic degeneration of the ventricular specialized conduction system with or without other associated forms of heart disease. RBBB may also occur in individuals with no other evidence of cardiac disease. LBBB tends to occur in patients with left ventricular disease, most often in patients with hypertension, arteriosclerotic cardiovascular disease, or cardiomyopathy. RBBB plus left anterior hemiblock may occur in patients with idiopathic degeneration of the ventricular specialized conduction system, or more frequently as the result of coronary artery disease with anteroseptal myocardial infarction. Left posterior hemiblock is generally the result of intrinsic degeneration of the conduction system or infiltrative cardiomyopathy. Hyperkalemia or quinidine or procainamide excess may prolong the QRS duration but rarely causes characteristic BBB.

Symptoms and Signs

Patients with IVCD are asymptomatic, unless their disease has progressed enough to cause periods of complete infranodal A-V block (see above). The commonest sign of RBBB on physical examination is wide splitting of the second sound which moves but never closes with expiration. In LBBB a paradoxic splitting of the second sound may be heard.

Mechanism and Diagnosis

An IVCD is readily diagnosed by ECG: it exists (by definition) if the QRS duration is >100 msec. In **RBBB,** because the right bundle impulse is conducted slowly or not at all, right ventricular activation occurs by muscle-to-muscle spread of the cardiac impulse. Since myocardial excitation is slower than excitation via the His-Purkinje system, right ventricular activation is delayed (causing delayed and slowed terminal forces on the ECG) and is dissynchronous with left ventricular activation. Characteristically, there is a large S wave in leads I and V_6 and an RR' is present in V_1 and V_2. Vectorially, in the frontal plane terminal forces are slowed and directed rightward, resulting in broad S waves in ECG leads I, aVL, V_6, and X. In the transverse plane, this delayed activation is seen anteriorly, corresponding anatomically to the right ventricle (FIG. 25–27). An rR' is seen in ECG leads V_1, V_2, and Z.

The **left bundle** is responsible for the programmed activation of the ventricular septum and the body of the left ventricle. Most authorities now agree that ventricular septal activation occurs primarily via branches of the left posterior division, and that the left anterior division activates the anterior left ventricular papillary muscle, the left ventricular outflow tract, and the base of the heart.

Several types of LBBB (formerly considered a single entity) are now recognized. FIG. 25–28 demonstrates **classic LBBB.** The posterior division of the left bundle branch is so abnormal that it fails to result in normal septal activation. The interventricular septum is therefore activated from right to left and the septal Q waves generally seen in leads I, aVL, and V_6 (X on the vector) are no longer inscribed. In addition, overall left ventricular activation is delayed and characteristic mid to terminal QRS notching is seen in these same leads. The normal mean QRS axis in the frontal plane (lying between +90 degrees and −30 degrees) is maintained because the left anterior division, although very diseased, still results in late activation of the anterior papillary muscle and base of the left ventricle. In most patients with LBBB, conduction within the right bundle is also delayed; although it is not as abnormal as conduction in the left bundle, it can prolong the H-V interval, as seen on the His bundle electrogram in FIG. 25–28.

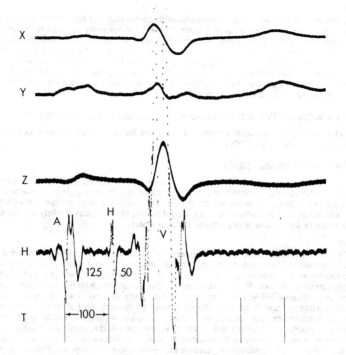

FIG. 25-27.   **Right bundle branch block (RBBB).**   Recorded are orthogonal vectorial leads X, Y, and Z (Frank system), a His bundle electrogram (H), and time marks at 100-msec intervals. Terminal rightward and anterior QRS slowing is shown, along with a normal H-V interval indicating that the remainder of the intraventricular conducting system is normal.

When conduction fails within the anterior as well as the posterior division of the left bundle branch (FIG. 25-29), ventricular activation occurs solely via the right bundle branch. This situation (akin to that seen with pacemakers implanted within the right ventricular apex) results in a superiorly directed QRS complex in the frontal plane. A QRS axis superiorly directed more than −45 degrees should suggest that both fascicles of the left bundle are no longer conducting.

When only the anterior fascicle of the left bundle fails to conduct, a characteristic ECG pattern referred to as **left anterior hemiblock (LAH)** results (FIG. 25-30). Ventricular septal activation is normal, as is depolarization of the right ventricle. Since the anterobasal portions of the left ventricle are activated by muscle-to-muscle excitation, their depolarization is delayed. QRS complexes are minimally widened (90 to 110 msec), but the mean QRS axis in the frontal plane is shifted superiorly and large S waves appear in the inferiorly directed ECG leads (II, III, aVF, and Y). Recently a form of incomplete LBBB has been described wherein only those portions of the left bundle responsible for septal activation fail to conduct. Only minimal QRS prolongation results but septal activation now proceeds from right to left and normal septal Q waves seen in I, L, and V_6 are lost. The H-V interval is prolonged since septal activation now occurs via the right bundle.

Although LBBB can result from disease of all three fascicles of the interventricular conducting system, more typically a bifascicular block is seen; i.e., RBBB combined with block in either the anterior-superior or posterior-inferior division of the left bundle branch. **RBBB with LAH** results in the combined ECG features of both (FIG. 25-31). The delayed right ventricular activation produces the typical large S waves seen in ECG leads I, aVL, V_6, and X, while the associated LAH shifts the mean QRS axis superiorly in the frontal plane, resulting in large S waves in the inferior ECG leads II, III, aVF, and Y. In almost two thirds of patients with RBBB plus LAH, trifascicular conduction system disease is present and can be detected by characteristic H-V interval prolongation on the His bundle electrogram. Subsequent paroxysmal complete infranodal A-V block is highly likely.

In **RBBB combined with left posterior hemiblock—RBBB with LPH**—a failure of conduction within the posterior division of the left bundle branch (FIG. 25-32a), all the characteristic features of RBBB are present but the terminal rightward vector is even more exaggerated; i.e., the terminal S waves in

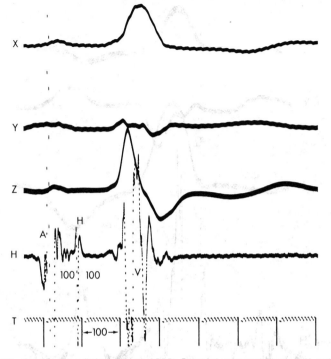

FIG. 25-28. Classic left bundle branch block (LBBB). Recorded are vectorial leads X, Y, and Z (Frank system), a His bundle electrogram (H), and time marks at 100-msec intervals. The typical mid to late leftward QRS slowing is seen in lead X. The normal mean QRS axis in the frontal plane (Y) and the prolonged H-V interval (100 msec) are characteristic in this form of LBBB, reflecting trifascicular conducting system disease.

leads I, aVL, V_6, and X are even deeper. In this condition ventricular activation is occurring solely via the anterior division of the left bundle branch; virtually all of the ventricular myocardium is being activated from left to right except the anterobasal portion of the left ventricle. The initial septal vector X (usually reflected by a small Q wave in leads I, aVL, and V_6) is lost. An initial Q wave seen in the inferiorly directed ECG leads (Y) may reflect a reversal of septal depolarization or, more likely, indicate that initial ventricular activation at the termination of the left anterior division is proceeding in a superior direction. Since the base of the left ventricle is activated first, the major QRS vector is inscribed in an inferior direction. This results in a characteristic open and inferiorly inscribed vector loop in the frontal plane (FIG. 25-32b), which results from the muscle-to-muscle spread of electrical activity first to the apex of the left and then the right ventricle.

   Nonspecific IVCDs are said to be present when the total QRS duration exceeds 100 msec and none of the criteria of classic BBB are met.

Prognosis and Treatment

   Although the prognosis of any BBB is primarily that of the cardiac disease underlying it, the presence of disease in two of the three fascicles of the ventricular conduction system predisposes to the development of intermittent complete infranodal A-V block and Stokes-Adams attacks. No specific therapy is indicated for IVCDs and the incidence with which these progress to complete infranodal IV block is only 2 to 3% per year.

VENTRICULAR PREEXCITATION

   Wolff-Parkinson-White (WPW) syndrome: *A form of accelerated A-V conduction, resulting from the existence of two A-V conduction pathways.* Conduction proceeds down the normal A-V nodal His-Purkinje pathway, but the ventricles are preexcited by an anomalous A-V connection between the atria and one of the ventricular muscle masses. Because two conduction pathways exist, QRS complexes really represent fusion complexes. The initial activation, being the result of muscle-to-

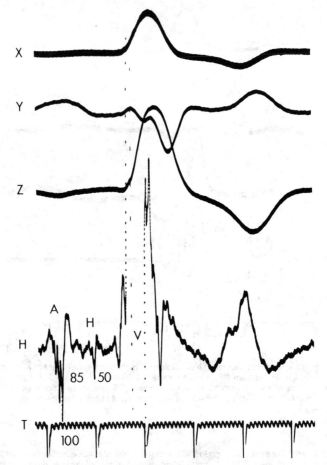

FIG. 25–29. **Left bundle branch block (LBBB) with a leftward mean QRS axis.** Recorded are vectorial leads X, Y, and Z (Frank system), a His bundle electrogram (H), and time marks at 100-msec intervals. The mean QRS axis in the frontal plane is terminally directed superiorly, resulting in a large S wave in lead Y. The H-V interval of 50 msec seen in this patient is the exception rather than the rule.

muscle spread, is slow, and results in a characteristic and pathognomonic delta wave at the onset of the QRS complex (FIG. 25–33a). The P-R interval is usually short (FIG. 25–33b). Although previously divided into Type A and B, electrophysiologic studies in the cardiac catheterization laboratory and at the time of open heart surgery have disclosed that accessory A-V corrections may occur anywhere around the fibrous rings of both mitral and tricuspid valves. The vector of the initial ventricular pre-excitation or delta wave is determined by the site of the bypass tract. The P-R interval is a function of the relative conduction velocity down the normal as opposed to the pre-excitation path.

Lown-Ganong-Levine (LGL) syndrome: *Ventricular preexcitation in which part or all of the normal A-V nodal conduction system is bypassed by an anomalous A-V connection between atrial muscle and the bundle of His.* This results in a short P-R interval and normal QRS complexes (FIG. 25–34a).

Symptoms, Signs, and Diagnosis

The ECG is diagnostic in both of these conditions. In ventricular pre-excitation of the WPW variety, the P-R interval is short and initial ventricular activation slowed resulting in a characteristic delta wave (FIG. 25–33). In partial A-V nodal bypass of the LGL type, the P-R interval is short but QRS duration is normal as is the initial ventricular activation sequence. They are entirely without symptoms and signs unless accompanied by paroxysmal atrial arrhythmias. A reentrant type of supraven-

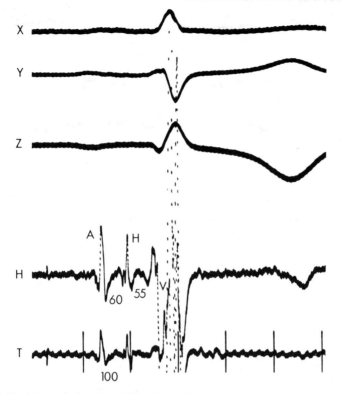

Fig. 25–30.   Left anterior hemiblock (LAH).   Recorded are vectorial leads X, Y, and Z (Frank system), a His bundle electrogram (H), and time marks at 100-msec intervals. Note the relatively normal QRS duration of 90 msec. The fact that the superiorly directed mean QRS axis in the frontal plane is more negative than -30 degrees is diagnostic. The slightly prolonged H-V interval (55 msec) may reflect minimal conduction delay in the left posterior division as well.

tricular tachycardia (SVT) is common. In this re-entrant arrhythmia, the initiating APB finds the accessory pathway refractory and conducts slowly down the normal A-V nodal conduction system. Having excited ventricular myocardium, the bypass tract has recovered excitability and is capable of conducting the impulse retrogradely to the atrium. The cycle is continued as an episode of SVT. It should be noted that because antegrade conduction proceeds down the normal A-V pathway, the delta wave is lost during episodes of SVT. Both atrial flutter and fibrillation occur in patients with both WPW and LGL syndromes. The symptoms and signs associated with these tachycardias may be severe in patients with anomalous A-V conduction (Fig. 25–34b). It has been recently recognized that the presence of an anomalous, rapidly conducting bypass tract may have dire consequences in the presence of atrial flutter or fibrillation. Extremely rapid ventricular rates (200 to 300/min) have resulted in ventricular fibrillation and sudden death.

Therapy

Therapy is directed at the prevention of episodes of SVT. Quinidine sulfate 200 to 400 mg orally t.i.d. or q.i.d. is most useful; procainamide and propranolol may also be used. Amiodarone and verapamil have been used to depress conduction in the bypass tract. Pacemaker therapy and surgical interruption of the anomalous pathways have been used with some success in patients with refractory and debilitating recurrent SVT. Surgical interruption of the bypass tract should be seriously considered when atrial fibrillation with extremely rapid ventricular responses is encountered.

MYOCARDIAL ISCHEMIC DISORDERS

CORONARY ARTERY DISEASE (CAD)

Most CAD is due to the subintimal deposition of atheromas in the large and medium-sized arteries serving the heart. Risk factors and the pathogenesis of atherosclerotic lesions and CAD are dis-

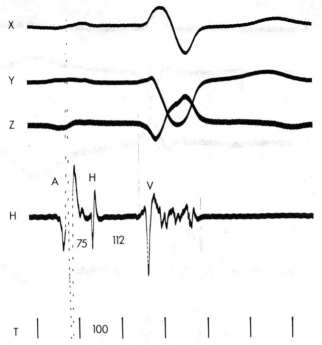

Fig. 25–31.   **Right bundle branch block (RBBB) plus left anterior hemiblock (LAH).** Recorded are vecto-rial leads X, Y, and Z (Frank system), a His bundle electrogram (H), and time marks at 100-msec intervals. The ECG features of both RBBB and LAH are combined. As in two thirds of cases, conduction in the left posterior division is also prolonged, giving rise to significant H-V interval prolongation (112 msec).

cussed under ARTERIOSCLEROSIS; ATHEROSCLEROSIS in Ch. 24. The process is characteristically insidi-ous in onset, often irregularly distributed in different vessels, and capable of abruptly interfering with blood flow to segments of the myocardium. The major complications of CAD are angina pectoris, myocardial infarction **(MI)**, and sudden cardiac death. Acute MI causes 35% of deaths in men be-tween ages 35 and 50 in the USA.

ANGINA PECTORIS

A clinical syndrome due to myocardial ischemia characterized by episodes of precordial discom-fort or pressure, typically precipitated by exertion and relieved by rest or sublingual nitroglycerin.

Etiology and Pathogenesis

Angina pectoris occurs when cardiac work and myocardial O_2 demand exceed the ability of the coronary arterial system to supply O_2. The pain of angina pectoris is believed to be a direct manifes-tation of myocardial ischemia. Presumably the accumulation of hypoxic metabolites during ischemia stimulates the sensory nerves encircling the heart, producing the deep visceral sensation of angina. Normally, myocardial metabolism is entirely aerobic, there being little capacity to maintain anaerobic metabolism. Objective proof of myocardial ischemia, seldom available clinically, would be a demon-stration of myocardial lactate production by sampling the coronary sinus during angina or stress. As the myocardium becomes ischemic, coronary sinus blood pH falls, cellular potassium loss occurs, lactate production replaces utilization, ECG abnormalities appear, and ventricular performance dete-riorates. Left ventricular diastolic pressure frequently rises during angina, at times to levels inducing pulmonary congestion and dyspnea.

The major determinants of myocardial O_2 consumption are heart rate, systolic tension or arterial pressure, and contractility. Any increase in these factors in a setting of reduced coronary blood flow may induce angina. During spontaneous angina the subjective awareness of pain is usually pre-ceded by modest increases in heart rate and a rise in BP that may at times be marked. If the angina is not relieved by medication, these changes represent a potentially disastrous positive biofeedback system: the higher the BP and the faster the heart rate, the greater the unmet myocardial O_2 need.

Patients with angina who succumb almost invariably have extensive coronary atherosclerosis and patchy myocardial fibrosis. Evidence of old MI may be present. Underlying disease other than athero-

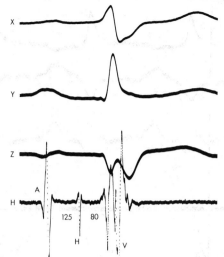

A. Recorded are vectorial leads X, Y, and Z (Frank system) and a His bundle electrogram (H). A deep S wave is inscribed in lead X, and the typical RR' pattern is seen in Z. The mean frontal plane QRS axis is shifted inferiorly (large R wave in Y) and an initial Q wave is seen in this inferiorly directed lead. The prolonged H-V interval (80 msec) indicates that disease exists within the anterior division of the left bundle branch as well, and that this patient has trifascicular conduction system disease.

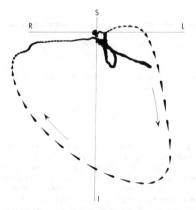

B. The frontal plane vector is shown, resulting from the display of leads X and Y in part A, above. The clockwise QRS loop shows the initial superior forces that result in the Q waves characteristically seen in the inferiorly directed ECG leads II, III, aVF, and Y. Thereafter, the loop moves rapidly inferiorly and then to the right. Terminal right-sided conduction delay is the result of the associated RBBB.

Fig. 25–32. **Right bundle branch block (RBBB) and left posterior hemiblock (LPH).**

sclerosis, such as calcific aortic stenosis, aortic insufficiency, syphilitic aortitis with coronary ostial constriction, and hypertrophic subaortic stenosis, may occasionally be present, either alone or coexisting with CAD. In these conditions either the coronary ostia are obstructed or myocardial work is markedly increased or both. An occasional patient with fatal MI is found to have essentially normal coronary arteries. Either coronary embolus or spasm may be postulated as causative (see below).

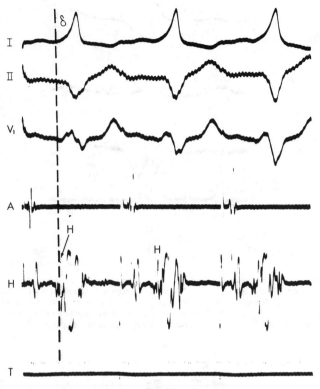

Fig. 25-33. Wolff-Parkinson-White syndrome (WPW).
A. Recorded are ECG leads I, II, and V₁, an atrial electrogram (A), a His bundle electrogram (H), and time marks at 10- and 100-msec intervals. Depolarization of the His bundle (H) occurs during inscription of the characteristic delta wave (δ). The QRS morphology represents the result of ventricular excitation via two independent pathways.

Symptoms and Signs

The discomfort of angina pectoris, highly variable, is most commonly felt beneath the sternum. It may be a vague, barely troublesome ache, or it may rapidly become a severe, intense precordial crushing sensation. Pain may radiate to the left shoulder and down the inside of the left arm, even to the fingers. It may radiate straight through to the back, into the throat, the jaws, the teeth, and occasionally even down the right arm. Anginal discomfort may be felt in the upper or lower abdomen. Since it is seldom felt in the region of the cardiac apex, the patient who points to that precise area or describes fleeting, sharp, or hot sensations usually does not have angina.

Angina pectoris is characteristically triggered by physical activity and usually persists no more than a few minutes, subsiding with rest. The response to exertion is usually predictable, but in some patients a given exercise may be tolerated one day and may precipitate angina the next. Angina is worsened when the exertion follows a meal. It is also exaggerated in cold weather, so that exertion without symptoms in the summer may induce angina in the winter. Walking into the wind or first contact with cold air on leaving a warm room may also precipitate an attack. Angina may occur at night **(nocturnal angina)** or when the patient is resting quietly and seemingly without stimulation **(angina decubitus).** Nocturnal angina is frequently preceded by a dream that may be accompanied by striking changes in respiration, pulse rate, and BP.

Attacks may vary in frequency from several/day to occasional seizures separated by symptom-free intervals of weeks, months, or years. They may increase in frequency to a fatal outcome or may gradually decrease or disappear if an adequate collateral coronary circulation develops, if the ischemic area becomes infarcted, or if congestive heart failure supervenes.

Since the characteristics of angina are usually constant for a given individual, any change in the pattern of angina—increased intensity of attacks, decreased threshold of stimulus, longer duration, or occurrence when the patient is sedentary or awakening from sleep—should be viewed as a

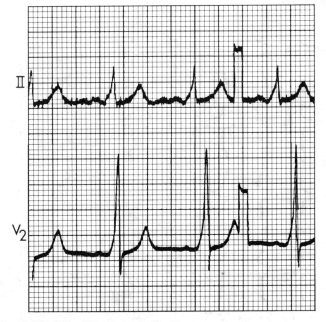

FIG. 25-33. **Wolff-Parkinson-White syndrome.** (*Cont'd*)
B. ECG leads II and V_2 are shown. The shortened P-R interval and characteristic initial slow ventricular depolarization result from preexcitation of the venctricles via the anomalous A-V conduction pathway.

serious increase in symptoms. Such changes are termed **unstable angina pectoris, acute coronary insufficiency, preinfarction angina,** or the **intermediate syndrome.** Unstable angina is the preferred term because it implies less judgment about prognosis. Unstable angina may be prodromal to acute MI; sudden death is less common. Prospective studies suggest that about 30% of patients with unstable angina will suffer an MI within 3 mo of onset.

Variant angina (Prinzmetal's angina) is characterized by pain *at rest* and by S-T segment elevation, not depression, during the attack. Between episodes, the ECG may be normal or may present a stable control pattern. Arrhythmia is not uncommon and the attacks tend to occur with regularity at certain times of the day. Recent observations during coronary arteriography confirm Prinzmetal's original suggestion that in many patients this form of angina is secondary to large vessel spasm. Injection of ergonovine IV has been used as a provocative test to induce spasm, but because of possible hazard should be done only in an experienced angiographic laboratory. Relief is usually prompt after sublingual nitroglycerin. Prognosis is variable. Newer vasodilators that act to block slow calcium movement such as verapamil and nifedipine appear to be highly effective.

Physical findings: Between attacks, and even during attacks, patients with angina pectoris may not have signs of organic heart disease. However, during the attack the heart rate usually rises, BP is frequently elevated, heart sounds become more distant, and the apical impulse is more diffuse. Palpation of the precordium may reveal a localized systolic bulging or paradoxic movement reflecting segmental myocardial ischemia in noncontracting myocardium. The 2nd heart sound may become paradoxic due to more prolonged left ventricular ejection during the ischemic episode. A 4th heart sound is common. In some individuals, a mid or late systolic apical murmur, rather shrill but not especially loud, may be heard. This murmur has been ascribed to localized papillary muscle dysfunction secondary to the ischemia.

Electrocardiogram: Recording an ECG continuously during an attack of chest pain thought to be angina is most helpful in evaluating the cause of the pain. A wide variety of changes may appear: characteristic S-T segment depression, hyperacute S-T segment elevation, decrease in R wave height, intraventricular or bundle branch conduction disturbances, and arrhythmia (usually ventricular extrasystoles). However, the ECG between episodes is entirely normal in about 30% of patients with a typical history of angina pectoris. In general, neither the extent nor the distribution of CAD can be predicted from the ECG. An abnormal resting ECG alone does not establish or refute the diagnosis of angina pectoris, which must be recognized from characteristic symptoms.

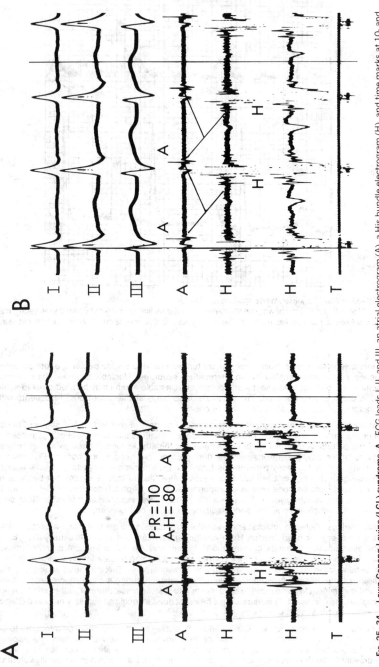

Fig. 25-34. Lown-Ganong-Levine (LGL) syndrome. A. ECG leads I, II, and III, an atrial electrogram (A), a His bundle electrogram (H), and time marks at 10- and 100-msec intervals are shown during *normal sinus rhythm*. The shortened P-R interval of 110 msec is a function of the short A-V nodal conduction time (A-H interval, 80 msec). B. Despite the short P-R interval during sinus rhythm, prolonged A-V nodal conduction (a long A-H interval) is responsible for the sustained reentrant tachycardia during *supraventricular tachycardia*.

Diagnosis

Angina pectoris is a *clinical diagnosis* which is based on a characteristic complaint of chest discomfort brought on by exertion and relieved by rest. Confirmation may be obtained by observing ischemic ECG changes during a spontaneous attack or by a test dose of sublingual nitroglycerin, which characteristically relieves angina pectoris within 1½ to 5 min. Failure to obtain prompt relief casts suspicion on a diagnosis of angina.

A positive exercise tolerance test (i.e., the development of ischemic ECG changes) does not confirm a diagnosis of angina pectoris unless the exact symptoms are produced during the exertion. Demonstration of CAD by angiography in the absence of symptoms also does not establish a diagnosis of angina pectoris, since the latter is a symptom reflecting myocardial ischemia and the former is an anatomic demonstration of deformed blood vessels.

Exercise tolerance tests: The level of cardiac work, BP, and heart rate required to induce angina in a given patient can usually be reproduced by the treadmill exercise test. Determining the cardiovascular response to exercise is an important tool in diagnosing and evaluating patients with possible coronary artery disease. However, the tests must be interpreted with due regard to their reliability and specificity, as with any other testing procedures.

Maximal heart rate during exercise is directly related to maximal O_2 consumption, with a linear relationship between heart rate and O_2 uptake by the body. The adequacy of an exercise test may thus be judged by the heart rate during stress. (Maximal heart rate attained during exercise declines with age; tables are available relating predicted maximal heart rate during exercise to sex and age.) Exercise may be limited by dyspnea, reduced endurance, fatigue, or chest pain.

The "ischemic" ECG response during or after exercise is characterized by a flat or downward-sloping S-T segment depression of > 0.1 millivolts (1 mm) lasting 0.08 seconds or more in a properly calibrated recording. J junction depression with an upward sloping S-T segment is difficult to interpret; it is associated with a high incidence of false-positive tests. Both sensitivity and reliability increase with the patient's age. Thus abnormal tests are falsely positive in 20% or more of patients under age 40, whereas over age 60 this may be reduced to $< 10\%$. A diagnosis of ischemic heart disease due to coronary artery abnormality as a result of a positive exercise test (due to ECG change) is almost always inferential. A positive test may mean that the heart is metabolically abnormal, but coronary angiography may show the large coronary arteries to be quite normal. False-negative tests also occur. In one recent large study 35% of patients with $> 70\%$ obstruction of one coronary artery (determined by angiography) had a normal (negative) treadmill exercise test. The frequency of positive tests increased with the number of coronary arteries obstructed, and greater degrees of S-T segment depression generally were correlated with more extensive disease. The test is most useful in men with chest pain thought to be due to angina and in these subjects has a specificity of 70% and a sensitivity of 90%. Exercise tests are more difficult to interpret in women under age 55; a high incidence of false-positive responses reduces the specificity.

When proper indications are present and the test is closely monitored, exercise tolerance in the patient with ischemia carries a remarkably low rate of risk, but a test is contraindicated when the resting ECG is unstable, suggesting acute ischemia or infarction. Patients with unstable angina or those in whom a recent diagnosis of MI is suspected should not be exercised. *A complete life support system including emergency drugs, airway, and defibrillator should always be immediately available for any patient undergoing exercise testing.*

Coronary arteriography: Controversy over the place of coronary arteriography in the management of patients with angina pectoris continues. However, angiography is indicated primarily for evaluation (1) of coronary artery anatomy in patients being considered for surgical bypass procedures and (2) of unusual, puzzling, or atypical chest pain possibly due to angina pectoris. Many experts believe that angiography is also indicated in selected young patients after first infarct and in survivors of unexpected cardiac arrest outside the hospital.

The coronary angiogram has shown correlation with postmortem findings, although the extent of disease is usually underestimated. Vessels as small as 1 mm may be visualized when high-quality imaging technics are used. CAD is recognized by narrowing, beading, or occlusion of the vessels. Obstruction is assumed to be physiologically significant when the lumen diameter is reduced $> 50\%$. Such findings frequently correlate well with the presence of angina pectoris, while lesser degrees of obstruction are not likely to result in ischemia. A left ventricular angiogram to evaluate wall motion is an essential part of the study. Two views at right angles to each other are obtained so that all portions of the free left ventricular wall and septum may be visualized. Analysis of left ventricular pressure and ejection fraction also provides useful information.

The major complications of coronary angiography are thrombosis at the arterial insertion site, MI secondary to catheter trauma, and death. Mortality rates $< 1:1000$ have been reported from many laboratories. High-grade mainstem left CAD appears to increase the risk of morbidity, and many angiographers routinely flush dye into the left coronary sinus for an initial evaluation to rule out left mainstem disease before engaging the orifice with the tip of the catheter.

In 5 to 10% of patients with apparent angina, coronary arteries are found to be normal. This condition occurs predominantly in young women. In some, the history seems typical; in others, the chest pain is atypical. That some patients with this syndrome have ischemia cannot be doubted; lactate production during spontaneous or induced pain has been observed. Reasons for the discrepancy between symptoms and angiography are not always clear. Many patients are heavy smokers. It is suggested that coronary artery spasm is part of a general vasospastic disorder because of its apparent association with migraine and Raynaud's phenomenon. Spasm may develop in normal coronary arteries or complicate extensive coronary artery atherosclerosis. The cause and mechanism of the spasm are not known.

Differential Diagnosis

Many conditions cause chest pain and must be considered in the differential diagnosis (e.g., abnormalities of the cervicodorsal spine, costochondral separation, and nonspecific chest wall pain). However, few truly mimic angina, and the syndrome of angina is so characteristic in most individuals that errors in diagnosis are usually the result of careless history taking. Differentiating GI disease from CAD may be difficult. The discomfort of angina is often ascribed to indigestion. It may indeed be accompanied by considerable bloating, belching, and abdominal stress; at times belching may give relief. Anginal discomfort felt in the upper or lower abdomen may be difficult to recognize. Peptic ulcer, hiatus hernia, and gallbladder disease may cause symptoms similar to angina pectoris or may precipitate attacks in patients with preexisting CAD. Thus, the possibility that a GI disorder and angina pectoris are both present must also be considered; the angina may be triggered, for example, by recurring episodes of esophagitis secondary to hiatus hernia. Nonspecific changes in the T waves and S-T segments have been reported in esophagitis, peptic ulcer disease, and cholecystitis—observations that complicate the task of unraveling the patient's complaints.

At times angina may be confused with dyspnea. In part this is explained by the striking alteration in ventricular function with a sharp and reversible rise in left ventricular filling pressure which often accompanies the attack of ischemia. The patient's description may be imprecise and whether he is suffering from angina, dyspnea, or both may be difficult to determine.

Prognosis

The prognosis in angina pectoris is better than has commonly been supposed and is improving with innovations in medical treatment. The major risks are sudden death or recurrent MI. Three major factors influence prognosis: age, extent of coronary disease (determined by angiography), and ventricular function. An annual mortality rate of 3% has been reported in single-vessel disease, of 6% in 2-vessel disease, and > 10% in 3-vessel disease. Significant lesions of the left main coronary artery or high in the anterior descending vessel carry a particularly high risk.

Clinically, an annual mortality rate of 1.4% has been reported in men with angina and no history of MI, a normal resting ECG, and normal BP. The rate rises to about 7.5% in those with systolic hypertension, to 8.4% when the ECG is abnormal, and to 12% if both risk factors are present.

Treatment

The underlying disease, usually atherosclerosis, must be delineated and treated and risk factors reduced (see ARTERIOSCLEROSIS; ATHEROSCLEROSIS in Ch. 24). Patients who smoke should discontinue the habit. Reduction of body overweight enhances well-being and reduces cardiac demand. Hypertension should be treated diligently, since even mild diastolic hypertension (90 to 100 mm Hg range) increases cardiac work. Angina sometimes improves markedly with treatment of mild left ventricular failure. Paradoxically, digitalis occasionally intensifies angina, presumably because the resultant increase in contractility critically raises the myocardial O_2 demand in the presence of fixed coronary blood flow.

Nitrates: For the **acute episode**, nitroglycerin 0.3 to 0.6 mg sublingually is the most effective agent. Within 1½ to 3 min, relief is usually dramatic and is complete by about 5 min. Large numbers of tablets may be taken daily without side effects other than an occasional headache. Patients with angina pectoris should carry nitroglycerin tablets with them at all times. Nitroglycerin may lose its potency unless stored in a tightly sealed glass container. Thus, it should be purchased in small amounts at frequent intervals.

Nitroglycerin is a potent smooth-muscle relaxer and vasodilator. In advanced CAD, however, probably has relatively little effect on the coronary blood vessels; its major site of action is in the peripheral vascular tree where it lowers systolic pressure, thus reducing myocardial wall tension one of the major determinants of myocardial O_2 need. Overall, the drug brings the myocardial O_2 supply and demand into more favorable balance, and pain is relieved.

Amyl nitrite, an extremely potent vasodilator, may be effective when severe angina is unresponsive to nitroglycerin and complicated by hypertension. An ampul containing 0.3 ml is crushed and its vapor briefly inhaled. Because of the drug's potency, only 2 or 3 inhalations are required; the patient should be lying down and in a well-ventilated room.

Selected **long-acting nitrates** are effective for long-term vasodilation or reduction of afterload. Serial exercise testing has shown improved exercise tolerance in patients taking these drugs. When sustained vasodilation or reduction of ventricular afterload is required, isosorbide dinitrate may be given sublingually (5 to 10 mg q 2 to 4 h) or orally (20 to 80 mg q 3 to 6 h). Objective improvement in exercise tolerance following ingestion of these drugs persists about 1 h. Another useful preparation is nitroglycerin paste, which may be applied to the chest wall q 4 to 6 h and is slowly absorbed.

β-Adrenergic blocking agents are most useful for therapy of angina pectoris. These drugs block sympathetic stimulation of the heart, reducing heart rate and contractility, thus reducing cardiac output and myocardial O_2 demand. Left ventricular end-diastolic pressure may rise, especially during exercise. Exercise tolerance is improved because of the reduction in systolic pressure, heart rate, and cardiac output, and hence in myocardial O_2 demand during stress. Tissue O_2 requirements are met by greater O_2 extraction from capillary blood; thus systemic arteriovenous O_2 difference is elevated.

Propranolol was the first β-blocker approved in the USA for treatment of angina. The clinically effective dose of propranolol varies. It is best to start with 40 to 60 mg/day in 3 divided doses and evaluate the response. Dosage may be gradually increased in increments of 30 to 50% until clinical effectiveness or troublesome side effects are encountered (optimum response usually occurs with a dose between 160 and 240 mg/day). It is useful to monitor the pulse rate when giving the drug; clinical effects are usually achieved when the resting pulse has dropped to 55 to 65 beats/min. Continued faster rates usually mean that more drug may be given. Excessive dosage may induce decreased exercise tolerance due to fatigue. Heart failure may develop with higher doses, but is readily handled by giving digitalis and diuretics, which may be instituted prior to initiating therapy with propranolol in selected cases. Because propranolol depresses the sinus node and blocks conduction at the A-V node, it is contraindicated in patients with advanced forms of heart block, prolonged P-R interval, intermittent A-V block, or sinus node disorders characterized by bradycardia. When propranolol is to be discontinued, the dose should be reduced slowly over several weeks because of clinical suspicion that sudden discontinuance of the drug increases the risk of MI.

Nadolol, a nonselective β-adrenergic blocker, has the advantage of long duration of action and is given only once daily. Usual doses are 40 mg/day initially which may be increased to 80 to 240 mg/day. Dosage should be adjusted in patients with impaired renal function. Metoprolol is a relatively cardioselective ($β_1$) adrenergic blocking drug whose half-life is about 3 h. Initial dose is 50 mg b.i.d. which may be increased to 300 to 450 mg/day.

Calcium antagonists, such as nifedipine and verapamil, are becoming first-line therapy of variant (vasospastic or Prinzmetal's) angina. They are also effective for many patients with angina of effort, generally being used, if necessary, after treatment with nitrates and β-blockers. Although some calcium antagonists can be advantageously combined with β-blockers, with verapamil there is a risk that additive effects on the A-V node may result in heart block.

Unstable angina is a medical emergency to be treated in a cardiac care unit with bed rest, sedation, and O_2. β-Adrenergic blockers may be indicated, and diuretics and digitalis are used if heart failure is present. During the acute phase the prognosis must be guarded; some patients progress to acute infarction despite intensive management. In the majority the condition subsides without evidence of myocardial damage.

The use of heparin has been advocated to prevent coronary arterial thrombosis in this situation, but its effect is not established. If medical stability is not soon achieved, aggressive management including early coronary arteriography and consideration for coronary artery bypass is usually indicated. Counterpulsation with the intra-aortic balloon is often highly effective when symptoms are severe and progressive.

Surgical treatment: Indications for surgical therapy of angina pectoris are continually being refined. The prognostic factors discussed above must be evaluated when coronary artery surgery is being considered. It is generally agreed that a coronary bypass procedure may be considered when the vessels are anatomically suitable in a patient whose angina pectoris is unresponsive to medical therapy and seriously interferes with normal activity. The "ideal" surgical candidate has severe angina pectoris, a normal-sized heart, no history of MI, localized disease suitable for bypass, normal ventricular function, and no adverse risk factors. In such patients elective surgery carries a 3 to 7% risk of perioperative MI and a 1 to 3% risk of mortality. About 85% of such patients have complete or dramatic relief of symptoms. At the end of 1 yr between 80 and 85% of surgical bypass grafts remain patent. Exercise testing shows a positive correlation between patency of the bypass graft and improvement in exercise tolerance, but some patients improve significantly despite closure of the bypass.

An increase in ventricular end-diastolic volume and a reduction in ejection fraction to < 50%, symptoms of heart failure, or extensive old MI significantly increase the risk of surgical mortality. Coronary bypass procedures generally do not improve ventricular function. Thus, persistent heart failure or disordered kinetics are not considered an indication for surgery, except in the presence of clear-cut ventricular aneurysm with decreased ventricular function; in such cases removal of the aneurysmal segment may sometimes result in clinical improvement.

While coronary bypass surgery improves the symptoms of angina pectoris, its effect on prognosis remains unclear. Coronary bypass procedures have improved the survival rate in patients with high-grade left mainstem CAD, but to date this is the only group in whom an improved prognosis has been demonstrated in a well-conducted study with patients randomized to medical or surgical treatment.

The NIH unstable angina study, a randomized comparison of medical and surgical treatment in patients with unstable angina, shows no difference in survival or the infarct rate in the 2 treatment groups, but symptomatic improvement has been significantly greater after surgery.

MYOCARDIAL INFARCTION (MI)

Ischemic myocardial necrosis usually resulting from abrupt reduction in coronary blood flow to a segment of myocardium. This clinical condition is characterized by precordial pain similar to (but usually more intense and prolonged than) angina pectoris and left ventricular dysfunction, ranging from moderate to severe; arrhythmias are common. Signs, symptoms, ECG abnormalities, and a rise in serum activity of enzymes released from myocardial cells reflect the cardiac damage.

Etiology and Pathogenesis

Atherosclerosis of the coronary arteries is the common denominator in most patients with MI. Whether or not the infarction is precipitated by acute coronary thrombosis remains controversial. Pathologic studies in patients who die from MI have suggested that thrombosis is usually the result of MI and not the initiating process. Thus, thrombi in the coronary arteries are observed in about 25% of individuals who die suddenly. When death occurs following prolonged heart failure and shock complicating MI, coronary thrombosis in the region supplying the damaged area is almost always observed. Angiographic studies in patients within hours of acute MI suggest that thrombosis is common.

Angiographic studies reveal that segmental abnormalities of myocardial contractility representing old infarction correlate reasonably well with disease of the artery supplying the area in question. Abnormalities in platelet aggregation in the patient with preexisting coronary disease may contribute to variable changes in coronary perfusion. However, infarction can occur without CAD or occlusion. Spasm may be a causative factor, or a coronary embolus secondary to rheumatic heart disease, endocarditis, or aortic stenosis may be indicated. If adequate collaterals are present, coronary occlusion can develop without subsequent infarction.

MI is predominantly a disease of the left ventricle but the area damaged may extend into the right ventricle or the atria. Right ventricular infarction is characterized by high right ventricular filling pressure, often with severe tricuspid regurgitation. **Transmural infarcts** involve the whole thickness of myocardium from epicardium to endocardium and are characterized by abnormal Q waves on the ECG. **Nontransmural infarcts** do not extend through the ventricular wall and cause only S-T segment and T wave abnormalities. **Subendocardial infarcts** usually involve the inner 1/3 of the myocardium where wall tension is highest and myocardial blood flow is most vulnerable to circulatory changes. Subendocardial infarctions tend to occur in 3-vessel coronary disease (involvement of anterior descending, right coronary, and circumflex vessels) and carry a high mortality. They may also occur following prolonged hypotension complicating hemorrhage, anesthesia, or extensive surgical procedures.

The ability of the heart to continue functioning as a pump is probably related directly to the extent of myocardial damage. Thus, pathologic studies have shown that patients who die with cardiogenic shock have an infarct, or a combination of scar and new infarct, of 50% or more of left ventricular mass.

Symptoms and Signs

The first symptom of acute MI usually is the development of deep, substernal, visceral pain described as aching or pressure, often with radiation to the back, the jaw, or the left arm. The pain is similar in character to that of angina pectoris but is usually more severe and relieved little, or only temporarily, by nitroglycerin. However, the discomfort may be very mild, and a significant percentage of acute infarctions are silent or unrecognized as illness by the patient. In severe episodes the patient becomes apprehensive and may develop a sense of impending doom. Symptoms of left ventricular failure, pulmonary edema, shock, or significant arrhythmia may develop and dominate the clinical picture.

On examination the patient is usually restless, apprehensive, pale, diaphoretic, and in severe pain. Peripheral or central cyanosis may be apparent and the skin is usually cool. The temperature is usually elevated. The pulse may be thready and the BP is variable, although most patients initially manifest some degree of hypertension unless cardiogenic shock is developing. Arrhythmia is common; bradycardia or extrasystoles may be observed early in the course of MI. The heart sounds are usually somewhat distant; the presence of a 4th heart sound is almost universal. There may be a soft systolic blowing apical murmur, a reflection of papillary muscle dysfunction, at the apex. The presence of a friction rub or more striking murmurs suggests the possibility of preexisting heart disease or another diagnosis. The detection of a friction rub within a few hours after the onset of symptoms of acute MI is distinctly unusual. Other physical signs may be present in relation to complications such as shock or pulmonary edema.

Laboratory Findings

Routine laboratory examination reveals abnormalities compatible with tissue necrosis. Thus the ESR is increased, the WBC is usually elevated, and differential blood count reveals a shift to the left.

The most helpful laboratory findings, however, are **serial measurements of blood enzyme activity** (see TABLE 25–4). In general, the extent of the rise of enzyme activity reflects the amount of myocardial damage. CPK is a relatively specific enzyme available for determination of myocardial tissue necrosis, rising to a peak within 24 h of muscle injury. Sampling of CPK for several days following the acute episode usually is sufficient to confirm the diagnosis. However, CPK originates from 3 sources: brain (BB isomer), skeletal muscle (MM isomer), and myocardium (MB isomer). While CPK from the

TABLE 25–4. SERUM ENZYMES IN MYOCARDIAL INFARCTION

Normal*	Elevations (days)			False Positives
	Onset	Peak	End	
CPK < 30	< 1	1–2	2–4	Muscle, brain disorders
AST (SGOT) < 45	1	1–2	3–4	Muscle, brain disorders
LDH < 600	2	4–5	7–8	Lung embolus, carcinoma, anemias
HBD < 300	2	5–6	10–12	Anemias

* CPK, creatine phosphokinase; AST, aspartate transferase; SGOT, serum glutamic oxaloacetic transaminase; LDH, lactic dehydrogenase; HBD, α-hydroxybutyric dehydrogenase.

brain does not ordinarily confuse the issue, either skeletal muscle injury or myocardial necrosis may cause an acute rise in serum CPK. IM injection of a wide variety of drugs (common practice in hospital emergency rooms) may cause sufficient skeletal muscle damage to increase serum CPK. Where the diagnosis is in doubt, analysis of MB-CPK is often helpful since normally serum does not contain significant MB isomer. AST (formerly SGOT) and ALT (formerly SGPT) are often useful in confirming the diagnosis of MI and evaluating the possible role of skeletal muscle damage, which contributes to AST rise, or of liver damage—which causes rises in AST and ALT, but not CPK. AST is elevated in almost all patients after an acute MI. It begins to rise in 12 h, reaches a peak of 2 to 4 times normal in 24 h, and returns to normal in 4 to 7 days. It may be elevated in other diseases when there is necrosis of heart muscle; e.g., in myocarditis of rheumatic, viral, bacterial, or metabolic etiology. AST is normal in pericardial effusion, arrhythmias, angina pectoris, coronary insufficiency, and cardiac failure unless accompanied by necrosis of heart muscle or by hepatic congestion and necrosis.

Serial ECGs: In **acute transmural MI** the initial ECG may be diagnostic, showing abnormal deep Q waves and elevated S-T segments in leads subtending the area of damage, or the ECG may be strikingly abnormal with elevated or depressed S-T segments and deeply inverted T waves without abnormal Q waves (see FIGS. 25–35 to 25–40). Serial tracings showing a gradual evolution toward a stable, more normal pattern, or the development of abnormal Q waves over the next few days tends to confirm the initial impression of acute MI. Since **nontransmural infarcts** are usually in the subendocardial or mid-myocardial layers, they are not associated with diagnostic Q waves on the ECG and commonly produce only varying degrees of S-T segment and T wave abnormality. In some patients the ECG abnormalities are less striking, variable, or nonspecific, and therefore difficult to interpret. Thus, the ECG may be diagnostic, supportive, or not helpful. However, a diagnosis of acute MI is probably not tenable when repeated ECGs are completely normal.

Myocardial imaging following IV injection of radioisotope and subsequent accumulation of indicator in heart muscle may be helpful in detecting infarcted or ischemic areas of myocardium. Currently 2 technics are available—"hot spot" and "cold spot." Technetium (^{99m}Tc) pyrophosphate precipitates as calcium accumulates in recently infarcted (hours to 3 to 4 days) myocardium, thus showing up as a hot spot when the precordium is scanned after injection of the tracer in a patient with recent myocardial damage. On the other hand, thallium (^{201}Tl) is distributed intracellularly in the manner of potassium. Its distribution is controlled by coronary blood flow. Precordial scanning after injection of the tracer in a patient with an old MI may reveal a cold spot or lack of image because of the scan. Thallium scanning is especially useful in diagnosing reversible ischemia during exercise testing when the tracer is injected at peak of exercise and the resulting image compared to resting control.

Cardiac catheterization (see also Ch. 23): Management of complications such as severe heart failure, hypoxia, or hypotension may be aided by measurement of right heart, pulmonary artery, and wedge pressures. Bedside technics for right heart catheterization utilizing balloon-tipped catheters that float into position (Swan-Ganz) are widely utilized in many centers. Analysis of right heart pressure and blood O_2 content may be helpful in evaluating complicated patients. Cardiac output can be determined with indicator dilution or other technics. Coronary arteriography is seldom if ever indicated in acute MI, according to current understanding. In acutely ill patients with MI complicated by acute mitral regurgitation or acquired ventricular septal defect, left ventricular angiography may be necessary to evaluate the possibility of surgical repairs.

Diagnosis

In a typical case the diagnosis is evident from the history, confirmed by the initial ECG and its subsequent evolution, and supported by the serial enzyme changes. In other instances the diagnosis is strongly suspected on the basis of history and ECG and confirmed by the typical rise and fall of serum CPK. A significant group of patients must be classified as having had a "possible" or "probable" MI because the clinical findings are typical or strongly suggestive, but objective confirmation from the ECG and enzyme assay is lacking. Some patients eventually prove to have other conditions,

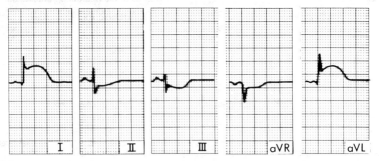

FIG. 25-35. Acute anterior left ventricular infarction—tracing obtained within a few hours of
the reciprocal depression

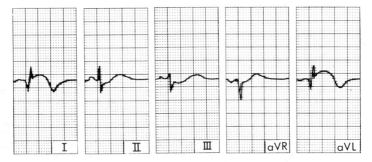

FIG. 25-36. Acute anterior left ventricular infarction—24 h later. Note that the S-T segments are
aVL, V₄,

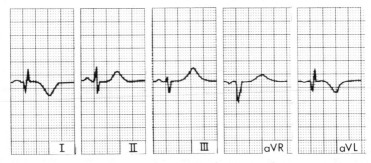

FIG. 25-37. Acute anterior left ventricular infarction—several days later. Significant Q waves and
probably only slowly change

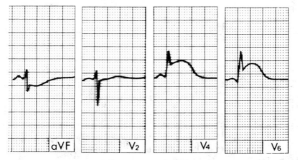

the onset of illness. Note the striking hyperacute S-T segment elevation in leads I, aVL, V_4, and V_6, and in the other leads.

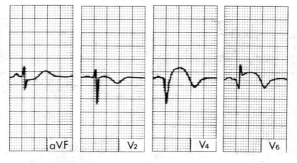

less elevated; also note the development of significant Q waves and the loss of the R wave in leads I, and V_6.

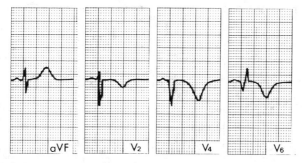

the loss of the R wave voltage persist. S-T segments are now essentially isoelectric. The ECG will over the next several months.

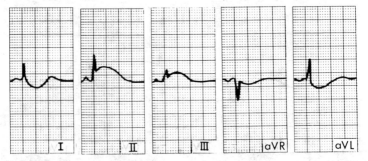

Fig. 25-38. Acute inferior diaphragmatic left ventricular infarction—tracing obtained within a few
the reciprocal depression

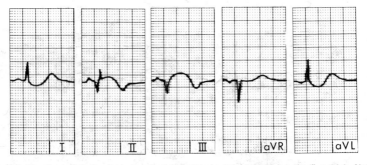

Fig. 25-39. Acute inferior diaphragmatic left ventricular infarction—after the first 24 h. Note the
in the

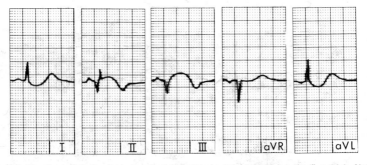

Fig. 25-40. Acute inferior diaphragmatic left ventricular infarction—several days later. S-T seg-
myocardial

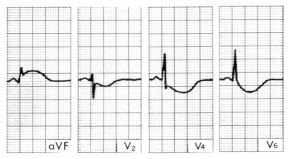

hours of the onset of illness. Note the hyperacute S-T segment elevation in leads II, III, and aVF, and in the other leads.

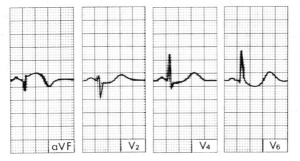

development of significant Q waves in leads II, III, and aVF, and the decreasing S-T segment elevation same leads.

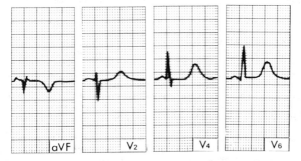

ments are now isoelectric. There are abnormal Q waves in leads II, III, and aVF, indicating that scars persist.

but if clinical suspicion was strongly based on a characteristic history, most will have suffered a small infarction.

Differential Diagnosis

Acute MI is so common in the Western world that it is wise to rule it out in all men over age 35 and all women over age 50 when the major complaint is chest pain. It must be differentiated from the pain of pneumonia, pulmonary embolism, pericarditis, rib fracture, costochondral separation, or chest muscle tenderness after trauma or exertion. Not infrequently the patient interprets the pain of infarct as indigestion, and evaluation may be difficult since many patients have coexisting hiatus hernia, peptic ulcer, or gallbladder disease. Some relief of the pain of infarction by belching or following antacid therapy is not uncommon, although such relief is usually brief or incomplete. Other conditions to be considered include acute aortic dissection, renal stone, splenic infarction, and a wide variety of abdominal disorders.

Treatment

Treatment is designed to: (1) relieve the patient's distress, (2) reduce cardiac work, (3) prevent complications, and (4) treat complications. (Complications are discussed separately, below.)

Prehospital treatment: Since 50% of all deaths from acute MI occur within 2½ h of onset of the clinical syndrome, the first few hours of management are critical. The major factor causing delay of treatment is the patient's denial that the symptoms represent a serious and potentially life-threatening illness. The immediate threats to life are ventricular arrhythmia or, occasionally, heart block. Optimal early treatment includes rapid diagnosis, alleviation of pain and apprehension, stabilization of heart rhythm and BP, and transportation to a hospital with a monitoring unit.

Morphine 10 to 15 mg IM or 4 to 6 mg IV repeated as needed is highly effective for the pain of MI. Morphine depresses respiration, reduces myocardial contractility, and is a potent vasodilator. Hypotension and bradycardia secondary to morphine can usually be overcome by prompt elevation of the lower extremities. Other narcotics, including meperidine, may be used; < 75 mg of meperidine is ineffective and 100 to 125 mg IM repeated as necessary may be required.

Extreme bradycardia with hypotension may respond to atropine sulfate 0.5 to 1 mg IV; it may be repeated after several minutes if the response is inadequate. It is best to give several small doses, because of the risk of inducing tachycardia from excessive doses. Ventricular premature beats are best treated with lidocaine 50 to 100 mg IV, repeated in 3 to 5 min if necessary. Lidocaine may also be given IM in a dose of 400 mg; antiarrhythmic blood levels are achieved in 10 to 15 min and maintained for as long as 1 h. Some advocate routine IM lidocaine administration prior to transporting the patient. This approach has little risk but has not been universally accepted. Moreover, during the first few days of illness, IM injection of any medication may confound diagnostic enzyme determinations.

Most patients are moderately hypertensive on arrival at the emergency room and the BP gradually falls over the next several hours. Severe hypotension or signs of shock are ominous and may be treated with vasopressors prior to arrival at the hospital; e.g., injection of metaraminol 2 to 10 mg IM or a carefully controlled IV drip of levarterenol in a concentration of 4 to 8 mg (of the base)/L. Both dopamine (5 mg/kg/min. increasing to 20 to 50 mg/kg/min.) and dobutamine (2.5 to 10 mg/min.) may be given by closely monitored IV drip when myocardial failure with consequent hypotension complicates MI.

Treatment in the hospital: Although some good-risk patients in Great Britain are sent home and carefully watched by the family physician, this approach remains controversial and would be difficult to manage in the average U.S. practice. Thus, a patient suspected of having acute MI should be admitted to a hospital with a cardiac care unit **(CCU)** as rapidly as possible. On arrival at the hospital, the patient should be monitored with portable equipment in the emergency room and a reliable IV route should be established. He should be promptly transferred to the CCU, without further diagnostic procedures in the emergency area. Despite the wide variety of electronic monitoring equipment available, the only body function which has consistently proved useful to monitor routinely and continuously is the rate and rhythm of the heart as revealed by the ECG. Qualified cardiac care nurses can interpret the ECG for arrhythmia and initiate prompt treatment following appropriate orders. All professional personnel should be prepared to apply cardiopulmonary resuscitation at an instant's notice. (See Cardiac Arrest and Cardiopulmonary Resuscitation, below.)

The CCU should be a quiet, calm, restful area. Single rooms are preferred and privacy consistent with monitoring functions should be assured. Usually visitors are restricted during the first few days of illness, and outside influences such as radios, newspapers, etc., are reduced to a minimum. A wall clock, a calendar, and an outside window help to orient the patient and prevent a sense of isolation.

Morphine may be given for pain as outlined above. Mood changes and apprehension during the acute illness are common, and a mild tranquilizer may be helpful; e.g., diazepam 2.5 to 5 mg orally t.i.d. or q.i.d.

Use of **anticoagulants** is elective, since deemphasis of bed rest and attention to passive and active exercises in bed have reduced the incidence of pulmonary embolism. Anticoagulants are often given to reduce the risk of pulmonary embolism in poor-risk patients requiring prolonged bed rest. An effective form of therapy is subcutaneous heparin 5000 u. q 8 or 12 h.

Antiarrhythmics: The usefulness of giving routine prophylactic lidocaine IV remains controversial. When nursing and monitoring facilities are limited, prophylactic lidocaine is probably indicated for the first 48 to 72 h since the drug is safe and highly effective. The major hazard is CNS depression due to overdosage.

Limiting the extent of ischemia: Cardiac performance after recovery depends essentially on the mass of functioning muscle surviving the acute episode. Reinfarction or extension of infarct during hospitalization is common. The use of increased inspired O_2 concentration is discussed under Hypoxia in COMPLICATIONS OF MYOCARDIAL INFARCTION, below. Recent animal studies suggest that reduction of the O_2 requirements of myocardium and an increase in coronary perfusion or reduction of afterload with vasodilators reduce the area of ischemic infarction. These observations need further evaluation, but, in selected patients, especially those with elevated arterial pressure, it appears to be appropriate in the acute stages of infarction to lower BP judiciously. Nitroglycerin, isosorbide dinitrate, trimethaphan, or nitroprusside has been used, but data demonstrating optimal safety and effectiveness are lacking. In general a quick-acting, readily-discontinued IV drug such as nitroprusside is probably preferable.

Long-term β-adrenergic blockade has been hypothesized to reduce mortality in patients surviving acute MI, but studies were inconclusive until a large multicenter double-blind randomized study in Norway was reported. Timolol maleate, a noncardioselective β-adrenergic blocking agent, was given, beginning on the 28th day following onset of MI symptoms and continued for up to 33 mo. Patients included varied from low- to high-risk and ranged in age from 20 to 75 yr. Patients with known contraindications to β-adrenergic blockade were excluded. Treatment resulted in a substantial reduction in mortality and reinfarction. The protective mechanisms and the pharmacologic properties of timolol that are responsible for these effects are not clarified nor was the optimal dose determined. The study protocol called for 5 mg b.i.d. for 2 days and 10 mg b.i.d. thereafter.

General measures include maintenance of normal bowel function and avoidance of straining at stool. Milk of magnesia 30 ml b.i.d. is an effective laxative; dioctyl sodium sulfosuccinate 100 mg b.i.d. may be added if necessary. Urinary retention is common in older patients, especially after several days of bed rest and atropine therapy. A catheter may be required, but it usually can be removed when the patient can stand or sit to void.

Smoking should be prohibited; a sojourn in a CCU is a potent motivation to discontinue smoking, and the physician should reinforce this attitude.

Acutely ill patients have little appetite for food, although modest amounts of tasty food are good for morale. Usually patients are offered a soft diet, somewhat reduced in calories, 1500 to 1800/day, with some reduction of sodium, 2 to 3 gm (87 to 130 mEq). Salt restriction is not required after the first 2 or 3 days for the patient who has no evidence of heart failure.

Rehabilitation: It is wise to keep the patient quiet in bed for the first 2 or 3 days until the course of the illness becomes reasonably evident. Bed rest for more than a short period of time results in rapid physical deconditioning with development of orthostatic hypotension, decreased work capacity, and increased heart rate during effort. Feelings of depression and helplessness are intensified. In recent years, the period of bed confinement and hospitalization in treatment of MI has been sharply curtailed. Patients without complications may be permitted chair rest, passive exercise, and a commode after 3 or 4 days. By 1 wk, walking to the bathroom and nonstressful paperwork or reading are allowed. Discharge from the hospital after 2 wk is reasonable and without significant hazard. Physical activity is gradually increased during the next 3 to 6 wk. Factors such as age, extent of injury, arrhythmia, heart failure, occupation, and personal ambition influence the rehabilitation program. Resumption of sexual activity is often of great concern and may be encouraged in parallel with other moderate physical activities. If cardiac function is well maintained 6 wk after acute infarction, most patients are able to return to their full range of normal activity and some establish more regular exercise programs than prior to their MI.

The impact of acute illness and treatment in the CCU provides strong motivation to both physician and patient for analysis and management of risk factors. Mortality after hospital discharge averages between 6 and 10% yearly, but survival for many decades is common. High-risk patients include those with recurrent ischemic attacks or persistent ventricular arrhythmia. Management of these challenging problems must be individualized. Frank discussion and thorough evaluation of the patient's physical and emotional status coupled with sound advice about smoking, diet, work and play habits, and exercise, together with effective treatment of hypertension, diabetes mellitus, obesity, and elevated blood lipids, may favorably alter the patient's long-term outlook and are important obligations of the physician providing continuous medical care.

Complications of Myocardial Infarction

Sudden Death

About 50% of patients with acute MI do not survive to receive medical attention or hospitalization. Mortality is greatest during the first hours; 50% of all deaths have occurred by $2\frac{1}{2}$ h after onset of pain. Primary ventricular fibrillation (fibrillation without warning from ventricular premature beats) probably accounts for the majority of cases of sudden death. In some patients, acute heart block or profound bradycardia with consequent hypotension may initiate cardiac arrest. (See also SUDDEN CARDIAC DEATH, below.)

Arrhythmia

Some form of arrhythmia with ventricular ectopic beats occurs in > 90% of patients with MI. Disturbances in conduction reflect damage to the sinus node, the A-V node, or the specialized conduction tissues. Recognition and management of arrhythmia are based on a thorough understanding of electrophysiology, electrocardiography, and pharmacology. A scheme of management of the commonly encountered arrhythmias is outlined in TABLE 25–5, and a summary of commonly used drugs is outlined in TABLE 25–6.

Sinus node disturbances are influenced by the origin of the artery to the sinus node (whether from the left or right coronary artery) and the possibility, especially in the older age group, of preexisting sinus node disease ("sick sinus syndrome"). Sinus bradycardia may be treated expectantly in most cases. However, when the heart rate falls below 55, treatment is usually indicated. IV atropine or a temporary transvenous pacemaker is usually effective. It is important to avoid overdose of atropine because unwanted tachycardia may occur, increasing cardiac work and risking extension of infarction.

Reversible changes in A-V conduction, Mobitz 1 conduction abnormalities with prolonged P-R time, or Wenckebach phenomenon are relatively common, particularly with an inferior-diaphragmatic infarction involving the blood supply to the posterior wall of the left ventricle with branches to the A-V node. These disturbances usually are self-limited and if the rate is well maintained do not merit treatment. Progression of Mobitz 1 to Mobitz 2 is unusual.

Life-threatening arrhythmias, major causes of mortality in MI in the first 72 h, include tachycardia from any focus rapid enough to reduce cardiac output and lower BP, frequent ventricular premature beats, Mobitz 2 heart block, ventricular tachycardia, and ventricular fibrillation. Complete heart block with failure of atrial impulses to capture the ventricle and slow ventricular rate is uncommon and usually denotes massive anterior infarction. Asystole is uncommon except as a terminal manifestation of progressive left ventricular failure and shock.

Persistent sinus tachycardia is generally an ominous sign, often reflecting left ventricular failure and low cardiac output. Atrial premature beats **(APBs),** atrial fibrillation, and atrial flutter occur in about 10% of patients with MI and may reflect left ventricular failure. Since APBs are often a forerunner of sustained atrial arrhythmia, prompt treatment is usually in order. Frequent APBs usually respond well to digitalis. Atrial flutter and fibrillation may be treated with digitalis or propranolol to slow the ventricular rate. If the rhythm persists and the patient develops heart failure or hypotension, precordial electric shock may be indicated. Precordial shock is not used as a first-line treatment because these arrhythmias frequently recur during the first few days of the acute illness. The aim of treatment is to slow the ventricular rate to acceptable levels. After several days the atrial flutter or fibrillation usually reverts spontaneously to a sinus mechanism. Paroxysmal atrial tachycardia is uncommon and usually occurs in patients who have had previous episodes.

It is important to make an exact electrocardiographic diagnosis of the mechanism of atrioventricular **(A-V)** block. Most Mobitz 1 arrhythmias may be treated expectantly. Occasionally, atropine or a pacemaker is required to maintain an adequate ventricular rate. True Mobitz 2 with dropped beats or A-V block with slow, wide QRS complexes is usually an ominous complication of massive anterior infarction. The rhythm and rate may be restored temporarily with isoproterenol infusion, but temporary transvenous pacemaking is the treatment of choice.

Ventricular premature beats **(VPBs)** occur in most patients with acute MI. VPBs, especially if closely coupled, multifocal, or in salvos, are important because they may initiate sustained ventricular arrhythmia, tachycardia, or fibrillation. Treatment is required if the VPBs are frequent, multifocal, or sufficiently premature to strike the vulnerable period of the diastolic repolarization phase of the cardiac cycle (during the ascending limb of the T wave). In most CCUs, > 3 VPBs/min are routinely treated with lidocaine IV. Since constant infusion with lidocaine requires several hours to reach equilibrium at therapeutic levels, it is important to initiate treatment with loading doses by bolus injection. An initial IV bolus of 50 to 100 mg is given, repeated 2 or 3 times at 3- to 5-min intervals, if necessary, until the arrhythmia has subsided. An infusion of 2 to 4 mg/min is then maintained, usually for 24 h, and then slowly discontinued. Recurrence of VPBs requires additional bolus doses of lidocaine and an increase in the infusion rate. In some instances ventricular arrhythmias persist despite large doses of lidocaine. Procainamide 250 to 500 mg orally q 2 to 6 h or quinidine 400 mg orally q 6 or 8 h may be required to control persistent VPBs. When large doses of these drugs are required, it is best to monitor their effectiveness with blood levels as an aid to avoiding toxicity. Causes of persistent arrhythmia such as hypoxia, hypokalemia, ventricular aneurysm, or digitalis toxicity should be diligently sought.

Cardiac arrest, when due to ventricular tachycardia or fibrillation, is treated by immediate defibrillation, or if equipment must be sent for, by cardiopulmonary resuscitation followed by defibrillation. Equipment in perfect working order should be immediately on hand in the emergency room and the CCU, and for transporting the patient to the CCU. Prophylactic antiarrhythmics are usually given after resuscitation.

TABLE 25-5. MANAGEMENT OF ARRHYTHMIAS IN ACUTE MYOCARDIAL
INFARCTION

Arrhythmia	First Choice	Second Choice	Comments
Atrial premature beats (APBs)	Digitalis	Quinidine	APBs are frequently forerunners of atrial fibrillation or flutter. CAUTION: *Avoid excessive dosage of digitalis because of increased susceptibility to arrhythmia in acute myocardial infarction*
Paroxysmal atrial tachycardia	Digitalis	Precordial DC shock	An uncommon complication of acute infarction. Avoid excessive digitalis.
Atrial fibrillation	Digitalis	Precordial DC shock Propranolol	Arrhythmia tends to recur, hence first aim of treatment is control of ventricular rate. If patient tolerates arrhythmia poorly, needs atrial "kick," or shows low stroke volume, immediate DC conversion may be necessary. Eventual spontaneous reversion is the rule. If rate is fast, small doses of propranolol orally or IV may increase A-V block and slow ventricular rate.
Atrial flutter	Digitalis	Precordial DC shock Propranolol	Comments above on atrial fibrillation are applicable to flutter. Some authorities recommend immediate DC shock in all instances of atrial flutter or fibrillation. If rate is fast, small doses of propranolol orally or IV may increase A-V block and slow ventricular rate.
Paroxysmal nodal tachycardia	Digitalis	Precordial DC shock	See atrial tachycardia. If rate is only moderately increased and associated with A-V dissociation, consider digitalis toxicity as causative.
Ventricular premature beats (VPBs)	Lidocaine	Quinidine Procainamide Disopyramide Phenytoin Overdriving with pacemaker	Decision to treat depends on setting. More than 5 VPBs/min, occurrence in salvos, or R on T phenomena (closely coupled) demands immediate and adequate treatment. Once VPBs are initially suppressed with lidocaine, a plan for long-term therapy with a longer-acting agent should be considered.
Ventricular tachycardia	Precordial DC shock	Lidocaine Quinidine Procainamide Disopyramide Phenytoin Overdriving with pacemaker	Forerunner of ventricular fibrillation. Best combination is immediate precordial shock followed by long-term administration of suppressive drugs. Slow rates without circulatory collapse may respond to lidocaine.
Ventricular fibrillation	Precordial DC shock	Closed-chest cardiac massage Intubation and ventilatory support	When cardiac arrest occurs in the CCU, precordial shock should be administered immediately. If unsuccessful, cardiopulmonary resuscitation may be necessary. The longer fibrillation persists, the less likely is survival.

Modified from T. Killip, *The Myocardium: Failure and Infarction,* edited by E. Braunwald. Copyright 1975 by HP Publishing Company, Inc. Used with permission.

Heart Failure

Heart failure occurs in about ⅔ of hospitalized patients with acute MI. Left ventricular dysfunction is usually predominant; hence the findings include dyspnea, inspiratory rales at the lung bases, and hypoxia. Clinical signs depend upon the size of the infarction, the elevation of left ventricular filling pressure, and the extent to which cardiac output is reduced. The mortality rate varies directly with

TABLE 25-6. CARDIAC DRUGS OF USE IN THE CORONARY CARE UNIT IN MANAGEMENT OF ARRHYTHMIAS

Drug	Dosage	Indications	Comments
Atropine	0.5–1 mg IV	Bradycardia due to sinus slowing; A-V dissociation	May be repeated 2 or 3 times. Urinary retention common. May rarely cause atropine psychosis or acute glaucoma. Excess dosage may cause sinus tachycardia.
Lidocaine	60–100 mg IV	Ventricular premature complexes	Effective in 3–5 min. May be repeated 3 times. Duration of action variable, usually 20–40 min. Bolus should be followed by steady infusion at 2–4 mg/min to maintain desired effect.
Quinidine*	200–400 mg orally q 6 h	Long-term suppression of ventricular arrhythmia	Aim is to achieve adequate blood level (3–6 mg/L) for effective suppression. May depress ventricular function, lower BP, or widen QRS.
Procainamide*	2–4 gm daily in divided doses q 3–6 h	Long-term suppression of ventricular arrhythmia	Aim is to achieve adequate blood level (5–8 mg/L) for effective suppression. May depress ventricular function, lower BP, or widen QRS.
Disopyramide*	Loading dose: 200–300 mg; then 100–200 mg q 6 h	Long-term suppression of ventricular arrhythmia	Electrophysiologic properties similar to quinidine procainamide. May cause hypotension, constipation, urinary retention, psychosis, other cholinergic effects. Occasionally causes severe myocardial depression. Severe exacerbation of heart failure uncommon.
Isoproterenol	1 mg in 500 ml 5% dextrose as a continuously regulated infusion	Bradycardia Sinus slowing A-V block Asystole	Provides short-term support until pacemaker or other definitive therapy is instituted. May induce ventricular arrhythmia. Markedly increases myocardial oxygen demand. Probably contraindicated in cardiogenic shock.
Propranolol	IV: 0.2–0.5 mg q 2 min; total dosage no more than 2–5 mg Orally: 5–20 mg q 6–8 h	Recurrent atrial fibrillation or flutter with rapid ventricular rate	IV: Use with great caution. May induce profound A-V block or systole. Reserve for special situations only. Orally: May depress contractility, slow sinus node, or induce high-degree A-V block.
Digoxin	0.5 mg IV, then 0.25 mg at 6 h, then 0.125 at 12 & 18 h Maintenance: 0.125 to 0.375 mg/day orally or IV	Congestive failure Supraventricular arrhythmias	Use cautiously in acute myocardial infarction because of apparent reduced toxic threshold. Excreted by kidneys, therefore reduce dose when BUN is elevated. Avoid hypokalemia.

* In general, quinidine, procainamide, and disopyramide are reserved for long-term suppression of ventricular arrhythmia after initial treatment with lidocaine. The problem is to give adequate dosage without incurring toxicity. Although "usual" dosage is often too little to achieve therapeutic blood levels, a higher dosage may suppress myocardial function. Idiosyncrasy to quinidine is well known. Procainamide may cause fever, leukopenia, or SLE. The anticholinergic effects of disopyramide may be troublesome. The electrophysiologic and toxic effects of quinidine, procainamide, and disopyramide differ from those of lidocaine and phenytoin. Propranolol is an antisympathetic and antiarrhythmic drug.

Modified from T. Killip, *The Myocardium: Failure and Infarction*, edited by E. Braunwald. Copyright 1975 by HP Publishing Company, Inc. Used with permission.

the severity of left ventricular failure. It is useful to classify patients according to the presence or absence of clinical evidence of left ventricular failure (see TABLE 25-7). Patients in Class 1 have a hospital mortality rate of 3 to 5%; those in Class 2, a rate of 6 to 10%. The rate is about 20 to 30% in patients in Class 3, and > 85% in patients in Class 4. See CONGESTIVE HEART FAILURE, above, for further discussion of this subject.

TABLE 25-7. CLINICAL CLASSIFICATION OF ACUTE MYOCARDIAL INFARCTION DETERMINED BY REPEATED EXAMINATION OF THE PATIENT DURING THE COURSE OF ILLNESS

Class 1.	No clinical evidence of left ventricular failure
Class 2.	Mild-moderate left ventricular failure Rales lower one-third lung fields, possible altered S_1 and S_2, possible S_3, arterial hypoxia
Class 3:	Severe left ventricular failure. Pulmonary edema
Class 4.	Cardiogenic shock. Hypotension, tachycardia, mental obtundation, cool extremities, oliguria, hypoxia

Modified from T. Killip and J. T. Kimball, "Treatment of Myocardial Infarction in a Coronary Care Unit. A Two-Year Experience with 250 Patients," in *The American Journal of Cardiology,* Vol. 20, pp. 457–464, Oct. 1967. Used with permission.

Hypoxia
Hypoxia is a common accompaniment of acute MI and is usually secondary to increased left atrial pressure with alteration of pulmonary ventilation-perfusion relationships, pulmonary interstitial edema, alveolar collapse, and increased physiologic shunting. Pa_{O2}, determined while the patient is breathing room air, is essentially normal in Class 1, slightly reduced in Class 2, and severely abnormal in Classes 3 and 4. In patients aged 50 to 70, normal Pa_{O2} at bed rest is about 82 ± 5 mm Hg. It is reasonable to give O_2 by nasal cannula in an attempt to maintain the Pa_{O2} at about 100 mm Hg. This may help to oxygenate the myocardium and may limit the extent of the infarction or the ischemic zone. In left ventricular failure, Pa_{O2} is invariably reduced when the patient is breathing room air. Determination of Pa_{O2} before and after response to a rapidly acting diuretic (such as furosemide 40 mg IV) may be helpful in establishing a diagnosis of left ventricular failure: the reduced Pa_{O2} should rise following diuresis.

Hypotension
When BP falls, the patient should be thoroughly evaluated and a treatable cause sought. If the patient remains alert, warm, and has good urine output, shock is not present and treatment may be expectant. Hypotension may be caused by drugs, especially narcotics, sedatives, or diuretics. The most common precipitating factor is the use of potent diuretic agents, especially in older patients; initial intensive diuresis may be followed hours later by hypovolemia and hypotension. Measurement of central venous pressure or preferably pulmonary arterial wedge pressure is helpful; in hypovolemia the pressures are low and respond to fluid infusion.

Cardiogenic Shock
The primary cause of cardiogenic shock in acute MI is inadequate performance of the left ventricle as a pump due to extensive damage. The incidence of cardiogenic shock appears to have decreased in recent years, perhaps due to early recognition and treatment of heart failure. However, despite intensive efforts, mortality when shock occurs remains in excess of 80% and has not changed in > 2 decades. Shock is diagnosed when systolic pressure is < 90 mm Hg, and when the patient is restless and has reduced mental awareness, cyanosis, oliguria (< 20 ml urine/h), and cool, moist extremities. Treatable causes such as cardiac tamponade, hypovolemia, GI bleeding, or arrhythmia should be sought and managed. See SHOCK in Ch. 24 for further discussion.

Functional Papillary Muscle Insufficiency
Functional papillary muscle insufficiency is common in MI, occurring in about 35% in one reported series. Frequent auscultation during the first few hours of infarction will often reveal a transient late apical systolic murmur thought to represent papillary muscle ischemia with failure of complete coaptation of the valve leaflets.

Myocardial Rupture
Three forms of rupture occur—tear of papillary muscle, development of a septal defect, and external rupture. **Rupture of the papillary muscle** is rare. It produces acute, severe mitral regurgitation and is characterized by the sudden appearance of a loud apical systolic murmur and thrill, usually accompanied by pulmonary edema. Emergency replacement of the mitral valve has been accomplished successfully. **Rupture of the intraventricular septum,** while rare, is 8 to 10 times more common than rupture of the papillary muscle. Sudden appearance of a loud systolic murmur and thrill medial to the apex along the left sternal border in the 3rd or 4th intercostal space, accompanied by

hypotension with or without signs of left ventricular failure, is characteristic. Diagnosis may be confirmed with a balloon-tipped catheter and comparison of blood O_2 saturation or P_{O2} of right atrial, right ventricular, and pulmonary artery samples. A significant step-up in the right ventricle is diagnostic. Although mortality is high, surgical repair of the defect has been accomplished in a number of instances. **External rupture,** characterized by sudden loss of arterial pressure with momentary persistence of sinus rhythm and often by signs of cardiac tamponade, is universally fatal.

Ventricular Asynergy

The hallmark of coronary artery disease is patchy left ventricular damage due to ischemia or infarction. Thus normal and abnormal myocardium are juxtaposed. A local noncontracting segment of left ventricle with no systolic inward motion, as revealed by angiography, is termed **akinetic.** **Hypokinetic** myocardium has reduced contractile excursion with partial impairment of inward motion. In an occasional patient, the myocardial hypokinesis is diffuse, and the term **ischemic myocardiopathy** is applied if presenting symptoms predominantly reflect low cardiac output and left heart failure with pulmonary congestion. A **dyskinetic** area shows systolic expansion or bulging (paradoxic motion).

Ventricular Aneurysm

Ventricular aneurysm is a not uncommon complication. Development is favored in the presence of a large transmural infarct and good residual myocardium. Aneurysms may develop in a few days or in weeks or months after the acute episode. They do not rupture, but may be associated with recurrent ventricular arrhythmias and low cardiac output. Mural thrombi and systemic embolization are distinct hazards. Diagnosis is suspected when paradoxic precordial movements are seen or felt, accompanied by persistent elevation of S-T segments on the ECG or a characteristic bulge of the cardiac shadow on x-ray. Ventriculography has revealed a high incidence of unsuspected left ventricular aneurysm. Surgical excision may be indicated when persistent left ventricular failure or arrhythmia complicates management in the presence of a functionally significant aneurysm.

Pericarditis

A pericardial friction rub may be detected in about 1/3 of patients with acute MI if auscultation is frequent. The friction rub indicates epicardial injury and is associated with transmural infarction. It is usually heard between 24 and 96 h after the onset of infarction. A friction rub earlier in the course of acute infarction is unusual and suggests the possibility of other diagnoses, such as acute pericarditis, although hemorrhagic pericarditis occasionally complicates the early phase of infarction. Acute tamponade is rare. Anticoagulants are generally contraindicated in acute MI in the presence of pericarditis. The pericarditis of MI usually subsides in 3 to 5 days.

Postmyocardial Infarction Syndrome (Dressler's Syndrome)

In a few patients, a syndrome develops several days to several weeks after acute MI and is characterized by fever, pericarditis with friction rub, pericardial effusion, pleurisy, pleural effusions, and joint pains. This syndrome is analogous to the **postpericardiotomy syndrome** and appears to be an autoimmune disorder secondary to damaged myocardium and pericardium. Differentiation from extension or recurrence of infarction may be difficult, but a significant rise in the cardiac enzymes does not occur. Patients usually respond satisfactorily to intensive aspirin therapy, 600 to 900 mg q 4 to 6 h. A short, intensive course of corticosteroids may be necessary in severe cases.

Emotional Difficulties

Anxiety, denial, and depression are common in patients with acute MI. Denial and unrealistic evaluation of symptoms may make it difficult to evaluate the patient in the early stages. Depression is common by the 3rd day of illness and is almost universal at some time during recovery. Once the acute phase of illness has subsided, the most important tasks are often management of depression, rehabilitation, and institution of long-term preventive programs. Overemphasis on bed rest, on inactivity, and on the seriousness of the illness reinforces depressive tendencies. A thorough explanation of the illness and an outline of a positive rehabilitation program in the setting of a thorough understanding of the patient's life situation and interpersonal adjustments will have an important positive impact.

Ventricular Arrhythmia Post-MI

Recent data suggest a significant risk of sudden death in the first 3 to 6 mo post-MI. Presence of frequent VPCs at discharge increases risk, as does persistent bundle branch block. Although some authorities advocate 24-h Holter monitoring prior to discharge and specific antiarrhythmic therapy, proof of effective therapy is lacking. Studies suggest that β-blockers (e.g., timolol) reduce the incidence of sudden death post-MI. A recent study concluded that sulfinpyrazone does also, but the conclusions have been challenged and the drug is not approved for such use by the FDA. Current knowledge supports the need to analyze carefully the patients at risk and individualize therapy.

SUDDEN CARDIAC DEATH (SCD)

SCD does not have a single, uniform definition. Broadly, it is *death due to a primary cardiac cause or mechanism occurring within 24 h of the onset of acute illness in a person thought to be free of heart disease or with symptomatically mild cardiac disease.* For many purposes the definition is restricted to a narrower time-span, such as instantaneous death, death within 1 h, 2 h, 6 h, etc., or simply prehospitalization death.

Etiology and Pathophysiology

In adults, > 90% of SCDs are due to coronary heart disease. Advanced coronary arteriosclerosis is found in 2 or 3 of the major coronary vessels in at least 75% of cases; 15% have a major narrowing of a single coronary vessel, and < 10% are free of substantial coronary artery disease. Evidence of old myocardial infarction is found in 50% of the patients, and 25% have small (< 1 cm in size) fibrotic scars in the myocardium. Acute coronary obstruction due to a ruptured plaque or thrombus is found in 40 or 50% of SCDs. Histologic changes of acute myocardial infarction are found in only 10 or 15% of cases since a minimum of 6 to 12 h of continued life after the onset of severe ischemia is required for such changes to become visible on light microscopy. However, in 5 or 10% of SCDs, the histologic age of such fresh infarcts antedates symptoms described retrospectively by relatives and close acquaintances.

Ventricular fibrillation is the most common cardiac rhythm observed immediately or shortly after the collapse of SCD victims, and cardiac standstill is found with increased frequency later following collapse. Little is known about antecedent rhythm disturbances. SCD can be due to ventricular fibrillation unassociated with acute myocardial infarction. Over 1/2 of the patients resuscitated from ventricular fibrillation outside the hospital do not develop clinical, ECG, or enzymatic characteristics of myocardial infarction.

In addition to arrhythmias, the pathophysiologic mechanisms that can result in sudden death include intrinsic pump failure due to loss of cardiac muscle; electromechanical dissociation; loss of valvular function due to perforation of a cusp or to rupture or incompetency of a papillary muscle; ventricular septal perforation with shunt development; extrinsic pump failure with pressure overload; cardiac rupture with or without tamponade; or emboli.

Other underlying diseases include rheumatic heart disease (especially aortic valvular disease), hypertensive heart disease, infiltrative and fibrotic processes involving the heart, cardiomyopathies, myocarditis, congenital heart diseases (especially those associated with cyanosis or aortic stenosis), cor pulmonale, bacterial endocarditis with cusp perforation, aneurysms with dissection or rupture, and emboli to the coronary or peripheral vessels. Ventricular fibrillation and SCD have been associated with the prolonged Q-T syndrome (which may be accompanied by deafness) and, on occasion, with the ballooning mitral valve syndrome. Some SCD seems to be neurally mediated, and sometimes the toxic effect of drugs prescribed to treat cardiovascular or other disease is causal.

Risk Factors

The risk factors for SCD are basically the same as for arteriosclerotic heart disease, but the most important risk factors are a history of myocardial infarction and the degree of its severity, particularly as manifested by residual impairment of cardiac function. This may be seen in residual S-T segment abnormalities in the ECG at rest, cardiomegaly, and heart failure. When associated with heart disease, ventricular arrhythmias of increasing frequency and severity—e.g., more than 10/h or 2/min, multifocal or coupled premature ventricular contractions, and ventricular tachycardia—are risk factors. However, ventricular arrhythmias without readily detectable heart disease carry little or no added risk for SCD.

Symptoms, Signs, and Clinical Course

By retrospectively questioning the family, new or modified symptoms of cardiovascular disease can be found in perhaps 2/3 of SCD victims—over several days, or sometimes for just hours or minutes. These may be a new chest discomfort, palpitations, an increase in anginal pain, breathlessness for no apparent reason, symptoms referrable to the musculoskeletal system or GI tract, overwhelming fatigue, or depression. Such symptoms are not specific for impending SCD, and the frequency with which SCD follows them is unknown.

It is often not possible to define the onset of acute illness precisely. The symptoms are often within the range of normal experience for the victim and represent premonitory symptoms of impending SCD only in retrospect. In other instances typical symptoms of acute myocardial infarction may progress rapidly to death. Denial of the significance of symptoms and the nonspecificity of many symptoms are 2 major impediments to the early recognition and adequate medical care of SCD victims. Half of those who die of ischemic heart disease die within 1 h of the onset of their acute illness, including the 25 to 33% who drop dead instantaneously or are found dead.

Laboratory Findings and Diagnosis

Diagnosis of SCD is best made from the clinical findings in association with autopsy confirmation of coronary or cardiac disease. Other illnesses that can cause death shortly after onset must be excluded; e.g., pulmonary emboli, deaths due to drugs, hepatic decompensation (especially with alcoholism), stroke, overwhelming infections (particularly pneumonias and infections of the CNS), and GI bleeding or perforation. Noncardiac causes must be carefully sought in victims whose death is unwitnessed or whose history is unreliable. The absence of ECG findings of infarction should not negate the diagnosis of SCD nor diminish appropriate treatment for patients with symptoms of acute cardiovascular disease.

Management

Management of SCD can be considered in the categories of chronic prophylactic therapy, the early therapy of acute cardiovascular symptoms, and cardiac resuscitation for patients who develop sudden cardiac arrest.

Although ventricular fibrillation may be the precipitating, and is certainly the final, event in most cases of SCD, long-term use of currently available antiarrhythmic drugs is rarely recommended for prophylaxis against SCD. Drugs that are most effective in abolishing and preventing ventricular arrhythmias can be parenterally administered in the hospital, but are usually not suitable for long-term oral administration. Orally effective drugs that reduce or prevent ventricular arrhythmias have not shown or have not been studied adequately enough to show efficacy in saving lives, except in the very small number of patients with recurrent ventricular fibrillation. They often have extensive side effects; some have to be taken q 3 to 6 h; and for optimal therapy the dose of some may have to be adjusted to achieve specific blood levels. Chronic antiarrhythmic therapy directed against ventricular arrhythmias is best restricted to patients who have significant symptoms from their arrhythmias. Effectiveness of a drug in reducing premature ventricular contractions should not be automatically equated with effectiveness in prophylaxis against SCD.

Procainamide is effective at blood levels of 4 to 8 µg/ml, which commonly require from 1.5 to 4 gm/day divided into q 3 to 6 h doses. The drug decreases the incidence of or totally abolishes ventricular arrhythmias in many patients, though its efficacy in lengthening life has not been proved. Because of side effects of migratory arthralgias, rashes, fevers, and a lupus-like syndrome, about 25% of patients must discontinue the drug within 1 mo, 50% of patients within 3 mo, and 75% by 18 mo. Most patients develop antinuclear antibodies. Discontinuing the drug reverses these effects.

Quinidine sulfate also is generally effective in abolishing ventricular arrhythmias. Its effective blood level is usually in the range of 3 to 6 µg/ml; this requires a typical oral dose of 200 to 400 mg q 6 h. Side effects include GI tract upset and the complete range of cinchonism, nervous system disturbances, thrombocytopenic purpura, and drug fever. Most importantly, it can provoke arrhythmias, including some that may be fatal.

Phenytoin has been used less extensively and with fewer side effects, but with little proof of effectiveness; suggested blood levels are 8 to 16 µg/ml, requiring 300 to 400 mg/day given orally in divided doses. Recent studies show no evidence of benefit against SCD from such a regimen.

Disopyramide 400 to 800 mg/day divided into 4 doses can be given. The claim that systemic side effects are less frequent than with other antiarrhythmic drugs is not generally accepted. Hypotension may develop with inadequately compensated congestive heart failure or in the presence of primary cardiomyopathy. As with quinidine, a propensity for Q-T prolongation and ventricular tachycardia and fibrillation is possible.

Some encouraging reports suggest that long-term administration of β-**adrenergic blocking agents** may reduce SCD in survivors of acute myocardial infarction; the data for **timolol maleate** are highly favorable, and this agent is available in the USA. The efficacy of propranolol as a long-term agent in the prevention of SCD is now being evaluated through large-scale clinical trial in the USA.

None of the above drugs should be used in patients with 2nd or 3rd degree atrioventricular block unless they have a cardiac pacemaker. For more detailed discussions of the administration, effects, and side effects of the above drugs, see CARDIAC ARRHYTHMIAS, and MYOCARDIAL INFARCTION, above.

A cardiac pacemaker, particularly the demand or standby type, may benefit patients who develop conduction disturbances that are likely to progress abruptly to complete heart block. There is some evidence that patients who develop bifascicular block, especially in association with peri-infarction block, during the course of acute myocardial infarction are at substantial risk for the subsequent abrupt development of complete heart block.

For profound bradycardias (heart rate < 50) or bradycardia associated with hypotension (heart rate < 60 with systolic BP < 100 mm Hg), the patient should be recumbent with his feet slightly elevated. Atropine 0.3, 0.6, or up to 1 mg IV or 2 or 3 mg IM is also generally needed. The IV dose may be repeated 2 or 3 times at 5 or 10 min intervals up to a maximum dose of 2 mg. The goal is to increase the heart rate to around 70/min and thereby augment cardiac output and BP.

Specific therapy for acute cardiac arrest follows directly.

CARDIAC ARREST AND CARDIOPULMONARY RESUSCITATION (CPR)

Arrest of circulation or serious depression of breathing is an urgent crisis that takes precedence over all others except control of massive external hemorrhage, which should be treated simultaneously. Either the heart or the lungs may fail first; the 2 events usually are closely related.

Cardiac arrest (*absent or inadequate heart contraction*) is manifested clinically by absent heart sounds, pulse, and BP, apnea, unconsciousness, and dilated pupils. It may be due to ventricular fibrillation (85%), cardiac standstill (10%), or circulatory collapse with sudden hypotension due to vasodilation or hypovolemia (5%). In **ventricular fibrillation** the contraction of the heart muscle fibers is uncoordinated and circulation ceases because cardiac output falls. It may be caused by low-voltage electric shock (110 to 220 volts for 2 to 3 seconds); sudden ionic imbalances (especially potassium) from hemolysis or fresh water drowning; sympathetic stimulation of a myocardium sensitized by chemical or anesthetic agents (epinephrine, cyclopropane); profound hypothermia; or, most typically, focal anoxia from coronary artery spasm or obstruction. **Cardiac standstill,** in which the ventricles are motionless and no blood is ejected from the right or left side of the heart, is usually caused by severe generalized anoxia or local myocardial O_2 lack. **Circulatory collapse** occurs when the heart beat, which may be rhythmic, is insufficient to produce a peripheral pulse or BP—as in syncope, vasomotor collapse, profound hypothermia, CNS damage, hypovolemic shock, electro-mechanical dissociation, serious hemorrhage, septicemia, and drug or anesthetic overdose.

Respiratory arrest may be caused by airway obstruction or respiratory depression, or it may be secondary to cardiac arrest. Cyanosis (except in CO poisoning) and eventually dilated pupils and cardiac arrest follow respiratory arrest. **Airway obstruction** may be partial or complete and may be due to blocking by the tongue, a foreign body, blood, mucus, or other substance; to spasm or edema of the vocal cords; or to inflammation, neoplasm, constriction, or trauma of the air passages. **Respiratory depression** implies inadequate ventilation and is diagnosed by obtaining an arterial blood gas which demonstrates hypoxemia and hypercapnia (hypercarbia). These phenomena progress to tissue or cellular hypoxia that further depresses breathing and circulation. Respiratory depression may be due to various factors acting on different components of the respiratory system: (1) **the CNS** (drug overdose, toxic gases, disease of or injury to the brain or spinal cord); (2) **upper and lower airways and the lungs** (submersion, strangulation, asphyxiation, aspiration); (3) **the lungs or chest wall,** thus disturbing the normal physiologic mechanisms of ventilation (pneumothorax, crushed chest, pulmonary edema); or (4) **the blood and circulatory system** (profound shock, CO or cyanide poisoning, electrocution, cardiac tamponade, severe hemorrhage).

TECHNICS OF CARDIOPULMONARY RESUSCITATION (CPR)

Successful CPR requires speed and efficiency. *Delay may be fatal!* Adequate amounts of O_2 must be distributed to the tissues constantly; tissue anoxia for > 4 to 6 min results in irreversible brain damage or death. CPR must be continued until the patient recovers or is pronounced dead. Breathing and heartbeat have been restored in humans after as long as 3 h of resuscitation.

The cause of the emergency—near-drowning, strangulation, suffocation, CO inhalation, electrocution, barbiturate intoxication, anesthetic overdose, insecticide poisoning, pulmonary embolism, or myocardial infarction—may require additional specific treatment, but the basic principles of heart-lung resuscitation apply to all field and hospital situations. The methods of artificial respiration described below are superior to the former manual resuscitation methods (e.g., back pressure or arm lift) and should be used in any situation except when severe facial injuries preclude the use of direct oronasal methods.

The A-B-C-D mnemonic (FIG. 25-41) is a simple, effective reminder of resuscitation situations and treatment. The exact time of arrest should be noted and assistance sought. If the patient is being monitored, a precordial thump, performed by raising a clenched fist 12 in. above the sternum and delivering a firm "thump," may be used initially, followed by the 4 A-B-C-D steps. In a non-monitored arrest, the 4 A-B-C-D steps are used initially. The 4 steps should be performed quickly, precisely, and in order. Sometimes spontaneous breathing resumes after **(A)—(A)irway is opened**—and further steps are not needed. Sometimes after **(B)—(B)reathing is restored,** circulation resumes spontaneously and cardiac compression is not needed.

(A)—(A)irway Opened

Restoration of adequate ventilation of the lungs is essential in both respiratory and circulatory arrest, and a **patent airway** is the first and most important requisite. In an unconscious subject, the neck flexes, the relaxed lower jaw drops down and backward, and the tongue obstructs the pharynx. The best manual maneuver to overcome this obstruction is to tilt the head back into maximum extension—thus stretching the neck muscles, lifting the jaw, and drawing the tongue away from the posterior pharyngeal wall. The technic is the same for patients of all ages. Place one hand behind the patient's neck and the other on top of his head. Then lift the neck and extend the head so that the chin points almost straight up (FIGS. 25-42a, 25-42b). Any dentures should be removed promptly.

(B)—(B)reathing Restored

If spontaneous breathing does not resume after the air passage has been opened, *artificial respiration should be started by mouth-to-mouth resuscitation* (expired-air ventilation, rescue breathing). The heel of one hand is pressed against the victim's forehead to keep his head extended backward, and his nostrils are pinched shut with the thumb and index finger of the same hand to prevent escape of air (FIG. 25-42b). (With experience and practice, his nose can be sealed with the rescuer's cheek.) The rescuer should open his own mouth widely, take a deep breath, place his mouth over the victim's (making a tight seal), and blow until he feels the lungs expand and sees the chest rise. The victim's passive exhalation should be heard when the rescuer removes his mouth. Initially, 4 quick breaths should be given in rapid succession without allowing time for complete deflation. Single breaths follow—about 12 times/min for adults, 20 times/min for children.

For adults, breaths of about 1 L each—i.e., twice the normal tidal volume—will maintain normal blood O_2 saturation and CO_2 elimination. Smaller breaths are required for children, and only small puffs from the rescuer's cheeks for small babies. Inhaled air contains about 21% O_2 and a trace of CO_2. Exhaled air, which contains about 16% O_2 and 4 to 5% CO_2, is more than adequate to maintain

HEART-LUNG RESUSCITATION

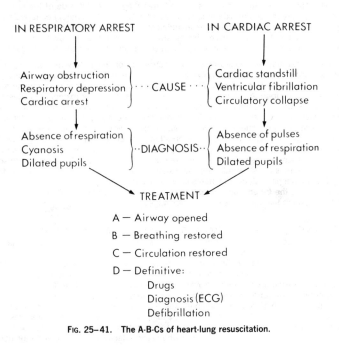

IN RESPIRATORY ARREST   IN CARDIAC ARREST

Airway obstruction   Cardiac standstill
Respiratory depression · · · CAUSE · · · Ventricular fibrillation
Cardiac arrest   Circulatory collapse

Absence of respiration   Absence of pulses
Cyanosis   · · DIAGNOSIS · · Absence of respiration
Dilated pupils   Dilated pupils

TREATMENT

A — Airway opened

B — Breathing restored

C — Circulation restored

D — Definitive:
      Drugs
      Diagnosis (ECG)
      Defibrillation

FIG. 25–41.   The A-B-Cs of heart-lung resuscitation.

a victim's blood O_2 and CO_2 at normal levels if the recommended rate and amplitude are used. If the rescuer develops hyperventilation alkalosis (manifested by dizziness, numbness, ringing in the ears, and paresthesias), the respiratory rate should be slower or the amplitude of each breath decreased.

After opening the airway and applying mouth-to-mouth or mouth-to-nose breathing, if the chest does not rise, the rescuer should assume that **the air passage is still blocked.** The blockage may be removed by sweeping a finger through the patient's mouth and pharynx. If this is not possible or if it does not relieve the obstruction, dislodging it should be tried. A small child can be picked up and inverted over the forearm. Firm blows should be delivered with the heel of one hand over the spine between the shoulder blades (FIG. 25–43a). If the patient is an adult or a large child, the **Heimlich maneuver** is the preferred treatment: the victim is rolled onto his stomach and, straddling his lower torso, the rescuer clasps both hands to form a fist just below the xiphoid process (the cartilage at the lower end of the sternum). A sudden rapid upward movement with the clenched hands causes intrapulmonary pressure to rise suddenly and expels the foreign body from the trachea. This can also be performed with the subject supine by applying pressure to the upper mid-abdomen. With progressive hypoxia the throat muscles relax, and this maneuver frequently will dislodge a supralaryngeal foreign body and CPR can be resumed quickly. If obstruction persists, a cricothyroidotomy or tracheostomy must be performed; in fact, high airway obstruction is almost the only indication for emergency tracheostomy today since oral airways or endotracheal tubes are preferred during resuscitation (see ESTABLISHMENT OF AN EMERGENCY AIRWAY in Ch. 31 for details of these procedures).

Mouth-to-nose resuscitation is done in essentially the same way as mouth-to-mouth resuscitation, except that the rescuer should hold the patient's lower jaw shut with one hand, seal the victim's mouth with his cheek, open his own mouth widely enough to assure a tight seal around the patient's nose, and inflate the lungs via the nostrils (FIG. 25–42d). **Combined mouth-and-nose resuscitation** is used for infants and small children. The mouth is placed over both mouth and nose and the lungs are inflated about 20 times/min, varying the amount of air according to the size of the child (FIG. 25–43d). In children and some adults the stomach may become excessively distended with air; only if the distention impairs respiration should one attempt to relieve it. If this happens, the head or entire body is turned to the side and the epigastrium compressed to eliminate the distention (FIG. 25–43e).

The most common errors in performing expired-air resuscitation are inadequate extension of the victim's head, inadequate opening of the rescuer's mouth, and an inadequate seal around the victim's mouth or nose. If the above methods fail to ventilate the victim adequately, endotracheal intubation and/or emergency tracheostomy should be performed. These procedures require experience

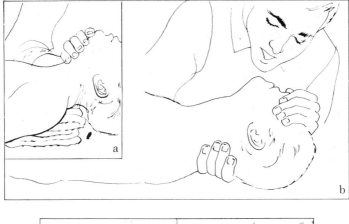

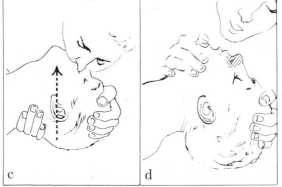

FIG. 25–42. **Expired air ventilation—adult. (a)** Position to open airway alone. **(b)** Proper position of hands and patient for opening the airway and mouth-to-mouth respiration. **(c)** Position of heads of resuscitator and patient for mouth to mouth respiration with cheek occluding nostrils. **(d)** Proper positioning for mouth-to-nose respiration.

and skill and should be used *only* if the above methods fail (see under ESTABLISHMENT OF AN EMERGENCY AIRWAY in Ch. 31).

(C)—(C)irculation Restored

This method of providing artificial circulation is called **external cardiac compression,** or **closed-chest cardiac compression.** Firm pressure on the lower sternum compresses the ventricles and results in a cardiac output shown by a palpable peripheral pulse, measurable BP and flow, and constriction of dilated pupils.

The victim is placed on a flat hard surface (e.g., floor, operating table, litter, bed-board). The heel of one hand is placed over the lower half of the sternum—*not* over the xiphoid process—and the other hand on top of the first. Then the rescuer should thrust straight downward, keeping his arms straight and using the weight of the upper part of his body to exert 80 to 100 lb of pressure; this should depress the sternum 1½ to 2 in. and hold for 0.5 seconds. The rescuer's hands should be kept in place while he releases the pressure. This cycle is repeated uniformly and smoothly about once/second, allowing equal time for compression and relaxation (systole and diastole). This smooth regular rhythm provides satisfactory blood flow, allows adequate time for cardiac refill, and avoids injuries from jerky, irregular efforts.

The heel of only one hand is used to perform external cardiac compression on children up to age 8 to 10 yr; the other hand can provide firm support beneath the chest. Only 2 fingertips are needed to compress the center of the sternum of a baby or very small child.

When properly performed, external cardiac compression should produce a BP of 80 mm Hg or higher, even though cardiac output is only about ⅓ to ½ of normal. This usually causes a palpable carotid pulse—a sign of adequate cerebral blood flow. However, the pupils frequently give the best

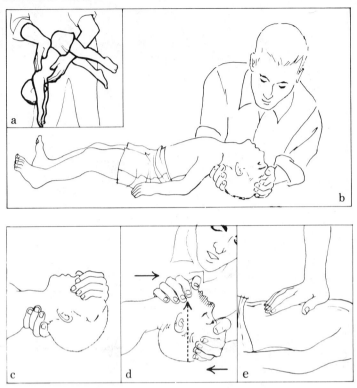

FIG. 25–43.   **Expired air ventilation—child. (a)** Dislodgement of foreign bodies from tracheobronchial tube. **(b)** Hyperextension of head to open the airway. **(c)** Position for mouth-to-mouth respiration. **(d)** Position for mouth-to-nose respiration. **(e)** Emptying of air from the stomach by pressure in left upper quadrant.

evidence of effective artificial circulation. Constricted pupils indicate adequate brain perfusion; dilated pupils indicate inadequate oxygenation of the brain and imminent death.

External cardiac compression alone does not ventilate the lungs; mouth-to-mouth resuscitation must be used for this. The combination constitutes **heart-lung (or cardiopulmonary) resuscitation.** A good routine is to follow the **Rule of 5:** Begin resuscitation in < **5** min; give the victim **5** breaths with mouth-to-mouth resuscitation; then start external cardiac compression and interpose 2 breaths between each 15 compressions; **never interrupt CPR for > 5 seconds until breathing and pulse have been restored.**

When 2 rescuers are present, a physiologically sound and practical technic is for one rescuer to interpose a breath between every 5 chest compressions by a 2nd rescuer. This avoids serious pauses in the circulation, allows continued chest compressions at about 60/min, and provides full lung inflations 12 times/min, thus assuring optimum oxygenation, BP, and blood flow.

If CPR is performed without assistance, the heart is compressed 15 times at a rate of 80/min, then the victim's head is quickly extended and the lungs are inflated twice, mouth-to-mouth. This cycle is repeated continuously. While this does not provide optimum ventilation and circulation, it is the best alternative until a 2nd rescuer arrives.

When CPR is carried out in a hospital, the adequacy of ventilation must be checked by obtaining an arterial blood sample (see under Therapy of Respiratory Failure in Ch. 32). Peripheral cyanosis is not a reliable guide to adequate oxygenation since it is influenced by local circulatory factors, lighting, and Hb content of blood.

External cardiac compression can cause injuries, but these should be minimal if the procedure is done properly. Practice and attention to detail will minimize trauma. **Costochondral separation** and **fractured ribs** may occur and sometimes cannot be avoided in pressing hard enough to produce a peripheral pulse; this type of injury is a small price for successful resuscitation. **Bone marrow emboli** have been reported after external cardiac compression, but evidence that they were a cause of death is lacking. External cardiac compression does not cause serious **heart damage** unless there is a preexisting ventricular aneurysm. **Lung damage** is rare but pneumothorax secondary to rib fracture can occur. **Laceration of the liver** is the most serious (sometimes fatal) complication and is usually caused by pressing too low on the sternum. *Do not press down on the xiphoid process!*

(D)—(D)efinitive Treatment

The cause of cardiac arrest—ventricular fibrillation, cardiac standstill, or circulatory collapse—can be diagnosed with assurance only from an ECG or its oscilloscope tracing. **Drugs** and **defibrillation equipment** should be made ready even before the ECG has been obtained because ventricular fibrillation causes at least 85% of the arrests in hospitalized patients and empiric therapy should be given. If unsuccessful an ECG will be necessary before further definitive measures are instituted. **Epinephrine** IV (5 to 10 ml of a 1:10,000 solution) may be given at the emergency site even before the diagnosis is established. It increases vasomotor tone, raises BP, and has a direct myocardial effect that improves the quality of ventricular contraction and promotes adequate cardiac output. The dosage is repeated q 3 to 5 min or as needed.

Blood rapidly becomes severely acidotic after cardiac arrest, despite effective CPR. One to two 50-ml ampules of 7.5% **sodium bicarbonate** (each containing 3.75 gm or 44.6 mEq) may be given *rapidly* IV and continued at a rate of 50 ml q 5 to 10 min if necessary (as indicated by arterial pH monitoring) to reverse the acidosis and improve myocardial function; this similarly assists in defibrillation and in restoring a normal heartbeat and cardiac output. In especially desperate situations, when myocardial action is weak and digitalis toxicity is not a risk, **calcium chloride** IV (10 ml of a 10% solution) may help to restore myocardial tone, pulse pressure, and cardiac output with a minimum of side effects. **Lidocaine** IV 50 to 100 mg as a bolus and 1 to 3 mg/min as an infusion (50 ml of 2% lidocaine in 1 L of 5% D/W) decreases myocardial irritability in recurrent or refractory ventricular tachycardia or fibrillation; repeated doses between defibrillation attempts are often needed. **Isoproterenol** given by IV infusion is frequently utilized for slow idioventricular rhythm until a pacemaker can be placed (a 5-ml ampul, containing 1 mg of isoproterenol, is diluted in 250 ml of 5% D/W). An ECG should be obtained immediately. The tracing will show ventricular fibrillation, absent ventricular activity, or, rarely, slow ventricular complexes of normal amplitude originating in an A-V junctional or ventricular pacemaker.

Ventricular fibrillation is treated with electrical countershock (precordial shock) with a direct-current capacitor discharge using a shock of 200 to 300 joules delivered energy. When defibrillation is unsuccessful, epinephrine 3 to 5 ml of a 1:10,000 solution (1:1000 solution diluted with 10 parts of normal saline) is given IV or, in the absence of effective circulation, down the endotracheal tube, and countershock is repeated. If weak, but inadequate, cardiac contractions return following defibrillation, 5 to 10 ml of 10% calcium chloride are given IV unless digitalis toxicity is a risk. When ventricular fibrillation is due to digitalis toxicity or results from the degeneration of ventricular tachycardia, rapid IV infusion of phenytoin 5 mg/kg IV at a rate of 50 mg/min up to 1 gm total dose or lidocaine 50 to 100 mg repeated 3 times at 1-min intervals IV will facilitate defibrillation and lessen the risk of relapse. Procainamide in 100-mg boluses followed by an infusion of 2 to 6 mg/min should be instituted if ventricular fibrillation recurs. Recurrent ventricular fibrillation may be controlled by continuous infusion of lidocaine 2 to 4 mg/min or procainamide 2 to 6 mg/min followed after 2 to 3 days with oral doses of quinidine 400 mg t.i.d. or q.i.d., procainamide 0.5 to 1.0 gm q 4 to 6 h, or phenytoin 100 mg q 6 h. In recurrent ventricular fibrillation or tachycardia unresponsive to these agents, bretylium tosylate should be administered. Hypotension may follow cardiac arrest, for which levarterenol (2 ampuls [8 mg] in 1 L of 5% D/W), metaraminol (200 mg in 1 L of 5% D/W), dopamine (200 mg in 500 ml of 5% D/W), or dobutamine (250 mg in 250 ml of 5% D/W) may be infused IV.

Following defibrillation, adequate cardiac output is not reliably indicated by a satisfactory ECG or oscilloscope tracing, but *only by the peripheral pulse or BP*. Sometimes CPR must be resumed after defibrillation and continued until breathing, peripheral pulse, and BP indicate restored cardiorespiratory function. Continued use of supportive drugs may be needed.

Cardiac standstill with absent ventricular complexes on the ECG is treated by the IV or intracardiac administration of epinephrine 3 to 5 ml of a 1:10,000 solution (or isoproterenol 2 mg). Calcium chloride (5 ml of a 10% solution) and atropine sulfate (0.5 to 1.0 mg) can be administered IV if rhythm is not restored. An **electrical catheter pacemaker** can be passed IV into the right ventricle. The stimulus of 3 to 10 milliamps is delivered at a rate of 70 to 80 times/min. Administration of calcium chloride 5 to 10 ml of a 10% solution IV may be tried if pacing failure persists.

Mechanical cardiac failure with satisfactory ventricular complexes on the ECG is a common complication of acute myocardial infarction. External cardiac compression, artificial respiration, IV infusion of sodium bicarbonate, electrical pacing, and infusion of epinephrine should be tried. Calcium chloride should be administered. Dopamine 4 μg/kg/min IV or isoproterenol (1 mg in 250 ml of 5% D/W, given at a rate of 10 to 20 drops/min) may also be used and increased if necessary. It is important to remember that cardiac tamponade can cause electro-mechanical dissociation and is readily treatable by pericardiocentesis. (For PERICARDIOCENTESIS, see PERICARDIAL DISEASE in Ch. 25.)

Special circumstances pertain when the ECG is already under observation at the time of cardiac arrest and when other electrical equipment is available for immediate use. If the delay is not > 90 seconds after the onset of arrest, a precordial thump is delivered. Countershock is given or electrical pacing is started (according to the ECG findings) before attempting resuscitation.

Caution is necessary to maintain both cardiac compression and pulmonary ventilation with the fewest and shortest interruptions possible. The distended ventricle should be emptied of blood by chest compression immediately before and after each procedure to ensure optimum conditions for contraction.

Treatment is terminated and the patient is pronounced dead if the pupils remain dilated and no sign of spontaneous respiration or cardiac contraction has appeared within 30 min. However, if a favorable change in these signs indicates that resuscitation may still be possible, treatment should be continued up to 60 to 90 min. Patients with hypothermia represent a special circumstance—CPR should continue until external warming has raised body temperature to normal, since successful resuscitation of the hypothermic patient has been reported after several hours of resuscitation (see also Ch. 217). Because the successfully resuscitated patient frequently relapses into cardiac arrest, it is important to monitor the ECG closely and keep other equipment in readiness until this danger has passed.

MECHANICAL RESUSCITATIVE DEVICES

Mechanical devices are not intended to and should not replace immediate mouth-to-mouth ventilation and manual external cardiac compression. They should be used only when available within seconds or to replace manual methods during sustained resuscitation or when the patient must be moved. Specialized equipment should be used only by experienced personnel.

Airway Adjuncts

The **face mask** may be a standard or modified anesthesia mask, available in children's and adults' sizes. A mask with a hand-compressible, self-inflating air bag attached is especially helpful. The victim's jaw must be kept elevated (FIGS. 25–42, 25–43) during its use and the mask held tightly over the nose and mouth. A collapsible plastic mask, which can be carried in a pocket, is also available.

The **double oropharyngeal airway** is more difficult to use, since the rescuer's fingers must seal the victim's lips around the tube while the thumbs clamp the nose. Muscle spasm may make insertion difficult or impossible for an inexperienced rescuer, and the airway in the victim's throat may stimulate vomiting as he regains consciousness. A simple **oral airway** or **breathing tube** that fits between the victim's teeth without a pharyngeal extension is preferable and easier to use. A new device, an **esophageal obturator airway**, consists of a tube with a balloon which is inserted into the esophagus. With this in place all air must pass into the trachea if it is not occluded. This device has been used extensively for resuscitations carried out in nonhospital environments.

Cuffed endotracheal tubes, either the orotracheal or the longer nasotracheal, secure the airway and prevent aspiration. Skill is required to place these tubes, especially in an uncooperative patient, and the unskilled should not attempt to use them in place of the mouth-to-mouth technic. A firm rubber nasotracheal airway will sometimes slip easily into the trachea, but the orotracheal tube requires a laryngoscope.

Mechanical Resuscitators

Mechanical respirators, resuscitators, inhalation therapy units, and anesthesia machines can be used to provide artificial respiration if the victim's head is properly positioned and an adequate airway is maintained. One must always be sure that the chest is moving since improper positioning of the head can cause airway obstruction and one may only inflate the stomach. Mechanical resuscitators are valuable for prolonged resuscitation, transportation of the patient, or O_2 therapy. They usually include an aspirator for removing mucus, blood, or vomitus from the airway and are discussed in Ch. 32.

Mechanical External Cardiac Compressors

Mechanical external cardiac compression devices activated by compressed air or O_2 can be used while transporting a victim of circulatory arrest. Some of these devices tilt the head backward and have a ventilation line supplying adjustable volume-cycled artificial respiration that can be used alone or interposed between chest compressions. With such equipment, only one rescuer is needed to hold the face mask and head. It should be used only by an experienced operator.

MYOCARDIAL DISEASE

Primary myocardial pathology is suspected when valvular, congenital, hypertensive, and pulmonary disease can be excluded, and there is no sign of myocardial ischemia to explain ventricular failure, cardiac enlargement, or other evidence of heart disease. Myocardial diseases that present mainly with ventricular failure include **myocarditis** and noninflammatory **cardiomyopathy. Hypertrophic cardiomyopathies** (idiopathic hypertrophic subaortic stenosis and idiopathic concentric hypertrophy) may present with syncope or sudden death. Some forms of cardiomyopathy mimic pericarditis. Myocardial involvement (including some forms of myocarditis) can also occur secondary to a number of systemic diseases.

MYOCARDITIS

Focal or diffuse inflammation of the myocardium which may be due to infectious agents, other causes of inflammation, or toxins.

A wide range of pathologic lesions can occur in myocarditis, including cellular infiltration, granulomatous lesions, myocardial necrosis, and interstitial fibrosis. In South America, **Chagas' disease** causes a chronic myocarditis with congestive heart failure; an acute form can be fatal. In addition to infectious causes, myocarditis may be due to sensitivity to drugs (e.g., emetine) or heterologous serum, toxic chemicals such as CO, or excessive radiation exposure. Myocarditis may also be seen in association with SLE, scleroderma, rheumatic fever, RA, or sarcoidosis. **Fiedler's myocarditis** is a rare and usually fatal condition in which the myocardial inflammation cannot be related to a previous or concurrent illness; a viral etiology has been postulated. Viral damage to the myocardium and the other structures of the heart seems to be fairly common. Some viruses are highly cardiotropic; e.g., the picornavirus group, which includes poliovirus, coxsackie-virus groups A and B, and the encephalomyocarditis (EMC) virus.

Symptoms, Signs, and Diagnosis

Myocarditis is difficult to diagnose clinically unless cardiovascular function is impaired. It presents with fatigue, dyspnea, palpitations, and occasionally precordial discomfort that occur during the first few weeks of a systemic infection, although diagnostic evidence of myocarditis may only become evident as the systemic infection is subsiding. Cardiac enlargement, a murmur or a pericardial friction rub, a gallop rhythm, or pulsus alternans may develop later. The first heart sound may be faint, and neck vein distention may appear when congestive heart failure develops. Persistent fever occurs, and the tachycardia is out of proportion to the degree of fever. Pulmonary or systemic emboli may occur, and nonspecific ECG abnormalities (supraventricular or ventricular arrhythmias, conduction defects, and ST-T abnormalities) are common. The earliest diagnostic changes to be noted are usually S-T segment and T wave abnormalities.

Diagnosis frequently depends on exclusion of other causes of cardiac disease, the presence of a specific systemic disorder, and identification of the physiologic abnormalities by routine measures and in some laboratories by cardiac catheterization and angiographic studies.

Course and Treatment

Myocarditis varies in severity. Recovery from mild myocarditis may ensue without residual cardiac insufficiency. With more severe involvement, heart failure may be fulminant and acute, and recurrent or chronic myocarditis may develop. Treatment includes managing the underlying infection or other condition, measures to decrease cardiac work, and control of ventricular failure, arrhythmias, and embolization that may occur. When myocarditis is suspected or apparent, complete bed rest and sedation, plus continued therapy of the underlying disease, are needed. O_2 is indicated for cyanosis or dyspnea.

Corticosteroids may be helpful in early acute myocarditis but should be used cautiously, since depression of immunologic defenses risks spread of systemic infection. Prednisone or prednisolone in minimal daily doses of 40 to 60 mg is given orally for 4 to 6 wk, then decreased (when response has been favorable) by 10 mg at 5-day intervals. Corticosteroids are discontinued after 8 to 12 wk if no clinical or laboratory signs of activity are still present. Rest must be continued until all evidence of cardiac involvement has disappeared.

CARDIOMYOPATHY

The cardiomyopathies include a variety of noninflammatory pathologic lesions of the myocardium. The term "cardiomyopathy" may refer to **primary cardiomyopathy,** which is idiopathic, or may be used literally to mean "heart muscle pathology" in the broadest sense, thus referring also to **secondary cardiomyopathy,** in which the etiology is known. Possible causes of secondary cardiomyopathy include viral infections, anemia, hypo- and hyperthyroidism, alcoholism, nutritional disorders, toxic agents, x-irradiation, bacterial infections, ischemia, the aging process, and many others. When found, any potential etiologic agent should be eliminated immediately to *prevent* the development of myocardial disease. Some causative agents are discussed below.

In obese patients with excess epicardial fat, **adipose tissue** may extend into the myocardium, causing atrophy of and replacing the muscle fibers. **Amyloid** may be deposited in the interstitium of the myocardium and conduction system, causing atrophy of encompassed myofibers. In patients with **Friedreich's ataxia,** focal destruction of myofibers, replacement fibrosis, infiltration with lymphocytes or occasionally with polymorphonuclear leukocytes, and hypertrophy of intact muscle cells may be found. Abnormal deposition of glycogen in myofibers has been observed in patients with a **deficiency of α-1,4-glucosidase.** In patients with **tuberous sclerosis,** deposition of glycogen may produce atrial or ventricular nodular lesions that may encroach on the lumena of the chambers. **Hemochromatosis** may include accumulation of hemosiderin within the myofibers, leading to focal scarring. The hearts of patients with **progressive muscular dystrophy** may show areas of fibrosis with atrophy of some muscle fibers and hypertrophy of others. Fatty changes, degeneration, and swelling of muscle fibers may accompany prolonged **hypervolemic shock, severe anemia,** or **thiamine deficiency.**

Endocardial fibroelastosis, a disorder of unknown cause, is a common form of primary myocardial disease in infancy and early childhood. Elastic tissue proliferates in the subendocardium, causing a diffuse, milky-white thickening of the endocardium and the subendocardium. Ventricular failure due to altered compliance develops, and most patients die before 2 yr of age. In infants or young children, differentiation from idiopathic cardiomyopathy or viral myocarditis is difficult. However, ECG evidence of left ventricular hypertrophy in an infant favors a diagnosis of endocardial fibroelastosis.

Whereas hypertrophy of muscle fibers may accompany most of the lesions described above, hypertrophy of the heart is striking in **idiopathic** or **primary cardiomyopathy.** This form of cardiomyopathy is usually not accompanied by other systemic manifestations. It is a common form of myocardial disease in the USA and Europe and usually occurs in young and middle-aged adults.

Symptoms, Signs, and Diagnosis

The earliest signs of myocardial damage are subtle S-T segment and T wave changes. Serial ECGs reveal progression or regression of the myocardial pathology. As the cardiomyopathy worsens, the patient develops fatigue, dyspnea, palpitations, and precordial discomfort. Ventricular failure with a gallop rhythm, and conduction disturbances including atrial and ventricular arrhythmias can be encountered in most forms of cardiomyopathy. Restriction of ventricular filling resulting from altered myocardial compliance has been observed in the cardiomyopathies associated with amyloidosis and hemochromatosis. Altered valvular function has been encountered in patients with mucopolysaccharidosis due to deposition of the substance in the valves and chordae tendineae. Obstruction to left ventricular outflow has been recorded in patients with glycogen storage disease as well as in those with the idiopathic form. Certain variants of idiopathic cardiomyopathy cause obstruction to left ventricular outflow as the hypertrophied ventricular septum abuts the anterior leaf of the mitral valve during systole.

Ideally, any type of cardiomyopathy must be diagnosed before the disease becomes so extensive that it is irreversible. The diagnosis usually depends on exclusion of other causes of cardiovascular disease, the presence of a specific systemic disorder, and identification of the physiologic abnormalities by routine measures and in some laboratories by echocardiography, cardiac catheterization, and angiocardiography.

Course and Treatment

Response to therapy is much more favorable when the myocardial damage is noted early and the etiologic agent is detected and removed. Absolute bedrest continuously over a prolonged period of time is the most rewarding therapy, permitting the myocardial lesions to heal while the myocardium is working at a reduced load.

Prognosis in idiopathic cardiomyopathy is poor, though temporary improvement may follow treatment of ventricular failure. The average length of life is 2 yr from onset of symptoms, though some patients survive 5 yr or longer. Mural thrombi with pulmonary and systemic embolization may develop during the later course of the disease. At autopsy, only cardiac enlargement is found grossly, but hypertrophy of muscle fibers, moderate fibrosis, and little, if any, inflammatory reaction are seen microscopically.

In most forms of cardiomyopathy, treatment is directed at control of arrhythmias and treatment of congestive phenomena whether due to ventricular failure or restriction of ventricular filling. Relief of subaortic stenosis in the idiopathic form has been accomplished by resection of hypertrophied muscle or the use of β-adrenergic blockers such as propranolol. Cardiotonics (e.g., digitalis, isoproterenol) and drugs that diminish venous return to the heart are *contraindicated* since they increase the degree of outflow obstruction.

HYPERTROPHIC MYOCARDIAL DISEASE

Primary myocardial disease characterized by hypertrophy of the myocardium with no significant cardiac dilation or inflammation.

Hypertrophic myocardial disease rarely presents with congestive heart failure; syncope or sudden death are more common presenting symptoms. Two types account for most cases—idiopathic concentric hypertrophy and idiopathic hypertrophic subaortic stenosis. Both are often familial, and both may manifest anginal pain and A-V and intraventricular conduction defects.

Concentric hypertrophy sometimes occurs early in cardiomyopathy but often presents alone in children or young adults. The patient may complain of chest pain, sometimes anginal, or mild dyspnea on exertion. There may be a history of syncope, palpitations, tachycardias or arrhythmias, or a family history of heart disease or sudden death. No characteristic murmur exists, but an atrial gallop is common. The only constant pathologic feature is hypertrophy of the myocardial cells; fibrosis is common and sometimes extensive.

In **idiopathic hypertrophic subaortic stenosis (IHSS, asymmetric ventricular hypertrophy, obstructive cardiomyopathy),** the hypertrophy affects the ventricular septum more than the rest of the myocardium. IHSS can be confused with valvular aortic stenosis since left ventricular hypertrophy and ejection systolic murmurs, though not maximal in the aortic area, are characteristic. Unlike valvular stenosis, the radial pulse in IHSS is quick and jerky. During systole, the hypertrophied interventricular septum abuts upon the anterior mitral leaflet, producing a functional obstruction to flow. Cardiac catheterization allows measurement of the pressure gradient between the left ventricular cavity and outflow tract, and the narrowing of the outflow tract during systole can be demonstrated by angiocardiography. Echocardiography allows measurement of the septal hypertrophy and visualization of the systolic movement of the anterior mitral leaflet. Right ventricular involvement, simulating pulmonary valvular stenosis, is rare.

Medical treatment involves primarily β-adrenergic blockers, e.g., propranolol. Calcium antagonists, such as verapamil and nifedipine, have recently been reported to be helpful. Obviously, the patient with obstructive hypertrophic myocardial disease, as with any form of cardiomyopathy, should be advised to rest, avoid strenuous activity, and follow proper diet and health measures. **Surgical resection of hypertrophied muscle** has been successful in some patients with progressive cardiac disability. Cardiotonics (e.g., digitalis, isoproterenol) or drugs that diminish venous return to the heart (e.g., nitroglycerin, amyl nitrite) are *contraindicated* since they increase the outflow obstruction.

VALVULAR HEART DISEASE

In the past, most cases of chronic valve disease either resulted from or were ascribed to previous rheumatic fever. With the declining incidence of acute rheumatic fever, other etiologies are increasingly recognized: congenital defects that may not become apparent until late childhood or adult years, myxomatous degeneration, infective endocarditis, syphilis, carcinoid, sclerosis, and calcification. Whatever the etiology, valve obstruction or regurgitation causes characteristic physical and laboratory findings. Echocardiography **(ECHO),** cardiac catheterization, and angiocardiography permit detailing of the structural defect. Secondary infective endocarditis is a continuing hazard for these patients. Antistreptococcal prophylaxis is advisable for those patients who have rheumatic valve disease.

MITRAL VALVE DISEASE

PROLAPSE OF THE MITRAL VALVE

Prolapse of the mitral valve is now recognized as a common and sometimes serious and progressive lesion. Prolapse of one cusp (usually the posterior) or both cusps back into the left atrium during ventricular systole may be **primary,** sometimes occurring in patients with Marfan's syndrome, or as an associated anomaly with atrial septal defect. It may be **secondary** to previous rheumatic fever, ischemic heart disease, cardiomyopathy, or ruptured chordae tendineae.

In the primary form there are protrusions of redundant mitral cusp tissue, frequently with myxomatous degeneration, causing a pleating or scalloping of the surface of the cusps. With increasing adult age, as the heart gets smaller, the valve tissue increasingly folds over and billows into the left atrium during ventricular systole. Sometimes excessive length of the chordae permits the cusp prolapse.

Symptoms, Signs, and Diagnosis

Most patients are asymptomatic. However, some may have chest pain (nonanginal), palpitations, fatigue, and/or dyspnea. A late systolic murmur and a midsystolic click, accentuated by standing and squatting, are clues to the lesion. Progressive mitral regurgitation may occur, causing left atrial and ventricular changes as occur with that lesion (see below). The ECHO shows diagnostic "hammocking," especially of the posterior mitral leaflet in late systole. Left ventriculography best demonstrates the cusp prolapse. Valve calcification, infective endocarditis, embolic cerebral vascular accidents, and paroxysmal tachycardia may be associated. Sudden death has been reported, usually in those who show T wave abnormalities in the ECG.

Treatment

Prophylaxis against SBE is indicated. Documented tachycardia should be treated as appropriate for the type present. Unrestricted activity is permitted asymptomatic patients unless significant mitral regurgitation is associated.

MITRAL REGURGITATION (Mitral Insufficiency)

Mitral regurgitation may result from rheumatic fever, mitral valve prolapse, endocardial fibroelastosis, dilation of the left ventricle due to severe anemia, myocarditis or myocardiopathy, and congenital valve abnormalities including endocardial cushion defects, double orifice mitral valve, and left-sided Ebstein's disease in cases with ventricular inversion.

Symptoms, Signs, and Diagnosis

With increasing regurgitation, fatigue, dyspnea, and ultimately frank congestive heart failure may occur. Arterial emboli may occur in patients with left atrial mural thrombi associated with atrial fibrillation. Physical findings including a strong apical impulse, blowing apical systolic murmur transmitted to the axilla, and, with increasing volume regurgitation, an apical low-pitched, early- to mid-diastolic murmur. Chest x-rays show enlargement of the left atrium and ventricle; a huge left atrium indicates marked regurgitation. The ECG shows variable degrees of left atrial and left ventricular hypertrophy and atrial arrhythmias if the atrial enlargement is severe. The ECHO shows increased left atrial and ventricular dimensions and permits evaluation of left ventricular function. Cardiac catheterization allows measurement of left atrial and pulmonary artery pressures. Left ventriculography defines the degree of regurgitation.

Treatment

Treatment depends on the severity of the mitral regurgitation. In cases with mild congestive heart failure, medical management may suffice. However, refractory congestive heart failure, progressive cardiomegaly, and pulmonary hypertension usually warrant surgery. A palliative mitral anuloplasty may be adequate and is preferred for young patients, but more often prosthetic or porcine hetero-graft valve replacement may be needed. Anticoagulation is needed for those with prosthetic valves. Continual prophylaxis against recurrent streptococcal pharyngitis (for rheumatics) and SBE is indicated. Prophylaxis against SBE is indicated at times of anticipated bacteremia, e.g., dental extraction.

MITRAL STENOSIS

Mitral stenosis is usually caused by previous rheumatic fever. It is the commonest form of rheumatic valvular heart disease in adults, but is rarely seen in children, since it takes years to develop enough fibrosis of the valve to cause obstruction. When mitral obstruction does occur in childhood, a congenital stenosis is usually present. Rarely, an atrial tumor may obstruct the valve orifice. When > 30% of the mitral orifice is obstructed, blood flow from the left atrium to the left ventricle is maintained only by a significant increase in left atrial pressure, which is reflected into the pulmonary veins and capillaries; eventually, pulmonary artery and right ventricular pressures rise.

Symptoms, Signs, and Diagnosis

The first symptom of mitral stenosis is exertional dyspnea; eventually paroxysmal nocturnal dyspnea develops. Exertion produces tachycardia with reduced ventricular filling time and, thus, reduced cardiac output. Blood accumulates in the left atrium and pulmonary veins, leading to congestion and dyspnea. Venous return to the heart, which is increased by recumbency, results in pulmonary congestion and dyspnea more noticeable at night. As stenosis progresses, pulmonary edema appears, often acutely after exertion. In some patients, the persistently elevated pulmonary vascular obstruction produces high pulmonary vascular resistance and, ultimately, right heart failure. Persistent pulmonary hypertension also causes anastomoses between the pulmonary and bronchial veins that may rupture, producing repeated hemoptysis.

Atrial fibrillation, which may develop from progressive left atrial enlargement, further impairs left ventricular filling and enhances the risk of cerebral, visceral, or peripheral emboli secondary to thrombus formation in the left atrium. Other complications of mitral stenosis include multiple pulmonary infections and SBE.

Physical findings include an opening snap, an apical presystolic rumble, and an accentuated 1st heart sound. In early stages of obstruction the rumble may occur in mid-diastole; it may be absent when cardiac output is markedly decreased, with atrial fibrillation, or when there is a large left atrial thrombus. An accentuated pulmonary valve closure sound signifies pulmonary hypertension. A soft decrescendo diastolic murmur heard along the left sternal border implies pulmonary valve incompetence secondary to pulmonary hypertension.

The **ECG** shows broad notched P waves (left atrial hypertrophy) and, with increasing pulmonary hypertension, right axis deviation and right ventricular hypertrophy. Atrial fibrillation may occur. The earliest **x-ray changes** include straightening of the left cardiac border due to dilated left atrial appendage, prominence of the pulmonary arteries, dilation of the upper lobe pulmonary veins, and posterior displacement of the esophagus by the enlarged left atrium. In severe stenosis, marked left atrial and right ventricular enlargement occur. The **ECHO** shows a flattening of the E-F slope of the mitral valve and an increased left atrial dimension (see also p. 237). **Right heart catheterization** with pulmonary artery wedge pressure determination (reflecting left atrial pressure) helps to distinguish mitral stenosis from structural pulmonary hypertension or multiple pulmonary embolizations. **Left heart catheterization** allows quantitation of the relative degree of stenosis and insufficiency of the mitral valve and any coexisting aortic lesion if present.

Treatment

Medical management consists of reduced activity, control of atrial fibrillation, treatment of congestive heart failure, and prevention of thromboembolic episodes, SBE, and streptococcal pharyngitis. If fibrillation is of recent origin, countershock or quinidine may effect a return to sinus rhythm that usually can be retained without carrying a risk of thromboembolism. When fibrillation has been present for some time, a return to sustained sinus rhythm is unlikely, and attempts to convert the rhythm to normal may carry a significant risk of thromboembolism. Following successful surgery, the probability of controlling the arrhythmia is increased. With persistent fibrillation, permanent anticoagulation therapy reduces the risk of serious thromboembolic complications.

Surgery should be considered when symptoms of exertional dyspnea persist despite optimal medical therapy. Surgical treatment of mitral stenosis varies with the type of pathology present. Closed valvulotomy, now rarely performed, is limited to a few patients with pure mitral stenosis without previous surgery, valve calcification, or left atrial thrombus. Open-heart surgery is recommended for most patients, especially for those undergoing repeat surgery and for complicated cases (e.g., associated mitral regurgitation or valvular calcification). Pregnancy is not a contraindication if the patient's symptoms are severe. Occasionally, mitral commissurotomy is feasible without inducing significant mitral regurgitation. More often, valve replacement is needed, especially when calcification is present. Either a prosthetic or a heterograft (usually porcine) valve is used for replacement. Considerable improvement usually follows, but the long-term prognosis is unknown. Anticoagulation is recommended with prosthetic valve replacement because of continuing risk of thromboembolism, especially in patients with atrial fibrillation. Other complications of prosthetic valve replacement include hemolytic anemia, prosthesis dysfunction, and infective endocarditis.

AORTIC VALVE DISEASE

AORTIC REGURGITATION (Aortic Insufficiency)

When the aortic valve cusps are distorted by rheumatic fibrosis, myxomatous degeneration, or a congenital defect, they do not appose competently during valve closure and blood regurgitates into the left ventricle. The stroke volume of blood expelled by the left ventricle in aortic insufficiency is increased, the increase equaling the volume that regurgitates. Left ventricular diastolic volume overload leads to dilation and hypertrophy of the left ventricle.

Symptoms, Signs, and Diagnosis

Many patients with mild aortic regurgitation are asymptomatic for decades. With progressive regurgitation, the patient may sense dyspnea and fatigue on mild exertion, syncope, chest pain, and eventually frank congestive heart failure. A high-pitched blowing decrescendo early diastolic murmur heard best at the 3rd and 4th left interspace along the sternal border is characteristic. Sometimes the murmur can be heard only in full expiration with the patient leaning forward. Many patients also have a systolic murmur, due to the increased stroke volume, which is heard at the right base and sometimes at the apex. An early low-pitched diastolic murmur (**Austin Flint**) may also be heard at the apex. Capillary pulsations may be seen at the base of the nail beds. A **water-hammer pulse** and **collapsing pulse** may be palpated at the wrist, while a **pistol-shot sound** and the **double Duroziez murmur** may be heard over the femoral artery. Arterial pulse pressure is widened with an elevated systolic pressure and a low diastolic pressure. Late in the disease, the diastolic pressure may rise because of an elevated left ventricular end-diastolic pressure. Chest x-ray shows left ventricular enlargement and aortic dilation. The ECG shows left ventricular hypertrophy and ST-T segment changes in the left precordial leads with advancing disease.

Treatment

For patients with dyspnea, fatigue, increasing heart size, left ventricular hypertrophy, and decreasing ejection fraction, valve surgery should be considered before frank congestive heart failure occurs. Aortic valvuloplasty is rarely successful; replacement of the aortic valve with a prosthetic or porcine valve is usually necessary. Good clinical improvement usually follows valve replacement unless irreversible left ventricular disease has occurred, but there is a postoperative risk of thromboembolism, infective endocarditis, and hemolytic anemia if a prosthetic valve is used. The long-term prognosis of valve replacement is unknown.

AORTIC STENOSIS

Aortic stenosis may result from fibrosis of the commissures years after acute rheumatic fever or from progressive stenosis of a congenitally diseased valve, often bicuspid. Some cases of combined aortic stenosis and insufficiency (**calcific aortic disease**) develop in middle or later life with no earlier history of rheumatic or congenital disease. Even the surgeon and pathologist may find it impossible to determine whether a distorted calcified obstructed aortic valve had an underlying congenital or rheumatic etiology.

Symptoms, Signs, and Diagnosis

Aortic stenosis is not clinically significant until the cross-section of the orifice has been reduced by at least 35% of its original size. Initially, commissural fusion or fibrosis occurs and is usually progressive; later, calcification may also occur, changing the valve into a rigid calcified mass. As a pressure gradient develops across the aortic valve, left ventricular hypertrophy and hypertension follow. Cardiac output and stroke volume at rest may be normal until late in the disease. Eventually, fatigue and exertional dyspnea appear. Angina may develop from poor coronary perfusion. Syncope on exertion, sometimes with loss of consciousness, is related to decreased cerebral blood flow secondary to inadequate cardiac output. As the disease progresses, left ventricular failure supervenes; this may be resistant to treatment. Angina, congestive failure, dizziness, and syncope are usually ominous signs.

The characteristic findings are a loud, rough, ejection systolic murmur over the 2nd right interspace, transmitted into the neck vessels with a corresponding thrill, and a diminished or absent 2nd aortic sound. An ejection sound at the left sternal border may be heard. The BP remains normal in the early stages of the disease; later, narrowing of the pulse pressure is usual. Calcification of the aortic cusps may be detected on x-ray. Left ventricular enlargement on x-ray may be absent until left ventricular failure occurs. The ECG usually demonstrates left ventricular hypertrophy when the obstruction is moderate and additional S-T and T wave abnormalities when the stenosis is severe. ECHO demonstrates a restricted valve orifice and dense valve echoes when severe fibrosis or calcification develops. Cardiac catheterization permits a precise measurement of the valve gradient, and angiography permits visualization of the site of obstruction and the coronary artery distribution, of great importance in surgical management.

Treatment

For the management of angina and congestive heart failure, see MYOCARDIAL ISCHEMIC DISORDERS and CONGESTIVE HEART FAILURE in Ch. 25. Strenuous activity is restricted for those with measured peak systolic valve gradients > 50 mm Hg, since sudden death may occur. For this group, surgery is strongly recommended. In young patients, considerable improvement may be effected by valvulotomy. However, most adults with severe aortic obstruction require valve replacement, utilizing a ball or disk prosthesis or a heterograft valve. Since there is some risk of postoperative thromboembolism in patients with valve prostheses, anticoagulants are usually advisable. Prophylactic antibiotics are prescribed at times of anticipated bacteremia (e.g., dental extraction) to prevent infection of the diseased or replaced valve.

TRICUSPID VALVE DISEASE

TRICUSPID REGURGITATION

Tricuspid regurgitation occurs when the valve leaflets cannot appose competently during right ventricular systole. It may be **primary,** due to rheumatic cusp distortion, congenital endocardial cushion defects, Ebstein's disease (downward displacement of one or more cusps into the right ventricle), or infective endocarditis. It may also be **secondary** to atrial fibrillation or to dilation of the right ventricle from any cause. Regurgitation induces a rise in right atrial pressure during ventricular systole. As the regurgitation progresses, there is increasing systemic venous congestion.

Symptoms, Signs, and Diagnosis

A pansystolic, blowing, medium-pitched murmur, accentuated by inspiration, is heard best in the 4th and 5th intercostal spaces over or close to the sternum. Neck vein distention, hepatomegaly, pleural effusion, ascites, and peripheral edema may occur. Cyanosis can develop if right-to-left shunting develops through a patent foramen ovale. The ECG shows right atrial and ventricular hypertrophy and sometimes a prolonged P-R interval. Chest x-ray demonstrates the right atrial and ventricular enlargement. ECHO shows an increased tricuspid valve excursion and right ventricular dimension. Cardiac catheterization documents an elevated right atrial V wave. Right ventriculography best demonstrates the regurgitation.

Treatment

Some patients require no treatment, since mild-to-moderate tricuspid regurgitation may be well tolerated for many years. However, increasing symptoms indicate the need for surgery. Occasionally, valve anuloplasty may be successful. More often, valve replacement is required.

TRICUSPID STENOSIS

Tricuspid stenosis may result from rheumatic valve fibrosis, occlusion of the valve orifice by tumor or thrombi, or rarely from a congenital defect. In the latter instance, it is usually associated with pulmonic stenosis and a hypoplastic right ventricle. Blood flow from the right atrium to ventricle is obstructed, with a resulting diastolic pressure gradient across the valve.

Symptoms, Signs, and Diagnosis

When associated with mitral stenosis, the symptoms of pulmonary congestion may be dominant. However, severe tricuspid stenosis causes distended neck veins and abdominal distention due to hepatic congestion, cirrhosis, and ascites. A low-pitched blowing presystolic murmur is heard along the lower right or left sternal border. ECG shows tall peaked P waves in leads II and V_1. Chest x-ray reveals a dilated right atrium and superior vena cava. Cardiac catheterization demonstrates a diastolic pressure gradient across the valve. Right atriography shows delayed emptying of a dilated right atrium through a constricted valve orifice.

Treatment

Medical and surgical management is similar to that for mitral stenosis (see above).

PULMONIC VALVE DISEASE

PULMONIC REGURGITATION

Pulmonic regurgitation is rarely a primary lesion except on a congenital basis when it is usually associated with ventricular septal defect. It frequently results from pulmonary artery dilation associated with severe pulmonary hypertension, as may occur with left heart failure, mitral valve obstruction, pulmonary vascular disease, or pulmonary fibrosis.

Symptoms, Signs, and Diagnosis

Symptoms are those caused by the associated disease. A high-pitched early decrescendo diastolic murmur is best heard at the 2nd and 3rd left intercostal space; it usually follows an accentuated pulmonic valve closure sound. Other physical findings as well as the ECG vary with the associated heart disease. The chest x-ray usually shows a dilated main pulmonary artery segment and right ventricular enlargement.

Treatment varies with the underlying disease process. In some instances valve replacement may be indicated if valve substance is deficient.

PULMONIC STENOSIS (See CONGENITAL HEART DISEASE in Vol. II, Ch. 21)

BACTERIAL ENDOCARDITIS

(Acute Bacterial Endocarditis; Subacute Bacterial Endocarditis)

Bacterial infection of the endocardium, characterized by symptoms of systemic infection, embolic phenomena, and endocardial vegetations. The course may be acute or subacute, depending on the virulence of the infecting organism.

Etiology

Acute bacterial endocarditis (ABE) is most commonly caused by enterococci and coagulase-positive staphylococci. The incidence of staphylococcal infections is related primarily to "hospital endemic" organisms and parenteral drug abuse. Pneumococcal endocarditis appears occasionally. Meningococci, gonococci, and *Hemophilus influenzae* are rare causes. Secondary implantation may follow cardiac surgery; the most common cause has been penicillin-resistant *Staphylococcus epidermidis*, but gram-negative bacilli and yeasts have also been recovered.

Subacute bacterial endocarditis (SBE) is usually due to α-hemolytic streptococci (*Streptococcus viridans*) and frequently follows a dental procedure. Other streptococci, such as enterococci, peptostreptococci, and microaerophilic streptococci, account for most other cases. Heart valves that are congenitally deformed or damaged by previous disease are predisposed to infection. Normal valves may be attacked in ABE but rarely in SBE.

Pathology

The basic lesion is a vegetation composed of fibrin masses and mesh, in which platelets, RBCs, polymorphonuclear leukocytes, and bacteria are entrapped. The valve is the usual primary site, but vegetations may start on or extend to the mural endocardium, especially at a site of trauma, injury, or anomaly. The valvular leaflets show signs of acute or subacute inflammation adjacent to the vegetation. Evidence of repair, bacterial action, and fibrin deposition are also seen in SBE. Signs of preexisting disease (scarring, distortion) with valvular malfunction are usual. Rupture or perforation of a cusp may occur, especially in ABE.

Symptoms and Signs

Onset of **SBE** is insidious and may mimic many systemic diseases without early signs of cardiac involvement. Fever, usually remittent, may be irregular or sustained; the daily peak is seldom > 39 C (102.2 F). Chills, malaise, and arthralgia are frequent complaints. Progressive anemia often intensifies the lassitude and anorexia due to the infection. Leukocytosis, petechiae, and embolic phenomena are common. **Janeway lesions** (erythematous macules on palms and soles) may be seen. Tender nodules 2 to 5 mm in diameter frequently develop about the tips of the digits **(Osler's nodes)**. Hemorrhages of various types in the ocular fundi, particularly **Roth's spots** (round or oval lesions with small white centers), are more common in ABE. Splenomegaly is frequent. Splenic infarcts produce acute upper left quadrant pain, often pleuritic, and an elevation in fever and WBCs. Massive peripheral embolization is rare.

Microscopic hematuria or diffuse glomerulonephritis is frequently due to petechial renal lesions, but gross hematuria from frank infarcts is rare. Two types of nephritis develop in bacterial endocarditis: (1) focal, caused by multiple small infarcts **("flea-bitten" kidney)**, and (2) diffuse, a true glomerular lesion. Rarely, the latter progresses to cause advanced or even fatal renal insufficiency.

Cardiac signs of the infection may be obscured at first by evidence of preexisting valvulitis; later, the character of the murmurs may change. As the disease progresses, congestive failure may develop.

In **ABE**, symptoms and signs are similar to those of SBE, but preexisting valvular heart disease is less likely and the course is more rapid. Acute endocarditis may complicate a frank staphylococcal or pneumococcal infection, heralded by a sudden worsening in the patient's condition with increasing signs of septicemia. An otherwise healthy individual with a seemingly inconsequential focal infection may suddenly develop chills, fever, and other evidence of systemic involvement due to endocarditis. The symptoms and signs of bacteremia eventually appear in either condition. Meningitis is rare in SBE, but ABE is frequently complicated by purulent meningitis, especially in pneumococcal endocarditis. SBE, on the other hand, may present with neurologic findings due to cerebral emboli, brain abscesses, or mycotic aneurysms.

Diagnosis

Endocarditis in its early stages may be confused with other infections: a low-grade fever may be ascribed to URI or urinary tract infection, especially in the aged; an elderly patient may have occult SBE obscured by refractory congestive heart failure; patients with rheumatic heart disease who develop fever and arthralgia from SBE may be suspected of having a recurrence of rheumatic fever. Symptoms of an infectious disease, bacteremia, and valvular involvement with or without changing murmurs, petechiae, and embolic phenomena usually point to the diagnosis. An unexplained fever in a patient with a heart murmur always should arouse suspicion of endocarditis. Most important is finding the organisms in blood culture—5 or 6 cultures usually suffice. Though the clinical picture may give clues about the causative organism, definitive information must be obtained from the blood culture, supported by antibiotic sensitivity tests. At times, special studies such as serum antibacterial activity will be necessary to guide the extent and duration of therapy.

Prognosis

Untreated, the disease is fatal. Antibiotic therapy has reduced mortality to about 15%, but heart failure due to valvular scarring and distortion may develop even after the infection is cured. Aortic valve damage may lead to rapid congestive failure and requires corrective surgery. Death may result from the associated cachexia and anemia, from cerebral or pulmonary embolism, or from cardiac or renal failure. Endocarditis after cardiac surgery generally has a poor prognosis, though patients have recovered following massive antibiotic therapy or reoperation.

Prophylaxis

Endocarditis sometimes follows operations on the oropharynx or genitourinary tract, which occasionally are associated with bacteremia. Patients with valvular or congenital heart disease should be given prophylactic procaine penicillin G 600,000 u. IM 1 h before surgery and then b.i.d. for 2 days or oral erythromycin 250 mg q.i.d. beginning 1 day before and continuing 2 days after surgery (e.g., dental extraction, tonsillectomy), or oral ampicillin 500 mg q.i.d. 1 day before until 2 days after cystoscopy or prostatectomy. New recommendations suggest a combination of penicillin plus streptomycin or gentamicin prior to dental procedures in patients with prosthetic heart valves.

Treatment

SBE caused by penicillin G-sensitive S. viridans or **anaerobic or γ-streptococcus:** These streptococci are inhibited by penicillin G concentrations < 0.2 μg/ml. Several regimens are recommended for the treatment of bacterial endocarditis caused by sensitive strains of streptococci. Successful therapy is assured when a bactericidal regimen is selected and treatment is begun early and continued over a long time. One of three regimens frequently is used: (1) penicillin G 2.4 to 6 million u./day in divided doses IM or IV for 4 wk; (2) penicillin G 2.4 million u./day in divided doses IM for 2 wk with streptomycin 500 mg IM q 12 h for the first week and 500 mg every day for the second week (Hunter regimen); or (3) penicillin V 750 mg orally q 4 h day and night, plus streptomycin 500 mg q 12 h IM for 2 wk. The superiority of one regimen over another has not been proved. Oral agents require careful monitoring.

Enterococcal endocarditis: Enterococci are relatively resistant to penicillin G, and high levels must be given. Some strains may be more sensitive to ampicillin. Penicillin G or ampicillin should be combined with streptomycin 500 mg IM q 12 h for 4 to 6 wk. The doses of penicillin G and ampicillin are not standard; penicillin G 10 to 40 million u./day IV or ampicillin 8 to 12 gm IV or IM is advised, with monitoring of the patient's serum for bactericidal activity. Gentamicin may be favored over streptomycin with some strains of enterococci.

Staphylococcal endocarditis: In infection with penicillin-sensitive staphylococci (i.e., staphylococci inhibited by < 1 μg/ml), penicillin G 10 to 40 million u./day IV should be given for 4 to 6 wk. For penicillin G-resistant staphylococci, methicillin 1.5 to 2 gm IV q 4 h or nafcillin 1 gm IV q 4 h should be given for 4 to 6 wk. Cloxacillin or dicloxacillin 1 to 1.5 gm orally q 4 h day and night may be substituted for IV methicillin or nafcillin after the 1st or 2nd wk if facilities for measurement of serum antistaphylococcal activity are available. Inhibitory titers of 1:8 to 1:16 are desired—i.e., the patient's serum diluted 1:8 or more, incubated for 24 h, and subcultured onto antibiotic-free medium should inhibit and preferably sterilize growth of the infecting staphylococcus.

Pneumococcal or Group A streptococcal endocarditis: Penicillin G 10 to 20 million u./day IV should be given for 3 to 4 wk.

Endocarditis in the presence of intracardiac prostheses: The mortality is high despite optimum management. S. epidermidis, which is coagulase-negative and penicillin-resistant, is the most common infecting organism. A few cases have been cured with methicillin or cloxacillin given for several weeks, some maintained in good health by "chronic suppression" with a penicillinase-resistant penicillin orally for 1 to 2 yr, and others cured only by surgical removal of the infected prosthesis.

Treatment of endocarditis in patients allergic to penicillin: Not all patients who give a history of penicillin sensitivity are truly sensitive, and tests for penicillin allergy are not always reliable. Penicillin or one of its derivatives is still the preferred and most dependable antibiotic for any kind of endocarditis caused by gram-positive cocci. Therefore, patients who are likely to show sensitivity to penicillin should be "desensitized" and if necessary given corticosteroids or be treated with an alternative bactericidal antibiotic; e.g., a cephalosporin or vancomycin.

In a suitable schedule for desensitization, penicillin G (sodium or potassium salt) is given at half-hour intervals as follows: (1) 10 u. intradermally, as a wheal, (2) then 100 u. subcutaneously, (3) then 1000 u. subcutaneously, (4) then 10,000 u. IM, and (5) finally 100,000 u. IM. Full therapeutic doses can then be given. No reaction will be observed in most instances. Urticaria may sometimes reappear later during the course of treatment. The physician should carry out this program himself and should have emergency drugs, equipment, and other personnel ready to deal with anaphylaxis.

Alternative bactericidal regimens for patients infected with penicillin-sensitive *S. viridans* include cephalothin 1 gm IV or IM q 6 h plus streptomycin 500 mg IM q 12 h for 2 wk. If signs of allergy appear, prednisone 5 mg orally q 6 h should be given during the remainder of the cephalosporin treatment. Vancomycin 500 mg IV t.i.d. for 10 to 14 days has been effective in enterococcal endocarditis in patients allergic to penicillin. Cephalosporins are *not* clinically effective against enterococci, even in combination with an aminoglycoside.

Response to treatment: Patients with *S. viridans* endocarditis usually feel better and their temperature approaches normal within 3 days of initiating therapy. Minor temperature elevations are unimportant. Enterococcal endocarditis may respond rapidly or slowly. Staphylococcal endocarditis usually responds slowly; fever and positive blood cultures may persist as long as 1 wk after the start of ultimately successful treatment. Response to treatment in pneumococcal and Group A streptococcal endocarditis is variable.

Petechiae may be seen during or after completion of antibiotic therapy. They are ordinarily sterile, associated with negative blood cultures, and do not call for different or additional antibiotics.

PERICARDIAL DISEASE

Etiology

The pericardium may be involved by inflammation, trauma, or neoplasms. **Inflammation** follows bacterial, viral, or fungal infection and sometimes accompanies systemic diseases (RA, SLE, scleroderma, uremia). It occasionally results from therapy; e.g., radiation or drugs such as procainamide, hydralazine, or anticoagulants. It also occurs without identifiable cause (idiopathic or nonspecific pericarditis), after pericardiotomy (postpericardiotomy syndrome), or as a consequence of myocardial infarction (postmyocardial infarction syndrome). **Trauma** to the pericardium may be due to penetrating or nonpenetrating chest injuries or may occur via the esophagus by swallowed foreign bodies. Saccular or dissecting aortic aneurysms may rupture into the pericardium, as may a myocardial aneurysm after infarction or trauma. Cardiac catheters occasionally penetrate the myocardium and enter the pericardial sac. Trauma can cause infection or hemopericardium. **Neoplasms** affecting the pericardium include carcinoma (especially of the lung or breast), sarcoma, and lymphomas; they may be an extension of thoracic tumors or metastases with or without serous hemorrhagic effusion. Neoplastic involvement may be focal or extensive; if extensive, cardiac performance may be hindered.

Pathology

Acute pericarditis may be fibrinous, serous, sanguineous, hemorrhagic, or purulent. The amount and quality of the cellular reaction depends on the inciting cause. The pericardial sac normally contains little fluid, but effusion develops in disease. The superficial layers of the subepicardial myocardium may be involved.

Fibrosis of the pericardium results from infection, trauma, or hemopericardium, or it may accompany collagen disease; often the cause is unknown. The fibrosis may be patchy or extensive and is frequently the site of calcific deposits. Adhesion of the visceral and parietal layers may partially or wholly obliterate the sac, or effusion may separate the 2 layers (effusive-constrictive pericarditis). Calcification and fibrosis may extend into the superficial layers of the myocardium.

Pathophysiology

Rapid but small—or slower, more massive—accumulation of pericardial fluid or decreased pericardial compliance due to fibrosis, calcification, or neoplasm may limit ventricular filling during diastole. This limitation is the most serious consequence of pericardial disease. The end-diastolic pressure in the ventricles is determined by the limiting effusion or thickened pericardium, and the diastolic pressures in the ventricles, atria, and venous beds become virtually the same. Systemic venous congestion increases and the hydrostatic pressure in systemic capillaries approaches osmotic pressure. Therefore, a further small increase in systemic venous and capillary pressure causes considerable transudation of fluid from the systemic capillaries. Signs of peripheral congestion in pericardial disease are more striking than those of pulmonary congestion, and frank pulmonary edema is rare despite massive fluid accumulation in the viscera and extremities.

Rising ventricular diastolic pressure, atrial, and venous pressures and falling stroke volume, cardiac output, and ultimately systemic arterial pressure follow abrupt fluid accumulation (**cardiac tamponade**). The resulting clinical findings are those of shock (decreased cardiac output and low systemic arterial pressure), together with dyspnea, orthopnea, and engorged neck veins. Cardiac tamponade is nearly always accompanied by an accentuation of the normal inspiratory decline in systemic systolic BP (**pulsus paradoxus**). A decline of 10 mm Hg or more is usually significant. The pulse may actually disappear during inspiration in advanced cases. Pulsus paradoxus can also occur in chronic obstructive lung disease, bronchial asthma, pulmonary embolism, right ventricular infarction, and clinical shock.

The effect of gradual pericardial scarring (**constrictive pericarditis**) on cardiac performance differs somewhat because the pace is slower. The only early abnormalities may be elevation of ventricular diastolic, atrial, and pulmonary and systemic venous pressures. Cardiac output and systemic arterial pressures may be maintained by tachycardia and systemic arteriolar vasoconstriction. Prolonged elevation of pulmonary venous pressure results in dyspnea and orthopnea; systemic venous hypertension produces hypervolemia, engorgement of neck veins, pleural effusion, hepatomegaly, ascites, and peripheral edema. Pulsus paradoxus occurs in the minority of instances, and is usually less severe than in tamponade.

Symptoms and Signs

Acute pericarditis may appear with pain, fever, pericardial rub, tamponade, ECG changes, or radiologic changes, or may be discovered incidentally in the course of a systemic illness. It begins abruptly or insidiously and is often preceded by dull or sharp precordial or substernal pain radiating to the neck, trapezius, or shoulders. Pain varies from mild to severe and is usually aggravated by thoracic motion, cough, and respiration; it is relieved by sitting up and leaning forward. Indolent pericarditis (often neoplastic, tuberculous, or uremic) may be painless. Usually pericardial pain can be distinguished from ischemic coronary pain because the latter is not aggravated by thoracic motion. Tachypnea and nonproductive cough may be present; fever, chills, and weakness are common.

When present, the dominant physical finding is a friction rub heard throughout the cardiac cycle. However, it is often intermittent and evanescent or it may be present only in systole or, less frequently, in diastole. Considerable pericardial fluid may muffle heart sounds, increase the area of cardiac dullness, and change the size and shape of the cardiac silhouette. However, cardiac tamponade may occur *without* any of these findings. The accumulation of even large amounts of fluid is usually sufficiently slow that the pericardium stretches and accommodates the fluid without interfering with cardiac performance. Other symptoms and signs such as pulsus paradoxus and those due to elevated venous pressure and falling cardiac output culminating in tamponade and shock are described in the discussion of pathophysiology, above.

Leukocytosis and a rapid ESR are common. Serial ECGs early in the disorder may show abnormalities confined to the S-T segments and T waves, generally involving all leads. The S-T segments in 2 or 3 of the standard leads become elevated but subsequently return to the baseline. Unlike in myocardial infarction, S-T segments do not show reciprocal depression (except in leads aVR and V_1), and there are no pathologic Q waves. The T waves may become flattened and then inverted throughout the ECG, except in lead aVR. With effusion, QRS voltage is usually decreased. Electrical alternans is uncommon, and is usually limited to occasional cases of cardiac tamponade. Sinus rhythm occurs in about 90% of cases. The cardiac silhouette on x-ray is not enlarged except with coexisting heart disease or effusion $>$ 250 ml.

Pericardial fibrosis or calcification is asymptomatic unless constrictive pericarditis is present; then symptoms and signs of peripheral congestion may appear along with an early diastolic sound **(pericardial knock)** and at times pulsus paradoxus. Pericardial calcification often is best seen in lateral chest films. The cardiac silhouette may be small, normal, or large. Nonspecific ECG changes may occur. The QRS voltage is usually low. T waves are usually abnormal. Atrial fibrillation (less commonly, atrial flutter) is present in perhaps 25% of patients with constrictive pericarditis.

Diagnosis

Pericarditis may be diagnosed solely from the history of pain and the characteristic ECG. A pericardial friction rub is also diagnostic. Pericarditis must be distinguished from causes of pleuritic pain and myocardial or pulmonary infarction. Pericardial effusion may be suspected by a rapid change in the cardiac silhouette on serial chest x-rays, especially when the lung fields remain clear. (When rapid changes in heart size are due to heart failure, pulmonary congestion is more likely.) The silhouette is often symmetrically enlarged, and the outlines of the individual cardiac chambers and great vessels are obliterated. Since considerable pericardial fluid may be present in myxedema or congestion secondary to ventricular failure, its presence does not necessarily imply pericarditis.

Tuberculous pericarditis is insidious in onset and may exist without pulmonary involvement. The PPD skin test is usually positive. Culture of pericardial fluid or tissue may be necessary for diagnosis or response to antituberculous therapy may confirm the diagnosis. Pericarditis from pyogenic, viral or mycotic infections or that associated with acute rheumatic fever, collagen disease, uremia, or acute myocardial infarction may be overlooked because of concern with other manifestations of the underlying disease; once recognized, its cause is usually identified.

Idiopathic pericarditis is frequently preceded by a URI. Other possible causes must be carefully excluded before idiopathic pericarditis is diagnosed. Blood cultures, skin tests for TB, examination of pericardial fluid or pericardial biopsy specimens for fungi, antinuclear antibody tests, histoplasmosis complement fixation tests, streptozyme tests, tests for neutralizing antibodies for coxsackievirus influenza virus, and ECHO virus, and search for LE cells in the blood should be among the diagnostic procedures. If pericardial fluid is recovered, it should be cultured and examined for tumor cells. Direct pericardial biopsy for culture and microscopic examination may be needed in recurrent or persistent pericardial effusion.

Postpericardiotomy and **postmyocardial infarction syndromes** may be difficult to identify and must be distinguished from pericardial infection following surgery and from a recent myocardial infarction or pulmonary embolus. Pain, friction rub, and fever appearing and recurring late after the known insult, and their rapid response to corticosteroids aid diagnosis. Trauma to the pericardium is usually suggested by the history and a rapid accumulation of blood in the sac precipitating tamponade.

The appearance of atrial arrhythmias and evidence of tamponade or constriction in neoplastic diseases suggest pericardial involvement.

Fibrosis of the pericardium is recognized by the demonstration of pericardial calcification (sometimes without pericardial constriction) or symptoms and signs of circulatory congestion. **Constrictive pericarditis** must be distinguished from myocardial or valvular disease or cirrhosis of the liver with congestion.

Special diagnostic technics may be required to differentiate effusion or constrictive pericarditis from a dilated heart. **Echocardiography**, which is safe, quick, and noninvasive, has a high degree of sensitivity and specificity for the recognition of pericardial fluid. It usually shows characteristic changes with tamponade, but the changes are not specific in constrictive pericarditis. The procedure discloses 2 echoes behind the left ventricle in the region of the posterior cardiac wall: one from the epicardium and the other from the pericardium. The interval between the echoes represents the fluid. CO_2 atrialgrams and radioisotope scanning of the heart are seldom used to recognize pericardial disease today.

Hemodynamic studies: Constrictive pericarditis may be suggested by the characteristic pressure records described below. The diagnosis may be confirmed by angiocardiography, which typically shows moderate pericardial thickening, as a thickened border between the cardiac chamber and the cardiac shadow, and straightening of the lateral right atrial border. These changes are not always present, and exploratory thoracotomy may be necessary.

The mean pulmonary wedge pressure, the pulmonary artery diastolic pressure, the right ventricular end-diastolic pressure, and the mean right atrial pressure are elevated and virtually identical in tamponade or constriction. The pulmonary arterial and right ventricular systolic pressures are only modestly elevated, so that pulse pressures are small. In the presence of constrictive pericarditis, atrial pressure curves may show accentuation of the X and Y descents, and ventricular pressure curves demonstrate a diastolic dip at the time of rapid ventricular filling. These changes in the pressure curves always occur in congestion due to constrictive pericarditis. In cardiac tamponade, there is no early diastolic dip in the ventricular pressure record. Although these hemodynamic abnormalities may also be found in severe congestive states due to myocardial diseases, their presence and angiocardiographic evidence of increased pericardial thickening or fluid around the opacified cardiac chambers is sufficient to establish the diagnosis of pericardial fluid or thickening.

Treatment

General: Aspirin 600 mg orally, codeine 15 to 60 mg orally, meperidine 50 to 100 mg orally or IM, or morphine 10 to 15 mg IM may be given q 4 h for pain. Anxiety or insomnia may respond to phenobarbital 15 to 30 mg orally t.i.d. or q.i.d. or pentobarbital 100 or 200 mg orally at bedtime. Anticoagulants are usually *contraindicated* in pericardial disease since they may cause intrapericardial bleeding and even fatal tamponade.

Specific: Pericarditis due to bacterial or mycotic infections is treated with specific antimicrobial agents. Tuberculous pericarditis may be treated with drug therapy (see under TUBERCULOUS PERICARDITIS in Ch. 8). The pericardial sac should be drained surgically if the pericarditis is due to a pyogenic infection. Pyogenic pericarditis is rare, but may occur with infective endocarditis, pneumonia, septicemia, or penetrating trauma, and in patients receiving immunosuppressive therapy.

Antibiotics are not indicated in idiopathic pericarditis nor in the postinfarction or postpericardiotomy syndromes, but corticosteroids may be required to control pain, fever, and effusion. Prednisone 20 to 60 mg/day orally in divided doses may be given for 3 to 4 days. The dose is gradually reduced if the response is satisfactory and may be discontinued in 7 to 14 days in some cases, but many months of treatment may be needed. Indomethacin 25 to 50 mg orally t.i.d. may control pain and effusion.

Therapy for pericarditis in rheumatic fever and the collagen diseases and for pericardial involvement in neoplastic diseases is directed at the underlying process. Surgical intervention is required in some instances of trauma to repair the injury and evacuate blood from the sac. Uremic pericarditis may respond to hemodialysis, aspiration, or systemic or local adrenal corticosteroid therapy.

Immediate **pericardiocentesis** may be required when tamponade develops; removal of even a small volume may be life-saving. Premedication with morphine 5 to 15 mg or meperidine 50 to 100 mg IM is desirable in non-urgent situations. The patient should be seated upright in a chair with his back supported. Some physicians prefer the patient recumbent with his back supported by a pillow for the subxiphoid approach. Under antiseptic conditions, the skin and subcutaneous tissues are infiltrated with lidocaine. A 3-in., short-beveled, 16-gauge needle is attached via a 3-way stopcock to a 30- or 50-ml syringe. The pericardial sac may be entered via the right or left xiphocostal angle or from the tip of the xiphoid process with the needle directed inward, upward, and close to the chest wall. An alternate approach is via the 5th left intercostal space 1 to 2 cm medial to the left border of cardiac flatness with the needle directed inward and slightly medially; if a distinct apical impulse is visible, the needle may be introduced 1 to 2 cm lateral to the impulse. The subxiphoid approach may be preferable for smaller effusions, and is now generally preferred for any pericardiocentesis. Cardiac impulses may be easily felt through the needle when the pericardial sac has been entered.

The needle is advanced with constant suction applied to the syringe. Fluid will be aspirated when the pericardial space is entered. Blood aspirated from the pericardial sac usually will not clot, while blood inadvertently aspirated from the cardiac chambers will. The needle should be clamped next to the skin to prevent it from entering farther than necessary and possibly puncturing the heart or injuring a coronary vessel. ECG monitoring is essential during the procedure to detect arrhythmias produced when the myocardium is touched or punctured. A plastic catheter may be passed through the needle into the sac and the needle withdrawn if repeated paracenteses are contemplated. Except in emergencies, pericardiocentesis, *a potentially lethal procedure*, should be performed under the supervision of a cardiologist or thoracic surgeon and in the cardiac catheterization laboratory. Thoracotomy is usually safer.

Congestion due to constrictive pericarditis may be alleviated with bed rest, salt restriction, and diuretics. Digitalis is indicated in atrial arrhythmias or myocardial failure. Recurrent or persistent effusions, with or without tamponade, and constrictive pericarditis usually require pericardiectomy. With specific infections, pericardiectomy is done preferably after specific antimicrobial therapy is begun. Patients with constrictive pericarditis who have mild symptoms, heavy calcification, or extensive myocardial damage, or who are elderly may be poor candidates for pericardial resection.

CARDIAC TUMORS

Tumors of the heart may be primary or secondary. Primary tumors are rare, being found in < 0.05% of autopsies; secondary tumors are 30 to 40 times more common. The tumors may be epicardial, myocardial, or endocardial, and their symptoms and signs may have localizing features. However, they mimic other heart diseases and are frequently diagnosed either by chance or because of a strong index of suspicion. Cardiac signs and symptoms may develop in a patient with extracardiac malignancies, which suggest that they have involved the heart.

PRIMARY CARDIAC TUMORS

Malignant cardiac tumors are rare, are seen predominantly in children, and may arise from any of the various heart tissues. Most common are the sarcomas, such as angiosarcoma, fibrosarcoma, rhabdomyosarcoma, and liposarcoma. They are associated with more acute and rapid deterioration than benign cardiac tumors. Sudden development of congestive heart failure, rapid accumulation of hemorrhagic pericardial effusion, often with tamponade, and various tachyarrhythmias or heart block may herald the tumor's presence. Metastases occur to spine, neighboring soft tissues, and major organs. Prognosis is poor and treatment is limited to irradiation, chemotherapy, and management of complications.

Benign cardiac tumors, including myxomas, rhabdomyomas, fibromas, lipomas, teratomas, and pericardial cysts, may have a ''malignant'' course and outcome if left untreated.

Myxoma is the most common intracavity cardiac tumor (comprising 50% of primary tumors). Seventy-five percent occur in the left atrium; the remainder are found mostly in the right atrium and rarely in the right and left ventricles. Myxomas are either semitransparent and gelatinous, with a lobular or villous surface, or appear as a round, firm mass. Myxoma cells resemble endothelial cells they are elongated and spindle-shaped with round or oval nuclei and prominent nucleoli. Cells and vessels are embedded in an amorphous matrix rich in acid mucopolysaccharide. The tumor mass is richly supplied with thin-walled capillaries. The tumor surface is usually endothelialized and may be coated with thrombi. Atrial tumors, especially right atrial myxomas, may contain calcium deposits visible on plain chest x-ray. Left atrial myxomas usually arise from the endocardium at the border of the fossa ovalis and are pedunculated; less commonly they are broad-based, sessile tumors. They are usually solid and when pedunculated may prolapse through the mitral valve orifice in diastole

Myxomas present the most varied clinical picture of all cardiac tumors. Three major syndromes may be encountered: (1) embolic phenomena, (2) obstruction to blood flow, and (3) constitutional syndromes. Tumor fragments or thrombotic material may embolize from right- or left-sided tumors to the lungs or periphery, respectively. Gelatinous myxomas are more friable and therefore more likely to embolize. The diagnosis may often be made by finding tumor cells in a surgically removed embolus. Obstruction to blood flow may occur at any valve orifice, most commonly at the mitral valve Interference with valve function by the tumor mimics signs and symptoms of valvular dysfunction due to rheumatic valve disease. Thus, left-atrial myxomas may cause pulmonary congestion and signs of mitral stenosis including the typical murmur, opening snap, and accentuated first heart sound. Murmurs of mitral insufficiency may also be present as a result of chronic damage to the valve leaflets or to the tumor's interference with proper valve closure. Clinical differentiation between left atrial tumor and primary mitral valve disease may be suggested by the influence of position on symptoms such as congestive failure and syncope and on the intensity of murmurs and the opening snap. Left atrial size is likely to be disproportionately smaller in relation to severity of the signs and symptoms in patients with tumor than with valvular disease. About 25% of patients with myxomas may have friction rubs the mechanism for this finding is not clear. Left atrial tumors can also produce a ''tumor plop'' sound as the pedunculated mass drops into the valve orifice during diastole. It differs from the opening snap of rheumatic mitral stenosis by its variability, timing, intensity, and character, sometimes having more than one component.

Constitutional symptoms that may be associated with myxomas are protean (see TABLE 25–8) and may mimic such disorders as bacterial endocarditis, collagen vascular disease, or occult malignancy.

TABLE 25–8. FINDINGS THAT MAY ACCOMPANY CARDIAC MYXOMAS

Fever	Elevated ESR
Weight loss	Elevated WBC count
Raynaud's phenomenon	Decreased platelet count
Clubbing of fingers	Positive C-reaction protein
Anemia	Abnormal serum proteins (usually increased γ-globulins)

Diagnosis is suspected from the symptoms and signs, is strongly suggested by an echocardiogram showing tumor echoes, and is confirmed by angiocardiography or gated radionuclide scanning. Surgical removal usually is curative.

Fibromas and **rhabdomyomas** arise within the myocardium or endocardium; **rhabdomyomas** are most frequent (comprising 20% of primary tumors). They are characterized by a large intracellular content of PAS-positive material, probably glycogen. Usually found in childhood or infancy, most cases are associated with tuberous sclerosis, adenoma sebaceum of the skin, kidney tumors, and arrhythmias. These tumors are predominantly intramural and lie in the interventricular septum or free wall of the left ventricle; multiple tumor nodules are the rule. Cardiac symptoms and signs include atrioventricular and intraventricular block, paroxysmal supraventricular and ventricular tachycardias, cardiomegaly, and manifestations of outflow tract obstruction of either ventricle, such as right- or left-sided congestive failure and murmurs of pulmonary or aortic stenosis. Association of these findings with features of tuberous sclerosis should suggest the diagnosis, which can be confirmed by angiocardiography. Surgical treatment of the multiple tumor nodules is usually ineffective and the prognosis is poor beyond the first year of life. Only 15% of a collected series of patients survived 5 yr.

Teratomas of the pericardium, often attached to the base of the great vessels, are rarer than **cysts** or **lipomas** and are usually seen in infants. They are generally asymptomatic and are often discovered on routine chest x-ray. Surgery is necessary only to rule out more serious tumors.

SECONDARY CARDIAC TUMORS

Malignant tumors that metastasize to the heart may involve any of the cardiac tissues. They include carcinomas, sarcomas, leukemias, and reticuloendothelial tumors. Lung and breast carcinomas invade the heart most frequently. As a group, melanosarcomas have one of the highest incidences of metastasis to the heart. Cardiac involvement by systemic malignancies is suggested by sudden cardiac enlargement, bizarre changes in cardiac contour on chest x-ray, cardiac tamponade, arrhythmias, or unexplained cardiac failure. Therapy is palliative, as with primary cardiac malignancies.

---

26. EXERCISE AND THE HEART

The constellation of physiologic response seen in individuals trained to perform endurance exercise is referred to as the "athletic heart syndrome." Sinus bradycardia is characteristic, and biventricular cardiac enlargement is readily apparent on x-ray. This syndrome should not be misdiagnosed as organic heart disease.

Physiology

Cardiac dilation and hypertrophy are characteristic of endurance-trained athletes, in contrast to the skeletal muscle and myocardial hypertrophy that occur in response to speed or strength (isometric) training. Hypertrophy and dilation in the endurance-trained athletes increase the pumping capability of the heart; increased O_2 delivery to the tissues, both at rest and with exercise, is due primarily to the increased stroke volume. The increase in diastolic filling time with bradycardia further augments the stroke volume and also increases coronary blood flow, which is predominantly a diastolic event. The total Hb and blood volume of endurance-trained athletes are also increased, further enhancing O_2 transport. Both resting heart rate and the heart rate at submaximal exercise decrease progressively with endurance training, primarily due to increased vagal tone, but decreased sympathetic stimulation also plays a role. Although the increased ventricular volume results in increased left ventricular stroke work, the O_2-sparing effect of the bradycardia predominates so that myocardial O_2 consumption decreases for the same amount of external work. Cardiac enlargement and bradycardia both characteristically regress when training is discontinued.

Untrained subjects increase cardiac output in response to exercise primarily by increasing the heart rate; the trained endurance athlete does so mainly by increasing stroke volume. Resting intracardiac pressures are normal in endurance-trained athletes, however, and their intracardiac pressures and pulmonary and peripheral vascular bed pressures respond normally to exercise. Ventricular work per minute is also normal.

Clinical Features

Sinus bradycardia, often with sinus arrhythmia, is characteristic. Atrial and ventricular arrhythmias may occur, and conduction and repolarization (ST-T) abnormalities are seen on the ECG. These arrhythmias are typically asymptomatic and may decrease or disappear with exercise, as the heart rate increases. QRS and T voltage are increased on the ECG, often with a prominent U wave, which is probably related to the bradycardia. Repolarization abnormalities are common. Systemic BP differs little between trained athletes and normal individuals. The heart is moderately enlarged, and the left ventricular impulse is hyperdynamic. A third heart sound is common, as is a left sternal border ejection systolic murmur. The cardiac silhouette is enlarged on chest x-ray; at fluoroscopy, cardiac pulsations are brisk and prominent. There is no correlation between the level of training or cardiovascular performance and the severity of the bradycardia, cardiac enlargement, or ECG abnormality.

There is no evidence that even the most strenuous physical activity is deleterious to the cardiovascular function of an individual with a normal heart. However, **sudden death**, both at rest and with exertion, occurs occasionally in apparently healthy young athletes, probably due to a cardiac arrhythmia. Although the increased ventricular refractory period with bradycardia favors the recurrence of ventricular ectopic rhythms, sudden death related to arrhythmia in athletes is most often due to previously undetected atherosclerotic coronary heart disease, hypertrophic cardiomyopathy, myocarditis, or congenital coronary artery or aortic valve anomalies.

---

27. DISEASES OF THE AORTA AND ITS BRANCHES

AORTITIS

Inflammation of the aorta.

Aortitis may present either by weakening of the aortic wall, leading to aneurysm formation, or by obstruction of the aortic lumen or of the openings of major branches, leading to symptoms and signs of ischemia. The aortic arch syndrome and syphilitic aortitis account for most cases, although other conditions, such as giant cell arteritis (temporal arteritis) and ankylosing spondylitis, may also involve the aorta.

In aortitis the adventitia is involved by chronic inflammation and fibrosis with endarteritis obliterans of the vasa vasorum. The media is involved by chronic inflammation and fibrosis and the intima is thickened by fibroblastic proliferation. As the name implies, giant cell arteritis is characterized by the prominence of giant cells in the inflammatory reaction.

Only the aortic arch syndrome will be discussed in this chapter; the other disorders are described elsewhere in this volume.

THE AORTIC ARCH SYNDROME (Pulseless Disease; Takayasu's Disease; Martorell's Disease; Reversed Coarctation; Young Oriental Female Disease)

A syndrome resulting from obliterative disease of one or more of the large branches of the aortic arch, commonly the innominate, the left common carotid, and the left subclavian arteries.

A variety of lesions can cause obliteration of the great branches of the aortic arch at or near their origins. The syndrome is usually the result of progression of arteriosclerosis and its complications; syphilitic aneurysms of the aortic arch also may cause obliteration of its branches. The age and sex distribution of the majority of patients with this condition is that of the underlying disease. There remains a group of patients (about 5%) with aortic arch syndrome in whom the disease results from a peculiar form of proliferative arteritis of unknown etiology. This occurs usually in young Oriental women 15 to 30 yr of age and is commonly referred to as Takayasu's disease, but it is also found among women and men of other races and at all ages.

Pathology

Maldevelopment of the embryonic branchial arterial arches can cause abnormal arterial pulses in the neck and upper extremities, but these should not be included as a part of this syndrome. The obliterative disease may affect all of the main arterial trunks from the aortic arch, or it may involve only one or two of them. Cases have been described secondary to blunt or penetrating intrathoracic trauma with contusion and intramural and perivascular hematoma. Some have been described secondary to syphilitic or arteriosclerotic aneurysms with intrasaccular thrombus projecting into the orifices of the branches of the aortic arch. Atheromas with thrombi obstructing the origins of the branches of the aortic arch have been found.

In **Takayasu's disease**, obliteration of the brachiocephalic, carotid, and subclavian arteries results from a peculiar panarteritis, or inflammatory involvement of all layers of the vessel wall, most intensely affecting the media and adventitia. Intimal proliferation encroaches upon the lumen and promotes thrombosis. Cellular infiltration by the lymphocytic series is found microscopically, and the frequency of giant cells has led to the term "giant cell arteritis." Elastic lamellae are disrupted, and this with patchy necrosis of the media weakens the wall of the aortic arch and sometimes results in aneurysm. The lesion resembles that of temporal arteritis and that seen in syphilis. The process typically involves the arch of the aorta and the origins of its principal branches; more distal involvement of these branches is generally secondary to thrombosis. Involvement of the abdominal aorta and the renal, coronary, or pulmonary arteries occurs infrequently. The etiology of the inflammatory process is unknown.

Symptoms and Signs

Patients present with symptoms of regional arterial insufficiency affecting the head and upper extremities. Other branches of the aorta are usually not involved. Gangrene is very rare. The symptoms vary according to the degree of involvement of the arterial trunks and to the extent of collateral circulation. Cerebral symptoms are common, secondary to involvement of the carotid and vertebral arteries. Syncope, sometimes with epileptiform seizures, may be a presenting symptom. Fainting related to turning of the head, as in the "carotid sinus syndrome," is often encountered. Temporary blindness, hemiplegia, aphasia, and loss of memory are frequent complaints. Progressive impairment of vision through early formation and rapid maturation of cataracts is found in some cases and corneal opacities may also develop. Occasionally, intermittent loss of visual acuity develops with muscular exercise, a "steal syndrome" referred to inaccurately as "intermittent visual claudication." Similarly, intermittent claudication develops in the muscles of mastication so that chewing becomes difficult. Degenerative and atrophic signs are detected in the face. The eyes are sunken and atrophy of facial skeletal muscles produces a hollow appearance of the cheeks so that the patient looks prematurely old.

Aching, cramping, numbness, and paresthesias in the arms are encountered with exercise, especially in the upstretched position. The brachial, radial, carotid, and superficial temporal pulses are weak or absent. Arterial pulses are normal in the lower extremities. The BP in the arms is low, but that in the legs is normal or elevated, hence the term "reversed coarctation of the aorta." The aortic disease rarely extends peripherally into the abdominal aorta and its bifurcation. Pulselessness and BP then are similar in all 4 extremities.

In some cases, examination of the eyegrounds shows vascular changes, the perimacular arteriovenous communications that attracted the attention of Takayasu who first described them in 1908. The optic disc may suggest atrophy of the optic nerve.

Collateral circulation develops as the obliterative disease progresses, and pulsation in collateral superficial arteries may be felt. Murmurs may be audible in the supraclavicular triangles. These are frequently both systolic and diastolic ("machinery murmurs") with systolic accentuation, and are easily distinguished from venous hums.

In acute phases or subacute pulseless disease secondary to panarteritis of the aortic arch and its branches, systemic effects may be observed: chills, fever, leukocytosis, and elevation of the ESR.

Diagnosis

The diagnosis is suggested by the symptoms and signs described above. It can be confirmed and the sites of the lesion can be identified with precision by aortic arch angiography. Visualization of the affected vessels and precise localization of the occlusive disease are essential if operative intervention is contemplated.

Examination of the peripheral blood shows abnormalities, especially in patients with acute and subacute panarteritis. The ESR is nearly always increased, the blood albumin and globulin may be abnormal, and LE cells may be present.

Treatment

There is no cure. Palliative therapy includes the use of vasodilators, anticoagulants, and corticosteroids, but most cases, especially those without active panarteritis, are not improved. Some success has been obtained with sympathetic denervation of the upper extremities. Endarterectomy with thrombectomy has had encouraging results in cases secondary to causes other than panarteritis, but the best results have been obtained by using tubular or compound "grafts" of synthetic fabrics to bypass the obstructing lesions. Resection and replacement of aortic arch aneurysms have been done successfully in highly selected patients.

AORTIC AND PERIPHERAL ANEURYSMS

Aneurysm: *A localized dilation of a blood vessel, usually an artery.* **Dissecting aneurysm:** *Longitudinal cleavage of the arterial media by a column of blood; the separation of the layers of the media usually does not completely encircle the lumen, but the entire length of the vessel may be involved.*

Etiology and Classification

True aneurysms result from focal weakness and distention of a blood vessel wall. Arteriosclerosis, often in conjunction with systolic hypertension, is commonly associated with varying degrees of elongation, tortuosity, and diffuse or localized dilation of the aorta (aneurysm). A **true aneurysm** contains all components of the vessel wall. Marfan's syndrome is associated with aneurysmal dilation of the first portion of the aorta, often leading to aortic valvular insufficiency. Syphilitic aneurysms most often occur in the ascending thoracic aorta. Abdominal aortic aneurysms are usually arteriosclerotic in origin, and calcification of the vessel wall may be seen on x-ray. These aneurysms may press upon and erode the vertebrae dorsally, or the aneurysm may rupture laterally or ventrally.

Congenital aneurysms of the intracranial carotid system or of the circle of Willis and its branches ("berry aneurysms") occur often in association with other vascular anomalies, such as coarctation of the aorta. They usually result from local weakness or absence of the arterial media. They are a common cause of subarachnoid and intracerebral hemorrhage in the adult (see SUBARACHNOID HEMORRHAGE in Ch. 122).

Mycotic aneurysms result from weakness of the vessel wall as the result of infection in it in patients with bacteremia or septicemia from bacterial endocarditis, enteric infections, or trauma. Mycotic aneurysms commonly occur in the peripheral arteries, but rare cases have also been described in the aorta.

Arteriovenous aneurysms occur as congenital vascular malformations, "portwine stains," "cirsoid" or "racemose" arteriovenous aneurysms, which may affect the head, tongue, cheek, or intracranial vessels. Pulmonary arteriovenous aneurysms (hemangioma of the lung) may be congenital and sometimes are associated with hereditary telangiectasia. Cyanosis, dyspnea, and cardiac failure may result from large lesions. Penetrating wounds (as from bullet, knife, or needle biopsy) may lead to arteriovenous aneurysms, particularly in iliac, brachial, or carotid regions, where an artery and vein are sheathed together. Arteriovenous communications are made surgically for access to hemodialysis in end-stage kidney disease.

Dissecting aneurysms are usually the result of or are associated with atherosclerosis, especially in the elderly. In young patients, however, a dissecting aneurysm is commonly due to one of two forms of medial necrosis: (1) cystic medial necrosis with cystic degeneration as in Marfan's syndrome or (2) necrosis with fibrotic repair but without cystic degeneration or notable vascular proliferation (Erdheim's necrosis). Two mechanisms have been proposed to account for the pathophysiology of dissecting aneurysms: (1) hemorrhage of the vasa vasorum produces an expanding intramedial hematoma, or (2) spontaneous intimal rupture initiates the dissection. Continuation of the dissection leads to complications and may cause death. Successful arrest of the acute process permits thrombosis of the false lumen so that the aorta is protected from expansion or rupture. Occasionally a dissecting aneurysm recanalizes, and the false channel is diverted back into the normal lumen. Experimentally, dissecting aneurysm has been produced by inducing lathyrism.

Clinically, dissecting aortic aneurysms are classified into 3 types according to anatomic and pathologic features. **Type I dissection** involves the ascending aorta and extends for a variable distance into the distal aorta and terminal branches; this is the most common type. **Type II dissections** are local dissections of the ascending aorta without distal extension; this is the rarest type and is more likely to be due to cystic medial necrosis of the aorta or Marfan's syndrome. **Type III dissections** begin at or just distal to the origin of the left subclavian artery and involve the descending aorta. These have the most favorable prognosis.

Symptoms and Signs

Symptoms of **intrathoracic aneurysms** include cough, hoarseness (from pressure on the recurrent laryngeal nerve), dyspnea, dysphagia, and pain that is either substernal or localized in the back from irritation of the thoracic vertebrae. Occasionally, bronchial or tracheal compression will cause a brassy cough that is constant, severe, and difficult to control by usual antitussive measures until the aneurysm is surgically repaired. Diagnosis may be suggested by the appearance of Horner's syndrome, deviation of the trachea, a tracheal tug, or inequality of the BP in the arms. Nonvascular tumors (e.g., goiter, thymoma, neurofibroma, teratoma, bronchogenic carcinoma) may be mistaken for aneurysms because of pulsation transmitted from the adjacent aorta.

Dissecting aortic aneurysms present with a variety of symptoms, but the onset of the dissection is usually associated with severe pain, often mimicking myocardial infarction. A dissecting aneurysm in an arteriosclerotic aorta commonly begins in the ascending aorta and may extend proximally, distally, or in both directions. The site of the pain may help to determine the site of dissection. If the pain starts anteriorly, the aneurysm is generally in the ascending aorta; if it is in the back, the aneurysm is probably distal to the left subclavian artery. If pain is located low in the back, the aneurysm is usually in the abdomen. Neck pain reflects dissection of the aortic arch. In some patients, dissecting aneurysms present initially with congestive heart failure secondary to valvular involvement and aortic insufficiency or with myocardial infarction due to encroachment on a coronary ostium. A few patients present in acute circulatory collapse due to rupture into the pericardium or into the pleural space. Carotid, brachial, or peripheral pulses may disappear or become unequal, and arterial pressures in the upper and lower extremities may differ. CNS symptoms are due to involvement of the origins of the vessels to the head and neck.

The pain of dissecting thoracic aortic aneurysm must be differentiated from that of myocardial infarction; measurement of cardiac enzymes as well as serial ECGs may help (see MYOCARDIAL INFARCTION under MYOCARDIAL ISCHEMIC DISORDERS in Ch. 25). The low BP in the legs that occurs with dissection is seen also in aortic saddle embolism, aortic coarctation, and the Leriche syndrome.

Abdominal aortic aneurysms of arteriosclerotic origin commonly pass unnoticed until they become of sufficient size to be palpable (4 to 6 cm) as a pulsating mass or become symptomatic. Pressure from the aneurysm upon lumbar vertebrae causes excruciating boring pain in the abdomen or back. Aneurysms usually are tender to palpation. The pain from leaking or bleeding abdominal aneurysm usually is felt in the left side, but may be felt anywhere within the abdomen. Significant leaking or rupture of aortic aneurysm is a frequent cause of vascular collapse and shock.

Popliteal aneurysms are dangerous lesions because they endanger the life of the affected limb. They are frequently not diagnosed until they thrombose, become painful and tender, and compromise the circulation. They may enlarge and compress the adjoining nerves and veins, or they may bleed. Small emboli may pass on from the aneurysm and lodge in the digital arteries resulting in gangrene of the digits, similar to embolization from subclavian aneurysms to the hands.

Arteriovenous aneurysms in the upper or lower extremities, if congenital or acquired prior to closure of the epiphyseal lines, result in an increased size of the ipsilateral limb. The venous component of the arteriovenous aneurysm, subjected as it is to arterial pressure, becomes hypertrophied and tortuous, and the walls may become calcified. Bacterial endarteritis with bacteremia may complicate the arteriovenous communication.

A patient with an arteriovenous aneurysm involving the carotids may be aware of a rhythmic, swishing noise synchronous with the heart beat. A large shunt will increase cardiac output, and may lead to heart failure. This complication is the more likely the nearer the heart is to the arteriovenous communication.

Diagnostic Studies

Radiology: Plain x-rays are useful for detecting and evaluating thoracic and abdominal aortic aneurysms, since they are visible as abnormal masses with or without calcification in the wall. In the thorax, a mediastinal mass suggesting an aneurysm may necessitate complete visualization of the thoracic aorta with contrast material to establish the diagnosis and evaluate its resectability. To evaluate an abdominal aneurysm, more than one view is desirable; an anterior-posterior view, right and left obliques, and an appropriate lateral view should be included. Calcification in the wall of the aorta is necessary to establish the exact dimensions and location of the aneurysm; if it is not present, aortography may be required to establish the diagnosis with certainty. Even aortography can be misleading if the aneurysmal sac is filled with laminated clot.

Invasive procedures include translumbar, retrograde femoral, or axillary aortography; the vessels of interest can be selectively catheterized, and direct needle puncture can be used to outline the course of single vessels. Selective technics can be used to visualize the aortic arch vessels, the intracranial arteries, the arteries to the abdominal viscera, and those to the lower extremities. Contrast studies are helpful in most cases before aortic surgery.

Ultrasound: Pulsed ultrasound can be used to define the size and location of abdominal aortic aneurysms. In contrast to arteriography, ultrasound is noninvasive and can depict an aneurysmal dilation without being limited to the moving bloodstream. By scanning the abdomen both longitudinally and transversely, ultrasonic images of the abdominal aorta from the level of the renal arteries to the aortic bifurcation can be generated. Since the technic is noninvasive, it can be used on a long-term basis to follow the progress of aortic aneurysms that are initially considered too small to require surgery.

Prognosis and Treatment

Prognosis of syphilitic aneurysms depends on the location and progression of the syphilitic process. Coronary ostial stenosis or aortic insufficiency associated with cardiac symptoms reduces life expectancy, but patients with relatively stabilized syphilitic lesions may survive many years. Adequate treatment of early syphilis prevents syphilitic aortitis and aneurysm. However, even after a syphilitic aneurysm has fully developed, antisyphilitic therapy may be helpful; procaine penicillin G 6 million to 10 million u., divided into daily IM injections over 1 to 2 wk, generally suffices. In Marfan's syndrome, survival is shortened when aortic insufficiency develops. Congestive heart failure due to aortic insufficiency must be treated appropriately.

Arteriosclerotic aneurysms of the abdominal aorta progress at variable rates. Once the diameter is > 6 cm, the hazard of rapid expansion and rupture is great, and surgical replacement is recommended. Patients with untreated aortic dissection often survive no more than hours or a few days; 44 to 89% of patients with dissecting aneurysms (Types I and II) die from rupture into the pericardial space. In exceptional cases reentry of the dissection into the main aortic lumen may prolong survival for several years.

Surgery is recommended for dissecting aneurysms of the ascending aorta and for patients admitted < 2 wk after the onset of dissection if the origin of the dissection can be identified on angiography and the patient is otherwise a good surgical risk. Complications of dissecting aneurysm such as overwhelming aortic insufficiency, localized leaking or impending rupture, or compromise of a major artery demand urgent surgical intervention. Overall, > 40% of patients may require surgery sometime after the acute dissection. Long-term medical therapy is used for patients in whom surgery is contraindicated because of advanced age or associated medical problems, for patients admitted to the hospital > 2 wk after the onset of symptoms of dissection, and for patients in whom the site of origin of the dissection cannot be positively identified by angiography. The mortality among patients with involvement of the ascending aorta when treated surgically is about 30%, as contrasted with about 70% for medically treated patients. The mortality rates of judicious medical and surgical treatment of descending aortic dissection (Type III) range from 10 to 20%.

All patients suspected of having a dissecting aneurysm should be admitted to an intensive care unit, and vital signs, venous pressure, urinary output, and clinical condition should be monitored. Hypertensive patients should receive medical therapy to lower the systemic BP and to reduce the velocity of contraction of the left ventricle, thereby decreasing the impact of ventricular systole against the aorta; systolic arterial pressure is reduced to 100 mm Hg and is maintained at that level to provide adequate renal, cerebral, and cardiac perfusion and to relieve pain. Initial control is achieved with trimethaphan, reserpine, guanethidine, and/or methyldopa. Trimethaphan is given IV in a concentration of 1 to 2 mg/ml (1 gm in 1000 ml or 500 ml of 5% D/W) as rapidly as necessary to achieve an adequate effect. Since tachyphylaxis to trimethaphan usually becomes evident within 48 h, the other antihypertensive agents must be started soon after hospitalization. Reserpine is given 0.5 to 2 mg IM q 6 h. Guanethidine may be given orally 25 to 50 mg b.i.d.; methyldopa may be given in doses of 1 to 3 gm/day orally or IV in 4 or 6 divided doses. Propranolol is used when not contraindicated in doses of 1 to 2 mg IV or 10 to 40 mg orally q 4 to 6 h. The head of the bed is elevated 35 to 40 degrees to obtain the orthostatic effect of the drugs. For long-term therapy, combinations of oral methyldopa, reserpine, propranolol, guanethidine, and a thiazide diuretic are used to control BP and ventricular contractility.

If the patient is not hypertensive on admission, the drug of choice is propranolol 20 to 40 mg orally q.i.d. After the initial reduction of arterial pressure, emergency aortography is obtained to confirm the diagnosis and to determine whether the ascending aorta is involved. Surgery for aneurysms of the ascending aorta requires cardiopulmonary bypass; the portion of the aorta with the intimal tear is resected, the dissected ends of the aorta are oversewn, and the resected area of aorta is replaced with a "graft." The aortic valve is replaced if necessary. Repair of the descending aorta is done with the patient on partial cardiopulmonary bypass.

The hazards of medical therapy include hypotension, which may be especially dangerous for the elderly. Acute tubular necrosis has occurred during therapy, and patients are often confused and disoriented. Peptic ulceration occurs in some patients receiving reserpine, and postural hypotension often develops when patients begin to ambulate but usually can be controlled by adjusting medications. Saccular aneurysms tend to develop late in the course of medical treatment; these aneurysms may rupture spontaneously and require surgical resection.

OCCLUSION OF THE ABDOMINAL AORTA AND ITS BRANCHES

Atherosclerosis of the aorta is usually asymptomatic unless occlusion occurs, plaques encroach on the ostia of one or more major branches, or embolization occurs to the periphery. Symptoms and signs relate to the organ or tissues in which clinically significant ischemia occurs and several characteristic syndromes may be seen, as indicated below. Aortic occlusive disease can also be caused by aortitis such as in Takayasu's disease or syphilitic aortitis.

SPLANCHNIC ARTERY OCCLUSION

Arteriosclerotic obliterative lesions and arteriosclerotic arterial aneurysms have been described involving all major visceral branches of the abdominal aorta, in particular the celiac and its branches, the superior mesenteric, renal, and inferior mesenteric. Obliterative lesions causing visceral ischemia can occur at the origins of these arteries or usually in their proximal portions. In most cases, when symptoms develop, all 3 arteries are partially obstructed, although the lesions in one may be predominant. Symptoms of visceral ischemia may also be caused by fibromuscular hyperplasia, aneurysms, and emboli, which are not uncommon, especially in the superior mesenteric artery or its branches. Rarely, partial and intermittent occlusion of the celiac and superior mesenteric arteries has been attributed to abdominal webs or bands near their origins. Embolism or acute thrombosis, often referred to as **intestinal apoplexy,** can have catastrophic results. Four fifths of patients who develop acute ischemic intestinal necrosis have either embolism or thrombosis, each accounting for 40% of the total cases.

In about 20% of patients who develop ischemic intestinal necrosis, usually fatal, no obstruction is found in the celiac or mesenteric vessels and their major branches. These patients are usually elderly and have, among other problems, arteriosclerotic heart disease. One possible explanation is that cardiac output temporarily has fallen, leading to a fall in pressure and collapse of the celiac and mesenteric arteries. However, since by Laplace's law, a much greater pressure is required to distend arteries whose diameter has decreased, the collapsed arteries cannot be distended to normal size or opened at all when cardiac output and BP return to normal. The splanchnic vascular bed remains ischemic, and intestinal necrosis occurs.

Chronic Intestinal Ischemia (Intestinal Claudication or Intestinal Angina)

As in atherosclerotic arterial disease elsewhere, the formation of obliterative lesions normally is accompanied by the development of collateral circulation usually adequate to fulfill basal metabolic requirements. Circulation in the GI tract is taxed by the increased work that must be performed during digestion. Meals therefore require an increased splanchnic circulation above basal, and if obliterative arterial disease makes this increase impossible, symptoms develop. These commonly are

(1) postprandial ($\frac{1}{2}$ to 1 h) mid-abdominal or upper abdominal cramp-like pain unrelated to the type of food eaten and unrelieved by usual therapeutic measures for peptic ulcer; (2) changed bowel habits (commonly constipation, seldom diarrhea); (3) occasional melena; (4) progressive weight loss and failure to gain weight by dietary measures; and (5) malabsorption syndrome. Steatorrhea is rare.

Acute Celiac, Splenic, and Mesenteric Occlusion

Occlusion of the **celiac axis** may be totally asymptomatic. Acute interruption of the hepatic branch, however, can produce hepatic necrosis with chills, fever, prostration, and death. Embolism and thrombosis of the hepatic artery are rare, but occasionally the right or common hepatic artery is interrupted at surgery. Infarction of the spleen may result from acute occlusion of the **splenic artery,** and small infarcts frequently occur in the spleen by embolization of branches of the splenic artery. These can produce severe pain by parietal peritoneal irritation. Splenectomy may be necessary.

Acute occlusion of the **superior mesenteric artery** is a common cause of catastrophic abdominal emergency. The pain is mid-abdominal or generalized, severe, and unrelenting, resembling that of acute hemorrhagic necrotizing pancreatitis or perforated gastric or duodenal ulcer. The pain is difficult to control. Nausea, vomiting, and prostration are typical. The physical examination reveals generalized abdominal spasm and shock. The shock is associated with hemoconcentration instead of hemodilution as in hemorrhagic shock and is difficult to correct by the usual means. Gross or occult blood is generally found in the stool. Abdominal x-rays can support the clinical impression of intestinal infarction in about $\frac{1}{3}$ of cases; the presumptive diagnosis can be based on characteristic x-ray changes: (1) pneumatosis intestinalis; (2) widening of the intestinal wall with ileus; (3) ileus with dilation of the small intestine and of the large intestine up to the splenic flexure. Fecal matter is seen in the colon in about 80% of cases with proved infarction secondary to mesenteric occlusion.

Acute occlusion and chronic obliterative disease of the **inferior mesenteric artery** are not likely to be symptomatic except when associated with occlusive disease of the superior mesenteric and other splanchnic arteries. The branches of this artery, through the sigmoidal arcades, have ready access to branches of the mid-colic and the middle and inferior hemorrhoidal arteries for collateral circulation.

The clinical **diagnosis** of vascular disease of the celiac and mesenteric arteries is made by arousal of strong suspicion based on history and physical examination. Plain x-rays of the abdomen may show calcific lesions in the aorta or in the distribution of some of its branches. Attempts to demonstrate diagnostic x-ray changes in the intestine have not been rewarding. Aortography and selective angiography enable precise visualization of the celiac artery and its branches, the mesenteric arteries, and the renal vessels. Obstruction of 80% or more of the lumen with or without post-stenotic dilation in these arteries confirms the clinical suspicion of abdominal angina and precisely localizes the offending artery and the actual site of the obstruction.

Mesenteric venous thrombosis also leads to intestinal necrosis. The symptoms and signs are similar to those of acute arterial occlusion but are less severe and dramatic. The intestinal necrosis is usually more limited and may be segmental. The length of intestine that must be resected is less extensive and the likelihood of survival is greater than after acute arterial mesenteric thrombosis.

RENAL ARTERY OCCLUSION

Among the causes of surgically correctable hypertension, occlusive disease of the renal arteries is the most common, occurring in about 5% of all hypertensive patients. Obliterative disease of the renal arteries is usually unilateral but often bilateral and is most commonly atherosclerotic. Obstructing plaques develop at the ostia of the renal arteries in the aorta or in the proximal portions of the arteries. Post-stenotic dilation of the renal artery is often observed distal to the obstructing lesion. Fibromuscular hyperplasia (or dysplasia) of the renal arterial walls is the second most frequent obstructive cause of renal hypertension. Narrowing of the renal artery is also caused by embolism or thrombosis, by renal arterial aneurysm with thrombosis or embolization, or by dissecting aneurysm. All of these lesions can cause diastolic hypertension. Their pathophysiologic relation to hypertension can be demonstrated by determining the renin activity of venous blood differentially collected from the 2 renal veins. The kidney, its circulation, and its excretory function can be studied by x-ray and by radionuclide excretion.

OCCLUSION AT THE BIFURCATION

Sudden occlusion at the aortic bifurcation is often a dramatic event resulting in absent femoral pulses, pain, weakness, and color and temperature changes in the lower extremities. Embolism commonly is the cause and the prognosis is that of the lesion which generated the embolus. Embolectomy nearly always is indicated and can be done easily transfemorally under local anesthesia.

Gradual occlusion of the terminal aorta may cause impotence in the male and intermittent claudication in the buttocks and thighs **(Leriche syndrome).** Claudication in the calves is due to narrowing or occlusion of the femoral arteries or their branches in addition to the occlusion of the bifurcation of the aorta. Gangrene of the toes also can occur.

28. PERIPHERAL VASCULAR DISORDERS

Vascular diseases of the extremities involve arteries, veins, and lymphatics. Since the extremities are readily accessible to examination, a correct clinical diagnosis can usually be made. Special instrumentation and angiography are rarely necessary to diagnose arterial insufficiency, but are helpful to document the location and extent of disease if surgical correction is contemplated. Noninvasive methods confirm the diagnosis and are useful in following the patient being treated medically or after revascularization. Noninvasive tests and/or venography are usually essential for diagnosing deep venous thrombosis.

OCCLUSIVE ARTERIAL DISEASES

PERIPHERAL ATHEROSCLEROTIC DISEASE (Arteriosclerosis Obliterans)

Occlusion of blood supply to the extremities by atherosclerotic plaques (atheroma).

By far, most patients with occlusive arterial disease have an underlying atherosclerotic process. The incidence, pathogenesis, risk factors, and prophylaxis of atherosclerosis are discussed in Ch. 24, above. Clinical syndromes depend upon the degree of encroachment and rapidity of development of the occlusive process and the particular vessel involved; various syndromes are discussed elsewhere in the text—e.g., in Ch. 27, under Myocardial Ischemic Disorders in Ch. 25, and in Ch. 122. The discussion here is limited to occlusive diseases of the extremities, both chronic (arteriosclerosis obliterans) and acute (thrombosis and embolism).

Symptoms and Signs

Chronic ischemia: Patients with arteriosclerosis obliterans have symptoms related to the slow, insidious development of tissue ischemia. The initial symptom is **intermittent claudication** due to a deficient blood supply in exercising muscle. The distress is described as a pain, ache, cramp, or tired feeling that occurs on walking; it occurs most commonly in the calf but also in the foot, thigh, hip, or buttocks. Relieved quickly by rest (usually in 2 to 5 min), the patient can walk the same distance again before pain recurs. Sitting is not necessary to obtain relief. The distress is worsened by walking rapidly or uphill, but it never occurs at rest. Progression of the disease is indicated by a lessening of the distance the patient can walk. Similar symptoms related to exertion occur with involvement of the upper extremity.

The occlusive disease may progress so that ischemic pain occurs at rest. **Rest pain** beginning in the most distal parts of the limb is a severe, unrelenting pain aggravated by elevation and often preventing sleep. To obtain relief, the patient will hang his foot over the side of the bed or will rest in a chair.

If intermittent claudication is the only symptom, the extremity may appear normal, but the pulses are reduced or absent. The level of arterial occlusion and the location of intermittent claudication are closely correlated. Aortoiliac disease frequently causes claudication in the buttocks and hips in addition to the calves, and femoral pulses are absent. In femoropopliteal disease, the claudication is characteristically in the calf, and all of the pulses below the femoral are absent. In patients with small vessel disease (e.g., Buerger's disease or diabetes mellitus) the femoral and popliteal pulses are present but foot pulses are absent. Helpful confirmatory signs of arterial insufficiency are pallor of the skin of the involved foot after 1 to 2 min of elevation, followed by rubor on dependency. Venous filling time following elevation is delayed beyond the normal limit of 15 seconds.

A severely ischemic foot is painful, cold, and often numb. The skin may be dry and scaly with poor nail and hair growth. As ischemia worsens, ulceration may appear, especially after local trauma. Ulcerations are characteristically on the toes or heel or occasionally on the leg. There is usually no edema, but a severely ischemic leg may be shrunken and atrophic.

More extensive obliterative disease may compromise the viability of tissues and lead to necrosis or gangrene.

Acute ischemia is caused by sudden arterial occlusion from an embolism in the heart, a proximal arteriosclerotic plaque, or an aneurysm or an acute thrombosis on preexisting atherosclerotic disease. The history includes sudden onset of severe pain, coldness, numbness, and pallor. The extremity is cold, either pale or cyanotic, and pulses are absent distal to the obstruction. In acute occlusion of the aorta (saddle embolus or thrombosis), all pulses normally in the lower extremities are absent. Characteristically, acute occlusions occur at bifurcations just distal to the last palpable pulse; thus, with occlusion at the common femoral bifurcation, the femoral pulse is palpable, and with occlusion at the popliteal bifurcation, the popliteal pulse is present. Acute occlusion may cause severe ischemia manifested by sensory and motor loss and induration of muscles on palpation.

The symptoms and signs of **vasospastic arterial disease** in Raynaud's disorders and scleroderma are discussed separately under Functional Peripheral Arterial Disorders, below.

Laboratory Evaluation

X-ray: Plain films of the extremities have no diagnostic value in occlusive disease. Intimal calcification merely confirms the presence of atherosclerosis, and medial calcification is not correlated with the occurrence of arteriosclerosis obliterans. **Angiography,** a prerequisite to surgical correction, provides details of the location and extent of lesions occluding the arterial system. Angiography should be complete and include aortography and bilateral femoral arteriography, visualizing the arteries as far distally as the feet. Methods include translumbar aortography combined with bilateral femoral arteriography, a method used by many vascular surgeons, or percutaneous catheterization via femoral artery or upper extremity.

Noninvasvie diagnostic instrumentation: A variety of noninvasvie instrumentation is available to evaluate arterial insufficiency. It is useful to confirm and document the arterial insufficiency found by clinical examination, to evaluate a patient for sympathectomy, revascularization, or amputation, and to follow the patient on conservative treatment or after surgery. These instruments are accurate, simple, portable, and relatively inexpensive.

The most widely used method is **Doppler ultrasound** (the principles and technics of ultrasound are discussed further in Ch. 226). Arterial stenosis and occlusion can be easily recognized by listening with the velocity detector (Doppler probe). The simplest method for estimating blood flow to the lower extremities is to measure the systolic BP at the level of the ankle and compare it to brachial systolic pressure. A BP cuff is applied to the ankle in the usual manner, inflated above brachial systolic pressure, and then deflated slowly. The ankle systolic pressure can be obtained accurately with a Doppler probe placed over the dorsalis pedis or posterior tibial arteries. The ankle systolic pressure normally is 90% or more of the brachial systolic pressure; with mild arterial insufficiency, it is between 70% and 90%; with moderate insufficiency, between 50% and 70%; and with severe insufficiency, below 50%.

Systolic pressures similarly obtained at the thigh and upper calf levels give additional information about the extent and location of the occlusive disease and the collateral blood flow. The above information can be supplemented by analyzing pulse volume waveforms obtained with a segmental plethysmograph (pulse volume recorder).

Treatment

Patients with intermittent claudication should walk 30 to 60 min daily; when discomfort occurs, they should stop, and then walk again. Because collateral circulation is developed, this mode of treatment usually improves the distance patients can walk without discomfort. Tobacco in all forms must be eliminated (see Ch. 48). Vasodilators are commonly prescribed, although there is no proof of their effectiveness. When a patient is sleeping, blocks should be used to elevate the head of the bed 4 to 6 in.

Prophylactic foot care is especially important: (1) Patients should inspect and feel their feet daily for cracks, fissures, calluses, corns, and ulcers. (2) Feet should be washed daily in lukewarm water, using mild soap; they should be dried gently and thoroughly. (3) A lubricant, such as lanolin, should be used for dry, scaly skin. (4) Bland, nonmedicated foot powders should be used for moist feet. (5) Toenails should be cut straight across, not too close to the skin. A podiatrist should do this if the patient's eyesight is poor. (6) Calluses or corns should be treated by a podiatrist. (7) Adhesive plasters and tape should not be used on skin. (8) Harsh chemicals or corn cures should not be used. (9) Patients should change stockings daily and avoid constricting garters. (10) Loose wool stockings can keep feet warm in cold weather, but hot water bottles or electric pads must not be used. (11) Shoes should fit well; they should be wide-toed without open heels or toes and should be changed frequently. (12) Special shoes should be prescribed if there is any foot deformity (e.g., previous toe amputation, hammer toe, bunion) in order to reduce trauma. (13) Walking barefoot should always be avoided.

In patients with diabetic neuropathic ulcers, weight bearing should be eliminated. Since most patients with this type ulcer have little or no occlusive disease, debridement, trimming of callus, and antibiotics frequently produce good healing. Drainage of infection may prevent major surgery later. After the ulcer has healed, appropriate inserts or special shoes should be prescribed. Refractory cases, especially if osteomyelitis is present, may require surgical removal of the metatarsal head (source of pressure), combined with amputation of the involved toe or a transmetatarsal amputation. A neuropathic joint may be satisfactorily managed with orthopedic appliances such as short leg braces, molded shoes, sponge-rubber arch supports, crutches, and prostheses. (See DIABETIC ARTERIOSCLEROTIC DISEASE in Ch. 24 for further discussion.)

In ischemic foot lesions, if revascularization is impossible, a therapeutic program may prevent amputation. Diabetes mellitus must be controlled as closely as possible, and complete bed rest with the head of the bed elevated on blocks is necessary. The lesion must be kept clean with daily soaks in mild soap or saline solution and then dressed with sterile dry dressings. A mild antibiotic ointment may be used. Irritating solutions should be avoided. An obvious infection should be cultured and appropriate antibiotics given systemically. Enzymatic debridement may be irritating and increase the pain. Surgical debridement when ischemia is severe does more harm than good and is very painful. Patients should be warned that healing may take a long time.

Reconstructive surgical procedures are well established valuable procedures. In properly selected patients, symptoms are relieved, ulcers healed, and amputations averted. The procedures are thromboendarterectomy, bypass graft (woven prosthetic tube or autogenous vein anastomosed end-to-side to the vessel above and below the obstruction), or resection with graft replacement (most often used in cases of abdominal aortic aneurysm and embolization of atheromatous material from a proximal site). Effective surgery depends on adequate angiography (aortography and bilateral femoral arteriography) that establishes the site of occlusion and the condition of the arteries above and below.

The success of a surgical procedure is directly related to the adequacy of blood flow into the graft (run in) and out of the graft (run off). Autogenous veins (usually the greater saphenous) are used most often to bypass occlusive lesions of the superficial femoral, popliteal, or tibial arteries. Thromboendarterectomy is used for short, localized lesions in the aorta, iliac, common femoral, or deep femoral arteries. Woven dacron for arterial prostheses is the preferred material to bypass disease in the aortoiliac area. PTFE (Gortex®) is the synthetic material of choice for femoropopliteal-tibial obstructions if saphenous vein is not available. The indications for arterial surgical procedures in the aortoiliac area are incapacitating (economic or avocational) intermittent claudication or severe ischemia due to associated distal disease. Surgery for femoropopliteal and/or tibial disease is reserved for patients who have severe ischemia with rest pain, ulceration, or minor gangrene. Patients with only intermittent claudication should always be treated conservatively at first; if the disease progresses to more severe ischemia, surgery is needed. In some cases, sympathectomy, which removes neurogenic vasoconstriction, can be very helpful and should be offered to selected patients with severe disease and those who are not candidates for revascularization. The value of these procedures is well established in terms of limb salvage and relieving claudication, but their reduction in mortality is small. The primary approach to treatment of atherosclerosis should be preventive.

Percutaneous transluminal angioplasty is a recent, promising development in treating localized occlusive arterial lesions due to atherosclerosis. The technic consists of dilating the diseased segment with the Grüntzig double lumen catheter, containing a balloon made of polyvinyl chloride. It can be inflated to 6 atmospheres pressure while maintaining a cylindrical balloon-shape to avoid overdilation. This flexible catheter can be made in small French size, allowing it to approach many arteries from many sites, such as renal, coronary, axillary, iliac, and superficial femoral-popliteal arteries.

The indications for percutaneous transluminal dilation of the peripheral arteries are (1) progressive and limiting intermittent claudication that prevents the patient from working, (2) rest pain, and (3) gangrene. Lesions suitable for this procedure are high-grade, short iliac stenoses and short, single or multiple stenoses of the superficial femoral-popliteal segment. Complete occlusions of the superficial femoral artery, 10 to 12 cm or less in length, have been successfully dilated. An excellent indication is dilation of a short, localized iliac stenosis prior to a distal femoropopliteal bypass operation. Contraindications are diffuse disease, long occlusions, stenosis at the takeoff of an essential collateral, and severe arterial calcification. Following the dilation, intra-arterial heparin is injected and the patient is maintained on heparin for at least 48 h. Following this, some workers have continued their patients on aspirin or another antiplatelet agent. Study in the noninvasive laboratory should be carried out before and after the dilation to document improvement and to follow-up the patient. A postdilation angiogram is usually done at the time of the procedure.

Complications that may require surgical intervention are thrombosis at the site of dilation, distal embolization, intimal dissection with occlusion by a flap, and possible complications from the heparin therapy. Various reports document success in the 90% and higher range.

When amputation is required for uncontrolled infection, unrelenting rest pain, and progressive gangrene, it should be kept as distal as possible; it is especially important to preserve the knee for optimal use of a prosthesis.

THROMBOANGIITIS OBLITERANS (Buerger's Disease)

An obliterative disease characterized by inflammatory changes in the small and medium-sized arteries and veins.

Etiology and Incidence

Buerger's disease occurs predominantly in men aged 20 to 40 who smoke cigarettes. The incidence has decreased drastically in recent years. A small number of investigators doubt that the disorder is a distinct clinical and pathologic entity and believe it is indistinguishable from occlusive disease due to atherosclerosis, systemic emboli, or idiopathic peripheral thromboses. The disagreement concerns the specificity of the pathologic lesion, but most clinicians agree that the clinical characteristics are sufficiently distinctive to consider thromboangiitis obliterans a discrete entity. The etiology is unknown, but the relationship of smoking to the occurrence and progression of the disease is apparent. There is no documented evidence that the condition occurs in nonsmokers implicating cigarette smoking as a primary etiologic factor.

Pathology and Pathophysiology

The disease involves the small and medium-sized arteries and, frequently, the superficial veins of the extremities in a segmental pattern. Rarely, in well advanced disease, vessels in other parts of the body are affected. The pathologic appearance is that of a nonsuppurative panarteritis or panphlebitis associated with thrombosis of the involved vessels. Proliferation of the endothelial cells and infiltration of the intimal layer with lymphocytes occurs in the acute lesion, but the internal elastic lamina is intact. The thrombus becomes organized and later is incompletely recanalized. The media is well preserved though it may be infiltrated with fibroblasts. Since the adventitia usually is more extensively infiltrated with fibroblasts, older lesions show periarterial fibrosis that may involve the adjacent vein and nerve as well.

Symptoms, Signs, and Diagnosis

Onset is gradual starting in the most distal vessels and progressing proximally, culminating in the development of distal gangrene. The symptoms and signs of thromboangiitis obliterans are those of arterial ischemia and of superficial phlebitis. A history of migratory phlebitis, usually in the superficial veins of the foot or leg, can be obtained in about 40% of cases. The patient may complain of coldness, numbness, tingling, or burning before objective evidence of disease is present. Raynaud's phenomenon is common. Intermittent claudication occurs in the involved extremity (usually the arch of the foot or the leg, but rarely the hand, arm, or thigh). Persistent pain is experienced with more severe ischemia, e.g., in the pregangrenous stage and when ulceration or gangrene is present.

Pulsations in one or more pedal arteries are impaired or absent in most cases, and in wrist arteries in about 40% of cases. Postural color changes (pallor on elevation and rubor on dependency) can frequently be demonstrated in affected hands, feet, or digits. Ischemic ulceration and gangrene, usually of one or more digits, may occur early in the disease but not acutely. Noninvasive studies show a severe decrease in blood flow and pressure in affected toes, foot, and fingers. The disease progresses proximally. Diagnosis can usually be established with clinical data. Arteriograms show segmental occlusions of the distal arteries, especially of hands and feet. Nonaffected arteries are smooth and of normal appearance. Collateral circulation forms around occlusions and may be more tortuous ("corkscrew" appearance) than collaterals associated with other occlusive diseases.

Prophylaxis and Treatment

Supportive care should be directed toward removing all factors that reduce the blood supply and using all possible means to increase it. Factors to be eliminated in addition to smoking include (1) thermal injury; (2) injury to tissues by chemical substances such as iodine, carbolic or salicylic acids, or other strong chemicals; (3) trauma, especially from poorly fitted footwear or minor surgery of digits; (4) fungal infections; and (5) vasoconstriction from exposure to cold or drugs.

Complete bed rest is necessary when gangrene, ulceration, or rest pain is present. The feet should be protected by bandaging with heel pads or foam rubber booties. Heat cradles should not be used unless thermostatically controlled to prevent the temperature from rising above body temperature. Gravity should be employed to assist arterial filling by elevating the head of the bed on 6- to 8-in. blocks. When there is no gangrene, ulceration, or rest pain, the patient should walk for 15 to 30 min twice/day.

Antibiotics, corticosteroids, and anticoagulants are ineffective, and vasodilators are of limited, if any, use.

Unremitting progression of the acute stage invariably occurs in the patient who continues to smoke and may produce so much tissue damage that amputation is required. The residual arterial insufficiency that is always present during a remission may be ameliorated by appropriate dorsal or lumbar sympathectomy providing the patient has given up smoking. Since large vessels such as the iliac, femoral, subclavian, and brachial arteries are rarely involved, bypass grafts are seldom applicable.

TEMPORAL ARTERITIS (Giant Cell Arteritis; Cranial Arteritis; Granulomatous Arteritis)

A chronic generalized inflammatory disease of the branches of the aortic arch; found principally in the temporal and occipital arteries, but may develop in almost any large artery. It is rarely seen in veins. The systemic symptoms are the same as those of **polymyalgia rheumatica**, to which it may be related or identical. Most cases occur in persons over age 50. The estimated incidence is 24:100,000, which rises considerably after age 80. The etiology is unknown, although recent data suggest that an autoimmune reaction is involved.

Pathology

Giant cell arteritis most often involves the arteries of the carotid system, particularly the cranial arteries; but segments of the aorta, its branches, the coronary arteries, and the peripheral arteries may also be affected. The histologic reaction is a granulomatous inflammation of the arteries; lymphocytes, epithelioid cells, and giant cells predominate. The inflammatory reaction causes a marked thickening of the intimal layer with narrowing and occlusion of the lumen.

Symptoms and Signs

The onset may be acute or gradual and may simulate an infection such as an influenza-like syndrome, with low-grade fever, malaise, anorexia, severe weakness, and weight loss. Polymyalgia is characterized by aching and stiffness involving mainly the trunk and proximal muscle groups such as the neck, shoulders, and the hip-pelvic area; occasionally the trunk is involved. Synovitis may occur especially in the knees. The characteristic headache, which may be uni- or bilateral, is a severe, throbbing, boring, or lancinating pain in the temporal area, with redness, swelling, tenderness, and nodulation of the temporal artery. Pulsations in the artery may be strong, weak, or absent. Serious complications include blindness, stroke, coronary occlusion, and arterial insufficiency of the upper and lower extremities. Half of the patients have ocular symptoms and 40% have visual loss. When visual loss occurs, it is bilateral in 75%. Keen awareness of the condition and early treatment may reduce the frequency of permanent visual loss to 5 to 10%. Less common symptoms include claudication of the muscles of mastication, the tongue, and the extremities. The aortic arch and its branches are involved in about 9% of cases. Angiograms show smooth, tapered occlusions or stenoses.

Diagnosis

The ESR is invariably elevated during the active phase of the disease. Leukocytosis and mild anemia may also be present. Because prolonged treatment is necessary, the clinical diagnosis should be confirmed by biopsy of an involved artery. Multiple biopsies of the temporal artery and its branches may be required to obtain positive pathologic findings. About 40% of patients with myalgia and negative findings on clinical examination of the temporal artery have positive findings on temporal artery biopsy. The temporal arteriogram shows areas of constriction and dilation interspersed with areas that appear normal; an arteriogram may help the surgeon choose the area to be biopsied. Muscle biopsies are useless because the arteries of muscles are not involved.

Treatment

To prevent blindness, treatment should start as soon as the diagnosis is suspected. High doses of corticosteroids initially control systemic and local symptoms. Prednisone 60 mg/day orally is given until symptoms and findings are gone and laboratory tests return to normal (usually 2 to 4 wk). Then the dosage is reduced to 40 mg/day for 4 to 6 wk. Thereafter, 5 to 10 mg/day should be given for up to 2 yr or longer to prevent relapse. The activity of the disease can be monitored by periodically determining the ESR. Relapse is characterized by recurrence of the symptoms of temporal arteritis or polymyalgia associated with a rise in the ESR.

FUNCTIONAL PERIPHERAL ARTERIAL DISORDERS

Vascular disorders that are functional in origin and may produce symptoms and signs of disturbance of the peripheral circulation in the absence of organic disease. They may be secondary to a local fault in the blood vessels or to disturbances in sympathetic nervous system activity, or they may accompany organic vascular disease.

RAYNAUD'S PHENOMENON AND DISEASE

Spasm of arterioles, especially in the digits (and occasionally other acral parts such as the nose and tongue), with intermittent pallor or cyanosis of the skin.

Etiology

Raynaud's phenomenon may be idiopathic (Raynaud's disease) or secondary to conditions such as connective tissue disorders (e.g., scleroderma, RA, SLE), neurogenic lesions (including the thoracic outlet syndromes), drug intoxications (ergot and methysergide), dysproteinemias, myxedema, primary pulmonary hypertension, and trauma. Idiopathic Raynaud's disease is most common in young women.

Pathology and Pathophysiology

Attacks of vasospasm of the digital arteries may last for minutes to hours but are rarely severe enough to cause gross tissue loss. In patients with longstanding Raynaud's disease, the skin of the digits may become smooth, shiny, and tight with loss of subcutaneous tissue **(sclerodactyly).** Small painful ulcers may appear on the tips of the digits. The vessels are histologically normal in the early stages, but in advanced cases the arterial intima may be thickened and thromboses may occur in small arteries. In secondary Raynaud's phenomenon the pathologic changes of the underlying disease are apparent.

Symptoms, Signs, and Diagnosis

Intermittent attacks of blanching or cyanosis of the digits is precipitated by exposure to cold or by emotional upsets. The color changes may be triphasic: pallor, cyanosis, redness (reactive hyperemia); or biphasic: cyanosis, then reactive hyperemia. Normal color and sensation are restored by rewarming the hands. Color changes are not present proximal to the metacarpophalangeal joints and rarely involve the thumb. Pain is uncommon, but paresthesias consisting of numbness, tingling, or burning are frequent during the attack.

Idiopathic Raynaud's disease is differentiated from secondary Raynaud's phenomenon by bilateral involvement and a history of symptoms for at least 2 yr with no progression of the symptoms and no evidence of an underlying cause. In idiopathic Raynaud's disease, trophic skin changes and gangrene are either absent or present only in minimal cutaneous areas. The symptoms and signs of the underlying disease usually become manifest within 2 yr, occasionally longer. In Raynaud's phenomenon associated with scleroderma, there may also be tightness or thickening of the skin of the hands, arms, or face, difficulty swallowing, and symptoms referable to other systems. Telangiectases may be found on the hands, face, and lips, and painful trophic ulcers may occur on the fingertips. The wrist pulses are usually present, but the Allen test frequently shows occlusion of the radial or ulnar artery distal to the wrist.

Treatment

Therapy of the secondary forms depends on recognition and treatment of the underlying disturbance. Mild cases of idiopathic Raynaud's disease may be controlled by protecting the body and extremities from cold and by using mild sedatives (e.g., phenobarbital 15 to 30 mg orally t.i.d. or q.i.d.). The patient must stop smoking since nicotine is a vasoconstrictor (see Ch. 48). Phenoxybenzamine 10 mg orally q.i.d. may be useful. Reserpine 0.25 mg orally 2 to 4 times/day may decrease the number and severity of attacks but side effects such as depression may prevent its use. Reserpine 1.0 mg in 5.0 ml of normal saline solution injected into the brachial artery at 3 monthly intervals may have a beneficial effect on the healing of ulcers. Methyldopa 1 to 2 gm/day or prazosin 4 to 8 mg/day may subjectively and objectively benefit patients with Raynaud's disease. Regional sympathectomy is reserved for patients with progressive disability; it often abolishes the symptoms, but the relief may last only 1 to 2 yr. Results from sympathectomy are generally better in patients with Raynaud's disease than in those with secondary Raynaud's phenomenon.

ACROCYANOSIS

Persistent, painless, symmetric cyanosis of the hands and, less commonly, the feet, caused by vasospasm of the smaller vessels of the skin. The etiology is unknown, but increased tone of the arterioles associated with dilation of capillaries and venules is thought to be the cause. The disorder usually occurs in women and is not associated with occlusive arterial disease. The digits and hands or feet are persistently cold, bluish, and sweat profusely; they may swell. The cyanosis is usually intensified by exposure to cold and lessened with warming. Trophic changes and ulceration do not occur, and pain is absent. **Diagnosis** is made from the persistent nature of the findings localized to the hands and feet in the presence of normal arterial pulsations. Except for reassurance and protection from cold, **treatment** is usually unnecessary. Vasodilators may be tried, but are usually ineffective. Sympathectomy is helpful but seldom warranted.

ERYTHROMELALGIA

A rare syndrome of paroxysmal vasodilation with burning pain, increased skin temperature, and redness of the feet and, less often, the hands. The etiology of primary erythromelalgia is unknown. Secondary erythromelalgia may occur in patients with myeloproliferative disorders, hypertension, venous insufficiency, or diabetes mellitus. The condition is characterized by attacks of burning pain in hot, red feet or hands. Distress is triggered by modest ambient temperatures usually varying between 29 and 32 C (84.2 and 89.6 F) in most patients. Trophic changes do not occur. Symptoms may remain mild for years or may become so severe that total disability results. **Diagnosis** is based on demonstration that the patient's complaints are related to objectively increased skin temperature. Secondary types should be differentiated from the rare primary disorder, since, in the former, correction of the underlying disorder may relieve the symptoms.

Treatment

Attacks can be avoided or aborted by rest, elevation of the extremity, and cold applications. Therapy is not always successful. Correction of the underlying disease in secondary forms is indicated. In primary erythromelalgia, modest doses of aspirin may produce prompt, prolonged relief; 600 mg may prevent attacks of pain for several days. Avoiding factors that produce vasodilation is usually helpful, and vasoconstrictors (e.g., ephedrine 25 mg orally, propranolol 10 to 40 mg orally q.i.d., or methysergide 1 to 4 mg orally q 4 h) may also produce relief.

VENOUS DISEASES

VENOUS THROMBOSIS (Thrombophlebitis; Phlebitis)

The presence of a thrombus in a vein.

The most common venous diseases that bring patients to a physician are deep venous thrombosis **(DVT), thrombophlebitis,** and its sequelae of **chronic venous insufficiency**—stasis pigmentation, stasis dermatitis, and stasis ulceration. These are usually readily diagnosed except for DVT of the calf, which requires venography or radioactive fibrinogen. Thrombophlebitis is an acute disease with symptoms that occur over a period of hours to 1 or 2 days. The disease process is usually self-limited and lasts between 1 and 2 wk, by which time the acute process subsides and the painful symptoms disappear.

The terms **phlegmasia alba dolens (milk leg)** and **phlegmasia cerulea dolens** are applied to extensive thrombosis of the involved extremity (depending on its color). The former term is archaic and is now referred to as **ileofemoral thrombophlebitis.** The latter term is still used and means a massive venous thrombosis often leading to venous gangrene and eventual death due to underlying disease, such as widespread malignancy. Eponyms are used to describe thrombosis of veins in specific anatomic areas: **Mondor's disease** refers to thrombosis of the superficial veins over the mammary gland or the adjacent chest wall; **Budd-Chiari syndrome** characterizes the results of hepatic vein thrombosis. **Phlebitis migrans** refers to recurrent venous thrombosis mainly in the superficial veins, but occasionally in deep veins of the extremities and other areas usually due to underlying malignancy. **Effort (strain) thrombosis** occurs in the subclavian vein secondary to trauma to the vein in the thoracic outlet during unusual physical effort in which the arm is fully abducted. **Chemical phlebitis** results from intimal injury induced by the introduction of catheters or noxious agents directly into a vein. "**Chronic thrombophlebitis**" does not exist. Pelvic vein, mesenteric vein, portal vein, renal vein, jugular-mesenteric vein thromboses, etc., are not discussed here.

Etiology

Multiple factors play a role in the etiology of venous thrombosis. Predominant are (1) injury to the epithelium of the vein, such as occurs with indwelling catheters, injection of irritating substances, thromboangiitis obliterans, and septic phlebitis; (2) hypercoagulability associated with malignant tumors, blood dyscrasias, oral contraceptives, and idiopathic thrombophlebitis; and (3) stasis which occurs in postoperative and postpartum states, varicose thrombophlebitis, and the thrombophlebitis that complicates prolonged bedrest of any chronic illness, congestive heart failure, stroke, and trauma.

It is likely that all of these factors play a role; i.e., endothelial injury exposes collagen, causing platelet aggregation and tissue thromboplastin release that, when stasis or hypercoagulability is present, trigger the coagulation mechanism.

Pathology

Most venous thrombi begin as a platelet nidus in the valve cusps of the deep calf veins. Tissue thromboplastin is released, forming thrombin and fibrin which trap RBCs and propagate proximally as a red thrombus. The red or fibrin thrombus is the predominant morphologic venous lesion; the white or platelet thrombus is the principal component of most arterial lesions. The fibrin thrombus can be prevented from forming or extending by anticoagulant drugs such as heparin or the coumarin compounds, but the platelet portion of the thrombus has not been shown to be influenced by these agents in usual therapeutic doses. Furthermore, antiplatelet agents, although under intensive study, have not been shown to be convincingly effective.

Symptoms and Signs

Deep venous thrombosis (DVT) may be asymptomatic or may manifest itself over the involved area by variable combinations of tenderness, pain, edema, warmth, bluish discoloration, or prominence of the superficial veins. In patients with deep thrombophlebitis involving the popliteal, femoral, and iliac segments, there may be tenderness, and a hard cord may be palpable over the involved vein in the femoral triangle in the groin, the medial thigh, or popliteal space. With ileofemoral venous thrombosis, dilated superficial collateral veins over the leg, thigh, and hip areas and lower abdomen usually appear. Bedside evaluation can determine the significance of these findings, but difficulties arise in the diagnosis of DVT of the calf. Since at least 3 main veins drain this area, thrombosis of one of them is not associated with swelling, cyanosis of the skin, or dilated superficial veins. The patient complains of soreness or of pain on standing and walking that is usually relieved by rest with the leg elevated. On examination, deep calf tenderness can be elicited, but differentiation from muscle pain is often difficult. Pain due to muscular causes is absent or minimal on dorsiflexion of the ankle with the knee flexed, and maximal on dorsiflexion of the ankle with the knee extended or during straight leg raising (**Homans' sign**); however, this is an unreliable indication of DVT. Loss of peripheral arterial pulses may occasionally accompany massive DVT, but venous thrombosis can also occur secondary to acute arterial occlusion.

Superficial thrombophlebitis: A thrombosed superficial vein always can be palpated as a linear, indurated cord; it may be associated with a variable inflammatory reaction manifested by pain, tenderness, erythema, and warmth. Palpation of a cord in the calf reflects occlusion of a superficial vein; the inference that this finding, per se, reflects DVT is not justified, since it seldom occurs.

Chronic venous insufficiency in the leg after deep thrombophlebitis is manifested by edema and dilated superficial veins. The patient may complain of fullness, aching, or tiredness in the leg or have no discomfort. This occurs during standing or walking and is relieved by rest and elevation. There is no tenderness over the deep veins to indicate an acute thrombophlebitis, but a history of a previous deep thrombophlebitis can usually be elicited. The **stasis syndrome** occurs in patients with chronic venous insufficiency if the edema is not controlled by an elastic support. With time, skin pigmentation appears on the medial and sometimes the lateral aspect of the ankle and lower leg. Further complications include **stasis dermatitis** and **stasis ulceration** in these areas. Patients with chronic venous insufficiency may develop **varicose veins**, but these are secondary to the DVT, are often mild, and are functioning as collateral vessels. They should not be surgically excised unless severe. The symptoms and signs of varicose veins are discussed separately, below.

Diagnosis

Physical examination usually can distinguish between acute arterial and venous obstruction. The dilemma can be resolved by noninvasive study or by arteriography or venography if necessary. A diagnosis of acute DVT cannot be made satisfactorily by local clinical findings > 50% of the time;

Homans' sign should not be relied upon for the diagnosis, and edema may be due to other causes. Specific limb findings, evidence of pulmonary embolism, and the overall clinical setting including the risk factors (mentioned under Etiology above) permit the physician to estimate the likelihood of the existence of DVT in the individual patient. If there is any doubt, a **venogram** should be obtained. Pulmonary embolism can be sought with lung scan or pulmonary arteriogram. Overlooking the presence of phlebitis may lead to death from pulmonary embolism, but treatment for venous thrombosis with anticoagulants in the absence of an intravascular thrombus demonstrable by venography or lung scan risks serious hemorrhage.

Localization of actively forming deep venous thrombi by injecting ^{125}I fibrinogen is a very sensitive screening test for deep calf, popliteal, and distal thigh thrombosis. Its limitations are that the thyroid gland must be blocked, which requires 24 to 36 h, and since the thrombus must be actively forming to incorporate the isotope, heparin must be withheld. Since ^{125}I fibrinogen appears in blood and exudate, it is not reliable when healing wounds or hematomas are present in the leg, and it cannot detect thrombi in the upper thigh or pelvis.

Isotope venography may be performed by injecting sodium pertechnetate Tc 99m into a peripheral vein and scanning the leg with a gamma camera. Although less painful and quicker, this method does not give the resolution of conventional venography. Noninvasive procedures are less accurate than venography but, in combination, can be diagnostic in 80 to 90% of cases.

Doppler ultrasound: (See Ch. 226 for additional discussion.) Recent complete obstruction of the proximal veins (popliteal and the veins proximal to it) of an extremity characteristically alters the spontaneous flow sounds heard in various segments of the extremity with the Doppler probe. The examiner listens over the femoral vein in the groin, the medial thigh, and the popliteal space. Normal sounds are similar to the "howling wind," which waxes and wanes with respirations. Below an obstruction, the respiratory phasicity disappears and abnormal sounds cannot be obliterated by Valsalva or augmented by release of Valsalva. Above an obstruction, augmentation of the venous sound by compressing muscle distally (lower thigh or calf) is lost. Reliable testing by this method requires considerable training. The test is not reliable in old disease with good collateral circulation. It does not detect thrombi in the calf or tributary veins since these do not cause obstruction to venous return. A negative ultrasound examination is not sufficient to exclude the diagnosis of DVT confidently in the presence of suspicious clinical findings.

Plethysmography can be used to diagnose thrombotic obstruction of major veins of the extremities with acceptable accuracy. Reductions in venous capacitance and outflow caused by an obstructing thrombus in a proximal vein causes changes in electrical impedance as well as volume and rate of outflow. These changes can be measured with approximately 90% accuracy with instruments based on these principles, i.e., Impedance Plethysmograph (IPG), Pulse Volume Recorder, phleborheoplethysmography, and mercury strain-gauge plethysmography. These methods are noninvasive, relatively inexpensive, require minimum cooperation by the patient, and can be performed well by a trained technician. They are frequently used in conjunction with Doppler ultrasound. These methods are not now sensitive enough to be relied upon for an accurate diagnosis. If their results are negative and the diagnosis of DVT is still suspected, venography should be done.

Prognosis

DVT is usually benign but occasionally terminates in lethal pulmonary embolism or chronic venous insufficiency. Superficial phlebitis alone, even when recurrent, does not cause either of these serious complications, although nonlethal pulmonary emboli have been rarely reported to have originated from superficial veins. The possibility of septic phlebitis exists whenever a septic process is present in the extremity distal to or at the level of the venous obstruction. Septic thrombi may form separately from the infectious focus or may occur by contiguity with the inflammatory area as part of a cellulitis.

Although there is a strong correlation between both superficial and deep phlebitis and cancer, the mechanism whereby malignancy may cause DVT is obscure. Most clinically recognized episodes of deep phlebitis are unassociated with cancer. However, when malignancy is the only risk factor in a patient with DVT, the malignant process is almost invariably advanced.

Prophylaxis (see Chs. 37 and 254)

Treatment

The objectives of therapy are to prevent pulmonary embolism (see Ch. 37) and chronic venous insufficiency. When acute DVT is diagnosed, the patient should be hospitalized and placed in bed with the foot of the bed elevated 6 in. Bathroom or commode privileges can be permitted immediately. Analgesics for pain should not include aspirin or other compounds that interfere with normal platelet function. Drugs such as phenylbutazone or corticosteroids are *not* indicated routinely, and antibiotics should be used only for a specific infection. Warm moist packs are comforting but optional in patients without arterial insufficiency.

Antithrombotic therapy should immediately be initiated with **heparin** if no absolute contraindications exist. Various treatment protocols have been recommended, but a simple and effective method follows: Calculate the dose of heparin on the basis of the patient's *ideal* weight (to avoid giving too much to an obese patient), using 500 u. of heparin/kg/24 h to determine the total daily dosage. This may then be given by continuous IV drip using a pump for accuracy or it may be given as an IV injection q 4 h (intermittent method). To guard against excessive effects, the partial thromboplastin time (PTT) is checked once a day. If the PTT is > 3 times normal, the dose of heparin is lowered accordingly (but the method of administration not changed). If the PTT is normal or lower than 2 to 3 times normal, the dose of heparin is not changed. The duration of heparin treatment varies, but is usually 7 to 14 days. Oral therapy with a coumarin preparation is initiated to overlap the use of heparin; e.g., warfarin sodium 10 to 20 mg/day may be given until the prothrombin time rises to a level 1.5 to 2.5 times control. When this is achieved, heparin is discontinued. The duration of oral anticoagulant therapy also varies, depending on the individual situation. A single episode of phlebitis subsiding clinically in 3 to 6 days in a young patient free of risk factors may require only 2 mo of therapy, but another patient with a demonstrable pulmonary embolus and persistent risk factors may require 6 mo of therapy.

The present status of other antithrombotic agents such as snake venoms, platelet antiaggregates, and thrombolytic compounds has not been established.

Thrombolytic therapy, using fibrinolytic agents for massive pulmonary embolism and extensive DVT as well as surgical interruption of the inferior vena cava are discussed in Ch. 37.

During the acute attack, the patient should be kept on bed rest with the legs elevated. Bathroom privileges are allowed once anticoagulant therapy is well established. When edema subsides, the patient should be measured for a firm below-knee elastic stocking to control the edema that will occur when the patient becomes ambulatory. This should be worn from the time the patient arises until bedtime to prevent the postphlebitic sequelae of chronic venous insufficiency: pain, edema, and skin pigmentation, and subsequent stasis and ulceration. When these complications occur, treatment with an Unna boot (see under STASIS DERMATITIS in Ch. 189) or bed rest in the hospital with elevation and compression dressings will heal most ulcers. Antibiotics are usually not indicated, except when the ulcer is surrounded by severe acute cellulitis. Saline dressings may help to loosen superficial exudate and slough. Large, refractory or recurrent ulcers may have to be excised, the incompetent perforating veins ligated, and the area covered with a split-thickness skin graft.

VARICOSE VEINS

Elongated, dilated, tortuous superficial veins, usually of the lower limb.

Etiology and Pathogenesis

Valved veins of the lower limb are of 3 types: (1) deep veins that drain venous sinusoids within the muscles, especially those of the calf, into the popliteal and femoral veins; (2) perforator veins, whose valves permit flow only from the superficial to the deep veins; and (3) superficial veins, forming a subcutaneous network that drains into the deep veins through perforators or the short and long saphenous veins, which enter the popliteal and femoral veins respectively. Venous flow is most efficient during muscular activity when the contracting muscles compress the sinusoids and deep veins, thereby pumping the blood toward the heart; the direction of flow is controlled by the venous valves.

The term varicose veins refers to those superficial veins whose valves are congenitally absent or scant or have become incompetent, permitting reversed flow in the dependent position. A family history is common. The site of the primary valvular incompetence is debated. To some the primary fault is valve failure at the saphenofemoral junction, permitting reflux into the saphenous vein with subsequent descending sequential valvular incompetence from the thigh to the calf. Others believe that the primary fault is in one or more perforator veins in the lower leg, resulting in high-pressure flow and increased volume from the deep to the superficial veins during muscular contraction. In time, the veins become dilated, separation of the valve cusps prevents their opposition, and flow reverses in the affected segment. As other perforator valves become incompetent, reflux occurs at additional sites. Progression of these factors proximally in the long saphenous vein causes secondary incompetence at the saphenofemoral junction.

Other etiologic factors include congenital arteriovenous fistulas, increased hydrostatic pressure due to hormonal changes during early pregnancy, pressure on the pelvic veins later in pregnancy, an abdominal tumor, or ascites. Occupations that require prolonged standing probably aggravate existing varicose veins, rather than being primary etiologic factors. Previous deep thrombophlebitis, with vein recanalization resulting in deep valve incompetency, leads to secondary incompetence of the perforator veins, and varicose veins develop.

Symptoms and Signs

Initially, superficial veins are tense and may be palpated but are not visible. Subsequently, they become visibly dilated or tortuous; the diagnosis is then obvious to the patient, who may seek medical advice at this stage. Patients with asymptomatic varicose veins often seek treatment for cosmetic reasons.

Symptoms are not necessarily related to the size or degree of varicosities; severely involved legs may be asymptomatic, whereas patients may point to small localized sites of varicosities as being painful. Varicose veins may be associated with aching, fatigue, or heat that is relieved by elevation of the leg or by compression hosiery. Symptoms tend to be worse during the menstrual period.

Diagnosis

The diagnosis of varicose veins is usually made by the patient, but their extent is accurately determined only by palpation with the patient standing, and is usually greater than can be determined by simple inspection. It is essential in symptomatic patients to rule out other possible causes. Lumbar nerve root irritation can cause an aching sensation in the calf. Osteoarthritis of the hip or knee or internal derangements of the knee must be excluded. Arterial insufficiency may present with intermittent claudication or rest pain with physical findings of trophic changes in the leg and diminution or absence of one or more pulses. A burning sensation may be due to peripheral neuritis from diabetic or alcoholic neuropathy. Probably the most significant feature of the history of pain of varicose veins is that it should be relieved when the leg is elevated.

Retrograde flow of blood past incompetent saphenous valves can be demonstrated by the **Trendelenburg test**. With the patient supine, the leg is raised above heart level to empty the veins and then a tourniquet is applied around the thigh to occlude the superficial veins. The patient then stands up quickly; if the superficial veins below the tourniquet fill quickly, the perforator or short saphenous veins are incompetent. If the veins remain empty until the tourniquet is released and then fill quickly from above, the long saphenous vein is incompetent. Using tourniquets simultaneously applied to the thigh and below the knee, short saphenous vein incompetency can be demonstrated. For more exact localization of perforators, however, multiple tourniquet tests or venography may be required.

Complications

When pigmentation (from RBC diapedesis), eczema, edema, subcutaneous induration, and ulceration occur, these findings suggest the presence of deep vein incompetence and the terms "**postphlebitic leg**" or "**stasis syndrome**" are applied. The ulceration is usually small, superficial, and very painful because of exposure of nerve endings if the ulcer is due to varicose veins (and not deep venous incompetence). Varicose veins may be seen or palpated very close to or in direct continuity with the ulcer. These ulcerations may start following minor trauma to an area of pigmentation, induration, eczema, or edema, and are usually chronic by the time they are seen.

Superficial thrombophlebitis presents with localized pain, cord-like induration, periphlebitis with reddish-brown discoloration, and fever; pulmonary embolism rarely occurs unless the deep veins become involved. Very thin-walled "**blow-outs**," more commonly seen in elderly patients, may rupture and hemorrhage with minimal trauma. Hyperesthesia may be associated with varicose veins, and subcutaneous calcification or ossification may occur in longstanding cases.

Treatment

Lightweight compression hosiery for small, mildly symptomatic varicose veins are helpful and often adequate. Heavier support elastic stockings, either knee length or thigh length, may be worn for more advanced cases by patients who prefer not to have active therapy or in whom it is contraindicated. Elastic bandages should not be advocated, because patients may wrap them too tightly, especially at the calf area, producing a tourniquet effect; even if correctly applied, they rapidly loosen and become ineffectual.

Since the advent of bypass grafting of the coronary and peripheral arteries, every effort is made to preserve the saphenous veins. When possible, local segmental excision of varices should be done. The saphenous veins should be stripped only if they are diseased throughout their course from ankle to groin. Localized varices are better treated by injection. When extensive surgery is indicated, it consists of ligation and stripping of the long and short saphenous veins, and the removal by dissection of as many of the tortuous and saccular varices as possible. Incompetent perforator veins must be ligated at or beneath the points where they emerge through the deep fascia, or the varices will recur. The patient must be forewarned that isolated recurrent varices may develop; these can often be obliterated by injections of sclerosing solution (see below).

Past attempts to produce fibrosis by chemical sclerotherapy were unsuccessful. Iatrogenic phlebitis and periphlebitis were painful and only a small percentage proceeded to the anticipated fibrosis required for a permanent cure. In most cases, thrombus formed, but subsequent lysis or contraction of the thrombus permitted recanalization and recurrence in addition to further damage to the venous valves. Additionally, with large varices, the thrombus could propagate into the deep veins via perforator veins with the possibility of becoming a pulmonary embolus. Therefore, the most common method of treatment became surgery.

Recent studies suggest that failure occurred because the resulting thrombus prevented the opposing walls of the inflamed vein from adhering and fusing. However, in experienced hands, current methods of injection sclerotherapy, with compression, give excellent results and require no hospitalization. *Successful sclerosing therapy requires total obliteration of the vein by fibrosis.* To accomplish this, the vein should be injected while it is as empty of blood as possible during and after the injection, using one of several "empty vein" technics. The preferred sclerosant is sodium tetradecylsulfate in 1 or 3% solution that damages the intima of the vein. Following injection and with the leg still elevated and appropriate rubber pads placed over the injected veins to compress them and maintain the opposing walls in contact, compression bandages are applied from the base of the toes to above the highest site of injection. The bandages remain on for a period of 3 wk, or longer if necessary, during which time the patient continues normal daily activities. Walking as much as possible is essential to activate the muscle pump and promote venous drainage from the lower limb. Adequate compression of the upper thigh veins may be difficult due to configuration of the thigh and the subcutaneous fat. In these cases, distal injection therapy is combined with proximal ligation of one or more thigh veins, or a full Trendelenburg ligation, under a local anesthetic. The patient requires no hospitalization and remains ambulatory and active. As with surgery, isolated varices may recur and require treatment.

Complications of injection therapy are few. Allergic reactions are rare and toxic effects have not been seen when no more than 4 ml of 3% solution (or the equivalent in 1% solution) are given. Extravascular injection can produce a slough of the overlying skin with subsequent scarring. Deep vein thrombosis with embolism is rare. Women should avoid taking oral contraceptives for at least 6 wk prior to treatment because of their potential thrombogenic effect. Patients should be advised that brown pigmentation of the skin may occur; this usually fades, but may be permanent.

Idiopathic telangiectases ("spider veins") are fine intracutaneous angiectases of no serious consequence, but they may be extensive and unsightly. Although usually asymptomatic, some patients describe burning or pain, and many women find even the smallest telangiectases cosmetically unacceptable. They can usually be eliminated by intracapillary injections of 1% solution of sodium tetradecyl-sulfate through a fine-bore needle. Care should be taken to avoid rupturing the fine capillaries and producing skin ulceration due to subcutaneous injection. Pigmentation may develop, but this subsides, often completely, and is rarely a cause for complaint. Best results are obtained with compression bandaging of the leg and ambulation, as described above, for at least 1 wk following the treatment.

ARTERIOVENOUS FISTULA

Arteriovenous fistulas, *abnormal communications between an artery and a vein*, may cause symptoms of arterial insufficiency, ulceration due to embolization and ischemia, or symptoms related to chronic venous insufficiency due to the high-pressure arterial flow within the involved veins. The affected part is usually enlarged and warm, with distended and often pulsating superficial veins. A thrill can be palpated over the fistula, and a continuous machinery murmur with accentuation during systole can be heard with the stethoscope. The altered hemodynamics may cause congestive heart failure if a significant portion of the cardiac output is diverted through the fistula. The treatment of choice is surgery, if feasible.

LYMPHEDEMA

Swelling of subcutaneous tissues due to obstruction, destruction, or hypoplasia of lymph vessels and accumulation of excessive lymph fluid.

Lymphedema may be primary or secondary. The **primary type** can be present from birth (congenital lymphedema) or may occur during puberty (lymphedema praecox) or less frequently later in life (lymphedema tarda). It is due to hypoplasia of the lymph vessels. Primary lymphedema occurs less frequently in men. The patient complains of swelling of the foot, leg, or entire extremity. It is usually unilateral and it is worse during warm weather, prior to menstrual periods, and after prolonged dependency. There is usually no discomfort. On examination the edema is diffuse, causes a typical mound of swelling on the dorsum of the foot (or hand), and is only partially pitting. There are usually no skin changes and no evidence of venous insufficiency.

Secondary lymphedema is often a result of infection, which, in the foot, most frequently results from dermatophytosis. The onset is explosive, with chills, high fever, toxicity, and a red, hot, swollen leg. Lymphangitic streaks may be seen in the skin, and lymph nodes in the groin are usually enlarged and tender. These features distinguish it from acute thrombophlebitis. The symptoms respond rapidly to anti-streptococcal antibiotics. Secondary lymphedema in older persons may be due to malignant disease in the pelvis or groin. Obliteration of lymphatic tissue by surgical excision or radiation therapy is another cause.

The goal of treatment is to eliminate the swelling by elevation or pneumatic compression and then to apply a firm elastic support to be worn from the time the patient arises until he retires. Occasionally diuretics are helpful.

LIPEDEMA

Lipedema is a syndrome of fatty, tender legs. The patient complains of swelling and tender tissues. On examination, most of the patient's fat is found to be distributed in the hips, thighs, and legs. Although the foot is spared, fatty tissue often hangs over the ankles. Tissue tenderness is generalized and is not over the course of the veins. The only treatment is for the patient to avoid further weight gain.

§4. PULMONARY DISORDERS

29. APPROACH TO THE PULMONARY PATIENT

The proper approach to diagnosis and treatment of pulmonary disorders requires the patient's history, a physical examination, a chest x-ray, an estimate of whether the disorder is acute or chronic, and a judgment as to whether the disorder is active or inactive. The relative importance of each of these elements in the appraisal varies from patient to patient. For example, the detection of an occupational lung disease, such as asbestosis, often requires a more detailed history to uncover the offending agent. In contrast, the physical examination may be most helpful in following the course of a patient with acute pneumococcal pneumonia. Occasionally, extrathoracic manifestations, such as distended neck veins, may provide the first clue to a mediastinal inflammatory process or tumor.

The chest x-ray is an essential supplement to the history and physical examination. Not infrequently, a routine, periodic film uncovers an occult, asymptomatic pulmonary lesion. It is useful, either per se or in conjunction with other indices, in determining whether a disorder is acute or chronic, active or inactive, and is a reliable means of tracing the evolution of a pulmonary disease and response to treatment. Usually, a series of chest x-rays, rather than a single one, is required to assess activity, prognosis, or response to treatment. Sometimes, a film taken years before the present illness helps with diagnosis and treatment.

Certain symptoms and signs that direct attention to the lungs as the focus of a clinical disorder are discussed below.

COUGH

An explosive expiration required for the self-cleansing of the lungs. It is a reflex act generally arising from stimulation of the mucosa of the airways. Many different stimuli can elicit a cough.

The sudden onset of a distressing cough that is part of an acute bronchitis or pneumonia is difficult for the patient to ignore, but, commonly, the patient with chronic cough either fails to notice the cough or takes it for granted. This is particularly true of the "smoker's cough" that many individuals come to accept as part of the waking up process each morning. Indeed, the patient with chronic bronchitis often *denies* cough until pressed for details. Nonetheless, the disregarded cough may have the same implications as a productive cough.

Cough should be characterized in terms of when and under what circumstances it occurs. For example, it may occur only when the patient is at work, triggered by noxious or allergenic materials, or it may occur in relation to changes in posture, as commonly seen in patients with chronic bronchitis or bronchiectasis when they lie down at night or get up in the morning.

Cough should be characterized with regard to whether it is nonproductive (dry) or productive of sputum. A productive cough that persists for months and tends to recur year after year is characteristic of chronic bronchitis. The gross and microscopic characteristics of sputum may be of important diagnostic help, and changes in sputum composition usually signify changes in the clinical course of the disorder. For example, relatively clear, nonviscous sputum may become thick and turn yellow, greenish, or brown, suggesting the presence of pus and the development of infection in the tracheobronchial tree in the lungs.

Microscopic examination of sputum is simple and rewarding. Selecting from a dense part of freshly collected sputum, a small drop can be placed on a glass slide and compressed with a cover slip. Low-power microscopic examination *without staining* will quickly reveal important data. The presence of squamous cells, which originate from above the larynx, suggests the presence of secretions that are not true sputum; the latter is characterized by the presence of alveolar macrophages or histiocytes. The presence of eosinophilia indicates that the disorder is noninfectious and probably allergic in nature; a predominance of neutrophils suggests the presence of infection. A Gram stain specimen of the sputum will confirm the presence of bacteria and begin their categorization.

DYSPNEA

Breathlessness; shortness of breath; the sensation of difficult, labored, or uncomfortable breathing. Dyspnea is a subjective complaint and represents the patient's perception that breathing is excessive, difficult, or uncomfortable. Usually it signifies an unpleasant sensation. Dyspnea is an important manifestation of disease when it occurs at a less strenuous level of activity than the individual normally tolerates. **Orthopnea** is breathlessness that occurs in the supine position and that is relieved by sitting or standing.

Pathophysiology

Dyspnea may refer to one or more sensations and may represent the subjective response to one or more mechanisms. Among the different sensations encompassed by the word "dyspnea" are the following: (1) the profound hyperpnea that occurs during and after severe exercise; (2) the sensation arising from bronchial or bronchiolar obstruction in patients with asthma and bronchitis; (3) the breathlessness that may occur with inappropriately slight exertion in patients with heart disease or severe anemia; and (4) the sensation that compels the subject to take the next breath after a period of breath-holding.

The afferent impulses that converge upon the brain to generate the sensation of dyspnea come from many different sites. Some come from the lungs, per se. Others seem to originate in the articulations of the chest cage. A role has been suggested for muscle spindles in the diaphragm, which transmit impulses via the phrenic nerve. The carotid and aortic bodies contribute by way of the peripheral chemoreceptors, and the respiratory centers in the medulla are strongly influenced by levels of CO_2 in blood and tissues. Other visceral, neural, and emotional stimuli may also be involved. An important issue currently being explored is the role of respiratory muscle fatigue in eliciting the sensation of dyspnea.

Although no single mechanism explains all instances of dyspnea, some useful relationships have emerged. Dyspnea depends on the disproportion between the amount of ventilation called for by the individual's physiologic state (resting, exercising, hypercapnic) and on the capability of his lungs and thorax to deliver this ventilation efficiently. The range of required ventilation varies from 5 L/min or less at rest to > 100 L/min during severe exercise. An individual's capability to breathe is reflected in his "maximum breathing capacity" (maximum voluntary ventilation). The maximum breathing capacity differs among normals and may be seriously compromised by pulmonary disease. A trained athlete may exceed 200 L/min whereas a patient with severe obstructive lung disease may not be able to attain even 20 L/min. Almost everybody will develop dyspnea when the required ventilation reaches about 1/3 of his maximum breathing capacity. Thus, dyspnea may result at high levels of ventilation even though breathing capacity is normal, or at lower levels of ventilation if the maximum breathing capacity is low. This relationship has proved useful in providing indices to predict when patients with pulmonary disease will become dyspneic.

Other factors relating to dyspnea are the work and energy cost of breathing. As indicated above, fatigue of the respiratory muscles, due to the effort involved in this extra work, is also being explored.

Types of Dyspnea

1. Physiologic: The most common type of breathlessness (dyspnea) is that associated with physical exertion. Ventilation is increased and maintained through an augmented respiratory stimulus provided by metabolic and other undefined factors. Dyspnea is also common during acute hypoxia, as at high altitude, where the increased respiratory stimulus is, in part, the effect of arterial hypoxemia on the carotid bodies. Dyspnea is also evoked by breathing high CO_2 concentrations in a closed space. However, when a person enters a closed space that is devoid of O_2 (e.g., containing 100% nitrogen), he may lose consciousness in about 30 seconds, before dyspnea warns of the danger. The sensation of dyspnea may also be minimal in cases of carbon monoxide poisoning.

2. Pulmonary: Dyspnea from pulmonary causes is usually either **restrictive** due to low compliance of the lungs or chest wall, or **obstructive** due to high airway resistance (partial airways obstruction). Patients with restrictive dyspnea (e.g., due to pulmonary fibrosis or chest deformities) are usually comfortable at rest but become intensely dyspneic when exertion causes pulmonary ventilation to approach their greatly limited breathing capacity. In obstructive dyspnea (e.g., as in obstructive emphysema or asthma), increased ventilatory effort induces dyspnea even at rest and breathing is labored and retarded, especially during expiration.

Diffuse pulmonary disease, with or without hypoxia, is often accompanied by hyperventilation and lowering of the Pa_{CO2}. Thus, it is possible to have a patient with dyspnea and a high Pa_{O2} and a low Pa_{CO2}, presumably due to heightened stimuli from the stretch receptors in diseased lungs.

3. Cardiac: In the early stages of heart failure, cardiac output fails to keep pace with increased metabolic need during exercise. As a result, the respiratory drive is increased largely because of tissues and cerebral acidosis; the patient therefore hyperventilates. Various reflex factors, including stretch receptors in the lungs, may also contribute to the hyperventilation. The shortness of breath is often accompanied by lassitude or a feeling of smothering or sternal oppression. In later stages of congestive failure, the lungs are congested and edematous, the ventilatory capacity of the stiff lungs is reduced, and ventilatory effort is increased. Reflex factors, particularly the juxtacapillary (J) receptors in the alveolar-capillary septa, contribute to the inordinate increase in pulmonary ventilation. **Cardiac asthma** is a state of acute respiratory insufficiency accompanying pulmonary and tracheobronchial asthma. Its manifestations may be indistinguishable from other types of asthma, but it originates in failure of the left ventricle. The airways obstruction is accompanied by hyperventilation. **Periodic** or **Cheyne-Stokes respiration** is characterized by alternate periods of apnea and hyperpnea, often including both neurologic and cardiologic components. In heart failure, slowing of the circulation is the predominant cause; acidosis and hypoxia in the respiratory centers contribute importantly.

Orthopnea is *the respiratory discomfort that occurs while the patient is supine* (thus impelling him to sit up). It is precipitated by an increase in venous return of blood to a left ventricle lacking the ability to meet the challenge of this increase in preload. Of lesser importance is the increase in the work of breathing in the supine position. Orthopnea, usually a manifestation of left ventricular failure, sometimes occurs in other cardiovascular disorders; e.g., pericardial effusion.

In **paroxysmal nocturnal dyspnea**, which may be dramatic and terrifying, the patient awakens gasping for breath and must sit or stand to get his breath. It may occur in mitral stenosis, aortic insufficiency, hypertension, or other conditions affecting the left ventricle. The same factors that cause orthopnea are involved, but they interact to produce a more urgent form of respiratory distress.

4. Circulatory: "Air hunger" (*acute dyspnea occurring in the terminal stages of exsanguinating hemorrhage*) is a grave sign calling for immediate transfusion. Dyspnea also occurs with chronic anemia, coming on only during exertion, except when the anemia is extreme.

5. Chemical: Diabetic acidosis (blood pH 7.2 to 6.95) induces a distinctive pattern of slow, deep respirations **(Kussmaul breathing).** However, the breathing capacity is well preserved, and the patient rarely complains of dyspnea. Conversely, in uremia the patient may complain of dyspnea because of severe panting brought about by a combination of acidosis, heart failure, pulmonary edema, and anemia.

6. Central: Cerebral lesions such as hemorrhage are often associated with intense hyperventilation that is sometimes noisy and stertorous and occasionally irregularly periodic **(Biot's respiration).**

7. Psychogenic: Hysterical types of overbreathing are commonest. In one type, there is continuous hyperventilation, sometimes leading to acute alkalosis from "blowing off" CO_2 (see also RESPIRATORY ALKALOSIS in Ch. 81), and positive Trousseau and Chvostek signs from lowered serum calcium ion levels. Another type is characterized by deep, sighing respirations, the patient breathing at maximal depth until respiration is "satisfactory," at which time the hyperventilatory impulse subsides. This is repeated at frequent intervals.

Treatment
Treatment of dyspnea is directed at the underlying conditions.

HEMOPTYSIS

Coughing up of blood as a result of bleeding from the respiratory tract.

Etiology
The source of hemoptysis may be either the pulmonary or bronchial circulation, or granulation tissue that contains vascular elements from both. About 95% of the pulmonary blood circulation is supplied by the pulmonary artery and its branches, a low-pressure system. The bronchial circulation, a high-pressure system, originates from the aorta and usually provides about 5% of the blood to the lungs, primarily to the airways and supporting structures. Bleeding may occur when branches of either system are disrupted, though bleeding usually arises from the bronchial circulation unless trauma or erosion by a granulomatous or calcified node or a tumor has occurred in a major pulmonary vessel. Pulmonary vascular bleeding may originate in the capillaries, small vessels (usually arteries), or major large vessels. Pulmonary venous bleeding is generally modest, and occurs primarily in association with pulmonary venous hypertension, particularly in association with left heart failure. Bronchial venous bleeding occasionally complicates "tight" mitral stenosis and may be life-threatening.

Blood-streaked sputum is a rather common complaint but is usually nonthreatening (e.g., a patient with a URI and bronchitis coughs up a few streaks of blood). Inflammatory causes account for 80 to 90% of cases of hemoptysis. Acute or chronic bronchitis is probably the commonest cause, bronchitis and bronchiectasis together causing about half of all cases. Recent infection in an old bronchiectatic sac, a healed cavity, or a cystic lesion causes vasodilation and engorgement of vessels and may be associated with bleeding ranging from a slow ooze to frank bleeding. Infestation of cavities by *Aspergillus* species (mycetoma, fungus ball) is an increasingly recognized cause of significant hemoptysis regardless of the cause of the cavity. TB accounts for 10 to 20% of cases. Tumors (especially carcinoma), perfused primarily by bronchial vessels, account for about 20% of cases; bronchogenic carcinoma must be strongly suspected in smokers who have hemoptysis and who are 40 yr old or more. Pulmonary infarction in association with thromboembolism and left heart failure (especially secondary to mitral stenosis) are less common causes of hemoptysis. Other less common causes (e.g., primary bronchial adenoma, arteriovenous malformations) are disproportionately important because of their tendency to cause severe bleeding. Metastatic cancer rarely causes hemoptysis. Hemoptysis of obscure origin on rare occasion occurs at the time of menstruation. See TABLE 29–1 for a list of conditions that may be responsible for hemoptysis.

Diagnosis
Hemoptysis, particularly of an appreciable quantity of blood or if recurrent, is a frightening and potentially fatal event and all diagnostic resources must be used to establish the etiology. More than 2 tsp of bright red blood is ominous because it suggests severe hemorrhage. Not only the quantity

TABLE 29-1. CONDITIONS ASSOCIATED WITH HEMOPTYSIS

Larynx and Pharynx
  Lymphoma
  Carcinoma
  Tuberculous ulceration

Trachea and Large Bronchi
  Benign or malignant primary tumor
  Telangiectasia
  Erosion by an aortic aneurysm
  Bronchogenic cyst
  Broncholithiasis
  Erosion by a caseocalcific node
  Erosion by a tumor from nodes, esophagus,
    or other mediastinal structures
  Severe acute bronchitis
  Trauma

Cardiovascular
  Left ventricular failure
  Mitral stenosis
  Pulmonary embolism/infarct
  Primary pulmonary hypertension
  Pulmonary arteriovenous fistula
  Atrial myxoma
  Fibrous mediastinitis with pulmonary vein
    obstruction
  Aortic aneurysm with leakage into the
    pulmonary parenchyma

Smaller Bronchial Structures
  Carcinoma
  Adenoma (carcinoid or cylindromatous)
  Acute bronchitis
  Bronchiectasis
  Bronchopulmonary sequestration
  Chronic bronchitis
  Trauma

Pulmonary Parenchyma
  Primary or metastatic tumor
  Infarct
  Abscess
  Active granulomatous disease (TB, fungal,
    parasitic, luetic)
  Fungus ball (*Aspergillus*) in an old cavity
  Acute pneumonia
  Idiopathic hemosiderosis
  Goodpasture's syndrome
  Trauma

Clotting Defects
  Thrombocytopenia
  Vitamin K-dependent factors: prothrombin (II),
    Stuart factor (X), Factor VII, Christmas
    factor (IX)
  Diffuse intravascular coagulation
  Heparin therapy
  Fibrinolytic therapy: urokinase
                        streptokinase
  Miscellaneous congenital coagulation defects

but the precise location of the bleeding must be determined. Hemoptysis must be differentiated from hematemesis and from blood or hemorrhagic exudate dripping into the tracheobronchial passages from the nose, mouth, or nasopharynx. The patient may be able to sense and tell the examiner where the bleeding is coming from, even specifying the side of the chest from which the hemoptysis stemmed. The history, physical examination, and chest x-ray usually define the more obvious causes of hemoptysis such as trauma, tumor, TB, bronchiectasis, heart failure, or pulmonary infarct/embolism.

A lung scan and pulmonary angiogram are useful for confirming the diagnosis of pulmonary embolism. Angiography will demonstrate an aortic aneurysm or a pulmonary arteriovenous fistula. Endoscopic examination is crucial during or shortly after an episode of acute bleeding, especially if the amount of bleeding is major. The fiberoptic bronchoscope causes less discomfort for the patient, but the rigid bronchoscope is the instrument of choice when bleeding is profuse. When the etiology is obscure, careful examination of the upper respiratory passages using a mirror and direct visualization, bronchography, and evaluation of the clotting mechanisms are indicated. Despite systematic and intensive search, the cause of the hemoptysis will not be found in 30 to 40% of all cases.

Treatment

The objectives are: (1) to prevent exsanguination; (2) to prevent asphyxiation in the exsanguinated blood; (3) to prevent blood clots from obstructing bronchi and causing segmental, lobar, or lung collapse, or hyperinflation of similar anatomic units; (4) to localize the area of aspirated blood as much as possible; (5) to control infection that may spread by aspiration of blood from an infected focus; (6) to stop the bleeding; and (7) to allay fear and anxiety.

Objective 1 (preventing exsanguination) requires careful clinical monitoring of the indicators of shock. The patient should be treated in an intensive care unit if bleeding is massive. Three or four units of blood should be cross-matched and available for use. IV fluids should be started and the Hct checked every 30 min if bleeding is brisk. Replacement of blood volume must be prompt and continued until bleeding stops either spontaneously or by surgical or medical therapy. Bleeding time, clotting time, platelet count, prothrombin time, and partial thromboplastin time should be assayed immediately to determine if there are any clotting abnormalities. *Narcotics should not be given.*

Objectives 2, 3, and 4 (preventing asphyxiation, airways obstruction, and spread to uninvolved lung) are accomplished by removing the extravascular blood from the lung. Coughing is the most efficient way to achieve this. The patient must be encouraged to cough and shown how to clear the secretions gently by slightly prolonging glottic closure before coughing. Inhalation of warm water vapor or mist helps to decrease throat irritation and ease the urge to cough explosively. The physician's reassurance, frequently repeated, is a very effective way to keep the patient coughing efficiently. Postural drainage may be helpful if bleeding is brisk. The patient should not be immobilized but should be encouraged to move about gently, keeping the side from which the bleeding is occurring (if known) dependent. If a major bronchus becomes obstructed by a clot or if evidence of atelectasis or progressive overinflation (check-valve effect of clot) develops, bronchoscopy should be performed immediately for clearance.

Objective 5 (preventing spread of infection) applies particularly to TB. If TB is suspected as the cause of the bleeding, antituberculosis therapy with at least 2 effective drugs (including INH or rifampin, or both) should be started at once. Penicillin should be given immediately if a lung abscess due to aspiration is suspected. When a fungal infection is the possible cause of the bleeding, amphotericin B therapy should be considered.

Objective 6 (stopping the bleeding) depends on the cause of the bleeding. If the bleeding is from a major vessel, little other than resection of the tissue or ligation of the vessel can be done, though these are usually measures of desperation and often useless. Collapse of the lung by artificial pneumothorax or pneumoperitoneum has been tried but is rarely helpful. Almost invariably, no intervention helps when bleeding is from the aorta. Bleeding from any large vessel requires early use of blood replacement; replacement will *not* encourage major vessel bleeding. Bleeding from smaller vessels usually stops spontaneously.

Since infection of bronchiectatic areas usually leads to bleeding, usually from subjacent enlarged bronchial arteries, treatment of the infection with appropriate antibiotics and postural drainage is essential.

If clotting abnormalities (see Ch. 95) are contributing to the bleeding, whole blood, specific deficient factors, or platelet transfusions are indicated. When a specific defect of vitamin K-dependent coagulation factors is present secondary to warfarin therapy, vitamin K_1 (phytonadione) should be given. (CAUTION: *See VITAMIN K DEFICIENCY in Ch. 78 for administration*) Only phytonadione is used since plasma derivatives run the risk of causing hepatitis. Protamine sulfate IV in a mg-for-mg equivalence is indicated for heparin overdosage.

When bleeding is precapillary in origin, conjugated estrogens 40 mg IV have been useful. If allergic vasculitis, Wegener's granulomatosis, or Goodpasture's syndrome is present, prednisone 80 to 100 mg/day may abruptly stop the bleeding. When diffuse intravascular coagulation is causing the bleeding, heparin in 5,000 to 10,000 u. doses has been used but success usually depends on control of the underlying disorder.

Early resection is indicated for such causes as bronchial adenoma or carcinoma. Broncholithiasis may require pulmonary resection—*never* endobronchial removal of the stone. Hemosiderosis may require multiple blood transfusions until the bleeding stops. Bleeding secondary to heart failure or mitral stenosis usually responds to specific therapy for the heart failure. Bleeding from pulmonary infarction is rarely massive and almost always ceases spontaneously. If emboli are recurrent and bleeding persists, anticoagulation may be contraindicated, with inferior vena cava ligation being the treatment of choice.

Objective 7 (allaying fear) is the most difficult for the physician, the nurse, and especially the patient. Sedatives and tranquilizers should be avoided if possible, but chlorpromazine 10 to 25 mg orally q 6 to 8 h may be given if absolutely necessary. Narcotics are **contraindicated.** The almost constant presence of a sympathetic and reassuring therapist is usually the best calmative. For minimal bleeding, a prompt, thorough diagnostic approach is most reassuring.

30. PULMONARY FUNCTION TESTS

Pulmonary function testing has progressed from simple spirometry to sophisticated physiologic testing over the past decade. This chapter will attempt to survey the major clinically applicable tests available and then will attempt to identify their role in clinical management, including recommendations for ordering tests.

In the normal respiratory system, the volume and pattern of ventilation are initiated by neural output from the respiratory center in the medulla of the brainstem. This output is influenced by afferent information from several sources, including higher centers in the brain, carotid chemoreceptors (Pa_{O2}), central chemoreceptors (Pa_{CO2} [H^+]), and neural impulses from moving tendons and joints. Nerve impulses travel via the spinal cord and peripheral nerves to the intercostal and diaphragmatic muscles where appropriate synchronous contraction generates negative intrapleural pressure. If the resulting inspiration is transmitted through structurally sound, unobstructed airways to patent, adequately perfused alveoli, then O_2 and CO_2 are respectively added to and removed from mixed venous blood. This feedback mechanism of control of breathing is normally very sensitive, so that alveolar ventilation is kept proportional to the metabolic rate and the arterial blood gas tensions are maintained within a very narrow range.

Malfunction of the respiratory system at any point in this pathway can result in deviation from this normal range, and consequent respiratory insufficiency. A disturbance at a given point can often be specifically measured if available tests and known patterns of pathophysiologic disturbances are understood. This chapter discusses tests of pulmonary function.

TABLE 30–1. PULMONARY FUNCTION ABBREVIATIONS

CC	Closing capacity	MMEF	Mean maximal expiratory flow (L/sec)
C_{dyn}	Dynamic lung compliance		
C_{STAT}	Static lung compliance	MVV	Maximal voluntary ventilation
CV	Closing volume (L)	Pa_{CO_2}	Arterial partial pressure of CO_2 (mm Hg)
DL_{CO}	Diffusing capacity for carbon monoxide (ml/min/mm Hg)	Pa_{O_2}	Arterial partial pressure of O_2 (mm Hg)
ERV	Expiratory reserve volume	PEF	Peak expiratory flow (L/sec)
FEV_1	Forced expiratory volume in 1 sec (L)	P_{TP}	Transpulmonary pressure (mm Hg)
FEV_3	Forced expiratory volume in 3 sec (L)	$\dot{Q}$	Perfusion (L/min)
FVC	Forced vital capacity	R_{AW}	Airway resistance
FRC	Functional residual capacity	RV	Residual volume
$[H^+]$	Concentration of hydrogen ions (nanomoles/L)	TLC	Total lung capacity
		V	Lung volume (L)
IRV	Inspiratory reserve volume	VC	Vital capacity
$MEF_{50\% \ VC}$	Mid-expiratory flow at 50% vital capacity (L/sec)	$\dot{V}$	Ventilation (L/min)
		$\dot{V}_A$	Alveolar ventilation (L/min)
$MIF_{50\% \ VC}$	Mid-inspiratory flow at 50% vital capacity (L/sec)	$\dot{V}_{CO_2}$	CO_2 production (L/min)
		$\dot{V}_{O_2}$	O_2 consumption (L/min)

Static Lung Volumes (see Fig. 30–1)

The **vital capacity (VC or "slow VC")** is the maximum volume of air that can be expired slowly and completely after a full inspiratory effort. This simply performed test is still one of the most valuable measurements of pulmonary function. It characteristically decreases progressively as restrictive lung disease increases in severity, and, along with the diffusing capacity, can be used to follow the course of a restrictive lung process and its response to therapy.

The **forced vital capacity (FVC)** is a similar maneuver utilizing a maximal forceful expiration. This is usually performed in concert with determination of expiratory flow-rates in simple spirometry (see Dynamic Lung Volumes and Flow Rates, below).

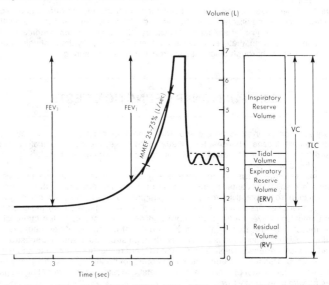

Fig. 30–1a.   **Normal.** RV ≅ 25% of TLC; FRC ≅ 40% of TLC. $FEV_1 = > 75\%$ of FVC; $FEV_3 = > 95\%$ of FVC.

Fig. 30–1.   **Spirograms and lung volumes.** FRC = RV + ERV. VC = TLC − RV.

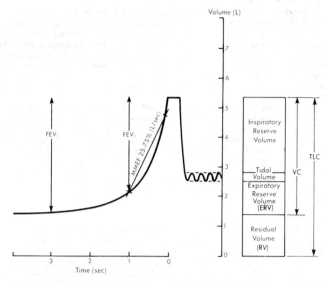

Fig. 30–1b.   **Restrictive disease.** Lung volumes are all diminished, the RV less so than the FRC, VC, and TLC. FEV_1 is normal or greater than normal. Tidal breathing is rapid and shallow.

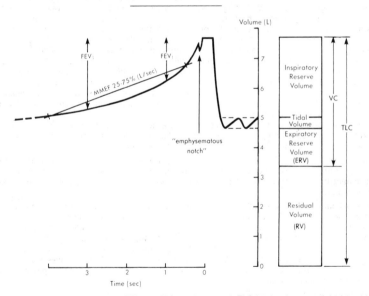

Fig. 30–1c.   **Obstructive disease.** RV and FRC are increased. TLC is also increased, but to a lesser degree, so that VC is decreased. There is prolongation of expiration. $FEV_1 = < 75\%$ of VC. Note the "emphysematous notch."

Fig. 30–1.   **Spirograms and lung volumes.** (*Cont'd*)

The (slow) VC can be considerably greater than the FVC in patients with airways obstruction. During the forceful expiratory maneuver, terminal airways can close prematurely (i.e., before the true residual volume is reached), and the distal gas is "trapped" and not measured by the spirometer.

Functional residual capacity (FRC) is physiologically the most important lung volume because it incorporates the normal tidal breathing range. It is defined as the volume of air in the lungs at the end of a normal expiration when all the respiratory muscles are relaxed. It is determined by the balance between the elastic forces (stiffness) of the chest wall, which tend to increase lung volume, and the elastic forces of the lungs, which tend to reduce it. These forces are normally equal and opposite at about 40% of **total lung capacity (TLC)**. Changes in the elastic properties of the lungs or of the chest wall result in changes in the FRC. The loss of elastic recoil of the lung seen in emphysema results in an increase in the FRC. Conversely, the increased lung stiffness of pulmonary edema, interstitial fibrosis, and other restrictive lung processes results in a decreased FRC. Kyphoscoliosis leads to a decrease in FRC and in the other lung volumes because the stiff, noncompliant chest wall restricts ventilation.

The FRC has 2 components, the **residual volume (RV)**, the volume of air remaining in the lungs at the end of a maximal expiration, and the **expiratory reserve volume** (FRC = RV + ERV).

The RV normally accounts for about 25% of the TLC. It changes with the FRC with 2 exceptions. In restrictive lung diseases, RV tends to remain nearer to normal than other lung volumes (shown in Fig. 30-1b). In small airways diseases, presumably because premature closure of the airways leads to air trapping, the RV may be elevated while the FRC and FEV_1 remain normal.

TLC equals the VC + the RV. In obstructive airways disease, RV increases more than does TLC, resulting in some decrease in VC, particularly in severe disease.

In obesity the ERV is characteristically diminished because of a markedly decreased FRC, and a relatively well-preserved RV.

Dynamic Lung Volumes and Flow Rates

Dynamic lung volumes reflect the nonelastic properties of the lungs, primarily the status of the airways. The spirogram (see Fig. 30-1a) records lung volume against time on a water or electronic spirometer during an FVC maneuver. The FEV_1 is the volume of air forcefully expired during the first second after a full breath and normally comprises > 75% of the VC. The mean maximal expiratory flow over the middle half of the FVC ($MMEF_{25-75\%}$) is the slope of the line that intersects the spirographic tracing at 25% and 75% of the VC. The MMEF is less effort-dependent than is the FEV_1 and is a more sensitive indicator of early airways obstruction.

Airway caliber (and therefore flow) is directly related to lung volume, being greatest at TLC, and decreasing progressively to RV. During a *forced* expiratory maneuver, the airways become further narrowed because of positive intrathoracic pressure. This "dynamic compression of the airways" limits maximum expiratory flow rates. The opposite effect is seen during an inspiratory maneuver, when negative intrathoracic pressure tends to maintain the caliber of the airways. The differences in airway diameter during inspiration and expiration thus result in greater flow rates during inspiration than expiration during much of the breathing cycle (see Fig. 30-2a). In chronic obstructive pulmonary disease **(COPD)** and asthma, prolongation of expiratory flow rates is further exaggerated because of airway narrowing (asthma), loss of structural integrity of the airways (bronchitis), and loss of lung elastic recoil (emphysema). In fixed obstruction of the trachea or larynx, flow is limited by the diameter of the stenotic segment rather than by dynamic compression, resulting in *equal* reduction of inspiratory and expiratory flows.

In restrictive lung disorders, the increased tissue elasticity tends to maintain airway diameter during expiration so that, at comparable lung volumes, flow rates are often greater than normal. (Tests of small airways function, however, may be abnormal—see below.)

Retesting of pulmonary function after inhalation of a bronchodilator aerosol (e.g., isoproterenol) provides information about the reversibility of an obstructive process (i.e., asthmatic component). Improvement in VC and/or $FEV_1(L)$ of > 10% is usually considered a significant response to a bronchodilator.

The **maximal voluntary ventilation (MVV)** is determined by encouraging the patient to breathe at maximal tidal volume and respiratory rate for 12 seconds; the amount of air expired is expressed in L/min. The MVV generally parallels the FEV_1 and can be used as a test of internal consistency and as an estimate of patient cooperation (MVV ≅ $FEV_1[L] \times 40$). The MVV decreases with respiratory muscle weakness and may be the only demonstrable pulmonary function abnormality in moderately severe neuromuscular disease. The MVV is considered an important preoperative test as it reflects the severity of airways obstruction as well as being an index of the patient's respiratory reserves, muscle strength, and motivation.

Flow-Volume Loop (see Fig. 30-2)

The disadvantage of the simple measurements discussed above is that they fragment the complex dynamic interrelationships of flow, volume, and pressure into simple dimensions for arbitrary measurement. The continuous analysis of these parameters during forced respiratory maneuvers is more physiologic and can be more revealing. An analogy in cardiology is the additional information obtained by vectorcardiography above that provided by the conventional ECG. For the flow-volume loop the patient breathes into an electronic spirometer and performs a forced inspiratory and expiratory VC maneuver while flow and volume are displayed continuously on an oscilloscope. The shape of the loop reflects the status of the lung volumes and of the airways throughout the respiratory cycle and can be diagnostic. Characteristic changes are seen in restrictive and in obstructive disorders. The loop is especially helpful in the assessment of laryngeal and tracheal lesions. It can distinguish between fixed (e.g., tracheal stenosis) and variable (e.g., tracheomalacia, vocal cord paralysis) obstruction. Fig. 30-2 illustrates some characteristic flow-volume loop abnormalities.

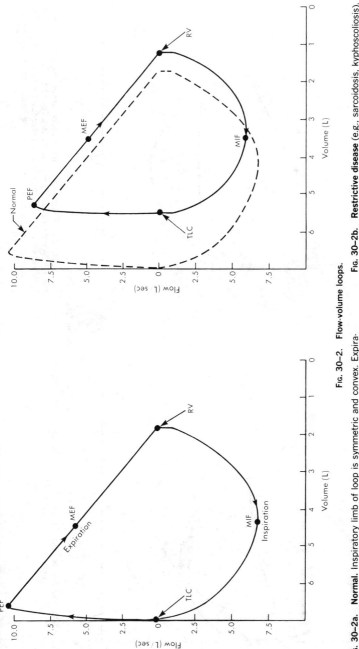

Fig. 30–2. Flow-volume loops.

Fig. 30–2a. Normal. Inspiratory limb of loop is symmetric and convex. Expiratory limb is linear. Flow rates at mid-point of vital capacity are often measured. Mid-inspiratory flow ($MIF_{50\%VC}$ or MIF) is greater than mid-expiratory flow ($MEF_{50\%VC}$ or MEF) because of dynamic compression of the airways. Peak expiratory flow is sometimes used to estimate degree of airways obstruction, but is very dependent on patient effort. Expiratory flow rates over lower 50% of VC (i.e., near RV) are sensitive indicators of small airways status.

Fig. 30–2b. Restrictive disease (e.g., sarcoidosis, kyphoscoliosis). Configuration of loop is narrowed because of diminished lung volumes, but shape is basically as in Fig. 30–2a. Flow rates are normal (actually greater than normal at comparable lung volumes because increased elastic recoil of lungs and/or chest wall holds airway open).

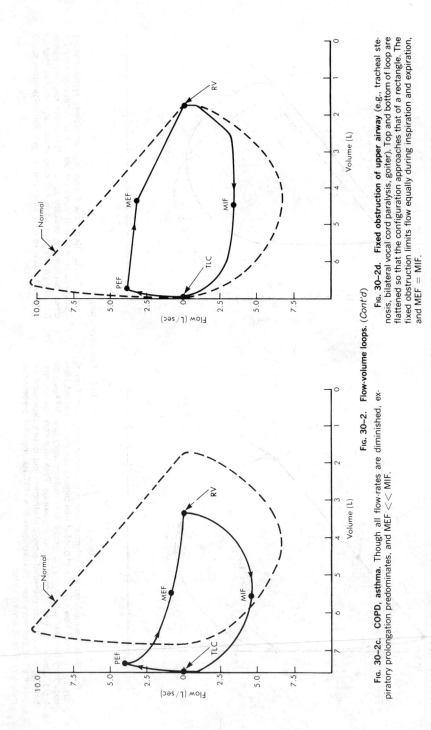

Fig. 30–2d.   **Fixed obstruction of upper airway** (e.g., tracheal stenosis, bilateral vocal cord paralysis, goiter). Top and bottom of loop are flattened so that the configuration approaches that of a rectangle. The fixed obstruction limits flow equally during inspiration and expiration, and MEF = MIF.

Fig. 30–2.   **Flow-volume loops.** (Cont'd)

Fig. 30–2c.   **COPD, asthma.** Though all flow-rates are diminished, expiratory prolongation predominates, and MEF << MIF.

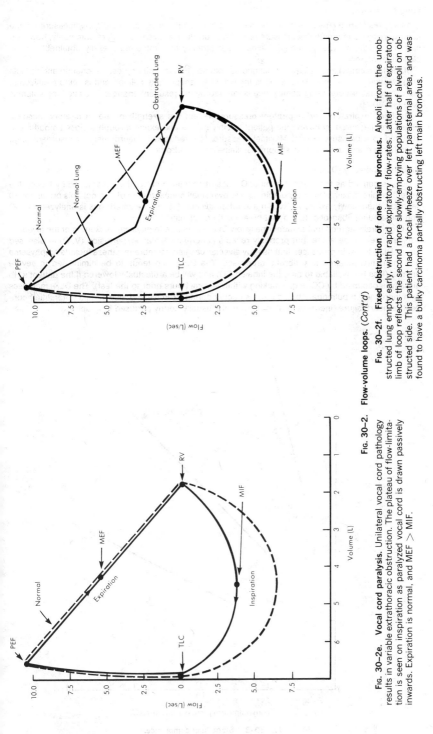

Fig. 30–2f. Flow-volume loops. (*Cont'd*)

Fig. 30–2f. Fixed obstruction of one main bronchus. Alveoli from the unobstructed lung empty early, with rapid expiratory flow-rates. Latter half of expiratory limb of loop reflects the second more slowly-emptying populations of alveoli on obstructed side. This patient had a focal wheeze over left parasternal area, and was found to have a bulky carcinoma partially obstructing left main bronchus.

Fig. 30–2.

Fig. 30–2e. Vocal cord paralysis. Unilateral vocal cord pathology results in variable extrathoracic obstruction. The plateau of flow-limitation is seen on inspiration as paralyzed vocal cord is drawn passively inwards. Expiration is normal, and MEF > MIF.

Lung Mechanics

Airway resistance (R_{AW}) can, with the help of a body plethysmograph, be directly measured in the laboratory by determining the pressure required to produce a given flow. More commonly, however, it is inferred from dynamic lung volumes and expiratory flow rates more easily obtainable in the clinical laboratory.

Static lung compliance (C_{STAT}) is defined as volume-change/unit of pressure-change and reflects lung elasticity or stiffness. This requires the use of an esophageal balloon and is seldom utilized in the clinical laboratory. Lung compliance is inferred by the resultant changes in static lung volumes (see Fig. 30–3).

Maximal inspiratory and expiratory pressures reflect the strength of the respiratory muscles. These are measured by having the patient forcibly inspire and expire through a closed mouthpiece attached to a pressure gauge. Maximal pressures are reduced in neuromuscular disorders (e.g., myasthenia gravis, muscular dystrophy, Guillain-Barré syndrome).

Diffusing Capacity (DL_{CO})

DL_{CO} is defined as the number of ml of CO absorbed/min/mm Hg. It is determined by having the patient inspire maximally a gas containing a known small concentration of CO, hold his breath for 10 seconds, then slowly expire to RV. An aliquot of alveolar (i.e., end-expired) gas is analyzed for CO and the amount absorbed during that breath is then calculated.

It is generally agreed that an abnormally low DL_{CO} is not due to physical thickening of the alveolar-capillary membrane alone, but probably reflects abnormal ventilation/perfusion ($\dot{V}/\dot{Q}$) in diseased lungs. DL_{CO} is low in processes that destroy alveolar-capillary membranes; these include emphysema and interstitial inflammatory fibrotic processes. The DL_{CO} also tends to be diminished in severe anemia (less Hb available to bind the inhaled CO) and will be artifactually lowered if the patient's Hb already is occupied by CO (e.g., smoking within several hours prior to the test). The DL_{CO} increases with increases in pulmonary blood flow as occurs during exercise and also in mild (interstitial) congestive heart failure (increase in blood flow to the usually poorly perfused lung apices).

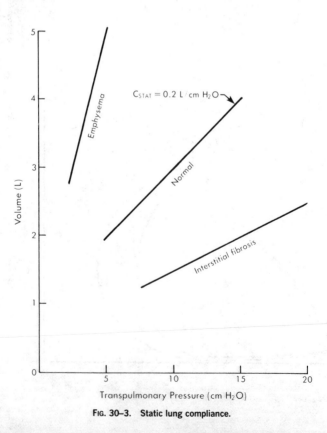

FIG. 30–3. Static lung compliance.

Distribution of Ventilation

The distribution of ventilation is studied by continuously recording the concentration of expired N_2 at the mouth following a single maximal inspiration of 100% O_2. If the distribution of ventilation is normal (i.e., the majority of alveoli fill and empty synchronously), there should be a $< 2\%$ increase in N concentration between 750 and 1250 ml of expired breath (see Fig. 30–4). A $> 2\%$ change implies asynchronous emptying of alveoli, which most commonly is due to airways obstruction. A more direct though more complex study involves lung scanning after the inhalation of radioactive xenon gas (the **ventilation lung scan** [see in Ch. 227]).

Peripheral "Small" Airways Studies

R_{AW} and FEV measurements reflect primarily the condition of the large airways. In the normal lung, bronchi < 2 mm in diameter contribute $< 10\%$ of the total airways resistance, yet their aggregate surface area is large. Disease affecting primarily the smaller airways can be very extensive and yet not affect the R_{AW} or any tests dependent on this such as the FEV_1. This is true of early obstructive lung disease and probably also of interstitial granulomatous, fibrotic, or inflammatory disorders. The status of the small airways is reflected by the MMEF and by expiratory flows in the last 25 to 50% of the FVC, best determined from the flow-volume loop (see Fig. 30–2a). More complex and sophisticated tests of small airways function have been devised. These include frequency-dependent changes in lung compliance (dynamic compliance), closing volume, and closing capacity. The latter can be determined by a modification of the N washout technic (see Distribution of Ventilation, above, and Fig. 30–3), but in general, measurement of these more complex tests adds little to those more readily available (see above) and has little place in the clinical laboratory.

Control of Breathing

Recent emphasis on the clinical importance of obstructive sleep apnea and central hypoventilation (pickwickian syndrome) has brought the study of the control of breathing to the clinical physiology laboratory.

Hypoxic drive (function of the carotid chemoreceptors) can be studied by plotting the ventilatory response to progressive decrements in inspired O_2.

CO_2 sensitivity (function of the central, medullary chemoreceptors) is reflected by the ventilatory response to progressive increments in inspired CO_2.

Central and obstructive sleep apnea can be distinguished by monitoring respiration during sleep. An ear oximeter monitors O_2 saturation. A CO_2 electrode placed in a nostril monitors P_{CO_2} and also serves as an indicator of air flow. Chest wall motion is monitored by a strain gauge or by impedance electrodes. In obstructive sleep apnea, air flow at the nose ceases despite continued excursion of the chest wall, O_2 saturation drops, and P_{CO_2} increases. In central apnea, chest wall motion and air flow cease simultaneously.

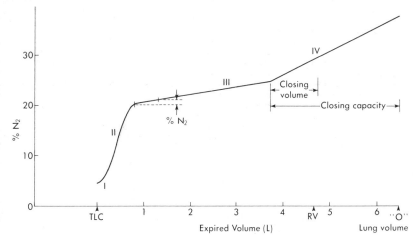

Fig. 30–4. Distribution of ventilation, and closing volume. The numbered phases of expiration refer to deadspace gas (I), mixed deadspace and alveolar gas (II), alveolar gas (III), and "airway closure" (IV). Normally, the CV is less than the FRC in both supine and sitting positions and all airways are open during tidal breathing. As the CV increases with progressive disease of the airways, more and more of the dependent airways become closed during part or all of tidal breathing, contributing to hypoxia. The % rise in nitrogen (N_2) between 750 and 1250 ml of expired gas is a reflection of the distribution of ventilation (see text).

How to Order and Interpret Pulmonary Function Tests

A "complete" set of pulmonary function tests in a good clinical laboratory includes determination of all lung volumes (VC, FRC, RV, TLC), spirometry (FVC, FEV_1, MMEF), diffusing capacity, flow-volume loop, MVV, and of maximum inspiratory and expiratory pressures. This extensive testing is tiring, time-consuming, expensive, and often not necessary for adequate clinical assessment.

Any physician who evaluates patients with pulmonary disorders should have access to simple spirometry in the office. Simple spirometry is the backbone of pulmonary function evaluation and usually provides sufficient information. A number of inexpensive electronic spirometers are now available capable of measuring VC, FEV_1, and PEF. The procedure is readily taught to both patient and operator and yields permanent, reproducible, and accurate data. While spirometry alone may not permit specific diagnosis, it can differentiate between obstructive and restrictive disorders and permits estimation of the severity of the process.

With a few simple guidelines, a great deal of useful information can be gathered from the simple spirogram. A low VC in association with normal flow rates ordinarily suggests restrictive disease (see Fig. 30-1b). COPD and asthma have the characteristic exponentially decreasing flows seen in Fig. 30-1c. In the patient with predominant emphysema, the airways can be intrinsically normal, and expiratory flow is limited by dynamic compression of the airways because of the loss of elastic supporting tissues. A finite amount of time is necessary for the airways (wide open at TLC) to snap shut after the onset of the FVC maneuver. Thus a transient of rapid flow is often reflected by a notch at the beginning of the tracing. The spirogram in Fig. 30-1c shows such an "emphysematous notch", and suggests that there has been substantial loss of lung elastic recoil; i.e., there is a significant component of emphysema present. In very severe COPD, expiratory flow can be so prolonged as to appear almost linear on visual analysis of the spirographic tracing. Since lung volume is a major determinant of airway caliber, the slope of the spirogram should continuously decrease from TLC to RV. A truly linear decrease in flow from TLC to RV is pathognomonic of fixed obstruction of the larynx or trachea (e.g., tracheal stenosis or tumor). The limitation to maximal flow here is no longer dynamic compression of airways but a fixed area of narrowing in the large airway.

The spirogram can occasionally be misleading in asthma because it may mimic restrictive disease if there is severe obstruction predominating in the smaller airways. Total occlusion of the airways precludes any air flow and much gas is trapped distally, thus underestimating the VC. The larger airways are patent, so the overall R_{AW} is not much increased and the FEV_1 is normal.

The severity of COPD and the potential for response to bronchodilator can be adequately assessed by simple spirometry (± flow-volume loop) before and after inhalation of bronchodilator. Simple spirometry with determination of the FVC, FEV_1, and MVV usually suffices as a general preoperative screen and should be performed in all smokers > 40 and in all patients with respiratory symptoms prior to chest or abdominal surgery. The response to treatment during an exacerbation of asthma can and should be monitored by portable (bedside) spirometry or by serial measurement of peak expiratory flow rates.

Patients with suspected laryngeal or tracheal pathology are adequately and specifically studied by a flow-volume loop (see Fig. 30-2d).

If weakness of the respiratory muscles is suspected, the MVV, maximal inspiratory and expiratory pressures, and VC are the appropriate tests.

Full tests should be requested when the clinical picture (history, physical examination, chest x-ray) does not coincide with the data obtained by simple spirometry, or when more complete characterization of an abnormal pulmonary process is desired. They are indicated prior to thoracotomy or extensive abdominal surgery (particularly in the patient with known or suspected pulmonary impairment) and to document the severity of interstitial pulmonary disorders. Periodic VCs and $DL_{CO}s$ usually suffice to follow the course of a restrictive process.

The following tables are intended as general guides to the interpretation of pulmonary function tests. TABLE 30-2 illustrates several simple patterns of pulmonary function abnormality. These are not necessarily mutually exclusive; a patient may have a combination of disorders (e.g., restrictive and obstructive disease), which complicates the interpretation. TABLE 30-3 details the expected changes in pulmonary function in restrictive and obstructive disorders of varying severity.

TABLE 30-2. CHARACTERISTIC CHANGES IN PULMONARY FUNCTION IN SEVERAL DISORDERS

Test	Restrictive Lung Diseases	Obstructive Airways Diseases Conventional‡	Obstructive Airways Diseases Central, Fixed§	Neuromuscular Disorders	Obesity
VC/FVC	↓*	N† or ↓	N	N or ↓	N or ↓
TLC	↓*	↑	N	N	↓
RV/FRC	↓/↓*	↑/↑*	N/N	N/N	N/↓*

* Distinctive features. ‡ E.g., COPD. (Continued)
† N = normal. § E.g., tracheal stenosis.

TABLE 30–2. CHARACTERISTIC CHANGES IN PULMONARY FUNCTION
IN SEVERAL DISORDERS *(Cont'd)*

Test	Restrictive Lung Diseases	Obstructive Airways Diseases		Neuromuscular Disorders	Obesity
		Conventional‡	Central, Fixed§		
FEV$_1$ (% VC)	N or ↑	↓*	↓	N	N
MMEF	↓	↓	↓	N	N
MVV	N	↓*	↓	↓*	N
MEF$_{50\% VC}$	N or ↓	↓	↓*	N	N
MIF$_{50\% VC}$	N	N	↓*	N	N
Inspiratory & expiratory pressures	N	N	N	↓*	N
Distribution of ventilation	N	abnormal*	N*	N	N
DL$_{CO}$	↓*	↓ emphysema N bronchitis	N	N	N or ↓

* Distinctive features.   ‡ E.g., COPD.
† N = normal.   § E.g., tracheal stenosis.

TABLE 30–3. CHARACTERISTIC CHANGES IN PULMONARY FUNCTION IN
RESTRICTIVE AND OBSTRUCTIVE DISEASE OF VARYING SEVERITY

Impairment	Restrictive Disease				
	None	Mild	Moderate	Severe	Very Severe
VC (% predicted)	>80	60–80	50–60	35–50	<35
FEV$_1$ (%VC)	>75	>75	>75	>75	>75
MVV (% predicted)	>80	>80	>80	60–80	<60
RV (% predicted)	80–120	80–120	70–80	60–70	<60
DL$_{CO}$	N	↓E	↓R	↓	↓↓
Arterial blood gases P$_{O_2}$: (during rest & exercise) P$_{CO_2}$:	N / N	N / N	↓E / ↓	↓ / ↓	↓↓ / ±↑
Dyspnea (severity)	0	+	+ +	+ + +	+ + + +
	Obstructive Disease				
VC (% predicted)	>80	>80	>80	↓	↓
FEV$_1$ (%VC)	>75	60–75	40–60	<40	<40
MVV (% predicted)	>80	65–80	45–65	30–45	<30
RV (% predicted)	80–120	120–150	150–175	>200	>200
DL$_{CO}$	N	N	N	↓	↓↓
Arterial blood gases P$_{O_2}$: (during rest & exercise) P$_{CO_2}$:	N / N	↓E / N	↓ / ↓	↓ / ↑E	↓↓ / ↑R
Dyspnea (severity)	0	+	+ +	+ + +	+ + + +

N = normal; R = rest; E = exercise.

31. SPECIAL PROCEDURES

ULTRASOUND

Details of ultrasound technic are discussed in Ch. 226. In thoracic diagnosis, the A-mode display is used, due to its cross-sectional presentation of the scanned area. Since air in the lungs is a poor conductor of high-frequency sound waves, deep structures are poorly discriminated by this technic. There are no medical contraindications or complications. With ultrasound, 3 lesions may be identified as fluid-containing or solid tissue: (1) pleural thickening, (2) masses close to the chest wall, and (3) mediastinal masses.

RADIONUCLIDE SCANNING OF THE LUNG

(See RADIONUCLIDE IMAGING METHODS in Ch. 227)

THORACENTESIS

Diagnostic indications: The presence of pleural fluid of undetermined etiology, the unanticipated recurrence of pleural fluid in the course of an illness, the occurrence of pleural fluid in patients with infectious disease when microbiologic diagnosis is not secure; the presence of pleural fluid in suspected malignant disease to help decide therapy, to establish the cell-type of a malignancy, to uncover a pleural hemorrhage or suppuration that requires more radical intervention.

Therapeutic indications: Relief of respiratory restriction due to large quantities of pleural fluid that compress lung or distort the mediastinum; to introduce antineoplastic or adhesion-inducing agents into the pleural space.

Relative contraindications include bleeding diatheses, hypersensitivity to local anesthetic agents, severe pulmonary insufficiency due to emphysema (life-threatening pneumothorax may occur if a bulla is inadvertently needled), suspicion of echinococcus cyst in the pleura (spill of the fluid can produce severe, possibly fatal, allergic reactions). The presence of cardiac arrhythmias imposes the need to monitor the patient and to premedicate him with atropine or other drugs.

Procedure

The upper level of the fluid is identified by physical examination and x-ray. The patient is given premedication of atropine 1 mg s.c. average for an adult plus an appropriate sedative, if necessary. He is seated comfortably, leaning on a support or, unusually, propped in such a position that the operator can gain access to a dependent position in relation to the fluid accumulation. The area to be aspirated is cleaned and draped. Local anesthetic, e.g., lidocaine, is used first to raise a skin wheal; the area of the puncture is then infiltrated down to the pleural surface. When aspiration (done before each injection to prevent inadvertent IV injection of the agent) yields fluid, the pleural space has been entered. Depending on the thickness of the chest wall, a 2- to 3-in. needle, 18-gauge, attached to a 30- to 50-ml syringe and a 3-way stopcock is introduced over the *upper* border of the rib which has been identified to be below the level of the fluid. If a larger bore needle is used, a small incision in the skin is advisable before introducing the needle. Introducing the needle over the upper border of the rib avoids traumatizing the intercostal vessels and nerve which are found in the costal groove in the under surface of each rib. In older patients the vessels may be tortuous, making this precaution even more important.

The first 20 ml of fluid are removed through the 3-way stopcock for culture, cell count, and sp gr, a small amount of heparin having been put into the tube collecting fluid for the latter examinations. A second 15- to 20-ml sample is taken for chemical analysis and, possibly, cytology. (Examination for malignant cells is best done on either a cell block of a large quantity of fluid that has been centrifuged or on the sediment obtained by filtering a large amount of fluid through a membrane filter.) Following these collections, the bulk of the remaining fluid is taken off either manually or with a vacuum bottle. No more than 1000 to 1200 ml are taken off at one time. Even less is removed if the patient complains of pressure, dizziness, or other symptoms of distress. The pulse is monitored during this procedure. If fluid cannot be obtained despite positioning, then thoracentesis under fluoroscopic guidance is recommended. After the procedure has been completed, P-A and lateral chest x-rays are required to record the change in quantity of fluid and any possible complications.

Diagnostic thoracentesis in very ill patients can be done by using a 21- to 23-gauge needle and removing only enough fluid for the few examinations required. Minimal preparation is necessary and only a simple syringe-needle setup is utilized. In place of a syringe-needle setup, an intracatheter may be inserted into the pleural space and the fluid withdrawn through it. This eliminates the danger of injuring the expanding lung with a needle.

Complications may be prevented or recognized early by careful clinical monitoring during and after the procedure and by the liberal use of x-rays. The major complication is hemorrhage—intrapleural, extrapleural, and intrapulmonary, secondary to trauma from the thoracentesis needle. Pneumothorax may occur from air leaks through the thoracentesis system or secondary to trauma to the surface of the lung. Air embolism from lung puncture is rare, but may be very serious if large. Trauma to either liver or spleen from the thoracentesis needle may occur if the needle is inserted below or through the diaphragm. Syncope may occur from vagal reflexes (including cardiac bradyarrhythmias secondary to fear, pain, or mediastinal shift), air embolus, or actual kinking of vessels secondary to shift of intrathoracic structures.

CLOSED PLEURAL BIOPSY

Indications are the same as those for diagnostic thoracentesis. For both malignant and infectious processes the diagnostic yield of closed pleural biopsy, when done with thoracentesis, is significantly greater than the yield from thoracentesis alone.

Contraindications are the same as for thoracentesis, except that the presence of bleeding diathesis is an absolute rather than a relative contraindication.

Procedure

Various needles are available. The technic described here will concentrate on the Abrams needle.

Local anesthesia, a small vertical incision at the insertion site at the upper border of a rib, and collection of fluid samples is performed first, as for a thoracentesis (see above). The needle with a syringe attached is pushed until its aperture enters the pleural space. During insertion the aperture of the needle is kept open so that entry into the pleural space will be immediately recognized. The needle is angled either laterally or down and gently pulled back until the tissues are "caught" by the aperture. The aperture is closed, a sharp blade being the occluding piece, which takes the sample of tissue and catches it in the barrel of the needle. The needle is then readmitted into the pleural fluid, the aperture opened with suction maintained by the syringe, and the small piece of pleura is sucked into the syringe along with a bit of the pleural fluid. The procedure is repeated several times in order to be sure that enough tissue has been taken. The aperture of the biopsy needle may be directed in any way except upward in order to prevent damage to the intercostal vessels and nerve as noted in Thoracentesis, above. When the biopsy procedure is completed, the thoracentesis may proceed as previously described. The biopsy specimens should be placed in sterile saline or on a sterile gauze pack in order to pick out a few pieces for microbiologic examination and the rest for morphologic study. After the procedure it is essential that P-A and lateral chest x-rays be obtained.

The Cope needle is constructed with a hook that pulls back into a shield and the biopsy procedure with it makes use of a hooking maneuver instead of the anchoring maneuver described for the Abrams needle. In all other respects the technic follows the same directions and constraints.

Complications are the same as for thoracentesis but the likelihood of hemorrhage or pneumothorax is greater. Careful clinical monitoring and x-ray follow-up permit early recognition and treatment of problems.

CLOSED TUBE THORACOTOMY

(Tube Drainage)

Indications: Pneumothorax, spontaneous and traumatic, is the condition most commonly treated with tube drainage. Massive and recurrent pleural effusions unmanageable by needle aspiration also require this treatment; the etiology may be infection, malignancy, chylothorax, etc. Other indications are empyema, hemothorax, and hemopneumothorax.

Contraindications: Adhesions which may prevent introduction of the tube, clotted hemothorax, and/or empyema with pachypleuritis preclude successful tube drainage and require a thoracotomy.

Procedure: The location is chosen for introduction of the tube. For pneumothorax, the anterior chest wall, 2nd or 3rd intercostal space, midclavicular line is used. For pleural effusion, hemothorax, empyema, etc., the axillary line is preferred in the 5th mid or posterior intercostal space. The skin and the intercostal space are infiltrated with 2% procaine or similar agent, a small incision is made, the intercostal muscles are separated, and the tube is introduced through a trocar or directly with the aid of a clamp. The tube is sutured to the skin and connected to an underwater drainage system. Sometimes drainage is promoted by the use of a pump that can generate up to 20 cm H_2O negative pressure.

Complications: Bleeding from an intercostal vessel injured by the trocar, subcutaneous emphysema if the side holes of the drainage tube are not properly placed inside the pleural space, infection of the local skin site, and pain are common.

THORACOSCOPY

Indication: To obtain a biopsy from a peripheral lesion of the lung or pleura under direct vision through a mediastinoscope or similar instrument.

Contraindications: Adhesions, central location of the lesions to be biopsied, bleeding tendency, or air leak.

Procedure: Under general anesthesia, the location is chosen in the anterior or lateral chest wall according to the location of the lesion. A small incision is made in the skin and the intercostal muscles. A mediastinoscope or a bronchoscope is introduced to explore the pleura and the lung. A biopsy is taken through the instrument with a forceps. The lung is then reinflated. Usually, a tube for drainage is left after the procedure.

Complications: Most are due to bleeding or air leak from the location of the biopsy. Infection of the pleural space in the course of the procedure is uncommon except when infected lesions are biopsied.

FIBERBRONCHOSCOPY

Direct visual examination of the tracheobronchial tree using a flexible tube (flexible bronchoscope; fiberbronchoscope) containing light-transmitting glass fibers that return a magnified image. Fiberbronchoscopes range in external diameter from 3 to 6 mm; the proper diameter depends on the size of the patient. The small caliber of the instrument makes it possible to enter segmental bronchi and to visualize subsegmental bronchi. The central channel of the scope is 2 to 2.5 mm in diameter and is used to aspirate secretions, to give anesthetic agents, to obtain brush or forceps biopsies, and to introduce bronchographic contrast material. It is also possible to obtain uncontaminated cultures through the channel. Lavage fluid, such as saline, acetylcysteine, and heparin can be introduced through the channel. Cuffing of the scope makes it possible to lavage a lobe via its lobar bronchus.

Diagnostic indications: It is used to explore the cause of an unexplained persistent cough, wheeze, or hemoptysis, or unresolved pneumonia or atelectasis, especially in a male smoker above age 30. The flexible bronchoscope is used for small hemoptysis, i.e., blood-tinged sputum or small quantities of blood; for large hemoptysis, rigid bronchoscopy is used. Fiberoptic bronchoscopy is also used to perform transbronchial lung biopsy and/or bronchial lavage in diffuse lung disease of obscure etiology, to investigate paralysis of the recurrent laryngeal or phrenic nerves, to search for the origin of positive cytology obtained from sputum or endobronchial aspiration or of any other suggestion of lung tumor, to determine the state of the tracheobronchial tree after acute inhalation injury, to determine the anatomy of the endobronchial tree, to visualize a bronchiectatic area, and postoperatively to evaluate the stump of a resected bronchus.

Therapeutic indications: Attempt to open atelectasis; attempt to drain lung abscess; assist a weakened patient to raise secretions; performing extensive suction through an endotracheal or tracheostomy tube; removal of certain foreign bodies; perform lung lavage after aspiration of acid or alkaline material especially; and identification of acute laryngeal obstruction to direct treatment. For removal of large amounts of secretions or foreign bodies, a rigid bronchoscope is generally preferred.

Contraindications depend, in part, on the clinical state. A few, such as an intractable bleeding disorder or severe cardiopulmonary failure, are usually absolute contraindications. But even in bleeding disorders, temporary correction of the defect by transfusion may sometimes allow enough time for visualization of the airways, although biopsy is avoided. An uncooperative patient can be made tractable by preoperative medication or general anesthesia. Cardiac arrhythmias, especially bradyarrhythmias, are contraindications unless they can be brought under control by premedication.

Procedure

The patient to be bronchoscoped fasts for at least 8 h before the procedure is done. P-A and lateral chest x-rays should be done within 24 h of the procedure. Clotting function should be known to be normal within 24 h of the procedure. Patients with a history of cardiac disease or arrhythmias or > 50 yr of age should be monitored using the ECG.

Premedication consists of atropine average dose 1 mg s.c. and morphine or valium in appropriate dose. Topical anesthesia is accomplished with 2 or 4% lidocaine by first spraying the mouth, throat, and tongue and then through the nose. The patient inhales with each spray and, after one nostril is well sprayed, the other is anesthetized. A nasal catheter is then placed through the least open nostril to the level of the uvula and O_2 4 to 6 L/min is given throughout the procedure.

Before inserting the fiberbronchoscope, lidocaine jelly is used as a lubricant to protect both the patient's mucosa and the fiberbronchoscope from abrasion. The scope may be inserted through the nose providing there is no block, and through the mouth providing a simple curved endotracheal tube is used both as guide and protection for the instrument. The fiberbronchoscope is advanced to the epiglottis and anesthesia of the glottis is completed through the bronchoscope. Additional anesthetic is administered through the fiberbronchoscope as sensitive areas are reached by injecting 1 to 2 ml of the agent through the open channel. It is important to avoid excessive anesthetic agent because of the increasing prospect of untoward reactions as dosage increases.

Insertion of the fiberbronchoscope through endotracheal tubes or tracheostomy tubes that are already in place is quite easy; the main concern is to ensure adequate ventilation of the patient while the procedure is going on. Attachments are available to enable ventilation to proceed during the examination.

The entire procedure can be done under general anesthesia if necessary. Even then topical anesthesia of the glottic structures is advised to minimize the possibility of laryngospasm during or after the procedure is completed.

Complications: The main complications include laryngospasm, cardiac arrhythmias (cardiac arrest is a particular threat in asthmatic patients), hemorrhage due either to biopsy or to injury of the bronchial mucosa by the bronchoscope, pneumothorax secondary to bronchial biopsy, arterial hypoxemia due either to obstruction of a major bronchus by the bronchoscope or to spillover in the course of bronchial lavage, allergic reactions either to premedication or to anesthetic agent, urinary retention or respiratory depression due to premedication, bronchospasm due to irritation of the mucosa by the bronchoscope, and infections of the tracheobronchial tree and lung introduced during the procedure.

One complication is potentially useful for cytologic or microbiologic studies—the almost invariable mild bronchitis that follows the procedure increases sputum production for a few days.

Since the patient's swallowing and cough reflexes are depressed for an hour or so, care must be taken to prevent aspiration by abstaining from eating or drinking for a few hours after the procedure.

MEDIASTINOSCOPY

Indications: The prime indication is the need to biopsy a tumor of the upper mediastinum or to determine whether lymph node metastases have occurred. In systemic diseases (e.g., Hodgkin's disease or lymphoma) both primary diagnosis and staging of the process may be achieved by mediastinoscopy and biopsy.

Contraindications: Superior vena cava syndrome, aneurysm of the aortic arch, and primary tuberculosis of the lung with lymph node involvement are the major conditions that militate against performing this operation. If the indication is urgent enough for the procedure to be performed, even these conditions are not absolute contraindications.

Procedure

Under general anesthesia in supine position with the neck extended, a transverse incision is made in the suprasternal notch. Because of anatomic limitations imposed by the aortic arch and the fascial compartments, the operator has easiest access to structures on the right side, particularly those in the same plane as the trachea and anterior to it. The mediastinoscope is introduced, the dissection is performed in the pretracheal fascia and extended under direct vision to the regional lymph nodes, where biopsy is performed. At the close of the procedure, the fascia and skin are sutured without drainage.

Complications are rare. Pneumothorax may occur if the pleura is opened. Local bleeding may be a problem, especially if superior vena caval obstruction exists. Infection is unusual. Arrhythmias may occur if the pericardium and the heart are touched.

MEDIASTINOTOMY

Indications: The same indications apply as for mediastinoscopy. This procedure is used to biopsy areas that cannot be reached by mediastinoscopy, especially the left side of the mediastinum, the subaortic glands, and structures at or below the level of the hili.

Contraindications are the same as for mediastinoscopy (see above).

Procedure

Under general anesthesia, the patient is placed in the supine position. A parasternal incision is made above the 3rd rib. The cartilage is excised. The approach is extrapleural. If a deeper approach is needed, a mediastinoscope is used. If the pleura is inadvertently entered during the procedure, drainage is established by leaving a catheter in the pleural space at the end of the procedure.

A lung biopsy may be performed through this approach. If indicated, the incision can be extended into a full thoracotomy for better exploration or excision.

Complications: Pneumothorax, bleeding from vessels such as the internal mammary arteries, intercostal arteries, etc., and infection occur infrequently.

SCALENE NODE BIOPSY

Indications: Biopsy of a scalene node may yield histologic evidence of metastatic bronchogenic carcinoma or of a systemic disease, e.g., sarcoidosis.

Contraindications: Without a palpable node, the procedure is usually unrewarding. Superior vena caval obstruction and other processes that cause congestion and edema of the supraclavicular area may preclude biopsy.

Procedure: The incision is made in the supraclavicular prescalene region, the sternocleidomastoid muscle is divided, the deep cervical fascia is opened, and the prescalene fat and node are removed.

Complications: Bleeding, pneumothorax and infection are uncommon complications. Even more unusual is lymph accumulation in the supraclavicular space.

LUNG BIOPSY

Indications: Either open or closed lung biopsy may be helpful in dealing with an unexplained diffuse process that primarily affects the interstitium or the alveoli; with an infectious process of obscure etiology, especially in immunosuppressed patients; with a pulmonary process which inexplicably worsens under treatment; and with solitary or multiple nodules when the diagnosis is unsettled.

Since lung biopsy is an invasive procedure, the decision to perform the biopsy is influenced by the general condition of the patient and by the likelihood that the information obtained may modify the outcome. It may be, however, more risky to treat a pulmonary problem without establishing a diagnosis histologically or microbiologically than to subject the patient to this invasive procedure.

Contraindications are relative, except for a bleeding diathesis. Even in this situation, especially if the need is extremely urgent, the administration of fresh blood or the specific replacement therapy may make it possible to perform the procedure. Other contraindications include respiratory insufficiency, emphysematous bullae (especially in the area to be biopsied), pulmonary hypertension, uncontrollable cough (for closed procedures), uncooperative patient (for closed procedures), and the lack of adequate laboratory facilities and trained personnel to handle the biopsy specimen.

Standard histologic examination is usually not enough. Microbiologic processing is a regular part of the procedure especially if infection is suspected, since, without culture, many infectious processes are indistinguishable one from the other; e.g., tuberculosis and histoplasmosis. If an allergic or immunologic process is suspected, provision must be on hand for immunologic studies. Special handling is also required for certain of the pneumoconioses.

Procedure

Transbronchial biopsy is often used for diffuse lung disease. It is particularly valuable for the diagnosis of sarcoidosis and miliary tuberculosis. However, for most other diffuse disorders, it has much less diagnostic value. It is usually done under fluoroscopic control but may be done blindly. A biopsy forceps is introduced through either a rigid or fiberbronchoscope into the bronchus leading to the area to be biopsied.

Drill biopsy involves pushing a trocar through the chest wall during inspiration and cutting out a piece of tissue with a high-speed trephine drill. At the same time that the rotating trephine removes a core of tissue, blood vessels are sealed off. Generally more than 1 piece of tissue can be obtained. A **percutaneous cutting needle** is used to biopsy peripheral lung nodules.

Aspiration biopsy: A "skinny" needle (22-, 23-, 24-gauge) is introduced into the lung. A large syringe is used to generate a sustained suction to aspirate lung fluid containing cells or microorganisms. This may be done several times. This procedure has proved useful in two circumstances: a peripheral nodule from which a cytologic diagnosis will be helpful, and an infectious disease of unknown etiology which urgently needs specific antimicrobial therapy.

Open biopsy permits the operator to visualize the surface of the lung, to select the optimum area for biopsy, and to obtain adequate tissue for the required studies. A small incision is made and the pleura is opened. Most of the biopsies are taken from the lingula on the left or from the middle lobe on the right side. After the biopsy, the lung is reexpanded and the chest is closed. A drain is left in place for 1 or 2 days postoperatively if the surgeon is concerned about the possibility of a pneumothorax. Repeated x-rays of the chest are used to check that the lung is fully expanded.

Complications: Hemorrhage, pneumothorax, cardiac arrest, and other vagal reflex disasters are possible in all of these procedures. Postoperative pain, especially in open biopsy, may be a problem. During closed procedures the possibility of air-embolus exists. Allergic reactions to the anesthetic agents occasionally occur during the closed procedures. Occasional deaths have occurred in the course of each of these procedures except for fine needle aspiration. Bronchopleural fistula with empyema is commoner after open biopsy than after the closed cutting procedures.

TRACHEAL ASPIRATION

Indications: Tracheal aspiration is indicated as a therapeutic measure when the patient is unable to cough up troublesome secretions. Diagnostic tracheal aspiration is performed to obtain for laboratory examination tracheobronchial secretions that are relatively uncontaminated by mouth, nose, and pharyngeal secretions.

The clinical situations most often associated with inadequate or absent cough are: (1) deep coma with absence of protective reflexes; (2) neuromuscular disorders (such as cervical spine injuries, myasthenia gravis, Guillain-Barré), chronic airways obstruction, bronchiectasis, cachexia; and (3) situations in which instability of the chest wall or severe pain prevents effective coughing, e.g., chest trauma with flail chest, postoperative pain from thoracic or abdominal surgery, or traumatic rib fractures.

Those patients who are apt to require tracheal aspirate for laboratory examination, especially special staining and cultures, include the immunosuppressed individual who develops a pulmonary infiltrate, the individual with a pulmonary infection who fails to respond to treatment or has a relapse while on previously effective antibiotic therapy, and the critically ill patient with pulmonary infiltrates whose life seems imminently threatened by the infection.

Contraindications: In the presence of laryngeal edema the use of any endotracheal instrumentation is contraindicated unless the need is life-threatening. Equipment for introducing an emergency airway must always be at hand. Laryngospasm may develop as a result of mechanical irritation of the vocal cords. Unconscious patients who lack a cough reflex may vomit during the suctioning, thereby further obstructing the air passages. Repeated suctioning should be avoided or postponed until an endotracheal tube has been placed.

In the patient who is subject to cardiac arrhythmias, vagal stimulation in the course of tracheal aspiration is a particular hazard. Small doses of atropine can be used to block vagal effects and to minimize the likelihood of arrhythmias. $Pa_{O_2} < 50$ Torr, digitalis excess, and electrolyte imbalances exaggerate the threat of arrhythmias.

Procedure

Tracheal aspiration through natural airways: Care is required to avoid trauma of the mucosa of the structures through which the catheter passes. For this reason it is best to use a relatively small size (No. 12 to 16 for adults), flexible, sterile, disposable, plastic catheter. It should have a side vent at its proximal end or be attached to a suction source with a "Y" connector and it must have a round distal end-opening with 2 to 3 extra holes on the side, to avoid trauma and invagination of mucosa during introduction and suctioning.

In the **transnasal approach,** the patient should be sitting upright against a support with neck slightly extended. The tongue is grasped with a piece of gauze and pulled firmly forward, and the catheter with side vent open is introduced into the pharynx through the nose. No suction is applied while the catheter is being positioned in the airway. As the patient inhales, the catheter is slipped gently through the vocal cords into the trachea; usually violent coughing ensues. When the coughing subsides, suction is applied *briefly and intermittently* (for about 5 to 10 seconds every 25 to 30 seconds) by occluding the side vent with the finger. The catheter is moved gently up and down in the trachea during the suction intervals. O_2 can be given by mask during suctioning.

Bronchial suctioning is usually done with tracheal aspiration. Both mainstem bronchi are aspirated. The patient's head is turned to the side opposite the bronchus to be aspirated and the catheter is advanced into the bronchus. The bronchus is suctioned while the catheter is rotated gently and withdrawn toward the trachea. Suction is released, the patient's head is turned to the opposite side, the catheter is slipped into the other bronchus, and suction is again applied.

Suctioning episodes must be brief, since they exhaust the patient; sterile catheters should be used each time. Although the nose is not sterile, it is good technic for the operator to use a sterile glove on the hand that holds the catheter to avoid adding organisms to the tracheobronchial tree of the patient.

The **transoral approach** is required when nasal passage cannot be accomplished because of obstruction. Proper positioning of the patient and of the head is essential. The patient usually sits in a chair, with head extended on the neck and the neck flexed on the thorax ("Nefertiti sniff" position); sometimes the supine position is used. A bite block is placed between the rear molars. The catheter is more readily dislodged by coughing during the transoral than during the transnasal approach. Also, bronchial suctioning is not practical in the transoral procedure.

Percutaneous transtracheal aspiration: The patient's head is extended. The skin of the anterior neck is disinfected, a local anesthetic is infiltrated, and a large-bore thin-walled needle attached to a syringe is inserted into the tracheal lumen in the midline (with the bevel pointing down) either through the cricothyroid membrane or a high intercartilaginous space. After air has been aspirated to ensure that the needle tip is within the lumen of the trachea, the syringe is removed, a sterile 30-cm polyethylene catheter is threaded through the needle into the trachea, and the needle is removed. Periodic instillation of small amounts of sterile saline induces coughing and raises secretions that are removed by nasopharyngeal suctioning. To obtain a specimen directly, a syringe is attached to the catheter and a specimen of secretion is aspirated into a sterile sputum collector. If secretions cannot be aspirated, a few ml of sterile saline are instilled and aspiration repeated. The catheter is withdrawn. In some situations (e.g., postoperative chest surgery) the catheter may be left in place for 24 to 48 h in order to stimulate cough until the patient is able to cough spontaneously.

Tracheal aspiration through an artificial airway, either an endotracheal tube or a tracheotomy, is performed using a sterile glove on one hand and a sterile catheter. The size of the soft plastic catheter is selected to allow $1/3$ of the endotracheal tube's lumen to remain free for air passage. A few ml of sterile saline are injected through the tracheal tube, an Ambu bag is immediately applied, and the patient is given a few high-volume ventilations (using the operator's ungloved hand) to loosen and mobilize sticky secretions. If a hypoxemic patient is being mechanically ventilated with supplemental O_2, an O_2 line should be attached to the Ambu bag and high concentrations of O_2 given for the few large-volume breaths. Immediately after this maneuver, the Ambu bag is removed and a sterile catheter inserted as deeply as possible. Suctioning is then performed by closing the side vent of the catheter, first in the trachea and then each major bronchus while turning the patient's head to the opposite side of the bronchus to be suctioned. Using a Teeman catheter will facilitate entering each main bronchus.

The catheter is withdrawn and the patient is ventilated. The catheter is washed through with sterile saline from a sterile cup. Each trial of repeated suctioning is preceded by the Ambu maneuver and introduction of a few ml of saline.

During suctioning, massive removal of air from the airway occurs, followed by reduction of lung volume or collapse, and arterial hypoxemia. Cardiac arrhythmias and/or arrest are more often due to hypoxia than to heightened vagal activity in response to irritation. Each trial of suctioning is limited to 15 to 30 seconds, and deep inflation with O_2 is used between trials. Severely hypoxic and apneic patients are suctioned through the T-opening of a swivel connector in order to provide a continuous flow of O_2 during the procedure.

Complications of tracheal suctioning include laryngospasm, cardiac arrhythmias and arrest, vomiting and aspiration of vomited material, trauma to the mucosa of the entire upper respiratory area through which the catheter is introduced, and infection of the area suctioned. Vigorous coughing generally produced by this maneuver may result in torn muscles and other musculoskeletal problems.

ESTABLISHMENT OF AN EMERGENCY AIRWAY

Indications

Occlusion of the airway is a medical emergency. After 4 to 5 min of anoxia severe or irreversible brain damage is likely to occur. Therefore prompt establishment of a patent airway and proper ventilation of the lungs are essential.

Acute respiratory arrest may follow a variety of conditions: (1) in comatose patients, upper airway obstruction from dropping back of the tongue, improper position of the lower jaw and head, vomitus, secretions, or foreign body; (2) acute laryngeal edema secondary to trauma or infection, especially if one or both vocal cords are paralyzed; (3) laryngospasm, usually reflex-induced; (4) severe, sudden, cardiac arrhythmia or arrest; (5) drowning or any other form of suffocation; (6) severe head trauma with acute respiratory center paralysis and coma; (7) penetrating chest trauma with consequent anoxia; (8) cervical spinal cord lesions; and (9) respiratory depression and apnea from drug overdose.

Chronic situations requiring establishment of an emergency airway are respiratory failure due to adult respiratory distress syndrome, acute respiratory insufficiency or chronic insufficiency due to chronic obstructive or restrictive lung disease, chronic neuromusculoskeletal diseases, exhaustion from any cause for which the patient needs mechanical ventilation, protection against gastric content aspiration, and effective removal of tracheobronchial secretions.

Contraindications: There is clearly no contraindication to maintaining a clear airway. When in doubt about intubating or tracheotomizing or not, the intervention should be given the benefit of the doubt. The decision to intervene promptly or to delay depends on the experience of the physician or other health professional on hand. Inexperienced individuals administering treatment should keep the airway open using proper positioning and ventilation of the patient by means of a mask and bag until more experienced help can take over.

Procedures

Check first for airway obstruction. Tilt the head, lift the lower jaw, prevent the tongue from obstructing the pharynx, remove secretions, foreign bodies, vomitus or blood; these simple procedures for establishing free air passage may be lifesaving. If the patient remains apneic, **provide mechanical insufflation** using mouth-to-mouth respiration or a mask and bag. In situations where aspiration of food is suspected, the Heimlich maneuver is appropriate. It is described, along with other noninvasive maneuvers, under Cardiac Arrest and Cardiopulmonary Resuscitation in Ch. 25. All these noninvasive measures should last no longer than 60 seconds. If they are insufficient to establish adequate air passage and ventilation, the following order of invasive procedures is suggested:

1. **An oropharyngeal airway** should be inserted over the tongue to relieve mechanical problems caused by a floppy tongue. The patient's head should remain tilted backward. Insertion of a soft rubber nasopharyngeal airway through a nostril may be successful in opening the airway when an oropharyngeal tube cannot be placed. Use of any such device is only a short-term measure.

2. **The esophageal obturator airway** has proved useful for paramedics and relatively untrained medical personnel. Patients with inadequate ventilation often thrash uncontrollably and become combative. If insufflation technics and upper airway clearing measures are not effective, invasive direct control will be necessary. In these patients, however, laryngoscopy and tracheal intubation may be technically impossible and surgical intervention difficult, particularly without experienced personnel. The same anatomic features of the pharynx (anterior location of the larynx and its small aperture) that make tracheal intubation difficult make it easy to intubate the esophagus. The esophageal obturator airway has been introduced for this purpose. This large tube, directly inserted through the mouth, tends to enter the posteriorly situated esophagus. Holes placed in the tube open into the oropharynx when the tube is properly positioned. The esophagus is "obturated" by inflating a balloon at the end of the tube. An airtight face mask is applied to the nose and mouth area; the tube is inserted into the mask by an airtight seal. Air delivered to the mask passes via the oropharynx only to the trachea, since the nose, mouth, and esophagus are completely closed off. A recent improvement in the apparatus enables venting of the distal esophageal lumen through the mask. Thus, air leaking around the esophageal balloon escapes to the atmosphere rather than to the stomach, avoiding gastric distention and vomiting.

3. **A large-caliber needle or trocar** (12- or 14-gauge) provides a rapid method of establishing an airway when the larynx is blocked. This simplest method of mechanical ventilation may save enough time to allow for more definitive control. It is a once-in-a-lifetime experience for most persons but is

only a temporizing measure to be used when all other attempts at establishing and securing an airway have failed and while awaiting experienced personnel and adequate equipment.

The trachea should be located and fixed with one hand and the needle then pushed percutaneously through the cricothyroid membrane into the tracheal lumen, pointing it toward the lungs. Satisfactory artificial ventilation can be achieved if such a needle can be connected via a 3-way stopcock or simple T-tube to a direct 50 lb/sq in. gas source (not a flow meter). The stopcock is turned intermittently, 16 to 20 times/min, to deliver gas; it is reversed to stop insufflation and permit passive expiration. Great care must be taken not to perforate the posterior wall of the trachea into the esophagus or to permit the needle to slip off the side of the trachea into one of the adjacent large blood vessels.

4. Emergencv cricothyrotomy (see FIG. 31–1): A tracheotomy is rarely necessary in an acute emergency, and use by an untrained person can rarely be justified. An emergency cricothyrotomy can be performed by a relatively untrained person with minimal and makeshift equipment, but it is hazardous. Since the patients involved are usually rather violent, the equipment scarce, and the personnel inexperienced, this approach can be advocated only as a last-ditch lifesaving measure. In severe face trauma, or if the patient has a clenched jaw obviating intubation, it may be the only alternative.

After extending the patient's neck, the operator should spread the skin over the trachea to make it taut, palpate the trachea with the finger, locate the cricothyroid membrane or the cricoid cartilage, and make a single vertical incision of about 0.5 cm ($^3/_{16}$ in.) through this membrane. The knife handle or some other blunt instrument is used to spread the edges of the incision, thereby establishing the lifesaving airway. Any small tube can be introduced through the incision to secure free air passage. As soon as this emergency airway is established and the patient is well-aerated, more definitive airway control should be effected.

5. Endotracheal intubation is indicated for all of the situations in which airway control or artificial ventilation are indicated if an oral airway fails to provide a free air passage. It remains the quickest, most efficient, and least traumatic technic for this purpose. Preparation for intubation requires the following:

1. Laryngoscope with the proper size and shape of blade. The Magill straight blade or the Macintosh curved blade can be used. For newborn infants and babies, the straight blade is preferable. Always precheck the laryngoscope light.

2. Proper size and weight cuffed endotracheal tube with fitted-in connector adjusted to fit the O_2 source. Always check the integrity of the tube's cuff before use.

3. Intubation (Magill) forceps.

4. Curved wire with a stopper (a guide).

5. Water soluble lubricant; laryngeal spray is arbitrary.

6. Proper-sized face mask.

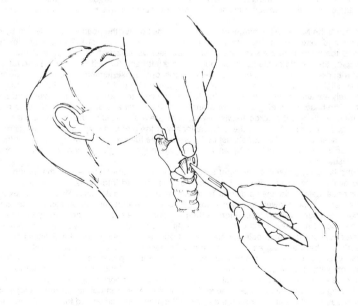

FIG. 31–1.   **Emergency tracheotomy (cricothyrotomy) technic.** (From PATIENT CARE, June 15, 1971. Copyright © 1971, Patient Care Publications, Inc., Darien, Conn. All rights reserved.)

7. Breathing bag, such as the Ambu bag.
8. O_2 source.
9. Suction apparatus.

Intubation may be done by either of 2 routes: transnasal or transoral.

Blind nasal intubation is indicated in all cases and may be more comfortable for an awake patient who has to tolerate prolonged intubation. It is also less likely that the tube will dislocate after nasal than after oral intubation. Disadvantages are that a longer tube is used than for the oral route (about 2 to 3 cm more for an adult), the tube diameter is smaller, suctioning is more difficult, and the procedure is more prolonged.

The largest possible tube diameter is selected according to the patient's nostrils. The patient lies with his head in the "sniff" position. Spray may be used for topical anesthesia; a drop of adrenalin is added to control bleeding.

A well-curved lubricated tube is advanced via the nostril into the nasopharynx. The lower jaw is then slightly elevated to lift the epiglottis. The opposite nostril is occluded and the patient, if cooperative, is asked to breathe deeply. The head should be slightly inclined to the side of the nostril used. The operator must place his ear near the proximal end of the tube, which is advanced so that breathing is maximally audible. This procedure is "led by the ear." The operator's free hand moves the larynx to meet the tube. As the tube passes between the cords, there is usually some breath-holding or cough, unless the patient is deeply unconscious. If, when advancing the tube, audible breathing sounds disappear, the tube should be pulled back and thrust down again. With the tube in the trachea, breath sounds through it will be free and inflation with a bag will expand the chest.

Blind nasal intubation may precipitate laryngospasm and vomiting; treatment facilities for these complications should be on hand.

Direct vision nasal intubation is used if blind intubation fails and a nasotracheal tube is desirable. The tube is passed through the nose as noted above. The mouth should be opened, either spontaneously or with some form of muscle relaxation, and the vocal cords visualized with the laryngoscope as noted under the orotracheal approach (see below). The tube tip is inserted into the hypopharynx and is guided between the cords either by slight movements or with the aid of Magill intubation forceps. An assistant gently pushes down the proximal end of the tube when the forceps is used.

Orotracheal direct vision intubation: This approach can be used in all cases except for patients with anatomic problems such as a short inflexible neck, micro- or macroprognathism, rabbit teeth, or ankylosis of the temporomandibular joint. In these patients, blind nasal intubation or tracheostomy is preferable.

For orotracheal intubation to be nontraumatic, reflexes must be absent and muscles should be relaxed. These conditions are easily induced in the operating room, but are much more difficult to arrange when emergency intubation is performed in less convenient settings. Unless the patient is relaxed and cooperative, the upper incisors and the vocal cords can be easily traumatized during the procedure.

When using the Macintosh laryngoscope, the best position for the head is slight flexion by means of a pillow and extension of the atlanto-occipital joint (sniffing position). This position brings the mouth and the pharynx into a straight line and facilitates visualization of the cords. A right-handed person holds the handle of the laryngoscope with the left hand (or switches hands) and introduces the tube with his right hand. The blade of the laryngoscope is inserted into the patient's mouth in the midline or slightly along the right side of the tongue pressing it to the left. The laryngoscope is progressively advanced over the base of the tongue in order to visualize first the uvula and then the epiglottis. The base of the epiglottis is now lifted with the distal end of the blade, avoiding pressure on the upper teeth, and the cords are visualized. They are recognized by their pallor and the triangular shape of the opening between them. Occasionally, if the glottis is very anterior, only its posterior part can be seen and then the tube must be inserted while fully curved by using the wire introducer. Pressure on the cricoid cartilage by an assistant will bring the glottis more posteriorly and thus facilitate visualization.

The tube is gently passed at the right side of the laryngoscope, adjacent to the mouth angle in order to avoid blocking the view and the light, and is inserted into the larynx and trachea. If the patient is not anesthetized, the cords may be in spasm or approximated as is often seen in expiration. The cords should be allowed to relax; if forced apart, the intubation is always traumatizing and complications result. Wait for inspiration as then the cords are maximally open; only then insert the tube. One should not persist if the intubation is difficult but should stop, ventilate the patient with mask and bag, consider the problem, obtain help if possible, and judge the effectiveness of noninvasive insufflation before trying again. With the tube in position, the laryngoscope is withdrawn and a gag, airway, or any other object is placed between the teeth to prevent the patient's biting the tube.

In patients with anatomical deformities of the neck, trauma of the face, or any other reason that intubation using a laryngoscope is technically or practically impossible, the intubation may be attempted using a fiberbronchoscope. The endotracheal tube is "run up" the bronchoscope and the bronchoscope inserted either through the nose or the mouth and advanced through the vocal cords into the trachea. The endotracheal tube is then "run down" the bronchoscope until it is in place in the trachea. The bronchoscope is then withdrawn.

Once the tube is between the vocal cords, ventilation must begin immediately in order to avoid arterial hypoxemia, but should be done gently—rupture of alveoli is possible by overinflation. If necessary this should be immediately followed by suctioning. Auscultation of both lungs while inflating them is essential immediately after tube insertion to prove bilateral air entry. Absence of breath sounds over both lungs and lack of chest expansion with inflation indicate esophageal intubation; in addition, gurgling of air passing the esophagus and stomach during inflation can be recognized. The tube should be pulled out, the patient oxygenated, and the tube reinserted properly. Absent or reduced breath sounds over one lung, most often the left, indicates one-lung intubation. The tube should be cautiously pulled back while auscultating the silent lung for return of breath sounds, meaning inflation and proper positioning of the tube.

Now fixation of the tube should be insured by use of adhesive tape or a hernia tape; the latter ties the tube around the neck of the patient. This is mandatory to prevent accidental tube displacement. If nasal intubation is used, a safety pin or an angle piece is placed at the proximal protruding end to prevent slipping of the tube into the nose.

The tube cuff should be inflated as soon as the tube is properly placed. This should be done just enough to prevent audible leakage of gas when compressing the reservoir bag with an appropriate volume. Overinflating the cuff more than normal capillary pressure (20 mm Hg) may cause ischemic damage of the tracheal mucosa. If a regular cuff is used for prolonged intubation, it must be deflated for 2 to 3 min q 2 h to minimize mucosal damage. Previous to any deflation of the cuff, efficient deep pharyngeal suctioning should be performed to remove any collected secretion above the cuff and thus avoid seeping of secretions down the trachea.

Prolonged ($>$ 2 to 3 days) intubation across the larynx was previously associated with an unacceptable incidence of complications, (e.g., granulomas, ulceration of the vocal cords, some glottic stenosis). However, these complications have been reduced by the use of low-pressure, high residual-volume occlusive cuffs, endotracheal tubes constructed of nontoxic materials which have been implant tested (marked I.T. or Z-79 designation), and good humidification. These cuffs need not be intermittently deflated. Endotracheal tubes have been left in place for several weeks without any increase in laryngeal lesions. However, prolonged intubation is associated with an increasing frequency of tracheal stenosis.

6. Tracheostomy as an emergency procedure has been replaced by endotracheal intubation as a proper emergency procedure in most cases. However, emergency tracheostomy is still indicated in trauma of the upper airway or cervical spinal cord, tumors involving the mouth or vocal cords, and some pharyngeal or laryngeal infections.

As a general rule, tracheostomy should be done electively. It is indicated to obtain long-term definitive airway control for prolonged ventilation of critically ill patients. It is used less often now than in previous years, reflecting refinements in therapy of respiratory failure and improvement in the technics, equipment, and sophistication of upper airway intervention. Though direct tracheal control of the airway by tracheotomy is appealing, there is a procedure-related mortality. Complications are common (see below). The procedure is preferably done with a naso- or orotracheal tube in place.

The trachea is entered by vertical incision of the 2nd and 3rd tracheal rings. Lower insertion of a tracheostomy tube may produce possible trauma of the innominate artery; higher incision may damage the larynx. Electrocautery simplifies dissection.

A silver tracheostomy tube with an inner removable cannula is used to keep the airway open. Plastic tracheostomy tubes, with soft low pressure cuffs, are used if ventilatory support is needed to relieve hypoxia, hypercarbia, or both. For a discussion of ventilatory support procedures (including positive end-expiratory pressure [PEEP]), see Ch. 32.

Plastic tracheostomy tubes with inflatable cuffs are preferable if the need for ventilatory support is anticipated. Changing of tracheostomy tubes during the early postoperative period should be avoided. It is a hazardous procedure since the tissue planes of the wound have not yet formed a sinus tract and there is a danger of inserting the replacement tube through a false route with all of the attendant complications.

Care should be taken to provide humidification, aseptic wound care, and sterile tracheal aspiration as well as to keep the tracheostomy tube in midline position and to prevent traumatizing the tracheal wall from the tube's tip.

Complications

Complications of introducing various tubes into the upper airways are many, but the most serious are immediate arterial hypoxemia due to airway obstruction during the procedure, cardiac arrhythmias resulting from reflex stimulation of the vagus from the pharynx and larynx, broken teeth, trauma, bleeding from a variety of sources, and aspiration of contents contained in the throat or mouth at the time the procedure is attempted or from emesis in the course of the intubation. Other acute complications are gastric distention and subsequent regurgitation, with evident or silent aspiration, and gastric rupture, which occasionally follows vigorous attempts at ventilation before the tube is in the trachea.

Further complications include injury to the vocal cords, ischemia, and pressure ulceration of tracheal mucosa followed by cicatricial stenosis of the upper airway within a few months. This complication occurs usually at the level of the inflated cuff and is seen after endotracheal intubation as well as after tracheostomy. The use of a soft high-compliance low-pressure cuff minimizes, but does not obviate, this complication. In addition, the endotracheal tube is a stimulus to increased tracheal and bronchial secretions which can complicate the pulmonary problems of the patient. Occlusion of endotracheal and tracheostomy tubes by secretions may occur and the situation, if not quickly recognized, may be life-threatening. Proper humidification and suctioning can prevent this complication. The endotracheal tube is an excellent portal of access for microorganisms and pulmonary infections, especially in debilitated patients. Additional serious problems can arise from an infected tracheostomy wound and mediastinal suppuration.

During tracheostomy, pneumothorax, recurrent laryngeal nerve paralysis, esophageal injury, and major vessel injury are all possible hazards. Later complications include tracheal stenosis following erroneous tracheal incision or even proper operative procedure, erosive tracheoesophageal fistula, or innominate artery erosion.

Special complications are particularly apt to occur with some of the specific, less popular, procedures mentioned above. When the esophageal obturator airway is used, bleeding and gastric distention are especially likely. With the insertion of a large needle or trocar into the trachea, perforation of the esophagus can occur due to penetration of the posterior wall of the trachea. Tearing of major blood vessels next to the trachea can lead to serious hemorrhage. High flow O_2 ventilation into a perforated vessel can result in air embolism.

Most of these complications can be prevented by anticipating their occurrence. Their treatment becomes obvious as soon as the diagnosis is made.

RESPIRATORY PHYSICAL THERAPY

Respiratory physical therapy falls into 2 major categories: (1) postural drainage with clapping and vibration, and (2) deep-breathing exercises. These specific modalities are applied by therapists, but the indications must be known to physicians who initiate them.

For postural drainage, the indications are (1) inability to raise pulmonary secretions due to weakness, paralysis, severe fatigue, or postoperative respiratory complications; (2) acute respiratory infections in those elderly who are too weak to cough effectively, in patients with neurologic diseases that compromise ability to cough, in patients with chronic airways obstruction (chronic bronchitis/emphysema), and in acute lung abscess; and (3) chronic inability to clear secretions from the lungs, e.g., in bronchiectasis, cystic fibrosis, and occasionally in patients with chronic airways obstruction without acute infections.

For deep breathing exercises, the indications are (1) before and after heart and lung surgery; the exercises should be taught preoperatively and used with vigor postoperatively in order to prevent major pulmonary complications. In upper abdominal surgery this approach may also be useful; and (2) in patients with chronic airways obstruction for whom special deep-breathing exercises have been endorsed by some as improving the patient's feeling of control over his breathing, especially in stressful situations. No proof exists that this is so. But in some patients, use of these exercises has been associated with improvement in exercise performance.

Contraindications: For postural drainage, clapping, and vibration the contraindications are (1) a recent acute myocardial infarction; (2) a recent spine injury or unstable intervertebral disc; (3) recent rib fracture(s) (although these generally preclude the procedure, some form of the technic may be used when raising secretions is a serious problem); (4) recent hemoptysis, unless the bleeding is caused by active infection associated with bronchiectasis (however, some form of postural drainage with or without clapping and vibration may be helpful to promote removal of clots from the tracheobronchial tree); and (5) severe osteoporosis.

Technic

Postural drainage is the positioning of the body so that there is drainage from a specific segment of the lungs to the main bronchi. **Clapping** is the technic used to assist secretions in flowing from the lung segment to the main bronchi so the patient can cough and expectorate more easily. Cupped hands are used with fingers held together in a relaxed position. The action comes from the wrist with alternate clapping of the hands. The force applied by clapping depends on the patient's tolerance. The patient's clothing should be removed. To avoid smarting or stinging of the skin it may be advisable to put a thin towel over the skin or the patient can wear a hospital gown. **Vibration** is done to aid in loosening tenacious secretions from the walls of the bronchi. This is performed with the hands held flat on the part being treated, and the therapist produces the vibrations with the whole arm starting at the shoulder. Treatment is given with the patient in proper postural drainage position. Clapping is done for 1 min and then vibrations are given on 5 exhalations. A patient may be asked to cough if he does not do so spontaneously.

Deep-breathing exercises are performed to increase distribution of ventilation and to prevent chest immobilization. The important factor in these exercises is prolonging expiration. The exercises are divided into segments: apical areas include the upper chest, costolateral areas include the lateral lower ribs and the diaphragm.

The therapist's hands are placed on the patient's apical area and the patient is instructed to inhale deeply through his nose expanding the upper chest only. The therapist may apply slight pressure as a stimulus. The patient is instructed to concentrate on this area only and not to use accessory neck muscles or his shoulders. He then exhales slowly through his mouth with slightly pursed lips. The therapist again may apply slight pressure on the area as to assist in exhalation. The exhalation is prolonged until the end of the breath.

The same procedure is used for costolateral areas. The lower ribs are to expand laterally and the upper chest and shoulders are not to be used. Exhalation is to be slow and prolonged to the end of the breath. For diaphragmatic breathing the patient is instructed to breathe causing the anterior lower ribs to flare out. Here, also, the therapist's hands are placed on the anterior lower ribs as if to assist in flaring the ribs on inhalation and slight pressure is given on exhalation.

These exercises are best taught with the patient sitting in front of a mirror so that he sees himself performing the exercises correctly. It is also helpful to have the patient put his hands on the specific segments giving slight pressure on inhalation and exhalation.

Complications of postural drainage, clapping, and vibration include rib fractures from too vigorous treatment or unrecognized osteoporosis or rib metastases, dizziness and syncope, exhaustion, and dyspnea. All of these except the dizziness and syncope may be prevented by careful monitoring of the patient during the procedure. When these complications occur, temporary discontinuation of treatment and simple symptomatic care will resolve the problem.

---

32. PULMONARY INSUFFICIENCY; RESPIRATORY FAILURE

Pulmonary insufficiency or some degree of respiratory failure occurs when the exchange of respiratory gases between the circulating blood and the ambient atmosphere is impaired. The terms are used synonymously though the term respiratory failure generally refers to more severe lung dysfunction. The gaseous composition of arterial blood with respect to O_2 and CO_2 pressures is normally maintained within restricted limits; pulmonary insufficiency occurs when the Pa_{O_2} is < 60 mm Hg and the Pa_{CO_2} is > 50 mm Hg, but pulmonary insufficiency or respiratory failure may be manifested by a reduced Pa_{O_2}, with a normal, low, or elevated Pa_{CO_2}.

There are 3 pathogenic categories of diseases of the respiratory apparatus: (1) those manifested mainly by airways obstruction; (2) those largely affecting the lung parenchyma but not the bronchi; and (3) those in which the lungs may be anatomically intact but the regulation of ventilation is defective because of abnormal musculoskeletal structure and function of the chest wall or primary dysfunction of the CNS respiratory center. The etiology and mechanisms of disease leading to the physiologic disturbances in each of these categories may differ, but the pattern of physiologic disturbance of lung function is quite similar. TABLE 32–1 lists the most commonly recognized chronic lung disorders in these categories. These and acute disorders (e.g., pulmonary edema, pneumonia, shock lung) which may lead to pulmonary insufficiency appear elsewhere in this volume.

Pathophysiologic Changes in Airways Obstruction

The diseases in this category induce an abnormally high resistance to airflow in the bronchial tree. The causes vary with the etiology but include secretions, bronchial mucosal edema, bronchial smooth muscle spasm, or structural weakness of bronchial wall supports. An abnormally high effort, and therefore energy expenditure, is required for ventilation to produce the necessary pressure differences between the mouth and alveoli during expiration and inspiration. The high resistance to airflow can profoundly affect the gas exchanging function of the lung in the alveoli by disturbing the distribution of ventilation to various parts of the lung with respect to regional perfusion by mixed venous blood.

The ventilation/perfusion ratio must be close to 1 for Pa_{O_2} and Pa_{CO_2} to remain normal (80 to 100 mm Hg for Pa_{O_2}; 40 ± 4 mm Hg for Pa_{CO_2}). Pa_{CO_2} is below normal if there is high alveolar ventilation for the level of perfusion; high regional perfusion with respect to ventilation reduces O_2 tension and content of pulmonary capillary blood, a more dire occurrence. The mixing of blood from such overperfused regions with blood from regions with a normal ventilation/perfusion ratio causes hypoxemia, which is determined quantitatively by the proportion and composition of blood mixing with the normally oxygenated blood. A true shunt of 50% of mixed venous blood (O_2 saturation 75%) mixing with a similar proportion of fully oxygenated blood results in an Sa_{O_2} of 87% or a Pa_{O_2} of 53 mm Hg. Hypercapnia or a high Pa_{CO_2} will not occur as long as regions of the lung are over-ventilated with respect to the regional perfusion (a high ventilation/perfusion ratio) so that CO_2 is expelled from the blood in large volumes and the regional capillary P_{CO_2} is below the normal 40 mm Hg. The net mixed Pa_{CO_2} remains normal in the presence of persistent hypoxemia. Arterial hypercapnia develops when total ventilation or regional ventilation is depressed so that regional hyperventilation sufficient to maintain the Pa_{CO_2} at normal can no longer occur. Hypercapnia may occur with exacerbations of bronchitis, pneumonia, or status asthmaticus, or suppression of total pulmonary ventilation due to pharmacologic depression of the respiratory center by such agents as codeine, morphine, barbiturates, or other sedatives.

TABLE 32–1. DISORDERS CAUSING CHRONIC PULMONARY INSUFFICIENCY:
PATHOGENIC CLASSIFICATION

1. **Airways Obstruction**
   Chronic bronchitis
   Emphysema
   Cystic fibrosis (mucoviscidosis)
   Asthma

2. **Abnormal Pulmonary Interstitium (Pulmonary Alveolitis, Interstitial Fibrosis)**
   Sarcoidosis
   Pneumoconiosis
   Progressive systemic sclerosis
   Rheumatoid lung
   Disseminated carcinoma
   Idiopathic fibrosis (Hamman-Rich syndrome)
   Drug sensitivity (hydralazine, busulfan, etc.)
   Hodgkin's disease
   Systemic lupus erythematosus
   Histiocytosis
   Radiation
   Leukemia (all cell types)

3. **Alveolar Hypoventilation Without Primary Bronchopulmonary Disease**
   Functional: Sleep, chronic exposure to CO_2, metabolic alkalosis
   Anatomic: Abnormal respiratory center (Ondine's curse), abnormal chest cage
                  (kyphoscoliosis, fibrothorax)
   Disordered neuromuscular function: Myasthenia gravis, infectious polyneuritis, muscular
                  dystrophy, poliomyelitis, polymyositis
   Obesity
   Hypothyroidism

The characteristic changes in lung volumes and ventilatory tests in intrathoracic airways obstruction are (1) reduced VC, (2) increased RV and FRC so that TLC may be normal or increased, and (3) reduced MVV, FEV_1, and airflow rates on expiration at all phases of the forced expiratory volume (see Ch. 30).

Diffuse Interstitial Fibrosis and Alveolitis

The pattern of physiologic abnormality in these diseases is strikingly different from that in airways obstruction. VC is reduced, usually with reduced RV, so that TLC is also reduced. However, tests of airways obstruction (e.g., the FEV_1 and the MVV) are usually normal. The Pa_{CO_2} is usually normal and often below normal because of hyperventilation, and is almost never elevated. The Pa_{O_2}, however, is mildly to moderately reduced at rest and more markedly reduced during exercise. The hypoxemia is caused by ventilation/perfusion imbalance and diffusion limitation by the structurally abnormal alveolar capillary membrane or by reduction in the total lung area for diffusion. Lung diffusing capacity for CO or O_2 is characteristically low at rest and during exercise.

Unlike the case in obstructive lung diseases, the major mechanical abnormality is increased lung stiffness (reduced lung compliance) with normal airway resistance. Ventilatory drive is also increased, frequently causing hyperventilation at rest and during exercise, with associated hypocapnia. The reduced lung compliance and the increased ventilatory drive and hypoxemia contribute to dyspnea, the outstanding symptom in this group of diseases.

Alveolar Hypoventilation Without Primary Bronchopulmonary Disease

Alveolar hypoventilation of this type occurs when pulmonary structure is intact but the regulatory function of ventilation in relation to whole body metabolism is disturbed. The pathognomonic manifestation of this imbalance between ventilatory and metabolic function is an elevated Pa_{CO_2} (normal = 40 ± 4 mm Hg) and a concomitantly reduced Pa_{O_2} (Pa_{O_2} falls as alveolar P_{CO_2} rises). Ventilation/perfusion imbalances are usual in addition to alveolar hypoventilation. The alveolar to arterial O_2 tension difference is therefore increased, contributing further to arterial hypoxemia. Sometimes (e.g., in central depression of the respiratory center), the elevated Pa_{CO_2} also results from a total alveolar hypoventilation; other times (e.g., in obesity and severe kyphoscoliosis), elevated Pa_{CO_2} may result from both ventilation/perfusion imbalance and reduced overall alveolar ventilation.

The pathologic basis of alveolar hypoventilation in the presence of normal lung structure (see TABLE 32–1) varies from weakness or paralysis of the ventilatory muscles (as in myasthenia gravis and infectious polyneuritis) to acquired or congenital damage to the medullary respiratory center. In most cases except obesity, lung compliance and airway resistance are unimpaired and voluntary hyperventilation usually markedly improves blood gas composition.

Consequences of Respiratory Failure

Depressed arterial and tissue O_2 tensions affect the cellular metabolism of all organs and, if severe, can cause irreversible damage in minutes. In addition, even moderate (< 60 mm Hg) alveolar hypoxia over days or weeks can induce pulmonary arteriolar vasoconstriction and increased pulmonary vascular resistance which leads to pulmonary hypertension, right ventricular hypertrophy (cor pulmonale), and eventually right ventricular failure.

Elevated arterial and tissue CO_2 tensions, however, affect mainly the CNS and the acid-base balance. Pa_{CO_2} elevations, usually > 70 mm Hg, are associated with marked cerebral vasodilation, increased CSF pressure, and changes in sensorium ranging from confusion to narcosis. Papilledema occurs at these levels of hypercapnia when they persist for many days; it is reversed on lowering of the Pa_{CO_2}.

Ventilatory responsiveness to CO_2 as a stimulus to breathing is diminished by persistent hypercapnia, largely due to the increase in blood and tissue buffers resulting from the generation of bicarbonate by the kidney in response to the elevated Pa_{CO_2}. The increased buffering capacity which also occurs in the CNS diminishes the decrease in pH which occurs with increases in plasma and tissue CO_2 levels. The contribution of pH to the ventilatory stimulus of CO_2 is therefore diminished. This can be seen in the relationship between pH, bicarbonate concentration, and Pa_{CO_2} in the Henderson-Hasselbalch equation. This effect on ventilatory responsiveness is reversed when the Pa_{CO_2} returns to normal.

Sudden rises in Pa_{CO_2} occur much faster than compensatory rises in extracellular buffer base; this causes marked acidosis (pH < 7.3), which additionally contributes to pulmonary arteriolar vasoconstriction, reduced myocardial contractility, hyperkalemia, hypotension, and cardiac irritability. This type of acidosis is rapidly reversed by increasing alveolar ventilation by mechanical hyperventilation if necessary and rapidly lowering Pa_{CO_2} to normal levels.

Therapy of Respiratory Failure

The detection of respiratory failure from any cause and its therapy depend on **analysis of arterial blood P_{O_2}, P_{CO_2}, and pH**; facilities for such analyses are essential for effective therapy.

When the Pa_{CO_2} is not elevated and only hypoxemia exists, the therapy of respiratory failure may be different than when both blood gas abnormalities are present. All available technics for reducing airways obstruction (i.e., bronchodilators, tracheal suction, moisturization, and chest physiotherapy) may be required in the treatment of respiratory failure. Ultimate recovery demands recognition of every factor leading to respiratory failure and use of therapeutic agents that can reverse these factors while the patient receives respiratory support by mechanical ventilation and high O_2 mixtures.

Oxygenation: The concentration of enriched O_2 selected to overcome hypoxemia should be the lowest concentration that will provide an acceptable Pa_{O_2}. Inspired O_2 concentrations exceeding 80% have significant toxic effects on the alveolar capillary endothelium and bronchi and should be avoided unless necessary for the patient's survival. Concentrations of inspired O_2 of $< 60\%$ are well tolerated for long periods without manifest toxicity. Most patients tolerate a $Pa_{O_2} > 55$ mm Hg quite well. However, Pa_{O_2} values in the range of 60 to 80 mm Hg are most desirable for adequate delivery of O_2 to tissues and prevention of increases in pulmonary artery pressure from alveolar hypoxia. Pa_{O_2} values between 55 and 80 mm Hg are acceptable. For pulmonary insufficiency resulting from ventilation/perfusion imbalances as associated with obstructive lung disease or with combined diffusion limitation and ventilation/perfusion imbalance, inspired O_2 concentrations of $> 40\%$ are usually *not* required. Most patients with these types of physiologic dysfunctions receive adequate oxygenation with 25 to 35% inspired O_2. Such concentrations can be given readily by face masks designed to deliver specific concentrations at the mouth, or by nasal cannulas. With face masks, the flow of O_2 required for a given percentage is predetermined by the mask design.

With nasal cannulas, the flow of O_2 can only be estimated. Such estimates require knowledge of the total minute ventilation of the patient in room air and the duration of inspiration and expiration. If the time in both phases of ventilation is equal, only half the flow of 100% O_2 from the O_2 reservoir can be assumed to be delivered to the patient. Thus, for a ventilatory rate of 10 L/min and a 4 L/min flow of 100% O_2 through nasal cannulas, the O_2 concentration delivered to the patient would be estimated at

$$\frac{(2 \times 100\%) + (8 \times 21\%)}{10 \text{ L}} = 37\% \ O_2.$$

If the minute ventilation rises and the O_2 flow is unchanged, the inspired concentration of O_2 decreases. Because of the uncertainties in such estimates (including the admixture of O_2 with room air, mouth breathing, varying respiratory rate), the actual Pa_{O_2} tension must be monitored regularly to determine the results of therapy.

When higher concentrations of O_2 must be delivered at the nose and mouth to achieve acceptable Pa_{O_2} levels (e.g., in severe pulmonary infection, shock lung, pulmonary edema), concentrations of O_2 delivered by nasal cannulas are inadequate and tight-fitting face masks capable of delivering up to 100% inspired O_2 may be necessary.

If adequate oxygenation by face mask requires continuous administration of O_2 concentrations of more than 80%, tracheal intubation and mechanical ventilation can usually provide adequate oxygenation with a lower concentration of inspired O_2, minimizing the risk of O_2 toxicity. This provides larger tidal volumes and a more favorable ventilation/perfusion ratio than does spontaneous breathing.

No matter which technic of O_2 delivery is used, the patient's comfort and bronchial clearance demand that the inspired gas be moisturized by passing it through a water trap.

Managing elevated Pa_{CO_2}: In airways obstruction or when the ventilatory apparatus or its CNS control fails, elevated blood and tissue P_{CO_2}, as well as hypoxemia, must be treated. The urgency and necessity of rapid lowering of an abnormally elevated arterial and tissue P_{CO_2} may be questioned when respiratory acidosis is compensated. Elevated Pa_{CO_2}, whatever the primary cause, indicates low alveolar ventilation with respect to body metabolism. A Pa_{CO_2} even to levels of 70 or 80 mm Hg is generally well tolerated as long as compensated by an increase in buffer base, which keeps arterial pH near normal; *the primary consideration must always be adequate oxygenation and the state of acidosis of the blood.* If supplying enriched O_2 during spontaneous ventilation leads to a continuously rising Pa_{CO_2} and acidosis, then mechanical ventilatory assistance is required to control the Pa_{CO_2}.

Mechanical ventilation: In nonacutely ill patients with respiratory failure, an IPPB apparatus can be applied by a mouthpiece and nose clip or a face mask for intermittent therapy throughout the day. This technic is not effective if respiratory failure is acute and severe. If continuous mechanical ventilatory assistance is required, the patient should have tracheal intubation through either the mouth or nose. Intubation allows easier suctioning and a wide variety of technics of mechanical ventilation to be applied as required. After the trachea is intubated, the tube may be left in place for as long as 10 to 14 days if necessary before a tracheostomy must be performed or the patient returns to spontaneous ventilation. Short-term tracheal intubation without tracheostomy may be adequate for treating acute episodes of respiratory failure due to pulmonary infection, severe left heart failure, pulmonary edema, inadvertent depression of ventilation by sedatives and analgesic agents, uncontrolled bronchospasm, pneumothorax, or combinations of the above.

Any mechanical ventilator, particularly if the driving pressure into the lung is high, may cause reduced venous return to the thorax, reduced cardiac output, and a consequent drop in systemic BP. This is particularly common when inspiratory positive pressures are high, hypovolemia is present, and vasomotor control is inadequate due to drugs, peripheral neuropathy, or muscle weakness.

There are 3 main types of mechanical ventilators for treating acute respiratory failure: (1) pressure-controlled, (2) volume-controlled, and (3) body-tank–type.

Intermittent positive pressure breathing (IPPB) apparatus: Ventilation is induced with a mechanical ventilator which delivers positive pressure during inspiration but allows the pressure in the airway to return to atmospheric pressure during the expiratory phase by spontaneous exhalation (see above). Various kinds of apparatus will introduce gas into the lungs by delivering the desired inspired mixture at a higher than atmospheric pressure through a face mask, mouthpiece, or intratracheal tube. All have similar features of control and performance. Ventilatory assistance is provided only during inspiration; expiration is passive. A slight inspiratory effort by the patient (about 1 cm H_2O negative pressure) opens a valve that initiates the flow of gas from the apparatus to the lungs. In most types of apparatus, a sensitivity control knob determines the ease with which inspiratory effort initiates inspiratory flow. Flow ceases when the pressure in the mouth or intratracheal tube reaches a positive pressure that has been preset by the pressure control on the apparatus. When inspiratory flow ceases, expiration occurs passively through an expiratory valve. The tidal volume delivered to the patient depends on the preset pressure at which the inspiratory flow ceases. In normal individuals, peak positive pressures of 15 cm H_2O usually provide tidal volumes of 800 to 1000 ml. If bronchial obstruction, obesity, stiff lungs, or thoracic deformity is present, positive pressures > 20 cm H_2O may be required to achieve normal tidal volumes. Newer devices can achieve inspiratory pressures of up to 60 cm H_2O. Such pressures may be required under circumstances of severely reduced lung compliance or increased airway resistance.

Moisture in the inspired gas or aerosol medications can be delivered by a nebulizer connected to the inspired gas flow.

Inspired gas **flow rates** of about 40 to 60 L/min are usually adequate, even in tachypneic states in which higher than normal flows are required. Excessively high flow rates may accentuate uneven distribution of inspired gas, especially in bronchial obstruction, and may result in high positive pressures in the proximal bronchi before an adequate tidal volume can be introduced. The inspiratory phase may then be unnecessarily short and the tidal volume inadequate for effective gas exchange.

In pressure-controlled ventilators, breathing frequency may be determined by allowing the patient to initiate the inspiratory effort and determine his own rate, or, when necessary, an automatic frequency control predetermines a rate and will initiate breathing automatically. The frequency control on most apparatus also allows automatic initiation of a tidal volume in a patient breathing spontaneously if a period of apnea longer than a preset duration occurs.

Volume-controlled ventilators: A preset tidal volume is delivered to the patient regardless of the pressure required to deliver the inspiratory volume. Expiration is passive. Controls vary the inspired O_2 mixture, inspiration and expiration time, and ventilatory frequency. Humidification and nebulization are provided. These ventilators are particularly useful for maintaining adequate alveolar ventilation regardless of rapid changes in the airway resistance or pulmonary compliance while the patient is being ventilated. Volume-controlled ventilators are in general selected most commonly for ventilatory support in the setting of intensive care.

Tank-type body ventilators: These can be used when ventilation is to be mechanically maintained for a prolonged period and when tracheostomy or tracheal intubation is not indicated. Such ventilators were commonly used prior to the availability of the mechanical ventilators discussed above. A new type of thoracic ventilator allows the patient to lie in a flexible plastic garment extending from the neck to the thighs with a rigid support overlying the thorax only, leaving the patient's arms free.

Positive end-expiratory pressure (PEEP): This term refers to ventilation in which a positive pressure is imposed in the airway at the end of expiration. Thus with PEEP, inspiration proceeds by imposing a positive pressure in the airway. After peak pressure and tidal volume are reached, expiration proceeds unobstructed. However, exhalation ceases at a preset expiration pressure that is set by an exhalation valve sensitive to pressure and placed in the exhalation part of the ventilator or tracheal tube. If a Pa_{O_2} of 50 to 70 mm Hg cannot be achieved with 60% inspired O_2 using positive pressure ventilatory assistance, a continuous PEEP of 3 to 15 cm H_2O may be tried to induce further expansion of the lung, improve the ventilation/perfusion ratio, and reduce shunting. Since the procedure is not innocuous and complications are directly related to the magnitude of the end-expiratory pressure, the lowest level of PEEP that achieves an adequate Pa_{O_2} should be applied. The major complications of PEEP are decreased venous return, reduced cardiac output, and pneumothorax. Application of PEEP to a severely ill patient is best done by an individual experienced with this technic.

Continuous positive airway pressure (CPAP): In this technic, during spontaneous breathing, a positive pressure is applied during the entire respiratory cycle (during inspiration and expiration). In this regard, exhalation bears some relationship to pursed-lip breathing. The technic may be applied by a head canopy that controls the ambient airway pressure with or without intubation. When the patient has an intratracheal tube, CPAP can be applied by a specially modified T piece in which a reservoir bag is placed in the expiratory line and the expiratory pressure is controlled by varying the degree of occlusion of the tailpiece of the bag. The term **continuous positive pressure breathing (CPPB)** is synonymous with CPAP and the term **continuous positive pressure ventilation (CPPV)** has been used instead of CPPB when ventilation is controlled by a mechanical ventilator rather than spontaneously.

Aerosols: When bronchospasm or bronchial edema is a factor, airway resistance can be reduced and ventilation/perfusion relationships improved by administering aerosolized bronchodilators. Such solutions may be given by a positive pressure breathing apparatus or by hand or mechanical nebulizers. Aerosolized bronchodilators are discussed in BRONCHIAL ASTHMA in Ch. 34.

Maintenance of clear airways: Clearing of secretions from upper and lower airways is crucial to treating respiratory failure. Since alveolar gas is 100% humidified at body temperature, room air or inspired gas delivered from a tank tends to dry out mucous membranes and add to the difficulty of raising secretions. The inspired stream delivered through a positive pressure breathing apparatus must be fully moisturized to ensure reduced viscosity of secretions. This can sometimes be achieved by heated nebulization, which highly moisturizes the inspiratory stream.

Physical therapy technics such as chest percussion several times/day in severely ill patients loosen secretions, allowing their removal by tracheal suction or spontaneous cough (see in Ch. 31).

Tracheal suction should be performed frequently through the mouth, nose, or tracheal tubes using sterile catheters and following other such precautions to minimize infection. In general, tracheal and lower airways suction without an intratracheal tube or tracheostomy by insertion of the suctioning catheter into the posterior pharynx is usually unsuccessful because of the difficulty of introducing the catheter past the vocal cords. Inadequate removal of secretions is an indication for tracheal intubation, which allows easy access to the upper and lower airways and minimizes the risk of aspiration of stomach contents.

---

33. ACUTE RESPIRATORY DISTRESS SYNDROME (ARDS)
(Adult Respiratory Distress Syndrome; Shock Lung; Wet Lung; Pump Lung)

Respiratory failure with life-threatening respiratory distress and hypoxemia, associated with various acute pulmonary injuries.

Etiology

This important and common medical emergency is precipitated by an acute illness or injury that directly or indirectly affects the lung, including direct chest trauma, prolonged or profound shock, fat embolism, massive blood transfusion, cardiopulmonary bypass, O_2 toxicity, sepsis, or acute hemorrhagic pancreatitis. Patients usually have not had previous lung disease. Using in-line filters to remove particulate matter from stored blood has decreased the severity of ARDS in patients undergoing massive blood transfusion or cardiopulmonary bypass.

Pathophysiology

When the pulmonary capillary endothelium and alveolar epithelium are injured, plasma and blood leak into the interstitial and intra-alveolar spaces. Alveolar atelectasis, capillary congestion, and early collagen formation may progress to acute interstitial fibrosis, resulting in decreased compliance. Surfactant activity may be low, and the functional residual capacity of the lungs is decreased. These pathologic changes lead to ventilation/perfusion maldistribution and hypoxemia.

Symptoms and Signs

Twelve to 24 h following the initial injury or illness or, more commonly, 5 to 10 days later following the onset of sepsis, convalescence is interrupted by progressive respiratory distress and failure. Dyspnea occurs initially, accompanied by tachypnea, hyperventilation, grunting expiration, and refractory hypoxemia. Intercostal and suprasternal retraction may be present on inspiration. Cyanosis is variable and may not improve with O_2 administration. Since edema is not present in the airways, auscultation often does not reveal rales, rhonchi, or wheezes. Chest x-rays show a diffuse bilateral alveolar infiltration similar to that seen in acute pulmonary edema of cardiac origin, except for the more peripheral distribution; the cardiac silhouette is usually normal. Arterial blood gas analysis shows low Pa_{O_2}, normal or low Pa_{CO_2}, and elevated pH reflecting mild to moderate respiratory alkalosis. Cardiac output is usually normal or elevated, except in patients with circulatory collapse.

Complications

Secondary bacterial invasion of the lung and persistent pulmonary sepsis, the most common complications, are associated with high morbidity and mortality. Gram-negative bacteria predominate in the lung, particularly *Klebsiella*, *Pseudomonas*, and *Proteus* spp. Pulmonary fibrosis may occur as a result of secondary infection, barotrauma, or O_2 toxicity. Antibiotics are not indicated prophylactically, but should be used to treat secondary infection as indicated by serial sputum cultures. Pneumothorax associated with the use of ventilators and positive end-expiratory pressure **(PEEP)** may occur suddenly. Prompt recognition and treatment are necessary to prevent sudden death. Pneumothorax occurring late in ARDS is an ominous sign, since it is usually associated with severe lung damage and need for high ventilatory pressures.

Diagnosis

Early diagnosis requires a high index of suspicion aroused by the onset of dyspnea following the known etiologic disorders, frequent examinations, x-rays, and serial arterial blood gas determinations. The initial finding is often a decreasing Pa_{O_2} in spite of a high inspired O_2 concentration. The characteristic symptoms, x-ray findings, and blood gas patterns confirm the diagnosis. When there is doubt about whether or not the syndrome is congestive heart failure, a Swan-Ganz catheter should be passed into the pulmonary artery. Low wedge pressures are characteristic of the lesion, high wedge pressures of congestive heart failure.

Prognosis

The survival rate is 60 to 70% with prompt early treatment; only 10 to 20% of patients survive without treatment. Patients who respond promptly to treatment have little or no residual pulmonary dysfunction or disability. Those requiring prolonged treatment, however, may develop restrictive lung disease.

Treatment

Despite different etiologies and probably different modes of pathogenesis, management principles are similar. Ventilation must be improved and the underlying cause of acute lung injury corrected.

Treatment of the underlying cause: Shock is treated aggressively to restore BP and urine output. Once vital signs have stabilized, monitoring of vascular volume is crucial. When ARDS develops, left- and right-sided heart pressures tend to disassociate due to increased resistance in the pulmonary vascular system. For this reason, if there is any question of the etiology of the problem, particularly if urinary output decreases, an index of left atrial pressures is crucial. A Swan-Ganz catheter generally is used to determine pulmonary artery wedge pressures and cardiac output. Poor skin perfusion and low urinary output ($<$ 0.5 ml/kg/h) with wedge pressure $<$ 15 mm Hg are indications for increasing fluids; pressure $>$ 15 mm Hg and poor skin perfusion are indications for cardiotonic drugs (isoproterenol 1 to 4 μg/min or dopamine 5 μg/kg/min) in an appropriate volume of IV fluid.

Sepsis should be vigorously treated with appropriate antibiotics and surgical drainage of closed-space infections. Frequent culturing of tracheal aspirates helps to detect pulmonary infection early and guide appropriate antibiotic therapy.

Treatment of the respiratory derangements: Most patients require intubation and assistance with a volume-controlled ventilator capable of delivering pressure up to 100 cm H_2O and of accurately metering the inspired O_2 concentration. Indications for tracheal intubation and positive-pressure ventilation are shown in TABLE 33–1. Large tidal volumes, 15 to 20 ml/kg, are often needed. Minute ventilation may range up to 20 to 30 L/min. PEEP is often necessary to increase the functional residual capacity of the lung and to improve oxygenation. It is usually instituted when inspired O_2 concentrations of $>$ 50% are required to maintain Pa_{O_2}. End-expiratory pressures of 5 to 10 cm of water are usually adequate, but 15 cm is occasionally required. PEEP may depress cardiac output and should be used cautiously in hypovolemic patients; correction of hypovolemia may allow safe

TABLE 33-1. INDICATIONS FOR CONTINUOUS MECHANICAL VENTILATION

Pulmonary (Parenchymal) Failure	Ventilatory Failure
Alveolar-arterial O_2 gradient $(A-a\Delta O_2) > 300$ torr $(FIO_2 = 1)$	Respiratory rate > 35 to 40/min
Right-to-left shunt fraction $(\dot{Q}_s/\dot{Q}_T) > 15$ to 20%	Inadequate alveolar ventilation with $Pa_{CO_2} > 48$ torr
Wasted ventilation $(V_D/V_T) > 0.6$	Vital capacity < 10 to 15 ml/kg
Compliance < 30 ml/cm H_2O	Maximal inspiratory force poorer than -25 cm H_2O

and effective use of PEEP. PEEP and positive-pressure ventilation may be discontinued when the criteria for ventilation shown in TABLE 33-1 have reversed. At this point, intermittent mandatory ventilation (IMV) should be introduced, with the patient taking 25%, then 50%, then 75% of his own breaths independent of the ventilator. This type of weaning should be initiated as early in the course of management as stability of the patient's condition permits. Finally, a "T" piece should be tried with the endotracheal tube in place and the patient allowed to breathe humidified O_2 spontaneously. If this is well tolerated, as confirmed by the above pulmonary function assessment for 3 to 4 h, the endotracheal tube can be removed. Fluid balance requires rigid monitoring. O_2 concentrations of $>$ 50% for 24 to 48 h may lead to O_2 toxicity and accentuation of the pulmonary injury.

See Ch. 32 for further discussion of pathophysiologic respiratory changes in respiratory failure and their management.

---

34. AIRWAYS OBSTRUCTION

BRONCHIAL ASTHMA

Reversible airways obstruction not due to any other disease.

Etiology

Bronchial asthma can occur secondarily to a variety of stimuli. Although the underlying mechanisms responsible for attacks of paroxysmal wheezing are unknown, inherited or acquired imbalance of adrenergic and cholinergic control of airway diameter has been implicated (see Pathophysiology and Pathology, below). Persons manifesting such imbalance have been shown to have hyperreactive bronchi. Moreover, in these individuals, bronchoconstriction may persist at subclinical levels even when they are asymptomatic. When individuals with hyperreactive bronchial trees are subjected to stresses of different kinds, overt asthma attacks may occur. Among the known stresses are viral respiratory infection, exercise, emotional upset, nonspecific factors (e.g., changes in barometric pressure or temperature), inhalation of cold air or such irritants as gasoline fumes, fresh paint and other noxious odors, or cigarette smoke, and exposure to specific allergens. Psychologic factors may aggravate an asthmatic attack but are not assigned a primary etiologic role.

Persons whose asthma is precipitated by allergenic exposure (most commonly airborne pollens and molds, house dust, animal danders), and whose symptoms are IgE-mediated, are said to have allergic or "extrinsic asthma." They account for only about 10 to 20% of the adult asthmatic population. In perhaps 30 to 50% of adult asthmatics, symptomatic episodes appear to be triggered by nonallergenic factors (infection, irritants, emotional factors). These patients are said to have nonallergic or "intrinsic asthma." In many individuals, both allergenic and nonallergenic factors appear to play significant triggering roles. Allergy is said to be more important in the etiology of asthma in infants and children than in adults, but the evidence is not entirely conclusive.

Pathophysiology and Pathology

Asthmatic attacks are characterized by narrowing of the large and small airways due to spasm of bronchial smooth muscle, edema and inflammation in the bronchial mucosal wall, and the production of tenacious mucus. Some areas of the lungs are hypoventilated due to the airways obstruction. Continued blood flow to underventilated areas of lung leads to a ventilation/perfusion imbalance resulting in hypoxia with little change in arterial pH or Pa_{CO_2}. Arterial hypoxemia is almost always present in attacks that are severe enough to require medical attention. Hyperventilation occurs early in the attack and results in a decrease in Pa_{CO_2}. With further progression of the attack, the patient's capacity to compensate by hyperventilation of unobstructed areas of the lung is further impaired by more extensive airway narrowing and muscular fatigue. Arterial hypoxemia worsens and Pa_{CO_2} begins to rise, leading to respiratory acidosis. At this stage, the patient is said to be in respiratory failure.

Early in the acute attack, there may be just a modest decrease in the maximum mid-expiratory flow (MMF). As the attack progresses, the forced vital capacity (FVC) and the volume expired during the first second of the FVC (FEV₁) progressively decrease and there is associated air trapping and increased residual volumes, resulting in hyperinflation of the lungs. Abnormalities in flow rates have been shown to persist for weeks to months after an acute attack despite otherwise normal pulmonary function tests.

The mechanisms underlying the bronchoconstriction described above are not well defined. However, an imbalance between β-adrenergic and cholinergic control of airway diameter has been proposed, based on some of the following facts. (1) Increased cholinergic responsiveness is suggested by the facts that most asthmatics respond excessively with bronchoconstriction after inhalation of cholinergic agents (e.g., methacholine) and that much irritant-induced bronchoconstriction can be partially blocked by atropine and its derivatives. (2) There is biochemical evidence of decreased β-adrenergic receptor responsiveness in many asthmatics. Recent studies have shown decreased numbers of β receptors in peripheral leukocytes of asthmatics compared to controls. The role that treatment with adrenergic drugs may play in the pathogenesis of these findings is still unclear. (3) In known asthmatics, an attack may be provoked by administration of the β-adrenergic blocking agent, propranolol.

The observed abnormalities in adrenergic and cholinergic functions in asthma appear to be controlled by the cyclic 3',5'-adenosine monophosphate (cyclic AMP [cAMP])—cyclic 3',5'-guanosine monophosphate (cyclic GMP) systems within various tissues, such as mast cells, smooth muscle, and mucus-secreting cells. The intracellular concentration of cAMP is a principal determinant of both smooth muscle relaxation and inhibition of IgE-induced release of several chemical mediators, such as (1) histamine, which causes bronchoconstriction (either directly or by cholinergic reflex action) and increases exocrine secretion; (2) slow-reacting substance of anaphylaxis (SRS-A), which has a slower onset of action and causes more prolonged bronchoconstriction; and (3) a low mol wt substance known as eosinophil chemotactic factor of anaphylaxis (ECF-A). Prostaglandins of the E series and drugs which stimulate β-adrenergic receptors lead to formation of intracellular cAMP and thus inhibit bronchoconstrictive mediator release and cause smooth muscle relaxation. By inhibiting cAMP phosphodiesterase (which hydrolyzes cAMP), methylxanthines such as theophylline permit intracellular cAMP to accumulate, thus decreasing both mediator release and smooth muscle tension. Cholinergic stimulation facilitates mediator release associated with increases in intracellular cyclic GMP.

The mechanisms described above appear to be sufficient to explain at least some of the pathophysiologic aberrations that occur in asthma. Although the relative importance of each mediator and the degree of autonomic imbalance cannot be defined in an individual asthmatic, it is important to understand these concepts since most of the drugs used in the therapy of asthma have profound effects on the cyclic nucleotide systems.

Pathologic findings in the airways of patients who have died of status asthmaticus have shown the presence of secretions, frequently in the form of extensive mucus plugs obstructing both large and small airways. The bronchial walls themselves show mucosal edema, thickening of the muscularis layer and basement membrane, and infiltration with eosinophils; mast cells are decreased.

Symptoms and Signs

Individuals with asthma differ greatly in the frequency and degree of their symptoms. Some have only an occasional symptomatic episode, mild in degree and of brief duration, and otherwise are entirely free of symptoms. Others have mild coughing and wheezing much of the time, punctuated by severe exacerbations of symptoms following exposure to known allergens, viral infections, exercise, or nonspecific irritants. Psychosocial stress alone may precipitate an attack or may be additive with these noxious exposures.

An asthma attack may begin acutely with paroxysms of wheezing, coughing, and shortness of breath, or insidiously with slowly increasing symptoms and signs of respiratory distress. In either case, the patient usually first notices the onset of dyspnea, tachypnea, cough, and tightness or pressure in the chest, and may even notice audible wheezes. All of this may subside quickly or persist for hours to days. Pulmonary function abnormalities (see under Diagnostic Tests, below), may persist for weeks to months after an acute attack, even in asymptomatic patients.

The cough during an acute attack sounds "tight" and is generally nonproductive of mucus. Except in young children, who rarely expectorate, tenacious mucoid sputum is produced as the attack subsides.

On physical examination during the acute asthmatic attack, the patient exhibits varying degrees of respiratory distress depending on the severity and duration of the episode. Tachypnea, anxiety, and audible wheezes are frequently present. Tachycardia and elevation of systolic BP are also common and are related to the primary disease, the effects of recent therapy, or both. Variable degrees of dehydration may be present in a patient with more prolonged episodes because of sweating and increased insensible water loss from the lungs secondary to tachypnea. The patient prefers to sit upright or even leans forward. Accessory muscles of respiration are used and the patient may appear to be struggling for air. Examination of the chest shows a prolonged expiratory phase with relatively high-pitched wheezes throughout most of expiration and through inspiration. The chest may appear to be quite hyperinflated due to air trapping. Although wheezes may be accompanied by coarse rhonchi, fine "wet" rales are not heard unless pneumonia, atelectasis, or cardiac decompensation is also present.

In more severe episodes, the patient may not be able to speak more than a few words at a time without having to stop for breath. Fatigue and severe distress are evident in the rapid, shallow, ineffectual respiratory movements. Cyanosis becomes evident as the attack worsens. Confusion and lethargy may indicate the onset of progressive respiratory failure with CO_2 narcosis. In such individuals, it is not unusual to hear *less* wheezing on auscultation. The chest may sound quiet because the combination of extensive mucous plugging of airways and patient fatigue has resulted in marked reduction of air flow and gas exchange. In an asthmatic with a quiet-sounding chest, an inexperienced examiner may incorrectly attribute the anxiety and respiratory distress to emotional factors or underestimate the severity of obstruction. Such a patient may actually have a more severe problem than a patient with audible wheezes. Extensive small airways obstruction may be present with few auscultatory findings.

Thus, the presence, absence, or prominence of wheezes does not correlate precisely with the severity of an asthma attack. The most reliable signs indicating a severe asthma attack include assessment of the degree of dyspnea at rest, difficulty in talking, pulsus paradoxus of > 20 to 30 mm, and the use of accessory muscles of respiration. The severity of an attack can be most precisely assessed by blood gas determinations.

Between acute attacks, physical examination may be normal during quiet respiration. However, sonorous or sibilant rales or fine wheezes may be heard during forced expiration or after the patient exercises. Low-grade to moderate wheezing may be heard at any time in some patients, even when the patient claims to be completely asymptomatic. With longstanding severe asthma, especially if dating from childhood, there may be evidence of secondary effects of chronic hyperinflation on the chest wall, such as a "squared off" thorax, anterior bowing of the sternum, and a depressed diaphragm.

Diagnostic Tests

Examination of the blood and the sputum of a patient with asthma commonly shows eosinophilia regardless of whether allergic factors can be shown to have an etiologic role in the disease. Blood eosinophilia > 250 to 400 cells/cu mm is the rule; in many asthmatics, the degree of the eosinophilia may correlate with the severity of the asthma. The extent to which blood eosinophilia can be suppressed with corticosteroids (as measured by total eosinophil counts) has been used as an index of the therapeutic efficacy of these agents.

The sputum in a patient with uncomplicated asthma is highly distinctive. Grossly, it is tenacious, rubbery, and whitish. In the presence of infection, particularly in adults, the sputum may be yellowish. Many eosinophils are found microscopically, frequently arranged in sheets; large numbers of histiocytes and polymorphonuclear leukocytes are also present. Eosinophilic granules from disrupted cells may be seen throughout the sputum smear. Elongated dipyramidal crystals **(Charcot-Leyden)** originating from eosinophils are commonly found. When infection is present, and particularly when there is a bronchitic element, polymorphonuclear leukocytes and bacteria predominate. In uncomplicated asthma, sputum cultures rarely reveal pathogenic bacteria.

Chest x-ray findings vary from normal to hyperinflation. Lung markings are commonly increased, particularly in chronic cases. Atelectasis, most often involving the right middle lobe, is common in children and may be a recurrent problem. Small segmental areas of atelectasis are frequently observed during acute exacerbations of asthma and may be misinterpreted as pneumonitis. The rapidity with which these areas clear, however, suggests atelectasis rather than pneumonitis. An esophogram should be considered part of the evaluation of an infant or young child with suspected asthma in order to rule out congenital anomalies, which might cause symptoms and signs of airways obstruction. Inspiratory and expiratory chest x-rays are helpful in diagnosing foreign-body aspiration as a cause of wheezing in children.

Pulmonary function tests are valuable not only in differential diagnosis, but also in known asthmatics for assessing the degree of airways obstruction and disturbance in gas exchange, for measuring the airway response to inhaled allergens and chemicals such as histamine and methacholine (bronchial provocation testing), for quantifying the response to therapeutic agents, and for long-term follow-up. Pulmonary function testing is most valuable diagnostically when performed before and after administering an aerosolized bronchodilator to determine the degree of reversibility of the airways obstruction.

Static lung volumes and capacities reveal various combinations of abnormalities; no abnormalities may be detected in mild cases in remission, however. Of the tests most often used clinically, total lung capacity **(TLC)**, functional residual capacity **(FRC)**, and residual volume **(RV)** are usually increased. Vital capacity may be normal or decreased.

Dynamic lung volumes and capacities provide an index of airways obstruction. They are reduced in asthmatics and return towards normal following administration of an aerosolized bronchodilator. In mild asthmatics during asymptomatic periods, tests of dynamic lung function may be within normal limits. Since expiratory flow is determined not only by the diameter of the airways but also by the elastic recoil forces of the lung, flow at high lung volumes will exceed flow at low lung volumes. Tests that measure flow at relatively large lung volumes (forced expiratory volume in 0.5 second [$FEV_{0.5}$], peak expiratory flow **[PEF]**, and flow between 200 and 1200 ml **[MEFR]**) are, to a considerable degree, effort-dependent and are less satisfactory than tests that measure flow over a larger range of lung volume. These include FEV_1 and the MMF, also known as the forced mid-expiratory flow **($FEF_{25\ to\ 75\%}$)** which measures flow between 25 and 75% of the FVC. The MMF is of particular value since it is considered to reflect small airways obstruction. Expiratory flow measurements at large lung volumes are insensitive to changes in peripheral airways resistance and reflect abnormalities principally in central airways. The expiratory flow-volume curve, in which expired lung volume is plotted against flow rate, is probably of greatest value. This flow-volume curve gives a clear, graphic picture of flow at large and small lung volumes and presumably, therefore, reveals abnormalities in both central and peripheral airways.

Because of airways obstruction, distribution of ventilation is frequently abnormal in patients with asthma; i.e., various lung units fill and empty asynchronously. Maldistribution of ventilation is quantified by the single-breath N test **(SBN_2)** and the 7-min N washout test. Closing volume (CV) is another test for detection of small airways disease; it is increased in asthmatics. Measurements of lung elasticity (lung compliance) in asthmatics, using an esophageal balloon to estimate pleural pressure, have shown a loss of elastic recoil, which is often reversible upon remission of the disease. Diffusing capacity for CO **(DL_{CO})** is generally normal in asthma; it is low in emphysema (in which there is loss of a functioning alveolar capillary bed with increased lung volume).

Other diagnostic tests: Allergy skin tests help identify environmental allergens which may play an etiologic role. Skin tests are customarily done to detect IgE antibody to inhalants (pollens, molds, epidermals, house dust) and other allergens (e.g., food) suggested by the patient's history. Specific IgE antibody to inhalants may also be detected by a **radioallergosorbent test (RAST)** on the patient's serum, but this test offers little advantage over properly done and interpreted skin tests. Measurement of total IgE may be useful in establishing the atopic constitution of the patient. **Inhalational bronchial challenge testing** has been used (a) with allergens to establish the clinical significance of positive skin tests, (b) with methacholine or histamine to assess the degree of airway hyperactivity in known asthmatics, or as a tool in establishing the diagnosis of asthma in instances where the symptoms are atypical. **Exercise testing** using a treadmill or bicycle ergometer has been used, particularly in childhood, to confirm the diagnosis of asthma in equivocal cases.

Determination of **arterial blood gases and pH** is essential to the adequate evaluation of a patient with symptomatic asthma. (See TABLE 34–1 and Ch. 32.)

Diagnosis and Staging

The diagnosis of asthma should be considered in any individual who wheezes. Asthma is the most likely diagnosis when typical paroxysmal wheezing starts in childhood or early adulthood and is interspersed with asymptomatic intervals. A family history of allergy or asthma can be elicited in more than half of asthmatics. Difficulties in diagnosis occur with the initial presentation of asthma, partic-

TABLE 34–1. STAGING OF THE SEVERITY OF AN ACUTE ASTHMA ATTACK

Stage	Symptoms and Signs	FEV_1 or FVC	pH	Pa_{O_2}	Pa_{CO_2}
I (mild)	Mild dyspnea; diffuse wheezes; adequate air exchange	50–80% of normal	N* or ↑	occasionally N or most often ↓	N or ↓
II (moderate)	Respiratory distress at rest; hyperpnea; marked wheezes; air exchange N or ↓	50% of normal	generally ↑	↓	generally ↓
III (severe)	Marked respiratory distress; marked wheezes or absent breath sounds; check for pulsus paradoxus > 10mm; sternocleidomastoid retraction	25% of normal	N or ↓	↓	N or ↑
IV (respiratory failure)	Severe respiratory distress; lethargy; confusion; prominent pulsus paradoxus; sternocleidomastoid retraction	10% of normal	↓↓	↓	↑↑

* N = normal.

ularly in individuals over age 50, or when atypical symptoms (e.g., cough without audible wheezing), physical findings, or x-rays are noted. It is necessary to consider and rule out other conditions in which wheezing is prominent.

Children with congenital malformations of the vascular system (vascular rings and slings) and of the GI and respiratory tracts (tracheoesophageal fistula) may present with wheezing. The presence of other congenital malformations, special attention to cases in which symptoms begin before age 1 yr, x-ray studies, and a high index of suspicion will lead to a diagnosis of congenital malformation as a cause of wheezing.

Foreign-body obstruction must be considered, particularly in children with unilateral wheezing or sudden onset of wheezing with no prior history of respiratory symptoms. Opaque foreign bodies are readily visible on x-ray. Nonopaque foreign bodies are more of a problem, but the diagnosis can be established by a history of sudden onset of cough and wheezing in a previously well child, combined with asymmetric diaphragmatic movement on inspiratory and expiratory chest x-rays.

Viral infections of the upper respiratory tract involving the epiglottis, glottis, and subglottis generally cause signs and symptoms of croup (inspiratory stridor, high-pitched cough, and hoarseness) that are distinct from the lower airways signs and symptoms of asthma. When epiglottitis is suspected, direct examination of the epiglottis should be performed with great care and with the capability for immediate intubation if acute airways obstruction develops during the examination. Primary bacterial infection of the lower airways, in the absence of underlying predisposing disease, is rare in infants and children. On the other hand, viral agents, particularly respiratory syncytial virus, can cause bronchiolitis with a clinical picture virtually indistinguishable from asthma during the first 2 yr of life. It is rare for an infant or young child to have > 1 to 2 episodes of infectious bronchiolitis; a history of recurrent episodes of obstructive airways disease should strongly suggest the diagnosis of asthma regardless of age. Chronic bronchitis as a primary diagnosis is rare in children and underlying disorders such as cystic fibrosis and immunologic deficiency disease should always be considered. These may be ruled out by a careful history, sweat test, and by in vivo and in vitro evaluation of immunologic competence.

In **adults,** symptoms and signs of airway obstruction due to upper airway involvement may be clarified by determination of a flow-volume curve. Chronic obstructive pulmonary disease and congestive heart failure are the main considerations in the differential diagnosis of wheezing, although multiple small pulmonary emboli frequently present with wheezing. Patients with hypersensitivity pneumonitis have a superficial clinical resemblance to asthmatics but generally have more constitutional symptoms after exposure to the offending substance and typically do not wheeze, except in allergic bronchopulmonary aspergillosis, discussed below. Patients with bronchial obstructions secondary to malignancy, aortic aneurysm, endobronchial tuberculosis, or sarcoidosis may occasionally present with wheezing.

Patients with allergic bronchopulmonary aspergillosis (see also ASPERGILLOSIS in Ch. 9) may present with typical asthmatic symptoms. The diagnosis of aspergillosis is confirmed by the finding of high peripheral blood eosinophilia, immediate skin test reactivity to *Aspergillus* antigen, precipitating antibodies against *Aspergillus* antigen, increased serum IgE concentrations (which appear to fluctuate with the activity of the disease), pulmonary infiltrates (transient or fixed), and a peculiar central type of bronchiectasis.

Other rare disorders in which signs and symptoms of asthma may be present include carcinoid syndrome, polyarteritis, and eosinophilic pneumonias (including tropical eosinophilia and other parasitic infestations that involve the lung during some phase of the disease). In all of these, the history is usually sufficiently atypical for asthma to suggest that another disorder is responsible for the airways obstruction.

Physical examination should stress a vigorous search for cardiac failure and the signs of chronic hypoxemia (clubbing of the fingers or pulmonary osteoarthropathy). Nasal polyposis should suggest aspirin intolerance. Unilateral wheezing should provoke a search for obstruction secondary to a foreign body, vascular malformation, aneurysm, or tumor. Listen for inspiratory wheeze over upper airway in tracheal obstruction.

Staging of the severity of the asthma attack is critical after the diagnosis is established. This is best accomplished by a combination of bedside evaluation of respiratory distress and monitoring of arterial blood gases, and bedside pulmonary function tests. TABLE 34–1 illustrates one method of staging asthma.

Assessment of etiologic factors is more difficult. Nonspecific irritant factors and evidence of infection (most often viral) should be carefully evaluated. Exacerbations related to environmental allergen exposures, history of rhinitis, or family history of atopic disorders suggests the strong likelihood of extrinsic allergic factors. Confirmation is best accomplished by an allergy evaluation that includes skin testing with allergy extracts (bronchodilators containing adrenergic agents should be discontinued for 12 h and antihistamines for 48 h, but corticosteroids may be continued in doses of up to 40 to 60 mg prednisone/day without interfering with the immediate skin test response). Negative skin test responses to a suitable battery of appropriate allergens strongly rule against an allergic component. However, positive skin tests indicate only the presence of a particular class (IgE) of antibodies and represent the potential for allergic reactivity to the allergens in question. Whether such potential sensitivities are clinically significant can be determined only when the results of the skin tests are correlated with the pattern of symptoms and are related to environmental exposures.

Complications

Pneumothorax may occur during an acute attack of asthma. It presents as a sudden worsening of the patient's respiratory distress, accompanied by sharp chest pains and, on physical examination, a shift of the mediastinum. X-ray examination confirms the diagnosis. **Mediastinal and subcutaneous emphysema** due to alveolar rupture and dissection of air along vessels is occasionally observed during an asthmatic attack. **Atelectasis,** usually involving the right middle lobe or even an entire lung, is more common. Unless the collapse involves a substantial amount of lung tissue, the atelectasis is usually only diagnosed as a result of x-ray examination. **Bronchiectasis** apparently was a complication of asthma in the preantibiotic days, but is now rare. While electrocardiographic evidence of acute **cor pulmonale** can occasionally be obtained during a severe episode of asthma, chronic cor pulmonale secondary to asthma is rare. Contrary to popular opinion, uncomplicated asthma rarely leads to chronic obstructive emphysema, especially in a nonsmoker.

General Principles of Treatment

The clinical approach to an asthmatic patient begins with the identification and control of exacerbating environmental or other factors. Drug therapy, as outlined below, is an important therapeutic modality and enables most patients to lead relatively normal lives with few adverse drug effects.

The detailed drug treatment approach described below is only one of a number that may be tried, but several general principles are important regardless of the exact drug or agent used. (1) Staging of the severity of the attack (see above) is highly important, especially if the attack has been prolonged (> 12 h) or if the patient is not well known to the examiner. (2) An orderly progression in the use of bronchodilator agents should be used, with the patient under close observation during initial therapeutic approaches. Treatment sufficient to alleviate acute respiratory distress but without maintenance follow-up treatment often results in a return of acute symptoms within the next 24 h. (3) Although some asthmatics may exhibit temporary benefit from inhalation of nebulized bronchodilators, many are unable to inhale the aerosol effectively and require IV and/or subcutaneous bronchodilator administration.

Rationale of Drug Therapy

There are 4 classes of drugs useful in the treatment of asthma. The first class is the β-**adrenergic agents,** including epinephrine, isoproterenol, ephedrine, and some more selective β_2-adrenergic agents (relatively more bronchodilatory β_2 effect and less cardiostimulatory β_1 effect). The most commonly used β_2-adrenergic agents include metaproterenol (orciprenaline), terbutaline, isoetharine, and salbutamol. The latter is not yet available in the USA. All of these agents cause bronchial smooth muscle relaxation and modulation of inhibition of mediator release, at least in part by stimulating the adenylate cyclase-cAMP system.

The second class of drugs includes **theophylline and its derivatives** (e.g., dihydroxypropyltheophylline). These cause bronchial smooth muscle relaxation and modulation of mediator release by inhibiting cAMP degradation by the enzyme phosphodiesterase (see Pathophysiology and Pathology, above). Theophylline appears to have an effect on calcium channels in cell membranes and part of its beneficial effect may be related to this property.

The third group of drugs is the **corticosteroids.** Their multiple mechanisms of action are not well understood. In addition to reducing edema and inflammation, very recent studies have shown that hydrocortisone is a very potent stimulus of B_2 receptor synthesis in several tissues.

Finally, **cromolyn sodium** (disodium cromoglycate—**DSCG**) represents a relatively new class of agents which appear to inhibit mediator release directly and independently of the cAMP system. The drug is used to prevent attacks.

In general, the adrenergic agents epinephrine and isoproterenol are most useful for treating the acute attack. Theophylline is a valuable adjunct to adrenergic drugs in the management of acute episodes; many, particularly in the USA, consider it to be the drug of choice for long-term continuous therapy. Because of their potentially dangerous long-term side effects, corticosteroids, while exceptionally effective, are withheld except for short-term use until all other treatments have failed. DSCG is primarily useful in children and some adults *for maintenance therapy only and has no place in treatment of the acute attack.* Opinions differ on the role of DSCG in treatment of chronic asthma. Some physicians believe it to be a first-line drug, while others prefer to use adrenergics and theophylline before turning to DSCG. Cost and problems with patient compliance appear to have limited the use of this drug in the USA.

Treatment of the Acute Attack

Drug therapy: Patients with acute asthma presenting in Stage I or II (see Table 34–1) without signs of severe distress may be effectively treated with epinephrine 1:1000 s.c. (0.05 to 0.2 ml in children; 0.3 to 0.5 ml in adults), repeated in 20 to 30 min if indicated. Alternatively, an aerosolized bronchodilator such as 5 drops of isoproterenol 1:200 or 10 drops of isoetharine 1% solution or salbutamol in 2 ml of water or saline may be tried, using compressed air for nebulization. If there is no response after two epinephrine injections, or if the attack worsens after the first injection, aminophylline should be given IV.

Different schedules for administration of aminophylline have been proposed with the understanding that individual patients may exhibit varying susceptibility to the beneficial or adverse effects of this drug. Monitoring blood theophylline levels so that levels of 10 to 20 μg/ml are achieved affords the most effective use of this drug. Most start with a loading dose of 6 mg/kg aminophylline (25 mg/ml, diluted 1:1 with IV fluids) for children or adults given over about 20 min through a pediatric soluset in the IV line. After the loading dose, about 6 mg/kg both in children and adults, a continuous infusion of 0.45 mg/kg/h in adults and 1.0 mg/kg/h in children < 12 yr of age is begun. When such continuous infusions of aminophylline are given, serum concentrations should be checked at least at 12-h intervals and appropriate adjustments made to maintain serum concentrations in the 10- to 20-μg/ml range. Should it not be possible for technical reasons to use the continuous infusion method, then the former practice of administering aminophylline IV in a dose of 4 to 6 mg/kg q 6 h is an acceptable but less desirable alternative. Arterial blood gases should be obtained whenever possible, but especially if there is no sign of prompt response (within about 30 min), if the patient is in severe distress or his condition is worsening, or if there is uncertainty as to what stage the patient is in.

With any patient presenting in Stage III, an arterial blood gas determination should be immediately obtained and aminophylline started IV. For a patient in severe distress, continuous infusion doses may be raised to no greater than 1 mg/kg/h in adults and 1.25 mg/kg/h in children. Monitoring of serum theophylline concentrations is essential to prevent theophylline toxicity. Greater caution should be exercised and lower (by 1/3 to 1/2) dosages should be used in patients who have congestive heart failure or liver disease or who are elderly.

Patients who present in Stage III and who show no improvement or whose signs and symptoms progress despite one dose of aminophylline should be started on IV corticosteroids. Criteria for hospitalization vary, but definite indications are failure to improve or relapse after 2 doses of aminophylline, and significant decrease in Pa_{O_2} (Pa_{O_2} < 50 mm) or increase in Pa_{CO_2} (Pa_{CO_2} > 50 mm), indicating progression to respiratory failure. Far too many patients with severe asthma attacks are sent home from hospital emergency rooms.

Any patient presenting in Stage IV or who reaches Stage IV should be immediately given hydrocortisone sodium succinate 4 mg/kg IV q 2 to 4 h or methylprednisolone 2 to 4 mg/kg IV q 4 h. IV corticosteroids in these doses (or double the maintenance dose, whichever is greater) are also indicated immediately for any acute asthmatic attack if the patient has been taking maintenance corticosteroids any time within the past 6 wk.

Patients in Stage IV who show no favorable response to aminophylline and who show evidence of fatigue and progressive deterioration in blood gases and pH should be considered candidates for endotracheal intubation and respiratory assistance. (See Ch. 32.) Such patients should be hospitalized in an intensive care unit.

Children in Stage III or IV have been given isoproterenol 0.08 to 2.7 μg/kg/min by continuous IV infusion with a Harvard pump. This procedure requires ECG and arterial blood gas monitoring in an intensive care unit (ICU) and supervision by clinicians experienced in ICU monitoring of asthmatic children. Because of arrhythmias, trials have not been successful in adults.

Once IV aminophylline and corticosteroids have been initiated in a hospitalized patient, they should be continued by this route until the patient's condition has stabilized and there is no danger of progression to respiratory failure. Drugs administered orally to a dehydrated, possibly nauseated patient may be erratically delivered to affected tissues. Nebulized bronchodilators may not be effective in a patient in acute respiratory distress because of the severity of the airways obstruction. However, in some patients, aerosolized bronchodilators (e.g., 5 drops of isoproterenol or 10 drops of isoetharine in 2 ml of saline or water) are very effective and may be given q 1 to 2 h as necessary. O_2, rather than room air, should be used as the aerosolizing gas. Antihistamines do not help and *may be harmful*. Sedatives and cough suppressants are **contraindicated** at this time.

Anxiety: Patients with respiratory distress may be extremely anxious because of hypoxia and the feeling of asphyxiation. Treatment of the underlying respiratory problems, including judicious use of O_2 therapy (see below), is the preferred approach to this problem, especially when conducted by calm, attentive, and supportive medical personnel.

Fluid and electrolyte therapy is required in the treatment of patients with status asthmaticus, especially when the episode lasts > 12 h, since these patients are usually dehydrated. Fluid therapy includes replacement of previous and current losses, not with any single arbitrary amount/24 h, but by constant infusion of fluid in amounts sufficient to result in a urine output adequate for the patient's age. Overhydration may cause pulmonary edema. In addition, humidification of inhaled air or gases may reduce excess respiratory tract loss, especially in hot or dry environments.

In a patient with a severe asthma attack with hypercapnea, respiratory acidosis may supervene. With progressive severity and duration of the episode, the arterial pH may drop alarmingly to ranges of pH 7 to 7.1. Most adults are intubated at this stage and started on assisted ventilation. It should be emphasized that the acidosis is mainly a reflection of a respiratory mechanical problem and treatment should be primarily directed toward alleviating this problem. Use of alkaline solutions in the IV fluid should be limited to maintaining the pH above 7.2, if feasible, since there is evidence of epinephrine resistance with acidosis. However, in administering alkaline solution, such as sodium bicarbonate, one should not attempt to convert pH levels to normal ranges because of the danger of inducing alkalosis, particularly as the asthma responds to therapy and increasing amounts of CO_2 are blown off by the lungs. This alkalosis is compensated for only slowly by renal mechanisms and, therefore, may persist for hours. Sodium bicarbonate should be given cautiously by drip infusion in doses of 20 to 40 mEq and there should be periodic arterial blood gas and pH monitoring so that no further alkali is given when pH levels reach > 7.3.

Potassium shifts occur with changes in arterial and tissue pH and fluid turnover in a dehydrated patient and may require that supplemental potassium be added to the infusion. In addition, the high doses of hydrocortisone given during therapy promote urinary potassium loss. This does not occur with methylprednisolone.

O_2 **therapy** is always indicated for severe asthmatics who require hospitalization since they are invariably hypoxemic. The inspired O_2 concentration **(FI_{O_2})** is guided by blood gas determinations; Pa_{O_2} should be maintained above 60 mm, preferably in the 70 to 90 mm range if possible. O_2 administration should be preceded by arterial blood gas determination. O_2 may be given effectively with a Venturi mask. In the occasional patient who will not tolerate any mask because of a "smothering" sensation, use of nasal prongs with low O_2 flow (2 to 4 L/min) may achieve the same result. Since O_2 may be very drying to the respiratory mucosa, it should always be humidified in the gas line.

Respiratory tract infections may play a major role in exacerbations of asthma attacks. These infections are predominantly viral; bacterial infections rarely play a significant role, especially in children. However, if the patient expectorates yellowish, green, or brown sputum, and Wright's stain of the sputum shows a predominance of polymorphonuclear leukocytes, antibacterial therapy is given empirically during an exacerbation. This is especially appropriate in adults with a known tendency to have chronic or recurrent bronchitis. In children, in whom most infections are viral, antibiotics are seldom needed. Antibiotic choice should be based on bacteriologic findings, but penicillin is usually most useful. If the patient is allergic to penicillin, erythromycin or tetracycline (the latter should not be given to young children) may be given. Gram stain of the sputum, noting intracellular bacteria, and chest x-rays are useful guides to therapy.

Chest x-ray is mandatory in all hospitalized asthmatic patients. Spontaneous pneumothorax and subcutaneous and mediastinal emphysema are complications of acute asthma, particularly in children. A large pneumothorax requires immediate treatment. Mediastinal and subcutaneous emphysema rarely cause difficulty, even when large. Rarely, compression of the glottis may occur with extreme extravasation of air into the soft tissues of the neck.

Treatment of Other Than the Acute Attack

Following an acute asthma attack, therapy should include oral medication for 2 to 4 wk even if the patient is asymptomatic. This is because pulmonary function abnormalities (particularly hypoxemia) may persist for at least this long. Several types of treatment are described below with the understanding that more than one approach may be used.

Cromolyn sodium, 1 capsule (20 mg) q 6 h via an inhaler, is most useful in children; its use may avoid the need to introduce corticosteroids or may enable a reduction in their maintenance dosage. While some physicians use cromolyn as a first-line maintenance drug for treatment of chronic asthma, in the USA it is often used in patients who do not respond satisfactorily to theophylline and adrenergic drugs and should be tried before starting corticosteroids. *The drug is not a bronchodilator, has no place in the treatment of an acute asthma attack, and is used only prophylactically.* It is effective in preventing exercise-induced asthma: administration immediately before exercise blocks an attack. Both extrinsic and intrinsic asthmatics may have a favorable response, although the likelihood is greater in extrinsic asthmatics. Most specialists recommend that the drug be stopped during an exacerbation of asthma since, in this instance, it may act as an airways irritant.

Bronchodilators: A variety of oral theophylline formulations are available in tablet, capsule, and liquid form. The amount of anhydrous theophylline base in the product is the therapeutically important dose. The development of sustained-release formulations of theophylline that maintain serum theophylline concentration in the therapeutic range when given t.i.d. and even b.i.d. represents a major advance in theophylline therapy. Since theophylline is a drug that is rapidly metabolized, particularly in children, serum theophylline concentration peaks (which may cause toxic symptoms) and troughs (which may be therapeutically ineffective) often occur with the conventional rapidly absorbed formulations. Sustained-release formulations overcome this problem. As with IV administration, toxic symptoms may be observed at concentrations > 20 μg/ml. Nausea, vomiting, and CNS stimulation should be watched for, serum theophylline measured, and the dose or dosing interval modified accordingly.

Several types of β-adrenergic agents are available. Ephedrine, which is a relatively weak β-agonist, was formerly a mainstay of therapy but frequently (particularly in children) caused undesirable side effects. There may be some additional bronchodilator effect when ephedrine is combined with theophylline, but this is paid for dearly with increased adverse effects. Aerosolized isoproterenol is useful for the acute attack, but the metered commercially available canisters can be abused, particularly by children, and the adverse effects of overuse must be carefully explained to patients. Five drops of isoproterenol 1:200 or isoetharine 1:100 in 2 ml of saline or water can be given at home with an external source of compressed air and nebulizer. Inhalation of this solution quickly relieves the acute attacks that many asthmatics experience during the night, and judicious use may help in long-term outpatient management.

While maintaining adequate doses of theophylline around the clock (usually q 6 h), further improvement can occasionally be obtained by adding one of the newer β_2 bronchodilators. Metaproterenol and salbutamol have a longer duration of action than isoproterenol; the dosage is two inhalations q 6 h between theophylline doses. Alternatively, terbutaline 2.5 to 5 mg can be given orally q 6 h to supplement theophylline therapy. Since adverse side effects of the β_2 selective agents are more evident when the drugs are given orally than when given by aerosol, the latter route of administration is preferred. However, hand tremor, the most commonly observed adverse β_2 effect, becomes much less troublesome with continuous administration of the drug. Both drugs should be used with caution in patients with a history of cardiac arrhythmias, or hyperthyroidism.

When there is no satisfactory response to theophylline and a β_2-adrenergic agent, corticosteroid therapy should be added. Short-term use of high doses of corticosteroids is frequently effective in relieving exacerbations. The aim is to discontinue corticosteroids wherever possible or to reduce to the lowest maintenance dose possible. A dosage of 40 to 60 mg of prednisone/day in adults or 1 to 2 mg/kg/day in children (either divided or given as a single dose in the early morning) should be maintained for 5 to 7 days, after which the patient is reevaluated. Some patients may require an additional 7 days to achieve maximum benefit, at which time the prednisone dose can be reduced by 50% decrements every 2 days until the drug is discontinued or the lowest dose that achieves a symptom-free state is reached. If prednisone cannot be discontinued without the appearance of an unacceptable degree of symptoms, it may be worthwhile to attempt alternate-day therapy with prednisone or another short-acting corticosteroid, beginning with double the previous daily dose given as a single dose before 8 AM every 48 h. If the patient does well, an attempt is made to reduce the dose by 5 mg every 10 to 14 days. Side effects are minimized with alternate-day therapy, but success may be difficult to achieve in adults; such attempts should be abandoned and daily doses reinstituted during an exacerbation of asthma.

Beclomethasone and triamcinolone acetonide are two of a new generation of aerosol corticosteroids with potent surface activity and represent a major advance in asthma therapy. They are most useful for chronic maintenance therapy; supplemental systemic corticosteroids are necessary for an acute attack. They control asthma, apparently without adverse effects, in doses from 400 to 800 μg/day. However, when chronic steroid-dependent asthmatics are converted to aerosols from systemic corticosteroids, an inadequate hypothalamic–pituitary–adrenal axis response to stress may occur and may require resumption of systemic corticosteroid treatment. Side effects include occasional flaring of allergic rhinitis or eczema—further evidence of a lack of systemic corticosteroid effect. *Candida albicans* has been cultured from the nasopharynx of patients on topical steroid aerosol therapy, but rarely causes disease.

Extrinsic factors (generally animal danders, dust, airborne molds, and pollens) should be rigorously investigated. If suspected, allergy skin tests should be done to confirm the history. Antigens that can be controlled by avoidance (animal danders, sometimes house dust) should be eliminated. Other antigens (dust, mold, and pollens) may be selected for a trial of hyposensitization therapy. Improvement may be noted 12 to 24 mo after beginning treatment. If no significant improvement is noted in this period, therapy should be discontinued. When improvement does occur, the optimum duration of therapy is unknown, but at least 3 yr is recommended.

Nonspecific exacerbating factors such as cigarette smoke, odors, irritant fumes, and changes in temperature, atmospheric pressure, and humidity should also be investigated and controlled when possible. Aspirin should be avoided, particularly by patients with nasal polyposis, because of a significant incidence of aspirin-induced asthma. Many aspirin-intolerant asthmatics also react adversely to indomethacin, and a lesser number to tartrazine (yellow No. 5).

Surgical procedures should be performed when the patient's pulmonary state is optimum, even if this requires introduction of corticosteroids. Their short-term administration is less hazardous postsurgically than a compromised respiratory status. Procedures involving nasal and tracheal manipulation are particularly troublesome and polypectomies in aspirin-sensitive asthmatics may require a week's pretreatment with 50 to 60 mg of prednisone/day.

ACUTE BRONCHITIS

Acute inflammation of the tracheobronchial tree, generally self-limited and with eventual complete healing and return of function. Though commonly mild, bronchitis may be serious in debilitated patients and in patients with chronic pulmonary or cardiac disease. Pneumonia is a critical complication.

Etiology

Acute infectious bronchitis, most prevalent in winter, is part of an acute URI. It may develop following the common cold or other viral infection of the nasopharynx, throat, or tracheobronchial tree, often with secondary bacterial infection. Exposure to air pollutants and, possibly chilling, fatigue, and malnutrition are predisposing or contributory factors. Recurrent attacks often complicate chronic bronchopulmonary diseases which impair bronchial clearance mechanisms. They may be associated with chronic sinusitis, bronchiectasis, bronchopulmonary allergy, or, in children, hypertrophied tonsils and adenoids.

Acute irritative bronchitis may be caused by various mineral and vegetable dusts; fumes from strong acids, ammonia, certain volatile organic solvents, chlorine, hydrogen sulfide, sulfur dioxide, or bromine; or tobacco or other smoke.

Pathology and Pathophysiology

Hyperemia of the mucous membranes is the earliest change, followed by desquamation, edema, leukocytic infiltration of the submucosa, and production of sticky or mucopurulent exudate. The protective functions of the bronchial ciliated epithelium, the phagocyte cells, and the lymphatics are disturbed and bacteria may invade the normally sterile bronchi with consequent accumulation of cellular debris and mucopurulent exudate. Cough, though distressing, is essential to the elimination of bronchial secretions. Airways obstruction may result as a consequence of edema of the bronchial walls, retained secretions, and, in some cases, spasm of bronchial muscles.

Symptoms and Signs

Acute infectious bronchitis is often preceded by symptoms of a URI: coryza, malaise, chilliness, slight fever, back and muscle pain, and sore throat. Onset of cough usually signals onset of bronchitis. The cough is initially dry and nonproductive, but small amounts of viscid sputum are raised after a few hours or days. The sputum later becomes more abundant and mucoid or mucopurulent. Frankly purulent sputum suggests superimposed bacterial infection. In a severe uncomplicated case, fever to 38.3 or 38.9 C (101 or 102 F) may be present for up to 3 to 5 days, following which acute symptoms subside (though cough may continue for 2 to 3 wk). Persistent fever suggests complicating pneumonia. Dyspnea may be noted secondary to the airways obstruction.

Pulmonary signs are few in uncomplicated acute bronchitis. Scattered sibilant or sonorous rhonchi may be heard, as well as occasional crackling or moist rales at the bases. Wheezing, especially after cough, is commonly noted. Persistent localized signs suggest development of bronchopneumonia.

Serious complications are usually seen only in patients with an underlying chronic respiratory disorder. In such patients, acute bronchitis may lead to severe blood gas abnormalities (acute respiratory failure).

Diagnosis

Diagnosis is usually possible on the basis of the symptoms and signs, but a chest x-ray to rule out other diseases or complications is indicated if symptoms are serious or prolonged. Arterial blood gases should be monitored when serious underlying chronic respiratory disease is present. In cases that do not respond to antibiotic therapy, or in special circumstances such as immunosuppression, Gram stain and culture of sputum should be done for specific etiologic diagnosis.

Treatment

General: Rest is indicated until fever subsides. Oral fluids (up to 3 or 4 L/day) are pushed during the febrile course. An antipyretic analgesic such as aspirin 600 mg q 4 to 8 h relieves malaise and reduces fever.

Local: A cough suppressant may be used if cough is troublesome and interferes with sleep, but extreme care should be used if the patient also has chronic obstructive lung disease. Steam inhalations may help. A vaporizer may be used for irritative cough. Bronchodilators may be indicated for asthmatic patients or when wheezing is prominent (see BRONCHIAL ASTHMA in Ch. 34).

Antibiotics are indicated when there is concomitant chronic obstructive lung disease, when purulent sputum is present, or when high fever persists and the patient is more than mildly ill. Oral tetracycline 250 mg q.i.d. is a reasonable first choice for most cases. When symptoms persist or recur, or in unusually severe disease, smear and culture of the sputum are indicated. Antibiotic therapy is then determined by the predominant organism and its sensitivity.

CHRONIC OBSTRUCTIVE PULMONARY DISEASE (COPD)

Clinically significant, irreversible, generalized airways obstruction associated with varying degrees of chronic bronchitis, abnormalities in small airways, and emphysema. The designation was introduced because chronic bronchitis, small airways abnormalities, and emphysema often coexist and it may be difficult in an individual case to decide which is the major factor producing the airways obstruction. When it is clear that the patient's entire disease can be explained by emphysematous changes in the lung, the diagnosis "**chronic obstructive emphysema**" is preferred to the more general designation COPD. Similarly, the diagnosis "**chronic obstructive bronchitis**" should be used when the obstructive abnormality is a direct result of an inflammatory process in the airways.

To avoid the semantic confusion often encountered in discussions of these disorders, the following definitions are provided. **Chronic bronchitis,** when unqualified, is defined as *a condition associated with prolonged exposure to nonspecific bronchial irritants and accompanied by mucus hypersecretion and certain structural alterations in the bronchi.* Clinically, it is characterized by chronic productive cough and is usually associated with cigarette smoking. **Pulmonary emphysema** is defined as *enlargement of the air spaces distal to the terminal nonrespiratory bronchioles, accompanied by destructive changes of the alveolar walls.* **Airways obstruction** is defined as *increased resistance to air flow during forced expiration.* It may result from narrowing or obliteration of the airways secondary to intrinsic bronchial disease or from excessive collapse of airways during forced expiration secondary to pulmonary emphysema.

The interrelationships between chronic bronchitis, pulmonary emphysema, and COPD are depicted in Fig. 34–1. Some degree of emphysematous change is extremely common in the general population, but not all patients with emphysema have sufficient airways obstructive problems to be considered as having COPD. Similarly, many cigarette smokers have evidence of chronic bronchitis, but only a minority have clinically significant airways obstruction, usually associated with marked changes in the small airways of the lung. As noted in Fig. 34–1, most patients with clinically significant irreversible airways obstruction (COPD) have some combination of chronic bronchitis and emphysema. It is uncertain, however, whether this overlap results from a common causal factor or whether emphysema and chronic bronchitis predispose to one another.

Etiology

The development of chronic bronchitis, emphysema, and chronic airways obstruction appears to be determined by a balance between individual susceptibility and exposure to provocative agents.

The basic lesion of **emphysema** apparently results from the effect of proteolytic enzymes on the alveolar wall. Such enzymes can be released from leukocytes participating in an inflammatory process. Thus, any factor leading to a chronic inflammatory reaction at the alveolar level encourages development of emphysematous lesions. Smoking presumably plays a role due to its adverse effects on lung defense mechanisms (particularly by impairing the function of the alveolar macrophage) permitting low-grade inflammatory reactions to develop with consequent recurrent or chronic release of leukocytic proteolytic enzymes (see Ch. 48). Fortunately, most people can neutralize such enzymes as a result of antiproteolytic activity of the α_1-globulin fraction of their sera. In a rare condition known as **homozygotic α_1-antitrypsin deficiency**, however, the seral antiproteolytic activity is markedly diminished. In such patients, emphysema may develop by middle age even in the absence of exposure to substances that interfere with lung defense mechanisms. In the absence of severe deficiency of α_1-globulin in the serum, however, the factors which make some cigarette smokers more susceptible to development of emphysema than others remain uncertain. It is also uncertain why persons with similar degrees of emphysema may have considerably varying degrees of severity of airways obstruction.

With sufficient exposure to bronchial irritants, particularly cigarette smoke, most persons develop some degree of **chronic bronchitis.** The lesion essential to development of severe airways obstruction is apparently located in the small airways and may be basically different from the ordinary large airways abnormality which leads to hypersecretion of mucus in most smokers. The reason why small airways abnormalities develop in some patients with chronic bronchitis is uncertain, but viral or bacterial pulmonary infections in childhood, an unidentified immunologic mechanism, a mildly impaired ability to inactivate proteolytic enzymes (as in heterozygotic α_1-antitrypsin deficiency), or unidentified genetic characteristics could be predisposing factors. While typical allergic bronchial asthma is not a common precursor of COPD, the exact interrelationships of these disorders are not known.

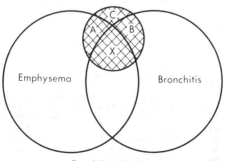

Total Population

FIG. 34–1. **The relationship of emphysema, bronchitis, and chronic obstructive pulmonary disease (COPD).** The cross-hatched circle represents patients with COPD. A—emphysematous (Type A) disease; B—bronchial (Type B) disease; X—mixed type disease; C—patients with COPD who have neither bronchitis nor anatomic emphysema. This diagram is not intended to depict precise quantitative relationships. (From Chronic Bronchitis and Emphysema, *Das Medizinische Prisma,* No. 4, p. 4, 1971, Boehringer Ingelheim. Used with permission.)

Prevalence

COPD is a major cause of disability and death. In the USA, it is second to heart disease as a cause of disability in Social Security statistics, and reported mortality rates have been doubling about every 5 yr. Its true mortality probably exceeds that from lung cancer. Some of this increase reflects the longer survival of patients who previously would have died of bacterial pneumonia before their COPD became known. Overall, it has been estimated that COPD affects as many as 15% of older men. Symptomatic COPD affects men 8 to 10 times more often than women, presumably as a result of the more frequent, prolonged, and heavier smoking in men; however, the incidence in women is now increasing.

Pathology

In patients with severe **emphysema,** the lungs are large and pale and often fail to collapse when the thorax is opened. Microscopic examination reveals "departitioning" of the lung due to loss of alveolar walls. Large bullae may be present in advanced disease. Changes may be most marked in the center of the secondary lobule **(centrilobular emphysema)** or more diffusely scattered throughout the lobule **(panacinar emphysema).** In all forms, the normal architecture is destroyed; rupture of septa results in air sacs of various sizes. The number of capillaries in the remaining alveolar walls is reduced, and the pulmonary arterial vessels may show sclerotic changes. These abnormalities lead not only to a reduction in the area of alveolar membrane available for gas exchange, but also to the perfusion of nonventilated areas and to the ventilation of nonperfused parts of the lung; i.e., **ventilation/perfusion abnormalities.** They also lead to poor support of the airways of the lung, accounting for excessive collapse of airways on expiration.

In **chronic bronchitis,** the bronchial walls are thickened, there is mucus in the lumen, and the number of goblet cells and mucous glands is increased. There may be purulent secretions and inflammatory changes in bronchial walls and surrounding lung parenchyma if infection is present. Such large airways changes do not account for severe airways obstruction, however, and in patients dying of COPD, narrowing or obliteration, or both, of small airways may be observed.

Right ventricular hypertrophy (cor pulmonale) is common in patients with advanced respiratory insufficiency.

Symptoms, Signs, and X-ray Findings

COPD is thought to begin early in life, though significant symptoms and disability usually do not occur until middle age. Mild ventilatory abnormalities may be discernible long before the onset of significant clinical symptoms. A mild "smoker's cough" is often present many years before onset of exertional dyspnea.

Gradually progressive exertional dyspnea is the most common presenting complaint. Patients may date the onset of dyspnea to an acute respiratory illness, but the acute infection may only unmask a preexisting subclinical chronic respiratory disorder. Cough, wheezing, recurrent respiratory infections, or, occasionally, weakness, weight loss, or lack of libido may also be initial manifestations. Rarely, initial complaints are related to congestive heart failure secondary to cor pulmonale, patients with such complaints apparently ignoring their cough and dyspnea prior to the onset of dependent edema and severe cyanosis.

Cough and sputum production are extremely variable. The patient may admit only to "clearing his chest" on awakening in the morning or after smoking the first cigarette of the day. Other patients may have severe disabling cough. Sputum varies from a few ml of clear viscid mucus to large bronchiectasis-like quantities of purulent material.

Wheezing also varies in character and intensity. Asthma-like episodes may occur with acute infections. A mild chronic wheeze that is most obvious on reclining may be noted. Many patients deny having any wheeze.

The physical findings in COPD are notoriously variable, especially in early cases. A consistent abnormality is obstruction to expiratory air flow manifested by a slowing of forced expiration. To demonstrate this, the patient is asked to take a deep breath and then empty his lungs as quickly and completely as possible. Forced expiration is normally virtually complete in < 4 seconds. This test, which should be part of every routine physical examination, may be abnormal even though the patient does not complain of dyspnea.

Other findings, including rhonchi, diminished vesicular breath sounds, tachycardia, distant heart tones, and decreased diaphragmatic motion, are not consistently present. The typical findings of gross pulmonary hyperinflation, prolonged expiration during quiet breathing, depressed diaphragm, pursed-lip breathing, stooped posture, calloused elbows from repeated assumption of the "tripod position," and marked use of accessory muscles of respiration are seen only in later stages of COPD. A barrel-chested appearance is an unreliable finding since it is often noted in elderly patients without significant respiratory problems. Late in the disease, there may be frank cyanosis from hypoxemia, a plethoric appearance associated with secondary erythrocytosis, and, in patients with severe cor pulmonale, signs of congestive heart failure. Mild, chronic, dependent edema is quite common and does not necessarily indicate heart failure. It may result from prolonged sitting, elevated intrathoracic pressures, and renal retention of salt secondary to blood gas abnormalities even in the absence of cor pulmonale.

X-ray findings are also variable. In early stages of the disease, the x-ray is often normal. Changes indicative of hyperinflation (e.g., depressed diaphragm, generalized radiolucency of the lung fields, increased retrosternal air space, and tenting of the diaphragm at the insertions to the ribs) are common and suggestive of emphysematous disease, but are not diagnostic. They may also be found in patients with asthma and occasionally in healthy persons. Localized radiolucency with attenuation of vascular markings is a more reliable indicator of emphysema.

Bullae are seen occasionally with COPD. Large bullae are generally well seen on ordinary x-rays, but small ones are more reliably detected with **planograms.** They may occur as part of a diffuse emphysematous process or as isolated phenomena and thus do not necessarily indicate a generalized lung disease.

Bronchitis itself does not have a characteristic appearance on ordinary chest x-ray, but **bronchograms** may reveal cylindrical dilation of bronchi on inspiration, bronchial collapse on forced expiration, and enlarged mucous ducts. Frank saccular bronchiectasis is unusual and generally occurs only in patients who have had a previous severe respiratory infection.

In patients with recurrent chest infections, a variety of nondescript postinflammatory abnormalities may be noted, such as localized fibrotic changes, honeycombing, or contraction atelectasis of a segment or lobe.

Isotopic lung scans generally demonstrate uneven ventilation and perfusion.

Diagnosis

COPD should be suspected in any patient with chronic productive cough or exertional dyspnea of uncertain etiology, or whose physical examination reveals evidence of slowing of forced expiration. Definite diagnosis depends on (1) demonstration of physiologic evidence of airways obstruction which persists despite intensive and maximum medical management, and (2) exclusion of any specific disease (e.g., silicosis, tuberculosis, or upper airway neoplasm) as a cause of this physiologic abnormality.

Spirometric testing reveals characteristic obstruction to expiratory air flow with slowing of forced expiration as manifested by a reduced 1-second forced expiratory volume (FEV_1) and a low maximum mid-expiratory flow. Slowing of forced expiration is also evident on flow-volume curves. The vital capacity (**VC**) and forced vital capacity (**FVC**) are somewhat impaired in patients with severe disease but are better maintained than the measures of the speed of expiration. For this reason, the FEV_1/VC and FEV_1/FVC ratios are regularly reduced to < 60% with clinically significant COPD. This degree of abnormality should persist despite prolonged, maximal therapy before a diagnosis of COPD is considered confirmed.

Maldistribution of ventilation and perfusion occurs in COPD and is manifested in several ways. An excessive physiologic deadspace ventilation indicates that there are areas of the lung in which ventilation is high relative to blood flow (a high ventilation/perfusion ratio), resulting in "wasted" ventilation. Physiologic shunting indicates the presence of alveoli with reduced ventilation in relation to blood flow (a low ventilation/perfusion ratio) which allows some of the pulmonary blood flow to reach the left heart without becoming fully oxygenated, resulting in hypoxemia. In late stages of the disease, overall alveolar underventilation with hypercapnia occurs, aggravating any hypoxemia present due to physiologic shunting. Chronic hypercapnia is usually well compensated, and pH levels are close to normal.

The pattern of physiologic abnormality in an individual case depends to some extent on the relative severity of intrinsic bronchial disease and anatomic emphysema. Diffusing capacity is regularly reduced in patients with severe anatomic emphysema, but is more variable in patients with airways obstruction associated with predominant intrinsic bronchial disease. In patients with severe emphysema, resting hypoxemia is usually mild and hypercapnia does not occur until terminal stages of the illness. In these patients, cardiac output may be quite low, but frank pulmonary hypertension and cor pulmonale are usually late developments. In patients with airways obstruction associated primarily with an intrinsic bronchial disorder, severe hypoxemia and hypercapnia may be noted relatively early. Such patients usually have a well-maintained cardiac output and tend to develop severe pulmonary hypertension with chronic cor pulmonale. The residual volume (RV) and total lung capacity (TLC) are markedly elevated in emphysematous patients, while pulmonary hyperinflation may be relatively slight in bronchitic COPD, but the ratio of RV to TLC tends to be elevated in both types of disease.

Detailed lung function measurements help to determine the severity of emphysema and intrinsic bronchial disease in an individual case, but are rarely needed for ordinary clinical evaluation. With severe emphysema, pressure-volume curves show a characteristic loss of recoil and increased compliance. Airways resistance measurements made in the body plethysmograph tend to reflect the severity of intrinsic bronchial narrowing.

In a few cases with severe emphysema but little bronchitis or with severe obstructive bronchitis but little, if any, emphysema, it is possible to distinguish **emphysematous type (Type A)** disease from **bronchial type (Type B)** disease on the basis of clinical and physiologic findings (see TABLE 34-2). Unfortunately, most patients appear to have a "mixed" syndrome, as shown in FIG. 34-1.

Specific parenchymal lung diseases which may lead to airways obstruction can usually be excluded by chest x-ray. Upper airway lesions (generally associated with stridor) and localized bronchial obstructions (often associated with a localized wheeze) must also be excluded. It is particularly important to exclude primary cardiac disease with congestive failure as a cause of the patient's respiratory insufficiency. A normal or small cardiac silhouette on chest x-ray is characteristic of

TABLE 34–2. CLINICAL TYPES OF CHRONIC OBSTRUCTIVE PULMONARY DISEASES

Characteristics	Emphysematous (Type A)	Bronchial (Type B)
Age at diagnosis	55–75	45–65
Cough onset	Often after onset of dyspnea	Usually before onset of dyspnea
Sputum	Scanty, mucoid	Copious, purulent
Recurrent infections	Occasional	Frequent
Chest x-ray	Normal or emphysematous	Normal or fibrotic
Pulmonary artery pressure	Normal or slightly high	Often very high
Chronic cor pulmonale	Unusual	Common
Lung compliance	Normal or high	Normal or low
Recoil pressure	Low	Normal or high
Airways resistance	Near normal	Elevated
Pulmonary overdistention	Marked	Mild or moderate
Diffusing capacity	Low	Variable
Chronic hypercapnia	Unusual	Common
Chronic hypoxemia	Mild or moderate	Often severe

COPD prior to development of frank cor pulmonale, but is most unusual in patients who are dyspneic as a result of a cardiac disorder.

Homozygotic α_1-antitrypsin deficiency should be suspected when there is a family history of obstructive airways disease, or when emphysema occurs in a woman, a relatively young man, or a nonsmoker. The diagnosis may be confirmed by measuring serum α_1-antitrypsin levels or by specific phenotyping.

Course and Prognosis

Some reversal of airways obstruction and considerable symptomatic improvement can often be obtained initially, but the long-term prognosis is less favorable in patients with persistent obstructive abnormality. After initial improvement, the FEV_1 generally falls 50 to 75 ml/yr, which is 2 to 3 times the rate of decline expected from aging alone. There is a concomitant slow progression of exertional dyspnea and disability. The course is punctuated by acute symptomatic exacerbations, generally related to superimposed bronchial infections.

Prognosis is closely related to the severity of expiratory slowing. When the FEV_1 exceeds 1.25 L, the 10-yr survival rate is about 50%; when the FEV_1 is 1 L, the average patient survives about 5 yr; when there is very severe expiratory slowing (FEV_1 about 0.5 L), survival for > 2 yr is unusual, particularly if the patient also has chronic hypercapnia or demonstrable cor pulmonale.

Treatment

Therapy does not result in cure, but provides symptomatic relief and controls potentially fatal exacerbations. It may also slow progression of the disorder, though this is unproved. Treatment is directed at alleviating conditions which cause symptoms and excessive disability (e.g., infection, bronchospasm, bronchial hypersecretion, hypoxemia, and unnecessary limitation of physical activity).

Infection: An attempt should be made to clear purulent sputum with a broad-spectrum antibiotic (e.g., tetracycline 250 mg q.i.d. for 10 days), the course repeated promptly at the first sign of recurrent bronchial infection or sputum purulence. Ampicillin or cephalothin may be used to treat severe exacerbations. Regular courses of a broad-spectrum antibiotic are indicated in patients with very frequent infectious exacerbations.

Bronchospasm: The degree of reversibility of airways obstruction can be assessed only by a vigorous and prolonged therapeutic trial of bronchodilators. See BRONCHIAL ASTHMA, above, for a detailed discussion of these drugs.

Corticosteroids have a very limited role in treating COPD, but a trial of these agents may be required to prove conclusively that the airways obstruction is not a result of potentially reversible bronchospasm. This is especially true when there is a past history suggesting asthma, eosinophilia, fluctuations in the severity of airways obstruction, or a good immediate response to inhalation of a bronchodilator. If a corticosteroid trial (e.g., prednisone 30 to 40 mg every morning for 3 wk) is undertaken, its usefulness should be documented by objective improvement in spirometric tests before long-term corticosteroid therapy is recommended, at which time the lowest maintenance dose which sustains improvement is used. In some patients, alternate-day therapy can be used for maintenance.

Bronchial secretions: Adequate systemic hydration is essential to prevent inspissation of secretions. In some patients bronchial hygiene may alsc be improved by inhalation of mist, postural drainage, and chest physical therapy, particularly following bronchodilator inhalation. Saturated solution of potassium iodide 10 drops in H_2O t.i.d. is used by some physicians in an attempt to thin bronchial secretions. Despite their wide use, IPPB machines have not been shown to improve the patient's ability to raise secretions or to affect favorably the overall condition of ambulatory patients with COPD.

Hypoxemia: Severe chronic hypoxemia, often associated with hypercapnia, accentuates pulmonary hypertension and leads to development of cor pulmonale in patients with COPD. Recurrent cardiac failure may develop and necessitate long-term O_2 therapy. Low flow (1 to 2 L/min) O_2 therapy via nasal prongs for 15 h or more/day (including sleeping hours) may be effective in reversing pulmonary hypertension and improving cardiac status. Around-the-clock O_2 supplementation has been shown to be preferable for patients with severe chronic hypoxemia (arterial O_2 tensions consistently < 55 mm Hg at rest) and appears to prolong survival. When instituting long-term O_2 therapy, it is important to monitor the blood gas responses. No more O_2 should be given than is needed to raise the arterial O_2 tension to 55 mm Hg. One should also be sure that chronic O_2 therapy does not lead to a progressive rise in CO_2 tension as a consequence of removing hypoxic ventilatory drive; in fact, this has rarely proved to be an important problem.

Even in patients without severe cor pulmonale, O_2 may be needed to correct severe exertional hypoxemia when the patient is started on a graded exercise program. Use of O_2 for symptomatic relief of dyspnea without verification of severe hypoxemia, however, is unjustified and potentially dangerous.

Hypercapnia: Patients with rapidly developing or worsening hypercapnia require immediate hospitalization and intensive therapy, but chronic well-compensated hypercapnia is generally well tolerated and requires no specific therapy.

Heart failure: The most important measure for controlling heart failure secondary to cor pulmonale is correction of excessive hypoxemia. Diuretic therapy and controlled sodium intake are important adjuncts. Digitalis must be used cautiously, if at all, since digitalis intoxication readily occurs in patients with COPD, probably as a result of fluctuating blood gas and electrolyte abnormalities.

Exercise tolerance: Prolonged inactivity leads to excessive disability in patients with COPD. As long as there is no severe cardiac disease, it is important to maintain a regular exercise program. This can usually be prescribed directly by the physician. If the patient is severely disabled, however, the program may be more effective if supervised by a trained physical therapist. The exercise program should have a specific meaningful goal (e.g., walking to the store, golfing) and should train those muscles needed for this specific activity. Breathing "exercises" (breathing training) may have a place in treating anxious patients who develop an excessively rapid ventilatory rate during exertion, but such exercises have not been shown to improve ventilatory capacity.

Depression: Periods of severe depression or marked anxiety are frequent in patients with COPD. A vigorous therapeutic program and an enthusiastic physician are most helpful. A nihilistic attitude toward management of this disease is inexcusable. The patient must understand the nature of the disease and the goals and expectations of therapy.

Exacerbations: Treat promptly; e.g., if sputum becomes purulent, prescribe a course of broad-spectrum antibiotics and a more intensive program of bronchodilation and bronchial hygiene (see above). Patients with increasing hypoxemia or hypercapnia should be hospitalized promptly for intensive therapy. *Sedatives and hypnotics should always be avoided* in patients with COPD, particularly during exacerbations, since they increase the risk of acute ventilatory failure.

---

35. BRONCHIECTASIS

A chronic congenital or acquired disease characterized by irreversible cylindrical, saccular, or varicose dilation of the bronchi, with secondary infection.

Etiology

Congenital bronchiectasis is a rare condition arising from agenesis of the alveoli with resultant cystic dilation of the terminal bronchi. The etiology of **acquired bronchiectasis** often is obscure. It can develop at any age, but most often begins in early childhood. It usually follows bronchial infection, most often a severe childhood pneumonia (commonly one complicating measles, pertussis, various immunologic deficiencies, aspirated foreign bodies, or erosion of bronchi by tuberculous lymph nodes), which destroys the supporting elastic and muscular components of the bronchial wall. The incidence of bronchiectasis has decreased dramatically with the widespread use of antibiotics and immunizations in pediatrics, but it is a common manifestation of cystic fibrosis and also occurs in **Kartagener's syndrome** (situs inversus, sinusitis, and bronchiectasis), a condition in which an abnormality in the cilial organelles results in defective mucociliary clearance that leads to suppurative bronchial infections and bronchiectasis. This etiology has also been identified in a few patients who do not have Kartagener's syndrome. In bronchopulmonary aspergillosis (see ALLERGIC BRONCHIAL ASPERGILLOSIS in Ch. 41), a characteristic dilation of intermediate bronchi is seen with normal-appearing bronchi proximal and distal to the dilated ones. This is an unusual bronchiectatic pattern. In adults, bronchiectasis also may develop following destructive inflammatory bronchial changes, necrotizing pneumonia, or lung abscess. It often is a prominent feature in cases of chronic pneumonia peripheral to an obstructing bronchogenic carcinoma.

The bronchi in areas of lung that have been extensively organized by fibrosing lung diseases (e.g., tuberculosis, silicosis) usually are foreshortened, widened, sometimes chronically inflamed, and occasionally described as bronchiectatic. In these diseases, however, there is probably less intrinsic disease of the bronchi and severe suppurative complications are less common.

Pathology

Bronchiectasis may be uni- or bilateral and is most common in the lower lobes, though the right middle lobe and the lingular portion of the left upper lobe also are frequently involved. It may be cylindrical, varicose, or saccular. In **cylindrical bronchiectasis**, the bronchi are slightly dilated and in bronchograms appear beaded and end abruptly without the usual branching pattern. The distal smaller bronchi cannot be seen on bronchograms but can be identified pathologically and are filled with inflammatory exudate. In **varicose bronchiectasis**, the bronchi are irregularly dilated and contracted. In **saccular bronchiectasis**, the dilated bronchi are much wider; only the first few branchings of the tracheobronchial tree are present. The bronchial walls show extensive microscopic evidence of inflammatory destruction, chronic inflammation, increased mucous secretion, and loss of cilia; there is extensive destruction and disappearance of adjacent interstitial and alveolar areas. These areas of parenchymal destruction may result in large areas of organization and fibrosis and in decreased volume.

Symptoms and Signs

The severity and characteristics of symptoms vary widely from patient to patient, and in some patients from time to time, depending largely on the extent of the disease and the amount of complicating chronic infection present. Chronic cough and sputum production are the most characteristic and common symptoms. These often begin insidiously, usually following a respiratory infection, and tend to worsen gradually over a period of years. A severe pneumonia with incomplete clearing of symptoms and residual persistence of cough and sputum production is a common mode of onset. As the condition progresses, the cough tends to become more productive and has a typical regularity, occurring in the morning on arising, late in the afternoon, and on retiring. Many patients are relatively free of cough during the intervening hours. The sputum usually is similar to that of bronchitis and is not characteristic. Less commonly, in longstanding cases, sputum may be abundant and may separate into three layers on standing: frothy at the top, greenish and turbid in the middle, and thick with pus at the bottom. Hemoptysis is common and may be the first and only symptom. Recurrent acute pneumonia is a common complication and its investigation may lead to the diagnosis of bronchiectasis.

Physical findings are not specific, but persistent rales over any portion of the lung suggest bronchiectasis. Clubbing of the fingers sometimes occurs when disease is advanced and there is persistent chronic infection. Pulmonary functional changes are those of any associated disease or of the pulmonary fibrosis that may complicate bronchiectasis. Ventilation/perfusion defects and mild reduction in Pa_{O_2} may be present if disease is extensive.

Diagnosis

Bronchiectasis must be suspected in all patients with the above symptoms and signs. Since the disorder is a morphologically defined entity, diagnosis is confirmed by bronchography, although this risks hypersensitivity to the iodine-containing contrast medium and a temporary worsening of pulmonary function. Bronchography should not be performed if the patient is sensitive to iodine-containing materials or has significant pulmonary functional impairment. The sputum should be cultured for aerobic and anaerobic pathogens before starting antimicrobial therapy. Tuberculosis, chronic bronchitis, and fungal infections must be ruled out. Tumor, foreign body, or other bronchial obstruction must also be ruled out, particularly when disease is unilateral or of recent onset or if the patient is over age 35.

Treatment

Therapy in most cases is directed at controlling infection with appropriate antibiotics and postural drainage. If a definite pathogen is not identified, procaine penicillin G is given IM in doses of at least 2 million u./day. Antibiotics usually decrease the volume and purulence of the sputum and should be continued until sputum is nonpurulent and less voluminous. Antibiotic therapy should be repeated at the first sign of returning infection, most often a change in the volume or purulence of the sputum. If infection recurs frequently, prolonged chemoprophylaxis with a broad-spectrum antibiotic (e.g., ampicillin, tetracycline) may be helpful. Postural drainage at least twice a day should be continued indefinitely, even when minimal or no secretions are produced (see in Respiratory Physical Therapy in Ch. 31). Some patients also may have diffuse chronic bronchitis and should be treated accordingly (see in Chronic Obstructive Pulmonary Disease in Ch. 34).

Resection is seldom necessary due to the effectiveness of antibiotics, but is indicated when the diseased area is localized and nonprogressive or when medical management is inadequate (as demonstrated by recurrent pneumonia or bronchial infection or by frequent hemoptysis).

36. ATELECTASIS

A shrunken and airless state of part or all of the lung; the disorder may be acute or chronic, complete or incomplete (partial atelectasis). Atelectasis is often accompanied by infection. The atelectatic lung or lobe is a complex mixture of airlessness, infection, bronchiectasis, destruction, and fibrosis.

Etiology

The chief cause of **acute or chronic atelectasis** in adults is bronchial obstruction (e.g., by plugs of tenacious bronchial exudate; foreign bodies; endobronchial tumors; tumors, lymph nodes, or an aneurysm compressing the bronchi; and bronchial distortions or kinkings). External pulmonary compression by pleural fluid or gas (e.g., due to pleural effusion, pneumothorax) may also cause atelectasis. Surfactant, a lipoprotein, covers the surface of the alveoli, reduces surface tension, and contributes to alveolar stability. Interference with its production may occur in O_2 toxicity, pulmonary edema, and other conditions that cause alveolar airlessness, and is probably important in the perpetuation of atelectasis.

Acute massive lung collapse is usually a postoperative complication, most frequently following surgery in the upper abdomen. Large doses of opiates and sedatives, very high O_2 concentrations during anesthesia, tight dressings, abdominal distention, and immobility of the body favor development of atelectasis, owing to limited respiratory movement, elevated diaphragm, accumulated viscid bronchial secretions, and suppressed cough reflex.

In the **middle lobe syndrome,** a form of chronic atelectasis, middle lobe collapse usually results from bronchial compression by surrounding lymph nodes. Partial bronchial obstruction in the presence of infection may also lead to chronic atelectasis and, ultimately, to chronic pneumonitis because of poor drainage of bronchial secretions. Acute pneumonia, usually with delayed and incomplete resolution, may also develop.

Pathology and Pathophysiology

Following obstruction of a bronchus, absorption of the gas in the peripheral alveoli by the circulating blood and consequent retraction of the lung produce the airless state within a few hours; lung shrinkage or collapse may be complete in the absence of infection. In the early stages, blood perfuses the airless lung, with consequent arterial hypoxia. Capillary and tissue hypoxia may result in transudation of fluid and pulmonary edema, filling the alveolar spaces with secretions and cells and preventing complete collapse of the atelectatic lung. The uninvolved surrounding lung distends, displacing the heart and mediastinum toward the atelectatic area; the diaphragm is elevated, and the chest wall flattens.

Hyperventilation and dyspnea are common. A decrease in Pa_{O_2} is usual and, if the atelectatic area is large, may be considerable; Pa_{O_2} often improves during and after the first 24 h, presumably as blood flow to the atelectatic area decreases. Pa_{CO_2} is usually normal or low as a result of the increased ventilation.

If the obstruction is removed, air enters the affected area, any complicating infection subsides, and the lung returns to its normal state in a variable length of time, depending on how much infection is present. If the obstruction is not removed and infection is present, airlessness and lack of circulation initiate changes that lead to development of fibrosis. If these conditions persist, the lung becomes fibrotic and bronchiectatic. In addition to bronchial obstruction, small areas of atelectasis may come about by inadequate regional ventilation and disturbances in surfactant formation from hypoxia, hyperoxia, and exposure to various toxins. Mild to severe disturbances in gas exchange may result.

Symptoms and Signs

Most of the symptoms and signs are determined by the rapidity with which the bronchial occlusion occurs, by the size of the area of lung affected, and by the presence or absence of complicating infection. **Rapid occlusion with massive collapse,** particularly if infection is present, causes pain on the affected side, sudden onset of dyspnea and cyanosis, a drop in BP, tachycardia, elevated temperature, and shock. Chest examination reveals dullness to flatness over the involved area and diminished or absent breath sounds. Chest excursion in the area is reduced or absent. The trachea and heart are deviated toward the affected side. The patient tends to lie with the atelectatic area dependent. **Slowly developing atelectasis** may be asymptomatic or cause only minor pulmonary symptoms. The **middle lobe syndrome** is also often asymptomatic, though a severe, hacking, nonproductive cough may be present because of irritation in the right lower and middle lobe bronchi. Physical examination discloses the same findings as in rapid occlusion.

Chest x-ray may show an airless area of lung, its size and location depending on the bronchus involved. If only segmental areas are affected, the shadow will be triangular, with its apex toward the hilum. When small areas are involved, distention of surrounding lung tissue causes the atelectatic area to appear curiously discoid in shape, particularly in subsegmental lower lobe atelectasis. If the atelectasis is lobar, the entire lobe is airless. The trachea, heart, and mediastinum are deviated toward the atelectatic area, the diaphragm on the affected side is elevated, and rib spaces are narrowed.

Diagnosis

Diagnosis is made from the clinical findings plus x-ray evidence of diminished lung size (indicated by retracted ribs, elevated diaphragm, and deviated mediastinum) and of a solid, airless mass. Bronchoscopy may reveal bronchial obstruction, but only a small number of bronchi are visualized, and examination may be negative unless the obstruction is in a main bronchus or in early divisions of the smaller bronchi.

Bronchogenic carcinoma, which may present with atelectasis, must be ruled out in all patients over age 35. Spontaneous pneumothorax produces clinical findings similar to those in atelectasis, but the percussion note is tympanitic, the heart and mediastinum are pushed to the opposite side, and x-rays are diagnostic. Massive effusion may also cause dyspnea, cyanosis, weakness, flatness over the involved area, and absent breath sounds, but the heart and mediastinum are deviated away from the involved area and the chest wall is not flattened.

Treatment

Acute atelectasis (including postoperative acute massive lung collapse) requires removal of the underlying cause. Acute massive atelectasis is best combated by prevention. Anesthetic agents with a long postanesthesia narcosis should be avoided, and narcotics should be used sparingly after surgery, since they depress the cough reflex. At the conclusion of anesthesia, the lungs should be left filled with air, not O_2. The patient must not be allowed to lie in one position for more than 1 h. Early ambulation is important. The patient should be encouraged to cough and breathe deeply. IPPB for 5 to 10 min/h during the postoperative period, using air and *not* O_2, may improve ventilation and bronchial drainage and prevent atelectasis. Nebulized bronchodilators and aerosols of water or saline may help to liquefy secretions and promote their easy removal. If bronchial obstruction is incipient, as indicated by wheezing or sharp, forced expirations, these measures are urgently required.

When a mechanically obstructed bronchus is suspected but relief is not obtained by cough or suction, bronchoscopy should be performed. Once bronchial obstruction is established, treatment is directed at the obstruction and at the infection invariably present. The patient should be (1) placed so that the uninvolved side is dependent, to promote increased drainage of the affected area, (2) given vigorous chest physiotherapy, and (3) encouraged to cough. If improvement is not evident in 1 or 2 h, bronchoscopy should be repeated to aspirate as much secretion as possible. Chest physiotherapy is then continued and the patient is encouraged to cough, move from side to side, and breathe deeply. Periodic use of IPPB may be helpful. Penicillin 600,000 u. IM t.i.d. or a broad-spectrum antibiotic such as ampicillin 0.5 gm orally q 6 h or tetracycline 0.5 gm orally q 6 h should be given at the outset and modified appropriately if a specific pathogen is isolated from sputum or bronchial secretions.

Chronic atelectasis is treated by segmental resection or lobectomy. Since secondary atelectasis usually becomes infected regardless of the cause of obstruction, a broad-spectrum antibiotic, penicillin, ampicillin, or tetracycline should be given. Obstruction of a major bronchus may cause severe hacking or spasmodic cough. Treatment resulting in too great a reduction in the cough reflex may produce further obstruction and should be avoided.

37. THROMBOEMBOLISM AND INFARCTION

Pulmonary embolism (thromboembolism): *Lodgement of a blood clot in a pulmonary artery with subsequent obstruction of blood supply to the lung parenchyma.* **Pulmonary infarction:** *Hemorrhagic consolidation (often followed by necrosis) of lung parenchyma resulting from thromboembolic pulmonary arterial occlusion.*

Etiology and Pathogenesis

The most common type of pulmonary embolus is a thrombus which usually has formed in the leg or pelvic veins. Most of those causing serious hemodynamic disturbances form in the iliofemoral veins, either de novo or by propagation from calf vein thrombi. Embolization of thrombi originating in the veins of the upper extremities or in the right cardiac chambers is infrequent. Amniotic fluid emboli and fat emboli following fractures are much less common types of pulmonary emboli in which the primary site of vascular obstruction is the pulmonary microcirculation (arterioles and capillaries rather than in the pulmonary arteries); the involvement of the microcirculation may result in the development of the so-called acute respiratory distress syndrome (see in Ch. 33).

Pulmonary infarction is an infrequent ($<$ 10% of cases) consequence of pulmonary embolism. It is sometimes due to thrombosis in situ of the pulmonary arteries as might occur in congenital heart disease associated with severe pulmonary hypertension or in hematologic disorders such as sickle cell anemia.

The pathogenesis of venous thrombosis involves stasis, increased blood coagulability, and vascular wall damage (Virchow's triad). Factors predisposing to thromboembolic disease include prolonged bed rest with immobility, chronic congestive heart failure, the postoperative state, pregnancy, hip fracture, use of oral contraceptives, chronic obstructive pulmonary disease, obesity, malignancy, hematologic disorders (e.g., polycythemia vera), vascular injuries resulting from minor trauma, and immobilization with stasis as may occur in chronic disease states. In many patients, no predisposing factor can be found.

Once released into the venous circulation, emboli are distributed to both lungs in about 65% of cases, to the right lung only in 20%, and to the left lung only in 10%. The lower lobes are involved 4 times more frequently than the upper lobes. Most thromboemboli lodge in the larger or intermediate (elastic or muscular) pulmonary arteries; 35% or fewer reach the smaller arteries.

Pathophysiology

The pathophysiologic changes which occur following pulmonary embolism are complex, involving alterations in pulmonary hemodynamics, gas exchange, and mechanics. The extent of alteration in cardiopulmonary function is determined by the degree of pulmonary arterial obstruction, which varies with the size and number of thrombi embolizing and obstructing the pulmonary arteries, and by the patient's preembolic cardiopulmonary status. A consideration of the pathophysiology of pulmonary embolism must include the mechanisms responsible for the following: (1) pulmonary hypertension, right ventricular failure, and shock; (2) dyspnea with tachypnea and hyperventilation; (3) arterial hypoxemia; and (4) pulmonary infarction.

1. **Pulmonary hypertension,** a most important physiologic alteration following embolization, results from increased pulmonary vascular resistance. As a consequence, the right ventricle must generate a higher pulmonary artery pressure to maintain normal cardiac output. Significant pulmonary hypertension ($>$ 20 mm Hg mean pressure) usually occurs only when $>$ 30 to 50% of the pulmonary arterial tree is occluded in the previously undiseased lung. Pulmonary hypertension may be further enhanced in the presence of preexisting cardiopulmonary disease, such as valvular dysfunction (e.g., mitral stenosis) or obstructive lung disease.

The primary mechanism of the increased resistance is obstruction of pulmonary arteries by the thrombi; i.e., a decrease in the total cross-sectional area of the pulmonary vascular bed. However, because some degree of pulmonary hypertension often develops with obstruction of $<$ 50% of the vascular bed, pulmonary vasoconstriction appears to play a definite, but secondary, role. Vasoconstriction is partly mediated by hypoxemia, by serotonin release from platelet aggregates on the thrombi, and possibly by other humoral substances, including prostaglandins.

If pulmonary vascular resistance increases to the extent that the right ventricle is unable to generate sufficient pressure (about 40 mm Hg mean pulmonary arterial pressure) to maintain cardiac output, **hypotension** (in which the central venous and right atrial mean pressures are increased) develops. This occurs only following massive embolization involving at least 50% and usually 75% or more of the pulmonary vascular bed in the absence of pre-existing cardiopulmonary disease. With severe hypotension and **shock,** mean central venous pressure tends to fall.

2. **Tachypnea,** often with **dyspnea,** almost always occurs following an embolic episode. It appears to be of reflex origin, most likely due to stimulation of intrapulmonary receptors in the alveoli (J receptors). This stimulation increases vagal afferent activity, which in turn stimulates medullary respiratory neurons. Consequent alveolar hyperventilation is manifested by a lowered arterial CO_2 tension.

Following pulmonary arterial occlusion, areas of the lung are ventilated but not perfused, resulting in "wasted ventilation" (the physiologic hallmark of pulmonary embolism). The degree of wasted ventilation can be estimated by measuring the physiologic deadspace or the arterial-alveolar CO_2 tension difference.

Alterations in lung mechanics with an increase in airway resistance and a decrease in lung compliance tend to occur. A decrease in the maximal expiratory flow rate results from diminished lung volume and possibly from bronchoconstriction. Heparin appears to lessen the degree of bronchoconstriction, when present, as evidenced by improved maximal expiratory flow rates. Reduced lung volume following thromboembolism sometimes is manifested on the chest x-ray by elevation of the diaphragm due to atelectatic infarcted segments. Since the changes in lung mechanics are usually transient and minor, they are unlikely to be important in the genesis of prolonged dyspnea. However, they probably contribute to development of arterial hypoxemia, described below.

3. **Arterial hypoxemia:** Arterial O_2 saturation is characteristically diminished (94 to 85% or lower), but may be normal. Hypoxemia is due to right-to-left shunting in areas of partial or complete atelec-

tasis; characteristically, this atelectasis can be partially corrected by deep breathing, either voluntary or induced by a positive pressure ventilator. Ventilation/perfusion ($\dot{V}_A/\dot{Q}$) imbalance probably also contributes to the hypoxemia. The mechanisms responsible for the $\dot{V}_A/\dot{Q}$ imbalance and atelectasis are not well defined. One explanation that has been offered is the release, after an embolic episode, of a humoral agent in the pulmonary arterioles that produces nonuniform constriction of distal airways and peripheral lung units with resultant underventilation of the units with respect to their perfusion; atelectasis results if these changes are severe. Tachypnea may augment the changes. In massive embolization, severe hypoxemia may result from right atrial hypertension that causes right-to-left shunting of blood through a patent foramen ovale.

4. Pulmonary infarction: Most pulmonary emboli do not produce infarction. When the bronchial circulation is intact and normal (i.e., in the absence of congestive heart failure or underlying chronic pulmonary disease), pulmonary infarction rarely develops. This suggests that collateral bronchial artery circulation adequately maintains viability of lung tissue despite the absence of pulmonary arterial flow. However, patients with previously abnormal pulmonary circulation are prone to develop pulmonary infarction. Pulmonary infarcts may heal by absorption and fibrosis, leaving a linear scar, or may resorb completely, leaving a normal lung (incomplete infarction).

Acute pulmonary thromboembolism is a dynamic process. The thrombi begin to lyse immediately after reaching the lung. Usually, complete clot lysis takes place within several weeks in the absence of preexisting cardiopulmonary disease, but, in some instances, even large thrombi may be lysed in a few days. The physiologic alterations lessen over hours or days as the pulmonary circulation becomes less obstructed. Massive emboli may cause death within a few minutes or hours without sufficient time for infarction to develop. Smaller emboli may produce infarction, which can heal with recanalization and restoration of blood flow through the occluded vessel. Infrequently, the embolic events recur for months or years, causing progressive pulmonary arterial obstruction with chronic pulmonary hypertension, increasing dyspnea, and cor pulmonale.

Symptoms and Signs

The clinical manifestations of pulmonary embolism are not specific. Diagnosis may be difficult without using special diagnostic procedures, the most important of which are radioisotope perfusion lung scans and pulmonary arteriography (see Diagnosis, below). The symptoms and signs vary in frequency and intensity depending on the extent of pulmonary vascular occlusion, the development of pulmonary infarction, and the patient's preembolic cardiopulmonary function. There may be no symptoms with small thromboemboli.

Embolism without infarction is manifested by breathlessness, which may be the only symptom if infarction does not develop. Tachypnea is a consistent and often striking feature. Anxiety and restlessness may be prominent.

Pulmonary hypertension, if severe, may cause dull substernal chest discomfort due to pulmonary artery distention or possibly myocardial ischemia. It may be manifested by an increase in the intensity of the pulmonary component of the basal 2nd sound or abnormal splitting (i.e., widened with less variation of splitting during inspiration) of the aortic and pulmonary components of the basal 2nd sound. If pulmonary vascular obstruction is massive, acute right ventricular insufficiency may supervene, with distended cervical veins, right ventricular heave, right ventricular (protodiastolic) gallop, sometimes with arterial hypotension and evidence of peripheral vasoconstriction. Lightheadedness, syncopal episodes, convulsive phenomena, and neurologic deficits may be the presenting events in a significant number of patients, usually reflecting a transient fall in cardiac output with secondary cerebral ischemia. Cyanosis is usual in patients with massive embolism, but not in patients with lesser obstruction.

Examination of the lungs is usually normal in the absence of pulmonary infarction. Wheezing may sometimes be heard, particularly if underlying bronchopulmonary or cardiac disease is present.

In addition to the above symptoms and signs, the manifestations of **pulmonary infarction** include cough, hemoptysis, pleuritic chest pain, fever, and signs of pulmonary consolidation or pleural fluid. A pleural friction rub may be heard. A small, peripheral embolus may cause infarction but not obstruct the pulmonary arteries to the extent that pulmonary hypertension develops.

The manifestations of embolization usually develop abruptly over a period of minutes; those of infarction over a period of hours. They often last several days, depending on the rate of clot lysis and other factors, but usually decrease in intensity every day. In those patients with chronic, recurrent emboli, the symptoms and signs of chronic cor pulmonale tend to develop insidiously over a period of weeks, months, or years.

Diagnosis

The diagnosis of pulmonary embolism with or without infarction is often difficult to establish. In patients with massive pulmonary embolism, the differential diagnosis includes bacteremic shock, acute myocardial infarction, peritonitis, and cardiac tamponade. In the absence of pulmonary infarction, the patient's symptoms and signs may be attributed to anxiety with hyperventilation because of the paucity of objective pulmonary findings. When infarction occurs, the differential diagnosis includes pneumonia, atelectasis, congestive heart failure, and pericarditis. A systematic approach to diagnosis is possible as outlined below.

1. **The clinical symptoms and signs** should suggest the diagnosis.

2. **Appropriate clinical diagnostic studies,** including chest x-ray, ECG, CBC, and serum enzyme (AST [formerly SGOT], LDH) and serum bilirubin determinations may be helpful. With infarction, the **chest x-ray** frequently shows a peripheral infiltrative lesion, often involving the costophrenic angle, with elevation of the diaphragm and pleural fluid on the affected side. Diminished pulmonary vascular markings in the embolized area may be noted in the absence of infarction. Dilation of the pulmonary arteries in the hilar area, the superior vena cava, and the azygos vein signal pulmonary hypertension and right ventricular strain. Since **ECG changes** are characteristically transient, serial tracings are often helpful in the diagnosis and in the exclusion of acute myocardial infarction. Changes most frequently seen in the ECG include P pulmonale, right bundle branch block, right axis deviation, and supraventricular arrhythmias. The sensitivity and specificity of **serum enzyme studies** have been disappointing and the studies are rarely helpful in diagnosis. The triad of elevated serum LDH and bilirubin and normal AST occurs in < 15% of patients with acute pulmonary embolism and infarction. Elevated LDH may be demonstrable in as many as 85% of patients with pulmonary infarction, but is not a specific finding, occurring also in cardiac failure, shock, pregnancy, renal and liver disease, anemia, pneumonia, carcinoma, and after surgical procedures. A profile of enzyme studies involving elevated LDH, normal CPK, and normal hydroxybutyrate dehydrogenase (HBD) is more specific in the diagnosis of pulmonary infarction and may differentiate acute myocardial infarction, but is of little value in diagnosing embolism without infarction. Blood levels of **fibrin split products** appear to rise rather consistently after pulmonary embolism whether infarction occurs or not, but the temporal relation of this rise to the onset of symptoms, and its time course, vary considerably. The specificity of this finding is also questionable since the incidence of elevation in other diseases is not well defined.

3. **Radioisotope perfusion lung scanning,** sometimes combined with **ventilation scanning,** is very valuable in establishing the diagnosis. These procedures are discussed in Radionuclide Imaging Methods in Ch. 227.

4. **Pulmonary arteriography:** Demonstration of emboli by angiography remains the most definitive diagnostic test. Angiography should be performed if the diagnosis is in doubt and appears urgent. The 2 primary criteria for arteriographic diagnosis of thromboembolism are intraarterial filling defects and complete obstruction (abrupt cutoff) of pulmonary arterial branches. Other frequent findings include partial obstruction of pulmonary arterial branches with increased caliber proximal and decreased caliber distal to the stenosis, and persistence of dye in the proximal portion of the artery during the late (venous) phase of the arteriograms. In those lung segments with obstructed arteries, pulmonary venous filling with contrast medium is delayed or absent.

5. **Additional diagnostic studies** to establish the presence or absence of iliofemoral venous thrombotic disease may be useful in the management of pulmonary embolism, particularly when signs of recurrent embolization despite anticoagulant therapy or contraindications to anticoagulant therapy make vena caval interruption an important therapeutic consideration. Contrast venography appears to be the most reliable means of establishing the diagnosis of iliofemoral venous thrombosis, though noninvasive measures such as impedance plethysmography of the leg and assessment of femoral venous flow velocity by externally applied Doppler ultrasound flow probe have been found to be about 75 to 90% as sensitive as phlebography. Intravascular injection of technetium-labelled albumin and ^{125}I fibrinogen with leg scanning may detect venous thrombi, but the latter technic is useful only in relation to deep veins of the calf.

Prognosis

Mortality following the initial thromboembolic event varies with the extent of embolization and the patient's preexisting cardiorespiratory status. A patient with markedly compromised cardiopulmonary function is at greater risk of developing thromboemboli, and the likelihood that he will die following significant embolization is high (probably > 25%). On the other hand, it is unlikely that a patient with normal cardiopulmonary status will die unless the degree of embolization is massive (i.e., the occlusive process involves > 50% of the pulmonary vascular bed). When the initial embolic event is fatal, death is often sudden, occurring within 1 to 2 h.

If a patient survives the initial embolic event but is not treated, the likelihood of a recurrent embolus is about 50%; as many as half of these recurrences may be fatal. Outcome is significantly modified by anticoagulant therapy, which reduces the rate of recurrence to about 5%; only about 20% of these will be fatal.

Prophylaxis

Pulmonary embolism can be prevented by preventing venous thrombosis. Therefore, the reduction of factors that predispose to venous thrombosis is of great importance, particularly those that minimize venous stasis. In postoperative (particularly elderly) patients, the use of elastic stockings to augment velocity of venous return in the legs, leg exercises, and early ambulation is widely used to lower the incidence of pulmonary embolism, but the usefulness of these measures has been questioned since they have little effect on the incidence of deep calf vein thrombosis. Intra- and postoperative pneumatic leg compression and electrical calf stimulation reduce the incidence of deep calf vein thrombosis, but their effects on iliofemoral vein thrombosis and pulmonary thromboembolic complications is not known.

Anticoagulant prophylaxis (see also Ch. 254) is effective in selected settings. Following hip or leg fracture in patients over age 50, immediate (preoperative) **oral anticoagulation** (using warfarin sodium), continued for 1 wk after the patient is ambulatory, significantly reduces the incidence of pulmonary embolism with about a 5% risk of hemorrhage. In the absence of contraindications to anticoagulant therapy, routine use of warfarin sodium has been advocated in patients (particularly the elderly) with congestive heart failure or debilitating disease of any kind that predisposes to immobility.

Low-dose heparin administration provides effective prophylaxis with reduced incidence of deep vein (calf) thrombosis and pulmonary embolism in patients undergoing a variety of major surgical procedures. At a blood level about 1/5 that required for therapeutic efficacy (prevention of thrombus propagation) heparin activates antithrombin III sufficiently to inhibit Factor X, which is required for conversion of prothrombin to thrombin at an early stage in the coagulation sequence. This results in preventing the initiation of clot formation, but is ineffective once Factor X has been activated and the coagulation process has started. No laboratory monitoring is required.

Heparin 5000 u. s.c. is given 2 h preoperatively and q 8 to 12 h (q 12 h appears to be equally effective and perhaps somewhat safer) thereafter for 7 days. The risk of major hemorrhage does not appear to be increased, though more wound hematomas have been observed. Low-dose heparin is usually recommended for patients undergoing thoracic, abdominal, urologic, or gynecologic surgery who are over age 40 to 50 yr, or who have risk factors such as prior thromboembolism, estrogen therapy, or obesity. Low-dose heparin prophylaxis is commonly employed for hospitalized patients with cardiac failure, acute myocardial infarction, stroke, paraplegia, or other debilitating disease, though its efficacy in these conditions is not clearly established. Use of low-dose heparin appears to be ineffective in patients undergoing hip surgery or abdominal prostatectomy, and is **contraindicated** in cerebral surgery.

Agents to prevent platelet aggregation (aspirin, dipyridamole) have been used to prevent venous thromboembolism, but results of these trials have been inconclusive or frankly negative. Dextran appears to be effective in reducing the incidence of thromboembolism in postoperative patients, but requires IV administration, is no more efficacious than warfarin, and has no fewer hemorrhagic complications.

Treatment

The management of pulmonary embolism involves treatment of the initial thromboembolic event and prevention of further thromboembolic episodes.

Treatment of the initial event is supportive. Analgesics are given if pleuritic pain is severe. Though anxiety is often prominent, sedation, particularly with barbiturates, should be undertaken with caution. O_2 therapy is indicated when appreciable arterial hypoxemia ($Pa_{O_2} < 50$ to 60 mm Hg) is present. Continuous O_2 should be given, usually by mask, in a concentration sufficient to raise arterial O_2 tension and saturation to normal (85 to 95 mm Hg, 95 to 98%) or as near normal levels as possible (at least > 50 to 60 mm Hg).

In patients with clinical findings suggestive of pulmonary hypertension and acute cor pulmonale, particularly pending diagnostic procedures such as lung scanning and/or arteriography, β-adrenergic stimulation may be helpful in maintaining tissue perfusion by virtue of its pulmonary vasodilator and cardiotonic effects. Isoproterenol 2 to 4 mg/L of 5% D/W may be infused at a rate sufficient to maintain systolic BP at 90 to 100 mm Hg under continuous ECG monitoring. Appropriate pharmacologic agents may be useful in aborting and preventing supraventricular tachyarrhythmias. Digitalis should be avoided during acute hypoxemia unless absolutely necessary; e.g., for serious arrhythmia or heart failure. When given IV, a modest initial dose is usually desirable (digoxin 0.25 to 0.5 mg; deslanoside 0.4 to 0.8 mg). Response to therapy in patients suspected of hemodynamic impairment with acute cor pulmonale may be monitored by serial measurement of arterial blood gases and hemodynamic parameters. Use of a flow-directed balloon (Swan-Ganz) catheter is valuable for determination of pulmonary artery and wedge pressures, as well as mixed venous blood O_2 saturation and/or content as an index of cardiac output.

Following **massive embolism**, particularly with hypotension, or submassive embolism and hypotension in patients with preexisting cardiorespiratory disease, 2 approaches to management may be considered: pulmonary embolectomy or thrombolytic therapy. In the event of cardiac arrest with massive embolism, the usual resuscitative measures are ineffective due to obstruction of blood flow through the lungs. In this setting, emergency partial (femoral venoarterial) bypass, pending pulmonary embolectomy, may be life-saving. In view of the considerable potential for diagnoses other than embolism, pulmonary angiography while on bypass is advisable in most cases prior to surgery.

Thrombolytic therapy may now be considered as an alternative to embolectomy when massive embolism is uncomplicated by hypotension or when systolic BP can be maintained at 90 to 100 mm Hg on moderate vasopressor dosage. Streptokinase and urokinase are equally effective fibrinolytic activators and exert their thrombolytic effect by enhancing conversion of plasminogen to plasmin, the active fibrinolytic enzyme. **Contraindications** to thrombolytic therapy include stroke within 2 mo, active bleeding from any source, preexisting hemorrhagic diathesis (as in severe liver or kidney disease), pregnancy, and surgery within the preceding 10 days—the latter representing a major limitation to its use. Therapy should be carried out within 3 days of the embolic episode, as organization of the thrombus will obviate the lytic effect.

Initially, a streptokinase resistance test is carried out, and if resistance levels are in excess of 1,000,000 IU, streptokinase should not be given. A loading dose of 250,000 IU streptokinase is given IV over a 30-min period, followed by a maintenance infusion of 100,000 IU/h for 24 h. Since antibodies to streptokinase develop, repeat administration should not be undertaken for 6 to 9 mo.

If the patient has been on heparin, prothrombin time should be permitted to fall to < 2 times control before initiating therapy. Similarly, for initiation of heparin therapy after thrombolytic treatment, it is desirable to wait until prothrombin time has fallen to < 2 times control. All patients on thrombolytic therapy have an increased bleeding risk, particularly from recent operative wounds, needle puncture sites, sites of invasive procedures, and the GI tract. Thus, invasive procedures should be avoided whenever possible; pressure dressings are usually required to stop oozing. Reversal of the fibrinolytic state is effectively brought about by giving ε-aminocaproic acid.

Preventing further thrombus formation with embolization then becomes the essence of treatment. Heparin may be given IV q 4 to 6 h, or by continuous IV drip with an infusion pump. Some evidence suggests that hemorrhagic complications are reduced by continuous infusion, which obviates the peaks and troughs of blood levels with bolus injection. By either method of administration, larger dosage may be required for the first 48 h.

Following a bolus loading dose of heparin 100 u./kg, it is given at a rate to keep the clotting time **(CT)** 2 to 2.5 times control or the partial thromboplastin time **(PTT)** 1.5 to 2 times control by checking the level 30 min prior to giving the next dose of heparin. The maintenance dose by continuous infusion is usually 10 to 50 u./kg/h. Once a therapeutic level is established with continuous infusion, CT and/or PTT need to be monitored only 1 to 2 times/day.

A hemorrhagic disorder or an active bleeding site is an **absolute contraindication** to heparin therapy; septic embolization is usually taken as a contraindication. Hemorrhagic complications of heparin therapy may require cessation of the drug; if severe, protamine sulfate may be given in an initial dose of 50 mg IV. Hemorrhagic complications are frequent in patients over age 65, particularly women, and heparin should be given to these patients only for short periods—usually no more than several days—before changing to an oral anticoagulant.

After 7 to 14 days, or when the patient becomes ambulatory, oral warfarin sodium is given in addition to heparin. The oral agent and heparin should overlap for 5 to 7 days, allowing the oral anticoagulant to take effect. Warfarin sodium may be given, usually in a dosage of 10 to 20 mg/day. When the prothrombin time rises to a level 1.5 to 2.5 times control, heparin is discontinued.

The use of any drug containing aspirin by patients taking anticoagulants should be avoided since aspirin can further impair hemostatic mechanisms. Drugs that interfere with protein binding or metabolism of the oral anticoagulants (e.g., barbiturates, quinine, phenylbutazone, clofibrate, chloral hydrate) should be used cautiously when given simultaneously with warfarin.

The duration of anticoagulation therapy is adjusted individually for each patient. In patients with a definable, reversible cause (e.g., the postoperative state), anticoagulation need be continued only until the condition is corrected (e.g., the patient is fully ambulatory). Otherwise, anticoagulation therapy may be continued empirically for 3 to 6 mo. A patient with a chronic medical disorder associated with high incidence of thromboembolism should be continued for long-term anticoagulant therapy.

Surgical venous interruption of the inferior vena cava should be considered in certain situations: (1) contraindications to anticoagulation, (2) recurrent emboli despite adequate anticoagulation, (3) septic pelvic thrombophlebitis with emboli, and (4) in conjunction with pulmonary embolectomy. Venous ligation at the femoral level is accompanied by unacceptable mortality from postoperative pulmonary embolism. The optimum site of interruption is the inferior vena cava just below the entry of the renal veins together with the spermatic or ovarian veins. Various procedures to interrupt the vena cava partially or completely are used. Patients who have had vena caval interruption require anticoagulation for at least 6 mo following the procedure. Morbidity following such procedures is significant (10 to 15%), and recurrent embolization may occur in as many as 50% of patients from the site of interruption or through large collateral (lumbar) veins if interruption is complete.

---

38. PNEUMONIA

An acute infection of the parenchyma (alveolar spaces and/or interstitial tissue) of the lung. Involvement of an entire lobe is called **lobar pneumonia;** of parts of the lobe only, **segmental** (or **lobular**) pneumonia; and of alveoli contiguous to bronchi, **bronchopneumonia.** It is most useful to refer to the pneumonia as bacterial or nonbacterial, or according to its specific etiologic agent, if known (e.g., pneumococcal, Friedländer's, mycoplasmal, viral, fungal, protozoal).

The microorganisms causing bacterial pneumonia include *Streptococcus pneumoniae* (pneumococci), *Staphylococcus aureus*, Group A hemolytic streptococci, *Klebsiella pneumoniae* (Friedländer's bacillus), *Hemophilus influenzae*, and *Francisella tularensis*. Pneumonia may also be caused by other bacterial pathogens, including the tubercle bacillus, or by viruses, rickettsias, or fungi. Pneumonia due to *Escherichia coli* and other gram-negative bacilli may complicate treatment with antimicrobial drugs inhibiting gram-positive bacteria, with immunosuppressive agents, or with both. Viral pneumonias may be more common than bacterial pneumonias in some populations, though demonstration of the causative agent requires special technics. For a description of etiologic agents and manifestations of bacterial pneumonia in newborns, see RESPIRATORY DISORDERS in Vol. II, Ch. 21.

Predisposing factors include the common cold, other acute viral respiratory infections, acute and chronic alcoholism, malnutrition, debility, exposure, coma, bronchial tumor, foreign matter in the respiratory tract (e.g., aspiration of vomitus or other material), treatment with immunosuppressive agents, and hypostasis.

PNEUMOCOCCAL PNEUMONIA

Pneumococcal pneumonia, the most common bacterial pneumonia, is usually lobar, but it may be segmental. Many of its features are similar to those of pneumonia caused by other organisms. The disease is generally sporadic but most frequent in winter. Healthy or convalescent carriers usually infect others, but there is no practical way to distinguish these carriers, especially from those with chronic bronchitis or bronchiectasis, to eliminate the organisms.

Pathology and Pathogenesis

Pneumococci reach the lungs via the respiratory passages. They lodge in the bronchioles and cause collapse of corresponding alveoli, where they proliferate and initiate an inflammatory process that begins with an outpouring of protein-rich fluid into the alveolar spaces. This fluid acts as a culture medium for the pneumococci and as a vehicle for their spread to other alveoli, segments (lobules), and lobes.

Pathologically, the early stage of pneumonia (the first 12 to 48 h) is called "**red hepatization**" because of the liver-like, reddish appearance of the consolidated lung that results from characteristic widespread dilation of pulmonary blood vessels and extravasation of erythrocytes into the alveoli.

A few hours after pulmonary capillaries dilate and edema fluid pours into the alveoli, polymorphonuclear leukocytes enter the alveolar spaces, rapidly fill the alveoli, and consolidate the lung ("**grey hepatization**"). "**Surface phagocytosis**" occurs (without antibodies) by leukocytic trapping of bacteria against an alveolar wall or other leukocytes; the process is more active when fibrin and large numbers of leukocytes are present. Tissue sections show few pneumococci in the consolidated lung but many in the advancing margin of the lesion, where edema fluid is abundant but leukocytes are sparse.

The "**macrophage reaction**" occurs next, as large mononuclear cells enter the alveoli, engulf any remaining pneumococci, and phagocytize the cellular debris of the exudate. This process continues until resolution is complete, indicated by physical examination and x-ray evidence that the lungs are clear.

The pathogenesis of other bacterial pneumonias resembles that of pneumococcal infections, but abscess formation may occur when infection is caused by organisms (e.g., staphylococci or gram-negative rods) that destroy pulmonary tissue.

Symptoms and Signs

Pneumonia often is preceded by URI. Onset usually is sudden, with a shaking chill, sharp pain in the involved hemithorax (**pleurisy**), cough with early sputum production, fever, and headache. All of these symptoms usually are present. Other presenting symptoms may include nausea and vomiting and, in children, a convulsion. Dyspnea is frequent; respiration is rapid (25 to 45/min) and painful due to pleuritic involvement; an expiratory grunt is characteristic. Delirium may occur, especially in alcoholic patients, when fever is high or cyanosis is marked. Often cyanotic and sweating profusely, the patient is acutely ill. The temperature rises rapidly to 38 to 40.5 C (100.4 to 105 F); the pulse accelerates to between 100 and 130. Signs of consolidation may be lacking during the first few hours, but fine rales and suppressed breath sounds soon are heard over the involved area. Frank consolidation, involving part of one or more lobes, is found later. A pleural friction rub often is heard in the early stages over the area of consolidation and at the site of the pain.

The cough is initially dry and hacking; however, if bronchitis preceded the pneumonia, coughing produces purulent sputum. Coughing usually occurs in extremely painful paroxysms. In later stages, the cough is more productive and usually painless. The sputum, pinkish or blood-flecked at first, becomes rusty at the height of the illness, then yellow and mucopurulent during resolution.

GI symptoms (abdominal distention, jaundice, diarrhea) often are present. In right-sided pneumonias involving the middle or lower lobes, tenderness and rigidity of the right side of the abdomen may suggest gallbladder disease, appendicitis, or peritonitis. Herpes infection often is present, usually on the lips and face.

Some cases have a more gradual, insidious onset, with URI and acute bronchitis, persisting or increasing fever, leukocytosis, and minimal physical signs (moist rales initially, with evidence of consolidation later).

Diagnosis

Pneumococcal pneumonia should be suspected in any patient with an acute febrile illness associated with chill, chest pain, and cough (especially cough with expectoration of viscid, rusty sputum, which is practically diagnostic by itself). Diagnosis is confirmed if physical examination discloses tachycardia, tachypnea, cyanosis, and signs of consolidation. Chest x-ray may provide further confirmation and, in early cases, may yield the only positive evidence of pulmonary consolidation. The WBC count may be normal or low but usually is elevated, and polymorphonuclear neutrophils predominate. The causative bacterium is determined by sputum smears and cultures and, in bacteremia, by blood cultures as well. Pneumococci are typed by the capsular swelling technic. Some laboratories now determine serotypes by counterimmunoelectrophoresis (CIE) of sputum, urine, or other body fluids (serum, pleural or cerebrospinal fluid) against type-specific antisera.

Prognosis

Of those treated, 90 to 95% of patients from age 2 to 50 survive; patients treated during the first 5 days of illness are most likely to recover. Any of the following factors makes the outlook less favorable and convalescence more prolonged: age < 1 yr or > 60 yr; a positive blood culture, especially if the number of colonies exceeds 100/ml; involvement of 2 or more lobes; WBC count < 5000; BUN > 70 mg/100 ml; underlying chronic disease; or development of an extrapulmonary focus of pneumococcal infection, such as meningitis or endocarditis. Complicating meningitis is the most serious adverse factor, but early recognition and treatment save many patients.

Treatment

Sputum and blood should be collected for culture before starting antimicrobial therapy. Pending demonstration of the pathogen by culture, specific therapy is based tentatively on the history, physical examination, Gram stain of the sputum, and capsular swelling test or CIE. A change in antibacterial therapy may be indicated by the results of the sputum and blood cultures. Penicillin G is the drug of choice if pneumococcal pneumonia is suspected, but the cephalosporins, tetracyclines, erythromycin, and lincomycin are also useful (see also PNEUMOCOCCAL INFECTIONS in Ch. 8).

Specific therapy: Crystalline penicillin G 600,000 u. is given IM q 12 h; it should be given IV q 6 h if the patient is in shock or if bacteremia is present or suspected. Patients without GI symptoms and signs who are not severely ill may be given potassium penicillin V 250 mg orally q 6 h and this regimen may be used when parenteral therapy is precluded or difficult. Decreased susceptibility of pneumococci has been reported (not in USA); where present, larger doses may be required. Tetracycline or erythromycin 500 mg q 6 h, or lincomycin or clindamycin 600 mg q 12 h, may be given parenterally or orally to penicillin-allergic patients, but sensitivity of the pneumococcus to these drugs must be confirmed if the patient fails to respond, since some strains are resistant to these agents. The cephalosporins (cephalothin or cefazolin 250 to 500 mg q 6 h, IM or IV) are also effective, but patients hypersensitive to penicillins should be considered potentially hypersensitive to cephalosporins. If meningitis is present or suspected, the dose of penicillin G should be 2 million u. q 2 h IV. Spinal fluid should be obtained for culture before such treatment is started. For pneumococcal **meningitis** in patients hypersensitive to penicillins, chloramphenicol 1 gm IV q 6 h (or tetracycline 1 gm IV q 12 h, except in infants and children) is the drug of choice; a cephalosporin should not be used because most do not enter the subarachnoid space.

Response to therapy is often prompt, but fever may persist for 4 days or longer in 50% of patients. Therapy need not be modified if steady though gradual improvement is evident. However, persisting fever without clinical improvement demands careful reexamination of the patient for extrapulmonary foci of infection, signs of hypersensitivity to medication, or evidence of superinfection; therapy should be modified according to the findings. In uncomplicated illness, antibiotic therapy is continued until the patient has been afebrile for at least 48 h.

Pleural empyema complicates about 5% of pneumococcal pneumonias. Diagnostic thoracentesis should be performed if there is pleural fluid, persistent fever, and leukocytosis. Pus, if present, should be aspirated and cultured; penicillin G 100,000 to 250,000 u. in 100 ml of sterile saline is injected into the pleural cavity. This procedure is repeated q 24 to 48 h until cultures of the pleural fluid are negative. If the exudate is very viscid, a large intercostal tube is inserted to facilitate drainage; surgery may be required if the empyema is loculated. The daily parenteral penicillin dose is increased to 10 million u./day if empyema is present.

Supportive measures must be instituted immediately: Complete bed rest, fluids, and, if needed, O_2 and analgesics should be given during the acute phase. O_2 is given to patients with cyanosis, marked dyspnea, circulatory disturbances, asthenia, or delirium. It may ameliorate cough and restlessness and prevent or relieve abdominal distention. The efficacy of O_2 therapy should be monitored by periodic determinations of blood gases, especially in patients with underlying emphysema or ventilatory disease. Patients who are treated during the first 2 days of illness and who respond rapidly may be allowed out of bed after they have been afebrile for 2 or 3 days. Longer periods of partial bed rest may be required for those who survive a stormy course.

Prophylaxis: A vaccine consisting of 14 of the 80-plus specific pneumococcal type-specific polysaccharides is available. The 14 types include about 80% of the pneumococci that cause serious infections: pneumonia, bacteremia, meningitis, empyema, and otitis media. Available data suggest that it is about 80% effective in preventing such serious infections with these types in persons > 2 yr old. There are insufficient data to evaluate the protection afforded infants and children < 2 yr old, splenectomized (asplenic) patients, those with sickle cell disease, and particularly people > 60 yr old, those with immunologic defects or chronic debilitating diseases and other predisposing illness, but some degree of protection has been noted in such individuals.

A single injection of vaccine containing 50 μg of each constituent, given IM, affords protection against most of the types in the vaccine up to 3 to 5 yr, and revaccination within that interval is not recommended. Reactions to the injection are infrequent, mild, and usually limited to local swelling, tenderness, and, infrequently, fever and general malaise. These reactions are more frequent and exaggerated after revaccination within 3 to 5 yr.

STAPHYLOCOCCAL PNEUMONIA

Etiology

Staphylococcal pneumonia is usually caused by coagulase-positive *Staphylococcus aureus*. It is often a complication of influenza, but may be primary, particularly in infants and the aged. It also occurs in hospitalized patients as a superinfection accompanying debility, surgery, tracheostomy, coma, or diseases or immunosuppressive therapy affecting host defenses against infection. Staphylococcal bacteremia complicating infections at other sites (furuncles, carbuncles) may cause hematogenous pulmonary involvement.

Symptoms and Signs

Some or all of the symptoms of pneumococcal pneumonia (pleural pain, dyspnea, cyanosis, productive cough) may be present in varying degrees of severity, and, in cases complicating influenza, may appear at any stage of the illness. Sputum may be copious and salmon-colored. Prostration is often marked. Physical examination of the lungs frequently demonstrates patchy involvement of several pulmonary segments, but lobar involvement may also occur. Pneumatoceles from < 1 cm to several cm in diameter, though common, may be difficult to detect by physical examination. Leukocytosis usually is present. Empyema is common in infancy. Furuncles are seen occasionally, and, if bacteremia occurs, metastatic abscesses may be found in the liver, kidneys, brain, or elsewhere.

Diagnosis

The symptoms and signs of pneumonia and a positive sputum (if the organism predominates) or blood culture are diagnostic. Gram stain of the sputum provides the earliest diagnostic clue and almost invariably contains myriads of gram-positive cocci resembling staphylococci. X-ray early in the disease shows many small, round areas of densities that later enlarge and coalesce to form abscesses and leave evidence of multiple cavities or pneumatoceles during resolution.

Prognosis and Treatment

Mortality is high, particularly in infants and in cases complicating influenza. The general principles of treatment for pneumococcal pneumonia (above) apply to staphylococcal pneumonia. Copious respiratory secretions or laryngeal involvement with diphtheritic-like membrane, however, may necessitate tracheostomy to maintain adequate toilet of the respiratory tract (especially when cough is ineffective and cyanosis is present). Because strains of staphylococci vary widely in sensitivity to antibacterial agents, the susceptibility of the infecting strain to all known potentially effective antibiotics must be assessed.

Until the sensitivity results are known, a penicillinase-resistant penicillin (oxacillin or nafcillin) or a cephalosporin should be given; the dose for each is 2 gm IV in saline over a 30-min period q 4 to 6 h or, to avoid the pain and discomfort of repeated injections, 8 to 12 gm/day by continuous IV infusion. Penicillin G 12 million u./day by continuous IV infusion is less expensive and may be substituted for the former antibiotics if the organism is penicillin-sensitive. Therapy is continued for 2 wk after the patient has become afebrile and the lungs have shown signs of clearing. Vancomycin 0.5 gm IV q 4 or 6 h is the drug of choice for patients allergic to penicillin and cephalosporin and for those not responding to other antistaphylococcal drugs. Vancomycin may be discontinued after the fever has subsided and staphylococci have been cleared from the sputum. Bacteremia that persists during several days of adequate antimicrobial therapy suggests endocarditis or other focal disease (osteomyelitis or multiple small brain abscesses) even in the absence of specific diagnostic signs and is an indication for continuing chemotherapy for an additional week or two.

STREPTOCOCCAL PNEUMONIA

Etiology

Hemolytic streptococci of Lancefield's Group A are the most common causative organisms, though other streptococci occasionally are responsible. The disease is now infrequently seen except as a complication of measles or influenza. Before modern chemotherapy, it commonly followed streptococcal sore throat or scarlet fever, but now rarely does.

Symptoms, Signs, and Diagnosis

The disease, which occurred in epidemics in military camps in both World Wars, usually begins with a sore throat, accompanied or followed by laryngitis and tracheobronchitis with presternal soreness and pain on coughing. It spreads by way of the bronchial and pleural lymphatics, producing bronchopneumonic lesions and pleural effusion. Toxemia is often pronounced. Early in the course of the pneumonia, presence of a large pleural effusion, frequently bloody, suggests Group A streptococcal pneumonia. A history of recent pharyngitis, measles, or influenza, with early development of empyema, is suggestive. Diagnosis is confirmed by demonstration of streptococci in sputum, blood, and pleural exudate. The gross appearance of sputum is not diagnostic, but stained smears may show chains of gram-positive cocci that can be identified by culture on blood agar.

Although **prognosis** has improved greatly since the introduction of chemotherapy, hemolytic streptococcal pneumonia may be a fulminant infection, especially when it complicates influenza or accompanies bacteremia, empyema, or both. Mild cases are seen occasionally.

Treatment

Penicillin G 1 million u. IM or IV q 4 or 6 h is the preferred drug for Group A streptococcal pneumonia. Cephalosporins (see PNEUMOCOCCAL PNEUMONIA, above) may be used for patients allergic to penicillin, but some patients hypersensitive to penicillin are also allergic to cephalosporins. In penicillin-allergic patients tetracycline or erythromycin may be given, but, since strains of Group A streptococci are often resistant to these drugs, the sensitivity of the isolated organism must be determined, and treatment is started promptly pending the results. Supportive therapy is the same as for pneumococcal pneumonia, above.

Empyema must always be anticipated and sought; exploratory thoracentesis should be performed to resolve any doubt. If pleural exudate is found, it should be aspirated and cultured. Penicillin G 250,000 or 500,000 u. in 25 or 50 ml of saline is instilled and the daily parenteral penicillin dosage is increased to 10 million u./day if empyema is present. Closed catheter drainage should be used if large amounts of fluid reaccumulate, and the catheter usually may be removed after 24 to 72 h. Plastic pleuritis rarely is seen.

PNEUMONIA CAUSED BY *Klebsiella* AND BY GRAM-NEGATIVE INTESTINAL BACILLI

Etiology and Pathology

Any of the more than 70 types of *Klebsiella pneumoniae* (Friedländer's bacillus) may cause pneumonia, though infection with Type 1 or 2 is most common. In *Klebsiella* pneumonia, the exudate is extremely viscid, necrosis and abscesses of the lung are common in the acute stage, and chronic abscess may complicate recovery. Pneumonia may also result from pulmonary infection with *Escherichia coli*, *Proteus* spp., *Salmonella* spp., *Pseudomonas aeruginosa*, anaerobic *Bacteroides* spp., and, in persons exposed in Southeast Asia, *Pseudomonas pseudomallei* (see also MELIOIDOSIS in Ch. 8).

Symptoms and Signs

The findings are similar to those of pneumococcal pneumonia, above, though onset may be more gradual and bronchopneumonia is the usual type of pulmonary involvement. Pleural involvement is common and the course often is fulminant. Signs of cavitation may develop and persist if the illness becomes chronic.

Diagnosis

Patients with pneumonia caused by klebsiellas or other enterobacteria usually are critically ill. The disease is suspected in any patient with unusually rapid spread of consolidation from one lobe to another. Predisposing conditions include alcoholism, diabetes mellitus, aspiration, immunosuppressive therapy, or suppression of the gram-positive respiratory tract flora by prior antimicrobial treatment. In Friedländer's pneumonia, the sputum is viscid and "ropy," and may be "brick-red" in color; stained smears typically show many encapsulated gram-negative bacilli. Mixed infection with *Pneumococcus* may occur. Blood culture frequently is positive. The pneumonic exudate may be sufficiently extensive to cause enlargement of the affected lobe, reflected in the x-ray by a downward curve of the horizontal interlobar fissure if the right upper lobe is involved. Areas of increased radiance within dense consolidation suggest cavitation. This finding, especially frequent in Friedländer's pneumonia, is not pathognomonic. In pneumonias caused by other gram-negative rods, the disease may develop and progress more slowly. Fever and cough are accompanied by purulent sputum containing large numbers of gram-negative rods, generally without the layer surrounding capsules characteristic of Friedländer's bacillus.

Prognosis

Mortality is high in Friedländer's and in other enterobacterial pneumonias, especially when treatment is delayed beyond the 2nd day of illness. Abscesses are common and may persist following recovery from the acute stage of the disease. Empyema may develop and require therapy as for empyema in pneumococcal pneumonia.

Treatment

Klebsiellas and other intestinal gram-negative bacilli vary widely in antibacterial susceptibility. The antibiotic sensitivity of the causative organism must be determined. Treatment may begin with a cephalosporin 8 to 12 gm/day IV and gentamicin 1 mg/kg IM or IV q 8 h until such information is available. Tetracycline 500 mg (or chloramphenicol 1 gm) may be given IV q 4 or 6 h in place of the cephalosporin, though chloramphenicol should be given only if suggested by the sensitivity tests. If the infection is not caused by *P. aeruginosa* and if the organism is sensitive, kanamycin 0.5 gm IM q 12 h may be given instead of gentamicin. In patients with impaired renal function, gentamicin and kanamycin dosages must be adjusted to avoid toxic effects. Pneumonia caused by sensitive strains of *P. aeruginosa* should be treated with carbenicillin 24 to 30 gm/day (or ticarcillin 10 to 16 gm/day) IV and gentamicin 1 to 1.5 mg/kg IM or IV q 8 h. Tobramycin 1 to 1.5 mg/kg, amikacin 5 mg/kg, or colistin 1 mg/kg IM q 8 h may be substituted for control of gentamicin-resistant organisms if sensitivity tests suggest use of either drug. In patients with reduced renal function (elevated serum creatinine) the doses should be appropriately adjusted downward. Infections caused by *P. pseudomallei* do not respond to polymyxins and are best treated with tetracycline, chloramphenicol, sulfadiazine, or kanamycin in varying combinations based on the sensitivities of the organism and the clinical severity of illness. The antimicrobial sensitivity of *Serratia* spp. and *Enterobacter* spp. should be determined in vitro; many strains sensitive to carbenicillin and gentamicin are resistant to colistin. Penicillin G 12 to 24 million u./day IV, clindamycin phosphate 2 gm/day IV, or chloramphenicol 4 gm/day IV may be given as initial treatment for pneumonia caused by *Bacteroides* spp., and changed depending on the organisms' in vitro sensitivity if the patient does not improve after 48 h. Empyema is treated by aspiration of fluid and, if indicated, by tube-drainage. Abscess is treated by postural drainage if x-ray shows a fluid level.

PNEUMONIA CAUSED BY *Hemophilus influenzae*

Etiology

Hemophilus influenzae was one of the principal bacterial causes of the pneumonias complicating the influenza pandemics of 1889 and 1918. Those pneumonias, rapidly lethal in a large percentage of cases, have not been encountered in subsequent epidemics of viral influenza; *H. influenzae* is now an infrequent cause of pneumonia. In infants and young children it is usually due to capsular Type B; it is most often associated with meningitis, and the organism may be cultured from blood. In older children and occasionally in adults, pneumonia occurs in patients with *H. influenzae* Type B, which may also cause acute epiglottitis. In older adults, pneumonia due to *H. influenzae* occurs predominantly in patients with chronic bronchitis and bronchiectasis and may be caused by any of several serotypes but predominantly by nonencapsulated, untypable strains. In these cases, sputum may yield both pneumococci and *H. influenzae*; though therapy with penicillin G or V, or with ampicillin or amoxicillin may produce clinical improvement and eradicate the pneumococci from the sputum, exacerbation of symptoms and signs may follow, with *H. influenzae* appearing in abundance in sputum. In such cases treatment with chloramphenicol is indicated.

Symptoms, Signs, and Diagnosis

H. influenzae pneumonia usually follows common viral URIs and is characterized by bronchopneumonia, bronchitis, and bronchiolitis (almost never by lobar pneumonia) with corresponding physical and x-ray findings. Symptoms include fever (to 99 F or sometimes higher), cough that may be croupy, malaise, myalgias, arthralgias (in adults), and increase in sputum, which may become yellow or greenish. Cyanosis may be marked, especially in infants and young children.

The characteristic small pleomorphic, gram-negative bacillus usually is seen in large numbers in gram-stained smears of sputum; satellite colonies are often seen around colonies of *Staphylococcus* on blood agar plates. Positive blood cultures confirm the diagnosis in some cases. Encapsulated strains may be typed by demonstrating capsular swelling with type-specific antiserum.

Prognosis and Treatment

Unless appropriate treatment is delayed until the bronchiolitis and pneumonia advance to produce severe cyanosis and anoxemia, most patients recover. Because penicillinase-producing strains of *H. influenzae* have appeared recently, sputum and pharyngeal swabs and blood should be obtained for culture, and therapy started with ampicillin 100 mg/kg/day IV *and* chloramphenicol 50 mg/kg/day IV in infants (orally when feasible). If the organism proves sensitive to ampicillin, the chloramphenicol is discontinued; if resistant, ampicillin is stopped.

PNEUMONIA OF LEGIONNAIRES' DISEASE

An acute bacterial infection caused by Legionella pneumophila *and characterized by pneumonia, high fever, relative bradycardia, dry cough, shaking chills, pleuritic pain, and diarrhea.*

Etiology and Epidemiology

Investigation of an outbreak of acute febrile respiratory illness occurring in members of the American Legion in Philadelphia in 1976 led to the discovery of a previously unrecognized bacterium. The name of the newly recognized bacterium is *Legionella pneumophila*. Human disease due to *L. pneumophila* has been retrospectively documented to have occurred as early as 1947, and outbreaks of the disease have occurred since at least 1965. More than 1000 cases have been reported throughout the USA, and additional cases have been recognized in England, Europe, Israel, and Australia.

Although apparently sporadic cases occur, there is a striking tendency for cases of Legionnaires' disease to appear in clusters. Outbreaks are typically associated with specific buildings (especially hospitals, hotels) or discrete geographic areas. *L. pneumophila* has been recovered from environmental water sources including lakes, creeks, cooling towers, evaporative condensers, ultrasonic nebulizers, showerheads, and hot water tanks. Mechanical devices (e.g., air conditioners) may serve as vectors of airborne spread.

Person-to-person transmission has not been demonstrated. The usual incubation period is 2 to 10 days. Most cases occur in summer or fall. The disease may occur at any age; however, most identified cases have occurred in middle-aged patients (mean age, 56 yr). There is a 2.5:1 male to female predominance. Identified risk factors include smoking, alcohol abuse, excavation adjacent to residence, construction work, and overnight travel during the incubation period. Underlying conditions, such as immunosuppressive therapy, cardiopulmonary, neoplastic, and renal disease, have been present in almost 50% of the reported cases. Renal transplant recipients appear to be at particular risk.

Symptoms and Signs

The manifestations of infecton with *L. pneumophila* range from asymptomatic seroconversion to severe, sometimes fatal, bronchopneumonia (Legionnaire's disease). A characteristic sign in patients with Legionnaires' disease is high fever with relative bradycardia. There is stepwise increase in temperature over several days with maximum temperature typically in excess of 39.4 C. The fever tends to be nonremitting. Physical examination of the chest shows rales early in the illness with consolidation noted as the disease progresses. Confusion, disorientation, and lethargy are noted in 1/3 of patients.

Anorexia, profound weakness, and malaise are almost universal symptoms. Cough occurs in > 90% of patients. Cough is typically dry and not troublesome. With progression of illness, minimally purulent, watery, frequently blood-tinged sputum may be produced. Recurrent shaking chills, pleuritic pain, and diarrhea are the other major symptoms. The diarrhea usually begins early in illness and is watery without blood or mucus. Small pleural effusions are common. Pulmonary cavitation has been observed but is unusual. Headache, nausea, vomiting, dyspnea, myalgia, and arthralgia may be present. Upper respiratory tract symptoms such as rhinitis and pharyngitis are distinctly unusual.

The term **Pontiac fever** refers to an illness that occurred during an outbreak in Pontiac, Michigan in 1968. It was characterized by fever, chills, headache, and myalgia, but was unassociated with pneumonia and/or mortality. Pontiac fever appears distinct from Legionnaires' disease; however, there is strong epidemiologic and bacteriologic evidence that Pontiac fever was caused by *L. pneumophila*. The full spectrum of disease caused by *L. pneumophila* remains to be defined.

Laboratory findings are nonspecific. Examination of sputum uncontaminated by oropharyngeal flora shows few to moderate polymorphonuclear leukocytes and no bacteria. Chest x-rays show patchy alveolar infiltrates, which progress to local consolidation and/or spread to involve other areas of lung.

Leukocytosis and elevation of the ESR are usual. Leukopenia may herald a poor prognosis. Disseminated intravascular coagulopathy may occur but is rare. Mild to moderate elevations of alkaline phosphatase, LDH, and AST (formerly SGOT), hyponatremia (in some instances due to the syndrome of inappropriate ADH secretion) and hypophosphatemia are frequent findings. Proteinuria is common. Hematuria and renal failure may occur. CSF examination is normal.

Diagnosis

L. pneumophila is a fastidious gram-negative bacterium. Six serogroups have been recognized. *L. pneumophila* has been cultured from lung tissue, transtracheal aspirate, pleural fluid, and blood. The solid media recommended for isolation is charcoal yeast extract agar.

The organism may be demonstrated in lung tissue and sputum by the use of special stains. The direct fluorescent antibody stain provides rapid, specific diagnosis. The Dieterle silver impregnation and Gimenez stains demonstrate the organism well, but are not specific. The Gram stain of clinical specimens is usually negative.

Serologic diagnosis is made by demonstration of a 4-fold rise in indirect fluorescent antibody titer to 1:128 or greater. Diagnostic rise in titer usually occurs 3 to 6 wk after onset of illness and, therefore is useful in retrospective diagnosis only. Sera should be obtained early in illness and at 3 and 6 wk after onset. A small percentage of patients with Legionnaires' disease do not develop a detectable antibody response.

The differential diagnosis of Legionnaires' disease includes pneumonia due to *Mycoplasma pneumoniae, Chlamydia psittaci, Coxiella burneti,* and viruses. The clinical presentation may also mimic pulmonary embolism.

Treatment and Prognosis

Erythromycin 500 mg to 1 gm orally or IV q 6 h is the drug of choice. The clinical response is often prompt, although progression on x-ray and persistent temperature elevation may be noted for several days. Therapy should be continued for 3 wk. Relapse and protracted convalescence have been noted in patients who have received shorter courses. Tetracycline 2 gm/day may be an effective alternative agent; however, experience is more limited than with erythromycin. Successful therapy with a combination of tetracycline and rifampin has been reported.

Mortality rates in patients with Legionnaires' disease are related to the underlying condition of the patient and to early specific therapy. In immunosuppressed patients who do not receive specific antimicrobial therapy, mortality may be as high as 80%.

TULAREMIC PNEUMONIA
(See TULAREMIA in Ch. 8)

PNEUMONIC PLAGUE
(See PLAGUE in Ch. 8)

MYCOPLASMAL PNEUMONIA

Etiology

Many illnesses formerly diagnosed as "primary atypical pneumonia" are caused by the pleuro-pneumonia-like organism *Mycoplasma pneumoniae* (Eaton agent). The disease occurs primarily in children and young adults; epidemics occur in schools and military populations and spread slowly. The incubation period is 10 to 14 days.

Pathology

Patchy areas of consolidation are observed on gross examination of the lungs. *M. pneumoniae* attaches to ciliated epithelium of the lower respiratory tract and, although it does not invade the epithelial cells, it causes destruction. This injury is accompanied by an acute interstitial pneumonitis with intense mononuclear cellular infiltration about the bronchioles; polymorphonuclear cells appear later in the disease in the bronchiolar lumena. The alveoli often are spared, although their septa may be congested and edematous, and they may contain many mononuclear cells (lymphocytes, plasma cells, monocytes, and desquamated alveolar lining cells).

Symptoms and Signs

In contrast to bacterial pneumonia, mycoplasmal pneumonia usually begins gradually. Headache, fever, malaise, and chilliness with frank rigors are common. Cough is often severe and initially nonproductive. Early in the disease, the sparse sputum contains some mononuclear cells but very few bacteria (normal mouth flora). As the illness evolves, mucopurulent, occasionally blood-tinged expectoration develops. Disparity between physical and x-ray chest findings is common during the first few days. Suppressed breath sounds and a few rales may identify the lesion in the absence of definitive x-ray changes, or physical examination may disclose no abnormality despite clearly evident infiltration in the chest x-ray. Pulse and respirations may be normal, even in the presence of fever.

Diagnosis

M. pneumoniae may be isolated by sputum culture on special media, though growth is slow. Various specific serologic tests, including CF, support a presumptive diagnosis. Cold hemagglutinins develop in a majority of the more severely ill patients, but may be delayed in appearance until the 3rd wk of the disease. The frequency of occurrence and range of titers vary widely in different series of cases reported. The WBC count usually is normal. Chest x-ray discloses pulmonary involvement with small round areas of density extending from the hilum at first and then spreading to involve areas within one or more lobes of one or both lungs. In severe cases the chest x-ray may resemble that of miliary TB.

Prognosis and Treatment

Death from mycoplasmal pneumonia is rare, though the illness may occasionally extend for several weeks. Tetracycline or erythromycin 500 mg orally q 6 h may hasten clinical improvement and should be given to severely ill patients, but these drugs may not eradicate the pathogen. Erythromycin-resistant mycoplasmas have been isolated from man. Symptomatic treatment is the same as for pneumococcal pneumonia. Inhalation of warm moist air may help to relieve bronchial irritation.

VIRAL PNEUMONIA

Etiology

Viral pneumonia may be caused by various agents: influenza and parainfluenza viruses; adenoviruses; respiratory syncytial virus; rhinoviruses; coxsackie-, echo-, and reovirus; cytomegalovirus; herpes simplex; and the viruses of the childhood exanthems. The pneumonia is primary, usually from exposure of a nonimmune individual to infected persons shedding virus, and may account for about 75% of all acute pulmonary infections in some populations (schools, military recruits).

Pathology

The trachea and bronchi may contain serosanguineous fluid; the affected areas of the lungs are congested and, at times, hemorrhagic. The ciliated epithelium of the bronchi usually is destroyed, with damage to the walls of the smaller bronchi and bronchioles. An intense inflammatory reaction surrounding these structures and their related blood vessels is composed of mononuclear cells, lymphocytes, and plasma cells in proportions that vary with the causative virus; this is in contrast to the marked predominance of polynuclear leukocytes in bacterial pneumonias. Thickened, edematous alveolar walls and alveoli may contain fibrin, predominantly mononuclear cells, and occasionally some polymorphonuclear leukocytes. In severe or fulminating influenza viral pneumonia, hyaline membranes are found in the alveoli. Characteristic intracellular viral inclusions may be seen in adenovirus, cytomegalovirus, respiratory syncytial virus, or varicella virus infections. Giant cells are typical of pneumonia caused by measles virus.

Symptoms and Signs

Most cases of viral pneumonia are mild, and pulmonary involvement often is undetected. Severe and even fatal illness may result, however, especially with influenza A virus. Pneumonias due to varicella or herpesvirus are associated with the disseminated form of these infections and may be extensive and severe. Symptoms vary widely from those of the common cold to those of rapidly progressive respiratory insufficiency. Constitutional symptoms may be pronounced, with severe headache, anorexia, fever, and myalgia. Sputum usually is mucopurulent, occasionally bloody, and often contains many mononuclear cells. Cough is common. Most viral lung infections are bronchopneumonic, frequently involving more than one pulmonary segment. In severe cases, confluence of lesions may consolidate an entire lobe. Initially, infiltration is less dense than that seen in bacterial pneumonia. The WBC count may be low, normal, or moderately elevated.

Diagnosis

Identifying the organism responsible for sporadic viral pneumonia is difficult, but may be important in institutional or communal outbreaks. The pneumonias complicating exanthematous infections (e.g., measles, herpes, varicella) may be identified tentatively by the morphology and other characteristics of the rash. Finding no bacterial pathogens in sputum cultures while finding mononuclear cells on smears of sputum suggests viral infection; however, the presence of bacteria, especially if only in small numbers, does not exclude it. Since isolation of viruses is still not feasible in many hospitals, the diagnosis of viral pneumonia is often based on clinical or epidemiologic findings and results of serologic tests. Serum should be obtained for serologic testing during both the acute and convalescent phases and sent to laboratories equipped to do the tests or to the public health laboratory to determine the presumptive cause of infection. The results of serologic tests are therefore not helpful in management of the cases.

Prognosis and Treatment

Prognosis varies widely with the causative virus, the extent of pulmonary involvement, the patient's age, and the presence or absence of underlying systemic disease. Treatment is symptomatic (see PNEUMOCOCCAL PNEUMONIA, above). Prophylactic vaccination with influenza A and B is available for those at high risk of serious infection and should be given to persons over age 50, those with chronic cardiac or pulmonary disease, and pregnant women. Amantadine 100 mg orally q 8 or 12 h, if given very early in the course of influenza A infection, may moderate the course of the disease.

RICKETTSIAL PNEUMONIA

(See Q FEVER in Ch. 10)

PSITTACOSIS

(Ornithosis; Parrot Fever)

An infectious atypical form of pneumonia caused by Chlamydia psittaci *and transmitted by certain birds.*

Etiology and Epidemiology

The agent responsible for psittacosis belongs to the genus *Chlamydia* (see Ch. 11). Psittacosis is found principally in the psittacine birds (parrots, parakeets, love-birds), less often in poultry, pigeons, and canaries (in whom it is often called ornithosis), and occasionally in the snowy egret and some seabirds (e.g., herring gulls, petrels, and fulmars). Human infection usually occurs by inhaling dust from feathers or excreta of infected birds; it may also be transmitted to man by a bite from an infected bird or, rarely, by cough droplets of infected patients. Man-to-man transmission may be associated with highly virulent avian strains, or the disease may be transmitted venereally. Pathologic changes are those of a pneumonitis with a mononuclear cell exudate, as in other "primary atypical" (viral and mycoplasmal, above, and rickettsial in Ch. 10) pneumonias.

Symptoms and Signs

Following a 1- to 3-wk incubation period, onset may be insidious or abrupt, with fever, chills, general malaise, and anorexia. The temperature gradually rises and cough develops, initially dry but at times becoming mucopurulent. Chest x-rays during the first week show pneumonitis radiating from the hilum; migratory lesions may be present. During the 2nd wk, pneumonia and frank consolidation may occur with secondary purulent lung infection. The temperature remains elevated for 2 to 3 wk, then falls slowly. The course may be mild or severe, depending on the age of the patient and the extent of pneumonia. A progressive, pronounced increase in pulse and respiratory rates is an ominous sign. Mortality may reach 30% in severe untreated cases, and even higher rates have been reported with virulent strains. Convalescence is gradual and may be prolonged, especially in severe cases.

Diagnosis and Laboratory Findings

Clinical differentiation from other atypical pneumonias is difficult. Initially, the disease may be confused with influenza, typhoid fever, mycoplasmal pneumonia, Legionnaires' disease, or Q fever. Psittacosis is suggested by a history of exposure to birds, and is confirmed by recovery of the agent or by serologic CF tests. In the USA, serum specimens obtained early in the disease and late in convalescence may be submitted to the Center for Disease Control through the State Laboratory Director.

Prophylaxis

Infected flocks of pigeons in the lofts of breeders (e.g., of racing or carrier pigeons) and dust from feathers and cage contents must be avoided; handling sick birds should be avoided. Spread by imported psittacine birds is controlled with a mandatory 45-day course of chlortetracycline-treated feed, which generally, but not always, eliminates any causative organisms from the birds' blood and feces. This may also be useful in controlling the disease in turkeys raised for market. Since cough droplets and sputum may infect other persons by inhalation, strict patient isolation should be instituted when the diagnosis is suspected on clinical and epidemiologic grounds (exposure to possible sources).

Treatment

Tetracycline 1 to 2 gm/day orally in divided doses given q 6 h is effective. Fever and other symptoms usually are controlled within 48 to 72 h, but the antibiotic should be continued for at least 10 days. Strict bed rest, O_2 when needed, and cough control with codeine 15 mg orally q 3 or 4 h are indicated.

FUNGAL PNEUMONIA

Primary fungal pneumonia is most commonly caused by *Histoplasma capsulatum* or *Coccidioides immitis*, and less commonly by species of *Candida*, *Cryptococcus*, or *Blastomyces* (see Ch. 9). Fungal pneumonia also may be a complication of antibacterial therapy, especially in patients with altered host defense mechanisms due to illness or immunosuppressive therapy (see Ch. 6).

PNEUMONIA CAUSED BY *Pneumocystis carinii*

Etiology

Pneumocystis carinii, probably a protozoan, may cause pneumonia in infants with immune deficiencies and in children of 1 to 4 yr who have acute lymphatic leukemia. It has been recognized with increasing frequency as a cause of pneumonia in patients of all ages who have immunologic deficiencies or who are undergoing immunosuppressive treatment (see Ch. 6).

Symptoms, Signs, and Diagnosis

Infection with *P. carinii* should be suspected in any patient receiving immunosuppressive therapy or having an immunologic deficiency who develops progressive pulmonary infiltration and respiratory insufficiency. Diffuse lung involvement, usually beginning in the lower lobes, and progressive respiratory insufficiency with increasing cyanosis are characteristic. The organism cannot be grown, and diagnosis is made by demonstrating it in Gram-Weigert–stained smears of expectorated or aspirated secretions (in occasional cases), but more reliably from stained sections of pulmonary tissue obtained by needle aspiration of open lung biopsy.

Prognosis and Treatment

Although the parasite in its various forms may occur in the body without evidence of infection, untreated acute and active infection usually progresses to death. The therapy of choice at present is trimethoprim/sulfamethoxazole 0.5 gm orally q 4 h until the lesion shows signs of clearing and clinical improvement occurs; it should thus be continued for 3 to 5 days or much longer if immunosuppressive therapy is continued.

POSTOPERATIVE AND POST-TRAUMATIC PNEUMONIAS

Etiology

Hypoventilation, impaired or inhibited cough reflex, bronchospasm, and dehydration may cause retention of bronchial secretions leading to segmental atelectasis and, in turn, to pulmonary infection. The incidence of such infection is higher in winter months and greatest in elderly or debilitated patients. About 60% of postoperative pulmonary infections follow abdominal operations, and about 20% occur after operations on the head and neck. These infections have also become frequent after thoracic operations involving the lung or esophagus. Pneumonia occurs equally after inhalation and spinal anesthesia; only about 10% of such infections follow operations performed under local or IV anesthesia. About 40% of post-traumatic pneumonias are complications of fractured ribs or trauma to the chest; the rest are divided about equally among skull fractures or other head injuries, other fractures, burns, or major contusions. Postoperative pneumonia differs from aspiration pneumonia by the absence of irritating gastric secretions, and anaerobic flora is not usually involved.

Bacteriologic studies of sputum and bronchial secretions show good correlations between profuse growth of pneumococci, *Hemophilus influenzae*, or both, and clinical evidence of pulmonary infection. Purulent sputum usually indicates infection, but scant or mucoid sputum with an abundance of organisms is sometimes found. Cultures yielding *Staphylococcus aureus*, coliform bacilli, or both, may be obtained from patients recently treated with antibiotics; such organisms, unless found in abundance in purulent sputum along with other evidence of clinical infection in the chest, are not an indication for antibacterial therapy.

Symptoms, Signs, and Diagnosis

These are the same as for other bacterial pneumonias caused by the same organisms. X-rays of the chest may show areas of atelectasis and sometimes evidence of pulmonary embolism and infarcts; the latter usually are associated with bloody expectoration (see Ch. 37).

Treatment and Prognosis

A brief period of hyperventilation by inhaling 5% CO_2 during recovery from anesthesia has been recommended to combat atelectasis and decrease bronchial secretion viscosity. After pulmonary infection has developed, a cephalosporin given parenterally is the antibiotic of choice and is likely to be effective, usually with a prompt response.

Prognosis depends on the underlying condition for which the operation was performed, the patient's age and prior health status, and on the nature, location, and extent of trauma. Complications resemble those of other pneumonias of the same bacterial etiology, but empyema may be more frequent in pneumonias that follow trauma or operations involving the lung and mediastinum.

Prevention

Routine use of prophylactic antibiotics preoperatively or immediately following trauma is not recommended. Nevertheless, ampicillin or, preferably, a cephalosporin may be given immediately preceding and after the operation and for not more than 48 h after operations on patients with chronic bronchitis, or following fractures of the skull (but penicillin is recommended to prevent meningitis) or of the ribs when the lungs are traumatized. However, results of prolonged prophylactic antibiotic usage have *not* been uniformly favorable.

ASPIRATION PNEUMONIA

Aspiration pneumonia may follow anesthesia, alcoholic intoxication, convulsive disorders, marked debility or disturbances of consciousness associated with vomiting, or immersion. Aspirated acid vomitus into the lower respiratory tract may cause **chemical pneumonitis.**

Treatment

Prompt treatment is important, with immediate aspiration of the tracheobronchial tree through an endotracheal tube or by bronchoscopy. Emergency therapy may involve artificial respiration similar to that used in victims of drowning. O_2 100% should be given under positive pressure, and, if necessary, the patient should be ventilated artificially. If aspiration of acid gastric contents or other chemical irritants (kerosene, gasoline) has occurred, hydrocortisone is recommended; 200 to 300 mg IM or IV is given initially and continued in doses of 100 mg IM q 6 h for 3 to 5 days. The value of prophylactic antimicrobials is uncertain. The patient should be observed closely for signs of pulmonary infection and the sputum examined by smear for evidence of pus cells and bacteria, and cultured repeatedly. Antimicrobial therapy should be based on the presence of fever, leukocytosis, pus and bacteria in sputum, and failure of the lesion to clear; the choice of therapy will depend on bacteriologic findings and should include a drug effective against anaerobes (penicillin, tetracycline, or clindamycin). Acidosis may develop in some patients and should be treated according to the chemical alterations in the blood.

---

39. LUNG ABSCESS

A localized, inflammatory lesion with necrosis of lung tissue and surrounding pneumonitis. The term "gangrene of the lung" denotes a similar though more diffuse and extensive process in which necrosis predominates. A lung abscess may be **putrid** (due to anaerobic bacteria) or **nonputrid** (due to anaerobes or aerobes).

Etiology and Pathology

Lung abscesses are usually due to aspiration of infected material from the upper airway by a patient unconscious or obtunded from alcoholism, CNS disease, general anesthesia, or excessive sedation. They are often associated with periodontal disease and are usually due to anaerobes; sometimes multiple organisms are acting synergistically. Bronchogenic carcinoma is a common cause of lung abscess in men over age 55 who smoke.

Pneumonia due to *Klebsiella pneumoniae* (Friedländer's bacillus), *Staphylococcus aureus*, *Actinomyces israelii*, or β-hemolytic streptococcus is sometimes complicated by abscess formation. Other less common causes of lung abscess include septic pulmonary emboli, secondary infection of pulmonary infarcts, and direct extension of amebic or bacterial abscesses from the liver through the diaphragm into the lower lobe of the lung. Caseating tuberculosis with cavity formation is not clinically considered a lung abscess.

In addition to the specific organisms mentioned above, the bacteria cultured from lung abscesses include other common pyogenic bacteria and nasopharyngeal flora, particularly anaerobes, spirochetes, fusiform bacilli, fungi, and saprophytic organisms. These may be primary or secondary invaders.

Single lung abscesses are most common. Multiple abscesses usually are unilateral and may develop simultaneously or spread from a single focus. In abscesses due to aspiration, the superior segment of the lower lobe and the posterior segment of the upper lobe of the right lung are affected most frequently, followed by the superior and posterior basal segments of the left lower lobe. The solitary abscess secondary to bronchial obstruction or an infected embolus starts as necrosis of the major portion of the involved bronchopulmonary segment. The base of the segment is usually adjacent to the chest wall, and the pleural space in the area is often obliterated by inflammatory adhesions. Hematogenous spread, which is rare, is usually diffuse.

In most instances, the abscess ruptures into a bronchus and its contents are expectorated, leaving an air-filled cavity with a fluid level in the lung. With adequate drainage, the walls of the abscess usually collapse and contract, eventually obliterating the cavity. If drainage is inadequate, the abscess wall becomes fibrotic and rigid and healing does not occur. Occasionally, an abscess ruptures into the pleural cavity, resulting in a sudden empyema, sometimes with bronchopleural fistula.

Bronchi or large blood vessels may be seen on x-ray as ridges on the cavity wall. Erosion of the vessels may cause serious hemorrhage. Rarely, septic emboli are carried through the pulmonary veins to the arterial system and initiate a secondary brain abscess. Bronchiectasis and amyloid disease are other late, but rare, complications.

Symptoms and Signs

Onset may be acute or insidious. Early symptoms are often those of pneumonia; i.e., malaise, anorexia, sputum-producing cough, sweats, chills, and fever. The sputum is purulent unless the abscess is completely walled off and it is frequently blood-streaked and sometimes foul-smelling (putrid). Severe prostration and a temperature of 39.4 C (103 F) or higher may be present. Chest pain, if present, indicates pleural involvement. Repeated chills in a patient with pneumonia suggest abscess formation.

Physical signs include a small area of dullness indicating localized pneumonic consolidation, and, usually, suppressed rather than bronchial breath sounds. Fine or medium moist rales may be present. Though unusual with current therapy, there may be tympany and amphoric breathing if the cavity is large.

An abscess may remain unsuspected until it perforates a bronchus, when a large amount of purulent sputum, fetid or nonfetid, may be expectorated over a few hours or several days. The sputum may contain gangrenous lung tissue. Fever, anorexia, weakness, and debility are usually present but are sometimes minimal if the disease is limited. Dyspnea occurs when the involvement is massive.

Failure of an area of pneumonia to resolve always suggests abscess formation, bronchial neoplasm, or both. The course must be followed by x-rays at 1- to 2-wk intervals in search of central areas of diminished density; bronchoscopic examination is indicated to rule out obstructive lesions if response to therapy is not prompt and complete.

With appropriate antibiotic therapy, signs of pulmonary suppuration generally disappear though this does not necessarily denote cure. If the abscess becomes chronic, weight loss, anemia, and hypertrophic pulmonary osteoarthropathy appear. Physical examination of the chest may be negative in the chronic phase, but rales and rhonchi are usually present.

Diagnosis

Initially, chest x-ray shows a segmental or lobar consolidation which becomes globular in shape as it distends with pus. Following rupture into a bronchus, a cavity with a fluid level appears on x-ray. This, with the symptoms and signs described above (particularly purulent, foul sputum), strongly suggests a lung abscess. If chest x-rays suggest an underlying lesion (e.g., bronchogenic carcinoma) and surgery is contemplated, tomograms may permit localization of the abscess.

Sputum should be examined by smear and culture for bacteria (including mycobacteria). Since the mouth normally contains anaerobic organisms and sputum may be contaminated on its way through the mouth, anaerobic cultures of sputum are likely to be of little value unless an unusual organism, such as *Clostridia,* is isolated. The attribution of disease to anaerobes usually requires that a specimen of bronchial secretions be obtained after bypassing the mouth; i.e., by transtracheal aspiration. Since this procedure is not completely innocuous, it should be reserved for cases that fail to respond to the usual antibiotic regimen (see below). Abscess due to anaerobes is often putrid; i.e., associated with a penetrating foul odor discernible at some distance from the patient. However, since some patients with abscesses due to anaerobes do not present this manifestation, the absence of a putrid odor does not permit a distinction between anaerobic and aerobic cases. On the other hand, a putrid odor is strong evidence of anaerobic causation and this simplifies the choice of antibiotic.

Bronchoscopy is not necessary if abscess resolution on x-ray is rapid and uneventful and if there is no reason to suspect a foreign body or tumor. If these must be ruled out, however, bronchoscopy can often be deferred until the patient's condition has been improved by antibiotics.

Lesions that simulate lung abscess include bronchogenic carcinoma, bronchiectasis, primary empyema with secondary bronchopleural fistula, TB, coccidioidomycosis, infected pulmonary bulla or air cyst, silicotic nodule with central necrosis, and subphrenic or hepatic (amebic or hydatid) abscess with perforation into a bronchus. Bacteriologic and cytologic study of the sputum, serial x-rays, CT, bronchoscopy, and mediastinoscopy as well as repeated clinical evaluation are important in differentiating these disorders from simple acute lung abscess.

Prognosis and Treatment

Prompt and complete healing of a lung abscess depends on adequate drainage through the bronchus into which it ruptures. With free drainage, resolution occurs; with inadequate drainage, the lesion is likely to become chronic, but this is very unusual with adequate antibiotic therapy. Almost all patients recover completely without surgery.

Treatment to eradicate infection and promote adequate drainage should be instituted as soon as sputum and blood have been collected for culture and sensitivity tests. The drug of choice is penicillin G 1.2 million u. (750 mg) orally q.i.d., or 300,000 to 600,000 u. IM q 6 to 8 h if the patient is unable to swallow medication. If there is no clinical response or defervescence in 4 to 7 days and a specific pathogen such as Klebsiella or Staphylococcus has not been isolated, tetracycline 500 mg orally q.i.d. should be substituted for the penicillin. If a gram-negative organism or Staphylococcus is isolated, the choice of an antibiotic depends on the results of sensitivity tests. Medical treatment should be continued until the pneumonitis has resolved and the cavity has disappeared or stabilized on serial x-rays, usually after 3 to 6 wk.

Postural drainage is instituted immediately. The daily sputum volume should be recorded as a measure of response to therapy. If the patient is weak or paralyzed, tracheostomy and suctioning may be necessary. Rarely, bronchoscopic aspiration may be required for thick, tenacious sputum. Surgical drainage is rarely necessary since lesions usually respond to antibiotics even when spontaneous drainage through the communicating bronchus is initially inadequate.

Pulmonary resection is the procedure of choice in an abscess resistant to medical therapy, particularly if bronchogenic carcinoma is suspected. Lobectomy is the most common procedure. Pneumonectomy may be necessary for multiple abscesses; segmental resection usually suffices for small lesions. The mortality rate following pneumonectomy is 5 to 10%; following lesser resections, much lower.

Planography and bronchography may demonstrate a persistent cavity or bronchiectatic changes despite antibiotic resolution of an acute abscess and only minimal residual shadows on routine x-ray, but these abnormalities are usually of no clinical significance in the absence of continued symptoms and signs. The opaque medium may not fill the cavity if there is residual inflammation of the bronchi. Bronchography should not be performed until at least 2 wk after the lesion has cleared or stabilized on x-ray. Residual bronchiectasis or cystic cavities require pulmonary resection only if symptoms of suppuration persist, infection recurs, or hemoptysis develops.

---

40. OCCUPATIONAL LUNG DISEASES

Lung disorders directly related to the inhalation of dust, fumes, vapors, and gases from the occupational environment.

The effects of an inhaled agent depend on a number of factors—its physical properties, its chemical properties, and the susceptibility of the exposed person (see TABLE 40-1). A particle is a solid particulate, a mist is a liquid particulate, a vapor is the gaseous form of substance that is normally a liquid, and gas is that physical state in which a substance has no fixed volume. In some instances, the inhaled material is deposited and retained in the lungs; if soluble, it is absorbed into the bloodstream. Insoluble particles and mists for the most part are removed by the body's defenses.

The physical state of the inhaled agent is of great importance. Particles are deposited in the respiratory tract as the result of 3 physical processes: sedimentation, inertial impaction, and diffusion. Sedimentation depends on Stokes' law, and is dependent on the particle's density and the square of its diameter. Inertial impaction occurs in bifurcating airways when the momentum of a particle is sufficient to carry it along in its original path so that it impinges on the bronchial wall. Diffusion is due to kinetic energy present in all small particles that causes them to move at random. Larger particles between 6 and 25 μ are deposited by sedimentation in the nose, and to a lesser extent in the conducting airways. Since they are too large to find their way into the lung parenchyma, they are known as the nonrespirable fraction. Particles of between 0.5 and 6 μ are known as the respirable fraction and are most prone to be deposited in the gas-exchanging portions of the lung. Particles between 1 and 2 μ are most often involved in the development of pneumoconiosis. Very

TABLE 40–1. FACTORS INFLUENCING EFFECTS OF INHALED AGENTS

Physical properties	Physical state (i.e., particle, mist, or gas; solubility, shape, density, penetrability, concentration, radioactivity)
Chemical properties	Acidity, alkalinity, fibrogenicity, antigenicity
Individual susceptibility	Integrity of body's defenses, immunologic status; i.e., atopy, tissue type (HLA type), airways geometry

small particles below 0.1 μ are deposited in the lung parenchyma due to diffusion. Other physical properties also influence the effects of deposited particles. Thus, those asbestos fibers with the greatest penetrability are more likely to migrate to the pleura and cause mesothelioma. The chemical properties of the inhaled agent are also important. While quartz is markedly fibrogenic, particles of coal, carbon, and tin oxide are far less so.

Individual susceptibility affects the development of occupational lung diseases, and there are marked variations in the rate of clearing of particles from the respiratory tract of different persons. Particles deposited in the dead space are removed by the mucociliary escalator more rapidly in some persons than in others; the clearance rate is genetically determined. Particles deposited in the lung parenchyma are taken up by alveolar macrophages, and the latter migrate with their engulfed particles to the terminal bronchioles where they catch the mucociliary escalator, or into the interstitium of the lungs where they are transported to the lymph nodes.

The site of deposition of the particle is of prime importance and to a large extent governs the lung's response (see TABLE 40–2). Deposition of particles in the nose may lead to hay fever, which may be regarded as occupationally related in an agricultural worker. Septal perforation may be seen in chrome workers, and nasal cancer in furniture workers. Deposition of particles in the trachea and bronchi may induce 3 responses. First, there may be bronchoconstriction, which can result from an antigen-antibody reaction; e.g., in some forms of occupational asthma. Second, as in byssinosis, the deposition of particles may (through pharmacologic mechanisms) cause the mast cells of the airways to produce bronchoconstrictors such as histamine and SRS-A. Next, the long-continued deposition of particles may induce mucus gland hypertrophy or bronchitis, which, in some instances, leads to a minor degree of chronic airflow obstruction. Finally, the deposition of asbestos fibers, and of dusts with radon daughters adsorbed to them, may lead to the development of lung cancer.

If particles deposited in the lung parenchyma are organic and antigenic, they may lead to the development of extrinsic allergic alveolitis (hypersensitivity pneumonia), an acute granulomatous process involving the alveoli and respiratory bronchioles (see Ch. 41). When the particle is inorganic, a fibrotic response may be seen that can be either focal and nodular as in typical silicosis, or diffuse and generalized as in asbestosis and berylliosis. Should the particle be inert (e.g., tin oxide), a benign pneumoconiosis without fibrosis develops. The inhalation of certain gases and vapors (e.g., mercury, cadmium, nitrogen dioxide) can cause acute pulmonary edema, acute alveolitis, and bronchiolitis obliterans.

TABLE 40–2. INFLUENCE OF SITE OF DEPOSITION OF THE RESPIRATORY TRACT

Site of Deposition	Clinical Response
Nose	Rhinitis, hay fever, septal perforation, nasal cancer

Trachea and bronchi	Bronchoconstriction
	  Antigen-antibody–mediated
	  Pharmacologically induced
	Bronchitis
	  Nonspecific response to inert dusts
	Lung cancer (radioactive dusts and gases)

Lung parenchyma	Extrinsic allergic alveolitis (organic dusts) Pneumoconiosis (mineral dusts) Acute pulmonary damage, bronchiolitis, pulmonary edema

DISEASES DUE TO INORGANIC (MINERAL) DUSTS

FIBROGENIC DUST DISEASES

SILICOSIS

A fibrogenic pneumoconiosis caused by inhaling crystalline free silica (quartz) dust; characterized by discrete nodular pulmonary fibrosis and, in more advanced stages, by conglomerate fibrosis and impaired respiratory function.

Etiology

Silicosis is the oldest known occupational lung disease. It usually follows long-term inhalation of small particles of free silica (silicon dioxide) in such industries as mining (lead, hard coal, copper, silver, gold), foundries, pottery making, and sandstone and granite cutting. Usually, 20 to 30 yr of exposure are necessary before the disease becomes apparent, though it develops in a much shorter time (< 10 yr) when the dust-dose is extremely high, as in such industries as tunneling, abrasive soap making, and sandblasting. The present standard for free silica in the industrial atmosphere is an 8-h time-weighted average based on the percent of silica in the dust. The formula for calculating this threshold limit value **(TLV)** for respirable dust is: TLV = (10 mg per cu meter/% SiO_2) + 2.

Pathology and Pathophysiology

Respirable particles of free silica ($< 5 \mu$ in diameter) are engulfed by alveolar macrophages. The macrophages ultimately die, hydrolytic enzymes are released, and fibrosis of the lung parenchyma occurs. The typical pathologic change initially is the formation of discrete hyalinized silicotic nodules distributed throughout the lungs. Later, coalescence of fibrosis results in conglomerate masses, contraction of the upper lung zones, and basilar emphysema with marked distortion of lung architecture. Ventilatory and gas exchange functions are affected, and ultimately there is reduced lung volume. This reduced lung volume distinguishes the overall physiologic pattern of silicosis from that of advanced chronic bronchitis or pulmonary emphysema. The striking pulmonary functional impairment occurs in association with progression to the severe late stages of silicosis. Respiratory failure is the ultimate consequence of silicosis, which may progress for some years even after exposure ceases.

When the dust-dose is extremely high and disease is accelerated, more uniform pathologic findings are found in the lung parenchyma. There is a diffuse interstitial reaction and, at times, filling of fine alveolar spaces with a proteinaceous material similar to that found in alveolar proteinosis.

Symptoms, Signs, and Clinical Course

Patients with **simple nodular silicosis** have no respiratory symptoms and usually no respiratory impairment. They may cough and raise sputum, but these symptoms are due to industrial bronchitis and occur equally frequently in subjects who have normal x-rays. Though simple silicosis has little effect on pulmonary function, occasionally categories 2 and 3 lead to a slight reduction of lung volumes, but the values are seldom outside the predicted range. **Conglomerate silicosis**, in contrast, leads to severe shortness of breath, cough, and sputum. The severity of the shortness of breath is related to the size of the conglomerate masses in the lungs; when they become extensive, the affected subject becomes completely disabled. As the masses encroaching on the vascular bed increase in size, pulmonary hypertension and right ventricular hypertrophy supervene. In advanced conglomerate silicosis, there may be signs of consolidation over the affected area and also of pulmonary hypertension. Eventually the person dies from cor pulmonale.

Pulmonary function abnormalities are frequent in complicated pneumoconiosis, especially in the later stages. These consist of decreased lung volumes and diffusing capacity, airways obstruction, and frequently pulmonary hypertension and desaturation. CO_2 retention is unusual. Populations exposed to silica have 3 times the risk of the development of TB; generally, the more silica present in the lungs, the greater the risk. **Silicotuberculosis** resembles conglomerate silicosis radiologically, and the distinction can be made only by culturing the sputum. The sera of many silicotics contain lung autoantibodies and antinuclear factor.

Diagnosis

Silicosis is diagnosed from characteristic x-ray changes and a history of exposure to free silica. Simple silicosis is recognized by the presence of multiple, small, rounded or regular opacities in the chest film, and is subdivided into categories 1, 2, and 3 according to their profusion. Conglomerate silicosis is recognized by the development of an opacity > 1 cm in diameter on a background of category 2 or 3 simple silicosis. Numerous other diseases may resemble simple silicosis, including miliary tuberculosis, welder's siderosis, hemosiderosis, and coal worker's pneumoconiosis. The presence of eggshell calcification does, however, distinguish silicosis from most other occupational lung diseases.

Prophylaxis

Silicosis is preventable with effective dust control methods. Since dust suppression cannot reduce the risk in sandblasting, external–air-supplied hoods should be used during sandblasting. Such protection may not be available to personnel performing other jobs in the area (e.g., painting, welding). For this reason, substitute abrasive materials should ultimately replace sand in this operation. Medical surveillance of all exposed workers should include periodic chest x-rays.

Treatment

No effective treatment is known for silicosis. Persons with airways obstruction accompanying silicosis should be treated as if they had chronic airflow obstruction (see CHRONIC OBSTRUCTIVE PULMONARY DISEASE in Ch. 34). Those who are exposed to silica and who have a positive tuberculin test should be given isoniazid for at least 1 yr. Some authorities recommend lifetime treatment because the alveolar macrophage function is permanently compromised by silica.

COAL WORKER'S PNEUMOCONIOSIS (CWP) (Coal Miner's Pneumoconiosis; Black Lung Disease; Anthracosis)

Diffuse nodular deposition of dust in the lungs as a result of long-term exposure to bituminous or anthracite coal dust in coal mining.

Pathology and Pathophysiology

In **simple CWP,** coal dust is widely deposited throughout the lungs, leading to the development of "coal macules" around the respiratory bronchioles. Later on mild dilation also occurs in the same region. This dilation is known as focal emphysema; however, it does not extend to the alveoli and is not associated with airflow obstruction. Because coal is relatively nonfibrogenic, distortion of lung architecture and functional impairment are minimal. However, a few miners with categories 2 or 3 simple CWP go on to develop **progressive massive fibrosis (PMF).** The latter is defined as *development of a large opacity > 1 cm on a background of relatively advanced simple CWP.* PMF may develop after exposure has ceased and may progress without further exposure, but not all subjects show progression. PMF encroaches on and destroys the vascular bed and airways, as does complicated silicosis, but this mass is amorphous and black. The development of PMF appears to be unrelated to the silica content of the coal; however, as in silicosis, antinuclear antibodies and lung autoantibodies may be present in the serum of the affected person.

Symptoms, Signs, and Diagnosis

CWP is not associated with any respiratory symptoms. Cough and sputum occur as frequently in men without x-ray evidence of this condition. When airways obstruction is present, then it is either due to coincident pulmonary emphysema from smoking, industrial bronchitis, or the presence of PMF, which is the only disabling form of CWP. A few minor abnormalities of the distribution of inspired gas are found in simple CWP, but these are not associated with respiratory symptoms. The diagnosis depends on a history of suitable exposure, usually at least 10 yr underground, and the characteristic x-ray pattern of small rounded opacities in both lung fields (simple CWP) or, in PMF, a shadow > 1 cm in diameter occurring on a background of at least category 2 or 3 simple CWP.

Prophylaxis and Treatment

CWP can be prevented by increasing the efficiency of dust suppression at the coal face. The development of PMF usually can be prevented by removing patients with x-ray changes typical of simple CWP from further coal dust exposure. There is no specific treatment; therapy is similar to that for nonspecific chronic obstructive disease (see CHRONIC OBSTRUCTIVE PULMONARY DISEASE in Ch. 34).

ASBESTOSIS

A diffuse fibrous pneumoconiosis resulting from the inhalation of asbestos dust (fibrous mineral silicates of different chemical compositions).

Etiology

Asbestosis is a consequence of long-term inhalation of asbestos fibers in the mining, milling, manufacturing, or application (e.g., of insulation) of asbestos products. The risk of developing asbestosis is related to the dose of asbestos dust to which the worker has been exposed. The incidence of lung cancer is also increased in asbestos-exposed workers. Although the asbestos exposure is usually less (asbestotic fibrosis is often absent), the risk is not entirely limited to cigarette smokers. Rare tumors of mesothelial lining surfaces **(pleural or peritoneal mesotheliomas)** have also been associated with asbestos exposure, though the exposure may have occurred many years earlier and may have been of very limited duration.

Pathology and Pathophysiology

Asbestos fibers continually divide along their long axes, their diameter ultimately becoming very small ($< 1 \mu$). These small fibers can be inhaled deep into the lung parenchyma where they produce diffuse alveolar, interstitial, and pleural fibrosis, resulting in reduced lung volumes and lung compliance (increased stiffness), and impaired gas transfer. Uncoated and coated (with an iron-protein complex) asbestos fibers (the latter are called **"asbestos bodies"**) may be present in lung tissue, with or without associated fibrosis. If there is no associated fibrosis, the presence of fibers in lung tissue indicates exposure only, not disease.

Symptoms and Signs

The patient characteristically notices the insidious onset of exertional dyspnea and reduced exercise tolerance. Symptoms of airways disease (cough, wheezing) are not usual but may occur in heavy smokers with associated chronic bronchitis. The chest x-ray reveals diffusely distributed irregular or linear small opacities, most prominent in the lower lung zones. Diffuse or local pleural thickening, with or without parenchymal disease, may also be visible. The process is progressive and symptoms become more severe in association with advancing x-ray and physiologic abnormalities. Ultimately, respiratory failure with marked impairment in oxygenation occurs.

Mesothelial tumors associated with asbestos exposure are invariably fatal. Bloody effusion with pain is often present. Spread is usually by local extension or, rarely, distant metastases.

Diagnosis

The diagnosis of asbestosis requires a history of occupational exposure, and x-ray, clinical, and physiologic evidence of diffuse pulmonary fibrosis. Histologic confirmation is rarely necessary or indicated. Mesothelioma is more difficult to diagnose and may be confirmed only by biopsy or autopsy. While the diagnosis of bronchogenic carcinoma can be made readily, the association with asbestos exposure in any individual case presents formidable medical and legal problems.

Prophylaxis and Treatment

Asbestosis is preventable, primarily by effective dust suppression in the work environment. Marked reduction in asbestos exposure has reduced the incidence of asbestosis, and further industrial hygiene advances are likely essentially to eliminate this disease. Once dust is controlled to a point where asbestosis is no longer a problem, evidence suggests that the excess risk of lung cancer in asbestos workers will decrease. The most effective preventive measure can be taken by the worker himself, however, by abstaining from cigarette smoking. Since the dose of asbestos exposure necessary for the development of mesothelioma is much less, the prevention of this tumor cannot be confidently predicted.

No specific therapy is available for asbestosis. Treatment is symptomatic (see CHRONIC OBSTRUCTIVE PULMONARY DISEASE in Ch. 34). Surgical resection occasionally produces cure for bronchogenic carcinoma, but is ineffective in treating mesothelioma.

BERYLLIOSIS (Beryllium Disease, Poisoning, or Granulomatosis)

A generalized granulomatous disease with pulmonary manifestations, caused by inhalation of dust or fumes containing beryllium compounds and products.

Etiology

Beryllium exposure used to be common in a wide variety of industries including beryllium mining and extracting, electronics, chemical plants, and the manufacture of fluorescent light bulbs. However, demand has dropped and beryllium finds its main use now in the aerospace industry. Berylliosis differs from most of the other pneumoconioses in that it appears to be a hypersensitivity disease and occurs only in a small proportion (about 2%) of those exposed. Exposure may be relatively brief, and the onset of the disease may be delayed as much as l0 or 20 yr. A few persons with berylliosis have been reported among those living in the vicinity of beryllium refineries.

Pathology and Pathophysiology

Acute berylliosis resembles a chemical pneumonitis, but other organs such as the skin and conjunctiva may be involved. Pathologic changes in the lung include nonspecific intra-alveolar edema and diffuse parenchymal inflammatory infiltrates. Early granuloma formation with mononuclear and giant cells may also occur. The hallmark of chronic berylliosis is a diffuse pulmonary and hilar lymph node granulomatous reaction histologically indistinguishable from sarcoidosis.

Symptoms, Signs, and Diagnosis

Patients with acute beryllium disease often have dyspnea, cough, weight loss, and a highly variable chest x-ray pattern, usually indicating diffuse alveolar consolidation. In chronic disease, patients complain of insidious and progressive exertional dyspnea. The chest x-ray shows a pattern of diffuse infiltrations, often with hilar adenopathy, resembling the pattern seen in sarcoidosis. Diagnosis depends on a history of exposure and the appropriate clinical manifestations. However, in most instances it is impossible to distinguish berylliosis from sarcoidosis in the absence of sophisticated immunologic technics.

Prognosis

Prognosis in the acute disease is good, but the chronic form often results in progressive loss of respiratory function. Right heart strain may result, with death from cor pulmonale.

Prophylaxis

The substitution of harmless compounds in the manufacture of fluorescent lamps has prevented many cases of the disease. Some exposure to fluorescent tubes manufactured prior to 1949 still occurs, often from tubes broken during salvage operations. Industrial dust suppression is the basis of prevention in other types of beryllium exposure, but its efficiency is imperfect. The disease (both acute and chronic) must be promptly recognized and affected workers removed from further beryllium exposure.

Treatment

Treatment of acute disease is generally symptomatic. The clinical manifestations are usually short-lived and completely reversible. Chronic beryllium disease may respond to corticosteroid therapy (e.g., full doses of prednisone 60 mg/day orally, gradually reducing the dose after 2 to 3 wk to maintenance levels of 10 to 15 mg/day, with complete tapering of medication once maximal improvement has resulted). Corticosteroids have been especially effective in relatively early chronic cases, resulting in remissions apparent not only clinically, but also physiologically and radiologically. Such improvement has been maintained for many years.

Less Common Causes of Pulmonary Fibrosis

Talc, tungsten carbide, and aluminum dust have been rarely associated with the development of diffuse pulmonary fibrosis. Clinical, x-ray, and physiologic changes are similar to those found in other diseases caused by dust inhalation and characterized by diffuse pulmonary fibrosis.

BENIGN PNEUMOCONIOSES

Several inert dusts, including iron oxide, barium, and tin, may produce conditions known respectively as **siderosis, baritosis,** and **stannosis.** These dusts are nonfibrogenic and the conditions which they produce should not be regarded as diseases since there is no functional impairment.

DISEASES DUE TO ORGANIC DUSTS

HYPERSENSITIVITY PNEUMONITIS (See in Ch. 41)

OCCUPATIONAL ASTHMA

Diffuse, intermittent, reversible airways obstruction caused by inhalation of irritant or allergenic particles or vapors from industrial processes.

Etiology

Numerous allergenic and nonallergenic materials in the occupational environment are recognized causes of reversible airways obstruction. Examples include castor bean, grain, proteolytic enzymes used in detergent manufacturing and beer- and leather-making industries, western red cedar wood, isocyanates, cotton, flax, formalin, epoxy resins, and hemp. The list is continually growing.

Pathophysiology

Although it is tempting to attribute most forms of asthma to either a Type I (IgE) or Type III (IgG) mediated immunologic response, such a simplistic approach is not justified. Thus, isocyanates and western red cedar sometimes cause bronchospasm up to 24 h following exposure, and the response may recur every night for a week or more in the absence of further exposure. Exposure to dusts of cotton, flax, or hemp may result in bronchoconstriction secondary to the liberation of bronchoconstrictors, leading to a condition known as **byssinosis**, which sometimes results in chronic irreversible airways obstruction. Unlike asthma, which gets worse with repeated exposure to allergens, byssinosis tends to improve during the work week with repeated exposures.

Symptoms, Signs, and Diagnosis

Patients generally complain of shortness of breath, chest tightness, wheezing, and cough, often in association with such upper respiratory symptoms as sneezing, rhinorrhea, and tearing. Symptoms may develop during work hours in association with specific dust or vapor exposure, but are often not apparent until some hours after leaving work, which makes the association with occupational exposure more difficult to establish. Nocturnal wheezing may be the only symptom of occupational asthma.

Diagnosis depends on recognition of causative agents in the working environment and on immunologic tests (e.g., skin tests) using the suspect antigen. In difficult cases, a positive, carefully controlled inhalation challenge test performed in the laboratory confirms the etiology of the airways obstruction. In byssinosis, respiratory symptoms characteristically worsen on the first day back at work following a weekend or holiday, and lessen during the work week. Pulmonary function tests show decreasing air flow during work and are further confirmation that occupational exposure is causative.

Prophylaxis and Treatment

Dust suppression is essential in industries where known allergens or bronchoconstrictor substances have been identified, though all instances of sensitization and clinical disease may not be eliminated. A highly susceptible individual must be removed from a setting known to produce his asthmatic symptoms.

Treatment for asthma (generally including an oral and aerosol bronchodilator, theophylline, and, in severe cases, corticosteroids) provides symptomatic improvement (see Bronchial Asthma in Ch. 34).

DISEASES DUE TO IRRITANT GASES AND CHEMICALS

ACUTE EXPOSURE

Etiology

Among the important irritant gases to which workers may be exposed in an industrial accident are chlorine, phosgene, sulfur dioxide, hydrogen sulfide, nitrogen dioxide, and ammonia. Acute heavy exposures may occur due to a faulty valve or pump or during transport of the gas.

Pathology and Pathophysiology

The respiratory damage is related to various factors, including the solubility of the gas. Relatively soluble gases (e.g., chlorine, ammonia) initially cause upper respiratory tract irritation and affect the lower, deep portions of the airways and lung parenchyma only if the victim's escape from the gas source is impeded. Less soluble gases (e.g., nitrogen dioxide) do not produce the warning signs of upper respiratory tract symptoms and are more likely to cause severe bronchiolitis, pulmonary edema, or both. In nitrogen dioxide intoxication **(silo fillers' disease)**, a lag of up to 12 h may occur before symptoms of pulmonary edema develop; occasionally, bronchiolitis obliterans progressing to respiratory failure is a late sequel.

Symptoms and Signs

The more soluble irritant gases cause severe burning and other manifestations of irritation of the eyes, nose, throat, trachea, and major bronchi. Marked cough, hemoptysis, wheezing, retching, and dyspnea are common, the severity of these symptoms being generally dose-related. In heavily exposed persons, patchy or confluent alveolar consolidation, seen on chest x-ray, indicates pulmonary edema. Most persons survive heavy acute exposure to irritant gases and generally make a full recovery. Bacterial infections, common during the acute phase, are the most serious complications.

Prophylaxis and Treatment

Care in handling these gases is the most effective preventive measure. The availability of adequate respiratory protection (e.g., gas masks with self-contained air supplies) is also of great importance should accidental exposure occur.

Treatment of heavy acute exposures is directed toward maintenance of vital gas exchange with assurance of adequate oxygenation and alveolar ventilation, at times requiring mechanical ventilation through an artificial airway (e.g., endotracheal tube). Bronchodilators, mild sedation, IV fluids and antibiotics, and nasal O_2 are required and may suffice in less severe cases. Adequate humidification of the inspired air must be assured. The efficacy of corticosteroid therapy (e.g., prednisone 45 to 60 mg for 1 to 2 wk) is difficult to prove, but corticosteroids are frequently used.

CHRONIC EXPOSURE

Chronic, low-level, continuous, or intermittent exposure to irritant gases or chemical vapors may be an important initiating or accelerating factor in the development of chronic bronchitis, though the role of such exposures in these diseases is difficult to substantiate. Exposure to carcinogenic chemicals is another important mechanism of disease. Though the route of entry into the body is via the lungs, lung tumors (as from exposure to bischloromethyl ether or certain metals) and tumors in other parts of the body (e.g., liver angiosarcomas following vinyl chloride monomer exposure) may result.

---

41. HYPERSENSITIVITY DISEASES OF THE LUNGS

(Allergic Pulmonary Diseases)

Hypersensitivity (allergic) diseases of the lungs include hypersensitivity pneumonitis (extrinsic allergic alveolitis), allergic bronchopulmonary aspergillosis, and many drug reactions. Other eosinophilic pneumonias and the pulmonary granulomatoses are of suspected allergic origin. Bronchial asthma is discussed in Ch. 34; OCCUPATIONAL ASTHMA, in Ch. 40.

Hypersensitivity reactions (see also Ch. 18) are classified into 4 types according to their pathogenetic mechanisms. **Type I (atopic or anaphylactic)** reactions (e.g., allergic [extrinsic] bronchial asthma) result from the release of pharmacologic agents (e.g., histamine) from IgE-sensitized basophils and mast cells after contact with antigen. **Type II (cytotoxic)** reactions (e.g., Goodpasture's syndrome) involve complement-fixing antibody with consequent cell lysis or antibody-dependent cellular cytotoxicity mechanisms. **Type III (immune-complex–mediated)** reactions (e.g., SLE) are associated with soluble antigen-antibody complexes, activated complement components, polymorphonuclear leukocyte chemotaxis, and subsequent vasculitis. **Type IV (cell-mediated or delayed)** reactions (e.g., tuberculosis) result from release of lymphokines (which affect other cells and lead to tissue damage) by sensitized lymphocytes following contact with antigen.

Hypersensitivity diseases of the lungs may involve mixed, rather than single, types of hypersensitivity reactions. For example, hypersensitivity pneumonitis may involve both Types III and IV; allergic bronchopulmonary aspergillosis, Types I and III.

HYPERSENSITIVITY PNEUMONITIS

(Extrinsic Allergic Alveolitis; Diffuse Hypersensitivity Pneumonia; Allergic Interstitial Pneumonitis; Organic Dust Pneumoconiosis)

A diffuse interstitial granulomatous lung disease caused by an allergic response to one of a variety of inhaled organic dusts. **Farmer's lung,** associated with repeated inhalation of dusts from hay containing thermophilic actinomycetes, is the prototype of numerous similar lung diseases that are associated with specific antigens.

Etiology and Pathogenesis

The number of specific organic dusts known to be capable of causing hypersensitivity pneumonitis is increasing. The dust is generally either a microorganism or a foreign animal or vegetable protein inhaled in considerable amounts. TABLE 41-1 lists the offending antigen associated with each form of the disease.

The disease is considered to be immunologically mediated. Precipitating antibodies to the offending antigen are usually demonstrated, suggesting a Type III allergic response, although vasculitis is not a common finding. Type IV hypersensitivity is suggested by the granulomatous primary tissue reaction.

Only a small proportion of exposed persons develop symptoms, and then only after the considerable period of exposure required for induction of sensitization. Chronic progressive parenchymal disease may result from continuous or frequent low-level exposure to the antigen. A history of previous allergic disease (e.g., asthma, hay fever) is uncommon and is not a predisposing factor. Indeed, patients with Type I sensitivity to the same material (e.g., asthmatics) can rarely tolerate the amount of exposure necessary to produce infiltrative disease.

TABLE 41-1. CAUSES OF HYPERSENSITIVITY PNEUMONITIS

Disease	Antigen	Source of Particles
Farmer's lung	*Micropolyspora faeni* or *Thermoactinomyces vulgaris*	Moldy hay
Bird fancier's lung; pigeon breeder's lung; hen worker's lung	Serum proteins and droppings	Parakeets; pigeons; hens
"Air-conditioner (or humidifier) lung"	*M. faeni, T. vulgaris,* etc.	Humidifiers, air conditioners
Bagassosis	*T. vulgaris* or *M. faeni*	Bagasse (sugar cane waste)
Mushroom worker's lung	*M. faeni* or *T. vulgaris*	Mushroom post-spawning compost
Suberosis (cork worker's lung)	Moldy cork dust	Moldy cork
Maple bark disease	*Cryptostroma corticale*	Infected maple bark
Malt worker's lung	*Aspergillus fumigatus* or *A. clavatus*	Moldy barley, malt
Sequoiosis	*Pullularia pullulans* or *Graphium* species	Moldy sawdust from redwoods
Cheesewasher's lung	*Penicillium* species	Moldy cheese
Wheat weevil disease	*Sitophilus granarius*	Infested wheat flour
Pituitary snuff taker's lung	Bovine and porcine serum protein and pituitary antigens	Heterologous pituitary snuff
Fishmeal worker's lung	Unknown	Fish meal
Coffee worker's lung	Coffee bean dust	Coffee beans
Furrier's lung	Animal hair or dander	Animal pelts
Thatched roof worker's lung	Unknown	Straw, reed, etc., used as roofing

Pathophysiology

A diffuse granulomatous interstitial pneumonitis is characteristic. Lymphocytes and plasma cells are present in thickened alveolar septa; the degree of fibrosis depends on the stage of the disease. Many cases of idiopathic pulmonary fibrosis may represent the end result of sensitization to an organic dust.

Symptoms and Signs

In **acute disease**, episodes of fever, chills, cough, and dyspnea occur in a previously sensitized individual, typically appearing 4 to 8 h after reexposure to the antigen. Anorexia, nausea, and vomiting may also be present. Fine to medium inspiratory rales may be heard on auscultation. Wheezing is unusual. With avoidance of the antigen, symptoms usually improve within hours, though complete recovery may take weeks and pulmonary fibrosis may follow repeated episodes. A **subacute form** may begin insidiously with cough and dyspnea over a period of days to weeks with progression requiring urgent hospitalization. In the **chronic form** of the disease, progressive exertional dyspnea, productive cough, fatigue, and weight loss may occur over months to years. The disease may progress to respiratory failure.

Chest x-ray findings range from normal to diffuse interstitial fibrosis. Bilateral patchy or nodular infiltrates and coarsening of bronchovascular markings, or a fine acinar pattern suggestive of pulmonary edema is commonly present. Hilar lymphadenopathy is rare. Pulmonary function studies show restrictive abnormalities: decreased lung volume, decreased CO diffusing capacity, hypoxemia, and abnormal ventilation/perfusion ratios. Airways obstruction is unusual in acute disease, but may develop in chronic disease. Eosinophilia is not expected.

Diagnosis

Diagnosis depends on a history of environmental exposure, compatible clinical features, chest x-ray, and pulmonary function tests. The demonstration of specific precipitating antibodies to the suspected antigen in the serum helps to confirm the diagnosis, though neither their presence nor their absence is definitive. Since symptoms are related to exposure to the antigen, the history may give excellent clues; e.g., persons exposed at work may become symptom-free every weekend; or symptoms may reappear 4 to 8 h after a reexposure. In puzzling cases or those without a history of environmental exposure, lung biopsy may be necessary. History of exposure to causative antigens may not be elicited easily, particularly in air conditioner or humidifier lung, and an environmental visit by the physician may prove helpful in difficult cases.

Hypersensitivity pneumonitis can be distinguished from psittacosis, viral pneumonia, and other infective pneumonias by cultures and serologic tests. Because of similar clinical features, x-rays, and pulmonary function tests, idiopathic interstitial pneumonitis or fibrosis (Hamman-Rich syndrome, cryptogenic fibrosing alveolitis, intrinsic allergic alveolitis) may be difficult to distinguish when the typical history of exposure followed by an acute episode cannot be elicited. Evidence of autoimmunity (positive anti-DNA antibody or latex fixation tests; presence of a collagen vascular disease) suggests idiopathic interstitial pneumonitis. Chronic eosinophilic pneumonias are usually accompanied by peripheral blood eosinophilia. Sarcoidosis often results in hilar and paratracheal lymph node enlargement and may involve other organs. Pulmonary angiitis-granulomatosis syndromes (Wegener's and allergic granulomatosis) are usually accompanied by upper respiratory tract or renal disease. Bronchial asthma and allergic bronchopulmonary aspergillosis present with eosinophilia and obstructive rather than restrictive pulmonary abnormalities.

Prophylaxis

Avoidance of the responsible antigen is necessary, but socioeconomic factors may make a change of environment difficult. Dust control or the use of protective masks to filter the offending dust particles in contaminated areas may be effective preventive measures. It may also be possible to prevent the growth of antigenic microorganisms (e.g., in bagasse or hay) by chemical means.

Treatment

The most effective treatment is cessation of further exposure. Acute disease is self-limiting if exposure to the antigen is avoided. Corticosteroids may be useful in severe acute or subacute cases, but may delay specific diagnosis by suppressing symptoms and signs if given before the cause is determined. Prednisone 60 mg/day is given orally in 4 divided doses for 1 to 2 wk, tapered over the next 2 wk to 20 mg/day in 1 dose, followed by weekly decrements of 2.5 mg until withdrawal is complete. A recurrence or progression of symptoms requires modification of this regimen. Precautions regarding the use of corticosteroids should be observed (see THE CORTICOSTEROIDS in Ch. 251). Antibiotics are not indicated unless there is a superimposed infection.

THE EOSINOPHILIC PNEUMONIAS

(P.I.E. [Pulmonary Infiltrates with Eosinophilia] Syndrome; Loeffler's Syndrome)

A group of diseases of both known and unknown etiology characterized by eosinophilic pulmonary infiltration and, commonly, peripheral blood eosinophilia.

Etiology and Pathogenesis

Parasites including roundworms, *Toxocara* larvae, and filariae; drugs such as penicillin, aminosalicylic acid, hydralazine, nitrofurantoin, chlorpropamide, sulfadimethoxine; chemical sensitizers such as nickel carbonyl inhaled as a vapor; and fungi such as *Aspergillus fumigatus* (causing allergic bronchopulmonary aspergillosis, discussed separately below) may be causative. Most eosinophilic pneumonias, however, are of unknown etiology, though a hypersensitivity mechanism is suspected. The eosinophilia suggests a Type I hypersensitivity reaction, while other features of the syndrome (vasculitis, round cell infiltrates) suggest Type III and possibly Type IV reactions.

Many patients have coexisting bronchial asthma. Eosinophilic pneumonias of unknown etiology associated with asthma are separable into three general groups: (1) extrinsic bronchial asthma with the P.I.E. syndrome, which often is in fact allergic bronchopulmonary aspergillosis; (2) intrinsic bronchial asthma with the P.I.E. syndrome, frequently with peculiar peripheral infiltrates on chest x-ray; and (3) allergic granulomatosis (Churg-Strauss syndrome, a variant of polyarteritis nodosa with a predilection for the lung).

A classification of the eosinophilic pneumonias based on clinical and pathologic characteristics is given in TABLE 41–2.

Pathology

Characteristic features include alveolar filling with eosinophils and large mononuclear cells, and septal infiltration with eosinophils, plasma cells, and large and small mononuclear cells. Mucus plugging of bronchioles and vascular infiltrations are also found.

Symptoms and Signs

Symptoms and signs may be mild or life-threatening. Simple pulmonary eosinophilia **(Loeffler's syndrome)** may be associated with low-grade fever, minimal (if any) respiratory symptoms, and prompt recovery. With other forms of the P.I.E. syndrome, there may be fever and symptoms of bronchial asthma, including cough and wheezing dyspnea at rest. Chronic eosinophilic pneumonia is often progressive and life-threatening without treatment.

Marked blood eosinophilia (between 20 and 40% and at times considerably higher) is usually striking. Chest x-rays reveal rapidly developing and disappearing infiltrates in various lobes depending upon the timing and frequency of the x-rays (migratory infiltrates).

Diagnosis

Helminthic infections should be sought depending on the patient's geographic location. Parasites and *A. fumigatus* may be found in the sputum. A careful drug history should be elicited. Differential diagnosis includes TB, sarcoidosis, Hodgkin's disease and other lymphoproliferative disorders, eosinophilic granuloma of the lung, desquamative interstitial pneumonitis, collagen vascular disease, and the hypereosinophilic syndrome ("eosinophilic leukemia"). Hypersensitivity pneumonitis and Wegener's granulomatosis are not usually associated with eosinophilia.

Treatment

The disease may be self-limited and benign, requiring no treatment. If the severity of the symptoms warrants it, however, treatment with corticosteroids (e.g., prednisone as for HYPERSENSITIVITY PNEUMONITIS, above) is usually dramatically effective and in idiopathic chronic eosinophilic pneumonia may be lifesaving. When bronchial asthma is present, the usual therapy is indicated (see BRONCHIAL ASTHMA in Ch. 34). In the presence of helminthic infections, appropriate vermifuges should be used (see in DISEASES CAUSED BY WORMS in Ch. 13).

ALLERGIC BRONCHOPULMONARY ASPERGILLOSIS

A noninvasive form of aspergillosis occurring in asthmatic patients as an eosinophilic pneumonia resulting from an allergic reaction to Aspergillus fumigatus.

Etiology, Pathology, and Pathogenesis

The presence of *A. fumigatus* growing in the bronchial lumen provokes an allergic response in the airways and parenchyma. Type I and Type III (and possibly Type IV) hypersensitivity reactions are involved in pathogenesis. The alveoli are packed with eosinophils. A granulomatous interstitial pneumonitis, showing peribronchial and alveolar septal infiltration with plasma cells, mononuclear cells, and numerous eosinophils, may be present. Bronchiolar mucous glands and goblet cells may be increased. A proximal bronchiectasis develops in advanced cases.

Symptoms and Signs

The patient usually presents with asthma-like symptoms (cough, wheezing, dyspnea) and intermittent low-grade fever. The sputum may be tenacious and purulent, and contains brown flecks or plugs. Signs of airways obstruction (prolonged expiration and wheezing) are found on chest examination and confirmed by pulmonary function tests.

Serial chest x-rays show transient shadows that may migrate from lobe to lobe. Mucus plugs may produce atelectasis. In chronic cases, bronchograms reveal bronchiectasis with a peculiar preference for proximal airways. Sputum examination may reveal small yellowish or brownish plugs containing *A. fumigatus* mycelia, Curschmann spirals, Charcot-Leyden crystals, mucus, and eosinophils. Sputum cultures may be positive for *Aspergillus* but are inconsistent and occasionally difficult to demonstrate. Pulmonary function studies show an obstructive pattern with decreased flow rates.

TABLE 41-2. CHARACTERISTICS OF THE EOSINOPHILIC PNEUMONIAS

Disease	Etiology	Association with Bronchial Asthma	Degree of Peripheral Eosinophilia	Systemic Involvement	Prognosis
Simple eosinophilic pneumonia (including idiopathic Loeffler's syndrome)	Unknown Drugs Parasites	Rare	Moderate	Rare	Excellent
Chronic eosinophilic pneumonia	Unknown Drugs Parasites	Usual	High	Rare	Good
Allergic bronchopulmonary aspergillosis (ABPA)	Aspergillus fumigatus	Always	High	None	Fair
Tropical eosinophilic	Parasites	Occasional	High	Occasional	Good
Allergic granulomatosis of Churg and Strauss	Unknown ? Drugs	Always	High	Common	Fair to poor

Blood eosinophilia is striking, occasionally > 50%. Serologic tests usually demonstrate precipitating antibodies to *A. fumigatus*. IgE levels may be extremely high in both total IgE and IgE antibody specific for *A. fumigatus*. Skin testing with *Aspergillus* antigen typically results in a biphasic positive reaction with an immediate Type I wheal-and-flare reaction, followed by a Type III Arthus reaction (erythema, edema, and tenderness that is maximum at 6 to 8 h). The significance of the late response is uncertain, however, and is both unnecessary and insufficient for the diagnosis.

Diagnosis

Though *Aspergillus* is a commensal of man, the combination of a positive sputum culture for *A. fumigatus*, the finding of serum-precipitating antibodies against *A. fumigatus*, and a positive wheal and flare skin test reaction is confirmatory in patients with consistent clinical features. Lung biopsy may be necessary in obscure cases.

Presenting features mimic simple bronchial asthma and may resemble allergic granulomatosis and other chronic eosinophilic pneumonias. In hypersensitivity pneumonitis, pulmonary abnormalities are restrictive rather than obstructive, and eosinophilia is rare. Invasive forms of aspergillosis (see Aspergillosis in Ch. 9) have different clinical features. Invasive aspergillosis usually occurs as a serious opportunistic pneumonia in immunosuppressed patients or after antibacterial or antifungal therapy in patients whose bronchi have been damaged by bronchitis, bronchiectasis, or TB. Aspergillomas may also occur in old cavitary disease such as TB, or, rarely, in the upper lobes of patients with rheumatoid spondylitis.

Treatment

A. fumigatus is ubiquitous and its avoidance is difficult. Treatment with corticosteroids and other antiasthmatic drugs (aminophylline, sympathomimetics, expectorants) is usually successful in allowing expectoration of the mucus plugs and, with them, the *Aspergillus*. The prednisone dosage regimen given above for Hypersensitivity Pneumonitis is appropriate, though 7.5 to 15 mg/day may be necessary for maintenance in long-term treatment. The success rate for maintenance therapy with inhaled beclomethasone diproprionate is not established. Immunotherapy and fungicidal or fungistatic agents are not recommended. Hyposensitization with extracts of *A. fumigatus* is *contraindicated* since it produces bothersome local reactions and may cause an exacerbation of symptoms.

A good prognostic sign and an indication of successful treatment is a sustained fall in serum IgE levels.

PULMONARY WEGENER'S GRANULOMATOSIS

A limited or variant form of Wegener's granulomatosis characterized by a necrotizing granulomatous angiitis involving the lungs. For a discussion of the progressive form of the disease characterized by generalized necrotizing granulomatous vasculitis involving the upper and lower respiratory tracts, the skin, the lung, and the kidneys, see Wegener's Granulomatosis in Ch. 104.

Etiology, Pathogenesis, and Pathophysiology

The etiology is unknown; Type III and Type IV hypersensitivity reactions may be involved. The characteristic pulmonary pathology consists of focal destruction and infiltration of veins and arteries, not explained by thromboembolism, accompanied by peripheral chronic necrotic lesions engulfed in granulation tissue containing plasma cells, lymphocytes, large mononuclear cells, and occasional epithelioid and giant cells. Limited forms of Wegener's granulomatosis involve the lung only; variant forms occur with atypical pathologic findings, including active lymphoreticular proliferation or bronchial rather than vascular localization.

Symptoms and Signs

Limited or variant forms of Wegener's granulomatosis may be asymptomatic or may present with fever, weight loss, malaise, cough, dyspnea, and chest pain. Symptoms and signs of generalized Wegener's granulomatosis are described in Ch. 104.

Chest x-rays reveal diffuse or nodular infiltrates, which may resemble malignant metastases. Necrotizing lesions are usually multiple and bilateral, occur in any part of the lung, and may cavitate. Hilar adenopathy is uncommon. Eosinophilia is *not* a feature of this disease. Serum complement levels are normal or elevated.

Diagnosis

Lung biopsy is usually necessary for definitive diagnosis when upper respiratory tract disease or typical skin lesions are absent. Differential diagnosis includes metastatic or primary neoplasm, lymphoma, infectious granulomas (e.g., tuberculosis), sarcoidosis, rheumatoid nodules, pulmonary infarction, lung abscess, aspiration pneumonia, and bronchiolitis obliterans.

Treatment

Although pulmonary disease may improve spontaneously, treatment is recommended as soon as the diagnosis is established. Therapy is described in Ch. 104. Limited Wegener's has been reported to respond more readily to adrenocorticosteroid therapy than does the full-blown disease, for which cyclophosphamide is the agent of choice.

42. GOODPASTURE'S SYNDROME

An uncommon Type II hypersensitivity disorder (see Ch. 18) of unknown etiology manifested by pulmonary hemorrhage with associated severe and progressive glomerulonephritis, and character-ized by circulating antiglomerular basement membrane antibodies in the blood and by linear deposi-tion of immunoglobulin and complement in the glomerular basement membrane.

Pathology

The changes observed at kidney biopsy are similar to those in any rapidly progressive glomerulo-nephritis, with epithelial cell crescents, glomerular adhesions, and interstitial inflammatory exudates. Intra-alveolar hemorrhages and septal fibrosis are present in the lungs. Immunofluorescent staining demonstrates linear deposition of immunoglobulin and complement in the glomular and, in some cases, in the alveolar-capillary basement membranes.

Symptoms, Signs, and Diagnosis

The patient, most often a young adult male, characteristically presents with severe hemoptysis, dyspnea, and rapidly progressive renal failure. Iron deficiency anemia is usual. Hematuria and pro-teinuria are common, and the urinary sediment usually contains cellular and granular casts. Chest x-rays may show progressive, migratory, asymmetric, bilateral, fluffy densities.

Though the combination of pulmonary hemorrhage and renal failure can also occur in idiopathic pulmonary hemosiderosis, certain collagen vascular diseases, acute glomerulonephritis with circula-tory congestion, Wegener's granulomatosis, and bacterial endocarditis, these diseases can often be excluded by their other distinguishing features and by renal biopsy. Linear deposition of immuno-globulin has been described in few cases of lupus nephritis and diabetic glomerulosclerosis, but antibody eluted from kidneys in these settings does not have antiglomerular basement membrane activity.

Prognosis and Treatment

The disease may be rapidly fatal. Corticosteroids alone or combined with azathioprine or mercap-topurine may prolong survival. Bilateral nephrectomy and renal transplantation have been associ-ated with cessation of life-threatening pulmonary hemorrhage, but their efficacy has not been established. Plasmapheresis with immunosuppressive agents has been used successfully in few patients.

43. IDIOPATHIC INFILTRATIVE DISEASES OF THE LUNGS

A spectrum of disorders with different etiologies but similar clinical features and diffuse pathologic changes that affect primarily interalveolar interstitial tissue. Interstitial infiltration is characterized in its acute phase by abnormal accumulation of histiocytes, lymphocytes, plasma cells, eosinophils, and proteinaceous exudate in alveoli and bronchioles. Hyperplasia of bronchiolar or alveolar epithe-lium may be present at a later stage. If the disorder progresses, the exudate may become organized, and necrosis, scarring, and reepithelialization of alveolar septae may take place. The whole process may ultimately lead to extensive fibrosis, progressive destruction of lung and formation of cysts ("honeycombing").

When a specific etiology can be defined, the pulmonary disease is classified accordingly and is discussed elsewhere in this section (e.g., occupational and hypersensitivity diseases of the lungs; sarcoidosis is discussed in Ch. 14).

Idiopathic pulmonary fibrosis (usual interstitial pneumonia [UIP], diffuse fibrosing alveolitis, Ham-man-Rich syndrome): when the etiology leading to pulmonary fibrosis cannot be defined (about 50% of cases), the term "idiopathic" is used.

Desquamative interstitial pneumonia (DIP) resembles idiopathic pulmonary fibrosis, but the histol-ogy tends to be more uniform: the cellular infiltrate is more sparse and less pleomorphic. There is striking hyperplasia of type II pneumocytes and filling of air spaces with macrophages. It has been argued that the separation of DIP from idiopathic pulmonary fibrosis is artificial because both histo-logic patterns can be found frequently in the same lung (probably representing different phases of the same process). However, the clinical recognition of DIP is important because the process is associated with a better prognosis and a better response to systemic corticosteroids.

Symptoms and Signs

Symptoms and signs vary with the extent of pulmonary infiltration, its rate of progress, and with the presence of complications such as pulmonary infections or cor pulmonale. Pulmonary symptoms may be few, but exertional dyspnea of insidious onset is almost invariably present. Cough is usually not prominent, but it is more likely to be present when there is secondary bronchial infection. Anorexia, weight loss, fatigue, weakness, and vague chest pains are common. Physical signs may be absent early in the course, but, as the disease progresses, tachypnea and labored breathing are observed and chest examination reveals prominent breath sounds and end-inspiratory crackles at lung bases. With progression, cyanosis, cor pulmonale, and clubbing may appear.

Laboratory Findings

Routine laboratory studies are not helpful. Polycythemia may be present secondary to chronic hypoxemia. **Chest x-rays** may be normal even in the presence of significant symptoms or functional abnormalities. X-ray changes tend to be more prominent at the bases and may include diffuse or patchy "ground-glass" haziness, linear markings, rounded opacities, small cystic lesions (honeycombing), evidence of reduced lung volumes, and signs of pulmonary hypertension. **Pulmonary function studies** reveal a restrictive ventilatory defect with reductions in both vital capacity and residual volume. The coefficient of retraction (maximum static transpulmonary pressure/total lung capacity) can be increased. Arterial blood gases show a low Pa_{CO_2}, denoting hyperventilation at rest and a decrease in Pa_{O_2}. The abnormal increase in $P(A-a)_{O_2}$ at rest may be exacerbated during exercise. The diffusing capacity for CO is usually reduced. These functional abnormalities can worsen as the disease progresses.

Diagnosis

Diagnosis is made by recognizing the clinical features, demonstrating the presence of a diffuse interstitial disorder, and excluding a specific etiology. Because the amount of tissue obtained by transbronchial biopsy is frequently insufficient, open lung biopsy is recommended for the identification of DIP. Open pulmonary biopsy is not indicated when there is radiographic honeycombing.

Prognosis

The outcome varies with the etiology and the rate of progression. Some patients may die within a month, while others survive many years. The mortality is smaller and the mean survival greater when histologic features of DIP are present on open lung biopsy.

Treatment

A trial of systemic corticosteroids is indicated in patients without evidence of extensive fibrosis. Prednisone 40 to 60 mg/day usually is given with gradual reduction of the dose to maintenance levels (10 to 30 mg every other day). The response to therapy is followed by serial chest x-rays and appropriate lung function tests. Gallium citrate Ga 67 lung scanning and serial analysis of cellular content of bronchoalveolar lavage fluid may prove to be useful to detect and follow the response of the inflammatory process to therapy. A few patients who have not improved on prednisone have shown improvement with azathioprine 3 mg/kg/day, but experience with this agent is limited. Other treatment is supportive and palliative. O_2 in high concentrations may help combat hypoxemia. Antibiotics are required if secondary bacterial infection occurs. Digitalis and diuretics are used to treat heart failure.

HISTIOCYTOSIS X

(Letterer-Siwe Disease; Hand-Schüller-Christian Syndrome; Eosinophilic Granuloma)

A group of disorders characterized by proliferation of histiocytes. Granulomatous lesions may occur in many organs, especially the lungs and bones. The etiology is unknown. Pathologically, the changes begin with progressive proliferation of histiocytes and infiltration with eosinophilic granulocytes. Fibrils are then formed, giant cells appear, and there may be lipoid phagocytosis. Xanthomas and foam cells appear. A fibrotic phase with little cellular infiltration finally supervenes. The lungs show varying degrees of granulomatosis, fibrosis, and honeycombing.

Letterer-Siwe disease occurs before age 3 yr and is usually fatal. Skin, lymph nodes, bone, liver, and spleen are frequently involved. **Hand-Schüller-Christian syndrome** most often begins in early childhood, but can appear even in late middle age. The lungs and bones are most frequently involved, though other organs may be affected. A triad of bone defects, exophthalmos, and diabetes insipidus occurs rarely. **Eosinophilic granuloma** occurs most commonly between ages 20 and 40 and characteristically involves bone, though about 20% of patients have lung infiltration and the lungs sometimes may be involved exclusively.

Without treatment, Letterer-Siwe disease is always fatal. Patients with Hand-Schüller-Christian syndrome or eosinophilic granuloma may recover spontaneously. If death ensues, it usually results from respiratory or cardiac failure. **Treatment** of the lung involvement in the 3 disorders is with corticosteroids.

IDIOPATHIC PULMONARY HEMOSIDEROSIS

A rare disease of unknown etiology characterized by episodes of hemoptysis, hemorrhage into the lung, pulmonary infiltration, and secondary iron deficiency anemia. It is most common in young children, but can occur in adults. Diffuse infiltration with hemosiderin-containing macrophages is characteristic, though hemosiderin deposition is found in many other disorders. Pulmonary hemorrhages, which determine the clinical course, vary from mild to severe but are most often mild and continuous. Blood in the interstitial spaces leads to pulmonary fibrosis. Patients may live for several years, developing pulmonary fibrosis and insufficiency along with chronic secondary anemia. **Treatment** is symptomatic and supportive. Death often occurs as a result of massive pulmonary hemorrhage.

44. PULMONARY ALVEOLAR PROTEINOSIS

A rare disease of unknown etiology characterized pathologically by filling of alveolar spaces with granular, periodic acid-Schiff (PAS)–positive material consisting mostly of protein and fat. Most cases appear between ages 20 and 50. Men are affected more often than women. The disease usually occurs in previously healthy people.

Pathology

Pathologic findings are limited to the lungs. Since the etiology is unknown, the earliest pathologic lesion has not been determined. Typically, the alveolar lining and interstitial cells are normal but the alveoli are plugged with amorphous PAS-positive granules containing lipoproteins and plasma proteins and other constituents of the blood. The lipid concentration of the alveolar spaces is very high, possibly because of abnormal clearance of alveolar phospholipids from these spaces. Interstitial fibrosis occurs rarely. The pathologic process may be diffuse or localized, and may progress, remain stable, or spontaneously clear. The basal and posterior lung regions are most commonly affected; occasionally only the anterior segments are involved. The pleura is not affected.

Symptoms and Signs

Clinical findings vary greatly. Some patients are asymptomatic; others have severe respiratory insufficiency. Most patients present with gradually progressive exertional dyspnea and nonproductive cough, though cough is occasionally productive, especially if the patient smokes cigarettes. Sputum characteristics are not helpful. Secondary infections occasionally develop, particularly with organisms such as *Nocardia*. Though the patient may have recently had a febrile illness or presented with one, persistent fever is rare unless secondary infection is present. Extrapulmonary symptoms are unusual. A few cases have occurred in patients with myeloproliferative disease but the significance of this association is unclear.

Physical findings are restricted to the lungs but may be absent despite diffuse parenchymal involvement visible on chest x-ray. Fine inspiratory rales are usually heard over the involved lung areas. The usual, though not invariable, x-ray appearance is a "butterfly" pattern of infiltrates resembling what is seen in pulmonary edema; the cardiac silhouette is normal. Hilar lymph node enlargement and pleural involvement are absent.

Vital capacity, residual volume, functional residual capacity, total lung capacity, and CO single-breath diffusing capacity are usually slightly reduced. Obstructive pulmonary disease is not a feature, and the FEV_1, $FEF_{25\ to\ 75\%}$, and MVV are normal. Hypoxemia may be present even at rest or, if disease is mild, only with mild to moderate exercise. The partial pressure of O_2 while breathing 100% O_2 is usually low, indicating an intrapulmonary right-to-left shunt.

Clinical Course

The natural history of this disease is unknown. Its gravity was initially overestimated since most of the original cases were diagnosed at autopsy. Disability from respiratory insufficiency is common, but death rarely occurs if the patient with significant symptoms is treated with bronchopulmonary lavage (see below). Spontaneous remissions may occur. Secondary infections, especially fungal, have occurred, though their true incidence is unclear.

Treatment

Therapy has remained largely empiric. A wide variety of agents has been employed with varying success, including potassium iodide, tyloxapol, and proteolytic enzymes such as streptokinase-streptodornase and trypsin. Systemic corticosteroids have been used unsuccessfully and may increase the possibility of secondary infection. The efficacy of any therapeutic regimen is difficult to evaluate because spontaneous remissions may occur and because the number of cases available for study by any one investigator is limited.

Bronchopulmonary lavage has recently been shown to be the most effective treatment, but it is indicated only in patients with significant symptoms and hypoxemia. Lavage with the patient under general anesthesia is usually performed on one lung at a time at 3- to 5-day intervals. Some patients require only one lavage and never have a recurrence of symptoms or infiltrates; others require lavage every 6 to 12 mo for many years.

Patients with minimal or no symptoms do not require treatment but should be watched for exacerbations which may lead to respiratory failure. Secondary infections should be promptly identified and treated.

45. PLEURAL DISORDERS

PLEURISY

Inflammation of the pleura.

Etiology

Pleurisy may occur as a result of (1) pleural injury by a process in the underlying lung (e.g., pneumonia, pulmonary infarction); (2) entry of an infectious agent or irritating substance into the pleural space (e.g., as in amebic empyema or pancreatitic pleurisy); (3) transport of an infectious or noxious agent or neoplastic cells directly to the pleura by the bloodstream or lymphatics (e.g., as in tuberculous pleural effusion, uremic pleurisy, or collagen vascular diseases such as SLE); (4) pleural trauma; (5) asbestos-related pleural disease in which the noxious agent (asbestos particles) reaches the pleura by traversing the conducting airways and respiratory tissues of the lungs; or (6) rarely, pleural effusion related to longstanding ingestion of dantrolene sodium.

Pathology

In the early stages of most cases of pleurisy, the pleura becomes edematous and congested, cellular infiltration occurs, and a fibrinous exudate develops on the pleural surface. The exudate may be reabsorbed or organized into fibrous tissue with resultant pleural adhesions. Some diseases, such as pleurodynia due to coxsackie B virus, may run their course without significant exudation of fluid from the inflamed pleura, the pleurisy remaining dry or fibrinous. More often, however, following this early stage, a pleural exudate develops due to an outpouring from damaged vessels of fluid rich in plasma protein. Occasionally, marked fibrous or even calcific thickening of pleura occurs without an antecedent acute pleurisy (e.g., asbestos pleural plaques, idiopathic pleural calcification).

Symptoms and Signs

Onset is usually sudden. Pain, the dominant symptom of fibrinous pleurisy, may vary from vague discomfort to an intense stabbing sensation. The pain is aggravated by breathing and coughing, or may be present only when the patient breathes deeply or coughs. The visceral pleura is insensitive; pain results from inflammation of the parietal pleura. Since the latter is innervated by the intercostal nerves, pain is usually felt over the site of the pleuritis, but pain may be referred to distant regions. Irritation of the posterior and peripheral portions of the diaphragmatic pleura, which are supplied by the lower 6 thoracic nerves, may cause pain referred to the lower chest wall or to the abdomen. As a result, diaphragmatic pleurisy may simulate intra-abdominal disease. The central portion of the diaphragmatic pleura is innervated by the phrenic nerves and involvement in this area causes pain referred to the neck and shoulder.

Respiration is usually rapid and shallow. Motion of the affected side may be limited. Breath sounds may be diminished. A pleural friction rub is the characteristic physical sign, though it is often absent and quite frequently is heard only 24 to 48 h after the onset of pain. The friction rub varies from a few intermittent sounds which may simulate crackles to a fully developed harsh grating, creaking, or leathery sound synchronous with respiration and usually heard on both inspiration and expiration. Friction sounds due to pleuritis adjacent to the heart (pleuropericardial rub) may vary with the heart beat as well as with respiration. It should be remembered that the clinical picture varies with the underlying disease.

When pleural effusion develops, pleuritic pain usually subsides. Percussion dullness, absent tactile fremitus, decreased or absent breath sounds, and egophony at the upper border of the fluid are then noticeable. The larger the pleural effusion, the more obvious the above signs. A large effusion may encroach on lung volume and produce or contribute to dyspnea.

Diagnosis

Fibrinous pleurisy is readily diagnosed because of the characteristic pleuritic pain. A pleural friction rub is pathognomonic. Diaphragmatic pleurisy may produce pain referred to the point of the shoulder. Basilar pleurisy may produce pain referred to the abdomen. Pleurisy is usually differentiated from acute inflammatory abdominal disease by x-ray and clinical evidence of a respiratory process; absence of nausea, vomiting, or disturbed bowel function; marked aggravation of pain by deep breathing or coughing; shallow rapid breathing; and tendency toward relief of pain by pressure on the abdomen. Intercostal neuritis may be confused with pleurisy, but the pain is rarely related to respiration and there is no friction rub. With herpetic neuritis, development of the characteristic herpetic eruption is diagnostic; pain may be present for months after the herpetic eruption subsides. Myocardial infarction, spontaneous pneumothorax, pericarditis, and chest wall lesions may simulate pleurisy. The friction rub of pericarditis may be confused with that of pleurisy, but usually is heard best over the left border of the sternum in the 3rd and 4th interspaces and characteristically is a "to-and-fro" sound synchronous with the heartbeat. Unlike the pleural friction rub, the pericardial rub is not influenced significantly by respiration, though there may be some variation in its intensity synchronous with respiration.

Chest x-rays are of limited value in diagnosing fibrinous pleurisy. The pleural lesion causes no shadow, but an associated pulmonary or chest wall lesion may. Chest x-rays are the most precise way of confirming physical findings and diagnosing the presence of pleural fluid. When there are no adhesions between the visceral and parietal pleura, fluid seeks the most dependent portion of the thorax. Because of the recoil force of the underlying lung, the upper border of the fluid is meniscus-shaped. With the patient in an upright position, the minimum amount of detectable fluid ranges from 300 to 500 ml. However, when frontal x-rays are taken with a horizontal x-ray beam and the patient lying on the affected side, < 100 ml of fluid is easily detectable; with careful positioning, as little as 10 to 15 ml of fluid can be seen. Large pleural effusions may result in complete opacification of the hemithorax and shift of the mediastinum to the contralateral side. Adhesions between visceral and parietal pleurae may result in atypical localization of pleural fluid (loculated pleural effusions). Obliteration of the costophrenic angle may denote a fibrosing and healing reaction or may remain permanent after healing is complete. Pleural plaques due to asbestos exposure present as localized areas of pleural thickening, usually in the lower 2/3 of the thorax.

Fibrosis of the pleura: Inflammatory reactions in the pleura heal by resolution and fibrosis. Even with long standing or severe pleural inflammations, the amount of scar tissue remaining after complete healing may be surprisingly slight. Occasionally, however, the lung becomes encased in a thick layer of fibrous tissue which limits chest wall motion, retracts the mediastinum toward the side of disease, and impairs pulmonary function. It may be impossible to differentiate localized pleural thickening from loculated pleural fluid except by thoracentesis.

Calcification of the pleura presents as focal, usually fenestrated, irregular plaques on the costal surfaces following intrapleural hemorrhage or infection, though a history of such an antecedent acute pleural lesion is often not obtainable. Focal plaque-like pleural fibrosis, at times with calcification, occurs many years after occupational exposure to asbestos, most often involving the diaphragmatic pleura.

When pleural fluid is present, pleural thoracentesis (see Ch. 31) should be almost always performed to confirm the presence of fluid and to determine its characteristics, including color and consistency. Clear yellow fluid is described as serous; bloody or blood-tinged fluid as sanguineous or serosanguineous; and translucent or thick fluid as purulent. Specimens should be taken for chemical, bacteriologic, and cytologic examination (the latter using tubes with heparin, 3 u./ml fluid, added). Microscopic examination of gram-stained pleural fluid sediment is essential with all purulent fluids when infection of the pleural space is a possibility. Fungi or actinomycetes may also be detected during the course of such an examination. Cultures for anaerobes should be sent to the laboratory in special transport media or in a capped syringe.

It is always important to determine whether serous fluid is a transudate or an exudate. Pleural fluid **transudates** generally have sp gr values < 1.015, total protein contents < 2.5 gm/100 ml, relatively low cell counts, pleural fluid to serum LDH ratios generally < 0.6, and pleural fluid LDH concentrations < 200 IU. Whenever the extravascular fluid space is increased, as in congestive heart failure, edematous renal disease, or myxedema, fluid tends to enter the pleural space. Peritoneal transudates may enter the pleural space more often on the right, directly through microscopic, mesothelial-lined communications which perforate the diaphragm. Such pleural fluid differs from that due to inflammation of the visceral or parietal pleura and subsides with control of the causative disease. Pleural **exudates** generally have sp gr values > 1.018, total protein contents > 3 gm/100 ml, and pleural fluid to serum LDH ratios > 0.6.

Total and differential cell counts should be obtained routinely except on grossly purulent pleural fluids. A predominance of polymorphonuclear leukocytes **(PMNs)** suggests an underlying pneumonia and a synpneumonic effusion which is usually sterile even with bacterial pneumonia. In the early stages of bacterial infection, fluid is not visibly purulent, there are many PMNs, and bacteria may be seen in a Gram stain. The presence of many small mature lymphocytes, particularly with few mesothelial cells, strongly suggests tuberculosis. Pleural fluid is commonly bloodstained in pulmonary infarction and pleural carcinomatosis. In pulmonary infarction, there is usually a mixture of lymphocytes and PMNs, and mesothelial cells are numerous. The presence of malignant cells in Papanicolaou-stained smears of pleural fluid is diagnostic of pleural carcinomatosis. LE cells may be seen in the pleural fluid in SLE. Glucose concentrations < 10 mg/100 ml are rare except in rheumatoid pleural effusion. Very high pleural fluid amylase values are characteristic of pancreatic pleural effusion; salivary amylase may gain access to the pleural space in rupture of the esophagus, but the clinical picture and acid pH of the fluid are usually enough to prevent misdiagnosis. Loculated pleural effusions tend to have pH values < 7.20. Eosinophils in the pleural fluid have no diagnostic significance. These laboratory tests on the pleural fluid are most useful when integrated with all of the clinical data and other appropriate clinical tests. For example, a tuberculin skin test is the key in the investigation of a patient with suspected tuberculous pleural effusion.

Needle biopsy of the parietal pleura (see Ch. 31), performed with a Cope or Abrams pleural biopsy needle, should be considered either at the time of the initial thoracentesis or soon after if the cause of the effusion is not readily apparent from the clinical findings and pleural fluid analysis. Culture of parietal pleural tissue often yields mycobacteria when the pleural fluid culture does not. The replacement of fluid by air and performance of thoracoscopy and visually directed parietal pleural biopsy using a fiberoptic endoscope may permit definitive diagnosis in obscure cases.

Hemothorax, *blood in the pleural space,* occurs most often from trauma, or, rarely, following rupture of a vessel in a parietopleural adhesion in association with spontaneous pneumothorax. Spontaneous hemothorax may also rarely be a complication of a coagulation defect. Pleural blood often does not clot and may be easily withdrawn through a needle or a water-sealed tube thoracotomy.

Chylothorax, *a milky or chylous pleural effusion,* is caused by traumatic or neoplastic (most often a lymphoma) injury to the thoracic duct. The lipid content of the fluid (neutral fat and fatty acids) is high; sudanophilic fat droplets are often seen microscopically. Cholesterol content is low.

Cholesterol effusion (chyliform or pseudochylous effusion): Rarely, golden, iridescent (due to the presence of light-reflecting cholesterol crystals) pleural fluid is obtained on thoracentesis. The crystals may be seen on microscopy; high concentrations (up to 1 gm/100 ml) of cholesterol may be measured, but neutral fat and fatty acid concentration is low. This type of effusion results from long standing chronic pleural effusion, as in tuberculous pleurisy or rheumatoid pleural effusion. The underlying disease should be carefully sought; cholesterol pleural effusion is not acceptable as a complete diagnosis.

Treatment

Treatment of the underlying disease is essential for fibrinous pleurisy and for pleural effusion. Pleural exudates due to underlying pulmonary disease (e.g., pneumonia, pulmonary infarction) and effusions secondary to a systemic disease (e.g., uremia or SLE) usually respond to such treatment.

Chest pain may be relieved by wrapping the entire chest with two or three 6-in. wide nonadhesive elastic bandages. Though these must be reapplied once or twice daily, the problem of skin irritation that results from applying adhesive strapping to the affected hemithorax is avoided and pain relief is comparable. Aspirin 0.6 gm orally q.i.d. is often all that is necessary. If not, codeine 30 to 60 mg orally or s.c. may be necessary, but its cough suppressant properties must be considered.

To prevent complicating pneumonia, adequate bronchial drainage must be provided. Coughing is often facilitated if additional temporary splinting of the chest wall is provided by having the patient or an attendant hold a pillow firmly against the painful chest wall. The patient taking narcotics should be urged to breathe deeply and cough when pain relief from the drug is maximal. Aqueous aerosol inhalation therapy with bronchodilators and antibiotic therapy should be considered for treatment of any associated bronchitis.

Thoracentesis often dramatically relieves dyspnea due to a large pleural effusion. Since cardiovascular collapse occurs rarely if several liters of pleural fluid are removed too quickly, fluid removal should be limited to 1200 to 1500 ml at one time. Pneumothorax may complicate thoracentesis if the visceral pleura is punctured or if air leaks into the pleural space (which is at subatmospheric pressure) as a result of a break in the continuity of the thoracentesis system used. Ultrasonography is of great assistance in the accurate localization of loculated pleural effusions and in their drainage by guided placement of a needle.

Indolent infection in the pleural space must be treated by a long course of appropriate antibiotic therapy. For example, tuberculous pleurisy responds to treatment with two simultaneously given antituberculosis drugs such as isoniazid and ethambutol; amphotericin B is effective in coccidioidal pleural effusion. Pleural fluid in such cases usually reabsorbs spontaneously.

Empyema (*purulent exudate in the pleural cavity*) is treated with high doses of parenteral antibiotics and drainage of the pleural space. One or two needle aspirations repeated daily may be adequate for small collections of thin pus, but water-sealed tube thoracotomy is usually preferable. When the empyema cavity is lined by a thick, organizing, fibrinous exudate or cortex, open drainage over weeks or months through a rib resection or intercostal tube may be necessary to obliterate the space. If the lung is partially collapsed by a thick cortex and the empyema space is large, thoracotomy and surgical decortication is the best way to expand the lung and obliterate the space. Surgery may also be necessary when bronchopleural fistula complicates empyema.

Treatment of pleural effusion due to **malignant pleural implants** is often difficult. Pleural fluid occasionally does not reaccumulate after the thorax has been tapped dry with a needle, especially if systemic antitumor therapy has been started, as in metastatic carcinoma of the breast. When fluid does reaccumulate, it generally responds to obliteration of the pleural space by instillation of a pleural irritant such as quinacrine or tetracycline. Adhesion of visceral and parietal pleurae (obliterating the pleural space) may be aided if the pleural space is kept empty after instilling the irritant by using water-sealed tube drainage for a few days. Specific chemotherapy of malignant pleural effusion with agents such as mechlorethamine (HN_2) *is not recommended* because they may cause bone marrow depression and are no more effective than the less toxic irritants.

For **hemothorax,** mixed enzymes (streptokinase-streptodornase) may be instilled to dissolve a clot and lyse fibrinous adhesions, but thoracotomy and decortication may be necessary to expand the lung and obliterate the pleural space.

Treatment of **chylothorax** is directed at the underlying cause of ductal damage.

Pleural fibrosis should be minimized by appropriate early therapy of pleural disease. Surgical decortication of pleural fibrous tissue does not usually improve lung function unless a sizable collection of air or fluid is removed simultaneously.

46. PNEUMOTHORAX

Free air in the pleural cavity, between the visceral and parietal pleurae.

Etiology and Pathophysiology

Traumatic pneumothorax: Normally, pressure in the pleural space is less than atmospheric because of lung recoil pressure. Following trauma, air may enter the pleural cavity in several ways. **Open pneumothorax** occurs when a penetrating chest wound creates a communication (pleurocutaneous fistula) between the outside air and the pleural space that permits air to rush in, thus causing the lung to collapse. In **closed pneumothorax**, the chest wall becomes airtight after penetration (e.g., by a thoracentesis needle or after a stab wound), or it may continue to receive air (e.g., when air leaks from a lung punctured by a fractured rib). Air may also leak from a ruptured bronchus or perforated esophagus into the mediastinum and then rupture into the pleural space. During thoracentesis, air may leak into the pleural space if the syringe and needle are not kept firmly sealed at all times. **Pulmonary barotrauma** is an important present-day cause of pneumomediastinum and pneumothorax in patients being mechanically ventilated. The complication occurs most often in the adult respiratory distress syndrome and is increased in frequency in patients with severe disease requiring high peak inspiratory pressure or positive end-expiratory pressure (**PEEP**) for management. Air may enter the pleural space because of breach of the parietal pleura or a pneumomediastinum may rupture through the mediastinal pleura into the pleural space.

Spontaneous pneumothorax: Air may enter the pleural space without antecedent trauma during the course of pulmonary disease or in a previously healthy person. Emphysema with rupture of a bulla is the most common underlying lung disorder. Asthma, eosinophilic granuloma, or lung abscess with bronchopleural fistula and empyema may also be causative. Active TB may rarely cause pneumothorax owing to perforation of a cavity into the pleural space; inactive TB may also be complicated by pneumothorax, owing to the presence of associated emphysema. Whatever the disease process, it is usually evident before the pneumothorax occurs.

The usual cause of spontaneous pneumothorax in an apparently healthy person, most frequently a man aged 20 to 40, and most commonly in the right lung, is rupture of an emphysematous bulla in the apex of the lung. The bulla may be undetectable by clinical examination. Most spontaneous pneumothoraces occur without associated exertion. Some have occurred during diving or high-altitude flying, apparently in association with the ambient pressure change which is unequally transmitted to different portions of the lung. A pneumothorax may also occur as a complication of interstitial pulmonary air leak and pneumomediastinum, which may be spontaneous or may complicate other processes such as spontaneous rupture of the esophagus or traumatic rupture of the bronchus.

In both traumatic and spontaneous pneumothorax, the communication between the bronchial tree and the pleural space (bronchopleural fistula) usually stops leaking and heals quickly as the lung collapses, but it may remain open.

A **tension (positive-pressure) pneumothorax** occurs when a check-valve mechanism in a bronchopleural fistula permits air to enter, but not leave, the pleural space, causing pressure within the space to rise above atmospheric; complete collapse of the lung and shift of the mediastinum to the opposite side result.

Induced pneumothorax: Artificial pneumothorax, formerly used extensively to treat tuberculosis, is rarely used as a diagnostic procedure to outline masses or replace fluid for better x-ray visualization of intrathoracic structures.

Symptoms and Signs

Symptoms vary greatly according to the size of the pneumothorax and the extent of disease in the lung. They range from minimal disturbance to severe dyspnea, shock, and life-threatening circulatory collapse. Sudden sharp chest pain, dyspnea, and, occasionally, a dry, hacking cough occur at onset. The pain may be referred to the corresponding shoulder, across the chest, or over the abdomen; it may simulate an acute coronary occlusion or an "acute abdomen." Symptoms tend to be less severe in a slowly developing pneumothorax and usually subside as accommodation to the altered physiologic state occurs.

Physical findings also depend on the size of the pneumothorax. With a small collection of air, there may be no detectable signs, or diminution of voice and breath sounds may be the only abnormality. With large or tension pneumothoraces, tympany on percussion, diminished or absent tactile fremitus and diminished motion on the affected side occur. Shift of the mediastinum may be detectable as displacement of the cardiac dullness and apex beat away from the affected side. Hypoxemia is minimal or absent in a previously well young person with spontaneous pneumothorax, but may be severe and associated with hypercapnia in a patient with diffuse underlying lung disease.

The chest x-ray is usually characteristic, showing air without lung markings peripherally, but limited by a sharp pleural margin with lung markings medially, indicating the position of the collapsed lung. A small pneumothorax may be overlooked on a routine inspiratory x-ray but is obvious on an expiratory x-ray. This is because the size and density of the lung (but not of the pleural air space) change during expiration. The mediastinum shifts to the contralateral side, especially with a large pneumothorax. Differential diagnosis includes emphysematous bullae and herniation of the stomach, the colon, or, much less commonly, the small bowel through the diaphragm.

Treatment

A small spontaneous pneumothorax requires no special treatment; the air is reabsorbed in a few days. Full absorption of a larger air space may take 2 to 4 wk, during which time there is uncertainty as to whether the pleural leak is closed and whether pleural fluid and epipleural fibrinous exudate will develop. The course can be shortened by introduction of a chest tube with water-sealed drainage, application of suction if there is a persistent bronchopleural fistula, and rapid expansion of the lung. This is desirable in all but the most minor degrees of lung collapse. If the fistula does not close, it should be surgically repaired or the involved lung segment should be removed.

In **tension pneumothorax,** *quick removal of air may be life-saving.* Air may be removed simply by inserting a 19-gauge or larger needle into the chest followed by use of a 3-way stopcock attached to a large syringe to withdraw air rapidly through the needle. The needle may be inserted anteriorly or laterally over a site displaying absent breath sounds and enhanced percussion note. If there is time for a chest x-ray, sites where the lung is held to the chest wall by adhesions should be avoided. Air is alternately withdrawn from the pleural space and expelled from the syringe into the room. This procedure is continued, as determined by the patient's clinical condition, until a tube thoracostomy has been done and water-sealed drainage of the hemithorax has been accomplished. The finger of a rubber glove or a piece of Penrose rubber drain tied to a needle or catheter inserted into the pleural space may serve as a check valve, preventing inspiratory air entry into the pleural space until a more sophisticated pleural drainage system is established.

Recurrent pneumothorax may cause considerable disability. Surgical intervention is generally indicated following two spontaneous pneumothoraces on the same side. The preferred procedures are thoracotomy with oversewing or excision of bullae and roughening of the pleura by rubbing with gauze, or, when bullous disease is extensive, parietal pleurectomy.

---

47. TUMORS OF THE LUNG

Etiology and Incidence

The lungs are the site of origin of primary benign and malignant tumors and receive metastases from many other organs and tissues. A strong dose-related statistical association exists between cigarette smoking and squamous cell and undifferentiated small (oat) cell bronchogenic carcinomas. The incidence of lung cancer is also increased in persons who work with asbestos, uranium ore, chromates, nickel dust, or bischloromethyl ether. Evidence also suggests that prolonged exposure to air pollution promotes lung neoplasms. Peripheral adenocarcinomas and alveolar cell (bronchiolar) carcinomas often occur in association with focal or diffuse lung scarring.

Primary carcinoma of the lung is the most common fatal cancer and its frequency is increasing. In 1969 to 1971, it accounted for 21.2% of cancer deaths in American men and 5.3% in American women. It most often occurs between ages 40 and 70.

Pathology

Four histologic types of bronchogenic carcinoma usually are distinguished: **(1) squamous cell,** frequently arising in the larger bronchi and commonly spreading by direct extension and lymph node metastasis; **(2) undifferentiated small (oat) cell,** producing early hematogenous metastases; **(3) undifferentiated large cell,** usually spreading through the bloodstream; and **(4) adenocarcinoma,** commonly peripheral, usually spreading through the bloodstream. **Alveolar cell (bronchiolar) carcinoma** consolidates air spaces, rarely extends beyond the lungs, and is distinguished from bronchogenic carcinoma by its multifocal origin. The lungs are often involved by **multifocal lymphomas.** Less common primary lung tumors include **bronchial adenoma** (sometimes malignant), **chondromatous hamartoma** (benign), **solitary lymphoma,** and **sarcoma** (malignant). **Metastases** to the lungs are common from primary cancers of the breast, colon, prostate, kidney, thyroid, testis, and bone.

Symptoms and Signs

Manifestations depend on the tumor's location and type of spread. Since most primary tumors are endobronchial, **cough** usually is present. In patients with chronic bronchitis, increased intensity and intractability of preexisting cough suggest a neoplasm. The **sputum** arising from an ulcerated bronchial tumor usually is not excessive (though it may be profuse and watery with alveolar cell carcinomas), but contains inflammatory exudate and is often blood-streaked. Copious **bleeding** (uncommon) strongly suggests invasion of large underlying blood vessels. Bronchial narrowing may cause air trapping with **localized wheezing,** and commonly causes **atelectasis** with mediastinal shift, diminished expansion, dullness to percussion, and loss of breath sounds. **Infection** of obstructed lung produces fever, chest pain, and weight loss. Persistent localized **chest pain** suggests neoplastic invasion of the chest wall. Peripheral nodular tumors are asymptomatic until they invade the pleura or chest wall and cause pain or metastasize to distant organs.

Late symptoms include weight loss and weakness. Serosanguineous pleural effusions are common and often large and recurrent. Horner's syndrome (due to invasion of the cervical thoracic sympathetic nerves) and infiltration of the brachial plexus and the neighboring ribs and vertebrae occur with apical (Pancoast) tumors. A tumor may extend directly into the esophagus, producing obstruction, sometimes complicated by a fistula. Phrenic nerve invasion may cause diaphragmatic paralysis. Superior vena cava obstruction and left recurrent laryngeal nerve paralysis (causing hoarseness) are produced by extension of tumor from neighboring lymph nodes. In the **superior vena cava syndrome (SVCS),** obstruction of venous drainage leads to dilation of collateral veins of the upper part of the chest and neck; edema and plethora of the face, neck, and upper part of the torso, including breasts; suffusion and edema of the conjunctiva; and CNS symptoms, such as headache, visual distortion, and disturbed states of consciousness. Intrapulmonary spread of primary and secondary cancer may cause lymphangitic carcinomatosis with subacute cor pulmonale. Hematogenous nodular metastases within the lungs are common, but bronchial invasion by a secondary tumor is rare. Hematogenous spread of primary lung neoplasms to the liver, brain, adrenals, and bone is common.

Extrapulmonary manifestations of lung cancer are numerous. In hypertrophic pulmonary osteoarthropathy, the best known, clubbing of the fingers and toes and periosteal elevation of the distal parts of the long bones occur. Other extrapulmonary manifestations (principally encephalopathy, subacute cerebellar degeneration, encephalomyelitis, and peripheral neuropathy) occur at all levels of the nervous system. Polymyositis and dermatomyositis may also occur. Metabolic syndromes due to production of substances with hormonal activity may develop. Oat cell carcinomas may secrete ectopic ACTH (resulting in Cushing's syndrome) or ADH (with water retention and hyponatremia) and are associated with the carcinoid syndrome (flushing, wheezing, diarrhea, and cardiac valvular lesions). Squamous cell tumors may secrete parathyroid-hormone–like substances that produce hypercalcemia. Other endocrine syndromes associated with primary lung carcinomas include gynecomastia, hyperglycemia, thyrotoxicosis, and skin pigmentation. Hematologic disorders, including thrombocytopenic purpura, leukemoid reaction, myelophthisic anemia, polycythemia, and marantic thrombosis may also occur.

Peripheral benign primary tumors usually are asymptomatic. **Benign endobronchial tumors** cause obstruction with distal infection.

Bronchial adenoma may be benign or malignant and occurs equally in both sexes. Its course is prolonged. The endobronchial portion of the adenoma dilates and obstructs the lumen of major bronchi. Brisk hemorrhage from the overlying mucous membrane often occurs. Recurrent pneumonia within the same lung zone and localized overlying pleural pain are common. Metastasis is infrequent.

Diagnosis

The principal sources of diagnostic information are the history, which raises the suspicion of tumor and provides early localizing information, and the chest x-ray, which visualizes and locates the lesion and demonstrates its anatomic effects. X-ray patterns correspond closely to the principal gross pathologic tumor types: major bronchial, segmental, and peripheral. In **asymptomatic** patients, a peripheral nodular mass can usually be seen. Previous x-rays are valuable to discern new growth. With smaller solitary nodules, overpenetrated x-rays and tomograms may demonstrate calcification, the amount of which must be more than a fleck to exclude scarring in association with cancer. Computed tomography is expensive but may demonstrate small lesions invisible to other technics.

In **symptomatic** patients, the chest x-ray may show bronchial narrowing and irregularity, parenchymal infiltration, and loss of air bronchogram in an atelectatic area of the lung. Breakdown of lung tissue may be visible in an obstructed area of lung or in association with a peripheral tumor. Obstructive emphysema is not common. Atelectasis in the middle lobe or in segments with small bronchi usually is produced by extension of a tumor arising in the neighboring lobar bronchus. Rarely, x-rays reveal zones of infiltration or obstruction in separate lobes that cannot be explained by a single neoplastic focus but are the result of diffuse submucous lymphatic permeation of the bronchial tree. Pleural effusions are often associated with infiltrating or peripheral tumors.

The presence of primary lung tumors and intrathoracic metastases can be indirectly demonstrated by bronchograms, radiophotoscans, lymphangiography, and interosseous azygography. Photoscans may show metastases in the liver, brain, and bones. The presence of primary tumors and metastases may be directly established by cytologic studies of the sputum and pleural fluid and by tissue biopsy. In rare cases, the sputum is positive for tumor cells when there is no demonstrable focus of disease.

In favorable cases without evident metastases, the principal methods used for visualization of bronchial tumors and for biopsy are rigid and flexible bronchoscopy. With a rigid bronchoscope, the visual field is limited to the major bronchi and their primary divisions, but the extent of the tumor can be effectively determined by carinal and random biopsy and the resistance produced by extrabronchial masses can be sensed. With bronchofiberoscopy (using the flexible bronchoscope), the subsegmental bronchi can be explored to demonstrate and sample tumors by washings and biopsy.

The resectability of the tumor and sometimes the diagnosis can be established by exploratory surgery, provided there are no obvious contraindications to exploration (e.g., distant or mediastinal metastases or cardiorespiratory insufficiency). Exploration can often be avoided when metastases are demonstrated by mediastinoscopy (which has largely replaced scalene node exploration) or by pleural or liver biopsy. Characteristic patterns of calcification seen on x-ray assist in diagnosing peripheral hamartoma and granuloma and usually make surgical exploration unnecessary. Palpable lymph nodes and skin nodules provide important diagnostic material.

Differential diagnosis includes foreign bodies, nonsegmental pneumonia, and endobronchial and focal pulmonary manifestations of tuberculosis, systemic mycoses, and autoimmune disease.

Prognosis and Treatment

The very poor prognosis for patients with **bronchogenic carcinoma** emphasizes the importance of prevention. Substances strongly associated with lung cancer, such as cigarette tobacco, should be avoided, and exposure to potentially carcinogenic substances in industry must be reduced below dangerous levels.

On the average, patients with untreated bronchogenic carcinoma survive 9 mo. Only about 25% of the tumors are resectable and the 5-yr survival rate for the total group is < 10%. In patients with well-circumscribed, slowly growing tumors, the 5-yr survival rate following excision ranges from 25 to 40%. Best results are obtained in patients with peripheral nodular lesions treated by lobectomy.

Endobronchial lesions usually require pneumonectomy to provide a safe plane of bronchial division proximal to the tumor. Pulmonary resection must be accompanied by removal of neighboring lymph nodes. Tumors extending into the chest wall can be removed en bloc; preoperative irradiation has been used in such cases and has been reported to be especially useful in resection of apical tumors.

Postoperative irradiation may be used to treat any remaining involved mediastinal lymph nodes. It is used often in managing painful metastases to bone and sometimes as a substitute for surgery when thoracotomy is contraindicated because of cardiorespiratory insufficiency or other serious disease. Irradiated patients should be carefully watched for signs of radiation pneumonitis, which may be controlled by prednisone 60 mg/day orally for about 1 mo before gradually tapering off the drug.

Despite many clinical trials of individual chemotherapeutic agents and groups of drugs, an effective specific drug regimen for bronchogenic carcinoma has not been established, though some improved results have been reported. In **oat cell carcinoma** surgical results are so poor that other forms of treatment have been advocated. The combination of multiple drug chemotherapy with radiotherapy has yielded higher survival rates than surgery for this tumor. Newer protocols have been reported to show more response, longer survival, and even some cures.

Anxiety and persistent pain are common in patients with incurable lung cancer. Sedatives, narcotics, and other drugs in combination are required (see NARCOTICS AND NARCOTIC ANTAGONISTS in Ch. 247).

Bronchodilator drugs and O_2 may be required for airways obstruction. Mechanical assistance (tracheal suction, mechanical ventilation) and physiotherapy may also be needed. Antibiotics are helpful in treating complicating infections.

Solitary metastases to the lungs have been excised after removal of the primary tumor. The 5-yr survival rate after excision is about 10%. **Benign bronchial tumors** should be resected because of the adverse effects of location, possible growth, and potential malignant transformation. Most **benign peripheral tumors** are undiagnosed before surgical exploration and excision.

---

48.   CIGARETTE SMOKING

Cigarette smokers are at an increased risk of premature death, usually from bronchopulmonary or cardiovascular disease. The life expectancy of an average 30-yr-old who smokes 15 cigarettes/day is shortened by > 5 yr. Although the health risks associated with smoking have been widely stressed, cigarette smoking still poses one of the greatest public health problems in the Western world.

Chemistry and Pharmacology

Tobacco smoke is a mixture of gases and minute droplets of tar; nearly 1000 components of tobacco smoke have been identified. Though some components are filtered off as the smoke is drawn through the unburned tobacco, they are redistilled as the burning ember advances, and the smoke in each successive puff becomes more concentrated. Since cigarette smoke is less irritating than pipe or cigar smoke, it is more likely to be inhaled. Cigarette smoking is thus more hazardous than pipe or cigar smoking, though the latter are not completely innocuous.

Substances of medical importance in smoke may be separated as follows:

1. **Carcinogens and cocarcinogens** are present in the tar. Carcinogens (principally polycyclic aromatic alcohols) initiate cancer formation. Cocarcinogens (including phenols, fatty acids, and free

fatty acids) accelerate the production of cancer by other initiators. Many cocarcinogens are also irritants.

2. Irritants cause immediate coughing and bronchoconstriction after smoke inhalation, inhibit cilial action in the bronchial epithelium, stimulate bronchial mucous secretion, suppress protease inhibition, and impair alveolar macrophage function.

3. Nicotine principally affects the nervous system and is probably responsible for a smoker's pharmacologic dependence on cigarettes. The effects are complex and include stimulation or sedation, depending on the dose and on the smoker's physical and psychologic states. Nicotine indirectly affects circulation by provoking catecholamine release which causes tachycardia, increased cardiac output, vasoconstriction, and increased BP. Nicotine also increases serum free fatty acids and platelet adhesiveness, and inhibits pancreatic bicarbonate secretion.

4. Toxic gases in cigarette smoke include CO, hydrogen sulfide, hydrocyanic acid, and oxides of nitrogen. The average carboxyhemoglobin level in people smoking one pack/day is about 5%, compared to $< 1\%$ in nonsmokers. This reduces the amount of Hb available for O_2 transport and shifts to the left the HbO_2–dissociation curve, impairing O_2 release to the tissues. Exposure to CO may also increase atheroma formation.

Diseases Related to Smoking

1. Lung cancer: Squamous cell and small (oat) cell lung carcinomas are associated with smoking. Epidemiologic studies have shown that men who smoke more than one pack/day are about 20 times more at risk of developing lung cancer than are nonsmokers. The risk is greatest in those who inhale, take more puffs/cigarette, relight half-smoked cigarettes, and start smoking at an early age. Filter tips may offer some protection. Laboratory experiments show that tobacco smoke condensate can produce skin cancer in animals and that animals inhaling cigarette smoke may develop cancer of the larynx or lung.

2. Chronic bronchitis and emphysema deaths are also about 20 times more frequent in people who smoke heavily. Both diseases can be produced in animals exposed to cigarette smoke. Pulmonary function tests often show airflow obstruction in the small airways even before chronic expectoration develops. The adverse effect of smoking on mucociliary clearance and on the normal balance between lung proteases and their inhibitors predisposes smokers to bronchopulmonary infection and emphysema.

3. Cardiovascular diseases: Cigarette smoking accelerates atherosclerosis and may double the risk of myocardial infarction. Smoking may precipitate an anginal attack or ischemic ECG changes in patients with coronary artery disease. The risk of developing cerebrovascular disease, peripheral vascular disease, or nonsyphilitic aortic aneurysm is also increased in smokers.

4. Pregnancy: The mean birth weight of infants born to mothers who smoke during pregnancy is 6 oz less than that of infants born to nonsmoking mothers. The incidence of spontaneous abortion, stillbirth, and neonatal death may also be increased in pregnant women who smoke.

5. Extrapulmonary cancers associated with cigarette smoking include cancer of the mouth, pharynx, larynx, esophagus, bladder, and pancreas.

6. Peptic (especially gastric) ulceration occurs more frequently and has a higher mortality rate in cigarette smokers than in nonsmokers. In addition, the effectiveness of medical treatment for peptic ulceration is reduced and the rate of ulcer healing is slowed.

7. Other conditions: Pulmonary TB is more common in smokers, perhaps due to activation of old tuberculous foci. **Tobacco amblyopia** may be caused by optic nerve damage due to the toxic action of cyanides in cigarette smoke in smokers with vitamin B_{12} deficiency. Smokers are also liable to develop **gingivitis** and require early **dental extractions.** Their **physical fitness** is reduced because of impaired pulmonary function and Hb transport of O_2 to the tissues.

8. Passive exposure to cigarette smoke may trigger bronchoconstriction in asthmatics and angina in patients with coronary artery disease. Respiratory disease is more common in children whose parents smoke.

Stopping Smoking

About 20% of cigarette smokers stop smoking. Although the mortality risk for people who stop smoking declines, even 15 yr later it is higher than in people who never smoked. Success in response to public health education is more likely in professional and managerial people and in those best able to understand the risks associated with smoking. Unfortunately, most smokers do not usually stop smoking until the onset of ill health. Withdrawal effects, possibly related to nicotine deprivation, include depression, anxiety, irritability, insomnia, weight gain, and GI symptoms. Hypnosis, aversion therapy, group therapy, and special smoking withdrawal clinics have helped individuals break the smoking habit, but the overall value of these aids is uncertain. Drugs such as lobeline and tranquilizers have been no more effective than placebos. Persons unable to stop cigarette smoking should be encouraged to change to a less dangerous method of smoking; e.g., a pipe or cigar, or filter-tipped cigarettes with a low tar and nicotine content. The risk may also be reduced by smoking fewer cigarettes, inhaling less, leaving a longer stub, and taking fewer puffs/cigarette. There is no evidence of addiction to other drugs in smokers who abandon the habit.

§5. GASTROINTESTINAL DISORDERS

49. INTRODUCTION

The study and treatment of GI disease has been profoundly modified by recent technologic developments. Diagnostic imaging, using the technics of radionuclide scanning, radioangiography, and computerized axial tomography, coupled with the continued development of the flexible fiberoptic endoscope, allow an amazing precision in diagnosis. Therapeutically, the H_2 antihistamine preparations, with their potent antacid effects, have changed the management of peptic ulcer disease. A vaccine for hepatitis B is now available. The discovery of the role of *Campylobacter*, *Yersinia*, and *Clostridium* organisms in inflammatory bowel disease has led to advances in treatment.

None of these advances, however, can replace a sound understanding of symptoms and signs and of the ways in which they may be presented to the physician. Only when an alert, concerned physician is buttressed with knowledge of the pathophysiology and natural history of a disease can new technology and modern therapeutics be wisely applied.

50. DISORDERS OF THE ESOPHAGUS

The human swallowing apparatus consists of the pharynx, upper esophageal (cricopharyngeal) sphincter, body of the esophagus, and lower esophageal sphincter. The upper third of the esophagus and structures proximal to it are composed of skeletal muscle; the distal esophagus and lower esophageal sphincter contain smooth muscle. This integrated system transports material from the mouth to the stomach and prevents reflux of the material into the esophagus.

COMMON SYMPTOMS AND SIGNS

Dysphagia

A subjective awareness of difficulty in swallowing due to impaired progression of matter from pharynx to stomach. The usual complaint is that food "gets stuck" on the way down. The feeling may be accompanied by pain. Dysphagia is the major symptom of esophageal transport disorders. The transport of liquids and solids may be impeded by organic lesions of the pharynx, esophagus, and adjacent organs, or by functional derangements of the nervous system and musculature. The cause of dysphagia, which may be a pre-esophageal or an esophageal abnormality, should always be carefully sought.

Pre-esophageal dysphagia: *Difficulty emptying material from the oral pharynx into the esophagus.* This symptom occurs with disorders proximal to the esophagus, most often in patients with generalized skeletal muscle or neurologic disorders such as dermatomyositis, myotonia dystrophica, myasthenia gravis, bulbar poliomyelitis, pseudobulbar palsy, and other CNS lesions, or may be associated with nasal regurgitation and tracheal aspiration followed by coughing.

Esophageal dysphagia may be due to **obstructive** or **motor disorders**. **Obstructive disorders** such as carcinoma, benign peptic stricture, and lower esophageal ring usually produce *dysphagia for solids alone* by mechanically reducing the esophageal lumen. Meat and bread are often singled out as the major offenders, but some patients can tolerate only liquids. The patient often points to the site of obstruction, but is inaccurate in about 20% of cases. In carcinoma of the esophagus, the dysphagia progresses rapidly over weeks or months. In peptic stricture, dysphagia progresses slowly over years and is preceded by a prominent history of gastroesophageal reflux. With a lower esophageal ring, dysphagia is intermittent.

Motor disorders causing esophageal dysfunction involve the smooth muscle of the esophagus. They produce *dysphagia for both solids and liquids* by impairing esophageal peristalsis and lower esophageal sphincter function, thus interrupting the smooth esophageal transport of a bolus. Achalasia, symptomatic diffuse esophageal spasm, and scleroderma are the most common motor disorders. From the onset of symptoms, the presence of dysphagia for *both* liquids and solids accurately distinguishes motor from obstructive causes.

Dysphagia should not be confused with **globus hystericus** (globus sensation), a feeling of having a lump in the throat that is unrelated to swallowing and occurs without impaired transport. Often noted in association with feelings of grief, globus hystericus is mainly emotional in etiology.

Chest Pain of Esophageal Origin

Chest or back pain, the second major symptom of esophageal disease, is classified as heartburn, pain during swallowing, or spontaneous esophageal motor disorder pain.

Heartburn, caused by reflux of gastric contents into the esophagus (gastroesophageal reflux; see below), is a substernal burning pain that rises in the chest and may radiate into the neck, throat, or even face. It usually occurs after meals or when the patient is lying down, and is frequently accompanied by regurgitation of gastric contents into the mouth.

Pain during swallowing (odynophagia) may occur with or without dysphagia and may be due to mucosal destruction as in esophagitis induced by gastroesophageal reflux, bacterial or mycotic infections, neoplasms, or chemicals, or to esophageal motor disorders such as achalasia and symptomatic diffuse esophageal spasm. The patient may describe the pain as a burning sensation or a substernal tightness typically elicited by very hot or very cold food or liquid. Onset is prompt on swallowing. Severe squeezing chest pain, brought on by swallowing cold beverages and invariably associated with dysphagia, is characteristic of esophageal motor disorders.

Spontaneous motor disorder pain is difficult to characterize apart from other esophageal symptoms. The diagnosis is one of exclusion and should be made only in patients with a definite history of dysphagia. Spontaneous esophageal chest pain may be severe and mimic angina pectoris, but the pain may radiate to the interscapular area of the back rather than to the jaw or left arm as in angina.

COMMON DIAGNOSTIC PROCEDURES

A **history** precisely detailing the patient's symptoms should establish an accurate diagnosis in about 80% of cases. The only **physical findings** in esophageal disease are: (1) cervical and clavicular lymphadenopathy due to metastatic spread of malignancy, (2) swellings in the neck from large pharyngeal diverticula, and (3) prolonged swallowing time (the time from the act of swallowing to the noise of the bolus of fluid and air entering the stomach, heard by auscultation with the stethoscope over the epigastrium and normally 12 seconds or less). Esophageal motor disorders are associated with prolonged swallowing times.

Laboratory Tests

X-ray studies: In addition to the standard barium meal, the advent of cinefluoroscopy has aided in detecting such disorders as esophageal webs and in assessing motor disorders such as cricopharyngeal spasm and achalasia.

Esophagoscopy has been greatly enhanced by the advent of the flexible fiberoptic esophagoscope.

Esophageal manometry determines the pressure in the upper and lower esophageal sphincters and the effectiveness and coordination of propulsive movements, and detects abnormal contractions. It is used in diagnosing achalasia, diffuse spasm, scleroderma, and lower esophageal sphincter hypo- and hypertension.

Esophageal pH monitoring, usually done in conjunction with esophageal manometry, demonstrates the reflux of gastric acid content and provides direct evidence of gastroesophageal reflux.

The Bernstein (acid perfusion) test is done by perfusing the esophagus through a nasogastric tube with solutions of isotonic saline or 0.1 N hydrochloric acid at a rate of 6 ml/min. The Bernstein test correlates closely with the complaint of heartburn. A patient may complain of heartburn and have a normal esophagus as demonstrated by esophagoscopy, but the Bernstein test will be positive, indicating that gastric acid reflux is cause for the complaint.

DISORDERS ASSOCIATED WITH PRE-ESOPHAGEAL DYSPHAGIA

In **cricopharyngeal incoordination,** the cricopharyngeal muscle (the upper esophageal sphincter) remains closed or opens in an uncoordinated way. It may cause a Zenker's diverticulum (see under ESOPHAGEAL DIVERTICULA, below); repeated aspirations of material from the diverticulum may lead to chronic lung disease. The condition may be **treated** by surgical section of the muscle.

Myasthenia gravis, myotonia, dysautonomia, and the oculogyric crises associated with phenothiazine therapy are other causes of pre-esophageal dysphagia and pseudo-bulbar palsies.

DISORDERS ASSOCIATED WITH ESOPHAGEAL DYSPHAGIA

OBSTRUCTIVE DISORDERS

EXTRINSIC OBSTRUCTION

The esophagus may be compressed by adjacent organs or extrinsic tumors. The symptom is dysphagia for solids, similar to intrinsic esophageal obstruction. Extrinsic obstruction may occur with an enlarged left atrium, aortic aneurysm, aberrant subclavian artery (see DYSPHAGIA LUSORIA below), substernal thyroid, bony exostosis, or extrinsic tumors—most commonly lung. The prognosis is based on the cause of the extrinsic obstruction. Diagnosis is usually made on x-ray.

CARCINOMA OF THE ESOPHAGUS

The most serious cause of dysphagia, carcinoma usually presents with progressive dysphagia for solids over several weeks, associated with marked weight loss. Carcinoma may occur in any portion of the esophagus and may appear as a stricture, mass, or plaque. The tumor is best diagnosed by x-ray, followed by endoscopy with biopsy and cytology. The yield on brush cytology is > 95% positive, while biopsy may be positive in about 70% of cases. Tumors are most frequently squamous cell carcinoma with about 5% of esophageal cancer being adenocarcinoma.

Conditions associated with an increased frequency of esophageal cancer are achalasia, lye stricture, Barrett's epithelium, and esophageal webs. The treatment of squamous cell carcinoma is either surgical resection or radiation therapy; adenocarcinoma is treated by surgery only. The overall prognosis is poor with < 5% long-term survival. Palliation for obstruction or esophageal fistulas consists of dilation procedures or insertion of a tube prosthesis.

LOWER ESOPHAGEAL RING (Schatzki's Ring)

A 2- to 4-mm submucosal structure, probably congenital, causing a ring-like narrowing of the distal esophagus at the squamocolumnar junction. Intermittent dysphagia for solids may occur when the narrowing is sufficient to produce obstruction, usually when the esophageal lumen is < 12 mm in diameter. The ring is usually demonstrated by barium x-ray studies if the distal esophagus is adequately distended with a solid bolus (barium tablet, bread, or marshmallow). Rings > 2.0 cm in diameter are usually asymptomatic and should not have symptoms attributed to them.

Instructing the patient to chew his food thoroughly is usually the only **treatment** required, but rings may be fractured endoscopically, by pneumatic dilation, or by resection.

ESOPHAGEAL WEBS (Plummer-Vinson or Paterson-Kelly Syndrome; Sideropenic Dysphagia)

A thin, membranous mucosal structure that grows across the lumen, usually in the upper esophagus. Esophageal webs may develop rarely in patients with untreated severe iron deficiency anemia or, even more rarely, without an overt anemia. They are usually located in the upper esophagus and produce dysphagia for solids; usually missed on ordinary barium swallow, they can be demonstrated best on cinefilms. The webs, composed of squamous epithelium, disappear with treatment of the anemia, but may be easily ruptured during esophagoscopy.

DYSPHAGIA LUSORIA

Dysphagia due to compression of the esophagus by a congenital vascular abnormality (usually an aberrant right subclavian artery arising from the left side of the aortic arch). The dysphagia may occur in childhood or may develop later due to arteriosclerotic changes in the aberrant vessel. Esophageal x-ray studies show the extrinsic compression above the aortic arch, at the third thoracic vertebra. Arteriography is necessary for absolute diagnosis. Surgical correction is only rarely indicated.

MOTOR DISORDERS

ACHALASIA (Cardiospasm; Esophageal Aperistalsis; Megaesophagus)

A neurogenic esophageal disorder of unknown etiology causing impairment of esophageal peristalsis and of lower esophageal sphincter relaxation. The condition may be due to a malfunction of the myenteric plexus of the esophagus that results in denervation of esophageal muscle.

Symptoms and Signs

Achalasia may occur at any age, but usually begins between ages 20 and 40. Dysphagia for both solids and liquids is the major symptom; onset is insidious and progression is gradual over many months or years. Increased pressure at the lower esophageal sphincter produces obstruction with secondary dilation of the esophagus and a tendency toward regurgitation and aspiration when the patient lies down. Nocturnal regurgitation of undigested food occurs in about 1/3 of the patients and may cause pulmonary aspiration with lung abscess, bronchiectasis, or pneumonia. Chest pain is less common, but may occur upon swallowing or spontaneously. Weight loss is usually mild to moderate but may become marked in untreated cases.

Diagnosis

X-ray studies of the esophagus demonstrate the absence of progressive peristaltic contractions during swallowing. The esophagus is dilated and frequently reaches enormous proportions, but is narrowed and beaklike at the lower esophageal sphincter. Esophageal manometry shows aperistalsis, increased lower esophageal sphincter pressure, and incomplete sphincteric relaxation with swallowing. Esophagoscopy reveals dilation but no organic obstructing lesion. The esophagoscope usually passes readily into the stomach. The denervated structures are more sensitive to pharmacologic stimuli; hence, methacholine s.c. (in graded doses of 1 to 2 mg) may dramatically increase intraesophageal pressure. Some patients are inordinately sensitive to methacholine and may develop severe cholinergic side effects (e.g., severe cardiac arrhythmias), but it is used with manometry as a diagnostic test.

Achalasia must be differentiated from a distal stenosing carcinoma and a peptic stricture; in the latter 2 conditions, the esophagoscope cannot be passed beyond the obstruction. Esophageal biopsy and cytology should be done in all cases to exclude carcinoma.

Prognosis

Pulmonary aspiration and secondary carcinoma are the determining factors in prognosis. Nocturnal regurgitation with coughing suggests possible aspiration. Pulmonary complications secondary to aspiration are difficult to manage. The incidence of esophageal carcinoma in patients with achalasia is about 5%.

Treatment

The aim of treatment is to reduce the pressure and thus the obstruction at the lower esophageal sphincter. Forceful or pneumatic dilation of the sphincter with a Mosher or Brown-McHardy dilating instrument is indicated initially, since results are satisfactory in about 80% of the patients; repeated dilations may be needed. Esophageal rupture and secondary mediastinitis requiring surgery occur in < 1% of the cases. A Heller myotomy, in which the muscular fibers in the lower esophageal sphincter are cut, is usually reserved for patients who fail to respond to pneumatic dilation and is successful about 85% of the time. Symptomatic gastroesophageal reflux follows surgery in about 15% of the patients.

SYMPTOMATIC DIFFUSE ESOPHAGEAL SPASM (Spastic Pseudodiverticulosis; Rosary Bead or Corkscrew Esophagus)

A generalized neurogenic disorder of esophageal motility in which normal peristalsis is replaced by phasic nonpropulsive contractions and, in some cases, by abnormal lower esophageal sphincter function.

Symptoms and Signs

Chest pain and dysphagia for both liquids and solids occur in close association. The pain, which may occur upon swallowing or spontaneously, is substernal and may mimic angina pectoris; it may awaken the patient from sleep. Nocturnal regurgitation and pulmonary aspiration are rare. Over many years, this disorder evolves rarely into achalasia.

Diagnosis

X-rays show nonperistaltic contractions and poor propulsion of a bolus; esophageal dilation is minimal or absent. Esophageal manometry demonstrates repetitive, high-amplitude, nonperistaltic contractions or spasms. Lower esophageal sphincter function is usually normal.

Treatment

The condition is difficult to treat. Nitroglycerin, long-acting nitrates, and anticholinergics have been used with limited success. Pneumatic dilation and bougienage have also been tried. Medical management is usually sufficient, but surgical myotomy along the full length of the esophagus may be helpful in intractable cases.

VARIANTS OF DIFFUSE SPASM AND ACHALASIA

Some patients show symptom complexes that do not fit either classic achalasia or classic diffuse spasm. Some of these have been called "**vigorous achalasia**" in that they have both the severe pain and spasm of diffuse spasm and the retention of fluid and aspiration of achalasia.

SCLERODERMA (See PROGRESSIVE SYSTEMIC SCLEROSIS in Ch. 104)

GASTROESOPHAGEAL REFLUX AND ITS COMPLICATIONS

Reflux of gastric contents into the esophagus.

Etiology

The functional and anatomic mechanisms that normally prevent gastroesophageal reflux include lower esophageal sphincter pressure, the angle of the cardioesophageal junction, the effect of gravity (except during recumbency), and, possibly, the action of the diaphragm. Gastroesophageal incompetence was previously attributed solely to a sliding hiatus hernia, but recent evidence indicates that the cause is lower esophageal sphincter incompetence. The sphincter may become weakened in the absence of a hiatus hernia, thus explaining the large number of asymptomatic patients with hiatus hernia and the increasing recognition of patients with marked reflux but no demonstrable hernia on x-ray.

Symptoms and Signs

Heartburn with or without regurgitation of gastric contents into the mouth is the most prominent symptom. Complications of gastroesophageal reflux include esophagitis, peptic esophageal stricture, and esophageal ulcer. Esophagitis may cause odynophagia and possibly massive, but usually limited, hemorrhage. Peptic stricture causes a gradually progressive dysphagia for solid foods. Peptic esophageal ulcers cause the same type of pain as do gastric or duodenal ulcers, but are usually localized to the xiphoid or high substernal region. They heal slowly, tend to recur, and usually leave a stricture upon healing.

Diagnosis

A careful history points to the diagnosis. X-ray studies, endoscopy, esophageal manometry, pH monitoring, and acid perfusion of the esophagus (Bernstein test) help to confirm the diagnosis and demonstrate possible complications. X-rays taken with the patient in the Trendelenburg position may show reflux of barium from the stomach into the esophagus. Abdominal compression may be used, but radiographic maneuvers are not usually sensitive indicators of gastroesophageal reflux. X-rays taken following a barium swallow readily demonstrate esophageal ulcers and peptic strictures, but are only rarely diagnostic in patients with hemorrhage due to esophagitis. Esophagoscopy provides accurate diagnosis of esophagitis with or without hemorrhage. Esophagoscopy in conjunction with cytologic washings and direct vision biopsy is essential for distinguishing benign peptic stricture from carcinoma of the esophagus. Barrett's epithelium is a term used to describe columnar meta-plastic epithelium that may occur in the lower esophagus following the chronic injury of peptic esophagitis. This epithelial change is associated with an increased frequency of esophageal adeno-carcinoma. Esophageal manometry, by determining pressure at the lower esophageal sphincter, indicates its strength and thereby distinguishes a normal from an incompetent sphincter. Esophageal pH monitoring shows the reflux of acid gastric contents into the esophagus and provides direct evidence of gastroesophageal reflux. The Bernstein test correlates closely with the presence of symptomatic gastroesophageal reflux; symptoms are promptly reproduced by acid perfusion and relieved by saline perfusion. Esophageal biopsy is an accurate indicator of gastroesophageal reflux, showing thinning of the squamous mucosal layer and basilar cell hyperplasia. These histologic changes may occur without evidence of gross esophagitis by endoscopy. A positive biopsy or a positive Bernstein test correlates best with esophageal symptoms of reflux regardless of endoscopic or x-ray findings.

Treatment

Uncomplicated gastroesophageal reflux may be tolerated for many years with good response to medical therapy. Management consists of (1) elevating the head of the bed 6 in.; (2) avoiding foods that are strong stimulants of acid secretion (e.g., coffee, alcohol); (3) avoiding certain drugs (e.g., anticholinergics), specific foods (fats, chocolate), and smoking, all of which reduce lower esopha-geal sphincter competence; (4) giving antacids 30 ml 1 h after meals and at bedtime to neutralize gastric acidity and possibly increase lower esophageal sphincter competence; and (5) possibly using bethanechol 25 mg orally t.i.d. to diminish gastroesophageal reflux. Metoclopramide (not yet ap-proved by the FDA) 15 mg orally 30 min before meals and at bedtime also will increase the lower esophageal sphincteric tone and prevent reflux. (6) Cimetidine 300 mg orally q.i.d. (30 min before meals and at bedtime) reduces acid secretion and improves heartburn.

Hemorrhage from esophagitis, unless massive, does not require emergency surgery, but it may recur.

Esophageal strictures are difficult to manage and require repeated dilation (e.g., with mercury-filled bougies) to achieve and maintain esophageal patency. If properly dilated, they do not seriously limit what the patient can eat.

New anti-reflux operations (Belsey, Hill, Nissen) are used in patients with serious esophagitis, hemorrhage, stricture, ulcer, or intractable symptoms, whether or not a hiatus hernia was present.

CORROSIVE ESOPHAGITIS AND STRICTURE

(See INGESTION OF CAUSTICS in Vol. II, Ch. 24)

MISCELLANEOUS DISORDERS

Congenital anomalies of the esophagus are discussed under GASTROINTESTINAL DEFECTS in Vol. II, Ch. 21.

ESOPHAGEAL DIVERTICULA

There are several types of esophageal diverticula, each of different etiology. A **pharyngeal diver-ticulum (Zenker's)** is an outpouching of the mucosa and submucosa posteriorly through the crico-pharyngeal muscle. It probably results from incoordination between pharyngeal propulsion and cricopharyngeal relaxation. **Mid-esophageal (traditionally called traction) diverticula** are either due to traction from mediastinal inflammatory lesions or secondary to motor disorders. An **epiphrenic diverticulum,** also probably of propulsive origin, occurs just above the diaphragm and usually ac-companies an esophageal motor disturbance (achalasia, diffuse esophageal spasm).

Symptoms, Signs, and Diagnosis

A Zenker's diverticulum fills with food which may be regurgitated when the patient bends or lies down. Aspiration pneumonitis may result if regurgitation is nocturnal. Rarely, the pouch becomes large and causes dysphagia. Traction and epiphrenic diverticula are rarely symptomatic in them-selves. All diverticula are diagnosed by barium-swallow x-ray.

Treatment

Specific treatment is usually not required, though surgical resection of the diverticulum is occasionally necessary.

HIATUS HERNIA

Protrusion of the stomach above the diaphragm.

Etiology and Pathology

Etiology is usually unknown, but a hiatus hernia may be a congenital abnormality or secondary to trauma. In a **sliding hiatus hernia**, the gastroesophageal junction and a portion of the stomach are above the diaphragm. One side of the herniated stomach is covered by peritoneum. In **paraesophageal hiatus hernia**, the gastroesophageal junction is in the normal location, but a portion of the stomach is adjacent to the esophagus.

Symptoms and Signs

A sliding hiatus hernia is common and may be seen by x-ray in > 40% of the population. Most patients are asymptomatic. Although gastroesophageal reflux occurs in a few patients, it is doubtful whether the hernia is the cause since reflux may also be found in patients with no demonstrable hernia on x-ray. Chest pain without gastroesophageal reflux can also occur. A paraesophageal hiatus hernia is generally asymptomatic, but, unlike a sliding hiatus hernia, may incarcerate and strangulate. Occult or massive GI hemorrhage may occur with either type of hiatus hernia.

Diagnosis

X-rays usually readily demonstrate hiatus hernia. Vigorous testing by applying abdominal compression may be required to show a sliding hiatus hernia.

Treatment

A sliding hiatus hernia usually requires no specific therapy, but any accompanying gastroesophageal reflux should be treated (see GASTROESOPHAGEAL REFLUX, above). A paraesophageal hernia of significant size should be reduced surgically because of the risk of strangulation.

ESOPHAGEAL LACERATION AND RUPTURE

Mallory-Weiss syndrome: *Laceration of the distal esophagus and proximal stomach during vomiting, retching, or hiccups.* GI hemorrhage from an arterial site is the usual clinical presentation. Initially described in alcoholics, the Mallory-Weiss syndrome is recognized in all types of patients. It frequently causes GI hemorrhage, comprising about 10% of patients with this disorder. **Diagnosis** is made during endoscopic evaluation or arteriography. The lesion is not seen on routine upper GI x-rays. Most episodes of bleeding stop spontaneously, but some patients require ligation of the laceration. Intra-arterial infusion of pitressin into the left gastric artery during angiography has also been shown to control bleeding.

The esophagus may be ruptured during endoscopic procedures or other instrumentations. **Boerhaave's syndrome,** *spontaneous esophageal rupture,* is a catastrophic illness with a high mortality. Perforation or rupture of the esophagus leads to mediastinitis and pleural effusion. Immediate surgical repair and drainage are required.

ESOPHAGEAL MONILIASIS

Infection with *Candida albicans* may extend from the mouth into the esophagus. It usually occurs in patients with chronic debilitating disease, or in those receiving corticosteroids, broad-spectrum antibiotics, or immunosuppressives. Patients may be asymptomatic, but usually odynophagia and, less frequently, dysphagia occur. Culture or histologic examination of the esophageal exudate shows clusters of spores and hyphae. On x-ray, the esophageal mucosa is irregular and ulcerated. **Treatment** consists of nystatin suspension 5 ml orally q.i.d. Nystatin lozenges have also been used to increase contact time with the involved area.

51. FUNCTIONAL DYSPEPSIA AND OTHER NONSPECIFIC GASTROINTESTINAL COMPLAINTS

Symptoms referred to the GI system in which a pathologic condition is not present, is poorly established, or, if present, does not entirely explain the clinical state. Patients with such complaints are very common in the primary care setting and account for 30 to 50% of the gastroenterologist's referral population. Both the referring physician and the GI specialist consider the illness atypical, as it does not fit within previously learned categories of disease. Uncertainty may lead to frustration judgmental attitudes toward the patients, and ordering inappropriate tests in a futile attempt to determine a biologic cause that explains the complaints.

Although functional or nonspecific symptoms may in part derive from medical disease (e.g., peptic ulcer, esophagitis), the contributory psychologic or cultural factors make diagnosis difficult and medical treatment alone insufficient. More often, histopathologic abnormalities are not established. Evidence may indicate altered physiologic activity (e.g., symptomatic diffuse esophageal spasm [see above], irritable bowel syndrome [see THE IRRITABLE BOWEL SYNDROME in Ch. 59]), the patient may be preoccupied with normal physiologic function (e.g., borborygmus in the hypochondriac), or psychologic illness may assume primary importance (conversion disorder, somatization in depression). In many cases, more than one of these factors is involved.

Regardless of the etiology, the experience and reporting of the symptoms vary, depending on the patient's personality, the psychologic meaning of the illness to him, and the influence of sociocultural patterns. Thus, symptoms of nausea and vomiting due to cholecystitis may be minimized or reported in an indirect, even bizarre fashion by the severely depressed patient, but presented with dramatic urgency by the histrionic patient. Although distressing, the patient's illness may satisfy certain psychologic needs; e.g., it may serve to avoid overt mental distress or lead to benefits derived from the attention and privileges of the sick role (removal from responsibilities, disability compensation). This helps to explain why many of these patients are noncompliant, have unexpected side effects to medication, and seem resistant to improvement. Finally, cultural influences may affect the reporting of symptoms. A bizarre idea, such as the patient's belief that illness is derived from evil spirits, may indicate a primary psychiatric disorder in an educated businessman, but be of little etiologic significance in the patient from a primitive cultural society.

Approach to the Patient

A patient-oriented clinical approach with appreciation of the psychosocial aspects of illness as outlined below should be followed in patients with inexplicable complaints.

1. **The history should be obtained by an open-ended interview style.** Questions that encourage the patient to respond spontaneously prevent physician bias from affecting the content of the history. The symptoms are then likely to be presented by the patient in relation to physiologic and psychosocial events that contribute to the illness. Leading questions or those that elicit "yes" or "no" answers should be avoided. To ask directly, "Is the pain relieved by food?" may get a falsely positive response, since the patient's wish to comply to the doctor's expectations overrides his intention to be accurate. However, an inquiry such as, "What makes the pain better or worse?" will minimize bias and may bring out important additional information that can be developed through specific questions to define the symptoms. The physician must elicit not only the location and quality of the symptoms but also their setting, the presence of aggravating and alleviating factors, and any associated symptoms. All information must then be synthesized to see how the complex of symptoms and related factors fit into diagnostic categories.

2. **The role of psychologic stress factors must be considered.** The experience of any event as stressful varies among individuals; e.g., divorce may sadden one person and relieve another. Such data are rarely obtained through direct inquiry. Rather, when the patient volunteers relevant information while discussing the setting of the symptoms, he should be encouraged to elaborate on these issues. A noncritical attitude must be maintained at all times.

3. **A behavioral ("functional") disorder does not preclude the presence or future development of medical disease.** Even though a history contains vague, dramatic, or bizarre symptoms, new and possibly significant complaints should not be minimized. Complete objectivity must guide the approach to each clinical problem. New physical findings or "hard" data suggesting pathologic changes (blood in the stool, fever, anemia, or metabolic disturbance) should prompt further evaluation.

4. **When in doubt, "don't just do something—stand there."** The tendency to order excess or unnecessary studies for the insistent patient with inexplicable complaints should be avoided; patients must often be managed with incomplete or nonspecific medical data. When a problem is not critical, the wise physician will temporize rather than embark upon an uncertain diagnostic or therapeutic plan. In time, new information may lead to directed evaluation and management.

5. **Diagnostic studies may not entirely explain a patient's clinical condition.** Endoscopy can establish the presence of a duodenal ulcer, but cannot clarify why one patient is asymptomatic and another disabled. Furthermore, the indications for and accuracy of all procedures selected must be considered. A negative medical evaluation does not entirely exclude physical disease. The appropriate study may not have been selected, the results may have been misinterpreted, or a false-negative result may have been obtained because of limitations of the study.

6. **Removal of the symptom is not always the goal of treatment.** The illness may have such adaptive value to the patient that the loss from giving up the "benefits" may be greater than the gain from relief of symptoms. Pain or suffering may substitute for more distressing feelings of guilt and sadness. The attention and privileges derived from being chronically ill may also be significant. When the patient overtly or covertly resists management, the illness can be assumed to fulfill certain needs. In these cases, the illness must be accepted and treatment should be oriented toward improving function *despite the continuation of the symptoms*. Although in this approach the physician seem-

ingly abandons his commitment to cure or remove disease, his frustration is reduced when the therapeutic goals are realistic; results in these patients are often favorable.

FUNCTIONAL DYSPEPSIA

Common discomfort often described as "indigestion," gaseousness, fullness, or pain that is gnawing or burning in quality and localized to the upper abdomen or chest.

These symptoms are not confined to a single organ or disease process and can have many etiologies. Correlating the symptoms of dyspepsia with pathophysiologic states is difficult. Endoscopic and radiographic detection of structural abnormalities that explain the symptoms varies so widely (from 14 to 87%) that estimates of incidence are meaningless. The studies may not be comparable because methods differ for population selection, analysis, and interpretation. Furthermore, an *association* between symptoms and pathophysiologic abnormalities does not necessarily mean *causation*. For example, histologic evidence of inflammatory gastritis can be found in 15 to 50% of *asymptomatic* healthy volunteers. Radiologic or pathologic "duodenitis," pyloric dysfunction with alkaline reflux, and cholelithiasis are other commonly described conditions with uncertain relationships to clinical symptoms.

Symptoms and Signs

Belching, abdominal distention, and borborygmus are often described in addition to epigastric or substernal pain. Eating may worsen or relieve the pain. Other associated symptoms may include anorexia, nausea, and change in bowel habits. Dysphoric states such as anxiety or depression may often be found.

Differential Diagnosis

Dyspepsia may be reported in cardiac ischemia (in which the discomfort is worsened by exertion), gastroesophageal reflux, diffuse esophageal spasm (particularly if dysphagia is present), peptic ulcer disease, and cholecystitis. Psychologic causes include anxiety with or without aerophagia, conversion disorder, somatization in depression, or hypochondriasis. Lactose intolerance may mimic these symptoms (see CARBOHYDRATE INTOLERANCE in Ch. 56). It is important to inquire about bowel habits. A history of alternating constipation and diarrhea suggests a generalized motility disorder as the etiology, such as the irritable bowel syndrome (see IRRITABLE BOWEL SYNDROME in Ch. 59).

No preplanned method of evaluation can be recommended. The history and complete examination will determine whether or not further studies are indicated. At a minimum, a CBC and tests for occult blood in the stool should be done. An upper GI series is usually required, particularly if the patient also has dysphagia, weight loss, vomiting, or change in the pattern of symptoms with eating. Upper esophagogastroduodenoscopy has been suggested for patients with continued unexplained symptoms and may be of additional value; it is more sensitive for detecting mucosal abnormalities. Caution is required in relating any nonspecific findings obtained as explanation for the symptoms. Esophageal manometry is indicated only if dysphagia, regurgitation, or evidence for aspiration suggests a motor disorder of the esophagus. Dyspepsia without other clinical findings is unlikely to be caused by cholelithiasis. In this situation, if oral cholecystography reveals gallstones in a functioning gallbladder, cholecystectomy may not relieve the dyspepsia. However, a compatible history and objective findings also suggestive of cholecystitis or choledocholithiasis (intermittent localizing right upper quadrant pain, vomiting after meals, fever, jaundice, or abnormal liver chemistries) require thorough evaluation of the biliary system and surgical intervention if disease is found.

Treatment

Dyspepsia with no evidence of underlying somatic disease usually calls first for reassurance and symptomatic management with observation over time. Treatment of reflux symptoms or epigastric discomfort may be tried with antacids.

Changes in the clinical state may require more extensive evaluation if new problems arise or if symptoms persist and become more disabling, but, for most patients with chronic nonspecific dyspepsia, continued observation with minimization of diagnostic studies suffices.

PSYCHOGENIC (FUNCTIONAL) NAUSEA AND VOMITING

Nausea: *The unpleasant feeling that one is about to vomit.* It may represent the patient's awareness of afferent stimuli to the medullary vomiting center. Nausea is associated with altered physiologic activity, including the gastric hypomotility and increased parasympathetic tone that precede and accompany vomiting. **Vomiting:** *The forceful expulsion of gastric contents produced by involuntary contraction of the abdominal musculature when the gastric fundus and lower esophageal sphincter are relaxed.* Vomiting should be distinguished from **regurgitation,** *the spitting up of gastric contents without associated nausea or forceful abdominal muscular contractions.*

Etiology and Psychophysiology

Vomiting may be considered part of a regulatory mechanism that allows for expulsion of potentially harmful substances. **Psychogenic vomiting** may be self-induced or may occur involuntarily in situations perceived by the patient to be anxiety-inducing, threatening, or in some way "distasteful." Common expressions referable to the digestive system express aversion. "I can't stomach that,"

"This is nauseating," "You make me want to throw up," and such thoughts can have physical representation. The psychologic factors leading to vomiting may be culturally determined, as occurs when eating exotic food considered repulsive in one's own cultural group. Vomiting may express hostility, as when a child vomits during a temper tantrum, or may be an attempt to represent a forbidden idea or wish, as with conversion disorders. For example, vomiting soon after or on the anniversary of an abortion or a hysterectomy can often be observed when a woman has unresolved conflicts related to the lost fetus or to her identity as a woman or mother. In this example of a conversion reaction, the patient's ambivalence leads to symptoms that represent both the experience of pregnancy (to retain symbolically what was lost) and its rejection.

"Rewards" such as exemption from school or work may reinforce vomiting, whatever its cause. In such situations the event removes or protects the patient, usually without his awareness, from a real or imagined threat that would otherwise produce mental distress. The physician will remain unaware of these factors unless he determines the meaning of the symptom to the patient.

Diagnosis

Elucidating the behavioral features that produce the vomiting in order to establish a psychogenic etiology may take more time than is available. Often this type of confirmation is never achieved and the physician must make inferences, working with indirect or suggestive data: (1) The history, physical examination, and initial laboratory data can often reasonably exclude significant physical disorders within the GI tract (cholecystitis, choledocholithiasis, intestinal obstruction, peptic ulcer disease, acute gastroenteritis, perforated viscus or other "acute abdomen," ingestion of noxious substances); derangements in other organ systems (e.g., acute pyelonephritis, myocardial infarction, acute hepatitis); toxic or metabolic disorders (systemic infection, radiation exposure, drug toxicity, diabetic ketoacidosis, cancer); or neurogenic causes (stimulation of the vestibular center, pain, meningitis, CNS trauma, or tumor). (2) The episodes may not follow any expected physiologic pattern; e.g., the vomiting may occur at the thought of food and may not be temporally related to eating. (3) Patients may have personal and family histories of functional nausea and vomiting, experiences that serve as models for the present symptoms. (4) With encouragement to describe the setting of the episodes, many patients will relate onset to a time of stress and will report recurrence and worsening during similar stressful periods; however, this association or even awareness of mental distress may not be acknowledged by the patient. (5) Despite the presence of symptoms for weeks or months, examination usually shows no weight loss, dehydration, or objective clinical abnormalities. However, patients with severe psychologic disturbance may develop malnutrition and metabolic abnormalities from protracted vomiting.

If history and examination do not exclude a physical disorder, further studies will depend upon clinical information already obtained. These include CBC, ESR, urinalysis, glucose, BUN, electrolytes, liver function tests, upper GI series with small bowel follow-through, and oral cholecystogram. If these are normal (i.e., having excluded upper GI, metabolic, and toxic diseases), psychogenic nausea and vomiting can be diagnosed with reasonable assurance.

Treatment

Comments such as "nothing is wrong" or "the problem is emotional" should be avoided. Therapeutic reassurance can indicate awareness of the patient's discomfort and express the desire to work toward his relief regardless of the etiology. Brief symptomatic treatment with antiemetics can be tried. Long-term management involves supportive, regular office visits, during which the patient may be helped to resolve his underlying problems.

GLOBUS SENSATION

("Lump in the Throat," Globus Hystericus)

The subjective sensation of a lump or mass in the throat. No specific etiology or physiologic mechanism has been established. Some studies suggest that elevated cricopharyngeal (upper esophageal sphincter) pressures or abnormal hypopharyngeal motility exist during the time of symptoms. The sensation may result from esophageal reflux or from frequent swallowing and drying of the throat associated with anxiety or other states of emotion. Globus is probably a physiologic manifestation of certain mood states. It is not associated with any specific psychiatric disorder or set of stress factors. Certain individuals may have an inherent or learned predisposition to respond in this manner.

The sensation resembles the normal reaction of being "choked up" during events that elicit feelings of grief, pride, or even happiness from mastery of hardship; suppression of sad feelings is most often implicated. Clinically, chronic symptoms may occur during states of unresolved or pathologic grief and be relieved by crying.

Diagnosis

Medical disorders that can be confused with globus sensation include cricopharyngeal or upper esophageal webs, symptomatic diffuse esophageal spasm, gastroesophageal reflux, skeletal muscle disorders (myasthenia gravis, myotonia dystrophica, polymyositis), or mass lesions in the neck or mediastinum causing esophageal compression. Most often, a careful history and physical examination can exclude these disorders. True dysphagia must be ruled out, for it would suggest a structural or motor disorder of the pharynx or esophagus. With globus, the symptoms occur during certain emotional states and do not worsen during swallowing. Food does not stick, and the symptom is often relieved with eating or drinking. There is no pain or weight loss.

If psychosocial features have been elicited and the physical examination is negative, the diagnosis is probable; if it is still in doubt, a CBC, plain or cine-esophagogram, chest x-ray, and esophageal manometric study as indicated by the clinical data may exclude other disorders.

Treatment

Treatment involves reassurance and sympathetic concern. No medication is of proven benefit. Underlying depression, anxiety, or other behavioral disturbances should be managed in a supportive manner with psychiatric referral if necessary. At times, indicating the association of symptoms to the patient's mood state can be beneficial.

ADULT RUMINATION

(Merycism)

The usually involuntary regurgitation of small amounts of food from the stomach (most often 15 to 30 min after eating), rechewing the material and, in most cases, again swallowing it. It is commonly observed in the infant. The true incidence in adults is unknown, as it seems to be a privately enjoyed act, but some individuals in the past offered public performances in which objects swallowed at random were selectively regurgitated. The pathophysiology is poorly understood. Only rarely have barium contrast studies been successful in showing the disturbance. The reverse peristalsis that occurs in animal ruminants has not been reported in humans. The few psychiatric studies available relate the act to an unconscious wish to attack or reject a threatening person or object.

Symptoms and Signs

Rumination is most often brought to the clinician's attention in patients with emotional disorders. During periods of stress, the patient may be less careful to conceal the act, and seeing this for the first time, others refer the patient to the physician. The patient reports no nausea, pain, or dysphagia.

Treatment

The general approach to the patient, as outlined in the introduction to this chapter, may disclose underlying emotional difficulties. An upper GI series and esophageal manometry are necessary to exclude disorders causing mechanical obstruction, a Zenker's diverticulum, or motility disturbances. Endoscopy usually adds little to the clinical evaluation. Although drug therapy generally does not help, metoclopramide, a new stimulant of intestinal motor activity, has had varied success. Psychiatric consultation is often required when food is continually expectorated, leading to weight loss.

HALITOSIS, REAL AND IMAGINED

An unpleasant odor to the breath. This may be produced by ingesting or inhaling substances that are in part excreted by the lungs, gingival or dental disease, fermentation of food particles in the mouth, or an association with diseases of other organ systems (e.g., hepatic encephalopathy, diabetic acidosis, infectious or neoplastic disease of the respiratory tract—see BREATH ODOR in Ch. 206). The esophagus is normally collapsed and separate from the airway. Although foul eructations may occur with gastric retention or gastric and esophageal tumors, GI disorders do not generally cause halitosis, and it is a fallacy that breath odor reflects the state of digestion and bowel function.

The response of others to halitosis is in part determined by acclimatization and social factors. Thus, an individual may be entirely unaware of his or her own bad breath, and what is unpleasant to a stranger may not be to a spouse or relative.

Psychogenic halitosis exists when an individual complains of bad breath that is not perceived by others. This may occur during anxiety states, as with a teenager on the first date. It may be reported by the hypochondriacal patient who commonly amplifies normal bodily sensations. At times the complaint may reflect a serious disorder of thinking. The obsessional patient may have a pervading sense of uncleanliness, or the paranoid individual may have the delusion that his organs are rotting.

Treatment

The removal or treatment of specific causes is effective. Further diagnostic evaluation should not be undertaken if the history and physical examination do not suggest an underlying disease. Attentive listening and reassurance help most patients. Persistence in this complaint despite reassurance may require psychiatric consultation.

52.   DISORDERS OF THE STOMACH AND DUODENUM

GASTROINTESTINAL BLEEDING

Vomiting of blood (**hematemesis**); *passage of black tarry stools* (**melena**); *passage of gross blood via the rectum* (**hematochezia**).

GI bleeding may be overt and obvious, or occult. **Overt bleeding** from the upper GI tract may be manifested by **hematemesis.** Slower bleeding in the upper tract permits gastric acid to convert red Hb to brown hematin, causing **"coffee ground" vomitus,** a form of bleeding often not recognized as such by a patient. In the absence of intestinal obstruction, hematemesis rarely arises from bleeding points distal to the ligament of Treitz. Swallowed blood from epistaxis or hemoptysis may result in the eventual vomiting of the blood and confusion as to the exact site of the bleeding.

Blood from an upper GI hemorrhage may pass through the intestine. If bleeding from the upper GI tract is copious and intestinal transit is rapid, the stools may contain red blood. Blood that passes through the intestine usually becomes black. About 50 to 300 ml of ingested blood are required to produce melena, which generally implies a bleeding source in the upper GI tract, but slowly bleeding lesions in the colon can be the cause at times. Melena may continue for several days after a large hemorrhage and does not necessarily indicate continued bleeding. Black stools may also be due to rapidly eliminated bile or to ingested iron, bismuth, berries, greens, or beets, and may mimic melena.

Hematochezia typically arises from lower intestinal sources but, as described above, may occur with rapid blood loss from the upper GI tract. If bleeding occurs in the distal colon at a site where feces are formed, the blood appears as streaks or clots on the surface of the stool. If bleeding is above this level, the stool may be red or mahogany throughout.

Occult bleeding manifests only as iron deficiency anemia, but may be detected chemically; e.g., by the guaiac test on a stool specimen. Up to 50 to 200 ml of blood can be lost daily without visible signs.

The causes of GI bleeding are listed in TABLE 52-1.

Symptoms and Signs

The manifestations of GI bleeding depend on the source of bleeding, the rate of blood loss, and the coexistence of other diseases. Weakness, easy fatigability, irritability, palpitations, pallor, headache, insomnia, and numbness and tingling in the extremities may result from anemia due to chronic bleeding. Shock and renal failure occur with massive hemorrhage. Vomiting of gross blood occurs with esophageal or rapid gastroduodenal bleeding. Slower bleeding in the upper tract permits the formation of coffee ground vomitus. For unknown reasons, an occasional patient with GI bleeding develops a craving to chew ice.

Other syndromes resulting from GI bleeding may be serious. **Prerenal azotemia** occurs when absorption of decomposed blood overloads renal and hepatic clearance mechanisms. Shock may compromise hepatic and renal functions, resulting in further azotemia. **Portal hypertension** causes shunting of absorbed metabolites away from the liver, resulting in elevated blood ammonia levels and, frequently, ammonia intoxication or coma **(hepatic encephalopathy).**

Diagnosis

The risk of mortality from GI bleeding increases when the patient is treated without a specific diagnosis. Early diagnosis (while the patient is still bleeding) increases diagnostic accuracy. All patients require a complete history and physical examination, blood studies to determine coagulation or liver malfunctions, and repeated monitoring of the Hct.

TABLE 52-1. CAUSES OF GASTROINTESTINAL BLEEDING

Common Causes

Peptic ulcer	Colonic carcinoma	Ulcerative colitis
Gastritis	Diverticulitis	Hemorrhoids
Gastroesophageal varices associated with portal hypertension	Gastric carcinoma Meckel's diverticulum Colonic polyps	Gastroesophageal lacerations in Mallory-Weiss syndrome
Gastric irritant medications (e.g., aspirin)		

Miscellaneous Causes (about 2% of cases)

Blood swallowed from oronasopharyngeal or respiratory passages or from external sources (e.g., as during birth)	Anticoagulant medications
	Lesions in small intestines (e.g., diverticula, regional enteritis, dysentery, intussusception, volvulus, mesenteric thrombosis, polyps)
Tumors or TB in any part of GI tract	
Hematobilia (usually posttraumatic)	Angiodysplasias, blood dyscrasias, coagulopathies
Postoperative bleeding	
Other esophageal or gastroduodenal lesions (e.g., esophagitis associated with hiatus hernia, diverticula, foreign bodies)	Uremia
	Blackwater fever
	Yellow fever
	Scurvy

Potential Source

Aortoduodenal fistula at an aortoprosthetic anastomosis (more frequent as more patients survive aortic surgery)

Confirming the site of active bleeding requires objective documentation. **Aspiration of gastric contents is the first and most important step in diagnosis;** all subsequent diagnostic maneuvers depend on the findings. Aspiration of a few "coffee grounds" from a patient reporting hematemesis usually indicates that bleeding has stopped and warrants watchful waiting rather than further and vigorous diagnostic procedures. The same finding and history in a patient with continuing melena and evidence of continuing blood volume depletion strongly suggests persisting hemorrhage from the area below the pylorus and above the ligament of Treitz, and warrants immediate esophagogas-troduodenoscopy. If aspiration instead yields a clot, lavage with iced saline is performed until the stomach is cleared. A No. 30 French Ewald tube may be needed instead of a Levin tube to remove a massive clot. Once the clot is cleared, the rate of continuing hemorrhage can be estimated from the nature of the aspirate, and this will determine whether immediate surgery, continuous monitoring by aspiration, further iced saline irrigation, endoscopy, radionuclide imaging, angiography, or hourly feedings are indicated.

If hematemesis has not occurred and gastric aspiration yields no blood, the bleeding must be presumed to be from a source below the pylorus. **Duodenoscopy** may be considered in patients with a history of duodenal ulcer, but **selective abdominal angiography** is the best diagnostic procedure in cases of active subpyloric bleeding. Radionuclide imaging with radioactive technetium offers a rapid, reliable method of localizing and proving active bleeding and is the best way to diagnose Meckel's diverticulum. The bleeding rate must be 2 to 5 ml/min for arteriography to demonstrate extravasation; vascular malformations may be shown even after bleeding stops. Angiography after proctoscopy is the diagnostic procedure of choice in colonic hemorrhage; **colonoscopy** is useful only when the bleeding rate is slow.

Where endoscopic, arteriographic, or scintiscan facilities are available, **barium studies** now have no place in the diagnosis of active GI bleeding because they obscure the field in subsequent angiographic assessment. When arteriographic facilities are not available and after endoscopy has failed to define a lesion, barium studies are sometimes useful in identifying possible bleeding sources.

Slow, chronic GI bleeding resulting in anemia requiring transfusion may defy all diagnostic studies; the source in such cases is often chronic gastritis or a vascular malformation. The **Bray-Hauser string test** has been useful in localizing some of these lesions.

Treatment

Every case of hematemesis, melena, or hematochezia should be considered an emergency until proved otherwise. Large-bore IV lines (size 16 or larger) should be installed and an appropriate solution started if hypovolemia is present. Blood should be drawn for hepatic, renal, coagulation, and hematologic studies, and for cross-matching. Central venous and bladder catheters for monitoring right atrial pressure and urine output should be used in patients who are in shock (see also SHOCK in Ch. 24), of advanced age, or debilitated. Unconscious or precomatose patients are more safely managed with endotracheal intubation in order to prevent aspiration and to ensure adequate ventilation. Active hemorrhage warrants prompt infusion of packed RBCs or whole blood. Fresh frozen plasma corrects most intrinsic or iatrogenic (due to medication or excessive transfusion) coagulopathies. Conversely, colloid solutions without coagulation factors should be used with caution in active bleeding, because significant dilution of these factors may occur if a contracted blood volume is rapidly expanded, e.g., with normal human serum albumin.

Specific treatment for GI bleeding depends mostly upon the nature and location of the responsible lesion and on the facilities available in the medical center involved. (See the appropriate chapters for details of treating specific lesions.) In torrential hemorrhage, however, some general principles can be applied. Resuscitation with massive infusion of colloid or even electrolyte solutions is the first consideration. Prompt and proper placement of an esophagogastric balloon tube may be lifesaving in patients with varices.

Where facilities exist, endoscopic and angiographic therapeutic as well as diagnostic methods should be employed following resuscitation of the patient. Pharmacoangiography with intra-arterial infusion of vasopressin into the identified bleeding vessel—or systemically in bleeding varices—may be useful in controlling some forms of bleeding, such as in gastritis, and in patients considered poor candidates for surgery but whose bleeding is too severe to be managed medically; e.g., patients with colonic hemorrhage, whose risk at surgery is greatly decreased if hemorrhage is stopped while the bowel is cleared with enemas and prepared with an oral antibiotic regimen—erythromycin base 1 gm and neomycin 1 gm or kanamycin 1 gm/h for 4 h, then 1 gm q 6 h for 36 to 72 h. Despite the availability of these newer diagnostic and therapeutic methods, their place in treatment remains to be established, and definitive surgery must not be delayed in a patient with massive hemorrhage.

In addition to the pharmacoangiography, embolization of the bleeding vessel with clotted blood or various foreign materials (e.g., detachable balloons, gelfoam) has been used. Endoscopically guided electrocoagulation, laser beam therapy, monomer glues, and injection sclerotherapy of varices have been used to stop bleeding. Cimetidine has been used to treat upper GI hemorrhage. Initial enthusiasm has been tempered by clinical trials; the exact value of cimetidine in therapy of upper GI hemorrhage is not yet clear.

If bleeding is minor or has stopped, the stomach may be aspirated with a tube for decompression and monitoring, or immediate treatment with milk and antacid feedings may be started. With gastritis, the diet should be advanced very gradually, since even slight stretching of the mucosa may restart bleeding.

GASTRITIS

Acute or chronic degeneration and/or inflammation of the gastric mucosa occurs in a wide variety of circumstances. The term gastritis is therefore an imprecise designation encompassing clinical, endoscopic, and pathologic findings that cannot be satisfactorily correlated. While nomenclature and data about these disorders remain controversial and in a state of flux, the following subject headings indicate a commonly used classification.

ACUTE GASTRITIS (Acute Erosive Gastritis; Acute Stress Erosion; Acute Hemorrhagic Gastritis)

Superficial, mucosal lesions of the corpus of the stomach that occur very rapidly in relation to a variety of stresses.

Etiology and Pathology

The most common provocative stresses are major burns ($>$ 25% BSA), trauma with multiple injuries, and major surgery, especially when complications of shock, sepsis, or renal or respiratory failure are present. Alcohol, corticosteroids, aspirin or other anti-inflammatory agents, food or drug allergens, or toxins (such as staphylococcus toxin) can generate gastritis. Gastritis may also accompany uremia and infectious diseases such as influenza. While a number of pathophysiologic factors appear to be involved, ischemia and impaired defenses against gastric acid are believed to be the most important. Lesions may be seen within hours of acute stress.

Pathologic findings include patchy or diffuse edema; hyperemia; inflammatory cell infiltration; epithelial cell degeneration and necrosis, particularly in the neck of the gastric glands; erosions (shallow ulcers not penetrating through the muscularis mucosa) or acute ulcers involving the full depth of the mucosa; and mucosal and submucosal hemorrhages.

Symptoms, Signs, and Diagnosis

Most often, there are no symptoms, but anorexia, nausea, vomiting, and postprandial epigastric distress may occur. Hemorrhage causes the greatest concern and can be massive. It occurs in about 10% of patients, is usually mild, and often follows the stressful event within 6 to 7 days. Hematemesis can be the only symptom of acute gastritis, although patients are commonly very ill as a result of the underlying disorder.

Endoscopy may show the characteristic hyperemia and erosions, but it must be performed early, since gastric mucosa heals rapidly and evidence of gastritis may be undetectable after several days. Biopsy confirms the diagnosis. X-ray studies are not helpful, since the lesion involves only the mucosa.

Prognosis and Treatment

Prevention of hemorrhage is often possible. The symptoms are usually mild; if severe bleeding requires surgery, mortality rates exceed 50%. Death results more often from the underlying disorder.

Treating the underlying disorder (e.g., shock, sepsis) or withdrawing the offending agent prompts the disorder to subside spontaneously. The use of antacids not only relieves pain, but may prevent hemorrhage. Their prophylactic use is recommended when predisposing conditions are apparent. Cimetidine 300 mg q 6 h is also being used with some success. Prochlorperazine 5 to 10 mg orally t.i.d. or q.i.d., or IM repeated q 3 to 4 h if necessary (but not exceeding 40 mg/day IM), may be given for nausea and vomiting. Hemorrhage occasionally requires transfusion. Ice water lavage using a No. 30 French tube and a Toomey syringe may stop the bleeding. Rarely, persistent severe hemorrhage must be stopped by emergency gastrectomy; in some cases, pharmacoangiography using intra-arterial vasopressin has been successful.

CORROSIVE GASTRITIS

Acute corrosive gastritis is caused by swallowing strong acids or alkalis, iodine, potassium permanganate, or heavy metal salts. The degree of injury and the symptoms depend upon the nature and amount of the ingested substance. Gastric damage may range from only a mild hyperemia and edema to severe necrosis of the mucosa, membrane formation, and a subsequent, possibly hemorrhagic, inflammatory reaction. Necrosis may extend to the deeper layers of the wall and result in perforation.

Ulcerations of the lips, tongue, mouth, and pharynx may suggest the diagnosis. Esophageal involvement may lead to dysphagia. Intense abdominal pain, hematemesis, melena, and shock may occur in severe cases. Esophageal and pyloric stricture are late complications.

Treatment

(See Ch. 258 and Ingestion of Caustics under Accidents and Poisonings in Vol. II, Ch. 24.)

ATROPHIC GASTRITIS

The condition is more common in the aged. The cause is unknown. Antibodies to gastric parietal cells can be demonstrated in some patients, but this may be a secondary phenomenon. Associations that are not fully explained have been noted between gastritis and gastric polyps, gastric carcinoma (usually with a diffuse gastritis), gastric ulcer (usually with a localized gastritis), and pernicious anemia (usually with gastric atrophy rather than gastritis, and possibly with genetic and/or immunologic mechanisms playing a role).

Pathology

Patchy or diffuse atrophy of the lamina propria and of the gastric glandular tubules, loss of parietal and chief cells, and inflammatory cell infiltration occur. Intestinal metaplasia, goblet cells, and lymphoid follicles may be present. Atrophy of the gastric mucosa, without cellular infiltration, may be seen in pernicious anemia.

Symptoms, Signs, and Diagnosis

No specific symptom pattern has been identified. Some patients complain of nausea, pain, and epigastric distress, especially after eating, but many are asymptomatic. Correlation of symptoms with pathologic findings is poor (see also Ch. 51). The condition may be detected during endoscopy performed to study otherwise unexplained digestive symptoms, or during a part of a workup for ulcer, cancer, anemia, or some other disorder.

Gastric analysis reveals hypochlorhydria if only sections of the gastric mucosa are involved or if parietal cell destruction is incomplete. If maximal stimulation reveals achlorhydria, atrophy involves the entire mucosa. Radiologically, the diagnosis is suggested by the absence of rugal markings on the greater curvature and fundus (a "bald" fundus) and by the presence of fine, thin gastric folds in the body of the stomach. Endoscopically, a pale mucosa with a visible submucosal vascular pattern suggests the characteristic thinning of the gastric mucosa. Endoscopic errors are common, however; biopsy establishes the diagnosis.

Treatment

Corticosteroids have been tried because some patients with atrophic gastritis have antibodies to parietal cells, and patients with pernicious anemia may have antibodies to intrinsic factor as well. However, the results of treatment with steroids have generally been disappointing and their routine use is not recommended. Antacids may relieve epigastric distress even though hypochlorhydria is present. Vitamin B_{12} 100 μg/mo IM should be given to prevent pernicious anemia.

GIANT HYPERTROPHIC GASTRITIS (Ménétrier's Disease; Giant Hypertrophy of the Gastric Mucosa; Hypertrophic Gastropathy)

A rare disorder, characterized by huge convoluted gastric rugae with a nodular and often polypoid surface in part of or throughout the entire fundus and body of the stomach. Microscopic examination may show mucosal hyperplasia. The gastric glands may be elongated, branching, or cystic, and may penetrate the muscularis mucosa. The glandular cells may be normal or metaplastic, and goblet cells may be present.

Symptoms, Signs, and Diagnosis

A variety of symptoms may be present, including upper abdominal discomfort or pain suggestive of ulcer, anorexia, nausea, and vomiting that may appear bilious. If exudation of protein into the gastric lumen occurs, it can result in hypoproteinemia with accompanying edema.

The diagnosis is usually first suspected when x-ray or endoscopic studies are performed to investigate the above symptoms. The x-rays show projecting, large, convoluted rugal folds; these are flexible but may be confused with carcinoma. The correct diagnosis is usually established by endoscopy and biopsy.

Endoscopy shows prominent rugae with surface nodulation, which, unlike normal prominent folds, are not obliterated when the stomach is distended with air. Biopsy may demonstrate gastric glandular abnormalities. Surgical exploration is occasionally necessary to exclude a diagnosis of carcinoma.

Treatment

Hypoproteinemia may require a high-protein diet and, rarely, gastric resection. Anticholinergics may reduce loss of serum protein into the stomach. Because of an increased incidence of gastric carcinoma with this disorder, patients should be reexamined periodically.

HYPERTROPHIC GASTRITIS

In many patients, mucosal nodularity and prominent rugae seen radiologically or endoscopically disappear when air distends the stomach. Although hyperemia, turgidity, and engorgement of the rugae are visible endoscopically in such patients, they may also be seen in patients with a normal stomach that is hypersecreting. Biopsy of the stomach wall usually shows no abnormality. Such hyperplastic mucosa has been described in patients with peptic ulcer and hyperchlorhydria and in patients with the Zollinger-Ellison syndrome. Peroral biopsy may be too superficial to identify the hyperplasia; a diagnosis of hypertrophic gastritis should be made cautiously, if at all.

OTHER TYPES OF GASTRITIS

Acute Suppurative Gastritis

This rare disease may occur as a complication of systemic pyogenic infection, ulcer, cancer, infarction, or surgical manipulation. Symptoms and signs include those of an acute abdominal emergency or sepsis, or both. **Diagnosis** is made at laparotomy, if not at autopsy. **Treatment** involves surgery and antibiotics.

Chronic Superficial Gastritis

The cause is unknown, but increasing evidence has implicated bile salts in the pathogenesis in some cases. Bile reflux into the stomach is commonly found in patients with gastric ulcer or prior gastric surgery, two conditions in which chronic gastritis is common. Pathologic findings may be patchy or diffuse, are often localized in the upper ⅓ of the mucosa, and include infiltration of the lamina propria with lymphocytes, plasma cells, and polymorphonuclear leukocytes, and necrobiosis of the neck cells of the gastric glands, with erosions. Endoscopy may show hemorrhagic areas, erosions, and adherent sticky mucus or exudate, or both. There is no consistent symptom pattern and the diagnosis may be suggested when endoscopy is performed to investigate nonspecific digestive symptoms. Hypochlorhydria may be present; achlorhydria is less common. Diagnosis is by biopsy. The disorder may be a precursor of atrophic gastritis, or it may heal without residual problems. No effective treatment is known.

Postoperative Gastritis

A chronic, often superficial gastritis is common postoperatively. It is frequently seen in association with bile reflux through a gastroenterostomy. Atrophy of the gastric mucosa may also occur frequently when the antrum (the gastrin-secreting area of the stomach) has been resected, perhaps because of loss of the trophic effect of gastrin. These pathologic changes may account for the hypo- or achlorhydria that often follows subtotal gastrectomy, but they are not clearly related to the chronic gastric symptoms that may develop after the surgery.

Antral Gastritis

While gastritis may be limited to the antrum, this term is usually used by a radiologist to describe a nonspecific deformity of the gastric antrum observed on x-ray. In fact, the deformity is usually *not* due to gastritis. Endoscopy is advisable, since the deformity may represent an unrecognized ulcer or cancer.

PEPTIC ULCER

A circumscribed ulceration of the mucous membrane penetrating through the muscularis mucosa and occurring in areas bathed by acid and pepsin.

Peptic ulcers occur most commonly in the first few centimeters of the duodenum, known as the duodenal bulb **(duodenal ulcers)**; they are also common along the lesser curvature of the stomach **(gastric ulcers)**. Less frequently, ulcers occur in the pyloric canal **(channel ulcers)**, in the duodenum just beyond the bulb **(postbulbar ulcers)**, or in a Meckel's diverticulum containing islets of secreting gastric mucosa. Following gastrojejunostomy, with or without partial gastrectomy, ulcers may develop in the stomach at the margin of the anastomosis **(marginal** or **stomal ulcers)**, or in the jejunum just beyond the anastomosis **(jejunal ulcers)**. Ulcers may also occur in the lower end of the esophagus, but a diffuse esophagitis is more usual. **Stress ulcers** appearing in severe illness or trauma are discussed in Acute Gastritis, above.

Etiology

Peptic ulcer occurs only if the stomach secretes acid. Most people secrete acid; some develop ulcers and others do not. There appears to be a balance between ulcer-promoting factors, such as the secretion of acid or pepsin into the stomach, and factors protecting the stomach's mucosal lining, such as mucus production, membrane barriers to permeability, and replacement of shed or damaged mucosal cells. Many influences can disturb this balance. Stress is implicated as a common precipitating factor. The causes of gastric and duodenal ulcers may differ; gastric ulcer, unlike duodenal ulcer, tends to develop later in life and is not associated with increased acid secretion. Certain drugs, such as aspirin and other nonsteroidal anti-inflammatory drugs, reserpine, and possibly corticosteroids predispose to formation of an ulcer, though not necessarily a true peptic ulcer. These ulcers tend to heal when the drug is discontinued and are unlikely to recur unless the drug is taken again. An ulcer penetrates the muscularis mucosa. If it does not, the lesion is an erosion. The drugs mentioned may be associated with erosion or ulcer.

Pathology

A single ulcer is most common, but two and occasionally more (duodenal, gastric, or both) are encountered. Gastric ulcers usually occur along the lesser curvature of the stomach where the pyloric glands border the oxyntic glands; they are usually 1 to 2.5 cm in diameter but vary from a few mm to several cm. Gastritis usually is present. Duodenal ulcers, usually found within 3 cm of the pylorus, also vary in size but tend to be smaller than gastric ulcers. They average about 1 cm, in diameter. Ulcers are usually round, oval, or elliptical, with sharp margins. The surrounding mucosa is often hyperemic and edematous. Ulcers penetrate into the submucosa or muscular layer. A thin layer of gray or white exudate usually covers the crater base which is composed of fibrinoid, granulation, and fibrous tissue layers. During healing, fibrous tissue in the base contracts the ulcer and may distort the surrounding tissue. Granulation tissue fills the base, and epithelium from the edges covers its surface.

Duodenal ulcers are almost always benign, but a gastric ulcer may be malignant. Clinical management of gastric ulcer involves determining whether the ulcer is malignant. Malignant degeneration within a benign gastric ulcer is a rare event. However, a malignant gastric ulcer may occasionally be mistaken for a benign gastric ulcer, and there may even be difficulty in determining whether a biopsy or pathologic specimen shows evidence of malignancy.

Symptoms and Signs

The usual peptic ulcer has a chronic, recurrent course. Symptoms vary with its location and the patient's age; complaints may be atypical in children and minimal in the elderly. Some ulcer patients may not have symptoms; others report them for the first time when a complication (e.g., hemorrhage or obstruction) develops. Only about ½ of the patients present with the characteristic pattern of symptoms. The typical pain is described as burning, gnawing, or aching, but the distress may also be described as soreness, an empty feeling, or hunger. The typical pain is steady, mild or moderately severe, located in a well-circumscribed area, and relieved by antacids or milk.

In patients with **duodenal ulcer**, typically, the pain tends to follow a consistent pattern; it is absent when the patient awakens, but appears in mid-morning. It is relieved by food, but recurs 2 or 3 h after a meal. Pain that awakens the patient at 1 or 2 AM is common and highly suggestive of ulcer. Frequently the pain occurs once or more each day for one to several weeks, and may then disappear without treatment. However, recurrence is usual, often within the first 2 yr, occasionally after several years. Patients often learn by experience when a recurrence is likely (e.g., commonly during the spring and fall or during episodes of emotional stress).

When patients present with a severe ulcer diathesis, especially when ulcers are noted in atypical locations, the presence of a gastrinoma and the Zollinger-Ellison syndrome should be considered. This subject is discussed in Ch. 53. The symptoms of **gastric ulcer** often do not follow the duodenal ulcer pattern, and eating may cause rather than relieve the pain. **Pyloric channel ulcer** is often associated with symptoms of obstruction, such as bloating after eating, or nausea and vomiting. The pain of **postbulbar ulcer** may be unrelated to meals. With **esophageal ulcer** or esophagitis, pain tends to occur when the patient swallows or lies down.

Complications of peptic ulcer are discussed below.

Diagnosis

Diagnosis is suggested by the symptoms and confirmed by the studies described below. Gastric cancer may present with similar manifestations and is discussed below in MALIGNANT NEOPLASMS OF THE STOMACH.

X-ray study with barium usually establishes the diagnosis of peptic ulcer. A crater is usually seen in profile as a projection beyond the normal barium-filled outline of the stomach or duodenum. Occasionally in the stomach and commonly in the duodenum, the crater appears "en face" as a collection of barium surrounded by a halo of radiolucency due to edema in the ulcer margin; multiple spot x-rays with compression over the area are often needed to demonstrate this. Fluoroscopy is important to distinguish craters from barium trapped between folds. In about ½ of the patients with duodenal ulcers, a crater cannot be shown. Deformity of the duodenal bulb is suggestive, but not conclusive evidence of an active duodenal ulcer, since the scarring of a healed ulcer, as well as edema and spasm secondary to an active ulcer, can cause deformity. Technics using air contrast have greatly improved the accuracy of x-ray studies.

Endoscopy using the fiberoptic gastroduodenoscope can help establish the diagnosis, particularly when x-ray studies are inconclusive or negative. Endoscopy, while associated with some discomfort and slight risk, often discloses craters in the duodenum, posterior wall of the stomach, and sites of surgical anastomosis not demonstrable by x-ray. Endoscopy in conjunction with multiple biopsies helps to identify malignant gastric ulcers. Some clinicians recommend endoscopy in preference to x-ray as the initial diagnostic procedure for patients with upper GI tract symptoms. The response of an ulcer to treatment can be followed endoscopically. Thus, lesions that are partially healed but no longer seen by x-ray may be visualized, and the cause of failure to heal, such as malignancy, may be identified. However, lesions may be missed by endoscopy because of blind spots in the field of view.

A **cytologic search** for tumor cells in gastric washings and with gastric brushing technics can be helpful in some laboratories to identify malignant gastric ulcers.

Esophagoscopy is often the only way to identify esophageal ulcers or esophagitis, since these lesions are usually too shallow to be identified by x-ray.

Gastric analysis: Gastric secretory studies may be useful to demonstrate achlorhydria or hypersecretion. To obtain reliable findings, the position of the aspirating tube is checked by fluoroscopy and the adequacy of drainage (of a continuous suction machine) is also checked by hand aspiration.

Benign peptic ulcer can be ruled out if the stomach does not secrete free hydrochloric acid as indicated by a drop of at least 1 pH u. after maximal stimulation (e.g., with betazole 1.5 mg/kg s.c. or pentagastrin 6 μg/kg s.c.). Secretion tends to be above normal with duodenal ulcer, and somewhat below normal with gastric ulcer. However, the amount of acid secreted either in the basal state or after stimulation varies widely among patients with an ulcer in either site. If there is marked hypersecretion, a gastrinoma and the Zollinger-Ellison syndrome should be considered.

Healing

Symptoms are usually relieved by treatment in a few days, but healing commonly requires from 2 to 6 wk and may require a longer time, particularly for large or longstanding ulcers. **Gastric ulcers** should be monitored by regular x-ray or endoscopic examination until healing is complete. If a gastric ulcer crater is not reduced to ½ its original size in 3 wk, a penetrating ulcer or malignancy must be suspected. Patients are maintained on the regimen of medication and diet described below until healing is confirmed by a repeat x-ray or endoscopy, because the ulcer can be only presumed to be benign until complete healing is certain. If complete healing does not occur, surgery should be considered to prevent complications or a prolonged, distressing course.

Duodenal ulcers also heal in 2 to 6 wk, but demonstration of healing is not as critical, since they are practically never malignant. Moreover, duodenal ulcer craters can be difficult to demonstrate and follow by x-ray. They are followed by barium x-ray or endoscopic examination to complete healing only when necessary for the patient's management. The remaining patients are advised to follow the regimen for the period that experience suggests is required for healing.

Recurrence

Within 2 yr of completing treatment, 50% or more of patients will have a recurrence. It has not been demonstrated that prescription of a prophylactic antacid regimen will prevent recurrence, perhaps because patients will not take antacid regularly, particularly when asymptomatic. Reports of the effectiveness of anticholinergics are inconsistent but a few studies report partial success. Several reports state that continued intake of cimetidine can prevent recurrence. However, when treatment is discontinued, usually after about 1 yr, there are recurrences. Although there is limited information on the long-term course of peptic ulcer, the evidence suggests that most patients can be expected to have some difficulty during a 10-yr follow-up. This suggests the necessity of following a prophylactic regimen for at least that long. Such a program is not commonly recommended because the drugs have side effects and with a relatively new drug such as cimetidine there may be as yet unrecognized toxic effects. Accordingly, many physicians institute treatment only when there is actual evidence of recurrence or at times such as during stress when the patient has developed an ulcer in the past.

Treatment

Treatment of gastric and duodenal ulcer is designed to neutralize or decrease gastric acidity, even though gastric acidity is usually normal in patients with gastric ulcer. With proper therapy, symptoms usually subside within a few days. Otherwise, the diagnosis may be incorrect; the patient may have a complication—often penetration; the therapeutic regimen may not be adequate; or the patient may not be following the regimen.

Evidence of anxiety or depression should be treated appropriately. Formal psychotherapy is not usually required, since the most potent "therapeutic agent" is the physician as a sympathetic listener and strong supportive figure. Sedatives or tranquilizers, e.g., chlordiazepoxide 5 to 10 mg 1 to 4 times/day, may be helpful. Prochlorperazine 5 mg 1 to 4 times/day may be given if nausea is a problem. These drugs should be given only after consideration of how they might influence the patient's effectiveness at work and while driving.

Aspirin and aspirin-containing drugs should be avoided, if possible, and another analgesic such as acetaminophen should be prescribed. Unless the ulcer is responding to medical management, indomethacin, phenylbutazone, corticosteroids, and reserpine should be discontinued, if possible.

Diet: No firm evidence proves that any diet speeds healing or prevents recurrence. Therefore, many physicians eliminate only foods that cause distress, such as fruit juices and spicy and fatty foods. Pepper, the only food that objective studies suggest is harmful, and coffee, tea, cocoa, and cola drinks, which contain caffeine that stimulates gastric acid secretion, are commonly prohibited. Decaffeinated coffee is allowed. The roles of alcohol and smoking are not yet established. Since alcohol can stimulate acid secretion, it is commonly restricted to small or moderate amounts. Evidence shows that ulcers heal more rapidly in patients who are admonished to stop smoking. Snacks between meals can be encouraged, but while food may neutralize acid, it also stimulates acid secretion.

Antacids give symptomatic relief, and recent studies indicate that they promote healing and reduce recurrences. In general, there are 2 types of antacids. (1) **Absorbable antacids:** Sodium bicarbonate and calcium carbonate, the most potent antacids, are occasionally taken for short-term or intermittent relief, but because they are absorbable, continuous use may cause alkalosis or the **milk-alkali syndrome.** Since symptoms of this complication are not distinctive (nausea, headache, weakness), the disorder may progress unrecognized to kidney damage. These soluble antacids should be used with particular caution by patients who have vomited or hemorrhaged, who are dehydrated, or who have hypertension or renal functional impairment. There is evidence that calcium salts increase acid secretion, perhaps by a local action on gastric mucosa.

(2) **Nonabsorbable antacids:** While absorbable antacids provide rapid and complete neutralization, the nonabsorbable antacids are more commonly used, particularly in ambulatory patients, because of fewer side effects. These antacids are relatively insoluble salts of weak bases. Their formulation determines their efficacy. Suspended antacids present a large surface area for interaction with hydrochloric acid; this activity forms nonabsorbed or poorly absorbed salts, thereby increasing gastric pH. The activity of pepsin diminishes as the pH rises above 2, and there is evidence that pepsin may be adsorbed by some antacids. Antacids may interfere with the absorption of other medications, such as tetracycline, digoxin, and iron.

Aluminum hydroxide is a relatively safe and very commonly used antacid. Phosphate depletion may rarely develop as a result of binding of phosphate by aluminum in the GI tract. Symptoms include anorexia, weakness, and malaise. Serum phosphorus and urine phosphorus levels fall. If there is bone resorption to compensate for phosphorus loss, urine calcium rises and there may be bone pain. If depletion is sufficiently severe and continues over years, osteomalacia may develop. Aluminum hydroxide also binds fluoride and this too may contribute to osteomalacia. However, the diet usually provides enough phosphorus in milk, meats, and legumes; phosphorus tends to correspond with protein in the diet. If dietary phosphorus is insufficient, a sodium potassium phosphate supplement can be given. The risk of phosphorus depletion increases in alcoholics and patients with renal disease, including those on hemodialysis. Aluminum hydroxide may cause constipation.

Magnesium salts may cause diarrhea. Since magnesium hydroxide is a more effective antacid than aluminum hydroxide and is a mild cathartic, many proprietary antacids contain both magnesium and aluminum hydroxides. A few preparations contain aluminum hydroxide and magnesium trisilicate. The latter tends to have less neutralizing potency. Bowel movements will usually be regular if 4 doses of 15 to 30 ml are taken daily. If patients take more than 4 doses, the increased amount of magnesium hydroxide may cause diarrhea; optimal bowel function may require titration with the individual antacids (i.e., aluminum hydroxide and the combination of aluminum and magnesium hydroxides) even for some patients taking only 4 doses/day. Since small amounts of magnesium are absorbed, magnesium preparations should be given cautiously to patients with renal damage.

Dosage regimens: Liquid preparations of aluminum hydroxide (with or without magnesium hydroxide) are usually given in a dose of 15 to 30 ml; in tablet form, 2 to 4 is the usual dose. Tablets tend to be more convenient but less effective than liquids. Preparations vary in their composition; in several, one tablet or 5 ml of liquid contains 200 mg of aluminum hydroxide and 200 mg of magnesium hydroxide. Preparations also vary in the form or "reactivity" of their components, and their in vitro neutralizing capacity varies with the method of measurement. The more effective liquid preparations tend to have a neutralizing capacity in vitro of at least 2 mEq/ml. However, the neutralizing capacity of a given preparation in vivo again varies with the method of measurement and also varies from patient to patient, and in the same patient from time to time. Ideally, since most of the antacid passes from the stomach within an hour, the patient should take antacids hourly while awake. Failing this, the optimal regimen appears to be 15 to 30 ml of liquid or 2 to 4 tablets 1 h and 3 h after each meal and at bedtime. Effectiveness, cost, and patient preference determine the choice of antacid.

Anticholinergics may be given to delay emptying of the stomach (usually rapid in uncomplicated duodenal ulcer) and thus prolong antacid retention, and, in adequate doses, to diminish acid secretion. Since anticholinergics are most potent in diminishing basal secretion, they are most useful at night when regular hourly intake of antacid is impractical. A larger than average dose may be given for greater effect and longer action. Sustained-release preparations can be used instead, but results are inconsistent. The most consistently effective approach, when warranted, is for the patient to be awakened about 2 AM for an extra dose.

Anticholinergics can cause dry mouth and blurred vision; the commonly used dose is just below that which produces these side effects, and varies from patient to patient. Common doses are poldine 4 mg, glycopyrrolate 1 mg, propantheline 7 to 15 mg, or isopropamide 5 mg. These medications are given orally before each meal and at bedtime. Occasionally, tincture of belladonna is used because the dose can be precisely titrated in drops; the dosage may range from 15 to 40 drops q.i.d. Tablet medications, though offering less flexibility of dosage, are often more convenient.

Difficulty urinating, enlarged prostate, evidence of acute narrow-angle glaucoma, or gastric retention **contraindicate** the use of anticholinergics. Complete pyloric obstruction may develop in patients with partial obstruction; urinary retention and glaucoma occur most often in patients over age 50.

Patients with esophageal ulcers or esophagitis should not be given anticholinergics and should abstain from smoking since these may impair the efficiency of the lower esophageal sphincter. Such patients should have the head of the bed elevated to prevent acid regurgitation.

Histamine H₂ receptor blocking agents (see also in Ch. 253): Many physicians use histamine H₂ receptor blocking agents in preference to other therapeutic agents. The largest experience to date has been with cimetidine, but similar drugs are under study. Cimetidine 300 mg with each meal and at bedtime lowers gastric acidity and promotes healing of duodenal and gastric ulcer. While symptoms are commonly relieved within the 1st wk, healing may take 2 to 8 wk and in a small proportion even longer. A fraction of duodenal and gastric ulcers do not heal with cimetidine treatment. With anastomotic and stomal ulcers, somewhat promising results need further evaluation. When cimetidine was used for 8 wk, serious toxicity was not seen. There have been slight elevations of transaminase and serum creatinine, and rare cases of gynecomastia; drowsiness, tiredness, dizziness, diarrhea, and rash, slightly more common in patients receiving cimetidine than placebo, were seen in $< 2\%$ of patients. Some abnormalities such as those of transaminase and creatinine may clear even while the patient continues the drug. When treatment is completed, some authorities suggest a gradual reduction in dosage rather than abrupt discontinuance of the drug.

Absorption of the drug is not impaired by antacids, hence both can be given concomitantly. Some investigators report that if low doses of an anticholinergic are given with cimetidine, the inhibitory effect on gastric secretion is enhanced. Thus, an antacid and/or an anticholinergic may be added to a cimetidine regimen in cases difficult to treat. The doses of other drugs being given should be reviewed because cimetidine may alter the metabolism or prolong the action of some drugs by decreasing hepatic microsomal enzyme activity (diazepam and warfarin are notable examples).

Nocturnal pain: An occasional patient awakens several hours after retiring despite control of day-time symptoms. Cimetidine 300 mg at bedtime may prevent nocturnal pain. Also helpful may be a large dose (30 to 60 ml) of a liquid nonabsorbable antacid and/or a large dose of an anticholinergic. Occasionally, fat in the form of cream 1/2 to 1 oz has been added to the bedtime antacid to delay gastric emptying. A hypnotic may be useful. If these simple measures fail, the patient may set an alarm in order to waken 30 min before the usual time of the pain, and then take an additional dose of antacid. Nocturnal pain not relieved by these measures suggests complications such as penetration or obstruction.

Carbenoxolone is reported to promote healing of gastric and duodenal ulcers. This is attributed to beneficial effects on the mucosa. However, treatment may be associated with sodium retention, edema, hypertension, and/or hypokalemia. The extent of these side effects tends to correspond with the dose and duration of treatment. They may thus be mild with the small but often effective dose of 150 mg/day. Further, these side effects can be treated with drugs such as spironolactone. However, caution should be exercised in patients with cardiovascular, pulmonary, or renal impairment. This drug is not on the US market because the FDA questions its effectiveness, side effects, and possible liver toxicity.

Certain prostaglandins seem promising because they inhibit gastric secretion and appear to protect gastric mucosa against damaging drugs (see Ch. 252).

Sucralfate is a sucrose- and aluminum-containing disaccharide. It is reported to combine with proteins and proteolytic enzymes (e.g., pepsin) and to form in the base of the ulcer a protective coating that promotes healing. **Additional agents,** mainly in use outside the USA, have also been reported to be effective in treatment of ulcers. These include sulpiride, said to act on the hypothalamus as a neuroleptic and to diminish vagally stimulated gastric secretion and thus promote healing, and several bismuth-containing preparations (including zolimidine and colloidal bismuth subcitrate) that have been described in Scandinavian and British literature.

Radiation therapy: Duodenal ulcer patients failing to respond to medical management, who are not candidates for surgery because of age or medical problems, and whose life expectancy is limited to a few years may be considered for radiation therapy. Up to 2000 rads may be given to the fundus in a 2-wk period. Significant but temporary reduction of gastric acidity with concomitant ulcer healing has been observed.

Hospitalization is recommended for patients who are not adequately relieved on an ambulatory regimen or who have complications. Hospitalization also expedites studies to detect malignancy of a gastric ulcer, ensures an adequate therapeutic trial, can temporarily remove the patient from a stressful environment, and offers patient and physician a special opportunity to consider psychosocial problems.

Surgery: Indications for peptic ulcer surgery are discussed below.

COMPLICATIONS OF PEPTIC ULCER

PENETRATION (Confined Perforation)

A peptic ulcer may penetrate the wall of the stomach or duodenum and enter an adjacent confined space or an organ such as the pancreas or liver. Adhesions prevent leakage into the free peritoneal cavity. Pain may be intense, persistent, referred to sites other than the abdomen (usually the back and due to penetration of a posterior duodenal ulcer into the pancreas), and modified by the patient's position. When medical therapy is unsuccessful in producing healing, surgery is required.

PERFORATION

Ulcers that perforate into the peritoneal cavity are usually located in the anterior wall of the duodenum, less commonly in the stomach. A free perforation usually presents as an acute abdominal emergency. The patient experiences sudden, intense, steady pain in the epigastrium which spreads rapidly throughout the abdomen, often becoming prominent in the right lower quadrant and at times being referred to one or both shoulders. The patient usually lies as still as possible, trying to avoid any movement, since even deep breathing can worsen the pain. The abdomen is tender, the abdominal muscles are rigid, and bowel sounds are diminished or absent. Liver dullness may be absent. *Symptoms and signs may be less striking in the aged, the moribund, or those on corticosteroids.* Perforation into the lesser sac and intermittent seepage occur rarely. They may be difficult to recognize.

Pain and abdominal rigidity may partially subside and the patient's condition appears to improve several hours after onset. Peritonitis with a temperature elevation may develop, however, and the patient's condition seriously deteriorates; shock, heralded by increased pulse rate and decreased BP, may then develop.

Diagnosis is confirmed by an upright or a lateral decubitus x-ray of the abdomen showing air in the peritoneal cavity, but it is not excluded if no air is seen.

Treatment

Acute perforation usually requires immediate surgery. The longer the delay, the poorer the prognosis. When surgery is clearly contraindicated, alternatives are continuous suction (preferably in an intensive care unit) and antibiotics.

HEMORRHAGE

Hemorrhage is a common complication. Symptoms include vomiting of fresh blood or "coffee ground" material; passage of bloody or tarry stools; and weakness, syncope, and diaphoresis due to blood loss. Ulcer must be considered as a possible cause of upper GI tract bleeding even if the patient denies having ulcer symptoms. In addition to what is discussed here, management requires location of the bleeding site (see GASTROINTESTINAL BLEEDING, above).

Treatment

Assessment and restoration of blood loss: Major blood loss is likely when the pulse rate is > 110, or the systolic BP is < 100 or shows an orthostatic drop of 16 mm or more. The Hct is a valuable index of blood loss, but may not be accurate if the bleeding has occurred over the preceding few hours, since complete restoration of blood volume by hemodilution may take 32 h. Transfusions are usually given to maintain the Hct at about 30 if there is risk of further hemorrhage, if complicating vascular disease is present, or if the patient is > 40 yr old. Packed RBCs may be used instead of whole blood when heart disease makes it important not to overload the circulation. After an adequate blood volume is restored, the patient must be observed closely for such evidence of further bleeding as an increase in pulse rate, a drop in BP, vomiting of fresh blood, or a recurrence of loose, tarry stools. Cessation of bleeding from gastric lesions may be determined by passing a nasogastric tube.

A **nasogastric tube** may be used for gastric lavage with up to several liters of ice water to slow or stop the bleeding. A large (Ewald) tube may be helpful in cleaning out the stomach if there are clots. Continuous gastric aspiration via a nasogastric tube may be used if the patient is vomiting.

Feedings of bland food such as milk may be started once nausea and vomiting subside. **Antacids** can be given hourly; if aluminum hydroxide is given, a cathartic salt such as magnesium hydroxide should be included, since aluminum hydroxide may cause fecal impaction following GI hemorrhage. Anticholinergics are usually *not* given during the acute phase, as they may alter the response of the circulatory system to hemorrhage. A sedative such as phenobarbital 15 mg q.i.d. can allay apprehension and control restlessness. Cimetidine 300 mg q.i.d. may be given; if the patient is nauseated or vomiting, it can be given IV.

Emergency surgery is usually indicated when (1) pulse rate, BP, and Hct indicate a deterioration in the patient's condition despite adequate treatment and transfusions; (2) more than 6 transfusions in 24 h have been needed to maintain a stable pulse and BP; and (3) bleeding stops but recurs.

OBSTRUCTION

Obstruction of the outlet of the stomach or duodenum may be due to scarring, to spasm and inflammatory swelling associated with an active ulcer, or, most commonly, to both.

Symptoms

Vomiting may occur with ulcer in the absence of obstruction and is therefore only suggestive of obstruction. However, gastric retention is suggested if the vomitus is of large volume or contains food eaten > 6 h previously, and is probable if it contains food from 2 or more meals. Bloating or fullness after eating, and loss of appetite are also suggestive. A prolonged period of vomiting may cause weight loss, dehydration, and alkalosis. Not uncommonly, a patient will have progressively cut his food intake and even have eliminated solid foods. Thus, he will present with marked weight loss and a history of either no vomiting or vomiting of only very recent onset. In other patients, as the obstruction continues, vomiting will become less frequent, decreasing to once/day, but the vomitus will be large in amount. Some patients with obstruction disregard or deny symptoms, coming to the doctor only when the obstruction is quite advanced.

Diagnosis

If the patient's history suggests obstruction, physical examination, gastric aspiration, or x-ray study may provide objective evidence of retention. Gastric retention is suggested if a succussion splash persists for 6 h after a meal, or if aspiration after an overnight fast yields > 200 ml of clear fluid contents or food residue or milk curds. If gastric aspiration shows marked gastric retention, x-ray studies should be deferred. If not, x-rays may be used to determine whether obstruction is present and to aid in determining the site, cause, and degree of obstruction. Obstruction is suggested if x-rays show more than a trace of barium in the stomach 6 h after its administration. If obstruction is severe with significant retention of barium or food for > 24 h, and particularly if the stomach is greatly enlarged, ulcer is the probable cause. Carcinoma of the stomach should be considered primarily with lesser degrees of obstruction and if there is no history of ulcer. After the stomach has been emptied, x-ray and endoscopy may be helpful in demonstrating whether the pylorus or duodenum is narrowed and in identifying the responsible lesion.

Treatment

Since the history and laboratory studies seldom indicate whether obstruction is due primarily to scarring or to edema and spasm, a trial of therapy is usually indicated. Obstruction that is due to edema and spasm from an active ulcer usually responds to conservative treatment. Mild retention may respond to routine ulcer therapy, but more marked obstruction requires continuous gastric suction. The decompression produced by suction allows the stomach to regain its tone, and the constant aspiration of acid and pepsin promotes healing of the ulcer with lessening of the associated edema and spasm. Continuous suction requires careful monitoring of electrolytes and fluid balance and administration of parenteral fluids in amounts adequate to compensate for the fluid and electrolytes aspirated as well as for normal fluid losses. Also, dehydration and electrolyte depletion may have developed from vomiting prior to treatment and must be corrected. If a patient has developed malnutrition that could increase the risk of surgery, parenteral hyperalimentation may be considered.

Gastric emptying should be tested after 2 or 3 days of continuous suction by monitoring emptying of normal secretions or by a saline load test. If adequate emptying is restored, hourly feedings of a liquid diet or milk can start; aspiration is performed q 4 h. Feedings may be increased if large volumes are not aspirated. The time interval between aspirations can be lengthened as evidence of retention subsides, but aspiration should continue at least once daily for several days, either at bedtime or in the morning, to determine whether retention recurs after a more liberal diet, and at further intervals until the patient eats a full regular diet.

SURGERY FOR PEPTIC ULCER

Indications for surgery include perforation; obstruction that does not respond to medical therapy or that recurs; two or more major hemorrhages; a gastric ulcer suspected of being malignant; and disabling recurrences of uncomplicated peptic ulcer. In the latter group, it is important to consider to what extent the disability is due to intractable disease and thus amenable to surgery.

The surgeon selects the operation on the basis of his own experience, the general condition of the patient, and the nature and severity of the ulcer disease. The more extensive the operation, the lower is the postoperative recurrence rate, but the greater is the frequency of side effects, and the greater the operative morbidity and mortality. In a highly selective vagotomy (also called parietal cell vagotomy or proximal vagotomy), only the vagal fibers to the gastric secretory cells are cut. Fibers to the antrum are not cut, thus preserving its motility, and possibly avoiding a drainage operation. While this operation may have a low incidence of side effects, it can be technically difficult to perform and, in some series, recurrences are fairly common. In selective vagotomy, all fibers to the stomach are cut, but those to the liver, gallbladder, and celiac plexus are spared. In truncal vagotomy, all vagal fibers below the esophagus are cut. With these operations, pyloroplasty or gastroenterostomy is required to facilitate drainage of gastric contents. In more extensive operations, vagotomy is combined with resection of the gastric antrum or even a hemigastrectomy. In subtotal gastric resection, about ¾ of the stomach may be removed, but vagotomy is not performed. Among the side effects of operations that involve vagotomy, diarrhea may be prominent, but it may subside with time.

A "dumping syndrome" may follow surgical drainage procedures, particularly with gastrectomy. Weakness, dizziness, sweating, nausea, vomiting, and palpitation occur soon after eating. Symptoms of hypoglycemia may occur about 2 h after a meal. A high-protein diet and adequate caloric intake, in the form of frequent small feedings of dry foods, are recommended. The patient should lie down after a large meal. Anticholinergics may be helpful (for doses, see under Treatment in PEPTIC ULCER, above).

Weight loss is common after subtotal gastrectomy, because the patient may limit food intake to prevent the dumping syndrome and other postprandial symptoms. If only a small gastric pouch is left, distention or discomfort may follow a meal of even moderate size. Anemia (usually from iron deficiency, but occasionally correctable with B_{12}) and osteomalacia may occur. Vitamin B_{12} 100 μg IM/mo is recommended for all patients with total gastrectomy as prophylaxis, but it may also be given to patients with subtotal gastrectomy if there is reason to suspect deficiency.

MALIGNANT NEOPLASMS OF THE STOMACH

This discussion is largely concerned with carcinoma, which accounts for 95% of malignant neoplasms of the stomach; less common are lymphomas (which may be localized primarily in the stomach) and leiomyosarcomas. The incidence of stomach cancer shows enormous differences in worldwide distribution, with extremely high levels in Japan, Chile, and Iceland. The disease has decreased in the USA to about 8:100,000, making it the 7th most common cause of death from cancer. It is most common in the North, in the poor, and in blacks. However, in Japan, where its incidence has also decreased, stomach cancer is still the most common form. Its incidence increases with age; < 25% of patients are under 50 yr.

Etiology and Pathogenesis

While its cause is unknown, stomach cancer is often associated with intestinal metaplasia of the gastric mucosa, which frequently occurs in patients with pernicious anemia, gastric atrophy, and atrophic gastritis. Gastric ulcer has been described as leading to cancer. If so, it occurs in a very small proportion of cases; in the vast majority of cases an undetected cancer was probably present from the beginning. Gastric polyps have also been cited as precursors of cancer; again it is more likely that a given polyp had an undetected focus of malignant cells than that it became malignant. Malignancy is particularly likely in a polyp > 2 cm in diameter or if there are several polyps. Cancer of the stomach is rare among patients with duodenal ulcer. However, after a partial gastrectomy, cancer of the gastric remnant becomes more common.

Pathology

Gastric carcinomas can be classified according to gross appearance: (1) **protruding** (polypoid or fungating); (2) **penetrating**—the tumor has a sharp, well-circumscribed border and may be ulcerated; (3) **spreading**, either superficially along the mucosa or infiltrating within the wall—if an ulcer is present, its edge tends to be ill-defined. If there is infiltration of the stomach wall by tumor and an associated fibrous reaction, a "leather bottle" stomach **(linitus plastica)** may be produced; (4) **miscellaneous**—those tumors that show characteristics of 2 of the other types. This is the largest group. Protruding tumors have a better prognosis than infiltrating tumors.

Another classification is based on histologic criteria: the extent to which the cells are arranged into normal-appearing tubular glands and the degree of differentiation of the cells. Grading based on these criteria correlates moderately with gross appearance and prognosis.

The Japanese Society for Gastroenterological Endoscopy (1962) developed a classification for Early Gastric Cancer, i.e., cancer limited to the mucosa and submucosa. Gross morphology provides the basis. **Three types are identified:** I, Protruded; II, Superficial—elevated, flat, or depressed; and III, Excavated.

Symptoms and Signs

In its early stages, cancer of the stomach may not cause symptoms that the patient recognizes or reports. Patients and physicians alike tend to dismiss symptoms present for a year or more. Since some cancers develop slowly over months or even years, symptoms of long duration should not be disregarded. Most people have subtle digestive symptoms at one time or another, and it may be difficult to be sure that a new pattern has developed; early symptoms may be dismissed as indigestion. Careful inquiry may detect a range of provocative clues. "Fullness" or slight pain after a large meal is a likely pattern if a cancer is in the pyloric region, a common site. Symptoms may suggest peptic ulcer, especially if a cancer involves the lesser curvature. A cancer in the cardiac region of the stomach may obstruct the esophageal inlet and cause dysphagia. Such cancers may be confused with esophageal cancer even after careful study. Loss of appetite or nausea may occur, especially with cancers involving the fundus. A patient may relate these symptoms to certain foods such as meat or the amount eaten, and adjustments in his diet will sometimes give him relief. Loss of weight, usually resulting from restriction of food intake, may bring the patient to the physician. Loss of strength also may be associated with restriction of food intake or with anemia. Any change in bowel habits with accompanying diarrhea or constipation can again result from changes in diet. Massive hematemesis or melena are uncommon, but secondary anemia may follow occult blood loss. Occasionally, the first symptoms and signs are due to metastases; the primary tumor in the stomach is "silent."

There are no specific early signs of the tumor. Later, loss of weight or a palpable mass may be present. Finally, spread of the tumor or metastases may lead to an enlarged liver, jaundice, ascites, skin nodules, and fractures.

Diagnosis

Differential diagnosis commonly involves peptic ulcer and its complications, which are considered above.

X-ray studies, a mainstay for detecting and diagnosing gastric cancer, have been unreliable in finding small, early lesions. However, by using double contrast technics that involve coating the mucosa with barium and inflating the stomach to bring out mucosal details, Japanese radiologists report carcinomas as small as 1 cm in diameter.

Endoscopy permits direct inspection of the stomach and biopsy of suspicious areas. Limitations in visualizing certain areas in the stomach and difficulty guiding the forceps to a precise area are diminishing with the development of better instruments and technics. It may be helpful to obtain several biopsies from an area under suspicion, but often it is not possible by inspection through the endoscope to be sure exactly where there is tumor. Occasionally, a biopsy limited to the mucosa will miss tumor tissue in the submucosa.

Cytological studies of gastric washings are helpful in some institutions; special technics, such as spraying the surface of the tumor with a jet of water during endoscopy or using devices that abrade the surface of the tumor may increase the yield of positive washings. In experienced hands, use of a brush, together with biopsy, improves results.

Gastric analysis is of limited value. The secretion of free acid does not rule out malignancy. If no free acid is secreted after a potent stimulant, and an ulcer is present, malignancy must be strongly suspected; but if there is not an ulcer, there is only a slightly increased chance of a malignancy.

Treatment

Excision of the tumor offers the only hope of cure, and the prognosis is good if the tumor is limited to the mucosa and submucosa. In the USA results are poor, because most patients have more extensive cancer when they come to surgery. Results with primary lymphoma of the stomach are better than those with carcinoma. There may be long survivals and even "cure," particularly with lymphosarcoma. X-ray therapy and chemotherapy are used to supplement surgery. With carcinoma, patients with malignant ulcers have the best results, probably because their symptoms bring them to the doctor early. However, among patients with other patterns of symptoms, those who have had symptoms for the longest periods tend to have the best prognosis, presumably because the tumors are growing slowly. Perhaps for the same reason, patients first seen when the tumor is large may have long survivals, even though they are not cured. Chemotherapy may have palliative value; x-ray therapy does not help. In Japan, where early cancers are detected by mass screening, the results of surgery are better than in the USA.

Surgery for cancer involves removal of most or all of the stomach. Frequently, lymph nodes draining the stomach are removed as well. The surgeon frequently discovers metastases or extensive tumor that precludes cure. The decision to perform a palliative procedure is difficult, because the effects of extensive gastric resection may require the patient to modify his lifestyle. He may have to curtail his food intake at any one time and modify dietary habits; he may then have less strength and have to change work habits; i.e., the inability to eat large quantities of food precludes heavy manual labor.

---

53. ACUTE ABDOMEN AND SURGICAL GASTROENTEROLOGY

ABDOMINAL PAIN

(See also PELVIC PAIN in Vol. II, Ch. 4)

At some time, most intra-abdominal disorders provoke pain. Characterizing and identifying the pain usually establish the diagnosis. The specificity theory states that pain is a separate sensory modality with its own specific neural apparatus. Primary sensory neurons for pain, both visceral and somatic, are mostly unmyelinated fiber (1 to 2 microns), but also some myelinated fibers (3 to 4 microns) are included. The so-called gate control theory may help explain the clinical observation that many physiological, physical, intellectual, social, and psychological variables determine the amount and quality of pain perceived. Specifically, modulation of nociceptive impulses occurs at the dorsal horn and at various levels of the ascending afferent systems.

The term "visceral afferents" denotes all afferent fibers from the viscera, including those which give rise to visceral reflexes, as well as those which subserve pain. Pain impulses from the abdominal cavity reach the CNS from the viscera via visceral afferents that travel with (1) the sympathetic nerves, (2) the parasympathetic nerves, and (3) from the parietal peritoneum, body wall, diaphragm, and the root of mesenteries via somatic afferents in the segmental spinal nerves or phrenic nerves.

Types of Pain

Three kinds of pain are distinguished: (1) visceral pain, (2) somatic pain, which includes superficial or cutaneous pain and deep pain from muscles, tendons, and joints, and (3) referred pain.

Visceral or splanchnic pain arises in abdominal organs invested with visceral peritoneum; impulses are conducted to the spinal cord over visceral afferents. Stimuli that produce visceral pain include increased tension in the wall of hollow viscera (either from distention or spastic contraction), stretching of the capsules of solid viscera, ischemia, and certain chemicals. Inflammation and ischemia lower the threshold for pain so that normal muscle contractions, ordinarily not felt, may produce pain. The role of chemical substances in visceral pain is not clear. Experimentally, pain can be produced by the intra-arterial injection of acid, alkaline, and hypertonic solutions, lactate, potassium ions, or bradykinin. Visceral pain tends to be diffuse and poorly localized, with a high threshold and a slow rate of adaptation. The patient feels "deep" pain in those cutaneous areas or zones that correspond roughly to the segmental distribution of somatic sensory fibers originating from the same segments of the cord as the visceral afferent fibers from the viscus in question. With severe visceral or deep somatic pain, concurrent responses due to autonomic reflexes may be prominent. These include sweating, nausea (sometimes with vomiting), tachycardia or bradycardia, fall in BP, cutaneous hyperalgesia, hyperesthesia or tenderness, and involuntary spastic contractions in the abdominal wall musculature. Muscular rigidity accompanying severe pain is most marked when the anterior peritoneal surface is involved; e.g., the board-like rigidity associated with a perforated ulcer.

Somatic pain is discomfort arising in the abdominal wall, particularly the parietal peritoneum, root of the mesenteries, and respiratory diaphragm; it is mediated by somatic afferents and segmental spinal nerves. Somatic pain is usually sharper than visceral pain and well localized close to the site of stimulation. When the source is on one side of the midline, the pain is generally lateralized. Acute appendicitis is a visceral disease that illustrates both visceral and somatic abdominal pain. The visceral pain of early appendicitis is perceived diffusely and dully in the periumbilical and lower epigastric regions, with little or no rigidity of musculature. Later, when the parietal peritoneum becomes involved in the inflammatory process, the somatic component of pain is more severe and sharply localized in the right lower quadrant. At this time there may be cutaneous hyperesthesia, tenderness, and muscular rigidity in the right lower quadrant.

Referred pain is perceived at a distance from the diseased viscus. The reference is usually to dermatomes, but on occasion the pain may be referred to the scar of a previous surgical operation, trauma, or localized pathologic process. Then it is called **"habitual,"** since one's prior pain experience influences its perception.

Etiology

Abdominal pain may be caused by a great variety of GI and intraperitoneal diseases, and because of overlapping nerve distribution, the pain may be secondary to extraperitoneal disorders. Pain of intra-abdominal origin (see TABLE 53–1) may emanate from the peritoneum, hollow viscera, solid viscera, mesentery, or pelvic organs, and may be caused by inflammation, mechanical processes such as obstruction or acute distention, or vascular disturbance. (See also BOWEL OBSTRUCTION, PERITONITIS, and PANCREATITIS below, and ACUTE AND CHRONIC CHOLECYSTITIS in Ch. 75.)

The extraperitoneal causes of abdominal pain are outlined in TABLE 53–2. Since their segmental distribution is similar, most intrathoracic diseases that cause abdominal pain are confused with upper abdominal disorders. Intraspinal diseases have pain patterns similar to the referred pain from abdominal pathologic conditions, but usually without abdominal tenderness or muscular rigidity. Before a lesion becomes apparent, tenderness and pain may accompany inflammation of peripheral nerves, e.g., herpes zoster. The pain often has a distribution similar to myocardial infarction or biliary tract disease, but awareness of the possibility, the relationship of pain location to the distribution of the affected nerves, and absent or atypical abdominal findings help avoid diagnostic error.

Differential Diagnosis

All patients not only perceive pain differently, but they vary in their ability to report and describe it. Thus, they may minimize, maximize, or distort their perceptions. Fortunately, certain *patterns of pain* occur with enough consistency to aid in making a diagnosis.

Abdominal pain of sudden onset usually results from a mechanical event, e.g., perforation, rupture or torsion and vascular embarrassment, hemorrhage into the peritoneum or retroperitoneum and even the abdominal wall, or primary vascular occlusion with consequent ischemia (see OCCLUSION OF THE ABDOMINAL AORTA AND ITS BRANCHES in Ch. 27). Common circumstances in which perforation occurs include duodenal ulcer, sigmoid diverticulitis, gastric ulcer, perforation associated with toxic megacolon, and obstructed bowel (particularly the sigmoid colon with consequent perforation of the cecum). Intraperitoneal abscesses, including ovarian and hepatic, may rupture and cause diffuse peritonitis. Ovarian cysts and hematomas may rupture. Torsion may involve the ovary, volvulus of the small or large bowel, and the omentum. Sudden onset of pain related to hemorrhage is most frequently caused by ectopic pregnancy, a leaking aneurysm, or traumatic rupture of the spleen or liver. Sudden onset of abdominal pain may also follow blockage of a hollow viscus like the ureter or the bile duct.

Abdominal pain of gradual onset that steadily increases suggests peritoneal irritation or continued increasing distention of the hollow organ. In this circumstance there may be no peritoneal irritation. When pain is described as crampy or colicky, it usually is related to intermittent peristalsis interrupted by an area of obstruction. Ureteral and biliary colic may be associated with crampy pain which also characterizes intestinal obstruction (see Ch. 75).

Abdominal pain that persists for 6 h is generally caused by conditions of surgical significance, but it is rare for any pain to be absolutely constant.

The location of pain should be described in terms of its original site, as well as shifting and radiation. Because of variations in location of organs and pathologic processes, as well as the vagueness of visceral pain, it is difficult to exclude diseases totally on the basis of location. However, certain relationships generally hold. Visceral pain usually is felt in the midportion of the abdomen, duodenal pain in the epigastrium, and pain for the remainder of the small intestine is characteristically referred to the region of the umbilicus. Pain originating in the large bowel is less well localized and frequently experienced in the hypogastrium. Sigmoid dilation may result in suprapubic or presacral pain.

Diffuse pain may be associated with peritonitis, leukemia, sickle cell crisis, pancreatitis, early appendicitis, mesenteric adenitis, mesenteric thrombosis, gastroenteritis, aneurysm, colitis, intestinal obstruction and metabolic, toxic, and bacterial causes.

TABLE 53–1. PAIN OF INTRA–ABDOMINAL ORIGIN

Mechanism	Origin	Pathologic Processes
Inflammation	Peritoneum	Chemical and nonbacterial peritonitis: perforated peptic ulcer, gallbladder, ruptured ovarian cyst, mittelschmerz Bacterial peritonitis Primary: pneumococcal, streptococcal, tuberculous Perforated hollow viscus: stomach, intestine, biliary tract
	Hollow intestinal organs	Appendicitis, cholecystitis, peptic ulcer, gastroenteritis, regional enteritis, Meckel's diverticulum, diverticulitis Colitis: ulcerative, bacterial, amebic
	Solid viscera	Pancreatitis, hepatitis, hepatic abscess, splenic abscess
	Mesentery	Lymphadenitis
	Pelvic organs	Pelvic inflammatory disease, tubo-ovarian abscess, endometritis
Mechanical (obstruction, acute distention)	Hollow intestinal organs	Intestinal obstruction: adhesions, hernia, tumor, volvulus, intussusception Biliary obstruction: calculi, tumor, choledochal cyst, hematobilia
	Solid viscera	Acute splenomegaly Acute hepatomegaly: cardiac failure, Budd-Chiari syndrome
	Mesentery	Omental torsion
	Pelvic organs	Ovarian cyst, torsion or degeneration of fibroid, ectopic pregnancy
Vascular	Intraperitoneal bleeding	Rupture: liver, spleen, mesentery, ectopic pregnancy; aortic, splenic, or hepatic aneurysm
	Ischemia	Mesenteric thrombosis, splenic infarction, omental ischemia Hepatic infarction: toxemia, purpura
Miscellaneous		Endometriosis

Modified from *Principles of Surgery*, by S. I. Schwartz, ed. 3. Copyright © 1979 by McGraw-Hill Book Company. Used with permission of McGraw-Hill Book Company and the author.

TABLE 53–2. EXTRAPERITONEAL CAUSES OF ABDOMINAL PAIN

Origin	Pathologic Processes
Cardiopulmonary	Pneumonia, empyema, myocardial ischemia, active rheumatic heart disease
Blood	Leukemia, sickle cell anemia
Neurogenic	Spinal cord tumor, osteomyelitis of the spine, tabes dorsalis, herpes zoster, abdominal epilepsy
Genitourinary	Nephritis, pyelitis, perinephric abscesses, ureteral obstruction (calculi, tumor), prostatitis, seminal vesiculitis, epidydimitis
Vascular	Dissection, rupture, or expansion of aortic aneurysm; periarteritis
Metabolic	Uremia, diabetic acidosis, porphyria, Addisonian crisis
Toxins	Bacterial (tetanus), insect bites, venoms, drugs, lead poisoning
Abdominal wall	Intramuscular hematoma
Psychogenic	Conversion reaction, hypochondriasis, somatic delusions

Modified from *Principles of Surgery*, by S. I. Schwartz, ed. 3. Copyright © 1979 by McGraw-Hill Book Company. Used with permission of McGraw-Hill Book Company and the author.

Right upper quadrant pain usually is caused by gallbladder, biliary tract disease, hepatitis, hepatic abscess, hepatomegaly due to congestive failure, peptic ulcer, pancreatitis, retrocecal appendicitis, renal pain, herpes zoster, myocardial ischemia, pericarditis, pneumonia, or empyema.

Right lower quadrant pain is characteristic of appendicitis, intestinal obstruction, regional enteritis, diverticulitis, cholecystitis, abdominal wall hematoma, ovarian cyst or torsion, salpingitis, mittelschmerz, endometriosis, ureteral calculi, renal pain, seminal vesiculitis, and psoas abscess.

Left upper quadrant pain is seen in gastritis, pancreatitis, splenic pathology, renal pain, herpes zoster, myocardial ischemia, pneumonia, or empyema. **Left lower quadrant pain** suggests diverticulitis, intestinal obstruction, appendicitis with the tip of the appendix located to the left of midline, leaking aneurysm, abdominal wall hematoma, ectopic pregnancy, mittleschmerz, ovarian cysts or torsion, salpingitis, endometriosis, ureteral calculi, renal pain, seminal vesiculitis, or psoas abscess.

Diagnostic Procedures

Laboratory studies of a patient who complains of abdominal pain should include Hct, WBC count and differential, platelet count, urinalysis, serum amylase, and, in certain cases, examination of the stool for ova and parasites.

Standard **x-rays** of the abdomen, including either upright or decubitus and flat film are useful to diagnose intestinal obstruction and/or perforation. An IVP may define renal or ureteral disease. Barium enema may confirm colonic obstruction and is particularly helpful to verify and treat pediatric intussusception. **Ultrasonography** is useful in defining calculi of the gallbladder, intra-abdominal abscesses, cysts (e.g., pancreas), aneurysms, dilated bile ducts and ureters. **Computed tomography** defines specific lesions and, by quantifying their density, helps to distinguish abscesses, hematomas, and solid tumors. **Angiography** is extremely helpful in defining vascular disease, the site of active bleeding, and the source of intraperitoneal bleeding caused by rupture of solid organs such as liver, spleen, or kidney.

BOWEL OBSTRUCTION

A condition in which the passage of intestinal contents is arrested or seriously impaired.

Etiology

The small or large intestine can be obstructed by mechanical blockage or cessation of bowel motility (peristalsis). **Mechanical blockage** occurs most often and may result from intra- or extraluminal or intramural barriers to the progression of bowel contents. Fibrous bands and adhesions (congenital or following surgery or inflammatory disease) and incarceration in a hernial sac are the most frequent causes. Primary or metastatic neoplasms, impacted feces, strictures from active or previous inflammatory disease of the bowel, intestinal worms, gallstones, Hirschsprung's disease, and volvulus are additional causes.

Adynamic (paralytic) ileus, resulting from failure of normal intestinal peristalsis, is most frequently associated with intra- or retroperitoneal infection. Ileus may be produced by ischemia from mesenteric artery embolism or mesenteric venous thrombosis, by retroperitoneal or intra-abdominal hematomas, after intra-abdominal surgery, in association with renal or thoracic disease, and by such metabolic disturbances as hypokalemia. Motility disturbances following abdominal surgery are largely a result of the change in colonic motility resulting from abdominal manipulation. The small intestine is largely unaffected and motility and absorption are normal within a few hours after operation. Stomach emptying is usually impaired for about 24 h, but the colon may remain inert for 48 to 72 h. This is confirmed by the fact that daily plain x-rays of the abdomen taken postoperatively show gas accumulating in the colon but not in the small bowel. Activity tends to return to the cecum before it returns to the sigmoid colon. If gas accumulates in the small intestine, it implies that some complication, such as obstruction or peritonitis, has developed.

Pathology

In **simple mechanical obstruction,** blockage occurs without vascular or neurologic compromise. Ingested fluid and food, digestive secretions, and gas accumulate, in excessive amounts if obstruction is complete. The proximal intestine distends and the distal segment collapses. The normal secretory and absorptive functions of the mucous membrane are altered and the bowel wall becomes edematous and congested. Severe intestinal distention is self-perpetuating and progressive, intensifying the peristaltic and secretory derangements and increasing the risks of dehydration, ischemia, necrosis, perforation, peritonitis, and death.

Strangulation or infarction of the bowel is most commonly associated with hernia, volvulus, intussusception, or vascular occlusion. Strangulation usually begins with venous obstruction, which may be followed by arterial occlusion resulting in rapid ischemia of the bowel wall. The bowel becomes edematous and infarcted, leading to gangrene and perforation.

In **closed-loop obstruction,** a loop of bowel is obstructed both proximally and distally (e.g., by a hernial sac). The same changes occur as in simple obstruction, but with a rapid rise in intraluminal pressure in the affected segment and early edema of the bowel wall, vascular occlusion produces gangrene and perforation.

Symptoms and Signs

Clinical features vary depending upon whether the obstruction is high or low in the intestinal tract, complete or incomplete, simple or strangulated, mechanical or paralytic. Vomiting, crampy pain, and abdominal distention occur; in general, the higher the obstruction, the less prominent the distention and the earlier and more severe the vomiting. With high obstructions of the proximal jejunum and above, vomiting causes early, substantial loss of electrolyte-rich intestinal fluid, which rapidly depletes the extracellular fluid and produces hypovolemic shock.

Complete mechanical obstruction of the small intestine causes severe, intermittent, crampy upper abdominal pain (colic) usually referred to the midline but sometimes radiating over the whole abdomen. Vomiting occurs and usually becomes malodorous and fecal in character. Constipation and failure to pass flatus are usually present from the outset, although small amounts of feces may be passed early in the course. Peristalsis above the obstruction may be visible. Bowel sounds are increased, high-pitched, and tinkling. Abdominal distention may not be prominent initially, but becomes conspicuous later when the obstruction is low in the small bowel. As the intestinal lumen proximal to the obstruction fills with electrolyte-containing intestinal fluid and gas, extracellular fluid dehydration develops. Increasing abdominal wall tenderness, muscle rigidity, and ileus suggest strangulation. **Partial obstruction of the small intestine** causes similar but less severe symptoms. Bowel actions may persist, usually with diarrhea.

Obstruction of the colon is usually insidious in onset. Abdominal distention with fullness of the flanks is more prominent, and is massive with volvulus of the colon. Vomiting tends to occur later in the course, and pain may be less severe than in small bowel obstruction. Constipation and failure to pass flatus are absolute if the obstruction is complete. Irregular bowel actions with passage of frequent small stools may occur with partial obstruction.

Paralytic ileus causes severe abdominal distention and distress. Bowel sounds are absent. The diagnosis may be overlooked since small amounts of flatus or liquid stools may be passed. Plain abdominal x-rays will show gas in the small intestine.

Strangulation may be difficult to differentiate from simple obstruction. Onset may be rapid with severe colicky pain. The symptoms and signs are initially those of mechanical obstruction, but gradually become those of ileus and peritonitis. Bowel sounds disappear; abdominal rigidity and acute, possibly localized, tenderness accompanied by marked shock may occur as a result of gangrenous change. The presence of a tender mass suggests the diagnosis. The WBC count is increased. Passage of blood from the rectum may occur, especially following vascular occlusion.

X-ray Findings

X-rays help to establish the diagnosis and locate the level of obstruction. Plain films show gaseous distention; in the small intestine this generally lies in the central area. Fluid levels are visible in x-rays taken with the patient upright. Loops of small bowel may be arranged in a stepladder pattern; mucosal folds may be prominent in the upper small bowel. The colon can be distinguished by haustral markings and by the distribution of the distended large bowel. Gas confined to the small bowel with multiple air-fluid levels ("J-loops") usually indicates a mechanical small bowel obstruction. Gas distributed throughout both the small and large intestines ("U-loops") occurs in paralytic ileus and obstruction due to vascular insufficiency. Barium enema radiography (using only 100 ml) may localize the site of an obstruction. Barium *should not be given by mouth* until it is known that the obstruction is not in the colon.

Diagnosis

Mechanical obstruction of the small intestine may simulate many acute abdominal conditions. Appendicitis, cholecystitis, salpingitis, ureteral colic, acute peptic ulcer, and acute pancreatitis must be included in the differential diagnosis. Serum amylase concentration is elevated in the acute pancreatitis.

Finding the cause of obstruction is important. A hernia should be sought and examined for evidence of incarceration. The presence of an operative scar suggests obstruction due to adhesions. Intussusception is suggested by rectal bleeding in a young child. Volvulus of the colon tends to occur later in life and is accompanied by the development of early, prominent distention.

Treatment

Obstruction must be relieved surgically at the earliest time consistent with safety; fluid, electrolyte, and hemodynamic balance must be restored; and the effects of the obstruction, including bowel distention and possible secondary infection, must be neutralized.

Nasogastric aspiration is performed by means of a Levin tube to remove intestinal contents regurgitating into the stomach. Long intestinal tubes such as the double-lumen Miller-Abbott tube or a Cantor tube may be passed to decompress the intestine directly. These tubes are often difficult to position, resulting in more distress to the patient. The Levin tube is almost always sufficient for this purpose.

Relief of intestinal obstruction usually requires surgical intervention; timing is important and immediate surgery may be necessary for strangulation or infarction, while celiotomy for relief of simple obstruction can usually be delayed until shock has been overcome and electrolyte balance has been reestablished.

Fluid and electrolyte losses require extracellular fluid replacement. The approximate loss may be gauged by the severity of vomiting and a clinical appraisal of the degree of dehydration. Pulse, BP, central venous pressure, and urine flow must be monitored. In dehydration, the Hb and Hct are elevated. The amount of fluid given depends in part on the level of the obstruction. During the first 24 h, sufficient lactated Ringer's solution or 0.9% sodium chloride should be given to restore urine flow and return the hemodynamic vital signs toward normal. A potassium deficit may require adding potassium chloride to the parenteral fluids after urine flow has been reestablished. Fluid output and balance charts should be maintained continuously and serum electrolyte levels determined daily so that fluid and electrolyte replacement can be related to losses after dehydration is corrected. Fluid replacement in patients with severe hepatic or cardiovascular disease must be done cautiously, and saline solution should normally not be given.

Analgesics may be given to control pain; sedation may also be necessary. Since morphine and its derivatives cause increased segmentation of the small intestine and may intensify nausea, meperidine 50 to 100 mg IM q 4 to 6 h is probably best. Confused or comatose patients should be given sedatives and analgesics cautiously. Parenteral antibiotics are indicated if peritonitis is present.

APPENDICITIS

Inflammation of the vermiform appendix.

Etiology, Incidence, and Pathology

Acute appendicitis results from bacterial invasion of the vermiform appendix. Contributory factors include intraluminal obstruction by a fecalith, parasites, a carcinoma tumor, or lymphoid hyperplasia. However, mucosal ulceration with bacterial invasion but no concomitant obstruction can mimic appendicitis. The condition is most common in adolescents and young adults, with a peak incidence between ages 15 and 24, and is also a common reason for intra-abdominal surgery in infants and children.

The inflammation causes edema and ischemia in all layers of the appendix and can progress to gangrene and perforation. Polymorphonuclear leukocytes and, possibly, micro-abscesses are present in the appendiceal lumen and wall. Loops of bowel, omentum, or parietal peritoneum may become adherent and an abscess may develop, either at the site of the appendix or elsewhere in the peritoneal cavity. Perforation may occur early in the course of the disease (within 24 to 48 h) and may produce either a localized or generalized peritonitis. Subsequently, abscesses may develop in areas of the peritoneal cavity remote from the appendix; e.g., pelvis, beneath the diaphragm, and the left side of the abdominal cavity. A mixed bacterial flora dominated by anaerobes and gram-negative bacilli is responsible for the infection.

Symptoms and Signs

Pain typically begins in the midepigastrium and moves to the right lower quadrant where it is persistent, steady, well localized, and accentuated by movement, deep respiration, coughing, or sneezing. Nausea and vomiting are common but not invariably present. Constipation of recent onset is characteristic, and the patient may not pass any rectal gas. A few patients have diarrhea, but this is more likely to be a sign of regional enteritis. There may be mild fever (up to 39 C [102.2 F]), which appears later than other signs, and a moderate leukocytosis.

When the appendix is in the normal position, tenderness and guarding are present over the right lower quadrant, typically at McBurney's point (1/3 the distance between the anterior superior iliac spine and the umbilicus). Tenderness may be localized to a spot lying under one finger. Rebound tenderness anywhere over the abdomen indicates peritoneal inflammation. The **psoas sign** (pain on passive hyperextension of the thigh) strongly suggests appendicitis.

Since the tip of the appendix may be located almost anywhere in the abdomen, findings may vary greatly. Abdominal muscle spasm and resistance may be absent with a retrocecal appendix. An appendix low in the pelvic cavity may cause tenderness on rectal and vaginal examination, without the usual marked abdominal tenderness; an appendix high in the pelvic cavity may cause less rectal tenderness. An appendix lying near the ureter may simulate ureteral colic, with pain radiating to the genitalia and burning on urination; hematuria from ureteral inflammation is occasionally seen. Other atypical sites may result in referral of symptoms to the right hypochondrium or to the left side of the abdomen.

Pain, fever, and leukocytosis are usually increased following perforation. Peritonitis causes generalized pain and tenderness; the abdomen is usually rigid and there may be protracted vomiting; ileus and subsequent shock are likely.

Appendiceal abscess usually develops 24 to 72 h following onset of symptoms; fever, leukocytosis, and local tenderness may be increased, and a mass may be palpable in the right ileal fossa.

Diagnosis

The diagnosis is often difficult in young children because it is a less likely age group and because vomiting may be the dominant symptom, overshadowing abdominal tenderness. Mesenteric adenitis is a common misdiagnosis in children, but pain and guarding are less prominent in this condition. In the elderly and in patients receiving corticosteroids, symptoms and signs may be muted, and in the elderly there are several additional possibilities to consider.

An elevated WBC count with a shift to the left is a useful diagnostic aid, although it may be absent or less evident in elderly patients. Pelvic inflammatory disease in females can usually be excluded by the history. Nausea and vomiting are prominent in acute gastroenteritis, and pain, when it occurs, is usually more generalized than in acute appendicitis. Appendicitis can also mimic other abdominal disorders, including pancreatitis, regional enteritis, cholecystitis, pyelonephritis, spastic colon, and, in children, volvulus and intussusception. Intrathoracic emergencies, including myocardial infarction and pulmonary embolus with diaphragmatic pleurisy, have occasionally been misdiagnosed as acute appendicitis.

Prognosis

With early operation, the mortality is low, the patient is usually discharged within 4 to 5 days, and convalescence is normally rapid and complete. With complications, the prognosis is more serious; if an appendiceal abscess develops, final resolution may take several weeks.

Treatment

With few exceptions, appendicitis is treated by operation. Occasionally, an early attack will subside spontaneously and will not show convincing signs of inflammation. After appendectomy for acute uncomplicated appendicitis, parenteral fluids usually are not required beyond the first day, and GI function returns promptly. Ambulation is desirable as soon as the patient recovers from the anesthetic. An appendiceal abscess requires drainage with or without appendectomy. When appendectomy is deferred under these circumstances, it may be performed a number of weeks after recovery from the acute process. The presence of an abscess or diffuse peritonitis resulting from rupture of the appendix dictates treatment for peritonitis (see that chapter, below, for further discussion of treatment).

Non-surgical treatment may be required in rare situations in which the facilities and the surgical team required for an operation are not available. In such cases, nasogastric suction, IV fluid replacement, ampicillin (IV dosages are as follows: adults, at least 500 mg q 6 h; infants < 1 wk, 50 mg/kg/day; infants of 1 to 4 wk, 100 mg/kg/day; infants of 4 wk to 2 yr, 200 mg/kg/day; children > 2 yr, 200 mg/kg/day) or another broad-spectrum antibiotic, and analgesics should be used.

MECKEL'S DIVERTICULUM

A congenital sacculation following incomplete obliteration of the vitello-intestinal duct. It may be found 30 to 150 cm (1 to 5 ft) proximal to the ileocecal valve in 1 to 2% of the population. Islands of gastric epithelium are occasionally found in a Meckel's diverticulum. Peptic ulceration may develop in this tissue with pain, perforation, or massive hemorrhage as complications of the ulcer. A Meckel's diverticulum may precipitate intussusception, particularly during childhood. The diverticulum may resemble the appendix with similar potential for obstruction or infection; thus, it may mimic appendicitis with similar complications and treatment (see APPENDICITIS, above). A chronic inflammatory process may lead to obstruction of the small intestine or to ileal stricture and the signs and symptoms of lower obstruction. **Treatment** is surgical.

PERITONITIS

Acute inflammation of the visceral and parietal peritoneum.

Etiology and Pathogenesis

Although chemical or mechanical stimuli can cause peritoneal irritation, the most common causes are the infecting bacteria *Escherichia coli* and *Streptococcus faecalis*; other pathogens and occasionally fungi have been identified. Organisms or irritants escape from the intestinal tract most often following perforation of the appendix or a peptic ulcer. Peritonitis may also complicate any operation in the abdominal cavity (e.g., due to leakage at a GI anastomosis), or may result from the spread of pelvic infection into the peritoneal cavity (e.g., from salpingitis) or from a hemoperitoneum due to injury or to rupture of an ectopic pregnancy. Cholecystitis, diverticulitis, colitis, and penetrating wounds of the abdomen are other common causes.

Peritoneal inflammation may be localized or diffuse, depending on the origin of the infection and the patient's defenses. Localized peritonitis frequently occurs in diverticulitis or early appendicitis, while a ruptured appendix or perforation of the colon or of a peptic ulcer usually causes widespread peritoneal contamination. Leakage of bile from the biliary tree produces a particularly severe peritonitis.

Symptoms, Signs, and Diagnosis

Clinical manifestations vary according to the cause and extent of the peritonitis. Onset is marked by severe localized or diffuse abdominal pain. In the early stages, as paralytic ileus develops, moderate abdominal distention is present, usually with nausea and vomiting and, occasionally, diarrhea. Direct abdominal tenderness, rebound tenderness, and marked muscle spasm are present; rebound tenderness may occur without direct tenderness. Later, the abdomen is silent to auscultation. Rectal examination discloses pelvic tenderness and may reveal a pelvic abscess. Plain x-rays of the abdomen may show patchy gaseous filling of the small and large bowel and the absence of well-defined loops. Free peritoneal fluid can often be seen between the coils, and the presence of intraperitoneal air is diagnostic of a perforation. A diagnostic tap or peritoneal lavage may demonstrate the type of exudate or allow culture of the bacteria.

Fever, tachycardia, chills, rapid breathing, and leukocytosis are signs of sepsis; shallow rapid respiration suggests diaphragmatic irritation with splinting. Hiccups and shoulder pain indicate diaphragmatic involvement. Vomiting, initially of reflex origin, usually persists, indicating ileus. As ileus progresses, distention increases and extracellular fluid loss into the intestinal lumen and the peritoneal cavity produces dehydration. Early leukocytosis may be followed by leukopenia in fulminant cases. Dehydration and acidosis develop if the disease is not treated. The eyes become sunken and the mouth becomes dry; circulatory collapse can be fatal; ultimately, the abdomen is tense and distended, and the typically shrunken "Hippocratic facies" appears.

Complications

Early, acute complications of peritonitis include shock, acute renal failure, acute respiratory insufficiency, and sometimes liver failure secondary to pylephlebitis and liver abscesses. Because the infection tends to loculate, abscess formation is typical. Abscesses most commonly are subdiaphragmatic, subhepatic, peritoneal, or pelvic, but they may occur anywhere in the peritoneal cavity. Pelvic abscesses, which are accompanied by diarrhea or increased urinary frequency, can be identified during pelvic examination by palpating a soft tender swelling that bulges into the anterior wall of the rectum. A subphrenic abscess may be obscure and may remain latent for weeks or years; it should be borne in mind, however, since severe toxemia and a high mortality rate may follow delayed treatment. Pain, which may be intermittent, is usually present in the upper abdomen; tenderness over the area of the abscess is an important localizing sign. Elevation and splinting of the diaphragm often occur, as well as small pleural effusions with basal rales.

Treatment

The cause must be eliminated, the infection treated, and the paralytic ileus and dehydration corrected. The source of peritoneal contamination usually must be eliminated by surgery (e.g., appendectomy, cholecystectomy, closure of a perforated peptic ulcer, resection of a gangrenous intestine, or exteriorization of a perforated colon).

Antibiotics (e.g., gentamicin, tetracycline, or cephalosporins) effective against the usual bacteria should be started early and revised if necessary once results of peritoneal fluid or blood cultures are known. Localized abscesses should be sought continuously until all local and systemic evidence of infection subsides; abscesses should be incised and drained.

The peritonitis and associated ileus require nasogastric decompression, IV fluids, and, when protracted, parenteral alimentation. Careful monitoring of urine flow, respiratory efficiency, and intravascular volume is necessary. Blood transfusion or plasma expanders are usually needed if the patient is in shock. The optimal initial replacement fluid is lactated Ringer's solution. Whole blood or packed RBCs are reserved for anemia. Treatment is continued until the gastric aspirate becomes clear and scanty, bowel sounds return to normal, and passage of flatus or feces occurs. Oral feedings should not be resumed too early; fully developed paralytic ileus rarely recovers within 48 h. Small doses of meperidine (10 to 20 mg IV) or morphine (2 to 4 mg IV) q 4 to 6 h may help to relieve pain.

PANCREATITIS

Inflammation of the pancreas. Pancreatitis is classified clinically and histologically as (1) **acute** or **acute relapsing**, in which pancreatic function and histology return to normal and symptoms disappear when the causes are eliminated; and (2) **chronic** or **chronic relapsing**, in which anatomic and functional changes persist even if the causes are removed. Classification may be difficult in a new patient. Diagnostic certainty evolves from the clinical course, laboratory findings, surgery, and histopathology.

ACUTE PANCREATITIS

Etiology and Pathogenesis

Biliary tract disease is the cause in about 1/2 of the patients. Surgery, particularly of the stomach and biliary tract, and alcoholism are other common causes. Infectious diseases (e.g., mumps), hyperlipoproteinemia (Types I and V), hyperparathyroidism, trauma, and drugs (azathioprine, corticosteroids, sulfasalazine, and possibly thiazide diuretics) are infrequent causes. The cause is undetermined in about 1/3 of the patients.

What precipitates most acute attacks is unknown. Attacks are temporally related to the passage of gallstones into the duodenum, but how this causes pancreatitis is unclear. Reflux of bile is unlikely because it causes only minimal inflammation unless infused at high pressures or unless there is pancreatic ischemia. Trauma or ischemia may precipitate attacks, since postoperative pancreatitis is most common after surgery on the stomach or biliary tree.

Gross pathologic changes include edema, hemorrhage, or necrosis, with morbidity and mortality increasing accordingly. Inflammation may be diffuse or spotty. An important factor in acute pancreatitis appears to be the liberation of plasma kinins that increase the permeability of blood vessels and cells and permit the interstitial accumulation of edema fluid and enzyme-rich pancreatic cell contents. Damage occurs if this edema fluid compresses blood vessels, causing ischemia, and if digestive enzymes such as trypsin, elastase, and phospholipase A are activated in the interstitial fluid, damaging normal tissue protein. Elastase, but not active trypsin, has been found in the pancreatic tissue of patients with pancreatitis. Elastase dissolves elastic fibers of blood vessels and may convert the pancreatitis from the edematous to the hemorrhagic form. Phospholipase A converts lecithin in bile to lysolecithin and may contribute to the inflammation.

The activated enzymes may diffuse from the pancreas and damage adjacent tissues (peritoneum, mesentery, spleen, kidney, and pleura). Injury to blood vessels may cause intestinal thrombosis, ischemia, or hemorrhage. **Pseudocysts** may develop because of tissue necrosis and liquefaction and may persist after the acute episode. They are most commonly found near the pancreas, but can also occur at sites as distant as the mediastinum. **Abscesses** are serious complications, usually caused by gram-negative organisms. Unknown mechanisms may trigger **fat necrosis** in the subcutaneous tissue and bone marrow.

Symptoms and Signs

The patient suffers severe abdominal pain. Usually generalized or in the upper quadrants, and often radiating to the back, it steadily increases, reaches a maximum in a few minutes or hours, and usually remains severe and steady, occasionally colicky, until it diminishes gradually over days or weeks as the inflammation subsides. Movement and sometimes respiration aggravate the pain; sitting up or flexion at the waist relieves it. Nausea and vomiting are common. Fever of 37.8 to 38.9 C (100 to 102 F) develops during the first few days. Shock may occur in severe attacks; BP is reduced, the pulse rate elevated, and the skin clammy.

Despite severe pain and tenderness, abdominal guarding and rigidity are present in only 30% of patients, and rebound tenderness in 15%. Diminished or absent bowel sounds and abdominal distention occur in 15% of patients. Common bile duct stones, or compression of the common bile duct by the swollen and inflamed pancreas may cause jaundice that diminishes as the inflammation subsides. Rectal examination is normal. After 1 to 2 days, faint ecchymoses may appear on the flanks **(Grey Turner's sign)** or about the umbilicus **(Cullen's sign)**; an epigastric mass may reflect diffuse extensive inflammation (phlegmon) or a pseudocyst. Massive upper GI bleeding, cardiovascular shock, hypocalcemia, Grey Turner's or Cullen's sign, or ascites suggests hemorrhagic pancreatitis. Pain persisting for > 5 days, with chills, fever, and an elevated WBC count, suggests development of either pancreatic abscess with bacteremia, or ascending cholangitis. Abscesses most commonly are detected 2 to 5 wk after the initial attack.

Laboratory Findings

Serum amylase concentration, the most valuable diagnostic test, usually increases to at least 500 Somogyi u./100 ml. Diagnostic certainty increases when the value is 1000 u. However, serum amylase may be increased with any abdominal inflammation (e.g., perforated viscus, mesenteric vascular occlusion, bowel obstruction) and in other conditions, such as mumps, renal failure, diabetic ketoacidosis, macroamylasemia, and, rarely, after morphine analogs. Serum amylase concentration usually peaks in 24 h and returns to normal in 3 to 10 days. Persistent high and elevated serum amylase concentrations (for a month or more) suggest the presence of carcinoma or a pseudocyst, which may be diagnosed with barium studies of the stomach and small and large intestine, with abdominal ultrasonography, or with CT. Urine amylase output measured over at least 2 h is often high even if the serum amylase concentration is normal. **Amylase/creatinine clearance ratio** increases in acute pancreatitis, but the sensitivity and specificity of the test remain unproved. A figure > 5.3% is abnormal. **Serum triglyceride concentration** may increase in acute pancreatitis, and if serum is milky, serum amylase concentration may be falsely reduced to normal values by a circulating inhibitor. **Serum lipase concentration** also increases and usually remains abnormal longer than the serum amylase. **Serum bilirubin concentrations** may increase in 25% of patients. **Hyperglycemia** may occur. The **serum calcium concentration** may decrease in 36 to 48 h because interstitial calcium forms salts with fatty acids liberated in the peripancreatic tissue; **parathormone concentration** may drop, and thyrocalcitonin concentration may increase. A reduction of calcium concentration to < 8 mg/dl implies marked inflammation. A poor prognosis is also suggested by lactic dehydrogenase concentrations > 700 u., serum aspartate transferase or AST (formerly SGOT) > 250 Sigma-Frankel units, and Pa_{O_2} < 60 mm Hg.

The WBC count may range from 12,000 to 20,000. The Hct may increase if serum exudes into the abdomen through the inflamed peritoneum, but more commonly the Hct decreases; a reduction > 10% in the first 2 days or a continued fall implies hemorrhagic pancreatitis.

Flat and upright plain films of the abdomen may help to establish the diagnosis if calcium (evidence of prior inflammation) is present in the pancreas. They may help to uncover calcified gallstones or the mottled appearance of an abscess. Localized ileus may be present in the left upper quadrant or central abdomen ("sentinel loop" or "colon cutoff" signs), but this finding is nonspecific. Because of ileus, barium studies of the upper GI tract are rarely used in the acute stage, but may be useful later to demonstrate pancreatic swelling or compression of a viscus by a pseudocyst. The chest x-ray may reveal atelectasis or a pleural effusion; when a pleural effusion is present, the amylase concentration in the pleural fluid may be elevated. Blood and necrotic debris in peritoneal fluid with a high amylase content suggest hemorrhagic pancreatitis. If the serum bilirubin is < 3 mg/100 ml, IV cholangiography may help to determine if the biliary tract is normal, although failure to visualize the common duct or gallbladder when the pancreas is inflamed does not necessarily indicate biliary disease. Ultrasonography (B-scan) or CT scan can also help to detect gallstones or enlarged biliary ducts indicating biliary tract obstruction, as well as to reveal an enlarged pancreas.

Differential Diagnosis

Acute pancreatitis should be considered in the differential diagnosis in every acute abdomen. Upper abdominal and lower thoracic inflammation due to common duct stones, acute cholelithiasis, perforated viscus, acute high intestinal obstruction, mesenteric infarction, ectopic pregnancy, and other causes must be excluded. A questionable diagnosis and increasing intra-abdominal inflammation justify an exploratory laparotomy.

Prognosis

The prognosis in acute hemorrhagic pancreatitis is poor; mortality may exceed 50%. In milder edematous pancreatitis, reported mortality is about 10%, but this rate, due to undiagnosed mild cases, may be too high. Diagnosis and treatment are of utmost urgency, since complications are severe; pancreatitis from alcoholism may become chronic and pancreatitis from gallstones may recur in a relapsing acute form (but pancreatitis following mumps, surgery, or trauma tends not to recur).

Treatment

Continuous gastric aspiration through a nasogastric tube reduces pain and may diminish stimulation of pancreatic secretion. Nothing is given by mouth. The value of anticholinergic agents (e.g., atropine) given to diminish gastric acid and pancreatic secretion is unproved, and these agents may increase ileus and cause urinary retention. Dehydration, hypokalemia, and alkalosis due to vomiting and gastric aspiration require correction of fluid and electrolyte balance. Shock (caused by pain, by loss of fluid into the peritoneal cavity, and perhaps by release of humoral agents from the damaged pancreas) must be treated with IV fluids, plasma, human serum albumin, or blood (see also SHOCK in Ch. 24). Hypoxemia, determined by measuring arterial blood gases, occurs frequently and should respond to O_2 via mask or nasal prongs. Pentazocine 30 to 60 mg or meperidine 75 to 150 mg IM q 3 to 4 h should be given for severe pain (not morphine because it contracts the sphincter of Oddi). Epidural or paravertebral anesthesia or splanchnic nerve block may reduce intractable pain. Calcium gluconate 10% solution, 10 to 20 ml IV q 4 h, should be given if hypocalcemia is present. Hyperglycemia should be treated with insulin. Antibiotics effective against fecal organisms (e.g., gentamicin 1 mg/kg IV or IM q 8 h for adults) should be given if there is evidence of secondary infection, but antibiotic prophylaxis is not justified. Abscesses require surgical drainage. Among other suggested treatments, the value of aprotinin, glucagon, peritoneal lavage, or hypothermia is unproved.

Oral feedings should be resumed when abdominal pain ceases, tenderness is minimal, ileus is absent, and the serum amylase or lipase concentrations are normal or nearly normal. One starts with clear liquids and progresses to a regular diet. If pain recurs or serum amylase increases, food is again withheld until the signs and symptoms of inflammation disappear. Parenteral nutrition is indicated if the course is prolonged. If pseudocysts are present and persist for 4 to 6 wk without diminution, they should be surgically drained.

While surgery is necessary for treating abscesses and unresolved pseudocysts, it remains undetermined whether patients having their first attack of gallstone pancreatitis should have emergency cholecystectomy (or cholecystostomy), or whether patients with severe pancreatitis benefit in the long run from draining the affected area.

An oral cholecystogram should be performed several weeks after the inflammation has subsided; the gallbladder should be removed if it fails to opacify during 2 "single dose" tests. Treatment of such causes of pancreatitis as hyperlipoproteinemia and hyperparathyroidism is discussed elsewhere in this volume.

CHRONIC PANCREATITIS

Etiology and Pathogenesis

Etiology is similar to that of acute pancreatitis. Chronic excessive alcohol ingestion, often associated with pancreatic calcification, appears to be the most common predisposing factor. Biliary tract disease follows in importance. A prolonged drinking bout may precipitate an attack in alcoholics. Other causes include obstruction of the main pancreatic duct due to stenosis, stones, or slowly growing cancers. Rarely, pancreatic duct damage from severe acute pancreatitis impairs drainage and causes chronic pancreatitis. Hereditary pancreatitis is rare.

In chronic calcific pancreatitis due to alcohol, protein plugs obstruct the smaller ducts and cause distal dilation of the ducts and acini and flattening of the epithelium. Scarring occurs initially at the site of the plug, then spreads diffusely when the main pancreatic duct becomes involved. Pseudocysts may form distal to the ductal obstruction.

Symptoms, Signs, and Diagnosis

Pain—persistent (chronic) or intermittent (chronic relapsing)—is usually localized to the upper abdomen, but may be generalized. It commonly radiates to the back, may be mild or severe, and may be described as aching, burning, gnawing, or stabbing. It usually lasts days or weeks, rarely for less than one day, and may be confused with the pain of peptic ulcer, gastritis, or biliary tract disease. When gas distends the bowel, as in adynamic ileus, passage of flatus may relieve the discomfort. Nausea and vomiting are common. Other clinical findings resemble those of acute pancreatitis. As the disease progresses, the number of functioning acinar cells that secrete pancreatic digestive enzymes diminishes. With reduced secretion of lipase, trypsin, and chymotrypsin, the patient develops steatorrhea and creatorrhea. Destruction of islet cells reduces insulin secretion and impairs glucose tolerance; some patients develop diabetes mellitus.

Diagnosis grows difficult as the disease progresses because insufficient amylase and lipase may be liberated to elevate the serum enzyme concentrations; 24-h urine amylase output may be elevated, however. When diagnosis is uncertain, measuring the volume and bicarbonate concentration of the duodenal contents after IV injection of secretin 1 clinical u./kg **(secretin test)** may indicate diminished pancreatic exocrine function, particularly if bicarbonate concentration in the duodenal aspirate does not rise above 70 mEq/L.

Evidence of pancreatic calcification on a plain x-ray film of the abdomen confirms prior inflammation and suggests an alcoholic etiology. Abdominal ultrasonography or CT is useful in detecting pancreatic swelling and in detecting and following the course of pseudocysts. Pancreatic angiography may show alternating arterial narrowing and dilation in extensive disease, but at this stage the diagnosis is usually apparent. Similarly, a pancreatic scan following injection of selenomethionine ^{75}Se is of doubtful value. Surgical exploration, operative cholangiography, and pancreatography are indicated for intractable pain or suspicion of biliary tract disease or a pseudocyst. Transduodenal endoscopic retrograde cholangiopancreatography (ERCP) may permit this assessment without a laparotomy.

Treatment

During relapse, treatment is the same as for acute pancreatitis. Aspirin or acetaminophen 600 to 900 mg q 4 h is often sufficient to relieve pain, but severe intermittent or unremitting pain often requires narcotic analgesics and frequently leads to drug addiction. Subtotal (95%) pancreatectomy or pancreaticojejunostomy may relieve pain intractable to medication. If gallstones are the cause, cholecystectomy prevents future attacks and may allow pancreatic morphology and function to return to normal.

Drinking alcohol is forbidden. Patients with steatorrhea benefit from a low-fat diet; medium-chain triglycerides may substitute for the usual dietary fat, but increased carbohydrate intake usually replaces the caloric loss. Pancreatic extract (pancreatin) 1.8 to 2.7 gm should accompany each meal. Pancreatin's effectiveness may be enhanced by 30 ml of an antacid, 0.5 gm sodium bicarbonate, or 300 mg cimetidine orally before meals. Vitamin supplements should include A, D, K, and folic acid; vitamin B_{12} 100 μg IM once/mo may be required. Calcium may be supplemented to prevent osteomalacia.

CANCER OF THE PANCREAS

EXOCRINE TUMORS

Ductal Adenocarcinoma

Symptoms and Signs

Adenocarcinomas of the exocrine pancreas arise from the duct cells 9 times more frequently than from acinar cells. Eighty percent occur in the head of the gland and may produce obstructive jaundice, while tumors located in the body and tail may cause splenic vein obstruction, splenomegaly, gastric and esophageal varices, and GI hemorrhage. Otherwise, symptoms are similar, regardless of the location of the cancer. Weight loss > 10% and abdominal pain are present in 90% of patients at the time of diagnosis. Severe upper abdominal pain usually radiates to the back. Relief may be obtained by bending forward, assuming the fetal position, or using aspirin. Symptoms occur late; in 90% of patients the tumor has spread beyond the gland or metastasized to liver or lung by the time of diagnosis.

Diagnosis

Tests used to detect pancreatic cancer are ultrasonography, CT, retrograde pancreatography, arteriography, and pancreatic function testing. Other scanning technics (e.g., radioselenium pancreatic scans—see under Pancreas in RADIONUCLIDE IMAGING METHODS, in Ch. 227) are either nonspecific or insensitive. Retrograde pancreatography and arteriography can distinguish pancreatitis from cancer and are relatively sensitive and specific, but (as with pancreatic function tests, which are valuable to detect pancreatic disease but cannot distinguish cancer from inflammatory disease) are invasive.

Thus, only ultrasonography and CT are relatively simple to perform and have acceptable sensitivity, specificity, predictive value, and wide applicability. In detecting pancreatic masses, their diagnostic accuracy is similar. Ultrasonography is the initial test because it is less expensive and does not utilize ionizing radiation. However, if the ultrasound study is negative or indeterminate, a CT scan should be done. If the CT scan is negative and a clinical suspicion of pancreatic neoplasm is still high, a normal retrograde pancreatogram or pancreatic function test, or both, would assure absence of disease with at least 90% confidence and help avoid laparotomy.

Patients who appear to have nonmetastatic resectable lesions or gastric or duodenal obstruction are submitted to operation for resection or palliation. Patients with liver metastasis should have a percutaneous liver biopsy for diagnosis. If an unresectable lesion is present, percutaneous CT or ultrasonic guided needle biopsy of the tumor is performed; if concomitant extrahepatic obstruction is present, this can be alleviated by percutaneously guiding a catheter through the liver, bile ducts, and into the duodenum under CT or ultrasound guidance.

Prognosis and Treatment

In the 10% of patients who have localized tumors, a total pancreatectomy or a Whipple procedure (pancreaticoduodenectomy) is performed. Five-year survival is < 2%. In most patients, only a palliative bypass procedure can be performed. The combination of 5FU and radiation therapy (6000 rads) may lengthen survival in ambulatory patients with locally unresectable lesions.

For control of pain, aspirin 0.65 gm alone or combined with codeine 30 to 120 mg orally q 4 h may be effective. Stronger oral or parenteral narcotics in dosages sufficient to relieve pain may be required. Percutaneous or operative splanchnic block can be remarkably effective. If palliative surgery has not relieved pruritus secondary to obstructive jaundice, it can be managed with cholestyramine 4 gm orally 1 to 4 times/day and phenothiazines.

Exocrine pancreatic insufficiency should be treated with pancreatin and diabetes mellitus should be carefully monitored and controlled.

CYSTADENOCARCINOMA

Cystadenocarcinomas are rare pancreatic tumors that present as upper abdominal pain and a palpable abdominal mass. They arise as a malignant degeneration of a mucus cystadenoma. Diagnosis by ultrasonography or CT scanning of the pancreas demonstrates a cystic mass of the pancreas with some debris within the cyst. Scans may be erroneously interpreted as demonstrating a necrotic adenocarcinoma.

In contrast to ductal adenocarcinomas, cystadenocarcinomas have a relatively good prognosis. Only 20% have metastasis at the time of operation, and complete excision of the tumor by either distal or total pancreatectomy or the Whipple procedure results in a 65% 5-yr survival.

ENDOCRINE TUMORS

Pancreatic islet cell tumors have 2 general presentations. **Nonfunctioning tumors** may cause obstructive symptoms of the biliary tract or duodenum, bleeding into the GI tract, or as abdominal masses. Hypersecretion of a particular hormone by **functioning tumors** may cause various syndromes; these include hypoglycemia (**insulinoma** hypersecretes insulin), Zollinger-Ellison syndrome (**gastrinoma** hypersecretes gastrin), hypokalemic diarrhea, called pancreatic cholera, (**gipoma** and **vipoma** cause changes in secretion of gastric inhibitory polypeptide or vasoactive intestinal peptide), carcinoid syndrome (caused by **carcinoid tumors**, which are difficult to distinguish histologically from islet-cell tumors), diabetes (**glucagonoma** hypersecretes glucagon), and **Cushing's syndrome** (from ACTH hypersecretion). These clinical syndromes also sometimes occur in **multiple endocrine adenomatosis** in which tumors or hyperplasia affect 2 or more endocrine glands, usually the parathyroid, pituitary, thyroid, or adrenals (see Ch. 89).

INSULINOMA

Symptoms and signs of hypoglycemia secondary to an insulinoma appear during fasting, are insidious, and may mimic a variety of psychiatric and neurologic disorders. CNS disturbances are characteristic: headache, confusion, visual disturbances, motor weakness, palsy, ataxia, marked personality changes, and possible progression to loss of consciousness, convulsions, and coma. Evidence of sympathetic stimulation (faintness, weakness, tremulousness, palpitation, diaphoresis, hunger, and nervousness) may occur, but is often absent.

Diagnosis

Correlation of excessive insulinemia, measured by insulin radioimmunoassay (IRI), with plasma glucose levels is mandatory to confirm the diagnosis. The most helpful procedure is a carefully supervised 72-h fast. Plasma insulin concentration falls progressively in normal individuals; in those with insulinoma, high insulin levels coexist with hypoglycemia. The possibility *must be considered* of surreptitious self-administration of insulin; it can be detected by demonstrating the presence of circulating insulin antibodies.

Usually within the first 24 h, hypoglycemia as the cause of the symptoms is established by Whipple's triad: (1) The attack comes during the fast, (2) symptoms occur in the presence of hypoglycemia (glucose < 40 mg/dl), and (3) ingestion of carbohydrates relieves the symptoms. Simultaneous hyperinsulinemia of > 6 μU/ml is diagnostic of insulin-mediated hypoglycemia.

If Whipple's triad is not observed after prolonged fasting, and the fasting plasma glucose after an overnight fast is more than 50 mg/dl, the tolbutamide test is useful. On the day of the test, sodium tolbutamide 1 gm is given IV over a 2-min period. Persistent hypoglycemia (blood glucose < 50 mg/dl, plasma glucose < 57 mg/dl) and hyperinsulinemia (IRI > 20 μU/ml) 2 to 3 h after tolbutamide administration is characteristic of insulinoma.

In difficult diagnostic problems, a C-peptide suppression test can be performed. During insulin infusion (0.1 u./kg/60 min) insulinoma patients fail to suppress C-peptide to normal levels ($\leq$ 1.2 ng/ml).

Angiography is the most reliable method for visualizing highly vascular islet-cell tumors of the pancreas. Preoperative localization can be achieved in 90% of cases. Celiac arterial injection followed by hepatic or splenic artery injection usually permits visualization of the tumor; occasionally, selective catheterization of pancreatic vessels is required. Stereoscopic filming in association with magnification and subtraction are almost routinely used.

Treatment

A small single adenoma at or near the surface of the pancreas can usually be enucleated. In the case of a single large or deep adenoma within the body or tail of the pancreas, multiple lesions in the body or tail (or both), or if no insulinoma is found (an unusual circumstance), a distal subtotal pancreatic resection is performed. In < 1% of cases, the insulinoma is ectopically located in peripancreatic sites of the duodenal wall or periduodenal area and can be found only by diligent search. Total pancreatectomy is reserved for resectable malignant lesions of the proximal pancreas, when medical therapy is ineffective, or if a previous subtotal resection proves inadequate.

Overall surgical cure rates should approach 90%, since only 10% of tumors are malignant. When hypoglycemia continues, diazoxide orally (200 to 800 mg/day) in conjunction with a natriuretic can be used. Streptozocin (1 gm/sq m BSA IV weekly for 4 wk), a broad spectrum antibiotic, may give measurable benefit in 50% of patients. Its use requires monitoring of renal function (urine proteins, serum creatinine), hepatic function, and potential hematopoietic toxicity (CBC).

ZOLLINGER-ELLISON SYNDROME (Z-E Syndrome; Gastrinoma)

A syndrome characterized by marked hypergastrinemia, gastric hypersecretion, and peptic ulceration. Usually there is an associated gastrin-producing tumor of the pancreas with cells of the non-β-type. Occasionally the tumors are at other sites particularly in the duodenal wall. Most patients have multiple tumors and > ½ of the tumors are malignant. Usually the tumors are small (< 1 cm in diameter) and their growth and spread are slow. They may be seen in patients who have abnormalities of other endocrine glands, particularly the parathyroids and, less often, the pituitary and adrenal glands. This polyglandular disorder, multiple endocrine adenomatosis, is discussed in Ch. 89.

Classically, the clinical presentation of Z-E syndrome is an aggressive peptic ulcer diathesis with ulcerations occurring in atypical locations (25% located distal to the duodenal bulb) or following surgical treatment. The complications of perforation, bleeding, and obstruction can be frequent and life-threatening. However, in > 50% of patients, clinical, x-ray, and endoscopic findings are indistinguishable from ordinary peptic ulcer disease. The Z-E syndrome should be suspected, however, if the ulcer is > 7.5 cm (3 in.) beyond the pylorus, is resistant to medical therapy, recurs after surgery, or if there is accompanying diarrhea. The diagnosis may not be suspected until after surgery and then may be more difficult to make. Therefore, serum gastrin should always be measured prior to surgery.

Diagnosis

Diagnosis is suspected in patients with a compatible clinical history, x-ray evidence of a duodenal or postbulbar ulcer associated with large edematous gastric and duodenal folds and large amounts of fluid in the stomach, and an excessive basal gastric acid secretory rate (one that exceeds 10 mEq/h in the unoperated patient or 5 mEq/h after a previous ulcer operation and is > 60% of the amount of acid secreted after a maximal stimulating dose of histamine, histalog, or pentagastrin). However, the most reliable test is the radioimmunoassay measurement of serum gastrin. All patients have > 150 pg/ml; markedly elevated levels of > 1000 pg/ml in a patient with compatible clinical features and gastric acid hypersecretion establishes the diagnosis. However, hypergastrinemia can be found in pernicious anemia, chronic gastritis, renal insufficiency, massive intestinal resection, and pheochromocytoma.

Provocative tests may be useful in patients without marked hypergastrinemia. In these tests, calcium (5 mg/kg/h IV for 3 h), secretin (1 to 2 u. GIH secretin/kg/h as a bolus IV injection), or a test meal is accompanied by measurements of serum gastrin. The characteristic responses in Z-E syndrome are marked increases in serum gastrin with calcium, a paradoxic increase with secretin, and a failure to increase $> 50\%$ after a standard meal. In antral G cell hyperplasia, the serum gastrin may not respond to calcium, is decreased with secretin, and increases markedly in response to a test meal. In idiopathic peptic ulcer disease, there is a small increase of serum gastrin in response to calcium, no paradoxic increase in response to secretin, and a moderate increase after a test meal.

Gastrinomas are visualized $< 50\%$ of the time by arteriography.

Treatment

Previously, to avoid complications and death from gastric hypersecretion, total gastrectomy was performed in all patients with Z-E syndrome. Since the advent of cimetidine, an H_2 receptor antagonist that markedly decreases gastric acid output, alleviates clinical symptoms, and promotes healing in patients with gastrinoma, several questions have been reopened. Do patients with gastrinoma require surgery and, if so, how aggressively should excision of the tumor be pursued? Because surgical cure (resection of tumor) is possible in 20% of patients with the nonfamilial type of Z-E syndrome, these patients should undergo exploratory laparotomy. Patients with multiple endocrine adenomatosis type I or metastatic tumors should not be explored. These patients, as well as patients with unresectable tumors, should be treated with cimetidine. The standard dose is 300 mg orally q.i.d. between meals, but some patients may require 3 to 4 gm/day in divided doses. The drug must be used indefinitely. Side effects such as gynecomastia and impotence have been reported. In refractory patients, the addition of anticholinergics (e.g., 15 to 30 mg propantheline bromide orally 30 min before meals) or antacids (e.g., magnesium-aluminum hydroxide gel 30 ml orally 1 and 3 h postprandially and at bedtime), or both, may also be helpful. If this treatment is unsuccessful, a total gastrectomy may be necessary. Total gastrectomy in Z-E syndrome is well tolerated without crippling nutritional complications, but patients need 100 μg vitamin B_{12} parenterally every month and iron and calcium supplements daily. In patients with metastatic disease, streptozocin may reduce tumor mass and serum gastrin concentration and be a useful adjunct to cimetidine therapy or total gastrectomy.

PANCREATIC CHOLERA (Verner-Morrison Syndrome; WDHA [Watery Diarrhea, Hypokalemia, Achlorhydria]; WDHH [Watery Diarrhea, Hypokalemia, Hypochlorhydria]; Vipoma Syndrome)

The major clinical features are prolonged massive watery diarrhea (fasting stool volume exceeds 750 to 1000 ml/day) and symptoms of hypokalemia and dehydration. Half of the patients have relatively constant diarrhea while the rest have alternating periods of severe and moderate diarrhea. One third have diarrhea < 1 yr prior to diagnosis, but in 25%, diarrhea is present for 5 yr or more prior to diagnosis. Lethargy, muscular weakness, nausea, vomiting, and crampy abdominal pain are frequent symptoms. During attacks of diarrhea, flushing similar to the carcinoid syndrome occurs rarely.

Diagnosis

Diagnosis requires the demonstration of a secretory diarrhea (twice the product of the sum of sodium and potassium stool concentrations accounts for all measured stool osmolality) without apparent cause. Other causes of secretory diarrhea and, in particular, laxative abuse must be excluded (see also DIARRHEA in Ch. 54). Arteriography and ultrasonography should be done but will not visualize the tumor in $^2/_3$ of patients. Circulating vasoactive intestinal peptide (**VIP**) by radioimmunoassay may be elevated but many false-positive and -negative results limit its usefulness. Gastric acid secretion is usually low, but normal values do not exclude the diagnosis. Pancreatic secretion, jejunal biopsy, and stool fat are normal or only mildly abnormal. In most cases, the diagnosis is established by finding a pancreatic tumor or a neurotumor at exploration.

Treatment

Initially, fluids and electrolytes must be replaced. To avoid acidosis, HCO_3 must be given to replace fecal loss of this ion. Because fecal losses of water and electrolytes increase as rehydration is achieved, continual IV replacement may become more difficult.

Resection of the tumor results in complete cure in $^1/_2$ of the patients. In patients with metastatic tumor, resection of all visible tumor may provide temporary relief of symptoms. Streptozocin has also been effective in reducing diarrhea and tumor mass. In $^1/_2$ of the patients with metastases, a corticosteroid (e.g., prednisone 20 mg/day orally) controls diarrhea.

CARCINOID

Symptoms and signs that encompass the carcinoid syndrome are often bizarre and include *diarrhea, abdominal cramps, borborygmi, episodic flushing, telangiectasia, cyanosis, pellagra-like skin lesions, bronchospasm, and valvular heart lesions.*

The constellation of typical clinical features, increased 5HIAA in a 24-h urine collection, and demonstration of liver metastasis by an abnormal liver scan may be sufficient to confirm the diagnosis without tissue confirmation by biopsy or laparotomy.

Treatment

Symptoms may be present several years before treatment is undertaken. Despite metastatic disease, 10- to 15-yr survivals are not unusual. Surgery rarely cures. Results of chemotherapy and irradiation are generally unrewarding and should not be undertaken unless there is evidence of rapid tumor growth. Other pharmacologic agents, although they do not affect tumor growth, are helpful. Niacin should be given to prevent pellagra. Flushing attacks can be controlled or diminished by using phenothiazines (prochlorperazine 5 to 10 mg orally or chlorpromazine 25 to 50 mg orally q 6 h) or the α-adrenergic blocker phenoxybenzamine 10 to 50 mg/day. In extreme cases, prednisone 10 to 40 mg/day can be used. Diarrhea and tenesmus are treated with diphenoxylate 2.5 to 5.0 mg orally q 4 h or tincture of opium 6 to 20 drops q 3 to 4 h. In intractable situations, specific serotonin antagonists, cyproheptadine 4 to 12 mg q 6 h or methysergide 2 to 4 mg t.i.d. or q.i.d., may be tried. The latter drug may be associated with development of fluid retention and retroperitoneal and cardiac fibrosis. A specific inhibitor of tryptophan hydroxylase, p-chlorophenylalanine 3 gm/day produces reduction or complete remission of diarrhea, but this drug produces allergic reactions in a majority of patients using it for > 6 wk.

GLUCAGONOMA

Pancreatic α-cell glucagon-secreting tumors are rare but similar to other islet cell tumors in that the primary and metastatic lesions are slow-growing; 15-yr survival times are common. The hypersecretion of glucagon is associated with diabetes mellitus (see p. 700). Frequently, weight loss and anemia are present but the most distinctive clinical feature is a chronic eruption involving the extremities that often is associated with a smooth shiny vermillion tongue. It is an exfoliating, brownish-red erythematous lesion, with superficial necrolysis and is termed **necrolytic migratory erythema.**

Diagnosis is made by demonstrating elevated levels of circulating immunoreactive glucagon in the presence of the typical angiographic appearance of an islet-cell tumor and proven by laparotomy.

Treatment by resection of the tumor will alleviate all symptoms. In the event of unresectability, metastasis, or recurrence, streptozocin may cause a decrease in the levels of circulating immunoreactive glucagon and symptomatic improvement.

---

54.   MANIFESTATIONS OF BOWEL DISEASE

DIARRHEA

(See also Ch. 55)

Increased volume, fluidity, or frequency of bowel movements relative to the usual pattern for a particular individual. Normal bowel habits vary considerably from one person to another, being modified by age and by social and cultural patterns. In an urban civilization, the normal frequency of bowel movements ranges from 2 to 3 movements/day to 2 to 3/wk. Increased stool frequency or fecal volume, changes in stool consistency, or blood, mucus, pus, or excess fatty material (oil, grease, or film) in the stool may indicate disease.

Pathophysiology

In healthy adults, stool weight ranges from 100 to 300 gm/day depending on the amount of nonabsorbable dietary material (mainly carbohydrate). Diarrhea occurs when stool weight is increased to > 300 gm/day, except in persons whose diet is rich in vegetable fiber, in whom daily stool weights > 300 gm are normal. Since 60 to 90% of stool weight is water, diarrhea is mainly due to excess fecal water. Categorizing diarrhea according to the major pathophysiologic cause of the increased stool weight may facilitate etiologic investigation and identify specific treatment.

1. **Osmotic diarrhea** occurs when excess nonabsorbable, water-soluble solutes are present in the bowel and retain water in the lumen. This occurs with lactose (lactase deficiency) and other sugar intolerances, and when poorly absorbed salts (magnesium sulfate, sodium phosphates) are prescribed as saline laxatives.

Ingestion of large amounts of the hexitols, sorbitol and mannitol, used as sugar substitutes in dietetic foods, candy, and chewing gum, causes diarrhea by a combination of slow absorption and rapid small-bowel motility ("dietetic food" or "chewing gum" diarrhea). The severity of symptoms is proportional to the amount consumed and body weight; the condition disappears as soon as intake stops.

2. **Secretory diarrhea:** The small and large bowel normally reabsorb salts (especially sodium chloride) and water which is ingested or which reach the lumen as a consequence of digestive secretions. Diarrhea may occur when the small and large bowel secrete rather than absorb electrolytes and water. Substances which induce secretion include bacterial toxins (e.g., as in cholera), bile acids (e.g., after ileal resection), unabsorbed dietary fat in steatorrhea, anthraquinone cathartics,

castor oil, and some hormones (e.g., secretin, calcitonin), drugs (e.g., prostaglandins), and vasoactive intestinal peptide (VIP) from a pancreatic tumor.

3. Malabsorption may produce diarrhea by either of the above mechanisms. If the unabsorbed material is abundant, water-soluble, and osmotically important (i.e., of low mol wt), the mechanism could be osmotic. Lipids are not appreciably water-soluble and cannot act this way; some (fatty acids, bile acids) act as secretagogues for electrolytes and water. In generalized malabsorption, as in nontropical sprue, fat malabsorption (causing colonic secretion) and carbohydrate malabsorption (causing osmotic diarrhea) can coexist.

4. Exudative diarrhea: Many mucosal diseases (e.g., regional enteritis, ulcerative colitis, TB, lymphoma, and carcinoma) cause an "exudative enteropathy." Mucosal inflammation, ulceration, or tumefaction may result in an outpouring of plasma, serum proteins, blood, and mucus, thereby increasing fecal bulk and fluidity. Involvement of the rectal mucosa may cause urgency and an increased frequency of bowel movements because the rectum is more sensitive to distention.

5. Altered intestinal transit: Chyme must be exposed to adequate absorptive surface of the GI tract for a sufficient amount of time if normal absorption is to occur. Factors which **decrease** exposure time include resection of the small or large bowel, gastric resection, surgery on the pyloric sphincter, vagotomy, surgical bypass of intestinal segments, and drugs or humoral agents (e.g., prostaglandins, serotonin) which speed transit by stimulating intestinal smooth muscle.

Malabsorption and diarrhea may also develop when the contact between chyme and mucosa is prolonged and fecal bacteria proliferate in the small intestine. Factors which **increase** exposure time include strictured segments, sclerodermatous intestinal disease, and stagnant loops created by surgery.

Consequences of Diarrhea

Electrolyte loss (sodium, potassium, magnesium, organic anions, and chloride), fluid loss with consequent dehydration, and vascular collapse may occur. **Collapse** may develop rapidly in patients who are very young, elderly, or debilitated, or who have severe diarrhea (e.g., those with cholera). **Metabolic acidosis** may develop due to bicarbonate loss. Serum sodium concentrations vary according to the composition of diarrheal losses relative to plasma. **Hypokalemia** may occur in severe or chronic diarrhea or if the stools contain excess mucus. Tetany due to **hypomagnesemia** following prolonged diarrhea has been observed.

Diagnosis

Clinical features vary greatly depending on the etiology, duration, and severity of the diarrhea, on the area of the bowel affected, and on the patient's general health. The history should note the time, place, and other circumstances of onset; duration and severity; associated abdominal pain or vomiting; presence of overt or occult blood in the stool; frequency and timing of bowel movements; evidence of steatorrhea (fatty, greasy, or oily stools with a foul odor); associated changes in weight or appetite; use of dietetic products (see Osmotic diarrhea, above); and presence of rectal tenesmus.

Macro- and microscopic examination of the stools may be helpful. The fluidity, volume, and presence of blood, pus, mucus, or excess fat should be noted. Generally, in diseases of the upper gut, the stools are voluminous and watery or fatty. In colonic disease, the movements are frequent, sometimes small in volume, and possibly accompanied by blood, pus, mucus, and abdominal discomfort. In diseases of the rectal mucosa, the rectum may be more sensitive to distention, and diarrhea may be characterized by frequent, small stools. Microscopy may confirm the presence of unabsorbed fat, meat fibers, or infestation with amebas, giardias, or other parasites. Stool pH, normally > 6.0, is decreased by bacterial fermentation of unabsorbed carbohydrate and protein in the colon.

Evidence of vascular collapse, dehydration, electrolyte depletion, or anemia should be sought. Abdominal examination and digital and proctoscopic rectal examination should be performed. Biopsy of the rectal mucosa and rectal swabbing for microscopic examination should be considered at proctoscopy.

Treatment

Diarrhea is only a symptom and the underlying disorder should be specifically treated if possible. Symptomatic treatment may also be necessary. Intestinal tone may be increased by diphenoxylate (2.5 to 5 mg as tablets or liquid, t.i.d. or q.i.d.), codeine phosphate 15 to 30 mg b.i.d. or t.i.d., or paregoric (camphorated opium tincture) 15 ml q 4 h. Peristalsis is decreased by anticholinergics such as belladonna tincture, atropine, or propantheline. Bulk is provided by a psyllium or methylcellulose compound; these bulking agents, though usually prescribed for constipation, also decrease the fluidity of liquid stools when given in small doses. Kaolin adsorbs fluid.

Severe acute diarrhea may require urgent fluid and electrolyte replacement to correct dehydration, electrolyte imbalance, and acidosis (see REGULATION OF WATER AND SODIUM HOMEOSTASIS in Ch. 81). An oral glucose-electrolyte solution may be given if nausea and vomiting are not severe. Fluids containing glucose (or sucrose, as table sugar), sodium chloride, and sodium bicarbonate are rapidly absorbed and easily prepared. Five ml (1 tsp) table salt, 5 ml (1 tsp) baking soda, 20 ml (4 tsp) table sugar, and flavoring are added to 1 L water (about 1 qt). Parenteral fluids are generally required for more severe diarrhea. If nausea or vomiting is present, oral intake should be restricted. However, when water and electrolytes must be replaced in massive amounts (e.g., in epidemic cholera), oral glucose-electrolyte supplements are sometimes given in addition to the more conventional IV therapy with electrolyte (bicarbonate) fluids (see CHOLERA in Ch. 8). Sodium chloride, potassium chloride, glucose, and fluids to counteract acidosis (sodium lactate, acetate, or bicarbonate) may be indicated. Fluid balance and estimates of body fluid composition must be monitored carefully. Associated vomiting or GI bleeding may require additional measures.

CONSTIPATION

(Constipation in children is discussed in BEHAVIORAL PROBLEMS in Vol. II, Ch. 24)

Difficult or infrequent passage of feces. Constipation can refer to hardness of stool, difficult defecation, a feeling of incomplete evacuation, or infrequent defecation. No body function is more variable and subject to extraneous influences than is defecation. Dietary, cultural, and individual physiologic factors modify normal bowel function. Normal frequency varies from 3 times/day to once/3 days.

Acute constipation represents a definite change *for that individual*, suggesting an organic cause. In patients complaining of constipation for only hours or a few days, mechanical bowel obstruction must be considered. A second organic cause is adynamic ileus, which often accompanies acute intra-abdominal disease (e.g., localized peritonitis, diverticulitis); it may complicate a variety of traumatic conditions (e.g., head injuries, spinal fractures) or may follow general anesthesia. Strong laxatives should be avoided in all of these circumstances. Less ominous, but often confusing, is the acute onset of constipation in bedridden patients (particularly the aged) or constipation related to side effects of drugs. A careful drug history should always be obtained, since constipation is caused by many agents, including those that act within the lumen (aluminum hydroxide, bismuth salts, iron salts, cholestyramine), anticholinergics, opiates, ganglionic blockers, and many tranquilizers and sedatives.

When the change of bowel habit persists for weeks or occurs intermittently with increasing frequency and/or severity, colonic tumors and other causes of partial obstruction should be suspected. Underlying causes must be identified and treated. Local conditions of the anorectum (e.g., anal fissures) that cause pain or bleeding should be sought; plain abdominal films with upright views, proctosigmoidoscopy, and possibly a barium enema examination may be required. If no disorder is found, treatment should be symptomatic (see below).

In **chronic constipation,** the common functional causes are those which hamper normal bowel movements because the storage, transporting, and evacuating mechanisms of the colon are deranged, sometimes by systemic disorders (e.g., debilitating infections, hypothyroidism, hypercalcemia, uremia, or porphyria), but more often by local neurogenic disorders—e.g., the irritable bowel syndrome (see THE IRRITABLE BOWEL SYNDROME in Ch. 59), inactive colon (see below), and megacolon (see HIRSCHSPRUNG'S DISEASE in Vol. II, Ch. 21). Certain neurologic disorders, such as Parkinson's disease, cerebral thrombosis, tumor, and injury to the spinal cord, are important extraintestinal causes. Psychogenic factors are most common. (See below under psychogenic constipation and under suggested treatments for specific disorders.)

Treatment

The patient's diet should contain sufficient residue to ensure adequate stool bulk. Vegetable fiber, which is largely indigestible and unabsorbable, increases stool bulk; certain components of fiber also adsorb fluid into the solid phase, making stools softer and thus facilitating their passage. Fruits and vegetables should be recommended or the diet can be supplemented by cereals containing bran, taken to tolerance. Unrefined miller's bran, taken as 2 to 3 tsp on fruit or cereal b.i.d. or t.i.d., may be preferred.

Bulking agents, such as bran, psyllium, and methyl cellulose, are the only laxatives that should be considered for chronic use. They act slowly and gently and are the safest medications for promoting stool elimination. Proper use involves gradually increasing the dose, best taken t.i.d. or q.i.d. and with sufficient liquid to prevent impaction of inspissated medication, until a softer, bulkier stool results. This approach produces "natural" effects and is not "habit-forming." **Psyllium** may fulfill the difficult qualifications of a "bi-directional normalizer." In constipation it promotes peristalsis and fecal elimination; in diarrheal states it decreases the number of watery stools.

Laxatives and cathartics should be used with care. They may interfere with absorption of various medications by binding the drugs chemically (tetracycline, calcium, and phosphate) or physically (digoxin on cellulose matrices); or rapid transit of the fecal stream may rush some drugs (and nutrients) beyond their optimal absorptive locus. Abdominal pain of unknown etiology, inflammatory bowel disorders, intestinal obstruction, GI bleeding, and fecal impactions are **contraindications** for their use. In addition to **bulking agents** (see above), laxatives and cathartics can be divided into several classes:

Wetting agents (detergent laxatives) soften stool by increasing the wetting ability of intestinal water. They have both hydrophilic and hydrophobic properties. These break down surface barriers, allowing water to enter the fecal mass, soften it, and increase its bulk. Increased fecal bulk may stimulate peristalsis and the softened stool moves more easily. **Mineral oil** softens fecal matter, resulting in more easily passed stool mass. Mineral oil itself may decrease absorption of fat-soluble vitamins. Mineral oil and detergent laxatives are slowly acting agents, and either may be useful following myocardial infarction or anorectal surgery, and in clinical situations requiring prolonged bed rest.

Osmotic agents or **saline cathartics** are used to prepare patients for some diagnostic bowel procedures and occasionally in the therapy of parasitic infestations. They contain poorly absorbed polyvalent ions (e.g., phosphate, magnesium, sulfate) and/or carbohydrates (e.g., lactulose, sorbitol). Since these substances remain in the bowel, they increase the intraluminal osmotic pressure, drawing water into the intestinal lumen. Stool volume increases and consistency decreases. The increased volume stimulates peristalsis, and the softened, watery stool moves easily through the bowel. These medications work rapidly, usually within 3 h. Magnesium and phosphate are partially absorbed and may be detrimental in some conditions (e.g., in renal insufficiency). Sodium (present in some preparations) may adversely affect congestive heart failure. These drugs may also upset fluid and electrolyte balance in patients without underlying disease who ingest large or frequent doses.

Secretory or stimulant cathartics, such as senna and its derivatives, cascara, phenolphthalein, bisacodyl, and castor oil, act by irritation of the intestinal mucosa or by direct neuronal (submucosal and myenteric plexus) stimulation. Some of these drugs are absorbed, metabolized by the liver, and returned to the bowel in the bile. Peristaltic movements and intraluminal fluid both increase, with cramping and passage of semisolid stool in 6 to 8 h. With continued use, melanosis coli, neuronal degeneration in the colon, "lazy bowel" syndrome, and serious fluid and electrolyte disturbances may occur. Stimulant-type cathartics are frequently helpful in preparing the bowel for diagnostic procedures.

PSYCHOGENIC CONSTIPATION

Many persons incorrectly believe that daily defecation is integral to normalcy and complain of constipation because the frequency of their bowel movements is not what they expect. Others may be concerned with a certain appearance (thin or pelletlike, color) or consistency of stools, though sometimes the major complaint is lack of satisfaction with the act of defecation. As a result of these beliefs, the colon is abused by laxatives, suppositories, and enemas. Overzealous treatment of an *imaginary* disorder can result in a *real* illness—the irritable bowel syndrome. This may be accompanied by **cathartic colon** (a "pipestem" colon lacking haustra on barium enema examination, thus mimicking ulcerative colitis) and **melanosis coli** (deposits of brown pigment in the mucosa, seen endoscopically and in colonic biopsies), both caused by long-term laxative ingestion.

Obsessive-compulsive people have problems of personal belief and also emotional need. Their anxiety is controlled by perfectionistic behavior, and their need to rid the body daily of "unclean" wastes may take on exaggerated importance. Failure to defecate daily may result in a vicious circle in which depression reduces defecatory frequency, and failure of defecation adds to the depression. Such people often become chronic cathartic users or spend excessive amounts of time on the toilet.

Treatment

Before advising or reassuring a patient concerning defecatory habits, the physician must exclude serious disease by rectal and proctoscopic examination, and by barium enema when indicated. Extraintestinal disease also should be excluded by appropriate tests. The psychologic needs of the individual should also be considered. It is neither kind nor useful to accuse an obsessive-compulsive patient of an abnormal attitude toward defecation, as one's psychophysiologic makeup cannot be altered, although psychotherapy may help to inculcate more rational ideas. On the other hand, when the problem is due to a mistaken belief, the physician must explain that daily bowel movements are not essential, that the bowel must be given a chance to function, that laxatives or enemas taken more often than once every 3 days deny the bowel that chance, and that the way to cure a stool that is "too thin" or "too green" is to avoid looking at it.

COLONIC INERTIA (Atonic Constipation; Colon Stasis; Inactive Colon)

Etiology

This constipation occurs in aged or invalid patients, especially the bedridden. Feces accumulate because the colon does not respond to the usual stimuli promoting evacuation, or because accessory stimuli provided by normal eating and physical activity are lacking. Use of other drugs for associated medical conditions frequently compounds the problem. It sometimes occurs in patients whose rectal sensitivity to the presence of fecal masses is dulled by habitual disregard of the urge to defecate, or by prolonged dependence on laxatives or enemas, often initiated in childhood.

Symptoms, Signs, and Diagnosis

The principal symptom, constipation, is unlike that seen in the irritable colon syndrome, since abdominal discomfort is absent or minimal and the stools are often putty-like or soft and not scybalous. Rectal examination frequently discloses an ampulla full of feces, yet the patient has no urge to defecate and is unable to do so effectively, even with effort. Proctoscopic and barium enema examinations are normal, though the contrast medium may sometimes be evacuated with difficulty and the colon may appear unusually redundant and capacious.

Fecal impaction may develop spontaneously or after barium has been given by mouth or enema. The patient has rectal pain and tenesmus and makes repeated but futile attempts to defecate. Cramps may occur and the patient may pass watery mucus or fecal material around the impacted mass, mimicking diarrhea. Rectal examination discloses a firm, sometimes rocklike, but often rubbery and putty-like mass.

Treatment

This is adapted to the general status of the patient. Since abdominal distress and other signs of bowel irritability are minimal, there is no harm in treating an elderly or invalid patient with osmotic laxatives (e.g., milk of magnesia 15 to 30 ml or sodium sulfate 15 gm in ½ glass of water). In the more chronic situation, the patient should try to have the bowel move at the same time daily, preferably 15 to 45 min after breakfast, since the food ingestion stimulates colonic motility. Initial efforts at regular, unhurried bowel movements may be aided by rectal instillation of 60 to 90 ml (2 to 3 oz) of warm (43.3 C [110 F]) olive oil or isotonic saline, or glycerin suppositories may be used.

Fecal impaction is treated by enemas of warm (43.3 C [110 F]) mineral or olive oil 60 to 120 ml (2 to 4 oz) followed by enemas of small (100 ml), commercially prepared, hypertonic solutions. If these fail, manual fragmentation and disimpaction of the mass are necessary. This procedure is painful, and peri- and intrarectal application of local anesthetics (e.g., lidocaine 5% ointment or dibucaine 1% ointment) is recommended. Some patients require general anesthesia.

---

55. GASTROENTERITIS: INFECTIVE AND TOXIC

A group of clinical syndromes predominantly manifested by upper GI tract symptoms (anorexia, nausea, or vomiting), diarrhea of variable severity, and abdominal discomfort. Subsequent losses of electrolytes and fluids from the body may be little more than an inconvenience to an otherwise healthy adult, but can be of grave significance to persons less able to withstand the stress (e.g., the aged, debilitated, or very young; see also ACUTE INFECTIOUS NEONATAL DIARRHEA in Vol. II, Ch. 21).

Etiology

Gastroenteritis, a generic term, often implies a nonspecific, uncertain, or unknown etiology. However, certain diseases of known bacterial, viral, parasitic, or toxic etiology can be included in the clinical definition. When a specific etiology can be identified, the less specific term (gastroenteritis) can be avoided. Some types of bacterial gastroenteritis, such as cholera, salmonellosis, and shigellosis, have established pathogenic mechanisms and can be considered prototypes for syndromes of lesser specificity.

Pathophysiology

1. Bacterial diarrheas due to exotoxins: Certain bacterial species elaborate exotoxins (enterotoxins) that impair intestinal absorption and can provoke secretion of electrolytes and water. In some instances (e.g., the enterotoxin of *Vibrio cholerae*), a chemically pure toxin has been characterized; pure toxin alone will produce the voluminous watery secretion from the small intestine seen clinically, thereby demonstrating an adequate pathogenic mechanism for the diarrhea. Enterotoxins probably explain other diarrhea syndromes previously attributed to nonspecific causes (e.g., *Escherichia coli* enterotoxin may cause some outbreaks of "nursery diarrhea" and "traveler's diarrhea").

2. Bacterial diarrheas due to mucosal invasion or ulceration: Some *Shigella*, *Salmonella*, and *E. coli* species penetrate the mucosa of the small bowel or colon and produce microscopic ulceration, bleeding, exudation of protein-rich fluid, and secretion of electrolytes and water. The invasive process and its results may occur whether or not the organism elaborates an enterotoxin.

Campylobacter infections are increasingly being recognized as a cause of gastroenteritis (see *Campylobacter fetus* INFECTIONS in Ch. 8).

3. Incompletely categorized gastroenteritis syndromes: This entity includes "intestinal flu" or "grippe" and some types of "traveler's diarrhea" (e.g., "turista"). Bacterial enterotoxins are the cause in some cases; viral infections in others.

Experiments with the "Norwalk agent" (a virus that causes transient symptoms in man) and with viruses isolated from the intestines of children with diarrhea have shown that both can cause jejunal mucosal damage and that electrolyte and fluid secretion occurs in infected animals. The incubation periods and self-limited courses of these experimental viral diseases suggest a similar pathogenesis for "intestinal flu."

4. Nonbacterial food poisonings: Gastroenteritis may follow ingestion of chemical toxins contained in plants (e.g., mushrooms, potatoes, garden flora), seafood (fish, clams, mussels), or contaminated food.

5. Miscellaneous causes: An inability to digest and absorb carbohydrate (e.g., lactose intolerance) may cause abdominal symptoms, possibly following milk ingestion and erroneously attributed to milk allergy (see CARBOHYDRATE INTOLERANCE in Ch. 56). True food allergy is rare and poorly understood. Heavy-metal (arsenic, lead, mercury, cadmium) ingestion may cause acute nausea, vomiting, and diarrhea. Many therapeutic agents, including broad-spectrum antibiotics, have major GI side effects.

General Symptoms and Signs

The character and severity of symptoms depend on the nature and dose of the irritant, the duration of its action, the resistance of the patient, and the extent of GI involvement. Onset is often sudden and sometimes dramatic, with anorexia, nausea, or vomiting; borborygmi; abdominal cramps; and diarrhea, with or without blood and mucus. Associated malaise, muscular aches, and prostration may occur.

Persistent vomiting and diarrhea result in severe dehydration and shock, with vascular collapse and oliguric renal failure. If vomiting causes excessive fluid loss, metabolic alkalosis with hypochloremia occurs; if diarrhea is more prominent, acidosis is more likely. Hypokalemia may result from either excessive vomiting or diarrhea. Hyponatremia may develop, particularly if nonelectrolyte fluids are used in replacement therapy. Severe dehydration and acid-base imbalance can produce headache and symptoms of muscular and nervous irritability.

The abdomen may be distended and tender; in severe cases, muscle guarding may be present. Gas-distended intestinal loops may be visible and palpable. Borborygmi are audible with the stethoscope, even without diarrhea (an important differential feature from paralytic ileus). The BP may be reduced, the pulse rapid, and the temperature elevated. Signs of extracellular fluid depletion (see in REGULATION OF WATER AND SODIUM HOMEOSTASIS in Ch. 81) may be present.

Diagnosis

A history of food allergy or intolerance, ingestion of potentially contaminated food or a known GI irritant, and recent travel habits may be important. An elevated total WBC count is of little diagnostic significance, but eosinophilia suggests allergy or parasitic infection. Stool examination and culture are indicated unless symptoms subside within 48 h. Sigmoidoscopy helps diagnose ulcerative colitis and amebic dysentery, though shigellosis may produce colonic lesions indistinguishable from those of ulcerative colitis. These and other differential diagnoses may require culture of food, vomitus, feces, urine, and blood; specific agglutination tests (positive after about 1 wk) may also be helpful.

The acute "surgical abdomen" is usually excluded by the history of frequent stools, a low WBC count, and the absence of muscle spasm and localized tenderness. However, diarrhea may occur at times in acute appendicitis, incomplete small bowel obstruction, other acute intra-abdominal emergencies, and colonic malignancy.

General Principles of Treatment

Supportive treatment is most important. Bed rest with convenient access to a bathroom, commode, or bedpan is desirable. When nausea or vomiting is mild or ended, fluids such as warm sweetened tea, "soda pop," oral glucose-electrolyte solutions (see DIARRHEA in Ch. 54), strained broth, cereal, gruel, or bouillon with added salt are taken. Nothing is taken by mouth while vomiting is present. If vomiting persists or dehydration is prominent, IV infusions of 5% dextrose are necessary, together with appropriate electrolyte replacements. The most dramatic example and a full discussion of the role of fluid therapy in gastroenteritis is in acute cholera (see CHOLERA in Ch. 8). Similar principles apply in other instances. Blood or a plasma expander is indicated in severe cases when shock occurs.

Vomiting can usually be helped by sedation with phenobarbital sodium 30 to 100 mg s.c. t.i.d. or q.i.d., alone or with scopolamine 0.5 mg s.c. Injections of an antiemetic (e.g., dimenhydrinate 50 mg IM q 4 h, or chlorpromazine 25 to 100 mg or more/day IM) or a prochlorperazine suppository (25 mg b.i.d.) may be beneficial. Meperidine 50 mg IM q 4 or 6 h if necessary, or an antispasmodic (e.g., propantheline 5 to 10 mg IM q 6 h) may be given for severe abdominal cramps. Morphine is best avoided because it increases intestinal muscle tone and may aggravate vomiting.

When the patient tolerates warm fluids, the diet gradually includes cooked bland cereals, gelatin, jellied consommé, simple puddings, soft-cooked eggs, and other bland foods. If after 12 to 24 h, moderate diarrhea persists in the absence of severe systemic symptoms, diphenoxylate 2.5 to 5 mg in tablet or liquid form t.i.d. or q.i.d., paregoric 5 ml orally q 4 h, codeine 15 to 30 mg orally t.i.d. or q.i.d., or a preparation containing bismuth, belladonna, and kaolin may be given.

Antibiotic therapy: The role of antibiotics is disputed, even for specific infectious diarrheas, but most authorities recommend treating symptomatic shigellosis. Antibiotics appropriate to sensitivity testing should be given when evidence shows systemic infection. However, antibiotics help neither those patients with simple gastroenteritis nor asymptomatic carriers to "clear" rapidly. In fact, antibiotics appear to favor and prolong the salmonellosis carrier state. Emergence of drug-resistant organisms may be related to indiscriminate use of antibiotics, which should be discouraged.

GASTROENTERITIS DUE TO BACTERIAL ENTEROTOXINS

CHOLERA AND NONCHOLERA VIBRIO DISEASE

(See CHOLERA and *Campylobacter fetus* AND VIBRIO INFECTIONS in Ch. 8)

NURSERY DIARRHEA DUE TO ESCHERICHIA COLI

(See under NEONATAL INFECTIONS in Vol. II, Ch. 21)

STAPHYLOCOCCAL FOOD POISONING

An acute syndrome of vomiting and diarrhea caused by the ingestion of food contaminated by Staphylococcus enterotoxin.

Etiology and Pathophysiology

Staphylococcus enterotoxin rather than the organism per se is one of the most common causes of food poisoning. The potential for outbreaks is high when food handlers with skin infections contaminate foods left at room temperature. Custards, cream-filled pastry, milk, processed meat, and fish provide media where coagulase-positive staphylococci grow and produce enterotoxin. There is no mucosal ulceration.

Symptoms and Signs

The incubation period is 2 to 8 h after ingesting food containing the toxin. Onset is usually abrupt, characteristically with severe nausea and vomiting. Other symptoms may include abdominal cramps, diarrhea, and occasionally headache and fever. Acid-base imbalance, prostration, and shock may ensue in severe cases. Stools occasionally contain blood and mucus. The attack is brief, most often lasting only 3 to 6 h, and recovery is usually complete. Rarely, fatalities occur, especially among the very young, the elderly, or those with chronic illness, as a result of fluid and metabolic stresses.

Diagnosis

Diagnosis hinges on recognizing the clinical syndrome described above. Usually, a number of persons are similarly affected, constituting a "point source" outbreak. Diagnostic confirmation requires isolating coagulase-positive staphylococci from the suspected food.

The syndrome should be distinguished from staphylococcal pseudomembranous enterocolitis arising from staphylococcal superinfection after oral administration of antibiotics (see Ch. 58).

Treatment

Treatment is supportive, as described above under General Principles of Treatment. Rapid replacement of fluid and electrolyte losses by IV infusion often brings dramatic relief.

BOTULISM

Neuromuscular poisoning from Clostridium botulinum *toxin.* Botulism occurs in 3 forms: foodborne, wound, and infant botulism.

Etiology and Pathophysiology

Seven types of antigenically distinct toxins are elaborated by the sporulating, anaerobic grampositive bacillus *C. botulinum.* Human poisoning is usually caused by Type A, B, E, or F toxin. Type A and B toxins are highly poisonous proteins resistant to digestion by GI enzymes. In foodborne botulism, toxin produced in contaminated food is ingested; but in wound and infant botulism, neurotoxin is elaborated in vivo by the growth of *C. botulinum* in infected tissue and in the GI tract, respectively. After absorption, the toxins interfere with the release of acetylcholine at peripheral nerve endings.

C. botulinum spores are highly heat-resistant; they may survive several hours at 100 C (212 F); however, exposure to moist heat at 120 C (248 F) for 30 min will kill the spores. The toxins, on the other hand, are readily destroyed by heat, and cooking food at 80 C (176 F) for 30 min safeguards against botulism. Toxin production (especially type E) can occur at temperatures as low as 3 C (37.4 F) and does not require strict anaerobic conditions. Between 1970 and 1977 in the USA, foodborne outbreaks were caused most often by type A toxin (51%), followed by type B (21%) and type E (12%); in 16% the toxin type was not identified. Type F outbreaks are very rare. Home-canned foods are the most common sources, but commercially prepared foods have been identified in about 10% of outbreaks. Vegetables, fish, fruits, and condiments are the most common vehicles, but beef, milk products, pork, poultry, and other foods have been involved. In outbreaks caused by marine products, type E accounted for about half, with types A and B causing the remainder.

Botulinus toxin types are distinctively distributed in the USA: Type A is seen predominantly west of the Mississippi River, type B in the Eastern states, and type E in Alaska and the Great Lakes area.

Symptoms and Signs

In foodborne botulism, onset is abrupt, usually 18 to 36 h after ingestion of the toxin, though the incubation period may vary from 4 h to 8 days. Neurologic symptoms are characteristically bilateral and symmetrical, beginning with the cranial nerves and following with descending weakness or paralysis. Common initial symptoms include dry mouth, diplopia, diminished acuity, blepharoptosis, loss of accommodation, and diminished or total loss of pupillary light reflex. Nausea, vomiting, abdominal cramps, and diarrhea frequently precede neurologic symptoms. Symptoms of bulbar paresis (dysarthria, dysphagia, nasal regurgitation) develop. Dysphagia can lead to aspiration pneumonia. The muscles of the extremities and trunk become weak. There are no sensory disturbances and the sensorium usually remains clear until shortly before death. Fever is absent and the pulse remains normal or slow unless intercurrent infection develops. Routine studies of the blood, urine, and CSF are usually normal. Constipation is frequent after neurologic impairment appears. **Major complications** include respiratory failure and pulmonary infections.

Wound botulism is manifested by the same symptoms of neurologic involvement as is seen in foodborne botulism, but there are no GI symptoms or epidemiologic evidence implicating food as a cause. Careful search should be made for breaks in the patient's skin.

Infant botulism, seen most frequently in infants 2 to 3 mo old, results from the ingestion of botulinal spores and their colonization in the GI tract and toxin production in vivo; unlike foodborne botulism, infant botulism is *not* caused by ingestion of preformed toxin. Constipation is present initially in 2/3 of cases and is followed by neuromuscular paralysis that begins with the cranial nerves and proceeds to peripheral and respiratory musculature. Cranial nerve deficits may be asymmetric and a spectrum based on severity may show variation from mild lethargy and slowed feeding to severe hypotonia and respiratory insufficiency. Affected infants have characteristically been normal before the onset of illness and have been either breast- or formula-fed. However, they have generally been exposed to foods other than milk, and spores are common in the environment. Cases have been related to the ingestion of honey, vacuum cleaner dust, and soil containing *C. botulinum.*

Diagnosis

The pattern of neuromuscular disturbances suggests the diagnosis of an isolated case; a likely food source provides an important clue. The simultaneous occurrence of 2 or more cases following ingestion of the same food simplifies the diagnosis. It is confirmed by demonstrating botulinus toxin in the serum or feces of the patient or by isolating the organism from feces. Finding *C. botulinum* **toxin** in suspect food identifies the source. Pets may develop botulism from eating the same contaminated food. Botulism may be confused with the Guillain-Barré syndrome, poliomyelitis, stroke, myasthenia gravis, tick paralysis, and poisoning due to curare or belladonna alkaloids.

In infant botulism, sepsis, congenital muscular dystrophy, hypothyroidism, and benign congenital hypotonia are additional considerations. Finding *C. botulinum* toxin or organisms in the feces establishes the diagnosis.

Special Precautions

Since even minute amounts of botulinus toxin acquired by ingestion, inhalation, or absorption through the eye or a break in the skin can cause serious illness, all materials suspected of containing toxin require special handling. Only experienced personnel, preferably immunized with botulinum toxoid should perform laboratory tests. Specimens should be placed in unbreakable, sterile, leak-proof containers, refrigerated (preferably not frozen), and examined as soon as possible. Wound specimens are an exception and should not be refrigerated. Further details regarding specimen collection and handling can be obtained from the Center for Disease Control, Atlanta, Georgia 30333.

Prophylaxis and Treatment

Proper home and commercial canning and adequate heating of food before serving are essential (see Etiology and Pathophysiology, above). Food showing any evidence of spoilage should be discarded. Infants < 1 yr of age should not be fed honey. Toxoids can be prepared for active immunization of persons working with *C. botulinum* or its toxins. Anyone known or thought to have been exposed to food contaminated with botulinus toxin must be carefully observed. Induction of vomiting, gastric lavage, and purgation in order to eliminate unabsorbed toxin is recommended.

The greatest threat to life is from respiratory impairment and its complications. All patients should be hospitalized and closely supervised; e.g., with serial measurements of vital capacity. Respiratory impairment requries management in an intensive care unit where intubation, tracheostomy, and the use of mechanical ventilators are readily available (see Ch. 32). IV alimentation may be required. Improvements in such supportive care have reduced mortality to < 10%.

Trivalent antitoxin (A, B, E) is available from the Center for Disease Control, which also stores a polyvalent antitoxin (A, B, C, D, E, F) for specific outbreaks due to C, D, or F botulism. Antitoxin should be given as soon as possible after the diagnosis of botulism has been made. The risks must be weighed against the potential benefits. It may, however, be beneficial even if given as late as several weeks after toxin ingestion, since circulating toxin has been detected in serum as late as 30 days after such ingestion. Antitoxin will not reverse the binding of already bound toxin and therefore will not reverse preexisting neurologic impairment; at best it will slow or halt further progression of the disease. Since these are horse serum antitoxins, there is a risk of anaphylaxis or serum sickness. For precautions in the use of horse serum antitoxin, see SERUM SICKNESS under DRUG HYPERSENSITIVITY and for treatment of reactions, see ANAPHYLAXIS under ATOPIC DISEASES, both in Ch. 19. The use of antitoxin in **infant botulism** has not been adequately studied, and at present is not generally recommended.

Guanidine is thought to increase acetylcholine release from terminal nerve endings and is advocated by some to treat patients with botulism. Reported results have been conflicting and the effectiveness of guanidine therapy for botulism remains unproven.

Clostridium perfringens FOOD POISONING

Acute gastroenteritis due to ingestion of an enterotoxin contained in food contaminated by C. perfringens.

Etiology

C. perfringens is widely distributed in feces, soil, air, and water. Contaminated meat has caused many outbreaks. The organisms form spores and generate a variably potent enterotoxin. The toxin produced by Type A strains causes a mild to moderate, self-limiting disease; that produced by Type C strains causes a severe, often fatal gastroenteritis. Some toxins are resistant and some are sensitive to heat of up to 100 C (212 F) for 1 h.

Symptoms, Signs, and Diagnosis

A mild gastroenteritis is most common, though a potentially fatal syndrome with severe diarrhea and abdominal pain, abdominal distention with gas, and collapse may occur. Diagnosis is based on epidemiologic evidence and the isolation of organisms from contaminated food.

Treatment

For supportive measures, see General Principles of Treatment at the beginning of this chapter. Penicillin (1 million u./day) may be helpful in severe cases. Necrosis of the small bowel may require surgical resection of the affected intestine.

SALMONELLOSIS (See SALMONELLA INFECTIONS in Ch. 8)

GASTROENTERITIS DUE TO INVASIVE ORGANISMS

These syndromes are largely due to *Shigella* infection (see SHIGELLOSIS in Ch. 8). Some types of enteropathogenic *E. coli* enteritis and salmonellosis may also be associated with mucosal invasion.

Certain intestinal parasites, notably *Giardia lamblia* (see GIARDIASIS in Ch. 13), invade the jejunal mucosa and cause nausea, vomiting, diarrhea, and general malaise. Giardiasis is endemic in some Alpine areas and in northern Russia. Large outbreaks have occurred in travelers. The disease can become chronic and can cause malabsorption syndrome (see Ch. 56).

GASTROENTERITIS OF UNCERTAIN ETIOLOGY

("Travelers Diarrhea"; "Intestinal Flu")

Sporadic cases of gastroenteritis in travelers ("turista") or of gastroenteritis affecting individuals or families ("intestinal flu," "grippe").

Etiology, Epidemiology, and Pathophysiology

Enteropathogenic *E. coli* and incompletely characterized enteric viruses (e.g., "Norwalk agent") are the most probable causes. Little is known of the epidemiology, though outbreaks may be sporadic or epidemic. The pathophysiology is uncertain, though enterotoxins and histologic alterations of the jejunal mucosa by viruses, with intestinal fluid secretion, have been suggested.

Symptoms, Signs, and Diagnosis

Nausea, vomiting, borborygmi, abdominal cramps, and diarrhea occur in highly variable combinations and degrees of severity. Most cases are mild and self-limited. The diagnosis is made clinically.

Prophylaxis and Treatment

Travelers should use restaurants with a reputation for safety and avoid foods from street vendors and school cafeterias. They should eat cooked foods, fruit that can be peeled, and drink bottled carbonated beverages; salads containing uncooked vegetables should be avoided. Bismuth subsalicylate suspensions are protective but must be taken in large doses (60 ml q.i.d.), which is inconvenient.

For supportive measures, see General Principles of Treatment, at the beginning of this chapter. Symptomatic treatment for diarrhea, and a bland diet are helpful. Iodochlorhydroxyquin *should not be used*, as it may cause neurologic damage. Travelers are advised to use common sense in eating and drinking. Antibiotics are **contraindicated**, as they may alter intestinal flora adversely and promote resistant organisms, but for severe cases trimethoprim/sulfamethoxazole is appropriate.

NONBACTERIAL FOOD POISONING

Poisoning due to ingestion of certain plants and animals containing a naturally occurring poison.

1. **Mushroom (toadstool) poisoning:** Two species of the *Amanita* genus are responsible for most cases. In **muscarine** poisoning due to *A. muscaria*, symptoms begin a few minutes to 2 h after ingestion. They consist of lacrimation, salivation, sweating, miosis, vomiting, abdominal cramps, diarrhea, vertigo, confusion, coma, and occasionally convulsions. Though patients may die in a few hours, complete recovery in 24 h is usual with appropriate therapy.

In **phalloidine** poisoning due to ingestion of *A. phalloides* and related species, symptoms occur after a 6- to 24-h interval. GI symptoms are similar to those of muscarine poisoning above, but oliguria and anuria may develop; jaundice due to liver damage is common and develops in 2 or 3 days. Remissions may occur, but eventual mortality is at least 50%, with death occurring in 5 to 8 days.

The potential for poisoning by mushrooms is unpredictable and may vary within the same species, at different times of the growing season, and with cooking. Alcohol ingestion may precipitate symptoms in some persons; disulfiram has been identified in some mushrooms.

2. Other poisonous plants: A large number of wild and domestic plants and shrubs contain poisonous substances in their leaves and fruit. Common examples include yew, morning glory, nightshade, castor bean, dieffenbachia (dumb cane), jequirity bean ("indian bean," "rosary pea"), tung nuts, horse chestnuts, and the bird-of-paradise flower (seeds or peapods). Fruit of the Koenig tree causes "vomiting sickness" of Jamaica. Green or sprouting tubers may contain solanine and produce acute nausea, vomiting, diarrhea, and prostration, usually of mild degree. Ingestion of fava beans by susceptible persons may precipitate acute hemolysis (favism). Ergot poisoning follows ingestion of grain contaminated with *Claviceps purpurea*, the ergot fungus. Specialized texts provide a full listing of recognized poisonous plants.

3. Fish poisoning: Most cases are caused by ingesting ichthyosarcotoxic fish; i.e., those that contain toxin in their musculature, viscera, skin, or mucus. The severity of attacks from ichthyosarcotoxism varies greatly and depends to some extent on the fish involved. Most important are the following: (1) **Ciguatera poisoning** can occur after eating any of $>$ 400 species of fish from the tropical reefs of Florida, the West Indies, or the Pacific where a dinoflagellate may supply a toxin that accumulates in the marine animal's flesh. Toxicity is greater in larger, older fish. Taste of the fish is not affected, and no known procedures of preparing the fish are protective. After abdominal cramps, nausea, vomiting, and diarrhea that lasts 6 to 17 h, pruritus, paresthesias, headache, myalgia, and face pain may occur. For months after, unusual sensory phenomena may keep a person from work; (2) **Tetraodon poisoning,** from the puffer fish, causes similar symptoms and signs; death may result from respiratory paralysis; (3) **Scombroid poisoning,** from the mackerel, tuna, bonito, or albacore, is due to bacterial decomposition after the fish is caught. The toxin is histamine-like and causes an immediate reaction with facial flushing as a characteristic symptom. It can also cause nausea, vomiting, epigastric pain, and urticaria within a few minutes of eating an affected fish. Symptoms usually last $<$ 24 h.

4. Paralytic shellfish poisoning: From June to October (especially on the Pacific and New England coasts), mussels, clams, oysters, and scallops may ingest a poisonous dinoflagellate ("red tide") which produces a neurotoxin that is not destroyed by cooking. The first symptoms appear 5 to 30 min after ingestion and consist of circumoral paresthesias. Nausea, vomiting, and abdominal cramps develop, followed by muscle weakness and peripheral paralysis. Respiratory failure may cause death.

Another shellfish poison, venerupin, was isolated in Japan following the ingestion of asari (*Venerupis semidecussata*) and oyster (*Ostrea gigas*). After a 24- to 48-h incubation period, GI symptoms, leukocytosis, retardation of blood coagulation, and liver function disturbances develop. Death occurs in about 1/3 of cases. The neurotropic effects of mussel poison are absent.

5. Contaminants: Chemical poisoning may follow ingestion of unwashed fruits and vegetables sprayed with arsenic, lead, or organic insecticides; acidic liquids served in lead-glazed pottery; or food stored in cadmium-lined containers. Symptoms are described in Ch. 258, under the chemical involved.

Treatment

General: Unless violent vomiting or diarrhea has occurred, or symptoms appeared several hours after the food was ingested, efforts should be made to remove the poison by gastric lavage. An emetic may be used. Apomorphine 5 mg s.c. is given only once. Alternatively, ipecac syrup 15 ml (1/2 oz) orally for children, up to 45 ml (1 1/2 oz) for adults, repeated once in 15 min if necessary, may be given, followed by about 200 ml of water. A saline cathartic (e.g., sodium sulfate 15 to 30 gm orally in water) may be required. If nausea and vomiting persist, fluids containing salts and dextrose should be given parenterally to combat dehydration and acid-base imbalance. Dextran, Normal Human Serum Albumin, or blood is indicated if shock threatens. Meperidine 50 to 100 mg IM q 4 to 6 h should be given for pain. Mechanical ventilation and intensive respiratory care may be required.

Specific: After eating an unidentified mushroom, the patient should be induced to vomit immediately; then identification of the mushroom species will aid further treatment. Atropine, 1 mg s.c. or IV q l to 2 h until symptoms are controlled, is a specific antagonist of parasympathetic overstimulation due to **muscarine** poisoning. In **phalloidine** poisoning, a high-carbohydrate diet (if tolerated) supplemented by IV administration of 10% dextrose and sodium chloride may help to combat the hypoglycemia of severe liver damage. In the treatment of **ergotism,** arterial spasm may be combated by amyl nitrite 0.3 ml by inhalation, nitroglycerin 0.4 mg sublingually, or papaverine 30 to 60 mg IM or IV. An anticonvulsive agent (e.g., sodium amobarbital 300 to 500 mg—more if required—slowly IV) should be used when indicated. Cholinesterase reactivators have been suggested as antidotes for **fish tox-ins.** For poisoning due to **food contamination** with arsenic, lead, cadmium, or organic insecticides, see Ch. 258.

MISCELLANEOUS CAUSES OF GASTROENTERITIS

DISACCHARIDASE DEFICIENCY AND GLUCOSE–GALACTOSE
MALABSORPTION (Alactasia) (See CARBOHYDRATE INTOLERANCE in Ch. 56)

FOOD ALLERGY (See GASTROINTESTINAL ALLERGY in Ch. 19)

ADVERSE EFFECTS OF DRUGS

Many therapeutic agents produce nausea, vomiting, and diarrhea as side effects. A detailed drug intake history must be obtained. In mild cases, cessation followed by reuse of the drug may establish a causal relationship. Commonly responsible agents include antacids containing magnesium as a major ingredient, antibiotics, anthelmintics, chemotherapeutic agents used in cancer therapy, colchicine, digitalis, heavy metals, laxatives, and radiation therapy. Specialized literature should also be consulted.

Iatrogenic, accidental, or intentional heavy-metal poisoning frequently produces nausea, vomiting, abdominal pain, and diarrhea.

Laxative abuse, sometimes denied by psychopathic individuals, may lead to weakness, vomiting, diarrhea, electrolyte depletion, and metabolic disturbances.

The **"Chinese-restaurant syndrome"** is a pharmacologic, not an allergic, phenomenon. The monosodium glutamate often used in Chinese food produces a dose-related syndrome of burning sensations throughout the body, facial pressure, and chest pain. The threshold dose varies considerably among individuals.

---

56. MALABSORPTION SYNDROMES

Syndromes resulting from impaired absorption of nutrients from the small bowel. Many different diseases or their consequences can cause malabsorption, either by means of impaired digestion or impaired absorption (see TABLE 56–1).

Clinical Presentation

Patients may present with 3 kinds of symptoms:

1. Symptoms directly attributable to malabsorption. These include diarrhea, abdominal distention, flatulence, abdominal bloating, and discomfort due to increased bulk of intestinal contents and gas production. Diarrhea is not always present. Sometimes steatorrhea occurs—pale, soft, bulky, malodorous stools that stick to the side of the toilet bowl or float and are difficult to flush away. This kind of stool is most likely to occur in celiac disease or tropical sprue. The stools in chronic pancreatic disease may appear greasy with free-floating globules of undigested dietary fat (triglyceride) because of pancreatic lipase deficiency. Steatorrhea can be present without florid abnormalities of the stool, and about 20% of patients may have no increase in fecal fat. Explosive diarrhea with abdominal bloating and gas after milk ingestion points to alactasia (lactase deficiency).

2. Symptoms due to deficiencies secondary to malabsorption. The range and severity of nutritional deficiencies relate to the severity of the primary disease and the area of the GI tract involved. Many patients with malabsorption are anemic, usually due to **deficiency of iron (microcytic anemia) and folic acid (megaloblastic anemia).** Vitamin B_{12} deficiency is uncommon, partly because body stores are considerable, and partly because few disorders cause B_{12} absorption to fall below the daily requirement. For pernicious anemia, see discussion of Vitamin B_{12} and Folic Acid Deficiencies in Ch. 92. B_{12} **deficiency** may occur in blind loop syndrome or many years after extensive resection of the distal small bowel. The usual 50-cm resection of the terminal ileum for ileocecal Crohn's disease seldom leads to significant B_{12} deficiency.

Calcium deficiency is common and is due partly to **vitamin D deficiency** with impaired absorption and partly to calcium binding with unabsorbed fatty acids. This may cause bone pain and tetany. Infantile rickets is rare but osteomalacia may occur in severe adult celiac disease. **Thiamine (vitamin B_1) deficiency** may cause paresthesia (so does B_{12} deficiency), and malabsorption of the mainly fat-soluble **vitamin K** can lead to hypoprothrombinemia with bruising and a bleeding tendency. Severe **riboflavin (vitamin B_2) deficiency** may cause a sore tongue and angular stomatitis, but **vitamin A, C, and niacin deficiencies** seldom cause clinical problems. **Protein malabsorption** may lead to hypo-

TABLE 56-1. DISEASE STATES ASSOCIATED WITH MALABSORPTION

	In the Presence of This Condition
Impaired digestion results from:	
Inadequate mixing	Gastroenterostomy Billroth II gastrectomy Gastrocolic fistula
Insufficient digestive agents	Chronic pancreatitis Cystic fibrosis Chronic liver failure Biliary obstruction Alactasia Sucrase-isomaltase deficiency
Improper milieu	Zollinger-Ellison syndrome (low duodenal pH) Bacterial overgrowth-blind loops (deconjugation of bile salts) Diverticula
Impaired absorption results from:	
Acute abnormal epithelium	Acute intestinal infections Neomycin Alcohol
Chronic abnormal epithelium	Celiac disease Tropical sprue Whipple's disease Amyloid Ischemia Crohn's disease
Short bowel	Intestinal resection for Crohn's disease Volvulus Intussusception Infarction
Impaired transport	Blocked lacteals—lymphoma Lymphangiectasia Addison's disease—? transport enzymes ? Abetalipoproteinemia

proteinemic edema, usually of the lower limbs. Dehydration, potassium loss, and muscle weakness can follow profuse diarrhea.

Secondary endocrine deficiencies may occur, and amenorrhea (primary or secondary) is an important presentation of celiac disease in young girls. Weight loss, an obvious consequence of malabsorption, is nonspecific. *Any combination of weight loss, diarrhea, and anemia should raise the suspicion of malabsorption.*

3. **Symptoms due to the disease which causes malabsorption.** Some diseases that cause malabsorption have distinctly different clinical presentations; e.g., the jaundice of biliary cirrhosis and pancreatic carcinoma; the abdominal angina of mesenteric ischemia; the boring central abdominal pain of chronic pancreatitis; and the severe, persistent ulcer dyspepsia of the Zollinger-Ellison syndrome.

Signs of malabsorption are weight loss, anemia, abdominal distention, hypoproteinemic edema, glossitis, stomatitis, carpopedal spasms, absent tendon reflexes, and cutaneous bruising. Dermatitis herpetiformis strongly points to a mild degree of celiac-like enteropathy.

Diagnostic Studies

Examination of the stool: Fecal fat excretion. Steatorrhea (flow of tallow), or excess stool fat, is absolute evidence of malabsorption when it is present. The measurement of fecal fat is the most reliable single test for establishing malabsorption. For an adult eating a normal diet with a daily fat intake of 50 to 150 gm, a fecal fat loss of 17 mEq or more/day is abnormal. Accuracy of stool collections during a period of typical daily routine is more important than strict balance studies. It is feasible and advantageous to perform fecal fat studies on ambulant outpatients. A 4-day collection is usually adequate. There is no completely satisfactory alternative to the direct measurement of fecal fat.

Inspection and microscopic examination of the stools are both of value. The typical stool appearances described above are unmistakable. The presence of fragments of undigested food suggests either extreme hypermotility or intestinal short circuits, such as gastrocolic fistula. Greasy stools from a jaundiced patient point to pancreatic cancer or primary biliary cirrhosis. Microscopic examination showing fat globules and undigested meat fiber suggests pancreatic insufficiency. Microscopy permits identification of ova or parasites.

Absorption tests: The oral glucose test is seldom used, since a significant proportion of normal subjects shows a flat absorption curve.

D-**Xylose absorption:** The D-xylose test is an indirect but relatively specific measure of proximal small bowel absorption. It is nearly always abnormal in primary jejunal disease, but rarely in other causes of malabsorption. D-Xylose 5 gm is given orally to the fasting patient, and urine is collected for the next 5 h. This dose is slightly less sensitive than a larger (25-gm) dose, but it does not cause nausea or diarrhea. Provided urine output is adequate and the GFR is normal, the test is unequivocally abnormal if < 1.2 gm of xylose is present in the 5-h collection. Values between 1.2 to 1.4 gm are borderline. The test is popular in pediatric practice, but because collecting complete urine samples in young children is difficult, some investigators prefer blood levels. However, the overlap between normal and abnormal levels is considerable unless the dose is calculated as 0.5 gm/kg, and even then the urinary level is more reliable.

Lactose absorption: See CARBOHYDRATE INTOLERANCE, below.

Iron absorption: Malabsorption of dietary iron can usually be inferred if a patient whose diet is adequate, and who has no chronic blood loss or thalassemia, has an iron deficiency state, indicated by low serum iron levels and diminished iron storage noted on bone marrow evaluation. It occurs mainly in celiac disease and postgastrectomy patients.

Folic acid absorption: Malabsorption of dietary folate can usually be inferred if a patient eating an adequate diet and not consuming excessive amounts of alcohol has a low serum and/or red cell folate level. Folate malabsorption occurs mainly in celiac disease and tropical sprue.

Vitamin B$_{12}$ absorption: The Schilling test can be used to evaluate malabsorption. Reduced urinary excretion ($< 5\%$) of radiolabeled B$_{12}$ indicates malabsorption of B$_{12}$, and when excretion is corrected to normal ($> 9\%$) with intrinsic factor bound radiolabeled B$_{12}$, the malabsorption is due to loss of gastric intrinsic factor activity (often true pernicious anemia). When intrinsic factor bound B$_{12}$ is not adequately absorbed, chronic pancreatitis, drugs, or small bowel disease (blind loops, jejunal diverticuli, or ileal disease) must be suspected.

^{14}**C-labeled glycocholic acid breath test:** Bile salts are deconjugated by intestinal bacteria. This occurs abnormally in small bowel disorders that cause stasis and bacterial overgrowth; e.g., blind loops, diverticula, and scleroderma. Excessive bile salt deconjugation can be demonstrated by the oral administration of ^{14}C-labeled glycocholic acid. If bacterial growth is excessive, ^{14}C-labeled glycine is split off, absorbed, and metabolized, and the labeled carbon is measured as breath $^{14}CO_2$. The test has limited usefulness.

Radiology: X-ray appearances may be nonspecific or diagnostic. An upper GI follow-through examination of the small bowel may show dilation of bowel loops, thickening of mucosal folds, and coarse fragmentation of the barium column, but these appearances only suggest malabsorption. On the other hand, radiology may show pancreatic calcification—a sign of chronic pancreatitis—fistulas, blind loops, or various inter-enteric anastomoses; jejunal diverticulosis; superior mesenteric artery occlusion; and mucosal patterns suggestive of intestinal lymphoma, scleroderma, or Crohn's disease.

Small bowel biopsy (see TABLE 56-2): Jejunal biopsy is a routine procedure; some modification of the Crosby capsule or the Rubin tube is used. Samples of jejunal juice can be taken at the same time for microbiologic testing of the intestinal flora. The mucosal sample can be examined grossly by hand lens or dissecting microscope and by light or electron microscopy, and tissue homogenates can be assayed for enzyme activity. The abnormalities demonstrated by these technics may be specific or nonspecific. Specific diagnoses include Whipple's disease, lymphosarcoma, intestinal lymphangiectasia, and giardiasis (in which the trophozoite may be seen in close association with the villus surface). Jejunal histology is also abnormal in celiac disease, tropical sprue, and dermatitis herpetiformis. The changes may be severe (subtotal villus atrophy), moderate (partial villus atrophy), or mild.

Pancreatic function: Two kinds of pancreatic function tests are currently in use, both of which require duodenal intubation: (1) In the Lundh test pancreatic secretion is *indirectly* stimulated by the oral intake of a formula diet, and lipase levels are measured in the duodenal aspirate; (2) pancreatic secretion is *directly* stimulated by injecting secretin IV, and the bicarbonate content of the duodenal aspirate is measured; average normal hourly secretion is about 15 mM in men and 12 mM in women. A double-lumen tube (Dreiling tube) is required that takes some experience to pass and position. Its main advantage is to permit sampling of "pure" pancreatic secretion, used also for cytologic examination.

Miscellaneous investigations: Special tests may be needed to diagnose less common causes of malabsorption; e.g., serum gastrin levels and gastric acid secretion in the Zollinger-Ellison syndrome, sweat chloride in cystic fibrosis, lipoprotein electrophoresis in abetalipoproteinemia, plasma cortisol in Addison's disease.

TABLE 56-2. JEJUNAL HISTOLOGY IN CERTAIN MALABSORPTIVE DISORDERS

Condition	Morphologic Characteristics
Normal	Finger-like villi with a villous-crypt ratio of about 4:1; columnar epithelial cells with numerous regular microvilli (brush border); mild round cell infiltration in the lamina propria
Untreated celiac disease	Virtual absence of villi and elongated crypts; increased round cells (especially plasma cells) in the lamina propria; cuboidal epithelial cells with scanty, irregular microvilli
Tropical sprue	*Mild* (minimal changes in villus height; moderate epithelial cell damage) *Severe* (similar to untreated celiac disease except lymphocytes predominate in the lamina propria)
Whipple's disease	Lamina propria densely infiltrated with periodic acid–Schiff-positive macrophages; villus structure may be obliterated in severe lesions
Intestinal lymphangiectasia	Dilation and telangiectasia of the intramucosal lymphatics

CELIAC DISEASE
(Nontropical Sprue; Gluten Enteropathy; Celiac Sprue)

A chronic intestinal malabsorption disorder caused by intolerance to gluten, characterized by a flat jejunal mucosa with clinical and/or histologic improvement following withdrawal of dietary gluten.

Etiology and Prevalence
This hereditary congenital disorder is caused by sensitivity to the gliadin fraction of gluten, a cereal protein found in wheat and rye, and to a lesser degree in barley and oats. Gliadin, acting as antigen, combines with antibodies to form an immune complex in the intestinal mucosa that promotes the aggregation of K (killer) lymphocytes. In some way these lymphocytes cause mucosal damage with loss of villi and proliferation of crypt cells. The prevalence of celiac disease varies from about 1:300 in Southwest Ireland to 1:5000 or more in North America. There is no single genetic marker for the condition.

Symptoms and Signs
Celiac disease may be symptomatic or asymptomatic. Family studies show that typical mucosal abnormalities appear in apparently healthy siblings of affected patients. The disease may present for the first time in infancy or adulthood, but it should not be assumed that an adult presentation is the first manifestation. Although the patient may have no knowledge of childhood disease, his mother may recall abdominal symptoms. If the adult patient is significantly smaller than his siblings, and has evidence of mild bowing deformities of the long bones, the likelihood of latent or undiagnosed childhood disease is increased.

In **infancy,** symptoms do not appear until the child eats food containing gluten. The child fails to thrive, begins to pass pale, malodorous, bulky stools, and suffers painful abdominal bloating. Iron deficiency anemia develops and, if hypoproteinemia is severe enough, edema appears. Celiac disease is strongly suspected in a pale, querulous child, with wasted buttocks and a pot belly, who has an adequate diet (thus ruling out protein-calorie malnutrition or kwashiorkor).

In **adults,** celiac disease is usually diagnosed when malabsorption is found in conjunction with a flat jejunal biopsy not due to some recognizable cause (e.g., tropical sprue, neomycin intake) and gluten is shown to be of etiologic significance. Family incidence is sometimes a valuable clue. It may present, apparently for the first time, up to the 6th decade. The average age of presentation in women is 10 to 15 yr earlier, because anemia in pregnancy and amenorrhea in young women may heighten clinical suspicion.

There is no single typical presentation. Many symptoms, such as anemia, weight loss, bone pain paresthesia, edema, and skin disorders, are secondary to deficiency states. If overt alimentary symptoms such as diarrhea, abdominal discomfort, and distention also occur, the real diagnosis is unlikely to be missed. Without these direct clues malabsorption may not be suspected.

Laboratory Findings
There tends to be iron deficiency anemia in children and folate deficiency anemia in adults. Depending on severity and duration, there can be any combination of low albumin, calcium, potassium and sodium, and elevated alkaline phosphatase and prothrombin time. The 5 gm D-xylose test (see

Diagnostic Studies, above) will usually be abnormal, and most patients will have steatorrhea that can range from mild to massive (20 to 150 mEq fatty acid/day).

In the immune protein system, levels of C_3 and C_4 are low in the untreated patient and rise with gluten withdrawal. The serum C_3 level is a possible screening test for celiac disease. The serum IgA level is usually normal or increased in untreated patients, and in $1/3$ to $1/2$, the IgM level is reduced.

Diagnosis

Diagnosis is suspected on the basis of the symptoms and signs, enhanced by the laboratory studies, and confirmed by biopsy showing a flat mucosa and clinical and histologic improvement on a gluten-free diet. Jejunal biopsy can be performed even in small infants, but to obviate the risk of bowel perforation, only an experienced investigator should do the test. If a biopsy cannot be done, the diagnosis may have to depend on the clinical and laboratory response (including xylose absorption) to a gluten-free diet.

Prognosis and Natural History

While gluten withdrawal has transformed the prognosis for celiac children and substantially improved it for adults, there is still some mortality from the disease, mainly among adults whose condition is severe from the beginning. An important cause of death is the development of lymphoreticular disease (especially intestinal lymphosarcoma). It is not known yet whether this risk is diminished by scrupulous adherence to a gluten-free diet. Some patients can tolerate the reintroduction of gluten into the diet. It is not certain whether this means that some mild cases can achieve complete remission (unlikely) or whether the gluten toxicity is a nonspecific effect on a mucosa previously damaged by an acute bacterial or viral enteritis. In any case, apparent clinical remission is often associated with histologic relapse that is only detected if review biopsies are performed.

Treatment

Dietary gluten must be excluded, as ingesting even small amounts may prevent remission or induce relapse. Gluten is so widely used in commercial soups, sauces, ice creams, hot dogs, and many other foods that patients need detailed lists of food-stuffs to avoid and expert advice from a dietitian familiar with the problems of celiac disease.

Supplementary vitamins, minerals, and hematinics may be given depending on the degree of deficiency. In mild cases no supplementation may be necessary. In severe cases comprehensive replacement may be required. For adults this includes ferrous sulfate 300 mg/day, folic acid 5 to 10 mg/day, calcium gluconate 5 to 10 gm/day, and any standard multivitamin preparation, all orally. Only if the prothrombin time is abnormal should vitamin K 10 mg IM be given. Proportional pediatric doses are given to children. Sometimes children, and rarely adults, who are seriously ill on first diagnosis may require a period of IV feeding. This should be carried out in accordance with the general principles of total parenteral nutrition (see PARENTERAL NUTRITION in Ch. 76).

A few patients respond poorly or not at all to gluten withdrawal, either because the diagnosis is incorrect or because the disease has entered a refractory phase. In the latter case, a response may be induced by a period of treatment with oral steroids, such as prednisone 10 to 20 mg b.i.d.

TROPICAL SPRUE

A disease of unknown etiology characterized by malabsorption, multiple nutritional deficiencies, and abnormalities in the small bowel mucosa.

Etiology and Incidence

Tropical sprue is an acquired disease related in some way to environmental and nutritional conditions. It occurs chiefly in the Caribbean, south India, and southeast Asia, affecting both the indigenous population and incomers. Some suggested causes are infection (bacterial or viral), parasitic infestation, vitamin deficiency (especially folic acid), or food toxin, such as might occur in rancid fats.

Symptoms, Signs, and Laboratory Findings

A common presentation is the triad of sore tongue, diarrhea, and weight loss. All features of the malabsorption syndrome (see above) may develop. Steatorrhea is common and D-xylose absorption is abnormal in > 90% of cases. Deficiencies of albumin, calcium, prothrombin, folic acid, vitamin B_{12}, and iron may occur. There is a megaloblastic anemia due to folic acid and vitamin B_{12} deficiency. Small bowel radiology shows the nonspecific changes of malabsorption—flocculation and segmentation of the barium column, with dilation of the lumen and thickening of the mucosal folds.

Diagnosis

The diagnosis should be suspected in an individual who has lived in an endemic area and who has megaloblastic anemia and symptoms and signs of the malabsorption syndrome. Celiac disease must be ruled out. Jejunal biopsy shows a varying degree of broadening and shortening of the villi and lengthening of the crypts with changes in the surface epithelium and an inflammatory cell infiltrate of lymphocytes, plasma cells, and eosinophils. In some patients changes may be minimal or absent, while in others there is subtotal villus atrophy. Biopsies must be compared with normal tissue from individuals in the same geographic region. What is a "mild" abnormality in the intestinal mucosa of

Europeans and North Americans is "normal" in areas of India, Africa, and southeast Asia. It is not yet clear whether this difference is racial or genetic, or whether it is due to environmental factors, e.g., chronic infection or infestation.

Treatment

The best treatment is folic acid (10 mg/day) and tetracycline or oxytetracycline (250 mg q.i.d.) for 1 or 2 mo, and then in half dosage for up to 6 mo, depending on the severity of the disease and the response to treatment. Other replacements are given as necessary. The condition should be reviewed histologically before stopping treatment.

WHIPPLE'S DISEASE

(Intestinal Lipodystrophy)

An uncommon illness occurring predominantly in males aged 30 to 60, characterized clinically by anemia, skin pigmentation, joint symptoms (arthralgia and arthritis), weight loss, diarrhea, and severe malabsorption. Though this systemic disorder affects many organs (e.g., heart, lung, brain serous cavities, joints, eye, GI tract), the small intestinal mucosa is always severely involved and the lesions observed in mucosal biopsies are specific and diagnostic.

Symptoms, Signs, and Diagnosis

The typical presentation is malabsorption in an adult male with additional features of polyarthritis, lymphadenopathy, and abnormal pigmentation. Abdominal pain is common. Cough and pleuritic pain may be accompanied by hilar adenopathy and pleural effusion. Symptoms of cardiac, hepatic and neuropsychiatric disease may also be present. Untreated, the disease is progressive and fatal Lymph node or intestinal biopsy establishes the diagnosis by showing foamy macrophages containing a glycoprotein that stains with the periodic acid-Schiff (PAS) reagent. Jejunal tissue may be otherwise normal or show clubbing of the villi, dilated lymphatics, or even partial villus atrophy Electron microscopy shows the PAS-positive material to be masses of rod-shaped bacilli.

Treatment

Many different types of antibiotics have been curative; e.g., chloramphenicol, tetracycline, chlortetracycline, sulfasalazine, ampicillin, and penicillin. One recommended regimen is procaine penicillin G 1,200,000 u. and streptomycin 1 gm daily for 10 to 14 days followed by tetracycline 250 mg orally q.i.d. for 10 to 12 mo. The streptomycin is often omitted. Clinical improvement occurs rapidly but histologic recovery may take up to 2 yr.

INTESTINAL LYMPHANGIECTASIA

(Idiopathic Hypoproteinemia)

A syndrome affecting children and young adults, characterized by telangiectasia of the intramucosal lymphatics of the small intestine. A congenital malformation of the lymphatics is most likely when onset occurs at birth. In acquired cases the defect may be secondary to retroperitoneal fibrosis or pancreatitis.

Symptoms, Signs, and Diagnosis

Early manifestations include massive, often asymmetric edema, and mild intermittent diarrhea with nausea, vomiting, and abdominal pain. Chylous effusions and ascites may be present. Lymphocytopenia occurs, as well as a marked reduction of serum albumin and immunoglobulins IgA and IgG Cholesterol may be low. A few patients have mild to moderate steatorrhea, but D-xylose absorption normal. Intestinal protein loss can be demonstrated using ^{131}I-labeled povidone or ^{51}Cr-labeled albumin. Jejunal biopsy shows the characteristic dilation and telangiectasia of the lymphatic vessel which distinguish this condition from other protein-losing disorders such as Crohn's and Whipple diseases.

Treatment

Some patients improve on a low-fat diet (< 30 gm/day), supplements of medium-chain triglycerides, and occasionally by resection, if the lesion is localized.

INFECTION AND INFESTATION

(For *Giardia lamblia, Diphyllobothrium latum* the fish tapeworm, *Ascaris lumbricoides* the round worm, and the hookworms *Ancylostoma duodenale*, or *Necator americanus*, see Ch. 13.)

Acute bacterial and viral infections may cause transient malabsorption, probably due to temporary superficial damage to the villi and microvilli. Chronic bacterial infections of the small bowel are uncommon apart from blind loops and diverticula. Intestinal bacteria may utilize dietary vitamin B perhaps interfere with enzyme systems, and cause areas of superficial inflammation.

CARBOHYDRATE INTOLERANCE
(Lactose Intolerance; Lactase Deficiency; Disaccharidase Deficiency; Glucose-Galactose
Malabsorption; Alactasia)

Diarrhea and abdominal distention caused by inability to digest carbohydrate because of a lack of one or more intestinal enzymes.

Pathophysiology

Disaccharides are normally split into monosaccharides by lactase, maltase, isomaltase, or sucrase (invertase) in the small intestine. Lactase splits lactose into glucose and galactose. Unsplit disaccharides remain in the lumen and osmotically retain fluid, causing diarrhea. Bacterial fermentation of sugar in the colon leads to gaseous, acidic stools. Since the enzymes are located in the brush border of mucosal cells, secondary deficiencies occur in diseases associated with morphologic alterations of the jejunal mucosa, e.g., celiac disease, tropical sprue, acute intestinal infections, neomycin toxicity. In infants, temporary secondary disaccharidase deficiency may complicate enteric infections or abdominal surgery.

The monosaccharides glucose and galactose are absorbed by an active transport process in the small bowel (fructose is absorbed passively). The **transport system** for these monosaccharides is lacking in the small bowel in glucose-galactose malabsorption, and symptoms develop after ingestion of most kinds of sugar.

Incidence

Lactase deficiency occurs *normally* in about 75% of adults in all ethnic groups except those of Northwest European origin for whom the incidence is < 20%. Although statistics are unreliable, the majority of nonwhites of North America gradually lose the ability to digest lactase between 10 and 20 yr. It affects 90% of Orientals, 75% of American blacks and Indians, with a high incidence among peoples from the Mediterranean area.

Glucose-galactose intolerance is an extremely rare congenital disorder, and deficiencies of other mucosal enzymes (sucrose, isomaltase, etc.) are also rare.

Symptoms and Signs

Symptoms and signs are similar, regardless of the specific enzyme deficiency. A child who cannot tolerate sugar will have diarrhea and fail to gain weight. An adult may have borborygmi, bloating, flatus, nausea, diarrhea, and abdominal cramps. Even when only lactose absorption is directly impaired by deficiency of the enzyme lactase, the resulting diarrhea may be severe enough to purge other nutrients before they can be absorbed. A clear history of milk intolerance may be obtained in patients with lactose intolerance. Some individuals recognize this early in life and consciously or unconsciously avoid ingesting dairy products, thus making a diagnostic history more obscure. In others, symptoms may simulate the irritable bowel syndrome or complicate a duodenal ulcer or gastrectomy.

Diagnosis

Lactase deficiency may be reliably ascertained by a breath-hydrogen test. The diagnosis may be suspected if acidic stools (pH < 6) are passed; it is further substantiated by a flat oral lactose tolerance test and absolutely confirmed by the finding of low lactase activity in a jejunal biopsy specimen. Glucose-galactose malabsorption is also diagnosed by demonstrating a flat oral tolerance test when the affected sugar is ingested.

The **lactose tolerance test** is specific for the clinical disorder of lactose intolerance. An oral dose of 50 gm of lactose causes diarrhea with abdominal bloating and discomfort, and there is a low or flat blood glucose curve. Equivalent amounts of glucose and galactose produce a normal rise in blood glucose without diarrhea. A rise in the blood glucose level of < 20 mg/100 ml is abnormal.

Treatment

The disorder is readily controlled by a lactose-free diet, or often simply by abstaining from milk drinks.

A child who lacks the transport enzyme can absorb fructose.

---

57. CHRONIC INFLAMMATORY DISEASES OF THE BOWEL

REGIONAL ENTERITIS
(Granulomatous Ileitis or Ileocolitis; Crohn's Disease)

A nonspecific granulomatous inflammatory disease usually affecting the lower ileum but often involving the colon and occasionally other parts of the GI tract.

Epidemiology

Most cases begin before age 40, with a peak incidence in the 20s. The disease occurs about equally in both sexes, is more common among (but not limited to) Jews, and shows a familial tendency.

Etiology and Pathology

The cause is unknown. The transmission of granulomas from tissue homogenates of ileitis patients to experimental animals and the recovery of viral particles and cell-wall–deficient bacteria from in vitro cultures of some of these homogenates suggest that a transmissible agent may be responsible.

The earliest macroscopic lesions of Crohn's disease appear to be tiny focal "aphthoid" ulcerations of the mucosa, usually with underlying nodules of lymphoid tissue. Sometimes these early aphthoid lesions regress, but in other cases, the inflammatory process progresses to involve all layers of the intestinal wall, which becomes greatly thickened. Changes are most marked in the submucosa, with lymphedema and lymphocytic infiltration occurring first, and extensive fibrosis later. Patchy ulcerations develop on the mucosa, and the combination of longitudinal and transverse ulcers with intervening mucosal edema frequently creates a characteristic "cobblestone" appearance. The attached mesentery is thickened and lymphedematous; mesenteric fat typically extends onto the serosal surface of the bowel. Mesenteric lymph nodes often enlarge. The transmural inflammation, deep ulceration, edema, and fibrosis are responsible for obstruction, deep sinus tract and fistula formation, and mesenteric abscesses, which are the major local complications.

Segments of diseased bowel are characteristically sharply demarcated from adjacent normal bowel—thus the name "regional" enteritis. Many segmental lesions may be separated by normal "skip areas." The ileum alone (ileitis) is involved in about 35% of cases; both ileum and colon (ileocolitis) in about 45%; and the colon alone (granulomatous colitis) in < 20%. Occasionally the entire small bowel (jejunoileitis) is involved, and rarely also the stomach or duodenum.

Sarcoid-type epithelioid granulomas in the intestinal wall and occasionally in the involved mesenteric nodes are characteristic, but may be absent in as many as half the cases and are not essential to the diagnosis. In contrast to intestinal tuberculosis, granulomas are not found in the lymph nodes unless they are also present in the bowel wall.

Symptoms and Signs

Chronic diarrhea associated with abdominal pain, fever, anorexia, weight loss, and an abdominal mass are the most common presenting features. However, many patients are first seen with an "acute abdomen" simulating acute appendicitis or intestinal obstruction, which must be ruled out. Four patterns of regional enteritis occur most often: (1) *inflammation*, characterized by right lower quadrant abdominal pain and tenderness, mimicking appendicitis when acute; (2) *obstruction*, in which intestinal stenosis causes recurrent partial obstruction with severe colic, abdominal distention, constipation, and vomiting; (3) *diffuse jejunoileitis*, with both inflammation and obstruction resulting in malnutrition and chronic debility; and (4) *abdominal fistulas and abscesses*, usually late developments, often causing fever, painful abdominal masses, and generalized wasting. Fistulas may be enteroenteric, enterovesical, retroperitoneal, or enterocutaneous. Obstruction, fistulization, and abscess formation are common complications of inflammation; intestinal bleeding, perforation, and small bowel cancer develop rarely. A history of perianal disease, especially fissures and fistulas, can be elicited in about 1/3 of patients.

Extraintestinal manifestations fall into 3 principal categories: (1) Complications often paralleling the activity of the intestinal disease and possibly representing acute immunologic or microbiologic concomitants of the bowel inflammation; these include peripheral arthritis, episcleritis, aphthous stomatitis, erythema nodosum, and pyoderma gangrenosum. These manifestations may be seen in over 1/3 of patients hospitalized with inflammatory bowel disease. They are twice as common when colitis is present as compared to when disease is confined to the small intestine. When extra intestinal manifestations occur, they are multiple in about 1/3 of cases. (2) Disorders associated with inflammatory bowel disease but running an independent course—ankylosing spondylitis, sacroiliitis, and uveitis. The genetic interrelationships among these syndromes, colitis (both ulcerative and granulomatous), and the HLA antigen B27 are discussed under the extracolonic complications of ulcerative colitis, below. (3) Complications relating directly to the disrupted physiology of the bowel itself. Chief among these are renal problems. Kidney stones result from disorders of uric acid metabolism, impairment of urinary dilution and alkalinization, and excessive oxalate absorption; urinary infections occur especially with fistulization into the urinary tract; and hydroureter and hydronephrosis may ensue from ureteral compression by retroperitoneal extension of the intestinal inflammatory process. Other bowel-related complications include malabsorption, especially in the face of extensive ileal resection or bacterial overgrowth from chronic small bowel obstruction or fistulization; gallstones, related to impaired ileal reabsorption of bile salts; and amyloidosis, secondary to longstanding inflammatory and suppurative disease.

In children, extraintestinal manifestations frequently predominate over GI symptoms. Arthritis, FUO, anemia, or growth retardation may be presenting symptoms; abdominal pain or diarrhea may be absent. Thus, evaluation of these systemic symptoms in young people must include barium studies of the small bowel and colon, since these may be the only presenting clues to the diagnosis of inflammatory bowel disease.

Laboratory findings are nonspecific and may include anemia, leukocytosis, increased ESR, and hypoalbuminemia.

Diagnosis

The diagnosis of regional enteritis is suspected in any patient with the inflammatory or obstructive symptoms described above, and in a patient without prominent GI symptoms who presents with perianal fistulas or abscesses or with otherwise unexplained arthritis, erythema nodosum, fever, anemia, or (in a child) stunted growth.

Definitive diagnosis is usually made radiologically. Barium enema x-ray may show reflux of barium into the terminal ileum with irregularity, nodularity, stiffness, thickening of the wall, and a narrowed ileal lumen. A small bowel series with spot x-rays of the terminal ileum usually most clearly demonstrates the nature and extent of the lesion. An upper GI series alone, without small bowel follow-through, will almost invariably miss the diagnosis.

When disease is limited to the colon (granulomatous colitis), differentiation from chronic ulcerative colitis may be difficult, though only about 10 to 20% of patients show this strictly colonic distribution. The diagnosis of granulomatous disease is more likely when there is no x-ray or sigmoidoscopic evidence of rectal involvement ("rectal sparing") and when rectal bleeding is absent. Asymmetric involvement of the bowel wall and segmental distribution of lesions on x-ray help to confirm the diagnosis. Severe perianal disease also suggests the presence of granulomatous and not ulcerative colitis. In active cases affecting the rectum, rectal biopsy is of little or no value in differentiating ulcerative from granulomatous colitis, since the pathognomonic granulomas of the latter disease are rarely found and since practically identical pathologic changes are seen in the active stages of both disorders.

Prognosis

Complete recovery may follow a single isolated attack of **acute ileitis.** This syndrome is usually unrelated to Crohn's disease; it is a benign self-limited ileal inflammation that occurs in young people, often with acute *Yersinia enterocolitica* infection. Established chronic regional enteritis with persistent structural abnormalities, usually incurable, is characterized by lifelong exacerbations. The disease rarely spreads spontaneously without surgical manipulation of the bowel. Fatal complications from free perforation, sepsis, inanition, or carcinoma are rare.

Treatment

No specific therapy is known. Anticholinergics and diphenoxylate 2.5 to 5 mg, loperamide 2 to 4 mg, deodorized opium tincture 10 to 15 drops, or codeine 15 to 30 mg, given orally up to q.i.d., may relieve cramps and diarrhea. Hydrophilic mucilloids such as methylcellulose or psyllium preparations sometimes help to prevent anal irritation by increasing stool firmness.

Antibacterials should be reserved for bacterial complications (e.g., abscesses, infected fistulas). Long-term sulfasalazine therapy is useful in suppressing or preventing relapses of chronic low-grade inflammatory activity, especially in the colon, but it is less useful in severe acute exacerbations. It has not been found helpful in preventing postoperative recurrence. Since GI intolerance is very common, the drug should be given with food, and dosage should be initially low (e.g., 0.5 gm orally t.i.d.) and gradually increased over a period of several days to 3 to 6 gm/day in divided doses.

Corticosteroid therapy is useful in the acute stages. It may dramatically reduce fever and diarrhea, relieve abdominal pain and tenderness, and improve the appetite and sense of well-being. Large doses of oral prednisone, 40 to 60 mg/day, should be given intially; the dosage is gradually reduced following a satisfactory response so that, at the end of 4 wk, the daily dosage does not exceed 10 or 20 mg. Chronic corticosteroid therapy is of less obvious benefit, but as little as 5 or 10 mg/day may help to control symptoms in some individuals.

Striking responses to **immunosuppressive drugs** have been reported in some patients, but their exact place in therapy has not been established. One large multicenter study demonstrated no benefit from azathioprine in Crohn's disease, although a longer-term investigation has suggested that 6-mercaptopurine significantly improved patients' overall clinical status, decreased their steroid requirements, and often healed fistulas. Other treatments that have been tried or proposed include metronidazole, levamisole, BCG vaccination, and even thymectomy, but no scientific studies of these measures have yet proved their efficacy. The wide variety of suggested approaches attests to the inadequacy of present-day therapy for this baffling disease.

Some patients with intestinal obstruction or fistula formation have improved on **elemental diets or hyperalimentation,** at least over a short term, and some children have achieved increased rates of growth. Thus, these measures may sometimes be valuable as preoperative or adjunctive therapy.

Surgery is usually necessary when recurrent intestinal obstruction or intractable abscesses or fistulas are present. Resection of the involved bowel or a bypass operation that totally excludes the diseased area may result in amelioration of symptoms indefinitely, but surgery is not curative. The recurrence rate after surgery is > 95%; ultimately, another operation is often required. Thus, surgery should not be performed unless specific complications or failure of medical therapy make it necessary. When operations have been required, the great majority of patients consider their quality of life to have been improved by surgery.

ULCERATIVE COLITIS

A chronic, nonspecific, inflammatory and ulcerative disease of the colon, characterized most often by bloody diarrhea. Any age may be affected, but the disease most frequently begins between ages 15 and 40. Although there is a familial tendency, the etiology is unknown.

The term "colitis" should be applied only to inflammatory disease of the colon (e.g., ulcerative, granulomatous, ischemic, or radiation colitis; bacillary or amebic dysentery). "Spastic" or "mucous" colitis is a functional disorder more properly described by the term "irritable bowel" (see THE IRRITABLE BOWEL SYNDROME in Ch. 59).

Pathology and Sigmoidoscopic Findings

The disease usually begins in the rectosigmoid area and may extend proximally, eventually involving the entire colon, or it may attack most of the large bowel at once. **Ulcerative proctitis,** a very common and more benign and limited form of the disease, usually remains localized to the rectum, although it too may undergo late proximal spread in about 10% of cases.

Pathologic change begins with degeneration of the reticulin fibers beneath the mucosal epithelium, occlusion of the subepithelial capillaries, and progressive infiltration of the lamina propria with plasma cells, eosinophils, lymphocytes, mast cells, and polymorphonuclear leukocytes. Crypt abscesses, epithelial necrosis, and mucosal ulceration ultimately develop.

Sigmoidoscopy provides a direct and immediate indication of the activity of the disease process. The mucous membrane is first seen as finely granular and friable, with loss of the normal vascular pattern, and often with scattered hemorrhagic areas; minimal trauma causes bleeding in multiple pinpoint spots. The mucosa soon breaks down into a red, spongy surface dotted with a myriad of tiny blood- and pus-oozing ulcerations. As the mucosa becomes progressively involved, the inflammatory and hemorrhagic processes extend into the muscular coats of the bowel. Large mucosal ulcerations with copious purulent exudate characterize severe disease. Islands of relatively normal or hyperplastic inflammatory mucosa (pseudopolyps) project above areas of ulcerated mucosa.

Even during asymptomatic intervals, the sigmoidoscopic appearance is rarely normal; some mild degree of friability or granularity almost always persists.

Symptoms and Signs

The usual manifestation is a series of attacks of bloody diarrhea varying in intensity and duration, interspersed with asymptomatic intervals. Onset of an attack may be acute and fulminant, with sudden violent diarrhea, high fever, signs of peritonitis, and profound toxemia. More often, an attack begins insidiously, with an increased urgency to defecate, mild lower abdominal cramps, and the appearance of blood and mucus in the stools.

When the ulcerative process is confined to the rectosigmoid area, the feces may be normal or hard and dry, but rectal discharges of mucus loaded with RBCs and WBCs accompany or occur between bowel movements. Systemic symptoms are mild or absent. If the process extends proximally, stools become looser and the patient may have 10 to 20 bowel movements/day, often with severe cramps and distressing rectal tenesmus, without respite at night. The stools may be watery and contain pus, blood, and mucus; they frequently consist almost entirely of blood and pus. Malaise, fever, anemia, anorexia, weight loss, leukocytosis, hypoalbuminemia, and elevated ESR may be present with extensive active colitis.

Complications

Hemorrhage is the most common local complication. In **toxic colitis,** a particularly severe local complication, transmural extension of the ulcerative process results in localized ileus and peritonitis. As the toxic colitis progresses, the colon loses muscular tone and within a matter of days or even hours begins to dilate. Plain x-rays of the abdomen show the loss of colonic tone and an accumulation of intraluminal gas over a long, continuous, paralyzed segment of colon which is distended to > 7 cm in diameter. Without effective treatment, massive colonic dilation (**toxic megacolon**) ultimately occurs and free perforation, generalized peritonitis, and septicemia may result. The severely ill patient has fever to 40 C (104 F), leukocytosis, abdominal pain, and rebound tenderness. The mortality rate is 10 to 30%.

Except for small **rectovaginal fistulas,** perirectal complications such as those seen in granulomatous colitis (e.g., major fistulas and abscesses) are not associated with ulcerative colitis. While minor changes in liver function tests are common, clinically apparent liver disease may occur in 1 to 3% of patients. The liver disease may manifest as fatty liver or more seriously as chronic active hepatitis, sclerosing cholangitis, or cirrhosis.

Extracolonic complications include peripheral arthritis, ankylosing spondylitis, sacroiliitis, posterior uveitis, erythema nodosum, pyoderma gangrenosum, episcleritis, and, in children, severely retarded growth and development. It is noteworthy that the arthritis, episcleritis, and skin complications often tend to fluctuate in tandem with the colitis, whereas the spondylitis, sacroiliitis, and uveitis usually follow a course independent of the bowel disease. Most colitis patients with spinal or sacroiliac involvement also have evidence of uveitis, and vice versa. In fact, these conditions may precede the colitis by many years and may even occur without coexisting bowel disease in relatives of colitis patients. Moreover, both ankylosing spondylitis and uveitis, whether they occur in the presence or absence of colitis, have a very strong association with the HLA antigen B27. These observations all seem to suggest some genetic overlaps among colitis, spondylitis, uveitis, and the B27 genotype

The risk of **colon cancer** is greatly increased in patients with ulcerative colitis (see Prognosis, below), and all patients require careful, frequent review for evidence of carcinoma. **Cancer of the biliary tract** is another risk, though rare, appearing late in the course of ulcerative colitis, even 20 yr after colectomy.

Diagnosis

The history and stool examination permit a presumptive diagnosis which almost always can be confirmed by sigmoidoscopy (see above). The severity and extent of the colitis should be established by barium enema x-ray studies except in active stages when risk of perforation contraindicates a barium enema. The x-ray examinations show mucosal edema, minute serrations, or gross ulcerations in severe cases; a shortened, rigid colon with an atrophic or pseudopolypoid mucosa is seen in cases of longer duration. In certain difficult cases, colonoscopy may aid in assessing the extent of disease, in evaluating the nature of a stricture, and in distinguishing ulcerative from Crohn's colitis. It has been suggested that colonoscopic biopsies could be valuable in detecting dysplastic changes that may be associated with carcinoma.

Differential Diagnosis

Severe perianal disease, sparing of the rectal mucosa, absence of bleeding, and asymmetric or segmental involvement of the colon suggest granulomatous colitis (see above) rather than ulcerative colitis. Amebic colitis may mimic ulcerative colitis in every clinical and radiologic detail. The presence of *Entamoeba histolytica* must be excluded by prompt examination of fresh, still-warm stool specimens, or of colonic mucus or exudate aspirated at the time of sigmoidoscopy. Especially in the male homosexual, specific proctitis (e.g., gonorrhea, herpes virus, chlamydia) is a problem (see Ch. 162). Also valuable are serologic tests, which are relatively sensitive and specific in invasive forms of amebiasis. Bacillary dysentery and acute salmonellosis are usually self-limited and identifiable by stool culture and by the presence of specific antibodies in the blood; *Campylobacter fetus* should also be ruled out by culture (see in Ch. 8). Colon cancer usually occurs in an older age group and seldom causes fever or purulent rectal discharge, but sigmoidoscopy and barium enema x-rays are needed to rule this out. Viral gastroenteritis is a brief illness without blood in the stools. Pseudomembranous enterocolitis can usually be related to an immediately antecedent surgical operation or administration of a broad-spectrum antibiotic.

Prognosis

A rapidly progressive initial attack may be fatal in nearly 10% of patients, usually due to exsanguinating hemorrhage, perforation, or sepsis and toxemia. Patients who first develop the disease after age 60 have a particularly poor prognosis; mortality from severe attacks is > 25%. Complete recovery after a single attack may occur in another 10% of all patients. In most cases, the disease is chronic, with repeated exacerbations and remissions.

The incidence of colon cancer is increased with involvement of the entire colon or with duration of disease for > 10 yr. The cumulative proportion of ulcerative colitis patients remaining at risk who develop colorectal cancer reaches 70% by the 4th decade of disease. Recent studies show that cancer risk increases measurably even when colitis does not involve the entire colon, but in such cases the cancers tend to develop at least a decade later than in patients with universal disease.

Primarily because of the increased cancer incidence, in childhood-onset ulcerative colitis, the mortality rate is 20% during each decade of continuing disease. Contrary to previous thinking, there appears to be no specifically higher cancer risk among patients with childhood-onset colitis, independent of their longer durations of disease. However, new studies show about 50% long-term survival after diagnosis of colitis-related cancer, a figure no worse than for colorectal cancer in the general (non-colitis) population.

Nearly ⅓ of all patients with extensive ulcerative colitis ultimately require surgery. Total proctocolectomy is permanently curative and, when performed in time, restores life expectancy to normal.

Patients with localized ulcerative proctitis have the best prognosis. Severe systemic manifestations, toxic complications, or malignant degeneration are unlikely, and late extension of the disease occurs in only about 10%. Surgery is rarely required and life expectancy is normal. However, since extensive ulcerative colitis may begin in the rectum and then spread proximally, it is not safe to assume that a proctitis will remain limited until it has stayed localized for at least 4 to 6 mo.

Treatment

Mild disease may be managed with nonspecific supportive measures—adequate physical and emotional relaxation; a normal diet but without raw fruits and vegetable roughage (and without milk for the ⅓ of patients who find it an irritant); and antidiarrheal medication. Anticholinergics and low doses of diphenoxylate (2.5 mg orally b.i.d. or t.i.d.) are indicated for relatively mild diarrhea; higher diphenoxylate doses (5 mg t.i.d. or q.i.d.), deodorized opium tincture (10 to 15 drops q 4 to 6 h), loperamide (2 mg after each loose movement), or codeine (15 to 30 mg q 4 to 6 h) may be used for more intense diarrhea. All these anti-diarrheal agents must be used with great caution in more severe cases, lest toxic dilation be precipitated.

Moderate disease may respond to sulfasalazine. To reduce GI side effects (nausea, dyspepsia, and anorexia), the drug should be taken with meals and the dosage should be increased gradually (e.g., from an initial 0.5 gm b.i.d. or t.i.d.) to therapeutic levels, usually 1 to 1.5 gm t.i.d. or q.i.d. Long-term sulfasalazine therapy (0.5 to 1 gm b.i.d. or t.i.d.) may help to maintain remissions and reduce the frequency of relapses.

In either **mild or moderate disease,** when the colitis does not extend proximally beyond the splenic flexure, remission may sometimes be achieved with instillation of hydrocortisone by enema instead of with oral corticosteroid therapy. Initially, hydrocortisone 100 mg in 60 ml of isotonic saline and methylcellulose is given rectally once or twice/day. It should be retained in the bowel as long as possible; instillation at night, with the foot of the bed elevated, may prolong retention. Treatment, if effective, should be continued daily for about 1 wk, then every other day for 1 to 2 wk, then discontinued gradually over 1 to 2 wk.

Moderately severe disease in ambulatory patients usually requires systemic corticosteroid therapy. Relatively intensive therapy with prednisone 10 to 15 mg orally t.i.d. or q.i.d. frequently induces dramatic remission. After 1 to 2 wk, the daily dose may be gradually reduced by about 5 to 10 mg every week or so. Sulfasalazine (2 to 4 gm/day in divided doses) may be added when the colitis is controlled by prednisone, about 20 mg/day; very gradual tapering off and ultimate withdrawal of the corticosteroid may then be possible.

Patients with chronic fecal blood loss may require iron to prevent anemia.

Severe disease requires hospitalization and parenteral corticosteroid or ACTH therapy. Response is usually prompt when hydrocortisone 300 mg/day or ACTH 75 to 120 u./day is given by continuous IV drip for 7 to 10 days. Studies comparing hydrocortisone with ACTH have not proved one superior to the other in severe ulcerative colitis, but in patients who have already been receiving long-term corticosteroids, pituitary-adrenal responsiveness might not be adequate to rely on ACTH alone. Unless dehydration due to diarrheal losses is imminent, it is usually advisable not to give hydrocortisone or ACTH in IV saline solution, since edema is then a frequent complication. The addition of potassium chloride 20 to 40 mEq/L to the IV fluids usually helps to prevent hypokalemia. Patients with heavy rectal bleeding often require blood transfusions to correct anemia.

Prednisone 15 mg q.i.d. orally may be substituted after remission has been achieved with the 7- to 10-day course of parenteral treatment. The patient who remains well on the oral regimen for 3 to 4 days may leave the hospital, and corticosteroid dosage may be gradually reduced at home under close medical supervision.

Azathioprine has been used in the treatment of ulcerative colitis, but its degree of efficacy has not been established.

Toxic colitis *is a grave emergency.* As soon as signs of toxic colitis or impending toxic megacolon are detected, the following steps should be instituted immediately: (1) discontinue all antidiarrheal medication; (2) give nothing by mouth and pass a long intestinal tube attached to intermittent suction; (3) give aggressive IV fluid and electrolyte therapy, with saline, potassium chloride, albumin, and blood as needed; (4) give ACTH 120 u./day or hydrocortisone 300 mg/day by continuous IV drip; (5) give antibiotics such as penicillin or ampicillin 2 gm IV q 4 to 6 h.

The patient must be watched closely for signs of progressive peritonitis or perforation. Percussion over the liver is important, since loss of hepatic dullness may be the first clinical sign of free perforation, especially in the patient whose peritoneal signs are suppressed by massive corticosteroid dosage. Abdominal x-rays should be obtained at least daily or even twice/day to follow the course of colonic distention. If the intensive medical measures do not produce dramatic improvement within 24 to 48 h, immediate subtotal colectomy and ileostomy are required or the patient may die.

Surgery: Emergency colectomy is indicated for massive hemorrhage, fulminating toxic colitis, or perforation. In the latter 2 conditions, subtotal colectomy with ileostomy and rectosigmoid mucous fistula is usually the procedure of choice, since total proctocolectomy with abdominoperineal resection is more than most critically ill patients can tolerate. The rectosigmoid stump is electively removed at a later date. Massive hemorrhage constitutes an exception to this principle of conservative operation in emergency situations. Here total proctocolectomy is required or else further bleeding from the retained rectum is likely.

Elective surgery is indicated for suspected carcinoma, growth retardation in children, or intractable chronic disease resulting in invalidism, and should always consist of a total proctocolectomy and ileostomy, since a retained rectum is a potential focus of relapse or malignant degeneration. Because of the high risk of carcinoma, elective prophylactic colectomy has been recommended for patients with total colonic involvement that began in childhood or adolescence and is of > 10 yr duration. Since this is a drastic approach to cancer prevention, however, technics are being sought to identify more specifically those patients at risk. So-called "dysplastic" changes in colonic or rectal mucosal biopsies show promise as an early warning signal of premalignant degeneration.

Total proctocolectomy permanently cures chronic ulcerative colitis, but permanent ileostomy is usually the requisite price, although various endorectal ileal "pull-through" procedures are currently under investigation. The **continent ileostomy** is a promising surgical technic that seems likely to improve patients' acceptance of an ileostomy. An internal reservoir pouch is fashioned out of the distal 40 cm of the patient's ileum and a one-way nipple valve keeps the pouch continent of both gas and stool. The patient empties the pouch several times/day by inserting a small plastic catheter through the valve. Although the cosmetic details of the ileostomy are less critical than the curative nature of proctocolectomy in a disease as serious as ulcerative colitis, the burden imposed by any form of ileostomy must be recognized, and care should be taken to see that the patient receives the instructions and psychologic support that are so necessary both before and after surgery. (See ILEOSTOMY CARE in Ch. 228.)

58. PSEUDOMEMBRANOUS ENTEROCOLITIS

An inflammatory bowel disorder in which membrane-like plaques of exudate replace necrotic intestinal mucosa. Several syndromes have been described.

Etiology and Pathology

An interplay of vascular and bacterial mechanisms appears responsible for a change in the balance of normal gut flora, allowing growth of pathogenic organisms, resulting in pseudomembranous enterocolitis. The patient commonly is debilitated, on broad-spectrum antibiotics, and has a history of vascular anoxia caused by GI surgery, postoperative shock, or drop in BP. Cardiovascular collapse, mercury poisoning, and uremia represent uncommon causes.

Whether the disease is neonatal, postoperative, or antibiotic-associated, gross pathologic examination shows raised plaques of yellowish exudate on the mucosa. Histologically, these pseudomembranous plaques consist of fibrin, mucin, leukocytes, and sloughed necrotic epithelial cells. The underlying mucosa manifests varying degrees of superficial necrosis, edema, lamina propria inflammatory infiltration, and submucosal vascular thrombosis. Toxin-producing strains of *Clostridium difficile* and its toxin have been identified in stools of most patients with typical pseudomembranous colitis after antibiotic exposure, and even in about 20% of cases of simple antibiotic-associated diarrhea without pseudomembranes.

Clinical Presentation and Diagnosis

Pseudomembranous enterocolitis comprises 3 entities, each with a somewhat different clinical and pathologic presentation. **Neonatal pseudomembranous enterocolitis** is discussed as NECROTIZING ENTEROCOLITIS under NEONATAL INFECTIONS in Vol. II, Ch. 21. **Postoperative pseudomembranous enterocolitis** affects the bowel and small intestine and sometimes the proximal colon. This syndrome typically appears 2 to 7 days following major GI surgery. The disease begins with colicky pain, nausea, and distention, followed by fever, and it often progresses abruptly to shock and death. Diarrhea is noted in $< 1/2$ of the cases. When it occurs, stools are profuse, watery, offensive, greenish-yellow, and sometimes bloody. In recent years, a substantial proportion of cases are associated with the use of antibiotics and may follow a more benign course.

Antibiotic-associated pseudomembranous colitis differs from the fulminating postoperative and neonatal forms in that it usually limits itself to the colon, necrosis is superficial, edema is prominent, diarrhea is almost universal, and the disease is usually self-limited and rarely fatal. Moreover, the disease may not appear until a week or two after antibiotic administration ceases. In fact, fully 30 to 50% of cases begin only after cessation of antibiotic treatment, so that the diagnosis must be suspected in anyone who develops diarrhea within 3 to 4 wk after exposure to antibiotics. Clinical manifestations vary widely. In the most common form of simple postantibiotic diarrhea, pseudomembranes are absent, and, in 80% of these cases, stool assays are negative for toxin-producing clostridia. Rarely, postantibiotic colitis resembles ulcerative colitis and may be fulminating or progress to a chronic phase. The best-defined variety, associated with typical pseudomembranes and toxin-producing clostridia, occurs most frequently with clindamycin or lincomycin but may sometimes occur after treatment with almost any other antibiotic, including ampicillin, cephalosporins, penicillin, amoxillin, tetracycline, chloramphenicol, or trimethoprim-sulfamethoxazole. Postantibiotic colitis is quite rare following erythromycin, and no cases have yet been attributed to vancomycin or parenteral aminoglycosides.

Sigmoidoscopy and plain films of the abdomen should be adequate to establish a diagnosis of pseudomembranous enterocolitis. Plain films may show the mucosal edema and nodularity typical of a colitis. In active or severe cases, barium enema examination is *contraindicated*.

Prophylaxis

While the incidence of clindamycin-induced colitis appears to be low, sometimes clusters of cases arise with alarming frequency—reaching > 20 to 30% for the uncomplicated diarrheal syndrome and up to 10% for documented pseudomembranous colitis. Although little can prevent the postoperative or neonatal varieties, the incidence of antibiotic-induced pseudomembranous enterocolitis can be minimized by reserving all antibiotics for suitable indication, by using only very short courses of systemic antibiotic prophylaxis for intestinal surgery, and particularly by reserving clindamycin for serious infections with *Bacteroides fragilis* or other anaerobes.

Treatment

If diarrhea occurs during antibiotic administration, antibiotics should be stopped immediately, unless their use is critically needed. Experience with toxigenic diarrheas and dysentery suggests that antiperistaltic drugs (e.g., diphenoxylate) be avoided.

Supportive measures are the mainstay of treatment. Fluid replacement is urgent; many liters/day may be required to sustain intravascular volume (see Treatment under CHOLERA in Ch. 8). Potassium and bicarbonate losses may have to be replaced as well as sodium, chloride, and water. Albumin infusion is sometimes needed when exudative protein loss and hypotension are prominent. Clinical and experimental reports suggest that cholestyramine (4 gm orally q.i.d.) or oral vancomycin (500 mg q 6 h) are safe and effective treatments for postantibiotic colitis associated with pseudomembranous and/or clostridial toxin. Simple postantibiotic diarrhea, without evidence of frank colitis on sigmoidoscopy and without signs of systemic toxicity, will usually subside spontaneously within 8 to 11 days once the offending antibiotic is discontinued. In fulminating toxic colitis, high-dose IV corticosteroid therapy has been used. Emergency colectomy may be life-saving, the judgment being made according to the same principles that govern the management of idiopathic ulcerative colitis (see Ch. 57).

---

59. FUNCTIONAL BOWEL DISEASE

THE IRRITABLE BOWEL SYNDROME
(Spastic Colon; Mucous Colitis)

A motility disorder involving the small intestine and large bowel and associated with variable degrees of abdominal pain, constipation, or diarrhea, apparently as a reaction to stress in a susceptible individual. This syndrome represents about 1/2 of all GI referrals or initial GI complaints in private and institutional care facilities. Women are more commonly affected than men, with a ratio of 3:1.

Etiology
No anatomic cause can be found. Emotional factors, diet, drugs, or hormones may precipitate or aggravate a heightened sensitivity to GI motility. Psychologically, many patients are obsessive-compulsive personalities. Feelings of anxiety, resentment, and guilt are most conducive to the onset of symptoms. Periods of stress and emotional conflict frequently result in depression frequently coincide with the onset and recurrences of the syndrome. Some common psychosocial stresses precipitating symptoms involve marital discord, anxiety related to children, loss of a loved one, and obsessional worries over trivial everyday problems. (See also Approach to the Patient in Ch. 51.)

Pathophysiology
The circular and longitudinal muscles of the small bowel and sigmoid colon are particularly susceptible to motor abnormalities. The proximal small bowel appears to be hyperreactive to the ingestion of food and parasympathomimetic drugs. In addition, when the normal segmentation mechanism of the sigmoid colon becomes hyperreactive, so-called spastic constipation results. Intraluminal pressure studies performed in the pelvic colon reveal that increased frequency and amplitude of contractions are associated with spastic constipation, in contrast to the diminished motor function associated with diarrheal episodes. Similar changes in the colon follow either the administration of parasympathomimetic agents or the ingestion of food. Mucorrhea may occur as a result of excessive parasympathomimetic stimulation or increased mechanical irritation of the colon.

A hypersensitivity to normal amounts of intraluminal gas exists, and also a heightened perception of pain in the presence of normal quantity and quality of intestinal gas. A hypersensitivity to the hormones gastrin and cholecystokinin is present. A common myoelectric pattern consisting of a greater frequency of basic electrical rhythm slow wave 3 cycle/min activity occurs. A dose of cholecystokinin or pentagastrin can reproduce this type of motor abnormality.

Symptoms and Signs
Symptoms include abdominal distress, erratic frequency of bowel action, and variation in stool consistency. Disagreeable abdominal sensations may also be associated with nonspecific symptoms, such as bloating, gas, nausea, headache, fatigue, lassitude, and flatulence.

Two major groups or clinical types of irritable bowel syndrome are recognized. In the first group, the **spastic colon type**, the bowel movements are variable. Most patients have pain of colonic origin over one or more areas of the colon in association with periodic constipation or diarrhea. The majority complain of lower abdominal pain or discomfort over the course of the sigmoid colon. The pain is either colicky and coming in bouts or a continuous dull ache. It may be relieved by a bowel movement. Symptoms are commonly triggered by ingesting food, though no specific food type is implicated. Patients may have either constipation or diarrhea; in some patients the two alternate. Mucorrhea occurs frequently. Nonspecific symptoms such as fatigue, depression, anxiety, and difficulty with mental concentration are common.

The second group primarily manifests **painless diarrhea**. The patient usually complains of urgent, precipitous diarrhea that occurs immediately upon arising or, more typically, during or immediately after a meal. Incontinence may occur. Nocturnal diarrhea is unusual.

On physical examination, patients with either variant generally appear to be in good health without evidence of significant organic disease. Palpation of the abdomen may reveal tenderness, particularly in the left lower quadrant, at times associated with a contracted tender colon.

Diagnosis

The diagnosis is based upon the characteristic clinical history and the exclusion of other disease processes. The stools of every patient must be cultured and carefully examined for occult blood, ova, and parasites. Proctosigmoidoscopic and barium enema examinations are necessary to rule out any more serious underlying disorder. In this syndrome, proctosigmoidoscopic examination is within normal limits, except for mild hyperemia and increased mucous. Conditions that may mimic irritable bowel syndrome include abuse of cathartics, amebiasis, allergic gastroenteropathy, lactase deficiency, and early ulcerative or granulomatous colitis. It may be difficult to differentiate the irritable bowel syndrome from diverticular disease of the colon, since the motor disturbance in both of these conditions is quite similar; in fact, irritable bowel syndrome may be the precursor of diverticular disease. It is imperative that patients with the irritable bowel syndrome be carefully reevaluated periodically to rule out any intercurrent pathologic process.

Treatment

The sympathetic understanding and guidance of the physician is of overriding importance. The patient must be reassured that no organic disease is present. Since psychologic stress, particularly a depressive reaction, may be a significant factor in this illness, it should be sought, evaluated, and treated. Regular physical activity helps to relieve symptoms of anxiety and assists in bowel function. In general, a normal diet should be followed. Beans, cabbage, and other foods containing fermentable carbohydrates may be eliminated if flatulence is a problem. Patients with diarrhea as the major symptomatic manifestation should avoid laxative foods. A bland bulk-producing agent such as psyllium hydrophilic mucilloid taken with 2 glasses of water tends to stabilize the water content of the bowel and provide bulk. These actions increase the diameter of the large bowel, particularly in the area of the sigmoid colon, thereby reducing lateral pressure. Unprocessed bran may help patients with spastic constipation.

It may be helpful to give anticholinergic agents (e.g., propantheline 7.5 to 15 mg) alone or in combination with a mild tranquilizer (e.g., chlordiazepoxide 5 to 10 mg) or sedative (e.g., phenobarbital 15 to 30 mg) t.i.d. orally 30 to 60 min before meals. In patients with more significant diarrhea, diphenoxylate 2.5 to 5 mg (1 to 2 tablets) may be given before meals. Loperamide 2 to 4 mg (1 to 2 capsules) may be an effective alternative. In depressed patients, amitriptyline 10 mg t.i.d. orally 30 to 60 min before meals has both antidepressant and anticholinergic effects and may be used without other anticholinergic therapy.

GAS

Physiology

Gas is present in the gut as a result of (1) air swallowing (aerophagia), (2) production in the lumen, or (3) diffusion from the blood into the lumen.

Aerophagia occurs normally in small amounts while swallowing food and liquids, but some people unconsciously swallow repeated boluses of air at other times, especially when anxious. Most swallowed air is subsequently eructated and only a small amount passes into the small bowel, the quantity apparently being influenced by posture. The esophagus empties into the posterior, cephalad aspect of the stomach. When the individual is upright, air rises above the liquid contents of the stomach, comes in contact with the gastroesophageal junction, and is readily eructated. When the individual is supine, air trapped below the fluid tends to be propelled into the duodenum. Excessive salivation may also lead to increased air swallowing and may be associated with various GI disorders (e.g., peptic ulcer) or with the nausea accompanying such disorders as uremia or liver disease. Belching in many patients may be associated with the use of such antacids as baking soda. Attributing the relief of ulcer symptoms to the belching rather than to the antacids, the patient continues habitual belching to relieve distress.

Gas is produced in the lumen by several mechanisms. Bacterial metabolism yields important volumes of hydrogen (H_2), methane (CH_4), and CO_2. Nearly all H_2 is produced by bacterial metabolism of *ingested* fermentable materials (carbohydrates and amino acids) in the colon and therefore is negligible after a prolonged fast or after a meal that is completely absorbed in the small bowel. H_2 is produced in large quantities after eating certain fruits and vegetables (e.g., baked beans) containing indigestible carbohydrates and by patients with malabsorption syndromes. Patients with disaccharidase deficiencies (most commonly lactose intolerance) pass large amounts of disaccharides into the colon which are fermented to H_2 (see CARBOHYDRATE INTOLERANCE in Ch. 56).

CH_4 is produced by bacterial metabolism of *endogenous* substances in the colon; the production rate is only minimally influenced by food ingestion. Some people consistently excrete large quantities of CH_4; others, little or none. Apparently familial, this trait appears during infancy and persists for life.

CO_2 may also be produced by bacterial metabolism, but a more important source is the reaction of bicarbonate and hydrogen ions in which 22.4 ml of CO_2 are released for each mEq of bicarbonate. Hydrogen ions, which may represent several hundred mEq of hydrogen ion, may be derived from gastric hydrochloric acid or the fatty acids released during digestion of the fats of a single meal. Theoretically, up to 4 L of CO_2 may be released into the duodenum following ingestion of a meal. The acid products released by bacterial fermentation of nonabsorbed carbohydrates in the colon may also react with bicarbonate to produce CO_2. Though bloating may occasionally occur, the rapid absorption of CO_2 into the blood prevents intolerable distention.

Gas diffuses between the lumen and the blood in a direction dependent upon the partial pressure difference between the two. The production of H_2, CO_2, and CH_4 may reduce the partial pressure of nitrogen in the lumen to a value far below that in the blood, possibly accounting for much of the nitrogen in the lumen.

Gas is eliminated by eructation, diffusion from the lumen into the blood with ultimate excretion by the lungs, bacterial catabolism, and passage through the anus. Antibiotics that selectively inhibit bacterial H_2 catabolism markedly increase H_2 excretion.

Symptoms and Signs

Excessive gas is commonly thought to cause eructation (belching), abdominal pain, bloating, distention, or passage of excessively voluminous or noxious flatus (farting). However, excessive intestinal gas has not been clearly linked to the above complaints; it is likely that many symptoms are incorrectly attributed to "too much gas." In most normal persons, 1 L of gas/hour can be infused into the gut with a minimum of symptoms, while patients with gas problems often cannot tolerate much smaller quantities. Thus, the basic abnormality in patients with bloating or distention may be an "irritable" intestine. Gas could be the inciting agent, or, perhaps, have no role in the pathogenesis of symptoms.

Repeated eructation indicates aerophagia. Some patients with this problem can readily produce a series of belches on command. In the splenic flexure syndrome, swallowed air becomes trapped in the splenic flexure and may cause diffuse abdominal distention. Left upper quadrant fullness and pressure radiating to the left side of the chest may result. There is increased tympany in the extreme left lateral aspect of the upper abdomen. Relief occurs with defecation or passage of flatus.

Among those who are flatulent, the quantity and frequency of gas passage can reach astounding proportions. One careful study noted a patient with daily flatus frequency as high as 141, including 70 passages in one 4-h period. This symptom, which can cause great psychosocial distress, has been unofficially and humorously described according to its salient characteristics: (1) the "slider" (crowded elevator type), which is released slowly and noiselessly, sometimes with devastating effect; (2) the open sphincter, or "pooh" type, which is said to be of higher temperature and more aromatic; and (3) the staccato or drum-beat type, pleasantly passed in privacy.

While questions of air pollution and degradation of air quality have been raised, no adequate studies have been performed. However, no hazard is likely to those working near open flames, and youngsters have even been known to make a game of expelling gas over a match-flame. Rarely, this usually distressing symptom has been turned to advantage, as with a Frenchman referred to as "Le Petomane," who became affluent as an effluent performer on the Moulin Rouge stage.

Treatment

Belching, bloating, and distention are difficult to relieve, since most complaints are due either to unconscious aerophagia or to exaggerated sensitivity to normal amounts of gas. An attempt must be made to reduce aerophagia. Since aerophagia may be due to excessive salivation, one must exclude such habits as excessive gum chewing or smoking, upper GI tract diseases such as peptic ulcer which may cause reflex hypersalivation, and disorders that may cause nausea and reflex salivation. When belching is associated with the use of carbonated beverages or antacids such as baking soda, these should be eliminated. The mechanism of repeated eructation should be explained and demonstrated. Clamping a pencil or other object between the teeth when aerophagia is troublesome may decrease the amount of involuntary or habit swallowing and break the cycle of aerophagia-discomfort-belch-relief. Foods containing nonabsorbable carbohydrates can be avoided. Milk-containing products should be excluded from the diet of patients with lactose intolerance.

There are few well-controlled studies demonstrating clear-cut benefit from any drug. Simethicone, an agent that breaks up small gas bubbles, has been incorporated into several preparations, and a variety of anticholinergic medications have also been used, all with variable results. Some patients with dyspepsia and postprandial upper abdominal fullness have benefited from antacids, metoclopramide (10 mg 30 min before meals), or bethanechol (5 to 25 mg 30 min before meals). These drugs work by increasing the rate of gastric emptying or increasing lower esophageal sphincter tone. Complaints of excessive flatus are treated with similar measures to try to minimize the volume of gas in the gut.

In general, symptoms of functional bloating, distention, and flatus run an intermittent, chronic course that is only partially relieved by therapy. Reassurance that these problems are not detrimental to health is important.

60.   DIVERTICULAR DISEASE

DIVERTICULOSIS

Diverticula, *small, saccular, mucosal herniations through the muscular wall of the colon*, may occur in any part of the colon, but most frequently in the sigmoid. They vary in diameter from 3 mm to > 3 cm and are present in 30 to 40% of persons over age 50, the incidence increasing with each subsequent decade of life. The diverticular wall consists of only a thin layer of mucosa and serosa. Diverticula are occasionally responsible for severe bleeding from the rectum, and often become inflamed, causing diverticulitis.

Etiology and Pathogenesis

Recent evidence suggests that a modern, highly refined low-residue diet plays an important role in the formation of diverticula. The lack of dietary bulk is associated with spasm of the colonic musculature, especially in the sigmoid. Intraluminal pressure builds up and the mucosa eventually pushes through the muscular coat at weak points, usually where the colonic blood vessels pierce the muscle to supply the mucosa. The diverticula become filled with inspissated feces, and ulceration of the attenuated mucosa and serosa may occur. Severe rectal hemorrhage may result if a small ulcer at the neck of the diverticulum erodes a branch of the colonic artery. Diverticula in the cecum or ascending colon are less numerous but more likely to ulcerate and bleed than those in the descending colon or sigmoid.

Symptoms, Signs, and Diagnosis

Most patients with diverticula are asymptomatic. When a barium enema x-ray examination shows diverticula in a patient with nonspecific abdominal distress (pain, flatulence) and disturbed bowel function, other causes should be excluded before symptoms are attributed to the diverticula. If rectal bleeding occurs, proctoscopic or colonoscopic examination and barium enema x-ray study should be performed to rule out other lesions, particularly polyps or carcinoma (see DIVERTICULITIS, below).

Treatment

A bland diet is *not* indicated for persons with diverticula. Sufficient dietary roughage is required to move the stool through the colon at a normal rate; bran fiber (whole wheat bread and 40 or 100% bran cereal) should therefore be added to the diet. Local heat application, rest, a diet with adequate bulk, and medication usually relieve symptoms. Small doses of phenobarbital (30 mg orally b.i.d.) and belladonna (e.g., 10 to 15 drops of the tincture orally b.i.d.) may relieve abdominal distress.

If severe bleeding occurs, immediate hospitalization, blood transfusions, and close observation are necessary. Surgery is occasionally required to prevent fatal hemorrhage. Since many diverticula are usually scattered throughout the colon, pinpointing the diverticulum responsible for the bleeding may be difficult. Colonoscopy and angiography can frequently localize the bleeding vessel, and resecting that segment of the colon controls the life-threatening complication. When the bleeding source cannot be determined, total colectomy is the safest procedure, since patients have died from secondary hemorrhage when only the sigmoid colon was removed. The operative risk in an elderly, rapidly bleeding patient can be reduced by staging the procedure. The colon is removed down to the low sigmoid to stop the bleeding; the ileum is exteriorized as an ileostomy and the low sigmoid colon as a colostomy; and intestinal continuity is later restored by ileorectal anastomosis.

DIVERTICULITIS

Inflammation of one or more diverticula, occasionally leading to potentially fatal obstruction or perforation, and to fistula formation.

Pathogenesis and Complications

A small, even minute, perforation of the thin-walled diverticulum due to inflammation or high colonic pressure leads to bacterial or possibly fecal contamination of the pericolic tissues. A small abscess develops and may be absorbed, may drain back into the bowel lumen, or may enlarge. The inflamed bowel segment (usually the sigmoid) often adheres to the bladder or other nearby pelvic organs (e.g., the vagina, especially after a hysterectomy), and a fistula may develop. With repeated inflammation, the colonic wall thickens, the lumen narrows, and acute obstruction may occur. One of the most dangerous complications is perforation into the free peritoneal cavity, resulting in leakage of purulent or fecal material and generalized peritonitis.

Symptoms and Signs

Pain and localized tenderness are present, most commonly in the left lower quadrant (since diverticula are most numerous in the sigmoid colon), but at times in the suprapubic area or low in the right lower quadrant where they closely simulate acute appendicitis. Pain is occasionally severe and associated with signs of spreading peritonitis. Crampy pain with abdominal distention suggests large or small bowel obstruction due to adherent jejunum or ileum. Aggravation of the pain by urination suggests adhesion of the inflamed bowel to the bladder. A change in bowel function to constipation (often interrupted by periods of diarrhea) is frequent. A mass is often palpable in the left lower quadrant. Fever and leukocytosis are usually present.

Differential Diagnosis

Pain and tenderness in the lower abdomen associated with disturbed bowel function and, perhaps, rectal bleeding suggest not only diverticulitis, but also *colon carcinoma, which must be ruled out before a diagnosis of diverticulitis is made.* Proctoscopic examination is usually negative in patients with diverticulitis, but must be performed to exclude carcinoma of the pelvic colon, particularly if rectal bleeding has occurred. A barium enema x-ray study is then done to rule out carcinoma of the sigmoid and to demonstrate diverticula and the presence of perforation, obstruction, or fistula. Proctoscopy and an initial barium enema x-ray study do not exclude cancer in 15 to 20% of patients; if a repeat barium enema 1 or 2 wk later or fiberoptic colonoscopy does not rule out malignancy, complete surgical removal of the lesion is indicated.

Prognosis

Morbidity and mortality (higher than they should be) can be reduced (mortality to < 3%) by early surgery before a serious complication develops, and by the use of a 2- or 3-stage operative procedure when primary resection is hazardous, particularly in elderly, poor-risk patients.

Treatment

For patients with acute diverticulitis, conservative therapy (hospitalization, bed rest, IV fluids, and nothing given orally) should be tried first. If the patient is febrile and has evidence of abscess formation, antibiotics (oral or IV) may be prescribed. Ampicillin is commonly used. The inflammatory process usually subsides, but signs of spreading peritonitis must be anticipated and sought. Emergency exteriorization of the perforated bowel segment must be considered if peritonitis develops. If the involved segment is too low for exteriorization, it is resected, the proximal colon brought out as a colostomy, and the rectal segment closed.

IV hyperalimentation has also been used to put the diseased bowel "at rest." If the acute inflammatory reaction (fever, pain, etc.) persists despite conservative treatment, resection of the inflamed segment of colon is indicated. In elderly or poor risk patients, or when distended colon, large abscesses, or peritonitis make resection and anastomosis hazardous, diversion of the fecal stream by a proximal transverse colostomy is first carried out. Usually, the inflammation gradually subsides and the diseased bowel can be resected with little risk 4 to 6 mo later, followed by closure of the temporary colostomy. Similar operative management is indicated when a fistula (e.g., colovesical) results in a severe pelvic inflammatory reaction.

In patients with recurrent diverticulitis or with symptoms suggesting an increasing degree of obstruction or early bladder involvement, early surgery often precludes the morbidity associated with 2 or 3 operative procedures plus many weeks of hospitalization. An adequate elective resection, done when the disease is quiescent and the colon has been well prepared preoperatively, is associated with little risk and few complications.

---

61. NEOPLASMS OF THE BOWEL

TUMORS OF THE SMALL INTESTINE

BENIGN TUMORS

Neoplasms of the jejunum and ileum comprise 1 to 5% of all tumors of the GI tract. They are predominantly benign and include leiomyomas, lipomas, neurofibromas, and fibromas; all may cause symptoms requiring surgery. Polyps occur in the small bowel but are more common in the colon (see below). Vascular tumors are multicentric in the small bowel in 55% of cases. **Hereditary hemorrhagic telangiectasia (Rendu-Osler-Weber syndrome)** is an inborn progressive tendency to form dilated endothelial spaces. Hemangiomas may bleed or intussuscept. Arteriography may help to locate the bleeding points. If a surgeon must operate without knowing the bleeding site, transillumination of the bowel or intraoperative endoscopy may help his search.

MALIGNANT TUMORS

Adenocarcinoma is uncommon. It usually arises in the proximal jejunum and causes minimal symptoms. **Primary malignant lymphoma** arising in the ileum may produce a long, rigid segment. Small intestinal lymphomas arise frequently in a setting of iliac sprue. The small bowel, particularly the ileum, is the second most common site (after the appendix) of **carcinoid tumors.** Multiple tumors are present in 50% of cases. Of those > 2 cm in diameter, 80% have metastasized by the time of operation. About 30% of small bowel carcinoids cause symptoms of obstruction, pain, bleeding, or the carcinoid syndrome (see Ch. 91). Treatment is surgical resection; repeated operations may be required.

TUMORS OF THE LARGE BOWEL

POLYPS OF THE COLON AND RECTUM

Polyp, a clinical term without pathologic significance, refers to *any mass of tissue that arises from the mucous membrane and protrudes into the lumen.* Polyps may be sessile or pedunculated and vary considerably in size. Such lesions are classified histologically as tubular (adenomatous) polyps, villous (papillary) adenomas (with or without adenocarcinoma), polypoid carcinomas, pseudopolyps, or other more uncommon tumors.

Incidence ranges from 7 to 50%; the higher figure includes very small polyps found at autopsy. Polyps are detected in about 5% of patients by routine barium enemas and with greater frequency by sigmoidoscopic and colonoscopic examination. They are often multiple, are most common in the rectum and sigmoid, and occur with decreasing frequency toward the cecum. About 25% of patients with cancer of the large bowel also have adenomatous polyps.

Villous adenomas become malignant in about 35% of cases. The question of premalignancy of tubular polyps is controversial, but the weight of evidence favors the view that they can become malignant.

Symptoms, Signs, and Diagnosis

Most polyps are asymptomatic. **Rectal bleeding** is the most frequent complaint. Large, sessile villous adenomas of the rectum may secrete copious amounts of mucus that may result in electrolyte imbalance. Occasionally a polyp on a long pedicle will prolapse through the anus. Rectal polyps may or may not be palpable by digital rectal examination and are disclosed only by sigmoidoscopic inspection. Since polyps are often multiple and may coexist with cancer, further investigation of the colon is mandatory even if a lesion is found by sigmoidoscopy.

On barium enema x-ray examination, a polyp appears as a rounded filling defect. Double contrast (pneumocolon) examination is of great value, but fiberoptic colonoscopy is the most reliable method of diagnosing colonic polyps.

Treatment

Polyps within reach of the proctosigmoidoscope should be removed completely with a snare or destroyed by fulguration. Large, sessile, soft, velvety, villous adenomas have a high malignant potential and must be excised completely. Lesions in the sigmoid and above should be removed with an electrocautery snare passed through the fiberoptic flexible colonoscope. Laparotomy should be considered if colonoscopy is unsuccessful. Colon resection is advisable if the polyp contains cancer that has invaded the muscularis mucosa.

FAMILIAL POLYPOSIS

A heterozygous, autosomal, dominant, inheritable disease of the colon in which multiple polyps carpet the colon and rectum. Malignancy develops before age 40 in nearly all untreated patients. Total proctocolectomy eliminates the risk of cancer, but rectal polyps often regress after abdominal colectomy and ileorectal anastomosis, and that operation is favored initially. New polyps that appear in the rectum must be fulgurated. If new polyps appear rapidly or in large numbers, the rectum should be excised and a permanent ileostomy established. Careful follow-up of the patient and his family is essential.

Gardner's syndrome is *a variant of a familial polyposis associated with desmoid tumors, osteomas of the skull or mandible, and sebaceous cysts.* **Peutz-Jeghers syndrome** is *an autosomal, dominant, congenital disease in which multiple polyps appear in the stomach, small bowel, and colon.* Affected individuals have melanotic pigmentation of the skin and mucous membranes, especially about the lips and gums. Histologically, these polyps are hamartomas.

OTHER POLYPS

Juvenile polyps occur in children, are non-neoplastic, and often autoamputate at puberty. Treatment is required only if bleeding or intussusception occurs. **Hyperplastic polyps,** also non-neoplastic, are common in the colon and rectum. **Pseudopolyps** that occur in chronic ulcerative colitis are discussed in Ch. 57.

CANCER OF THE COLON AND RECTUM

In Western countries the colon and rectum account for more cases of cancer than any other anatomic site except the skin. In the USA approximately 49,000 people die of this disease each year. About 75% of these cancers occur in the rectum and sigmoid colon, and 95% are adenocarcinomas. Cancer of the colon and rectum is the most frequent cause of death among visceral malignancies that affect both sexes. The incidence increases with age, beginning to rise at age 40 and reaching a peak at 60 to 75 yr. Carcinoma of the colon is commoner in females, and carcinoma of the rectum is commoner in males. Synchronous colonic cancers—i.e., more than one cancer—are found in 5% of patients. There is a low genetic predisposition to cancer of the large bowel. Other predisposing factors include chronic ulcerative colitis, granulomatous colitis, and familial polyposis. Populations with a high incidence of colorectal cancer consume diets containing less fiber and more animal protein, fat, and refined carbohydrates than populations with a low incidence of this disease. Carcinogenic substances may be ingested in the diet, but it seems more likely that carcinogens are produced endogenously from dietary substances or intestinal secretions, probably by bacterial action. The exact role of dietary factors is not established.

Cancer of the colon and rectum spreads by (1) direct extension through the wall of the bowel, (2) hematogenous metastasis, (3) regional lymph node metastasis, (4) perineural spread, and (5) intraluminal metastasis.

Symptoms, Signs, and Diagnosis

Adenocarcinoma of the colon and rectum has a slow growth rate and a correspondingly long interval before reaching symptom-producing size. During this asymptomatic phase, diagnosis depends on routine examination. When symptoms develop, they depend on the location of the lesion, its type, extent, and complications. The **right colon** has a large caliber, a thin wall, and a fluid content, and carcinomas here are usually fungating. They may grow large and may be palpable through the abdominal wall. Fatigue and weakness due to severe anemia may be the only complaints. Gross blood may not be visible in the stool, but occult blood may be detected. Because of the liquid content, large caliber, and fungating lesions, symptoms associated with obstruction (e.g., change in bowel habit) may be a late finding. The **left colon** has a smaller lumen, the feces are semisolid, and cancer here tends to encircle the bowel, causing alternating constipation and frequency of stool. Partial obstruction with colicky abdominal pain or complete obstruction may be the presenting picture. The stool may be streaked or mixed with blood. In cancer of the **rectum** the most common presenting symptom is the passage of blood with a bowel movement. Whenever rectal bleeding occurs, even with obvious hemorrhoids, coexisting cancer must be ruled out. There may be tenesmus or a sensation of incomplete evacuation. Pain is noticeably absent.

About 65% of cancer of the colon and rectum are within reach of the examining finger or the sigmoidoscope. Sigmoidoscopy should be performed in every patient with suspected cancer of any portion of the bowel, and biopsies taken of tumors. Barium enema x-ray examination is unreliable in detecting cancer of the rectum, but is the most important means of diagnosing cancer of the colon. Barium should not be administered by mouth, since it may precipitate acute large-bowel obstruction. Colonoscopy need be performed only when x-ray diagnosis is inconclusive. Simple, inexpensive testing of the stool for occult blood may be done by asymptomatic patients themselves as part of general physical examinations. When positive, further studies should be done. Elevated serum carcinoembryonic antigen **(CEA)** is not specifically associated with colorectal cancer, but CEA levels are high in 70% of patients. Following CEA is helpful in detecting recurrence after surgical resection.

Treatment and Prognosis

Treatment of cancer of the colon consists of wide surgical resection of the lesion and its regional lymphatic drainage after preparation of the bowel. For cancer of the rectum, the choice of operation depends upon its distance from the anus and gross extent. Abdominoperineal resection of the rectum requires a permanent sigmoidostomy. Low anterior resection, with anastomosis of the sigmoid colon to the rectum, is the curative procedure of choice only if a margin of 5 cm of normal bowel can be resected below the lesion and if the operation is technically possible. Other limited palliative operations are indicated at times.

An attempt at surgical cure is possible in 70% of patients. The 5-yr survival rate after curative operation with cancer limited to the mucosa is 90%; with positive lymph nodes, 30%. Some tumors can be controlled locally by electrocoagulation. Preliminary results of studies of postoperative radiation therapy, chemotherapy, and immunotherapy are promising.

---

62. ANORECTAL DISORDERS

Introduction

The anal canal is derived from an invagination of the ectoderm, the rectum from entoderm. The resultant anatomic differences are important considerations in evaluating and treating anorectal disorders. The **lining** of the rectum consists of red, glistening glandular mucosa; the anal canal is lined with anoderm, a continuation of the external skin. For their **nerve supply,** the anal canal and adjacent external skin are generously supplied with somatic sensory nerves and are highly susceptible to painful stimuli; the rectal mucosa has an autonomic nerve supply and is relatively insensitive to pain. **Venous drainage** above the anorectal juncture is through the portal system; the anal canal is drained through the caval system. The **lymphatic return** from the rectum is along the superior hemorrhoidal vascular pedicle to the inferior mesenteric and aortic nodes, but the lymphatics from the anal canal pass to the internal iliac nodes, the posterior vaginal wall, and the inguinal nodes. The venous and lymphatic distributions determine how malignant disease and infection spread and how hemorrhoids are formed.

At the superior boundary of the anal canal is the anorectal juncture (pectinate line, mucocutaneous juncture, or dentate line) where there are 8 to 12 anal crypts and 5 to 8 tiny papillae. Anorectal abscesses and fistulas originate in the crypts.

The sphincteric ring encircles the anal canal. It is composed of the fusion of the internal sphincter, longitudinal muscle, the central portion of the levators, and the components of the external sphincter. Anteriorly it is more vulnerable to trauma, which can result in incontinence. The puborectalis forms a muscular sling around the rectum for support and assistance in defecation.

In diagnosing anorectal disorders, the **history** should include the details of bleeding, pain, protrusion, discharge, swelling, abnormal sensations, bowel actions, nature of the stool, use of cathartics and enemas, and abdominal and urinary symptoms. **Examination** should be gentle and requires good lighting. It consists of external inspection, perianal and intrarectal digital palpation, rectovaginal bi-digital palpation in the female, anoscopy and sigmoidoscopy to 25 cm above the anal verge, as well as examination of the abdomen. Inspection, palpation, and anoscopy are best done with the patient in the left lateral Sims' position, and the sigmoidoscopy with the patient in the knee-chest position or inverted on a tilt-table. With painful anal lesions, topical or even general anesthesia may be required. A flexible, fiberoptic sigmoidoscope, 65 cm long, can usually reach the upper sigmoid colon. Preexamination enemas or laxatives are usually unnecessary and may actually interfere with interpreting the findings. Biopsies, smears, and cultures may be taken and x-ray examination ordered if indicated.

HEMORRHOIDS

(Piles)

Varicosities of the veins of the hemorrhoidal plexuses. Internal hemorrhoids lie beneath the mucosa just above the anal canal; external hemorrhoids lie beneath the anoderm or external skin. Combined (internal-external) hemorrhoids may occur. Hemorrhoids are found in the right anterior, right posterior, and left lateroposterior positions.

Etiology

Since the superior hemorrhoidal plexus drains into the valveless portal venous system, the erect position of man predisposes to hemorrhoidal disease. Pregnancy is a common cause of hemorrhoids. Sedentary occupations, straining at work, sitting on hard, cold surfaces, prolonged standing, constipation, and diarrhea are no longer believed to cause hemorrhoids, but such factors may produce **thrombosed external hemorrhoids** (see below).

Symptoms, Signs, and Diagnosis

Bright red rectal bleeding, unmixed with the stool, is usually the first symptom. Protracted bleeding may cause marked secondary anemia. Prolapse occurs at first only with defecation and spontaneously reduces itself. Later, the protrusion must be reduced manually or may become permanently prolapsed. Mucoid discharge is most marked when the hemorrhoids are constantly protruding and may cause skin irritation. However, persistent pruritus ani is not a symptom of hemorrhoids. Pain occurs only when there is an acute attack of prolapse with inflammation and edema or when there is a coexisting painful lesion, such as a fissure.

The hemorrhoids may prolapse and become incarcerated. They may then appear dark because of intravascular thrombosis, but the mucosa will still be viable. Gangrene follows occlusion of the nutrient arteries supplying the hemorrhoids. The mucosa becomes black, loses its sheen, and appears dead.

The subcutaneous external varices may be seen on inspection. Unless internal hemorrhoids are prolapsed, anoscopy must be used to detect them. Proctosigmoidoscopy is needed to detect inflammatory or malignant disease at a higher level that may be responsible for the bleeding or other symptoms attributed to the hemorrhoids. Barium enema x-ray studies should be done in all patients over age 40 who have rectal bleeding.

Treatment

Straining at stool and diarrhea should be avoided. Suppositories and rectal ointments offer only transient anesthetic and astringent effects. Reducible prolapsed hemorrhoids should be replaced within the rectum by gentle pressure. The patient should lie down to reduce the protrusion whenever necessary. In the acute stage of prolapse, the patient should remain in bed, and cold compresses of either water or witch hazel should be applied. After the acute reaction has subsided, warm compresses or warm sitz baths are helpful. Sedatives should be taken as required.

Prolapsed, irreducible, inflamed, or gangrenous hemorrhoids may be treated conservatively or by immediate operation. Surgery offers the most rapid relief of symptoms and the shortest convalescence.

Early, uncomplicated, symptomatic internal hemorrhoids may be treated by sclerotherapy in which an irritating chemical solution is injected into the areolar tissue surrounding the hemorrhoidal varices. Phenol 5% in sesame oil or quinine urea hydrochloride, 5% aqueous solution, are effective sclerosing agents.

The rubber band method of treatment has become popular, especially in treating patients who are poor operative risks. This method uses a special instrument to place a rubber band around the base of the hemorrhoid to strangulate it.

Hemorrhoids may be destroyed by cryosurgery using liquid nitrogen or CO_2 to create an extremely low temperature in a probe that is applied to the hemorrhoid. This method usually does not require anesthesia or hospitalization, but it is cumbersome, less precise in application than surgery, and often produces copious, prolonged drainage and delayed bleeding.

Surgical excision of all redundant mucosa and hemorrhoidal tissue produces an excellent long-term result.

THROMBOSED EXTERNAL HEMORRHOID

(Perianal Hematoma)

A painful, subcutaneous, para- or intra-anal hematoma.

This common lesion is not a true hemorrhoid but rather a hematoma due to rupture of an external hemorrhoidal vein. The thrombosis follows a sudden increase in intravenous pressure and usually occurs after heavy lifting, coughing, sneezing, exercise, straining at stool, or parturition. The disorder occurs most frequently in otherwise healthy young people and is not related to internal hemorrhoidal disease. Recurrence is frequent.

The lesion is a very painful, tense, smooth, bluish elevation beneath the skin. The pain is greatest at the onset and gradually subsides in 2 to 3 days. Spontaneous rupture frequently occurs, with disgorgement of the thrombus and considerable bleeding. The lesion must be differentiated from a prolapsed internal hemorrhoid.

Symptoms may be eased by warm sitz baths and mild sedation. During the first 48 h, evacuation of the thrombus or complete excision under local anesthesia may give immediate relief. Spontaneous resolution will occur without treatment.

ANAL FISSURE

(Fissure in Ano; Anal Ulcer)

An acute longitudinal tear or a chronic ovoid ulcer in the stratified squamous epithelium of the anal canal.

Etiology, Symptoms, and Signs

Acute, linear fissure may be caused by passage of large stools, childbirth trauma, diarrhea, or iatrogenic trauma. Infants may develop acute fissures. **Chronic fissure** is actually a chronic, elliptic, or round ulcer which follows fibrosis due to chronic infection. The fissure usually lies in the posterior midline, but may occur in the anterior midline. An external skin tag (the **"sentinel pile"**) may be present at the lower end of the fissure and an enlarged ("hypertrophic") papilla at the upper end. Chronic fissures must be differentiated from carcinoma, primary lesions of syphilis, TB, and ulceration associated with granulomatous enteritis.

Fissures are extremely painful, especially during defecation, and cause marked spasm of the anal sphincters. Examination must be very gentle and may only require spreading the anus apart.

Treatment

Fissures often respond to conservative measures, including stool softeners and local anesthetic ointments (e.g., 5% lidocaine ointment) used before and after defecation. Warm (not hot) sitz baths for 10 or 15 min after each bowel movement or as often as necessary to ease discomfort will give temporary relief. Topical application of 50% phenol in oil is anesthetic and may interrupt the pain-spasm-pain cycle.

When conservative measures fail, surgery is required. Subcutaneous division of the stenotic internal sphincter in a lateral quadrant of the anal canal, with removal of the hypertrophic papilla and sentinel pile but without removal of the fissure itself, is usually curative. Removing the fissure and an adjacent crypt and anoplasty may also be necessary.

ANORECTAL ABSCESS

Etiology, Symptoms, and Signs

Anorectal abscess results from bacterial invasion of the pararectal spaces, usually extending from an anal crypt. A mixed infection usually occurs; *Escherichia coli*, *Proteus vulgaris*, streptococci, staphylococci, and bacteroides are predominant causes. The abscess may be subcutaneous, ischiorectal, retrorectal, submucous, pelvirectal (supralevator), or intramuscular.

Superficial abscesses are the most painful; swelling, redness, and tenderness are characteristic. Deeper abscesses cause toxic symptoms, but localized pain is less severe. External swelling does not occur, but digital rectal examination reveals tender swelling. High pelvirectal abscesses may cause no rectal symptoms and may be associated with lower abdominal pain and FUO. It must be remembered that inflammatory bowel disease (e.g., regional enteritis) is sometimes found in association with anorectal abscess.

Treatment

Prompt incision and adequate drainage are required; one should not wait until the abscess points externally. Suppuration is almost always present when the diagnosis is made. Antibiotics are of limited value. Persistent anorectal fistula may occur following drainage.

ANORECTAL FISTULA

(Fistula in Ano)

A tube-like tract with one opening in the anal canal and the other opening usually in the perianal skin.

Etiology

Fistulas are usually due to spontaneous or surgical drainage of pyogenic abscesses or, less commonly, to granulomatous disease of the intestine (see REGIONAL ENTERITIS in Ch. 57) or TB. Most fistulas originate in the anorectal crypts; others may result from diverticulitis, neoplasm, or trauma. Fistulas in infants are congenital and are more common in boys. Rectovaginal fistulas may be congenital or may follow radiotherapy, pelvic surgery, childbirth, or malignancy.

Symptoms, Signs, and Diagnosis

A history of recurrent abscess followed by intermittent or constant discharge is usual. On inspection, one or more secondary openings can be seen. In TB or granulomatous disease, the discharge may be watery and the margins of the opening violaceous. A cord-like tract can often be palpated. A probe can be inserted into the tract to determine its depth and direction. Anoscopic examination of the crypts may reveal the primary opening. Sigmoidoscopy is required. Roentgen fistulography in fistulas suspected of being noncryptogenic or extensive is of diagnostic value. Hidradenitis suppurativa, pilonidal sinus, dermal suppurative sinuses, and urethroperineal fistulas must be differentiated from cryptogenic fistulas.

Treatment

The only effective treatment is fistulotomy. The primary opening and the entire tract must be unroofed and converted into a "ditch." Partial division of the sphincters may be necessary. Some degree of incontinence may occur if a considerable portion of the sphincteric ring is divided. Fistulotomy is inadvisable in the presence of diarrhea, active ulcerative colitis, or active granulomatous enterocolitis since delayed wound healing may present a severe problem.

PROCTITIS

(See Chs. 57 and 162)

PILONIDAL DISEASE

Acute abscess or chronic draining sinuses in the sacrococcygeal area.

Pilonidal disease usually occurs in young, hirsute whites, and is more common in males. One or several midline or eccentric pits or sinuses occur in the skin of the sacral region and may lead to a cavity, often containing hair. The lesion is usually asymptomatic unless it becomes acutely infected.

Treatment of acute abscesses is by incision and drainage. As a rule, one or more chronic draining sinuses persist and must then be surgically extirpated by excision and primary closure or, preferably, by an open technic and marsupialization.

RECTAL PROLAPSE AND PROCIDENTIA

Protrusion of the rectum through the anus.

Transient, minor prolapse of just the rectal mucosa frequently occurs in otherwise normal infants. In adults, however, mucosal prolapse is persistent and may progressively worsen.

Procidentia consists of complete prolapse of the entire thickness of the rectum along with the peritoneum as a sliding hernia. Abnormal anterior displacement of the rectum due to elongation of the mesorectum is probably the primary cause.

The patient should be examined while standing or squatting, and straining, to determine the full extent of the prolapse. Sigmoidoscopy and barium enema x-rays of the colon must be done to search for intrinsic disease. Primary neurologic disorders must be ruled out.

Treatment

In infants and children conservative treatment is most satisfactory. Underlying nutritional disorders should be corrected and causes of straining eliminated. Strapping the buttocks together firmly between bowel movements usually facilitates spontaneous resolution of the prolapse. For simple mucosal prolapse in adults, the excess mucosa can be excised. For complete procidentia, an abdominal operation with elevation and posterior fixation of the rectum to the sacrum to correct its anterior displacement has been most successful. In patients who are very old or in poor general condition, a wire loop can be inserted which encircles the sphincteric ring (Thiersch procedure).

MALIGNANT TUMORS OF THE ANORECTUM

(See also Ch. 61)

Epidermoid (squamous cell) carcinoma of the anorectum comprises 3 to 5% of rectal and anal cancers. Leukoplakia, lymphogranuloma venereum, chronic fistulas, and irradiated anal skin are predisposing causes. Metastasis is along the lymphatics of the rectum as well as in the inguinal lymph nodes. Basal cell carcinoma, Bowen's disease (intradermal carcinoma), extramammary Paget's disease, cloacogenic carcinoma, and malignant melanoma are less common. Surgery is the **treatment** of choice.

FECAL INCONTINENCE

Loss of voluntary control of defecation.

Anal incontinence may result from injuries or diseases of the spinal cord, congenital abnormalities, accidental injuries to the rectum and anus, procidentia, senility, fecal impaction, extensive inflammatory processes, tumors, and deformities following dilation and obstetric and operative procedures.

Treatment for mild degrees of incontinence is a low-residue diet, anticholinergic drugs to reduce intestinal motility, enemas q 1 to 3 days with a device that allows retention of the irrigating fluid, and daily exercises of sphincteric contraction. Surgery, if required for repair, obtains good results if performed before atony of the muscle occurs. In treating fecal incontinence, biofeedback conditioning or direct electric stimulation may be of value if the sphincters are intact.

PRURITUS ANI

Anal and perianal itching.

Etiology

The perianal skin has a maximum "readiness to itch," and pruritus ani has many causes: (1) **dermatologic disorders** (e.g., psoriasis, atopic dermatitis); (2) **allergic reactions** such as contact dermatitis due to local anesthetics (especially the "-caine" preparations), various ointments, or aromatic and other chemicals used in soap; and eczema following the ingestion of certain foods (it is doubtful, however, that true allergy is a causative agent); (3) **microbes** such as fungi (e.g., dermatophytosis, candidiasis) and bacteria (secondary infection due to scratching); (4) **parasites** (pinworms and, less commonly, scabies or pediculosis); (5) **oral antibiotic therapy** (especially tetracyclines); (6) **disease processes** such as systemic diseases (e.g., diabetes mellitus, liver disease), proctologic disorders (e.g., skin tags, cryptitis, draining fistulas), and neoplasms (e.g., Bowen's disease, extramammary Paget's disease); (7) **hygiene**, either poor with residual irritating feces or overmeticulous with excessive use of soap and rubbing; (8) **warmth and hyperhidrosis**, due to tight body stocking, jockey shorts, warm bed clothing, obesity, climate; and (9) **psychogenic response** (the importance of the anxiety-itch-anxiety cycle varies from trivial to overwhelming). Hemorrhoids do not cause pruritus ani.

Skin changes may be characteristic or minimal and may be masked by excoriation due to scratching and secondary infection.

Treatment

Eating spices (especially peppers) and citrus fruits (especially grapefruit) should be avoided. Clothing should be loose and bed clothing light. Soft, moistened paper tissue or cotton or soft cloth impregnated with glycerin and witch hazel should be used to clean after bowel movements. Soap applied directly to the perianal area during bathing, self-medication with anesthetic ointments, and scratching and rubbing with harsh toilet tissue are interdicted. Liberal and frequent dusting with nonmedicated talcum powder may combat moisture. Hydrocortisone acetate 1% in emulsion base, applied sparingly q.i.d., is usually most effective. Iodochlorhydroxyquin 3% may be added as a fungicide. Systemic causes and parasitic infestations must be treated specifically. Biopsies should be taken in refractory lesions to detect malignancy. X-ray treatment and surgery or injections to create permanent local anesthesia are rarely if ever indicated.

FOREIGN BODIES IN THE RECTUM

Swallowed foreign bodies, gallstones, or fecaliths may lodge at the anorectal juncture. Urinary calculi, vaginal pessaries, or surgical sponges or instruments may erode into the rectum. Foreign bodies, some bizarre, may be introduced intentionally into the rectum; enema tips and thermometers, broken or intact, are among the most common.

Sudden, excruciating pain during defecation should arouse suspicion of a penetrating foreign body, which is usually lodged at the anorectal juncture. Other manifestations depend upon the size and shape of the foreign body, its duration in situ, and the presence of infection or perforation.

Digital rectal and proctoscopic examinations are usually diagnostic. X-ray examination is helpful only when the foreign body is radiopaque.

Treatment

Smaller objects may be removed through an endoscope. Larger ones often are more difficult to grasp and extract as they tend to slip through the tight sphincteric ring into the commodious ampulla. Special procedures for removal include using gauze covering, rubber tubing, a corkscrew, or a tonsil snare. A hole may be bored through the foreign body or a catheter passed beside it in order to overcome the suction which opposes withdrawal. Simultaneous pressure upon the abdomen is sometimes helpful. Extractions usually require spinal anesthesia. Sphincterotomy may be necessary.

63.   INTRODUCTION

The liver, the largest and metabolically the most complex organ in the body, consists of myriads of individual functional units known as **hepatic acini**. The organ has a remarkable capacity for regeneration in response to injury. Even extensive patchy necrosis usually resolves completely, as in acute viral hepatitis. Incomplete regeneration with fibrosis, however, results from confluent necrosis which bridges entire acini, or from less pronounced but ongoing chronic damage.

For clinical purposes the liver can be considered in terms of blood supply, parenchymal cells, Kupffer cells, and biliary passages. Specific diseases tend to affect these components in predictable patterns, often with characteristic clinical and biochemical consequences. Symptoms of liver disease usually reflect parenchymal cell necrosis or impaired bile secretion, rather than fibrosis.

The liver receives its **blood supply** from both the portal vein and the hepatic artery; the former provides about 75% of the total 1500 ml/min flow. Small branches of each vessel, the terminal portal venule and terminal hepatic arteriole, enter each acinus at the portal triad (zone 1 of Rappaport). The then pooled blood flows through sinusoids between plates of parenchymal cells. Nutrients are exchanged across the spaces of Disse which separate parenchymal cells from the porous sinusoidal lining. Sinusoidal flow from adjacent acini merges at the terminal hepatic venule (central vein, zone 3). These tiny vessels coalesce and eventually form the hepatic vein which carries all efferent blood into the inferior vena cava. A rich supply of lymphatic vessels also drains the liver. Interference with the hepatic blood supply is common in cirrhosis and other chronic diseases and is usually manifested by portal hypertension (see Ch. 73).

Hepatic parenchymal cells comprise the bulk of the organ. These polygonal cells lie next to the blood-filled sinusoids and are arranged in sheets or plates which radiate from each portal triad toward adjacent central veins. Parenchymal cells carry out exquisitely complex metabolic processes and are responsible for the liver's central role in metabolism. Their more important functions include the formation and excretion of bile; regulation of carbohydrate homeostasis; lipid synthesis and secretion of plasma lipoproteins; control of cholesterol metabolism; formation of urea, serum albumin, clotting factors, enzymes, and numerous other proteins; and metabolism or detoxification of drugs and other foreign substances. In most hepatic diseases parenchymal cell dysfunction occurs to some degree and produces various clinical and laboratory abnormalities (discussed below).

Kupffer cells line the hepatic sinusoids and are an important part of the body's reticuloendothelial system. These spindle-shaped cells filter out minute foreign particles and bacteria, and play a role in immune processes involving the liver. Because of its Kupffer cells and rich blood supply, the liver is often secondarily involved in infections and other systemic illnesses.

The **biliary passages** begin as tiny bile canaliculi formed by adjacent parenchymal cells. These microvilli-lined structures progressively coalesce into ductules, interlobular bile ducts, and larger hepatic ducts. Outside the porta hepatis, the main hepatic duct joins the cystic duct from the gallbladder to form the common bile duct, which drains into the duodenum. Interference with the flow of bile anywhere along this route produces the characteristic clinical and biochemical picture of cholestasis (see Ch. 64).

64.   CLINICAL FEATURES OF LIVER DISEASE

Symptoms and signs of hepatic dysfunction are numerous; only the major clinical features are discussed here. Some abnormalities occur only in chronic disease; others are seen in either acute or chronic disorders.

JAUNDICE

A yellow discoloration of the skin, sclerae, and other tissues due to excess circulating bilirubin. Serum bilirubin is normally < 1 mg/100 ml, with the conjugated or direct-reacting fraction not > 0.3 mg/100 ml. Jaundice becomes apparent if levels exceed 2 to 2.5 mg/100 ml. Mild jaundice is best seen by examining the sclerae in natural light.

BILIRUBIN METABOLISM

The catabolism of heme yields bile pigments; sources include the Hb of degenerating RBCs, RBC precursors in the marrow, and heme proteins of liver and other tissues. There is no evidence for the direct synthesis of bilirubin from heme precursors. Bilirubin is a pigmented organic anion closely related to porphyrins and other tetrapyrroles. As an insoluble waste product, it must be converted to water-soluble forms for excretion. This transformation is the overall purpose of bilirubin metabolism, which takes place in 5 major steps:

1. **Formation:** About 250 to 350 mg of bilirubin forms daily; 75 to 80% is derived from the break-down of senescent RBCs. The remaining 20 to 25%, the **early-labeled bilirubin,** comes from other heme proteins located primarily in the bone marrow and liver. The heme moiety of Hb is degraded to iron and the intermediate product biliverdin by the enzyme heme oxygenase. Biliverdin is converted to bilirubin via another enzyme, biliverdin reductase. These steps occur primarily in cells of the reticuloendothelial system.

Enhanced destruction of RBCs (hemolysis) is the most important cause of increased bilirubin formation. Increased production of early-labeled bilirubin occurs in some hematologic disorders with ineffective erythropoiesis, but usually is not clinically important.

2. **Plasma transport:** Bilirubin, which is insoluble in water, is transported in the plasma bound to albumin. The binding weakens under certain conditions, such as acidosis, and there is competition for the binding sites, e.g., by certain antibiotics and salicylates. Because this circulating **unconjugated** ("indirect-reacting") bilirubin cannot cross cell membranes other than those in the liver, it does not appear in the urine.

3. **Hepatic uptake:** The details of bilirubin uptake by the liver have not been worked out. The process is rapid and probably involves active transport, but does not include uptake of the attached serum albumin. The importance of intracellular binding proteins (ligandin or Y protein, etc.) is still unclear.

4. **Conjugation:** Free bilirubin is concentrated in the liver, then conjugated with glucuronic acid to form bilirubin diglucuronide or **conjugated** ("direct-reacting") bilirubin. This reaction, catalyzed by the microsomal enzyme glucuronyl transferase, renders the pigment water-soluble. Recent evidence suggests that glucuronyl transferase forms only bilirubin monoglucuronide, with the second glucuronic acid moiety being added at the bile canaliculus via a different enzyme system. Bilirubin conjugates other than the diglucuronide are also formed, but their significance is uncertain.

5. **Biliary excretion:** Conjugated bilirubin is secreted into the bile canaliculus with other bile constituents. Other organic anions or drugs can affect this complex process. In the gut, bacterial flora deconjugate and reduce the pigment to various compounds called **stercobilinogens.** Most of these are excreted in the feces and impart the brown color to stool, although substantial amounts are absorbed and re-excreted in the bile; small amounts reach the urine as **urobilinogen.** The kidney can also excrete bilirubin diglucuronide, but not unconjugated bilirubin. This explains the dark urine characteristic of hepatocellular or cholestatic jaundice, whereas urinary bile is absent in hemolytic jaundice.

DISORDERS OF BILIRUBIN METABOLISM

At any of the above steps, abnormalities can result in jaundice. Increased formation, impaired hepatic uptake, or decreased conjugation all cause unconjugated hyperbilirubinemia. Impaired biliary excretion produces conjugated hyperbilirubinemia. In practice, however, hepatic disease and biliary obstruction create multiple defects, resulting in a mixed hyperbilirubinemia. Therefore, in most patients with obvious hepatobiliary disease, bilirubin fractionation is of little diagnostic value, and in particular will not differentiate hepatocellular from obstructive jaundice. Fractionation is useful if one of the disorders discussed below is suspected; these produce jaundice in the absence of demonstrable liver disease.

Unconjugated Hyperbilirubinemia

Hemolysis: Increased formation of bilirubin occurs in hemolysis and may exceed the liver's capacity to handle it, even though the normal liver can handle considerably more bilirubin than the normal load. Because the hyperbilirubinemia is unconjugated, bile is absent from the urine. Even in brisk hemolysis, serum bilirubin rarely exceeds 3 to 5 mg/100 ml unless hepatic damage also exists. The combination of modest hemolysis and mild liver disease, however, may result in surprisingly severe jaundice; in these circumstances the hyperbilirubinemia is mixed. Hemolytic anemia is discussed in Ch. 92.

Gilbert's syndrome: Previously considered rare, but by far the commonest of the benign chronic hyperbilirubinemias, this disorder may affect as much as 3 to 5% of the population. Its pathogenesis is uncertain. There appear to be complex defects in the hepatic uptake of bilirubin. In addition, glucuronyl transferase activity is low; therefore, the disorder may be related to the much rarer Type II Crigler-Najjar syndrome (see below). Many patients also have mildly diminished RBC survival, but this is insufficient to explain the hyperbilirubinemia.

Mild unconjugated hyperbilirubinemia is the only significant abnormality. The disorder, presumably lifelong, is most often detected in young adults with vague nonspecific complaints. Bilirubin usually fluctuates between 2 and 5 mg/100 ml and tends to increase with fasting and other stresses. In some cases family members are affected, but a clear genetic pattern is often difficult to establish.

This disorder is significant clinically only because it is often misdiagnosed as chronic hepatitis. However, it can be easily differentiated by normal liver function tests, absence of urinary bile, and characteristic bilirubin fractionation. Hemolysis is differentiated by the absence of anemia or reticulocytosis. Liver histology is normal, but biopsy is not needed to make the diagnosis. Patients with Gilbert's syndrome should be reassured that they do not have liver disease.

Crigler-Najjar syndrome: This rare inherited disorder is associated with a deficiency of glucuronyl transferase and occurs in 2 forms: Patients with Type I (complete) disease, which is autosomal recessive, have severe hyperbilirubinemia and usually die of kernicterus within the first year of life. Patients with Type II (partial) disease, which appears to be an autosomal dominant trait, have less severe hyperbilirubinemia ($<$ 20 mg/100 ml) and usually survive into adulthood without neurologic damage. Phenobarbital, which induces the partially deficient glucuronyl transferase, can diminish the jaundice.

Breast milk jaundice: In this rare disease of infants, hyperbilirubinemia is induced by breast feeding. Inhibition of glucuronyl transferase by a steroid present in the milk has been blamed, but this is unproven. A similar, but probably unrelated disorder, has been described in which bilirubin conjugation is inhibited by an unknown serum factor (the Lucey-Driscoll syndrome).

Primary shunt hyperbilirubinemia: This is a rare, familial benign condition associated with overproduction of early-labeled bilirubin.

Noncholestatic Conjugated Hyperbilirubinemia

Dubin-Johnson syndrome: Asymptomatic mild jaundice characterizes this rare autosomal recessive disorder. In contrast to Gilbert's syndrome, the hyperbilirubinemia is conjugated and bile appears in the urine. The liver is deeply pigmented due to an intracellular melanin-like substance, but is otherwise histologically normal. The cause of the pigment deposition is unknown. The basic defect involves impaired excretion of various organic anions, including BSP and cholecystographic dyes as well as bilirubin. Transaminase and alkaline phosphatase levels are usually normal, and bile salt excretion is not impaired. For unknown reasons, derangements in urinary coproporphyrin excretion accompany this syndrome.

Rotor syndrome: This rare disease is similar to the Dubin-Johnson syndrome, but the liver is not pigmented and there are other subtle metabolic differences.

CLINICAL APPROACH TO JAUNDICE

The differential diagnosis of jaundice involves attempting to answer specific questions which narrow the possibilities. The first question should be whether the jaundice is due to hemolysis (uncommon), hepatocellular dysfunction (common), or biliary obstruction (intermediate). If hepatobiliary disease is present, other important questions follow: Is the condition acute or chronic? Is it due to primary hepatic disease or to a systemic disorder involving the liver? Are alcohol or other drugs responsible? Is cholestasis of intra- or extrahepatic origin? Will surgical therapy be needed? Are complications present? These questions are approached by clinical, functional, and morphologic assessment.

Clinical Evaluation

Diagnostic errors usually result from an inadequate history and physical examination with undue reliance on laboratory data.

Jaundice without dark urine suggests unconjugated hyperbilirubinemia due to hemolysis or Gilbert's syndrome rather than hepatobiliary disease. See other signs and symptoms below for clinical features that suggest a parenchymal or cholestatic disorder. Ascites, signs of portal hypertension, or cutaneous and endocrine features usually imply a chronic rather than an acute process. Patients frequently notice dark urine before skin discoloration, and its onset therefore provides a better guide to the duration of jaundice. Sudden nausea and vomiting preceding jaundice most often indicate acute hepatitis or common duct obstruction by stone; abdominal pain or rigors favor the latter. More insidious anorexia and malaise occur in many conditions, but particularly suggest alcoholic liver disease or chronic hepatitis.

A systemic disorder rather than primary liver disease should be sought. For example, distended jugular veins are an important clue to congestive heart failure or constrictive pericarditis in a patient with hepatomegaly and ascites. Cachexia and an unusually hard or lumpy liver are more often due to metastatic tumor than to cirrhosis. Diffuse lymphadenopathy suggests infectious mononucleosis in an acutely jaundiced patient and lymphoma or leukemia in a chronic illness. Hepatosplenomegaly without other signs of chronic liver disease may be due to an infiltrative disorder such as lymphoma or amyloidosis; schistosomiasis and malaria commonly give this picture in endemic areas.

Other diagnostic features and the approach to cholestatic jaundice are discussed below.

Functional Evaluation

Liver function tests are discussed in more detail in Ch. 65. They are usually helpful but should never replace clinical judgment.

Mild hyperbilirubinemia with normal transaminase and alkaline phosphatase levels usually reflects hemolysis or Gilbert's syndrome rather than liver disease; bilirubin fractionation settles the issue. By contrast, the depth of jaundice and bilirubin fractionation does not help to differentiate hepatocellular from cholestatic jaundice. Striking transaminase elevations suggest a hepatitis or an acute hypoxic episode, and disproportionate increases of alkaline phosphatase a cholestatic or infiltrative disorder. In the latter, bilirubin is typically normal or only slightly increased. Bilirubin levels > 25 to 30 mg/100 ml are usually due to hemolysis or to renal dysfunction superimposed on severe hepatobiliary disease, as the latter alone rarely causes such deep jaundice. Low albumin and high globulin levels indicate chronic rather than acute liver disease. Improvement of an elevated prothrombin time after vitamin K administration (5 to 10 mg IM for 2 to 3 days) favors a cholestatic over a hepatocellular process. This fact, however, has limited diagnostic value, since patients with hepatocellular disease may improve when given vitamin K.

X-rays and other ancillary investigations are discussed in Ch. 65.

Morphologic Evaluation

Percutaneous liver biopsy has great diagnostic value but is not required in most cases of jaundice. **Peritoneoscopy** (laparoscopy) permits direct inspection of the liver and gallbladder without the trauma of a full laparotomy, and is useful in selected cases of jaundice. **Diagnostic laparotomy** may be needed in some patients with cholestatic jaundice or unexplained hepatosplenomegaly. These procedures are discussed more fully in Ch. 66.

CHOLESTASIS

A clinical and biochemical syndrome that results when bile flow is impaired. The term "cholestasis" is preferred to "obstructive jaundice" because a mechanical obstruction is not always present.

Etiology

Bile flow may be impaired at any point from the liver cell canaliculus to the ampulla of Vater. For clinical purposes a distinction between intra- and extrahepatic causes is crucial.

The commonest **intrahepatic** causes are viral or other hepatitis (see Ch. 69), drugs (see Ch. 70), and alcoholic liver disease (see Ch. 71). Some less common etiologies are primary biliary cirrhosis (see Ch. 68), cholestasis of pregnancy (see HEPATIC DISORDERS IN PREGNANCY in Vol. II, Ch. 16), metastatic carcinoma, pericholangitis secondary to ulcerative colitis, and numerous rare disorders.

Extrahepatic cholestasis is most often due to a common duct stone or pancreatic carcinoma. Less frequently, benign stricture of the common duct (usually related to previous surgery), ductal carcinoma, pancreatitis or pancreatic pseudocyst, and sclerosing cholangitis are causes.

Cholestasis in infants, caused by neonatal hepatitis and biliary atresia, are discussed under GASTROINTESTINAL DEFECTS and under NEONATAL INFECTIONS in Vol. II, Ch. 21.

Pathophysiology and Clinical Findings

Cholestasis reflects **bile secretory failure;** the mechanisms are complex, even in mechanical obstruction. Contributing factors may include interference with microsomal hydroxylating enzymes, which leads to the formation of poorly soluble bile acids; impaired activity of Na^+, K^+-ATPase, necessary for canalicular bile flow; interference with the function of microfilaments, thought to be important for canalicular function; and enhanced ductular reabsorption of bile constituents.

The pathophysiologic effects of cholestasis are independent of the underlying etiology, and reflect 2 general consequences: bile constituents back up into the systemic circulation and fail to enter the gut for excretion. Bilirubin, bile salts, alkaline phosphatase, cholesterol, and phospholipids are the most important constituents affected.

Retention of bilirubin produces jaundice with mixed hyperbilirubinemia; dark urine results from urinary excretion of conjugated bilirubin. Less bilirubin in the gut causes pale stools. An excess of circulating bile salts is thought to produce intense pruritus due to skin irritation, although correlation with blood or cutaneous levels of bile salts is poor; failure to excrete bile salts results in steatorrhea and an elevated prothrombin time, because fat and vitamin K cannot be absorbed. The increased prothrombin time may lead to a bleeding tendency.

The most characteristic laboratory abnormality is a disproportionately high serum alkaline phosphatase level; this is primarily due to increased hepatic synthesis rather than impaired excretion. High serum cholesterol and phospholipid levels result from impaired biliary excretion of these lipids, although increased hepatic synthesis and decreased plasma esterification of cholesterol also contribute. The lipids circulate as a unique, abnormal, low-density lipoprotein called lipoprotein-X.

In **chronic cholestasis** muddy skin pigmentation, excoriations from pruritus, and cutaneous lipid deposits such as xanthelasmas or xanthomas may develop. Malabsorption of calcium and vitamin D may eventually result in osteomalacia, osteoporosis, and bone pain.

Any systemic symptoms (anorexia, vomiting, fever, etc.) reflect the underlying cause rather than cholestasis itself.

Diagnosis

Intra- and extrahepatic cholestasis must be differentiated. A detailed **history** and **physical examination** are especially important, since most diagnostic errors result from inadequate clinical study and over-reliance on laboratory data. Intrahepatic cholestasis is favored by symptoms of hepatitis; heavy alcohol ingestion; recent use of new drugs; or signs of chronic parenchymal disease such as spider nevi, splenomegaly, or ascites. Extrahepatic cholestasis is suggested by biliary or pancreatic pain, rigors, or a palpable gallbladder.

Laboratory tests are of limited diagnostic value. Serum bilirubin and alkaline phosphatase levels may reflect the severity of cholestasis but not its cause. Marked serum transaminase elevations suggest a hepatocellular process but are occasionally seen in extrahepatic cholestasis, especially with acute obstruction due to a common duct stone. High serum amylase levels usually indicate extrahepatic obstruction. After vitamin K is given, an improved prothrombin time favors extrahepatic obstruction, but parenchymal disorders may also respond. The presence of antimitochondrial antibody will help to distinguish primary biliary cirrhosis from extrahepatic obstruction.

X-rays of the biliary tract are often essential, but the liver cannot excrete contrast media in significant cholestasis of any cause. Oral cholecystography or IV cholangiography may be tried if the serum bilirubin level is < 3 to 4 mg/100 ml, but nonvisualization does not always indicate an extrahepatic condition. Barium swallow may show a pancreatic mass, but usually is not helpful.

The most valuable radiologic technics unfortunately require specialized expertise and equipment and are not widely available. Transhepatic and retrograde cholangiography provide direct visualization of the biliary tract and are the most accurate, but they involve some risk to the patient. *Ultrasound and computed tomography scanning are noninvasive and reliably reveal dilated bile ducts, which implies mechanical obstruction;* however, absence of this sign does not necessarily indicate intrahepatic cholestasis.

Although **liver biopsy** usually clarifies the diagnosis, errors may arise, especially in drug cholestasis or early extrahepatic obstruction. Biopsy is safe in most cholestatic patients but relatively hazardous with severe or longstanding extrahepatic obstruction.

Except in patients with suppurative cholangitis, cholestasis is not an emergency. The approach to diagnosis should be based on clinical judgment plus the local availability of specialized technics. If the diagnosis is initially uncertain, serial liver function tests should be used to monitor the patient. In general, liver biopsy is preferable if clinical judgment favors an intrahepatic cause; assessment of the biliary tree is required if mechanical obstruction is thought to be more likely. In the latter case, cholestasis that is improving should first be evaluated by noninvasive x-rays or ultrasound studies of the biliary tract. Patients with progressive disease may need direct cholangiography (transhepatic or retrograde). **Diagnostic laparotomy** is indicated if cholestasis worsens and simpler tests are not helpful.

Treatment

Extrahepatic biliary obstruction usually requires surgical therapy, which is contraindicated in intrahepatic cholestasis. Treating the underlying cause usually suffices. Pruritus in irreversible disorders such as primary biliary cirrhosis usually responds to cholestyramine (8 to 16 gm/day given in 2 to 4 divided doses), which binds bile salts in the intestine. Hypoprothrombinemia improves after phytonadione (vitamin K_1); 5 to 10 mg/day IM is given for 2 to 3 days, unless severe hepatocellular damage is present. Supplements of calcium and fat-soluble vitamins A and D may be needed in longstanding cases, and severe steatorrhea can be minimized by partial replacement of dietary fat with medium-chain triglycerides.

HEPATOMEGALY

Enlargement of the liver indicates either primary or secondary liver disease, but absence of hepatomegaly does not exclude a serious disorder. When the liver is palpable, its upper border should be percussed to ensure that the organ is not merely low-lying. The lower border of a normal liver is often palpable at or slightly below the right costal margin. Serial determinations of liver size may be of prognostic value; e.g., a rapidly shrinking liver in fulminant hepatitis implies a poor outcome, as does a rapidly enlarging organ in metastatic carcinoma.

Equally as important as liver size is its quality on palpation. The normal liver has a rubbery-soft, sharp, smooth edge. This consistency is often maintained in enlargement due to acute hepatitis, fatty infiltration, passive congestion, and early biliary obstruction. The cirrhotic liver edge is usually firm, blunt, and irregular; individual cirrhotic nodules are rarely palpable, and discernible lumps suggest malignant infiltration. Audible friction rubs or bruits over the liver, though rare, are other valuable clues to tumor.

Hepatic tenderness is overdiagnosed, usually because of the patient's anxiety when the liver edge is palpated. True tenderness, a deep-seated aching sensation, is best elicited by punch percussion or compression of the rib cage. It is felt in acute hepatitis, passive congestion, and malignancy.

ASCITES

The presence of free fluid in the peritoneal cavity.

Etiology

In liver disease, ascites indicates a chronic or subacute disorder and is not seen in acute conditions such as uncomplicated viral hepatitis, drug reactions, or biliary obstruction. The commonest cause is cirrhosis, especially of alcoholic etiology. Other hepatic causes include chronic active hepatitis, severe alcoholic hepatitis without cirrhosis, and hepatic vein obstruction. Portal vein thrombosis does not usually produce ascites unless parenchymal damage is also present.

Nonhepatic causes of ascites include generalized fluid retention due to systemic disease such as congestive heart failure, nephrotic syndrome, severe hypoalbuminemia, or constrictive pericarditis; and intra-abdominal causes such as carcinomatosis or tuberculous peritonitis. Hypothyroidism occasionally causes marked ascites, and pancreatitis rarely produces surprisingly large amounts of fluid ("pancreatic ascites"). Patients with renal failure, especially those on hemodialysis, occasionally develop unexplained intra-abdominal fluid ("nephrogenic ascites").

Pathophysiology

The mechanisms that produce ascites are complex and incompletely understood. Two important factors in liver disease are low serum osmotic pressure due to hypoalbuminemia and high portal venous pressure; these appear to act synergistically by altering the Starling forces that govern fluid exchange across the peritoneal membrane. Hepatic lymphatic obstruction may also be involved. Circulating blood volume is usually normal or high, yet the kidney behaves as if it were low and avidly retains sodium; urinary sodium concentration is typically < 5 mEq/L. This has led to the concept that renal sodium retention is due to decreased "effective" circulating volume secondary to the ascites. Other evidence, however, suggests that the kidney plays a primary role in initiating the process, perhaps by a neural or humoral mechanism, and that the ascites is a result rather than the cause of the sodium retention (the "overflow" theory of ascites). Increased circulating aldosterone probably contributes to renal sodium retention and is due both to enhanced production and to decreased metabolism.

Symptoms, Signs, and Diagnosis

Nonspecific abdominal discomfort and dyspnea may occur with massive ascites, but lesser amounts are usually asymptomatic. Diagnosis is made by detecting shifting dullness on abdominal percussion. In advanced cases the belly is taut, the umbilicus is flat or everted, and a fluid wave can be elicited. Differentiation from obesity, gaseous distention, pregnancy, or ovarian tumors and other intra-abdominal masses usually is easily made by clinical examination, but diagnostic paracentesis may be required. In liver disease or in intra-abdominal disorders, ascites is usually isolated or out of proportion to peripheral edema; in systemic disease, the reverse is usually true.

If the cause is uncertain, a **diagnostic paracentesis** should be done. From 50 to 100 ml of fluid is removed and, as clinically indicated, is assessed for gross appearance, protein content, blood cells, cytology, culture, acid-fast stain, or amylase. In most disorders the fluid is clear and straw-colored. Turbidity and a high WBC count suggest infection, while sanguineous fluid usually signals neoplasm or tuberculosis. The rare milky (chylous) ascites is most common with lymphoma. A protein concentration of < 3 gm/100 ml favors liver disease or a systemic disorder; a higher protein content suggests an exudative cause such as tumor or infection, but ascitic protein in cirrhosis occasionally exceeds 4 gm/100 ml.

Treatment

Bed rest and dietary sodium restriction are the mainstays of therapy. A 20- to 40-mEq/day sodium diet, though unpalatable, usually initiates diuresis within a few days and rarely causes serious electrolyte derangements. Diuretics should be used if rigid sodium restriction fails. Spironolactone 100 to 200 mg/day or triamterene 300 mg/day orally in 2 or 3 divided doses is usually effective without causing the marked potassium loss often associated with thiazides or related diuretics. Fluid restriction is not needed unless serum sodium falls below 130 mEq/L and oral fluid intake is high. Unless massive ascites causes respiratory embarrassment, therapeutic paracentesis should not be done, because it depletes the body of needed protein and may impair circulating volume. Technics for the autologous infusion of ascites, such as the LeVeen peritoneovenous shunt, are associated with complications; their role in managing resistant ascites is controversial.

Changes in body weight and urinary sodium determinations measure response to treatment. Weight loss of about 0.5 kg/day is optimum, as the ascitic compartment cannot be mobilized much more rapidly. Harsh diuresis produces fluid loss at the expense of the intravascular compartment and may cause renal failure or electrolyte imbalance, such as hypokalemia, which may precipitate hepatic encephalopathy. Inadequate dietary sodium restriction is the usual reason for persistent ascites.

PORTAL–SYSTEMIC ENCEPHALOPATHY

(Hepatic Encephalopathy; Hepatic Coma)

A neuropsychiatric syndrome due to liver disease and usually associated with portal-systemic shunting of venous blood. The term "portal-systemic encephalopathy" is more descriptive of the pathophysiology than "hepatic encephalopathy" or "hepatic coma," but clinically all 3 are used interchangeably.

Etiology

Portal-systemic encephalopathy may be seen in fulminant acute hepatitis due to viruses, drugs, or toxins, but more commonly occurs in cirrhosis or other chronic disorders where extensive portal-systemic collaterals have developed. The syndrome also follows portacaval shunt or similar surgical procedures which create portal-systemic connections.

In patients with chronic liver disease, encephalopathy is usually precipitated by specific, potentially reversible stresses, such as GI bleeding; infection; electrolyte imbalance, especially hypokalemia; alcoholic debauches; or iatrogenically by tranquilizers, sedatives, analgesics, and diuretics.

Pathogenesis

The liver metabolizes and detoxifies digestive products brought from the gut by the portal vein. In hepatic disease these products escape into the systemic circulation if portal blood bypasses parenchymal cells or if the function of these cells is severely impaired. The resulting toxic effect on the brain produces the clinical picture.

The offending toxic substances are not precisely known, and the syndrome is probably multifactorial. Ammonia, a product of protein digestion, probably plays an important role, but biogenic amines, short-chain fatty acids, and other enteric products may also be responsible or may act with ammonia. Aromatic amino acid levels in serum are usually high and branched chain levels low, but whether this is causal is unclear. The pathogenesis of the cerebral toxicity is also uncertain. Alterations in cerebrovascular permeability and cellular integrity may play a role, especially in fulminant hepatitis. The brains of patients with liver disease appear abnormally sensitive to metabolic stresses. Interference with cerebral energy metabolism and inhibition of neural impulses by toxic amines acting as false neurotransmitters may occur.

Pathologic changes are usually confined to hyperplasia of astrocytes, with little or no neuronal damage, but in fulminant hepatitis, cerebral edema is common.

Symptoms, Signs, and Diagnosis

Personality changes, e.g., inappropriate behavior, altered mood, and impaired judgment, are common early manifestations and may antedate any apparent change in consciousness. Sophisticated psychomotor tests in cirrhotic patients can often detect such abnormalities not suspected clinically. Usually, **impaired consciousness** occurs. Initially, subtle sleep pattern changes or sluggish movement and speech may be present. Drowsiness, confusion, stupor, and frank coma indicate increasingly advanced encephalopathy. **Constructional apraxia**, in which the patient cannot reproduce simple designs such as a star, is a characteristic early sign. A typical musty sweet odor of the breath, **fetor hepaticus**, frequently occurs. A peculiar and characteristic flapping tremor, **asterixis**, is elicited when the patient holds his arms outstretched with wrists dorsiflexed; as coma progresses, this sign disappears and **hyperreflexia** and the **Babinski response** may be seen. **Agitation** or **mania** may occur in fulminant cases and in children, but is otherwise uncommon. **Seizures** and **localizing neurologic signs** are also uncommon. Their presence should suggest another cause of coma such as subdural hematoma.

The diagnosis should be possible on clinical grounds. There is no correlation with liver function tests. An **EEG** shows diffuse slow-wave activity even in mild cases, and may be useful in questionable early encephalopathy. The **CSF** is unremarkable except for mild protein elevation. **Blood ammonia levels** are usually elevated, but values correlate poorly with clinical status; bedside judgment is a better guide.

Prognosis

Encephalopathy due to chronic liver disease usually responds to treatment, especially if the precipitating cause is reversible. In most such cases the syndrome completely regresses without permanent neurologic sequelae. Some patients, especially those with surgical portacaval shunts, require continuous therapy, and irreversible extrapyramidal signs or spastic paraparesis may eventually develop; this is rare. Coma associated with fulminant hepatitis is fatal in up to 80% of cases despite intensive therapy, and patients with advanced chronic liver failure often die in hepatic coma.

Treatment

Precipitating causes should be sought; treating the cause may be sufficient in mild cases. Eliminating toxic enteric products is the other main therapy: (1) The bowels should be cleared with enemas. (2) Dietary protein should be eliminated (20 to 40 gm/day may be allowed in mild cases). Oral or IV carbohydrate will supply the lost calories. (3) Oral neomycin, 4 to 6 gm/day in 4 divided doses, helps to minimize bacteria-formed toxins, and can be tube-fed in liquid form to comatose patients. Parenteral antibiotics are usually ineffective. (4) Oral lactulose is a useful alternative to neomycin, especially in cases of mild or chronic encephalopathy. This synthetic disaccharide syrup alters colonic pH and flora, and also acts as an osmotic cathartic. The initial dosage, 30 to 45 ml t.i.d., should be adjusted to maintain 2 or 3 soft stools daily.

Sedation deepens the coma and should be avoided, even if the patient is agitated. Treating coma due to fulminant hepatitis by exchange transfusion and other complex procedures designed to remove circulating toxins has not been proved valuable. High-dose corticosteroids should not be used, because in controlled trials they have proved ineffective. Other treatment under study includes L-dopa, a precursor of normal neurotransmitters; bromocriptine, a dopamine agonist; infusions of branched chain amino acids or of keto-analogs of essential amino acids; and development of an "artificial liver." Of these, amino acid preparations show the greatest promise for routine management of encephalopathy.

PORTAL HYPERTENSION
(See Ch. 73)

OTHER SYMPTOMS AND SIGNS

SYSTEMIC ABNORMALITIES

Anorexia, fatigue, and weakness are common features of liver disease due to parenchymal dysfunction. Fever may occur, especially in viral or alcoholic hepatitis, but rigors are rare and in a jaundiced patient suggest biliary obstruction with cholangitis. Profound anorexia and nausea are especially common in viral and alcoholic hepatitis. Marked deterioration of general health and development of a "cirrhotic habitus" with wasted extremities and protuberant belly often signal advanced cirrhosis.

SKIN AND ENDOCRINE CHANGES

Patients with chronic liver disease can develop several cutaneous and endocrine abnormalities. Spider nevi (vascular spiders), palmar erythema, gynecomastia, testicular atrophy, impotence, and amenorrhea or other menstrual irregularities are probably caused by altered hormone metabolism in the diseased liver. Parotid gland enlargement and Dupuytren's contractures may also occur, especially in alcoholic cirrhosis. In hemochromatosis, deposition of iron and melanin makes the skin slate gray or bronze. Chronic cholestasis often causes muddy skin pigmentation, excoriations from constant pruritus, and cutaneous lipid deposits (xanthelasmas or xanthomas).

Glucose intolerance, hyperinsulinism, insulin resistance, and hyperglucagonemia are common in cirrhosis; the elevated insulin levels may be ascribed to decreased hepatic degradation rather than increased secretion, while the opposite is true for glucagon. Thyroid function tests must be interpreted with caution because of altered hepatic handling of thyroid hormones. Complex derangements occur in the metabolism of sex hormones. In male cirrhotics, estrogen levels are generally high and testosterone levels low, possibly in part due to a direct toxic effect of alcohol on the gonads.

HEMATOLOGIC DISTURBANCES

Multiple hematologic abnormalities are associated with liver disease. Anemia is frequent. Its pathogenesis may involve blood loss, nutritional folate deficiency, hemolysis, marrow suppression by alcohol, and chronic liver disease per se. Leukopenia and thrombocytopenia often accompany portal hypertension, while leukocytosis is seen in cholangitis, tumor, and fulminant hepatitis.

Coagulation disturbances are common and complex. Impaired hepatic synthesis of clotting factors is frequent and may be due to parenchymal dysfunction and to inadequate absorption of vitamin K, which is required for the hepatic synthesis of factors II, VII, IX, and X. An abnormal prothrombin time results and, depending on the severity of hepatocellular dysfunction, may respond to parenteral phytonadione (vitamin K_1) 5 to 10 mg/day given for 2 to 3 days. Thrombocytopenia, disseminated intravascular coagulation, and dysfibrinogenemia also contribute to clotting disturbances in many patients.

RENAL AND ELECTROLYTE ABNORMALITIES

Renal and electrolyte disorders are common, especially in chronic disease with ascites. **Hypokalemia** is caused by excess urinary potassium loss from increased circulating aldosterone, renal retention of ammonium ion in exchange for potassium, secondary renal tubular acidosis, and diuretic therapy. Management consists of giving oral potassium supplements and avoiding potassium-losing diuretics. The kidney may avidly retain sodium (see under ASCITES, above). Nevertheless **hyponatremia** is common; it usually reflects advanced parenchymal disease and is difficult to correct. Total body sodium depletion is much less often responsible than relative **water overload;** potassium depletion may also contribute. Appropriate water restriction and potassium supplements may be helpful; use of diuretics that increase free water clearance is controversial. Intravenous saline is rarely useful unless hyponatremia is life-threatening or good evidence exists for total body Na depletion; it should be avoided in cirrhotics with fluid retention, as it exacerbates ascites and has only a transitory effect on serum sodium levels. Variable metabolic and respiratory derangements may produce **alkalosis** or **acidosis** in advanced liver failure. **Blood urea concentrations** are often low because of impaired hepatic synthesis; superimposed GI bleeding causes elevations because of an increased enteric load rather than true renal impairment, since creatinine values usually remain normal.

Kidney failure in hepatic disease may reflect (1) disease directly affecting both organs, such as carbon tetrachloride toxicity (rare); (2) circulatory failure with decreased renal perfusion; or (3) functional renal failure (often called **"hepatorenal syndrome,"** a term that should be abandoned because it lacks a uniform meaning). This type of kidney failure, a progressive disorder with no apparent anatomic abnormality in the kidney, usually occurs in fulminant hepatitis or advanced cirrhosis with ascites. Its unknown pathogenesis may involve neural or humoral alterations of renocortical blood flow. Insidiously progressive oliguria and azotemia herald its onset. A low urinary sodium concentration and benign sediment usually distinguish it from tubular necrosis, but prerenal azotemia may be more difficult to differentiate; in doubtful cases, response to a volume load should be attempted. Renal failure is almost invariably progressive and fatal. Terminal hypotension with tubular necrosis may complicate the picture, but the kidneys are characteristically unremarkable at autopsy.

CIRCULATORY CHANGES

A hyperkinetic circulatory state with increased cardiac output and tachycardia may accompany acute liver failure or advanced cirrhosis. Cirrhotic patients with collateral anastomoses may also develop arterial desaturation and clubbing of the fingers. Hypotension usually occurs in advanced liver failure and may contribute to the development of renal dysfunction. The pathogenesis of these circulatory derangements is poorly understood.

Specific disorders of hepatic circulation (e.g., Budd-Chiari syndrome, portal hypertension) are discussed in Ch. 73.

---

65. LABORATORY EVALUATION OF THE LIVER AND BILIARY SYSTEM

It is impractical to try to isolate hepatocytic, mesenchymal, and biliary tree functions, since they are so interdependent in this complex organ. Because of this, and because interpretation of most biochemical studies used in the routine investigation of liver disorders is so imperfect, no attempt will be made to categorize or isolate the various functions and the tests that may or may not reflect their disorders. In general, too many laboratory tests are available and too few are interpreted adequately; relatively few improve patient care.

The few tests so useful that they should be part of the routine evaluation of liver disease include serum bilirubin, alkaline phosphatase, aminotransferase, and prothrombin time determinations. A few other tests are practical in particular circumstances. These include various viral antigens and antibodies in patients suspected of having viral hepatitis, serum copper and ceruloplasmin in suspected cases of Wilson's disease, serum protein electrophoresis in possible α_1-antitrypsin deficiency, serum mitochondrial antibodies in possible primary biliary cirrhosis, dye elimination studies in some patients with congenital hyperbilirubinemia, and α-fetoprotein levels in possible hepatocellular carcinoma. Most other biochemical tests are either redundant or applicable only to research. Numerous radiologic tests may be useful. Blood collection for these tests is discussed in Ch. 230; discussion here is limited to their practical application in evaluating liver disorders.

Tests Useful for Routine Evaluation

Serum bilirubin: Hyperbilirubinemia is discussed in detail in JAUNDICE in Ch. 64. Determination of the serum bilirubin is a necessary part of the routine evaluation of liver disease. Fractionation into total- and direct-reacting bilirubin is performed much too frequently in light of its clinical value. Estimation of the reserve bilirubin binding capacity of the serum can be important in the attempt to prevent kernicterus (see METABOLIC CONDITIONS in Vol. II, Ch. 21).

Serum alkaline phosphatase: Alkaline phosphatase is elevated in diseases of the liver, pancreas, lung, and bone; in some malignancies without metastases; and in pregnancy. It is composed of a group of enzymes which hydrolyze organic phosphate ester bonds in vitro, at alkaline pH. The physiologic function of these enzymes is unknown, though they may be involved in transport, since they are associated with the outer membrane of cells.

The alkaline phosphatase level varies with age. In the first 4 wk of life, it rises rapidly to 5 or 6 times above normal values. It then decreases slowly until puberty, when there is another increase, followed by a decrease to adult levels at 16 to 20 yr of age. It is slightly increased in older people. The level rises twofold during the 3rd trimester of pregnancy, threefold during labor, and returns to normal 2 to 3 wk after delivery.

Alkaline phosphatase is elevated in obstructive and hepatocellular liver disease and moderately to markedly elevated in obstructive jaundice, biliary cirrhosis, cholangiolitic hepatitis, occlusion of one hepatic duct, and space-occupying lesions in the liver. It is slightly to moderately elevated in viral hepatitis, infectious mononucleosis, cirrhosis, and destructive lesions of the lung. It is markedly elevated in osteitis deformans; moderately elevated in rickets, osteomalacia, hyperparathyroidism, and metastatic bone disease, and slightly elevated in healing fractures.

Alkaline phosphatase may be fractionated by heat denaturation under controlled conditions into **bone, intestinal,** or **placental fractions.** Serum electrophoresis may also separate the various isoenzymes for qualitative estimation. The heat-stable component is of placental origin. The **Regan isoenzyme** associated with some neoplasms is also heat-stable. The more specific origin of alkalin phosphatase elevations is sometimes used to establish the existence of metastases.

There are many conditions, drugs, and chemicals that affect alkaline phosphatase determinations. It is therefore important to collect and prepare the specimen carefully, and to interpret the result in the light of the patient's clinical and therapeutic drug history.

5'-Nucleotidase: The 5'-nucleotidases are phosphatases that differ from the alkaline phosphatases because they are inhibited by nickel ions. They are apparently restricted to the plasma membranes of the liver cell. Determination of their activity in the serum can be useful in distinguishing between increased alkaline phosphatase activity of hepatic and nonhepatic origin. In practice the test is useful only in assessing the anicteric patient.

Serum aminotransferase: Increase in the serum activity of certain hepatocellular enzymes is common in all kinds of liver disorders. The enzyme most widely studied in this regard is the aspartate transferase **(AST)**, formerly SGOT. Elevations of its activity are found in myocardial infarction, circulatory congestion, muscle injury, CNS disease, and other nonhepatic disorders. While nonspecific, this test is reliable and economical to use in routine screening for liver disorders. Values of > 400 u./ml are abnormal and highly suggestive of acute viral or toxic hepatitis.

The alanine transferase **(ALT)**, formerly SGPT, is equally sensitive and possibly more specific for liver disease than the AST, but since it usually adds nothing to one's understanding of liver disorders, it is not recommended in addition to the AST. The same advice applies to the lactic and isocitric dehydrogenases.

Prothrombin time: Although the liver manufactures most of the plasma coagulation factors and influences blood coagulation by several other mechanisms, bleeding is rarely the direct cause of death in liver failure. More frequently the multifactorial coagulation abnormalities in liver disease serve only to increase blood loss from the GI tract or elsewhere, or to prevent diagnostic procedures such as liver biopsy.

The test is of little diagnostic use in terms of hepatocellular function because most of the analytical procedures involved are relatively insensitive to small reductions in the concentration of the vitamin K-dependent coagulation factors. However, because the biologic half-lives of the proteins involved are relatively short, a matter of hours to a very few days, hypoprothrombinemia can be the first sign of *fulminant hepatic failure*. Determining the prothrombin time after excluding vitamin K deficiency is the single most useful test to follow the patient with severe acute hepatitis.

Tests Useful in Special Circumstances

γ-**Glutamyl transpeptidase:** Estimation of the serum activity of this enzyme provides a highly sensitive index of alcohol and drug hepatotoxicity, of infiltrative lesions of the liver, and of biliary tract obstruction. It is normal in the presence of bone disease; thus it renders the rather complex estimation of alkaline phosphatase isoenzymes unnecessary in most of the few cases where confusion may exist. Although it is perhaps more sensitive than some other routine tests, because it shares their lack of specificity, its precise contribution remains undefined.

Glutamate dehydrogenase is a mitochondrial enzyme whose increased activity in the serum may provide a sensitive index of hepatocellular necrosis, especially in the alcoholic.

Serum albumin: Serum albumin is a transport vehicle for numerous substances and the main determinant of plasma osmotic pressure. Its concentration in the serum is determined by its distribution between the intra- and extravascular beds, by the relative rates of its synthesis and degradation, and by plasma volume. Although the normal human liver produces 10 to 15 gm (0.2 mM)/day of this important protein, determination of its concentration in the serum is usually of little value as an index of hepatocellular function in acute liver disease because the biologic half-life of the protein is about 20 days. The test itself is insensitive and not specific.

The concentration of serum albumin is frequently decreased in patients with advanced chronic liver disease. This does give some quantitative information about hepatocellular function in these patients, but there is poor correlation between its rate of synthesis and its concentration in the serum. Serum albumin is also decreased in some renal diseases, chronic infections, intestinal malabsorption, third-degree burns, and water intoxication. The decrease is due, respectively, to urinary loss of albumin, impaired hepatic synthesis of albumin, direct loss of albumin through the burned skin, or dilution of the albumin by hydration.

Serum immunoglobulins: Most of the serum γ-globulins consist of immunoglobulins produced in response to specific antigenic stimulation. Levels of serum γ-globulin can be elevated in acute liver disease and are usually elevated in chronic liver disease, regardless of etiology. Knowledge of the serum γ-globulin concentration adds little to the evaluation of most patients. While serum IgM may be elevated in acute viral hepatitis A and in primary biliary cirrhosis, and IgG may be elevated in chronic active hepatitis, the response is both variable and nonspecific; therefore, quantitation of the individual serum immunoglobulins is of no diagnostic value.

Viral antigens and antibodies: (See VIRAL HEPATITIS in Ch. 69.) Other viruses, such as the Epstein-Barr virus, can produce hepatitis (see INFECTIOUS MONONUCLEOSIS in Vol. II, Ch. 27).

Antimitochondrial antibodies: Antibodies directed against mitochondria are present in $> 90\%$ of patients with primary biliary cirrhosis. The test is particularly valuable because needle biopsy of the liver may not provide diagnostic tissue. Although there is some overlap with chronic active hepatitis, and a low titer of antibodies can be found in some cases of drug-induced hepatotoxicity, a high titer of antimitochondrial antibodies in the appropriate clinical situation is usually accepted as diagnostic of primary biliary cirrhosis.

Other antibodies: Smooth muscle, microsomal, and nuclear antibodies are nonspecific, of little diagnostic value, and unnecessary when properly interpreted liver biopsies are available.

α-**Fetoprotein:** This serum protein, normally synthesized by the hepatocytes, can be elevated in the newborn, in the patient with hepatocellular carcinoma, and in the patient recovering from massive hepatic necrosis. However, judging from reports of its secretion by nonhepatic primitive mesenchymal cell tumors, the response cannot be considered specific. Testing for α-fetoprotein is probably of value in screening patients for hepatocellular carcinoma and may prove of prognostic value in the patient with fulminant hepatic failure. Immunoelectrophoresis appears to be an adequate method for screening, but the considerably more sensitive radioimmunoassay may be necessary in certain clinical situations involving response to therapy.

Dye elimination tests: Tests that measure the removal of various endogenous and exogenous substances from the blood are highly sensitive indicators of hepatic functional integrity. In fact, they are too sensitive for routine clinical use; furthermore, they are nonspecific and can be both complex and time-consuming.

The standard **BSP retention test** is widely used. Since the test is not quantitative, it need not be done if the patient has other evidence of liver disease. *Not without danger,* it is rarely indicated in clinical practice. However, it can play a role in the evaluation of **Gilbert's syndrome,** in which it is usually normal, and of the **Dubin-Johnson syndrome,** when regurgitation of conjugated dye into the bloodstream can be demonstrated at 90 to 120 min.

With care to avoid extravasation of dye, a 5% aqueous solution of BSP (5 mg/kg) is injected IV over a period of 30 seconds. The patient should be fasting and should not have obvious liver disease. After 45 min, the BSP concentration in venous blood *obtained from the opposite arm* is determined spectrophotometrically. The upper limit of normal is 5% retention of dye at 45 min.

More elaborate dye studies, involving measurement of the percentage disappearance rate from plasma, hepatic transport maximum (T_m), and relative storage capacities, provide better information concerning hepatic excretory function, but are useful only as research tools.

Indocyanine green, which is metabolized differently than BSP, has been less studied. Although measurable by ear-piece densitometry, apparently less toxic than BSP, and not subject to extrahepatic uptake, renal excretion, or an enterohepatic circulation, the dye is unlikely to gain widespread use. It is expensive and shares the same limitations as BSP in terms of clinical practice.

Rose bengal may have a useful clinical role in evaluating cholestasis in infants. After thyroid uptake has been blocked with Lugol's solution, the infant is given ^{131}I rose bengal 1 to 3 μCi/kg IV. During the next 72 h, > 75% of the injected dose is normally excreted in the feces. In patients with complete biliary atresia, fecal excretion is usually < 5% of the injected dose.

Bile acid studies: Bile acid metabolism is extremely complex and methods available for analyses are undergoing rapid evolution. The measurement of serum bile acids may prove to be useful in monitoring liver function, but further comparisons with more conventional tests are needed. A definite possibility is that serum can be used instead of duodenal bile to monitor patients undergoing bile acid therapy for gallstone disease. Analysis of fecal and urine bile acids is difficult, of undetermined clinical value, and restricted to special research units.

Bile pigment excretion: The study of bile pigments in the urine is simple and of some clinical importance. The appearance of bilirubin in the urine can be the earliest sign of hepatobiliary disease; commercially prepared tablets are available for the detection of bilirubin and provide the most sensitive and satisfactory test for evaluating the anicteric patient.

Normal urine contains trace amounts of urobilinogen and no bilirubin. While the urobilinuria can increase with hemolysis and hepatobiliary disease, the test for urobilin is too sensitive, and the response too nonspecific to be of any diagnostic value. Disappearance of urobilin from the urine can be a feature of the cholestatic phase of acute hepatitis or of complete mechanical obstruction of the extrahepatic biliary system. In neither case does this information add substantially to clinical evaluation and management. Quantitative analysis of urine pigments is of no diagnostic significance; the value of their quantitative evaluation in feces is restricted to research units.

The quantitative estimation of coproporphyrin I and III is also restricted to research units and will likely remain so. The diagnostic significance of coproporphyrin isomer excretion in hepatobiliary disease is probably limited to study of the Dubin-Johnson syndrome. Analysis of δ-aminolevulinic acid and porphobilinogen is required for evaluating certain metabolic diseases of the liver.

X-rays of the Liver and Biliary Tree

Plain x-ray of the abdomen is of limited clinical usefulness; however, calcifications of the liver, hemochromatosis, opaque dye deposits, the presence of air in the biliary tree, and radiopaque biliary calculi can be identified. This examination usually provides an accurate assessment of spleen size, as the lower margin of the spleen is almost always visible. An enlarged spleen causes downward displacement of the splenic flexure of the colon and medial displacement of the fundus of the stomach.

Oral cholecystogram: This examination is simple, reliable, and relatively undemanding of the patient, who fasts after a fat-free meal in the evening prior to examination. At least 3 different views of the gallbladder region are obtained 12 to 16 h after ingestion of a standard dose (3 gm) of an iodine-containing contrast agent (such as iopanoic acid or sodium tyropanoate). The gallbladder is stimulated to contract with a fatty meal or cholecystokinin, and in 70 to 80% of cases, views of the common bile duct can be obtained. In 95% of properly prepared patients without vomiting, diarrhea, pyloric obstruction, malabsorption, or significant hepatocellular dysfunction, failure to visualize the gallbladder indicates gallbladder disease, usually with stones. If the results are not definite, a repeat examination with the same or greater dose of contrast agent is carried out the following day.

This test is indicated in the diagnosis of cholelithiasis, chronic cholecystitis, and tumors of the gallbladder. It is useful in the differential diagnosis of opacities or masses in the right upper quadrant of the abdomen. Nausea, vomiting, and diarrhea can occur in about 20% of patients receiving the contrast agent, but the side effects are usually mild. Iodine sensitivity reactions and acute renal failure are the only serious complications that may occur. Ultrasonography (see below) will probably replace cholecystography as the primary procedure to detect gallstones and other biliary tract diseases.

IV cholangiography: Although the gallbladder can sometimes be visualized by this technic when oral cholecystography has failed, the use of IV cholangiography is usually restricted to those patients with symptoms suggestive of biliary duct disease. Only the standard technic is discussed here, although infusion technics and other modifications are used.

A film of the right upper quadrant is taken. The fasting patient is then given 1 ml of an iodinated contrast agent such as meglumine iodipamide IV. If no reaction occurs in 3 min, the remainder of the dose, usually a total of 20 ml, is injected over a 10-min period. Prone, left oblique, and anterior views are taken at 10-min intervals until optimal visualization of the common bile duct is obtained. This usually occurs within 40 min of the start of the injection. Repeat films are taken at 60 and 120 min if cholecystectomy has not been done. Tomography should be used. The common bile duct will be visualized in > 90% of noncholestatic, anicteric patients but in only about 10% of those with a serum bilirubin > 4 mg/100 ml. The common bile duct has a diameter up to 14 mm under normal circumstances and may be somewhat larger when gallbladder disease is present and/or following cholecystectomy. Small calculi can easily be missed; intrahepatic calculi are rarely seen. Although partial biliary obstruction sometimes promotes a greater density of dye in the ducts at 120 min than at 60 min, the IV cholangiogram is really useful only for anatomic information. The side effects and contraindications are similar to those of oral cholecystography but the side effects are more frequent and dangerous. The indications for IV cholangiography have been sharply reduced since the advent of ultrasonography (see below).

Operative cholangiography: A direct approach to the biliary tree with injection of dye into the cystic duct or common bile duct at laparotomy provides excellent visualization of the duct system and is both quicker and more accurate than IV cholangiography. While indications remain controversial, this procedure is recommended in any patient who is jaundiced on the basis of calculus disease of the biliary tree or who gives a history suggestive of choledocholithiasis. This diagnostic approach will be less used as operative choledochoscopy becomes more widely available.

Endoscopic retrograde cholangiopancreatography (ERCP): This technic has developed into an invaluable diagnostic and therapeutic procedure. It provides precise definition of biliary and pancreatic anatomy, and with its associated surgical technics, it has substantially reduced the morbidity, mortality, and economic cost of biliary tract disease.

The initial endoscopic examination often provides information concerning upper GI tract pathology and can identify ampullary and periampullary pathology. The pancreatogram may identify a pancreatic neoplasm or pancreatitis. It will also define the pancreatic duct anatomy, providing information that may be useful when subsequent biliary tract manipulation is attempted. The cholangiogram will visualize the intrahepatic and entire extrahepatic biliary tree. Cystic duct obstruction, stones, strictures, and tumors will be identified. Pus can be drained, small common bile duct stones disrupted or flushed from the bile duct, and a large common bile duct stone removed by basket extraction or endoscopic papillotomy. Although hemorrhage and pancreatitis have been encountered, the incidence of significant side effects is remarkably low. The immediate future of endoscopic biliary surgery is secure.

Percutaneous transhepatic cholangiography: This technic is useful in defining the site, and possibly the nature, of mechanical obstruction to the biliary tree. The technic is usually employed after ultrasound examination has identified mechanical obstruction on the basis of dilated intra- or extrahepatic bile ducts.

The basic technic is similar to that of liver biopsy. Either an anterior subcostal or lateral intercostal approach is used. The liver is punctured under fluoroscopic control with a 6- to 8-in. plastic-sheathed needle. The needle is removed and the sheath then slowly withdrawn while maintaining suction. When bile is aspirated, withdrawal is stopped and water-soluble radiopaque material is injected under fluoroscopic control. If no bile is aspirated on three or four passes into the liver, the bile ducts are probably not dilated and no mechanical obstruction exists. Bleeding and bile peritonitis are encountered rarely, so the study does not have to be performed immediately preoperatively. The technic is used to introduce decompressing catheters into the biliary tree in a particularly useful adjunct to the management of complete mechanical biliary tract obstruction. The technic is restricted to specialized centers, with most surgeons still preferring operative cholangiography for localizing the obstruction site. Even in specialized centers, it tends to play a secondary role to ERCP. Although percutaneous transhepatic cholangiography is simple, it has a greater complication rate and lesser applicability than ERCP.

Radionuclide scanning can determine the shape and location of the liver, follow its size and function during the course of therapy, define right upper quadrant masses, direct the approach for liver biopsy, and investigate space-occupying lesions of the liver. The reticuloendothelial system is probed and hepatic blood flow and the biliary system assessed, using IV radiocolloids such as Technetium 99m labelled substituted iminodiacetic acid compound **(HIDA)**. Hepatobiliary imaging with labeled HIDA also provides functional information regarding cystic duct patency and is both highly sensitive and specific in the diagnosis of acute cholecystitis. Hepatocellular function, apart from bile production, has been evaluated by studying the uptake of radioactive selenomethionine and vitamin B_{12}. Radionuclide rapid sequence flow studies and blood pool images have been used to assess hepatic blood flow and especially the vascularity of space-occupying lesions. Although liver scans lack specificity and have relatively low limits of resolution, they are rapid, simple, convenient, and relatively noninvasive. For these reasons, they are excellent screening procedures for investigation of liver diseases.

Ultrasound (US)

US uses non-ionizing sound waves and demonstrates echoes from the interfaces between tissues of different densities and elasticities. This technic is exceptionally useful in evaluating lesions of the abdomen. The development of gray scale signal processing permits amplification and processing of very low amplitude echoes into a visual display in shades of gray. An additional stimulus to its applicability is the development of rapid viewing (real time) systems that permit sequential presentation of images as moving structures. US data are morphologic and independent of physiologic and pathologic considerations.

US is useful in evaluating cholestatic jaundice. The bile ducts stand out as echo-free tubular structures. The technic is $> 95\%$ accurate in differentiating surgical from medical jaundice. US can locate the site of biliary obstruction in 85% of cases and can frequently determine the cause of obstruction.

US defines cystic lesions of the liver, bile ducts, and pancreas as echo-free lesions with sharp borders and strong posterior echoes. Abscesses and hematomas can be defined and the technic is about 90% accurate in detecting liver tumors. US is more accurate than radionuclide scanning in detecting liver tumors, more specific in differentiating solid from cystic lesions, and has a lower false-positive rate. Because lesions can be localized accurately in 3 dimensions, aspiration or biopsy needles can be precisely guided.

US is not particularly sensitive to changes resulting from diffuse hepatocellular disease, but may show parenchymal changes in advanced disease. US can detect small amounts of ascites and can define some vascular abnormalities associated with portal hypertension. By integrating the cross-sectional areas of serial planes of analysis, one can determine the volume of the liver and spleen with reasonable accuracy. US will probably become the initial diagnostic approach to lesions of the gallbladder and biliary tree. It is already the screening procedure of choice for pancreatic disease. The normal pancreas can be visualized in 70% of examinations and its overall accuracy in designating a normal pancreas from one with an abnormality approaches 90%. Although limited by fat, bone, and intestinal gas, and dependent upon the expertise of the operator and interpreter, US is both versatile and economical.

Computerized Tomography (CT)

Using x-rays to demonstrate the density of tissues has proved useful in the clinical evaluation of the liver, biliary tree, and pancreas. Although not limited by intestinal gas, bone, or fat and much less dependent than US on operator and interpreter expertise, the current accuracy of CT is not significantly greater than that of gray scale US. Furthermore, CT uses radiation and highly complex equipment, its planes of scanning restrict its versatility, it is much more expensive and it is less widely available. CT may succeed where US fails because of intestinal gas or obesity, and it complements US in investigating abdominal lesions.

66. MORPHOLOGIC EVALUATION OF LIVER DISEASE

Percutaneous Needle Biopsy

Valuable diagnostic and prognostic information at relatively small risk is provided by percutaneous needle biopsy. Done at the bedside under local anesthesia, the procedure usually causes minimal patient discomfort. The Menghini aspiration technic is simple and safe to use, but the procedure requires a trained operator. In expert hands the incidence of serious complications is about 0.2%.

Electron microscopy of liver biopsies has greatly advanced the knowledge of hepatic pathophysiology but is of little diagnostic value clinically.

Indications include (1) jaundice or hepatosplenomegaly of unknown cause, (2) unexplained liver function abnormalities, (3) diagnosis and staging of alcoholic liver disease (findings are usually characteristic, and the extent of irreversible fibrosis vs. reversible inflammation can be determined), (4) atypical hepatitis (biopsy is not needed in ordinary acute viral hepatitis but should be done if the diagnosis is uncertain or the clinical course atypical), (5) evaluation of chronic hepatitis, (biopsy is essential for diagnosis and follow-up; unsuspected alcoholic liver disease and other alternate disorders are detected often enough to justify biopsy in most patients with chronic parenchymal disease), (6) differential diagnosis of cholestasis, (7) suspected malignancy (biopsy detects metastatic carcinoma in about ²/₃ of cases and may establish the diagnosis despite negative liver scan; cytologic examination of the biopsy fluid yields positive findings in an additional 10% or so of cases; results are less valuable in lymphoma and correlate poorly with the clinical impression of hepatic involvement), and (8) fever of unknown origin (obscure cases are often clarified, especially if elevated alkaline phosphatase or other liver function test abnormalities are present; biopsy is particularly valuable in detecting tuberculosis and other granulomatous infiltrations).

Limitations of the procedure include (1) need for a skilled interpreter (many pathologists have little experience with needle specimens), (2) sampling error (collecting tissue from a nonrepresentative area of the liver seldom occurs in hepatitis and other diffuse conditions but may be a problem in cirrhosis and malignancy), (3) inability to differentiate hepatitis etiologically (e.g., viral vs. drug-induced), and (4) occasional errors or uncertainty in cases of cholestasis.

Contraindications include a clinical bleeding tendency, prothrombin time more than 2 to 3 seconds over control values despite administration of vitamin K, severe thrombocytopenia, marked ascites, high-grade biliary obstruction, and subphrenic or right pleural infection.

The most frequent **complications** are intra-abdominal bleeding and bile peritonitis. These hazards are minimized by appropriate selection of cases, anticipatory coagulation studies, blood typing, and bed rest with observation for 24 h post biopsy. Rare complications include hemobilia, intrahepatic hematoma, transient bacteremia, and hepatic arteriovenous fistula.

Peritoneoscopy (Laparoscopy)

This procedure is used often in Europe, but in North America experience is limited. A pneumoperitoneum is created under general or local anesthesia, then the laparoscope is introduced into the peritoneal cavity through the anterior abdominal wall. The instrument allows direct inspection of the peritoneum, liver, and other organs, and biopsy can be done under direct vision. However, peritoneoscopy is more complex than percutaneous biopsy, and requires more skill. Adhesions from previous surgery may preclude adequate visualization. In addition to anesthetic risks, **complications** include tissue emphysema, bowel perforation, and intraperitoneal or abdominal wall bleeding.

Laparotomy

Surgical wedge or needle biopsy provides better specimens and less sampling error than percutaneous needle specimens. Unexplained hepatosplenomegaly, fever of unknown origin, and lymphoma may require laparotomy for clarification. More commonly, laparotomy establishes the cause of cholestatic jaundice when simpler tests fail. Diagnostic laparotomy should be avoided in patients with severe hepatocellular dysfunction because of the risk of precipitating acute liver failure.

Open liver biopsy through a small incision can be combined with portal venography and cholangiography ("minilap"). The diagnostic role of minilap remains to be established.

67. FATTY LIVER

The abnormal accumulation of fat in hepatocytes, said to occur in 25% of individuals and to be the commonest response of the liver to injury.

Etiology

Diffuse fatty change of the liver, often zonal in distribution, is associated with many clinical situations. In the neonatal period it can occur in a familial or idiopathic manner, in Wolman's disease, in cystic fibrosis of the pancreas, and in association with inborn errors of glycogen, galactose, tyrosine, and homocystine metabolism. Later it can be found in Reye's syndrome, phytanic acid storage disease (Refsum's disease), Wilson's disease, hemochromatosis, abetalipoproteinemia, obesity, and diabetes. It can be a complication of a diet deficient in proteins or involving amino acid imbalances and it can be caused by a wide variety of chemicals and drugs, including carbon tetrachloride, yellow phosphorus, alcohol, corticosteroids, and tetracyclines. Diffuse fatty metamorphosis can complicate both small-bowel bypass surgery and pregnancy.

Focal fatty change is much less common and less well recognized. Occurring in nodular form and usually subcapsular in location, focal fatty change can be important in the differential diagnosis of space-occupying lesions of the liver.

Pathology

If lipid deposit is marked, the liver tends to be grossly enlarged, smooth, and pale. Microscopically, the general architecture can be normal. In the form of triglycerides, the fat tends to appear as large droplets that coalesce and displace the cell nucleus to the periphery. In Wolman's disease, triglyceride collects with cholesterol esters in lysosomes that do not fuse. Lipid accumulation, presumably as triglyceride, also occurs in small droplet form in tetracycline and aflatoxin hepatotoxicity. Fat that gathers as free fatty acids, cholesterol, cholesterol esters, and phospholipids tends to collect in a microvesicular form in secondary lysosomes that do not fuse. The hepatocytes feature a foamy cytoplasm and a central nucleus.

Free fatty acids collect in acute fatty liver of pregnancy and probably in Reye's syndrome. Cholesterol esters gather in familial high density lipoprotein deficiency (Tangier disease), cholesterol ester storage disease, and Wolman's disease. Phospholipids accumulate under the influence of certain drugs and in several rare inborn errors of phospholipid metabolism.

With hepatotoxins primarily affecting protein synthesis or with protein malnutrition, the lipid tends to collect in Zone I. With other hepatotoxins and with diets deficient in factors other than amino acids, the fat tends to collect in Zone 3. In acute fatty liver of pregnancy, the fine droplet fatty change is diffuse but usually spares those hepatocytes in Zone I, immediately around the portal tracts. In contrast, the fat accumulation in Reye's syndrome is predominantly in Zone I.

Unusual lysosomes, called lipolysosomes, featuring a limiting membrane, containing fat, and exhibiting acid phosphatase activity are usually associated with the fatty liver and may play a major role in metabolizing storage lipid.

Pathogenesis

The liver occupies a central position in lipid metabolism. Nonesterified fatty acids (NEFA), absorbed from the diet or released into the blood from chylomicrons or adipose sites, comprise a small but rapidly used pool that accommodates almost all energy requirements of a fasting animal. Some NEFA are taken up by the liver to join the hepatic pool of free fatty acids, a portion of which is synthesized by the liver. Some hepatocytic NEFA are oxidized for energy, but most are rapidly incorporated into complex lipids, such as triglycerides, phospholipids, glycolipids, cholesterol, and cholesterol esters. Some of these complex lipids enter a slowly used pool that comprises the structural lipids of the cell and the site for storage of the lipid. The remaining complex lipids enter an active pool that is used to synthesize lipoproteins. Most lipoproteins are secreted into the plasma where they provide the main source of lipid for the peripheral tissues in a fasting animal.

Except for specific inborn errors of lipid metabolism and for poorly understood conditions such as acute fatty liver of pregnancy and Reye's syndrome, the lipid that collects in the liver is mainly triglyceride. This is so because hepatic triglycerides have the highest turnover rate of all hepatic fatty acid esters and because no feedback inhibition regulates the uptake of fatty acids by the liver.

Triglyceride accumulation in the liver results from either increased synthesis or decreased elimination of triglyceride from the hepatocytes. Increased triglyceride synthesis may be associated with an increase in the activity of triglyceride synthetase or an increased concentration of NEFA as a result of increased uptake, increased synthesis from acetyl CoA, or decreased oxidation by the hepatocytes. Decreased elimination of NEFA may involve decreased hydrolysis by lysosomal lipases, decreased lipoprotein secretion, or decreased synthesis of lipids other than triglycerides.

The several possible mechanisms involved in the pathogenesis of the fatty liver may operate alone or together. Increased hepatic uptake of NEFA seems to contribute to the fatty liver induced by carbon tetrachloride, phosphorus, isopropanol, and various inhibitors of protein synthesis. Increased synthesis of NEFA from acetyl CoA seems to contribute to the fatty liver caused by essential fatty acid deficiency, acute ethanol poisoning, and phenobarbital treatment. Decreased oxidation of fatty acids may contribute to the fatty liver induced by carbon tetrachloride, phosphorus, hypoxia, and certain vitamin deficiencies (niacin, riboflavin, and pantothenic acid). A block in the hepatocytic production and secretion of lipoproteins is often the main cause of triglyceride accumulation in the liver. A block in apolipoprotein synthesis appears to be the most important pathogenetic factor in several types of toxic fatty liver and in the fatty liver produced by diets deficient in protein (Kwashiorkor) or imbalances in amino acids. Toxic inhibition of protein synthesis can lead to a fatty liver through inhibition of mRNA synthesis (aflatoxin, amanita phalloides toxins, D-galactosamine and dimethylnitrosamine), through inhibition of amino acyl transfer RNA synthesis, or binding to ribosomes (puromycin, tetracycline), through inhibition of mRNA translation (cycloheximide, emetine) or through inhibition of initiation of protein synthesis (carbon tetrachloride, phosphorus). In spite of much research, the pathogenesis of most cases remains poorly understood.

Symptoms, Signs, and Diagnosis

It most often is discovered on physical examination as nontender hepatomegaly and is usually asymptomatic. However, it can present with right upper quadrant pain and jaundice or can be the only physical abnormality found after sudden, unexpected, and presumably metabolic death.

There is a poor association between fatty liver and abnormalities of the commonly used biochemical tests for liver disease. Although BSP retention is almost always present, the test is nonspecific and should not be performed. The diagnosis of fatty liver can be made only on histologic grounds.

Fatty liver is potentially reversible and usually is not in itself harmful. However, since it may indicate the action of a hepatotoxin or the presence of an unrecognized disease or metabolic abnormality, the diagnosis calls for further evaluation of the patient.

Treatment

No specific therapy is known except to eliminate the cause or treat the underlying disorder. Anabolic steroids can augment the release of hepatic triglycerides from the fatty liver, but their use is rarely indicated.

68.   FIBROSIS AND CIRRHOSIS

FIBROSIS

Excess fibrous tissue in the liver resulting passively from collapse and condensation of preexisting fibers or actively through the synthesis of new fibers by fibroblasts.

Etiology

Fibrosis is a common response to parenchymal cell injury induced by a wide variety of agents, including numerous chemicals and drugs such as alcohol, methotrexate, arsenicals, isoniazid, oxyphenisatin, methyldopa, polyvinylchloride, and thorium dioxide. The deposition of endogenous and exogenous substances in the liver, as in myeloid metaplasia, Gaucher's disease, certain glycogen storage diseases, Wilson's disease, and the iron overload syndromes, is associated with fibrosis. Various infections of the liver—viral, bacterial, spirochetal, and parasitic—can cause hepatic fibrosis, as can chronic obstruction to bile flow and various disturbances of the hepatic circulation.

Pathogenesis

Active fibroplasia is usually associated with inflammation. It may be located around hepatocytes, proliferated bile ductules, or macrophages, and in the portal tracts. Many cell types appear to be capable of collagen synthesis, but in the liver, interest has focused mainly on the lipocytes or Ito cells which lie in the perisinusoidal recesses and may represent inactive fibroblasts. Collagen can be removed as well as synthesized; regression of liver fibrosis is possible after removal of the offending agent.

The influence of fibrosis on hepatic structure and function depends upon its localization: pericellular fibrosis leads to hepatocellular atrophy; fibrosis around the terminal hepatic venules leads to venous outflow block; periportal fibrosis leads to portal hypertension on the basis of portal venous inflow block; and periductular fibrosis leads to cholestasis. Extensive fibrosis can result in the formation of septa, which can interfere significantly with hepatic circulation. Lobular fibrosis such as that found in some granulomatous diseases is often associated only with abnormalities of certain serum enzyme activities (e.g., alkaline phosphatase) and with BSP retention. Congenital hepatic fibrosis, a variant of congenital cystic liver disease, features excess portal and periportal connective tissue that is mature and interferes with portal venous blood flow. The condition presents as portal hypertension with excellent hepatocellular function and no cirrhosis.

Diagnosis

The fibrosis that accompanies many hepatic disorders is rarely the main characteristic of the disease. The diagnosis depends upon histologic examination of the liver. Aniline blue or trichrome stains are particularly useful. Silver impregnation of the reticulin can be used to distinguish passive from active fibrosis.

Treatment

Management includes treating the underlying cause and complications of fibrosis (e.g., portal hypertension) and is discussed below in relation to these subjects. New therapeutic approaches focus on inhibiting collagen synthesis and maturation by proline analogs, colchicine, penicillamine, and lathyrogenic agents.

CIRRHOSIS

The disorganization of liver architecture by widespread fibrosis and nodule formation. The nodules are portions of parenchyma demarcated by connective tissue. In cirrhosis all parts of the liver must be involved, but large nodules can contain intact architecture. Fibrosis is not synonymous with cirrhosis; nodule formation with fibrosis is not cirrhosis. **Partial nodular transformation of the liver** and the solitary hyperplastic nodule or **focal cirrhosis** are not examples of a true cirrhosis. These lesions consist of isolated areas of fibrosis and nodularity in an otherwise normal organ.

Etiology and Incidence

Cirrhosis is exceeded only by heart disease, cancer, and cerebrovascular disease as a cause of death in the 45 to 65 age group in the USA; the vast majority of cases are secondary to chronic alcohol abuse. In many parts of Asia and Africa, cirrhosis due to chronic viral hepatitis is a major cause of death.

Congenital causes of cirrhosis include hereditary hemorrhagic telangiectasia and inborn errors of metabolism such as galactosemia, certain glycogen storage diseases, tyrosinosis, fructose intolerance, α_1-antitrypsin deficiency, thalassemia, Wilson's disease, and hemochromatosis. Cirrhosis can be induced by **chemicals**, e.g., alcohol, methotrexate, halothane, and oxyphenisatin. Cirrhosis can follow **infections** such as viral hepatitis Type B and congenital syphilis, and can develop after **intestinal bypass operations, biliary obstruction** (either primary or extrahepatic), or prolonged **passive congestion** of the liver associated with tricuspid insufficiency, constrictive pericarditis, or hepatic vein thrombosis. In many instances, no etiology can be established, and the term **cryptogenic cirrhosis** is applied. Primary biliary cirrhosis is discussed separately below.

Classification and Pathogenesis

The morphologic classification of cirrhosis is difficult because each cirrhotic liver has a different configuration, the end result of the interplay of many independent factors. Furthermore, cirrhosis is not a static lesion. The traditional classification of cirrhosis as portal, postnecrotic, posthepatitic, and biliary blends morphologic, pathologic and etiologic terms and makes no sense conceptually. The initiating lesion in portal cirrhosis is usually in Zone 3 and all cirrhosis follows cellular necrosis (postnecrotic) and inflammatory change (posthepatitic). A current tendency avoids classifying cirrhosis and accepts instead a morphologic description of the pathology. Much more important than its classification are the activity, stage of development, and complications of the disease process. Cirrhosis either is or is not present. However, to accommodate those committed to classifications, the following one is reasonably practicable:

Micronodular cirrhosis is characterized by thin, regular bands of connective tissue and by small nodules that vary little in size and, characteristically, terminal hepatic veins or portal spaces cannot be identified.

Macronodular cirrhosis is characterized by connective tissue bands of varying thickness and by nodules that vary in size and contain portal spaces and terminal hepatic veins. The concentration of portal spaces in the fibrous scars demonstrates previous collapse.

Mixed cirrhosis combines micro- and macronodular cirrhosis.

Regardless of the classification, the pathogenesis of cirrhosis is important. Cirrhosis results when the liver reacts normally to injury, whatever the cause, and the varieties of cirrhosis are related not to the causative agent but to the form of the injury and to the liver's reaction to it. The liver may be injured severely and all at once, as in submassive necrosis with hepatitis; moderately over months or a few years, as in biliary tract obstruction and chronic active hepatitis; or modestly, but continuously and chronically, as in alcohol abuse. Fibrosis and parenchymal regeneration result as the natural but modifiable reactions to this injury.

Restoration of intrahepatic circulatory pathways is an essential part of the repair process. New vessel formation follows intact pathways to connect hepatic artery and portal vein with the hepatic venules. The interconnecting vessels, contained in fibrous sheaths around the surviving parenchymal nodules, receive the sinusoidal flow of these nodules. However, these new passageways provide a high-pressure, relatively low-volume sinusoidal drainage system that is much less efficient than normal. The result is an increase in portal vein pressure **(portal hypertension)**. Disordered blood flow to the nodules and compression of hepatic venules by regenerating nodules also contribute to portal hypertension.

Many complications of cirrhosis are related to portal hypertension, since it leads to the development of collateral flow from the portal system to the systemic circulation. Collateral vessels form commonly around the stomach and lower esophagus, producing esophageal varices. Rarely, severe hemorrhoidal disease occurs after similar portal-systemic shunting. Bleeding from esophageal, gastric, or other varices is caused in part by high pressure in the portal circulation. In addition, ascites and portal-systemic encephalopathy are related to the build-up of pressure in the portal system and the functional bypass of the liver by the portal-systemic shunting (see also PORTAL HYPERTENSION in Ch. 73).

Symptoms and Signs

Many patients with cirrhosis are asymptomatic and well-nourished, making the diagnosis difficult and somewhat surprising. Generalized weakness, anorexia, malaise, weight loss, and loss of libido are common. In the malnourished patient, other problems may exist, e.g., paresthesiae and glossitis.

A palpable, firm, smooth liver with a blunt edge is characteristic. Ordinary cirrhotic nodules are rarely if ever palpable. Evidence of collateral venous circulation, ascites, and splenomegaly may occur with portal hypertension. Other signs of chronic liver disease include muscular wasting, palmar erythema, vascular spiders, gynecomastia, parotid gland enlargement, hair loss, testicular atrophy, and peripheral neuropathy. Clubbing of the fingers, Dupuytren's palmar contracture, pleural effusions, dilated abdominal wall collateral veins, and hepatic fetor are not uncommon.

Laboratory Diagnosis

None, any, or all routine biochemical tests of liver function may be abnormal, including serum bilirubin, AST (previously called SGOT), ALT (previously called SGPT), γGTP, and serum alkaline phosphatase. These tend to reflect hepatocellular insufficiency rather than cirrhosis. However, a prolonged prothrombin time, increased serum γ-globulin, and decreased serum albumin suggest cirrhosis. Anemia and various morphologic abnormalities of the erythrocytes are common and usually multifactorial in nature, due to deficient intake of iron and folic acid, chronic blood loss, and hypersplenism.

Scintiscanning characteristically reveals decreased uptake of isotope with an irregular pattern of labeling in the liver and uptake of label by the spleen and bone marrow. Ultrasound examination is not particularly helpful in uncomplicated cirrhosis. The diagnosis of cirrhosis is a pathologic one best documented by biopsy. Even needle biopsy specimens are usually diagnostic.

Complications

Most of the severe complications of cirrhosis are secondary to portal hypertension and the portal-systemic shunting of blood discussed above. They include GI hemorrhage (see also Ch. 52); portal-systemic encephalopathy, ascites, and renal failure (see Ch. 64). Hepatocellular carcinoma frequently complicates cirrhosis, especially that associated with chronic viral hepatitis B.

Prognosis

If the patient has experienced major complications, such as hematemesis, hepatic coma, ascites, and jaundice, the prognosis is grave; e.g., a 1-yr survival of < 50% can be expected in such a patient with alcohol-induced liver disease who continues to consume excess alcohol. However, even with severe signs, a patient may respond to treatment, especially if the offending agent (alcohol, copper, etc.) can be removed.

Treatment

Treatment of cirrhosis is based upon the etiology involved and the management of specific complications. Abstinence from alcohol, a nutritious diet containing protein as tolerated, reasonable rest, and therapeutic multivitamins are indicated for the patient with alcohol-induced liver disease. The use of corticosteroids remains controversial but may aid the treatment of chronic active hepatitis even when cirrhosis has developed. The treatment of cirrhosis is discussed further under specific etiologic diseases (see Etiology of Cirrhosis, above).

BILIARY CIRRHOSIS

PRIMARY BILIARY CIRRHOSIS

A disease of unknown etiology characterized by chronic obstructive jaundice. It is commonly associated with autoimmune disorders, but the precise significance of this association is not yet known.

Pathogenesis

The early course of primary biliary cirrhosis features a chronic nonsuppurative destructive inflammation of the intrahepatic bile radicles. Only later does a true cirrhosis develop.

Although 4 typical stages in its evolution have been defined, the disease is focal with considerable overlap between the stages in any one case. The initial lesion involves inflammation of the medium-sized bile ducts associated with chronic inflammation of the portal tracts. Granuloma may be found. In the smaller portal tracts, bile ducts may be conspicuously absent. Parenchymal changes are minimal and histologic cholestasis unusual. As destruction of the medium-sized bile ducts progresses, the portal tracts become distorted, inflammation spreads into the parenchyma, bile ducts proliferate intensely, and periportal fibrosis develops. By this time most portal tracts are affected. Progressive scarring continues with less bile duct proliferation and less inflammation. Fibrous bands link the portal tracts, and Zone I cholestasis and Mallory hyaline become evident. Although often slow, progression is inevitable, with the end product a firm, regular, intensely bile-stained cirrhosis. It can be difficult to distinguish primary biliary cirrhosis from other cirrhotic processes microscopically in the absence of granuloma and the pathognomonic bile duct lesions.

Symptoms, Signs, and Diagnosis

Although it can affect both sexes and a broad age spectrum, the disease most commonly affects females between the ages of 35 and 60. It usually presents insidiously with pruritus that can precede jaundice and other manifestations by many months. The patient is usually pigmented from the outset, tanned as a result of melanocyte stimulation. The liver is usually enlarged, nontender, and firm, and the spleen is usually enlarged. Other signs include skin xanthomas, xanthelasma, steatorrhea, osteomalacia, and osteoporosis. Pain in the fingers and toes may occur due to xanthomatous peripheral neuropathy. As the disease progresses, all the features and complications of cirrhosis can develop. Primary biliary cirrhosis is associated with many other conditions, especially the collagen diseases. It has been associated with RA, scleroderma, sicca complex, and autoimmune thyroiditis.

Early laboratory findings are those of cholestasis with elevation of the serum alkaline phosphatase disproportionately greater than any increase in the serum bilirubin and aminotransferases. In fact the serum bilirubin can be normal early in the course of the disease. The concentration of serum bile acids is elevated, as are the serum activities of the γGTP and 5′-nucleotidase. The serum cholesterol concentration may be increased and the serum total lipids usually are increased. The serum lipoproteins are increased mainly because lipoprotein-X is present. Serum albumin is normal early in the course of the disease, but the globulins usually increase, the serum IgM often to very high values. Antibodies against a component of the inner membrane of mitochondria are present in 85 to 95% of cases and are of considerable diagnostic value. Such mitochondrial antibodies can also be found in some patients with HBsAg-negative chronic active hepatitis and sometimes it can be very difficult to distinguish between these problems.

The differential diagnosis includes extrahepatic biliary obstruction, chronic active hepatitis, primary sclerosing cholangitis, drug-induced cholestasis, and the cholangitic lesions associated with inflammatory bowel disease. Potentially curable extrahepatic biliary obstruction must be ruled out early. Liver biopsy can be diagnostic but is often nonspecific. Intravenous cholangiography is often negative because of cholestasis. Retrograde cannulation of the biliary tract (ERCP) is currently the most satisfactory method for ruling out extrahepatic bile duct obstruction. Ultrasound examination of the liver and percutaneous transhepatic cholangiography provide alternate approaches. Diagnostic laparotomy is rarely necessary.

Treatment

No specific treatment is known. Satisfactory results have been reported with prednisone and azathioprine, either alone or in combination, but their value is controversial. The same comment must also apply to penicillamine therapy. The slow progress of the disease is compatible with prolonged survival. Pruritus may be controlled with cholestyramine 6 to 12 gm/day orally in divided doses. Bile salt insufficiency associated with steatorrhea may require supplements with vitamins A, D, and K to prevent deficiencies. Calcium deficiency may also occur and calcitrol may be of particular therapeutic value. Because of the occurrence of large immune complexes in the serum, therapeutic approaches to their dissolution are currently under study. The treatment of the complications of primary biliary cirrhosis is similar to that for other types of cirrhosis.

OBSTRUCTIVE BILIARY CIRRHOSIS

Cirrhosis caused by obstruction of the extrahepatic bile ducts by stone, tumor, scar, or congenital atresia. Intrahepatic bile ducts are usually dilated and are surrounded by inflammatory reaction. Connective tissue is increased near the portal areas, but lobular structure is well preserved initially. Later, portal-to-portal bridging fibrosis occurs and distorts the architecture of the liver.

Symptoms and Signs

Intermittent or chronic jaundice usually occurs over a period of months to years. It is obstructive in type, with increased serum alkaline phosphatase and hypercholesterolemia. The skin has a green, bronzed appearance and frequently shows xanthomatous deposits. Hepatocellular failure develops slowly, as does portal hypertension with its associated ascites, portal systemic encephalopathy, and GI tract hemorrhage.

Treatment

Early diagnosis is essential, with ERCP, percutaneous transhepatic cholangiography and liver biopsy as the most useful aids. Potentially correctable extrahepatic obstruction must be treated surgically. Medical treatment is similar to that for primary biliary cirrhosis.

---

69. HEPATITIS

An inflammatory process in the liver characterized by diffuse or patchy hepatocellular necrosis affecting all acini.

The 3 major causes of hepatitis are Types A, B, and non-A, non-B viruses; alcohol; and drugs. Rarer etiologies include infectious mononucleosis, yellow fever, cytomegalovirus, other specific viral infections, and leptospirosis.

Parasitic infections such as schistosomiasis, malaria, and amebiasis affect the liver but do not cause a true hepatitis. Pyogenic infections and abscesses are also generally considered to be separate problems. Involvement of the liver with tuberculosis and other granulomatous infiltrations is sometimes called "granulomatous hepatitis" but produces different clinical, biochemical, and histologic features than diffuse hepatitis.

A variety of systemic infections and other illnesses may produce small focal areas of hepatic necrosis and inflammation. This nonspecific reactive hepatitis causes minor liver function abnormalities but is usually asymptomatic.

Noninfectious hepatitis and some of the hepatic infections are described under their specific topic headings, and in part are summarized in TABLE 69–1, below. Hepatitis due to drugs and alcohol is discussed in Chs. 70 and 71, respectively.

Tᴀʙʟᴇ 69–1. SELECTED INFLAMMATORY CONDITIONS OF THE LIVER

Disease or Organism	Comments
Viruses	
Epstein-Barr	Infectious mononucleosis. Clinical hepatitis with jaundice, 5–10%; subclinical liver involvement in remainder. Important cause of acute hepatitis in young adults.
Yellow fever	Jaundice with systemic toxicity, bleeding. Liver necrosis with little inflammatory reaction.
Cytomegalovirus	*Neonatal:* hepatomegaly, jaundice, congenital defects. *Adult:* mononucleosis-like illness with hepatitis; may occur posttransfusion.
Other	Hepatitis occasionally, from herpes simplex, ECHO, coxsackie, rubeola, rubella, varicella.
Bacteria	
Tuberculosis	Hepatic involvement common. Granulomatous infiltration. Usually subclinical; jaundice rare. Disproportionate ↑ alkaline phosphatase. Liver biopsy valuable.
Actinomycosis	Granulomatous reaction with progressive necrotizing abscesses.
Pyogenic abscess	Serious infection acquired via portal pyemia, cholangitis, hematogenous or direct spread. Various organisms, especially gram-negative & anaerobic. Patient ill, toxic, yet only mild liver dysfunction. Differentiate from amebic abscess, drain surgically.
Other	Minor focal hepatitis common in numerous systemic infections. Usually subclinical.
Fungi	
Histoplasmosis	Granulomas in liver & spleen, usually subclinical; heal with calcification.
Other	Granulomatous infiltration sometimes in cryptococcosis, coccidioidomycosis, blastomycosis, etc.
Protozoa	
Amebiasis	Important disease, often without obvious dysentery. Usually large single abscess with liquefaction. Patient ill, tender hepatomegaly, surpisingly mild liver dysfunction. Differentiate from pyogenic abscess.
Malaria	Major cause of hepatosplenomegaly in endemic areas. Jaundice absent or mild unless active hemolysis.
Toxoplasmosis	Transplacental infection. Neonatal jaundice, CNS & other systemic manifestations.
Kala-azar	Infiltration of reticuloendothelial system by parasite. Hepatosplenomegaly.
Helminths	
Schistosomiasis	Important disease. Periportal reaction to ova with progressive hepatosplenomegaly, "pipestem" fibrosis, portal hypertension, varices. Parenchymal function preserved; not true cirrhosis.
Clonorchiasis	Biliary tract infestation; cholangitis, stones, cholangiocarcinoma.
Fascioliasis	*Acute:* tender hepatomegaly, fever, eosinophilia. *Chronic:* biliary fibrosis, cholangitis.
Echinococcosis	One or more hydatid cysts, usually calcified rim. May be large but often asymptomatic; liver function preserved. Can rupture into peritoneum or biliary tract.
Ascariasis	Biliary obstruction by adult worms, parenchymal granulomas from larvae.
Toxocariasis	Visceral larva migrans syndrome. Hepatomegaly with granulomas, eosinophilia.
Spirochetes	
Leptospirosis	Acute fever, prostration, jaundice, bleeding, renal injury. Liver necrosis often mild despite severe jaundice.
Syphilis	*Congenital:* neonatal hepatosplenomegaly, fibrosis. *Acquired:* variable hepatitis in secondary stage, gummas with irregular scarring in tertiary stage.
Relapsing fever	Borrelia infestation. Systemic symptoms, hepatomegaly, sometimes jaundice.

TABLE 69-1. SELECTED INFLAMMATORY CONDITIONS OF THE LIVER
(Cont'd)

Disease or Organism	Comments
Unknown	
Sarcoidosis	Granulomatous infiltration common. Usually subclinical; jaundice rare. Occasionally progressive inflammation with scarring, portal hypertension. Liver biopsy valuable.
Idiopathic granulomatous hepatitis	Active chronic granulomatous inflammation not due to known causes (sarcoid variant?). Systemic symptoms may dominate with fever, malaise. Corticosteroids suppress symptoms.
Ulcerative colitis Crohn's disease	Spectrum of hepatic disease, especially in ulcerative colitis. Includes periportal inflammation ("pericholangitis"), sclerosing cholangitis, cholangiocarcinoma, ↑ incidence of chronic active hepatitis. Poor correlation with activity or treatment of bowel disorder.

ACUTE VIRAL HEPATITIS

(See also NEONATAL HEPATITIS B VIRUS INFECTION in Vol. II, Ch. 21)

Diffuse hepatocellular inflammatory disease caused by at least 3 different viral agents.

This is a common and important worldwide disease. Older terms that should be abandoned include infectious hepatitis (IH) and short-incubation hepatitis for Type A disease; and serum hepatitis (SH), posttransfusion hepatitis, and long-incubation hepatitis for virus B infection.

Etiology and Viral Characteristics

At least 3 distinct viruses are responsible—viruses A, B, and non-A, non-B; the latter is probably more than one agent. Liver infections due to other specific viruses such as cytomegalovirus, yellow fever virus, etc., are considered separate disorders and are not included in general usage of the term *acute viral hepatitis*.

Hepatitis B virus: This is the most thoroughly characterized. The infective ("Dane") particle consists of an inner core plus an outer surface coat. The former contains DNA and DNA polymerase, and replicates within the nuclei of infected hepatocytes. Surface coat is added in the cytoplasm, and for unknown reasons is produced in great excess; it can be detected in serum by immunologic means as hepatitis B surface antigen (see below).

The B virus is associated with a wide spectrum of liver disease, from a subclinical carrier state to acute hepatitis, chronic hepatitis, postnecrotic (posthepatitic) cirrhosis, and hepatocellular carcinoma. It also has a poorly understood association with several primarily nonhepatic disorders including polyarteritis nodosa and other collagen vascular diseases, membranous glomerulonephritis, essential mixed cryoglobulinemia, and papular acrodermatitis of childhood. The pathogenetic role of the virus in these disorders is not clear, but in some patients tissue deposition of immune complexes contains viral antigen.

At least 3 distinct antigen-antibody systems are intimately related to the hepatitis B virus: (1) Hepatitis B surface antigen (**HBsAg,** Australia antigen) is associated with the viral surface coat; its presence in serum indicates active B infection and implies infectivity of the blood. Several antigenetic subtypes of HBsAg exist that are of epidemiologic interest but have little clinical significance. Circulating HBsAg provides the first evidence of acute hepatitis B infection. It characteristically appears during the incubation period, usually 1 to 6 wk before clinical or biochemical illness develops, and disappears during convalescence. The corresponding antibody (anti-HBs) appears only weeks or months later, after clinical recovery, and usually persists for life; its detection therefore implies hepatitis B infection in the past and relative protection against future infection. In up to 10% of cases HBsAg persists following acute infection and anti-HBs does not develop; these patients can develop chronic hepatitis or become asymptomatic carriers of the virus. (2) Core antigen (**HBcAg**) is associated with the viral inner core. It can be found in infected liver cells but is not detectable in serum except by special technics which disrupt the Dane particle. Antibody to the core (anti-HBc) is thought to reflect active viral replication and generally appears at the onset of clinical illness, with gradually diminishing titer thereafter. It is regularly found in chronic hepatitis B carriers, who do not mount an anti-HBs response, and occasionally may be the only marker of active B infection. (3) The e antigen (**HBeAg**) is closely associated with virus B, but its exact origin is still unknown. Found only in HBsAg-positive serum, its presence may be associated with greater infectivity of the blood and a greater likelihood of progression to chronic liver disease, though this is still debated. In contrast, presence of the corresponding antibody (anti-HBe) may point to lesser infectivity and usually portends a benign outcome.

Hepatitis A virus: This is a smaller particle than virus B and is an enterovirus-like RNA virus. Viral antigen (HAAg) is found in serum, stool, and liver only during acute infection. IgM antibody appears early in the disease but disappears within a few weeks, followed by the development of IgG antibody which persists, probably for life (anti-HA). Thus IgM antibody is a marker of acute infection, while IgG anti-HA indicates previous exposure to virus A and immunity to recurrent infection. Unlike hepatitis B, there is no known chronic carrier state for hepatitis A, and the agent appears to play little or no role in the production of chronic liver disease.

Non-A, non-B virus(es): Little is known about the identity of this agent or agents, though increasing evidence points to at least 2 separate viruses. In general the biologic and clinical behavior appears akin to that of hepatitis B.

Epidemiology

Virus A spreads primarily by fecal-oral contact, though blood and possibly secretions are also infectious. Fecal shedding of the virus occurs during the incubation period and usually ceases a few days after symptoms begin; thus infectivity often has already passed when the diagnosis is made. Water- and food-borne epidemics are common, especially in underdeveloped countries. Ingestion of contaminated raw shellfish can be responsible. Sporadic cases are usually due to person-to-person contact. Most infections are subclinical or unrecognized, and population surveys of anti-HA have revealed remarkably widespread exposure to the virus. This varies with age, socioeconomic class, geography, and other factors, but in some countries more than 3/4 of the adult population appears to have been previously exposed.

Virus B is mainly transmitted parenterally. Transfusion of contaminated blood or blood products is the typical source, although the sharing of needles by drug abusers is often responsible. An increased risk to patients and personnel in renal dialysis units has also been identified. Nonparenteral spread can also occur, e.g., between sexual partners, but infectivity is far lower than for virus A and the means of acquisition in many cases is unknown. The role of transmission by insects that bite is unclear. Surveys of anti-HBs have shown that unrecognized infection with virus B is common, though less widespread than with hepatitis A. Chronic carriers provide a worldwide reservoir. Carrier prevalence varies widely with geographic and other factors, from < 0.5% of the population in North America and northern Europe to > 10% in some regions of the Far East. Vertical transmission from mother to infant is partly responsible (see HEPATIC DISORDERS IN PREGNANCY in Vol. II, Ch. 16). Figures are higher among residents of closed institutions, drug abusers, homosexuals, and other subgroups than for the general population.

Little is known about the epidemiology of non-A, non-B viruses. They can be transmitted parenterally and are responsible for many cases of sporadic acute hepatitis. A chronic carrier state also appears to exist.

The epidemiology of posttransfusion hepatitis has changed since the advent of donor screening for HBsAg. Non-A, non-B hepatitis is now by far the commonest cause, though virus B is still responsible for a significant minority of cases. The remainder are mainly due to cytomegalovirus and Epstein-Barr virus; virus A causation is now deemed very rare.

Virus A infection has an incubation period of about 2 to 6 wk; virus B and probably virus(es) non-A, non-B, about 4 to 25 wk. All age groups are affected, though hepatitis A is most common in children and young adults.

Pathology

All liver acini are affected by patchy necrosis and mononuclear inflammatory infiltrate. Histologic evidence of regeneration is also present, even in early cases. The underlying reticulin framework is usually preserved and complete histologic recovery is the rule, unless extensive necrosis bridges entire acini.

Symptoms and Signs

Hepatitis varies from a minor flu-like illness to fulminant, fatal liver failure, depending on the patient's immune response and other poorly understood virus-host factors. The following applies to a typical case; variants are discussed below.

The **prodromal phase** begins suddenly with anorexia, malaise, nausea and vomiting, and fever. Distaste for cigarettes is a characteristic early manifestation of profound anorexia. Urticarial eruptions and arthralgias may occur, especially in Type B infection. After 3 to 10 days the **icteric phase** is ushered in by the appearance of dark urine, followed by jaundice. Systemic symptoms typically regress at this point, and the patient feels better despite worsening jaundice. Features of cholestasis may develop. Jaundice usually peaks within 1 to 2 wk, then fades during a 2- to 4-wk **recovery phase.**

Physical examination shows variable jaundice. The liver is usually enlarged and is often tender, but the edge remains soft and smooth. Mild splenomegaly is present in 15 to 20% of patients. Signs of chronic liver disease are not seen in uncomplicated cases.

Laboratory Findings

Striking transaminase elevations are the hallmark of the disease. High values appear early in the prodromal phase, peak before jaundice is maximal, and slowly fall during the recovery phase. The aspartate transferase (**AST**) or alanine transferase (**ALT**) (previously called SGOT or SGPT respectively) are typically 1000 to 3000 u., but correlation with clinical severity is poor. The ALT is typically more elevated than the AST, but this is only of limited value in differentiation from alcoholic or obstructive liver disease. Urinary bile appears before jaundice; its early detection provides a valuable clue to the diagnosis. The degree of hyperbilirubinemia is variable and fractionation is of little clinical value. Alkaline phosphatase is only modestly raised unless cholestasis is severe. Major prolongation of the prothrombin time is not common. The WBC count is usually low-normal, and blood smear often shows a few atypical lymphocytes.

Diagnosis

In the prodromal phase, hepatitis mimics a variety of flu-like illnesses and is difficult to diagnose. Approach to the diagnosis of jaundice is considered in Ch. 64. Drug or toxic hepatitis is distinguished primarily by history. Prodromal sore throat, diffuse adenopathy, and marked atypical lymphocytosis favor infectious mononucleosis. Alcoholic hepatitis is suggested by history of ingestion, more gradual onset of symptoms, and presence of spider nevi or other signs of chronic parenchymal disease. Extrahepatic obstruction and neoplasm are usually easily distinguished from hepatitis but occasionally are more difficult to rule out. Liver biopsy is not needed in most cases but should be considered if the diagnosis is uncertain; if the clinical course is atypical or unduly prolonged; if spider nevi, palmar erythema, or other clues to chronic liver disease are present; or if complications such as encephalopathy or fluid retention develop.

For specific etiology, Type B is diagnosed by identifying HBsAg in serum; further studies are needed to clarify the additional diagnostic value of anti-HBc and HBeAg. Failure to detect HBsAg does not entirely exclude virus B, as antigenemia may be transient. At the moment, hepatitis A is usually diagnosed indirectly by detecting antibody of the IgM type; better routine tests should soon be available. Non-A, non-B causation is currently diagnosed by exclusion.

Prognosis

Hepatitis resolves spontaneously in the large majority of cases, with the total illness usually lasting 4 to 8 wk. Atypical courses are discussed below. A favorable prognosis in hepatitis B is less certain than in virus A infection, especially in the elderly and in posttransfusion cases, where mortality may reach 10 to 15%. Non-A, non-B cases appear more likely to have a fluctuating clinical course and progression to chronic disease, especially if acquired via transfusion.

Prophylaxis

Personal hygiene helps to prevent spread of hepatitis A. Blood of patients with acute hepatitis must be handled with care, and in type A disease, stool should also be considered infectious. However, isolation of patients has been overemphasized; it does little to prevent spread of virus A and is of no value in type B or non-A, non-B disease. Posttransfusion infection is minimized by avoiding unnecessary transfusions, using volunteers rather than paid blood donors, and screening all donors for HBsAg. The latter is now almost universally available and has significantly decreased, though not eliminated, iatrogenic hepatitis B.

The value of prophylaxis with γ-globulin preparations is still debated; inadequately designed clinical trials and variable antibody titers underlie much of the uncertainty. Standard **immune serum globulin (ISG)** provides good protection against clinically apparent hepatitis A and should be administered to the household contacts of index cases and to travelers planning a prolonged visit to endemic areas; 0.02 ml/kg given IM is generally recommended but some experts advise 0.06 ml/kg (3 to 5 ml for adults). ISG is less clearly efficacious against hepatitis B and non-A, non-B but should probably be given at the higher dosage to regular sexual contacts of index cases; other household contacts need not be treated. Recently available, **hepatitis B immune globulin (HBIG)** contains much higher antibody titers against virus B. However, it is uncertain how much better it is clinically than ISG, and its cost limits its use. HBIG should be given to subjects with accidental "needle stick" exposure to HBsAg-positive blood, and possibly to infants born of HBsAg-positive mothers. On present evidence ISG or HBIG need not be given routinely to recipients of blood transfusion, contacts of HBsAg carriers or patients with chronic hepatitis, or patients and staff in dialysis units.

A **vaccine** for active immunization against hepatitis B is available. Preliminary testing showed an almost universal anti-HBs response in susceptible recipients and a dramatic reduction of about 90% in the incidence of hepatitis B infection. Vaccination is anticipated to have a major worldwide impact on the disease and may eventually diminish hepatocellular carcinoma, known to be associated with chronic virus B infection (see Ch. 74).

Treatment

In most cases no special treatment is required. Appetite usually returns after the first few days, and patients need not be confined to bed. Undue restrictions on diet or activity are without scientific basis. Vitamin supplements are rarely required. Corticosteroids are contraindicated in ordinary cases. Most patients may safely return to work before jaundice completely resolves and before AST or ALT are normal.

VARIANTS OF ACUTE VIRAL HEPATITIS

Anicteric hepatitis, a minor flu-like illness without jaundice, may be the only clinical manifestation of acute hepatitis, especially in children. There is evidence that this far exceeds "typical" hepatitis in frequency, but the diagnosis is usually overlooked unless the characteristic elevations in AST and ALT are sought.

Recrudescent hepatitis occurs in a minority of patients during the recovery phase. The prognosis remains good and chronic hepatitis rarely follows.

Despite general regression of the inflammatory process, **cholestatic hepatitis** occasionally persists with jaundice, elevated alkaline phosphatase, and pruritus. Differentiation from extrahepatic biliary obstruction may be difficult. Eventual resolution is the rule. Cholestyramine 8 to 16 gm/day can relieve itching.

Fulminant hepatitis, a rare syndrome, is usually seen in hepatitis B, non-A, non-B infection, or drug injury; virus A is rarely responsible. Rapid clinical deterioration with the onset of hepatic encephalopathy presages a serious illness; in some cases coma develops within hours. There is massive necrosis of liver parenchyma and a decrease in liver size ("acute yellow atrophy"). Bleeding is common, resulting from parenchymal failure and disseminated intravascular coagulation. Increasing prothrombin time is a bad prognostic sign. Functional renal failure often develops and usually portends a fatal outcome.

Survival in adults is uncommon despite heroic measures; the prognosis for children is less grim. Meticulous nursing care and careful management of specific complications provide the best hope for recovery. Therapeutic measures such as massive doses of corticosteroids or exchange transfusions have not proved effective. Remarkably, survivors usually recover completely with no permanent hepatic damage.

Bridging necrosis, an uncommon variant, is characterized histologically by zones of collapse which bridge adjacent portal and/or central areas. Clinically it may be indistinguishable from ordinary viral hepatitis, but is suggested by an insidious rather than sudden onset and by the development of fluid retention or mild encephalopathy. The prognostic implication of bridging is debated; patients with chronic active hepatitis may largely arise from this subgroup, though most patients with bridging do recover fully. Corticosteroid therapy is controversial.

CHRONIC HEPATITIS

A spectrum of disorders that merge into acute hepatitis on the one hand and cirrhosis on the other. Hepatitis lasting for 6 mo is generally defined as "chronic," though this is arbitrary. Complex terminology has created confusion about chronic hepatitis; most cases, however, can be classified into chronic persistent or chronic active forms.

Chronic Persistent Hepatitis (Persistent Hepatitis)

This *benign* disorder usually follows typical acute hepatitis but may be detected de novo, especially in young drug abusers. Persistently high transaminase values with vague or no symptoms are characteristic. Other liver function tests are usually unremarkable and jaundice is uncommon. Clinical signs of chronic liver disease are absent.

The **diagnosis** depends on needle biopsy, which shows portal mononuclear infiltrate without significant fibrosis or acinar disarray. Overlap with chronic active hepatitis occurs but is uncommon. Occasionally, diffuse lobular inflammation is superimposed, with features of persisting acute hepatitis (chronic lobular hepatitis). Eventual recovery is usual, though the disorder may persist for years. Treatment is not necessary, and neither diet nor activity should be restricted.

Chronic Active (Aggressive) Hepatitis

This *serious* disorder often results in liver failure and/or cirrhosis. It is best regarded as a group of closely related conditions rather than a single disease. In most patients the **etiology** is unknown. Hepatitis B virus causes a minority of cases, but virus A is not thought responsible; the role of non-A, non-B virus(es) is not known. Drugs (e.g., methyldopa and isoniazid) are occasionally responsible. Wilson's disease may present as chronic active hepatitis and should be considered in children and young adults with the disorder. The **pathogenesis** is obscure, but considerable evidence favors an abnormal immune response to the causative agents. Some cases appear to have antibodies directed against a liver membrane antigen, but firm proof of a true autoimmune mechanism is still lacking.

Clinical features vary. About ⅓ of the cases follow acute hepatitis, but most develop insidiously de novo. Nonspecific malaise, anorexia, and fatigue often dominate the clinical picture. Jaundice is variable and is not always present. Signs of chronic liver disease such as splenomegaly, spider nevi, and fluid retention usually develop. Multisystemic or "immune" manifestations often occur, especially in young women and in cases of idiopathic origin. These can affect virtually any body system and include acne, amenorrhea, arthralgia, ulcerative colitis, pulmonary fibrosis, nephritis, and hemolytic anemia.

Laboratory abnormalities are those of an active hepatitis plus the frequent presence of "immune" abnormalities. These may include high γ-globulin levels (especially IgG), antinuclear factor, LE cells, and smooth-muscle antibodies. HBsAg, if present, indicates virus B as the etiology and is usually not associated with the above "immune" manifestations.

In **diagnosis,** the disorder must be differentiated from alcoholic liver disease, recrudescent viral hepatitis, chronic persistent hepatitis, and primary biliary cirrhosis. Clinical and laboratory features are helpful but *liver biopsy is essential for definitive diagnosis.* Biopsy shows periportal necrosis with lymphocytic and plasma cell infiltrates (so-called "piecemeal necrosis"); the acinar architecture is usually distorted by zones of collapse and fibrosis, and frank cirrhosis often coexists with the signs of ongoing hepatitis.

Treatment includes cessation of causative drugs, management of complications, and the use of corticosteroids and, sometimes, azathioprine. Controlled trials have demonstrated clinical, biochemical, and histologic improvement with these drugs, which suppress the inflammatory reaction, in a significant percentage of cases. Recent reports suggest that nonviral chronic active hepatitis responds, particularly when autoimmunity is evident, while cases due to viral infection do not. Dosage adjustment should be supervised by a specialist. Recent evidence suggests that steroids may harm rather than benefit HBsAg-associated cases; this patient subgroup should therefore be treated cautiously until the issue is clarified.

The **prognosis** is highly variable. With drug etiology, the disease may regress completely when the offending agent is withdrawn. Cases associated with HBsAg tend to be relatively resistant to steroid suppression; those with dominant "immune" features, relatively sensitive. With adequate therapy patients usually live several years, but hepatocellular failure, cirrhosis, or both eventually develop in most cases.

70. DRUGS AND THE LIVER

The liver metabolizes many drugs and toxins, most commonly by processes of oxidation, reduction, or conjugation. Interaction between drugs and the liver can be divided into 3 basic categories: (1) hepatic enzyme induction; (2) effects of liver disease on drug metabolism; and (3) liver damage due to drugs.

Enzyme Induction

Hepatic enzymes responsible for drug transformation are often induced (stimulated) by the agents they metabolize; hence many drugs stimulate their own catabolism. This effect is usually nonspecific so that transformation of other drugs is also enhanced. Important clinical consequences may result. For example, a patient on both oral anticoagulants and phenobarbital may suddenly bleed if the latter, a potent enzyme inducer, is discontinued. Ethanol also acts as a drug in this respect, which accounts for the well-known tolerance of alcoholics to sedatives and other agents. (See also Ch. 241.)

Influence of Liver Disease on Drug Metabolism

Complex effects on drug clearance and biotransformation can occur in liver disease, depending on alterations in plasma binding capacity, hepatic blood flow, extraction capacity, cellular transformation pathways, biliary excretion, etc. Net results for an individual drug are unpredictable and do not correlate well with the type of liver damage, its severity, or liver function tests. Thus, no general rules can be used to modify drug dosage in patients with liver disease.

Cerebral sensitivity to narcotics and sedatives is often enhanced in liver disease, so that seemingly small doses may precipitate hepatic encephalopathy.

Liver Damage Due to Drugs

Drugs are an important cause of hepatic disease. The mechanisms are variable, complex, and in most instances poorly understood. Some agents act as direct cellular toxins; injury from these is generally predictable, dose-related, and characteristic for the particular agent. Others produce damage only rarely in particularly susceptible individuals; injury from these is generally unpredictable and not dose-related. Although the latter is often termed a hypersensitivity, evidence for a true allergic reaction is usually lacking; idiosyncratic response is a preferable term. Moreover, the distinction between direct toxicity and idiosyncrasy seems less clear than previously thought. For example, in susceptible patients some drugs previously considered allergens appear to damage cell membranes directly via toxic intermediate metabolites.

No classification of drug jaundice is completely satisfactory, but most acute cases can be divided into hemolytic, hepatocellular, cholestatic, and miscellaneous reactions. Some drugs can produce chronic damage, including neoplasms.

Hemolysis: Drugs cause hemolysis by a variety of mechanisms. Mild jaundice may result from unconjugated hyperbilirubinemia, but no true hepatic damage occurs and liver function tests are normal.

Hepatocellular necrosis is conceptually divided into direct toxicity and idiosyncrasy, though as noted above this distinction may be artificial.

Direct toxicity: Most direct hepatotoxins produce dose-related liver necrosis, often with effects on other organs such as the kidneys. Damage can take several forms; e.g., carbon tetrachloride and related hydrocarbons cause severe centrolobular necrosis and fatty infiltration; phosphorus produces primarily periportal damage; ingestion of various *Amanita* mushrooms results in fatal hemorrhagic necrosis; and high-dose IV tetracycline, especially in pregnant women, produces diffuse fine-droplet fatty infiltration with a hepatitis-like clinical picture.

Acute overdosage of the mild analgesic **acetaminophen (paracetamol)** is an important cause of fulminant liver failure in Great Britain and is likely to become increasingly common in North America. Doses exceeding 10 to 15 gm deplete the liver of glutathione, which normally detoxifies the drug by binding potentially hazardous intermediate metabolites. When this mechanism is saturated, the resulting free intermediates bind to liver macromolecules and produce centrizonal necrosis. Liver damage is often not apparent until 3 to 5 days after ingestion, when the picture of acute hepatic failure develops. Mortality climbs as ingestion exceeds 25 gm. Early treatment with agents which replete glutathione appear beneficial, including cysteamine, L-methionine, and N-acetylcysteine; the latter is now generally preferred, as it can be given orally and is nontoxic. A loading dose of 140 mg/kg orally followed by 70 mg/kg q 4 h for 3 days will prevent major liver damage if started within 12 to 16 h of poisoning. Recent evidence also incriminates acetaminophen in chronic liver damage (see below).

Idiosyncrasy: Drugs can produce acute hepatocellular necrosis which is clinically, biochemically, and histologically indistinguishable from viral hepatitis. This type of reaction appears to differ from the above forms of toxic necrosis and is generally considered idiosyncratic; however, the mechanism is uncertain and probably varies with the specific drug. Offending agents are numerous and include isoniazid (INH), methyldopa, monoamine oxidase inhibitors, indomethacin, propylthiouracil, phenytoin, and the anesthetic agent halothane. Of these, INH and halothane have been most thoroughly studied.

INH causes minor, usually transient transaminase elevations in up to 20% of patients. Frank hepatitis occurs in 1 to 2% *and can be fatal.* Subjects over age 35 and rapid acetylators of the drug appear more susceptible. Unlike most similar drug hepatitis, which appears within a few weeks of starting the agent, INH injury may be delayed up to a year and the association may therefore be overlooked. Chronic active hepatitis and cirrhosis can develop if the drug is not stopped. Whether the reaction is due to a hypersensitivity mechanism or to hepatotoxic metabolites is debated, but most evidence favors the latter.

The existence of **halothane-related hepatitis** is still doubted in some quarters but is almost universally accepted among hepatologists. Repeated exposure to the anesthetic at relatively short intervals is a common antecedent; unexplained postoperative fever after the preceding exposure may provide a warning signal. The mechanism of injury is still unclear. Obesity seems a risk factor, possibly because halothane metabolites are stored in adipose tissue. Hepatitis typically develops within a few days to 2 wk after operation, is heralded by fever, and is often severe. Distinction from posttransfusion viral hepatitis is aided by a shorter latent period, absence of hepatitis antigens in serum, occasional presence of eosinophilia or skin rash, and sometimes subtle histologic differences. Mortality is high but surviving patients usually recover completely.

Cholestasis: A variety of agents can produce a primarily cholestatic reaction. In most instances the pathogenesis is poorly understood, but there are at least 2 clinically distinct forms of cholestatic injury.

The **phenothiazine type** is a periportal inflammatory reaction often associated with acute clinical onset, fever, and high transaminase as well as alkaline phosphatase levels. Differentiation from extrahepatic obstruction may be difficult, even by liver biopsy. The reaction seems due to individual idiosyncrasy, and in some cases eosinophilia and other evidence of a sensitivity reaction occurs. Other evidence, however, points to a direct toxic action on hepatic canaliculi, possibly via interference with membrane ATPase. This type of cholestasis occurs in about 1% of patients given chlorpromazine, less often with other phenothiazines. Complete resolution is usual, though rarely progression to a chronic biliary cirrhosis-like illness can occur even if the drug is withdrawn. A similar picture can be produced by tricyclic antidepressants, chlorpropamide, phenylbutazone, erythromycin estolate, and other drugs, though these have been less thoroughly studied and progression to chronic liver damage has not been established.

The **steroid type** is a pure cholestatic reaction with little or no hepatocellular inflammation. Gradual onset of cholestasis without systemic symptoms is usual. Alkaline phosphatase is elevated but transaminase levels are usually unimpressive, and liver biopsy shows only centrolobular bile stasis with little portal reaction or parenchymal disarray. Complete resolution follows cessation of the offending steroid. This type of cholestasis is produced by oral contraceptives, methyltestosterone, and related drugs, most of which are C-17 alkylated steroids. About 1 to 2% of women taking oral contraceptives develop the syndrome; figures vary around the world, possibly because of genetic factors. The reaction appears to be an exaggeration of the physiologic effect of sex hormones on hepatic bile formation, rather than an immunologic sensitivity or membrane cytotoxicity. Interference with canalicular water flow and microfilament function may be responsible, although the exact mechanism of impaired bile transport is still uncertain. The syndrome is closely related to cholestasis of pregnancy (see Vol. II, Ch. 16); women with the latter condition often develop cholestasis when given oral contraceptives, and vice versa.

Miscellaneous reactions: Some drugs produce variable forms of hepatic dysfunction that are difficult to classify. Responsible agents include aminosalicylic acid (PAS), sulfonamides, several other antibiotics, quinidine, allopurinol, and aspirin. Many anti-neoplastic drugs also cause hepatic damage; mechanisms vary.

Chronic Liver Disease

Ongoing liver damage indistinguishable from chronic active hepatitis can be produced by the laxative oxyphenisatin (no longer marketed), INH, and methyldopa. In some instances the illness begins as an acute hepatitis, in others more insidiously; progression to cirrhosis may occur. A chronic active hepatitis-like picture with scarring has recently been reported in patients using acetaminophen long-term in doses as low as 3 gm daily.

As noted above, chlorpromazine can rarely produce chronic cholestasis with progressive biliary fibrosis. Methotrexate induces insidiously progressive hepatocellular damage and scarring, often with unremarkable liver function tests; occasional biopsy is advisable in patients on long-term use of the drug, usually for psoriasis. Arsenicals can produce non-cirrhotic hepatic fibrosis with portal hypertension, and chronic scarring is also occasionally seen in health faddists who ingest enormous amounts of vitamin A or niacin. In many tropical and subtropical countries, chronic liver disease and hepatocellular carcinoma are believed to result from ingestion of fungal products known as aflatoxins in food.

In addition to the above-noted cholestasis, considerable recent evidence associates the use of oral contraceptives with the occasional development of benign hepatic adenomas, focal nodular hyperplasia (an unusual adenoma-like condition of the liver), and rarely, hepatocellular carcinoma (see Ch. 74). The adenomas are often subclinical but may present with sudden intraperitoneal rupture and hemorrhage requiring emergency laparotomy. Hepatic vein thrombosis with Budd-Chiari syndrome may also occur in women on oral contraceptives, as part of a general increased clotting tendency. These drugs also enhance the lithogenicity of bile, with a resultant increased incidence of gallstones.

---

71. LIVER DISEASE DUE TO ALCOHOL

A spectrum of clinical syndromes and pathologic changes of the liver caused by alcohol. It constitutes a major and potentially preventable health problem.

Pathogenesis

In general, a linear correlation exists between the severity of liver damage and the intensity of alcohol abuse as measured by duration and dose. However, the mechanisms by which alcohol actually damages the liver have not yet been adequately defined.

By providing calories without essential nutrients, decreasing the appetite, and causing malabsorption through its toxic effects on the gut and pancreas, ethanol promotes malnutrition. Ethanol is also a hepatotoxin whose metabolism creates profound derangements of the liver cell. Apparent variations in the susceptibility of individuals and the greater susceptibility of females to alcoholic liver disease suggest that other factors are also significant. Family clustering of alcoholic liver disease occurs frequently enough that the influence of genetic factors cannot be dismissed. Although the data are controversial, and many abnormalities no doubt are secondary rather than primary, various immunologic abnormalities in patients with alcoholic liver disease suggest that one's immunologic status may play a major role in determining susceptibility to alcohol.

Metabolism of Ethanol

Ethanol is readily absorbed from the GI tract and $> 90\%$ of it is metabolized by the liver through oxidative mechanisms involving mainly alcohol dehydrogenase and certain microsomal enzymes. Acetaldehyde, the major product of oxidation, is in turn oxidized. Although details of its subsequent metabolism are not entirely clear, acetaldehyde itself may be implicated in some of the untoward effects of alcohol on the liver and other organs. The conversion of ethanol to acetaldehyde and of the latter to either acetate or acetyl coenzyme A involves the production of reduced nicotinamide adenine dinucleotide (NAD). Therefore, ethanol metabolism promotes a reduced intracellular state that interferes with carbohydrate, lipid, and other aspects of intermediary metabolism. The oxidation of ethanol is coupled with the reduction of pyruvate to lactic acid, which promotes hyperuricemia, hypoglycemia, and acidosis (see HYPOGLYCEMIA in Ch. 90). Ethanol oxidation is also coupled with the reduction of oxaloacetic acid to malate. This may explain the reduced activity of the citric acid cycle, reduced gluconeogenesis, and increased fatty acid synthesis associated with ethanol metabolism. An increase in α-glycerophosphate after ethanol administration is well documented; the glycerol thus produced may promote increased triglyceride synthesis. Although O_2 consumption is normal after ethanol, there is a metabolic shift from O_2 consumption during the breakdown of fatty acids to that consumed during the oxidation of alcohol to acetate. This shift may explain the reduced lipid oxidation and increased ketone formation recorded after ethanol ingestion. There is also evidence that alcohol metabolism induces a local hypermetabolic state in the liver, promoting hypoxic damage in Zone 3, that area around the terminal hepatic venules.

Although the hypothesis that alcoholics metabolize ethanol differently than non-alcoholics remains under study, there is no doubt that chronic ingestion of ethanol leads to adaptation by the liver with hypertrophy of the smooth endoplasmic reticulum and increased activity of the hepatic drug metabolizing enzymes. This fact is of clinical importance, since the alcohol abuser develops an increased tolerance to alcohol and to a variety of drugs including sedatives, tranquilizers, and antibiotics.

Pathology

The spectrum of hepatic pathology associated with prolonged alcohol consumption ranges from the simple accumulation of neutral fat in hepatocytes to cirrhosis and hepatocellular carcinoma. The widely accepted fatty liver-alcoholic hepatitis-cirrhosis spectrum is a concept of convenience. The findings usually overlap and many patients present features of the entire spectrum. The key lesion may well be fibrosis around the terminal hepatic venules. From the pathologic point of view, it is better to make a diagnosis of alcoholic liver disease and describe the specific findings in each patient.

Fatty liver appears to be the initial change associated with alcoholic liver disease and is the most common hepatic abnormality in hospitalized alcoholics. Usually asymptomatic, it may produce painful, tender hepatomegaly or even intrahepatic obstructive jaundice. It has also been associated with portal hypertension and acute hepatocellular failure. Its pathogenesis is not clear. Fat droplets of varying size are found in most hepatocytes except in regenerating areas. The droplets tend to coalesce, forming large globules which frequently occupy the entire cytoplasm. Fatty cysts probably represent late stages of the fatty change. These cysts are usually located periportally and ultrastructural evidence suggests that they form through fusion of the fat content of several hepatocytes (see also Ch. 67).

Hydropic change is prevalent in the early stages of alcoholic liver injury. Although insufficiently explained, ethanol does affect the membrane transport of cations, increasing intracellular sodium and water. It can also be associated with the intracellular accumulation of excess protein. **Mallory's alcoholic hyaline** is a fibrillar protein of uncertain origin and significance. It appears as dense acidophilic masses of variable size and shape near the nuclei of cells containing little or no fat. The cells are obviously damaged and neutrophils infiltrate the adjacent sinusoids. Mallory's alcoholic hyaline is characteristic of alcoholic liver disease, but it is also found in some cases of Wilson's disease, Indian childhood cirrhosis, the cirrhosis that follows small-intestine bypass surgery, primary biliary cirrhosis, hepatocellular carcinoma, and focal nodular hyperplasia. In association with this hyaline change, one usually finds a laying down of connective tissue in the sinusoids and around individual hepatocytes, especially in Zone 3 of the liver acinus. A subgroup of patients have prominent sclerosis around the terminal hepatic venules. This lesion, called **sclerosing hyaline necrosis** or **central hyaline sclerosis**, can lead to portal hypertension *before* the development of cirrhosis, and may be the earliest manifestation of the tendency to develop cirrhosis.

Focal liver necrosis is frequently found in biopsy specimens; these patients have no specific clinical or laboratory abnormalities. However, patients with **diffuse inflammation and necrosis** have **alcoholic hepatitis.** They have enlarged, smooth, yellow livers which microscopically feature necrosis, inflammation, and sclerosis. Alcoholic hepatitis is considered to be the precursor of **cirrhosis**, and the progression of alcoholic hepatitis to cirrhosis has been documented. About 20% of heavy drinkers will develop cirrhosis in which the liver is finely nodular with its architecture disorganized by thin fibrous septa and nodules. If drinking stops and the liver undergoes a constructive regenerative response, the picture can be that of a mixed cirrhosis (see Ch. 68).

Increased liver **iron** is seen in alcoholics with normal, fatty, or cirrhotic livers, but the incidence is < 10%. The underlying mechanisms are obscure, but there appears to be no relationship with the amount of iron consumed in the alcohol or with the length of drinking history. The distribution of iron found in hepatocytes and Kupffer cells is not pathognomonic. This iron elicits a meager inflammatory response and its role in hepatocellular damage is controversial.

Symptoms, Signs, and Diagnosis

Variations in drinking patterns, individual susceptibility to hepatotoxic effects of alcohol, and the many kinds of tissue damage noted above promote a highly variable clinical picture. For a long time, there may be no symptoms and no signs referable to the liver. In general, symptoms can be related to the amount of alcohol ingested and the overall duration of alcohol ingestion. Thus, symptoms usually become apparent in the 30s and severe problems tend to appear in the 40s.

Patients with only a fatty liver are usually asymptomatic but may have an enlarged, smooth, and occasionally tender liver. Routine biochemical studies are often within normal limits.

The diagnosis of alcoholic hepatitis should not be made on clinical grounds, since the diagnosis is a pathologic one and the histologic lesion can be found in all parts of the clinical spectrum of alcoholic liver disease. Patients with alcoholic hepatitis may present with fever, jaundice, right upper quadrant pain, leukocytosis, and hepatomegaly, but so also may patients with sepsis, cholecystitis, or mechanical extrahepatic biliary obstruction. Patients with cirrhosis, portal hypertension, portal systemic encephalopathy, or hepatocellular carcinoma often present clinical features of these problems (see under the appropriate headings).

Laboratory Investigation

The laboratory can be remarkably *un*helpful in establishing the diagnosis of alcoholic liver disease. Although sometimes suggestive, routine hematologic and biochemical tests are nonspecific and do not permit a definitive diagnosis. In alcoholic liver disease one can find various abnormalities of erythrocyte morphology, including target cells, macrocytes, spur cells, and stomatocytes. One may find that the activity of the serum alanine aminotransferase (formerly SGPT) is depressed relative to that of the serum aspartate aminotransferase (formerly SGOT). The activity of the serum γ-glutamyl transpeptidase may be helpful in detecting alcohol consumption, the value of the enzyme lying not in its specificity but in its sensitivity to changes in liver status. An increase in the plasma concentration of α-amino-N-butyric acid may indicate chronic alcohol consumption. The activity of the serum glutamate dehydrogenase may be helpful in detecting liver cell necrosis, the value of this enzyme lying in its specificity as a mitochondrial enzyme localized predominantly in Zone 3, the region of the liver acinus most susceptible to alcohol damage. Hepatic collagen synthesis and hepatic prolyl hydroxylase activity are correlated and the activity of the latter may prove to be of prognostic value. Liver scans and ultrasound examinations are frequently performed. All of the above may be helpful, but in the final analysis, one depends on documentation of the liver morphology. While blind needle biopsy is usually sufficient, guided biopsy at laparoscopy is more reliable.

Treatment

In theory the treatment of this condition is simple and straightforward; in practice it is difficult: *the patient must stop drinking alcohol.* Following severe bouts of illness and major adverse social consequences (e.g., job loss and threat of divorce) and a review of the facts by a physician who establishes rapport, many will stop drinking. It helps to point out that much of alcoholic liver disease is reversible. Otherwise, management is nonspecific and focuses on general supportive care (see also DEPENDENCE ON ALCOHOL in Ch. 136).

Although still controversial, it is unlikely that corticosteroids have any role to play in the treatment of alcoholic liver disease. There is much interest in therapeutic measures directed against hepatic fibrogenesis, but the use of colchicine, penicillamine, and proline analogs must still be restricted to carefully designed and executed clinical trials. The same comment must be applied to propylthiouracil, a drug currently under study to reduce the local hypermetabolic state induced in the liver by alcohol. Trauma, infection, malignant degeneration, GI bleeding, nutritional deficiencies, fluid retention, and portal systemic encephalopathy require specific attention.

Prognosis

Nonfibrotic liver damage may be reversed with abstinence. The reversibility of sclerosing hyaline necrosis is under study. The significance of alcoholic hepatitis appears to be determined by the degree of associated fibrosis and liver cell necrosis. The survival of patients with alcoholic hepatitis, fibrosis, and cirrhosis improves if drinking stops.

---

72. POSTOPERATIVE HEPATIC DISORDERS

Mild liver function derangements sometimes occur after major surgery and reflect poorly understood effects of anesthetic and operative stress. Patients with underlying liver disease may develop more severe dysfunction postoperatively; for example, laparotomy may precipitate acute liver failure in the patient with viral or alcoholic hepatitis.

Transient hypotension and circulatory failure can cause acute centrolobular necrosis with marked transaminase elevations. Jaundice, when present, is mild and enzyme elevations are usually transient unless the pigment load on the liver is increased by concomitant factors such as blood transfusions, hemolysis, resorption of hematomas, and sepsis. In these circumstances the hyperbilirubinemia is mixed and may be severe, although liver failure is uncommon and complete resolution is usual. This multifactorial type of jaundice is especially frequent after cardiovascular or major abdominal surgery that requires numerous transfusions.

True postoperative hepatitis is usually due to viral transmission via transfusion, and must be differentiated from the above abnormalities. The latter are usually maximal within a few days of operation, whereas viral hepatitis rarely develops before 2 wk. Halothane anesthesia may also produce postoperative hepatitis and should be suspected if hepatitis develops within 10 days of surgery, especially if preceded by unexplained fever (see Ch. 70).

Cholestatic reactions are most often due either to biliary obstruction from intra-abdominal complications or to drugs prescribed postoperatively (see Ch. 70). Obscure intrahepatic cholestasis occasionally develops after major surgery; the cause is unknown, but gradual recovery is usual.

73.   VASCULAR LESIONS OF THE LIVER

Thrombotic, occlusive, and inflammatory lesions of arteries and veins within and adjoining the liver.

LESIONS OF THE HEPATIC ARTERY

Congenital anomalies of the hepatic artery are common; 45% are variations on the conventional textbook picture. The main variants are replacement of the left or right hepatic artery, an accessory left or right hepatic artery, or a common hepatic artery originating from the superior mesenteric artery. Usually of no clinical significance, these anomalies can be important to the surgeon and interesting to the angiographer.

Hepatic artery occlusion is usually caused by thrombosis, embolism, or surgical ligation. The occlusion may produce an ischemic infarct of the liver but results are unpredictable because of individual differences in hepatic vasculature and the extent of collateral circulation. The underlying problem is usually part of a systemic process. The hepatic artery and its branches are involved in approximately 60% of cases of polyarteritis nodosa, and thrombotic occlusion leading to hepatic infarction has been documented in 15% of cases. A necrotizing hepatic arteritis has been described in drug addicts.

Aneurysms of the hepatic artery occur secondarily to infection, arteriosclerosis, trauma, and polyarteritis nodosa. They are often multiple and, although rare, they are dangerous because they tend to rupture into the peritoneal cavity, common bile duct, or adjacent hollow viscera. Accordingly, the ruptured hepatic artery aneurysm can present with upper abdominal colic, obstructive jaundice, or GI tract hemorrhage. When identified, hepatic artery aneurysms should be excised if possible. Otherwise hepatic artery ligation is indicated.

LESIONS OF THE HEPATIC VENOUS SYSTEM

Veno-occlusive disease (VOD) involves an obliterative lesion of the terminal hepatic venules and the small tributaries of the hepatic venous system. The larger branches of the hepatic veins are not involved. The lesion is basically ischemic, with fibrin and platelet aggregates surrounding the veins and obstructing the flow of blood from the hepatic sinusoids. This in turn leads to hepatocellular and sinusoidal cell damage. The lesion has been produced experimentally by alkaloids from crotalaria and Senecio plants, by other hepatotoxins (dimethylnitrosamine, aflatoxin, and azathioprine), and by radiation. It has also been reported in a family featuring immune deficiencies.

VOD is endemic in Jamaica, where tea is made from Senecio leaves, and it is reported from many other countries. It presents in an acute manner with the sudden onset of ascites and tender, smooth hepatomegaly. Although patients of all age groups are affected, it involves primarily children ages 1.5 to 3 yr. Characteristically, the patient recovers promptly with or without treatment, but some die with acute hepatic failure, and others present at a later date with portal hypertension with or without cirrhosis. There is no specific therapy apart from withdrawal of any offending toxin. Treatment of the associated portal hypertension is similar to that for the Budd-Chiari syndrome (see below).

BUDD-CHIARI SYNDROME

A rare syndrome resulting from thrombosis of the major hepatic veins. It affects both sexes and all age groups but especially those between ages 20 and 40 yr.

Etiology

Although usually no cause is confirmed, disorders of blood coagulation are often incriminated. Abnormal coagulation may be involved in cases associated with polycythemia vera and other myeloproliferative disorders, with sickle cell anemia, and with the use of oral contraceptives. Malignant disease in the region of hepatic veins and especially renal cell carcinoma have been implicated, as have abdominal trauma, paroxysmal nocturnal hemoglobinuria, pregnancy, congenital absence of the hepatic venous ostia, and various suppurative lesions of the liver.

Pathology

Hepatic vein occlusion occurs either in the intrahepatic portion of the inferior vena cava, or more often in the large hepatic veins near their entrance to the inferior vena cava. The obstruction is usually caused by thrombi, sometimes by fibrous cords, webs, or membranes that presumably are the residue of thrombi. Hepatic veins may be obscured by surrounding fibrosis, and the parenchyma of the liver features severe sinusoidal congestion, atrophy, and/or destruction of the hepatocytes in Zone 3. In chronic cases, perivascular fibrosis develops and nodular regeneration with subsequent loss of normal architecture may occur. Portal hypertension develops with splenomegaly and portal systemic anastomoses. Secondary portal vein thrombosis occurs in approximately 20% of cases and spontaneous rupture of the liver has been reported.

Symptoms and Signs

Patients usually present with abdominal pain, tender smooth hepatomegaly, gross and therapeuti-cally resistant ascites, and mild jaundice. The onset can be acute and devastating but it is usually subacute, with a delay of weeks or months before the complete picture of portal hypertension and liver cell failure becomes apparent. The prognosis is poor; < ⅓ of patients survive for 1 yr.

Diagnosis

Routine biochemical testing is of little value, but hepatic scintiscanning can be diagnostic. The isotope becomes concentrated in the caudate lobe, which is drained by veins that empty directly into the vena cava and which are often unaffected in patients with thrombosis of the main hepatic veins. Hepatic venography defines the extent of the thrombosis and any involvement of the vena cava. Liver biopsy can reveal the changes mentioned above.

Treatment

Side-to-side portacaval decompressive surgery should be considered early in the treatment of cases with a patent portal vein and inferior vena cava, but the perioperative mortality is high. Con-servative management employing anticoagulant or fibrinolysin therapy should be considered only in patients with incomplete obstruction of the hepatic veins and should be continued only if clinical improvement is rapid and associated with demonstrable clearing of the thrombosis.

LESIONS OF THE PORTAL VEIN

Congenital anomalies of the portal vein include aplasia and stricture. Cavernous transformation of the portal vein may represent a congenital malformation but is usually the end result of postpartum thrombosis followed by recanalization and new vessel formation. **Portal phlebosclerosis**, probably a congenital disorder, is recognized as a thickening of the intima of the portal veins with collagenous proliferation.

Portal vein thrombosis may occur at any point in its course. No etiological factor can be identified in > ½ of cases but it may be associated with inflammatory processes such as suppurative pyelo-phlebitis, cholangitis, adjacent suppurative lymphadenitis and hepatic abscess. It is rare in cirrhosis without cancer, but it frequently complicates hepatocellular carcinoma. Portal vein thrombosis oc-curs in pregnancy, especially in eclampsia.

The clinical effect of portal vein thrombosis depends on the location and extent of the thrombosis and the nature of any underlying liver disease. It may lead to infarction of the liver **(Zahn's infarct)** or segmental atrophy, i.e., left lobe atrophy. If associated with mesenteric vein thrombosis, it is acutely fatal. If the portal vein thrombosis develops slowly, then collaterals may form and portal vein recanal-ization occurs. Nevertheless, **portal hypertension** is the end result (see below).

Biochemical tests are usually normal although the alkaline phosphatase can be elevated. The major clinical problem is bleeding varices. Recurring hemorrhage tends to be well tolerated because liver cell function is usually normal. If the splenic vein is patent, the treatment of choice is a spleno-renal shunt; if not, a mesocaval shunt should be performed. Since small veins promote shunt throm-bosis, shunting procedures in a child should be delayed as long as possible. Endoscopic sclerosis of esophageal varices has been advocated in this situation.

LESIONS OF THE SINUSOIDS

Sinusoidal portal hypertension with normal portal veins and without clinical evidence of postsinus-oidal portal hypertension has been reported. Pathologically, the liver features marked Kupffer cell hypertrophy with narrowing of the sinusoidal lumena and a perisinusoidal fibrosis with obliteration of the space of Disse.

Peliosis hepatis is an uncommon lesion characterized by multiple small blood-filled cystic spaces distributed in an apparently random manner in the liver parenchyma. The pathogenesis of the lesion remains obscure but focal parenchymal cell necrosis with hemorrhage is the most generally ac-cepted concept. Peliosis hepatis is associated with chronic wasting disorders, especially advanced pulmonary TB, with a number of different malignant neoplasms, and with the administration of ana-bolic androgenic steroids and oral contraceptives. Peliosis hepatis is usually asymptomatic and diag-nosed incidentally, but it can cause hepatic failure and the lesions can rupture.

Sinusoidal dilation without peliosis has been associated with corticosteroid therapy and with space-occupying lesions of the liver. In the latter case the lesion may reflect local mechanical ob-struction of the microcirculation.

PORTAL HYPERTENSION

Increased portal vein pressure caused by extrahepatic portal vein obstruction, increased hepatic blood inflow, or increased resistance to hepatic blood outflow. The veins of the portal venous system carry all blood from the abdominal GI tract, spleen, pancreas, and gallbladder back to the heart through the liver. The portal vein is formed posterior to the head of the pancreas at the level of the 2nd lumbar vertebra by union of the splenic and superior mesenteric veins. At the porta hepatis it divides into two main branches; its intrahepatic distribution is segmental, with terminal portal venules draining into the sinusoids. The portal vein carries about 1000 to 1200 ml of blood/min and 70% of the O_2 supplied to the liver. The portal venous system is valveless; its pressure, produced and maintained by the volume of inflow and resistance to outflow, is normally < 13 mm Hg. Portal venous inflow includes everything up to the level of the sinusoids. It is controlled by the sympathetic nervous system and is therefore responsive to certain vasoactive drugs and hormones. The venous outflow tracts, the hepatic venules and veins, are passive conduits unreactive to neurogenic and other stimulation. The normal portal vein pressure is therefore controlled chiefly by variations in inflow.

Portal hypertension depends on increased inflow and/or increased resistance to outflow. However, the response of the portal venous pressure to increases in hepatic blood flow is not linear. Furthermore it is limited, and the portal vein pressure does not usually rise above 25 mm Hg. Therefore, most cases of portal hypertension not caused by extrahepatic portal vein obstruction are thought to be caused by increased resistance to hepatic blood outflow.

Pathogenesis

The creation of arteriovenous or venous-venous anastomoses, the creation of abnormal and conflicting inflow currents, and mechanical compression and distortion of effluent channels by fibrous septa and parenchymal nodules are sufficient to explain the portal hypertension of cirrhosis (see Ch. 68). However, the basis for the postsinusoidal portal hypertension of partial nodular transformation, biliary cirrhosis, the late stages of a hepatic artery-portal vein fistula, or the late stages of schistosomiasis remains unexplained.

Most consequences of portal hypertension are associated with the development of portal-systemic anastomoses formed in order to return splanchnic blood to the heart. These collateral vessels develop along the falciform ligament and into the left renal vein via the splenic, diaphragmatic, or pancreatic veins, where protective epithelium adjoins absorptive epithelium, as in the cardia of the stomach, and where abdominal organs contact retroperitoneal tissues or adhere to the abdominal wall. Blood therefore returns to the heart via the azygos-hemiazygos system, the inferior vena cava, or the pulmonary veins. The metabolic effects of this collateral circulation are not yet fully understood, but they include the development of portal-systemic encephalopathy (see Ch. 64), gastric acid hypersecretion, and reduced uptake of O_2, metabolites, and drugs by the liver.

Symptoms and Signs

Clinically, portal hypertension is most often associated with cirrhosis and presents with splenomegaly, ascites, GI bleeding, or portal-systemic encephalopathy.

A plain x-ray of the abdomen may show calcification of the portal vein or hepatosplenomegaly. Tomograms of the mediastinum may show an enlarged azygos vein. Esophageal varices are visualized indirectly by radiologic technics or directly by endoscopy. The combined approach is often needed.

Diagnostic Tests

In any candidate for portal decompressive surgery, the patency of the portal vein must be determined by splenoportography, omphaloportography, or the venous phase of celiac angiography.

Portal venous pressure is measured by several approaches. **Intrasplenic pressure** can be measured by percutaneous insertion of a catheter into the red pulp of the spleen. This procedure, simple, safe, and repeatable, is the most common approach. Pressure in the **portal vein** itself can be measured at operation or by omphaloportography. The latter approach, which involves cannulation of the left branch of the portal vein via the veins in the round ligament, provides more physiologic data and is safer than percutaneous splenic puncture. While some morbidity is associated with the procedure, good pressure readings and visualization of the portal venous system are possible in most cases. **Intrahepatic pressure**, obtained by percutaneous liver puncture, also reflects portal vein pressure but is rarely used. The **wedged hepatic vein pressure**, obtained by insertion of a catheter into a hepatic vein until it can be advanced no further, is easy, safe, and reliable, but does not usually provide information concerning the patency of the portal vein. The sinusoidal or postsinusoidal pressure thus obtained reflects the portal venous pressure in most cases of chronic liver disease.

The combination of the wedged hepatic vein pressure and one of the prehepatic measurements of portal vein pressure permits the classification of portal hypertension into presinusoidal and postsinusoidal hypertension. In **presinusoidal portal hypertension,** only the prehepatic portal vein pressure is elevated; in **postsinusoidal portal hypertension**, both the prehepatic portal vein and the wedged hepatic vein pressures are elevated. **Intrahepatic presinusoidal portal hypertension** occurs, for example, in the early stages of schistosomiasis, congenital hepatic fibrosis, granulomatous infiltrations, myeloproliferative disease of the liver, acute alcoholic fatty liver, and acute viral hepatitis. **Extrahepatic presinusoidal portal hypertension** results from a block to the portal or splenic vein. **Intrahepatic postsinusoidal portal hypertension** is associated with the later stages of schistosomiasis, veno-occlusive disease of the liver, partial nodular transformation of the liver, and almost all cases of cirrhosis. **Extrahepatic postsinusoidal portal hypertension** is caused by hepatic vein outflow block and can be found with prolonged tricuspid insufficiency or constrictive pericarditis and with diseases of the hepatic venous system, as in the Budd-Chiari syndrome, veno-occlusive disease, and sickle cell anemia.

Treatment

The patient with portal hypertension presenting with an acute upper GI hemorrhage should be hospitalized regardless of the size of the hemorrhage (see also Ch. 52). Encephalopathy should be anticipated and no sedatives administered. The patient should be given a reduced protein intake, neomycin or lactulose orally, cleansing enemas, and blood transfusions as clinically indicated. Vitamin K_1, though often ineffective in the presence of severe parenchymal cell disease, should be given parenterally to the patient.

Vasopressin lowers the portal pressure at least temporarily in many cases and should be the initial routine treatment of bleeding esophageal varices. It can be given as 20 u. in 100 ml glucose IV over 10 min with the patient sitting on a bedpan and forewarned of abdominal pain. It can also be given as an infusion into the splanchnic circulation. A satisfactory response in terms of bleeding is not specific for variceal bleeding, since erosive gastritis and peptic ulceration can also respond to the mesenteric vasoconstriction induced by vasopressin. Reduction in hepatic artery flow is undesirable, but at present no alternative method of lowering portal pressure is available. Furthermore, vasopressin causes coronary vasoconstriction, and evidence of myocardial ischemia is a *contraindication* to its use. Vasopressin may be repeated q 3 to 4 h if rebleeding occurs, but its efficacy usually diminishes with continued use. The ultimate failure of this agent to control hemorrhage reflects the degree of liver failure rather than the treatment.

Esophageal tamponade by means of a Sengstaken-Blakemore tube should be attempted if vasopressin fails, but its use is associated with such a high complication rate that it should be restricted to specialized centers. **Gastric cooling** is better tolerated than esophageal tamponade but also needs special apparatus and a great deal of attention.

Every patient with an upper GI hemorrhage should be under the care of a surgeon as well as a physician from the time of admission to the hospital. Most centers still prefer to submit the patient with cirrhosis complicated by variceal bleeding to elective rather than emergency surgery. Insufficient evidence exists to justify the claim that the selective decompression of gastroesophageal varices achieved through a distal splenorenal shunt provides somewhat better long-term control than either the classic portacaval or splenorenal shunt. Complications associated with portal decompressive surgery include deterioration of liver function, the development of disabling portal-systemic encephalopathy, transverse myelopathy, and hemosiderosis. Portacaval decompression usually prevents repeat hemorrhage from the varices; other long-term benefits to the patient remain to be established. A promising development is that of identifying those patients in whom portal diversion will produce a low residual intrahepatic venous pressure and either early death or chronic encephalopathy. *These patients are not candidates for portal decompressive surgery of any kind.*

Widespread dissatisfaction with the safety and efficacy of portal decompressive surgery has led to the introduction of other approaches to variceal hemorrhages. These approaches, none of them studied in a prospective and adequately controlled manner, include transhepatic obliteration of the varices, endoscopic sclerotherapy of the varices, laser coagulation of the varices, and esophageal transection.

VASCULAR DISORDERS OF THE LIVER ASSOCIATED WITH SYSTEMIC DISEASE

Circulatory Failure

In **acute heart failure**, ischemic changes of the liver are common. Histologically, the liver features necrosis of the hepatocytes and congestion in Zone 3. The inflammatory response is usually modest and the lobular architecture retained.

With **chronic cardiac failure** the liver is usually firm. Its nutmeg appearance on cross-section is produced by the association of the dark congested Zone 3 areas and the pale, sometimes fatty, Zone I areas. Fibrosis is frequent but cirrhosis is rare; its pathogenesis requires repeated and prolonged episodes of heart failure. Histologically one finds congestion and loss of hepatocytes in Zone 3. The areas of necrosis can join and in severe cases Zone 3 to Zone 3 bridging can be found. The lobular reticulin framework can be destroyed and new collagen forms around the terminal hepatic veins.

Diagnostically, acute cardiac decompensation can present with elevations of the aminotransferases to ranges suggesting acute hepatitis. **Therapeutically,** efforts are directed toward the underlying cardiac disease.

Sickle Cell Disease (see Vol. II, Ch. 25)

Liver damage due to impaired sinusoidal blood flow is common in sickle cell disease. Aggregates of erythrocytes and thrombi obstruct the sinusoids, especially in Zone 3 and lead to sinusoidal congestion and focal necrosis. The Kupffer cells are enlarged and contain ceroid, hemosiderin, and phagocytosed erythrocytes.

Rendu-Osler-Weber Disease (see Ch. 95)

In hereditary hemorrhagic telangiectasia one may find telangiectasia, hemangioma, fibrosis, and cirrhosis of the liver. The associated arteriovenous shunting can produce an enlarged liver with a palpable thrill and continuous bruit. High output cardiac failure can be severe and can further compromise the integrity of the liver.

74. HEPATIC NEOPLASMS

BENIGN

Benign liver tumors are relatively uncommon. Many are subclinical and are detected incidentally at laparotomy or autopsy. Others are discovered because of hepatomegaly, right upper quadrant discomfort, or intraperitoneal hemorrhage. Liver function tests are normal or only trivially elevated. The diagnosis is usually established only at laparotomy, although scanning technics and arteriography may provide preoperative clues.

Hepatocellular adenoma is the most important. Seen primarily in women of childbearing age, its prevalence has increased due to the widespread use of oral contraceptives, which appear to play a role in pathogenesis (see also Chs. 70 and Vol. II, Ch. 11). It most commonly presents as an acute surgical abdominal problem due to abrupt rupture and bleeding into the peritoneal cavity. Though not generally considered precancerous, a few cases with malignant transformation have recently been described. Contraceptive-related adenomas sometimes regress if the drug is stopped. **Focal nodular hyperplasia** is a similar localized tumorlike disorder which histologically may resemble macronodular cirrhosis and is probably a hamartoma rather than a true neoplasm. Oral contraceptives have been implicated. Related variants exist, and histopathologic overlap with adenoma may occur; terminology is confusing. **Hemangiomas** may become apparent because of associated consumption coagulopathy or hemodynamic disturbances, especially in infants. **Bile duct adenomas** and a variety of rare **mesenchymal neoplasms** also occur.

MALIGNANT

METASTATIC CARCINOMA

This is by far the most common form of hepatic tumor. The liver provides a fertile bed for blood-borne metastases; lung, breast, colon, pancreas, and stomach are the most frequent primary sites, though virtually any source may be responsible. Hepatic spread is not uncommonly the initial clinical manifestation of cancer elsewhere.

Clinically, nonspecific evidence of malignancy is frequent, such as weight loss, anorexia, and fever. The liver is characteristically enlarged and hard, and may be tender; massive hepatomegaly with easily palpable lumps signifies advanced disease. Hepatic bruits and pleuritic-like pain with an overlying friction rub are uncommon but characteristic signs. Splenomegaly is occasionally present, especially with a primary pancreatic cancer. Concomitant ascites is frequent; jaundice is usually absent or mild until the late stages unless biliary obstruction by tumor coexists. In the earliest stages abnormal BSP retention may be the only biochemical manifestation, though alkaline phosphatase, and sometimes LDH, typically increase earlier or to a greater degree than other liver function tests. Bilirubin and transaminase levels are variable.

Diagnosis of hepatic metastases is best made by percutaneous liver biopsy, which gives positive results in about 2/3 of cases; an additional 10% can be identified by cytologic examination of the aspirating fluid. Some authors prefer biopsy under direct vision through a laparoscope, though this is more complex. Isotopic scanning is widely used in diagnosis (see also Chs. 65 and 227); though often suggestive, it cannot detect small metastases or reliably discriminate tumor from cirrhosis and other benign causes of impaired uptake. Ultrasound, CT, and other nonhistologic investigations may help but are also nonspecific. **Treatment** is usually futile.

HEMATOLOGIC MALIGNANCIES

Hepatic involvement in **leukemia** and related disorders is common, due to infiltration with the abnormal cells. The diagnosis is usually apparent from hematologic assessment, and liver biopsy is not needed. Diagnosing **hepatic lymphoma,** especially Hodgkin's disease, is more complex. Knowledge of liver involvement is important for staging and therapeutic decisions, but unfortunately there is poor correlation among clinical, biochemical, and histologic findings. Hepatomegaly and abnormal liver function tests may reflect a nonspecific reaction to Hodgkin's disease elsewhere rather than true liver involvement, and biopsy often shows nondescript focal mononuclear infiltrates or granulomas of uncertain significance. The role of periteonoscopy or open biopsy is still debated.

PRIMARY CANCER

HEPATOCELLULAR CARCINOMA (Hepatoma)

Hepatocellular carcinoma is much less common than metastatic disease in most areas of the world, but is an important cause of death in certain areas of Africa and Southeast Asia. About half the patients have underlying cirrhosis; alcoholic, postnecrotic, and especially hemochromatotic cirrhosis all have a propensity to malignant transformation. Environmental carcinogens may play a role; e.g., ingestion of food contaminated with fungal aflatoxins is believed by many to contribute to the high incidence in subtropical regions. Increasing evidence incriminates chronic infection with hepatitis B virus, although whether the virus is directly oncogenic is not known. The association is particularly impressive in areas of high prevalence but also exists in some European and North American patients who do not have underlying alcoholic cirrhosis.

Symptoms, Signs, and Diagnosis

Abdominal pain, weight loss, a right upper quadrant mass, or unexplained deterioration in a previously stable patient with cirrhosis are the most common clinical presentations. Fever is relatively frequent and may simulate infection. Interesting systemic metabolic manifestations occasionally occur, including hypoglycemia, erythrocytosis, hypercalcemia, and hyperlipidemia. Scanning technics, hepatic arteriography, and especially biopsy are useful diagnostic aids. Biochemical tests are usually of little help except for the characteristic presence of α-fetoprotein in serum. This substance reflects hepatocellular dedifferentiation and is detectable by radioassay in most cases; less sensitive technics eliminate false-positives from other conditions with lower α-fetoprotein titers, but have a lesser yield.

Prognosis and Treatment

The prognosis for hepatocellular carcinoma is grim and treatment is generally unsatisfactory; survival may follow aggressive surgery in selected cases.

OTHER PRIMARY CANCERS

Cholangiocarcinoma, tumor arising from intrahepatic biliary epithelium, is common in the Orient where underlying infestation with liver flukes is believed partially responsible. Elsewhere it is less frequent than hepatocellular carcinoma. Histologic overlap between the two may occur. Patients with longstanding ulcerative colitis occasionally develop cholangiocarcinoma. **Hepatoblastoma** is one of the commoner cancers of infants; it occasionally presents with precocious puberty due to ectopic gonadotropin production, but is usually detected because of failing systemic health and a right upper quadrant mass. The rare **angiosarcoma** has recently attracted attention because of an association with industrial exposure to vinyl chloride. For all these tumors, diagnosis is based on histologic assessment. Therapy is usually of little value, and the prognosis is poor.

---

75. EXTRAHEPATIC BILIARY DISORDERS

INTRODUCTION

The bile ducts, cystic duct, and gallbladder comprise the biliary tract, whose structure is so variable that there is no "normal anatomy" of this system. The principal function of the biliary tract is to transport bile from the liver into the duodenum. **Cholelithiasis** (gallstones) is the primary abnormality of the biliary tract. About a half million people are hospitalized in the USA each year because of gallbladder disorders. Symptoms and signs of biliary tract abnormalities are quite variable and depend on the extent of the disease and the presence of complications. For laboratory studies used in the diagnosis of gallbladder disease, see Ch. 65. Since biliary tract abnormalities are mechanical in nature, they are almost always treated surgically.

ABNORMALITIES OF THE GALLBLADDER

BILE ACID METABOLISM

Bile acids are steroid compounds derived from cholesterol and formed exclusively in the liver. The bile acid pool of the body, weighing 3 to 4 gm, undergoes enterohepatic circulation about 10 times/day; therefore, the perfusion rate in the liver and small bowel is about 35 gm of bile acids/day. Bile acids probably account for most of the water entering the bile canaliculus; because they are detergents and form micelles, they keep otherwise insoluble constituents of the bile and intestinal contents in solution, facilitating their transport and absorption.

The two primary bile acids—cholic and chenodeoxycholic acids—constitute $> 80\%$ of the bile acids in man. Cholic acid conversion from cholesterol is restricted to a single major pathway, while chenodeoxycholic acid may be formed along several pathways. The identification and proper sequence of all intermediate compounds involved in their synthesis are not yet known. Prior to their secretion into the bile, bile acids are conjugated, primarily with glycine and taurine. The enteric phase of bile acid metabolism is complex. While there may be some proximal absorption, bile acids are primarily absorbed in the terminal ileum. Those that are not absorbed pass into the large bowel where bacteria metabolize them, producing secondary bile acids (deoxycholic and lithocholic), some of which are absorbed and return to the liver via the portal vein. The normal liver efficiently extracts bile acids from the portal blood, and the bile acid pool is largely confined to this enterohepatic circulation. Bile acids returning to the liver via the portal vein are subject to further chemical modification and re-excreted into the bile.

Although disorders of bile acid metabolism have been incriminated in the pathogenesis of certain forms of chronic liver disease, gastritis, diarrhea, and the malabsorption syndrome, and in the rare familial cerebrotendinous xanthomatosis, their role in the pathogenesis of cholesterol cholelithiasis provides the current focus of interest.

CHOLELITHIASIS (Gallstones)

Concretions in the gallbladder. Ten percent of the general population of the USA and 20% of those > 40 yr of age have gallstones. The problem is commoner in women, in Oriental, Latin American, and Indian peoples, and in those with cirrhosis of the liver and certain diseases of the small intestine.

Etiology

Cholesterol is a water-insoluble lipid normally solubilized in bile by virtue of its incorporation into mixed micelles of bile acids and phospholipids. The limits of cholesterol solubility determined in model systems simulating bile apply to the bile of patients with cholesterol gallstones. The molar ratio of cholesterol to bile acids plus phospholipids appears to determine whether cholesterol will remain in aqueous micellar solution or tend to precipitate and form stones; a bile saturated or supersaturated with cholesterol appears to be essential for cholesterol gallstone formation. Data suggest that patients with this disease have both a relative increase in cholesterol biosynthesis and a relative decrease in bile acid biosynthesis. But such conditions are not sufficient for stone formation and other factors are necessary; e.g., gallbladder stasis, quantitative and qualitative alterations in bile mucus, increased biliary bilirubin concentrations, biliary tract infection, and dietary, endocrine, and genetic factors. Those factors which promote nidus formation and retention and those which encourage structural organization and enlargement of the stone are still not well understood. Several kinds of metabolic defects may lead to cholesterol gallstone formation. Furthermore, cholesterol gallstones vary in their morphology, and it is uncertain whether or not they represent a single disease entity. Many gallstones are mixed gallstones that contain quantities of calcium and bilirubin with cholesterol. Patients with hemolytic anemias may have pure bilirubin stones; those with gout may have uric acid stones.

Symptoms and Signs

Patients with uncomplicated gallstones usually are asymptomatic but may complain of upper abdominal discomfort, bloating, belching, and food intolerance. Because these symptoms are also found in common conditions such as functional dyspepsia (see Ch. 51), considerable controversy exists as to whether they should be attributed to the gallstones (see CHRONIC CHOLECYSTITIS, below). Symptoms and signs depend upon the size, number, and location of gallstones. Multiple small stones often cause intermittent episodes of abrupt, severe pain when a small stone passes into the common bile duct. Large stones may cause pain by intermittent obstruction of the outlet of the gallbladder.

Complications of gallstones include acute and chronic cholecystitis, cholangitis, internal biliary fistula, choledocholithiasis, pancreatitis, and cancer of the gallbladder.

Prognosis, Treatment, and Prophylaxis

Despite the prevalence of gallstones, their natural history is not well understood or fully defined. In terms of morbidity, > 60% of patients with cholelithiasis will experience no, or only one, attack of biliary pain; most of the remaining patients will have only episodic pain. Nevertheless, the incidence of serious complications is high enough that cholecystectomy is often advocated as the treatment of choice, unless other serious illness contraindicates surgery. Multiple small stones are likely to cause complications, e.g., obstruction of the cystic duct, choledocholithiasis, and pancreatitis. Elderly and obese patients require special consideration as to the threat of biliary disease versus the increased complications of surgery.

Gallstones may be dissolved in vivo by giving bile acids orally for many months. The secondary bile acid, chenodeoxycholic acid, also promotes cholesterol unsaturation of bile and has been the most widely studied agent to date. Present evidence suggests that this treatment is safe and effective and may prove to be a useful therapeutic approach to the elderly or other poor-risk patients with gallstones. Chenodeoxycholic acid 15 mg/kg/day is given orally, ½ of the dose with each morning and evening meal. Patients should start on a smaller dose and gradually increase it to a fixed dose of 750 to 1000 mg/day. Of all patients with radiolucent gallstones, 50 to 75% of those who complete up to 3 yr of continuous therapy will have complete dissolution of gallstones. Therapy is ineffective when there is nonvisualization of the gallbladder or calcified stones on oral cholecystogram. The risk of side effects may be increased in patients with active ulcer disease, inflammatory bowel disease, active liver disease, and in women capable of becoming pregnant. The side effects are diarrhea, development of acute biliary complications during treatment, and liver function abnormalities. Theoretical concerns are body cholesterol accumulation, hepatotoxicity, precipitation of acute symptoms as stones become smaller, increased risk of colon cancer, and fetal toxicity. A limiting factor is that some, if not most, patients will form stones again if therapy is stopped after dissolution.

CHRONIC CHOLECYSTITIS

Chronic inflammatory reaction of the gallbladder—the commonest type of gallbladder disease.

Etiology and Pathology

The etiologic factors are similar to those for gallstones, but a specific bacterium (e.g., *Salmonella typhosa*) has occasionally been incriminated.

Chronic cholecystitis usually develops insidiously without a definite preceding attack of acute cholecystitis. The gallbladder has a chronic inflammatory reaction that may vary in degree from a few scattered lymphocytes in epithelial folds forming deep crevices (Rokitansky-Aschoff sinuses) to a very thick fibrous wall. Cholelithiasis is also usually present and controversy persists as to which of these disorders occurs first.

Symptoms and Signs

The symptoms and signs can be ill-defined and are not unique to gallbladder pathology. They vary with the extent of the disease, the presence and location of gallstones, and the presence of complications. Many patients complain only of flatulence with occasional nausea or other functional dyspeptic symptoms (see Ch. 51). Most have episodes of epigastric and right upper quadrant pain that radiates to the back below the tip of the right scapula. The pain is mild to excruciating. It is usually steady and not the frequently described "biliary colic." This pain often occurs after a meal or awakens the patient at night; symptoms are frequently related to the ingestion of fatty foods. The physical examination will at times reveal tenderness to deep pressure in the right upper quadrant of the abdomen.

Complications include acute cholecystitis, internal biliary fistula, choledocholithiasis, pancreatitis, and perhaps carcinoma of the gallbladder.

Diagnosis

Chronic cholecystitis is usually suspected from the symptoms and confirmed by nonvisualization of the gallbladder on oral cholecystography. If the history is atypical or if there is reason to believe that the dye was not absorbed from the GI tract or excreted from the liver, the cholecystogram should be repeated to substantiate the findings prior to surgery. Ultrasound will often prove the existence of gallstones in patients with nonvisualization of the gallbladder on cholecystogram. Laboratory studies are not helpful unless complications occur. Even if gallbladder stones are present, they may not be the cause of the patient's symptoms; peptic ulcer disease, diaphragmatic esophageal hiatus hernia, pancreatitis, and functional bowel disease should be excluded.

Treatment

Cholecystectomy is the treatment of choice unless other serious illness contraindicates surgery. See treatment with chenodeoxycholic acid, above.

ACUTE CHOLECYSTITIS

Acute inflammation of the gallbladder.

Etiology

In most instances acute cholecystitis is caused by a gallstone which occludes the outlet of the gallbladder or cystic duct. Inflammation of the gallbladder can occur without stones and bacterial infection; chemical irritation and the digestive activities of certain enzymes may play a contributing role.

Pathology

The findings depend upon the extent of the acute process. In gross appearance the gallbladder varies from being moderately enlarged, edematous, and erythematous to being fiery red or covered with exudate. Microscopically, there may be moderate edema, polymorphonuclear cells or ulcerations, or even necrosis of the mucosa and wall. As pathologic changes progress, lymphatic and venous blockage results and gangrene may develop (see below).

Symptoms and Signs

In acute cholecystitis, pain often occurring at night or in the early morning is a prominent symptom. The pain usually is well localized to the right upper quadrant of the abdomen, but associated epigastric pain and pain radiating through to the tip of the right shoulder blade are frequent. Whether the onset is sudden or gradual, the pain reaches a plateau that is maintained with little fluctuation and is usually quite severe. Causes of the pain may include contraction of the gallbladder against the blocked cystic duct, irritation of the overlying parietal peritoneum, and stimulation of nerves in the mesentery and gastrohepatic ligaments around the bile ducts. Parenteral analgesia is often required for relief. Nausea, vomiting, and flatulence are frequent. Temperature elevation is usually slight; if it is marked or associated with chills, cholangitis is usually present. If jaundice occurs, choledocholithiasis or pancreatitis is more often the cause. On physical examination, the right upper quadrant musculature is often rigid with pronounced, localized tenderness and there is splinting of respiration (**Murphy's sign**). The liver edge is tender, and in about half the cases a mass can be palpated in the region of the gallbladder. When complications of acute cholecystitis are present, these findings will be extended and exaggerated.

Diagnosis

The diagnosis usually is based on the symptoms and physical examination of the patient. In a few patients, x-rays of the abdomen will reveal opaque gallstones. The gallbladder will not be visualized on oral cholecystogram, but IV cholangiography may be helpful by showing nonvisualization of the gallbladder with visualization of the bile ducts. Diagnostic ultrasound will identify gallstones in about 75% of affected patients. Acute cholecystitis without stones occurs in a significant number of patients; thus, the absence of stones on ultrasound does not exclude acute cholecystitis. **Radionuclide scanning with labeled HIDA** (see in Ch. 65) provides functional information regarding cystic duct patency and is both highly sensitive and specific in the diagnosis of acute cholecystitis. It is a noninvasive technic that reliably confirms or refutes a diagnosis of cholecystitis. Laboratory studies usually reveal a moderate elevation of the WBC count, with a shift to the left; serum amylase is elevated in 15% of patients. The differential diagnosis includes acute appendicitis, intestinal obstruction, perforated peptic ulcer, acute pancreatitis, diaphragmatic pleurisy, and myocardial ischemia.

Treatment

Most physicians recommend cholecystectomy, but the decision must be individualized. It is rarely necessary to rush a patient to surgery because of acute cholecystitis. When the diagnosis is in doubt and a surgical emergency is not indicated by severe peritoneal irritation or increasing toxic signs, the patient can be treated medically and a cholecystogram should be obtained at a later date. Patients with concomitant serious illnesses should be closely observed; if the acute process subsides, surgery should be delayed for 6 wk to 2 mo.

COMPLICATIONS ASSOCIATED WITH ACUTE CHOLECYSTITIS

Empyema of the Gallbladder

Frank infection in which the acutely inflamed gallbladder contains thick purulent material. In most instances, bacterial invasion of the gallbladder is secondary to the stasis and embarrassed blood supply. *Escherichia coli* is the most common cause; *Bacillus aerogenes*, enterococci, *Klebsiella*, *Proteus vulgaris*, *Staphylococcus*, and *Clostridium* are implicated less often.

Empyema of the gallbladder is an intra-abdominal abscess. Pain, tenderness, temperature elevation, and WBC are exaggerated and early surgical treatment is mandatory.

Gangrene of the Gallbladder

Complete necrosis of a portion of the gallbladder in one or more areas. Edema of the gallbladder in acute cholecystitis can lead to venous stasis and loss of arterial supply. Pain, tenderness, temperature elevation, and WBC are usually exaggerated; without surgical intervention, perforation of the gallbladder is likely.

Perforation of the Gallbladder

Perforation most often results from gangrene and probably occurs in 10% of patients with acute cholecystitis. When perforation occurs, the pain and tenderness of the abdomen become more generalized. The pulse rate usually increases markedly. Hypotension and other signs of shock ensue. The incidence is much higher in older patients. Often the gallbladder area is sealed off by the omentum and surrounding structures and perforation results in a pericholecystic abscess. Morbidity and mortality are high, and surgery is mandatory.

Postoperative Acute Cholecystitis

A distinct type of acute cholecystitis that occurs after surgery for other diseases, most frequently after GI surgery, but that may follow any surgical procedure. The etiology is not understood, the diagnosis is difficult due to the pain and tenderness of recent surgery, and morbidity and mortality are extremely high.

Internal Biliary Fistula

Communication of the gallbladder or bile ducts with surrounding hollow viscera. Most internal biliary fistulas follow acute cholecystitis with adherence of the gallbladder to the hollow viscera and erosion of a stone into the structure. A few are attributed to peptic ulcers. The **symptoms and signs** depend upon the presence of acute cholecystitis, pericholecystic abscess, obstruction of the bile ducts, and the hollow viscera involved. The history of most patients indicates longstanding biliary disease; most have had recurring right upper quadrant pain, often associated with chills, fever, vomiting, jaundice, and weight loss. Patients with "**gallstone ileus**" often have intermittent obstruction, followed by complete obstruction. The **diagnosis** can usually be made from the x-ray findings of air in the gallbladder or biliary tree on plain films or barium entering the gallbladder or biliary tree during an upper GI series. Close observation of the right upper quadrant for air in the gallbladder or biliary tree should be made in all patients, especially the elderly, with intestinal obstruction. The **treatment** is surgical; the type of operation depends upon the location of the fistula, the presence of obstruction of the bile ducts or intestinal obstruction, and the patient's general condition.

CHOLESTEROLOSIS OF THE GALLBLADDER

Deposition of cholesterol in the epithelial cells and in histiocytes found in the mucosal folds and stroma of the gallbladder. The etiology is unknown. The appearance of yellow flecks due to cholesterol on a background of reddish mucosa has resulted in the name "**strawberry gallbladder.**" There is no relationship to the serum cholesterol or systemic metabolic changes. Some authorities believe that the symptoms are like those of chronic cholecystitis and cholelithiasis, while others state that cholesterolosis alone produces no symptoms. Unless chronic cholecystitis and cholelithiasis are present, there are no distinctive changes on the cholecystogram. Usually, the diagnosis is made by the pathologist after removal of the gallbladder. Some authorities advise cholecystectomy in patients with typical symptoms of gallbladder disease and a normal cholecystogram, believing that many of these patients will have cholesterolosis, but the results of surgery are generally poor in such cases.

DIVERTICULOSIS OF THE GALLBLADDER

Invagination of mucosa forming generalized large cystic spaces, which may be exaggerated (Rokitansky-Aschoff sinuses), in the wall of the gallbladder. Some believe that it is similar microscopically to an adenomyoma and call it **adenomyomatosis** of the gallbladder. The symptoms and signs are the same as those of chronic cholecystitis. The diagnosis is usually confirmed by a cholecystogram, which shows the irregularity of the mucosa and cystic spaces in the wall of the gallbladder. The treatment is cholecystectomy.

BENIGN TUMORS OF THE GALLBLADDER

A reported increase in benign tumors of the gallbladder, found in about 1% of gallbladders removed at surgery, is probably due to improvements in cholecystography. Benign neoplasms of the gallbladder include adenoma, cystadenoma, fibroadenoma, adenomyoma, and hamartoma. Nonneoplastic tumors are inflammatory, cholesterol, and ectopic tissue processes. Symptoms and signs are vague or nonexistent. If present, they mimic chronic cholecystitis. The diagnosis is made by demonstration of a filling defect in the gallbladder on a cholecystogram. Authorities disagree as to whether or not these tumors may be premalignant; most recommend cholecystectomy.

CARCINOMA OF THE GALLBLADDER

The incidence of carcinoma of the gallbladder has been reported from 0.2 to 5% in various series on cholecystectomies. It ranks fifth among carcinomas of the GI tract and allied glands. Most patients are females between 60 and 70 yr.

The frequent association of gallstones and cancer of the gallbladder has been accepted by many as indicating a causal relationship, leading to the advice that early cholecystectomy for patients with gallstones may prevent carcinoma of the gallbladder.

Many patients with carcinoma of the gallbladder have intermittent pain and dyspepsia similar to that seen in cholecystitis and cholelithiasis for several years. Unfortunately, the symptoms of more severe pain, recent weight loss, and jaundice appear only in the late stages of the disease. A firm tender mass is often palpable in the right upper quadrant.

Oral cholecystograms usually show poor or no visualization of the gallbladder. With the advent of ultrasound and CT, the diagnosis should be made more frequently prior to surgery.

Only 30% of cases of carcinoma of the gallbladder are resectable at operation. Cholecystectomy, resection of the adjacent liver, and skeletinization of the bile ducts is the treatment of choice. More radical operations have not improved the dismal outlook for these patients.

ABNORMALITIES OF THE BILE DUCTS

CHOLEDOCHOLITHIASIS

Calculi in the common bile duct.

Etiology

Although stones in the bile ducts usually come from the gallbladder, they may be formed in the intra- or extrahepatic bile ducts. There is usually inflammation or partial obstruction of the bile ducts when stones are formed there.

Symptoms, Signs, and Complications

Most common bile duct stones can pass into the duodenum, especially if they are < 5 mm in diameter, and do not cause major clinical problems. The patient can remain asymptomatic even if the stones are not passed. If, however, the stones produce pancreatitis or acute obstructive cholangitis, the effects can be devastating. Pain will occur in the right upper quadrant and epigastrium of the abdomen. It is of the typical biliary colic type in only 1/3 of patients. Nausea and vomiting are frequent. Temperature elevation usually denotes the presence of cholangitis. Tenderness is usually slight unless there is an associated acute cholecystitis or cholangitis. Jaundice is often intermittent or rapidly disappears. More subtle and chronic complications include biliary stricture and biliary cirrhosis.

Diagnosis

The diagnosis can be difficult to establish. Choledocholithiasis must be considered in all patients with jaundice and pain in the epigastrium or the right upper quadrant of the abdomen. When the serum bilirubin is < 3 mg/100 ml, an IV cholangiogram may reveal a stone in the ducts. **Ultrasound** may identify gallstones; it is also helpful in differentiating obstructive jaundice from hepatocellular disease by revealing dilation of the bile ducts. Oral cholecystograms and IV cholangiograms are usually of no value due to the elevated serum bilirubin. Percutaneous transhepatic cholangiograms, ultrasound, and CT are useful in diagnosis and valuable in differentiating obstruction due to stones from obstruction caused by tumors of the bile ducts or pancreas or due to pancreatitis. Otherwise, the diagnosis is suggested by an elevated serum bilirubin and alkaline phosphatase and confirmed by exploratory surgery.

Prognosis and Treatment

In general, the prognosis for choledocholithiasis is good. The stones will be passed spontaneously in 20% of patients; otherwise, surgical removal of the stones and correction of bile duct obstruction are required. When treatment is nonsurgical, the patient should remain under close medical supervision until the stones are passed.

CHOLANGITIS

Inflammation of the bile ducts.

Etiology

Bacteria, most often *E. coli*, enter the bile ducts via the lymphatic system or bloodstream, or by regurgitation of intestinal contents. Obstruction of the bile ducts by stones or tumor is usually present. Gram-negative septicemia with endotoxic shock (see SHOCK in Ch. 24) may be a complication.

Symptoms and Signs

Charcot's triad of right upper abdominal pain, jaundice, and fever with chills are characteristic symptoms. Intermittent and colicky pain can be severe. The jaundice is usually mild, cholestatic, and variable, because the bile duct obstruction is rarely complete. Fever is frequent, often intermittent, and may be low-grade but often is quite high. The patient is usually very ill and has only moderate tenderness to palpation in the right upper quadrant of the abdomen.

Diagnosis

The diagnosis is usually made by the symptoms and signs and is supported by an increase in serum bilirubin. Other laboratory findings include a conjugated hyperbilirubinemia and leukocytosis with a left shift. Serum amylase activity will be elevated if the pancreas is involved in the pathologic process. The activity of the serum alkaline phosphatase and serum transaminases may also be elevated. Multiple blood cultures should be obtained. A cholecystogram or IV cholangiogram may be helpful after the acute process subsides.

Treatment

Antibiotics (e.g., tetracycline or ampicillin) and fluid replacement are required initially. High doses of antibiotics may be required, but their efficacy will be short-lived if the bile ducts remain obstructed. Acute obstructive cholangitis is a surgical emergency when a patient is deteriorating despite medical treatment. A patient in shock requires emergency decompression of the biliary tree.

HELMINTHIASIS OF THE BILE DUCTS

Ascaris lumbricoides and *C. sinensis* are the two main parasites that may inhabit the bile ducts. *A. lumbricoides* has been reported in almost all parts of the world, but *C. sinensis* is confined almost entirely to the Orient.

BENIGN TUMORS OF THE EXTRAHEPATIC BILE DUCTS

Although unusual, benign tumors of the bile ducts are not rare; papilloma and adenoma are the commonest. Fibroadenoma, adenomyoma, leiomyoma, granular cell myoblastoma, neurinoma, and hamartoma also occur. Jaundice, often intermittent, and pain are the predominant symptoms. The treatment of choice is local excision.

CARCINOMA OF THE EXTRAHEPATIC BILE DUCTS

These infrequent tumors challenge diagnosis and treatment. Anatomic considerations make it necessary to divide carcinoma of the extrahepatic bile ducts into 3 categories: upper, middle, and lower (periampullary). The upper parts of the ducts are intimately related to the liver, the middle parts to the portal vein and hepatic artery, and the lower parts to the pancreas and duodenum.

Due to the location of these tumors, there is usually a rapid onset of symptoms. Nearly all patients have jaundice and >50% have pain. Other symptoms in order of frequency are weight loss, vomiting, anorexia, fever, diarrhea, constipation, nausea, and, rarely, chills.

Ultrasound and CT are valuable in evaluation. Percutaneous transhepatic cholangiography and endoscopic retrograde cholangiopancreatography with cannulation of the major papilla with cholangiography are important in making the diagnosis and localizing the tumor for the surgeon.

Both palliative measures and resections for cure depend on the location of the tumor. Carcinoma in the proximal portion of the bile duct system requires complex liver and duct resections with very few long-term survivors. Palliation may be accomplished by forcibly dilating the ducts and inserting a "T" tube or "Y" tube. Resectable tumors of the central portion of the bile ducts are treated by local or block excision. Bile drainage is re-established by hepaticojejunostomy. In nonresectable tumors in this area, palliation is accomplished by hepaticojejunostomy. Radical resection by pancreatoduodenectomy for carcinomas of the distal duct system has been more promising. Five-year survival rates of 20 to 30% have been reported for resectable tumors. Choledochoduodenostomy or choledocho- or hepaticojejunostomy is used for palliation in this area. Although some carcinomas of the bile ducts are very slow growing and not resectable, palliative procedures are worthwhile.

76. NUTRITION—GENERAL CONSIDERATIONS

NUTRITION

Nutriment, that part of food which nourishes the body, consists of micro- and macronutrients. **Micronutrients** (see TABLE 76–1) include **vitamins** and some **elements.** They are essential for health, generally are consumed in small amounts ($<$ 1 gm/day), usually are absorbed unchanged, and have catalytic functions. **Vitamins** are classified as fat-soluble (A, D, E, and K) or water-soluble (B group and C). The former and vitamin B_{12} tend to be stored in the body. Other B vitamins and vitamin C are not stored in the body and function as coenzymes.

Many **elements** present in food are essential for health (see Ch. 79). Some, such as calcium, phosphorus, and potassium, occur in the body in concentrations $>$ 0.005%. Others, termed **trace elements,** such as iron, zinc, and iodine, occur in much smaller concentrations ($<$ 0.005%). Some elements (e.g., barium, strontium) are suspected of being essential, but definite proof is lacking. Other elements found in the body (e.g., gold, silver) have no known metabolic role.

Carbohydrates, fats, and **proteins** are **macronutrients** and upon digestion yield, respectively, glucose and other monosaccharides, fatty acids and glycerol, and peptides and amino acids. Amino acids have structural roles; enzymes are proteins. Macronutrients are interchangeable sources of energy; fat yields 9 kcal/gm, protein or carbohydrate yields 4 kcal/gm, and ethanol yields 7 kcal/gm.

Carbohydrate and fat spare tissue protein. If sufficient nonprotein calories are not available, from either dietary sources or tissue stores (particularly of fat), efficient use of protein for tissue maintenance, replacement, or growth does not occur and considerably more dietary protein is required for positive nitrogen balance.

The polyunsaturated fatty acids, **linoleic** (9,12-octadecadienoic), **linolenic** (9,12,15-octadecatrienoic), and **arachidonic** (5,8,11,14-eicosatetraenoic), are termed **essential fatty acids (EFA)** and unlike all other lipids must be provided by the diet. Arachidonic acid can be made in the body from linoleic acid. The EFA are precursors of prostaglandins, and vitamin B_6 is involved in their metabolism.

Dietary requirements depend on age, sex, height, weight, and activity (metabolic and physical). The objective of a proper diet is to achieve and maintain the desirable body composition. Recommended dietary allowances (which include a significant safety factor) are given in TABLE 76–2. In adults, body weight in relation to height, frame, and sex is useful as an indication of overall nutritional status. Generally, up to about age 25, body weight progressively increases.

A wide variety of foods in the diet tends to ensure adequate intake of all essential nutrients. Persons on a "general" diet should be encouraged to include at least a minimum of certain types of foods recommended in a basic dietary plan (see TABLE 76–3, below). The remainder of the diet can be built freely around these foods, with caloric values as needed. Supplemental vitamin, mineral, and caloric requirements, associated with increased physiologic need, may be met by additional portions from the food groups listed in the table or by taking extra nutrients in concentrated or pure form. Intake of foods supplying only energy should be limited.

Prenatal diets are discussed in Vol. II, Ch. 13 and **diets for infants** in NUTRITION in Vol. II, Ch. 23.

Fiber, mainly a complex mixture of indigestible carbohydrate material, is a natural and hitherto much-neglected component of the normal diet. The typical Western diet is low in fiber, due to the prevailing consumption of highly refined wheat flour and a low intake of fruit and vegetables. The role of fiber in the prevention of constipation and the management of diverticular disease (see Ch. 60) is well established. Other possible effects of fiber being investigated include an influence on the development of cardiovascular disease through modification of bile acid metabolism; a relationship to carcinoma of the colon, and a satiety-producing effect; and the control of obesity.

The body is about 60% water and balance is vital for normal metabolism (see Ch. 81).

NUTRITION IN CLINICAL MEDICINE

The importance of nutrition in clinical medicine is being increasingly acknowledged. This is partly due to the recognition that malnutrition frequently accompanies prolonged illness and may accompany acute injury and complicated surgical and medical procedures. Many genetic metabolic disorders require special diets for their management. There is also an increased understanding of the role of nutritional factors in degenerative disorders. Deficiency states such as marasmus, kwashiorkor, and xerophthalmia continue to form a major part of clinical practice in developing countries, but these and other deficiencies may occur anywhere under conditions of deprivation.

TABLE 76–1. THE PRINCIPAL MICRONUTRIENTS (VITAMINS AND MINERALS)

Micronutrient	Principal Sources	Functions	Effects of Deficiency and Toxicity	Usual Therapeutic Dosage
Vitamin A	Fish liver oils, liver, egg yolk, butter, cream, vitamin A-fortified margarine, green leafy or yellow vegetables	Photoceptor mechanism of retina; integrity of epithelia; lysosome stability; glycoprotein synthesis	*Deficiency:* Night blindness; perifollicular hyperkeratosis; xerophthalmia; keratomalacia *Toxicity:* Headache; peeling of skin; hepatosplenomegaly; bone thickening	10,000–20,000 µg (30,000–60,000 IU)/day; see Ch. 78 for higher dosage)
Vitamin D	Fortified milk is main dietary source: fish liver oils, butter, egg yolk, liver, ultraviolet irradiation	Calcium and phosphorus absorption; resorption, mineralization, & collagen maturation of bone; tubular reabsorption of phosphorus (?)	*Deficiency:* Rickets (tetany sometimes associated): osteomalacia *Toxicity:* Anorexia; renal failure; metastatic calcification	*Primary Deficiency:* 10–40 µg (1400–1600 IU)/day *Metabolic Deficiency:* 1–2 µg/day 1,25-$(OH)_2D_3$ or 1α-$(OH)D_3$
Vitamin E group	Vegetable oil, wheat germ, leafy vegetables, egg yolk, margarine, legumes	Intracellular antioxidant; stability of biologic membranes	*Deficiency:* RBC hemolysis; creatinuria; ceroid deposition in muscle	30–100 mg/day
Vitamin K (activity) **Vitamin K₁** (phytonadione) **Vitamin K₂**	Leafy vegetables, pork, liver, vegetable oils, intestinal flora after newborn period	Prothrombin formation; normal blood coagulation	*Deficiency:* Hemorrhage from deficient prothrombin *Toxicity:* Kernicterus	In situations conducive to neonatal hemorrhage, 2–5 mg during labor or daily for 1 wk prior; or 1–2 mg to newborn (see Ch. 78)
Essential fatty acids (linoleic, linolenic, arachidonic acids)	Vegetable seed oils (corn, sunflower, safflower); margarines blended with vegetable oils	Synthesis of prostaglandins, membrane structure	Growth cessation, dermatosis	Up to 10 gm/day
Thiamine (vitamin B₁)	Dried yeast; whole grains; meat (especially pork, liver); enriched cereal products; nuts; legumes; potatoes	Carbohydrate metabolism; central & peripheral nerve cell function; myocardial function	Beriberi; infantile & adult (peripheral neuropathy, cardiac failure; Wernicke-Korsakoff syndrome)	30–100 mg/day

Riboflavin (vitamin B₂)	Milk, cheese, liver, meat, eggs, enriched cereal products	Many aspects of energy & protein metabolism; integrity of mucous membranes	Cheilosis; angular stomatitis; corneal vascularization; amblyopia; sebaceous dermatosis	10–30 mg/day
Niacin (nicotinic acid, niacinamide)	Dried yeast, liver, meat, fish, legumes, whole-grain enriched cereal products	Oxidation-reduction reactions; carbohydrate metabolism	Pellagra (dermatosis, glossitis, GI & CNS dysfunction)	Niacinamide 100–1000 mg/day
Vitamin B₆ group (pyridoxine)	Dried yeast, liver, organ meats, whole-grain cereals, fish, legumes	Many aspects of nitrogen metabolism, e.g., transaminations, porphyrin & heme synthesis, tryptophan conversion to niacin. Linoleic acid metabolism	Convulsions in infancy; anemias; neuropathy; seborrhea-like skin lesions. Dependency states (see Ch. 78)	25–100 mg/day
Folic acid	Fresh green leafy vegetables, fruit, organ meats, liver, dried yeast	Maturation of RBCs; synthesis of purines & pyrimidines	Pancytopenia: megaloblastosis (especially pregnancy, infancy, malabsorption)	1 mg/day
Vitamin B₁₂ (cobalamins)	Liver; meats (especially beef, pork, organ meats); eggs; milk & milk products	Maturation of RBCs; neural function; DNA synthesis, related to folate coenzymes; methionine & acetate synthesis	Pernicious anemia: fish tapeworm & vegan anemias; some psychiatric syndromes; nutritional amblyopia. Dependency states (see ch. 78)	In pernicious anemia 50 μg/day IM first 2 wk, 100 μg twice/wk next 2 mo, thereafter 100 μg/mo
Biotin	Liver, kidney, egg yolk, yeast, cauliflower, nuts, legumes	Carboxylation & decarboxylation of oxalocetic acid; amino acid & fatty acid metabolism	Dermatitis, glossitis. Dependency states (see ch. 78)	150–300 μg/day
Vitamin C (ascorbic acid)	Citrus fruits, tomatoes, potatoes, cabbage, green peppers	Essential to osteoid tissue; collagen formation; vascular function; tissue respiration & wound healing	Scurvy (hemorrhages, loose teeth, gingivitis)	100–1000 mg/day
Sodium	Wide distribution—beef, pork, sardines, cheese, green olives, corn bread, potato chips, sauerkraut	Acid-base balance; osmotic pressure; pH blood: muscle contractility; nerve transmission; sodium pumps	*Deficiency:* Hyponatremia. *Toxicity:* Hypernatremia; confusion, coma	See in Ch. 81

(Continued)

TABLE 76–1. THE PRINCIPAL MICRONUTRIENTS (VITAMINS AND MINERALS) (Cont'd)

Micronutrient	Principal Sources	Functions	Effects of Deficiency and Toxicity	Usual Therapeutic Dosage
Potassium	Wide distribution—whole and skim milk, bananas, prunes, raisins	Muscle activity, nerve transmission; intracellular acid-base balance and water retention	*Deficiency:* Hypokalemia: paralysis, cardiac disturbances *Toxicity:* Hyperkalemia: paralysis, cardiac disturbances	See in Ch. 81
Calcium	Milk and milk products, meat, fish, eggs, cereal products, beans, fruits, vegetables	Bone and tooth formation; blood coagulation; neuromuscular irritability; muscle contractility; myocardial conduction	*Deficiency:* Hypocalcemia and tetany; neuromuscular hyperexcitability *Toxicity:* Hypercalcemia: GI atony; renal failure; psychosis	10–30 ml 10% calcium gluconate soln IV in 24 h
Phosphorus	Milk, cheese, meat, poultry, fish, cereals, nuts, legumes	Bone and tooth formation, acid-base balance, component of nucleic acids, energy production	*Deficiency:* Irritability; weakness; blood cell disorders; GI tract & renal dysfunction *Toxicity:* Hyperphosphatemia in renal failure	Potassium acid and dibasic phosphate parenteral 600 mg (18.8 mEq)/day
Magnesium	Green leaves, nuts, cereal grains, seafoods	Bone and tooth formation; nerve conduction; muscle contraction; enzyme activation	*Deficiency:* Hypomagnesemia; neuromuscular irritability *Toxicity:* Hypermagnesemia; hypotension, respiratory failure, cardiac disturbances	2–4 ml 50% magnesium sulfate soln./day IM
Iron	Wide distribution (except dairy products)—soybean flour, beef, kidney, liver, beans, clams, peaches Much unavailable (<20% absorbed)	Hemoglobin, myoglobin formation, enzymes	*Deficiency:* Anemia; dysphagia; koilonychia; enteropathy *Toxicity:* Hemochromatosis; cirrhosis; diabetes mellitus; skin pigmentation	Ferrous sulfate or gluconate 300 mg orally t.i.d.

Element	Sources	Functions	Deficiency/Toxicity	Supplementation
Iodine	Seafoods, iodized salt, dairy products Water variable	Thyroxine (T_4) & tri-iodothyronine (T_3) formation and energy control mechanisms	*Deficiency:* Simple (colloid, endemic) goiter; cretinism; deaf-mutism *Toxicity:* occasional myxedema	150 µg iodine/day as potassium iodide added to salt 1:10–40,000 ppm
Fluorine	Wide distribution—tea, coffee Fluoridation of water supplies with sodium fluoride 1.0–2.0 ppm	Bone and tooth formation	*Deficiency:* Predisposition to dental caries; osteoporosis (?) *Toxicity:* Fluorosis, mottling, pitting of permanent teeth; exostoses of spine	Sodium fluoride 1.1–2.2 mg/day orally
Zinc	Wide distribution—vegetable sources Much unavailable	Component of enzymes and insulin; wound healing; growth	*Deficiency:* Growth retardation; hypogonadism; hyogeusia: in cirrhosis; acrodermatitis enteropathica	30–150 mg zinc sulfate/day orally
Copper	Wide distribution—organ meat, oysters, nuts, dried legumes, whole-grain cereals	Enzyme component	*Deficiency:* Anemia in malnourished children; Menkes' kinky hair syndrome *Toxicity:* Hepatolenticular degeneration; some biliary cirrhosis (?)	0.3 mg/kg/day copper sulfate, orally
Cobalt	Green leafy vegetables	Part of vitamin B_{12} molecule	*Deficiency:* Anemia in children (?) *Toxicity:* Beer-drinker's cardiomyopathy	20–30 mg/day cobaltous chloride, orally
Chromium	Wide distribution—brewer's yeast	Part of glucose tolerance factor (GTF)	*Deficiency:* Impaired glucose tolerance in malnourished children; some diabetics (?)	----

TABLE 76-2. RECOMMENDED DAILY
FOOD AND NUTRITION BOARD, NATIONAL ACADEMY

	AGE (yr)	WEIGHT kg (lb)	HEIGHT cm (in.)	PROTEIN (gm)	VITAMIN A ACTIVITY (RE) †	VITAMIN D (µg) ‡	VITAMIN E§ (mg α T.E.)
Infants	0.0-0.5	6 (13)	60 (24)	kg × 2.2	420	10	3
	0.5-1.0	9 (20)	71 (28)	kg × 2.0	400	10	4
Children	1-3	13 (29)	90 (35)	23	400	10	5
	4-6	20 (44)	112 (44)	30	500	10	6
	7-10	28 (62)	132 (52)	34	700	10	7
Males	11-14	45 (99)	157 (62)	45	1000	10	8
	15-18	66 (145)	176 (69)	56	1000	10	10
	19-22	70 (154)	177 (70)	56	1000	7.5	10
	23-50	70 (154)	178 (70)	56	1000	5	10
	51+	70 (154)	178 (70)	56	1000	5	10
Females	11-14	46 (101)	157 (62)	46	800	10	8
	15-18	55 (120)	163 (64)	46	800	10	8
	19-22	55 (120)	163 (64)	44	800	7.5	8
	23-50	55 (120)	163 (64)	44	800	5	8
	51+	55 (120)	163 (64)	44	800	5	8
Pregnant				+30	+200	+5	+2
Lactating				+20	+400	+5	+3

* The allowances are intended to provide for individual variations among most normal persons as they live in the USA under usual environmental stresses. Diets should be based on a variety of common foods in order to provide other nutrients for which human requirements have been less well defined.

† Retinol equivalents. 1 Retinol equivalent = 1 µg retinol or 6 µg β carotene.

‡ As cholecalciferol. 10 µg cholecalciferol = 400 IU vitamin D.

§ α-tocopherol equivalents. 1 mg d-α-tocopherol = 1α T.E.

** The folacin allowances refer to dietary sources as determined by *Lactobacillus casei* assay after treatment with enzymes ("conjugases") to make polyglutamyl forms of the vitamin available to the test organism.

†† 1 N.E. (niacin equivalent) is equal to 1 mg of niacin or 60 mg of dietary tryptophan.

MALNUTRITION

Malnutrition is any disorder of nutrition and may be categorized as follows:
1. Cause: primary (exogenous); secondary (endogenous).
2. Type: excess, toxicity (overnutrition); deficiency (undernutrition).
3. Nutrient: vitamins, elements, protein, energy sources.
4. Degree: mild, moderate, severe.
5. Consequences: depleted stores, biochemical lesion, functional change, structural lesion.
6. Duration: acute, subacute, chronic.
7. Outcome: reversible, irreversible.

Primary malnutrition is caused by inappropriate dietary intake, inadequate or excessive. **Secondary malnutrition** arises from inappropriate digestion, absorption, transport, storage, metabolism, or elimination of nutrients. Primary and secondary malnutrition often occur together.

ELEMENTAL OR DEFINED FORMULA DIETS

These diets provide essential nutrients in a readily assimilated form, require little or no active digestion, and have minimal residue. When a portion of functional intestine is available for absorption, this is a safer and less expensive alternative to total parenteral nutrition (see below) for patients who cannot be fed orally.

These diets are usually unsuitable for oral feeding; they are unpalatable, only small amounts (10 to 150 ml) can be tolerated at a time, and it is difficult to monitor amounts given and prevent hyperosmolar dehydration.

DIETARY ALLOWANCES,* Revised 1980
OF Sciences—National Research Council

	WATER-SOLUBLE VITAMINS						MINERALS					
ASCORBIC ACID (mg)	FOLACIN** (µg)	NIACIN†† (mg N.E.)	RIBOFLAVIN (mg)	THIAMINE (mg)	VITAMIN B_6 (mg)	VITAMIN B_{12}‡‡ (µg)	CALCIUM (mg)	PHOSPHORUS (mg)	IODINE (µg)	IRON (mg)	MAGNESIUM (mg)	ZINC (mg)
35	30	6	0.4	0.3	0.3	0.5	360	240	40	10	50	3
35	45	8	0.6	0.5	0.6	1.5	540	360	50	15	70	5
45	100	9	0.8	0.7	0.9	2.0	800	800	70	15	150	10
45	200	11	1.0	0.9	1.3	2.5	800	800	90	10	200	10
45	300	16	1.4	1.2	1.6	3.0	800	800	120	10	250	10
50	400	18	1.6	1.4	1.8	3.0	1200	1200	150	18	350	15
60	400	18	1.7	1.4	2.0	3.0	1200	1200	150	18	400	15
60	400	19	1.7	1.4	2.2	3.0	800	800	150	10	350	15
60	400	18	1.6	1.4	2.2	3.0	800	800	150	10	350	15
60	400	16	1.4	1.2	2.2	3.0	800	800	150	10	350	15
50	400	15	1.3	1.1	1.8	3.0	1200	1200	150	18	300	15
60	400	14	1.3	1.1	2.0	3.0	1200	1200	150	18	300	15
60	400	14	1.3	1.1	2.0	3.0	800	800	150	18	300	15
60	400	13	1.2	1.0	2.0	3.0	800	800	150	18	300	15
60	400	13	1.2	1.0	2.0	3.0	800	800	150	10	300	15
+20	+400	+2	+0.3	+0.4	+0.6	+1.0	+400	+400	+25	§§	+150	+5
+40	+100	+	+0.5	+0.5	+0.5	+1.0	+400	+400	+50	§§	+150	+10

‡‡ The RDA for vitamin B_{12} in infants is based on average concentration of the vitamin in human milk. The allowances after weaning are based on energy intake (as recommended by the American Academy of Pediatrics) and consideration of other factors such as intestinal absorption.

§§ The increased requirement during pregnancy cannot be met by the iron content of habitual American diets nor by the existing iron stores of many women; therefore the use of 30–60 mg of supplemental iron is recommended. Iron needs during lactation are not substantially different from those of non-pregnant women, but continued supplementation of the mother for 2–3 months after parturition is advisable in order to replenish stores depleted by pregnancy.

Reproduced from "Recommended Dietary Allowances," 9th ed., 1980, by permission of the National Academy of Sciences, Washington, D.C.

TABLE 76-3. BASIC DAILY DIETARY PLAN*

Milk group: (Whole milk unless skim is desirable)
   Children to age 12 . . . . 3 to 4 cups
   Teenagers . . . . 4 cups
   Adults . . . . 2 cups
   Pregnant women . . . . 4 cups
   Nursing mothers . . . . 6 cups
   (Cheese, ice cream, and other milk products can replace all or part of the fluid milk. Butter and margarine and other fats and oils are included, consistent with caloric requirements.)

Meat group: 2 or more servings
   Beef, veal, pork, lamb, poultry, or fish (3 oz edible portion = 1 serving); eggs, preferably not > 4/wk; nuts and dried beans or peas as alternates (1 cup, cooked = 1 serving)

Vegetable-fruit group: 4 or more servings (3½ oz or ½ cup = 1 serving)
   A dark green or deep yellow vegetable (important source of vitamin A) at least every other day
   A citrus fruit or other fruit or vegetable rich in vitamin C daily
   Other fruits and vegetables including potatoes

Bread-cereal group: 4 or more servings (bread, 1 slice = 1 serving; cereals, cooked or prepared, 1 cup = 1 serving)
   Whole-grain, enriched, or restored products

* Provides approximately 1600 kcal.

Nasogastric feeding is preferred, using a 16-gauge, 24-in. polyethylene catheter. Starting with a 25% wt/vol solution, 1 kcal/ml is fed at a rate of 50 ml/h and increased by 25 ml/h to a total of 125 ml/h (3000 kcal/24 h). With jejunostomy feeding, a 16-gauge, 36-in. polyethylene catheter is used, starting with a 10% wt/vol solution at 50 ml/h and increased by 25 ml/h/day up to the daily fluid requirements. Concentration is thereafter increased by 5% wt/vol/day until maximum tolerance is achieved (usually 20% wt/vol concentration; 0.8 kcal/ml, at 125 ml/h for 2400 kcal/day).

Components of a selection of elemental diets are listed in TABLE 76–4.

PARENTERAL NUTRITION

Although not a new method of therapy, only recently has parenteral nutrition been widely practiced. Its use is accompanied by certain dangers, such as infection, thrombosis, catheter and air embolization, and metabolic problems (see below). It should only be used when oral and tube feeding, including the use of elemental diets, are contraindicated or inadequate.

Indications: Less than 5% of all acute hospital admissions require **total parenteral nutrition (TPN)** for any length of time. Mortality from acute alimentary failure, as in enterocutaneous fistula, has been considerably reduced by TPN. Patients who have had extensive intestinal resection for such conditions as Crohn's disease and ulcerative colitis have maintained good health at home for up to 10 yr on TPN. It reduces the risks accompanying surgery in undernourished patients, and promotes tissue repair and immune response following major surgery, trauma, and especially burns or multiple fractures with sepsis. Short-term (5 to 10 days) TPN has been lifesaving in comatose patients and in intractable anorexia nervosa. Support with parenteral nutrition has permitted chemotherapy and radiation therapy in patients with cancer otherwise considered unsuitable for any treatment. In infancy, protracted diarrhea and major alimentary tract surgery in the newborn are the main indications.

Regimens: When parenteral nutrition is required to supplement inadequate oral or tube feeding for periods < 10 days, a peripheral vein may be used. When support is necessary for longer periods, or feeding must be entirely by the IV route, or when nutritional requirements are increased, then a central venous catheter should be used.

A wide variety of IV feeding regimens are in current use, but with increasing experience a certain degree of standardization is emerging. Alternatives to dextrose, such as fructose, sorbitol, xylitol, and ethanol, as carbohydrate sources of energy have been found to give rise to various metabolic problems (see below) and are not in common use. Fat emulsions containing soybean or safflower oil are commercially available. Besides being a concentrated source of energy, they prevent EFA deficiency in long-term TPN. Energy should be provided at 40 to 45 kcal/kg and between 30 and 60% of total calories can be given as fat.

Nitrogen (N) is provided from a wide range of amino acid solutions. Protein hydrolysates containing fibrin or casein derivatives may be administered IV. Synthetic crystalline amino acid solutions have a better defined amino acid profile and have largely replaced protein hydrolysates in TPN in the USA. They are particularly useful in special situations in the young, in renal failure, and in hepatic failure. Amino acid solutions should provide 30% of their N as essential amino acid N for adults, and about 40% for infants. The nitrogen/nonprotein calorie ratio should be about 1 gm N/150 kcal.

Requirements for electrolytes and other elements and vitamins are met by addition to the IV solutions. Phosphate depletion has resulted when phosphate has not been specially added. Clinical folate, zinc, selenium, and chromium deficiencies have also been reported. Toxicity of fat-soluble vitamins must be guarded against in prolonged administration.

These general principles are followed in the regimen advocated by Wretlind; see TABLE 76–5, which gives the composition of 3 solutions designed for use in adults, with the amounts to be given daily. TABLE 76–6 provides details of the amounts of nutrients supplied daily.

Precautions: Solutions must be prepared aseptically under a laminar-flow, filtered-air hood. Catheter insertion and maintenance must be performed with strict surgical and aseptic technics. The nutrient solution is generally delivered to the patient from a bottle or plastic bag by gravity, with an in-line Millipore® filter about 2.5 mm diameter between the infusion tubing and catheter. A filter with porosity of 0.22 μ provides sterility but a peristaltic pump is then necessary. This creates a risk of air embolization and close supervision is necessary. This porosity is too small for use with fat emulsions. Millipore® filters of 0.45 μ porosity may then be used, but while the passage of particulate matter and some microorganisms is prevented, sterility is not assured.

Monitoring: Fluid balance, metabolic balance, temperature, daily weight, serum electrolytes (daily initially), fat-clearing capacity, serum P, Ca, Mg (every 3rd day), blood sugar (at least daily initially), liver function (twice weekly), Hb, Hct, MCV, urinary urea and electrolytes, urine and serum osmolality, and acid-base balance should all be monitored together with specific tests dictated by the presenting illness.

Metabolic complications: These may be related to (1) inappropriate use of energy substrates exemplified by excessive amounts of glucose without adequate insulin cover resulting in lactic acidosis, and excessive fat emulsion beyond a patient's clearing capacity; (2) inappropriate energy

TABLE 76–4. COMPARISON OF COMPONENTS OF ELEMENTAL OR CHEMICALLY DEFINED DIETS

Component	Vivonex®	Vivonex HN®	Vital®	Precision LR®	Precision HN®	Precision Isotonic®	Flexical®
Carbohydrate							
gm/1000 kcal	230	211	188	223	205	150	152
% cal	90.5	86.5	74	89.2	82.2	59.9	61
Type	Glucose Oligosaccharides	Glucose Oligosaccharides	Hydrolized corn syrup solids Sucrose	Maltodextrin Sucrose citrate	Maltodextrin Sucrose citrate	Glucose Oligosaccharides Sucrose citrate	Corn syrup solids Modified tapioca starch
Lactose	None	None	None	None	None	None	None
Fat							
gm/1000 kcal	1.5	0.9	10.8	1.4	1.2	31.3	34
% cal	1.3	0.8	9.3	1.3	1.1	28.1	30
Type	Safflower oil	Safflower oil	Med. chain triglycerides Safflower oil	Med. chain triglycerides Soy oil	Med. chain triglycerides Soy oil	Soy oil	Soy oil MCT oil
Essential fatty acids (% total fat)	80	80					26.5
Amino acids							
gm/1000 kcal	20.6	43.3	41.7	24	41.7	30	22.5
% cal	8.2	17.7	16.7	9.5	16.7	12	9
Type	Pure crystalline amino acids	Pure crystalline amino acids	Hydrolized soy, whey, & meat. Free amino acids.	Egg albumin (pasteurized egg white solids)	Egg albumin (pasteurized egg white solids)	Egg albumin (pasteurized egg white solids) Sodium caseinate	Hydrolyzed casein plus free amino acids—Met., Try., Trp.
Osmolality mOsm/kg (at standard dilution)	550	810	460	525 (Orange)	557	300	550 (Plain)

Modified from CLINICAL NUTRITION: A physiologic approach, by M. H. Overton and B. P. Lukert. Copyright © 1977 by Yearbook Publishers, Inc., Chicago. Used with permission of Year Book Publishers, Inc., and the authors.

TABLE 76–5. INFUSION SOLUTIONS WITH ADDITIONS FOR ADULTS ON
INTRAVENOUS NUTRITION*

Solution	Amount (ml/day)
Solution 1	
Solution of crystalline amino acids (7%) and carbohydrates (10%) (Vamin, Vitrum) with the addition of*	1,000
Solution of electrolytes (Vitrum) containing 5 mM of Ca, 1.5 mM of Mg, 50 μmol of Fe, 20 μmol of Zn, 40 μmol of Mn, 5 μmol of Cu, 50 μmol of F, 1 μmol of I, and 13.3 mM of Cl	10
Solution 2	
Fat emulsion (Intralipid 20%)** with the addition of an	500
Emulsion of fat-soluble vitamins (Vitrum) containing 0.75 mg of retinol, 3 μg of cholecalciferol, and 0.15 mg of vitamin K_1	10
Solution 3	
Glucose solution 10% for intravenous nutrition with the addition of*	1,000
Solution of lyophilized water-soluble vitamins (Vitrum) containing 1.2 mg of thiamine, 1.8 mg of riboflavin, 10 mg of nicotinamide, 2 mg of pyridoxine, 0.2 mg of folic acid, 2 μg of cyanocobalamin, 10 mg of pantothenic acid, 0.3 mg of biotin, and 30 mg of ascorbic acid and	10
Potassium phosphate solution (Addex-Kalium, Pharmacia) containing 30 mM of K, 6 mM of P, and 21 mM of acetate	15

  * The given amounts are intended to cover a basal requirement. When greater amounts are demanded, 1.5 to 2 times the cited volumes should be given.
  ** Intralipid 10% may be used in an amount of 1,000 ml and with 500 ml of glucose solution 20%, if no increase of total water volume is desired.
  From A. Wretlind, *Total Parenteral Nutrition*, edited by J. Fischer. Copyright 1976 by Little, Brown and Company. Used with permission.

substrates such as fructose, sorbitol, xylitol, or ethanol that may cause hyperuricemia, hyperbilirubinemia, lactic acidosis, and folate deficiency; (3) inadequate monitoring that may result in electrolyte imbalance, hyperosmolar dehydration syndrome, hypophosphatemia, acid-base imbalance, and hyperlipidemia; (4) failure to balance constituents (e.g., nitrogen/nonprotein calorie ratio—see above) defeating the objectives of TPN; (5) deficiency syndromes or, rarely, toxicity resulting from inappropriate amounts of vitamins and trace elements (see above); and (6) malfunction of certain organs such as liver, kidneys, lungs, and microcirculation. Hepatic and renal failure necessitate the use of crystalline amino acid solutions, although none generally available appears to be ideal. Earlier suggestions that fat emulsion is contraindicated in acute pancreatitis and that it impairs pulmonary ventilation perfusion have not been confirmed.

NUTRIENT–DRUG INTERACTIONS

Nutritional deficiency may impair the metabolism of drugs. Energy and protein deficiencies reduce enzyme levels in tissues including those involved in the metabolism of drugs. Response to drugs may be affected by impaired absorption due to changes in the GI tract and by disturbed liver function. Deficiency of minerals such as Ca, Zn, and Mg impairs drug metabolism. Potassium depletion from the use of diuretics, especially those of the thiazide group, and adrenal steroids increases the risk of digitalis-induced cardiac arrhythmias. Vitamin C deficiency is associated with decreased activity of drug-metabolizing enzymes. The frequency of adverse drug reactions in the elderly may be related to their frequent low vitamin C status.

Many drugs affect appetite, absorption, and glucose, lipid and protein metabolism. Some of the most important of these are listed in TABLE 76–7. Those drugs that are used specifically to produce such an effect are not included.

Other drugs affect mineral metabolism. Potassium depletion may also result from the regular use of purgatives. Na and water retention is marked, at least temporarily, with cortisone, deoxycorticosterone, and aldosterone; much less with prednisone, prednisolone, and the newer steroid analogs. It also occurs with estrogen-progestogen oral contraceptives and phenylbutazone and oxyphenbutazone. Non-heme iron absorption is either impaired or facilitated by a number of dietary substances.

TABLE 76-6. AMOUNTS OF NUTRIENTS IN INTRAVENOUS NUTRITION
SOLUTIONS (See TABLE 76-5) GIVEN TO ADULTS

Energy and Nutrients	Amount/day			
	Solution 1 (1,010 ml)	Solution 2 (510 ml)	Solution 3 (1,025 ml)	Total
Water	0.94 L	0.38 L	0.97 L	2.3 L
Energy	650 kcal	1,000 kcal	410 kcal	2,060 kcal
Amino acids	70 gm	—	—	70 gm
Glucose or fructose	100 gm	12.5 gm*	100 gm	213 gm
Fat	—	106 gm**	—	106 gm
Sodium	50 mM	—	—	50 mM
Potassium	20 mM	—	30 mM	50 mM
Calcium	7.5 mM	—	—	7.5 mM
Magnesium	3.0 mM	—	—	3.0 mM
Iron	50 μmol	—	—	50 μmol
Zinc	20 μmol	—	—	40 μmol
Manganese	40 μmol	—	—	40 μmol
Copper	5 μmol	—	—	5 μmol
Chloride	68.3 mM	—	—	68.3 mM
Phosphorus	—	7.5 mM	6 mM	13.5 mM
Fluoride	50 μmol	—	—	50 μmol
Iodide	1 μmol	—	—	1 μmol
Thiamine	—	—	1.2 mg	1.2 mg
Riboflavin	—	—	1.8 mg	1.8 mg
Nicotinamide	—	—	10 mg	10 mg
Vitamin B_6	—	—	2 mg	2 mg
Folic acid	—	—	0.2 mg	0.2 mg
Vitamin B_{12}	—	—	2 μg	2 μg
Pantothenic acid	—	—	10 mg	10 mg
Biotin	—	—	0.3 mg	0.3 mg
Ascorbic acid	—	—	30 mg	30 mg
Vitamin A	—	0.75 mg	—	0.75 mg
Vitamin D	—	3 μg	—	3 μg
Vitamin K_1	—	0.15 mg	—	0.15 mg
Tocopherol	—	100 mg	—	100 mg

* Glycerol.
** 6 gm of phosphatides.
From A. Wretlind, *Total Parenteral Nutrition*, edited by J. Fischer. Copyright 1976 by Little, Brown and Company. Used with permission.

Other effects include impaired thyroid uptake or release of iodine by sulfonylureas, phenylbutazone, cobalt, and lithium; lowered plasma Zn and elevated Cu by oral contraceptives; and osteoporosis from prolonged use of adrenal steroids the cause of which is unclear.

The metabolism of many vitamins is affected. Ethanol impairs thiamine absorption and isoniazid is a niacin and pyridoxine antagonist. Complaints of depression in women taking oral contraceptives are usually associated with high progestogen content. These patients have a disturbance of tryptophan metabolism that is responsive to 20 mg pyridoxine t.i.d. The disturbance is due to induction of tryptophan pyrrolase, a rate-limiting enzyme affecting niacin metabolism, resulting in the use of pyridoxine for niacin synthesis at the expense of 5-hydroxytryptamine neurotransmitter formation. Folic acid absorption is inhibited by ethanol and oral contraceptives. Most patients receiving phenytoin, phenobarbital, primidone, or phenothiazines for long-term anticonvulsant therapy develop low serum and erythrocyte folate levels and occasionally megaloblastic anemia, probably as an effect on hepatic microsomal drug metabolizing enzymes. Administration of folic acid interferes with the anticonvulsant action, but regular yeast tablet supplements raise folate levels without this effect. Vitamin B_{12} malabsorption has been reported with aminosalicylic acid, slow-release potassium iodide, colchicine, trifluoperazine, ethanol, and oral contraceptives. Anticonvulsant-induced vitamin D deficiency is well-recognized.

FOOD ADDITIVES AND CONTAMINANTS

The addition of chemicals to foodstuffs to preserve them or to improve taste, and the elimination or control of natural and artificial contaminants of food are subject to increasingly stringent legislation

TABLE 76-7. EXAMPLES OF SIDE EFFECTS OF DRUGS ON NUTRITIONAL STATUS

Effect	Drugs
Appetite increased	Alcohol, insulin, steroids, thyroid hormone, sulfonylureas, psychotropic drugs, antihistamines
Appetite decreased	Bulk agents (methyl cellulose, guar gum), mazindol, glucagon, indomethacin, morphine, cyclophosphamide, digitalis
Malabsorption	Neomycin, kanamycin, chlortetracycline, phenindione p-aminosalicylic acid, indomethacin, methotrexate, liquid paraffin
Glucose metabolism	
Hyperglycemia	Narcotic analgesics, phenothiazines, benzothiadiazine diuretics, probenecid, phenytoin, coumarins
Hypoglycemia	Sulfonamides, aspirin, phenacetin, β-adrenergic blockers, monoamine oxidase inhibitors, phenylbutazone, barbiturates
Lipid metabolism	
Plasma lipids reduced	Aspirin and p-aminosalicylic acid, L-asparaginase, chlortetracycline, colchicine, dextrans, fenfluramine, glucagon, phenindione, sulfinpyrazone, trifluperidol
Plasma lipids increased	Oral contraceptives (estrogen-progestogen type), adrenal corticosteroids, chlorpromazine, ethanol, thiouracil, growth hormone, vitamin D
Protein metabolism	Tetracycline, chloramphenicol

and control. Only those additives that have been passed as safe at specified "action levels" after exacting laboratory testing are permitted. Poisonous or deleterious contaminants, such as pesticide residues, are subject to similar control.

The use of additives reduces the wastage of foods and food raw materials, prevents spoilage of many perishable foods, and provides the public with a greater variety of attractive foods than would otherwise be possible. Against these benefits have to be set the known risks. The issues involved are frequently difficult to resolve. The use of nitrite in cured meats may be taken as an example of the complexity of the problem. Nitrite inhibits the growth of *C. botulinum* and imparts a desired flavor. However, there is evidence that nitrite is converted in the body to nitrosamines, which are known carcinogens in animals. This issue is not resolved. Another example is sweetening agents. Cyclamates have been banned because they are carcinogenic in high doses in animals. Similar studies are being carried out on saccharin.

The complete elimination of contaminants from certain foodstuffs cannot be achieved without damaging the foodstuff. Action levels are set which may vary for different foodstuffs. Thus the residual tolerance for aldrin and dieldrin is 0.03 ppm for eggs but 0.3 ppm for butter, fish (smoked, frozen, canned), and milk. Aflatoxin, a known liver carcinogen in animals, has a residual tolerance level of 20 ppb for peanuts and peanut products but 0.5 ppb for milk. A level of 0.5 ppm has been set for lead in evaporated milk and of 1.0 ppm for mercury in fish, oysters, clams, mussels, and wheat.

In summary, demonstrated health problems arising from food additives have been trivial except for isolated incidents. Long-term effects of contaminants such as mycotoxins and heavy metals are difficult to assess.

77. UNDERNUTRITION

STARVATION—INANITION

Structural and functional changes due to inadequate intake of nutrients and energy sources.

Etiology

Primary inanition results from inadequate intake of all nutrients, which may be involuntary as in famine, imprisonment, shipwreck, and other circumstances of privation, and severe anorectic disease; or voluntary as in fasting and anorexia nervosa.

Secondary inanition may be caused by (1) impaired digestion in gastric and pancreatic disease, (2) disordered absorption in malabsorption syndromes, (3) impaired utilization in endocrine dysfunction, metabolic disorders, severe infections, or degenerative diseases, (4) increased nutritional requirements in thyrotoxicosis, surgical procedures, injuries, burns, and convalescence, and (5) loss of body fluids as in hemorrhage, burns, draining wounds, large-scale removal of fluids from body cavities, transudation from traumatized tissue, or of protein in protein-losing enteropathy and nephrosis.

Symptoms and Signs

Weight loss is characteristic and may reach 50% in adults and even more in children. The loss is greatest in the liver and intestines, moderate in the heart and kidney, and least in the nervous system. Emaciation is most obvious where normally prominent fat depots and muscle masses waste and bones protrude. The skin becomes thin, dry, inelastic, pale, and cold. A patchy brown pigmentation may occur. Perifollicular keratosis is not infrequent. The hair is dry and sparse and falls out easily.

Most systems are affected. Achlorhydria and diarrhea are frequent, the latter often being terminal. Heart size and output are reduced. There is bradycardia and lowered systolic, diastolic, and venous pressure. Respiratory rate, minute volume, and vital capacity are all reduced. The main endocrine disturbance is gonadal atrophy with loss of libido (there is amenorrhea in the female). Intellect remains clear but apathy and irritability are common. Work capacity is diminished due to muscle destruction and eventual anemia and cardiorespiratory failure. Hypothermia frequently contributes to death. Anemia is usually mild, normochromic, and normocytic. In famine edema, serum proteins are normal, but due to loss of fat, extracellular water is relatively increased, tissue tension is low, and the skin is inelastic.

Laboratory Findings

Plasma levels of total amino acids and fatty acids are elevated, indicating catabolism of tissue protein and triglyceride, respectively. Individual amino acids follow different patterns; e.g., alanine falls progressively; glycine shows a delayed rise; and valine rises over 10 days and then progressively falls. Plasma insulin is low, glucagon may be high, and albumin is normal or slightly reduced despite edema. Urinary nitrogen excretion progressively falls, mainly due to diminished urea output.

Treatment

In the early stages of rehabilitation, food intake must be limited until GI function has been restored. Food should be bland and feedings limited initially to about 100 ml to avoid diarrhea. A recommended formula consists of 42% dried skim milk, 32% edible oil, 25% sucrose plus K, Mg, and vitamin supplements, reconstituted to give 10- to 15%-strength dried skim milk. Intake is gradually increased until about 5000 kcal/day may be consumed and weekly weight gain of 1.5 to 2.0 kg attained. If diarrhea persists in the absence of infections, temporary lactose intolerance may be suspected. Yogurt, in which lactose is partially hydrolyzed to glucose and galactose, is well tolerated. Severely debilitated patients require feeding by nasogastric tube. In acute deficiency, replacement should be suited to the loss; i.e., blood transfusion for acute blood loss, human albumin or plasma to replace plasma protein loss. Pooled human plasma may transmit hepatitis virus and should be *avoided*. Elemental diets or parenteral nutrition is required for those who cannot be fed orally (see Ch. 76).

Detailed dietary instruction, not merely a prescribed balanced diet, is needed for correction of deficiencies that are often multiple. When the diet is inadequate because of such factors as allergy, GI disease, dietary fads, or poor eating habits, or when there is impaired utilization of, or abnormal requirement for, one or more nutrients, nutritional supplements are needed.

Vitamin deficiencies may be corrected by individual or polyvitamin supplements. For patients with increased protein requirements, eating appropriate foods is the method of choice.

Mineral deficiencies on a nutritional basis are rare except for Fe. For discussion and treatment of these and other specific nutritional deficiencies, see Chs. 78 and 79. For daily caloric requirements, recommended daily mineral and vitamin allowances, etc., see Ch. 76.

PROTEIN-CALORIE MALNUTRITION

(PCM; Protein-Energy Malnutrition)

Etiology and Epidemiology

Protein provides the amino acids essential for tissue repair and growth, particularly in early life and pregnancy. If energy requirements exceed intake, catabolism of body tissue, including protein, will exceed synthesis. If energy intake is adequate but protein lacking, a pure protein deficiency will result. In practice, varying degrees of energy and protein deficiency occur, usually combined.

In the adult, general inanition is the most common manifestation. In the infant and young child, dietary deficiency of energy and protein results in a spectrum of disease termed **protein-calorie malnutrition**. Mild PCM is evidenced only by retarded growth; moderate cases may additionally show early biochemical changes. Severe cases are classified by clinical and biochemical findings into **marasmus**, due mainly to energy (calorie) deficiency, and **kwashiorkor** (Ga language of Ghana; "the disease the first child gets when the second is on the way") in which protein deficiency predominates. Intermediate forms with mixed etiology and symptoms are called **marasmic kwashiorkor**.

Marasmus is widespread in children under 3 yr of age living in developing countries and commonly follows early weaning, unhygienic bottle feeding with diluted formulas, repeated gastroenteritis, and "therapeutic" starvation. Kwashiorkor is predominant in areas of Africa, Asia, and Latin America, where the child is weaned late onto starchy food lacking in protein, and is often precipitated between ages 1 to 4 by measles or some other acute infection.

Pathophysiology

When there is a deficit in energy intake, the body draws on its own stores to maintain blood glucose, about ⅔ of which is utilized by the brain. Liver glycogen is depleted within a few hours, and thereafter skeletal muscle protein is utilized by **gluconeogenesis** to maintain adequate plasma glucose. Most of the nitrogen is transported to the liver as alanine and glutamine. At the same time triglycerides from fat depots are converted to free fatty acids, meeting the energy needs of tissues other than nerve. In prolonged starvation, increased lipolysis tends to protect body protein, and fatty acids yield ketone bodies that the brain can use as an alternative energy source.

Total body protein synthesis is about 300 gm/day in the average adult male. The daily obligatory loss is only about 30 to 90 gm, as 80 to 90% is reutilized. The daily allowance of protein recommended for an adult is about 0.8 gm/kg body wt (see TABLE 76–2). Of this dietary protein, about 20% of the constituent amino acids should be essential amino acids (see TABLE 77–1), since these cannot be synthesized in adequate amounts by the body and must be present in the diet. The degree to which the essential amino acid pattern of the dietary protein approximates that of the body's requirement determines **protein quality.**

In protein deficiency, adaptive enzyme changes occur in the liver, amino acid synthetases increase, and urea formation diminishes, thus conserving nitrogen and reducing its loss in the urine. Homeostatic mechanisms initially operate to maintain the level of plasma albumin. The rate of synthesis and catabolism soon decrease. Albumin shifts from the extravascular to the intravascular compartment. Eventually plasma albumin concentration falls, leading to reduced oncotic pressure and edema. Growth, immune response, repair, and production of enzymes and hormones are all impaired in severe protein deficiency.

Symptoms and Signs

Mild and moderate PCM may be classified by calculating weight as a percentage of expected weight/length (normal, 90 to 110%; mild PCM, 85 to 90%; moderate, 75 to 85%; severe, < 75%) using international standards.

Marasmic infants show gross weight loss, growth retardation, and wasting of subcutaneous fat and muscle. Kwashiorkor is characterized by generalized edema, "flaky paint" dermatosis, thinning and decoloration of the hair, enlarged fatty liver, and petulant apathy in addition to retarded growth.

Laboratory Findings

Mild or moderately severe cases of PCM may show slight depression of plasma albumin and a lowering of the urinary urea/creatinine and hydroxyproline/creatinine ratios. Increased urinary 3-methylhistidine reflects muscle breakdown. In both marasmus and kwashiorkor the percent body water, extracellular water, and plasma volume are increased. Electrolyte depletion (especially K and Mg), anemia (usually Fe deficiency), low levels of some enzymes and circulating lipids, falling blood urea, and metabolic acidosis are also present. Diarrhea is sometimes related to intestinal disaccharidase deficiency, especially lactase. Kwashiorkor is characterized by low plasma levels of albumin, transferrin, essential amino acids (especially the branched-chain), β-lipoprotein, and glucose, and an "overflow" aminoaciduria. Plasma cortisol, insulin, and growth hormone levels are high.

Diagnosis

Differential diagnosis includes secondary growth failure due to malabsorption, congenital defects, or deprivation. The skin changes of kwashiorkor differ from those of pellagra in which they occur on parts exposed to light and are symmetrical. Edema in nephritis, nephrosis, and cardiac failure is accompanied by features of these diseases. Hepatomegaly from disorders of glycogen metabolism and cystic fibrosis must be differentiated.

TABLE 77–1. ESTIMATED ESSENTIAL AMINO ACID REQUIREMENTS

Amino Acid	Daily Requirements (mg/kg)		
	Adult	Infant	Child (10–12 yr)
Histidine	16	28	20
Isoleucine	10	70	30
Leucine	14	161	45
Lysine	12	103	60
Methionine & cystine	13	58	27
Phenylalanine & tyrosine	14	125	27
Threonine	7	87	35
Tryptophan	3.5	17	4
Valine	10	93	33

Modified from Energy and Protein Requirements; Report of a Joint FAO/WHO *Ad Hoc* Expert Committee. *WHO Technical Report Series* No. 522. Copyright 1973 by FAO and WHO. Used with permission.

Treatment

Fluid and electrolyte balance should be restored and maintained. All but the most severely ill respond to a diet based on milk; dilute milk feedings can usually be introduced after 24 h. For treatment of shock superimposed on established dehydration, see SHOCK in Ch. 24.

Low-lactose formulas have been helpful in some cases in controlling excessive diarrhea caused by lack of disaccharidases. Lactic acid-fortified milk (0.125 ml/oz of milk) is preferred by some. Sufficient milk should be given to infants and small children to supply 2 to 5 gm of protein/kg/day. At this stage, more calories in the form of sugar and cereal may be added to the milk diet to provide 150 to 250 kcal/kg/day. Increased dietary allowances soon become possible and the diet is supplemented with high-energy foods such as candies, cake, puddings, meats, eggs, and fruit juices. Prepared nutritional supplements are available commercially. Bulky or low-caloric vegetables or fruits should be avoided and those containing 10 to 20% carbohydrate used. Supplementary vitamins may be advisable. Small, frequent feedings around the clock are tolerated best in the early stages of recovery. Antibiotics may be indicated. Unless urgent, treatment of malaria or other parasitic infections should be postponed until the patient is clinically improved. Blood transfusion is **contraindicated** unless the Hb is < 4 gm/100 ml.

Prognosis

Mortality varies between 15 and 40%. Death in the first days of treatment is usually due to electrolyte imbalance, infection, hypothermia, or circulatory failure. Stupor, jaundice, petechiae, low serum Na, and low serum vitamin A are ominous signs. Recovery is more rapid in kwashiorkor than in marasmus; disappearance of apathy, edema, and anorexia are favorable signs.

Long-term effects of malnutrition in childhood are not fully understood. In the adequately treated case the liver probably recovers fully without subsequent cirrhosis, but some GI malabsorption and pancreatic deficiency may remain. Persistent chromosomal breaks observed in malnourished children have not been shown to be due to the malnutrition per se. Humoral immunity is usually unimpaired. Cell-mediated immunocompetence is markedly compromised in the acute phase but is restored with recovery. Behavioral development may be markedly retarded in the severely malnourished child. The degree of mental impairment is related to the duration of malnutrition and to the age of onset. The young infant with marasmus is more severely affected than the older child with kwashiorkor. Prospective studies suggest that a relatively mild degree of mental retardation persists into school age.

78. VITAMIN DEFICIENCY, TOXICITY, AND DEPENDENCY

VITAMIN A (RETINOL) DEFICIENCY

(Night Blindness; Xerophthalmia; Keratomalacia)

Vitamin A (retinol) is fat-soluble and is found mainly in fish liver oils, liver, egg yolk, butter, and cream. Green leafy and yellow vegetables contain β-**carotene** and other provitamin carotenoids that undergo central fission of the molecule in the mucosal cells of the small intestine to form retinol, which is then esterified. Most of the body's vitamin A is stored in the liver as **retinyl palmitate**. It is released into the circulation as retinol, bound to a specific protein, retinol-binding protein **(RBP)**, and is also attached to tryptophan-rich prealbumin **(TRPA)**. The 11-*cis* isomer of retinal (vitamin A_1 aldehyde), combined with a protein moiety, forms the prosthetic group of photoreceptor pigments in the retina that are involved in night, day, and color vision. Vitamin A is also concerned with the maintenance of normal epithelial tissue. TABLES 76–1 and 76–2 give sources and recommended daily allowances. Equivalents, for diets with different proportions of retinol and β-carotene, are as follows: 1 USP u. equals 1 IU; 1 IU equals 0.3 μg of retinol; 1 μg of β-carotene equals 0.167 μg of retinol; other provitamin carotenoids are half as active as β-carotene. Inadequate intake or utilization of vitamin A can impair dark adaptation and cause night blindness; xerosis of the conjunctiva and cornea; xerophthalmia and keratomalacia; keratinization of lung, GI tract, and urinary tract epithelia; and increased susceptibility to infections. Impaired hue discrimination, defective taste and smell, and anemia that may be masked by hemoconcentration have also been reported.

Etiology

Primary vitamin A deficiency is usually caused by prolonged dietary deprivation. It is endemic in areas such as southern and eastern Asia where rice, devoid of carotene, is the staple. Secondary deficiency may be due to inadequate conversion of carotene, or to interference with absorption, storage, or transport of vitamin A. Interference with absorption or storage is likely in celiac disease, sprue, cystic fibrosis, operations on the pancreas, duodenal bypass, congenital partial obstruction of the jejunum, obstruction of the bile ducts, giardiasis, and cirrhosis of the liver. Vitamin A deficiency is common in protein-calorie malnutrition (marasmus or kwashiorkor) not only because the diet is deficient but also because vitamin A storage and transport are defective. Liver stores are depleted in deficiency before plasma levels begin to fall, followed later by retinal dysfunction, and finally by epithelial structural changes.

Symptoms and Signs

The severity of the effects of vitamin A deficiency is inversely related to age. Growth retardation is a common sign in children. Increased susceptibility to infection occurs at all ages. Pathognomonic changes are confined to the eye. Perifollicular hyperkeratosis of the skin is nonspecific and sporadic. The earliest, rod dysfunction, can be detected by dark adaptometry, rod scotometry, or electroretinography. These tests require cooperative subjects. Xerosis of the bulbar conjunctiva consists of drying, thickening, wrinkling, and muddy pigmentation. In advanced deficiency, **Bitot's spots** (superficial, foamy patches composed of epithelial debris and secretions on the exposed bulbar conjunctiva) are most likely due to vitamin A deficiency when they are large and occur in young children with other evidence of hypovitaminosis A. The cornea becomes xerotic, infiltrated, and hazy at an early stage. Keratomalacia rapidly supervenes with liquefaction of part or all of the cornea, leading to rupture, with extrusion of the eye contents and subsequent shrinking of the globe **(phthisis bulbi)**, or to anterior bulging **(corneal ectasia** and **anterior staphyloma)**, and blindness. Mortality in advanced cases is high (50% or more).

Diagnosis and Laboratory Findings

Evidence of depletion is unobtainable in the preclinical stage except for a history of inadequate intake. Plasma retinol 1evels fall when liver stores are exhausted. The normal range is 20 to 50 μg/100 ml; 10 to 19 μg is low, and < 10 μg is deficient. Mean plasma RBP is 47 μg/ml for adult males and 42 μg for females. Up to the age of 10 yr the range is 20 to 30 μg. Plasma vitamin A and RBP fall in deficiency and in acute infections. Other causes of night blindness (e.g., retinitis pigmentosa) must be excluded. Secondary infection may complicate the corneal changes. Trial with therapeutic doses of vitamin A will assist in the diagnosis.

Prophylaxis

Xerophthalmia remains the major cause of blindness in young children in most developing countries, where prophylactic doses of 200,000 IU (66,000 μg) of oily vitamin A palmitate orally once every 3 to 6 mo are advised for all children 1 to 4 (half the dose for those under 1). The diet should include green leafy vegetables. Bread, sugar, and monosodium glutamate are being fortified with vitamin A. Vitamin A supplements should be given routinely in secondary deficiency. Infants suspected of being allergic to milk should receive adequate vitamin A in the substitute formula.

Treatment

The cause should be corrected, and vitamin A given in therapeutic doses at once, followed by maintenance doses as required. Eye lesions and accompanying systemic changes are a threat to vision and to life. Vitamin A palmitate in oil given orally 200,000 IU (66,000 μg) daily for 2 days and once before discharge from hospital is usually effective. In the presence of vomiting or malabsorption, water-miscible vitamin A must be given IM, as oil preparations are not utilized by this route. Thereafter, 25,000 to 50,000 IU (8,000 to 16,000 μg) may be given orally until response is adequate. Maintenance therapy, or treatment of mild or suspected deficiency, includes 10,000 to 20,000 IU (3000 to 6000 μg)/day orally in 3 divided doses as cod-liver oil, red palm oil, or other concentrate. Prolonged daily administration of large doses, especially to infants, is to be **avoided** as hypervitaminosis (see below) may result.

HYPERVITAMINOSIS A

Excessive intake of vitamin A may be either acute or chronic. **Acute toxicity** in children has resulted from taking large doses ($> 300,000$ IU or 100,000 μg) and manifests as increased intracranial pressure and vomiting. Recovery is spontaneous with no residual damage; no fatalities have been reported. Arctic explorers, after ingesting several million units of vitamin A in polar bear or seal liver, have developed drowsiness, irritability, headache, and vomiting a few hours later, with subsequent peeling of the skin. Tablets containing vitamin A, sold for the prevention and relief of sunburn, have occasionally induced acute hypervitaminosis even when taken in accordance with the manufacturer's directions.

Chronic poisoning in older children and adults usually develops after doses above 100,000 IU (33,000 μg)/day have been taken for months. Infants may develop evidence of toxicity within a few weeks when given 20,000 to 60,000 IU (6,000 to 20,000 μg)/day of water-dispersible vitamin A.

Clinical Findings

Sparse coarse hair, alopecia of the eyebrows, dry rough skin, and cracked lips are early signs. Severe headache, **pseudotumor cerebri**, and generalized weakness are prominent later. Cortical hyperostoses and arthralgia are common, especially in children. Hepatomegaly and splenomegaly may occur.

Excessive ingestion of carotene does not cause hypervitaminosis A but produces high carotene blood levels (> 250 μg/100 ml) **(carotenemia)** which, while usually asymptomatic, may lead to **carotenosis** wherein the skin (but not the sclera) becomes deep yellow, especially on the palms and soles. Carotenosis may also occur in diabetes mellitus, myxedema, and anorexia nervosa possibly from a defect in conversion of carotene to vitamin A.

Diagnosis

Normal plasma vitamin A values range from 20 to 50 $\mu g/100$ ml. In hypervitaminosis A, fasting blood levels may exceed 100 $\mu g/100$ ml and have been as high as 2000 $\mu g/100$ ml. Differential diagnosis may be difficult as symptoms are varied and bizarre.

Prognosis and Treatment

Prognosis is excellent. Symptoms and signs usually disappear within 1 to 4 wk after stopping vitamin A ingestion.

VITAMIN D DEFICIENCY—RICKETS AND OSTEOMALACIA

This fat-soluble vitamin occurs mainly in 2 forms: **ergocalciferol** (activated ergosterol, calciferol, **vitamin D₂**), found in irradiated yeast; and **cholecalciferol** (activated 7-dehydrocholesterol, **vitamin D₃**), formed in human skin by exposure to sunlight (ultraviolet radiation) and found chiefly in fish liver oils and egg yolks. Milk is fortified with both forms. Synthesis in the skin is normally the major source. For recommended daily allowances see TABLE 76–2; 1 μg vitamin D equals 40 IU.

Vitamin D can be considered to be a prohormone with several active metabolites that behave as hormones. It is converted in the liver to $25\text{-}(OH)D_3$, the major circulating form. It undergoes enterohepatic circulation and is reabsorbed from the gut. In the kidney it is further hydroxylation to the much more metabolically active form $1,25\text{-}(OH)_2D_3$ (1,25-DHCC; calcitriol) whose main function is to increase Ca absorption from the intestine. Another metabolite, $24,25\text{-}(OH)_2D_3$, may have a specific effect in promoting normal bone formation and mineralization. The critical 1-hydroxylation of $25\text{-}(OH)D_3$ is strongly stimulated by PTH and, independently of PTH, by hypophosphatemia.

Metabolic bone disease resulting from vitamin D deficiency is called **rickets** in children and **osteomalacia** in adults. These diseases result from common pathogenetic factors but differ in their clinical and pathologic expression owing to differences between growing and formed bones.

Inadequate exposure to sunlight and poor dietary intake are usually necessary for clinical vitamin D deficiency to develop. Rickets is not uncommon in the tropics, due to swaddling of infants and confinement of women and children to the home. Nutritional rickets is very rare in the USA but still occurs in Britain, where milk is not fortified with vitamin D, and where immigrants of Asiatic origin shun sunlight.

All the features of rickets and osteomalacia may become evident when the supply of vitamin D is inadequate, its metabolism is abnormal, or tissues are resistant to its action (see TABLE 78–1). As this classification shows, most conditions associated with rickets nowadays are unrelated to vitamin D deficiency.

The actions of vitamin D, or more appropriately its metabolites, are summarized in TABLE 78–2.

Etiology

An etiologic classification of rickets and osteomalacia is important in relation to the manifestations of disease and to effective treatment. Some diseases interfere with the absorption of vitamin D or with the formation of its active metabolites. In these circumstances, the manifestations of these diseases will be superimposed upon those described below. If there is deficiency of vitamin D me-

TABLE 78–1. CLASSIFICATION OF RICKETS AND OSTEOMALACIA

Deficiency of vitamin D

Dietary lack, high phytate or phosphate intake, lack of sunlight, malabsorption syndromes

Defective production of $25\text{-}(OH)D_3$

Liver disease (advanced parenchymal and cholestatic disease)

Anticonvulsants (prolonged use of phenobarbital, phenytoin, increased catabolism of $25\text{-}(OH)D_3$

Defective production of $1,25\text{-}(OH)_2D_3$

Vitamin D-dependent rickets, type I (defective 1-hydroxylation)

Vitamin D-dependent rickets, type II (end organ resistance to $1,25\text{-}(OH)_2D_3$)

? Familial hypophosphatemic (vitamin D-resistant) rickets (renal tubular defect in phosphate transport)

? Acquired hypophosphatemic rickets (often associated with soft tissue tumors—"oncogenic osteomalacia"

? Chronic renal failure (renal osteodystrophy)

? Fanconi syndrome

? Renal tubular acidosis

? Diabetes mellitus (increased incidence of osteopenia, osteoporosis, and some fractures)

? Pseudohypoparathyroidism

TABLE 78–2. ACTIONS OF VITAMIN D AND ITS METABOLITES

Intestine
  Enhances Ca transport (absorption), the main function of 1,25-$(OH)_2D_3$
  Enhances PO_4 transport (absorption)

Bone
  Enhances bone resorption (PTH-like effect)
  Stimulates normal mineralization
  Affects collagen maturation

Muscle
  Restores normal function (? mechanism)

Parathyroid glands
  ? Inhibits PTH secretion

tabolites, vitamin D-resistant states occur that may be overcome to a varying extent (but often with undesirable side effects) by massive doses of vitamin D. Some of these states are now better treated with very small doses of metabolite or synthetic analog (see below).

Pathology

Changes in children include defective calcification of growing bone and hypertrophy of the epiphyseal cartilages. Epiphyseal cartilage cells cease to degenerate but new cartilage continues to form, so that the epiphyseal cartilage becomes irregularly increased in width. Calcification then stops and osteoid material accumulates around the capillaries of the diaphysis. The cancellous bone of the diaphysis and of cortical bone may be resorbed in chronic deficiency.

Adequate treatment with vitamin D permits Ca and PO_4 deposition through degeneration of the cartilage cells within 24 h and penetration by a vascular network within 48 h. Osteoid material at the diaphysis ceases to form, and normal endochondral production of new bone is resumed. The changes in adults are similar but not confined to the ends of the long bones.

Symptoms and Signs

In the neonatal period metaphyseal lesions and tetany accompany maternal osteomalacia. Young infants are restless, sleep poorly, and have reduced mineralization of the skull **(craniotabes)** away from the sutures. In older infants, sitting and crawling are delayed and there is bossing of the skull, costochondral beading **(rachitic rosary)** and delayed fontanelle closure. From 1 to 4 yr, there is enlargement of epiphyseal cartilages at the lower ends of the radius, ulna, tibia, and fibula; delay in walking, bowlegs, and kyphoscoliosis. In older children and adolescents there is pain on walking, and the development of such deformities as bowlegs and knock-knees in extreme cases.

Rachitic tetany is caused by hypocalcemia and may accompany either infantile or adult vitamin D deficiency. The clinical findings are discussed under HYPOCALCEMIA in DISTURBANCES IN CALCIUM METABOLISM in Ch. 81.

X-ray changes precede clinical signs, becoming evident in the 3rd or 4th mo of life—even at birth if the mother is vitamin D-deficient. Bone changes in rickets are most evident at the lower ends of the radius and ulna. The diaphyseal ends lose their sharp, clear outline, are cup-shaped, and show a spotty or fringy rarefaction. Later, the distance between the ends of the radius and ulna and the metacarpal bones appears increased, since the true ends are noncalcified and invisible. The shadows cast by the shaft decrease in density, and the network formed by laminas becomes coarse. Characteristic deformities are produced by bending of the bones at the cartilage-shaft junction due to weakness in the substance of the shaft. As healing begins, a thin white line of calcification appears at the epiphysis, becoming denser and thicker as calcification proceeds. Later, lime salts are deposited beneath the periosteum, the shaft casts a denser shadow, and the lamellas disappear.

In adults, demineralization **(osteomalacia)** occurs, particularly in the spine, pelvis, and lower extremities; the fibrous lamellas become visible by x-ray, and incomplete ribbon-like demineralizations appear in the cortex (pseudofractures, Looser's zones, Milkman's fractures). Pseudofractures are rare in osteomalacia but, when present, are pathognomonic. As the bones soften, weight may cause bowing of the long bones, vertical shortening of the vertebrae, and flattening of the pelvic bones, which contracts the pelvic outlet.

Laboratory Findings

With identification of specific binding proteins for vitamin D metabolites, 25-$(OH)D_3$ and other vitamin D sterols may be measured in plasma. Reported values for healthy subjects are 25 to 40 ng/ml for 25-$(OH)D_3$ and 20 to 45 pg/ml for 1,25-$(OH)_2D_3$. In rickets 25-$(OH)D_3$ values are very low and 1,25-$(OH)_2D_3$ is undetectable. A low serum phosphorus (normal 3.0 to 4.5 mg/100 ml) and a high serum alkaline phosphatase are characteristic. The serum Ca is low or normal, depending on the effectiveness of the secondary hyperparathyroidism in restoring the serum Ca to normal. The serum

PTH is elevated, and urinary Ca is low in all forms of the disease except those associated with acidosis.

Diagnosis

A history of inadequate vitamin D intake suggests rickets and helps to distinguish it from infantile scurvy (see under VITAMIN C DEFICIENCY, below) and other conditions. Congenital syphilis can be identified by serologic and other tests; chondrodystrophy, by the large head, short extremities, and thick bones, and by normal serum Ca, P, and phosphatase values.

Osteogenesis imperfecta, cretinism, congenital dislocation of the hip, hydrocephalus, and polio-myelitis should be readily distinguishable. Manifest tetany in infantile rickets must be differentiated from convulsions due to other causes. Rickets refractory to vitamin D may be caused by severe renal damage or in renal tubular acidosis, sex-linked hypophosphatemia, and Fanconi's syndrome.

Osteomalacia must be differentiated from other causes of widespread bone decalcification (e.g., hyperparathyroidism, senile or postmenopausal osteoporosis, the osteoporosis of hyperthyroidism, Cushing's syndrome, multiple myeloma, and atrophy of disuse). Serum Ca, PO_4, alkaline phosphatase, and 25-$(OH)D_3$ levels, together with x-ray findings, confirm the diagnosis.

Treatment

With adequate calcium and phosphorus intake, adult osteomalacia and uncomplicated rickets can be cured by intake of vitamin D 1600 IU (40 μg)/day. Serum 25-$(OH)D_3$ and 1,25-$(OH)_2D_3$ begin to rise within 1 or 2 days. Serum P rises in about 10 days, followed in the 3rd wk by x-ray signs of Ca and P deposition in the osseous tissues. After about 1 mo of therapy, the dose can be reduced gradually to normal levels. If tetany is present, treatment should be supplemented during the 1st wk with IV calcium salts (see HYPOCALCEMIA under DISTURBANCES IN CALCIUM METABOLISM in Ch. 81).

Those forms of rickets and osteomalacia that result from defective production of vitamin D metabolites (see TABLE 78–1) do not respond to the usual doses effective in nutritional rickets. Some of these conditions respond to massive doses but toxicity may result. In some of the conditions in which there is evidence of defective 25-$(OH)D_3$ production, 50 μg/day of 25-$(OH)D_3$ will augment plasma levels and result in clinical improvement.

Hereditary vitamin D-dependent rickets, type I, an autosomal recessive syndrome, characterized by severe rickets, low or normal serum Ca, hypophosphatemia and generalized aminoaciduria, responds to physiologic quantities of 1,25-$(OH_2)D_3$ (1 to 2 μg/day) IV or orally. This is the only form of rickets in which defective vitamin D metabolism has been definitely established as the cause of the disease.

Familial hypophosphatemic (vitamin D-resistant) rickets, an X-linked dominant disorder, responds to oral phosphate (1 to 4 gm/day in 5 divided doses). Long-term treatment with 1,25-$(OH)_2D_3$ has been shown to be effective in restoring bone dynamics toward normal.

In **chronic renal failure (renal osteodystrophy),** treatment with 1,25-$(OH)_2D_3$ (1.5 to 2 μg/day) is highly effective in increasing Ca absorption, promoting positive Ca and P balances, increasing serum Ca, reducing serum alkaline phosphatase and iPTH (immuno-reactive parathyroid hormone), and improving skeletal x-ray and bony architecture.

Prevention

Health education, including dietary advice, should be given to susceptible communities. A weekly capsule of vitamin D (75 μg) gives complete protection. Vitamin D fortification of chappati flour (125 μg/kg) has proved effective among Asian immigrants in Britain.

HYPERVITAMINOSIS D

Vitamin D 40,000 IU (1000 μg)/day produces toxicity within 1 to 4 mo in infants; toxic effects have been observed in adults receiving 100,000 IU (2500 μg)/day for several months. Elevated serum Ca levels of 12 to 16 mg/100 ml are a constant finding when toxic symptoms occur (normal values are 8.5 to 10.5 mg/100 ml). *Frequent determinations of serum calcium (weekly at first and then monthly) should be made in all patients receiving large doses of vitamin D.*

The first symptoms are anorexia, nausea, and vomiting, followed by polyuria, polydipsia, weakness, nervousness, and pruritus. Renal function is impaired, as evidenced by low specific gravity urine, proteinuria, casts, and azotemia. Metastatic calcifications may occur, particularly in the kidneys. Serum Ca is markedly elevated, plasma 25-$(OH)D_3$ is elevated while 1,25-$(OH)_2D_3$, surprisingly, is normal.

A history of excessive vitamin D intake is critical in differentiating this condition from all other hypercalcemic states. Vitamin D toxicity occurs commonly during the treatment of hypoparathyroidism. So-called **"hypercalcemia in infancy, with failure to thrive"** has been seen with daily vitamin D intakes less than 2000 IU or 50 μg (as low as 1000 IU or 25 μg); in these cases there may be hypersensitivity to the vitamin. In the **supravalvular aortic stenosis-infantile hypercalcemia syndrome** there is evidence of a genetically predetermined hypersensitivity to vitamin D.

As the new, highly active forms of vitamin D are being increasingly used, possible toxic effects of long-term therapy will need to be watched for.

Treatment consists of discontinuing the vitamin, a low-calcium diet, keeping the urine acid, and corticosteroids. If kidney damage or metastatic calcification has occurred, it may be irreversible.

VITAMIN E (TOCOPHEROL) DEFICIENCY

The vitamin E group includes the α, β, γ, and δ tocopherols; α is the most active. Vegetable oils and wheat germ are good sources of this fat-soluble vitamin. Vitamin E is an antioxidant that appears to act by maintaining the stability of membranes complexed with polyunsaturated phospholipids. In deficiency, activity of an enzyme, δ-aminolevulinic acid dehydratase, involved in heme synthesis is diminished. Vitamin E has close metabolic relationships with selenium (see in Ch. 79). Deficiency in man causes RBC hemolysis, creatinuria, and deposition of ceroid in muscle. (For sources and daily allowances, see TABLES 76-1 and 76-2.)

Etiology

Primary deficiency may occur in early infancy, especially with infant formulas high in unsaturated oils. Protein-calorie malnourished children often have low vitamin E status. Adult males have required many months on experimental diets to evidence vitamin E deficiency. Secondary deficiency may be expected in any malabsorption syndrome, especially with steatorrhea (as in sprue, celiac disease, cystic fibrosis, or biliary atresia) and in abetalipoproteinemia due to transport dysfunction.

Diagnosis and Laboratory Findings

Shortened length of RBC life has been attributed to vitamin E deficiency in adults. Edema and flaky dermatitis have been associated with low plasma E and increased peroxide hemolysis in premature infants on formulas containing vegetable oil. The deficiency state may be diagnosed when the plasma tocopherol level is low (< 0.8 mg/100 ml in the adult). RBC susceptibility to hydrogen peroxide is increased with levels < 0.5 mg/100 ml; this is reversed by vitamin E. Excessive creatinuria and increased plasma creatine phosphokinase levels are present on a creatine-free diet.

Treatment

If there is malabsorption in overt deficiency, vitamin E 30 to 100 mg/day should be given as dl-α-tocopheryl acetate IM. For infants, who are especially susceptible, a minimum daily allowance of 0.5 mg/kg (the amount usually obtained from human milk) is recommended.

VITAMIN K DEFICIENCY

Vitamin K activity is present in 2-methyl-1,4-naphthoquinones substituted at the 3 position with a phytyl group (phylloquinone or vitamin K_1 including synthetic **menadione** and **phytonadione**) or a multiprenyl side chain (the menaquinone or vitamin K_2 series). Vitamin K controls the formation in the liver of factor II (prothrombin), factors VII (proconvertin), IX (Christmas factor), and X (Stuart factor) as well as a fifth, recently identified, coagulation factor. Prothrombin contains a newly discovered amino acid, γ-carboxyglutamic acid, and vitamin K is probably required for de novo protein synthesis or at a post-translational level by the liver. The recent isolation of this amino acid from bone and kidney suggests that vitamin K may act here also. Deficiency causes *hypoprothrombinemia, manifested by defective coagulation of the blood and hemorrhage*. The adult daily requirement is about 2 mg.

Etiology

Vitamin K is usually formed in the body from intestinal bacterial synthesis. Lack of intestinal bacterial flora probably explains the hypoprothrombinemia observed during the first 3 to 5 days of life. Therapy with nonabsorbable sulfonamides or oral antibiotics may interfere with vitamin K synthesis in the intestines.

Secondary deficiency often results from impaired absorption due to lack of bile salts in patients with external biliary fistulas or obstructive jaundice and other GI conditions causing malabsorption. Excessive amounts of mineral oil may also prevent absorption. Severe liver disease may inhibit prothrombin synthesis, a condition unresponsive to vitamin K therapy. Coumarin anticoagulants produce hypoprothrombinemia, since they act as antimetabolites for vitamin K.

Symptoms and Signs

Symptoms are those of hypoprothrombinemia superimposed on the conditioning disease. In obstructive jaundice, hemorrhage, if it occurs, usually begins after the 4th to 5th day. It may begin as a slow ooze from a surgical wound, the gums, nose, or GI mucosa, or it may be massive into the GI tract. Some intracranial hemorrhages at birth and other hemorrhagic disorders are traceable to the hypoprothrombinemia of the first few days of life. Breast-fed infants who have not received vitamin K are especially susceptible, as human milk is a poor source of the vitamin.

Laboratory Findings

All vitamin K-dependent plasma glycoproteins—factors II, VII, IX, X, and a fifth, recently discovered—are significantly depressed. Reduction of quantitative prothrombin to 80% of normal or below is abnormal, and reduction to 20% or less is associated with an increasing incidence of active bleeding. Bleeding and coagulation times are usually not altered significantly until the prothrombin level has fallen to below 20%.

Diagnosis

Hypoprothrombinemia may result from anticoagulant or salicylate therapy, failure to absorb vitamin K, severe liver damage, or an unknown cause. Liver pathology can usually be ruled out if 2 to 5 mg of water-soluble synthetic vitamin K, given IV, produces a significant increase in prothrombin levels within 2 to 6 h. Many diseases, such as scurvy, allergic purpura, leukemia, and thrombocytopenia, can produce hemorrhagic symptoms without hypoprothrombinemia.

Treatment

Phytonadione (vitamin K_1) is the preparation of choice. It may be used in any hypoprothrombinemia, particularly that caused by the vitamin K antagonists derived from coumarin or indandione. Menadione sodium bisulfite is not effective against these antagonists. Whenever possible, phytonadione should be given s.c. or IM. The usual adult dose is 10 mg IM. *In emergencies*, from 10 to 50 mg of phytonadione dissolved in 5% dextrose or 0.9% sodium chloride should be given IV **at a rate not to exceed 1 mg/min.** This may be repeated in 6 to 8 h if the prothrombin time has not been shortened satisfactorily. The counteractive effect is detectable within an hour or 2 and, in most cases, is effective within 3 to 6 h. Oral phytonadione 5 to 20 mg is indicated for nonemergency control of hypoprothrombinemia in patients taking anticoagulants. Beneficial effects are usually apparent within 6 to 10 h after starting therapy.

Vitamin K_1 1 to 2 mg IM is commonly recommended for the newborn to prevent hypoprothrombinemia, to reduce the incidence of intracranial hemorrhage incidental to birth trauma, and prophylactically when surgery is contemplated. Recommended alternative procedures are: (1) vitamin K_1 given to the mother in prophylactic dosages (2 to 5 mg orally/day) for 1 wk prior to expected confinement, or (2) vitamin K_1 solution (2 to 5 mg IM) given to the mother 6 to 24 h before delivery.

HYPERVITAMINOSIS K

Menadione and its water-soluble analogs can cause hemolysis in persons with G6PD deficiency and in others when large doses are used. **In the newborn,** large doses of menadione have produced anemia with Heinz bodies, hyperbilirubinemia, and kernicterus (especially in premature infants with erythroblastosis). The dose should be limited: 2 to 5 mg for women in labor; 1 to 2 mg for newborn babies.

ESSENTIAL FATTY ACID DEFICIENCY

Full-term babies fed a skim-milk formula low in linoleic acid suffered growth failure and a dermatosis; the condition was reversed when linoleic acid was added. Deficiency is unlikely to occur on natural diets, although cow's milk has only about ¼ the amount present in human milk. While total fat intake in many developing countries is very low, much of it is of vegetable origin and rich in linoleic acid. Essential fatty acid deficiency has been a hazard of long-term fat-free parenteral nutrition in the past, but fat emulsions, now coming into general use, are alleviating this (see PARENTERAL NUTRITION in Ch. 76). A 10% soybean oil emulsion contains about 56 gm/L linoleic acid.

Early in deficiency, plasma levels of linoleic and arachidonic acids are low and the abnormal presence of 5,8,11-eicosatrienoic acid occurs from lack of inhibition of its synthesis from oleic acid.

THIAMINE (VITAMIN B_1) DEFICIENCY

(Beriberi)

The coenzyme thiamine pyrophosphate **(TPP)** participates in carbohydrate metabolism through decarboxylation of α-keto acids. Thiamine also acts as coenzyme to the apoenzyme transketolase in the pentose monophosphate pathway for glucose. (For sources and daily allowances of thiamine, see TABLES 76–1 and 76–2.) Deficiency causes **beriberi** with peripheral neurologic, cerebral, and cardiovascular manifestations.

Etiology

Primary thiamine deficiency arises from inadequate intake, particularly in people subsisting on highly polished rice. Milling removes the husk, which contains most of the thiamine, but boiling before husking disperses the vitamin throughout the grain, thus preventing its loss. Secondary deficiency arises from (1) increased requirement, as in hyperthyroidism, pregnancy, lactation, and fever; (2) impaired absorption, as in long-continued diarrheas; and (3) impaired utilization, as in severe liver disease. A combination of decreased intake, impaired absorption and utilization, and increased requirements occurs in alcoholism. Frequent, long-continued, or highly concentrated dextrose infusions, coupled with low thiamine intake, may precipitate thiamine deficiency.

Pathology

The most advanced neural changes occur in the peripheral nerves, particularly of the legs. The distal segments are characteristically affected earliest and most severely. Degeneration of the medullary sheath has been demonstrated in all tracts of the cord, especially in the posterior columns and in the anterior and posterior nerve roots. Changes are noted also in the anterior horn and posterior ganglion cells. Lesions of hemorrhagic polioencephalitis occur in the brain when deficiency is severe.

The heart is dilated and enlarged; muscle fibers are swollen, fragmented, and vacuolized, with interstitial spaces dilated by fluid. Edema and serous effusions may develop, even in patients without congestive heart failure.

Symptoms and Signs

Early deficiency produces fatigue, irritation, poor memory, sleep disturbances, precordial pain, anorexia, abdominal discomfort, and constipation.

Peripheral neurologic changes (dry beriberi) are bilateral and symmetric, involving predominantly the lower extremities, and are ushered in by paresthesias of the toes, burning of the feet (particularly severe at night) calf muscle cramps, and pains in the legs. Calf muscle tenderness, difficulty in rising from a squatting position, a quantitative diminution in the vibratory sensation in the toes, and plantar dysesthesia are early signs. A diagnosis of mild peripheral neuropathy can be made when ankle jerks are absent. Continued deficiency causes loss of knee jerk, loss of vibratory and position sensation in the toes, atrophy of the calf and thigh muscles, and finally foot-drop and toe-drop. The arms may become involved after leg signs are well established.

Cerebral beriberi (Wernicke-Korsakoff syndrome; acute hemorrhagic polioencephalitis) results from severe and acute deficiency superimposed on chronic deficiency. Mental confusion, aphonia, and confabulation constitute the early stage called **Korsakoff psychosis.** Cerebral blood flow is markedly reduced and vascular resistance increased. Nystagmus, total ophthalmoplegia, coma, and death in the untreated case is **Wernicke's encephalopathy.**

Cardiovascular beriberi: Biventricular congestive failure and pulmonary congestion result in edema, anasarca, and dyspnea. Three major derangements occur: peripheral vasodilation leading to a high output state, biventricular myocardial failure, and retention of Na and water.

Infantile beriberi occurs in infants breast-fed by thiamine-deficient mothers, usually between the 2nd and 4th mo of life. Cardiac failure, aphonia, and absent deep tendon reflexes are characteristic.

Laboratory Findings

Elevated blood pyruvate and diminished urinary thiamine excretion (< 50 μg/day) are consistent but late changes. Erythrocyte transketolase activity diminishes before and increases after addition of thiamine pyrophosphate (TPP effect), and is more sensitive. Variations in apoenzyme levels in some diseases may complicate interpretation.

Diagnosis

A form of polyneuropathy, which does not respond to thiamine, occurs in uncontrolled or long-continued diabetes mellitus and is clinically similar to that of thiamine deficiency. Other forms of bilateral symmetric polyneuropathy beginning in the legs are infrequent. Single-nerve neuritides and those beginning elsewhere are unlikely to be due to thiamine deficiency.

Edema of cardiovascular beriberi responds to bed rest as well as or better than the edema of most other forms of heart disease but responds poorly to digitalis. Response to a therapeutic trial of thiamine in uncomplicated cardiovascular or cerebral beriberi is usually prompt and complete. Diagnosis is difficult when complicated by hypertensive, degenerative, or infectious heart disease.

Treatment

In mild polyneuropathies, 10 to 20 mg/day of thiamine is given in divided doses. The dose is 20 to 30 mg/day in moderate or advanced neuropathy. In cardiovascular beriberi and in Wernicke-Korsakoff syndrome, 50 to 100 mg s.c. or IV b.i.d. is usually given; these doses should be continued until a therapeutic response is obtained or until a strong odor of thiamine in the urine indicates saturation. Basic therapy should then be resumed.

Rarely, fatal anaphylactic reactions unrelated to dose size have followed IV injection. The possibility of such reactions must be considered, particularly in patients who have previously received thiamine parenterally, if an interval has elapsed without treatment.

RIBOFLAVIN (VITAMIN B₂) DEFICIENCY

Riboflavin is a water-soluble vitamin, essential for proper growth and tissue function. Sources and recommended daily allowances are listed in TABLES 76–1 and 76–2. Deficiency results in oral, ocular, cutaneous, and genital lesions.

Etiology

Primary riboflavin deficiency is associated with inadequate consumption of milk and other animal protein. Conditioned deficiencies are most frequent in chronic diarrheas, liver disease, chronic alcoholism, and when postoperative nutrient infusions lack supplementary vitamins.

Symptoms, Signs, and Laboratory Findings

The commonest signs consist of pallor and maceration of the mucosa in the angles of the mouth (**angular stomatitis**) and vermilion surfaces of the lips (cheilosis), followed by superficial linear fissures that may leave scars on healing. When these lesions are infected by *Candida albicans*, grayish white exuberant lesions, termed **perlèche**, result. The tongue may have a magenta hue. Cutaneous **manifestations** usually affect the nasolabial folds, alae nasi, ears, eyelids, scrotum, and labia majora. These areas become red, scaly, and greasy, and sebaceous material accumulates in hair follicles, producing **dyssebacea** or **shark skin.**

The **eye** may rarely show neovascularization of the cornea and epithelial keratitis, resulting in lacrimation and photophobia. Nutritional amblyopia may respond to riboflavin.

Urinary excretion of < 30 μg of riboflavin/gm of creatinine is associated with clinical signs of riboflavin deficiency. Increased activation of RBC glutathione reductase by riboflavin is an early sign.

Diagnosis

The lesions described are not found solely in riboflavin deficiency. Cheilosis may result from vitamin B_6 deficiency, edentulism, or ill-fitting dentures. Seborrheic dermatitis and ocular lesions may be produced by a number of conditions. Therefore, diagnosis of riboflavin deficiency cannot depend on the history and presence of suggestive lesions alone. Laboratory tests, elimination of other causes, and a therapeutic trial may be necessary.

Treatment

Riboflavin 10 to 30 mg/day orally in divided doses is given until a response is evident; then 2 to 4 mg/day until recovery. Riboflavin can be given IM 5 to 20 mg/day, in single or divided doses.

NIACIN (NICOTINIC ACID) DEFICIENCY

(Pellagra)

This water-soluble B vitamin is found in many foods that also contain thiamine (see TABLE 76–1). Through the role of nicotine-adenine dinucleotide (**NAD,** coenzyme I) and nicotine-adenine dinucleotide phosphate (**NADP,** coenzyme II) in oxidation-reduction reactions, niacin derivatives play a vital function in cell metabolism. (For daily allowances, see TABLE 76–2.)

Etiology

Severe niacin deficiency is a principal cause of **pellagra.** Primary deficiency usually occurs in areas where maize (Indian corn) forms a major part of the diet. Bound niacin, found in maize, is not assimilated in the intestinal tract unless it has been previously alkali-treated (as in the preparation of tortillas). Corn protein is also deficient in tryptophan, a precursor from which the body can synthesize niacin. Amino acid imbalance may also play a part, as pellagra is common in India among those who eat a millet with a high leucine content. Secondary deficiencies are seen in diarrheal disease, cirrhosis of the liver, and alcoholism, and following extensive postoperative use of nutrient infusions lacking vitamins. Pellagra may also complicate prolonged isoniazid (INH) therapy (the drug replaces niacinamide in NAD); malignant carcinoid tumor (tryptophan is diverted to form 5-hydroxytryptamine); and Hartnup disease (see in Ch. 153).

Symptoms and Signs

Pellagra is characterized by cutaneous, mucous membrane, CNS, and GI symptoms. The complete syndrome of advanced deficiency includes scarlet stomatitis and glossitis, diarrhea, dermatitis, and mental aberrations. Symptoms may appear alone or in combination.

Four types of **cutaneous lesions,** usually bilaterally symmetric, are recognized: (1) acute, consisting of erythema followed by vesiculation, bullae, crusting, and desquamation; secondary infection is common, notably following exposure to sunlight (actinic trauma); (2) intertrigo, also an acute lesion, characterized by redness, maceration, abrasion, and secondary infection in the intertriginous areas; (3) chronic hypertrophy, in which the skin is thickened, inelastic, fissured, and deeply pigmented over pressure points; secondary infection often develops, and the lesion shows a sharply defined pearly border of regenerating epithelium when healing begins; and (4) chronic atrophic lesions, with dry, scaly, inelastic skin too large for the part it covers (seen in older pellagrins). Distribution of the above lesions, which occur at trauma points, is more characteristic than their form. Sunlight causes Casal's necklace and butterfly-shaped lesions on the face.

Changes in the **mucous membranes** primarily involve the mouth but may also affect the vagina and urethra. Scarlet glossitis and stomatitis are characteristic of acute deficiency. The tip and margins of the tongue and the mucosa around Stensen's duct are affected first. As the lesion progresses, the entire tongue and oral mucous membranes become a bright scarlet color, followed by sore mouth, increased salivation, and edema of the tongue. Ulcerations may appear, especially under the tongue, on the mucosa of the lower lip, and opposite the molar teeth. They are often covered by a grayish slough containing Vincent's organisms.

Gastrointestinal symptoms, which are indeterminate in early cases, include burning of the mouth, pharynx, and esophagus, and abdominal discomfort and distention. Later, nausea, vomiting, and diarrhea may occur. Diarrhea, often bloody because of gastrointestinal hyperemia and ulceration, is serious.

CNS involvement includes (1) organic psychosis, characterized by memory impairment, disorientation, confusion, and confabulation (excitement, depression, mania, and delirium predominate in some patients; in others, the reaction is paranoid), and (2) **"encephalopathic syndrome,"** characterized by clouding of consciousness, cogwheel rigidity of the extremities, and uncontrollable sucking and grasping reflexes. Differentiation from the CNS changes in thiamine deficiency is difficult.

Diagnosis

Niacin deficiency must be distinguished from other causes of stomatitis, glossitis, diarrhea, and dementia. Diagnosis is easy when the clinical findings include skin and mouth lesions, diarrhea, delirium, and dementia. More often, the condition is less fully developed. In these cases, history of a diet lacking niacin and tryptophan is significant. Urinary excretion of N′-methylniacinamide and pyridone is decreased.

Treatment

Multiple deficiencies of B vitamins and protein often occur together; therefore, the diet should be balanced. Supplemental niacinamide 300 to 1000 mg/day should be given orally in divided doses. In most cases, 300 to 500 mg is sufficient. Niacinamide is generally used in deficiency states, since niacin can cause flushing, itching, burning, or tingling sensations and niacinamide does not; however, niacinamide does not possess hypolipidemic or vasodilating properties as does niacin. When oral therapy is precluded, due to lack of patient cooperation or diarrhea, 100 to 250 mg should be injected s.c. 2 to 3 times/day. In encephalopathic states, 1000 mg orally plus 100 to 250 mg parenterally is recommended.

VITAMIN B₆ (PYRIDOXINE) DEFICIENCY AND DEPENDENCY

Deficiency: *A state in which the tissue pool of pyridoxal phosphate is depleted.*

Dependency: *A state in which the coenzyme pool is adequate, but the ability of a protein apoenzyme to bind the coenzyme is defective.* The resulting imbalance can be overcome by increased pyridoxine intake.

Vitamin B₆ comprises a group of closely related compounds: **pyridoxine, pyridoxal,** and **pyridoxamine.** They are phosphorylated in the body to pyridoxal phosphate, which functions as a coenzyme in many reactions, including decarboxylation and transamination of amino acids, deamination of hydroxyamino acids and cysteine, conversion of tryptophan to niacin, and metabolism of fatty acids. Consequently, the vitamin complex is important in blood, CNS, and skin metabolism. (For sources and daily allowances, see TABLES 76–1 and 76–2.)

Etiology

Primary deficiency is rare, since most foods contain the vitamin, but an outbreak of convulsions in infants did follow the destruction of vitamin B₆ in artificial milk. Secondary deficiencies may result from malabsorption, chemical inactivation by drugs (e.g., isonicotinic acid hydrazide, hydralazine, DL-penicillamine), excessive loss, and increased metabolic activity.

Symptoms and Signs

Deficiency: The vitamin B₆ antagonist **deoxypyridoxine** produces seborrheic dermatosis, glossitis, cheilosis, peripheral neuropathy, and lymphopenia. Vitamin B₆ deficiency can cause convulsions in infants and anemia in adults (usually normoblastic but occasionally megaloblastic).

Dependency: Several recessive or X-linked states have been described, affecting different apoenzymes and producing symptoms such as convulsions, mental deficiency, and cystathioninuria; iron overload anemia, urticaria, and asthma; and xanthurenicaciduria.

Diagnosis and Laboratory Findings

The symptoms of vitamin B₆ **deficiency** are not characteristic, and therapeutic trial is often necessary. Direct measurement of the coenzyme pool is not possible. In deficiency the tryptophan load test (50 mg/kg for children and 2 gm for adults) shows increased urinary excretion of xanthurenic acid (> 50 mg/day in the adult) and other intermediates on the niacin pathway. Plasma pyridoxine falls (< 25 ng/ml) as do urinary excretion of pyridoxine (< 20 μg/gm creatinine) and 4-pyridoxic acid (< 0.5 mg/day). Erythrocyte glutamic pyruvate and oxaloacetic transaminase activities are increased. Early recognition of **dependency** is necessary to prevent death or mental retardation. Correction of convulsions by a parenteral dose of about 20 mg of pyridoxine is diagnostic. This should be complemented by tests for aminoaciduria and an apoenzyme.

Treatment

Deficiency in the adult usually responds to pyridoxine 50 to 100 mg/day orally. Underlying causes such as use of pyridoxine inactivating drugs (anticonvulsants, corticosteroids, estrogens, isoniazid, penicillamine, and hydralazine) or malabsorption should be corrected. Conditions that increase metabolic demand require amounts in excess of the recommended allowance. In **dependency** in the infant the daily requirement (normally 0.4 mg) is increased many times (up to 10 mg). As much as 200 to 600 mg daily of pyridoxine may be needed for treatment of adults.

FOLIC ACID DEFICIENCY

Many plant and animal tissues contain folic acid **(pteroylglutamic acid, folacin)** as reduced methyl or formyl polyglutamates. They are unstable, and 50 to 90% may be destroyed by boiling or canning. (See TABLES 76–1 and 76–2 for sources and daily allowances.) In the tetrahydro form, folates act as coenzymes for processes in which there is transfer of a one-carbon unit, as in purine and pyrimidine nucleotide biosynthesis, amino acid conversions such as histidine to glutamic acid through formiminoglutamic acid **(FIGLU)**, and generation and use of formate.

Absorption takes place in the small intestine. In the epithelial cells polyglutamates are reduced to dihydro- and tetrahydrofolates. They are bound to protein and transported as methyl tetrahydrofolate. Plasma levels vary from 3 to 21 ng/ml and closely reflect dietary intake. Red cell folate (normal 160 to 640 ng/ml whole blood, corrected to packed cell volume of 45%) is a better indicator of status. The total body folate is about 70 mg, 1/3 of which is found in the liver. About 20% of ingested folate is excreted unabsorbed together with 60 to 90 μg/day not reabsorbed from bile.

Folate deficiency causes megaloblastic anemia and other hematologic changes (see ANEMIA DUE TO FOLIC ACID DEFICIENCY under MEGALOBLASTIC ANEMIAS in Ch. 92). Infertility and GI disturbances such as glossitis, stomatitis, and intestinal malabsorption also occur. Deficiency has been reported in association with the following conditions but has not been proved to be their cause: skin disorders (psoriasis, dermatitis herpetiformis, rosacea, eczema, exfoliative dermatitis); obstetric disorders (toxemia of pregnancy, abortion, abruptio placentae, congenital malformations); neuropathy; and psychiatric disorders. Possible causes of folic acid deficiency are given in TABLE 78–3. See TABLE 76–1 for usual therapeutic dosage.

VITAMIN B_{12} DEFICIENCY

The vitamin B_{12} molecule consists of the nucleotide 5,6-dimethylbenzimidazole linked at right angles to a four-pyrrole ring with a cobalt atom (the corrin nucleus). Several different **cobalamins**, which vary only in the ligand attached to the cobalt atom, occur in nature. (See TABLES 76–1 and 76–2 for sources and recommended daily allowances.) Strict vegetarians may obtain cobalamin from legume nodules where it is synthesized by microorganisms.

Intrinsic factor, secreted by parietal cells of the gastric mucosa, probably has two binding sites: one for free cobalamin and the other for ileal microvilli, which require a neutral pH and the presence of free calcium and are readily saturated. Vitamin B_{12} alone passes into the mucosal cell. Little cobalamin is absorbed passively throughout the length of the GI tract.

Vitamin B_{12} is present in plasma as methylcobalamin, 5'-deoxyadenosylcobalamin, and hydroxocobalamin bound to specific proteins, transcobalamin I and II. The normal range of vitamin B_{12} plasma concentration is 150 to 750 pg/ml, which represents only about 0.1% of the total body content, most of which is in the liver. Excretion is mainly through the bile and to a lesser extent via the kidneys. The total daily loss is 2 to 5 μg. Vitamin B_{12} and folic acid are both involved in nucleoprotein synthesis, probably facilitating the reduction of the ribose moiety of uridylic acid, before methylation of uracil to thymine in the synthesis of DNA.

Because of its slow rate of utilization and considerable stores, vitamin B_{12} deficiency (a fall in tissue stores below 0.1 mg and a plasma level below 100 pg/ml) usually takes many months to appear. However, hematologic and neurologic changes have been reported recently in the breastfed baby of a vegan. The hematologic changes due to vitamin B_{12} deficiency are discussed in Ch. 92; the neurologic changes of combined system disease are discussed in Ch. 129. Psychoses and optic atrophy may also occur. In one form of the latter, **tobacco amblyopia**, the cyanide in tobacco smoke may be detoxified by hydroxocobalamin which is converted to the more readily excreted congener cyanocobalamin, thereby causing a deficiency in vitamin B_{12}. It is also postulated that vitamin B_{12} deficiency could result in deficiency of a sulfur donor, necessary for the conversion of cyanide to thiocyanate, by its known role as methylcobalamin in the transmethylation of homocysteine to methionine. TABLE 78–4 lists the main causes of vitamin B_{12} deficiency. See TABLE 76–1 for usual therapeutic dosage and Ch. 92 for treatment of anemia due to vitamin B_{12} deficiency.

TABLE 78–3. CAUSES OF FOLIC ACID DEFICIENCY

Primary deficiency
  Poor diet: lacking fresh, slightly cooked food; chronic alcoholism

Secondary deficiency
  Inadequate absorption: malabsorption syndromes (esp. celiac disease, sprue), drugs (phenytoin, primidone, barbiturates, cycloserine, oral contraceptives?), specific malabsorption for folate (congenital, acquired), blind loop syndrome
  Inadequate utilization: folic acid antagonists (methotrexate, pyrimethamine, triamterene, diamidine compounds, trimethoprim), anticonvulsants?, enzyme deficiency (congenital, acquired), vitamin B_{12} deficiency, alcohol, scurvy
  Increased requirement: pregnancy, infancy, malignancy (esp. lymphoproliferative), increased hematopoiesis, increased metabolism
  Increased excretion: vitamin B_{12} dependency?, liver disease?

Modified from V. Herbert: "The Five Possible Causes of all Nutrient Deficiency: Illustrated by Deficiencies of Vitamin B_{12} and Folic Acid," *The American Journal of Clinical Nutrition*, Vol. 26, pp. 77–86, Jan. 1973. Copyright American Society for Clinical Nutrition, Inc. Used with permission of the Society and the author.

TABLE 78–4. CAUSES OF VITAMIN B$_{12}$ DEFICIENCY

Primary deficiency
  Inadequate diet: veganism, chronic alcoholism (rare), dietary faddism

Secondary deficiency
  Inadequate absorption: lack of intrinsic factor (pernicious anemia, destruction of gastric mucosa, endocrinopathy), intrinsic factor inhibition, small intestine disorders (celiac disease, sprue, malignancy, drugs, specific malabsorption for vitamin B$_{12}$), competition for vitamin B$_{12}$ (fish tapeworm, blind loop syndrome)
  Inadequate utilization: antagonists, enzyme deficiencies, organ disease (liver, kidney, malignancy, malnutrition), transport protein abnormality
  Increased requirement: hyperthyroidism, infancy, parasitic infestation
  Increased excretion: inadequate binding in serum, liver disease, renal disease

Modified from V. Herbert: "The Five Possible Causes of all Nutrient Deficiency: Illustrated by Deficiencies of Vitamin B$_{12}$ and Folic Acid," *The American Journal of Clinical Nutrition,* Vol. 26, pp. 77–86, Jan. 1973. Copyright American Society for Clinical Nutrition, Inc. Used with permission of the Society and the author.

VITAMIN B$_{12}$ DEPENDENCY

Several specific disorders of cobalamin-dependent metabolism have been reported. In each there is some ill-understood defect either in (1) cellular uptake of the vitamin precursor, (2) conversion of the vitamin to the coenzyme form, or (3) coenzyme-apoenzyme interaction. The metabolism of methylmalonic acid is usually affected, with large amounts excreted in the urine. These disorders usually respond to massive doses of vitamin B$_{12}$ (1000 µg/day IM).

BIOTIN DEFICIENCY AND DEPENDENCY

Raw egg white contains a biotin antagonist, avidin, and high and prolonged consumption has resulted in dermatitis and glossitis responding rapidly to 150 to 300 µg biotin daily.

Dependency: Retarded physical and mental development, alopecia, keratoconjunctivitis, and defects in T cell and B cell immunity have been reported in children with deficiencies of biotin-dependent carboxylases. Urinary excretion of various organic acids assists diagnosis; response has been complete to large doses of biotin (10 mg) daily.

VITAMIN C (ASCORBIC ACID) DEFICIENCY
(Scurvy)

Vitamin C is essential to collagen formation and helps to maintain the integrity of substances of mesenchymal origin, such as connective tissue, osteoid tissue of bone, and dentin of teeth. It is essential for wound healing and facilitates recovery from burns. It is a strong reducing agent and is reversibly oxidized and reduced readily in the body (it is presumed to function as a redox system in the cell). It is involved in the metabolism of phenylalanine and tyrosine and, as a reductant (with oxygen, ferrous iron, and a 2-ketoacid) activates enzymes that hydroxylate protocollagen proline and lysine to collagen hydroxyproline and hydroxylysine. Synthesis of an elastin, which becomes increasingly deficient in hydroxyproline, occurs in scorbutic animals. Vitamin C protects folic acid reductase, which converts folic acid to folinic acid. It may participate in the release of free folic acid from its conjugates in food and it facilitates the absorption of iron. Severe deficiency results in **scurvy,** *an acute or chronic disease characterized by hemorrhagic manifestations and abnormal osteoid and dentin formation.* (For sources and daily allowances of vitamin C, see TABLES 76–1 and 76–2.)

Etiology

Primary deficiency in infants is due to lack of supplementary vitamin C. In adults it is usually due to food idiosyncrasies or improper diet. Deficiencies occur in GI disease, especially when the patient is on an "ulcer diet." Pregnancy, lactation, and thyrotoxicosis increase the vitamin C requirement. Diarrhea increases fecal loss, and achlorhydria decreases the amount of vitamin absorbed. Acute and chronic inflammatory diseases, surgical operations, and burns can significantly increase the body requirements. Cold increases urinary excretion of vitamin C.

Pathology

Formation of intercellular cement substances in connective tissues, bones, and dentin is defective, resulting in weakening of capillaries with subsequent hemorrhage and defects in bone and related structures. Hemorrhagic areas are organized avascularly, so that wounds heal poorly and break open easily. Bone lesions result from cessation of endochondral growth due to failure of the osteoblasts to form osteoid tissue. Instead, a fibrous union is formed between the diaphysis and the epiphysis, and costochondral junctions enlarge. Densely calcified fragments of cartilage are embedded in this fibrous tissue. Small ecchymotic hemorrhages within or along the bone, or large subperiosteal hemorrhages due to small fractures just shaftward of the white line, complicate these lesions.

Symptoms and Signs

Infantile scurvy usually occurs between the 6th and 12th mo of life. Early symptoms include irritability, anorexia, and failure to gain weight. The child screams when moved and may keep his legs motionless because of pain from subperiosteal hemorrhage. Advanced cases show angular enlargements of the costochondral junctions (scorbutic rosary), swelling over the ends of the long bones (especially at the lower end of the femur), and a tendency to hemorrhage, as shown by swollen hemorrhagic gums surrounding erupting teeth. Hemorrhages into the skin at this age are rare, and gingivitis does not develop until teeth have erupted. Fever, anemia, and increased pulse and respiration rates are common. The anemia is usually caused by an iron deficiency; however, macrocytosis and a megaloblastic bone marrow may be seen due to a combined deficiency of vitamin C and folic acid.

X-ray findings are characteristic. The ends of the long bones show a transverse thickening and increased density—the **white line.** Immediately shaftward of the white line is a localized area of rarefaction, first evident at the lateral margins and appearing in the x-ray as a small fracture. The trabecular markings of the shaft become indistinct, giving it a ground-glass appearance. After 7 to 10 days of therapy, some calcification results; x-ray shows a club-like swelling extending from the white line to the middle of the shaft (never into the joint). The blood is resorbed, and the bone resumes its normal shape as treatment proceeds.

In adults, scurvy remains latent for 3 to 12 mo following onset of severe vitamin C deficiency. Overt scorbutic symptoms are preceded by lassitude, weakness, irritability, weight loss, and vague myalgias and arthralgias. Multiple splinter hemorrhages may form a crescent near the distal ends of the nail and are more extensive than those in bacterial endocarditis. The gums become swollen, purple, spongy, and friable, and bleed readily in extreme deficiency. Secondary infection, gangrene, and loosening of teeth eventually occur. Gum changes occur only with natural teeth or hidden roots. Old scars break down, new wounds fail to heal, and spontaneous hemorrhages may occur in any part of the body, especially as perifollicular petechiae and ecchymoses into the skin of the lower limbs. (These changes in old age are not necessarily scorbutic.) Bone lesions, except for subperiosteal hemorrhage, do not occur.

Other symptoms and signs of scurvy include bulbar conjunctival hemorrhage, Sjögren's syndrome, femoral neuropathy from hemorrhage into femoral sheaths, oliguria, edema of the lower extremities, impaired vascular reactivity, and arthritis resembling rheumatoid arthritis. Bleeding gums are not the most characteristic feature of scurvy. The hyperkeratotic hair follicle with surrounding hyperemia or hemorrhage is almost pathognomonic.

Laboratory Findings

Usually the plasma ascorbic acid content is nearly nonexistent in manifest scurvy, but this is not always diagnostic; low levels may also be found in nonscorbutic persons. *Ascorbic acid levels in the WBC-platelet layer of centrifuged blood are more significant;* levels < 0.1 mg/100 ml are closely correlated with scurvy. When vitamin C stores are depleted, little appears in the urine following a test dose. A positive capillary fragility test is an almost constant finding, and anemia not due to blood loss is common. Bleeding, coagulation, and prothrombin times are normal.

Diagnosis

Infantile scurvy must be differentiated from rickets, poliomyelitis, osteomyelitis, rheumatic fever, and from hemorrhagic disorders (e.g., blood diseases, severe anemias, allergic purpuras). Rickets often occurs before the 5th mo, scurvy almost never before the 6th. The diseases may occur simultaneously. Hemorrhagic manifestations are absent in rickets. The costochondral junctions are enlarged in either condition, but in scurvy the swellings are angular while in rickets they tend to be rounded. Poliomyelitis is often considered because the baby does not move his legs and cries when moved; in scurvy, the absence of neurologic changes, the presence of bleeding, and bone changes permit differentiation. Joint involvement may suggest rheumatic fever, but this disease is uncommon before age 2. The bone swellings in scurvy never extend into the joint. Other diseases that cause bleeding can usually be excluded by their characteristic tests (see Ch. 95). In doubtful cases, a therapeutic trial of ascorbic acid 300 to 500 mg orally will stop the pain of infantile scurvy within 24 to 48 h and will decrease gingival swelling and bleeding within 72 h.

Adult scurvy must be differentiated from arthritis, hemorrhagic diseases, and gingivitis. Joint symptoms are due to bleeding around or into the joint. The presence of hemorrhage elsewhere, plus blood studies, aids in diagnosis.

Prophylaxis

Infants should be given unboiled orange juice daily, beginning with 1 tsp in the 2nd to 4th wk of life, with progressive increases until at 5 mo the intake is 2 to 3 oz. If tomato juice is used, 3 times as much should be given. If the infant reacts unfavorably, ascorbic acid 25 to 30 mg/day should be given up to the age of 3 mo, and 50 to 75 mg thereafter. Most nutritionists believe that huge doses of vitamin C (about 10 gm/day) do not decrease the incidence or severity of the common cold (see in Ch. 12) or influence the progress of malignant disease.

Treatment

Ascorbic acid 50 mg q.i.d. should be given orally for 1 wk in **infantile scurvy**, then 50 mg t.i.d. for 1 mo, with prophylactic doses thereafter, supplemented by orange or tomato juice. The total dose of ascorbic acid may be given as 4 to 8 oz of orange juice or 12 to 24 oz of tomato juice/day. These doses can be halved within 1 or 2 wk, and prophylactic amounts can be used after 1 mo. In vomiting or diarrhea, one half the recommended oral dose may be given IM or IV as sodium ascorbate.

For **adult scurvy**, ascorbic acid 250 mg q.i.d. orally is recommended until signs have disappeared. The usual maintenance doses can then be given. When parenteral therapy is required, sodium ascorbate can be given at the same dosage. Ascorbic acid 300 to 500 mg/day orally in divided doses should be given for several months in chronic scurvy with gingivitis, repeated hemorrhagic manifestations, or joint symptoms. Superimposed infection and calcareous deposits prevent rapid response in chronic scorbutic gingivitis.

79. ELEMENT DEFICIENCY AND TOXICITY

There are 15 trace elements presently recognized as necessary for warm-blooded animals. They occur in concentrations less than 0.005% body wt. In order of demonstrated need, they are iron, iodine, copper, manganese, zinc, cobalt, molybdenum, selenium, chromium, tin, vanadium, fluorine, silicon, nickel, and arsenic. Disturbances in metabolism of the macroelements sodium, potassium, calcium, and magnesium are considered in Ch. 81.

Except for iron and iodine, it is uncommon for element deficiencies to develop spontaneously in man, however bizarre the diet. The introduction of synthetic diets as treatment for inborn errors of metabolism, the development of IV feeding, and the advent of renal dialysis present iatrogenic risks that emphasize the nutritional importance of these elements. As methods for their assay have been developed and their physiology studied, new errors of metabolism have been discovered. With increasing pollution and development of synthetic foods, excessive intake may occur, producing signs of toxicity only after many years. Many lay periodicals and "health food" stores promote dolomite as a good source of calcium and magnesium, and it is widely used. However, recent reports indicate that dolomite may also contain potentially toxic metals, including iron, chromium, phosphorus, nickel, silicon, zinc, and cadmium.

PHOSPHATE DEPLETION

The risk of phosphate depletion has increased following chronic hemodialysis (in which patients may be dialyzed with P-free solutions while ingesting large amounts of P-binding antacids), chronic renal failure, and renal transplantation. Total parenteral nutrition regimes are often low in P, as are the diets of acute and chronic alcoholics.

As in other hypophosphatemic states (see also Chs. 78 and 81), there is osteomalacia; blood Ca is normal or raised and there is marked parathyroid hyposecretion. Renal clearance of P is markedly reduced; of Ca, greatly elevated.

Soft tissue symptoms, not seen in other conditions with low plasma P, include confusion, dysarthria, parasthesias, peripheral neuropathy; muscle weakness, true myopathy; red cell rigidity and overt hemolytic anemia, impaired O_2 release due to red cell deficiency of 2,3-diphosphoglycerate; abnormal liver function tests; profound anorexia, nausea and vomiting; and renal tubular dysfunction (see TABLE 76–1).

DISTURBANCES IN IRON METABOLISM

The total body Fe in healthy adult males is about 3.45 gm and in females about 2.45 gm. About 61% in males and 71% in females occur in Hb; 10 and 12% respectively occur in tissues as myoglobin and enzymes; and 29% in males and 16% in females occur as storage Fe in liver, spleen and bone marrow. Serum ferritin accurately reflects Fe stores (normal male 94 ng/ml, female 34 ng/ml).

The main features of Fe metabolism are described in FIG. 79–1 and its legend.

Non-heme Fe occurs in food in both organic and inorganic forms; each must be reduced to the ferrous state and released from conjugation by gastric and other secretions. The absorption of non-heme Fe in any food is affected by the composition of the meal; for example, when eggs and bread were eaten separately absorption was 1 to 2% and 30% respectively, but 5 and 5.3% respectively when eaten together. Phytate reduces absorption, as do Ca and P together; tea forms insoluble Fe tannate complexes. EDTA (ethylenediaminetetraacetic acid) is added to food to prevent oxidation by free metals. FDA regulations permit EDTA in certain foods at levels ranging from 25 to 800 mg/kg. Diets containing as much as 50 to 100 mg of EDTA have been shown to cause significant reduction of non-heme Fe absorption. Conversely, ascorbic acid maintains Fe in a reduced, more soluble form

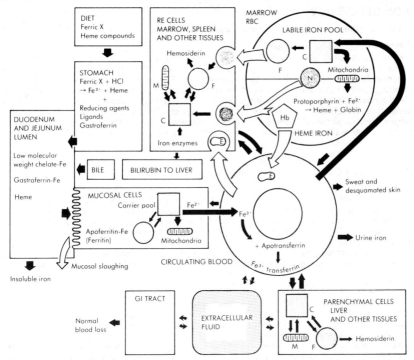

FIG. 79-1. **Iron metabolism.** Ingested heme compounds and organic chelates, when subjected to the action of hydrochloric acid (low pH) in the stomach, are broken down to form heme molecules and ferric ions. The ferric ions react with reducing agents, ligands, and gastroferrin. Only iron kept soluble, either as heme molecules or by binding to low–molecular-weight chelates or gastroferrin, can undergo absorption, which occurs chiefly in the duodenum and proximal jejunum. Luminal iron incorporated into the mucosal cell enters the carrier pool (C). Most of this iron is deposited as ferritin (F) or utilized by mitochondria (M) for enzyme synthesis and then is lost by sloughing. The remainder is absorbed by being transferred from the carrier pool to the plasma, where it is bound tightly in the ferric state to the β_1-globulin transferrin. Iron leaves the plasma primarily by entering the labile iron pool of the erythroid series, from which there is considerable feedback of iron into the plasma, mainly via reticuloendothelial (RE) cells. Within the developing erythroid cells of the bone marrow, ferrous ions combine with protoporphyrin to form the porphyrin heme, which in turn combines with globulin to form hemoglobin. Hemoglobin is released into the circulation within circulating red cells (E) that have an average life span of 117 days. At the time of their disintegration, these cells are removed from the circulation by the spleen and other reticuloendothelial tissues with excretion of the split porphyrin as bilirubin in the bile and conservation of almost all the iron, which reenters the plasma and is bound once more to transferrin. These phagocytic RE cells normally are the chief source of iron entering the plasma. About 2/3 of normal total body iron loss (1.0 mg/day) occurs as the result of the GI blood loss of 1.2 ml/day (0.6 mg Fe/day). About 18% of the iron leaving and entering the plasma does so in equilibration with extracellular fluid transferrin; the formation and breakdown of myoglobulin and the heme enzymes; iron absorption; and iron storage. Arrows are not quantitative. (From J. B. Stanbury, J. B. Wyngaarden, and D. S. Fredrickson, *The Metabolic Basis of Inherited Disease*, ed. 4, 1978. Copyright © by McGraw-Hill, Inc. Used with permission of McGraw-Hill Book Co.)

and greatly enhances non-heme Fe absorption. Dosing with 200 mg/day increases Fe absorption 2- to 3-fold. The long-term effect on Fe status of these and larger doses of ascorbic acid for prophylaxis against the common cold (see Ch. 12) deserves further study.

A smaller fraction of dietary Fe is in the form of heme. This is absorbed as an intact porphyrin complex into the mucosal cell and absorption is neither inhibited nor enhanced by the substances mentioned above. Regular consumption of meat may account for as much as 1/3 of the total Fe absorbed daily. Dual radioiron tags are available to measure Fe absorption from a complete meal. In one study in males, non-heme Fe averaged 5.3% absorption and heme Fe 37%.

Daily Fe requirements (see TABLE 76-2) are 10 mg for the adult male and 18 mg for the female. In health, average intakes have been shown to be 16 mg for the male and 11 mg for the female. Absorption in the male was 0.9 mg (6%) but 1.3 mg (12%) in the female.

IRON DEFICIENCY

Etiology, pathophysiology, symptoms and signs, diagnosis, and treatment are dealt with in Ch. 92.

Prevention

Fe is absorbed with difficulty and most people barely meet their daily requirements. Additional losses due to pregnancy (0.5 to 0.8 mg/day), lactation (0.4 mg/day), and blood loss due to disease or accident readily lead to Fe deficiency. Proposals by the FDA to increase the level of Fe fortification of food (at present 33 mg/kg) to protect these vulnerable groups have met with strong opposition on the grounds that those segments of the population not requiring additional Fe may be put at risk of developing Fe overload. The conflict is unresolved. It is clear that an available Fe salt will have the same absorption as the non-heme Fe of the diet, regardless of the vehicle. However, some presently employed salts are less well absorbed. Ferrous sulfate and reduced Fe of small particle size are the best.

IRON OVERLOAD (Hemosiderosis; Hemochromatosis)

For acute iron poisoning, see TABLE 258-4. Iron overload is characterized by greater than normal focal or generalized deposition of iron within body tissues **(hemosiderosis).** When such deposition is associated with tissue injury, with total body Fe > 15 gm, it is known as **hemochromatosis.** TABLE 79-1 presents a classification of these conditions. The differential diagnosis is difficult but depends on the history of Fe administration, examination of relatives, degree of Fe overload, and presence or absence of localizing signs.

Primary hemochromatosis is an uncommon, slowly progressive entity in which the cause of the increased iron absorption is not known, but a high familial incidence of iron overload may be demonstrated.

Symptoms, Signs, and Diagnosis

Hemochromatosis is rare before middle age. The typical manifestations are cirrhosis of the liver, a peculiar bronze pigmentation of the skin, diabetes mellitus (overt in 50 to 60% of patients), and cardiomyopathy, manifested by cardiomegaly, congestive failure, and arrhythmias or conduction disturbances. Pituitary failure is not uncommon and may be the cause of the frequently observed testicular atrophy and loss of libido. Abdominal pain, arthritis, and chondrocalcinosis occur less often. Presumably, all of these changes are due to parenchymal iron deposition, although an increased familial incidence of diabetes mellitus suggests that factors other than pancreatic siderosis may play a role. Hepatomas occur with increased frequency in patients with longstanding hemochromatosis.

The plasma iron is > 200 μg/100 ml and the transferrin saturation is > 70%. Urinary iron excretion is markedly increased (> 2 mg/24 h) by the chelating agent deferoxamine 500 to 1000 mg IM. Demonstration of hepatic siderosis and cirrhosis by liver biopsy confirms the diagnosis. Family members should be screened for evidence of iron overload.

TABLE 79-1. CLASSIFICATION OF HEMOSIDEROSIS AND HEMOCHROMATOSIS

Primary (idiopathic) hemochromatosis. Genetically determined error with increased absorption of Fe from a normal diet, including atransferrinemia, thalassemia major and Y-linked hypochromic anemia

Secondary hemosiderosis or hemochromatosis

1. Increased parenteral Fe intake; repeated transfusions, Fe dextran IM.
2. Increased Fe absorption
   a. Increased Fe ingestion
      (1) African Bantu (alcoholic beverages) or Ethiopian (tef cereal) hemosiderosis with hemochromatosis
      (2) Alcoholic cirrhosis with hemosiderosis or hemochromatosis
      (3) Oral Fe therapy with hemosiderosis or hemochromatosis
      (4) Kaschin-Beck disease with hemosiderosis
   b. Increased Fe absorption from a normal amount of dietary Fe; anemia with erythroid hyperplasia

Focal hemosiderosis

1. Idiopathic pulmonary hemosiderosis
2. Renal hemosiderosis
3. Porphyria cutanea tarda with hepatic hemosiderosis

Treatment

Phlebotomy removes excess iron from the body and improves survival, though without altering the incidence of hepatoma. Phlebotomy should be instituted prior to the development of advanced liver disease. About 500 ml of blood (about 250 mg iron) is removed weekly until plasma iron levels are normal, then every 3 to 4 mo as necessary to maintain plasma iron below 150 micrograms /100 ml. Repeat liver biopsy may be a more reliable way of monitoring tissue iron deposits. Anemia occasionally develops during venesection treatment. In such cases, deferoxamine 500 to 1000 mg/day IM may permit further reduction of iron stores without producing anemia. Diabetes mellitus, cardiac abnormalities, and other secondary manifestations are treated as indicated.

Focal hemosiderosis chiefly occurs in the lungs and kidneys. Pulmonary hemosiderosis due to recurrent pulmonary hemorrhage occurs as an idiopathic entity, as part of Goodpasture's syndrome, and in mitral stenosis. Occasionally the iron loss into the lungs is severe enough to cause iron-deficiency anemia. Renal hemosiderosis results from extensive intravascular hemolysis due to trauma (e.g., fragmentation of RBCs in association with prosthetic aortic valves) or in paroxysmal nocturnal hemoglobinuria. Free Hb is filtered at the glomerulus, and renal iron deposition occurs with saturation of haptoglobin. No damage to the renal parenchyma occurs, but unusually heavy hemosiderinuria may cause iron deficiency.

Treatment is predominantly supportive. In acute episodes, blood transfusion may be required, but otherwise anemia responds to oral Fe. Results with splenectomy and with ACTH or cortisone have been variable.

IODINE

Nearly 80% of the total iodine present in the body is found in the thyroid, almost all as **thyroglobulin,** the storage form of thyroid hormone. Marine foods are rich dietary sources. Drinking water, which supplies a relatively small proportion of the intake, reflects the soil content of locally grown foods.

Iodine deficiency results in colloid or endemic goiter (see Euthyroid Goiter in Ch. 86), and should be corrected with iodized salt, not with Lugol's solution (see Table 76–1).

Chronic toxicity results when daily requirements are exceeded about 20-fold ($>$ 2000 μg). Increased uptake of I by the thyroid leads to inhibition of organic I formation **(Wolff-Chaikoff effect),** and eventually iodide-goiter or myxedema especially in patients with pre-existing Hashimoto's thyroiditis.

FLUORINE

Bones and teeth contain most of the body's fluorine. Sea fish and tea are rich sources, but intake is mainly from drinking water. Fluoridation of water that contains less than the ideal level of 1 ppm significantly reduces the incidence of dental caries in the community.

Excess accumulation of fluorine **(fluorosis)** occurs in teeth and bone in proportion to the level and duration of intake. Communities where the level in drinking water exceeds 10 ppm are commonly affected. Fluorosis is most evident in permanent teeth that develop during high fluorine intake. Deciduous teeth are affected only at very high levels of intake. The earliest changes, chalky-white, irregularly distributed patches on the surface of the enamel, become infiltrated by yellow or brown staining, giving rise to the characteristic "mottled" appearance. Severe fluorosis weakens the enamel, resulting in surface pitting. Bony changes, characterized by osteosclerosis and exostoses of the spine and genu valgum, usually are seen only after prolonged high intake in adults.

ZINC

The body contains 1 to 2.5 gm of zinc, found mainly in bones, teeth, hair (which can be used to assess zinc status), skin, liver, muscle, and testes. In the plasma, $1/3$ is attached loosely to albumin, and about $2/3$ is firmly bound to globulins. Plasma levels relate closely to dietary intake, but various diseases may cause low levels. Zinc is also present in RBCs, mainly as carbonic anhydrase, and in WBCs and platelets. For estimated dietary requirements, see Table 76–2.

Chelation of dietary zinc by high fiber and phytate content of whole-meal bread, geophagia, and parasitism may be factors leading to reduced absorption and deficiency problems. In several studies in the USA and elsewhere a small proportion of children over age 4 yr had low zinc status, associated with poor appetite, poor growth, and impaired taste (hypogeusia). With zinc treatment, appetite improved, taste became normal, and catch-up growth occurred. High milk consumption, poor in zinc, may have been responsible. A syndrome of dwarfism and hypogonadism with low zinc status, seen in the Middle East, has been shown to respond to zinc supplementation.

Acrodermatitis enteropathica, an inherited, previously fatal disorder has been shown to result from malabsorption of zinc. It is characterized by psoriasiform dermatitis, hair loss, paronychia, growth retardation, and diarrhea. Zinc sulfate 30 to 150 mg/day results in complete remission.

DISTURBANCES IN COPPER METABOLISM

The normal adult body contains about l00 to l50 mg of copper, 90% of which is found in muscle, bone, and liver. In the blood, more than 90% is found in the plasma associated with **ceruloplasmin** (an α_2-globulin that transports copper), with the remainder bound to albumin and in the RBCs. The plasma copper concentration is elevated during pregnancy and estrogen therapy because the rise in plasma protein levels includes ceruloplasmin.

The copper content of an ordinary diet is about 2 to 5 mg/day. Absorption occurs mainly in the proximal small intestine and is regulated by bodily needs and affected by dietary form. Some copper may be complexed and rendered unavailable. Albumin-bound copper is transported to the liver, bone marrow, and other sites. It is readily dissociable, making free copper available for excretion in the urine. The major route of excretion, however, is by way of the bile. Copper is removed from the blood by hepatic uptake, partially excreted in the bile (35 to 205 μg/100 ml), and partially returned to the blood associated with ceruloplasmin, which is synthesized in the liver.

Copper is a component of mitochondrial (e.g., cytochrome oxidase), cytoplasmic (e.g., tyrosinase), and nuclear enzyme systems. Copper-deficient animals exhibit diminished activity of such cuproenzymes.

COPPER DEFICIENCY

Copper deficiency is a rare cause of anemia in adults, although hypocupremia is found in states characterized by depressed serum protein levels, such as kwashiorkor, sprue, and nephrotic syndrome. The significance of this hypocupremia is not known. In "dysproteinemia" of infancy, hypocupremia is associated with some features similar to copper deficiency in animals (e.g., anemia associated with depressed serum iron) (see Ch. 92).

Menke's kinky hair syndrome is a sex-linked abnormality caused by a defect in intestinal copper absorption. Affected infants have low levels of copper and ceruloplasmin that lead to progressive cerebral degeneration, retarded growth, abnormally sparse and brittle hair, arterial lesions, and scurvy-like bone changes. Copper given IV early in infancy (200 μg/kg/day) has alleviated this condition.

COPPER EXCESS

Copper excess may result from hereditary disorders of copper metabolism (see WILSON'S DISEASE, below), excessive intake of copper, or exposure to hemodialysis solutions contaminated with copper. Manifestations of acute copper intoxication include nausea, vomiting, abdominal pain, diarrhea, and diffuse myalgias. In some instances, abnormal mental states progressing to coma and death are associated with profound metabolic acidosis and necrotizing pancreatitis. However, the most consistent feature is severe hemolytic anemia, associated with increased Heinz bodies, abnormal autohemolysis, Hb thermolability, and depressed levels of RBC G6PD and glutathione reductase. Direct damage to the RBC membrane may contribute to the hemolysis, the severity of which correlates better with the erythrocyte (whole blood) level than with the serum copper level.

WILSON'S DISEASE (Hepatolenticular Degeneration)

This uncommon familial disease is inherited as an autosomal recessive trait and occurs most often in children of consanguineous marriages.

Etiology and Pathogenesis

The disease is manifested in individuals homozygous for the abnormal gene. The observed alterations result from progressive accumulation of copper within the body tissues, particularly the erythrocytes, kidney, liver, and brain. Copper absorption appears to be accelerated, and although the urinary excretion of free copper is usually increased, affected individuals are in positive copper balance from birth. Defective synthesis of ceruloplasmin is an associated defect in both homozygous affected patients and heterozygous carriers, but the significance of the depressed ceruloplasmin concentration is uncertain.

Symptoms, Signs, and Diagnosis

Asymptomatic hepatic copper accumulation occurs early in the disease. After about 5 yr, hepatic copper binding sites are saturated, copper is released from the liver, and rapid uptake of copper into erythrocytes may produce acute hemolytic anemia that may be severe and recurrent. Hepatic insufficiency may subsequently develop. In 30 to 50% of patients, hepatocellular necrosis develops during the stage of hepatic copper release, producing cirrhosis with ascites, edema, and progressive hepatic failure. Alternatively, the hepatic manifestations may resolve. The serum copper may be depressed, normal, or increased; ceruloplasmin levels usually are decreased but may be increased or normal. Hypercupriuria frequently is present. The **Kayser-Fleischer ring** (a golden-brown or gray-green pigment ring at the corneal limbus due to copper deposition in Descemet's membrane) is present in about 50% of patients at this stage. Radiating brownish spokes of copper carbonate on the anterior or posterior lens capsule less commonly form the characteristic **sunflower cataract**. If the patient survives these early stages, he again becomes asymptomatic. Positive copper balance continues, but subsequent copper deposition is extrahepatic.

When cerebral copper accumulation is sufficient to destroy the nerve cells (especially in the putamen and caudate nuclei, the dentate nuclei, and cerebral cortex), the neurologic syndrome begins. The most common features include tremor of one or both upper extremities (volitional at first, and later at rest as well), choreoathetoid movements, rigidity of skeletal muscles (occasionally resulting in permanent contractures), dysarthria, and personality changes progressing to dementia. In this stage, the triad of cirrhosis, basal ganglia disease, and Kayser-Fleischer rings are found. The serum copper and ceruloplasmin levels are abnormally low in association with hypercupriuria.

Many patients also exhibit renal dysfunction due to intrarenal copper deposition. While GFR may be reduced, the most common abnormalities are tubular. Proximal tubular dysfunction results in Fanconi's syndrome with generalized aminoaciduria, glycosuria, hyperuricosuria, and phosphaturia. Distal renal tubular acidosis may produce medullary nephrocalcinosis, and a urinary concentrating defect may be present. Osteomalacia may result from phosphate wasting.

The **diagnosis** of Wilson's disease is obvious in the fully developed disease but should be considered in patients with otherwise unexplained manifestations such as those described above. The sequence of pathologic change is not necessarily reflected in the appearance of clinical manifestations and often neurologic disease is the first symptom. A decreased ceruloplasmin level with hypocupremia and with compatible clinical changes, confirms the diagnosis. Since heterozygotes, normal newborn infants, and some patients with hypoproteinemia may exhibit hypocupremia and hypoceruloplasminemia, liver biopsy occasionally is necessary to establish the diagnosis by demonstration of elevated hepatic copper content ($> 100 \mu g/gm$ wet tissue). Asymptomatic siblings of patients should have periodic determinations of serum copper and ceruloplasmin. If hypocupremia or hypoceruloplasminemia is found without other manifestations, such as hemolytic anemia, liver biopsy should be performed.

Treatment

The untreated disease is invariably fatal, with death usually resulting from hepatic failure or infection. Prevention of further copper accumulation is achieved by avoiding foods high in copper (organ meats, shellfish, nuts, dried legumes, chocolate, whole-grain cereals, etc.). With the added use of the oral copper binder penicillamine, a negative copper balance may be achieved in treating asymptomatic patients, either in the early hepatic accumulation stage or after reduction of tissue copper stores.

D-Penicillamine 250 mg once/day orally is given initially, with increments every 1 or 2 wk up to a maintenance dose of 2 to 4 gm/day given in divided doses on an empty stomach. With clinical improvement (usually after several months) or with reduction of free plasma copper to normal levels, the dose is reduced to 1.5 gm/day. Pyridoxine 25 to 50 mg/day is given to prevent pyridoxine deficiency; serum iron concentrations should be monitored, since iron may also be chelated. Acute toxic reactions to penicillamine (e.g., fever, rash, leukopenia, or thrombocytopenia) occur in about 1/3 of patients, but often it is possible to discontinue the drug temporarily and restart therapy with concomitant administration of corticosteroids. Platelet and WBC counts should be obtained every 1 to 2 wk for several weeks, with monthly counts thereafter. Occasionally, the start of treatment exacerbates neurologic symptoms, but these usually subside with temporary cessation of the drug. Chronic administration rarely is associated with toxic side effects other than easily preventable or correctable vitamin B_6 and iron deficiency. Proteinuria usually does not occur during penicillamine treatment. However, frequent urinalyses should be obtained during therapy, as penicillamine may rarely precipitate Goodpasture's syndrome. Although not accepted universally, prevailing opinion is that lifelong penicillamine therapy is indicated in conjunction with a low-copper diet.

Indian childhood cirrhosis is a rapidly progressive disorder and an important cause of death in the Asian subcontinent. A recent study there demonstrated prolific orcein-staining material in hepatocytes, suggesting accumulation of copper-binding protein as in Wilson's disease. Similar deposits have been reported in liver and renal tubules in an infant of Asian immigrants to Britain.

OTHER TRACE ELEMENTS

Cobalt

The significance of cobalt in health and nutrition is confined, as far as is known, to its presence in the cobalamin (vitamin B_{12}) molecule. Dietary deficiency in man has not been proved.

Cobaltous chloride in large doses (20 to 30 mg/day) has been advocated in addition to iron in the treatment of iron-deficiency in chronic renal failure, but should be used only if cobalt deficiency is suspected, as it is potentially toxic. Overdosing in infants may cause hypothyroidism and congestive heart failure.

Chromium

Chromium is now recognized as an essential trace element. In addition to being part of several enzyme systems, it is associated with a low-molecular weight organic complex termed **glucose tolerance factor (GTF)** that acts with insulin in promoting normal glucose utilization. Brewer's yeast, which is rich in GTF, has been shown to improve glucose tolerance, lower serum cholesterol and triglycerides in some elderly subjects, and to reduce insulin requirements in some diabetics. Glucose tolerance is usually impaired in protein-calorie malnutrition, especially in kwashiorkor, and some cases have shown a dramatic response to trivalent chromium. Deficiency has been reported in patients on prolonged parenteral feeding.

Selenium

Selenium is involved in the reoxidation of reduced glutathione and has close metabolic interrelationships with vitamin E. It is part of the enzyme glutathione peroxidase, which is thought to destroy peroxides derived from unsaturated fatty acids. Deficiency has occurred in patients on long-term parenteral feeding. In China a childhood cardiomyopathy has been attributed to selenium deficiency and protection claimed for prophyactic dosing with 1 mg/wk of sodium selenite.

Manganese

Manganese is a component of several enzyme systems and is essential for normal bone structure. Intake varies greatly, depending mainly upon the consumption of rich sources such as unrefined cereals, green leafy vegetables, and tea. Human deficiency has not been reported. Manganese poisoning is usually limited to those who mine and refine ore; prolonged exposure causes neurologic symptoms resembling parkinsonism or Wilson's disease.

80. OBESITY

Obesity is characterized by excessive accumulation of body fat. A body weight 20% over that given in standard height/weight tables is arbitrarily considered obesity. Except for heavily muscled persons, this presumption is usually correct.

Obesity is not a condition for which a precise definition is particularly useful. Unlike many "real" diseases (and like hypertension), obesity represents one arm of a distribution curve of body fat or body weight, with no sharp cut-off point. Its importance lies in the many, often serious, complications to which obese people are subject. It is these complications that warrant undertaking a treatment that is so often unsuccessful.

Etiology

The cause of obesity is simple—consuming more calories than are expended as energy. However, we usually do not know why persons consume more calories than they expend. At least 7 factors may contribute to obesity.

Social factors may be the most important known determinants of obesity and they have made endocrine and psychologic influences appear less important, as causes of obesity, than had been thought. For example, obesity is 6 times more prevalent among lower-class women than among upper-class women. This relationship between social class and obesity is more than correlational; it is also causal. The social class of one's parents is almost as closely linked to obesity as is one's own social class. Although obesity can, and does, influence one's own social class (lowering it), it cannot have influenced the social class of one's parents, suggesting that the social class into which a person is born is a powerful determinant of obesity. This conclusion is strengthened by the finding that obesity is far more common among lower-class children than upper-class children; significant differences are already apparent by age 6. Other social factors, particularly ethnic and religious, are also closely linked to obesity. How these factors lead to obesity, or its control, has not been established, but differences in life style, and particularly dietary and exercise patterns, probably play a major role.

Endocrine factors: A number of metabolic abnormalities have been studied relative to obesity, but they are usually the consequences rather than causes. An exception is adipose tissue proliferation in hyperadrenocorticism, where increased production of adrenal corticosteroids leads to increased gluconeogenesis and a correspondingly greater demand for insulin. The pancreatic β cells respond and the resulting overproduction of insulin stimulates lipogenesis. Even in this special condition more calories are consumed during the period of weight gain than are expended as energy.

Psychologic factors: Many obese persons report that they overeat when emotionally upset, but it has proved difficult to achieve a precise understanding of the factors linking emotions and obesity. Many nonobese persons also overeat when emotionally upset, and there have been no controlled studies demonstrating the influence of psychologic factors on obesity. Two deviant eating patterns apparently based on stress and emotional disturbance, however, may contribute to the obesity of a few persons. **Bulimia** is *the sudden, compulsive ingestion of very large amounts of food in a very short time, usually followed by agitation, self-condemnation, and often by self-induced vomiting.* The **night-eating syndrome** *consists of morning anorexia, evening hyperphagia, and insomnia.* Attempts at weight reduction in these 2 conditions are usually unsuccessful and may cause the patient unnecessary distress.

Genetic factors: It is widely recognized that obesity runs in families: 80% of the offspring of 2 obese parents are obese, compared with 40% of the children of 1 obese parent and only 10% of the offspring of 2 nonobese parents. This finding, plus the existence of several forms of experimental obesity of clearly genetic origin have led some to conclude that genetics plays a major role in human obesity. But children acquire their eating habits as well as their genes from their parents, and there are forms of experimental obesity of clearly environmental origin. The fact is that the relative contribution of genetic and environmental factors and their interactions have not been determined.

Developmental factors: The increased adipose tissue mass in obesity can result from either an increase in size of fat cells **(hypertrophic obesity),** from an increase in the number of fat cells **(hyperplastic obesity),** or from an increase in both **(hypertrophic-hyperplastic obesity).** Most persons whose obesity began in adult life suffer from hypertrophic obesity. They lose weight solely by a decrease in the size of their fat cells; the number of fat cells does not change.

Persons whose obesity began in childhood are more likely to suffer from hyperplastic obesity, usually of the combined hypertrophic-hyperplastic type. They may have up to 5 times as many fat cells as either persons of normal weight or those suffering from pure hypertrophic obesity. As a result, they may be able to reach a normal body weight only by marked depletion of the lipid content of each fat cell. Such depletion, and particularly the associated events at the cell membrane, may set a biologic limit to weight reduction among persons with hyperplastic obesity and may help to explain their difficulty in reducing to normal weight as well as their proclivity to regain weight. The early years of life are particularly important in the genesis of hyperplastic obesity. Thus, there are compelling anatomic as well as psychologic reasons for the prevention of childhood obesity.

Another developmental factor, not related to fat cell number, is the tendency to accumulate body fat with age. The prevalence of obesity more than doubles between 20 and 50 (animals also become fatter with age). This is usually ascribed to the persistence of high-caloric intake despite reduced caloric expenditure.

Physical activity: Decreased physical activity in affluent societies is often cited as a major factor in the rise of obesity; e.g., the prevalence of obesity in the USA has more than doubled since the turn of the century, despite a 10% decrease in daily caloric intake.

Caloric requirements are lower among persons with a sedentary life style, but animal experiments suggest that physical inactivity contributes to obesity also by a paradoxic effect on food intake. Although food intake increases with increasing energy expenditure, food intake may not decrease proportionately when such activity falls below a minimum level; restricting physical activity may actually increase food intake in some people.

Brain damage: Brain damage, particularly to the hypothalamus, can lead to obesity, although it is a very rare cause in humans and is the subject of only isolated case reports. Its major significance is as a reminder that whatever the social and metabolic determinants of obesity, the final common pathway to caloric balance lies through behavior mediated by the CNS.

Physical Signs

The signs of obesity are an increase in body weight and the evident mass of fatty tissue. Pressure on the thorax from the encompassing sheath of fatty tissue combined with pressure on the diaphragm from below by large intra-abdominal accumulations of fat may occasionally be life-threatening. The resulting reduced respiratory capacity may produce dyspnea on even minimal exertion. In the massively obese this condition may progress to the **pickwickian syndrome,** characterized by hypoventilation, retention of CO_2 leading to decreased effects of CO_2 as a respiratory stimulant and resultant hypoxia and somnolence. Progesterone and its derivatives have been used to increase ventilation with some success.

Obesity may lead to a variety of orthopedic disturbances, including low back pain, aggravation of osteoarthritis, particularly of the knees and ankles, and often huge calluses on the feet and heels. Even mild degrees of obesity may be associated with amenorrhea and other menstrual disturbances. BP is frequently elevated in the obese and hypertension is commoner among them than among the nonobese. However, masses of subcutaneous tissue between the BP cuff and the brachial artery can cause false elevated readings when a standard size cuff is used. The remedy is to use a wide cuff long enough to completely encircle the arm with the bladder containing air. Skin disorders are particularly common among the obese. Their lower ratio of body surface to body mass results in impaired heat loss and an increase in sweating, particularly after meals. This sweat becomes trapped with skin secretions in the thick folds of skin to produce a culture medium that is particularly conducive to bacterial growth. Pathogenic bacteria can produce infections that are resistant to treatment. Every motion produces friction between the skin folds that further macerates the skin and adds to the pain and discomfort. Mild to moderate edema of the feet and ankles is common. All of these complications can easily be controlled by weight reduction.

Diagnosis

Obesity is apparent on observation and can be quantified by weight and height measurements. Attention should be paid to special distributions of fat; e.g., a truncal distribution with a buffalo hump is suggestive of hyperadrenocorticism, although generalized obesity is also seen in this disease. The peculiar accumulation of fluid of the hypothyroid patient should be kept in mind, since mild obesity can be confused with hypothyroidism.

Complications

Obesity adversely affects morbidity and mortality, primarily through cardiovascular complications. The death rate from many diseases, from accidents, and from surgery, is significantly higher among the obese, increasing with the magnitude of the obesity. Sudden death is also more common. Although recent reports suggest that the dangers of mild obesity may have been overstated, there is no question of the ill effects of degrees of overweight in excess of 35% or of any degree of overweight among diabetics and hypertensives.

A common problem in obesity is impaired glucose tolerance and fasting hyperglycemia, even in persons without a family history of diabetes. Obesity imposes marked resistance to the action of insulin, increasing insulin requirements and resulting in hyperinsulinism. Histologic examination of the pancreatic islets shows an increased number of enlarged islets. Blood immunoreactive insulin assays demonstrate not only increased fasting levels of insulin, proportional to the degree of obesity, but also excessive responses to glucose or amino acid challenges. This hyperinsulinism responds well to weight reduction, disappearing completely unless diabetes is present.

Three of the most potent risk factors for coronary artery disease—hypertension, adult-onset diabetes, and hyperlipidemia—are far more prevalent among the obese than among slim subjects. Furthermore, these conditions are markedly improved by weight reduction, suggesting that obesity may play a role in their genesis. Weight reduction may allow 75% of adult-onset diabetics to discontinue medication, and the BP of most hypertensives will be reduced.

While carefully controlled studies show little difference in overall psychopathology between obese and nonobese persons when taken as a group, for a small number of obese persons psychopathology may be closely linked to their obesity. Obese young women of upper and middle socioeconomic classes are particularly vulnerable. They may manifest disordered eating patterns and are at high risk for another troublesome syndrome— disparagement of the body image. Characteristically, they feel that their bodies are grotesque and loathsome and that others view them with hostility and contempt. This results in self-consciousness and impaired social functioning. Such disturbances are relatively uncommon, and occur almost exclusively in persons who have been obese since childhood.

Attempts to lose weight may cause complications; symptoms of anxiety and depression may appear in as many as half of patients undergoing medical treatment for obesity.

Prognosis and Treatment

The prognosis for obesity is poor, particularly for obese children, and the course tends to progress throughout life. The odds against an obese child becoming a normal-weight adult are about 4:1. For those who have not reduced by the end of adolescence, the odds may reach 28:1. Obesity is a chronic condition resistant to treatment and prone to relapse. Most obese persons will not participate in outpatient treatment, and those who do will not lose a significant amount of weight. Most of those who do lose weight will regain it. These results are poor, not because of failure to implement any therapy of known effectiveness, but because no simple or generally effective therapy exists. The numerous people who try to reduce without medical assistance, on diets and advice from magazines, may have more success.

The basis of weight reduction in all treatment regimens is to establish a caloric deficit by reducing intake below output.

Diet: The simplest way to reduce caloric intake is with a low-calorie diet. Optimal long-term effects are achieved with a balanced diet containing readily available foods. For most people, the best reducing diet consists of their usual foods in amounts limited with the aid of standard tables of food values. Such a diet gives the best chance of long-term maintenance of the weight loss, although it is the most difficult diet to follow during weight reduction. Consequently, many people turn to novel or even bizarre diets, of which there are many. The effectiveness of these diets, if any, results, in large part, from monotony—nearly everyone will tire of almost any food if that is all they get to eat. Consequently, when they stop the diet and return to their usual fare, the incentives to overeat are increased.

Fasting has had considerable vogue as a treatment for obesity, but it is now rarely used. Most patients promptly regain most of the weight they lose. Since fasting is not without complications, it should be carried out in a hospital. The expense required for such limited benefits warrants the use of fasting in exceptional circumstances only.

An outgrowth of therapeutic fasting is the so-called "protein-sparing modified fasting," designed to maintain nitrogen balance with amounts of protein small enough to have only a negligible effect upon weight loss. One such diet, for example, contains no more than 320 kcal/day (45 gm of egg albumin and 30 gm of glucose), whereas another recommends only slightly larger amounts: 1.4 gm of protein/kg of lean body mass. Vitamin and mineral supplements are necessary. These diets appear to be safe and can be carried out on an outpatient basis. The major problem with these diets, like that of all conservative treatments for obesity, is failure to maintain weight loss.

An important distinction must be made between the carefully studied "protein-sparing modified fast" and the commercially exploited "liquid protein diets." These "liquid proteins" are of low bio-

logic quality and their use has resulted in a number of deaths. They have no place in the treatment of obesity.

Medications: Drug treatment of obesity has been profoundly altered by progressively restrictive governmental regulation of the use of amphetamines as appetite suppressants. Various agents are taking the place of the amphetamines: diethylpropion, fenfluramine, and mazindol. Their efficacy and side effects seem comparable and their potential for abuse limited. However, to an even greater degree than after other conservative treatment, weight is regained after drug treatment and the use of appetite suppressants is currently out of favor.

The eating binges of a significant percentage of obese and nonobese bulimic patients have been markedly decreased during short-term trials of phenytoin in oral doses of 300 mg/day. Thyroid or thyroid analogs are indicated only for the occasional obese person with hypothyroidism. Bulk producers may help control the constipation that follows decreased food intake, but their effectiveness in weight reduction is doubtful. Chorionic gonadotropin has been found ineffective for weight reduction.

Physical activity is frequently recommended in weight-reduction regimens and its usefulness has probably been underestimated even by its proponents. Since caloric expenditure in most forms of physical activity is directly proportional to body weight, with the same amount of activity obese persons expend more calories than do those of normal weight.

Surgery: Radical surgical treatment may offer some hope to persons with morbid obesity (100% overweight) *in whom all other treatments have failed.* These treatments produce extensive weight loss in most patients—from 80 to 150 lb—and far better maintenance of this loss than is achieved by conservative treatments. Complications of obesity such as impaired glucose tolerance, hypertension, and hyperlipidemia are usually greatly mitigated. Food intake is significantly reduced and many patients report less anxiety and depression than during weight reduction by other means, normalization of their eating patterns, and improved psychosocial functioning.

Against these benefits must be placed the dangers and complications of surgery. Problems are particularly common and severe following **jejunoileal bypass surgery,** which is designed to reduce the absorbtive surface of the intestine by bypassing all but 18 in. of it. Jejunoileal bypass is regularly associated with severe and often longlasting diarrhea, electrolyte disturbances, liver failure, calcium deposits in the renal parenchyma, urinary calculi, and polyarthritis. Mortality rates as high as 10% have been reported in institutions with little experience with the procedure. The severity of these problems and the appearance of new problems for years after surgery persuaded the 1978 Consensus Conference of the National Institutes of Health that continuation of jejunoileal bypass surgery is probably not warranted.

The Conference was undoubtedly influenced toward this negative view of jejunoileal bypass by early reports on **gastric bypass** and **gastric stapling** indicating that these procedures are followed by far fewer complications. Gastric bypass is a modified Billroth-II operation designed to produce a 60-ml pouch that markedly restricts the amount of food that can be consumed at one time. Gastric stapling is designed to produce the same effect by means of a row of staples across most of the gastric fundus. Studies now under way should soon determine the indications, benefits, and costs of these procedures.

Jaw wiring has achieved something of a vogue in recent years as a means of producing rapid weight loss, but it, too, is followed by rapid regaining of weight once the wires that hold the jaws together are removed. The procedure may have limited usefulness in preparing morbidly obese persons for surgical procedures, but otherwise has no place in the treatment of obesity.

Behavior modification is a promising new treatment with better results than traditional outpatient treatment for mild to moderate obesity. Based upon principles of learning combined with pragmatic measures, behavior modification is notable for its efforts to design a comprehensive weight control program. This program includes measures for controlling the purchase, storage, preparation, serving, and consumption of food; for increasing physical activity; for modifying maladaptive attitudes; and for rewarding appropriate behaviors. The procedures can be clearly specified and readily taught. As a result, they are being increasingly utilized by non-physicians, such as nurses and dietitians in the doctor's office, and by the burgeoning self-help movement.

Behavior modification has substantially reduced the high rate of dropouts from treatment and the incidence of emotional complications of dieting. Weight losses, however, tend to be modest and are maintained only somewhat better than those achieved by other conservative measures.

Self-help organization: The largest self-help organizations are the non-profit TOPS (Take Off Pounds Sensibly) and the commercial Weight Watchers®, which together treat nearly a million people a week, half of whom receive some form of behavior modification. Costs for attending meetings are small and many people find the group support and the frequent weighings helpful. There is merit in this provision of readily accessible assistance, which makes few demands upon the participants and permits them to leave and rejoin without penalties. However, dropout rates are very high and little is known about the weight losses of representative samples of participants.

81.　DISTURBANCES IN WATER, ELECTROLYTE, MINERAL, AND ACID-BASE METABOLISM

In health, the composition and volume of body fluids remain remarkably constant despite wide ranges of dietary intake and metabolic activity. The mechanisms responsible for maintaining this homeostasis are closely interrelated. Thus many disorders of water, electrolyte, and acid-base metabolism are mixed disturbances. This discussion summarizes aspects of the pathophysiology, recognition, and management of commonly encountered fluid and electrolyte abnormalities.

This topic as it relates to infants and children is discussed separately in Vol. II, Chs. 21 and 22.

REGULATION OF WATER AND SODIUM HOMEOSTASIS

Water

The total body water (TBW) content of adult men varies from 55% of body wt in the obese to 65% in thin individuals. Values for adult women average about 10% less. About $2/3$ of TBW is intracellular and $1/3$ extracellular. The plasma volume comprises about $1/4$ of the total extracellular fluid (ECF). TBW content is normally regulated by a combination of factors, including the thirst mechanism, elaboration of antidiuretic hormone (ADH) by the posterior pituitary gland, and the kidneys. The major physiologic controls for thirst and ADH secretion are the osmolality and volume of TBW. Normally, body fluid osmolality is maintained within narrow limits, a 2% increase (or decrease) leading to release (or complete suppression) of ADH. However, when the volume of body fluid is sufficiently reduced, ADH release may lead to water conservation at the expense of tonicity. Pain, stress, and drugs such as narcotics and barbiturates may also cause ADH secretion.

In addition to ingested water, another 200 to 300 ml/day is formed in the body by tissue catabolism. Water losses via the kidney can be reduced to as little as 300 to 500 ml/day in the absence of renal disease or other factors affecting the renal concentrating mechanism. Insensible water losses, via expired air and the skin (without sweating), constitute about 0.4 to 0.5 ml/h/kg body wt or about 650 to 850 ml/24 h in a 70-kg man. In the presence of fever, an additional 50 to 75 ml/day may be lost for each degree of temperature elevation above normal. Losses via sweat vary from negligible to large amounts. GI water losses are negligible in health but can be significant in diarrhea or vomiting.

Since cell membranes in general are freely permeable to water, the osmolality of the ECF (290 mOsm/kg water) is about equal to that of the intracellular fluid (ICF). Therefore, the plasma osmolality is a convenient and accurate guide to intracellular osmolality. One may approximate body fluid osmolality by using the formula

Plasma osmolality (mOsm/kg) =

$$2 \, ([Na] + [K]) \, \text{plasma} + \frac{[BUN]}{2.8} + \frac{[Glucose]}{18}$$

where sodium (Na) and potassium (K) are given as mEq/L and blood urea nitrogen (BUN) and glucose concentrations are in mg/100 ml.

Plasma hypertonicity (hypernatremia) indicates cellular dehydration, and plasma hypotonicity (hyponatremia) indicates cellular swelling. This relationship may not hold with significant azotemia, hyperglycemia, or hyperlipidemia. Urea penetrates readily into cells; since the intracellular urea concentration equals the extracellular urea concentration, no significant change in cell volume occurs. Thus, in azotemia, although the plasma osmolality is increased, the "effective" plasma osmolality is not changed and approximately equals twice the plasma sodium concentration. In marked hyperglycemia, ECF osmolality rises and exceeds ICF osmolality (since glucose penetrates cell membranes slowly), prompting a shift of water from ICF to ECF. Thus, the plasma Na concentration falls in proportion to the dilution of the ECF. Finally, apparent hyponatremia with normal plasma osmolality may occur in hyperlipidemia and extreme hyperglobulinemia, since the lipid or protein forms a significant part of the plasma taken for analysis, but the Na concentration/L of plasma water is normal.

Sodium

The total body Na content is regulated by a balance between dietary intake and renal Na excretion. Because renal Na excretion can be adjusted to wide ranges of Na intake, significant Na depletion does not occur unless renal Na conservation is abnormal (e.g., from primary renal disease or adrenal insufficiency) or when extrarenal losses (e.g., GI losses) are combined with inadequate intake. Similarly, Na overload implies defective renal Na excretion.

Renal Na excretion is controlled by a number of variables, which include (1) glomerular filtration rate (GFR) and the filtered load of Na, (2) the rate of adrenal glucocorticoid and mineralocorticoid (primarily aldosterone) secretion, and (3) a complex of hemodynamic and possibly humoral adjustments. The latter (known as "third factor") diminishes proximal tubular Na reabsorption in response to ECF volume expansion. The role of "third factor" in disorders characterized by Na retention and edema formation remains uncertain.

The ECF volume is regulated by the total body Na content. Thus disorders of Na balance are manifested by changes in the ECF and plasma volume, and the best clinical guide to Na needs is the ECF volume. In contrast, the plasma Na concentration and osmolality best reflect water balance with respect to body fluid solute. Serum Na levels are usually determined by flame photometry or by the use of an ion-specific electrode.

Water metabolism here refers to *excretion or retention of water independent of Na*. Although isotonic fluid losses constitute the loss of both water and Na, the clinical manifestations of such disorders are referable primarily to ECF volume depletion and resultant hemodynamic disturbances. In contrast, both hypotonicity and hypertonicity of body fluids are manifested primarily as mental disturbances. The term **"disorders of water balance"** is restricted here to *disturbances in osmolality*. It should be noted that mixed disorders of salt and water homeostasis are frequent. Thus depletion of total body fluid content due to renal losses of Na and water may be found in adrenal insufficiency, and a disorder of water balance exists only if body fluid osmolality is altered (i.e., if hyponatremia or hypernatremia is present).

CLINICAL DISORDERS OF WATER AND SODIUM METABOLISM

Although conditions of pure Na depletion or excess and water depletion (dehydration) or excess can exist, most clinical disturbances of Na and water balance are mixed. Deficits or excesses of water are shared by the ICF and ECF in approximate proportions of 2/3 ICF and 1/3 ECF. As a result, clinical signs of ECF and plasma volume alteration usually are absent or not prominent. Instead, abnormalities of the CNS (due to osmotically mediated changes in cell volume) are the most frequent clinical changes. These vary from subtle changes in mental status and personality to irritability, hyperreflexia, seizures, coma, and death.

In contrast, Na depletion is characterized by signs of ECF and plasma volume depletion. When mild, the only alterations may be diminished skin turgor or intraocular tension; both are unreliable signs. When ECF volume has diminished by about 5% or greater, evidence of plasma volume deficit is present in the form of orthostatic tachycardia and/or hypotension (decrease of systolic pressure of 10 mm Hg or greater) and decreased central venous pressure **(CVP).** The latter often can be estimated by observing the height of the internal jugular venous pulsation above the 2nd intercostal space; this height in cm + 5 is approximately equal to the CVP. Na excess expands the ECF volume and, when severe, causes edema. About 3 L of fluid must accumulate in an average 70-kg man before edema becomes evident. If local causes of edema are excluded, its presence is a reliable sign of Na excess. Additional manifestations of Na excess depend largely upon cardiac status and the distribution of ECF between the vascular and interstitial spaces.

PRINCIPLES OF FLUID THERAPY

Fluid and electrolyte therapy consists of providing maintenance requirements and replacing any deficits and ongoing abnormal losses. The approximate composition and volume of some common losses are given in TABLE 81–1. In the presence of normal renal function, the provision of mainte-nance and other requirements is quite simple, since the kidney retains what is needed and excretes any excess. When renal function is abnormal and/or when there are large abnormal losses, it is necessary to measure the volume and electrolyte content of all significant losses and to tailor admin-istered fluids to the individual patient. Deficits of Na may be estimated initially from the change in body wt. In any event, it is best to monitor volume parameters carefully (BP, pulse, Hct, and CVP or pulmonary artery pressure) during the administration of saline solutions, especially if large amounts of fluid are given rapidly or if renal or cardiac disease is present. The type of solution given to replace ECF volume deficits depends upon the initial plasma Na concentration. If the latter is < 115 to 120 mEq/L, 3% or 5% sodium chloride is given (see Treatment under HYPONATREMIA, below). Likewise, if there is severe hypernatremia, salt replacement must consist of hypotonic solutions such as 0.45% sodium chloride.

In states characterized by renal retention of Na, intake must be restricted, based upon the rate of renal Na excretion and the degree of ECF volume expansion.

Water needs are determined by estimates of maintenance requirements and the serum Na concen-tration. If renal function is seriously impaired or if a disturbance of water metabolism is present, major adjustments must be made in water intake. For example, when severe hyponatremia exists due to water retention, restriction of water intake to 1000 ml or less/24 h may be mandatory. Additional modifications of electrolyte content must be made in the presence of disturbances of acid-base and K metabolism, which will be discussed separately.

As a rule of thumb, 1/2 of calculated deficits, plus maintenance and projected losses, may be given during the first 24 h of treatment. About 1/2 of the total 24-h volume is given in the first 8 h. In shock, it may be necessary to give fluid at faster rates, and careful attention must be given to volume parameters and the K content of such fluids.

TABLE 81-1. FLUID LOSSES IN ADULTS

Type of Loss	Composition	Volume/24 h
Maintenance (predicted needs in absence of disease)		
Insensible	Water	12 ml/kg body wt
Sweat	Na^+ 50 mEq/L K^+ 7 mEq/L Cl^- 40 mEq/L	Variable; should be estimated when sweating is severe
Urine	Variable; average 24-h loss of: Na^+ 75–170 mEq* K^+ 40– 60 mEq Cl^- 115–145 mEq	Variable; average volume, 1000–1500 ml
Abnormal losses		
Nasogastric suction	Na^+ varies directly with pH: 20–116 mEq/L (60)** K^+ 5– 32 mEq/L (9) Cl^- 50–154 mEq/L (100)	Measure
Diarrheal stool	Na^+ 50–100 mEq/L K^+ 20– 40 mEq/L Cl^- 40– 80 mEq/L	Measure

* Note that urinary Na content normally varies directly with dietary Na intake.
** Numbers in parentheses indicate average values.

COMBINED SODIUM AND WATER DEFICITS

A loss of sodium and water, producing extracellular fluid volume depletion.

Losses of Na from the body are always combined with water losses. The end result of Na depletion is ECF volume depletion; whether it is hypotonic, isotonic, or hypertonic depends largely upon the route of loss (e.g., GI, renal) and the type of fluid ingested by or given to the individual. Other factors, such as the activation of ADH secretion or impaired solute delivery to the distal tubule with resultant water retention, may also affect the final serum Na concentration. The common causes of ECF volume depletion are listed in TABLE 81-2.

Clinical Features and Diagnosis

ECF volume depletion should be suspected in patients with a history of inadequate fluid intake (especially in comatose or disoriented patients), vomiting, diarrhea (or iatrogenic GI losses; e.g., nasogastric suction, ileostomy, or colostomy), diuretic therapy, symptoms of diabetes mellitus, or renal or adrenal disease. A history of weight loss over a short period of time is useful. Physical signs, such as diminished skin turgor, intraocular tension, and dry shrunken tongue, are often unreliable, especially in the elderly or "mouth-breathers." More reliable signs include a low CVP (measured or estimated from the neck veins), postural hypotension, or tachycardia (the last 2 signs may occur in bedridden patients without ECF volume depletion). When depletion is severe, disorientation and

TABLE 81-2. PRINCIPAL CAUSES OF ECF VOLUME DEPLETION

I. Extra-renal
    A. GI: vomiting, diarrhea, GI suction
    B. Skin: sweating
    C. Dialysis: hemodialysis, peritoneal dialysis

II. Renal/Adrenal
    A. Chronic renal failure; salt-wasting renal disease (medullary cystic disease; Interstitial nephritis; less frequently, pyelonephritis, myeloma)
    B. Acute renal failure: recovery phase
    C. Diuretic therapy
    D. Bartter's syndrome
    E. Adrenal disease: Addison's disease (glucocorticoid deficiency), hypoaldosteronism

overt shock may be present. The Hct is often increased but is valueless unless the baseline level is known or it is disproportionately high for the underlying disease (e.g., renal failure).

If renal function is sufficiently intact and losses are extrarenal, the urine Na concentration is usually < 10 to 15 mEq/L and urine osmolality is often elevated. In the presence of metabolic alkalosis the urine Na concentration may be high; a low urine chloride concentration (< 5 mEq/L) indicates ECF volume depletion in this instance. If the Na loss is due to renal disease or adrenal insufficiency, the urine Na concentration generally exceeds 20 mEq/L. Significant ECF volume depletion frequently produces mild to moderate rises in the BUN and plasma creatinine levels (prerenal azotemia).

Treatment

Mild to moderate ECF volume depletion may be corrected by increased oral intake of Na and water in the conscious patient with no GI dysfunction. When depletion is severe and accompanied by hypotension or when oral fluid administration is impractical, IV saline is infused, following the precautions outlined under PRINCIPLES OF FLUID THERAPY, above. When renal excretion of water is normal, Na and water deficits may be safely replaced with isotonic (0.9%) saline. When there is an associated disturbance in water metabolism, replacement fluids are modified as discussed in the following sections.

HYPONATREMIA

A decrease in the serum sodium concentration below the normal range (136 to 145 mEq/L), usually indicative of hypo-osmolality of body fluid due to an excess of water relative to solute.

Clinical Features and Diagnosis

The principal causes of hyponatremia are shown in TABLE 81–3. With the exception of the artifactual (hyperlipidemia) and osmotic varieties, hyponatremia results from renal retention of water. In Na-depleted patients, the manifestations are primarily those of ECF volume depletion, unless water intake is excessive and resultant hyponatremia severe.

Dilutional hyponatremia with expansion of TBW usually is associated with an elevated total body Na content. In edematous states (e.g., congestive heart failure, cirrhosis, nephrotic syndrome, acute glomerular disease, and idiopathic edema syndrome), the kidney is unusually salt-acquisitive, presumably because of a diminished effective circulating blood volume. The kidney responds by retaining salt and water as if the individual were ECF volume-depleted. The urine Na concentration generally is very low (< 10 mEq/L). Hyponatremia results from volume-mediated ADH release (urine osmolality elevated) or partially from diminished Na delivery to the distal tubules (e.g., severe congestive heart failure). The clinical features are those of the underlying disease plus low urinary Na excretion and, frequently, a concentrated urine with respect to plasma.

Dilutional hyponatremia may also result from excessive water intake without Na retention in the presence of renal failure, Addison's disease, myxedema, or nonosmotic ADH secretion (e.g., postoperative states, drugs such as narcotics, vincristine, and chlorpropamide). All involve defective water excretion. Rarely, massive water ingestion (> 20 to 25 L/day) may produce hyponatremia in the presence of normal renal water excretion.

The **syndrome of inappropriate ADH secretion** occurs in association with oat cell carcinoma of the lung, a variety of pulmonary and CNS disorders, or acute intermittent porphyria; or it may be idiopathic. It is due to sustained ADH elaboration that is inappropriate with respect to body fluid osmolality. Typically, there are (1) inappropriately hypertonic urine with respect to plasma, even when hyponatremia is marked; (2) normal GFR; (3) hyponatremia and hypo-osmolality of body fluids; (4) expansion of TBW without edema; and (5) urinary Na wasting that increases with salt-loading. The syndrome is identical to that produced by chronic administration of exogenous vasopressin in indi-

TABLE 81–3. PRINCIPAL CAUSES OF HYPONATREMIA

I. Sodium depletion in excess of water depletion or replacement of sodium losses with water alone (may occur in many of conditions listed in TABLE 81-2)

II. Dilutional hyponatremia (water intake in excess of output; always implies impaired water excretion)

   A. Primary dilutional hyponatremia: renal failure; states characterized by elevated output of ADH, e.g., postoperative narcotic administration; syndrome of inappropriate ADH secretion (SIADH), e.g., with pulmonary neoplasms or infections (tuberculosis), CNS infections (meningitis, encephalitis), trauma, acute intermittent porphyria

   B. Neuroendocrine: adrenal and pituitary insufficiency, myxedema

   C. Associated with sodium retention and edema (congestive heart failure; hepatic cirrhosis; renal sodium acquisitive states such as nephrotic syndrome, acute glomerulonephritis, toxemia of pregnancy)

   D. Osmotic hyponatremia: severe hyperglycemia

viduals allowed free access to water. Both the hyponatremia and urinary Na wasting can be corrected by water restriction. This syndrome must be distinguished from other hyponatremic states with identifiable causes of ADH secretion, especially Addison's disease.

Water intoxication may result when the effective plasma osmolality falls to 240 mOsm/kg or less, irrespective of the underlying cause. However, the rate of fall of osmolality may be as important as the absolute magnitude of the decrease; symptoms may occur at somewhat higher plasma osmolalities if the change is rapid. Experimentally, brain water content is elevated both in acute and chronic hyponatremia. However, as a result of decreased brain electrolyte content (primarily K) in the chronic setting, the increase in brain water content is less than would be expected from the level of plasma osmolality. The development of subtle changes in mental status, lethargy, and confusion in a clinical setting associated with impaired water excretion suggests water intoxication. If intoxication is progressive, stupor, neuromuscular hyperexcitability, convulsions, prolonged coma, and death may result. Evidence of volume expansion is not prominent unless there is an associated disturbance of Na metabolism, since the expansion of body water is predominantly ($2/3$) intracellular.

Treatment

Management of hyponatremia depends upon its severity and the underlying cause. The presence of hyponatremia, hyperkalemia, and hypotension should suggest adrenal insufficiency and the need for IV glucocorticoid administration (100 to 200 mg of soluble hydrocortisone in 1 L of 5% glucose in 0.9% saline is given rapidly over 4 h in acute adrenal insufficiency). When adrenal function is normal, the correction of hyponatremia associated with ECF volume depletion usually requires salt (0.9% saline) administration alone. If the underlying disorder is slow to respond or hyponatremia is marked, water restriction (500 to 1500 ml/24 h, depending on the severity of the disturbance) is prudent. If the syndrome of inappropriate ADH release is present, severe water restriction is required; i.e., 25 to 50% of maintenance. Lasting correction depends upon successful correction of the basic disease. In cases where the ADH excess is untreatable (tumor, some idiopathic cases), the use of the tetracycline derivative demeclocycline 900 to 1200 mg/day has been helpful. However, nephrotoxicity has resulted from demeclocycline administration to patients with hepatic cirrhosis. Prudence dictates that the drug be used with caution until further experience is obtained.

When symptoms of water intoxication are present or imminent (e.g., serum Na < 120 mEq/L; effective osmolality < 240 mOsm/kg), it is necessary to give hypertonic (3% or 5%) sodium chloride. A 3% sodium chloride solution provides 0.51 mEq of Na/ml; a 5% solution, 0.86 mEq/ml. An amount of Na sufficient to raise the serum Na concentration to about 120 to 125 mEq/L is given over 12 h in conjunction with water restriction. The amount of Na (mEq/L) necessary to raise the serum Na level to 125 mEq/L can be approximated by multiplying the deficit (125 mEq/L-measured serum value in mEq/L) by the TBW. Although the Na given will remain in the extracellular compartment, it will behave as if it were distributed in the TBW, owing to its osmotic effect. In patients with concomitant ECF volume expansion or incipient congestive heart failure, the administration of a potent loop diuretic such as furosemide or ethacrynic acid may be combined with replacement of urine electrolyte losses by isotonic or hypertonic saline plus potassium chloride. If the likelihood of renal response to a diuretic is small, or if the hyponatremia is particularly severe (e.g., serum Na < 105 mEq/L), dialysis may be necessary.

HYPERNATREMIA

An elevation of the serum sodium concentration above the normal range (136 to 145 mEq/L), indicative of a deficit in body water relative to sodium.

Pathogenesis

Hypernatremia generally results when water losses exceed Na losses in conjunction with inadequate water intake. Water losses may be due to impaired renal water conservation or to excessive extrarenal losses. Rarely, hypernatremia may result from a grossly elevated Na intake (without concurrent water loss) in association with limited access to water (e.g., in infants or unconscious adults). The principal causes of hypernatremia are listed in TABLE 81–4.

Clinical Features and Diagnosis

As in pure water excess, the major clinical feature of water deficit is CNS dysfunction resulting from brain cell shrinkage. Confusion, neuromuscular excitability, seizures, or coma may result. Experimentally, brain solute is elevated in response to chronic hypernatremia (due to the accumulation of "idiogenic" osmoles). Excretion of a large volume of hypotonic urine is characteristic of patients with abnormal renal water conservation. When losses are extrarenal, the route of water loss is often evident (e.g., diarrhea, excessive sweating) and the urine is highly concentrated and of low volume.

The syndrome of hyperglycemic (hyperosmolar) nonketotic coma is recognized by the combination of marked hyperglycemia, hyperosmolality, and absence of ketosis, usually associated with combined Na and water depletion.

Treatment

The initial aim is water replacement and, in those patients with associated Na depletion, restoration of ECF volume. Water replacement can be accomplished orally in the conscious patient without GI disturbance, or by IV infusion in patients unable to swallow. Although most patients may be given 5%

TABLE 81–4. PRINCIPAL CAUSES OF HYPERNATREMIA

I. Abnormal renal wasting of water with inadequate intake of water
   A. Diabetes insipidus
      1. Pituitary ADH deficiency
      2. Nephrogenic (ADH unresponsive)
   B. Osmotic diuresis: marked glycosuria, mannitol diuresis, urea diuresis due to high-protein tube feedings (high sodium load contributory), chronic renal failure
   C. Recovery phase of acute renal failure
   D. Hypercalcemia, hypokalemia

II. Water depletion with normal renal conservation of water but inadequate intake of water
   A. Excessive sweating and insensible losses (often infants, comatose or disoriented patients without access to water)
   B. Diarrheal disorders (especially in children)
   C. Disordered thirst mechanism

III. Grossly excessive intake of sodium with limited access to water

---

D/W, too rapid infusion may produce glycosuria, thereby increasing salt-free water excretion and increased hypertonicity of body fluids. However, in patients with the hyperglycemic, hyperosmolar syndrome, or associated Na deficits, 0.45% sodium chloride is preferable. If volume disturbances are severe enough to produce shock, colloid and isotonic (0.9%) saline may be required before turning to hypotonic saline. The hypernatremia should be corrected over a period of 24 to 48 h in order to avoid cerebral edema due to the presence of excess brain solute.

When renal water losses are due to pituitary diabetes insipidus, use of vasopressin (lypressin) nasal spray (q 2 to 6 h) or vasopressin tannate in oil (0.5 to 1 ml s.c. or IM q 24 to 72 h) stops the renal water loss. (CAUTION: *Vasopressin tannate in oil must be shaken thoroughly immediately before use.*) In pituitary and nephrogenic diabetes insipidus, administration of a thiazide diuretic along with modest Na restriction reduces free water loss. Patients with hyperosmolar, hyperglycemic coma should receive regular insulin in a dose of 10 u. for every 100 mg/100 ml of blood glucose. Insulin is given (½ s.c., ½ IV) q 2 h until the blood glucose falls below 250 mg/100 ml. Glucose 5% in 0.45% or 0.9% saline is then given with appropriate insulin coverage. The blood glucose concentration should be measured q 2 h during treatment, since the total insulin requirement may be as little as 40 u., or > 500 u.

DISTURBANCES IN POTASSIUM METABOLISM

Potassium (K) is primarily an intracellular cation, only about 2% of total body K being extracellular. Since most intracellular K is contained within muscle cells, total body K is roughly proportional to lean body mass. A 70-kg man contains about 3500 mEq of K. In health, and in states of simple K deficiency or excess, the serum K level provides a reasonable estimate of total body K content with respect to capacity; that is, serum K rises when total K content exceeds capacity and falls when total body K is depleted with respect to intracellular capacity. Serum K levels may be determined by flame photometry or by the use of an ion-specific electrode.

Assuming no change in pH, a 1 mEq/L decrease in serum K concentration, when the initial level is 4 mEq/L or greater, indicates a deficit of 100 to 200 mEq of K. A fall in serum K to < 3 mEq/L indicates a deficit in total body K of about 200 to 400 mEq. However, when disease states alter membrane function (permeability or active transport), when acid-base disturbances exist, and when lean body mass is significantly diminished (as in prolonged starvation), the serum K level is an unreliable guide to total body K content.

The serum K concentration is affected significantly by serum pH. Acidosis is associated with movement of K from cells into the extracellular space, and alkalosis with transfer of K in the opposite direction, independent of the total body K/capacity relationship. A 0.1 change in pH results in about a 0.6 mEq/L inverse change in serum K concentration. Thus, serum K increases with acute acidosis and falls with acute alkalosis; this implies that a low or normal serum K level in the presence of significant acidosis indicates K depletion.

Dietary intake of K normally varies between 40 and 150 mEq/day. In the steady state, urinary and fecal K excretion equals K input into the ECF. When the ingested or administered K load increases acutely, the rise in serum K may be blunted by increased endogenous insulin secretion or mineralocorticoid secretion promoting intracellular transfer of K. If elevated intake continues, renal K excretion rises, probably due to K-stimulated aldosterone secretion. In addition, stool K content may rise. The renal response to K restriction is relatively slow in developing, and when urinary K excretion is reduced to 15 to 20 mEq/24 h, significant K depletion is present. Thus, the renal conservation mechanism for K is far less efficient than that for Na.

Most of the K from the glomerular filtrate is reabsorbed in the proximal tubule and loop of Henle; excreted K is secreted into the filtrate in the distal tubule. K excretion is regulated by aldosterone and the electrical potential difference in the distal and collecting tubules. Aldosterone secretion leads to kaliuresis, and aldosterone deficit or suppression impairs renal K excretion. Actions that increase the luminal negativity of the distal tubule favor secretion of K; a similar change in the collecting tubule limits back-diffusion of K into the renal interstitium. Physiologically, the most important variable governing luminal negativity is the presence of Na ions. Thus, states characterized by diminished distal Na delivery (e.g., congestive failure) may be attended by impaired renal K excretion. Conversely, increased distal Na delivery may be associated with increased K excretion if K depletion is not present. The relationship of K and hydrogen ion excretion is discussed under DISTURBANCES IN ACID-BASE METABOLISM, below).

POTASSIUM DEFICIT AND HYPOKALEMIA

Etiology and Pathogenesis

K depletion usually is due to excessive losses of K in the urine or stool. **Kaliuresis** occurs in adrenal steroid excess; in association with diuretics (e.g., thiazides, furosemide, ethacrynic acid, but not spironolactone or triamterene); in osmotic diuresis (e.g., diabetic ketoacidosis); in renal tubular disease, such as renal tubular acidosis, Fanconi's syndrome, and, rarely, pyelonephritis; with excessive licorice ingestion; and with carbenicillin or high-dose penicillin treatment. **Gastrointestinal losses** usually are due to diarrhea, chronic laxative abuse or clay ingestion, vomiting or suction (renal K wasting with developing metabolic alkalosis is of primary importance), and bowel diversion. Villous adenoma of the colon is a rare cause of K loss from the GI tract. The **transfer of extracellular K into cells** may also cause hypokalemia, as in glycogenesis (total parenteral nutrition or administration of insulin to patients with diabetes mellitus), familial periodic paralysis, and acute alkalosis. **Other causes** include decreased intake, as in starvation and failure to give K in IV solutions, and losses in sweat, as in cystic fibrosis.

Symptoms, Signs, and Diagnosis

Severe hypokalemia (serum K < 3 mEq/L) may produce muscular weakness and lead to paralysis and respiratory failure. Muscular malfunction may result in respiratory hypoventilation, paralytic ileus, hypotension, muscle twitches, and tetany. K nephropathy impairs the concentrating mechanism, producing polyuria and decreased maximal urinary concentrating ability with secondary polydipsia.

Cardiac effects usually are minimal until serum K levels are < 3 mEq/L, *except in patients receiving digitalis*. The characteristic ECG changes of S-T segment depression, increased U wave amplitude, and T wave amplitude < U wave amplitude (in same lead) are shown in FIG. 81–1. Severe hypokalemia may produce premature ventricular and atrial contractions and ventricular and atrial tachyarrhythmias, as well as advanced disturbances of atrioventricular conduction in patients not receiving digitalis. Similar disturbances occur at less severe degrees of hypokalemia in the presence of digitalis.

Hypokalemia

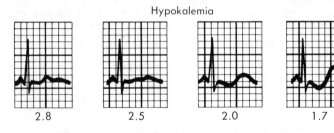

| 2.8 | 2.5 | 2.0 | 1.7 |

Hyperkalemia

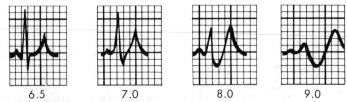

| 6.5 | 7.0 | 8.0 | 9.0 |

FIG. 81–1. **ECG patterns in hypokalemia and in hyperkalemia.** (Serum potassium in mEq/L)

Laboratory Findings

The serum K level is < 3.8 mEq/L. Metabolic alkalosis is often present unless the hypokalemia results from diarrhea or renal tubular acidosis, both of which cause metabolic acidosis. Severe depletion of K impairs the response of the tubule to ADH and may result in isosthenuria or a state resembling nephrogenic diabetes insipidus. Generally, the creatinine clearance and serum creatinine are normal and urine sediment changes are nonspecific. The concentrating defect is reversible with repletion of K.

Treatment

Correction of the underlying cause may suffice when hypokalemia is minimal. When deficits and hypokalemia are more severe (serum K < 3 mEq/L) or when continued therapy with K-depleting agents is necessary, potassium chloride is given orally (10% KCl) or IV. Usually 20 to 80 mEq/day in excess of losses given in divided doses is sufficient to correct deficits over a period of several days. Enteric-coated K preparations should be *avoided* as they may lead to small-bowel ulceration. A wax impregnated KCl preparation containing 8 mEq/tablet appears to be a safe alternative to 10% KCl. One should attempt to ensure that oral food intake contains sufficient quantities of K. Routine K replacement is not necessary in most patients receiving diuretics. Addition of triamterene 100 mg/day or spironolactone 25 mg q.i.d. may be useful in occasional patients who become hypokalemic with diuretic therapy, but should be avoided in patients with renal failure. Correction of K deficiency should be carried out with particular care in patients with renal insufficiency.

When K deficits must be replaced parenterally, the rate of correction of hypokalemia is limited because of the slow rate of transfer of K from the extra- to intracellular compartments. If serum K is high (states of acidemia) even though total body K is low, one should wait until the serum K starts to fall before administering IV K. Even when K deficits are severe, it is rarely necessary to give > 80 to 100 mEq of K in excess of continuing losses in a 24-h period. In most situations, the K concentration of IV solutions should not exceed 40 mEq/L and infusion rates should not exceed 10 mEq/h. Rarely, it may be necessary to give K solutions IV at a more rapid rate in order to prevent progressive severe hypokalemia. Infusion of > 40 mEq potassium chloride/h should be undertaken *only with continuous monitoring of the ECG and hourly serum K determinations in order to avoid severe hyperkalemia and cardiac arrest.* Glucose solutions containing K may cause transient worsening of hypokalemia and should be avoided if possible, particularly in patients receiving digitalis. In the presence of acidosis or chloride excess, potassium phosphate is an attractive alternative parenteral preparation.

POTASSIUM EXCESS AND HYPERKALEMIA

Hyperkalemia (serum K > 4.7 mEq/L) may occur when acidosis produces a shift of K out of cells into the ECF or as a consequence of K excess. Since the kidneys normally excrete K loads rapidly, the occurrence of hyperkalemia usually is associated with diminished renal function. K excess is particularly common in acute oliguric states (especially acute renal failure) associated with severe crush injuries, burns, bleeding into soft tissue or the GI tract, or adrenal insufficiency. In chronic renal failure, hyperkalemia is uncommon until uremia supervenes, unless K loads are excessive (e.g., dietary, GI bleeding, salt-substitutes, oral or parenteral K therapy, or K-sparing diuretics). An exception is the occurrence of hyperkalemia in patients with diabetic nephropathy (or interstitial renal disease), hyporeninemia, and hypoaldosteronism despite creatinine clearances often > 10 ml/min. If sufficient potassium chloride is ingested orally, or rapidly given parenterally, severe hyperkalemia may result, even with normal renal function.

Symptoms, Signs, and Diagnosis

Although flaccid paralysis occasionally occurs, hyperkalemia is usually asymptomatic until cardiac toxicity supervenes (Fig. 81–1). The earliest ECG changes are shortening of the Q-T interval and tall, peaked T waves (serum K > 5.5 mEq/L). Progressive hyperkalemia produces nodal and ventricular arrhythmias, widening of the QRS complex (serum K > 6.5 mEq/L), P-R interval prolongation and disappearance of the P wave, and, finally, degeneration of the QRS complex to a sine wave pattern and ventricular asystole or fibrillation.

Laboratory Findings

The serum K level is > 4.7 mEq/L. Artifactual hyperkalemia may be seen when K is measured in the serum of patients with thrombocytosis due to release of K from platelets during clotting; the plasma K level is normal. Hemolysis of blood samples may also produce spurious elevations of blood K levels.

Treatment

Mild hyperkalemia may respond to diminished K intake or discontinuance of K-sparing diuretics. A serum K of 6 mEq/L requires aggressive therapy. However, in acute or chronic renal failure (especially in the presence of hypercatabolism or tissue injury), treatment should be initiated when the serum K level exceeds 5 mEq/L.

If no ECG abnormalities are present and the serum K is < 6 mEq/L, sodium polystyrene sulfonate, a sodium-cycle cation exchange resin, is given in 70% sorbitol to ensure rapid passage through the GI tract; 15 to 30 gm for adults (1 gm/kg/day in divided doses for infants or young children) in 30 to 70 ml of 70% sorbitol may be given orally q 4 to 6 h. Patients unable to take oral medications because of ileus or other reasons may be given similar treatment by rectal retention enema. About 1 mEq of K is removed/gm of resin given. Resin therapy is slow and often fails to lower serum K significantly in hypercatabolic states. Since Na is exchanged for K when sodium polystyrene sulfonate is used, Na overload may be iatrogenically produced.

In emergencies (cardiac toxicity or serum K level > 6 mEq/L) the following measures are instituted immediately and followed by sodium polystyrene sulfonate administration:

1. Sodium bicarbonate 88 to 176 mEq is given to adults by rapid IV push and repeated as needed, especially if the patient is acidotic. **In infants and young children,** sodium bicarbonate 3 mEq/kg may be given over 30 to 60 min.

2. IV administration of 10 to 20 ml of 10% calcium gluconate over 15 to 30 min (hazardous in patients on digitalis) in adults may reverse the ECG changes without changing serum K level. When the ECG has deteriorated to a sine wave or worse, the calcium gluconate may be given by IV push (5 to 10 ml over 2 min). **In infants and young children,** myocardial contractility is stabilized by giving 0.25 ml/kg of calcium gluceptate over 2 to 3 min with ECG monitoring.

3. IV administration of 100 to 300 ml of 50% glucose containing 1 u. of regular insulin/3 gm glucose over a 30-min period may lower serum K for 4 to 6 h. Effects may not occur for 30 to 60 min. In extreme emergencies 15 u. of regular insulin may be given by IV push and covered with 50% glucose or continuous infusion of 10% D/W. **In infants and young children,** similar effects may be accomplished by giving a continuous infusion of 10 or 20% glucose to which is added 0.5 u. of insulin/gm of glucose.

4. Hemodialysis should be instituted promptly after emergency measures in patients with renal failure or if emergency treatment is not effective. Peritoneal dialysis is relatively inefficient with respect to K removal but may benefit the acidotic patient, especially if volume overload is likely to occur with sodium bicarbonate.

DISTURBANCES IN CALCIUM METABOLISM

Normal serum calcium **(Ca)** levels range between 8.8 and 10.4 mg/100 ml. Approximately 40% of the total blood Ca is bound to serum proteins (about 0.8 mg Ca bound/gm protein) while the remaining 60% is ultrafilterable and includes ionized Ca plus Ca complexed with phosphate and citrate. The ionized Ca fraction (about 50% of the total blood Ca) is influenced by pH changes. Acidosis is associated with decreased protein-binding and increased ionized Ca and alkalosis with a fall in ionized Ca due to increased protein-binding. These pH-induced changes in ionized Ca occur independently of any change in total blood Ca concentration.

In the laboratory determination of serum Ca, only total serum Ca is usually measured (atomic absorption spectrophotometry is the most accurate method). Ideally, the ionized serum Ca should be determined, since it is the physiologically active form, but such a test is not available for routine use. However, development of ion-specific electrodes for Ca has facilitated the determination of ionized Ca.

Maintenance of the blood Ca level is partially dependent upon dietary Ca intake (0.5 gm to 1 gm/day), GI absorption of Ca, and renal Ca excretion. The major factor preserving the constancy of the blood Ca concentration is the bone Ca reservoir. About 99% of body Ca is in bone, of which 1% is freely exchangeable with ECF.

Parathyroid hormone (PTH), an 84-amino acid, single-chain polypeptide (mol wt 9500), is secreted by the parathyroid glands. PTH and vitamin D (now also considered to be a hormone) are the principal regulators of Ca and phosphorus **(P)** homeostasis; their metabolic actions are interrelated. PTH promotes renal formation of the active metabolite of vitamin D. Conversely, with a deficiency of the vitamin or any resistance to its action, some of the effects of the hormone are blunted.

The most important actions of PTH are (1) increasing the rate of bone resorption with mobilization of Ca and P from bone, (2) increasing renal tubular reabsorption of Ca, (3) increasing intestinal absorption of Ca (mediated by an action on the metabolism of vitamin D), and (4) decreasing renal tubular reabsorption of phosphate (PO_4). These actions account for most of the important clinical manifestations of PTH excess or deficiency.

The percentage of dietary Ca absorbed via the intestine increases with a fall in Ca intake and decreases when dietary Ca is increased. The mechanism is vitamin D-dependent. The active metabolite of vitamin D (1,25-dihydroxycholecalciferol; 1,25-DHCC) enhances small-intestine Ca transport by mediating synthesis of mucosal Ca-binding proteins. PTH also enhances intestinal Ca absorption, but this action appears to be due to PTH-mediated formation of 1,25-DHCC in the kidney. Renal Ca excretion generally parallels Na excretion and is influenced by many of the factors that govern Na transport in the proximal tubule. Independently of Na (and vitamin D), PTH enhances renal distal tubular Ca absorption and increases renal PO_4 excretion. PTH causes an efflux of bone Ca into the ECF within minutes after glandular release, probably by stimulating osteocytic osteolysis. Long-term increases in PTH secretion promote osteoclastic osteolysis. PTH activates adenyl cyclase in bone and kidney, leading to formation of cAMP. The role of cAMP in the target organ effects of PTH is not entirely clear. The physiologic effects of PTH upon bone are importantly influenced by normal levels of active vitamin D, which acts in a permissive fashion to enhance osteolysis. See VITAMIN D DEFICIENCY in Ch. 78.

Physiological tests of parathyroid function largely have been supplanted by the measurement of circulating PTH levels in the plasma or serum by radioimmunoassay **(RIA)**, and by the measurement of total or nephrogenous cAMP excretion in the urine.

Most clinically available RIAs for PTH detect the carboxy-terminal (C-terminal) segment of the PTH molecule and react both with the secreted hormone and biologically inactive C-terminal cleavage fragments. C-terminal assays correlate highly with the number of osteoclasts and are useful in the diagnosis of primary hyperparathyroidism. Since C-terminal fragments accumulate in the plasma with declining renal function, PTH levels measured by a C-terminal assay will increase progressively with decreasing renal function, limiting the usefulness of the assay. However, the C-terminal assay generally reflects the long-term activity of the parathyroid glands in patients on chronic dialysis; in this instance, the metabolic clearance of C-terminal fragments is delayed but constant. Immunoassays directed at the amino-terminal (N-terminal) site are more suitable for detecting rapid changes in PTH secretion in response to acute changes in ionized Ca. Whatever the RIA utilized, clinical interpretation of the PTH level is possible only in the context of the concomitantly measured serum Ca level. Since the sensitivity of some assays is poor, some normal individuals will exhibit undetectable levels of PTH.

Cyclic AMP excreted in the urine is derived both from filtered cAMP and tubular secretion of cAMP in response to PTH. The nephrogenous component of urinary cAMP constitutes up to 50% of the total urinary cAMP excreted. Total urinary cAMP, when factored by GFR or per unit creatinine excretion and related to plasma Ca level, provides reasonable diagnostic separation and reflects acute changes in PTH secretion in response to acute changes in the ionized Ca level. Thus it may be superior to C-terminal PTH assays in acute stimulation or suppression tests of parathyroid function.

HYPOCALCEMIA (Hypocalcemia in neonates is discussed in Vol. II, Ch. 21)

Total serum calcium < 8.8 mg/100 ml in the presence of normal serum proteins.

Etiology and Pathogenesis

Hypocalcemia is an infrequent laboratory finding. It occurs as the result of:

(1) **Deficiency or absence of parathyroid hormone: Hypoparathyroidism** *(a tendency to hypocalcemia, often associated with chronic tetany, resulting from hormone deficiency, characterized chemically by low serum calcium and high serum phosphorus levels)* usually follows accidental removal of or damage to several parathyroid glands during thyroidectomy. Although transient hypoparathyroidism is common following subtotal thyroidectomy, the disease occurs permanently in < 3% of expertly performed thyroidectomies. Manifestations begin about 24 h postoperatively. Parathyroid deficiency is more common after radical thyroidectomies for cancer. **Idiopathic hypoparathyroidism**, in which the parathyroids are absent or atrophied, is uncommon. It may occur sporadically as an isolated or inherited condition, or in association with the DiGeorge syndrome. It also occurs as part of a genetic syndrome of hypoparathyroidism, Addison's disease, and mucocutaneous candidiasis. Although antiparathyroid antibodies may be detectable, there is no evidence that such antibodies are responsible for the hypoparathyroidism. In contrast to the postoperative and idiopathic forms, **pseudohypoparathyroidism** is characterized not by deficiency of PTH but by target organ (bone and kidney) unresponsiveness to its action. This is a sex-linked inherited disorder and often is associated with short metacarpal and metatarsal bones, short stature, and mental retardation. In some patients with hypoparathyroidism and pseudohypoparathyroidism, subnormal formation of 1,25-DHCC may contribute to the relative refractoriness of hypocalcemia to correction by vitamin D.

(2) **Vitamin D deficiency,** due to inadequate dietary intake, decreased exposure to sunlight, or intestinal malabsorption and associated with rickets or osteomalacia. Functional vitamin D deficiency may occur during prolonged anticonvulsant therapy with barbiturates and phenytoin presumably the result of increased catabolism of 25-(OH)D$_3$. (See also p. 591.)

(3) **Vitamin D dependency,** in which formation of 1,25-DHCC is defective, and familial hypophosphatemic rickets.

(4) **Renal tubular disease,** including the Fanconi syndrome due to nephrotoxins (e.g., heavy metals) and distal renal tubular acidosis.

(5) **Renal failure,** where diminished formation of 1,25-DHCC coupled with hyperphosphatemia produces hypocalcemia.

(6) **Magnesium depletion** occurring with intestinal malabsorption or dietary deficiency, which causes hypocalcemia by relatively deficient secretion of PTH, as well as end-organ resistance to its action.

(7) **Acute pancreatitis,** which lowers serum Ca levels when Ca is chelated by lipolytic products.

(8) **Hypoproteinemia** of any cause with reduction in protein-bound Ca (e.g., nephrotic syndrome, cirrhosis, protein-losing enteropathy). Hypocalcemia due to diminished protein-binding is asymptomatic, since the ionized Ca fraction is unaltered and the effects of Ca upon membrane excitability are produced by the ionized fraction.

(9) **During periods of increased Ca utilization** coupled with inadequate intake (e.g., after surgical correction of hyperparathyroidism with healing bone lesions), hypocalcemia can also develop. It may complicate childhood leukemia and may develop in oxalic acid poisoning and during sodium edetate therapy.

Although excessive secretion of calcitonin might be expected to cause hypocalcemia, low serum Ca levels are rare in patients with medullary carcinoma of the thyroid, a tumor that typically secretes large amounts of calcitonin.

Symptoms, Signs, and Diagnosis

Hypocalcemia is frequently asymptomatic and is often suggested by the clinical manifestations of the underlying disorder (e.g., cataracts, basal ganglia calcification, and chronic moniliasis in some patients with **idiopathic hypoparathyroidism**).

The clinical manifestations of hypocalcemia are primarily neurologic. Slowly developing, insidious hypocalcemia may produce mild, diffuse encephalopathy and thus should be suspected in any patient with unexplained dementia, depression, or psychosis. Papilledema occasionally may be present and cataracts may develop after prolonged hypocalcemia. Severe hypocalcemia (serum Ca < 7 mg/100 ml) may cause laryngospasm and generalized convulsions.

The most characteristic syndrome is **tetany,** resulting from severe hypocalcemia or a reduction in the serum ionized Ca fraction without marked hypocalcemia (e.g., in respiratory or metabolic alkalosis). Tetany is characterized by (1) sensory symptoms consisting of paresthesias of the lips, tongue, fingers, and feet; (2) carpopedal spasm, which may be prolonged or painful; (3) generalized muscle aching; and (4) spasm of facial musculature. Tetany may be overt (spontaneous symptoms) or latent. In **latent tetany** (generally present at serum Ca levels of 7 to 8 mg/100 ml), the neuromuscular instability frequently is brought out by provocative tests. **Chvostek's sign** is contraction of the facial muscles, elicited by a light tapping of the facial nerve. It occasionally is present in normal individuals and is often absent in chronic hypocalcemia. **Trousseau's sign** is carpopedal spasm caused by reduction of the blood supply to the hand when a tourniquet or blood pressure cuff above systolic pressure is applied to the forearm for 3 min. It also occurs in alkalotic states, hypomagnesemia, hypokalemia, and hyperkalemia, and in about 6% of normal persons. Latent tetany may become overt due to hyperventilation or administration of sodium bicarbonate or Ca-depleting diuretics (e.g., furosemide). All of the manifestations of hypocalcemic tetany may be masked by concomitant hypokalemia. The ECG typically shows prolongation of the Q-T interval.

Diagnosis

The serum Ca level is < 8.8 mg/100 ml and is usually 7 mg/100 ml or less when tetany is present (unless it is induced by alkalosis). The characteristic abnormalities of respiratory and metabolic alkalosis are discussed in Disturbances in Acid-Base Metabolism, below. **Parathyroid deficiency** is characterized by low serum Ca, high serum PO_4, normal alkaline phosphatase, and low or absent urinary Ca. Immunoreactive circulating PTH is immeasurably low in patients with idiopathic hypoparathyroidism. This disorder becomes manifest in childhood and may be associated with Addison's disease, steatorrhea, and moniliasis. Hyperphosphatemia is present when hypocalcemia results from hypoparathyroidism or renal failure. The 2 are easily differentiated by the presence of marked azotemia in renal failure. **Type I pseudohypoparathyroidism** can be distinguished by the frequent presence of some skeletal abnormalities (most frequently shortening of the 1st, 4th, and 5th metacarpals), the absence of phosphaturia, the failure of plasma and urinary cAMP to increase normally following injection of parathyroid extract, and the presence of immunoreactive hormone in the circulation.

Increased stool weight and fat content, along with a low serum carotene level, are characteristic of **intestinal malabsorption.** Steatorrhea frequently is associated with **hypomagnesemia** (e.g., < 1.6 mEq/L). In **osteomalacia** or **rickets** the plasma PO_4 level often is mildly reduced and alkaline phosphatase is elevated.

Treatment

Acute severe hypocalcemic tetany is treated initially with IV infusion of Ca salts. Ten ml of 10% calcium gluconate may be given IV over 15 to 30 min, but the effect lasts for only a few hours. Therefore, it may be necessary to repeat infusions and/or to add 20 to 30 ml of 10% calcium gluconate to 1 L of 5% D/W and infuse it over 12 to 24 h. Infusions of Ca are *hazardous in patients receiving digitalis and should be given slowly with continuous ECG monitoring.* Calcium chloride causes thrombophlebitis when given IV and is highly irritating if extravasated. IM injection of calcium gluconate likewise is contraindicated because it can cause local necrosis. When tetany is due to hypomagnesemia, it may respond transiently to Ca or K administration but is permanently relieved by magnesium repletion (see Hypomagnesemia, below).

In **transient hypoparathyroidism after thyroidectomy or excision of a parathyroid adenoma,** supplemental oral Ca may be sufficient to prevent hypocalcemia. However, hypocalcemia may be particularly severe and prolonged following subtotal parathyroidectomy in patients with chronic renal failure. The marked hypocalcemia and elevated serum alkaline phosphatase in such settings may be due to the rapid uptake of Ca into bone. Prolonged parenteral administration of Ca may be necessary to avoid serious hypocalcemia in the postoperative period; as much as 1 gm of Ca/day may be required for 5 to 10 days, before oral Ca and vitamin D are sufficient to maintain adequate blood Ca levels.

In **chronic hypocalcemia,** as in hypoparathyroidism or renal failure, Ca usually is given orally with vitamin D. Ca may be given as calcium gluconate (l gm $\cong$ 90 mg Ca) or calcium carbonate (1 gm $\cong$ 400 mg Ca) to provide 1 to 2 gm of Ca/day. Although any vitamin D preparation may suffice, 1-hydroxylated compounds such as calcitriol (1,25-DHCC), and "pseudo" 1-hydroxylated analogs such as dihydrotachysterol, offer the advantage of more rapid onset of action and more rapid clearance from the body. Calcitriol is particularly useful in renal failure, since it requires no metabolic alteration; it is the drug of choice in hereditary vitamin D dependent rickets, which responds to physiologic doses of 0.25 to 0.5 μg/day orally. Patients with hypoparathyroidism and pseudohypoparathyroidism usually respond, respectively, to calcitriol in oral dosages of 0.5 to 2 μg and 1 to 3 μg/day.

In all instances, *vitamin D intoxication with severe symptomatic hypercalcemia can be a serious complication.* Adequate dietary or supplemental Ca (1 to 2 gm/day) and phosphorus must be supplied. Effective therapy is indicated by absence of symptoms and normal or near-normal Ca. The latter should be checked frequently (e.g., weekly) at first, and at 1- to 3-mo intervals after the patient's condition has stabilized. In most instances, the maintenance dose of calcitriol will decrease with time.

Treatment of hypocalcemia in patients with renal failure must be combined with dietary phosphorus restriction and phosphate-binding agents, such as aluminum hydroxide gel, in order to prevent hyperphosphatemia and metastatic calcification. *Vitamin D administration is hazardous in renal failure* and should be limited to individuals with symptomatic osteomalacia or secondary hyperparathyroidism (serum Ca < 11 mg/dl) or to patients with postparathyroidectomy hypocalcemia. The efficacy and relatively short duration of action of calcitriol (and other 1-hydroxylated analogs that may become available in the future) makes it the drug of choice in such patients. Simple osteomalacia may respond to as little as 0.25 to 0.5 μg/day, while correction of postparathyroidectomy hypocalcemia may require prolonged administration of as much as 2 μg of calcitriol/day and 2 gm or more of Ca/day.

Vitamin D-deficiency rickets responds to as little as 400 IU/day; in **osteomalacia** 5000 IU/day of vitamin D_2 or D_3 is given for 6 to 12 wk and then reduced to 400 IU/day. Provision of 2 gm of Ca/day is desirable, at least during the early stages of treatment. **Vitamin D-refractory, familial and nonfamilial, hypophosphatemic rickets** are treated with inorganic phosphate (1 to 3 gm/day). Additionally, high doses of vitamin D (50,000 to 100,000 IU/day) are given to treat the familial variety. Treatment with vitamin D requires monitoring of the serum Ca level and should be discontinued if hypercalcemia develops. **Alkalosis-induced tetany** is treated by correction of the underlying disturbance.

HYPERCALCEMIA

Total serum calcium > 10.5 mg/100 ml.

Etiology and Pathogenesis

The principal causes of hypercalcemia are listed in Table 81-5. Most frequently, hypercalcemia is due to excessive bone resorption with respect to new bone formation and release of Ca into the ECF.

Hyperparathyroidism is *a generalized disorder resulting from excessive secretion of parathyroid hormone by one or more parathyroid glands; it is usually characterized by hypercalcemia, hypophosphatemia, and abnormal bone metabolism. Nephrolithiasis and reduction of bone mass are common.* The cause is unknown; it may be the end result of long-term stimulation of parathyroid secretion by a variety of stimuli. Histologic examination usually reveals a marked enlargement of one of the parathyroid glands (adenoma of a single gland). Enlargement (hyperplasia) of 2 or more parathyroid glands is being recognized with increasing frequency, probably because of more efficient and earlier diagnosis and treatment. Conditions that can lower the serum Ca, such as renal insufficiency and intestinal malabsorption syndromes in which increased secretion of the hormone represents an adaptive response to a normal stimulus, are termed **secondary hyperparathyroidism** and are characterized by normocalcemia or mild hypocalcemia. Where secondary hyperparathyroidism has been established for some time, glandular hyperplasia may become so pronounced that hypersecretion of PTH becomes relatively autonomous, leading to so-called **tertiary hyperparathyroidism.** The syndromes of **familial multiple endocrine neoplasia (MEN-Types I and II)** are commonly associated with hyperparathyroidism. These syndromes are discussed in Ch. 89.

Ectopic hyperparathyroidism ("humoral hypercalcemia of malignancy") occurs with certain cancers (e.g., bronchogenic carcinoma, hypernephroma, hepatoma), producing a PTH-like substance that can be detected by radioimmunoassay, while others have hypercalcemia in the absence of detectable PTH-like material or bony metastases. In some instances, elaboration of prostaglandin-like substances accounts for the hypercalcemia. Tumors (e.g., multiple myeloma) that metastasize to bone probably produce hypercalcemia by stimulating osteoclastic resorption.

Vitamin D in pharmacologic doses produces excessive bone resorption as well as increased intestinal Ca absorption. (See p. 593.)

TABLE 81–5. PRINCIPAL CAUSES OF HYPERCALCEMIA

I. Excessive osteolysis

   A. Parathyroid hormone excess; e.g., primary hyperparathyroidism, parathyroid carcinoma, advanced secondary hyperparathyroidism (especially after renal transplantation)
   B. Ectopic hyperparathyroidism ("humoral hypercalcemia of malignancy"); e.g., malignancy, with or without elevated levels of PTH, in absence of bone metastases
   C. Malignancy with bone metastases; e.g., carcinoma, leukemias, lymphomas, myeloma
   D. Hyperthyroidism
   E. Vitamin D intoxication
   F. Immobilization (in patients with rapid bone remodeling—e.g., young, growing individuals or those with Paget's disease; elderly patients with osteoporosis)

II. Excessive GI calcium absorption and/or intake

   A. Milk-alkali syndrome
   B. Vitamin D intoxication
   C. Sarcoidosis

III. Elevated concentration of plasma proteins

IV. Uncertain mechanism

   A. Myxedema, Addison's disease, postoperative Cushing's disease
   B. Thiazide diuretic treatment
   C. Infantile hypercalcemia

V. Factitious

   A. Prolonged venous stasis while obtaining blood sample
   B. Exposure of blood to cork stoppers or contaminated glassware

In the **milk-alkali syndrome,** excessive amounts of Ca and absorbable alkali are ingested, usually during peptic ulcer therapy, resulting in increased Ca absorption and hypercalcemia.

Symptoms and Signs

The underlying cause of hypercalcemia (see TABLE 81–5) is often apparent from the history and associated clinical findings (e.g., excessive ingestion of Ca and alkali, widespread malignancy, or overt Addison's disease). Radiographic evidence of bone disease may suggest the diagnosis (e.g., hyperparathyroidism, Paget's disease, osteolytic or osteoblastic lesions in myeloma).

Many patients with mild hypercalcemia are asymptomatic, and the condition is discovered accidentally during routine laboratory screening. The clinical manifestations of hypercalcemia include constipation, anorexia, and nausea and vomiting with abdominal pain and ileus. Reversible impairment of the renal concentrating mechanism leads to polyuria, nocturia, and polydipsia. More severe elevation of serum Ca (usually > 12 mg/100 ml) is associated with emotional lability, confusion, delirium, psychosis, stupor, and coma. Myopathy may cause prominent skeletal muscle weakness. Seizures are rare. Hypercalciuria with nephrolithiasis or urolithiasis is common. Less often, prolonged or severe hypercalcemia may produce reversible acute renal failure or irreversible renal damage, due to precipitation of Ca salts within the kidney parenchyma **(nephrocalcinosis).** Peptic ulcers and pancreatitis may also be associated with hyperparathyroidism, but the relationship between these conditions and the parathyroid dysfunction remains obscure. Renal damage may result in azotemia and hypertension. **Osteitis fibrosa cystica,** in which increased osteoclastic activity causes rarefying osteitis with fibrous degeneration, the formation of cysts, and the development of fibrous nodules in the affected bone, may develop when hyperparathyroidism is severe or of long duration. Once common, osteitis fibrosa cystica is now rarely seen, except in chronic dialysis patients with secondary hyperparathyroidism, and only a few patients show one or more features of bone disease that are readily recognized by x-ray examination (bone cysts, "salt-and-pepper" appearance of the skull, subperiosteal resorption of bone in the phalanges and distal clavicles). Hyperparathyroid bone disease often is associated with increased serum alkaline phosphatase. The Q-T interval in the ECG is shortened in severe hypercalcemia. Hypercalcemia that exceeds 18 mg/100 ml may result in shock, renal failure, and death.

Laboratory Findings and Diagnosis

In **hyperparathyroidism** the ionized serum Ca concentration is elevated, although the level may fluctuate. A low serum PO_4 level suggests primary or ectopic hyperparathyroidism, especially when coupled with an elevated PO_4 clearance (depressed tubular reabsorption of PO_4) and mild hyperchloremic acidosis. The serum Ca is rarely > 12 mg/100 ml in primary hyperparathyroidism. A serum Ca > 12 mg/100 ml usually is due to tumors or other causes of hypercalcemia. It may be difficult to distinguish primary from secondary hyperparathyroidism in the presence of renal insufficiency. A high serum Ca and normal serum PO_4 suggest primary hyperparathyroidism, especially in the nondialyzed patient.

The **milk-alkali syndrome** is recognized by history and by the combination of hypercalcemia, metabolic alkalosis, and, frequently, azotemia with hypocalciuria. With cessation of Ca and alkali ingestion, the blood Ca level rapidly returns to normal.

Myeloma should be suggested by the syndrome of anemia, azotemia, and hypercalcemia. This diagnosis is confirmed by bone marrow examination or finding a monoclonal gammopathy or free light chains in the serum or urine on immunoelectrophoresis. In **other endocrine causes** of hypercalcemia (e.g., thyrotoxicosis, Addison's disease), the typical laboratory findings of the underlying disorder help to establish the diagnosis. Hypercalciuria is found in most disorders causing hypercalcemia, except milk-alkali syndrome, Addison's disease, thiazide therapy, and renal failure.

Circulating PTH (C-terminal assay) usually is elevated in patients with hyperparathyroidism, and is suppressed in patients with vitamin D intoxication, the milk-alkali syndrome, and sarcoidosis. There are immunologic differences between PTHs secreted in ordinary hyperparathyroidism and those secreted in ectopic hyperparathyroidism. Immunoassays capable of detecting these differences may provide decisive information in the differentiation of primary and ectopic hyperparathyroidism. Measurement of urinary total or nephrogenous cAMP is useful as a biologic marker of PTH action in difficult cases, particularly when measured in response to Ca loading in patients with Ca urolithiasis or in patients with hypercalcemia of unknown origin. Increased basal excretion of cAMP in the presence of hypercalcemia is indicative of hyperparathyroidism.

Treatment

The management of hypercalcemia depends upon the severity of Ca elevation and the underlying cause. When the blood Ca is < 11.5 mg/100 ml, correction of the underlying disturbance often is sufficient.

The mainstay of therapy of *severe* hypercalcemia is extracellular volume expansion with IV saline to promote calciuria. The aim is to attain a urine volume of 3 L/day. Preexisting volume deficits should be replaced prior to beginning the diuresis with the infusion of isotonic (0.9%) saline and administration of furosemide in patients with sufficient renal function. One to 2 L of IV isotonic saline are followed by furosemide 80 to 100 mg IV q 2 h for 24 h. Urine losses are replaced with isotonic saline and 5% D/W in a ratio of 4:1 plus sufficient potassium chloride (20 mEq/L) to prevent hypokalemia. Fluid intake and output and serum and urine electrolytes must be monitored carefully.

When the serum Ca exceeds 15 mg/100 ml, rapid reduction is necessary. While there is no completely safe means by which severe hypercalcemia can be corrected, acute hemodialysis (with low or calcium-free dialysis fluid) is probably the safest and most reliable method. Similarly, in **patients with advanced renal failure**, dialysis (either peritoneal or hemodialysis) is the method of choice to promptly control hypercalcemia.

A more hazardous approach is the IV administration of 1 L of disodium and monopotassium phosphate (0.081 mole disodium phosphate + 0.019 mole monopotassium phosphate to provide a solution of pH 7.4). Each liter contains 3.1 gm of phosphorus. No more than 0.5 to 1.0 gm should be given IV in 24 h; usually 1 or 2 doses in 2 days are sufficient to lower serum Ca for 10 to 15 days. Lowering of serum Ca with such treatment is associated with diminished urinary Ca content. Soft-tissue calcification is the major complication, and acute renal failure may occur. The IV infusion of an isotonic solution of sodium sulfate decahydrate (38 gm/L), given at 1 to 2 L/24 h *is even more hazardous and less effective than phosphate administration and should not be utilized in patients with marginal cardiac or renal function.*

Long-term control of hypercalcemia may be achieved by oral phosphate administration. The equivalent of 1 to 1.5 gm/day of elemental phosphorus may be given in divided doses. Diarrhea is the limiting factor in oral phosphate therapy.

The addition of prednisone 20 to 40 mg/day orally will effectively control hypercalcemia in most patients with vitamin D intoxication and sarcoidosis, while some patients with myeloma or metastatic malignancy respond to 80 to 120 mg/day of prednisone. However, since the response to steroid therapy takes several days and since many causes of hypercalcemia fail to respond to steroids, it is usually necessary to seek other treatment modalities.

In patients with metastatic malignancy, mithramycin 25 to 50 μg/kg body wt IV is extraordinarily effective, producing a prompt, prolonged lowering of serum Ca. It should be used *cautiously* in patients already receiving cytotoxic drugs (e.g., melphalan or cyclophosphamide in patients with myeloma), in order to avoid profound hypocalcemia. Toxic effects of mithramycin include thrombocytopenia, hepatotoxicity, and renal damage. Since mithramycin probably depresses osteolytic activity, theoretically it should be useful in any form of hypercalcemia due to osteolysis. However, it should be used only for severe hypercalcemia that is refractory to safer alternative modes of treatment.

Indomethacin, 75 to 150 mg/24 h, may lower serum Ca levels in patients with **prostaglandin-induced hypercalcemia.**

Calcitonin (thyrocalcitonin): *The rapidly acting peptide hormone of the parafollicular cells (thyroid "C" cells) of ultimobranchial origin.* The ultimobranchial bodies, which fuse with the thyroid in mammals, remain as separate structures in lower species. Calcitonin is secreted in response to hypercalcemia, which it reduces by inhibiting osteoclastic activity and thus the rate of Ca release from bone. Human, porcine, and piscine preparations differ structurally and immunologically.

A commercial preparation of salmon calcitonin is available; it is most useful in the treatment of Paget's disease. Calcitonin is effective in certain other forms of hypercalcemia; its limited hypocalcemic effect has the virtue of ensuring that serious hypocalcemia cannot result from its use.

In **hyperparathyroidism,** treatment is surgical if the disease is symptomatic or progressive. Chances of cure depend on successful removal of all excess functioning tissue and on reversibility of renal damage; renal insufficiency may progress despite cure of the underlying disease. Abnormally functioning parathyroid glands may be found in unusual locations and experience is required to find them. Preoperative localization of abnormally functioning parathyroid tissue is possible by immunoassay of the thyroid venous drainage. This procedure is indicated in all patients having had previous unsuccessful parathyroid surgery.

When hyperparathyroidism is mild, no special postoperative precautions are required. The elevated serum Ca level drops to just below normal within 24 to 48 h after surgery. In patients with severe osteitis fibrosa cystica, prolonged symptomatic hypocalcemia may occur and require large doses of Ca together with vitamin D, usually for 1 to 3 mo (see HYPOCALCEMIA, above).

HYPOPHOSPHATEMIA

The incidence of hypophosphatemia (serum concentration < 2.5 mg/100 ml) in hospitalized patients ranges between 2 and 10%. Most (85%) of the 500 to 700 gm of body PO_4 is contained in bone, while the remainder is predominantly intracellular. Phosphorus is an important component of nucleic acids and cellular and subcellular membranes and is intimately involved in aerobic and anaerobic energy metabolism.

The causes of hypophosphatemia are many but clinically significant hypophosphatemia commonly occurs in relatively fewer settings. Chronic hypophosphatemia most often results from a fall in renal PO_4 reabsorption and is not associated with intracellular PO_4 depletion. Causes include hyperparathyroidism, hormonal disturbances, renal tubular defects (intrinsic and acquired, as with hypomagnesemia and hypokalemia), and chronic diuretic administration. Though hypophosphatemia usually is asymptomatic, muscle weakness and osteomalacia can occur if PO_4 depletion is present.

Similarly, chronic starvation, malabsorption, or deficient dietary intake of phosphorus may cause hypophosphatemia but are uncommon as sole causes of phosphate depletion. Mild chronic hypophosphatemia of any etiology may predispose to the development of severe acute or chronic hypophosphatemia. Severe chronic hypophosphatemia usually results from a prolonged negative PO_4 balance and leads to PO_4 depletion, anorexia, muscle weakness, and osteomalacia with bone pain. Causes include chronic starvation or malabsorption, especially if combined with vomiting or copious diarrhea; chronic malnutrition; or chronic ingestion of large amounts of aluminum hydroxide antacid. The latter is particularly prone to produce PO_4 depletion when combined with decreased dietary intake and dialysis losses of PO_4 in patients with chronic renal failure.

Acute severe hypophosphatemia *(serum phosphorus < 1 to 1.5 mg/100 ml)* is most often due to transcellular shifts of phosphorus, often superimposed upon chronic hypophosphatemia and PO_4 depletion. Serious neuromuscular disturbances may occur, including progressive encephalopathy, coma, and death. Profound muscle weakness may be accompanied by rhabdomyolysis, especially in acute alcoholism. Hematological disturbances include hemolytic anemia, decreased release of O_2 from Hb, and impaired leukocyte and thrombocyte function. These acute syndromes presumably result from depletion of intracellular ATP or decreased red cell 2,3-diphosphoglycerate and diminished delivery of O_2 to tissues. The most common clinical settings of acute severe hypophosphatemia include the recovery phase of diabetic ketoacidosis and acute alcoholism, and total parenteral nutrition **(TPN).**

Treatment is empiric and is dictated by the underlying cause and the severity of hypophosphatemia. In mild to moderate chronic phosphate depletion, supplemental oral phosphate (0.08 to 0.16 mM/kg body wt, b.i.d. to t.i.d.) may be given but usually is poorly tolerated due to diarrhea. Ingestion of 1 qt of low fat or skim milk will provide 1 gm of phosphorus (32 mM) and may be more acceptable. Removal of the cause of hypophosphatemia (e.g., cessation of phosphate-binding antacids or diuretics, correction of hypomagnesemia) is preferable when possible. **When hypophosphatemia is anticipated,** as in diabetic ketoacidosis, acute alcoholism, and TPN, the administration of IV monobasic potassium phosphate in appropriate dosage is relatively safe as long as renal function is well preserved. The usual maintenance dose in TPN is 15 mM/day, while alcoholics may require up to 30 mM/day during the course of parenteral nutrition. In diabetic ketoacidosis, 50 mM or more may be required in the first 24 h; supplemental PO_4 is discontinued when oral intake is resumed. In each instance, but particularly when PO_4 is given IV or to patients with impaired renal function, it is advisable to monitor serum Ca and phosphorus levels during therapy. Sodium phosphate preparations generally should be used in patients with impaired renal function.

When the serum phosphorus concentration falls below 1.0 to 1.5 mg/100 ml, PO_4 should be given IV in larger amounts. In most cases, no more than 0.25 mM/kg of body wt (17.5 mM for a 70 kg adult) should be given over 6 h. Hypocalcemia, hyperphosphatemia, and hypokalemia may be avoided by careful monitoring and avoidance of more rapid rates of PO_4 administration.

DISTURBANCES IN MAGNESIUM METABOLISM

Magnesium **(Mg)** is the 4th most plentiful cation in the body (total body content about 2000 mEq in a 70-kg man), but only 1% exists in the ECF. About 50% of the total body Mg is found in bone and is not readily exchangeable with Mg in ECF; the remainder is intracellular. Plasma Mg concentration is maintained between 1.6 and 2.1 mEq/L. Observations in Mg-depleted individuals suggest that maintenance of plasma Mg concentration largely is a function of dietary intake and extremely effective renal and intestinal conservation, possibly regulated in part by PTH. Within 7 days of initiation of a Mg-deficient diet, renal and fecal Mg excretion fall to about 1 mEq/24 h each. The intestinal response is impaired if dietary intake of Ca and PO_4 is high.

About 70% of plasma Mg is ultrafilterable (roughly 55% free or ionized); the remainder is bound to protein. Like Ca, protein-binding of Mg is pH-dependent. Plasma Mg concentration and either total body Mg or intracellular Mg content are not closely related. However, plasma hypomagnesemia may reflect diminished body stores of Mg.

A wide variety of enzymes including phosphatases (e.g., adenosine triphosphatase and alkaline phosphatase) are Mg-activated or -dependent. Mg is required for thiamine pyrophosphate cofactor activity and appears to stabilize macromolecular structure (e.g., DNA and RNA). Mg is also related to Ca and K metabolism in an intimate but poorly understood fashion (see HYPOMAGNESEMIA, below).

HYPOMAGNESEMIA

Plasma magnesium concentration < 1.6 mEq/L.

Hypomagnesemia often is equated with Mg depletion. However, serum Mg concentration, even if free Mg ion is measured, may not reflect the status of intracellular or bone Mg stores.

Etiology and Pathogenesis

Magnesium depletion usually results from inadequate intake plus impairment of renal or gut absorption. It has been described in association with (1) **prolonged parenteral feeding,** usually in combination with loss of body fluids via gastric suction or diarrhea; (2) **lactation** (increased requirement for Mg); and (3) **conditions of abnormal renal conservation** of Mg, such as hypersecretion of aldosterone, ADH, or thyroid hormone, hypercalcemia, diabetic acidosis, and diuretic therapy.

Clinically significant Mg deficiency most commonly is associated with (1) **malabsorption syndromes** from all causes, in which elevated fecal Mg is probably related to the level of steatorrhea rather than to deficient bowel absorptive sites per se; (2) **protein-calorie malnutrition** (e.g., kwashiorkor); (3) **parathyroid disease,** in which hypomagnesemia is seen after removal of a parathyroid tumor, especially if severe osteitis fibrosa is present (presumably, Mg is transferred to rapidly mineralizing bone and Mg deficiency may account for the resistance of hypocalcemia to correction with vitamin D in occasional patients with hypoparathyroidism); and (4) **chronic alcoholism,** in which hypomagnesemia probably is due to both inadequate intake and excessive renal excretion.

Neonatal hypomagnesemia occurs in normal premature infants, in DiGeorge's syndrome, in familial hypoparathyroidism, after exchange transfusion, and in infants of mothers having diabetes mellitus, toxemia, hyperparathyroidism, and Mg deficiency. It often is associated with hypocalcemia and hypophosphatemia.

Symptoms, Signs, and Diagnosis

The disorders associated with Mg deficiency are complex and usually accompanied by multiple metabolic and nutritional disturbances. Furthermore, since the curare-like action of Mg ion is well known, response of neuromuscular irritability to Mg administration is not necessarily proof that Mg deficiency caused the neuromuscular irritability.

The clinical manifestations of Mg deficiency are most reliably described by experimental Mg depletion in human volunteers. In this setting, anorexia, nausea, vomiting, lethargy, weakness, personality change, tetany (e.g., positive Trousseau's or Chvostek's sign, or spontaneous carpopedal spasm), tremor, and muscle fasciculations may be present. The neurologic signs, particularly tetany, correlate with the development of hypocalcemia and hypokalemia. Myopathic potentials are found on electromyography. Any changes in the ECG are also compatible with hypocalcemia or hypokalemia. Although not observed experimentally, it is likely that severe hypomagnesemia may produce generalized tonic-clonic seizures, especially in children.

Laboratory Findings

Hypomagnesemia is often present when Mg depletion is associated with protein-calorie malnutrition. Hypocalcemia and hypocalciuria are common in patients with steatorrhea and alcoholism. In these settings, hypocalcemia responds to Mg repletion and is resistant to Ca administration. Hypokalemia, with increased urinary K excretion and metabolic alkalosis, may be present. Thus, the presence of unexplained hypocalcemia and hypokalemia should suggest the possibility of Mg depletion.

Treatment

Treatment with Mg salts (sulfate or chloride) is indicated when Mg deficiency is symptomatic or associated with severe, persistent hypomagnesemia (e.g., < 1 mEq/L). In such settings, a deficit of 1 to 2 mEq/kg may exist. The amount given should be twice the estimated deficit (if renal function is normal), since about 50% of the administered Mg will be excreted in the urine. In emergencies (e.g., seizures) or when serum Mg is < 1 mEq/L, magnesium sulfate heptahydrate is given IV at a rate not exceeding 1.5 ml of a 10% solution/min (magnesium sulfate heptahydrate contains about 8.1 mEq of Mg/gm of the salt). Usually, half of the deficit is given in the first 24 h and the remainder over the next several days. Alternatively, magnesium chloride 2 mEq/kg body wt may be given IV over 4 h. In less severe instances, gradual repletion is achieved by parenteral administration of 0.25 to 0.5 mEq/kg/day. Mg salts also may be given orally and are well tolerated, even in patients with steatorrhea. During Mg therapy, the serum Mg level should be monitored frequently, particularly in patients with renal insufficiency. Treatment is continued until a normal serum Mg level is achieved.

In **emergencies involving neonates,** 0.25 to 1 ml of 50% magnesium sulfate injection IM or IV is given over 10 to 15 min with careful ECG monitoring. This dose may be repeated 2 to 3 times/day. Close monitoring of the serum Mg and the patient's clinical status is essential. If prolonged oral therapy is necessary, twice the maintenance dose of 10 to 20 mg/kg of Mg as magnesium sulfate heptahydrate (1 ml 50% solution contains 500 mg Mg) may be given initially and adjusted upward.

HYPERMAGNESEMIA

Plasma magnesium > 2.1 mEq/L.

Symptomatic hypermagnesemia is common in patients with renal failure who receive Mg salts or ingest Mg-containing drugs such as antacids or purgatives.

Hypermagnesemia leads to generalized impairment of neuromuscular transmission, probably as the result of inhibition of acetylcholine release at the neuromuscular junction. At serum concentrations of 5 to 10 mEq/L, the ECG shows prolongation of the P-R interval, widening of the QRS complex, and increased T wave amplitude. Deep tendon reflexes disappear as the serum Mg level approaches 10 mEq/L; hypotension, respiratory depression, and narcosis develop with progression of the hypermagnesemia. Cardiac arrest may occur as the result of a high blood Mg concentration (about 25 mEq/L). **Treatment** of severe Mg intoxication consists of circulatory and respiratory support, with IV administration of 10 to 20 ml of 10% calcium gluconate. The latter may reverse many of the Mg-induced changes, including the respiratory depression. The administration of IV furosemide or ethacrynic acid increases Mg excretion, if continuous and adequate hydration is maintained. Hemodialysis may be of value in severe hypermagnesemia if BP can be maintained, since a relatively large fraction (about 70% of blood Mg) is ultrafilterable. When hemodialysis is impractical, peritoneal dialysis may be effective.

DISTURBANCES IN ACID-BASE METABOLISM

The pH of ECF in health is maintained at about 7.40 (range, 7.35 to 7.45). Acute changes in pH due to acid or alkali loads (or deficits) are immediately damped by interaction with extracellular and intracellular buffer systems. In the absence of pulmonary disease, respiratory compensation further diminishes pH aberrations. Ultimately, however, the kidneys maintain pH homeostasis by excretion or retention of hydrogen ions and regeneration of lost buffers.

The bicarbonate (**HCO$_3^-$**) buffer system, one of several body buffers, is of singular importance. The **Henderson-Hasselbalch** equation, expressed in terms of the HCO$_3^-$ system, reads:

$$pH = 6.1 + \log \frac{HCO_3^-}{\alpha(Pa_{CO2})}$$

where $\alpha = .03$ mM/L/mm Hg at 38 C

At a pH of 7.4, the ratio of HCO$_3^-$ to α (Pa$_{CO2}$) is 20:l. Their *ratio,* rather than their concentrations, determines blood pH. The physiologic importance of this buffer system derives from the fact that 2 mechanisms (renal and respiratory) exist for adjusting the ratio of this major ECF buffer pair, and thus the pH of the ECF. The denominator α(Pa$_{CO2}$) can be modified rapidly by changes in respiratory minute ventilation, while the numerator (HCO$_3^-$) is subject to renal regulation.

Renal regulation of the HCO$_3^-$ concentration of ECF is accomplished in several ways. Hydrogen (H) ion may be secreted into the renal tubular lumen in exchange for Na; for each H ion secreted, a HCO$_3^-$ ion is added to the ECF. Thus, net reabsorption of filtered HCO$_3^-$ occurs. Since the pH of the fluid leaving the proximal tubule is about 6.5, most filtered HCO$_3^-$ is reabsorbed in the proximal tubule. In the distal tubule, H ion secretion is partially dependent upon aldosterone-mediated Na reabsorption and can lower the pH to as low as 4.5 to 5. Throughout the nephron, secreted H ion is buffered by urinary buffers such as PO$_4$ (titratable acid) and ammonia. In this manner, filtered HCO$_3^-$ operationally is reabsorbed, and also new HCO$_3^-$ can be generated to replace that lost in body buffer reactions. Since filtered Na is reabsorbed either in association with an anion (i.e., chloride) or by cationic exchange (i.e., with H ion and, to a lesser extent, K), the total Na reabsorbed approximates the sum of the chloride reabsorbed and H ion secreted. Thus, there is an inverse relationship between chloride reabsorption and H ion secretion. This relationship is highly dependent upon the existing level of Na reabsorption.

Renal HCO$_3^-$ reabsorption also is influenced by body potassium stores. There is a general reciprocal relationship between intracellular potassium content and hydrogen ion secretion. Thus, potassium depletion is associated with increased hydrogen ion secretion and attendant HCO_3^- generation, leading to an HCO_3^- increase in ECF and metabolic alkalosis. Finally, renal HCO_3^- reabsorption is influenced by the Pa_{CO2} and the state of ECF volume. An increased Pa_{CO2} leads to increased HCO_3^- reabsorption, and a decreased ECF volume leads to increased Na reabsorption and HCO_3^- generation; e.g., in the proximal tubule.

Clinical disturbances of acid-base metabolism classically are defined in terms of the HCO_3^- buffer system (see Henderson-Hasselbalch equation, above). Rises or falls of the numerator (HCO_3^-) are termed, respectively, **metabolic alkalosis or acidosis;** rises or falls in the denominator ($\alpha[Pa_{CO2}]$) define, respectively, **respiratory acidosis and alkalosis. Simple disturbances** include both the primary alteration and the expected compensation (e.g., in metabolic acidosis there is a primary fall in the HCO_3^- concentration of the ECF and a secondary fall in the Pa_{CO2} due to compensatory hyperventilation). Compensation may be classified as uncompensated, partial, or complete. **Mixed disturbances** are more complex disorders in which 2 or more primary alterations coexist (e.g., respiratory acidosis with superimposed diuretic-induced metabolic alkalosis).

It may be necessary to refer to a nomogram in order to distinguish simple from mixed disorders. However, measurement of the pH of arterial (or arterialized venous) blood, the Pa_{CO2}, and the CO_2 combining power **(CO_2CP)** of venous blood (or calculation of HCO_3^-) along with recognition of a disease entity known to produce an acid-base derangement and knowledge of the expected responses of the blood gases and buffers, including compensatory changes, are usually sufficient to correctly identify most clinical acid-base problems (see TABLE 81-6).

METABOLIC ACIDOSIS

A primary fall in extracellular fluid bicarbonate concentration; pH and carbon dioxide combining power are reduced.

Etiology and Pathogenesis

The principal causes of metabolic acidosis are shown in TABLE 81-7.

Excessive acid production or ingestion: A common form is diabetic ketoacidosis with increased production of acetoacetic and β-hydroxybutyric acid. Occasionally, diabetic acidosis may be associated with an altered NADH/NAD ratio leading to lactic acidosis and elevated levels of β-hydroxybutyric acid. The plasma ketone level is not increased when measured by the usual methods that detect only acetoacetic acid. Lactic acidosis may develop in any state of diminished tissue oxygenation (e.g., vascular shock), with phenformin administration, or ethanol ingestion. Rarely it occurs idiopathically. In salicylate, methanol, or ethylene glycol poisoning, interference with normal intermediary metabolism or accumulation of exogenous organic anions may cause metabolic acidosis.

TABLE 81-6. CHEMICAL FINDINGS IN THE PLASMA OF PATIENTS
WITH ACID-BASE DISTURBANCES

Disturbance	pH	Pa_{CO2}	CO_2 Combining Power
Normal	7.34–7.38 (venous) 7.38–7.42 (arterial)	43 mm Hg (venous) 40 mm Hg (arterial)	21–28 mEq/L
Metabolic alkalosis	↑	↑**	↑*
Metabolic acidosis	↓*	↓**	↓*
Respiratory alkalosis	↑*	↓*	↓**
Respiratory acidosis	↓*	↑*	↑**
Mixed metabolic and respiratory acidosis	↓	↑	↓
Mixed metabolic and respiratory alkalosis	↑	↓	↑
Mixed metabolic acidosis and respiratory alkalosis	↑↓	↓	↓
Mixed metabolic alkalosis and respiratory acidosis	↑↓	↑	↑

* Primary change
** Compensatory change

Impaired renal excretion of acid occurs in acute or advanced chronic renal failure due to reduced hydrogen ion excretion. In chronic renal failure, the major defect is insufficient ammonia production (and thus decreased ammonium ion excretion) as the result of progressive diminution in functioning renal mass. In renal tubular acidosis (RTA) with a relatively normal filtration rate, the defect is either proximal tubular HCO_3^- wasting (proximal RTA) or an inability to generate an acid urine (gradient-limited or distal RTA).

Symptoms, Signs, and Diagnosis

The major symptoms and signs of acidosis are often obscured by or difficult to separate from those of the underlying disease. Mild acidosis may be asymptomatic or may be accompanied by vague lassitude, nausea, and vomiting. The most characteristic finding in severe metabolic acidosis (e.g., pH < 7.2 and CO_2 CP < 10 mEq/L) is hyperpnea, manifested by an early increase in depth and, later, frequency of respiration (Kussmaul breathing). Signs of ECF volume depletion may also be present, especially in patients with diabetic acidosis or GI alkali loss. Severe acidosis may cause circulatory shock, due to impaired myocardial contractility and peripheral vascular response to cate-cholamines, and progressive obtundation.

Laboratory Findings

The urine pH is < 5.5 when the plasma HCO_3^- concentration falls to low levels with severe acidosis. The blood pH is < 7.35 and CO_2 CP < 21 mEq/L. In the absence of pulmonary disease, the Pa_{CO2} is < 40 mm Hg. Many forms of metabolic acidosis are characterized by an abnormal anion gap (TABLE 81–7). The anion gap (representing undetermined plasma anions) is estimated by subtracting the sum of the chloride concentration and CO_2 CP from the plasma Na concentration (normal up to 15 mEq/L). When metabolic acidosis is associated with the accumulation of unmeasured anions, such as sulfate in renal failure, ketones in diabetic or alcoholic ketoacidosis, lactate or exogenous toxins such as ethylene glycol or salicylates, the anion gap is > 15 mEq/L. Metabolic acidosis associated with a normal anion gap (hyperchloremic metabolic acidosis) usually results from primary bicarbonate loss, either via the GI tract or in the urine (e.g., renal tubular acidosis). Diabetic acidosis usually is characterized by the presence of hyperglycemia and ketonemia. In diabetic patients with hyperglycemia and nonketotic acidosis, blood lactic acid and/or β-hydroxybutyric acid levels are elevated. Ethylene glycol poisoning should be suspected in individuals having unexplained acidosis and oxalate crystals in the urine. Salicylate poisoning is characterized early by respiratory alkalosis with metabolic acidosis developing later; blood levels of salicylate are usually > 30 to 40 mg/100 ml.

Since volume depletion often accompanies acidosis, mild azotemia (BUN 30 to 60 mg/100 ml) is common. Greater elevations of the BUN, especially in conjunction with hypocalcemia and hyper-phosphatemia, suggest renal failure as the cause of the acidosis. Changes in the serum K during acidosis were discussed earlier in this chapter.

Treatment

Therapy of chronic renal acidosis is discussed under ANOMALIES IN KIDNEY TRANSPORT in Ch. 153. The treatment of metabolic acidosis consists of therapy of the underlying disease (e.g., insulin in diabetic acidosis) and IV administration of sodium bicarbonate when acidosis is severe (pH < 7.2). This can be given by adding varying amounts of sodium bicarbonate (44 to 88 mEq) to either 5% D/W or hypotonic saline (one-fourth or one-half isotonic saline), or by using 5% sodium bicarbonate solutions, depending on the clinical setting and attendant water and volume disturbances. The goal

TABLE 81–7. PRINCIPAL CAUSES OF METABOLIC ACIDOSIS
AND METABOLIC ALKALOSIS

I. **Metabolic Acidosis**
   A. With elevated "anion gap"
      1. Renal failure
      2. Diabetic ketoacidosis
      3. Lactic acidosis
      4. Exogenous poisons (ethylene glycol, salicylates, methanol, paraldehyde)
   B. With normal "anion gap"
      1. GI alkali loss (diarrhea, ileostomy, colostomy)
      2. Renal tubular acidosis
      3. Interstitial renal disease (e.g., "selective hypoaldosteronism")
      4. Ureterosigmoid loop
      5. Ingestion of acetazolamide or ammonium chloride

II. **Metabolic Alkalosis**
   A. Diuretic therapy (thiazides, ethacrynic acid, furosemide)
   B. Vomiting or gastric drainage
   C. Hyperadrenocorticism (Cushing's syndrome, aldosteronism, exogenous corticosteroid administration)

of HCO_3^- therapy is to raise the CO_2 CP to about 10 to 12 mEq/L. The amount of sodium bicarbonate necessary can be approximated by the formula:

$$\text{mEq of } NaHCO_3 \text{ required} = (CO_2 \text{ CP desired} - CO_2 \text{ CP observed}) \times 25\% \text{ TBW}$$

The apparent distribution space of HCO_3^- is > 25% of TBW, due to continuing transfer of intracellularly buffered H ion out of cells into the ECF. However, it is best to raise the pH of the ECF only to a safe level, such as 7.2, while other measures are instituted to correct the cause of the acidosis, thereby averting some of the **complications of alkali treatment.** These include volume overload in patients with cardiac and renal disease and the precipitation of acute tetany in patients with renal failure. Too rapid correction of acidosis may also result in a rise in the Pa_{CO2} at a time when CSF bicarbonate levels are still low, thus inducing a "relative CSF acidosis." Occasionally, this may be associated with obtundation, coma, or death. In patients with marked overproduction of H ions (e.g., lactic acidosis), it may be necessary to give very large quantities of sodium bicarbonate IV in conjunction with dialysis to minimize ECF volume expansion.

RESPIRATORY ACIDOSIS

A primary increase in arterial carbon dioxide pressure; pH is low and carbon dioxide combining power increases if renal function is intact.

Etiology and Pathogenesis

Respiratory acidosis is the result of alveolar hypoventilation leading to pulmonary CO_2 retention. It occurs with (1) depression of the central respiratory center caused by drugs, anesthesia, neurologic disease, abnormal sensitivity to CO_2 (e.g., cardiopulmonary obesity syndrome); (2) abnormalities of the chest bellows (e.g., poliomyelitis, myasthenia gravis, Guillain-Barré syndrome, crush injuries of the thorax); (3) severe reduction of alveolar surface area for gas exchange (conditions characterized by ventilation/perfusion imbalance; e.g., chronic obstructive pulmonary disease [emphysema, chronic bronchitis], severe pneumonia, pulmonary edema, asthma, or pneumothorax]; and (4) laryngeal or tracheal obstruction. Neurologic changes with CO_2 retention may depend upon the development of CSF acidosis or intracellular acidosis in the brain. Hypoxemia and metabolic alkalosis frequently accompany respiratory acidosis and may contribute to the neurologic abnormalities.

Symptoms, Signs, and Diagnosis

The most characteristic change is metabolic encephalopathy with headache and drowsiness progressing to stupor and coma. It usually develops slowly with advancing respiratory failure, but abrupt, full-blown encephalopathy may be precipitated by sedatives or pulmonary infection in patients with advanced respiratory insufficiency. Asterixis and multifocal myoclonus are generally present; in some patients, dilation of retinal venules and papilledema result from increased intracranial pressure. The encephalopathy may be reversible if hypoxic brain damage has not occurred.

Laboratory Findings

In acute respiratory acidosis, the low pH is due to the acute elevation in Pa_{CO2}. The CO_2 CP may be normal or slightly increased. When renal compensation is fully developed, as in chronic respiratory acidosis, the fall in pH is blunted due to renal HCO_3^- retention and elevation of the CO_2 CP. If diuretic therapy (e.g., for chronic cor pulmonale) causes superimposed metabolic alkalosis, the high Pa_{CO2} may be associated with a high CO_2 CP, hypochloremia, and a normal or alkaline blood pH.

Treatment

The treatment must improve the underlying pulmonary disturbance. Severe respiratory failure with marked hypoxemia often requires mechanically assisted ventilation. Sedative drugs (narcotics, hypnotics) should be avoided except as necessary to facilitate mechanical ventilation. Although most patients with chronic CO_2 retention and hypoxia tolerate modest O_2 enrichment of inspired air, some patients respond with a significant fall in respiratory minute volume and further acute elevation of the Pa_{CO2}. Presumably, such patients have adapted to chronic hypercapnia (CO_2 narcosis) so that their major respiratory stimulus is hypoxemia. Therefore the lowest O_2 concentration required to elevate the Pa_{O2} to acceptable levels (> 50 mm Hg) should be given. This can be accomplished with O_2 administration by a Ventimask®, beginning with a 24% O_2 concentration. The Pa_{CO2} should be carefully monitored and, if it rises to dangerous levels (> 50 to 55 mm Hg), mechanical ventilation must be considered.

If mechanical ventilation is used in patients with chronic respiratory failure, the Pa_{CO2} should be lowered slowly, especially if concomitant metabolic alkalosis (high CO_2 CP and normal or alkaline pH) is present. Rapid lowering of the Pa_{CO2} will cause severe metabolic alkalosis (pH > 7.5). The resultant leftward shift of the oxyhemoglobin dissociation curve and cerebral vasoconstriction may lead to seizures and death. Providing adequate inspired O_2, lowering the Pa_{CO2} more slowly, and repairing potassium or chloride deficits will prevent such neurologic consequences.

METABOLIC ALKALOSIS

A primary increase in blood bicarbonate; pH and carbon dioxide combining power are elevated.

Etiology and Pathogenesis

Metabolic alkalosis develops as the consequence of loss of acid from the ECF; e.g., loss of acid-containing gastric juice, loss of acid via the urine or stool, transfer of H ions into cells, excessive loads of HCO_3^- (e.g., alkali administration to patients with renal failure), or rapid contraction of the extracellular space (e.g., with potent diuretics). Whatever the cause, the kidney tends to correct the alkalosis rapidly by excreting excess HCO_3^-, unless other factors, such as volume contraction, result in both a Na-acquisitive state and increased HCO_3^- reabsorption. Thus, a diminished effective arterial volume, K deficiency, and persistent adrenal steroid excess are common clinical settings for chronic metabolic alkalosis (TABLE 81–7). Perhaps the most frequent and important of these settings is ECF volume contraction and avid renal sodium reabsorption.

Diuretics cause metabolic alkalosis by several mechanisms, including (1) acute contraction of the ECF volume (sodium chloride excretion without HCO_3^-), thereby increasing the concentration of HCO_3^- in the ECF; (2) diuretic-induced K and chloride depletion, and (3) secondary aldosteronism. Continued use of the diuretic or either of the latter 2 factors may maintain the alkalosis.

The loss of gastric hydrochloric acid by suction or vomiting produces metabolic alkalosis that is perpetuated by concomitant ECF volume contraction (sodium chloride loss in gastric juice) and development of K deficiency, due to secondary aldosteronism and K loss in gastric juice.

In states of persistent adrenal steroid excess, alkalosis results from steroid-mediated reabsorption of Na in the distal tubule in exchange for H ion. Sodium chloride reabsorption in the distal tubule leads to ECF volume expansion and decreased proximal Na reabsorption. Thus, a continuing supply of Na is delivered distally for exchange with H and K ions. Potassium depletion then leads to persistence of the alkalosis.

Symptoms, Signs, and Diagnosis

Metabolic alkalosis should be suspected in the above clinical settings. The most common clinical manifestations are irritability and neuromuscular hyperexcitability, perhaps due to hypoxia from a transient leftward shift of the oxyhemoglobin dissociation curve. When severe, the ionized Ca fraction may fall low enough to provoke tetany, although total serum Ca is unchanged (see HYPOCALCEMIA, above). Muscular weakness, impaired GI motility (e.g., gastric retention, ileus), and polyuria should suggest K depletion.

Laboratory Findings

The blood pH and CO_2 CP are elevated. Striking increases in the Pa_{CO2} to levels as high as 50 to 60 mm Hg may occur with compensatory hypoventilation, especially in patients with mild renal insufficiency. The urine is alkaline except in the presence of severe K depletion, in which case it may be acid (**"paradoxic aciduria"**). Hypochloremia and hypokalemia are usual. When metabolic alkalosis is associated with ECF volume depletion, the urine chloride is almost always low (< 10 mEq/L), while the urine Na may exceed 20 mEq/L in the early stages. Conversely, metabolic alkalosis associated with primary adrenal steroid excess and volume expansion is characterized by high urine chloride.

Treatment

Correction of the underlying disturbance is desirable, when possible. Metabolic alkalosis usually resolves when ECF volume deficits are replaced with oral or IV sodium chloride. However, when K deficiency is severe, or in patients with adrenal steroid excess, the alkalosis cannot be corrected until the K deficit is repaired (**saline-resistant alkalosis**). In the post-hypercapnic state, persistent metabolic alkalosis responds to chloride, given as potassium chloride, sodium chloride (if volume depletion is present), or ammonium chloride. When mild, metabolic alkalosis usually requires no specific therapy. It should be corrected promptly, however, in patients with myocardial irritability and those with neuromuscular hyperexcitability. In such instances, ammonium chloride administration may be desirable along with other measures (e.g., correction of hypokalemia).

RESPIRATORY ALKALOSIS

A primary decrease in carbon dioxide pressure; blood pH is increased and carbon dioxide combining power is reduced.

Etiology and Pathogenesis

Hyperventilation, leading to excessive loss of CO_2 in expired air, results in respiratory alkalosis. The Pa_{CO2} and cerebral tissue P_{CO2} fall, and both plasma and cerebral tissue pH rise. Cerebral vasoconstriction results and, along with the Bohr effect, may produce cerebral hypoxia and the characteristic symptom complex. The common causes are anxiety (**"hyperventilation syndrome"**), overventilation of patients on assisted ventilation, primary CNS disorders, salicylism, hepatic cirrhosis, hepatic coma, hypoxemia, fever, and gram-negative septicemia.

Symptoms, Signs, and Diagnosis

Obvious hyperventilation is usually present, particularly when respiratory alkalosis is due to cerebral or metabolic disorders. The breathing pattern in the anxiety-induced syndrome varies from frequent, deep, sighing respirations to sustained, obvious rapid, deep breathing. Patients tend to complain of anxiety, often expressing fear of cardiac disease, and are often surprisingly unaware of their hyperventilation. When symptoms are referable to respirations, the complaint is usually of inability to "catch my breath" or "get enough air," despite the fact that unimpaired overbreathing is taking place. Tetany, circumoral paresthesias, acroparesthesias, giddiness or lightheadedness, and syncope may occur. In such patients, the symptoms often can be reproduced by voluntary overventilation. Blood lactate and pyruvate levels increase and ionized calcium falls. In all situations, the diagnosis of hyperventilation is confirmed by finding a low Pa_{CO2}.

Treatment

Respiratory alkalosis due to anxiety resolves on rebreathing expired CO_2 from a *paper* bag (plastic bags may cause accidental suffocation). Other measures aimed at amelioration of chronic anxiety may be helpful (e.g., sedative or tranquilizing drugs). Overventilation with mechanical respirators can be corrected by diminishing minute ventilation, when excessive, or by adding dead space. When hyperventilation is due to hypoxemia, O_2 enrichment of inspired air and treatment aimed at correction of abnormal pulmonary gas exchange is appropriate. Correction of respiratory alkalosis by increasing the inspired CO_2 concentration may be dangerous in patients with CNS disturbances (which may be associated with a low CSF pH). The treatment of salicylism is given in Vol. II, Ch. 24.

---

82. METABOLIC ANOMALIES

ANOMALIES IN PIGMENT METABOLISM

THE PORPHYRIAS

A group of inborn errors of metabolism caused by mutations in genes that code for various enzymes of the heme biosynthetic pathway. One type of porphyria (porphyria cutanea tarda) can also be caused by certain toxic agents such as hexachlorobenzene.

The specific enzymes affected by the mutations and the diseases that are caused by each mutation are best understood after examination of the heme biosynthetic pathway, shown in Fig. 82–1. The pathway can be considered to consist of 8 basic steps, starting with the condensation of glycine and succinyl coenzyme A **(CoA)** to form δ-aminolevulinic acid **(ALA)**, the aliphatic precursor of heme. The ALA undergoes self-condensation to form porphobilinogen **(PBG)** in step 2, which is followed by polymerization of PBG to uroporphyrinogen III in steps 3 and 4. This intermediate is the reduced (hexhydro-) form of uroporphyrin and differs from the porphyrin in that it is colorless, non-fluorescent, and nonphotosensitizing (it is readily oxidized to the porphyrin in the presence of light and O_2). In step 5, the four acetic acid side chains are sequentially decarboxylated to form methyl groups, and in the process uroporphyrinogen III is converted to coproporphyrinogen III. Both propionic acid side chains of pyrrole rings A and B undergo oxidative decarboxylation to vinyl groups in the conversion of coproporphyrinogen III to protoporphyrinogen in step 6. Protoporphyrinogen is then oxidized to protoporphyrin by removal of 6 hydrogen atoms. The final step involves chelation of ferrous iron by protoporphyrin to form heme, which is then utilized in various hemoproteins.

Mutations that decrease enzyme activity have been described for all enzymes of the heme biosynthetic pathway except ALA synthetase. The diseases that correspond to the various mutations are presented in TABLE 82–1. The mutation involving ALA dehydrase was discovered accidentally in an asymptomatic individual. There is no known disease produced by this mutation. The classification of the porphyrias as shown in TABLE 82–2 is based on the organ from which the excess porphyrins or porphyrin precursors originate.

CONGENITAL ERYTHROPOIETIC PORPHYRIA (Erythropoietic Uroporphyria; Günther's Disease)

This disease is characterized by *severe cutaneous lesions on exposed areas of the body, hemolytic anemia, and large amounts of uroporphyrin I in the urine.*

Etiology, Genetics, and Incidence

The great increase of serum and urinary uroporphyrin has been attributed to decreased tissue uroporphyrinogen III cosynthetase (enzyme 4 of the heme biosynthetic pathway), but opinion concerning this conclusion is divided. The disease occurs in all races, but is rare. Approximately 70 authenticated cases were reported up to 1968. Males and females are equally affected. The disease is transmitted by a Mendelian recessive mode.

Symptoms and Signs

Clinically this disease presents cutaneous lesions and hemolytic anemia. The onset of symptoms is often in the first year and almost always before age 5. Skin lesions appear as vesicles or bullae on exposed portions of the body. Ulceration and sometimes secondary infection, followed by healing,

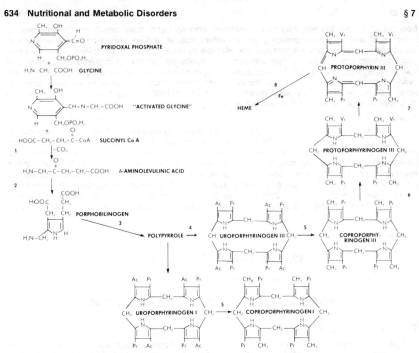

FIG. 82–1. **Heme biosynthetic pathway.** (From *Duncan's Diseases of Metabolism,* ed. 8, 1980, edited by P. K. Bondy and L. E. Rosenberg. Copyright 1980 by W. B. Saunders Company. Used with permission.)

leads to scarring. This ultimately may produce severe deformities of the nose, ears, eyes, and fingers, with areas of alopecia, pigmentation, and depigmentation. Hypertrichosis may develop on the limbs and face. The skin lesions are related to the photosensitizing action of the excess porphyrin, but the cause of the hypertrichosis remains unknown. Most patients experience hemolysis and ineffective erythropoiesis, but some compensate sufficiently by increased RBC production to prevent the normochromic anemia which occurs in others. Splenomegaly develops in some patients and occasionally thrombocytopenia, which has been attributed to hypersplenism. With rare exceptions, these patients have not survived beyond middle age. The cause of death is not always clear, but some have died of renal failure, hepatic failure, or bleeding of uncertain etiology.

TABLE 82–1. DISEASES THAT CORRESPOND TO VARIOUS MUTATIONS IN HEME SYNTHESIS

Step of Pathway Affected by Mutation	Name of Enzyme Involved	Name of Disease	Genetic Mode of Transmission
2	ALA dehydrase	No disease	See text
3	Uroporphyrinogen I synthetase	Acute intermittent porphyria	Dominant
4	Uroporphyrinogen III cosynthetase	Congenital erythropoietic porphyria	Recessive
5	Uroporphyrinogen decarboxylase	Porphyria cutanea tarda	Dominant or acquired
6	Coproporphyrinogen oxidase	Hereditary coproporphyria	Dominant
7	Protoporphyrinogen oxidase	Variegate porphyria	Dominant
8	Ferrochelatase	Erythrohepatic porphyria (erythropoietic protoporphyria)	Dominant

TABLE 82-2. CLASSIFICATION OF THE PORPHYRIAS

Erythropoietic
Congenital erythropoietic porphyria (Günther's disease, erythropoietic uroporphyria)

Erythrohepatic porphyria (erythropoietic protoporphyria)

Hepatic porphyria

Acute intermittent porphyria	Hereditary coproporphyria
Variegate porphyria (mixed porphyria)	Porphyria cutanea tarda

Laboratory Findings

The basic defect causes a huge increase of uroporphyrin I and an increase of coproporphyrin I (produced by the non-enzymatic oxidation of the corresponding porphyrinogens) that produce a red ("port wine") urine. Uroporphyrin excretion may reach 50 mg/day, i.e., more than 1000 times the normal excretion rate. Fecal coproporphyrin I is increased but fecal protoporphyrin is usually not significantly increased. Plasma and erythrocyte uroporphyrin I and coproporphyrin I levels are increased. Erythrocyte-free protoporphyrin levels usually do not exceed those seen in other hemolytic anemias. Urinary porphyrin precursor excretion is not increased, and the Watson-Schwartz test (for porphobilinogen) is negative.

Normoblastic hyperplasia is usually seen in marrow samples. Fluorescence microscopy shows fluorescent normoblasts (the nucleus is most evident). In the peripheral blood, some of the circulating red cells fluoresce and reticulocytosis is often seen. There may be poikilocytosis, anisocytosis, and polychromatophilia.

Diagnosis

The appearance of dark urine and severe cutaneous photosensitivity in early life, usually accompanied by hemolytic anemia and erythrodontia, suggests the diagnosis. This is confirmed by demonstration of high levels of uroporphyrin I (by direct measurement) and fluorescence of red cells and marrow normoblasts. If erythrodontia is not obvious, red fluorescence of the teeth should be sought.

Treatment

The skin should be shielded from light by means of protective clothing. The creams and lotions used for sunburn prophylaxis are of little value in this disease, because they do not absorb the Soret band of wavelengths (those in the violet portion of the spectrum [about 400 nm]) that are absorbed by porphyrins and cause the skin damage. Beta-carotene, taken orally, has been used successfully to protect against acute photosensitivity reactions in erythrohepatic porphyria (see details below) and in a preliminary study of 1 patient with congenital erythropoietic porphyria there was a significant decrease in photosensitivity and slight improvement in hemolytic anemia. Another approach has been the topical application of dihydroxyacetone and lawsone (Duoshield®, Rowell Labs, Inc., Baudett., Minn.), which produces a sun-screen filter that is chemically induced in the skin.

Hemolysis can augment photosensitivity, since stimulation of erythropoiesis by hemolysis also increases porphyrin production (which is responsible for the photosensitivity). Splenectomy has sometimes been followed by decreased hemolysis and porphyrin excretion, but some patients have experienced recurrence of anemia. Likewise, steroid (prednisone) therapy has produced variable results in treatment of the hemolysis. Transfusions have decreased urinary porphyrin excretion as much as 90%, presumably by suppressing erythropoiesis. Recent investigations have shown IV hematin administration to diminish red cell, plasma, and urinary uroporphyrin levels. Further studies are necessary to determine the possible value of hematin therapy in this disease.

ERYTHROHEPATIC PORPHYRIA (Erythropoietic Protoporphyria)

A dominantly transmitted mendelian disorder characterized by acute photosensitivity reactions, no urine abnormalities, and, in some patients, serious liver disease.

Etiology, Genetics, and Incidence

A deficiency of ferrochelatase (the final enzyme of the heme biosynthetic pathway) has been shown in bone marrow, peripheral blood reticulocytes, liver, and fibroblasts, resulting in accumulation of protoporphyrin. The measured enzyme activity usually ranges between 8 to 25% of normal. Enzyme and other chemical studies show that one parent is normal and the other bears the mutation. This is in keeping with the dominant mode of inheritance of the disease, but measurements showing the enzyme decrease to greatly exceed 50% of normal constitute an unexplained paradox. The fact that the genetically affected parent is sometimes asymptomatic, along with other considerations, has raised some question concerning a simple mendelian dominant mode of transmission of this disease. The exact prevalence is not known, but is probably 4 or higher per 100,000 population, as high or higher than acute intermittent porphyria. Current evidence indicates that excess protoporphyrin can originate in both liver and marrow cells. The disease is therefore more properly named erythro-hepatic porphyria.

Symptoms and Signs

Cutaneous symptoms almost always begin before age 13 and usually involve (in decreasing order of frequency) burning, swelling, itching, and redness of the skin. Itching and burning may occur without redness, swelling, and scarring. This lack of objective findings may suggest psychiatric problems. Since window glass transmits the Soret band of wavelengths that are responsible for the photosensitization, the burning can occur indoors, as well as outdoors. Symptoms may begin after just a few minutes of exposure or may require hours. The burning may be mild or severe and persist for days. Some patients develop erythema and edema of the involved areas; the edema occasionally persists for weeks. Bullae and purpura may occur in children and occasionally in adults. These lesions may produce crusts and heal with superficial scars. There may be chronic skin lesions with thickening and scarring of the skin of the nose, cheek, and back of the hands and fingers. These are usually mild, but in tropical areas papular thickening of the skin may produce a "cobblestone" appearance. The erythrondontia and fluorescence of teeth, characteristic of congenital erythropoietic porphyria, are *not* seen in this disease. Hirsutism and hyperpigmentation are rare in erythrohepatic porphyria.

There is an increased incidence of gallstones, sometimes at an early age, with high levels of protoporphyrin in the gallstones. Deposition of protoporphyrin in the liver is thought to be the basis for the development of liver disease. Liver function tests are generally normal until shortly before clinical evidence of hepatic disease appears. Jaundice is followed by a downhill course over a period of months. At least 11 deaths from liver failure have been reported in this disease. Jaundice, increased serum transaminase levels, BSP retention, hepatosplenomegaly, hepatic encephalopathy, and portal hypertension with bleeding esophageal varices have been reported during the liver failure of erythrohepatic porphyria.

Some patients have a mild to moderate microcytic and normochromic anemia. Occasionally a mild hemolytic anemia occurs.

Laboratory Findings

Urinary porphyrins and porphyrin precursors are not increased. The 3 patterns of chemical abnormalities seen in patients or their asymptomatic relatives are (I) increased protoporphyrin in erythrocytes, plasma, and feces, (II) increased erythrocyte protoporphyrin with no increase of fecal protoporphyrin, and (III) increased fecal protoporphyrin with no increase of erythrocyte protoporphyrin. Pattern III is unusual and has been seen in some asymptomatic relatives of symptomatic patients; some increase of coproporphyrin occurs with the increased protoporphyrin. The increase of red cell protoporphyrin is usually not accompanied by an increased fecal protoporphyrin excretion and hence pattern II above is the most commonly observed finding in symptomatic patients.

Although morphology of the marrow is normal, there is fluorescence of a variable fraction of normoblasts and circulating red cells. A brown pigment, which has been identified as protoporphyrin, is present in the cytoplasm of hepatocytes, the lysosomes of Kupffer cells, portal histiocytes, and sometimes in bile ducts and canaliculi. Micronodular cirrhosis is seen in some patients. A distinct finding by polarization microscopy is the birefringence of the porphyrin crystals observable as Maltese crosses.

Diagnosis

A history of acute photosensitivity reactions and increased red cell protoporphyrin levels are the most important findings for the diagnosis. Increased erythrocyte protoporphyrin levels occur in other disorders, such as iron deficiency, lead intoxication, and hemolysis, but these do not cause photosensitivity. Since photosensitivity occurs in other conditions, neither acute photosensitivity nor increased erythrocyte protoporphyrin alone is sufficient to prove the diagnosis. If other causes of increased erythrocyte protoporphyrin levels are ruled out, the diagnosis is justified in the presence of the 2 basic findings characteristic of the disease. A positive family history is helpful, but may be negative. If liver disease is evident or suspected, fluorescence and polarization microscopy is valuable in demonstrating protoporphyrin crystals in liver biopsy samples. The most definitive diagnostic test for this disease would be demonstration of decreased tissue levels of ferrochelatase, but this complicated measurement is available only in certain research laboratories at present.

Treatment

Administration of beta-carotene 15 to 180 mg/day orally usually increases tolerance to light, beginning 1 to 2 mo (sometimes 3 mo) after initiation of therapy. Blood levels of 400 to 600 μg/100 ml are usually adequate, but if these do not provide sufficient protection, beta-carotene can be administered in a dose of 180 mg/day for 3 mo before considering this agent a failure. At these doses blood levels are often in the range of 800 μg/100 ml. Some patients have been treated with doses of 250 mg/day without apparent toxicity. This agent can produce skin discoloration, but no serious side effects have been reported in these patients. While beta-carotene can provide protection against photosensitivity, it does not alter the fundamental biochemical abnormalities, since red cell, plasma, and fecal porphyrin levels are unaffected. Although prevention and treatment of liver disease are important considerations in this disorder, experience is limited in treatment and nonexistent in prevention. Both the erythron and liver may be sources of excess protoporphyrin in this disorder. A high carbohydrate intake has been shown to lower fecal protoporphyrin excretion in some patients, presumably by repression of hepatic ALA synthetase. Accumulation of hepatic protoporphyrin may result from flux through the liver of protoporphyrin originating in the erythron, as well as that originating in the liver. The latter component might be decreased by a high carbohydrate intake in patients in whom excess protoporphyrin originates in the liver. Attempts to diminish hepatic protoporphyrin by interrupting its enterohepatic circulation with cholestyramine and by repression of hepatic ALA synthetase using IV hematin are being studied.

ACUTE INTERMITTENT PORPHYRIA

This disease can exist in latent form indefinitely or acute attacks of neurologic dysfunction can be precipitated by various environmental and endogenous factors. It does not produce cutaneous disease.

Etiology, Genetics, and Incidence

The basic enzyme defect in this disease is a 50% decrease of uroporphyrinogen I synthetase (enzyme 3 of the heme biosynthetic pathway). This defect is transmitted by an autosomal dominant mode of inheritance. The manifest disease is more frequent in women and occurs in all races. The prevalence in the USA is estimated to be at least 3 to 4 per 100,000 population.

The disease exists in latent form until an attack of acute neurologic dysfunction is precipitated. Four groups of precipitating factors have been described. These include drugs, starvation, sex hormones, and infection. Some attacks of acute porphyria occur in individuals in whom no exogenous precipitating factor can be found. Drugs that have been implicated in precipitating attacks of acute porphyria include barbiturates, sulfonamides, griseofulvin, phenytoin, methsuximide, chlordiazepoxide, meprobamate, isopropylmeprobamate, dichloralphenazone, glutethimide, amidopyrine, antipyrine, isopropylantipyrine, dipyrone, methprylon, imipramine, ergot preparations, methyldopa, chloramphenicol, chlorpropamide, pentazocine, eucalyptol, and danazol.

Safe and probably safe drugs include morphine, codeine, methadone, hyoscine, chloral hydrate, meperidine, penicillins, streptomycin, tetracyclines, nitrofurantoin, mandelamine, corticosteroids, rauwolfia alkaloids, guanethidine, diphenhydramine, promethazine, promazine, chlorpromazine, trifluoperazine, prochlorperazine, meclizine, digoxin, mersalyl, atropine, prostigmine, neostigmine, tetraethylammonium bromide, propoxyphene, diazepam, ketamine, propanidid, acetylsalicylic acid, ether, nitrous oxide, dicumarol, and propranolol.

Starvation and crash dieting have precipitated attacks of porphyria. In animals a high carbohydrate intake decreases and starvation increases experimental porphyria caused by certain compounds. The effects of diet relate to the ability of glucose and certain other carbohydrates to block the induction of hepatic ALA synthetase.

Female sex hormones have been implicated in precipitating acute attacks of porphyria as evidenced by the facts that (a) biochemical and clinical manifestations almost always occur after puberty, (b) the manifest disease is more frequent in females, and (c) a certain fraction of women with this disease experience a cyclic pattern of recurrent attacks in relation to menstrual periods, often beginning about 3 days before menstruation. Pregnancy has also been implicated in precipitating some attacks of acute porphyria, but probably less than 5% of women with known latent acute intermittent porphyria will experience significant activity of the disease during pregnancy, particularly if they avoid the known precipitating factors.

Both bacterial and viral infections have been followed by acute attacks of porphyria, but the mechanism is unknown.

Symptoms and Signs

Symptoms of the acute attack result from nervous system damage. *Any part of the nervous system can be involved and the specific clinical findings depend on which areas are affected.* **Autonomic neuropathy** is common and causes abdominal pain, which may be mild or severe. The pain may be localized or general and is often accompanied by vomiting and constipation. It may be constant or colicky and may be accompanied by abdominal tenderness. Low grade fever and mild leukocytosis, along with the pain, can suggest a number of other diagnoses. Other autonomic manifestations include labile hypertension, sinus tachycardia, postural hypotension, sweating, and vascular spasm in the retina or skin of the extremities.

Peripheral neuropathy may be sensory or motor. Low back and leg pain may occur as a chronic pain syndrome without other significant neurologic manifestations or it may precede motor neuropathy. Paresthesias are occasionally seen, but sensory neuropathy is usually not accompanied by objective findings. All motor nerves are subject to porphyric neuropathy, which may be asymmetric and may progress at a highly variable rate. Flaccid paralysis may develop within days or weeks.

CNS involvement can produce an organic brain syndrome (hallucinations, coma, etc.), seizures, cerebellar and basal ganglion manifestations, hypothalamic dysfunction, and bulbar paralysis. Respiratory paralysis may require assisted respiration and is associated with a high mortality rate.

During acute attacks some patients develop **hyponatremia**, which may be profound (serum Na less than 100 mEq/L). This may be caused by GI loss of Na, inappropriate release of ADH, and probably primary renal loss of Na. Some patients who have many of the classical findings of inappropriate

ADH release are found to be hypovolemic and probably are experiencing primary renal loss of Na. Thus, hypothalamic pathology may cause hyponatremia, but the other causes should also be considered carefully, since treatment for inappropriate ADH release differs from that for primary Na loss.

The most frequent **psychiatric manifestations** are depression and an organic brain syndrome. In patients who are not experiencing other activity of the disease, it is difficult to estimate the role of porphyria in producing depression.

The outcome of the acute attack can vary through a spectrum from death to complete recovery. Some patients who recover may retain varying types of neurologic deficit.

Laboratory Findings

The characteristic finding of this disease is increased porphyrin precursor excretion in the urine. During asymptomatic periods some patients do not excrete increased amounts of either ALA or PBG, some excrete increased amounts of PBG with no increase of ALA, and others excrete increased amounts of both precursors. During the acute attack, however, all patients excrete increased amounts of PBG. Since the mutation of this disease causes a decrease of the enzyme that converts PBG to uroporphyrinogen, there is no increase of enzymatically produced porphyrins. When urine PBG excretion is high, an increase of urinary uroporphyrin may be evident. This is thought to result from polymerization of PBG, particularly in acid urine.

BSP retention, increased thyroxin-binding globulin, hypercholesterolemia, and hyperbetalipoproteinemia may be found in some patients.

Diagnosis

Abdominal pain of obscure origin, unexplained peripheral neuropathy, or unexplained cerebral lesions should raise the question of an attack of porphyria. Tachycardia, hypertension, dark urine, and a positive family history are further helpful findings. However, the diagnosis of an attack of acute intermittent, variegate, or hereditary coproporphyria cannot be made with certainty unless increased urinary PBG is demonstrated. This can be done by the qualitative Watson-Schwartz or Hoesch tests or by quantitative chromatographic methods, which should always be used to confirm positive qualitative tests. Lead intoxication can be mistaken for acute porphyria and vice versa, but lead intoxication is accompanied by increased ALA excretion without a significant increase in PBG excretion.

Measurement of erythrocyte uroporphyrinogen I synthetase has provided an enzyme test for acute intermittent porphyria. This is useful in detecting the presence of the mutation, but is not capable of distinguishing between the acute attack and asymptomatic periods. Furthermore, while the mean value of the enzyme in a population of patients with acute intermittent porphyria is $1/2$ the mean of a non-porphyric population, there is some overlap in the range of values of the 2 groups, producing a "gray zone" of values, which are not diagnostic.

Differentiation of acute intermittent porphyria from variegate and hereditary coproporphyria is largely academic, since each can produce the same types of neurologic disease. However, the latter 2 disorders can produce cutaneous lesions, which are not seen in acute intermittent porphyria. In addition to the enzyme test, acute intermittent porphyria is distinguished from the other porphyrias by a characteristic pattern of metabolite excretion. Porphyrin precursor excretion is usually, but not always, increased during asymptomatic periods and increases with attacks of acute intermittent porphyria. Although urinary coproporphyrin may be increased, freshly voided urine may not contain increased amounts of uroporphyrin.

There is no major increase of fecal protoporphyrin, as seen in variegate porphyria during both remission and active phases of the disease, and no great increase of fecal coproporphyrin, as usually seen in hereditary coproporphyria.

Treatment

Management involves prevention of attacks, treatment of symptoms, and attempts to reverse the fundamental disease process. Prevention of attacks entails instructing the patient to avoid the known precipitating factors as listed above. An example would be avoidance of sodium thiopental for oral or other surgery. This is very important and could be lifesaving. Other members of the patient's family should also be tested, first by urine measurements and then, if urine tests are negative, by the enzyme test.

Pain control is the first step in the management of symptoms. In some patients, phenothiazines are useful for control of abdominal pain, presumably by their effect on decreasing autonomic outflow. The dose required varies with each patient and should be started at low levels and increased until abdominal pain is controlled. In some patients meperidine is also required. An extrapyramidal syndrome produced by phenothiazines should not be confused with activity of porphyria. Careful analysis of the physiologic mechanism that produces hyponatremia determines the type of treatment for this complication. Propranolol has been useful in treating tachycardia and hypertension. Management of infections and other complications that are not specific for porphyria are discussed elsewhere in this volume.

Of the many methods that have been used in attempts to reverse the basic disease process, only 2 will be discussed. The first involves a high carbohydrate intake of 300 to 400 or more grams/day. Liquid supplements containing sugar are useful. There is a spectrum of responsiveness which varies from a large decrease of porphyrin precursor excretion and dramatic clinical improvement to no significant response biochemically or clinically. The reason for this variation is unknown. Since there is virtually no risk in this treatment, it should be attempted in all patients experiencing an acute attack. A second approach currently under study is IV hematin administration (3 mg/kg given once a day over 20 min). This lowers porphyrin precursor excretion and appears promising clinically. At the above dose no clinically significant toxicity has been seen (except for occasional venous irritation), but at much higher doses, reversible anuria has occurred. In women experiencing regular cyclic attacks related to menstrual periods, oral contraceptives (given cyclically) have been valuable in preventing the attacks. Some of the new preparations are too low in estrogen content and require additional estrogen supplements. Experience with the cyclic pattern of attacks is limited and patients suffering from them must be carefully supervised. Patients who do not have the cyclic pattern of attacks should not receive hormone therapy.

VARIEGATE PORPHYRIA

This disease is identical to acute intermittent porphyria but can also produce cutaneous disease on exposed portions of the body.

Etiology, Genetics, and Incidence

Although there have been claims of decreased ferrochelatase activity in this disease, recent studies show a decrease of protoporphyrinogen oxidase as the fundamental defect. Variegate porphyria is transmitted as an autosomal dominant disorder. It probably has a lower prevalence than acute intermittent porphyria in the USA, but in South Africa it has been estimated at 300 per 100,000 in the white population.

Symptoms and Signs

This disease can produce neurologic and cutaneous disease, either simultaneously or separately. The skin lesions resemble those of porphyria cutanea tarda (see below). There may be bullae, erosions, scarring, and pigmentation involving skin that is exposed to light. Acute photosensitivity is uncommon, and increased skin fragility is of much greater significance. Hypertrichosis may be evident. The acute attack of neurologic dysfunction is similar to that of acute intermittent porphyria described above.

Laboratory Findings

Fecal protoporphyrin is increased during both asymptomatic periods and acute attacks of neurologic disease. Porphyrin precursor excretion is often normal or slightly increased during asymptomatic periods, but increases during acute attacks. Increased urinary PBG can be detected by the Watson-Schwartz or Hoesch tests, but should be confirmed by a quantitative determination. Urine uroporphyrin and coproporphyrin are increased, with coproporphyrin usually exceeding uroporphyrin during asymptomatic periods. During acute attacks, uroporphyrin increases and usually exceeds coproporphyrin.

Diagnosis

The differential diagnosis of the acute attack (in which increased PBG excretion must be demonstrated) is the same as that for acute intermittent porphyria. If typical skin lesions on the exposed portions of the body are or have been present, a diagnosis of variegate porphyria should be considered. Increased fecal protoporphyrin excretion must be demonstrated along with the characteristic urinary findings before the diagnosis is certain. Although the enzyme defect has been demonstrated in cultured fibroblasts, no practical diagnostic enzyme test is available at present.

Treatment

The acute attack is treated as described for acute intermittent porphyria. Whether carotenoid therapy, as described in the treatment of erythropoietic protoporphyria, will prove useful in managing the cutaneous problems of variegate porphyria is not yet known.

HEREDITARY COPROPORPHYRIA

Etiology, Genetics, and Incidence

A decrease of about 50% of coproporphyrinogen oxidase activity is the fundamental defect in this disease. It is transmitted as an autosomal dominant disorder. The incidence is unknown, but data on at least 111 cases have been reported by one author.

Symptoms and Signs

The disease can produce neurologic dysfunction as in acute intermittent porphyria, and also can cause photosensitivity, which usually does not extend beyond the acute attack.

Laboratory Findings

During asymptomatic periods the urine may be normal or there may be an increase of urinary coproporphyrin. Fecal coproporphyrin is increased during both symptomatic and asymptomatic periods. During acute attacks porphyrin precursor excretion is increased.

Diagnosis and Treatment

Findings are similar to those of acute intermittent porphyria. The diagnosis of an acute attack must be substantiated by demonstration of increased urinary PBG. A positive Watson-Schwartz or Hoesch test should be confirmed by quantitative determination of urinary PBG. The high fecal coproporphyrin excretion differentiates this disease from acute intermittent porphyria. It is not known whether treatment of photosensitivity by beta-carotene, as described for erythropoietic protoporphyria, will be successful in this disease. **Treatment** of the acute attack is the same as in acute intermittent porphyria.

PORPHYRIA CUTANEA TARDA

This disease produces cutaneous lesions on exposed portions of the body, but no neurologic disease. Liver disease occurs in some patients.

Etiology, Genetics, and Incidence

The basic defect is a decrease of uroporphyrinogen decarboxylase activity, which is transmitted as an autosomal dominant defect. The prevalence is not known, but the disease is probably as common or more common than acute intermittent porphyria.

The factors that can activate this disease are alcohol, excess iron intake, and estrogen or oral contraceptives. Iron overload appears to be a major activating factor. This disease was formerly very uncommon in menstruating women, but as ingestion of all of the above precipitating factors increases, a number of young menstruating women are now victims of the active disease. In men, most cases occur after age 35. The effect of estrogen in men is seen in the number of cases of porphyria cutanea tarda that are reported in men receiving estrogen for carcinoma of the prostate.

Symptoms and Signs

The cutaneous manifestations begin as areas of erythema with vesicles or bullae that occur on exposed portions of the body, usually following minor trauma. Crusts and scabs develop, followed by scarring. Hirsutism, areas of pigmentation and depigmentation, and sclerodermoid changes may be evident as chronic lesions. The vesicles and bullae are usually most evident in sunny weather, particularly in late summer and autumn. Acute photosensitivity reactions are not common in this disease. In severe untreated cases, disfiguring changes can occur in the ears, nose, and fingers.

Liver disease is present in many patients with porphyria cutanea tarda. Histologically, the most frequent findings are siderosis and evidence of recurring liver damage. Some patients have frank cirrhosis. Liver fluorescence may be demonstrable. Chloroquine produces a reaction in this disease that can include fever, headache, malaise, abdominal pain, vomiting, and red urine. The latter results from a great increase of uroporphyrin excretion.

Laboratory Findings

Urinary uroporphyrin is considerably increased. Coproporphyrin is also increased in the urine, but usually not to the level seen with uroporphyrin. Some increase of ALA may occur, but there is no increase of PBG excretion. Porphyrins with 7, 6, and 5 carboxyl groups are also demonstrable in the urine. In recent years a group of tetracarboxylated porphyrins, the isocoproporphyrins, have been demonstrated in the feces in this disorder. In some patients there is an increase of serum iron and abnormal liver function tests.

Diagnosis

Vesicles, bullae, erosions, crusting, and chronic changes on exposed portions of the skin should raise the possibility of porphyria cutanea tarda. The skin lesions cannot be distinguished clinically from those of variegate porphyria. A high urinary uroporphyrin (which usually exceeds coproporphyrin) is present in porphyria cutanea tarda, and levels in this disease (untreated) are usually higher than the urinary uroporphyrin levels in patients with only cutaneous manifestations of variegate porphyria (where coproporphyrin often exceeds uroporphyrin). Because treatment and prophylaxis of these diseases are different, it is important to make the distinction between them. Variegate porphyria is accompanied by a high fecal protoporphyrin, which is not seen in porphyria cutanea tarda. Increased urinary PBG rules out porphyria cutanea tarda, but a slight increase of ALA does not. Two other measurements are specific for porphyria cutanea tarda, but are not yet widely available. These are decreased erythrocyte uroporphyrinogen decarboxylase and increased fecal isocoproporphyrin.

Treatment

The disease responds clinically and biochemically to iron removal by means of phlebotomy. If there are no contraindications to phlebotomy, 300 to 500 ml blood can be removed about every 3 wk while Hb and urine porphyrin levels are monitored. If Hb decreases to < 11 gm%, phlebotomy is stopped until the level increases. Phlebotomy is then continued until urine uroporphyrin excretion is < 500 to 600 μg/day. In one study the mean amount of blood that had to be removed in order to produce a remission was 6.8 L (range: 2 to 14 L). Remissions usually last for years and recurrences can be retreated.

Since chloroquine can mobilize tissue porphyrins, it has been used to treat this disease. Only low doses can be used (125 mg twice a week) over a long time period (8 to 18 mo) because of the acute reaction to chloroquine described above. Occasionally, after a year of the above drug therapy, the dosage must be doubled to 250 mg twice a week, in order to achieve a remission. Phlebotomy is quicker in producing a remission and is the preferred method of treatment. Patients should be urged to avoid the precipitating factors mentioned above.

ANOMALIES IN AMINO ACID METABOLISM

Anomalies of amino acid metabolism may be categorized as those of transport and those of catabolism. Both are genetically determined. Although the latter are usually considered the only true metabolic anomalies, defects in amino acid transport in the renal tubule or GI mucosa are also metabolic, since they are caused by enzyme defects. Abnormalities in plasma levels of various metabolites occur in the catabolic group, but are absent in the transport group. Newly discovered entities and recognition of variations in many of the original or classic types are leading to the definition of increasing numbers of catabolic disorders.

The salient features of catabolic amino acid metabolic diseases are listed in TABLE 82-3. Phenylketonuria as a prototype is discussed in greater detail below, since it was the first of the group to be described and is the commonest.

PHENYLKETONURIA (PKU; Phenylalaninemia; Phenylpyruvic Oligophrenia)

An inborn error of metabolism, characterized by a virtual absence of phenylalanine hydroxylase activity and an elevation of plasma phenylalanine, that frequently results in mental retardation.

Etiology and Incidence

Excess phenylalanine, an essential amino acid, is normally eliminated from the body by hydroxylation to tyrosine. The enzyme **phenylalanine hydroxylase** is essential for this reaction. If it is inactive, phenylalanine accumulates in the blood and is excreted in excess in the urine; some is transaminated to phenylpyruvic acid, which may be further metabolized to phenylacetic, phenyllactic, and o-hydroxyphenylacetic acids; all are excreted in the urine. The exact etiology of the mental retardation is not known, but it is the consequence of the biochemical defect. This enzyme defect, transmitted as an autosomal recessive trait, is found in most population groups but is rare in Ashkenazi Jews and in blacks. Incidence in the USA of the typical variety is approximately 1:16,000 live births.

Clinical Features

Clinical symptoms of PKU are usually absent in the newborn period, hence *laboratory screening tests are mandatory for its detection.* Rarely, an infant may be lethargic or may feed poorly. Mental retardation is the most important symptom; the majority of untreated patients manifest some degree of mental retardation, usually severe. They tend to have lighter colored skin, hair, and eyes than unaffected family members. Some infants may have a rash similar to infantile eczema.

Many neurologic symptoms and signs, especially affecting reflexes, occur. Both petit and grand mal seizures are common in older children, and the incidence of abnormal EEGs is 75 to 90%. Children manifest extreme hyperactivity and psychotic states, and often exhibit an unpleasant "mousy" body odor which is caused by phenylacetic acid in the urine and sweat.

Diagnosis

Early diagnosis depends on detecting a high plasma phenylalanine level together with a normal or low plasma tyrosine. The exact plasma level which serves as a cut-off point between classic PKU and the variants of this disease cannot be fixed, although 20 mg/100 ml (1.2 mM/L) has been proposed. Better methods of differentiation are required.

After the newborn has consumed a moderate amount of milk (the source of phenylalanine) for at least 48 h, he should be screened for PKU. The **Guthrie inhibition assay test** is usually used. A strain of phenylalanine-dependent *Bacillus subtilis* is cultured in a medium on which is placed a filter paper disc impregnated with several drops of capillary blood and other discs containing varying amounts of phenylalanine (controls). The zone of growth around the disc containing the blood sample is proportional to the phenylalanine content. After 4 to 6 wk of age, abnormal levels of phenylalanine metabolites may appear in the urine, including phenylpyruvic acid, phenyllactic acid, phenylacetic acid, and o-hydroxyphenylacetic acid. **Another screening test** involves the addition of a few drops of 10% ferric chloride solution to a urine sample or wet diaper (a paper test strip is commercially available). A deep bluish green color indicates the presence of phenylpyruvic acid in the urine. Urine testing is done *after* the neonatal period and should be repeated at regular intervals for 1 yr if the infant has a family history of PKU. The results of all screening must be confirmed by more exact tests using fluorimetric methods or ion exchange column chromatography.

Variants

Screening programs have detected a number of infants with abnormally high phenylalanine levels. In many, the finding is secondary to neonatal (developmental) tyrosinemia, which can be distinguished by abnormal plasma tyrosine levels. The remaining cases can be divided into classic PKU and mild and severe forms of "**hyperphenylalaninemia.**" Mild forms usually exhibit plasma levels of below 8 to 10 mg/100 ml while on a normal diet; the severe forms are associated with greater elevations. The distinction between severe hyperphenylalaninemia and classic PKU cannot be made by plasma phenylalanine measurements alone. Exact differentiation requires assay of liver phenylalanine hydroxylase activity, which is virtually absent in classic PKU and present in amounts varying from 5 to 15% of normal in the hyperphenylalaninemias. The liver is normally the only place where measurable quantities of phenylalanine hydroxylase may be found.

No sequelae to the mild variants are expected. The consequences of the more severe forms are not known and these patients should be treated the same as those with classic PKU until more information is available.

TABLE 82-3. ANOMALIES IN AMINO ACID METABOLISM

Disease	Amino Acid Affected	Enzyme Defect	Clinical Features	Treatment
Phenylketonuria	Phenylalanine	Phenylalanine hydroxylase	Neurologic symptoms; mental retardation	Controlled phenylalanine intake
Tyrosinosis (Medes)	Tyrosine	Tyrosine α-ketoglutarate aminotransferase (?)	One reported case, probably benign	
Tyrosinemia	Tyrosine	Tyrosine aminotransferase	Mental retardation, keratitis, dermatitis	Controlled phenylalanine and tyrosine intake
Tyrosinemia	Tyrosine and methionine	p-Hydroxyphenylpyruvic acid hydroxylase—may be secondary to another defect	Fanconi's syndrome, hepatic cirrhosis, fulminating hepatic failure	Controlled phenylalanine, tyrosine, and methionine intake
Albinism	Tyrosine	Tyrosinase	Absent pigment in skin, hair, eyes	Protection of skin & eyes from actinic radiation
Alkaptonuria	Tyrosine	Homogentisic oxidase	Arthritis, dark urine	
Histidinemia Classic	Histidine	L-Histidine ammonia lyase (liver and skin)	Retardation, neurologic manifestations; frequently benign	Low-protein diet, controlled histidine intake
Variant	Histidine	L-Histidine ammonia lyase (liver only)	As above	As above
Maple syrup urine disease (branched chain ketoaciduria) Classic	Leucine Isoleucine Valine Alloisoleucine	Branched chain keto-acid decarboxylase	Reflex changes, hypertonicity, odor of urine and perspiration, convulsions, coma, death	Controlled intake of branched chain amino acids, exchange transfusion and peritoneal dialysis for acute episodes
Intermittent	Same	Same, but some activity	Symptoms only with stress (fever, infection)	Same for acute episodes, none necessary between episodes
Intermediate	Same	Degree of activity between classic and intermittent	Retardation, neurologic symptoms; full-blown picture develops with stress	Protein intake limited to requirement
Thiamine-responsive	Same	Same, presumably cofactor deficiency	Similar to mild picture of intermediate	Thiamine—large doses
Valinemia	Valine	Valine aminotransferase	Retardation	Controlled valine intake

Isovaleric acidemia	Leucine	Isovaleryl CoA dehydrogenase	Vomiting, lethargy, acidosis, retardation, odor of sweaty feet, neonatal death	Controlled leucine intake; glycine
β-Hydroxyisovaleric aciduria	Leucine	β-Methylcrotonyl-CoA carboxylase	Retardation, muscle atrophy, unpleasant urine odor	Controlled leucine intake
α-Methylacetoacetate accumulation	Isoleucine	Acetyl-CoA thialase (?)	Episodes of acidosis, coma; retardation	Low-protein diet, controlled isoleucine intake
Homocystinemia	Methionine	Cystathionine synthetase (1) Pyridoxine-responsive (2) Non-pyridoxine-responsive	Skeletal abnormalities, ectopia lentis, retardation, thromboembolic disease	(1) Massive doses of pyridoxine (2) Controlled intake of methionine and cystine supplementation, also folic acid supplementation
Cystinosis	Cystine	Unknown	Cystine accumulation throughout RE system, WBC, cornea; Fanconi's syndrome, renal failure	Symptomatic for Fanconi's syndrome; renal transplant for failure
Cystathioninemia	Methionine	Cystathionase	Retardation (?), large number of individuals have no clinical symptoms—benign trait	Large doses of pyridoxine
Glycinemia (non-ketotic)	Glycine	Glycine cleavage enzyme system	Convulsions, retardation	Low-protein diet, strychnine (?)
Methylmalonic acidemia (form of ketotic glycinemia)	Isoleucine Valine Threonine Methionine	Methylmalonyl-CoA mutase (1) Apoenzyme deficiency (2) Vitamin B_{12} cofactor deficiency	Acidosis, lethargy, coma, mental and physical retardation	(1) Low-protein diet, controlled isoleucine, valine, threonine intake (2) Massive doses of vitamin B_{12}
	Same	Methylmalonyl-CoA racemase	Same	Same as (1) above
Propionicacidemia (form of ketotic glycinemia)	Threonine Isoleucine Methionine	Propionyl-CoA carboxylase (1) Apoenzyme deficiency (2) Coenzyme deficiency	Acidosis, lethargy, coma, mental and physical retardation	(1) Low-protein diet, controlled intake of threonine, isoleucine, and methionine (2) Large doses of biotin
Sarcosinemia	Sarcosine	Sarcosine dehydrogenase	Mental retardation (?), no symptoms	May be benign trait, no treatment indicated

(Continued)

TABLE 82-3. ANOMALIES IN AMINO ACID METABOLISM (Cont'd)

Disease	Amino Acid Affected	Enzyme Defect	Clinical Features	Treatment
β-Alaninemia	β-Alanine	β-Alanine-α-ketoglutarate amino transferase	Seizures, somnolence, death	Pyridoxine (?)
Prolinemia, Type I	Proline	Proline oxidase	Hereditary nephritis, nerve deafness (?)	May be benign trait
Prolinemia, Type II	Proline	Δ¹Pyrroline-5-carboxylate dehydrogenase	Convulsions, mental retardation	Low-protein diet, low proline & glutamic acid
Hydroxyprolinemia	Hydroxyproline	Hydroxyproline oxidase	Mental retardation, CNS symptoms	Low-protein diet (?) Benign (?)
Lysinemia	Lysine	Lysine-ketoglutarate reductase	Muscle weakness, retardation, benign in some instances	Controlled lysine intake (?)
Lysine intolerance	Lysine Arginine	Lysine: NAD oxidoreductase (deaminating)	Vomiting, coma	Low-protein diet, controlled lysine intake
Saccharopinuria	Lysine	Aminoadipic semialdehyde – glutamate reductase	Retardation	Controlled lysine intake
Pipecolicacidemia	Lysine	Pipecolate oxidase	Retardation	Controlled lysine intake
Hyperammonemia Type I	Ammonia	Carbamylphosphate synthetase	Vomiting, lethargy, acidosis, death	Low-protein diet; essential amino acid mixture, ketoacid analogs of amino acids; arginine
Hyperammonemia Type II	Ammonia	Ornithine transcarbamylase	Recurrent vomiting, irritability, lethargy, coma, seizures, X-linked, lethal in the male	Low-protein diet; essential amino acid mixture, ketoacid analogs of amino acids; arginine
Ornithinemia	Ornithine	Ornithine keto-acid transaminase	Gyrate atrophy of choroid & retina	Low-protein diet (?)

	Ornithine Ammonia Homocitrulline	Transport defect into mitochondria (?)	Seizures, retardation	Low-protein diet
Syndrome of hyperornithinemia, hyperammonemia, & homocitrullinemia				
Citrullinemia	Citrulline	Argininosuccinic acid synthetase	Vomiting, coma, convulsions	Low-protein diet; essential amino acid mixture, ketoacid analogs of amino acids; arginine
Argininosuccinic-acidemia	Argininosuccinic acid	Argininosuccinase	Seizures, retardation	Low-protein diet; essential amino acid mixture, ketoacid analogs of amino acids; arginine
Argininemia	Arginine	Arginase	Retardation, seizures, spasticity	Low-protein diet; essential amino acid mixture, ketoacid analogs of amino acids
Glutamicacidemia	Glutamic acid	?	Mental and physical retardation, seizures, trichorrhexis nodosa	?
Pyroglutamic acidemia	Pyroglutamic acid	?	Episodic vomiting, retardation	?

Elevated plasma phenylalanine levels may also occur as a result of **tetrahydrobiopterin deficiency.** Dietary therapy can correct the abnormal plasma phenylalanine level but severe neurologic deterioration continues. This occurs because tetrahydrobiopterin is a cofactor in the synthesis of dopamine, norepinephrine, and serotonin; deficiency of these neurotransmitters may account for the neurologic symptoms. Tetrahydrobiopterin deficiency may occur either as a result of a defect in the synthesis of biopterin or a deficiency of dihydropteridine reductase, which reduces biopterin to its active form, tetrahydrobiopterin. Substitution therapy with levodopa, carbidopa, and 5-OH tryptophan, in addition to dietary treatment, may have a beneficial effect on these variants if started early in life.

Treatment

Treatment consists in limiting the phenylalanine intake of the child so that his essential amino acid requirement is met but not exceeded. This allows normal growth and development but prevents accumulation in the body of phenylalanine and its abnormal end products. Monitoring of the child and his plasma phenylalanine levels is required. Since all natural protein contains about 4% phenylalanine, it is impossible to satisfy the protein requirement without exceeding the phenylalanine requirement. Hence, casein hydrolysates (treated to remove the phenylalanine) or mixtures of amino acids should constitute the protein moiety of the diet. Lofenalac®, a widely used product in the USA, is a complete food except for its phenylalanine content and is used in place of the usual milk in the diet. Low-protein natural foods, such as fruits, vegetables, certain cereals, etc., are allowed. The phenylalanine requirement is supplied by measured quantities of natural protein and the residual phenylalanine content of Lofenalac® (80 mg/100 gm of dry powder). The requirement in terms of body wt decreases with age; it varies from 60 to 90 mg/kg/day during the first months of life and decreases to 20 to 30 mg/kg/day by the end of the first year. A new dietary product, completely free of phenylalanine, is now available in the USA (Mead Johnson Phenyl-free).

Treatment must be initiated during the first days of life to prevent mental retardation. Treatment started after 2 to 3 yr of age may be effective only in controlling the extreme hyperactivity and intractable seizures. The length of time that treatment must be continued is unknown. Some clinicians believe that it must be continued for life; others think that it may be terminated when myelinization of the brain is virtually complete, at about 5 yr of age.

Prognosis

With untreated PKU, prognosis, while not life-threatening, is poor for intellectual development. Early and well-maintained treatment makes normal development possible and prevents CNS involvement.

ANOMALIES IN CARBOHYDRATE METABOLISM

(See Ch. 90 in this volume and Vol. II, Ch. 25)

ANOMALIES IN LIPID METABOLISM

Abnormal levels of blood or tissue lipids resulting from metabolic disorders which may be inborn or due to endocrinopathy, specific organ failure, or external causes.

HYPERLIPOPROTEINEMIA (Hyperlipidemia)

The major plasma lipids, including cholesterol and the triglycerides, do not circulate free in solution in the plasma, but are bound to proteins and transported as macromolecular complexes called lipoproteins. The major lipoprotein families— chylomicrons, very low-density (prebeta) lipoproteins **(VLDL)**, low-density (β-) lipoproteins **(LDL)**, and high-density (α-) lipoproteins **(HDL)**—although closely interrelated, usually are classified operationally in terms of their physicochemical properties, such as electrophoretic mobility, or density when separated in the ultracentrifuge. Triglycerides are the major lipids transported through the blood. Between 70 and 150 gm of triglycerides enter and leave the plasma each day as compared to 1 to 2 gm of cholesterol or phospholipid. Chylomicrons, the largest lipoproteins, carry exogenous glyceride from the intestine via the thoracic duct to the venous system. In the capillaries of adipose tissue and muscle, 90% of chylomicron glyceride is removed by a specific group of lipases. Fatty acids and glycerol, derived from hydrolysis of chylomicrons, enter the cells for energy utilization or storage. The remnant chylomicron particles are then removed by the liver. VLDL carry endogenous glyceride primarily from the liver to the same peripheral sites for storage or utilization and are quickly degraded by lipases similar to those that act on chylomicrons. This endogenous VLDL rapidly becomes a lipoprotein intermediate shorn of much of its glyceride and surface apoproteins. Within 2 to 6 h this lipoprotein intermediate is degraded further through the removal of more glyceride to LDL which, in turn, has a plasma half-life of 3 to 4 days. VLDL is the main source of plasma LDL. The fate of LDL is unclear, but active receptor sites that specifically bind LDL and thereby remove it from the circulation have been found on the surface of fibroblasts and other cells.

Normal Levels of Serum Cholesterol and Triglycerides

It is difficult to define the normal level of serum cholesterol, since prospective studies have shown that the incidence of coronary heart disease rises in linear fashion with the level of serum cholesterol, and values that are generally accepted as within normal ranges in the USA are higher than those found among comparable individuals in populations with a low incidence of atherosclerosis.

The optimal serum cholesterol for the middle-aged American man is probably 200 mg/100 ml, or less. For practical purposes hypercholesterolemia is defined as a value above the 95th percentile for the population, which in Americans ranges from 230 mg/100 ml in individuals < 20 yr old, to > 300 in individuals > 60 yr old. However, these limits are clearly excessive because of the known cardiovascular risk of cholesterol values at these levels, and a convenient rule of thumb is that any level of serum cholesterol > 200 mg/100 ml plus the person's age should be considered abnormal. Even these limits may be too high. In contrast to serum cholesterol, it is not clear that serum triglycerides are independent risk variables. Triglyceride levels, like cholesterol, do vary with age and it is reasonable to consider that a serum triglyceride concentration of > 250 mg/100 ml is abnormal.

As indicated below, even more information can be obtained about coronary risk by viewing the plasma cholesterol in terms of the units of lipid transport—the lipoproteins—than by a simple measurement of total cholesterol. Sixty to 75% of total plasma cholesterol is transported on LDL, the levels of which are directly related to cardiovascular risk. HDL, which normally accounts for 20 to 25% of the total plasma cholesterol, is inversely associated with cardiovascular risk. HDL levels are positively correlated with exercise and moderate alcohol intake and inversely related to smoking, obesity and the use of progestin-containing contraceptives.

Studies show CHD prevalence at HDL levels of 30 mg/100 ml to be more than double that at 60 mg/100 ml and familial excesses of HDL or deficiency of LDL have been associated with decreased CHD risk. These findings provide a cogent reason to determine whether elevated cholesterol levels are due to increases in LDL or the "benevolent" HDL.

Laboratory Methods

Serum cholesterol may be determined by colorimetric, gas-liquid chromatographic, or enzymatic methods. Other automated "direct" methods have been developed.

The serum triglyceride concentration usually is measured by determining the glycerol content either colorimetrically, enzymatically, or fluorometrically by way of its conversion to formaldehyde.

Lipoprotein electrophoresis is only useful where hyperlipidemia exists and should be accompanied by measurement of serum triglyceride and cholesterol values. It is not a screening test and should be done only if triglycerides or cholesterol are elevated or abnormally low.

Translating Hyperlipidemia to Hyperlipoproteinemia

Hyperlipidemia is the sign of a heterogeneous group of disorders differing in clinical features, prognosis, and response to therapy. Sufficient elevation in the concentration of any of the lipoproteins can result in hypercholesterolemia. Similarly, hypertriglyceridemia may result from increased concentrations of chylomicrons or VLDL alone or in combination. This lack of specificity makes translation of hyperlipidemia into hyperlipoproteinemia (HLP) useful. Table 82–4 describes 5 types of hyperlipoproteinemia. Each represents a shorthand or jargon term for the lipoproteins increased in the plasma. Since each of the lipoprotein families has a relatively fixed composition with respect to cholesterol and triglycerides, and since the 2 largest (chylomicrons and VLDL) refract light and cause plasma turbidity, defining hyperlipoproteinemia usually can be done simply by observation of standing plasma (24 h storage at 4 C) and by an accurate cholesterol and triglyceride determination. Electrophoresis usually is not required for the translation of hyperlipidemia into HLP.

Defining the lipoprotein pattern does not conclude the diagnostic process, since no HLP can be regarded as unique. Each may be *secondary* to other disorders that must be ruled out, such as hypothyroidism, alcoholism, and renal disease, or may be *primary*, in which case family screening should be performed. Primary HLP may be familial, and family screening often leads to identification of other (often asymptomatic) hyperlipoproteinemic subjects.

If measurement of lipid or lipoprotein levels is to be useful, one must be aware of the following: (1) The concentrations of lipids and lipoproteins increase with age. A value acceptable for a middle-aged adult might be alarmingly high in a child of 10. (2) Chylomicrons normally appear in the blood 2 to 10 h after a meal; a fasting specimen (12 to 16 h) should therefore be used. (3) Lipoprotein concentrations are under dynamic metabolic control and are readily affected by diet, illness, drugs, and weight change. Samples for lipid analysis should be taken during a steady state. If abnormal, at least 2 confirmatory samples should be taken before selecting therapy (always dietary first). (4) When HLP is secondary to another disorder, treatment of that disorder usually will correct the HLP.

Type I Hyperlipoproteinemia (Exogenous Hypertriglyceridemia; Familial "Fat-Induced" Lipemia; Hyperchylomicronemia)

A relatively rare disorder due to either a congenital deficiency of lipoprotein lipase (LPL) activity or the congenital absence of the lipase activating protein apolipoprotein C-II. In both cases the ability to remove or "clear" chylomicrons from the blood is impaired.

TABLE 82–4. CHARACTERISTICS OF

Type	Other Names	Genetic Form	Plasma Cholesterol Level	Plasma Triglyceride Level
I	Exogenous hypertriglyceridemia Familial hyperglyceridemia Familial chylomicronemia Fat-induced hyperlipidemia Hyperchylomicronemia	Autosomal recessive; rare	Normal or slightly increased	Very greatly increased
II	Familial hypercholesterolemia Familial hyperbetalipo- proteinemia Familial hypercholesterolemic xanthomatosis	Autosomal dominant; common	Greatly increased	(a) Normal (b) Slightly increased
III	Broad beta disease Familial dysbetalipoproteinemia Floating betalipoproteinemia	Mode of inheritance unclear; uncommon but not rare	Greatly increased	Greatly increased
IV	Endogenous hypertri- glyceridemia Familial hyperprebetalipo- proteinemia Carbohydrate-induced triglyceridemia	Common, often sporadic when familial; genetically heterogeneous	Normal or slightly increased	Greatly increased
V	Mixed hypertriglyceridemia Combined exogenous and endogenous hypertri- glyceridemia Mixed hyperlipemia	Uncommon but not rare; genetically heterogeneous	Normal or slightly increased	Very greatly increased

Symptoms, Signs, and Diagnosis

This disease is manifested in children or young adults by pancreatitis-like abdominal pains; pinkish-yellow papular cutaneous deposits of fat (eruptive xanthomas), especially over pressure points and extensor surfaces; lipemia retinalis; and hepatosplenomegaly.

Symptoms and signs are exacerbated by increased amounts of dietary (exogenous) fat, which accumulates in the circulation as chylomicrons, sometimes reaching spectacular triglyceride levels and causing marked lactescence. Chylomicrons not only refract light and produce lactescence but also cream up on standing overnight in the cold. A cream layer overlying an otherwise clear plasma is often diagnostic, as is the failure of the lipoprotein lipase activity to increase after injection of IV heparin (**PHLA**, post-heparin lipolytic activity).

Prognosis

Pancreatitis is the principal sequela. Recurrent bouts of abdominal pain during periods of fat indulgence may be marked by episodes of severe and sometimes fatal hemorrhagic pancreatitis. Avoidance of dietary fat will prevent serious sequelae and allow for an otherwise normal life. There is no evidence that this form of HLP predisposes to atherosclerosis.

Treatment

The goal is reduction of circulating chylomicrons to avoid episodes of acute abdominal pain and pancreatitis. A diet markedly restricted in all common sources of fat is effective. Caloric supplementation can be offered and diet palatability enhanced by using 20 to 40 gm of medium chain triglycerides (**MCT**)/day. These fatty acids (C_{12} or less) are not transported via chylomicron formation but are bound to albumin and pass directly through the portal system to the liver.

THE PRIMARY HYPERLIPOPROTEINEMIAS

Risk Factor in Atherosclerosis	Major Secondary Causes	Clinical Presentation	Treatment
Risk not apparently increased	SLE; dysgamma globulinemia; insulinopenic diabetes mellitus	Pancreatitis Eruptive xanthomas Hepatosplenomegaly Lipemia retinalis	Dietary: low intake of fat; no alcohol; weight reduction
Very strong risk factor, especially for coronary atherosclerosis	Excess dietary cholesterol; hypothyroidism; nephrosis; multiple myeloma; porphyria; obstructive liver disease	Accelerated atherosclerosis Xanthelasma Tendon and tuberous xanthomas Juvenile corneal arcus	Dietary: low-cholesterol, low-fat diet consisting mainly of polyunsaturated fats Drugs: cholestyramine; colestipol; niacin; probucol Possible surgery
Very strong risk factor for atherosclerosis, especially in peripheral circulation	Dysgamma-globulinemia; hypothyroidism	Accelerated atherosclerosis of coronary and peripheral vessels Planar xanthomas Tuboeruptive and tendon xanthomas	Dietary: reduction to ideal weight; maintenance of low-cholesterol, balanced diet Drugs: clofibrate; niacin
Probable risk factor, especially for coronary atherosclerosis	Excess alcohol consumption; oral contraceptives; diabetes mellitus; glycogen storage disease; pregnancy; nephrotic syndrome; stress	Possible accelerated atherosclerosis Glucose intolerance Hyperuricemia	Weight reduction; low-carbohydrate diet; no alcohol Drugs; niacin
Risk of athero-sclerosis not clearly increased	Alcoholism; insulin-dependent diabetes mellitus; nephrosis; dysgamma-globulinemia	Pancreatitis Eruptive xanthomas Hepatosplenomegaly Sensory neuropathy Lipemia retinalis Hyperuricemia Glucose intolerance	Weight reduction; low-fat diet; no alcohol Drugs: niacin

TYPE II HYPERLIPOPROTEINEMIA (Familial Hypercholesterolemia; Hyperbetalipoproteinemia; Familial Hypercholesterolemic Xanthomatosis)

A genetic disorder of lipid metabolism characterized by an elevated serum cholesterol in association with xanthelasma, tendon and tuberous xanthomas, arcus juvenilis, accelerated atherosclerosis, and early death from myocardial infarction. This disorder occurs most frequently with a familial distribution in the pattern of a dominant gene with complete penetrance. It appears to be caused by absent or defective LDL cell receptors resulting in delayed LDL clearance, increased levels of plasma LDL, and accumulation of LDL over joints, pressure points, and in blood vessels.

Symptoms, Signs, and Diagnosis

The patient may be asymptomatic or any of the aforementioned manifestations may be present. Xanthomas are usually in the Achilles, patellar, and digital extensor tendons. Sometimes a family history of premature coronary heart disease (before age 55) is present.

The serum cholesterol elevation in the presumed heterozygote may be as much as 2 to 3 times normal, all secondary to increased LDL. The plasma is usually translucent and triglyceride levels normal, since LDL does not refract light, regardless of its concentration. In the rare presumed homozygote with this disorder, cholesterol levels of 500 to 1200 mg/100 ml occur and are usually associated with xanthomas before age 10. A normal free cholesterol to cholesterol ester ratio and phospholipid level differentiate this disorder from the marked hypercholesterolemia (with clear plasma) seen in obstructive liver disease (see below and in CHOLESTASIS in Ch. 64).

Prognosis

The incidence of xanthomas and other external stigmas will increase with each decade in the presumed heterozygote with this disorder. Sometimes, especially in females, an Achilles tendonitis will recur. Atherosclerosis, especially of the coronary vessels, is markedly accelerated, particularly in males. One of 6 Type II males will have had a heart attack by age 40, and by age 60 the ratio increases to 2 of 3. Homozygotes with this disorder may develop and succumb to coronary atherosclerosis and its sequelae before age 20.

Treatment

With effective cholesterol lowering, an unsightly xanthoma will cease growing and regress or disappear. The major reason these patients are subjected to cholesterol-lowering drugs and diets is not cosmetic, but rather the presumption that therapy will decelerate the premature development of atherosclerosis and lessen the likelihood of an acute myocardial infarction.

The most effective dietary means of lowering serum LDL levels and hence cholesterol has been strict avoidance of foods containing cholesterol and saturated fatty acids. Meat (especially organ meats and obvious fat), eggs, whole milk, cream, butter, lard, and other saturated cooking fats are eliminated and replaced with foods low in saturated fat and cholesterol (e.g., fish, vegetables, poultry) and supplemented when necessary with polyunsaturated oils and margarines.

Cholestyramine and colestipol, bile acid sequestrants, effectively lower serum cholesterol, especially when coupled with diet. A dosage of 12 to 32 gm in 2 to 4 divided daily doses will lower LDL levels (by increasing LDL removal) by 25 to 50%. In some instances sequestrants are associated with side effects, such as constipation and unpalatability, that may limit general patient acceptance. Niacin may also be useful in Type II HLP, but the high dosage required (3 to 9 gm/day in divided doses with meals) coupled with its side effects of gastric irritability, hyperuricemia, hyperglycemia, flushing, and pruritus, restricts its general use. Niacin is most effective when combined with cholestyramine in the Type II homozygote or severe heterozygote. Probucol 500 mg b.i.d. may lower LDL levels 10 to 15% more when added to diet. However, probucol often lowers HDL levels. Thyroid analogs like D-thyroxine effectively lower LDL levels but are contraindicated in patients with suspected or proved heart disease. Clofibrate has little effect on serum cholesterol or LDL levels in this disorder, may produce gallstones and other metabolic problems, and usually is not indicated. Other agents are generally less effective than strict dietary management.

SECONDARY HYPERCHOLESTEROLEMIA

Hypercholesterolemia is common in **biliary cirrhosis**, as is a marked increase in the serum phospholipids and an abundant free cholesterol to cholesterol ester ratio. The serum is not lactescent because the overabundant lipoproteins (lipoproteins-x) are small and do not scatter light. Planar xanthomas and xanthelasma are common with prolonged and severe lipemia.

Hypercholesterolemia due to increased concentrations of LDL may be associated with **endocrinopathies** (hypothyroidism, hypopituitarism, diabetes mellitus) and usually is reversed by hormone therapy. Hypoproteinemias as seen in the **nephrotic syndrome**, metabolic aberrations such as **acute porphyria**, or **dietary excesses** with cholesterol-containing foods may also produce hyperbetalipoproteinemia. Cholesterol levels may be elevated secondary to increased concentrations of HDL in postmenopausal women or younger females taking oral contraceptives primarily containing estrogen.

TYPE III HYPERLIPOPROTEINEMIA (Broad Beta Disease; Dysbetalipoproteinemia)

A less common familial disorder characterized by the accumulation in serum of a beta-migrating very low-density lipoprotein, rich in triglycerides and cholesterol, associated with tuboeruptive and pathognomonic planar (palmar) xanthomas and a marked predisposition to severe premature atherosclerosis. It appears to result from a defect in the conversion of triglyceride-rich VLDL to LDL.

Symptoms, Signs, and Diagnosis

The disorder usually does not appear until early adulthood in males and is further delayed 10 to 15 yr in females. Peripheral vascular disease manifested by claudication or tuboeruptive xanthomas on the elbows and knees may be the first symptoms.

Serum may be cloudy to grossly turbid, often with a slight chylomicron layer. Both cholesterol and triglyceride levels are elevated, often equally. Precise definition of this abnormality requires ultracentrifugation and electrophoresis with the demonstration of a cholesterol-rich, beta-migrating VLDL. A mild abnormality in glucose tolerance and hyperuricemia may be present. Though usually familial this type of HLP may be seen in dysproteinemias.

Prognosis

This disorder is associated with a marked predilection for early and severe coronary and peripheral artery disease. With treatment, the peripheral vessel disease may abate and the hyperlipidemia can nearly always be reduced to normal.

Treatment

Therapy is particularly gratifying, since marked reductions of both cholesterol and triglyceride levels will occur along with marked regression of all xanthomas. Dietary measures alone with the emphasis on weight reduction to ideal body weight and then restriction of dietary cholesterol and carbohydrate may suffice. The addition of clofibrate 2 gm/day or niacin 2 to 3 gm/day is most effective and usually normalizes the blood lipid levels.

TYPE IV HYPERLIPOPROTEINEMIA (Endogenous Hypertriglyceridemia; Hyperprebetalipoproteinemia)

A common disorder, often with a familial distribution, characterized by variable elevations of serum triglycerides, contained predominantly in very low-density (prebeta) lipoproteins and a possible predisposition to atherosclerosis. Depending on the level of endogenous triglyceride used to define Type IV HLP, the disorder is common in adult American middle-aged males.

Symptoms, Signs, and Diagnosis

This disorder is usually recognized in adults and is frequently associated with mildly abnormal glucose tolerance curves and obesity. This type of lipemia may be exaggerated when dietary fat is restricted and carbohydrate added reciprocally (with caloric intake kept constant). Serum is turbid and triglyceride levels disproportionately elevated. Cholesterol may be normal or slightly increased. It is frequently seen secondary to stress, alcoholism, and dietary indiscretion, and may be associated with hyperuricemia.

Prognosis

The prognosis is uncertain. It may be associated with a predisposition to premature coronary artery disease.

Treatment

Weight reduction, when applicable, is the most effective treatment. Often this alone will normalize the blood lipid levels. Long-term maintenance of body weight and dietary restriction of carbohydrate and alcohol are important. Niacin 3 gm/day orally or clofibrate 2 gm/day in divided doses will further reduce the lipemia in those not controlled by diet alone. However, both drugs have troublesome side effects.

TYPE V HYPERLIPOPROTEINEMIA (Mixed Hypertriglyceridemia; Mixed Hyperlipidemia; Hyperprebetalipoproteinemia with Chylomicronemia)

An uncommon disorder, sometimes familial, associated with defective clearance of exogenous and endogenous triglycerides and the risk of life-threatening pancreatitis.

Symptoms, Signs, and Diagnosis

This disorder usually first appears in early adulthood with showers of eruptive xanthomas over the extensor surfaces of the extremities, lipemia retinalis, hepatosplenomegaly, and abdominal pain. Symptoms are exacerbated by ingestion of increased amounts of dietary fats. Serum triglyceride levels usually are markedly elevated with only modest elevations in cholesterol. Serum is turbid to cloudy with a distinct cream layer on top. Levels of lipoprotein lipase are usually normal. Hyperuricemia, glucose intolerance, and obesity are common. This pattern may be secondary to alcoholism, nephrosis, starvation with refeeding, or severe insulinopenic diabetes.

Prognosis

The main risk is pancreatitis. Recurrent bouts may occur with fat indulgence and lead to pseudocyst formation, hemorrhage, and death. Peripheral neuropathy characterized primarily by dysthesia may occur and together with pancreatitis can usually be prevented by fat restriction. This form of HLP, like Type I, shows little predilection to atherosclerosis.

Treatment

Weight reduction is extremely effective, as in Types III and IV, and should be followed with a maintenance diet restricting all fats to < 50 gm/day together with alcohol restriction. Niacin 3 to 6 gm/day is effective. Clofibrate 2 gm/day may also be helpful.

SECONDARY HYPERTRIGLYCERIDEMIA

The most common forms of hypertriglyceridemia seen in clinical practice are not the primary (familial) types but those secondary to other disorders such as acute alcoholism, chronic severe uncontrolled diabetes mellitus (diabetic lipemia), nephrosis, and glycogenosis, and to drugs (estrogens, oral contraceptives, thiazides, corticosteroids, etc.). Any of the abnormal familial lipoprotein abnormalities may be mimicked or exacerbated. **Treatment** depends on reversal of the underlying disorder or withdrawal of the offending drug.

FAMILIAL LECITHIN CHOLESTEROL ACYLTRANSFERASE DEFICIENCY (LCAT Deficiency)

This is a rare inheritable disorder transmitted as a recessive trait. It is characterized by absence of the enzyme that normally esterifies cholesterol in the plasma and is manifested by marked hypercholesterolemia and hyperphospholipidemia (free cholesterol and lecithin) together with hypertriglyceridemia. Renal and liver failure, anemia, and lens opacities are common. Treatment with a fat-restricted diet reduces the concentration of lipoprotein complexes in plasma and may be of value in preventing kidney damage. Renal transplantation has been successfully performed for renal failure.

HYPOLIPOPROTEINEMIA (Hypolipemia)

Low lipoprotein levels in the serum seen as rare familial disorders, or secondary to hyperthyroidism, anemia, malabsorption, and malnutrition.

HYPOBETALIPOPROTEINEMIA

A rare inheritable disorder transmitted as a simple mendelian dominant trait and characterized by reduced levels of beta-lipoprotein (LDL). There are usually no other clinical signs or symptoms. Serum lipids are low with plasma cholesterol levels in the 70 to 120 mg/100 ml range despite normal food intake. Absorption of fat is normal. No treatment is required.

ABETALIPOPROTEINEMIA (Acanthocytosis; Bassen-Kornzweig Syndrome)

A rare congenital disorder usually transmitted as a recessive trait and characterized by the complete absence of beta-lipoproteins and by steatorrhea, acanthocytes (erythrocytes with spiny projections of the membrane), retinitis pigmentosa, ataxia, and mental retardation. Absorption of fat is markedly impaired. Neither chylomicrons or VLDL are formed. All serum lipids are significantly reduced and no postprandial lipemia can be demonstrated. There is no specific **treatment.** Parenteral and oral administration of massive doses of vitamins E and A may delay or retard the neurologic sequelae. (See also Vol. II, Ch. 25.)

TANGIER DISEASE (Familial Alpha-Lipoprotein Deficiency)

A rare familial disorder characterized by recurrent polyneuropathy, lymphadenopathy, orange-yellow tonsillar hyperplasia, and hepatosplenomegaly (storage of cholesterol esters in reticuloendothelial cells) associated with a marked decrease in high-density lipoproteins. Serum cholesterol is very low; triglycerides are normal or elevated. The disorder may manifest first in adult life with hepatosplenomegaly or recurrent polyneuropathy. There is no treatment.

LIPIDOSES

GAUCHER'S DISEASE (Glucosyl Cerebroside Lipidosis)

A rare familial disorder of lipid metabolism resulting in an accumulation of abnormal glucocerebrosides in reticuloendothelial cells, and manifested clinically by hepatosplenomegaly, skin pigmentation, skeletal lesions, and pingueculae. The underlying defect appears to be a lack of glucocerebrosidase activity, which normally hydrolyzes glucocerebroside to glucose and ceramide.

Etiology and Pathology

Inheritance is recessive. The condition usually appears in childhood, but onset may be in infancy or adult life. The characteristic pathologic finding is widespread reticulum cell hyperplasia. The cells are filled with glucocerebroside and a fibrillar cytoplasm. They are 20 to 80 μ in diameter, round, oval, or spindle-shaped, with one or several small eccentrically placed nuclei. They are found in the liver, spleen, lymph nodes, and bone marrow.

Symptoms, Signs, Diagnosis, and Prognosis

Splenomegaly is the outstanding finding. Hepatomegaly and occasionally lymphadenopathy occur. Bone involvement may result in pain, and swelling of adjacent joints sometimes appears. Pingueculae and brown pigmentation of the skin may be present. Onset is more acute in infants (cerebral form); nuchal rigidity and opisthotonos may be noted. Splenic and marrow involvement frequently leads to pancytopenia. Epistaxis or other hemorrhages due to thrombocytopenia may occur. X-rays show flaring of the ends of the long bones and thinning of the cortex. Diagnosis clinically is based on demonstration of the characteristic cells in bone marrow, splenic aspiration, or liver biopsy specimens. It may be confirmed by demonstrating the absence of glucocerebrosidase activity in cell culture. There are several forms of this disorder due to differential cellular enzyme deficiency. Infants usually die within a year. Patients who survive to adolescence may live for many years.

Treatment

Splenectomy may be indicated in cases with anemia, leukopenia, or thrombocytopenia, or when the size of the spleen causes discomfort. Blood transfusions may be given for the anemia. Enzyme replacement by administration of glucocerebrosidase may be useful; however, this procedure is still experimental.

NIEMANN-PICK DISEASE (Sphingomyelin Lipidosis)

A familial disorder of lipid metabolism in which sphingomyelin accumulates in the reticuloendothelial cells. There are at least 5 different forms of this lipidosis characterized by different levels of sphingomyelinase. The enzyme is absent in the severe juvenile form. This abnormality of lipid metabolism may be accompanied by demyelination and neurologic symptoms. The infantile and juvenile forms are inherited as recessive traits, appearing most often in Jewish families. Patients may show xanthomas, pigmentation, hepatosplenomegaly, lymphadenopathy, and mental retardation. Pancytopenia is a common finding. Diagnosis may be made by tissue biopsy. Absence of the sphingomyelin-cleaving enzyme can be demonstrated in both biopsy specimens and tissue culture. Serum lipids usually are normal. **Treatment** at present is supportive; there is no specific therapy.

FABRY'S DISEASE (Angiokeratoma Corporis Diffusum Universale; α-Galactosidase Deficiency)

A rare, familial, sex-linked disorder of lipid metabolism in which glycolipid (galactosylgalactosylglucosyl ceramide) accumulates in many tissues. The metabolic abnormality is due to the absence of the lysosomal enzyme α-galactosidase A needed for the normal catabolism of trihexosyl ceramide. Clinical recognition in males results from characteristic skin lesions (angiokeratomas) over the lower trunk. Patients may show ocular deposits, febrile episodes, and burning pain in the extremities. Death results from renal failure, or cardiac or cerebral complications of hypertension or other vascular disease. Heterozygous females may exhibit the disorder in an attenuated form; they are most likely to show corneal opacities. Enzymatic replacement of the deficient enzyme by transfusion has been accomplished but is not practical. Treatment is otherwise supportive, especially during periods of pain and fever.

WOLMAN'S DISEASE (Acid Cholesteryl Ester Hydrolase Deficiency)

Manifested in the first weeks of life, this familial condition is characterized by hepatosplenomegaly, steatorrhea, and adrenal calcification. Large amounts of neutral lipids, particularly cholesterol esters and glycerides, accumulate in the body tissues. Deficiency of an acid lipase has been described. There is no specific therapy, and death usually occurs by 6 mo of age.

CHOLESTERYL ESTER STORAGE DISEASE

An extremely rare familial disease characterized by hepatomegaly and accumulation of cholesterol esters and triglycerides mainly in lysosomes in the liver, spleen, lymph nodes and other tissues. A deficiency in cholesteryl ester hydrolase has been described. Patients may be asymptomatic. Diagnosis is made by liver biopsy. There is no treatment.

VAN BOGAERT'S DISEASE (Cerebrotendinous Xanthomatosis)

A rare recessive familial disorder characterized by progressive ataxia, dementia, cataracts, and tendon xanthomas. Cholestanol (5α-cholestan-3β-ol), which is usually barely detectable in the body, is found in increased concentrations in the nervous system, lungs, blood, and xanthomas. Though plasma cholesterol levels are usually low or normal, premature atherosclerosis also occurs. Disability is progressive though often not manifested until after age 30. Defective cholesterol catabolism and bile acid formation have been demonstrated. No specific treatment has proved effective. Treatment with chenodeoxycholic acid (0.5 to 1.5 gm/day) has been suggested.

β-SITOSTEROLEMIA AND XANTHOMATOSIS

A rare recessive familial disease characterized by the accumulation of plant sterols in the blood and tissues and by the occurrence of tendon xanthomas. The prognosis of the disease is unknown. Increased intestinal absorption of dietary β-sitosterol has been demonstrated. Treatment at present is dietary and involves a diet low in plant sterol content.

REFSUM'S SYNDROME (Phytanic Acid Storage Disease)

A rare recessive familial disorder of lipid metabolism characterized clinically by peripheral neuropathy, ataxia, retinitis pigmentosa, and bone and skin changes. It is associated with marked accumulation of phytanic acid in the plasma and tissues. (See also TABLE 25–19 in Vol. II, Ch. 25.) The disorder is believed to be due to the absence of phytanic acid hydroxylase, an enzyme needed for the metabolism of phytanic acid. Prolonged treatment with a diet deficient in phytanic acid is beneficial.

OTHER LIPIDOSES

Several rare inheritable lipidoses have been demonstrated using sophisticated technics of tissue culture and enzyme analysis. The more common ones are:

Tay-Sachs disease (G_{M2} gangliosidosis) is characterized by very early onset, progressive retardation in development, paralysis, dementia, blindness, cherry red retinal spots, and death by age 3 or 4.

This recessive disorder is most common in families of Eastern European Jewish origin and is caused by deficiency of the enzyme hexosaminidase A, resulting in accumulation of sphyngolipids in the brain. An infantile disorder often fatal by age 2 is **generalized (G$_{M1}$) gangliosidosis** in which the ganglioside G$_{M1}$ accumulates in the nervous system. In **sulfatide lipidosis (metachromatic leukodystrophy)** there is a deficiency of the enzyme cerebroside sulfatase, causing metachromatic lipids to accumulate in the white matter of the CNS, peripheral nerves, kidney, spleen, and other visceral organs. It is characterized by progressive paralysis and dementia usually beginning before age 2 and fatal by age 10. **Galactosyl ceramide lipidosis,** also known as **Krabbe's disease** or **globoid leukodystrophy,** is a fatal infantile disorder characterized by progressive retardation, paralysis, blindness, deafness, and pseudobulbar palsy. This familial condition appears to be secondary to a deficiency of galactocerobroside β-galactosidase. **Diagnosis** of these disorders may be made *prenatally* from amniotic fluid. No treatment is known.

83. AMYLOIDOSIS

Accumulation in the tissues of the fibrillar protein amyloid usually (but not always) in amounts sufficient to impair normal function.

Pathophysiology and Classification

The cause of amyloid production and its deposition in tissues is unknown. Immunologic derangements have been implicated—B cell activation, T cell suppression, macrophage involvement—but to date all such abnormalities have been nonspecific. Under light microscopy amyloid is a homogeneous, highly refractile substance with an affinity for Congo red dye, both in fixed tissues and in vivo. On electron microscopy amyloid consists of 100 Å fibrils; on x-ray diffraction it has a cross beta pattern. Biochemically, however, 2 major types of amyloid and several less common forms have been defined. One has an N-terminal sequence that is homologous with a portion of the variable region of an immunoglobulin light chain termed AL; the other has a unique N-terminal sequence of a nonimmunoglobulin protein called AA protein. The chemical structure of amyloid associated with aging, with familial amyloid polyneuropathy, and with endocrine organs may represent other biochemical forms of amyloid.

Chemical analyses relating to various forms of amyloidosis may therefore lead to a new classification. At present, 2 major clinical forms are recognized, though differentiation is not always clearcut. Amyloidosis is classified as **primary** when there is no associated disease and **secondary** when associated with chronic diseases, either infectious (tuberculosis, bronchiectasis, osteomyelitis, leprosy) or inflammatory (rheumatoid arthritis, granulomatous ileitis). Amyloid is also found in association with multiple myeloma, Hodgkin's disease, other tumors, and familial Mediterranean fever. It may accompany aging and appear in familial forms unassociated with other disease, often with distinctive types of neuropathy, nephropathy, and cardiopathy. Patients with the primary type and that associated with multiple myeloma usually have the immunoglobulin light-chain form of amyloid fibrils (AL). Patients with secondary amyloidosis have demonstrated the presence of AA protein.

In **primary amyloidosis,** the heart, lung, skin, tongue, thyroid gland, and intestinal tract may be involved. Localized amyloid "tumors" may be found in the respiratory tract or other sites. Parenchymal organs (liver, spleen, kidney) and the vascular system are frequently involved.

Secondary amyloidosis shows a predilection for the spleen, liver, kidney, adrenals, and lymph nodes. However, no organ system is spared and vascular involvement may be widespread. The liver and spleen are often enlarged, firm, and rubbery. The kidneys are usually enlarged. Sections of the spleen show large, translucent, waxy areas where the normal malpighian bodies are replaced by pale amyloid, producing the "sago" spleen.

Amyloid associated with certain tumors (multiple myeloma) may be widespread and show unique sites of involvement. Amyloid may have a strictly local occurrence in association with some malignancies (e.g., medullary carcinoma of the thyroid gland). It has a high association in the pancreas with adult onset diabetes mellitus.

Symptoms and Signs

Manifestations are nonspecific and are determined by the organ or system affected. Often they are obscured by the underlying disease, which may be fatal before secondary amyloidosis is suspected. The nephrotic syndrome is the most striking manifestation. In the early stages only slight proteinuria may be noted; later the distinctive symptom complex develops with anasarca, hypoproteinemia, and massive proteinuria. Amyloid disease of the liver produces hepatomegaly, but rarely jaundice. Liver function tests usually are normal, although abnormal BSP excretion or elevated alkaline phosphatase may be observed. Occasionally, portal hypertension may occur with esophageal varices and ascites. Massive hepatomegaly (liver weight > 7 kg) has been reported. Skin lesions may be waxy or translucent; purpura may result from amyloidosis of small cutaneous vessels. Cardiac involvement is common and may manifest itself as cardiomegaly, intractable heart failure, or any of the common arrhythmias. Atrial standstill has been found in several kinships. GI amyloid may cause esophageal motility abnormalities, gastric atony, small and large intestinal motility abnormalities, malabsorption, bleeding, or pseudo-obstruction. Macroglossia is common in primary and myeloma-related amyloid. A firm, symmetric, nontender goiter resembling Hashimoto's or Riedel's struma may result from amyloidosis of the thyroid gland. Amyloid arthropathy may mimic RA in some cases of multiple myeloma. Peripheral neuropathy is seen in some cases of primary or myeloma-associated amyloid. It is common in some familial amyloidoses. Lung involvement may be characterized by focal pulmonary nodules, tracheobronchial lesions, or diffuse alveolar deposits.

Diagnosis

Amyloidosis can be diagnosed only by biopsy. Secondary amyloidosis should be suspected when the condition of a patient with a chronic suppurative disease progressively deteriorates and the common manifestations of amyloidosis, such as hepatomegaly, splenomegaly, or albuminuria, appear. Biopsy of rectal mucosa is the best screening test. Other useful biopsy sites are gingiva, skin, nerve, kidney, and liver. Tissue sections should be stained with Congo red dye and observed with a polarizing microscope for the green birefringence that is characteristic of amyloid.

Prognosis

In secondary amyloidosis, prognosis depends on successful treatment of the underlying disease. All forms of amyloid renal involvement carry a poor prognosis, but with supportive therapy (e.g., eradication of pyelonephritis), patients may remain stable and even improve. Amyloidosis associated with multiple myeloma has the poorest prognosis, early death within 1 to 2 yr being common. However, localized amyloid tumors may be removed without recurrence. Myocardial amyloidosis may cause death from arrhythmias or intractable cardiac failure. Prognosis in familial amyloidoses varies with each kinship.

Treatment

Therapy is directed first to the underlying cause. If this can be controlled, amyloidosis may be arrested. Management of amyloidosis itself is generally symptomatic. Kidney transplantation has been performed in a few patients with renal amyloid; however, it is technically difficult due to the potential for bleeding. Amyloid will ultimately recur in a donor kidney, but several recipients have done very well and lived up to 10 yr. Corticosteroids or immunosuppressive agents are not of proven value. Digitalis should be used with care in amyloid heart disease, since it may precipitate arrhythmias. Colchicine has been utilized to prevent the acute attacks of familial Mediterranean fever and it has been suggested that patients so treated develop no new amyloid. No proof yet exists that colchicine alleviates primary or secondary amyloid, but clinical trials are in progress.

§8. ENDOCRINE DISORDERS

84. HYPOTHALAMIC–PITUITARY RELATIONSHIPS

The hypothalamus modulates the activity of the pituitary gland (hypophysis) via 2 distinct routes, one to the posterior and the other to the anterior pituitary. The hypothalamus is connected with the posterior pituitary (neurohypophysis) by the supraopticohypophyseal nerve tract (peptidergic neurons). No nervous connection with the anterior pituitary (adenohypophysis) exists, but blood coursing through the hypothalamus gathers into a portal venous system which traverses the anterior pituitary and thus serves as a channel for direct transmission of hypothalamic neurohormones. By these 2 routes, the hypothalamus is able to stimulate or release pituitary hormones.

The hypothalamic nerve centers are also connected by neurons with the cortex, midbrain, hindbrain, and spinal cord. Thus, neurotransmitters (serotonin, norepinephrine, and dopamine) released by these neurons terminating in the hypothalamus can trigger production of neurohormones by hypothalamic neurosecretory cells, providing a coordinated mechanism linking stimuli of a visceral or intellectual nature to the function of the hypothalamus and, therefore, of the pituitary gland (see Fig. 84–1). Other neurotransmitters released by the peptidergic neurons are epinephrine, acetylcholine, and the neuropeptides such as substance P, neurotensin, and endorphins.

Neurohypophyseal Function

The supraoptic and paraventricular nuclei of the hypothalamus secrete 2 octapeptide hormones—vasopressin and oxytocin. **Vasopressin (antidiuretic hormone, ADH)** regulates water balance by stimulating resorption in the distal renal tubule. The 2 major controls of vasopressin release are increased osmotic pressure and decreased effective plasma volume. The former seems to be a direct hypothalamic response, while plasma volume changes are detected by receptors in peripheral blood vessels. Vasopressin release is also mediated by neural stimuli (e.g., in response to stress).

Lesions damaging the hypothalamic or pituitary infundibular portions of the system cause deficient secretion of vasopressin, resulting in **diabetes insipidus** (see Ch. 85).

Oxytocin, structurally similar to vasopressin, has 2 known functions. It can stimulate uterine contractions, more so as pregnancy progresses; however, hypophysectomized women may go into labor spontaneously, making the physiologic importance of this action uncertain. Oxytocin release is stimulated by suckling and causes the myoepithelial cells of the breast to contract, expressing milk into the ducts (the "letdown" reflex of nursing mothers).

Both oxytocin and vasopressin are produced in the hypothalamus, are transported down axons bound as granules to carrier proteins **(neurophysins),** and are stored in the nerve endings of the posterior pituitary. They are released from these endings into the general circulation, where the granules dissociate, releasing free hormone and neurophysin.

The neurosecretory cells of the neurohypophyseal tract respond to neurotransmitters, being activated by cholinergic and inhibited by adrenergic stimuli. They therefore represent a type of neuroendocrine transducer, transforming neural input into hormone release.

Adenohypophyseal Function

The hypothalamus controls the secretion of **releasing** or **inhibiting hormones** into the hypothalamic-pituitary portal venous system through which they are carried to the anterior pituitary. Here, they bind to specific cell membrane receptors, altering cAMP production in the cells and stimulating formation and release of pituitary hormones into the general circulation.

Thyrotropin-releasing hormone (TRH) is a potent releaser of pituitary thyroid-stimulating hormone **(TSH)** and also causes release of prolactin. Whether TRH is a physiologic releasing factor for prolactin has yet to be established. **Gonadotropin-releasing hormone (GnRH)** causes an increase of both luteinizing hormone **(LH)** and follicle-stimulating hormone **(FSH).** These relationships are described in Vol. II, Ch. 2. TRH and GnRH have been characterized and synthesized. Both are polypeptides with few amino acids (3 and 10 amino acids respectively). Corticotropin-or ACTH-releasing factor **(CRF)** has not been characterized but is probably a similar substance. Other releasing factors or hormones may be present for growth hormone and possibly for prolactin. Still other factors *inhibit* release of pituitary hormones; the most clearly established of these are **somatostatin,** which inhibits secretion of growth hormone **(GH),** and prolactin-inhibiting factor **(PIF,** a substance thought to be dopamine), which inhibits secretion of prolactin. Inhibiting factors may exist for other hormones also.

Secretion of releasing hormones by the hypothalamus is controlled by several mechanisms. It is postulated that CRF secretion, for example, is stimulated by stress, by falling plasma corticosteroid concentrations, and by the time of day. Secretion is felt to be more active in the late hours of sleep and less active in the late afternoon and evening—a rhythm reflected in similar changes in plasma cortisol concentration. The rhythmicity is dependent on light and can be reversed by transposing of the light-dark cycle. CRF is inhibited by rising plasma concentrations of corticosteroids and ACTH. CRF is released in spurts of varying duration, rather than at a constant slow rate, and other releasing

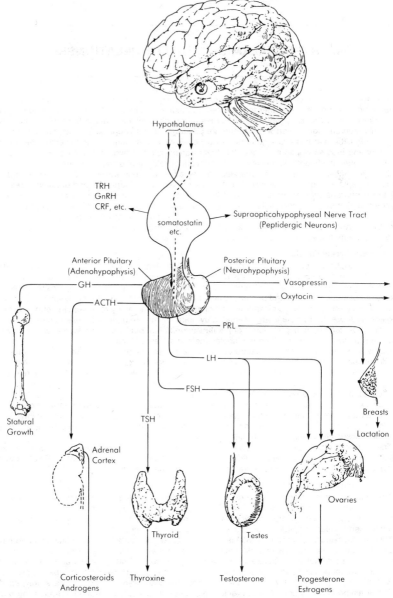

FIG. 84–1. **Interrelationship between the pituitary gland, the hypothalamus, and target organs.** The stimulating hormones and factors entering the pituitary are indicated by a solid line, while a broken line shows the inhibiting hormones and factors. (Modified from "The Hormones of the Hypothalamus," by R. Guillermin and R. Burgus, *Scientific American* 227 (5), p. 26, Nov. 1972. Copyright © 1972 by Scientific American, Inc. All rights reserved.)

hormones apparently exhibit a similar pattern. The release of GnRH depends on the concentration of estrogen in a complex relationship between the hypothalamus, pituitary, and ovaries, which is described in detail in Vol. II, Ch. 2.

Diseases of the hypothalamus, including tumors, encephalitis, and other inflammatory lesions, may reduce the hypothalamic secretion of hypophysiotropic hormones and thus affect pituitary activity.

This may be inhibitory, by decreasing releasing hormone levels, or facilitative, by reducing the secretion of inhibiting hormones. Since hypothalamic factors originate in different regions of the hypothalamus, it is not uncommon for secretory defects in hypothalamic disease to involve only a single releasing hormone and produce a single defect of pituitary hormone secretion; e.g., **Kallman's syndrome,** characterized by deficiency of GnRH and secondary hypogonadism. On the other hand, by reducing secretion of PIF, hypothalamic lesions may produce lactation associated with **hyperprolactinemia.** Other hypothalamic lesions are likely to produce decreased secretion of TSH or ACTH from the pituitary, producing **secondary hypopituitarism.** The availability of TRH in clinical quantities makes it possible in some instances to distinguish between hypopituitarism of hypothalamic origin (secondary) and hypopituitarism due to disease of the pituitary (primary).

*Hyper*secretion of hypothalamic releasing hormones is not definitely established, but there is reason to suspect that it occurs in certain types of **acromegaly** and in **Cushing's syndrome.** The rare inherited disease **lipoatrophic diabetes** is associated with excessive plasma levels of releasing factors for growth hormone and ACTH. The disease is characterized by loss of body fat, insulin-resistant diabetes mellitus, excessive growth (often segmental), hypertrophied muscles, and acanthosis nigricans. However, the relationship between these findings and excessive secretion of releasing factors is not clear, since hypophysectomy does not improve the clinical picture.

Clinical syndromes that occur as a result of hypothalamic lesions become manifest as aberrations of pituitary hormone function and are discussed in detail in Ch. 85 and in Vol. II, Ch. 25.

85. PITUITARY

The pituitary is composed of functionally and anatomically distinct anterior and posterior parts. Oxytocin and vasopressin (antidiuretic hormone—**ADH**) are synthesized in the hypothalamus and stored in peptidergic neurons terminating in the median eminence, the pituitary stalk, and the posterior pituitary lobe. They are described in Ch. 84. The cells of the anterior pituitary lobe synthesize and release several polypeptide and protein hormones. These influence a variety of metabolic processes essential for normal growth and development; they also maintain the normal structure and activity of several target glands. Release and inhibition of the anterior pituitary hormones is regulated by neurohormones elaborated by neurosecretory cells in the hypothalamus (see Ch. 84).

Corticotropin (ACTH) maintains the normal morphology of the adrenal cortex and stimulates secretion of (1) cortisol, the major glucocorticoid, and (2) certain corticosteroids with weak androgenic (17-KS) activity. The adrenal cortex atrophies in the absence of ACTH, and secretion of cortisol and adrenal 17-KS virtually ceases. Similarly, **thyroid-stimulating hormone (TSH)** influences structural characteristics of the thyroid gland and stimulates secretion of thyroid hormones; in the absence of TSH, uptake of iodine by the thyroid and synthesis and release of thyroid hormones are markedly diminished. **Follicle-stimulating hormone (FSH),** in the female, brings about maturation of the ovarian follicle, and **luteinizing hormone (LH)** is involved in ovulation and the development of the corpus luteum; these gonadotropins also influence the ovarian secretion of steroid hormones (estrogens, progestins). FSH, in the male, is involved principally in the maintenance of spermatogenesis, while LH (also referred to as interstitial-cell-stimulating hormone or **ICSH**) stimulates the secretion of testosterone by the testicular interstitial (Leydig) cells. Lack of the gonadotropic hormones, FSH and LH, leads to gonadal atrophy and impairment in both the reproductive and the steroid secretory functions of the gonads.

Growth hormone (GH), also called **somatotropin,** exerts a multitude of effects, playing an important role in regulating the growth of the skeleton, connective tissue, and a wide variety of viscera. These effects probably reflect the stimulatory action of the hormone on nucleic acid and protein synthesis. GH also has a lipolytic action in fat cells, and is involved in glucose homeostasis, tending to elevate blood glucose by impairing glucose metabolism by tissues such as muscle and fat. Some of the effects of GH, particularly those on the skeleton, are mediated by circulating small molecular weight peptide plasma factors referred to as **somatomedins,** the synthesis of which is believed to be induced by GH in the liver. Normal plasma somatomedin levels are 0.7 to 1.3 u./ml.

The pituitary produces a lactogenic hormone called **prolactin (PRL).** GH and PRL probably arise from separate acidophil cells of the anterior pituitary, while TSH, FSH, and LH arise from basophils. In disorders where hyperpigmentation is associated with elevated ACTH levels (e.g., Addison's disease or Nelson's disease) increased melanophore-stimulating activity can also be demonstrated and is principally responsible for changes in pigmentation. Recent studies suggest that ACTH and the peptide causing this activity (in the past called "**MSH**") originate in common basophilic cells in the pituitary and are part of a single larger polypeptide, β-lipotropin (also referred to as β-lipotropic hormone or β-**LPH**), which is composed of ACTH and also the endorphins and enkephalins—these latter 2 parts of β-lipotropins are thought of as endogenous opioides, since they bind to and activate receptors for morphine and other narcotics. Circulating MSH activity is caused by β-LPH.

ANTERIOR LOBE DISORDERS

HYPOFUNCTION OF THE ANTERIOR PITUITARY

HYPOPITUITARISM IN THE ADULT

Etiology

Hypopituitarism may result from space-occupying or infiltrative lesions involving the sella turcica, including craniopharyngiomas (probably the most common); chromophobe or acidophil adenomas of the pituitary; metastatic carcinomas (e.g., from the breast); sarcoidosis; histiocytosis X, autoimmune hypophysitis; internal carotid artery aneurysms; and, rarely, tuberculosis or fungus infections affecting the meninges, with subsequent spread to the pituitary. Hypopituitarism may also result from infarction of the pituitary, usually associated with postpartum hemorrhage or shock **(Sheehan's syndrome)**. More rarely it is associated with shock in patients with extensive cerebrovascular disease (particularly patients with diabetes mellitus). Anterior pituitary hypofunction may also be due to lesions involving the hypothalamus, such as metastatic neoplasms, craniopharyngiomas, pinealomas, meningiomas, histiocytosis, or ependymomas.

Symptoms and Signs

The number of deficient pituitary hormones and the degree of deficiency depend on the nature of the underlying pathologic process and the stage of the disease at which the patient is seen. An *isolated* deficiency of gonadotropins or ACTH may occur; these disorders are described separately below. The function of all target glands will decrease when all hormones are deficient **(panhypopituitarism)**, and evidence of hormone deficiency usually occurs in sequence, beginning with the gonadotropins, then GH, TSH, and, finally, ACTH. Lack of FSH and LH in the female leads to infertility, amenorrhea, and decreased secondary sexual characteristics; lack of FSH and LH in the male leads to testicular atrophy, decreased spermatogenesis with consequent infertility, and a decrease in secondary sexual characteristics; GH deficiency, perhaps in conjunction with lack of cortisol, may lead to hypoglycemia; TSH deficiency leads to hypothyroidism; and ACTH deficiency leads to hypofunction of the adrenal cortex with attendant hypotension and intolerance to stress and infection. Postpartum lactation may not occur in Sheehan's syndrome, and hypopituitarism may develop slowly.

Other clinical manifestations of hypopituitarism must also be considered in the light of the underlying process. For example, chromophobe or acidophil adenomas or craniopharyngiomas may produce severe headaches. The tumor may extend beyond the sella turcica to involve the optic chiasm, producing unilateral or bitemporal hemianopia. Tumors (particularly craniopharyngiomas) may involve the hypothalamus, causing diabetes insipidus, and may affect the appetite center with consequent obesity.

Differential Diagnosis

X-rays of the sella turcica to exclude a tumor are essential in hypopituitarism. The walls of the sella may be demineralized, irregular, or ballooned. The visual fields should also be examined. In patients with an enlarged sella suspected of harboring a tumor, it is important to determine whether the tumor has extended beyond the boundaries of the sella. Computerized tomography **(CT)** is used to document superior and lateral suprasellar extension of the tumor and excludes the possibility of an aneurysm eroding the sella. CT can also rule out the **empty sella syndrome** in which the sella is enlarged, filled with CSF, but *without* a tumor.

Pituitary deficiency secondary to a relative lack of hypophysiotropic factors **(hypothalamic hypopituitarism)** is often suggested by the presence of diabetes insipidus, mildly *elevated* prolactin levels, and *reduced* levels of TSH, GH, and FSH.

To distinguish hypothalamic hypopituitarism from primary pituitary deficiency, several provocative tests are available. The TRH test usually differentiates the disorders adequately. TRH is administered IV (200 μg) and TSH levels are determined at time 0, 15, 30 min, 1 h, and 2 h. The patient with hypothalamic hypopituitarism (and/or hypothalamic hypothyroidism) will have a marked response, while in true hypopituitarism no release of TSH will be seen. Similar tests may be available soon for LH and FSH.

Hypothyroidism will be reflected in subnormal thyroid function tests. In the patient with hypothyroidism, measurement of plasma TSH best distinguishes primary hypothyroidism (plasma TSH increased) from hypopituitarism (TSH decreased)—(see HYPOTHYROIDISM in Ch. 86). Plasma FSH and LH will be low in hypopituitarism, in contrast to the findings in patients with primary hypogonadism in whom plasma gonadotropins are elevated; estrogen levels are low in both instances.

Because plasma **GH levels** are low or undetectable under normal conditions, it is necessary to demonstrate a failure to respond to appropriate stimuli. The standard stimulus, by which other stress-related hormones are evaluated, is insulin-induced hypoglycemia **(insulin tolerance test).** Regular insulin 0.1 u./kg is given IV and blood sugar, cortisol, and GH are measured at 15-min intervals for 120 min. As the blood sugar will fall by at least 50%, *symptomatic hypoglycemia, not without risk, is induced; therefore, careful patient monitoring is mandatory.* A normal patient responds to this stimulus with a peak GH of at least 10 ng/ml, as measured by radioimmunoassay. Less dangerous, but also less reliable, tests of GH release use IV arginine infusion (500 mg/kg given over 30 min) or oral L-dopa administration.

ACTH deficiency will be reflected in urinary 17-OHCS of < 3 mg/24 h and urinary 17-KS of < 5 mg/24 h. Giving cosyntropin 25 μg IM or IV will produce a distinct increase in plasma cortisol (measured at time 0, 30, and 60 min post injection) in contrast to the findings in patients with **primary adrenal insufficiency (Addison's disease),** where no stimulation will occur. Occasionally, the patient with hypopituitarism will secrete sufficient ACTH to maintain urinary 17-OHCS in the normal range, but will be unable to increase ACTH secretion and plasma cortisol in response to various stimuli (limited ACTH reserve). This can be demonstrated either with the insulin tolerance test (see above) or with the **metyrapone test:** Preferably, 2 baseline 24-h urines are collected for 17-OHCS assays; metyrapone 750 mg orally q 4 h is then given for 6 doses on the 3rd day, during which a 24-h urine is again collected; and a 4th 24-h urine is collected on the day following administration of the drug. In normal individuals, metyrapone will produce a 2- to 4-fold increase in urinary 17-OHCS above baseline on the day of, or the day after, metyrapone administration; this will fail to occur in patients with limited ACTH reserve. An insulin tolerance test (see above) will also fail to stimulate plasma cortisol to normal levels in response to the induced hypoglycemia, but will not differentiate between primary (Addison's) or secondary (hypopituitarism) adrenal insufficiency.

Some authors have proposed ways in which the reserve capacity of the anterior pituitary to secrete various hormones might be tested simultaneously. For example, the simultaneous injection of insulin (0.1 u./kg *with careful monitoring and glucose at hand*), TRH (200 μg), and gonadotropin-releasing hormone **(GnRH)** (100 μg) has been proposed, with the measurement in the ensuing 3 h of plasma pituitary hormone levels by radioimmunoassay. Insulin-induced hypoglycemia stimulates release of GH and ACTH, TRH brings about release of TSH and prolactin, and GnRH stimulates release of the gonadotropins.

Since pituitary function tests may be abnormal in **anorexia nervosa,** it is often difficult to distinguish this condition from hypopituitarism. However, patients with anorexia nervosa (usually female) often have marked cachexia (rare in hypopituitarism), maintain secondary sexual characteristics (although amenorrheic), and have a history of psychiatric disturbance. In contrast to patients with hypopituitarism, patients with anorexia nervosa may exhibit *increased* plasma GH levels. The TRH test often shows a "hypothalamic" pattern of TSH release in these patients.

Treatment

Treatment is directed toward replacing the hormones *of the hypofunctioning target glands* as discussed in the pertinent chapters in this section and in Vol. II. When hypopituitarism is due to a pituitary tumor, specific treatment must be directed at the tumor. If there are no signs of extension of the tumor beyond the sella, pituitary supervoltage irradiation may be employed; however, transsphenoidal surgery is the treatment of choice. When progressive extrasellar extension is suspected (e.g., reflected in visual field defects), surgical removal of the tumor is necessary, usually through a transphenoidal approach; occasionally a transfrontal approach is used. These patients usually receive supervoltage irradiation as well, since it is often impossible to ensure complete extirpation of the tumor.

PITUITARY DWARFISM (See Vol. II, Ch. 25)

SELECTIVE PITUITARY HORMONE DEFICIENCIES (See Vol. II, Ch. 25)

HYPERSECRETION OF ANTERIOR PITUITARY HORMONES

ACROMEGALY AND GIGANTISM

Etiology

Acromegaly or gigantism results from the excessive secretion of GH caused by an acidophilic adenoma of the pituitary, less commonly by a chromophobe adenoma, and rarely by a histologically normal pituitary. A few cases of ectopic GH-producing tumors have also been described.

Symptoms and Signs

Hypersecretion of GH prior to closure of epiphyses leads to proportional growth of bone; both length and width of bone are increased. Height may be more than 7 or 8 ft, hence the term **pituitary gigantism.** GH hypersecretion after closure of epiphyses leads to periosteal overgrowth and cortical thickening. Overgrowth of the mandible leads to protrusion of the jaw (prognathism). There is an overbite and the teeth become separated. Bone overgrowth and soft tissue thickening lead to characteristic coarsening of the facial features. The hands are widened and the fingers become broad, requiring a larger ring size. Similar changes in the feet require a larger shoe size. This increase in dimension of the acral parts has led to the term **acromegaly.** The heart and kidney may also become enlarged, and renal clearance of phosphate is frequently impaired.

Erosion of articular surfaces takes place, and joint complaints are common. The skin is thickened, with increased sweating, and females may note hypertrichosis. Galactorrhea may be present, and the occurrence of hypertension is not uncommon.

A pituitary adenoma will not only produce signs of GH excess, but also may induce signs of deficiency of other pituitary hormones by compression of nontumorous pituitary tissue. Signs of hypogonadism may appear with decreased libido in either sex and with menstrual disturbances in women. Headaches are common. The tumor may produce signs of extrasellar extension, such as loss in visual fields (e.g., a bitemporal hemianopia).

Diagnosis

This can be made from the characteristic clinical findings. Skull x-rays disclose cortical thickening, enlargement of the frontal sinuses, and enlargement and erosion of the sella turcica. X-rays of the hands show tufting of the terminal phalanges and soft tissue thickening. Glucose tolerance usually is abnormal. Elevated serum inorganic PO_4 has been used as an index of active acromegaly, but is now recognized as an imprecise reflection of growth hormone levels.

The measurement of plasma GH concentrations by radioimmunoassay is probably the most direct and precise means of assessing the hypersecretion of GH. Patients with acromegaly or gigantism generally have fasting, recumbent levels considerably in excess of 10 ng/ml. Furthermore, plasma GH is not suppressed during a glucose tolerance test as in normal persons. The measurement of plasma GH levels also is useful in assessing the efficacy of various treatments. The measurement of somatomedin C by radioimmunoassay correlates well with the activity of the disease.

Treatment

Supervoltage irradiation, delivering about 5000 R to the pituitary, has been used to treat acromegaly and gigantism. There is controversy, however, over the efficacy of this treatment, which often fails to correct GH hypersecretion. This therapy generally does not induce hypopituitarism or other undesired effects. **Heavy particle irradiation** allows delivery of large doses to the pituitary. It appears not only to normalize GH secretion in a larger percentage of patients, but also may induce hypopituitarism. **Cryohypophysectomy** has been utilized as a means of ablating the pituitary gland, but has been replaced by surgical hypophysectomy because it is believed to correct pituitary hyperfunction more predictably; **transphenoidal resection** is the method of choice. A combined surgery/radiation approach is indicated in patients with signs of progressive extrasellar involvement by a pituitary tumor. The difficulty of totally ablating GH-secreting pituitary tissue is shown by the persistence of circulating GH in some cases, sometimes even at elevated levels, after surgery. If surgical and/or radiation therapy is unsuccessful in restoring GH levels to normal, **bromocriptine mesylate** 15 mg/day orally in divided doses may be used. It is effective in about 75% of cases.

CUSHING'S SYNDROME (See under ADRENAL CORTICAL HYPERFUNCTION in Ch. 88)

GALACTORRHEA

A syndrome of galactorrhea and amenorrhea in females has been described, some of whom have a chromophobe adenoma of the pituitary **(Forbes-Albright syndrome).** Galactorrhea may also occur in men. It has been shown that the pituitary secretes excessive quantities of prolactin in these patients. Persistent galactorrhea and amenorrhea may also occur after pregnancy **(Chiari-Frommel syndrome),** again presumably due to excessive pituitary prolactin and to deficient gonadotropins.

The differential diagnosis of galactorrhea also includes its occurrence in association with nonendocrine tumors, as well as its occurrence in association with ingestion of certain drugs, such as the phenothiazines (which have a stimulatory effect on pituitary prolactin secretion) and morphinergic agents (i.e., methadone). Primary hypothyroidism must be ruled out, since the elevation in prolactin seen with this disease is secondary to the elevated TRH levels as reflected in high TSH concentration (see also SECONDARY AMENORRHEA in Vol. II, Ch. 3).

The diagnostic evaluation of the patient with galactorrhea should include skull x-rays, AP and lateral cone-down views, to exclude a large pituitary tumor. Visual field examination should be performed. CT is used to detect smaller pituitary and suprasellar tumors, and to rule out empty sella syndrome. Prolactin levels should be measured and, although there is considerable controversy, most investigators feel that these levels reflect the relative size of the sella lesion. Tumors are never malignant and most women with elevated prolactin have no significant functional impairment except for menstrual irregularities and decreased libido. In men, decreased libido, impotence, and diminished sperm may be seen with or without galactorrhea.

Surgical resection becomes the therapy of choice in suprasellar involvement by a tumor. The use of bromocriptine is now considered the treatment of choice for galactorrhea syndromes where prolactin levels are below 200 ng/ml and there is no radiographic evidence of a significant intrasellar mass or suprasellar extension. Recent evidence suggests that the preoperative use of bromocriptine can reduce the size of large tumors permitting a more satisfactory surgical result.

POSTERIOR LOBE DISORDERS

DIABETES INSIPIDUS

A temporary or chronic disorder of the neurohypophyseal system, due to deficiency of vasopressin (ADH) and characterized by excretion of excessive quantities of very dilute (but otherwise normal) urine and by excessive thirst.

This disorder is termed **vasopressin-sensitive diabetes insipidus (DI)** to distinguish it from **nephrogenic diabetes insipidus (NDI)** in which the kidney is vasopressin-resistant. The disturbance in water metabolism is similar in both and is characterized by the daily production of a very large volume of dilute urine (sp gr usually < 1.005 or osmolality < 200 mOsm/L). DI may be complete, partial, permanent, or temporary. All of the pathologic lesions associated with DI involve the hypothalamic nuclei (supraoptic and paraventricular) or a major portion of the pituitary stalk. Simple destruction of the posterior lobe, although associated with temporary DI, does not produce the sustained disorder. The posterior lobe is the major site for ADH storage and release but is not involved in its synthesis. In its absence, newly synthesized hormone can still be released into the circulation as long as the hypothalamic nuclei and part of the neurohypophyseal tract are intact.

Cases of DI may be separated into two main groups: (1) primary or idiopathic, involving about 50% of the cases, and due to a marked decrease in the hypothalamic nuclei of the neurohypophyseal system, and (2) secondary or acquired, due to a variety of pathologic lesions. The acquired lesions which produce DI (in decreasing order of frequency) are (1) posthypophysectomy, (2) cranial injuries, particularly basal skull fractures, (3) suprasellar and intrasellar tumors (primary or metastatic), (4) histiocytosis, (5) granulomas (sarcoidosis or tuberculosis), (6) vascular lesions (aneurysm, thrombosis), and (7) infections (encephalitis or meningitis).

Symptoms and Signs

Onset may be insidious or abrupt and may occur at any age. Enormous quantities of fluid may be ingested and excreted (3 to 30 L/day). Nocturia is usually present in DI and in NDI. Dehydration develops rapidly if urinary losses are not continuously replaced (e.g., if the patient becomes unconscious).

The only symptoms in the idiopathic form are polydipsia and polyuria. In the secondary type, symptoms and signs of the associated lesions are also present.

Diagnosis

DI must be differentiated from other causes of polyuria (TABLE 85-1). The diagnosis is established after demonstrating that one or more stimuli for secretion of ADH (e.g., water deprivation, hypertonic saline infusion, or nicotine administration) do not cause a significant reduction in the polyuria and concentration of urine, even though the kidney is responsive to exogenous ADH. The most reliable method of demonstrating endogenous secretion of ADH is by **complete water deprivation**, *a test that may be hazardous and should be performed only with the patient under constant direct supervision.* The test is initiated by weighing the patient and measuring *serum* Na concentration and osmolality. Voided urine is collected hourly and its sp gr or osmolarity (preferable) is measured. Dehydration is continued until (1) orthostatic hypotension and postural tachycardia appear, (2) 4 to 5% of the initial body weight has been lost, or (3) urinary concentration does not change > 0.001 sp gr or 30 mOsm/L with sequentially voided specimens. At the end of the test, the serum Na concentration and osmolarity are again determined, and 10 u. of *aqueous* vasopressin are given by IM injection. Hourly urine samples are again collected and sp gr or osmolarity measured for 2 h post injection. The patient also must be kept under direct supervision during the test to prevent inadvertent fluid intake.

Three types of response are common: (1) The urine concentrates with a sp gr of > 1.020 or 700 mOsm/L with no further concentration following administration of ADH. These findings demonstrate normal response of the neurohypophyseal and renal system. In addition to normal subjects it may be found in some cases of psychogenic polydipsia. (2) The urine concentration is less than noted above following dehydration, and a significant increase in urinary concentration follows administration of ADH. This pattern reflects failure of ADH secretion and is found in patients with DI. (3) Normal urinary concentrations are not achieved after either dehydration or vasopressin administration. Such results are consistent with NDI of the acquired or idiopathic variety.

Psychogenic (compulsive) polydipsia may present a difficult problem in differential diagnosis. These patients, who may ingest and excrete up to 6 L of fluid/day, are often obviously emotionally

TABLE 85-1. COMMON CAUSES OF POLYURIA

I.	Vasopressin-sensitive polyuria
	A. Decreased synthesis of ADH* (idiopathic or acquired diabetes insipidus)
	B. Decreased release of ADH (compulsive polydipsia)
II.	Vasopressin-resistant polyuria
	A. Congenital nephrogenic diabetes insipidus
	B. Acquired nephrogenic diabetes insipidus
	1. Chronic renal disease
	2. Systemic or metabolic disease (e.g., myeloma, amyloid, hypercalcemic or hypokalemic nephropathy, sickle cell disease)
	C. Osmotic diuresis
	1. Glucose (diabetes mellitus)
	2. Poorly resorbed solutes (mannitol, sorbitol, urea)

* Antidiuretic hormone (vasopressin)

disturbed. Unlike patients with DI and NDI, they do not usually have nocturia, nor does their thirst awaken them at night. Although some have a normal response to fluid deprivation, in others prolonged polydipsia produces impaired renal tubular function and inability to concentrate the urine, which may persist for weeks after fluid intake has been reduced to normal. Under these circumstances, patients respond poorly both to restricted fluid intake and to vasopressin, and therefore resemble patients with NDI. After prolonged restriction of fluid intake to 2 L or less/day, concentrating ability returns.

Treatment

Hormonal therapy: If a causative factor can be found, eradication should be attempted. Otherwise, effective control of DI may be obtained with several preparations of ADH which are available. (1) Lypressin, a synthetic vasopressin as a nasal spray is the simplest form for self-administration. Applications q 2 to 6 h are usually required. Desmopressin acetate (a longer-acting synthetic ADH substitute) may be inhaled or blown high into the nasal passage with an insufflator. In most patients nasal irritation is a frequent limiting factor with the powders. (2) An IM (*never IV*) injection of vasopressin tannate in oil in a dose of 0.3 to 1 ml (1.5 to 5 u.) usually controls polyuria and thirst for 1 to 3 days. (3) Aqueous posterior pituitary injection has little use in chronic treatment, but 5 to 10 u. s.c. or IM will give an antidiuretic response that usually lasts 6 h or less.

Nonhormonal therapy: Two types of drugs have been found useful in reducing polyuria: (1) various diuretics, primarily thiazides, and (2) ADH-releasing drugs such as chlorpropamide, carbamazepine, and clofibrate. The thiazide drugs paradoxically reduce urine volume in DI and NDI, primarily as a consequence of reducing extracellular fluid volume and increasing proximal tubular resorption. Urine volumes may fall by 25 to 50% during the daily administration of customary doses of thiazides (e.g., 15 to 25 mg/kg body wt of chlorothiazide). On the other hand, none of the other drugs are effective in NDI and are effective only in partial DI when residual ADH is present.

Chlorpropamide, carbamazepine, or clofibrate is capable of reducing or entirely eliminating the need for vasopressin in some patients. Chlorpropamide not only causes some release of ADH but also potentiates the action of ADH on the kidney. The dose of chlorpropamide is usually 3 to 5 mg/kg body wt orally once or twice/day. Hypoglycemia may be a significant adverse reaction of chlorpropamide treatment. If this occurs, partial or total substitution with clofibrate or carbamazepine is suggested. Clofibrate 500 to 1000 mg orally b.i.d. or carbamazepine 100 to 400 mg orally b.i.d. is recommended for adults only. Because the effects of chlorpropamide, carbamazepine, and clofibrate differ from those of the thiazides, the use of one of these agents with a diuretic may show additive effects and complement each other therapeutically.

---

86. THYROID

THYROID HORMONE FORMATION

The general scheme of thyroid hormone biosynthesis is depicted in FIG. 86–1. Iodide, ingested in food and water, is actively concentrated by the thyroid gland, converted to organic iodine by peroxidase, and incorporated into tyrosine in **thyroglobulin.** The tyrosines are iodinated at either one (monoiodotyrosine, MIT) or two (diiodotyrosine, DIT) sites and then coupled to form the active hormones (diiodotyrosine + diiodotyrosine → tetraiodothyronine **[thyroxine, T$_4$];** diiodotyrosine + monoiodotyrosine → **triiodothyronine [T$_3$]**). Thyroglobulin, a glycoprotein containing T$_3$ and T$_4$ within its matrix, is taken up as colloid droplets by the thyroid cells. Lysosomes containing proteases cleave T$_3$ and T$_4$ from thyroglobulin, resulting in release of free T$_3$ and T$_4$. The iodotyrosines (MIT and DIT) are also released from thyroglobulin but do not reach the bloodstream. They are deiodinated by intracellular deiodinases and their iodine utilized by the thyroid gland.

Although some of the free T$_3$ and T$_4$ is deiodinated in the thyroid gland with the iodine reentering the thyroid iodine pool, most diffuses into the bloodstream where it is bound to certain serum proteins for transport. The major thyroid transport protein is **thyroxine-binding globulin (TBG),** which normally accounts for about 80% of the bound thyroid hormone. Other thyroid-binding proteins, including **thyroxine-binding prealbumin (TBPA)** and **albumin,** account for the remainder of the bound serum thyroid hormone (20%). About 0.05% of the total serum T$_4$ and 0.5% of the total serum T$_3$ remain free but in equilibrium with the bound hormone.

All reactions necessary for T$_3$ and T$_4$ formation are influenced and controlled by pituitary **thyroid-stimulating hormone (TSH).** TSH binds to its thyroid plasma membrane receptor on the external cell surface and activates the enzyme adenylate cyclase, increasing the formation of cyclic AMP, the nucleotide that serves as a messenger to mediate the intracellular effects of TSH. Pituitary TSH secretion is controlled by a negative feedback mechanism modulated by the circulating level of free T$_3$ (and probably free T$_4$). Increased levels of free T$_3$ and free T$_4$ inhibit TSH secretion by the pituitary, whereas decreased levels of free T$_3$ or free T$_4$ increase TSH release from the pituitary. TSH secretion is also influenced by **thyrotropin-releasing hormone (TRH),** a 3-amino acid peptide synthesized in

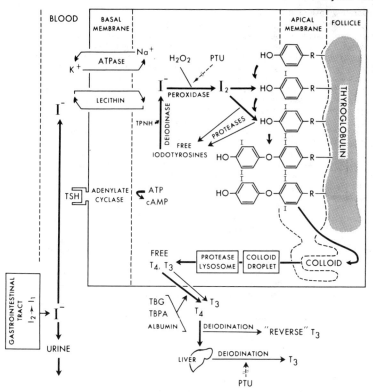

FIG. 86–1. Biosynthesis of thyroid hormones.

the hypothalamus. TRH, released into the portal system between the hypothalamus and pituitary, binds to the thyrotropic cells of the anterior pituitary and causes the subsequent release of TSH. The precise regulation of TRH synthesis and release has not been completely elucidated.

About 15% of the circulating T_3 is produced by the thyroid. The remainder is produced by mono-deiodination of the outer ring of T_4, mainly in the liver. Monodeiodination of the inner ring of T_4 also occurs, possibly in extrahepatic sites, to yield $3,3',5'-T_3$ (reverse T_3 or rT_3). This compound has minimal metabolic activity but is present in normal human serum and thyroglobulin. In many instances in which serum T_3 declines (e.g., chronic liver and renal disease, acute illness, starvation, and carbohydrate-deficient diets), rT_3 levels increase, suggesting that peripheral deiodination pathways shift to produce rT_3.

Observations pertaining to rT_3 metabolism in fetal life are of great importance. Total amniotic T_4 and T_3 are low, in contrast to levels in maternal serum. Fetal rT_3 levels in amniotic fluid are much higher than the corresponding values in maternal serum throughout pregnancy (15 to 42 wk). These data imply that rT_3 derives primarily from the fetus and that it may be possible to diagnose fetal hypothyroidism as early as the 15th wk of pregnancy, utilizing radioimmunoassay for rT_3. These levels appear to decrease after 30 wk gestation and may serve as a useful index of pregnancies of $<$ 30 wk duration.

Physiologic Effects of Thyroid Hormone

Thyroid hormones have 2 major physiologic effects. They increase protein synthesis in virtually every body tissue (the mechanism has not been precisely defined, but it is known that T_3 and T_4 enter cells, bind to discrete nuclear receptors, and influence the formation of mRNA), and they increase O_2 consumption. Thyroid hormones increase O_2 consumption by increasing the activity of the Na-K ATPase (Na pump), primarily in tissues responsible for basal O_2 consumption (i.e., liver, kidney, heart, and skeletal muscle). The increased activity of Na-K ATPase is secondary to increased synthesis of this enzyme; therefore, the increased O_2 consumption is also probably related to the nuclear binding of thyroid hormone.

Laboratory Testing of Thyroid Function

   1. Protein-bound iodine (PBI):   The measurement of PBI permits an estimate of the circulating thyroid hormone level, but direct measurement of T_3 and T_4 is more accurate and has replaced it. However, PBI determination may be useful in Hashimoto's thyroiditis.

   2. Serum total T_4 (serum total thyroxine) is measured by radioimmunoassay **(RIA)** involving a specific antigen-antibody reaction. A double antibody technic is used. RIA measures total T_4, both bound and free. It may also be measured by competitive protein-binding or by column chromatography. The tests are simple, inexpensive, and rapid. Total T_4 is a direct measurement of thyroxine, unaffected by contaminating non-T_4 iodine. However, changes in serum-binding protein levels produce corresponding changes in total T_4, even though the physiologically active free T_4 is unchanged. Thus, a patient may be physiologically normal but have an abnormal total T_4. **TBG is increased** in pregnancy, by estrogen therapy or oral contraceptives, in the acute phase of infectious hepatitis, in cirrhosis, hypothyroidism, carcinoma of the breast, acute intermittent porphyria, and prolonged perphenazine therapy. It may also be increased genetically or idiopathically. **TBG is decreased** by large protein losses (as in the nephrotic syndrome), by anabolic steroids including testosterone, by cortisol, and by the growth hormone excess in acromegaly. TBG may also be decreased genetically or idiopathically. Finally, large amounts of phenytoin and aspirin displace T_4 from its binding sites on TBG, thereby falsely lowering the serum total T_4 level.

   3. T_3 resin uptake: This test circumvents the problem of variations in serum TBG levels and reflects the **unsaturated** thyroid hormone-binding sites on TBG. It is *not* a measurement of circulating T_3. In normal subjects, 25 to 35% of the TBG binding sites are occupied by thyroid hormone. When ^{131}I-T_3 is added to the patient's serum, in vitro, a portion binds to unoccupied TBG sites. After equilibration, a resin is added which binds the remaining unbound ^{131}I-T_3. The value obtained is expressed as a ratio or percentage; some laboratories report as % unbound, while others report as % bound.

   Thus, in hypothyroidism, characterized by decreased levels of circulating thyroid hormone, there are less occupied and more unoccupied TBG binding sites. More ^{131}I-T_3 is bound to TBG, resulting in *less* uptake of ^{131}I-T_3 by the resin. The converse pertains in hyperthyroidism. The T_3 resin uptake test is most useful when there is a stable change in the TBG level and the concentration of free thyroxine is unchanged. For example, when TBG is increased (as in pregnancy), *both* occupied and unoccupied binding sites on TBG are increased. The total T_4 is increased because the TBG sites tend to remain 25 to 35% occupied regardless of the TBG level. Since 99.5% of circulating T_4 is bound to transport proteins, total T_4 is increased in a euthyroid patient with a normal free T_4. However, the T_3 resin uptake reflects the unoccupied sites on the increased amount of TBG, therefore more ^{131}I-T_3 is bound, resulting in a *decreased* resin uptake. Thus, when TBG is increased in the euthyroid patient, the total T_4 is increased and the T_3 resin uptake is decreased; when TBG is decreased in the euthyroid patient, the total T_4 is decreased and the T_3 resin uptake is increased.

   Performance of the serum total T_4 assay and the T_3 resin uptake test permits a valid interpretation of thyroid status in virtually all patients (see TABLE 86–1).

   4. Free thyroxine (T_4) index: The product of the value of the T_3 resin uptake and the serum total thyroxine concentration is known as the free thyroxine index and provides an estimate of the concentration of free T_4.

TABLE 86–1. LABORATORY EVALUATION OF THYROID FUNCTION IN VARIOUS THYROID DISORDERS

Physiologic State	Serum T_4 (Thyroxine)	Serum T_3 (Triiodothyronine)	Resin T_3 (Triiodothyronine Uptake)	24-h Radioiodine Uptake (Thyroid)	Basal Metabolic Rate
Hyperthyroidism, untreated	High	High	High	High	High
Hyperthyroidism, T_3 toxicosis	Normal	High	Normal	Normal	High
Hypothyroidism, untreated	Low	Low	Low	Low	Low
Euthyroid, on iodine	Normal	Normal	Normal	Low	Normal
Euthyroid, on exogenous thyroid hormone	High, on T_4 Low, on T_3	High, on T_3 Normal, on T_4	Normal	Low	Normal
Euthyroid, on estrogen	High	High	Low	Normal	Normal
Euthyroid, on phenytoin	Low	Low	High	Normal	Normal

5. Free thyroxine: Theoretically, this determination is the optimum test, since it most accurately reflects thyroid status. However, the measurement of free thyroxine is difficult, has many technical pitfalls, and is not readily available.

6. Serum total T_3 (serum total triiodothyronine): Measurement of serum T_3 is performed by RIA. Since T_3 is also bound to circulating serum proteins such as TBG, TBPA, and albumin, alterations in serum proteins alter the total T_3 levels in a manner identical to that observed for T_4.

7. Serum thyroid-stimulating hormone (TSH): This hormone, measured by RIA, is the best test for demonstrating primary hypothyroidism and for distinguishing between primary and secondary hypothyroidism. In primary hypothyroidism TSH is elevated, whereas in secondary hypothyroidism it is usually undetectable. It should be noted that some patients, following partial thyroidectomy or ^{131}I treatment, have increased serum TSH but may have sufficient thyroid secretory rates to maintain a normal T_4.

8. Thyrotropin-releasing hormone (TRH) test: Serum TSH is determined before and after an IV injection of 500 μg of synthetic TRH. Normally, there is a rapid rise in TSH of 5 to 35 μU/ml, reaching a peak in 30 min and returning to normal by 120 min. The rise is exaggerated in primary hypothyroidism. The TRH test is useful in distinguishing pituitary from hypothalamic hypothyroidism. Hypothyroid patients secondary to a pituitary deficiency do not release TSH in response to TRH. It is assumed that patients with a hypothalamic disorder having deficient TRH reserve and a normal pituitary reserve will usually release TSH in response to TRH. However, it is not certain that this is always the case and probably depends on other associated hormonal abnormalities. The test may also be useful in the diagnosis of hyperthyroidism in which TSH release remains suppressed, even in response to injected TRH, because of the inhibitory effects of the elevated free T_4 and free T_3 on the pituitary thyrotroph cell.

9. Radioactive iodine uptake (RAI): This test has disadvantages in cost, time, patient inconvenience, and radiation exposure. It is of value in the diagnosis of hyperthyroidism in which the RAI uptake is elevated, but is useless in the diagnosis of hypothyroidism, since the normal 24-h RAI uptake may be as low as 1% due to the large iodine intake in our diet. RAI uptake is particularly useful in the context of a T_3 suppression test and calculation of the dose of ^{131}I when it is selected as the treatment modality.

10. Thyroid scanning with radioiodine or ^{99m}technetium is not a routine test. It is useful in delineating structural abnormalities of the thyroid; e.g., to distinguish Graves' disease from multinodular goiter and a single toxic adenoma or to determine the functional state of a single nodule ("hot" vs "cold"). For a detailed discussion of radioisotope scanning of the thyroid see RADIONUCLIDE IMAGING METHODS in Ch. 227.

HYPERTHYROIDISM

(Thyrotoxicosis; Toxic Diffuse Goiter; Graves' Disease; Basedow's Disease; Toxic Nodular Goiter; Plummer's Disease)

See TABLE 86-2 for types of hyperthyroidism.

Graves' Disease (Toxic Diffuse Goiter)

Graves' disease *consists of hyperthyroidism, but also is characterized by one or more of the following: goiter, exophthalmos, and pretibial myxedema.* The cause of the hyperthyroidism is not completely understood but is probably immunologic. Patients with Graves' disease have a circulating thyroid stimulator in their serum known as **long-acting thyroid stimulator (LATS)**, which is a 7S γ-globulin with characteristics of an antibody. However, LATS is not demonstrable in at least 20 to 40% of patients with Graves' disease. Due to the large percentage of LATS-negative patients with Graves' disease, the search has continued for other immunoglobulins with thyroid stimulatory activity. One of these, called "Human Thyroid Stimulator" (also called "LATS-protector"), is of particular interest because it specifically stimulates human thyroid. It appears likely that a family of immunoglobulins that are antibodies to the TSH receptor, including LATS and Human Thyroid Stimulator, can bind to the receptor site, stimulate the thyroid, and cause hyperthyroidism. TSH is *not* a cause of Graves' disease.

TABLE 86-2. TYPES OF HYPERTHYROIDISM

Most Common	Very Rare
Graves' disease (toxic diffuse goiter)	TSH-producing tumor of the pituitary
Toxic multinodular goiter	Metastic embryonal carcinoma of the testis
Toxic adenoma	Choriocarcinoma
Thyrotoxicosis factitia	Struma ovarii
Subacute thyroiditis	
Silent thyroiditis	

Symptoms and Signs

Many symptoms and signs are associated with hyperthyroidism. They are the same for all forms of hyperthyroidism with some exceptions, such as infiltrative ophthalmopathy and dermopathy, which are confined to Graves' disease. The clinical presentation may be dramatic or subtle. **The more common signs are:** (1) goiter, (2) tachycardia, (3) widened pulse pressure, (4) warm, fine, moist skin, (5) tremor, (6) eye signs (see below), and (7) atrial fibrillation. **The most frequent symptoms are:** (1) nervousness and increased activity, (2) increased sweating, (3) hypersensitivity to heat, (4) palpitations, (5) fatigue, (6) increased appetite, (7) weight loss, (8) tachycardia, (9) insomnia, (10) weakness, and (11) frequent bowel movements (occasionally diarrhea). Many symptoms of hyperthyroidism are similar to those of adrenergic excess. There is a marked increase in adrenergic activity in hyperthyroidism, and many agents that block stimulation of the adrenergic nervous system relieve the symptoms of hyperthyroidism (see Treatment). However, the mechanism of the augmented adrenergic activity in hyperthyroidism is uncertain and further puzzling, since serum catecholamine levels are decreased. Older persons, particularly those with toxic nodular goiter, may present atypically with an **apathetic** or **masked** (monosymptomatic) form (see Ch. 232).

Eye signs noted in patients with thyrotoxicosis include stare, lid lag, lid retraction, and mild degrees of conjunctival injection or edema-producing symptoms including orbital pain, lacrimation, irritation, and photophobia. These eye signs are largely due to excessive adrenergic stimulation and remit promptly upon successful treatment of the thyrotoxicosis. **Infiltrative ophthalmopathy** is a more serious development and is specific for Graves' disease. It is characterized by increased retro-orbital tissue, producing exophthalmos, and by lymphocytic infiltration of the extraocular muscles, producing a spectrum of ocular muscle weakness frequently leading to blurred and double vision. The pathogenesis of infiltrative ophthalmopathy is poorly understood. It may occur before the onset of hyperthyroidism or as late as 15 to 20 yr afterwards and frequently worsens or improves independent of the clinical course of hyperthyroidism. Infiltrative ophthalmopathy results from autoimmune phenomena distinct from those initiating Graves'-type hyperthyroidism, and in the presence of normal thyroid function is known as **euthyroid Graves' disease**.

Infiltrative dermopathy, also known as pretibial myxedema (a confusing term, since myxedema suggests hypothyroidism), is characterized by nonpitting infiltration of mucinous ground substance, usually in the pretibial area. The lesion is very pruritic and erythematous in its early stages and subsequently becomes brawny. Like ophthalmopathy, infiltrative dermopathy may appear years before or after the hyperthyroidism. LATS and other thyroid-stimulating immunoglobulins are invariably present. Topical steroids can sometimes relieve the pruritus. The dermopathy usually spontaneously remits after months or years.

Other Forms of Hyperthyroidism

Thyroid storm is characterized by abrupt onset of more florid symptoms of thyrotoxicosis, with some exacerbated symptoms and signs atypical of uncomplicated Graves' disease. Included are fever; marked weakness and muscle-wasting; extreme restlessness with wide emotional swings; confusion, psychosis, or even coma; and hepatomegaly with mild jaundice. The patient may present with cardiovascular collapse and shock. Thyroid storm results from untreated or inadequately treated thyrotoxicosis and may be precipitated by infection, trauma, surgery, embolism, diabetic acidosis, fright, toxemia of pregnancy or labor, discontinuance of antithyroid medication, or radiation thyroiditis.

It is rare in children. *Thyroid storm is a life-threatening emergency requiring prompt and specific treatment* (see Treatment and TABLE 86–6, below). The mortality rate in treated cases is about 25%.

T_3 **toxicosis:** Both T_3 and T_4 are regularly increased in patients with hyperthyroidism. Increases in serum T_3 are usually somewhat greater proportionally compared to T_4, probably because of both increased thyroidal secretion of T_3 and increased peripheral conversion of T_4 to T_3. In some thyrotoxic patients, only T_3 is elevated; this condition is called "T_3 toxicosis." It is difficult to diagnose because T_3 is not measured by the ordinary thyroid function tests, but requires a specific RIA. The criteria to establish the diagnosis are (1) symptoms and signs of hyperthyroidism, (2) normal T_4 and ^{131}I uptake, (3) nonsuppressible ^{131}I uptake, (4) failure to release TSH in response to TRH (see TRH test above), or (5) elevated serum T_3.

T_3 toxicosis may be seen in any of the natural disorders producing hyperthyroidism, including Graves' disease, multinodular goiter, and the autonomously functioning solitary thyroid nodule. If T_3 toxicosis continues untreated, the patient eventually develops the typical laboratory abnormalities of hyperthyroidism; i.e., elevated T_4 and ^{131}I uptake. This suggests that T_3 toxicosis is an early manifestation of ordinary hyperthyroidism and should be treated as such.

Toxic adenoma and toxic multinodular goiter (Plummer's disease): One or more thyroid nodules occasionally hyperfunction autonomously for unknown reasons. The excess T_3 and T_4 inhibit the hypothalamic-pituitary axis, stopping TSH production and decreasing production of hormone in the rest of the thyroid. RAI uptake in the hyperfunctioning nodule is increased while, in the rest of the gland, it is decreased. Multinodular goiter with or without hyperthyroidism is more common in older people. Neither toxic multinodular goiter nor toxic adenoma is associated with LATS, exophthalmos, or the pretibial myxedema found in Graves' disease. Since nodules often produce selective increases in T_3 levels, determination of serum total T_3 should be included in the thyroid function tests selected for evaluation of nodular goiter.

Toxic adenoma and multinodular goiter are treated surgically or with radioiodine.

Thyrotoxicosis factitia: This syndrome of hyperthyroidism results from self-administration of thyroid hormone; patients (commonly medical or paramedical personnel) may be surreptitiously taking T_4 or T_3. Laboratory evaluation will vary accordingly. If the disorder is caused by ingestion of preparations containing T_4, the serum T_4 will be elevated. When ingestion of T_3 is the cause, serum T_4 will be below normal. In either case, serum T_3 levels will be increased, particularly when preparations containing T_3 are the causative agents; there will be no goiter.

Silent thyroiditis: Silent thyroiditis is characterized by a variable but mild degree of thyroid enlargement, absence of thyroid tenderness, normal or slightly elevated sedimentation rate, normal WBC count, and a self-limited hyperthyroid phase of several weeks to several months, often followed by transient hypothyroidism but with eventual recovery to the euthyroid state. Although the etiology of silent thyroiditis is obscure, recent evidence suggests an autoimmune component. Biopsies reveal evidence of lymphocytic infiltration as is seen in Hashimoto's thyroiditis. Human antithyroglobulin antibodies measured by a RIA are sometimes elevated in silent thyroiditis and may remain so for up to 9 mo; thus, silent thyroiditis would appear to be a variant of Hashimoto's thyroiditis. However, unlike the hyperthyroidism occasionally seen with Hashimoto's thyroiditis, the elevated thyroid hormone levels of silent thyroiditis occur in association with a very low RAI uptake. The combination of a high serum thyroid hormone concentration and a low RAI uptake can also be seen with subacute thyroiditis, factitious hyperthyroidism, and iodine ingestion. Since this is a self-limited transient disorder of one to several months, treatment is conservative, usually only requiring β-adrenergic blockade with propranolol (see below). Surgery and radioactive iodine therapy are contraindicated.

Excess TSH produced by a pituitary tumor can cause secondary hyperthyroidism through overproduction of thyroid hormone. Hypothyroidism secondary to metastatic embryonal carcinoma or choriocarcinoma is due to the TSH-like properties of human chorionic gonadotropin (HCG). **Struma ovarii** is a generally benign ovarian teratoma containing predominantly thyroid tissue. Approximately 5% of the patients with struma ovarii develop hyperthyroidism. Treatment involves removal of the teratoma.

Diagnosis

The diagnosis of hyperthyroidism is usually straightforward and depends on a careful clinical history and physical examination, a high index of suspicion, and routine thyroid hormone determinations. A serum T_4 assay and a T_3 resin uptake test are a highly accurate combination of initial tests for assessing thyroid status and are relatively inexpensive. Occasionally, a serum T_3 determination is required (see above, T_3 Toxicosis). The determination of free thyroxine is less often required and is not as easily available. If the diagnosis of hyperthyroidism remains unclear after these initial tests, more expensive, sophisticated, and time-consuming tests may be required. For example, a TRH test or a T_3 **suppression test** may have to be performed. For the latter, a RAI uptake test is performed initially and after 7 days of treatment with 25 μg of liothyronine (triiodothyronine) t.i.d. orally. The usual response is a fall in RAI uptake of *50% or more*. In patients with hyperthyroidism (regardless of type) uptake is decreased by < 50%. Occasional exceptions to this rule include some patients with euthyroid multinodular goiter and patients with euthyroid Graves' ophthalmopathy.

Treatment of Hyperthyroidism

A number of approaches are utilized for the treatment of hyperthyroidism (see TABLE 86–3).

Iodine in pharmacologic doses inhibits the release of T_3 and T_4 within a few hours and inhibits the organification of iodine, a transitory effect lasting from a few days to a week. It is used for the emergency management of thyroid storm, for thyrotoxic patients undergoing emergency surgery, and (since it also decreases the vascularity of the thyroid gland) for the preoperative preparation of thyrotoxic patients selected for subtotal thyroidectomy. Iodine is generally *not* used for routine treatment of hyperthyroidism. The usual dosage is several drops of potassium iodide solution t.i.d. or q.i.d. orally or 0.5 gm sodium iodide in 1 L isotonic (0.9%) saline given IV slowly q 12 h. Complications of iodine therapy include inflammation of the salivary glands, conjunctivitis, skin rashes, and induction of hyperthyroidism **(Jod-Basedow phenomenon).**

Propylthiouracil and methimazole are antithyroid agents that decrease organification and impair the coupling reaction. There is no "escape" phenomenon as there is with iodine. Propylthiouracil

TABLE 86–3. TREATMENT OF HYPERTHYROIDISM

Iodine
Propylthiouracil and methimazole
Radioactive iodine
Surgery
Propranolol—adjunctive, usually not used alone except for special, short-
    term circumstances

(but not methimazole) also inhibits the peripheral conversion of T_4 to T_3. The usual starting dosage for propylthiouracil is 100 to 150 mg orally q 8 h, and for methimazole 10 to 15 mg orally q 8 h. When the patient becomes euthyroid the dosage is decreased to the lowest effective amount, usually 100 to 150 mg propylthiouracil or 10 to 15 mg methimazole daily in 2 or 3 divided doses. In general, control can be achieved within 6 wk to 3 mo. More rapid control can be achieved by increasing the dose of propylthiouracil to 450 to 600 mg/day (at the risk of increasing the incidence of side effects). Doses of propylthiouracil of this magnitude or greater (800 to 1200 mg/day) are generally reserved for the more seriously ill patients including those with thyrotoxic storm. Maintenance doses can be continued for one year or many years depending on the clinical circumstances. Although the statistics vary, it appears that 16 to 40% of the patients will enter remission anywhere from 1 mo to 2 yr after induction of the euthyroid state with antithyroid drugs. At the present time there is no clear benefit in using high doses of antithyroid drugs concomitantly with replacement doses of thyroid hormone.

Adverse effects include allergic reactions, nausea, loss of taste, and, in < 1% of patients, a reversible agranulocytosis. If the patient is allergic to one agent, it is acceptable to switch to the other. In case of agranulocytosis, it is unacceptable to switch to another agent, and more definitive therapy should be invoked, such as radioiodine or surgery.

The disappearance or marked decrease in gland size and the redevelopment of suppressible thyroid function, as determined by T_3 suppression test or TRH test, may be evidence that the patient is undergoing remission.

Radioactive iodine ^{131}I is generally used in patients past their childbearing years, because it is not clear what the effects may be on their progeny. There has been no proven increased incidence of tumors, leukemia, or carcinoma of the thyroid and some use this therapy in younger patients. Radioiodine is the treatment of choice for Graves' disease in patients > 40 yr of age. Dosage of ^{131}I is difficult to gauge and the response of the gland cannot be predicted. If enough ^{131}I is given to produce euthyroidism, 1 yr later 25% of the patients will have hypothyroidism, and the incidence continues to increase at a regular rate for up to 20 yr or more thereafter. On the other hand, if smaller doses are used, there is a high incidence of recurrence of hyperthyroidism.

Surgery is used in patients < 21 yr who should not receive radioiodine; in individuals who cannot tolerate other agents because of hypersensitivity or other problems; in patients with very large goiters (100 to 400 gm [normal thyroid weighs 20 gm]), and in some patients with toxic adenoma and multinodular goiter.

Surgery offers a good prospect for recovery. In expert hands, postoperative recurrences vary between 2 and 9%; hypothyroidism occurs in about 3% of patients the first year and in about 2% with each succeeding year. Vocal cord paralysis and hypoparathyroidism are uncommon complications, but difficult to treat. In preparing the patient for surgery, iodine (saturated solution of potassium iodide 3 drops orally t.i.d.) should be given for 2 wk before the operation to reduce the vascularity of the gland and facilitate surgery. Propylthiouracil must be given prior to surgery, since the patient should be euthyroid before surgery. Surgical procedures are more difficult in patients who previously have undergone thyroidectomy or radioiodine therapy.

Propranolol: Symptoms and signs of hyperthyroidism due to adrenergic stimulation may respond to β-adrenergic blocking agents, e.g., propranolol. Phenomena that improve and that do not improve with propranolol are shown in TABLES 86–4 and 86–5. Propranolol is not as useful for stare and lid retraction as once thought, suggesting that these may be predominantly α-effects (or at least a mixture of α- and β-effects). It should be noted that propranolol decreases myocardial contractility through a non-β-adrenergic mechanism. Because propranolol is a direct myocardial depressant, there are some difficulties that accompany its use (see below).

Propranolol is indicated in thyroid storm. It rapidly decreases heart rate, usually within 2 to 3 h when given orally, and in minutes when given IV. It may bring about rapid defervescence of fever in thyroid storm. Propranolol is also indicated for the prompt management of troublesome tachycardia found in other forms of hyperthyroidism (including thyroiditis) and especially in older patients with no history of congestive heart failure, since it ordinarily takes several weeks to get relief from antithyroid agents. However, propranolol should not be used routinely in all types of hyperthyroidism. For details concerning propranolol therapy see ADRENERGIC BLOCKING DRUGS in Ch. 248.

A treatment regimen for **thyroid storm** listing all of the above-mentioned therapies is shown in TABLE 86–6.

TABLE 86–4. PHENOMENA IMPROVED BY PROPRANOLOL

Tachycardia	Diarrhea (occasional)
Tremor	Proximal myopathy
Mental symptoms	(occasional)
Heat intolerance and sweating	Serum T_3 (decreased about
(occasional)	50%)

TABLE 86–5. PHENOMENA NOT IMPROVED BY PROPRANOLOL

Oxygen consumption—although excess catecholamines (as in patients with pheochromocytoma) increase O_2 consumption, the major stimulus to O_2 consumption is thyroid hormone increase of $Na^+ \cdot K^+ \cdot ATPase$ activity
Goiter
Bruit
Circulating thyroxine levels
Weight loss (may be stabilized, but not improved)
Exophthalmos
Myocardial contractility

HYPOTHYROIDISM

(Myxedema)

The characteristic reaction to thyroid hormone deficiency in the adult.

Primary hypothyroidism, the most common form, is probably an autoimmune disease, usually occurring as a sequel to Hashimoto's thyroiditis. It results in a shrunken fibrotic thyroid gland with little or no function. The second most common form is **post-therapeutic hypothyroidism,** especially following RAI therapy or surgery for hyperthyroidism. Hypothyroidism during therapy with propylthiouracil, methimazole, and iodides usually abates after cessation of therapy.

Most patients with goiters are either euthyroid or have hyperthyroidism, but **goitrous hypothyroidism** may occur in endemic goiter. Iodine deficiency decreases thyroid hormonogenesis; TSH is released, the thyroid gland enlarges under the TSH stimulus and traps iodine avidly, and goiter ensues. If iodine deficiency is severe, the patient becomes hypothyroid, but this disease is virtually extinct in the USA since the advent of iodized salt. **Endemic cretinism** may occur in the offspring of parents with endemic goitrous hypothyroidism.

Rare inherited enzymatic defects can alter the synthesis of thyroid hormone. **Congenital goiters** with or without hypothyroidism have been classified into 4 types. *Type 1* involves a defect in iodide transport probably secondary to an alteration in synthesis of cell surface proteins necessary for transport. *Type 2* is associated with several defects in iodination mechanisms within the thyroid. One involves the absence of the enzyme peroxidase, necessary for the organification of iodine, which can result in goitrous cretinism. Another appears to involve a defect of hydrogen peroxide generation, and is associated with deaf mutism, a complex known as **Pendred's syndrome.** Patients with Pendred's syndrome are usually euthyroid, and the deafness is not secondary to the hypothyroidism. The defect is inherited as autosomal recessive. A third defect, associated with abnormal peroxidase, allows sufficient compensation for maintenance of a euthyroid state. *Type 3* congenital goiters are found in patients with dehalogenase defects. Although the precise biochemical abnormality is unclear, patients have complete or partial deiodination defects of MIT and DIT within thyroglobulin. *Type 4* congenital goiters are associated with defects in the synthesis of thyroglobulin. **Athyreotic cretinism** is found in children born without a thyroid gland.

Secondary hypothyroidism occurs when there is failure of the hypothalamic-pituitary axis, either due to deficient secretion of TRH from the hypothalamus or lack of secretion of TSH from the pituitary.

TABLE 86–6. TREATMENT OF THYROID STORM

Iodine—30 drops Lugol's solution/day orally in 3 or 4 divided doses; or 1 to 2 gm sodium iodide slowly by IV drip
Prophylthiouracil—900 to 1200 mg/day orally or by gastric tube
Propranolol—160 mg/day orally in 4 divided doses; or 1 to 2 mg *slowly* IV q 4 h under careful monitoring
IV glucose solutions
Correction of dehydration and electrolyte imbalance
Cooling blanket for hyperthermia
Digitalis if necessary
Treatment of underlying disease such as infection
Adrenal steroids—100 to 300 mg hydrocortisone/day IV or IM

Definitive therapy after control of the crisis consists of ablation of the thyroid gland with ^{131}I or surgery.

Symptoms and Signs

The symptoms and signs of primary hypothyroidism are generally in striking contrast to those of hyperthyroidism and may be quite subtle and insidious in onset. The facial expression is dull; there is puffiness and periorbital swelling caused by infiltration with the mucopolysaccharides, hyaluronic acid and chondroitin sulfate; eyelids droop because of decreased adrenergic drive; hair is sparse, coarse, and dry; and the skin is coarse, dry, scaly, and thick. Patients are forgetful, and show other evidence of intellectual impairment with a gradual change in personality. There may be frank psychosis ("**myxedema madness**").

There is often carotenemia, particularly notable on the palms and soles, caused by deposition of carotene in the lipid-rich epidermal layers. Deposition of mucinous ground substance in the tongue may produce macroglossia. There is bradycardia due to a decrease in both thyroid hormone and adrenergic stimulation. The heart is enlarged due, in large measure, to accumulation of a serous effusion of high protein content in the pericardial sac. There may also be pleural or abdominal effusions. The pericardial and pleural effusions develop slowly, and only infrequently result in respiratory or hemodynamic distress. Patients generally note constipation, which may be severe. Paresthesias of the hands and feet are common, due to carpal-tarsal tunnel syndrome caused by deposition of mucinous ground substance in the ligaments around the wrist and ankle, producing nerve compression. The reflexes may be very helpful diagnostically because of the brisk contraction and the slow relaxation time. There is often menorrhagia, in contrast to the hypomenorrhea of hyperthyroidism. Hypothermia is commonly noted if the temperature is measured rectally. Anemia is often present, usually normocytic normochromic in character and of unknown etiology; but it may be hypochromic due to menorrhagia, and sometimes is macrocytic because of impaired B_{12} absorption related to decreased intrinsic factor synthesis.

Myxedema coma: This life-threatening complication of hypothyroidism is extremely rare in warm climates, but not uncommon in cold areas. Its characteristics include a background of longstanding hypothyroidism, coma with extreme hypothermia (temperatures 24 to 32.2 C [75.2 to 90 F]), areflexia, seizures, CO_2 retention, and respiratory depression caused by decreased cerebral blood flow. Severe hypothermia may be missed unless temperatures are recorded using special low-reading thermometers. Rapid diagnosis (based on clinical judgment, history, and physical examination) is imperative because early death is likely. Precipitating factors include exposure to cold, infection, trauma, and drugs that suppress the CNS. See below for treatment.

Hypothyroidism in the young produces other symptoms and signs: **Neonatal hypothyroidism (cretinism)** is characterized by respiratory distress, cyanosis, jaundice, poor feeding, hoarse cry, umbilical hernia, and retardation of bone growth. Diagnosis requires a high index of suspicion and is greatly aided by routine determination of serum T_4 and TSH in umbilical cord blood, or filter paper blood spots taken at 2 to 5 days of age. Prompt treatment (preferably *in utero* or no later than the first week to 10 days of the postnatal period) prevents or markedly reduces abnormalities in mental development. **Childhood (juvenile) hypothyroidism** is characterized by growth retardation, delayed dentition, and mental deficiency. The symptoms and signs of **adolescent hypothyroidism** are similar to those of adults; additionally there may be short stature and precocious puberty with an enlarged sella turcica.

Diagnosis of Primary vs. Secondary Hypothyroidism

It is important to differentiate secondary from primary hypothyroidism, because, while secondary hypothyroidism is not common, it often involves other endocrine organs affected by the hypothalamic-pituitary axis. The clues to secondary hypothyroidism are a history of amenorrhea rather than menorrhagia in a woman with known hypothyroidism and some suggestive differences on physical examination. In secondary hypothyroidism, the skin and hair are dry but not as coarse; skin depigmentation is often noted; macroglossia is not as prominent; breasts are atrophic; the heart is small without accumulation of the serous effusions in the pericardial sac; BP is low; and hypoglycemia is often found because of concomitant adrenal insufficiency or growth hormone deficiency.

Laboratory evaluation shows a *low* level of circulating TSH in secondary hypothyroidism, whereas in primary hypothyroidism there is no feedback inhibition of the intact pituitary and serum levels of TSH are *very high*. The serum TSH is the most simple and sensitive test for the diagnosis of primary hypothyroidism. Serum cholesterol is generally low in secondary hypothyroidism, but high in primary hypothyroidism. Other pituitary hormones and their corresponding target tissue hormones may be low in secondary hypothyroidism.

The TRH test (see thyroid function testing above) is useful in distinguishing between hypothyroidism secondary to pituitary failure and hypothyroidism due to hypothalamic failure. In the former, TSH is not released in response to TRH, whereas in the latter TSH is released.

The **TSH stimulation test** was used to distinguish between primary and secondary hypothyroidism before the serum TSH immunoassay became available but is only occasionally used today. The test is performed by carrying out an initial RAI uptake for a 24-h period. On the next 3 days, 5 USP units of TSH are given IM. On the 4th day, the 2nd RAI uptake is performed. Patients with primary hypothyroidism will not respond; patients with secondary hypothyroidism will have a brisk response unless they have had longstanding secondary hypothyroidism (e.g., for 15 or 20 yr). The test has 3 disadvantages: (1) it requires administration of radioactive iodine on two occasions, with its associated radiation exposure; (2) it is expensive and time-consuming for the patient; and (3) allergic reactions to the bovine TSH used in the test are not infrequent. There are also certain risks associated with TSH stimulation. If the patient has arteriosclerotic heart disease, a sudden increase in heart rate may lead to angina or myocardial infarction. Patients with secondary hypothyroidism may have adrenal insufficiency, and an increase in metabolic rate can precipitate adrenal crisis unless glucocorticoid therapy is given. Finally, in rare cases, there may be enlargement of the thyroid as a result of TSH stimulation which, if the gland is located substernally, may result in respiratory distress.

The **determination of serum total T_3 levels** in hypothyroidism deserves special mention. The numerous conditions associated with decreased circulating levels of total T_3 include (1) hypothyroidism, both primary and secondary; (2) decreased serum TBG; and (3) chronic liver and renal disease, acute and chronic illness, starvation, and low carbohydrate diets. In the 3rd group the decrease in T_3 concentration is related to decreased peripheral conversion of T_4 to T_3. "Reverse" T_3 levels rise, indicating a shift in the peripheral monodeiodination pathways.

Generally, both serum T_3 and T_4 levels are decreased in hypothyroidism. Curiously, perhaps as many as 25% of patients with primary hypothyroidism (elevated serum TSH, low serum T_4) may have normal circulating levels of T_3. This remains unexplained, but may result from sustained TSH stimulation of the suboptimally functioning thyroid and incorporation of the trapped iodine preferentially into the pathway responsible for synthesizing the more potent thyroid hormone, T_3.

Treatment of Hypothyroidism

A variety of thyroid hormone preparations are available for replacement therapy, including synthetic preparations of thyroxine, liothyronine (triiodothyronine), combinations of the 2 synthetic hormones, and desiccated animal thyroid. Synthetic preparations of L-thyroxine are preferred; the *average* maintenance dosage is 150 to 200 µg/day orally. Absorption is fairly constant at about 60% of the dose. T_3 is generated from the T_4 by the liver. In infants and young children the average maintenance dose of L-thyroxine is 2.5 µg/kg/day.

T_3 **(liothyronine sodium)** should not be used alone for long-term replacement because its rapid turnover requires that it be taken b.i.d. or t.i.d. T_3 is used mainly in starting therapy because the rapid excretion is useful in the initial titration of a patient with longstanding hypothyroidism in whom cardiac arrhythmias may occur in the early stages of replacement. In addition, administration of standard replacement amounts of T_3 (25 to 75 µg/day) results in rapid increases in serum T_3 levels (300 to 1000 ng) within 2 to 4 h, returning to normal by 24 h. Therefore, when assessing serum T_3 levels in patients on this particular regimen, it is important for the physician to be aware of the time of prior administration of the hormone. In addition, it appears that patients receiving T_3 are chemically hyperthyroid for at least several hours a day and thus are exposed to greater cardiac risks. Similar patterns of serum T_3 concentrations are seen when mixtures of T_3 and T_4 are taken orally, although the peak levels of T_3 are somewhat lower. Replacement regimens with synthetic preparations of T_4 reflect a different pattern of serum T_3 response. Increases in serum T_3 occur gradually over weeks, finally reaching a normal value at about 8 wk after initiation of therapy.

Treatment of myxedema coma consists of large doses of IV T_4 (500 µg IV bolus) or T_3 if available (40 µg IV), because TBG must be saturated before any free hormone is available for response. The maintenance dose for T_4 is 50 µg/day IV, and for T_3, 10 to 20 µg/day IV until the hormone can be given orally. The patient should *not* be rewarmed rapidly because of the threat of cardiac arrhythmias. If alveolar ventilation is compromised, immediate mechanical ventilatory assistance is required.

THYROIDITIS

HASHIMOTO'S THYROIDITIS

(Chronic Lymphocytic Thyroiditis; Hashimoto's Struma; Autoimmune Thyroiditis)

This autoimmune disorder is thought to be the most common cause of primary hypothyroidism. It is more prevalent (8:1) in women than men and most frequent between the ages of 30 and 50. A family history of thyroid disorders is common and incidence is increased in patients with chromosomal disorders, including Turner's, Down's, and Klinefelter's syndromes. Histologic studies reveal extensive infiltration of lymphocytes in the thyroid.

Patients complain of painless enlargement of the gland or fullness in the throat. On examination there is a nontender goiter, smooth or nodular, and more rubbery in consistency than the normal thyroid; 20% of patients have hypothyroidism when first seen. Other forms of autoimmune disease are common, including pernicious anemia, RA, SLE, and Sjögren's syndrome. Frequent coexistence with other endocrine disorders, including Addison's disease (adrenal insufficiency), hypoparathyroidism, and diabetes mellitus, all of which may be autoimmune in nature, is also observed. There may be an increased incidence of thyroid neoplasia, particularly papillary carcinoma, possibly because of increased TSH stimulation.

Laboratory findings early in the disease consist of a normal T_4 but an increased PBI, due to production of abnormal iodinated proteins, and high titers of antithyroid antibodies. Similarly, RAI uptake is increased early because of a defect in organification in conjunction with a gland continuing to trap iodine. Late in the disease, the patient develops hypothyroidism with a decrease in T_4 and in RAI uptake. Antibodies in this stage are usually no longer detectable.

Treatment of Hashimoto's thyroiditis requires lifelong replacement with thyroid hormone to correct and prevent hypothyroidism. The average oral replacement dose with L-thyroxine is 150 to 200 μg/day.

SUBACUTE THYROIDITIS (Granulomatous, Giant-Cell, or DeQuervain's Thyroiditis)

This type of thyroiditis is probably virus-induced. Frequently, there is a history of mumps, and it has been described following a wide variety of URIs. Histologic studies do not show lymphocyte infiltration of the gland, as in Hashimoto's disease, but there is a characteristic giant-cell infiltration.

Clinical features are the sudden onset of "sore throat" (in reality, neck pain) with tenderness of progressive intensity in the neck and low-grade fever (37.8 to 38.3 C [100 to 101 F]). The neck pain shifts characteristically from one side to the other and finally settles in one area. It often radiates to the jaw and ears, is often confused with dental problems, pharyngitis or otitis, and is aggravated by swallowing or turning the head. Hyperthyroidism is common in the early stages of the disease because of release of hormone from the markedly inflamed gland. Additionally, there is lassitude and prostration not seen with other thyroid disorders. On physical examination, the thyroid is assymetrically enlarged, firm, and tender. The process is self-limited, generally subsiding in a few months; occasionally it recurs, and only rarely results in hypothyroidism.

Laboratory findings early in the disease include an increase in T_4, a decrease in RAI uptake (often 0), leukocytosis, and a high sedimentation rate. After several weeks, the T_4 is decreased and the radioiodine uptake remains low. Full recovery is the rule; rarely, patients may become hypothyroid.

Treatment consists of aspirin 600 mg q 4 h and, only as a last resort, glucocorticoids such as prednisone 5 mg orally q 6 h. On discontinuance of the latter, there is often a severe rebound in symptoms.

EUTHYROID GOITER

(Simple, Endemic, Nontoxic Diffuse, or Nontoxic Nodular Goiter)

An enlargement of the thyroid gland due to diminished thyroid hormone production but without clinical hypothyroidism. If the deficiency is caused by inadequate dietary intake of iodine, it is called **endemic (colloid) goiter.** Euthyroid goiter is the most common form of thyroid enlargement and is frequently noted at the onset of puberty, during pregnancy, and at menopause. Numerous other causes include intrinsic thyroid hormone production defects or the ingestion of goitrogens (such as turnips) that contain antithyroid substances similar to thiouracil. Many drugs, including aminosalicylic acid (PAS), sulfonylureas, lithium, and even iodine in large doses, may block the synthesis of thyroid hormone. Compensatory TSH elevations occur, preventing hypothyroidism, but the TSH stimulation results in goiter formation. Persistent stimulation and involution may result in nontoxic nodular goiters.

Symptoms, Signs, and Diagnosis

In the early stages, diagnosis depends on the presence of a soft, symmetric, smooth goiter. There may be a history of low iodine intake or ingestion of goitrogens. Thyroidal radioiodine uptake may be normal or high, with a normal thyroid scan. The serum T_4 concentration and the T_3-resin uptake are usually normal. Later, multiple nodules and cysts may appear.

Treatment

The cause should be identified. Iodine deficiency is rare in the USA today, but if present, iodine is given. If a goitrogen is being ingested, it should be discontinued. In other instances, suppression of the hypothalamic-pituitary axis with thyroid hormone will block the TSH stimulation that leads to goiter formation. Full replacement doses are necessary; i.e., sodium levothyroxine 150 to 200 μg/day orally or desiccated thyroid 90 to 120 mg/day orally. Large goiters occasionally require surgery to prevent interference with respiration or to correct cosmetic problems.

THYROID CANCERS

Usually, either the patient or the doctor notices an otherwise symptomless lump in the neck. Rarely, metastases from a small thyroid cancer may lead to presenting complaints due to lymph node enlargement, pulmonary symptoms, or a destructive bone lesion. Most thyroid nodules are benign and, as a rule, thyroid cancers are not highly malignant and generally are compatible with normal life expectancy, *if treated properly.* There are 5 types of thyroid cancer: papillary, follicular, mixed (most common), medullary (solid, with amyloid struma), and anaplastic (rare).

The suspicion that the patient has cancer is increased by the following factors: (1) age (the young are more susceptible); (2) sex, if the patient is a man (more women have thyroid cancer by a ratio of 2:1, but women have more thyroid disease by a ratio of about 8:1; thus, a man with a nodule should be regarded with greater suspicion); (3) a solitary nodule (multinodular lesions are usually multinodular goiter); (4) a cold nodule on RAI uptake scanning (hot nodules are seldom cancer); (5) a history of radiation exposure to the head, neck, or chest (e.g., for an enlarged thymus or tonsils, for acne or Hodgkin's disease, etc.); (6) if there is radiographic evidence of fine, stippled "psammomatous" calcification (papillary carcinoma) or dense, homogeneous calcification (medullary carcinoma); (7) recent or rapid enlargement; and (8) "stony-hard" consistency. Biopsy is of some use in distinguishing benign from malignant nodules when one has the technic available and the pathologist to read the samples. It is not clear whether fine-needle biopsy or Vim-Silverman is preferred.

Papillary carcinoma is the most common thyroid malignancy. Females are affected 2 to 3 times more often than males. It is more frequent in the young, but it takes a more malignant course in the elderly. It is often associated with a history of radiation exposure and spreads via the lymphatics. Lateral aberrant thyroid rests may be found that are actually occult metastases with a benign histologic appearance. Papillary thyroid carcinoma is highly TSH-dependent and may develop in hypothyroid glands secondary to Hashimoto's thyroiditis. **Treatment** for small, encapsulated tumors localized to one lobe is lobectomy. Thyroid hormone may minimize growth or produce regression of papillary carcinoma. Large or diffusely spreading tumors require total or near-total thyroidectomy with postoperative radioiodine ablation of residual thyroid tissue with 150 mCi ^{131}I. Replacement doses of L-thyroxine are given afterwards at an average oral dose of 150 to 200 μg/day.

Follicular carcinoma accounts for about 25% of thyroid cancer and is more common in the elderly. It is more malignant than papillary carcinoma, spreading hematogenously with distant metastases. It also is often associated with a history of radiation exposure and is more frequent in females than in males. Treatment is the same as for papillary cancer. Metastases appear to be more amenable to radioiodine therapy.

Anaplastic carcinoma accounts for 10% or less of thyroid cancer and occurs mostly in elderly patients, females slightly more than males. The tumor is characterized by rapid and painful enlargement and is almost always fatal within 1 yr of diagnosis.

Medullary (solid) carcinoma of the thyroid may occur as a sporadic form (usually unilateral) or as a familial form (frequently bilateral), transmitted as an autosomal dominant. Patients are usually $>$ 15 yr of age. Pathologically there is a proliferation of parafollicular cells (C cells) that produce excessive calcitonin, a hormone that can lower serum Ca and PO$_4$, and there are characteristic amyloid deposits that stain with Congo red. Metastases are via lymphatics to cervical and mediastinal nodes, but there may also be metastases to liver, lungs, and bone, with dense calcifications.

Medullary carcinoma of the thyroid may have a dramatic biochemical presentation when it is associated with ectopic endocrinopathies such as Cushing's syndrome with excess ACTH, prostaglandin elevations, and increased serotonin production. This disease is also associated with **Sipple's syndrome** (medullary carcinoma of the thyroid, pheochromocytoma, and hyperparathyroidism). However, all 3 are not always present in the same patient. Pheochromocytoma is present in 50 to 75%; hyperparathyroidism, in 50%. Additional findings not regularly present with this syndrome include disorders of the neural ectoderm, including mucosal neuromas; megacolon associated with neural disturbances; diarrhea, probably secondary to prostaglandin production; pectus excavatum; poorly developed musculature; and marfanoid appearance, with long arms and fingers.

Laboratory evaluation: RAI scan shows a nonfunctioning, cold nodule which does not concentrate radioiodine (see also RADIONUCLIDE IMAGING METHODS in Ch. 227). X-rays show a dense, homogenous, conglomerate calcification. The best diagnostic test for medullary carcinoma is assay for excess calcitonin, since only rarely is the serum level normal. A challenge with calcium, glucagon, or pentagastrin provokes output of abnormal amounts of this hormone. The histaminase level is increased in 50% of patients and usually indicates metastatic disease. Increased histaminase levels occasionally may be found without metastases and also may be seen in pregnancy, subacute thyroiditis, and after heparin injection. As a clinical test, intradermal injection of histamine is used; in medullary carcinoma patients, no flare occurs. Inhibitors of histaminase have no effect on the tumor.

Treatment of medullary carcinoma consists of total thyroidectomy, even if bilateral involvement is not obvious. Lymph node and radical neck dissection may also be performed if metastases are found. If hyperparathyroidism is present, removal of hyperplastic or adenomatous parathyroids is required. If pheochromocytoma occurs, it is usually bilateral, and anterior abdominal surgery is the preferred approach. *Pheochromocytomas should be removed before thyroidectomy* because of the danger of provoking hypertensive crisis during surgery. Suppression of thyroid hormone production is rarely effective.

Because of the familial incidence of medullary carcinoma of the thyroid, it is important to screen relatives by periodically determining the levels of serum calcitonin, Ca, PO$_4$, and urinary catecholamines.

Implications for Thyroid Cancer of External Irradiation to the Head, Neck, and Upper Thorax in Infancy and Childhood

External irradiation to the head, neck, or upper thorax was administered in the past to treat a variety of conditions, including recurrent tonsillitis, adenoiditis, acne, tinea capitis, and thymic enlargement. The thyroid was incidentally irradiated by these procedures.

Although not appreciated at the time, relatively small doses of radiation during infancy and childhood increase the risk of developing benign and malignant thyroid neoplasms. It requires about 5 yr after exposure to develop a thyroid abnormality, but the patient remains at increased risk for at least 30 to 40 yr after exposure. Probably no more than 1/3 of those irradiated develop a thyroid neoplasm; most are benign. However, about 7% of the irradiated group develop thyroid carcinoma; most are papillary, mixed follicular-papillary, or follicular, and are generally slow-growing and relatively non-aggressive. The tumors are frequently multicentric and the thyroid scan does not always reflect areas of involvement. In a number of instances microscopic foci of cancer have been observed in areas considered normal.

Initial evaluation of all patients having received external irradiation to the thyroid gland should include examination of the thyroid gland for any palpable abnormality and a radioisotope scan, preferably using 99mtechnetium in combination with a gamma counter and a pinhole collimator. In the absence of any abnormality, many physicians recommend physiologic replacement therapy with thyroid hormone with the aim of suppressing thyroid function and thyrotropin secretion to decrease the chance of developing a thyroid neoplasm. The presence of a scan abnormality in the absence of a palpable abnormality requires clinical judgment as to whether a period of suppressive therapy with thyroid hormone is required or whether or not there should be surgery. Additionally, all patients should have a determination of thyroid autoantibodies in the initial evaluation, since diffuse or irregular enlargement of the thyroid gland may be due to Hashimoto's (lymphocytic) thyroiditis. Physical examination of the neck should be performed yearly. Scanning is *not* repeated routinely.

Near-total thyroidectomy is the treatment of choice when operative intervention is required. The operation must be performed by a surgeon with proven expertise in thyroid surgery because of the risks inherent in such a procedure, including hypoparathyroidism and destruction of the recurrent laryngeal nerve.

---

87. PARATHYROID

(See DISTURBANCES IN CALCIUM METABOLISM in Ch. 81)

---

88. ADRENAL

The adrenal cortex produces androgens, glucocorticoids (e.g., cortisol), and mineralocorticoids (e.g., aldosterone). The effects of the adrenocortical hormones and the physiology of the pituitary-adrenal system are described in Chs. 84 and 85. The distinct clinical syndromes produced by **hypofunction** or **hyperfunction** of the cortex are discussed below.

ADRENAL HYPOFUNCTION

ADDISON'S DISEASE (Primary or Chronic Adrenocortical Insufficiency)

An insidious and usually progressive disease resulting from adrenocortical hypofunction.

Etiology and Incidence

About 70% of cases are due to idiopathic atrophy of the adrenal cortex, the remainder to partial destruction of the gland by granuloma (e.g., tuberculosis), neoplasm, amyloidosis, or inflammatory necrosis. The incidence is about 4:100,000. Addison's disease occurs in all age groups, about equally in each sex, and tends to become clinically apparent during metabolic stress or trauma.

Pathophysiology

The principal hormones produced by the adrenal cortex are cortisol (hydrocortisone), aldosterone, and dehydroisoandrosterone (dehydroepiandrosterone). Adults secrete about 20 mg of cortisol, 2 mg of corticosterone (which has similar activity), and 0.2 mg of aldosterone daily. Although considerable quantities of androgens (primarily dehydroisoandrosterone and androstenedione) are normally produced by the adrenal cortex, these exert their chief physiologic activity after conversion to testosterone and dihydrotestosterone.

In Addison's disease, there is increased excretion of Na and decreased excretion of K chiefly in the urine, but also in the sweat, saliva, and GI tract. Low blood concentrations of Na and Cl and high serum K result. These changes in electrolyte balance produce increased water excretion with severe dehydration, increased plasma concentration, decreased circulatory volume, hypotension, and circulatory collapse.

Cortisol deficiency contributes to the hypotension and produces disturbances in carbohydrate, fat, and protein metabolism, and severe insulin sensitivity. In the absence of cortisol, insufficient carbohydrate is formed from protein; hypoglycemia and diminished liver glycogen result. Weakness, due in part to deficient neuromuscular function, follows. Resistance to infection, trauma, and other stress is diminished because of reduced adrenal output. Cardiac output is reduced and circulatory failure can occur. Reduced cortisol blood levels result in increased pituitary ACTH production and an increase in β-lipotropin, which has melanocyte-stimulating activity and produces the hyperpigmentation of skin and mucous membranes characteristic of Addison's disease.

Symptoms and Signs

Weakness, fatigue, and orthostatic hypotension are early symptoms. Pigmentation is usually increased except in adrenal insufficiency secondary to pituitary failure. Increased pigmentation is characterized by diffuse tanning of both exposed and nonexposed portions of the body, especially on pressure points (bony prominences), skin folds, scars, and extensor surfaces. Black freckles over the forehead, face, neck, and shoulders; areas of vitiligo; and bluish-black discolorations of the areolas and of the mucous membranes of the lips, mouth, rectum, and vagina are common. Weight loss, dehydration, hypotension, and small heart size are characteristic in the later stages of the disease. Anorexia, nausea, vomiting, and diarrhea often occur. Decreased cold tolerance, with hypometabolism, may be noted. Dizziness and syncopal attacks may occur. The ECG may show decreased voltage and prolonged P-R and Q-T intervals. The EEG shows a generalized slowing of the α-rhythm.

An **adrenal crisis** is characterized by profound asthenia; severe pains in the abdomen, lower back, or legs; peripheral vascular collapse; and, finally, renal shutdown with azotemia. Body temperature may be subnormal, though severe hyperthermia due to infection is often seen. Crisis is precipitated most often by acute infection (especially with septicemia), trauma, operative procedures, and salt loss due to excessive sweating during hot weather.

Laboratory Findings

A low serum Na level (< 130 mEq/L), a high serum K level (> 5 mEq/L), and an elevated BUN, together with a characteristic clinical picture, suggest the possibility of Addison's disease (see TABLE 88-1).

Diagnostic Tests

Adrenal insufficiency can be specifically diagnosed by demonstrating failure to increase plasma cortisol levels, or urinary 17-hydroxycorticosteroid (17-OHCS) or 17-ketogenic steroid (17-KGS) excretion, upon administration of corticotropin (ACTH). Urinary 17-KGS or 17-OHCS excretion, in the absence of endogenous ACTH stimulation, is unreliable as an index of adrenocortical functional capacity, since baseline excretion does not adequately separate low-normal from the abnormally low value. A single determination of plasma cortisol or 24-h urinary 17-OHCS or 17-KGS excretion is not useful and may be misleading in diagnosing adrenal insufficiency. However, if the patient is severely stressed or in shock, a single depressed plasma cortisol determination is highly suggestive. An elevated plasma ACTH level in association with a low plasma cortisol level is highly diagnostic.

Testing of adrenal function is performed as follows:

The single-dose metyrapone test is useful in diagnosis. About 30 mg/kg metyrapone is given orally at midnight with a small amount of food to avoid gastric irritation. At 8 AM the following morning, plasma is drawn for cortisol and substance S (11-desoxycortisol) determinations. A normal increase in substance S in the plasma is 7 to 22 μg/dl. A low plasma cortisol with failure of the substance S to increase suggests adrenal insufficiency of primary or secondary type. An increased plasma ACTH indicates the disease is primary to the adrenal gland.

Cosyntropin, a synthetic ACTH that has fewer side effects than the natural preparations, may be given at a dose of 0.25 mg IM. Blood samples are taken and plasma cortisol is measured before the injection and after 60 and 90 min. In healthy adults, plasma cortisol ranges from 4 to 25 μg/100 ml; following administration of ACTH, it should more than double in 60 to 90 min. In patients with Addi-

TABLE 88–1. LABORATORY FINDINGS SUGGESTING ADDISON'S DISEASE

Blood chemistry	Low serum Na* (< 130 mEq/L)
	High serum K* (> 5 mEq/L)
	Ratio of serum Na:K (< 30:1)
	Low fasting blood sugar (< 50 mg/100 ml)
	Decrease in CO_2 combining power (< 28 mEq/L)
	Elevated BUN (> 20 mg/100 ml)
Hematology	Elevated hematocrit
	Low WBC count
	Relative lymphocytosis
	Increased eosinophils
X-ray.	Evidence of:
	Small heart
	Calcifications in the adrenal areas
	Renal tuberculosis
	Pulmonary tuberculosis

* Na = sodium; K = potassium.

son's disease, cortisol levels remain low. Such patients should be tested further to determine if the low levels are due to primary adrenal insufficiency or secondary adrenal insufficiency caused by pituitary disease.

To distinguish between primary and secondary adrenal insufficiency, when plasma ACTH determination is not available, 0.25 mg of cosyntropin may be infused IV (after dilution with dextrose or sodium chloride solution) over a period of 8 h daily for 2 days. Patients with primary adrenocortical insufficiency will show little or no increase in plasma cortisol or 24-h urinary corticosteroid levels. Those with secondary adrenocortical insufficiency will have a significant increase in plasma cortisol or 24-h urinary corticosteroid levels.

Dexamethasone 0.5 mg orally t.i.d. should be given during testing with ACTH, beginning on the day before the test. This ensures that treatment will not be delayed and the patient is protected against vascular collapse and reactions to ACTH. The excretory products of 1.5 mg of dexamethasone are insufficient to interfere with the test.

Plasma and urinary cortisol levels are usually determined by radioimmunoassay. Urinary 17-OHCS may be determined by reacting phenylhydrazine with C-21 adrenocorticoids having the dihydroxyacetone group (17,21-dihydroxy-20 ketone). This is known as the **Porter-Silber reaction.** This reaction does not measure all of the 17-hydroxycorticoids, and thus a more inclusive method may be used to assess total adrenocortical activity. Borohydride reduction followed by periodate oxidation converts 17-oxygenated steroids to C-19 17-ketosteroids that are then measured as 17-KGS by the colorimetric (Zimmerman) reaction.

Diagnosis

Addison's disease is usually suspected following the discovery of hyperpigmentation, although in some patients this may be minimal. In the early stages of the disease, weakness, although prominent, is benefited by rest, unlike neuropsychiatric weaknesses that are often worse in the morning than after activity. Most myopathies can be differentiated by their distribution and the lack of pigmentation and characteristic laboratory findings. Patients with hypoglycemia due to oversecretion of insulin may have attacks at any time, usually have increased appetite with weight gain, and have normal adrenal function. Patients with adrenal insufficiency develop hypoglycemia following fasting, due to their decreased ability to carry out gluconeogenesis. The low serum Na must be differentiated from edematous patients (particularly those on diuretics), the dilutional hyponatremia of inappropriate ADH syndrome, and the rare salt-losing nephritis. These patients are not likely to show hyperpigmentation, hyperkalemia, and increased BUN, which are characteristic of adrenal insufficiency. Hyperpigmentation due to bronchogenic carcinoma, ingestion of heavy metals such as iron or silver, chronic skin conditions, or hemochromatosis should be considered. The characteristic pigmentation of the buccal and rectal mucosa seen in Peutz-Jeghers syndrome should not cause confusion. The frequent presence of vitiligo in association with hyperpigmentation may be a helpful indication, although this may also occur with hyperpigmentation due to other causes.

Prognosis

With continued substitution therapy, the prognosis is excellent and a patient with Addison's disease should be able to lead a full life.

Treatment

In addition to appropriate treatment of complicating infections (e.g., tuberculosis), therapy should include the following.

Treatment of acute adrenal insufficiency: Therapy should be instituted immediately once a provisional diagnosis of adrenocortical failure has been made. If the patient is acutely ill, confirmation by an ACTH response test should be postponed until recovery is achieved. Hydrocortisone 100 mg as a water-soluble ester (usually the succinate or phosphate) is injected IV over 30 seconds, followed by an infusion of 1 L of a 5% glucose-in-saline solution containing 100 mg hydrocortisone ester given over 2 h. Additional saline is given until dehydration and hyponatremia are corrected. Hydrocortisone therapy is given continuously to a total dosage in 24 h of > 300 mg. Mineralocorticoids are not required when high-dose hydrocortisone is given. Restoration of BP and general improvement may be expected within 1 h or less after the initial dose of hydrocortisone. Vasopressor agents may be needed until the full effect of hydrocortisone is apparent. An IV infusion of metaraminol bitartrate, 100 mg in 500 ml of sodium chloride injection, may be given at a rate adjusted to maintain BP. (CAUTION: *In acute addisonian crisis, a delay in instituting corticosteroid therapy may result in the patient's death, particularly if hypoglycemia and hypotension are present.*) A total dose of hydrocortisone 150 mg is usually given over the second 24-h period if the patient is markedly improved, and 75 mg is given on the third day. Maintenance oral doses of hydrocortisone (30 mg) and fludrocortisone acetate (0.1 mg) are given daily thereafter. Recovery depends upon treatment of the underlying cause (e.g., infection, trauma, metabolic stress) and adequate hydrocortisone therapy.

Recognition of patients with Addison's disease is not difficult. However, a significant number of patients with "limited" adrenocortical reserve who appear healthy experience acute adrenocortical insufficiency when under stress. Shock and fever may be the only signs observed. Treatment should not be delayed until the diagnosis is certain, but hydrocortisone should be given as described above. Salt and water requirements may be considerably less than in cases with total deficiency.

Treatment of complications: These include hyperpyrexia and psychotic reactions. Fever > 40.6 C (105 F) orally occasionally accompanies the rehydration process. Except in the presence of a falling BP, antipyretics (e.g., aspirin 600 mg) may be given orally with caution q 30 min until the temperature begins to fall. If psychotic reactions occur after the first 12 h of therapy, hydrocortisone dosage should be reduced to the lowest level consistent with maintenance of BP and good cardiovascular function.

Treatment of chronic adrenal insufficiency: Normal hydration and absence of orthostatic hypotension are criteria of adequate replacement therapy. Hydrocortisone 20 mg orally is usually given in the morning and 10 mg in the afternoon. A daily dosage of 40 mg may be required. Night doses should be avoided, as they may produce insomnia. Normally, hydrocortisone is secreted maximally in the early morning hours, little being secreted at night. Additionally, fludrocortisone 0.1 mg to 0.2 mg orally once/day is recommended. This mineralocorticoid replaces aldosterone that is normally secreted in healthy individuals. It is often necessary to reduce the dose of fludrocortisone to 0.05 mg every 2nd day on initial institution of therapy because of ankle edema, but the patient usually adjusts and can then take the larger doses. Fludrocortisone produces hypertension in some patients. This should be treated by reducing the dosage rather than using diuretics. Intercurrent illnesses (e.g., infections) should be regarded as potentially serious and the patient should double his hydrocortisone dosage until he is well. If nausea and vomiting preclude oral therapy, medical attention should be sought immediately and parenteral therapy started. Patients living or traveling in areas where medical care is not readily available should be instructed in self-administration of parenteral hydrocortisone.

In **coexisting diabetes mellitus and Addison's disease,** hydrocortisone dosage usually should not be > 30 mg/day; otherwise, insulin requirements are increased. Complete control of glycosuria is often difficult in this syndrome. In coexisting thyrotoxicosis and Addison's disease, definitive therapy should be given early. **Following total bilateral adrenalectomy** for hyperadrenocorticism, carcinoma of the breast, or hypertension, the patient should be maintained on oral hydrocortisone 20 to 30 mg/day. In addition, a mineralocorticoid may be given (for dosage, see Treatment of chronic adrenal insufficiency, above).

SECONDARY ADRENAL INSUFFICIENCY

Adrenal hypofunction due to a lack of ACTH may occur in panhypopituitarism, in patients receiving corticosteroids, or for a period of time after discontinuing corticosteroid therapy. Panhypopituitarism occurs most commonly in women with Sheehan's syndrome, but may also occur secondary to chromophobe adenomas, craniopharyngioma in younger persons, and a variety of tumors, granulomas, and, rarely, infections or trauma which lead to destruction of pituitary tissue. Patients receiving corticosteroids, or who have discontinued their use for a period of weeks to months, may have insufficient ACTH secretion during metabolic stress to stimulate the adrenals to produce adequate quantities of corticosteroids; or they may have atrophic adrenals that are unresponsive to ACTH. Isolated ACTH deficiency is idiopathic and extremely rare.

Symptoms and Signs

Patients with secondary adrenal insufficiency are not hyperpigmented as are those with Addison's disease. They have relatively normal electrolyte values. Hyperkalemia and elevated BUN are generally not present because of the near-normal secretion of aldosterone in these patients. Hyponatremia may occur on a dilutional basis. Those with panhypopituitarism, however, have depressed thyroid and gonadal function and hypoglycemia, and coma may supervene when symptomatic secondary adrenal insufficiency occurs. Tests to differentiate primary and secondary adrenal insufficiency are discussed under Addison's disease, above.

Treatment

Treatment of secondary adrenal insufficiency is similar to that described above for Addison's disease. Each case varies with regard to the type and degree of specific adrenocortical hormone deficiencies. Generally, fludrocortisone is not required, since aldosterone is produced. These patients may do better on lower doses of hydrocortisone than patients with primary insufficiency. During acute febrile illness or following trauma, patients receiving corticosteroids for nonendocrine disorders may require supplemental doses to augment their endogenous hydrocortisone production. In panhypopituitarism, other pituitary deficiencies should be treated appropriately.

ADRENAL CORTICAL HYPERFUNCTION

Hypersecretion of one or more adrenocortical hormones produces distinct clinical syndromes. Excessive production of androgens results in adrenal virilism; hypersecretion of glucocorticoids produces Cushing's syndrome; and excess aldosterone output results in aldosteronism. These syndromes frequently have overlapping features. Adrenal hyperfunction may be compensatory as in congenital adrenal hyperplasia, or may be due to acquired hyperplasia, adenomas, or adenocarcinomas.

CONGENITAL ADRENAL HYPERPLASIA (See Vol. II, Ch. 25)

ADRENAL VIRILISM (Adrenogenital Syndrome)

Any syndrome, congenital or acquired, in which excessive output of adrenal androgens causes virilization. The effects depend on the sex and age of the patient when the disease begins and are more marked in women than men. In adult women, this syndrome is caused by adrenal hyperplasia or by an adrenal tumor. In either case, symptoms and signs include hirsutism, baldness, acne, deepening of the voice, amenorrhea, atrophy of the uterus, clitoral hypertrophy, decreased breast size, and increased muscularity. An increase in libido may occur. Hirsutism may be the only feature in mild cases.

Delayed virilizing adrenal hyperplasia is a variant of the congenital variety (above), and both are caused by a defect in hydroxylation of cortisol precursors. Urinary 17-KS are elevated, pregnanetriol excretion is often increased, and cortisol or 17-OHCS excretion is diminished. Plasma testosterone and androstenedione are elevated. Suppression of 17-KS excretion with dexamethasone 0.5 mg orally q 6 h confirms the diagnosis. Dexamethasone 0.5 to 1 mg orally at bedtime is the recommended treatment, but even these small doses may produce signs of Cushing's syndrome in some patients. Though most symptoms and signs of virilism disappear, the hirsutism and baldness disappear slowly and the voice may remain deep.

With **virilizing adenomas** or **adenocarcinomas**, in contrast to adrenal hyperplasia, dexamethasone administration either does not suppress or only partially suppresses androgen excretion. The tumor site may be determined by CT scan. **Treatment** requires adrenalectomy. In some cases, the tumor secretes both excess androgens and cortisol, resulting in Cushing's syndrome with suppression of ACTH secretion and atrophy of the contralateral adrenal. If this is the case, hydrocortisone should be given pre- and postoperatively as described below. Mild hirsutism and virilization with hypomenorrhea and elevated plasma testosterone may be seen in the **Stein-Leventhal syndrome.**

Feminizing adrenal tumors are rare and usually malignant. Most occur in men. Presenting symptoms and signs include gynecomastia and feminization. Prognosis is poor. Treatment requires surgical removal of the tumor. The use of *o,p'* DDD (mitotane) may be helpful if total removal cannot be obtained surgically.

CUSHING'S SYNDROME

A constellation of clinical abnormalities due to chronic exposure to excesses of cortisol (the major adrenocorticoid) or related corticosteroids.

Etiology

Hyperfunction of the adrenal cortex may be ACTH-dependent or it may be independent of ACTH regulation. The production of cortisol by an adrenocortical adenoma or carcinoma is found in the latter. The administration of supraphysiologic quantities of exogenous cortisol or related synthetic analogs suppresses adrenocortical function and mimics ACTH-independent hyperfunction. ACTH-dependent hyperfunction of the adrenal cortex may be due to (1) hypersecretion of ACTH by the pituitary, (2) secretion of ACTH by a nonpituitary tumor such as an oat cell carcinoma of the lung (the **ectopic ACTH syndrome**), or (3) administration of exogenous ACTH. While the term **Cushing's syndrome** has been applied to the clinical picture resulting from cortisol excess regardless of the cause, hyperfunction of the adrenal cortex resulting from pituitary ACTH excess has frequently been referred to as **Cushing's disease,** implying a particular physiologic abnormality. Patients with Cushing's disease may have a basophilic adenoma of the pituitary, or a chromophobe adenoma. In some cases, no histologic abnormality is found in the pituitary despite clear evidence of ACTH overproduction. Microadenomas, which are difficult to visualize radiographically, are often the cause.

Symptoms and Signs

Clinical manifestations include rounded "moon" facies with a plethoric appearance. There is truncal obesity with prominent supraclavicular and dorsal cervical fat pads (buffalo hump); the distal extremities and fingers are usually quite slender. Muscle wasting and weakness are present. The skin is thin and atrophic, with poor wound healing and easy bruising. Purple striae may appear on the abdomen. Hypertension, renal calculi, osteoporosis, glucose intolerance, and psychiatric disturbances are common. Cessation of linear growth is characteristic in children. Females usually have menstrual irregularities. An increased production of androgens, in addition to cortisol, may lead to hypertrichosis, temporal balding, and other signs of virilism in the female.

Diagnosis

Plasma cortisol is normally 10 to 25 μg/dl in the early morning hours (6 to 8 AM) and declines gradually to < 10 in the evening (6 PM and later). Patients with Cushing's syndrome usually have elevated morning cortisol levels and lack the normal diurnal decline in cortisol production, so that evening plasma cortisol levels are above normal and total 24-h cortisol production is elevated. Single cortisol samples may be difficult to interpret due to the episodic secretion that produces the wide range in normal values.

About ⅓ of the secreted cortisol is metabolized to 17-OHCS that are measured in the urine. Urinary 17-OHCS are influenced by body size and weight; obese patients may have relatively elevated values. Normal urinary 17-OHCS range between 3 and 10 mg/24 h. Urinary 17-KGS measure a somewhat larger proportion of cortisol metabolites; normal secretion is 5 to 16 mg/24 h. Patients with Cushing's syndrome have higher values. Urinary 17-KS may also be elevated to > 20 mg/24 h in men and to > 15 in women. Free urinary cortisol is elevated and less subject to increase in obese patients (normal 10 to 100 μg/24 h).

Dexamethasone test: the administration of 1 mg of dexamethasone orally at 11 to 12 PM with measurement of plasma cortisol at 7 to 8 AM the following morning is a good screening test for Cushing's syndrome. Most normal patients will suppress their morning plasma cortisol to 5 μg/dl or less following this procedure, whereas most patients with Cushing's syndrome will continue to secrete undiminished quantities of cortisol.

Giving oral dexamethasone 0.5 mg q 6 h for 2 days to normal subjects leads to inhibition of ACTH secretion. Consequently, urinary 17-OHCS will usually decrease to < 3 mg/24 h on the 2nd day. In patients with Cushing's disease, pituitary ACTH secretion is relatively resistant to suppression and therefore urinary 17-OHCS will not decrease in a normal fashion. In patients with adrenal tumors, cortisol production is independent of ACTH and therefore dexamethasone will have no suppressive effect. In patients with the ectopic ACTH syndrome, the production of ACTH by the nonpituitary tumor is almost always unaffected by dexamethasone; hence urinary 17-OHCS remain unchanged. The production of ACTH by the pituitary in Cushing's disease is only *relatively* resistant to suppression. Hence, when the oral dose of dexamethasone is increased to 2 mg q 6 h for 2 days, urinary 17-OHCS will usually decrease by at least 50% from the baseline values. In contrast, urinary 17-OHCS or cortisol will not be suppressed in most patients with an adrenal tumor or with the ectopic ACTH syndrome. This test distinguishes patients with a pituitary abnormality from other forms of Cushing's syndrome.

If the dexamethasone test points to an adrenal tumor or the ectopic ACTH syndrome, these two possibilities can be separated by determining the plasma ACTH concentration. The plasma ACTH level will be markedly elevated in the ectopic ACTH syndrome (usually > 500 pg/ml) and will be unmeasurable in Cushing's syndrome due to an adrenal tumor. Patients with Cushing's disease usually have moderately elevated plasma ACTH values (75 to 200 pg/ml).

The overnight **metyrapone test** will often give useful information in determining the etiology of the Cushing's syndrome. Patients with pituitary dependent Cushing's disease have a marked increase in plasma substance S (11-desoxycortisol), but patients with adrenal tumors fail to show this increase. The total amount of steroid produced (as metyrapone blocks 11-hydroxylation of cortisol) must be determined. Therefore, total cortisol and substance S levels are measured to see that an increase in total steroid has occurred, and not just that 11-desoxycortisol has replaced cortisol in the plasma.

A less useful test in evaluating patients with Cushing's syndrome is the **ACTH stimulation test.** Infusion of ACTH 50 u. over an 8-h period produces a 2- to 5-fold increase in urinary 17-OHCS in patients with Cushing's disease, where the adrenals show bilateral hyperplasia and hyperresponsiveness due to chronic endogenous ACTH excess. In about 50% of cases of adrenal adenoma, ACTH stimulation will produce a clear and sometimes marked increase in plasma cortisol and urinary 17-OHCS. Adrenal carcinomas are generally unresponsive to ACTH.

The evaluation of the patient with Cushing's syndrome, after adrenal hyperfunction is established, should also include radiologic examination for a pituitary tumor and a careful search for signs of a nonpituitary, ACTH-producing neoplasm. An IVP may show depression of a kidney by an adrenal tumor. Adrenal scanning, after ingestion of iodinated cholesterol, may differentiate hyperplasia and adenoma or carcinoma. If computerized scanning is available, it is the procedure of choice if biochemical tests suggest the presence of an adrenal tumor.

Treatment

Therapy is directed at correcting the hyperfunction of the pituitary gland or the adrenal cortex; the precise approach depends on the underlying physiologic abnormality.

If clinical manifestations are severe and definitive correction is immediately required, either suppression of excess cortisol production with aminoglutethimide followed by bilateral adrenalectomy, or removal of a pituitary adenoma will be the treatment of choice. Transphenoidal hypophysectomy is usually successful when carried out by an experienced neurosurgeon. While the majority of patients may be cured by this operation and normal pituitary function will remain intact, recurrences occur and may appear months or years after the operation. Adrenalectomized patients require steroid replacement analogous to those with Addison's disease.

If clinical manifestations are not severe, pituitary irradiation may be tried initially. Supervoltage technics and delivery of 4000 to 5000 R to the pituitary will cause remission in about 30% of cases. With heavy particle irradiation, there will be a higher response rate, but hypopituitarism is more likely to occur. If there is no response to pituitary irradiation after 6 mo, adrenalectomy is indicated.

In 5 to 10% of patients who have undergone adrenalectomy for Cushing's disease, the pituitary gland will continue to expand, causing a marked increase in ACTH and β-MSH secretion, resulting in severe hyperpigmentation **(Nelson's syndrome).** Although continued pituitary growth may be arrested in these patients by irradiation, many have also required hypophysectomy. The indications for hypophysectomy are the same as for any pituitary tumor—an increase in size such that it encroaches upon surrounding structures, producing visual field defects, pressure upon the hypothalamus, or other complications. Routine irradiation after hypophysectomy is often carried out.

Adrenocortical neoplasms are treated by surgical removal of the tumor. Patients must receive supplementary cortisol during surgery and in the postoperative period, since their nontumorous adrenal cortex will be atrophic and suppressed. Where possible, treatment of the ectopic ACTH syndrome consists of removing the nonpituitary tumor producing the ACTH. However, in most cases, the tumor is disseminated and cannot be excised. Adrenal inhibitors such as metyrapone, mitotane (o,p'-DDD), and aminoglutethimide may then be used to control severe metabolic disturbances (e.g., hypokalemia) resulting from hyperfunction of the adrenal cortex.

HYPERALDOSTERONISM

Aldosterone is the most potent mineralocorticoid produced by the adrenals. It causes Na retention and K loss. In the kidney, aldosterone causes transfer of Na from the lumen of the distal tubule into the tubular cells in exchange for K and H. The same effect occurs in the salivary glands, sweat glands, and cells of the intestinal mucosa, and in exchanges between intra- and extracellular fluids.

Aldosterone secretion is regulated by the **renin-angiotensin mechanism,** and to a lesser extent by ACTH. Renin, a proteolytic enzyme, is stored in the juxtaglomerular cells of the kidney. Reduction in blood volume and flow in the afferent renal arterioles induces secretion of renin. Renin causes transformation of **angiotensinogen** (an α_2-globulin) in the liver to **angiotensin I,** a 10-amino acid polypeptide, which is converted to **angiotensin II,** an 8-amino acid polypeptide. Angiotensin II causes secretion of aldosterone and, to a much lesser extent, of cortisol and desoxycorticosterone. The Na and water retention resulting from increased aldosterone secretion increases the blood volume and reduces renin secretion. Aldosterone is measured by radioimmunoassay.

Primary aldosteronism (Conn's syndrome) is due to an adenoma, usually unilateral, of the glomerulosa cells of the adrenal cortex or, more rarely, to an adrenal carcinoma or hyperplasia. Hypersecretion of aldosterone may result in hypernatremia, hyperchlorhydria, hypervolemia, and a hypokalemic alkalosis manifested by episodic weakness, paresthesias, transient paralysis, and tetany. Diastolic hypertension and a hypokalemic nephropathy with polyuria and polydipsia are common. Aldosterone excretion on a high Na intake ($>$ 10 gm/day) is usually $>$ 200 μg/day if a tumor is present. Deprivation of Na causes K retention. Personality disturbances and hyperglycemia and glycosuria are occasionally seen. In many cases, the only manifestation may be mild to moderate hypertension.

A helpful test is to give spironolactone 200 to 400 mg/day orally, which reverses the manifestations of the disease, including hypertension, within 5 to 8 wk (this may also occur in patients with hypertension not due to increased aldosterone). Measurement of plasma renin is helpful in the diagnosis. This is usually carried out by obtaining a recumbent plasma renin value in the morning, giving furosemide 80 mg orally, and then repeating the renin determination after the patient has remained upright for 3 h. Normal individuals will have a marked increase in renin in the upright position, while the patient with hyperaldosteronism will not. About 20% of patients with essential hypertension, who do not necessarily have hyperaldosteronism, have a low renin that does not respond to the upright position. Measurements of plasma aldosterone, either peripherally or following catheterization of the adrenal veins, may be helpful. Diagnosis is thus dependent upon demonstrating elevated secretion of aldosterone in urine or blood, expansion of the extracellular space as demonstrated by lack of increase in plasma renin in the upright posture, and the K abnormalities noted. A CT scan will often demonstrate a small adenoma in these cases.

Secondary aldosteronism, an increased production of aldosterone by the adrenal cortex caused by stimuli originating outside the adrenal, mimics the primary condition and is related to hypertension and edematous disorders (e.g., cardiac failure, cirrhosis with ascites, the nephrotic syndrome). Secondary aldosteronism seen with the accelerated phase of hypertension is believed to be due to renin hypersecretion secondary to renal vasoconstriction. Hyperaldosteronism is also seen in hypertension due to obstructive renal artery disease (e.g., atheroma, stenosis). This is caused by reduced blood flow in the affected kidney. Hypovolemia, which is common in edematous disorders, particularly during diuretic therapy, stimulates the renin-angiotensin mechanism with hypersecretion of aldosterone. Secretion rates may be normal in cardiac failure, but hepatic blood flow and aldosterone metabolism are reduced so that circulating levels of the hormone are high.

The principal differences between primary and secondary aldosteronism are shown in TABLE 88-2.

Treatment

Once the diagnosis of primary aldosteronism is made, both adrenal glands should be explored for possible multiple adenomas. It may be necessary to dissect the gland to demonstrate a tumor. The prognosis is good in overt aldosteronism when a solitary adenoma can be defined. Following removal of an aldosterone-producing adenoma, all patients have lowering of BP; complete remission occurs in about 70%. With adrenal hyperplasia and hyperaldosteronism, about 70% remain hypertensive although there is reduction of BP in most patients. If bilateral adrenalectomy is necessary, permanent postoperative corticosteroid therapy must be maintained. In normokalemic aldosteronism, diagnosis and definition are difficult, and surgical exploration may be unrewarding.

TABLE 88-2. ALDOSTERONISM—DIFFERENTIAL DIAGNOSIS

Clinical Finding	Primary Aldosteronism	Secondary Aldosteronism	
		Hypertension	Edema
Blood pressure	↑	↑↑	N,↓
Edema	0	0	+
Serum sodium	↑,N	↓,N	↓,N
Serum potassium	↓	↓	N,↓
Plasma-renin activity	↓↓	↑↑	↑
Aldosterone	↑	↑↑	↑

↑ = increased; ↓ = decreased; 0 = absent; N = normal; ↑↑ = significantly increased; ↓↓ = significantly decreased; + = present.

Modified from *Harrison's Principles of Internal Medicine,* ed. 6, edited by M. M. Wintrobe et al. Copyright © 1970 by McGraw-Hill, Inc. Used with permission of McGraw-Hill Book Company.

PHEOCHROMOCYTOMA

A tumor of chromaffin cells that secrete catecholamines, causing hypertension. In about 80% of cases, pheochromocytomas are found in the adrenal medulla, but may also be found in other tissues derived from neural crest cells (see Pathology, below). They appear equally in both sexes, are bilateral in 10% of cases (20% in children), and are usually benign (95%). Although pheochromocytomas may occur at any age, the maximum incidence is between the third and fifth decades.

Pathology

Pheochromocytomas vary in size but average only 5 to 6 cm in diameter. Rarely, they are large enough to be palpated or cause symptoms due to pressure or obstruction. The tumor is usually a well-encapsulated nest of chromaffin cells that appear malignant upon microscopic examination. The cells have multiple bizarre shapes with pyknotic, large, or multiple nuclei. The tumor may be considered benign if it has not invaded the capsule and if no metastases are found. In addition to the adrenals, tumors may be found in the paraganglia of the sympathetic chain, retroperitoneally along the course of the aorta, in the carotid body, in the organ of Zuckerkandl (at the aortic bifurcation), in the GU system, in the brain, and in dermoid cysts.

Pheochromocytomas are part of the **syndrome of familial multiple endocrine adenomatoses — Type II (Sipple's syndrome),** and may be found along or associated with medullary thyroid carcinoma and parathyroid adenomata (see Ch. 89). A **Type III syndrome** has been described which includes pheochromocytoma, mucosal (oral and ocular) neuroma, and medullary thyroid carcinoma. There is a significant association (10%) with **neurofibromatosis (von Recklinghausen's disease)** and it may be found with hemangiomas, as in **von Hippel-Lindau disease.**

Symptoms and Signs

The most prominent feature is hypertension, which may be paroxysmal (45%) or persistent (50%) and is rarely absent. It is due to secretion of one or more of the catecholamine hormones or precursors: norepinephrine, epinephrine, dopamine, or dopa. Additionally, tachycardia, diaphoresis, postural hypotension, tachypnea, flushing, cold and clammy skin, severe headache, angina, palpitation, nausea, vomiting, epigastric pain, visual disturbances, dyspnea, paresthesias, constipation, and a sense of impending doom are common; some or all of these symptoms and signs may occur in any patient. Paroxysmal attacks may be provoked by palpation of the tumor, postural changes, abdominal compression or massage, induction of anesthesia, emotional trauma, β-adrenergic blocking agents, and, rarely, micturition.

Physical examination, except for the common finding of hypertension, usually is normal, unless performed during a paroxysmal attack. The severity of retinopathy and cardiomegaly is often less extensive than might be expected for the degree of hypertension present.

Diagnosis

The principal urinary metabolic products of epinephrine and norepinephrine are the **metanephrines** and **vanillylmandelic acid (VMA).** Normal persons excrete only very small amounts of these substances in the urine. Normal values for 24 h are: free epinephrine and norepinephrine < 100 µg; total metanephrine < 1.3 mg; and VMA < 10 mg. In pheochromocytoma and neuroblastoma, there is an increased urinary excretion of epinephrine, norepinephrine, and their metabolic products. Excretion of these compounds may also be elevated in coma or extreme stress states. All of these compounds may be measured in the same urine specimen. The methods for detection of VMA and metanephrines depend upon the conversion to vanillin, the extraction of vanillin into toluene, and the final spectrophotometric determination of vanillin at 360 mµ. These values may be exceeded in patients being treated with rauwolfia alkaloids, methyldopa, or catecholamines, or following ingestion of foods containing large quantities of vanilla, especially if renal insufficiency is present.

Catecholamines (mainly epinephrine and norepinephrine) are measured fluorimetrically after extraction and adsorption on alumina gel. Interference from epinephrine-like drugs, antihypertensives (e.g., methyldopa), and other drugs that produce fluorescence (e.g., tetracycline and quinine) must be considered in the evaluation of abnormal results. Radioenzymatic procedures are also available.

Plasma catecholamine determinations are usually valueless unless collected during a paroxysm or following a drug such as glucagon that is known to provoke the release of catecholamines.

Because of their hyperkinetic states, these patients may have an elevated BMR despite being euthyroid. Although the BMR is rarely measured, these patients appear hyperkinetic. Blood volume is reported to be constricted. Hyperglycemia, glycosuria, or overt diabetes mellitus may be present with elevated fasting levels of plasma free fatty acid and glycerol. Plasma insulin concentrations are inappropriately low for the simultaneously collected plasma glucose values.

Provocative tests with histamine or tyramine *are hazardous and should not be used.* Glucagon (0.5 to 1 mg injected rapidly IV) will provoke a rise in blood pressure exceeding 35/25 mm Hg within 2 min in normotensive patients with pheochromocytoma. *Phentolamine mesylate must be available to terminate any hypertensive crisis.* If a patient with pheochromocytoma is hypertensive, phentolamine 5 mg injected IV will cause a fall in blood pressure exceeding 35/25 mm Hg within 2 min. False-positive results occur in patients with uremia, stroke, and malignant hypertension, and in those taking certain pharmacologic agents. A modification of this test has been developed which takes advantage of catecholamine inhibition of insulin release. An IV infusion of 10% glucose in water is begun (2 ml/min) 30 min prior to the injection of phentolamine (blood is sampled twice for measurement of glucose and insulin prior to the injection). Following the administration of phentolamine, each time the BP is measured, blood is again sampled. Pheochromocytoma is present if there is a significant fall in BP, a fall in glucose exceeding 18 mg/100 ml, or a rise in insulin exceeding 13 μu./ml.

Attempts at localizing tumors by x-ray should be limited to multiple views of the chest and abdomen and IV pyelography with tomography of the perirenal areas. Phlebography has been recommended by certain radiologists as safe and effective in the localization of these tumors; others feel that phlebography, aortography, and retroperitoneal gas insufflation are contraindicated as they may induce a serious or fatal paroxysm. Localization of the level of the tumor by repeated sampling of plasma catecholamine concentrations during catheterization of the vena cava has been accomplished, but is also a potentially dangerous procedure. Recently, computerized tomography (CT) scanning has been successfully used to localize the tumors in 10 of 11 patients where the tumor exceeded 2 cm in diameter. An isotope with specific affinity for the adrenal medulla or cortex, to improve noninvasive adrenal imaging, is not yet available.

Treatment

Surgical removal of the tumor is the treatment of choice. It is usually possible to delay surgery until the patient is in optimum physical condition by the use of a combination of α- and β-adrenergic blocking agents (phenoxybenzamine 40 to 160 mg/day and propranolol 30 to 60 mg/day, respectively, orally in divided doses) and the infusion of trimethaphan camsylate or sodium nitroprusside.

A new agent, **metyrosine** (see also below) may be used alone or in combination with an α-adrenergic blocking agent (phenoxybenzamine); the optimally effective dosage of metyrosine should be given for at least 5 to 7 days before surgery.

An anterior abdominal approach should be used by the surgeon, even if the tumor has been localized in the renal area, so that a search for other pheochromocytomas can be made. It is essential that BP be continuously monitored via an intra-arterial catheter. Anesthesia should be induced with a nonarrhythmic agent such as a thiobarbiturate and continued with methoxyflurane. During surgery, paroxysms of hypertension should be controlled with IV boluses of phentolamine 1 to 5 mg, and tachyarrhythmias with propranolol 1 to 5 mg IV. If a muscle relaxant is needed, pancuronium, which does not release histamine, is the agent of choice. Blood should be given prior to the removal of the tumor; the patient should receive 1 to 2 u. in anticipation of probable operative loss. A levarterenol infusion of 4 to 12 mg/L should be started any time hypotension appears. Some patients whose hypotension responds poorly to levarterenol may benefit by the addition of hydrocortisone 100 mg IV.

Malignant metastatic pheochromocytoma should be treated with α- and β-adrenergic blocking agents and with metyrosine. The latter agent inhibits tyrosine hydroxylase, which catalyzes the first transformation in catecholamine biosynthesis. Thus, levels of VMA and blood pressure fall. It is possible to control the blood pressure even though the tumor growth continues and will eventually cause death.

NONFUNCTIONAL ADRENAL MASSES

Spontaneous neonatal adrenal hemorrhage may produce large suprarenal masses, simulating neuroblastoma or Wilms' tumor. Adrenal insufficiency is rarely observed unless both glands are involved. **Benign adrenal cysts** are observed in the elderly and may be due to cystic degeneration, vascular accidents, bacterial infections, or parasitic infestations (*Echinococcus*). Rare **nonfunctional adrenal carcinoma** produces a diffuse and infiltrating retroperitoneal process that usually manifests as metastatic disease and is not amenable to surgery, though mitotane may afford chemotherapeutic control when used in association with supportive exogenous corticosteroids. **Tuberculosis of the adrenal** is a blood-borne disease which may cause calcification and adrenal insufficiency (Addison's disease).

89. MULTIPLE ENDOCRINE NEOPLASIA (MEN) SYNDROMES
(Multiple Endocrine Adenomatosis [MEA]; Familial Endocrine Adenomatosis)

A group of genetically distinct familial diseases involving adenomatous hyperplasia and malignant tumor formation in several endocrine glands. Three distinct syndromes have been identified; all 3 appear to be inherited as an autosomal dominant trait with a high degree of penetrance, variable expressivity, and significant pleiotropism. The relationship between the genetic abnormality and the pathogenesis of the various tumors is not understood. Clinical manifestations may be noted as early as the 1st or as late as the 7th decade of life. The clinical features depend upon the type of endocrine tumors present. Proper management includes the early identification of affected members within a kindred and surgical removal of the tumors where possible.

MULTIPLE ENDOCRINE NEOPLASIA, TYPE I (MEN-I)
(Multiple Endocrine Adenomatosis, Type I [MEA-I]; Wermer's Syndrome)

The MEN-I syndrome is characterized by tumors of the parathyroid glands, pancreatic islets, and the pituitary.

Hyperparathyroidism is present in almost 90% of affected patients. Asymptomatic hypercalcemia is the commonest manifestation; about 25% of patients have evidence of nephrolithiasis or nephrocalcinosis. In contrast to sporadic cases of hyperparathyroidism, diffuse hyperplasia or multiple adenomas are found more frequently than solitary adenomas.

Islet cell tumors of the pancreas have been reported in about 80% of affected patients. About 40% of these tumors originate from the β-cell, secrete insulin, and are associated with fasting hypoglycemia. In about 60% of cases they are derived from non–β-cell elements. Gastrin is the hormone most commonly secreted by the non–β-cell tumors and is associated with intractable and complicated peptic ulceration **(Zollinger-Ellison syndrome**—see p. 497). Over 1/2 of affected MEN-I patients have peptic ulcer disease; in the majority of cases the ulcers are multiple or atypical in location and the incidence of hemorrhage, perforation, and obstruction is correspondingly high. The extreme hypersecretion of gastric acid in these patients may be associated with inactivation of pancreatic lipase, resulting in diarrhea and steatorrhea. In patients presenting initially with the Zollinger-Ellison syndrome, further investigation commonly reveals evidence of the MEN-I complex.

In other cases, non–β-cell islet tumors have been associated with a severe secretory diarrhea that results in fluid and electrolyte depletion. This complex, referred to as the "watery diarrhea, hypokalemia, and achlorhydria syndrome" **(WDHA; pancreatic cholera**—see p. 498) has been ascribed to vasoactive intestinal peptide **(VIP)** in some patients, although other intestinal hormones or secretogogues, including prostaglandins, may contribute. Hypersecretion of glucagon and the ectopic secretion of ACTH (with the production of Cushing's syndrome) has also been noted in some patients with non–β-cell tumors.

Both the β- and non–β-cell tumors are usually multicentric in origin, and multiple adenomas or diffuse islet cell hyperplasia commonly occur. In about 30% of cases the islet cell tumors are malignant, with local or distant metastases. The incidence of malignancy appears to be higher in the non–β-cell tumors. Malignant islet cell tumors within the MEN-I syndrome often follow a more benign course than sporadic islet cell carcinomas.

Pituitary tumors have been noted in about 65% of patients with the MEN-I syndrome. About 25% of those with pituitary tumor have acromegaly, which is clinically indistinguishable from the sporadic form of the disease. The remainder appear to have chromophobe adenomas; although initially these were believed to be nonfunctioning, recent evidence suggests that many of the chromophobe tumors secrete prolactin. Local expansion of the tumor may cause visual disturbance and headache as well as *hypo*pituitarism.

Adenomas and adenomatous hyperplasia of the thyroid and adrenal glands have been described less often in patients with the MEN-I syndrome. These have rarely been functional and their significance within the MEN-I complex is uncertain. **Carcinoid tumors,** particularly those derived from the embryologic foregut, have been reported in isolated cases of the MEN-I syndrome. Multiple subcutaneous and visceral **lipomas** may be associated as well.

Diagnosis
The clinical features of the MEN-I syndrome depend upon the pattern of tumor involvement in the individual case. About 40% of reported cases have had tumors of the parathyroids, pancreas, and

pituitary. Almost any combination of tumors and symptom complexes outlined above is possible. A patient in an affected kindred manifesting any one of the classic features of the syndrome is at risk for the development of the other associated tumors. *Periodic screening of both affected individuals and unaffected relatives is, therefore, essential.* This should usually include the following: review of the history for symptoms suggestive of peptic ulcer disease, diarrhea, nephrolithiasis, hypoglycemia, and hypopituitarism; physical examination for features of acromegaly and subcutaneous lipomas; x-ray of the sella turcica; measurement of serum Ca, PO_4, gastrin, and prolactin. The diagnosis of insulin-secreting β-cell tumor of the pancreas is established by demonstrating fasting hypoglycemia in conjunction with an elevated plasma insulin level; gastrin-secreting non–β-cell tumor of the pancreas is established by demonstrating elevated basal plasma gastrin levels, an exaggerated gastrin response to infused Ca, and a paradoxic rise in gastrin level after infusion of secretin. The diagnosis of acromegaly is established by elevated growth hormone levels that are not suppressed by glucose administration.

Treatment

Treatment of the parathyroid and pituitary lesions is primarily surgical, although in some cases pituitary irradiation may suffice. Islet cell tumors are more difficult to manage, since the lesions are often small and difficult to find and multiple lesions commonly exist. If a single tumor cannot be found, total pancreatectomy may be required for adequate control of hyperinsulinism. Diazoxide and/or streptozocin may be useful therapeutic adjuncts in the treatment of hypoglycemia. The therapy of gastrin-secreting non–β-cell tumors is total gastrectomy, rather than removal of the pancreatic lesions. Cimetidine (H_2 receptor-antagonist) may be useful for symptomatic control of intractable ulcer disease, and may offer an alternative to surgery in some patients.

MULTIPLE ENDOCRINE NEOPLASIA, TYPE II (MEN-II)

(MEN-IIA; Multiple Endocrine Adenomatosis, Type II [MEA-II]; Sipple's Syndrome)

The MEN-II syndrome is characterized by medullary carcinoma of the thyroid, pheochromocytoma, and hyperparathyroidism. The clinical features of MEN-II depend upon the type of tumor present.

Medullary carcinoma of the thyroid is a malignant neoplasm derived from the calcitonin producing parafollicular or C cells. The tumors contain and secrete large amounts of calcitonin, which is useful in establishing the diagnosis and following the course of the disease. Almost all patients with the MEN-II syndrome will have medullary carcinoma of the thyroid. The usual presentation is that of an asymptomatic thyroid nodule, although many cases are now diagnosed during routine screening of affected MEN-II kindreds before palpable tumor develops. Diarrhea may be present in advanced cases, presumably on the basis of a humoral product such as calcitonin or ectopically produced substances such as kallikreins, serotonin, or prostaglandins. Ectopic production of ACTH with Cushing's syndrome has been noted as well. Medullary carcinoma of the thyroid begins as C-cell hyperplasia, is almost always bilateral and multicentric, and may be associated with the local production of amyloid; fibrosis and calcification within the tumor are commonly noted. Although very high levels of calcitonin are the rule in advanced medullary carcinoma of the thyroid, hypocalcemia is extremely rare. Occasionally, symptoms secondary to metastatic disease lead to diagnosis. The tumor metastasizes to cervical lymph nodes, liver, lung, and bone, and although metastases may occur early, long-term survival is common with 2/3 of affected patients alive at the end of 10 yr.

Pheochromocytoma occurs in about 50% of affected patients within an MEN-II kindred and in some kindreds accounts for 30% of the deaths. As compared with sporadic cases of pheochromocytoma, the familial variety within the MEN-II syndrome begins with adrenal medullary hyperplasia and is multicentric and bilateral in > 50% of cases; extra-adrenal pheochromocytomas are rare in conjunction with MEN-II. The pheochromocytomas are usually epinephrine-producing and increased epinephrine excretion may be the only abnormality early in the course of the disease. Hypertensive crisis secondary to pheochromocytoma is a common presentation, and many of the reported kindreds have first come to medical attention after the diagnosis of bilateral pheochromocytomas in the proband. The hypertension in patients with pheochromocytoma in MEN-II syndrome is more often paroxysmal than sustained, in contrast to the usual sporadic case. The pheochromocytomas are almost always benign, but a tendency for local recurrence has been noted in some of the reported kindreds.

Hyperparathyroidism is present less commonly than medullary carcinoma of the thyroid or pheochromocytoma. About 25% of affected patients within an MEN-II kindred have clinical evidence of hyperparathyroidism (which may be longstanding), with hypercalcemia, nephrolithiasis, nephrocalcinosis, or renal failure. In an additional 25%, without clinical or biochemical evidence of hyperparathyroidism, parathyroid hyperplasia is noted incidentally during thyroid surgery for medullary carcinoma. As in the MEN-I syndrome, the hyperparathyroidism frequently involves multiple glands either as diffuse hyperplasia or multiple adenomas.

On rare occasions clinical features typical of MEN-I, such as the Zollinger-Ellison syndrome, may appear in patients with the MEN-II syndrome; generally, however, the MEN syndromes are distinct.

Diagnosis

Since pheochromocytoma may be asymptomatic in MEN-II patients, excluding pheochromocytoma with certainty may be difficult. Measurement of free catecholamines in a 24-h urine specimen with a specific analysis for epinephrine is the most sensitive way of establishing the diagnosis. VMA excretion is often normal early in the course of disease. CT scan is useful in localizing the pheochromocytoma or establishing the presence of bilateral lesions. Medullary carcinoma of the thyroid is diagnosed by measurement of plasma calcitonin after provocative infusion of pentagastrin and calcium; plasma Ca and PO_4 should be measured. In most patients basal calcitonin levels are elevated, but in some the basal levels are normal and the medullary carcinoma can be diagnosed only by an exaggerated response to calcium and pentagastrin.

Family members in affected kindreds should be screened periodically as follows: review of the history for paroxysmal symptoms suggestive of pheochromocytoma (headache, sweating, palpitations) and renal colic; the BP should be checked and the thyroid carefully palpated. Laboratory studies are performed as described above for suspected probands.

Treatment

Pheochromocytoma should be removed first, since, even if asymptomatic, it greatly increases the risk of surgery for medullary carcinoma or hyperparathyroidism. Since medullary carcinoma of the thyroid is ultimately fatal if untreated, *any patient within an MEN-II kindred displaying pheochromocytoma or hyperparathyroidism should have a total thyroidectomy* even if the diagnosis of medullary carcinoma of the thyroid cannot be established preoperatively.

MULTIPLE ENDOCRINE NEOPLASIA, TYPE III (MEN-III)

(MEN-IIB; Multiple Endocrine Adenomatosis, Type III [MEA-III]; Mucosal Neuroma Syndrome)

MEN-III consists of multiple mucosal neuromas, medullary carcinoma of the thyroid, and pheochromocytoma, often associated with a marfanoid habitus. Although about 50% of the reported cases have been sporadic rather than familial, it is not clear that families were thoroughly screened in all the reported cases; the true incidence, therefore, of sporadic MEN-III syndrome is unknown. In distinction to MEN-I or II, hyperparathyroidism does not appear to be a feature of the MEN-III syndrome.

The distinctive feature of this syndrome is the presence of mucosal neuromas in most, if not all, affected subjects. The neuromas present as small glistening bumps about the lips, tongue, and buccal mucosa. The eyelids, conjunctiva, and cornea are also commonly involved. Thickened eyelids and diffusely hypertrophied lips are also characteristic. Although the neuromas and facial characteristics are present at an early age, the syndrome is often not recognized until the presentation of medullary carcinoma of the thyroid or pheochromocytoma in later life. GI abnormalities related to altered motility (constipation, diarrhea, and, occasionally, megacolon) are common, and are thought to result from diffuse intestinal ganglioneuromatosis.

About half the reported cases show the complete syndrome with mucosal neuromas, pheochromocytomas, and medullary carcinoma of the thyroid. Less than 10% have neuromas and pheochromocytomas alone, while the remainder have neuromas and medullary carcinoma of the thyroid without pheochromocytoma.

Medullary carcinoma of the thyroid and pheochromocytoma closely resemble the corresponding disorders in the MEN-II syndrome; both tend to be bilateral and multicentric. The implications for diagnosis, family screening, and treatment are the same as described above for the MEN-II syndrome. *All affected patients should have a total thyroidectomy as soon as the diagnosis is established.* Pheochromocytoma, if present, should be removed prior to the medullary carcinoma.

90. DISORDERS OF CARBOHYDRATE METABOLISM

DIABETES MELLITUS

A syndrome resulting from a variable interaction of hereditary and environmental factors, and characterized by abnormal insulin secretion and a variety of metabolic and vascular manifestations reflected in a tendency toward inappropriately elevated blood glucose levels, accelerated nonspecific atherosclerosis, neuropathy, and thickened capillary basal lamina causing renal and retinal impairment.

The syndrome has no distinct etiology, pathogenesis, invariable set of clinical findings, specific laboratory tests, or definitive and curative therapy, although it is nearly always associated with fasting hyperglycemia and decreased glucose tolerance. The complete clinical syndrome of diabetes mellitus involves hyperglycemia, large-vessel disease, microvascular disease (retina and kidney), and neuropathy.

A new classification of diabetes mellitus developed by the National Diabetes Data Group (NDDG) from the National Institutes of Health distinguishes the following subclasses: (1) **Insulin-dependent diabetes mellitus (IDDM or Type I)**, a ketosis-prone type of diabetes associated with certain histocompatibility antigens (HLA) on chromosome 6 and with islet cell antibodies. (2) **Noninsulin-dependent diabetes mellitus (NIDDM or Type II)**, a nonketosis-prone type of diabetes not secondary to other diseases or conditions. This subclass of diabetes has been subdivided into **obese NIDDM** and **nonobese NIDDM**. (3) **Diabetes associated with certain conditions and symptoms** such as pancreatic disease, changes in other hormones besides insulin, the administration of various drugs and chemical agents, insulin receptor abnormalities, genetic syndromes, and malnourished populations. (4) **Gestational diabetes**, where glucose intolerance develops or is discovered during pregnancy, is considered as a separate class. (5) **Impaired glucose tolerance (IGT)** is present when individuals have plasma glucose levels intermediate between normal and those considered diabetic. Terms such as chemical, latent, borderline, subclinical, and asymptomatic diabetes should be abandoned, since the use of the term diabetes invokes social, psychologic, and economic sanctions that are unjustified in light of the lack of severity of the glucose intolerance.

Pathophysiology

Hyperglycemia: A relative or absolute lack of insulin secretion associated with an excess of circulating stress hormones (including glucagon, catecholamines, and cortisol) is responsible for inappropriate elevation of blood glucose and associated alterations in lipid metabolism characterizing the metabolic syndrome. Depending upon the severity of insulin secretion impairment, patients usually can be categorized as IDDM or NIDDM. The differing characteristics of these 2 categories are listed in TABLE 90–1.

Large vessel disease: Diabetics have an increased incidence, earlier onset, and increased severity of atherosclerosis in the intima and calcification in the media of the arterial wall. This is discussed in detail in ARTERIOSCLEROSIS; ATHEROSCLEROSIS in Ch. 24. Diabetes mellitus usually is present when such calcification is seen in patients under 40. Peripheral vascular disease is 50 to 100 times more common in diabetics than in normals.

Microvascular disease: Diabetics have an abnormality of the capillary basal lamina (basement membrane) that is characterized by added layers and consequent increased thickness of the lamina and is easily demonstrable in the major capillary beds of skin and skeletal muscle. It is not a diffuse generalized process but is regional (e.g., more frequent in the legs than the abdominal wall) and focal (involving one segment of a capillary but not the next). Clinically, the most important sites of microvascular involvement are the retina and the renal glomeruli. The process is also observed in the renal medulla, nervous system, pancreas, and heart, but apparently spares the lungs. A similar process involving capillaries is seen in aging, though to a lesser degree. A thickened basal lamina has been observed in hypothyroidism and myositis, but is not present in all conditions with elevated blood glucose (e.g., many patients with Cushing's syndrome).

Neuropathy: Segmental injury to nerves, associated with demyelination and Schwann cell degeneration, involves sensory and motor peripheral nerves, nerve roots, the spinal cord, and the autonomic nervous system. It is characterized by temporary changes with nerve repair evident both microscopically and clinically. Affected nerves show basal lamina thickening similar to the capillary abnormalities. Clinical neuropathy may precede symptoms or signs of carbohydrate or vascular abnormalities, and the presence of unexplained neuropathy should lead to investigations of other components of the syndrome.

Ketoacidosis: Important physiologic aspects are discussed below.

Symptoms and Signs

The earliest symptom of elevated blood glucose is polyuria from the osmotic diuretic effect of glucose. Continued hyperglycemia and glucosuria may lead to thirst, hunger, and weight loss. Glucosuria is also associated with an increased incidence of monilial vaginitis and itching. It is uncertain whether the incidence of other infections (e.g., pyelonephritis, cystitis) is increased as a *direct* result of hyperglycemia. Accelerated fat catabolism in the untreated insulin-dependent patient produces ketoacidosis leading to anorexia, nausea, vomiting, air hunger, and, if untreated, coma and death. Onset tends to be abrupt in children and insidious in older patients.

The symptoms and signs of large-vessel atherosclerosis in the diabetic are the same as in nondiabetic patients. The symptoms and signs of microvascular disease are those of renal failure if the glomerular capillaries are involved, or visual loss if the retinal capillaries are affected. Proteinuria usually is the first indication of nephropathy, and it may reach nephrotic levels. The greater the proteinuria, the more rapid is the development of renal failure. Hematuria and sterile pyuria are frequent and early findings, whereas hypertension occurs late. Renal failure is seen in 50% of IDDM patients after 20 to 30 yr of diabetes. Diabetic retinopathy is usually first detected 5 yr or more after the diagnosis of diabetes mellitus is made, but is present to some degree by 10 yr in 50% of patients (see Ch. 214).

A bilateral, comparatively symmetric, distal polyneuropathy (predominantly sensory) is the most frequent form of diabetic neuropathy. Symptoms generally appear earlier and more severely in the feet, occasionally with sensory loss in a "glove and stocking" distribution or with the appearance of painless penetrating plantar ulcers. Nerve involvement may be characterized by lancinating pain in the distribution of a single dermatome, or the posterior columns of the spinal cord may be affected,

TABLE 90–1. GENERAL CHARACTERISTICS OF TWO MAJOR CLINICAL TYPES OF DIABETES MELLITUS

Characteristic	Insulin-Dependent (Type I)	Non–Insulin-Dependent (Type II)
Age of onset	Often < 25	Often > 40
Body build	Almost always lean	90% are obese
Ketoacidosis develops off insulin	Yes	No
Endogenous insulin secretion	Insulinopenia	Variable insulin levels
Predominant vascular disease	Microangiopathy	Atherosclerosis
Histocompatibility antigens (HLA) and islet cell antibodies	Present	Absent
Family history	Minor	Marked
Twin concordance	Low	High
Islet cell morphology	Loss	Hyperplasia

producing loss of position sense and deep tendon reflexes with a positive Romberg sign. Major nerve trunks may be involved, with pain, sensory loss, motor weakness, and deprivation of sympathetic innervation in the distribution of a major spinal or cranial nerve. The 3rd and 6th cranial nerves are most often involved. Diabetic amyotrophy is found characteristically in elderly men, producing a predominant muscle weakness around the hip and upper leg. While the appearance resembles other neuropathies and myopathies, these symptoms in diabetics may be reversible, often improving within 1 to 2 yr. The autonomic nervous system may be involved diffusely, and autonomic insufficiency often occurs early as sweating disturbances or postural hypotension with significant symptoms. Sexual impotence in the male may be the most common symptom (50 to 60%) of neuropathy in diabetes mellitus; over a period of 6 mo to 1 yr, there is a gradual onset of decreasing firmness of erection. While constipation is perhaps the most common intestinal manifestation of diabetic autonomic neuropathy, it tends to be overshadowed by diarrhea, which is usually intermittent, watery, and frequently worse at night. Severe continuous steatorrhea suggests the possibility of coexisting celiac disease or pancreatic carcinoma.

Clinical course: Some diabetics deteriorate rapidly with a course complicated by episodes of ketoacidosis and vascular manifestations, while others go through life with mild nonprogressing glucose intolerance and few other manifestations of the syndrome. The presence of large- and small-vessel disease, as well as neuropathy, seems unrelated to the degree of glucose intolerance or to the amount of insulin required. The only reliable direct correlate with serious vascular manifestations is the duration of diabetes mellitus. The longer the disease is present, the more likely are such manifestations.

Diagnosis of Diabetes Mellitus

Despite the importance of neuropathy, microangiopathy, and large-vessel disease to the diabetic syndrome, they do not conclusively establish the diagnosis. The absence of a precise diagnostic marker for diabetes mellitus continues to be a problem. The diagnosis, according to the NDDG, should be based on (1) unequivocal elevation of plasma glucose concentration, together with the typical symptoms of polyuria, polydipsia, ketonuria, and rapid weight loss; or (2) fasting plasma glucose concentration ≥ 140 mg/dl on more than one occasion (without the presence of other factors such as fasting, complicating illness, pregnancy, certain drugs or stress that are known to elevate plasma glucose); or (3) elevated plasma glucose concentration after an oral glucose challenge on more than one occasion.

Although glucose tolerance testing has been used in an attempt to detect the diabetic syndrome at an early stage, many factors that elevate fasting glucose levels (e.g., stress, starvation, drugs, or hormones—see TABLE 90–2) can alter glucose tolerance. Erroneous diagnoses of diabetes mellitus may be made in patients who demonstrate hyperglycemia, glucosuria, and abnormal glucose tolerance when hospitalized with severe stress such as is associated with stroke, myocardial infarction, or systemic infection. Such patients may even require insulin temporarily to control hyperglycemia, but they become normoglycemic as the stressful situation subsides.

The procedure for administering the **oral glucose tolerance test (OGTT)**, recommended by the NDDG, is to perform the test in the morning after at least 3 days of unrestricted diet (≥ 150 gm carbohydrate) and normal physical activity. The subject should then fast for at least 10 h but no more than 16 h (water is permitted). During the test the subject should remain seated and not smoke, and the adverse influences of the drugs and hormones listed in TABLE 90–2 must be avoided. The dose of

TABLE 90–2. DRUGS AND HORMONES ASSOCIATED WITH IMPAIRED GLUCOSE TOLERANCE

Diuretics and antihypertensive agents Chlorthalidone Clonidine Diazoxide Furosemide Metolazone Thiazides	**Psychoactive agents** Chlorprothixene Haloperidol Lithium carbonate Phenothiazines Tricyclic antidepressants
Hormones and hormonally active agents Catecholamines Mineralocorticoids Progestins } Estrogens } Oral contraceptives Growth hormone Glucagon Glucocorticoids (natural and synthetic) Thyroid hormones (toxic levels)	**Neurologically active agents** Phenytoin Isoproterenol Levodopa **Antineoplastic agents** Alloxan L-Asparaginase Streptozocin
Analgesic, antipyretic, and antiinflammatory agents Indomethacin	**Miscellaneous** Isoniazid Niacin

glucose administered should be 1.75 gm/kg ideal body weight but not more than 75 gm. A commercially prepared carbohydrate load equivalent to this dose is also acceptable.

A fasting blood sample is then collected, after which glucose, in a concentration not exceeding 25 gm/dl in flavored water, is drunk in about 5 min. Zero time is when drinking starts, and blood samples are collected at 30-min intervals for 2 h. Diabetes is diagnosed (by the OGTT) in nonpregnant adults and children if, after the glucose load, both the 2-h sample and another sample within the 2-h period show a venous plasma glucose ≥ 200 mg/dl. Impaired glucose tolerance is present if values are between these and normal glucose levels (see TABLE 90–3).

Gestational diabetes is diagnosed in pregnant women, who were not diabetic before pregnancy, whose plasma glucose levels meet or exceed the levels in TABLE 90–3 for 2 or more values following a 100-gm oral glucose load.

An OGTT is primarily important for diagnosing (1) postprandial reactive hypoglycemia (see under HYPOGLYCEMIA below), (2) diabetes mellitus in pregnancy, when special measures may affect fetal survival (see DIABETES MELLITUS in Vol. II, Ch. 18 and DISTURBANCES OF THE NEWBORN in Vol II, Ch. 21), (3) diabetes mellitus in the presence of other metabolic abnormalities (e.g., hyperlipidemia or hyperuricemia) that might be helped by treatment of hyperglycemia, and (4) diabetes mellitus in the unexplained presence of neuropathy, retinopathy, or peripheral vascular disease. In addition, an abnormal test may help persuade a coronary-prone patient to lose weight or stop smoking. When the

TABLE 90–3. DIAGNOSTIC CRITERIA OF THE NATIONAL DIABETES DATA GROUP

Criteria for Diagnosis of Diabetes Mellitus and Impaired Glucose Tolerance (All plasma glucose values in mg/dl)						Criteria for Diagnosis of Gestational Diabetes (100 gm OGTT)**
	Normal		Diabetes Mellitus		Impaired Glucose Tolerance	Venous Plasma Glucose
	Adult	Child	Adult	Child	Adult	Child	
FPG* OGTT**	< 115 < 140	< 130 < 140	≥ 140 ≥ 200	≥ 140 ≥ 200	115–139 140–199	130–139 140–199	Fasting ≥ 105 mg/dl 1 h ≥ 190 mg/dl 2 h ≥ 165 mg/dl 3 h ≥ 145 mg/dl

* Fasting Plasma Glucose
** Oral Glucose Tolerance Test (at least 2 values)

From "Classification and Diagnosis of Diabetes Mellitus and Other Categories of Glucose Intolerance," by the National Diabetes Data Group, *Diabetes*, vol. 28, page 1049, December 1979. Reproduced with permission of the American Diabetes Association, Inc., and the National Institutes of Health.

fasting plasma glucose concentration is in the diabetic range more than once, an OGTT is not necessary for the diagnosis.

Diagnosis of Ketoacidosis and Hyperosmolar Coma

The possibility of ketoacidosis is suggested by (1) confusion or coma, the patient almost always appearing extremely ill and often with changes in sensorium; (2) air hunger (an attempt to compensate for metabolic acidosis); (3) fruity acetone odor on the breath; (4) nausea and vomiting (almost always present); (5) abdominal tenderness, a complaint of nearly 1/3 of patients, which, with nausea and vomiting, may mimic viral gastroenteritis or an acute abdomen; (6) extreme thirst and dry mucous membranes, reflecting water depletion; (7) weight loss; and (8) a diabetic history, present in about 90% of patients.

Differentiation of ketoacidotic coma from insulin shock (hypoglycemia), and rapid bedside confirmation of a clinical impression without delaying treatment are outlined in Table 90-4. Hyperglycemia can be diagnosed at the bedside using commercially available blood glucose test strips (Dextrostix® or Chemstrip® bG), and a rough quantitation of plasma or serum ketones can be made using either Ketostix® reagent strips or Acetest® reagent tablets. Serum or plasma is serially diluted with tap water using test tubes and a syringe providing 1 in 2, 1 in 4, 1 in 8, and 1 in 16 dilutions. The presence of hyperglycemia plus a "large" amount of ketones in the serum 1 in 2 dilution confirms the diagnosis of diabetic ketoacidosis, and therapy can be started at once. Occasionally, lactic acid and β-hydroxybutyric acid can contribute significantly to the low pH without reacting to the ketone strips or tablets. More precise determinations of blood or plasma glucose, serum bicarbonate, pH, serum electrolytes, and BUN help in the patient's management but are not necessary for initial diagnosis and emergency treatment.

TABLE 90-4. DIFFERENTIAL DIAGNOSIS: KETOACIDOTIC COMA AND INSULIN SHOCK

Diagnostic Factors	Ketoacidotic Coma	Insulin Shock
History:		
Food intake	Normal or excessive	May be insufficient
Insulin	Insufficient	Excessive
Onset	Gradual (days)	Sudden (more gradual with long-acting insulins)
Preceding febrile illness or other stress	Frequent	Absent
Physical examination:		
Appearance	Extremely ill	Very weak
Skin	Dry and flushed	Moist and pale
Infection	Frequent	Absent
Fever	Frequent	Absent (hypothermia may be present)
GI symptoms:		
Mouth	Dry	Drooling
Thirst	Intense	Absent
Hunger	Absent	Occasional
Vomiting	Common	Rare
Abdominal pain	Frequent	Absent
Respiration	Exaggerated, air hunger	Normal or shallow
Breath (acetone odor)	Present	Rare
Blood pressure	Low	Normal
Pulse	Weak and rapid	Full and bounding
Eyeballs	Soft	Normal
Laboratory findings:		
Urine glucose (bedside)	High	Absent in 2nd specimen
Urine ketones (bedside)	High	Absent in 2nd specimen
Blood glucose (bedside)	High	< 60 mg/dl
Serum ketones (bedside)	Large in undiluted specimen	Absent to trace
Serum bicarbonate	< 10 mEq/L	> 22 mEq/L
Response to treatment	Gradual (6 to 12 h following use of insulin)	Rapid, following carbohydrate administration or glucagon injection

Ketoacidosis also occurs in **nondiabetic alcoholic patients.** There is chronic heavy drinking until 1 to 3 days before presentation when persistent anorexia, abdominal pain, nausea, and vomiting commence with consequent food abstention. Hydrogen ion formation by alcohol metabolism leads to increased production of β-hydroxybutyrate (not measurable by the standard nitroprusside test), increased lactate formation, and decreased gluconeogenesis. Metabolic acidosis with variable plasma glucose levels (hypoglycemic to mildly hyperglycemic) in a patient with a history of alcoholism suggests the diagnosis. Alcoholic diabetics may present with a complex mixture of alcohol and diabetic acidosis. (For treatment of ketoacidosis, see below).

Hyperglycemic-hyperosmolar nonketotic coma occurs in the setting of insulin deficiency and renal and cerebral impairment, largely in elderly, mildly obese patients who often present a history of previous mild diabetes mellitus. Hyperglycemia from insulin deficiency leads to osmotic diuresis and decreased renal perfusion, which exaggerates the hyperglycemia and hyperosmolality. Cerebral impairment decreases fluid intake, which again exacerbates the dehydration, renal impairment, and hyperosmolality, culminating in frank coma, acute renal shutdown, thrombosis, vascular collapse, and lactic acidosis. The patient's serum osmolality, either directly measured or reflected by combined elevation of the serum Na and glucose, exceeds 360 mOsm/L. (For treatment, see below.)

Treatment of Diabetes Mellitus—General Considerations

The primary objective is to achieve the patient's optimal health and nutrition. Whether treatment of asymptomatic hyperglycemia decreases morbidity and mortality is unknown, and there is significant risk of hypoglycemia in elderly patients given oral hypoglycemic agents or insulin therapy. Therefore, it appears best not to use drug therapy in elderly patients with impaired glucose tolerance or asymptomatic fasting hyperglycemia.

Whether a more physiologic approach to insulin replacement will significantly reduce morbidity and mortality in patients taking insulin is still unknown. Efforts in this direction include the use of an insulin pump worn on the belt that constantly infuses a low dose of rapid-acting (regular or crystalline) insulin s.c. or IV with additional boluses of insulin pumped in immediately prior to meals. Alternatively, 3 daily premeal injections of insulin injection may be given through an indwelling subcutaneous needle in addition to a low daily dose of prolonged-acting insulin. It is hoped that these attempts to emulate normal pancreatic function may be associated with a clearly demonstrable improvement in the morbidity and mortality from the vascular and neural manifestations of diabetes.

The objectives of symptom control are (1) to avoid ketoacidosis and (2) to control symptoms resulting from hyperglycemia and glucosuria.

Symptom control begins with the measurement of urine glucose as an index of plasma glucose levels. In starting therapy, it is best to analyze the urine prior to each meal and at bedtime. The timing of the collections and the method of testing must be understood. Collecting "double-void" urine specimens immediately prior to meals helps avoid testing urine stored in the bladder since the preceding meal. The patient is instructed to void about 30 min before the meal, drink 2 or 3 glasses of water, and then void again immediately prior to the meal; the latter specimen is then tested for glucose. An atonic bladder or a prostatic obstruction may prevent complete emptying of the bladder before the test collection and reduce the reliability of the test. The method for testing for urine glucose is chosen on the basis of whether the patient normally spills glucose in the urine or not. Tes-Tape® and Clinistix® are excellent for screening glucosuria, but provide poor quantitation. Clinitest® kits and Diastix®, while slightly more expensive, provide semiquantitation of glucosuria and should be used in patients who normally spill some glucose, to detect changes in urine glucose levels that will influence treatment or warn of impending ketoacidosis. For occasional patients, particularly juveniles with a low renal glucose threshold, the 2-drop Clinitest® method may give a better range of quantitation than the standard 5-drop method (NOTE: A special 2-drop color chart must be used). All urine glucose results should be recorded as "per cent" readings; the "plus" scales indicate different glucose concentrations with different methods. The patient is asked to keep a chart of the urine glucose test results.

Occasional plasma glucose determinations by the laboratory can be timed on the basis of urine test and hypoglycemic symptom reports. The lowest plasma glucose values, usually before meals and at bedtime when the urine is negative for glucose, are generally most useful in regulating the drug and dietary regimens. They help to determine renal glucose threshold and guide interpretation of urine tests. Occasionally, in difficult cases, determination of total 24-h urinary glucose excretion to document the overall glucose loss under a prescribed regimen will be helpful in making therapeutic decisions.

More precise control of blood glucose is possible with patients determining their own blood glucose levels using Chemstrip® bG visual measurements or Dextrostix® measurements with a reflectance meter. Such tests are primarily useful for insulin-dependent diabetics and can determine quickly whether nonspecific symptoms are caused by hyper- or hypoglycemia. These measurements are inexpensive and sufficiently accurate for clinical use. Generally, reduced blood glucose levels result from improvement in patient motivation and understanding of their disease. A spring-loaded lancet holder such as the Autolet® may increase patient acceptance. The Chemstrip® color is stable and test results can be verified by the nurse or physician from strips submitted by the patient on a weekly basis. One approach is to have a patient measure his blood glucose 7 times a day: before each meal, 1 h after each meal, and at bedtime. Such a profile is obtained no more frequently than twice a week and may be needed rarely with a stable, well-controlled patient.

Types of Insulin Available

The 7 forms of insulin currently available in the USA have different rates of onset of effectiveness and duration of action. These insulins may be classified as fast-, intermediate-, and long-acting; their properties are listed in TABLE 90–5. All are available in 10-ml bottles, at concentrations of 100 u. and 40 u./ml. The previously available 80 u./ml insulin has been removed from the market in the USA to avoid confusion. Syringes for U-100 and for U-40 insulin indicate directly on the syringe the number of insulin units. To simplify insulin use and to reduce patient error, only U-100 insulin should be prescribed, with U-40 given rarely for patients on low doses. Insulins are available in 2 series: Lente (Lente®, Semilente® and Ultralente®) and protamine (crystalline-zinc, NPH, and protamine zinc).

All of these insulins contain pancreatic impurities, including glucagon, somatostatin, pancreatic polypeptide, and proinsulin. The comparative degree of purity is reflected in the parts per million (ppm) of proinsulin. Improved Squibb insulin has < 25 ppm and Squibb purified insulin has < 10 ppm. Lilly's Iletin I® has < 50 ppm, while its more purified Iletin II® has < 10 ppm. The insulins marketed by Nordisk and Novo have < 1 ppm. Whether or not increased purity is worth the additional cost is unclear, but a trial of a purer insulin is suggested when insulin allergy, insulin resistance, or lipoatrophy is encountered (see Complications of Insulin Treatment, below). *Care must be taken in switching to a purer insulin preparation,* as patients may require lower or higher doses. An initial dosage reduction of 20% at the time of switching will usually prevent hypoglycemia. Monospecies pork insulins (as opposed to beef or beef/pork insulins) are less immunogenic in human subjects.

Human insulin has been produced biosynthetically and recently became available for the treatment of diabetes mellitus.

Insulin injection (crystalline-zinc insulin, regular insulin) and **prompt insulin zinc suspension** (Semilente®, Semitard®) have a rapid onset and short duration of action. *Insulin injection is the only insulin that may be given IV* and is the insulin used for the initial emergency treatment of diabetic ketoacidosis and marked hyperglycemia. Both of the rapid-acting insulins are used when early onset of action is desired, generally supplementing intermediate-acting insulins.

Intermediate-acting insulins include **isophane insulin suspension (NPH insulin, Insulatard®, Leo Retard RI®), insulin zinc suspension** (Lente®, Monotard®, Lentard®), and **globin zinc insulin injection.** These preparations have sufficiently rapid onset of action to control post-breakfast blood glucose levels, and activity lasts long enough to continue control to the following morning. In the absence of ketoacidosis or other acute complications, most diabetics can be controlled with a single

TABLE 90–5. CHARACTERISTICS OF VARIOUS INSULINS

Action	Preparation	Appearance	Protein Modifier	Peak Effect (Hours)	Duration of Action (Hours)
Rapid	Insulin injection (regular, crystalline-zinc, Actrapid®, Velosulin Quick®)	Clear solution	None	2–3	5–7
	Prompt insulin zinc suspension (Semilente®, Semitard®)	Cloudy suspension	None	3–6	12–16
Intermediate	Isophane insulin suspension (NPH, Insulatard®, Leo Retard RI®)	Cloudy suspension	Protamine	4–12	18–28
	Insulin zinc suspension (Lente®, Monotard,® Lentard®)	Cloudy suspension	None	$6^{1}/_{2}$–$14^{1}/_{2}$	18–24
	Globin zinc insulin injection	Clear solution	Globin	8–16	18–24
Prolonged	Protamine zinc insulin suspension (PZI)	Cloudy suspension	Protamine	14–20	30–36
	Extended insulin zinc suspension (Ultralente®, Ultratard®)	Cloudy suspension	None	16–18	36 +

daily injection of 20 to 60 u. of an intermediate-acting insulin given s.c. before breakfast. Initially, 10 to 20 u./day may be given. Thereafter, on the basis of glucose determinations on pre-meal, double-void urine samples and of symptoms of hypoglycemia, the dose may be adjusted by 2 to 10 u./day until satisfactory control is obtained. Patient blood glucose monitoring may be very helpful here. As optimum control is approached, it is advisable to continue a given dose for 3 successive days before changing it. If adequate control cannot be obtained with a single daily dose of an intermediate-acting insulin, the addition of a small amount of fast-acting insulin of the same series to the morning injection may be required. Alternatively, the dose of intermediate-acting insulin may be divided; approximately $2/3$ of the total dose should be given in the morning, and the remainder just before the evening meal.

Protamine zinc insulin suspension and **extended insulin zinc suspension** (Ultralente®, Ultratard®) are long-acting insulins which may be given as a single daily dose 30 to 90 min before breakfast to some patients with mild to moderately severe stable diabetes mellitus. However, since stability of the patient is difficult to achieve with long-acting preparations, they are rarely used alone.

Management of Difficult-to-Control ("Brittle") Diabetics

Some insulin-requiring patients demonstrate rapid swings between heavy glucosuria and symptomatic hypoglycemic reactions. Seven principles are helpful in managing these patients:

1. Patient monitoring of a profile of blood glucose levels at home using commercially available blood test strips (see above), may help both patient and physician analyze the precise nature of the "brittleness" and take appropriate steps towards its correction.

2. The patient's dietary, insulin, and emotional baselines should be stabilized and daily exercise should remain relatively constant. The time of day and caloric content of breakfast, lunch, dinner, and additional scheduled snacks should be stable from day to day.

3. On the basis of either hypoglycemic reactions and premeal glucosuria or of a self-monitored blood glucose profile, the morning insulin dose may be adjusted and supplemented with either the short-acting or long-acting preparation of the same series, as indicated. Under these circumstances, the Lente® insulins are a little easier to use; protamine zinc insulin added in the same syringe to isophane or insulin injection inordinately prolongs the effect of the combination.

4. Between-meal and bedtime snacks, representing a shift in mealtime calories but not an increase in total daily caloric intake, match caloric intake more closely to the intermediate insulin action curves.

5. Giving $1/3$ of the total daily insulin dose before the evening meal is helpful.

6. Rarely, unstable ketoacidosis-prone patients require multiple injections of rapid-acting insulin. The insulin is given in divided portions before meals based on the results of blood or urine tests.

7. Some diabetics demonstrate brittleness, with wide swings of plasma glucose from daytime hyperglycemia and glucosuria to nighttime hypoglycemic reactions. It is important to document such swings with blood glucose self-monitoring strips. Such patients often benefit by having their insulin dose reduced by 30 to 70%, and then gradually increased over several days; they often stabilize at a lower dose level.

Complications of Insulin Treatment

Insulin shock (hypoglycemia) may occur if too much insulin or too little food is taken. (See Hypoglycemia, below, for diagnosis and therapy.) All patients receiving insulin, and their families, must be instructed concerning the symptoms and immediate treatment of hypoglycemia. A patient receiving insulin should always carry sugar or candy to be eaten immediately if epinephrine-like symptoms are felt (see Symptoms and Signs under Hypoglycemia, below). Carrying an identification card or engraved metallic emblem on a bracelet or necklace (Medic Alert Foundation, Turlock, California 95380) stating that the patient has diabetes mellitus and is taking insulin will help in case of accident or emergency illness.

Local reactions to insulin injections, often occurring during the first few weeks of insulin therapy, most commonly consist of stinging or itching at the injection site, possibly followed by heat, induration, erythema, and an urticarial reaction. The new more purified insulin preparations may reduce the incidence of local reactions. Treatment may consist of switching from the beef-pork insulin combination to pure pork (or occasionally pure beef) insulin. Systemic allergic reactions are uncommon; they include hives, urticaria, cardiopulmonary or GI symptoms, and, rarely, anaphylaxis. Systemic treatment with antihistamines, corticosteroids, and even epinephrine injection may be required.

Patients occasionally develop **insulin resistance** and require > 200 u. daily to control hyperglycemia. Shifting to a more purified insulin preparation may lower insulin requirements, as may the *cautious* addition of tolbutamide to the insulin regimen. Lilly's concentrated regular pork insulin preparation (Iletin II®, U–500) is designed for insulin-resistant patients.

The s.c. injection of insulin in certain susceptible patients may rarely result in either atrophy or hypertrophy of the local fat tissue. Nearly all patients with atrophy show improvement when their daily dose of one of the newer purified insulins is injected directly into the affected area. No specific treatment for injection site hypertrophy is effective; careful injection site rotation is recommended.

Oral Hypoglycemic Agents

Several sulfonylureas that can lower the blood glucose level when given orally may be used to treat a limited number of selected patients. These are tolbutamide, chlorpropamide, acetohexamide, and tolazamide. Oral agents should not be used as a substitute for insulin in the insulin-dependent patient; although their mechanisms of action are not clear, they are not oral forms of insulin. Their biologic half-lives following oral administration cannot be measured accurately, making the selection of dose and timing of administration somewhat haphazard.

The **University Group Diabetes Program (UGDP)** attempted to evaluate various types of therapy in non–insulin-dependent diabetic patients, comparing tolbutamide or phenformin (a biguanide, since withdrawn from general use in the USA) treatment with diet alone and with 2 insulin treatment regimens. The study has led to 2 major conclusions: (1) The combination of diet and tolbutamide or diet and phenformin therapy in the treatment of mild non–insulin-dependent diabetics is no more effective than diet alone in prolonging life, at least in the dosages of phenformin and tolbutamide that were used. (2) Tolbutamide plus diet, or phenformin plus diet, may be less effective than diet alone or than diet plus insulin insofar as minimizing cardiovascular mortality.

The UGDP study raised genuine controversy about whether increased cardiovascular mortality is associated with the use of sulfonylureas. However, after 17 yr, the investigators reported that, in their non–insulin-dependent diabetics, there was no evidence that insulin, or any other drug that lowered plasma glucose levels, altered the course of vascular complications. Furthermore, only a variable insulin dose program showed reliable and sustained reduction of plasma glucose levels.

For the symptomatic non–insulin-dependent patient, who cannot physically administer or receive insulin injections (e.g., arthritis or blindness) and whose need for control is of relatively short duration, the sulfonylureas may lower plasma glucose levels and control symptoms. Such a situation accounts for a very small number of non–insulin-dependent diabetics. For the remaining symptomatic patients, insulin is indicated. For the asymptomatic non–insulin-dependent patients, weight control and reduction of other atherosclerotic risks is the best therapy.

Acute toxic effects following the use of oral hypoglycemic agents appear to be relatively rare. Following either an initial dose or months of therapy with one of the sulfonylureas, cholestatic jaundice or severe hypoglycemia has occurred. The latter at times may last for several days. Chlorpropamide has been associated with symptomatic hyponatremia and water intoxication due to potentiation of antidiuretic hormone action on renal tubules.

If a sulfonylurea is tried, a given dose should be continued for 4 to 6 wk before determining that the drug is a success or failure at symptom control. Doses of the sulfonylureas generally should not exceed 3 gm/day of tolbutamide, 500 mg/day of chlorpropamide, 1.5 gm/day of acetohexamide, and 1 gm/day of tolazamide.

Treatment of Ketoacidosis

Ketoacidosis is associated with 5 physiologic abnormalities that must be immediately evaluated and corrected:

1. Hyperglycemia: With normal renal circulation, blood glucose concentrations rarely exceed 400 mg/dl. With fluid loss and compromised renal perfusion, however, higher values are found.

2. Acidosis is the result of lipid mobilization and breakdown of free fatty acids in the liver to acetoacetic and β-hydroxybutyric acids.

3. Low blood volume is due to loss of both fluid and electrolytes. Hct, postural BP changes, neck vein observation, and central venous pressure can reflect the severity of this depletion.

4. Hyperosmolality is also a potential contributing factor in coma as a result of renal water loss and water depletion due to sweating, nausea, and vomiting. Significant osmolal elevation generally is reflected by hyperglycemia > 500 mg/dl and suggests inadequate renal perfusion. Occasionally hyperosmolality alone can cause hyperglycemic-hyperosmolar nonketotic coma (see above).

5. Potassium loss: Although total body K is depleted, the serum K in the presence of acidosis is often deceptively sustained in the normal range.

Immediate treatment: The cornerstones of ketoacidosis therapy, required in all patients, are insulin and IV fluids. **Insulin** is given immediately. The choice of insulin regimen should be based on the experience of the therapeutic team; the objective in all approaches is to achieve optimally effective levels of circulating insulin and maintain them until there is evidence of biochemical recovery. An ideal rate of blood glucose lowering is 75 to 100 mg/dl/h. A more rapid drop may lead to osmotically induced fluid shifts, manifested by confusion or other evidence of CNS deterioration. One approach is to give a continuous IV infusion of insulin injection in saline at a rate of 10 u./h or, alternatively, to give the same dose via intermittent IM (not s.c.) injection. Because circulatory insufficiency is common in ketoacidosis, absorption from s.c. sites is unpredictable; therefore, insulins other than insulin injection (regular or crystalline-zinc insulin) are never used. The IV infusion can be administered through an infusion pump or a pediatric infusion set. This "low-dose" approach is as safe and effective as previous high-dose regimens and provides greater ease in avoiding hypoglycemia and hypokalemia. Any method of treatment, however, requires close clinical supervision.

IV fluids should also be started at once. The first liter of isotonic saline should be given over 20 to 60 min, depending upon the severity of extracellular volume depletion. Hypotonic solutions are less effective in restoring renal perfusion. Glucose solutions do not help correct the electrolyte and pH disturbances and are withheld until plasma glucose begins to fall. Low blood volume and shock usually respond to vigorous infusion of saline but may require plasma or plasma expanders (see SHOCK in Ch. 24). If serum K is low, addition of KCl to the first bottle of IV fluid should be considered.

Two other immediate measures which may be required include **nasogastric intubation** (for intractable vomiting, abdominal distention, and gastric dilation, or to avoid aspiration in a comatose patient) and **bladder catheterization** (to monitor urine output in severely ill or comatose patients).

Continuing treatment: Hourly blood glucose determinations and semiquantitation of serum ketones by serum serial dilution will reflect patient improvement. Patients without a 10% drop in plasma glucose after 2 h should have the insulin dose doubled each hour until a response occurs. After the blood glucose falls to 250 mg/dl, an infusion containing glucose helps to avoid late hypoglycemia.

Bicarbonate may be added to the IV solution during the first 2 or 3 h *only* if acidosis is severe (blood pH < 7.1, bicarbonate < 10 mEq/L). It is seldom required, and the administration rate should not exceed 100 mEq/h. Excessive bicarbonate therapy may be paradoxically associated with CSF acidosis and inhibition of hemoglobin O_2 transport and tissue oxygenation.

Potassium loss is estimated from the serum K level interpreted in light of the degree of acidosis. Initially, serum K should be measured hourly; *failure to assess K accurately is the commonest cause of death during treatment of ketoacidosis.* As soon as urine flow is known to be adequate, K can be added to the infusion at the rate of 20 mEq/h or less. Faster rates in the presence of severe depletion require extreme caution with careful monitoring to avoid hyperkalemic cardiac arrest. If the initial serum K is very low, replacement should be started even before adequate urine flow is confirmed.

Marked improvement should occur within 8 h. Reevaluation at that time of the 5 areas of physiologic abnormalities (listed above) should direct therapy to any significant remaining imbalances. Treatment is continued until the patient is able to take fluid freely by mouth. As soon as food is tolerated, oral fluids followed by the patient's diet and insulin therapy should be resumed.

An underlying cause for the ketoacidosis must always be sought; common problems include omitted insulin dose, infection, GI upset, alcoholism, myocardial infarction, CVA, or previously undiagnosed diabetes mellitus. Since a leukocytosis of 15,000 to 30,000 is common in ketoacidosis, this is not helpful in indicating infection.

Treatment of **alcoholic ketoacidosis** is by IV infusion of glucose in saline or water. Insulin may also be required if hyperglycemia suggests diabetes is present. **Hyperglycemic-hyperosmolar nonketotic coma** is treated by giving 1 or 2 L of 0.9% saline IV initially to restore intravascular volume and BP followed by 5 or 6 L of 0.45% saline over the next 24 h to replace free water loss. The patient's clinical state will determine the exact volume and rate of administration. IV insulin is administered cautiously (10 to 30 u. insulin injection q 2 to 3 h as a bolus or by constant infusion) until plasma glucose approaches 250 mg/dl. Lower values during the first 24 to 48 h may cause or aggravate cerebral edema. Supplements of K are also indicated as in the treatment of ketoacidosis. In spite of attentive therapy, mortality is 40 to 70%, with 1/3 of the deaths occurring within the first 24 h.

PREGNANCY IN THE DIABETIC PATIENT

Diabetes mellitus is associated with increased maternal, fetal, and neonatal morbidity and mortality. These problems and their management are discussed in Vol II, Ch. 18 and Vol. II, Ch. 21.

CARE OF THE INSULIN-REQUIRING DIABETIC DURING SURGERY

The aim of diabetic treatment is to prevent ketoacidosis and minimize osmotic diuresis and hypoglycemic reactions. Because of the insulin-antagonizing action of high plasma cortisol levels associated with surgical stress, it is safe to give 1/3 to 1/2 of the patient's normal daily dose of insulin in the morning prior to the operation. Five percent glucose in either water or salt solution is infused during the operation and continued postoperatively to provide 50 gm of glucose q 8 h until oral feeding is resumed. After the patient begins to recover from anesthesia, the preoperative insulin dose may be repeated. Serum glucose and ketone levels should be obtained 4 h and 8 h postoperatively. Additional insulin injection is indicated only if hyperglycemia is > 250 mg/dl or if ketone concentration becomes "large" in the undiluted serum specimen. Serum glucose levels < 100 mg/dl indicate a need for more glucose infusion. As oral feeding is tolerated and activity increases, the patient may, over a few days, resume his preoperative insulin dose. Emergency nonelective surgical procedures with greater associated stress, or patients who develop early postoperative complications, require more frequent monitoring of serum glucose and ketones.

Patients who normally do not require insulin can usually be managed without supplemental insulin, but some may temporarily require small doses of insulin injection (10 to 12 u. once or twice/day) to control the hyperglycemia and glucosuria associated with surgical stress.

DIET FOR DIABETES

Beyond the basic requirements to provide adequate calories and necessary nutrients, there are marked differences in diet therapy for the 2 major types of diabetics: insulin-dependent nonobese patients and non–insulin-dependent patients, most of whom are obese. Patients who require insulin must schedule their meals to provide regular caloric intake. In overweight patients, special attention must be given to total caloric consumption. An understanding of the differing goals, strategies, and priorities of diet therapy in these 2 types of diabetic patients is essential in the proper treatment of this disease. Dietary differences are so marked that teaching sessions should not include both types of patients simultaneously (see TABLE 90–6).

TABLE 90–6. DIETARY STRATEGIES FOR THE TWO MAIN TYPES OF DIABETES MELLITUS

Dietary Strategy	Insulin-Dependent Nonobese Patients	Non–Insulin-Dependent Obese Patients
Decrease calories	No	Yes
Increase frequency of feedings	Yes	No
Day-to-day consistency of intake of calories, carbohydrate, protein, and fat	Very important	Not necessary if average caloric intake remains in low range
Day-to-day consistency of the ratios of carbohydrate, protein, and fat for each of the feedings	Desirable*	Not necessary
Consistency of timing of meals	Very important	Not necessary
Extra food for unusual exercise	Usually appropriate	Not usually appropriate
Use of food to treat, abort, or prevent hypoglycemia	Important	Not neccesary

* The total daily insulin requirement is apparently not much affected when dietary constituents are changed under isocaloric conditions, but insulin requirement immediately after a high-carbohydrate meal is higher than immediately after a low-carbohydrate meal, even if the meal is isocaloric.

Adapted from K. M. West, *Postgraduate Medicine* Vol. 60, pp. 209–216, Sept. 1976. Used with permission.

Diets for diabetic patients should be neither insufficiently detailed nor unnecessarily complex and should be tailored to fit the propensities and lifestyle of the patient. Sociologic, cultural, and economic barriers to patient adherence to a prescribed diet should be considered and avoided.

Insulin-dependent nonobese patients: These are usually young diabetics. Diet is chosen to provide adequate calories to achieve desirable weight, adequate nutrients for normal growth and development, and adequate design to encourage patient compliance. Meal planning is necessary to avoid alternating periods of feasting and fasting and consequent high or low blood glucose levels. Regular spacing of food intake will avert episodes of hypoglycemia as injected insulin continues to work between meals. Peaks of hyperglycemia and glucosuria due to excessive ingestion of simple sugars (candies, table sugar, pastries, etc.) should be minimized in all diabetic patients. Exercise, particularly strenuous sports, requires diet adjustment to avoid the hypoglycemia of associated increased insulin absorption from subcutaneous sites leading predominantly in turn to decreased hepatic glucose release.

Obese patients who do not require insulin: Most diabetic patients who do not require insulin are overweight. Provision of a nutritionally adequate diet restricted in calories is the single most important objective in treatment. A balanced intake of at least 1200 kcal is usually recommended to minimize catabolism of lean tissue and to provide adequate vitamins, minerals, and other nutrients. Although weight reduction is the most important challenge in therapy of these patients, it is a difficult objective to achieve (see Ch. 80).

Diet composition: There is no need to disproportionately restrict the intake of carbohydrates in the diet of most diabetics. Flexibility in diet design helps many patients to adhere to an effective program. Lowering of fat consumption may reduce risk factors of coronary heart disease, the most important cause of death and debility in the diabetic. One third of diabetic patients in clinical surveys have hyperlipidemia, suggesting the need for reducing dietary fat. The standard diets and food exchange lists revised in 1976 by the American Diabetes Association are somewhat restricted in fat (about 35% of calories).

One approach to diabetic dietary management involves a system of food exchanges that can provide a variable menu while maintaining consistent distribution of daily calorie intake, especially for patients taking daily insulin. For non–insulin-dependent patients (diabetic or nondiabetic) needing to lose weight, the exchange list system may be helpful in reaching this goal.

The exchange list system involves the grouping of foods with similar fat, carbohydrate, and protein content into lists allowing the exchange of a portion of one food on a list with another on the same list when composing a menu. An exchange list system has been prepared by committees of the American Diabetes Association and American Dietetic Association in cooperation with the National Institutes of Health, and published in 1976. While the lists assist in controlling total calories and provide information on the amount and type of fat present in various foods, the varieties of foods listed are of necessity quite limited. For example, fast foods (burgers and shakes), combination foods (pizza, macaroni and cheese), convenience foods (soups, TV dinners), and ethnic foods are omitted from these lists. These "Exchange Lists for Meal Planning" may be acquired from the American Diabetes Association, the American Dietetic Association, or local Diabetes Association affiliate offices. In addition, "A Guide for Professionals: The Effective Application of Exchange Lists for Meal Planning" (1977) is available from these same sources.

Unfortunately the exchange list system will not be suitable for all patients. Adherence to a dietary program clearly must be individualized to take into account the preferences and life-style of each patient. Many patients on insulin can be instructed to eat regular meals of about the same size, at about the same time of day, and will do well without further specification. Special diet foods are not recommended for diabetics except for water-packed fruits and artificially sweetened soft drinks. Other "diabetic foods" are often more expensive and may have nearly the same calories as regular foods.

More complicated dietary problems, especially attempts at weight loss, can benefit from guidance provided by a registered dietitian or other qualified diet counselor who will work closely with the individual patient. Many physicians lack adequate background and time to instruct a patient properly about diet. Furthermore, single encounters between a diet counselor and patient cannot alter lifelong habits, nor can generalized preprinted meal lists and diets be effective in meeting the challenge. Most successful educational programs for diabetics involve a team including a dietitian, nurse, and physician in which each member of the team educates the patient in his or her area of expertise. The patient's role with the team must be emphasized, for without the patient's cooperation, even the best plans will fail. A single lesson in diet or in any other principle of diabetic management is useless. The educational plan for the diabetic must be a continuing lifelong process.

HYPOGLYCEMIA

An abnormally low blood glucose level.

Etiology

The causes of hypoglycemia may be divided into 2 categories: (1) reactive hypoglycemia in response to a meal, specific nutrients, or drugs, and (2) spontaneous hypoglycemia in the fasting state.

Reactive hypoglycemia following a meal is the most common type and is characterized by the development of symptomatic hypoglycemia 2 to 4 h after eating. A very rapid absorption of glucose into the circulation and a subsequent outpouring of a corresponding excess of insulin appear in **alimentary or postgastrectomy hypoglycemia**, often, but not always, seen after gastric resection. A similar reactive hypoglycemia due to delayed insulin response is seen in some mild maturity-onset diabetic patients after a carbohydrate load and may be one of the first indications of diabetes mellitus. Another type of reactive hypoglycemia which follows a carbohydrate load is known as **"functional" hypoglycemia** and its mechanism is unknown.

Other types of reactive hypoglycemia may be caused by the administration of excess insulin, less frequently by oral hypoglycemic agents, and in some patients after ingestion of alcohol or other drugs (see TABLE 90–7).

Alcohol-induced hypoglycemia is metabolically related to alcoholic ketoacidosis (see above) and either may occur separately or together in alcohol abusers. Neither requires impaired liver function and both occur 1 to 3 days after anorexia, nausea and vomiting, and consequent starvation have terminated a period of chronic alcohol abuse. Hypoglycemia results from a combination of starvation and impaired hepatic gluconeogenesis.

Spontaneous hypoglycemia in the fasting state may be due to failure of glucose production (extensive hepatic disease) or, rarely, the inability of normal production to keep up with excessive glucose consumption (vigorous exercise or pregnancy). Hypoglycemia in the fasting state can also result from excess glucose utilization through insulin overproduction from an islet cell tumor or, rarely, from an extrapancreatic neoplasm. Occasionally a large tumor such as a sarcoma may consume enormous amounts of glucose, leading to hypoglycemia. Other less common causes of hypoglycemia are included in TABLE 90–7.

Symptoms and Signs

The symptoms and signs of hypoglycemia may be grouped into 2 categories: (1) faintness, weakness, tremulousness, palpitation, diaphoresis, hunger, and nervousness, such as may result from epinephrine administration (acute hypoglycemia with epinephrine-like symptoms indicates that endogenous epinephrine-induced glycogen mobilization has already started), and (2) a pattern of CNS symptoms including headache, confusion, visual disturbances, motor weakness, palsy, ataxia, and marked personality changes. These CNS disturbances may progress to loss of consciousness, convulsions, and coma. With recurring episodes of hypoglycemia in the same patient, the symptoms may be repetitive, although the tempo and severity of an attack may vary.

Symptoms of anxiety, including sweating, headaches, hunger, tachycardia, weakness, and occasionally seizures and coma may suggest hypoglycemia, but most patients with such symptoms are not hypoglycemic.

Diagnosis

The documentation of low plasma glucose ($<$ 50 mg/dl) specifically associated with objective signs or subjective symptoms, which are relieved by the ingestion of sugar or other food, are the

TABLE 90-7. CLINICAL CLASSIFICATION OF HYPOGLYCEMIC DISORDERS

I. Reactive causes (following administration of exogenous factors)
    A. Meals (carbohydrate)
        1. Excessive insulin action or defective counter-regulatory response to normal insulin action
            a. Alimentary (postgastrectomy) hypoglycemia
            b. Late hypoglycemia of early maturity-onset diabetes mellitus
        2. Mechanism unknown (probably similar)
            a. "Functional" hypoglycemia (essential, idiopathic)
    B. Specific nutrients (inhibit hepatic glucose output)
        1. Fructose: hereditary fructose intolerance (fructose-1-phosphate aldolase deficiency)
        2. Galactose: galactosemia (galactose-1-phosphate uridyl transferase deficiency)
        3. Leucine: leucine hypersensitivity of infancy and childhood; branched-chain ketonuria (maple syrup urine disease)
    C. Drugs
        1. Excess glucose utilization
            a. Exogenous insulin administration (factitious, iatrogenic)
            b. Insulin plus:
                        Propranolol
                        Oxytetracycline
                        EDTA (ethylenediaminetetraacetic acid)
                        Mebanazine* (monoamine oxidase inhibitor)
                        Manganese
            c. Sulfonylurea
            d. Sulfonylurea plus:
                        Sulfisoxazole
                        Dicumarol
                        Phenylbutazone
                        Alcohol
            e. Phenformin*
        2. Deficient glucose production
            a. Alcohol
            b. Unripened ackee fruit ("Jamaican vomiting sickness")
            c. Salicylates
            d. Aminobenzoic acid
            e. Haloperidol
            f. Propoxyphene
            g. Chlorpromazine

II. Spontaneous causes (endogenous metabolic processes) producing hypoglycemia in the fasting state
    A. Excessive glucose utilization
        1. Excessive insulin effect
            a. Insulinoma
            b. Deficiency of contrainsulin hormones:
                        Glucagon   Epinephrine
                        Cortisol   Thyroid hormones
                        Growth hormone
            c. Neonatal hypoglycemia in infants of diabetic mothers
            d. Treated erythroblastosis fetalis in neonates
        2. Other mechanisms increasing glucose utilization
            a. Exercise
            b. Fever
            c. Pregnancy
            d. Renal glycosuria
            e. Large tumor (e.g., sarcoma)
    B. Deficient glucose production
        1. Diffuse liver disease (hepatomas, acute necrosis—rarely cirrhosis)
        2. Specific hepatic enzyme defects for:
            a. Glycogen mobilization (glycogen storage disease)
            b. Glucose release (glucose-6-phosphatase deficiency)
            c. Gluconeogenetic renewal of glucose-6-phosphate from smaller fragments (fructose-1, 6-diphosphatase deficiency)
        3. Nonpancreatic neoplasms—release substance(s) inhibiting hepatic glucose production (occasionally tumors demonstrate excessive glucose utilization)
        4. Ketotic hypoglycemia of childhood (deficient gluconeogenetic substrate alanine)

* Not used in USA.

essentials for diagnosing hypoglycemia. Lower plasma glucose levels are often seen in normals. While normal men fasting for 72 h rarely drop their plasma glucose levels below 55 mg/dl, normal women demonstrate lower levels during a similar fast, more than half showing levels < 50 mg/dl. During 5-h OGTT, 25% of normal individuals demonstrate plasma glucose levels < 50 mg/dl at some time following glucose ingestion, and occasional individuals have values below 35 mg/dl without symptoms.

Once hypoglycemia has been diagnosed, careful consideration of onset time and symptom pattern leads rapidly to appropriate tests to establish the cause. The first factor for diagnostic discrimination is to determine whether the hypoglycemia occurs within 4 h of a meal (carbohydrate load) or whether it is brought on by a fast, either overnight or more prolonged. Epinephrine-like symptoms are more typically associated with the former, reactive category.

In fasting hypoglycemia, it is important to rule out an **islet cell tumor (insulinoma)** which may be surgically correctable. Symptoms from insulinoma hypoglycemia usually appear insidiously and can mimic a variety of psychiatric and neurologic disorders. The symptoms are characterized by CNS disturbances (e.g., headache, confusion, and coma), while evidence of sympathetic stimulation is often absent. Since excessive insulin release is a manifestation of this disease, the correlation of the **insulin radioimmunoassay** with plasma glucose levels is mandatory in confirming the diagnosis. A carefully supervised fast, which in normal individuals is associated with a progressive fall in plasma insulin concentration, will reveal inappropriately high tumor-sustained insulin levels in the presence of hypoglycemia. The ratio of immunoreactive insulin (μU/ml) to glucose (mg/dl) in the plasma rarely exceeds 0.3 in the absence of an insulinoma. Where elevated insulin levels are associated with hypoglycemia, however, the possibility that the insulin was exogenously given rather than endogenously produced must be considered. Measurement of C-peptide, a by-product of endogenous insulin production and absent in exogenous insulin, may aid in differentiation of these 2 causes of hypoglycemia.

Treatment

Acute or severe episodes of hypoglycemia with epinephrine-like or CNS symptoms may be relieved by ingestion of oral glucose or sucrose. In an attack characterized primarily by CNS symptoms (suggesting that the corrective action of epinephrine is inoperative), glucose should be given promptly. One convenient method is to stir 2 or 3 tbsp of granulated sugar into a glass of fruit juice or water. If the patient is unable to swallow, the immediate parenteral administration of glucagon (see under GLUCAGON, below) will often arouse the patient from coma and permit oral therapy. Failing this, IV glucose must be given.

The treatment of spontaneous hypoglycemia in the fasting state involves removing or controlling the cause whenever possible. An operable insulinoma must be ruled out.

Hypoglycemic symptoms from inoperable tumors may be controlled with drugs such as diazoxide or streptozocin. Reactive hypoglycemia following ingestion of drugs or specific nutrients is similarly treated by avoiding or controlling the causative agent. Treatment of hypoglycemia following meals, on the other hand, is often complex. "Functional" hypoglycemia may occasionally be treated successfully by relieving emotional stress. The single most useful treatment regimen for all 3 reactive hypoglycemias that follow meals is a diet high in protein and restricted in carbohydrate. Not all patients will be completely relieved on this regimen, but many will have amelioration of their attacks.

Diabetic patients taking insulin should always carry sugar lumps or candy with them, and the patient's family and friends should be instructed in recognizing the symptoms of hypoglycemia and in giving the emergency treatment mentioned above.

Before a patient receives definitive treatment for hypoglycemia (excluding emergency treatment), *all* of the following should be present: (1) documented occurrence of low blood glucose level; (2) symptoms shown to occur when the blood glucose is low; (3) demonstration that the symptoms are relieved specifically by the ingestion of sugar or other food; and (4) identification of the particular type of hypoglycemia that is causing the symptoms.

GLUCAGON

Glucagon is a single-chain polypeptide hormone produced by alpha cells in the pancreatic islets of Langerhans and in the wall of the stomach and duodenum. The plasma concentration of alpha-cell glucagon can be measured by radioimmunoassay **(RIA)**. The GI tract and probably other sites also secrete several other substances with glucagon-like immunoreactivity, but these differ in physicochemical and biologic properties from alpha-cell glucagon. While these substances interfered with the earlier RIA determinations, the development of a more specific antiserum for circulating alpha-cell glucagon now allows more precise measurement.

Glucagon has a hyperglycemic action. It mobilizes glucose and raises the blood glucose level by both stimulating glycogenolysis and augmenting glucose formation from amino acids. It also accelerates free fatty acid release from adipose tissue. Thus, glucagon is a regulator of nutrient mobilization, as insulin is a regulator of nutrient storage.

Glucagonomas are infrequently occurring glucagon-secreting tumors of the islet alpha cells. Patients may present with glucose intolerance, an erythematous, eczematous dermatitis, glossitis, stomatitis, vaginitis, and unexplained weight loss. These tumors are more likely to be malignant than insulinomas and frequently metastasize to the liver (see also GLUCAGONOMA in Ch. 53).

Glucagon is used pharmacologically primarily to counteract severe hypoglycemic reactions in diabetic patients taking insulin. It has also been used in psychiatric patients during insulin shock therapy. The ability of glucagon to counteract hypoglycemia depends upon the availability of liver glycogen. It is virtually useless in starvation, adrenal insufficiency, or chronic hypoglycemia, and may be ineffective in a number of diabetic patients with hypoglycemia severe enough to require hospitalization. However, it is the drug of choice for the initial urgent counteraction of hypoglycemia in comatose patients unable to take oral glucose solution and for whom IV glucose is not immediately available. Insulin-requiring diabetics with a tendency toward hypoglycemic reactions should have glucagon available in their home for family members to administer in case of a hypoglycemic emergency. Instruction in the preparation and parenteral administration of glucagon should be given before an emergency arises.

Glucagon is available commercially in vials containing 1 mg of dried powder accompanied by a vial of diluting solution for parenteral administration. It can be stored without refrigeration for 4 or 5 yr. The usual dose is 0.5 to 1 mg, which may be given s.c. (using an insulin syringe), IM, or IV. There is generally no advantage in giving > 1 mg of glucagon. If the patient does not awaken from coma within 20 min, IV glucose must be given immediately and the diagnosis of the cause of coma must be reconsidered. Oral carbohydrate should be given as soon as the patient responds. The most frequent side effects are nausea and vomiting.

A diabetic in coma from acidosis rather than from insulin reaction will not respond to glucose or glucagon, but will require immediate appropriate therapy as indicated in DIABETES MELLITUS, above.

GENETIC ABNORMALITIES OF CARBOHYDRATE METABOLISM

GALACTOSEMIA

A metabolic inability, inherited as an autosomal recessive trait, to convert galactose to glucose because of absence of the enzyme galactose-1-phosphate uridyl transferase. The incidence in Great Britain is about 1 in 80,000 births. The infant appears normal at birth, but within a few days or weeks of milk feeding develops anorexia, vomiting, jaundice, hepatomegaly, aminoaciduria, proteinuria, growth failure, and ultimately ascites, and edema, and may die from wasting and inanition. Untreated survivors are usually stunted and mentally retarded, and many have cataracts; however, mild cases may occur without serious impairment. The diagnosis is suspected from the presence of non–glucose-reducing substances (galactose and galactose-1-phosphate) in the urine and confirmed by the absence of galactose-l-phosphate uridyl transferase activity in erythrocytes, leukocytes, or skin fibroblasts. The diagnosis can be made at birth in a drop of cord blood. Prenatal diagnosis by amniocentesis is also possible by assaying enzymes from cultured amniotic cells, but cannot be justified ethically.

Treatment

If the mother has high blood galactose levels, the fetus may be damaged, whether or not it is deficient in galactose-1-P-uridyl transferase. Amniocentesis will not reveal whether the fetus' brain development has been impaired.

Milk, which contains galactose and lactose (a disaccharide which on hydrolysis yields glucose and galactose), should be eliminated from the diet at once, preferably during pregnancy in women who are known carriers of the trait, since galactose presented to the fetus in utero can produce permanent mental damage. Synthetic galactose- and lactose-free milk substitutes and foods are available. Strict dietary restriction should be maintained until the patient is at least 2 yr old and preferably 6 yr old. Prognosis is good if galactose has been eliminated before birth and until age 6. Prevention is through genetic counseling.

GALACTOKINASE DEFICIENCY

An inability to metabolize galactose due to a deficiency of the enzyme galactokinase, inherited as an autosomal recessive defect. As in the more common galactosemia, plasma and urinary galactose concentrations are elevated, but no GI or brain disturbances occur. Unless galactose is removed from the diet, cataracts develop rapidly. Enzyme tests for galactose-1-phosphate uridyl transferase are normal, but galactokinase activity is absent in the erythrocytes. **Treatment** is as for galactosemia.

GLYCOGEN STORAGE DISEASES (Glycogenoses)

A group of hereditary disorders caused by lack of a specific enzyme involved in glycogen synthesis or breakdown, and characterized by the deposition of abnormal amounts or types of glycogen in the tissues (see TABLE 90–8). The incidence of all forms of glycogen storage diseases is about 1 in 40,000. Inheritance is autosomal recessive, except in Type IX, which is X-linked. Types O, I, IV, and VI mainly affect the liver. Types II and III involve most tissues. Types V and VII are restricted to skeletal muscle (see GLYCOGEN STORAGE DISEASE OF MUSCLE in Ch. 138); Type II also affects the myocardium. Diagnosis is by demonstrating absence of the specific enzyme in a biopsy of the affected tissue. **Treatment** in Types O, I, and III is directed toward preventing hypoglycemia and ketosis by frequent small carbohydrate feedings and a high protein intake during the day and continuous overnight intragastric feeding of a high dextrin preparation (e.g., Vivonex®). Limiting exercise reduces the muscle cramps of Type V. No effective treatment is known for the other types.

TABLE 90–8. CHARACTERISTICS OF THE GLYCOGENOSES

Type	Enzyme Missing	Organs Involved	Clinical Symptoms	Eponym
0	UDPG-glycogen transferase	Liver, muscle	Large fatty liver	––––––
I	Glucose-6-phosphatase	Liver, kidney, intestine	Large liver and kidney; dwarfism; hypoglycemia; acidosis; hyperlipemia	von Gierke
II	Lysosomal glucosidase	All organs	Cardiomegaly; hepatomegaly	Pompe
III	Debrancher system	Liver, muscle, heart	Hepatomegaly; normal ECG, lipids, glucose	Forbes, Cori
IV	Brancher enzyme	Generalized amylopectin	Hepatosplenomegaly; ascites; cirrhosis; liver failure	Andersen
V	Muscle phosphorylase	Skeletal muscle	Weakness, cramps on exercise with no blood lactate rise	McArdle
VI	Liver phosphorylase	Liver	Hepatomegaly; normal spleen, glucose, lipids; no acidosis	Hers
VII	Phosphofructokinase	Skeletal muscle	As for Type V	Tarui

VIII, IX, X: Rare disorders of the control mechanism for phosphorylase

HEREDITARY FRUCTOSE INTOLERANCE

A metabolic inability to utilize fructose, caused by absence of the enzyme 1-phosphofructoaldolase, and transmitted as an autosomal recessive trait. The intake of considerable amounts of fructose induces hypoglycemia, with nausea, vomiting, malaise, substernal pain, excessive sweating, tremors, confusion, coma, and convulsions. Smaller doses can cause proximal renal tubular acidosis. Excessive phosphate, glucose, uric acid, and bicarbonate appear in the urine, and the ability to acidify the urine is lost. Prolonged chronic fructose intake may lead to cirrhosis and mental deterioration. Patients develop a strong dislike for sweets and fruit. There is no intellectual impairment.

Diagnosis is confirmed by demonstrating a fall in blood glucose 5 to 40 min after giving fructose 250 mg/kg IV. **Treatment** is to exclude fructose (found chiefly in sweet fruits), sucrose, and sorbitol from the diet. Attacks of fructose-induced hypoglycemia are treated with glucose.

FRUCTOSURIA

A harmless excretion of fructose in the urine, caused by an autosomal recessive lack of the enzyme fructokinase. The incidence in the general population is about 1 in 130,000. This benign asymptomatic defect prevents normal utilization of ingested fructose, resulting in abnormal levels in the blood and urine. Fructosuria may lead to an incorrect diagnosis of diabetes mellitus (fructose will reduce copper sulfate, but will not react with glucose oxidase). No treatment is required.

PENTOSURIA

A harmless autosomal recessive metabolic derangement characterized by the excretion of L-xylulose in the urine due to absence of the enzyme L-xylulose dehydrogenase. It occurs almost exclusively in Jews, with an incidence of 1 in 2500 in American Jews. As with fructosuria, its only importance is the danger that the presence of xylulose in the urine may lead to an erroneous diagnosis of diabetes mellitus. Treatment is not required.

RENAL GLUCOSURIA (See Ch. 153)

DISACCHARIDASE DEFICIENCY AND GLUCOSE-GALACTOSE

MALABSORPTION (See CARBOHYDRATE INTOLERANCE in Ch. 56)

91. CARCINOID SYNDROME

A syndrome of episodic cutaneous flushing, diarrhea, valvular heart disease, and, less commonly, asthma, usually caused by metastatic carcinoid tumors that secrete excessive amounts of vasoactive substances, including serotonin, bradykinin, histamine, prostaglandins, and polypeptide hormones.

Etiology and Pathophysiology

Tumors of the diffuse peripheral endocrine system (as described by Feyrter) produce various polypeptides and biogenic amines, with corresponding clinical presentations. The carcinoid syndrome is usually associated with functioning malignant tumors arising from endocrine cells situated in the ileum, but can arise from anywhere in the GI tract, the pancreas, the gonads, or in the bronchi. A primary intestinal carcinoid tumor does not produce the syndrome unless hepatic metastases have occurred, since metabolic products released by the tumor are rapidly destroyed by blood and liver enzymes in the portal circulation—serotonin (5-hydroxytryptamine [5-HT]), for example, by hepatic monoamine oxidase. Hepatic metastases, however, release these substances via the hepatic veins directly into the systemic circulation. Primary pulmonary and ovarian carcinoids bypass the portal route and may induce symptoms directly. Serotonin acts on smooth muscle to produce diarrhea, colic, and malabsorption; histamine and bradykinin, through their vasodilator effects, are responsible for flushing. The role of prostaglandins and of the various polypeptide hormones, which may be produced by enterochromaffin or other paracrine cells, awaits further investigation.

Symptoms and Signs

The most common and often earliest manifestation is cutaneous flushing, typically of the head and neck, often precipitated by emotion or the ingestion of food or alcohol; striking color changes ranging from pallor or erythema to cyanosis may occur. Abdominal cramps with recurrent diarrhea develop and are often the major complaint. Many patients develop right-sided endocardial fibrosis, producing pulmonary stenosis and tricuspid regurgitation; left heart lesions are rare because 5-HT is destroyed during passage through the lung. A few patients have asthmatic wheezing; some have decreased libido and impotence.

Diagnosis

Diagnosis is confirmed by demonstrating an increased urinary excretion of the serotonin metabolite, 5-hydroxyindoleacetic acid (5-HIAA). A colorimetric test is carried out after the patient has abstained from serotonin-containing foods (such as bananas, tomatoes, plums, avocados, pineapples, eggplant, and walnuts) for 3 days to avoid false-positive results. Certain drugs, including guaifenesin, methocarbamol, and phenothiazines, also interfere with the test. On the 3rd day a 24-h urine sample is collected for assay. Normal excretion of 5-HIAA is < 10 mg/day; in patients with carcinoid syndrome it is usually > 50 mg/day.

Provocative tests have been proposed in which either calcium gluconate or epinephrine is used IV to induce flushing. Localization of the tumor may require an extensive evaluation, including laparotomy. Rarely, certain highly malignant tumors, including oat cell carcinoma of the lung, carcinoma of the pancreas, and carcinoma of the thyroid (probably medullary carcinoma) may also produce the syndrome and must be excluded by appropriate examinations.

Treatment

Curative resection of primary lung carcinoids is possible. For patients with hepatic metastases, surgery is diagnostic or palliative only, and x-ray treatment is unsuccessful. No convincing combination of chemotherapy has been established, but regimens including doxorubicin appear to be the most promising. Niacin and an adequate protein intake are needed because dietary tryptophan is diverted to serotonin by the tumor; pellagra may result. Diarrhea may be controlled by codeine phosphate 15 mg orally q 4 to 6 h, tincture of opium 10 to 20 drops q 6 h, or diphenoxylate 2.5 mg orally 1 to 3 times/day, or by peripheral serotonin antagonists such as cyproheptadine 4 to 8 mg orally q 6 h, or methysergide 1 to 2 mg q.i.d. Enzyme inhibitors that prevent the conversion of 5-hydroxytryptophan to serotonin include methyldopa 250 to 500 mg orally q 6 h, or phenoxybenzamine 10 mg/day. Flushing may be treated with phenothiazines (e.g., prochlorperazine 5 to 10 mg or chlorpromazine 25 to 50 mg orally q 6 h). Phentolamine 5 to 15 mg (an α-adrenergic blocking agent) has prevented experimentally induced flushes. Anti-inflammatory corticosteroids (e.g., prednisone 5 mg orally q 6 h) are particularly useful for the severe flushing caused by bronchial carcinoids.

§9. HEMATOLOGIC DISORDERS

92. ANEMIAS

Circumstances in which RBC and/or Hb content decreases because of blood loss, impaired production, or destruction of RBCs. The RBC count, Hb, and/or Hct diminish. A presentation of the anemias follows their etiologic classification. Anemias due to defective hemoglobin synthesis are discussed in Vol. II, Ch. 25.

Classification and Terminology of Anemias

I. Anemias Due to Excessive Blood Loss
  A. Acute Posthemorrhagic
  B. Chronic Posthemorrhagic
II. Anemias Due to Deficient Red Cell Production
  A. Hypochromic Microcytic Anemias
    1. Iron-Deficiency Anemia
    2. Atransferrinemic Anemia (Iron Transport Deficiency)
    3. Iron Utilization Anemias (Sideroblastic Anemias)
    4. Iron Reutilization Anemias (Anemia of Chronic Disease)
  B. Normochromic Normocytic Anemias
    1. Hypoproliferative Anemias
      a. Anemia of Renal Disease
      b. Anemia of Endocrine Failure (Myxedema and Hypopituitarism)
      c. Anemia of Protein Depletion
    2. Hypoplastic (Aplastic) Anemias
    3. Myelophthisic Anemias
  C. Megaloblastic Anemias
    1. Anemia Due to Vitamin B_{12} Deficiency
    2. Anemia Due to Folic Acid Deficiency
    3. Anemia Due to Copper Deficiency
    4. Anemia Due to Ascorbic Acid Deficiency
III. Anemias Due to Excessive Red Cell Destruction—Hemolytic Anemias
  A. Hemolytic Anemias Due to Extrinsic Red Cell Defects
    1. Anemias Due to Reticuloendothelial Hyperactivity
      Hypersplenism-Congestive Splenomegaly
    2. Anemias Due to Immunologic Abnormalities
      a. Isoimmune (Isoagglutinin) Hemolytic Anemia
      b. Autoimmune Hemolytic Anemia
        (1) Warm Antibody Hemolytic Anemia
          (Coombs-Positive Hemolytic Anemia)
        (2) Cold Antibody Disease
          (a) Cold Agglutinin Disease
          (b) Paroxysmal Cold Hemoglobinuria
      c. Complement-Sensitive Associated Anemia
        Paroxysmal Nocturnal Hemoglobinuria
    3. Anemias Due to Mechanical Injury
      a. Traumatic Hemolytic Anemias (Microangiopathic Hemolytic Anemia)
      b. Hemolysis Due to Infectious Agents
  B. Hemolytic Anemias Due to Intrinsic Red Cell Defects
    1. Anemias Due to Alterations of Red Cell Membrane
      a. Congenital
        (1) Congenital Erythropoietic Porphyria
        (2) Hereditary Spherocytosis
        (3) Hereditary Elliptocytosis
      b. Acquired
        (1) Stomatocytosis
        (2) Anemia Due to Hypophosphatemia
    2. Anemias Due to Abnormalities of Red Cell Metabolism (Hereditary Enzyme Deficiencies)
      a. Embden-Meyerhof Pathway Defects
      b. Hexose Monophosphate Shunt Defects (Glucose-6-Phosphate Dehydrogenase Deficiency)
    3. Anemias Due to Defective Hemoglobin Synthesis (Hemoglobinopathies)
      a. Sickle Cell Anemia
      b. Hemoglobin C Disease
      c. Hemoglobin S-C Disease
      d. Thalassemias
      e. Hemoglobin S-Beta Thalassemia Disease

General Symptoms and Signs

Anemia is a clinical sign or symptom; its use as a *diagnostic* term requires an understanding of its mechanism or essential nature. Its clinical expression results from tissue hypoxia, and its specific signs represent cardiovascular-pulmonary compensatory responses to that hypoxia. Its clinical symptoms depend upon the severity and duration of the anemia. Severe anemia can be associated with weakness, vertigo, headache, tinnitus, spots before the eyes, ease of fatigue, drowsiness, irritability, and even bizarre behavior. Amenorrhea, loss of libido, GI complaints, and, sometimes, jaundice and splenomegaly can occur. Finally, congestive heart failure or shock can result. (See TABLE 92–1, below.)

Laboratory Evaluation

Laboratory tests quantitate the degree of the anemia and provide data to aid in understanding its cause (see NORMAL LABORATORY VALUES in Ch. 230). The basic evaluation requires a CBC, which includes RBC indices, reticulocyte count or estimate of polychromatophilia, platelet count, and a review of cellular morphology on the peripheral blood smear.

The normal range of RBCs at sea level is 5.4 million/cu mm (μl) ($\pm$ 0.8) for men and 4.8 million ($\pm$ 0.6) for women. At birth, the blood count is slightly higher; by the 3rd mo it falls to levels of about 4.5 million ($\pm$ 0.7), slowly increasing after age 4 through puberty.

The normal life span of an erythrocyte is 120 days; therefore, 1/120 of the total red cell mass must be replaced daily. This newly released population (40,000 to 50,000/cu mm [μl]) represents 0.8 to 1% of the total red count and can be identified as polychromatophilic cells on routine stains or "reticulocytes" when supravital staining technics are used. Since the reticulocyte represents the release of a young cell population, it is an important criterion of marrow activity. The presence of reticulocytes can be considered a response to a need for red cells. This response is characteristic in hemolytic anemias and in acute and severe bleeding. Reticulocytosis is also seen in response to specific treatment of vitamin B_{12}, folic acid, and iron deficiencies, and may indicate the onset of remission in aplastic anemia or leukemia. A "normal" reticulocyte count in anemia indicates failure of the bone marrow to respond fully.

Reticulocyte count: A few drops of blood are initially stained with fresh methylene blue, counterstained with Wright's stain, and then counted under oil immersion. One thousand consecutive RBCs are counted and the number having a blue-staining reticulum are expressed as a percentage. The normal range is 0.5 to 1.5%. These may also be counted using automated differential counters

Iron and iron-binding capacity: Serum iron determination and iron-binding capacity should both be performed, since the relationship between their values is important. In iron deficiency, the serum iron is low and the iron-binding capacity high. Both values are decreased in various chronic disorders, such as inflammatory diseases. The serum iron is elevated and may equal the iron-binding capacity in severe hemolysis, megaloblastic anemias, aplastic anemias, and hemochromatosis. Though serum iron may be normal in patients with treated iron deficiency, iron-binding capacity usually remains elevated for several weeks.

The **normal Hb level** for men is 16 ($\pm$ 2) gm/dl and 14 ($\pm$ 2) gm/dl for women. The Hct, which is the volume of packed red cells is 47 ($\pm$ 5) % for men and 42 ($\pm$ 5) % for women.

The diagnostic criteria for anemia in men are an RBC < 4.5 million/cu mm (μl), a Hb < 14 gm/dl or a Hct < 42 gm/100 ml; for women these criteria are an RBC < 4 million/cu mm (μl), Hb < 12 gm/dl, or a Hct < 37 gm/100 ml.

Other features of circulating RBCs help to indicate the type of anemia present. The **red cell indices** (the mean corpuscular volume **[MCV]**, mean corpuscular Hb **[MCH]**, and mean corpuscular Hb concentration **[MCHC]**) derived from the quantitative data, denote the volume and character of the Hb content. Thus, RBC populations with MCVs < 80 μm^3/RBC (femtoliter) are termed **microcytic** and those with MCV > 99 fl are termed **macrocytic**. The term **hypochromia** refers to populations of cells with MCH content < 27 pg/RBC or a MCHC < 30%. These quantitative relationships can usually be recognized on a peripheral blood smear and, *together with the indices, permit a classification of anemias that correlates well with etiologic classification (see TABLE 92–1) and greatly aids diagnostic evaluation.*

In addition, variations in size **(anisocytosis)** and shape **(poikilocytosis)** may be seen. Evidence of RBC injury may be identified directly from RBC fragments or portions of disrupted cells **(schistocytes)**, as well as evidence of significant membrane alterations from oval-shaped cells **(ovalocytes**, or spherocytic cells. **"Target" cells,** which represent cells with either an inadequate amount of Hb or an excess of membrane, appear as thin cells with a central dot of Hb. **Polychromatophilia** refers to bluish cells that owe their tint to remnants of RNA that can be seen with classic metachromatic stains (Wrights' or Giemsa stain, etc.). These young reticulocyte cells can be further characterized by supravital stains that recognize the reticular material within them.

By most of the automated technics, the Hb, RBC count, and MCV are electronically and therefore reliably measured. The Hct, MCH, and MCHC, by contrast, are calculated. Thus the MCV is an important index in recognizing the microcytic hypochromic states. (In the past and in most texts the determined MCHC was used as an important criterion of these hypochromic microcytic states. For instance, a decreasing MCHC was seen in developing iron deficiency; probably the amount of trapped plasma in the measured Hct was greater in such states. Since plasma trapping is not a issue in the electronically calculated Hct, the MCHC has become a trivial parameter in differential diagnosis.) Reliance upon the Hct and the indices is therefore of less value, since they are derived numbers. Nevertheless, even derived values may help; for instance, increased MCHC values ($> 36\%$) are often a clue to the presence of significant spherocytosis or cold-agglutinin disease.

Bone marrow aspiration and biopsy are important technics which clarify the mechanisms of some anemias.

General Considerations

Rather than a diagnosis, anemia is an expression of a symptom complex. Defining its pathophysiologic mechanism provides the basis for planning appropriate therapy. A serious error would be to ignore the need to investigate a mild anemia; its presence indicates an underlying disorder, but the degree of its severity offers little information about its genesis or clinical significance.

Some general diagnostic patterns can be used to expedite the differential diagnosis. Hemorrhage should be an initial consideration. Once it is ruled out, the only other mechanisms are decreased production or increased destruction (i.e., hemolysis). Since RBC survival is 120 days, maintenance of steady populations requires renewal of $1/120$ of the cells each day. Complete cessation of production results in a decline of about 10%/wk of the control value. Production defects result in a relative or absolute reticulocytopenia. When RBC values fall at a rate $> 10\%$ (i.e., 500,000 RBC/cu mm [μl]) without hemorrhage, hemolysis is established as a causative factor.

A convenient approach to most anemias that result from production defects is to examine cellular changes. Thus, microcytic (MCV < 80 μm^3/RBC [femtoliter]) and hypochromic RBCs provide evidence that the production defect results from defects in heme and/or globin synthesis (e.g., iron deficiency, thalassemia and related Hb synthesis defects, or the anemia of chronic disease). By contrast, the normochromic normocytic anemias with a defective production pose a hypoproliferative or hypoplastic mechanism. Finally, some anemias provide the hallmark of large (MCV > 100 μm^3/RBC [femtoliter]) RBCs or macrocytes which suggests a defect in DNA synthesis. These are usually due either to defective vitamin B_{12} or folate metabolism, or to an interference with DNA synthesis by cytoreductive chemotherapeutic agents.

Similarly, a few common mechanisms of increased destruction such as sequestration by spleen, antibody-mediated destruction, defective RBC membrane function, and an abnormal Hb provide a rapid focus for differential diagnosis of hemolytic anemias.

One of the most critical clinical lessons in the management of anemias is that therapy should be specific and this infers that an appropriate diagnosis be made. Indeed, the response to therapeutic intervention serves to corroborate the diagnosis. While treatment with multiple agents (i.e., "shotgun therapy") may at times provide transient repair of the anemia, because it risks serious sequelae, such therapy is not justifiable.

Transfusions of RBCs provide a form of "instant" repair that should be reserved for patients with cardiopulmonary symptoms or signs, active uncontrollable bleeding, or some form of hypoxemic end-organ failure. Transfusion procedures and blood components are discussed in detail in Chapter 93 below.

ANEMIAS DUE TO EXCESSIVE BLOOD LOSS

ACUTE POSTHEMORRHAGIC ANEMIA

Anemia caused by the rapid loss of a large amount of blood.

Etiology and Pathogenesis

Since the marrow reserve is limited, anemia may result from any massive hemorrhage, which may be due to spontaneous or traumatic rupture or incision of a large blood vessel, erosion of an artery by lesions such as peptic ulcer or a neoplastic process, or failure of normal hemostatic processes. Immediate effects depend on the duration and amount of hemorrhage. Sudden loss of $1/3$ of the blood volume may be fatal, but as much as $2/3$ may be lost slowly over a 24-h period without such risk. Symptoms are due to a sudden decrease in blood volume and to subsequent hemodilution, with a decrease in the O_2-carrying capacity of the blood.

Symptoms and Signs

The pace of the anemia determines the degree of symptoms. Faintness, dizziness, thirst, sweating, weak and rapid pulse, and rapid respiration (at first deep, then shallow) may occur. Orthostatic hypotension is common. BP may at first rise slightly because of reflex arteriolar constriction, then gradually fall. If bleeding continues, BP may fall and death may ensue (see also SHOCK in Ch. 24).

Laboratory Findings

During and immediately after hemorrhage, the RBC count, Hb, and Hct are deceptively high because of vasoconstriction. Within a few hours, tissue fluid begins to enter the circulation, resulting in hemodilution and a drop in the RBC count and Hb proportional to the severity of bleeding. The resultant anemia is normocytic. Polymorphonuclear leukocytosis and a rise in platelet count may occur within the first few hours. Several days after the bleeding event, evidence of regeneration appears: blood smears may disclose polychromatophilia, reticulocytosis, slight macrocytosis; if the hemorrhage was massive and acute, occasional normoblasts and immature WBCs may be seen.

TABLE 92–1. CHARACTERISTICS OF COMMON ANEMIAS

Etiology or Type	Morphologic Changes	Special Features
Acute blood loss	Normochromic, normocytic; marrow hyperplastic	In severe hemorrhage may be nucleated RBCs & left shift of WBCs; also leukocytosis
Chronic blood loss	*See* Anemia Due to Iron Deficiency; may show features of Acute Blood Loss if recent severe hemorrhage has supervened	
Iron deficiency	Hypochromic, microcytic, aniso- & poikilocytosis; marrow hyperplastic, with delayed hemoglobinization	Achlorhydria, smooth tongue, & spoon nails may be present; stainable marrow iron absent; serum iron low; total iron-binding capacity increased
Vitamin B$_{12}$ deficiency	Oval macrocytes; megaloblastic marrow; granular leukocytes hypersegmented	Serum B$_{12}$ level < 150 pg/ml; frequent GI & CNS involvement; Schilling test positive; indirect serum bilirubin elevated; cholesterol decreased
Folic acid deficiency	Same as vitamin B$_{12}$ deficiency	Serum folate < 5 ng/ml; nutritional deficiency & malabsorption (sprue, pregnancy, infancy, alcoholism)
Marrow failure	Normochromic, normocytic; marrow aspiration often fails or may show hypoplasia of erythroid series or of all elements	Occasionally idiopathic, but usually a history of exposure to toxic drugs or chemicals (e.g., chloramphenicol, atabrine, hydantoins, insecticides)
Pyridoxine-responsive anemia	Usually hypochromic; rarely normocytic or macrocytic; marrow hyperplastic, with delayed hemoglobinization; siderocytes may be present	Inborn or acquired metabolic defect; stainable marrow iron plentiful; response to pyridoxine partial, rarely complete
Acute hemolysis	Normochromic, normocytic; marrow, normoblastic hyperplasia	Increased serum bilirubin (indirect) & increased stool & urine urobilinogen; hemoglobinuria in fulminating cases

Condition	Blood Findings	Other Findings
Chronic hemolysis	Normochromic, normocytic; marrow, normoblastic hyperplasia; basophilic stippling (especially in lead poisoning)	Survival studies show shortened RBC life span; radio-iron turnover increased
Hereditary spherocytosis (congenital hemolytic jaundice)	Spheroidal microcytes in smear	Erythrocytes show increased osmotic fragility; shortened survival of labeled RBCs; radioactivity buildup over spleen
Paroxysmal nocturnal hemoglobinuria	Normocytic (may be hypochromic due to iron deficiency)	Dark morning urine; hemosiderin present; positive acid hemolysis & sugar-water tests; reticulocytes may be decreased
Paroxysmal cold hemoglobinuria	Normocytic, normochromic	Follows exposure to cold; due to a cold agglutinin. Usually associated with congenital or acquired syphilis
Sickle cell anemia	Aniso- & poikilocytosis; some sickle cells in smear; all sickle in wet preparation	Limited to blacks; electrophoresis shows S Hb; painful crises & leg ulcers may occur; bony changes shown by x-ray
Thalassemia	Hypochromic, microcytic; thin cells; target cells; basophilic stippling; aniso- & poikilocytosis; nucleated RBCs in homozygotes	Decreased osmotic fragility; elevated A_2 & F Hb; Mediterranean ancestry; homozygotes anemic from infancy; splenomegaly; bony changes on x-ray
Infection or chronic inflammation	Normochromic, normocytic; marrow normoblastic; iron plentiful	Serum iron decreased; total iron-binding capacity decreased
Marrow replacement (myelophthisis)	Aniso- & poikilocytosis; nucleated RBCs; early granulocyte precursors; marrow aspiration may fail, or show leukemia, myeloma, or metastatic cells	Liver and spleen may be enlarged; bone changes may be demonstrable; radio-iron uptake greater over spleen and liver than sacrum; reticulocytes may be slightly increased if many normoblasts in blood

Treatment

Immediate therapy consists of hemostasis, restoration of blood volume, and treatment of shock (see also SHOCK in Ch. 24). Blood transfusion, the only reliable means of rapidly restoring blood volume, is indicated for severe bleeding with threatening vascular collapse. Plasma is presently the most satisfactory temporary substitute for blood. Parenthetically, recent trials with chemical agents (primarily perfluorochemicals) capable of transporting O_2 has shown significant promise; at least one such agent (FLUOSOL-DA®) is currently in clinical trials and appears capable of providing O_2-carrying capacity for up to 72 h. Saline or dextrose infusions have only a transient beneficial effect. Absolute rest, fluids by mouth as tolerated, and other standard measures for treating shock are indicated.

Subsequent therapy can include iron to replace that lost with bleeding.

CHRONIC POSTHEMORRHAGIC ANEMIA

A hypochromic microcytic anemia caused by prolonged moderate blood loss, as from a chronically bleeding GI tract lesion (e.g., peptic ulcer or hemorrhoids), urologic, or gynecologic site. The clinical features and treatment of this condition are discussed below, under IRON–DEFICIENCY ANEMIA.

ANEMIAS DUE TO DEFICIENT RED CELL PRODUCTION

In the presence of anemia, adequate response of the marrow is evidenced by reticulocytosis or polychromatophilia.

HYPOCHROMIC MICROCYTIC ANEMIAS

Deficient or defective heme or globin synthesis produces a small-sized RBC (microcytic) population that is inadequately filled with Hb (hypochromic). However, early changes may be minimal. Four pathophysiologic mechanisms can produce these changes: iron deficiency, defects in iron transport or iron utilization, or iron reutilization.

IRON–DEFICIENCY ANEMIA (Anemia of Chronic Blood Loss; Hypochromic Microcytic Anemia; Chlorosis; Hypochromic Anemia of Pregnancy, Infancy, and Childhood)

Chronic anemia characterized by small, pale RBCs and depletion of iron stores.

Etiology (See also DISTURBANCES IN IRON METABOLISM in Ch. 79)

Iron deficiency, the commonest cause of anemia, may be due to increased iron requirement, diminished iron absorption, or both. Iron deficiency is likely during the first 2 yr of life because of demands of rapid growth without adequate iron in the diet. Adolescent girls may become iron-deficient from growth requirements, inadequate diet, and added loss from menstruation. In adult males, the most frequent cause is chronic occult hemorrhage, usually from the GI tract. The most important lesson concerning iron deficiency is that hemorrhage must be the foremost consideration in any adult. In women, pregnancy causes iron deficiency unless supplemental iron is given. Other bases for anemia may be decreased absorption of iron after gastrectomy, upper small-bowel malabsorption syndromes, and occasionally some forms of pica (primarily clay), but such mechanisms are rare compared to hemorrhage. Most forms of pica (starch, ice, etc.) are associated with decreased intake due to caloric substitution rather than with decreased absorption.

Pathophysiology

The **first stage** of iron-deficiency anemia is iron depletion: iron loss exceeds the gain, storage iron (represented by bone marrow iron content) is progressively depleted, but Hb and plasma iron remain normal. As storage iron decreases, there is a compensatory increase in absorption of dietary iron and in the concentration of transferrin (represented by a rise in iron binding capacity measurement). In the **second stage,** exhausted stores have insufficient iron available to meet the needs of the erythroid marrow. While the plasma transferrin level increases, the plasma iron concentration declines, leading to a progressive decrease in iron available for RBC formation. When the plasma iron falls to $< 50~\mu g/100$ ml and the transferrin saturation to $< 16\%$, erythropoiesis is impaired, and the **third stage** is defined by an anemia with normal appearing RBCs and indices. In the **fourth stage,** microcytosis precedes hypochromia. Finally, in the **fifth stage,** the symptoms and signs of tissue iron deficiency appear.

Symptoms and Signs

In addition to the usual signs and symptoms of anemia, in chronic severe iron deficiency, a person may crave dirt or paint (**pica**) or ice (**pagophagia**), and, in rare advanced cases, have dysphagia associated with a postcricoid esophageal web (**Plummer-Vinson syndrome**). The signs of far-advanced iron-deficiency anemia may include **glossitis, cheilosis,** and **koilonychia.** Glossitis and cheilosis, which are not specific for iron-deficiency anemia, will develop only when the anemia is severe. Finally, fatigue and loss of stamina can occur through a separate effect on the tissues (perhaps cellular enzyme dysfunction).

Diagnosis

Although pica and especially pagophagia suggest iron lack as the mechanism in the differential diagnosis of the hypochromic microcytic states, actually no specific symptoms or signs exist. Therefore, laboratory characteristics (see TABLE 92-2) serve as critical diagnostic features. The classical criterion of iron-deficient erythropoiesis is absence of marrow iron stores. Other laboratory findings follow a predictive pattern of the pathophysiologic stages. Serum ferritin concentration provides a useful measure of body iron stores. A low serum ferritin concentration (< 12 ng/ml) identifies iron deficiency and currently represents the best non-invasive test of iron status. Unfortunately, ferritin values are elevated in the presence of liver injury and in some neoplasms and must be interpreted with care.

Iron-deficiency anemia in the adult almost always indicates hemorrhage which must be ruled out. Iron therapy without pursuit of its cause is poor practice; a mild degree of anemia must never be used as an excuse for failure to seek the site of bleeding. In circumstances of chronic intravascular hemolysis (e.g., paroxysmal nocturnal hemoglobinuria, chronic disseminated intravascular coagulation, etc.), RBC fragmentation (recognizable on a peripheral smear) may produce iron lack by chronic hemoglobinuria and hemosiderinuria.

Treatment

Iron can be provided by ferrous sulfate or ferrous gluconate 300 mg orally t.i.d. Oral iron is safer than parenteral iron; the rate of response is the same with either route. Parenteral iron should be reserved for those who do not tolerate or will not take oral iron, or for patients who lose large amounts of blood steadily due to capillary or vascular disorders (e.g., hereditary hemorrhagic telangiectasia). Iron in enteric-coated capsules is not well absorbed and has no place in therapy.

A maximal reticulocyte response usually occurs 7 to 10 days after iron replacement begins. For 2 wk, the Hb rises little, but thereafter the rise should be 0.7 to 1 gm/100 ml/wk in severe anemia. A subnormal response may result from continued hemorrhage, underlying infection or malignancy, insufficient intake of iron, or, very rarely, malabsorption of oral iron. As the Hb approaches normal, its pace tapers; the anemia should be corrected within 2 mo. Therapy should continue for at least 6 mo to replenish tissue stores.

ATRANSFERRINEMIC ANEMIA (Iron Transport Deficiency)

This exceedingly rare anemia appears when iron cannot move from storage sites (mucosal cells, liver, etc.) to the erythron (developing red cells). The presumed mechanism is either absence of the iron transport protein transferrin or the presence of a defective transferrin molecule. In addition to the anemia, hemosiderosis of lymphoid tissue, especially along the GI tract, is prominent.

TABLE 92-2. DIFFERENTIAL DIAGNOSIS OF THE HYPOCHROMIC–MICROCYTIC STATES

	Deficiency	Transferrin Defect	Defect in Iron Utilization	Defect in Iron Re-utilization
Peripheral Blood				
Microcytosis (*M*) vs. hypochromia (*H*)	M > H	M > H	M > H	M < H
Polychromatophilic targeted cells	Absent	Absent	Present	Absent
Stippled red cells	Absent	Absent	Present	Absent
Serum Iron				
Serum iron: Iron-binding capacity	↓ : ↑	↓ : ↓	↑ : Normal	↓ : ↓
% Saturation of Transferrin	< 10%	0	> 50%	> 10%
Serum ferritin (normal 30–300 ng/ml)	< 12	(No data available)	> 400	30–400
Bone marrow				
Erythrocyte-granulocyte ratio (normal 1:3 to 1:5)	1:1—1:2	1:1—1:2	1:1—5:1	1:1—1:2
Marrow iron	Absent	Present	Increased	Present
Ringed sideroblasts	Absent	Absent	Present	Absent

Adapted from "The Differential Diagnosis of the Hypochromic Microcytic States," by E.P. Frenkel, in *The Medical Journal of St. Joseph Hospital*, Vol. 11, June, 1976. Copyright by *The Medical Journal of St. Joseph Hospital*, Houston. Used with permission of the *Journal* and the author.

Iron Utilization Anemias (Sideroblastic Anemias)

These anemias are due to inadequate or abnormal utilization of intracellular iron for Hb synthesis, despite adequate or increased amounts of iron within the mitochondria of the developing red cell precursors. This defect includes 2 clinical subgroups: first, hemoglobinopathies, primarily of the thalassemic type; and, second, sideroblastic (or iron overload) anemias. Since other clinical-laboratory characteristics help define circumstances of thalassemia, the term sideroblastic is generally applied to the second subset.

Although sideroblastic anemia is commonly microcytic and hypochromic, a dimorphic (both large- and small-sized) population of circulating cells is usually recognizable. An important clue to defective heme synthesis in the peripheral blood is the presence of polychromatophilic stippled, targeted RBCs. Other laboratory features include increases in serum iron and serum ferritin concentrations and saturation of transferrin. Erythroid hyperplasia is present in the bone marrow; iron stain reveals the pathognomonic morphologic feature of iron-engorged paranuclear mitochondria in the developing RBCs called ringed sideroblasts.

Ineffective erythropoiesis can be defined clinically as anemia and reticulocytopenia in the presence of erythroid hyperplasia. Radiolabeled iron transfers rapidly from plasma transferrin to the marrow, but it fails to reappear normally in circulating RBCs at a normal rate. Ferrokinetic studies provide evidence of ineffective erythropoiesis, inferring intramedullary death of RBCs.

Etiology and Pathophysiology

Clinical correlates (Table 92–3) have been made in some cases of sideroblastic anemia; but clear etiologic and pathophysiologic mechanisms are unknown. The list of diseases known to be associated occasionally with sideroblastosis is formidable and virtually all of them commonly produce other more typical defects in RBC production.

Treatment and Prognosis

The best results follow recognition and removal of a specific cause (especially alcohol). Although rare congenital cases have responded to pyridoxine 50 mg t.i.d. orally, complete correction of the anemia does not result. Similar trials in acquired cases have had weak responses. Rare responses to androgens also are recorded. In general, idiopathic cases must be managed supportively. If anemia produces cardiopulmonary symptoms, packed RBC transfusions may be necessary. Because of the already significant iron burden, such transfusions hasten the advent of clinical symptoms secondary to hemosiderosis, and iron chelation therapy should be considered.

A subset of idiopathic cases progresses to frank leukemia (usually acute granulocytic leukemia). Early occurrence of leukopenia and thrombocytopenia seems to suggest such a likelihood. Since the leukemic transition may take up to 10 yr and since early therapy (with currently available cytoreductive agents) of the "pre-leukemic" phase does not result in improved survival, no special therapy is indicated.

Iron Reutilization Anemia (Anemia of Chronic Disease)

This is the second commonest form of anemia in the world. The RBCs are normocytic to microcytic (see Table 92–2) and the marrow erythroid mass fails to expand in response to the anemia.

Table 92–3. TYPES OF IRON UTILIZATION DEFECTS

Defects in hemoglobin synthesis
Thalassemias
Other related hemoglobinopathies
Sideroblastic anemias
Congenital
Sex-linked
Pyridoxine responsive
Non-pyridoxine responsive
Autosomal
Acquired
Primary (Idiopathic)
Secondary
Drugs (e.g., anti-TB agents, chloramphenicol)
Alcohol
Occasional incidence (e.g., granulomatous diseases, neoplasms, RA)

Adapted from "The Differential Diagnosis of the Hypochromic Microcytic States," by E.P. Frenkel, in *The Medical Journal of St. Joseph Hospital,* Vol. 11, June, 1976. Copyright by *The Medical Journal of St. Joseph Hospital,* Houston. Used with permission of the *Journal* and the author.

Etiology and Pathogenesis

This type of anemia was thought to occur with a long-term disorder of which infections, inflammatory disease (especially RA), and cancer are most frequently identified. However, the underlying disease need not be chronic, since the pathophysiologic features of this anemia appear during virtually any infection or inflammation. The induced defect is one of decreased RBC production. With a RBC loss of about 1%/day, the anemia is not clinically evident before 1 to 3 wk. The underlying pathophysiologic mechanism is that senescent RBC iron fails to be released by the reticulum cells for Hb synthesis by the erythron. Man uses about 25 mg/day of iron for normal erythropoiesis. Only 1 to 2 mg of iron is available from dietary sources, but a highly efficient recycling of iron derived from senescent RBCs provides a critical iron balance mechanism. In chronic disease, reticulum cells tenaciously retain iron from senescent RBCs, making it unavailable for reuse. In some respects, the circumstance has the pattern of an "internal" iron deficiency to which the normal compensatory responses are blunted. There is a reticulocytopenia and a failure to compensate for the anemia with erythroid hyperplasia. A decrease in erythropoietic activity may be a partial factor in the anemia. The iron studies are as shown in TABLE 92–2 with the failure of compensatory production of transferrin. Thus, the primary pattern is one in which a barrier or defect in the movement of storage iron (in reticuloendothelial cells) to plasma (and hence the erythron) exists and in which the usual compensatory mechanisms fail to generate a response. That some potential for response exists has been documented by the ability to generate RBC production following hemorrhage or hypoxia; i.e., circumstances of markedly enhanced erythropoietic production.

Symptoms, Signs, and Laboratory Findings

The clinical findings are usually those of the underlying disease (whether infectious, inflammatory, or neoplastic). The laboratory findings are shown in TABLE 92–2. In general, the anemia is of moderate severity, rarely with a Hb < 8 gm/dl unless a secondary complicating mechanism is also present. The serum ferritin determination helps to differentiate iron deficiency from the anemias of chronic disease. If iron deficiency is present in addition to the anemias of chronic disease, the serum ferritin does not increase (remaining below 65 ng/ml), and, in the clinical setting of infection, inflammation, or cancer, such a value suggests a combined mechanism.

Treatment

The only therapy is that of the underlying disease. Hematemics have no value. Since these anemias are of modest severity and generally not progressive, blood transfusions are rarely required.

NORMOCHROMIC NORMOCYTIC ANEMIAS

Decreased RBC production, termed bone marrow failure, results in normochromic normocytic anemias. The mechanisms involved are **hypoproliferation,** in which the normal humoral stimulus (erythropoietin) is lacking; **hypoplasia,** in which RBC precursors are lost, either from a defect in stem cell pool or an injury to the microenvironment that supports the marrow, and **myelophthisis,** in which the normal marrow space is infiltrated and replaced by abnormal or nonhematopoietic cells.

HYPOPROLIFERATIVE ANEMIAS

Normochromic normocytic anemias are characterized by a reticulocytopenia (i.e., decreased delivery of cells) and a failure of the erythroid mass to expand in response to the anemia. Studies with radiolabeled iron reveal a sluggish production of RBCs. The pathophysiologic mechanism appears to be a relative or absolute decreased production of erythropoietin or a hypometabolic state with resultant failure to respond to erythropoietin. As noted above, the anemias of iron deficiency and lack of iron reutilization are also hypoproliferative, since they have restricted erythroid hyperplasia and decreased erythropoietinemia; nonetheless, the primary mechanistic defect is altered iron metabolism, and the proliferative failure appears to be an epiphenomenon of unknown basis. Hypoproliferation is commonly associated with anemias of renal disease, of hypometabolic states (e.g., myxedema), and of protein deprivation, which may cause hypometabolism.

Anemia of Renal Disease

The severity of the anemia that occurs in renal failure correlates roughly with the extent of renal dysfunction. Thus, the secretory function of the kidney in producing the hormone erythropoietin in general parallels the excretory function, and anemia occurs when the creatinine clearance falls to < 45 ml/min. Decreased erythropoietin production, resulting in inadequate humoral stimulus of RBC production, is expressed as a peripheral reticulocytopenia and a subnormal marrow response (absence of erythroid hyperplasia). Renal lesions primarily in the glomerular region (amyloidosis, diabetic nephropathy, etc.) generally result in the most severe anemia for their degree of excretory failure.

Other mechanisms may compound the severity of this disorder. In uremia, a mild added hemolytic component (a shortened RBC survival) is common; its basis is uncertain, but it is related to the retained "metabolic debris of uremia" that somehow injures RBCs. Less common, but more easily recognizable, is the anemia associated with RBC fragmentation, called microangiopathic hemolytic anemia, that occurs when the renal vascular endothelium is injured (e.g., in malignant hypertension, polyarteritis nodosum, or acute cortical necrosis). In children, this can be an acute, often fatal illness called the hemolytic-uremic syndrome (HUS—see under THROMBOCYTOPENIA in Ch. 95). Recognition of these hemolytic mechanisms helps in the clinical approach to the renal lesion as well as the anemia; the term *anemia of renal failure* applies only to the hypoproliferative hypoerythropoietinemic mechanism.

Laboratory Findings

No specific features identify this form of hypoproliferative anemia (see above). A superimposed, microangiopathic hemolysis can be recognized on peripheral blood smear by RBC fragmentation and (usually) thrombocytopenia.

Treatment

Therapy is directed at the underlying renal disease. If adequate renal function is reestablished, the anemia is relieved. In patients treated with long-term dialysis, increased erythropoiesis has been seen, but it rarely returns to normal. Androgens have been used to stimulate erythropoiesis; in general, they raise the peripheral venous Hct about 10%, a degree almost too modest to warrant their problems and risks. Transfusions are rarely indicated, except when cardiopulmonary symptoms or signs develop.

Anemia of Endocrine Failure (Myxedema; Hypopituitarism)

The exact pathophysiologic basis for this anemia is uncertain. Decreased metabolism may result from decreased tissue responsiveness to normal stimuli (i.e., erythropoietin). In general, the anemia is rarely severe (Hb > 9 gm/dl). As the hypometabolic state is repaired, the anemia subsides. Complete repair may require 6 to 9 mo of a normal metabolic status; the reasons for such a slow response are not clear.

The laboratory data may be confusing, since the disorder may be compounded by iron deficiency secondary to the hyper- and polymenorrhagia seen in myxedema, by megaloblastic changes secondary to malabsorption of vitamin B_{12}, or by an admixture of these mechanisms.

Anemia of Protein Depletion

The clinical and laboratory findings in protein depletion mimic those in the hypometabolic states. Its mechanism has been related to general hypometabolism without actual supportive data. In animals, protein depletion results in decreased erythropoietin production. The exact role of protein in hematopoiesis in man is not clear.

HYPOPLASTIC (APLASTIC) ANEMIAS

These normochromic normocytic anemias often have borderline high MCV values. By definition, the marrow mass is decreased (hypoplastic). Commonly the term hypoplastic (aplastic) anemia is used to imply a panhypoplasia of the marrow with associated leukopenia and thrombocytopenia. That confusion in nomenclature has led to the term *pure red cell aplasia* to define the selective marked reduction or absence of erythroid precursors.

Etiology and Pathogenesis

About 1/2 of cases of aplastic anemia are idiopathic; they are commonest in adolescents and young adults. In the remainder, the cause can be a chemical agent (e.g., benzene, inorganic arsenic), radiation, or drugs (e.g., antineoplastic agents). Many drugs (antibiotics, anti-inflammatory drugs, anticonvulsants, etc.) have been implicated in individual cases. The mechanism of such events is unknown, but a selective (perhaps genetic) hypersensitivity appears to be the basis. A very rare form of aplastic anemia, **Fanconi's anemia** (a type of familial aplastic anemia with bone abnormalities, microcephaly, hypogenitalism, and brown pigmentation of skin), occurs in children with abnormal chromosomes.

Pure RBC aplasia, on the other hand, implies a mechanism selectively destructive to the erythroid precursors; other hematopoietic elements are unaffected. Clinical correlations exist with some cases of RBC aplasia but the pathophysiologic mechanisms are unknown. Thus, acute erythroblastopenia is well known to be a brief reversible disappearance of RBC precursors in the marrow during a variety of acute viral illnesses, especially in children. Indeed, this may be recognized fortuitously, since the sequela of the aplasia (i.e., the anemia) requires a duration greater than usually exists with the acute episode. **Chronic RBC aplasia** has been associated with thymomas, immunologic injury, and less often with drugs (tranquilizers, anticonvulsants, etc.), toxins (organic phosphates), riboflavin deficiency, and chronic lymphocytic leukemia. A rare congenital form, Blackfan–Diamond syndrome, is described. Erythroid aplasia may occur transiently during various infections and hemolytic disorders (aregenerative crisis, acute erythroblastopenia), and in association with tumors of the thymus.

Symptoms and Signs

The clinical onset is usually insidious, often occurring over weeks or months after exposure to a toxin. However, it is occasionally explosive. Signs vary with the severity of the pancytopenia. General symptoms of anemia are usually severe. Waxy pallor of skin and mucous membranes is characteristic. Chronic cases may show considerable brown skin pigmentation.

In aplastic anemia severe thrombocytopenia may occur, with bleeding into the mucous membranes and skin. Hemorrhages into the ocular fundi are frequent. Agranulocytosis with life-threatening infections is common. Splenomegaly is absent, unless induced by transfusion hemosiderosis.

The clinical presentation of pure RBC asplasia is generally milder. The symptoms relate to the anemia, or the underlying concomitant clinical problem.

Laboratory Findings

The anemia is normochromic and normocytic (rarely, macrocytic). A WBC count of 1500 or lower is common, the reduction occurring chiefly in the granulocytes. Platelets are often markedly reduced. Reticulocytes are decreased, even when coexistent with hemolysis. The aspirated bone marrow is acellular. The serum iron is elevated. In pure RBC aplasia, the marrow cellularity and maturation may be normal except for a complete absence of erythroid precursors.

Treatment

The only known effective therapy for aplastic anemia is bone marrow transplantation. The initial approach is to evaluate siblings for HLA compatibility and arrange for the transplantation. Blood transfusions represent a risk to the subsequent successful transplant, and blood products should be used only when absolutely essential. Androgens have been tried in nontransplant candidates, but response to these hormones is rare.

Pure RBC aplasia has been successfully managed with immunosuppressive therapy (prednisone and cyclophosphamide), especially when an immunologic basis is implicated. Most patients with an identified thymoma improve following thymectomy, and the response rate merits such an approach.

MYELOPHTHISIC ANEMIAS

In addition to being normochromic, the hallmarks of these anemias are anisocytosis, poikilocytosis, and the presence of nucleated RBCs in the smear. Immature myeloid cells are also seen. These findings occur when there is replacement of the marrow by infiltrative neoplasms, granulomatous diseases, (lipid) storage disease, or fibrosis.

Etiology and Pathogenesis

In general, this form of anemia is assumed to be the logical sequela of a decreased amount of functioning hematopoietic tissue. Attractive as this may be, the hypothesis is unproved. Measurements of RBC production rates have yielded normal or increased values in some cases. RBC life span is often reduced. A metabolic fault related to the underlying disease and, in some cases, erythrophagocytosis have been considered pathogenetic factors, but never demonstrated.

The most common cause is carcinoma metastasizing to bone marrow from primary tumors, most often located in the breast, prostate, kidney, lung, or adrenal or thyroid gland. Another frequent cause is myelofibrosis, which may be of undetermined origin, or, in some instances, a late stage of polycythemia vera, or chronic granulocytic leukemia. In children a rare cause is marble-bone disease of Albers-Schönberg.

Unfortunately, assorted terms are confusing. **Myeloid metaplasia** refers to the extramedullary hematopoiesis in the liver and spleen that may accompany myelophthisis from any cause. **Myelofibrosis,** the replacement of marrow by fibroblastic cells, may be idiopathic or secondary. An old term, **agnogenic myeloid metaplasia,** indicates primary myelofibrosis and extramedullary hematopoiesis, but myelofibrosis may be present with little or no extramedullary hematopoiesis. In some cases, **myelosclerosis** (new bone formation) occurs.

Symptoms and Signs

In severe cases, the usual symptoms of anemia may be present, as well as symptoms referable to the underlying disease. Splenomegaly, sometimes massive, occurs and associated hepatomegaly is common; symptoms of pressure from splenomegaly may be the presenting complaint.

Laboratory Findings

The anemia, usually of moderate severity, is characteristically normocytic but may be slightly macrocytic. Morphologic alterations in the erythrocytes may be extreme, with wide variation in size and shape. Another outstanding feature is the presence in the blood of nucleated RBCs, mostly normoblasts, and immature WBCs. In the peripheral blood, the term *leukoerythroblastic* has been applied to this cellular pattern, a picture resulting from either a disruption of the marrow sinusoids or hematopoiesis in extramedullary sites. Polychromatophilia and reticulocytosis are often present. Reticulocytosis that may be due to premature release of reticulocytes from the marrow or extramedullary sites is not necessarily an index of increased blood regeneration. The WBC count may be normal, reduced, or increased. The platelet count is often low, and giant, bizarre-shaped platelets may be seen.

Kinetic studies with labeled iron may indicate hematopoietic activity in the spleen and/or the liver. The marrow may be difficult to obtain by aspiration; findings vary according to the underlying disease. Marrow trephine biopsy is usually necessary to establish the diagnosis.

X-rays of the skeletal system may disclose bony lesions (myelosclerosis) characteristic of long-standing myelofibrosis or other osseous changes (i.e., lytic lesions of a neoplasm) suggesting the underlying cause of the anemia.

Treatment

Therapy is that of the underlying disorder. In idiopathic cases, management is supportive. Blood transfusions are indicated if the anemia produces cardiovascular symptoms. In primary myelofibrosis, androgens and/or corticosteroids have been used in an attempt to increase RBC production or decrease their destruction; modest responses have been observed.

MEGALOBLASTIC ANEMIAS

Megaloblastic states result when defective deoxyribonucleic acid (DNA) synthesis is present. The result of defective DNA synthesis is continued ribonucleic acid synthesis with an increase in cytoplasmic mass and maturation. This results in the delivery of macro-ovalocytic RBCs to the circulation and disordered maturation (dyspoiesis) of all cells so that cytoplasmic maturity is greater than nuclear maturity, producing the "megaloblast" in the marrow. Interference with normal cellular maturation increases intramedullary cell death (ineffective erythropoiesis) with resultant indirect hyperbilirubinemia and hyperuricemia. All cell lines are affected so that leukopenia and thrombocytopenia as well as the anemia may occur. Other hallmarks include reticulocytopenia, since there is defective RBC production. Hypersegmentation of polymorphonuclear leukocytes is a standard finding in megaloblastic states; the mechanism of their production is unknown.

The etiologic mechanisms for the megaloblastic states include deficiency or defective utilization of vitamin B_{12} or folic acid, cytotoxic agents (generally antitumor or immunosuppressive drugs) that interfere with DNA synthesis, and a rare autonomous form, the **Di Guglielmo syndrome**. Elucidation of the etiologic basis as well as the pathophysiologic mechanisms are crucial in megaloblastic anemias.

ANEMIA DUE TO VITAMIN B_{12} DEFICIENCY (Pernicious Anemia)

Vitamin B_{12} is present in meat and other animal protein foods. Absorption occurs in the terminal ileum and requires the presence of intrinsic factor, a specific secretion of the gastric parietal cells in the fundus and body of the stomach, to transport the vitamin across the intestinal mucosa. B_{12} is stored in the liver in sufficient quantities to sustain physiologic needs for 3 to 5 yr.

Etiology and Pathophysiology

Decreased B_{12} absorption is the major pathophysiologic mechanism that may be due to one of several factors (see also VITAMIN B_{12} DEFICIENCY in Ch. 78 and Clinical Presentation in Ch. 56). In pernicious anemia, the most common cause of B_{12} deficiency, the atrophic gastric mucosa fails to secrete intrinsic factor. Gastrectomy, chronic atrophic gastritis, and myxedema may also cause similar deficient intrinsic factor secretion. Deficiency of intrinsic factor is rarely congenital. Competition for available B_{12} and cleavage of the intrinsic factor may occur in the blind loop syndrome (because of bacterial utilization of B_{12}) or in fish tapeworm infestation. Ileal absorptive sites may be congenitally absent or destroyed by inflammatory regional enteritis or surgical resection. Less common causes of decreased B_{12} absorption include chronic pancreatitis, malabsorption syndromes, and administration of certain drugs (e.g., oral calcium chelating agents, aminosalicylic acid, biguanides). Inadequate B_{12} intake in vegans, or, very rarely, increased B_{12} utilization in longstanding hyperthyroidism may also be causative.

Symptoms and Signs

In most patients, anemia develops insidiously and progressively as the large hepatic stores of B_{12} are depleted. It is often more profound than would be expected from the symptoms, since physiologic adaptation can occur with its slow evolution. Splenomegaly and hepatomegaly may occasionally be seen. Various GI manifestations may be present, including anorexia, intermittent constipation and diarrhea, and poorly localized abdominal pain. Glossitis, usually described as "burning of the tongue," may be an early symptom. Considerable weight loss is common.

Neurologic involvement (see also COMBINED SYSTEM DISEASE in Ch. 129) may be present *even in the absence of anemia*. The most common involvement is that of peripheral nerves. Second to this is spinal cord involvement beginning in the dorsal column with loss of vibratory sensation in the lower extremities, loss of position sense, and ataxia; lateral column involvement follows, with spasticity, hyperactive reflexes, and a Babinski's sign. Some also have irritability, mild depression, or actual paranoia (megaloblastic madness). Yellow-blue color blindness occurs rarely.

Among the rare signs may be a fever of unknown origin that responds promptly to B_{12} therapy. Endocrine deficiencies, especially of the thyroid and adrenal glands, if they are associated with pernicious anemia, suggest an autoimmune basis for gastric mucosal atrophy. Hypogammaglobulinemia may be associated with pernicious anemia.

Laboratory Diagnosis

The anemia is macrocytic, with an MCV > 100. The smear shows macro-ovalocytosis, aniso- and poikilocytosis, and basophilic stippling of the RBCs. Howell-Jolly bodies (residual fragments of the nucleus) are common. Unless the patient has been treated, there is a reticulocytopenia. Hypersegmentation of the granular leukocytes is one of the earliest findings; leukopenia develops later. Thrombocytopenia is observed in about $1/2$ of severe cases, and the platelets are often bizarre in size and shape. The bone marrow demonstrates erythroid hyperplasia and megaloblastic changes. Serum bilirubin may be elevated because of the ineffective erythropoiesis.

The commonest method to establish that B_{12} deficiency is the cause of the megaloblastosis is by serum vitamin B_{12} assay with either microbiologic or radioisotopic method. The former is specific but tedious, subject to interference by a variety of drugs, and now rarely done. Radioisotopic assays have suffered from problems in specificity. In general, low values (< 150 pg/ml) are reliable indications of B_{12} deficiency. In borderline circumstances (150 to 250 pg/ml) clinical judgment and other tests must supplement the radioassay. Tissue deficiency of B_{12} results in methylmalonic (and propionic) aciduria. Autoantibodies to gastric parietal cells can be identified in 80 to 90% of patients with pernicious anemia and in 40 to 50% of those with intrinsic factor deficiency.

Achlorhydria is present in most patients with pernicious anemia. Gastric analysis demonstrates a small volume of gastric secretions (achylia gastrica) with a pH > 6.5; achlorhydria is confirmed if the pH rises to between 6.8 and 7.2 following histamine administration. Absent gastric intrinsic factor secretion occurs with pernicious anemia.

The **Schilling test** measures the absorption of radioactive B_{12} with and without intrinsic factor. It is particularly useful in establishing the diagnosis in patients who have been treated and are in remission. The Schilling is most expediently done by a dual isotope label. B_{12} labeled with one isotope is attached to a purified intrinsic factor extract; B_{12} is also labeled with a different isotope but one free of intrinsic factor. After these are given orally, a flushing dose of B_{12} is given parenterally. Urine is collected over the next 24 h. Normally each labeled fractional excretion will exceed 9% of the doses. Decreased excretion of the radiolabeled B_{12} ($< 5\%$) and normal excretion of the labeled B_{12}-bound to intrinsic factor establishes a defect in intrinsic factor production (generally pernicious anemia). Subnormal absorption of B_{12}, uncorrected by intrinsic factor, is seen in sprue and other malabsorption syndromes. Since the test provides B_{12} repletion, it should be performed after completion of all studies and planned therapeutic trials.

Because of the increased incidence of gastric cancer in patients with pernicious anemia, GI x-rays should be taken in every patient with this diagnosis. These may also disclose other causes of megaloblastic anemia (e.g., intestinal diverticula or blind loops, or abnormal small-bowel patterns characteristic of sprue).

Treatment

The amount of B_{12} retained by the body is in proportion to the amount given. Calculation of the specific amount of therapeutic B_{12} required is difficult, since repletion must include restoration of hepatic stores, normally 3,000 to 10,000 μg, and B_{12} retention declines as restoration of stores is achieved. Vitamin B_{12} 1000 μg is given IM 2 to 4 times/wk until the hematologic abnormalities are corrected, and then is given once monthly. Although hematologic correction usually occurs within 6 wk, neural improvement may take up to 18 mo. Folic acid administration (instead of B_{12}) to anyone in the B_{12}-deprived state is *contraindicated*, since it may result in fulminant neurologic deficit. Oral iron therapy is given if iron deficiency is diagnosed by an absence of stainable iron in the bone marrow prior to B_{12} treatment.

B_{12} maintenance therapy must be given for life unless the pathophysiologic mechanism for the deficiency is corrected.

ANEMIA DUE TO FOLIC ACID DEFICIENCY

Etiology and Pathophysiology

The metabolism, several pathophysiologic mechanisms, and causes of folate deprivation are also discussed in Ch. 78.

Long-term cooking destroys folic acid, which is abundant in foods such as green leafy vegetables, yeast, liver, and mushrooms. Folate is absorbed in the duodenum and upper jejunum. Hepatic storage is limited, providing only a 2- to 4-mo supply in the absence of intake. Borderline dietary intake of folic acid is common. Alcohol interferes with its intermediate metabolism and probably absorption as well. Therefore, persons living on a marginal subsistence diet ("tea-and-toasters") and chronic alcoholics are prone to develop macrocytic anemia from folic acid deficiency, as are those with chronic liver disease. Infants deficient in vitamin C may have "megaloblastic anemia of infancy." Since the fetus obtains its folic acid from maternal supplies, pregnant women are susceptible to developing a megaloblastic anemia.

Intestinal malabsorption is another common cause of folate deficiency (see in Ch. 56). In tropical sprue, the malabsorption itself is secondary to the atrophy of intestinal mucosa resulting from lack of folic acid. Even minute doses will correct both the anemia and the steatorrhea in most of these patients.

Folic acid deficiency may develop in patients on long-term anticonvulsant therapy or oral contraceptives due to decreased absorption, or antimetabolites (methotrexate) and antimicrobial agents (e.g., trimethoprim–sulfamethoxazole) that interfere with folate metabolism.

Finally, increased demand for folate occurs in pregnancy and lactation, with long-term dialysis, chronic hemolytic anemias, and psoriasis.

Diagnosis

The clinical features of folate deficiency are those of the anemia. Neurologic lesions such as those seen in B_{12} deficiency do not occur. The primary laboratory feature that differentiates this from other forms of megaloblastic anemia is measurable folate depletion. The peripheral blood and bone marrow findings are exactly those described under B_{12} deficiency. Serum folic acid levels < 5 ng/ml suggest a deficiency. Erythrocyte folate levels are low (normal, 90 to 450 ng/ml) and are diagnostic of deficiency. (The range of "normal" depends upon the laboratory method used.)

Treatment

Folic acid 1 mg/day is given orally to repair tissue depletion. The patient's awareness of the importance of adequate intake of folic acid is critical; approximately 50 μg of folate is required daily, with 2 to 3 times that amount required in pregnancy and childhood.

ANEMIA DUE TO COPPER DEFICIENCY (See also COPPER DEFICIENCY in Ch. 79)

Lessons from earlier animal models suggested that copper deficiency was rare clinically and that it produced a hypochromic microcytic anemia. Recent clinical evidence in man in hyperalimentation programs indicates that the development of copper deficiency, commonest in infants and children, is an important potential clinical risk. In addition, the anemia is primarily megaloblastic with remarkable toxic vascularization in the cytoplasm of developing RBCs. If severe, marrow hypoplasia may occur, an uncommon event in megaloblastic states unless they are secondary to anticancer chemotherapeutic agents. Copper supplements (copper sulfate) completely correct the anemia.

Parenthetically, it should be noted that copper excess has been associated with an acute hemolytic anemia which appears mediated by the potent oxidizing effect of the free copper (cupric ion) on the RBC membrane. Such episodes of copper excess have been seen primarily during hemodialysis when water containing excess copper salts was utilized.

ANEMIA DUE TO ASCORBIC ACID (VITAMIN C) DEFICIENCY

Deficiency of ascorbic acid is often associated with anemia. This is hypochromic and may be normocytic microcytic (if there has been longstanding blood loss) or, occasionally, macrocytic. When macrocytic, investigation will demonstrate associated folic acid deficiency. Correction then requires both vitamin C (500 mg/day) and folic acid (as noted above).

ANEMIAS DUE TO EXCESSIVE RED CELL DESTRUCTION—HEMOLYTIC ANEMIAS

The normal life span of RBCs is about 120 days. As they age, RBCs are removed by components of the reticuloendothelial system, principally in the spleen, where Hb catabolism takes place. The essential feature of hemolysis is a shortened RBC life span; a hemolytic anemia results when bone marrow production can no longer compensate for RBC destruction. General aspects of hemolytic anemias will be discussed below, followed by a description of specific disorders.

Pathogenesis

Most hemolysis occurs **extravascularly;** i.e., in the phagocytic cells of the spleen, liver, and bone marrow. Hemolysis is usually due to (1) abnormalities within the RBC contents (Hb or enzymes); (2) abnormalities of the RBC membrane (permeability, structure, or lipid content); or (3) abnormalities extrinsic to the RBC (serum antibodies, trauma in the circulation, or infectious agents). The spleen is usually involved, and if splenomegaly results, it reduces RBC survival by destroying mildly abnormal RBCs or warm antibody-coated cells. Severely abnormal RBCs or those with cold antibodies or complement coating are destroyed within the circulation or in the liver, which (because of its large blood flow) is efficient in removing damaged cells.

Intravascular hemolysis is uncommon; it results in hemoglobinuria when the Hb released into plasma exceeds the Hb-binding capacity of plasma haptoglobin. Hb is reabsorbed into renal tubular cells where the iron is converted to hemosiderin, part of which is assimilated for reutilization and part of which reaches the urine when the tubular cells slough.

Clinical Laboratory Manifestations

The systemic manifestations of hemolytic anemias resemble those of other anemias. Hemolysis may be acute, chronic, or episodic. Acute severe hemolysis **(hemolytic crisis)** is uncommon; it may be accompanied by chills, fever, pain in the back and abdomen, prostration, and shock. Severe hemolysis is also accompanied by increased RBC destruction (jaundice, splenomegaly, and, in certain types of hemolysis, hemoglobinuria and hemosiderinuria), and increased RBC production (reticulocytosis and hyperactive bone marrow). Anemia in chronic hemolytic states may be exacerbated by a temporary failure of RBC production **(aplastic crisis);** this is usually related to an infection.

Jaundice occurs when the conversion of Hb to bilirubin exceeds the liver's capacity to form bilirubin glucuronide and to excrete it into bile (see also JAUNDICE in Ch. 64). Thus, unconjugated (indirect) bilirubin accumulates. Increased pigment catabolism is also manifested by increased stercobilin in the stool and urobilinogen in the urine. Pigment gallstones frequently complicate chronic hemolysis. Hemolysis can usually be identified by the simple criteria described. Nevertheless, the definitive criterion of the hemolytic process is a measure of RBC survival, preferably with a nonreutilizable label such as radiochromium (^{51}Cr). The measured survival of radiolabeled cells establishes not only the hemolytic state but, with surface counting, one can also identify sites of RBC sequestration, thereby providing diagnostic and therapeutic implications. In general, a half-life (for ^{51}Cr-labeled RBCs) of 18 days or greater (normal 28 to 32 days) indicates hemolysis mild enough that a normally responsive marrow should be capable of maintaining normal RBC values. When the marrow does respond appropriately, producing near-normal RBC values, the term "**compensated**" hemolytic anemia is used. Selective splenic sequestration with expected repair following splenectomy can be anticipated when surface count ratios reveal a spleen to liver ratio in excess of 3:1 (normal 1:1).

Other tests of RBC destruction (increased indirect hyperbilirubinemia, increased fecal urobilinogen or carbon monoxide production) or evidence of repair (reticulocytosis) support but do not establish the hemolytic state.

The RBC morphologic examination may show evidence of cell destruction (fragmentation, spherocytes, etc.) or erythrophagocytosis; these help establish the diagnosis and the mechanism. Other tests of mechanisms of hemolysis include Hb electrophoresis, RBC enzyme assays, osmotic fragility, Coombs test, cold agglutinins, and acid hemolysis or sucrose lysis tests.

Morphologic clues, so important in diagnosing most anemias, are of limited value in the hemolytic anemias. The common classification into intrinsic RBC defects and lesions extrinsic to the RBC is sometimes difficult to utilize clinically because the application of laboratory methods to resolve these forms often involves a battery of tests. An alternative approach to the differential diagnosis is to consider the population at risk (i.e., geographic, genetic, underlying disease, etc.) and then proceed through the likely potential mechanisms. In general, these can be divided into (1) RBC sequestration due to alterations in vascular complex (i.e., hypersplenism); (2) immunologic injury (warm or cold antibody mediated); (3) mechanical injury (RBC fragmentation); (4) alterations of RBC structure (abnormal membranes) or metabolism (enzymopathies); and (5) abnormal Hbs.

Treatment is individualized to specific hemolytic disorders. Hemoglobinuria may necessitate iron replacement therapy. Splenectomy is beneficial when the RBC defect is associated with selective splenic sequestration.

HEMOLYTIC ANEMIAS DUE TO ABNORMALITIES EXTRINSIC TO THE RED CELL

Donor cells are destroyed at a rate equal to autologous cells. No abnormality of the RBC can be identified or implicated in RBC destruction.

ANEMIAS DUE TO RETICULOENDOTHELIAL HYPERACTIVITY

Hypersplenism-Congestive Splenomegaly (See also HYPERSPLENISM in Ch. 100)

Hypersplenism is characterized by a mechanism that produces splenic enlargement with associated increased filtering and phagocytic function. Often other cytopenias (leukopenia, thrombocytopenia) occur with the anemia. Although the primary mechanism is a mechanical sieve-like action resulting in RBC sequestration, another mechanism compounding the degree of anemia is that splenic enlargement is associated with plasma volume expansion resulting in a dilutional component. In addition, in some immune-mediated conditions, the spleen may serve not only as the site of RBC sequestration but may be also a site of antibody production, thereby superimposing an immune basis upon that of congestion.

Etiology and Pathogenesis

In general, the degree of anemia relates to the size of the spleen. Thus, diseases associated with reticuloendothelial hyperplasia and splenomegaly are most likely to produce hypersplenism, but any disease that can produce splenomegaly can produce hypersplenism. The term indicates the presence of peripheral cytopenia(s) with bone marrow hyperplasia of the elements reduced in the circulation as due to splenic overfunction and by implication repairable by splenectomy. The anemia is primarily due to splenic sequestration with an added dilutional component. Radiolabeled autologous or donor RBCs can be shown to sequester in the spleen.

Symptoms and Signs

The clinical findings are usually based upon the underlying disease state causing the congestive splenomegaly. Unless other mechanisms coexist to compound their severity, the anemia and other cytopenias are modest and asymptomatic. Splenomegaly is the hallmark of hypersplenism, and spleen size correlates directly with the degree of anemia.

Laboratory Findings

Since the anemia is produced by splenic sequestration, no particular RBC morphology exists. The diagnosis may be suggested by the presence of other cytopenias (platelet counts range between 50,000 to 100,000/ml; WBC in range of 2500 to 4000/ml with normal WBC differential count). ^{51}Cr-radiolabeled RBC survival studies show accelerated destruction and selective splenic sequestration. A measurable expanded plasma volume is common.

Treatment

Therapy is directed at the cause of congestive splenomegaly. Since the anemia is mild, splenectomy is rarely indicated for the hypersplenism itself.

ANEMIAS DUE TO IMMUNOLOGIC ABNORMALITIES

Isoimmune (Isoagglutinin) Hemolytic Anemia

Reactions to incompatible blood: (See Ch. 93.)

Autoimmune Hemolytic Anemia

Warm antibody hemolytic anemias: RBCs coated with IgG (auto-) antibodies are removed by the reticuloendothelial system. These antibodies may arise spontaneously, or in association with certain diseases (SLE, lymphoma, chronic lymphocytic leukemia), or after stimulation by a drug (α-methyldopa, L-dopa, etc.). *The laboratory hallmark is a positive Coombs test,* and the autoantibodies may be related to a portion of the Rh locus. High-dose penicillin or cephalosporins may result in an antibody directed against an antibiotic-RBC membrane complex; cessation of the drug results in disappearance of the accelerated destruction.

Clinical Laboratory Features

Autoimmune hemolytic anemia affects women more often than men, and most commonly those under age 50. Splenomegaly is usual. This potentially lethal anemia is usually severe. A thrombotic tendency often accompanies the hemolysis. Since RBC destruction is primarily in the spleen, hemoglobinuria and hemosiderinuria are rare. A direct Coombs test demonstrates antibody coating the RBC surface. The blood smear frequently reveals spherocytes.

Treatment

In all drug-induced hemolytic anemias, withdrawal of the drug decreases the hemolytic rate. With α-methyldopa and related drugs, hemolysis usually ceases within 3 wk; however, the positive Coombs test may persist for > 1 yr. Corticosteroids occasionally are used if hemolysis is very severe. With penicillin and analogous drugs, hemolysis ceases as soon as the drug is cleared from the plasma.

In idiopathic cases, the anemia responds to corticosteroids, but frequently relapses on withdrawal of the steroid; splenectomy is frequently required to control the hemolytic process. Immunosuppressive agents have been used in patients refractory to steroids and splenectomy.

Cold antibody disease (cold agglutinin disease): Patients with lymphoproliferative diseases, infectious mononucleosis, or *Mycoplasma pneumoniae* may develop IgM antibodies directed against the I or i antigen of RBCs. Agglutination occurs at low temperatures, but only minimally above 30 C (86 F). With agglutination, complement fixation results. Intravascular hemolysis is seldom enough to cause hemoglobinuria and hemosiderinuria, but their presence is an important diagnostic aid. In general, hemolysis is mild.

No underlying cause is found in some patients. This idiopathic form is generally seen in older people. *Mycoplasma pneumoniae* is a common cause in younger people. Regardless of cause, the primary site of destruction is the liver.

Therapy is of only modest effect. Avoidance of cold exposure is often quite helpful. Splenectomy is of no value. Immunosuppressive agents have often been effective. Blood transfusions should be given with caution. The blood should be warmed via an on-line warmer. Autologous cell survival may be better than that of transfused cells because administered blood becomes antibody-coated; autologous cells have already "survived" the antibody effect on the RBCs, and effete complement fragments (C3d) on their surface do not affect RBC survival.

Paroxysmal cold hemoglobinuria (PCH; Donath-Landsteiner syndrome): In this rare disease, hemolysis occurs minutes to hours after exposure to cold; exposure may be localized (e.g., drinking cold water, handwashing in cold water). Intravascular hemolysis is caused by an autohemolysin that unites with RBCs at low temperatures and lyses them only after warming. The cold hemolysin is a 7S immunoglobulin. PCH due to such a cold-activated autohemolysin occurs in some patients with congenital or acquired syphilis, and antisyphilitic therapy may cure the PCH. Most however, occur after a nonspecific "viral" illness or in patients previously well.

Symptoms include severe pain in the back and legs, headache, vomiting, diarrhea, and passage of dark brown urine. Findings include hemoglobinuria, mild anemia, and moderate reticulocytosis. There may be temporary hepatosplenomegaly. Mild hyperbilirubinemia may follow the attack.

Therapy consists of strict measures to avoid cold exposure. Splenectomy is of no value. Immunosuppressive therapy has been effective, but its trial should be restricted to the nonlimited or idiopathic cases.

Complement-Sensitive Associated Anemia

Paroxysmal nocturnal hemoglobinuria (PNH; Marchiafava-Micheli syndrome): This rare disorder of the hematopoietic system is characterized by episodes of hemolysis and hemoglobinemia, the latter accentuated during sleep. The cause is unknown, but it seems that defective RBCs are unusually susceptible to normal complement in plasma. Thus, PNH is an acquired membrane defect with sensitivity to a serum component. PNH is commonest in men in their 20s, but it occurs at any age. Crises may be precipitated by infection, administration of iron or vaccines, or, in women, menstruation.

Abdominal and lumbar pain may occur, along with splenomegaly, hemoglobinemia, hemoglobinuria, and symptoms of severe anemia. The anemia is normocytic and normochromic. Protracted urinary Hb loss may result in iron deficiency even though some organs, particularly the kidneys, may be saturated with hemosiderin. Leukopenia and thrombocytopenia are common. Gross hemoglobinuria is common during crises, and the urine may contain hemosiderin. Affected patients are strongly predisposed to both venous and arterial thrombi, a common cause of death.

Diagnostic tests include the acid hemolysis test in which hemolysis usually occurs if blood is acidified with CO_2, incubated for 1 h, and centrifuged. Also useful is the sugar-water test of Hartman, which is dependent on the enhanced hemolysis of complement-dependent systems in isotonic solutions of low ionic strength. Bone marrow hypoplasia may be present.

Treatment is symptomatic. Empiric use of adrenal steroids (prednisone 20 to 40 mg/day) has resulted sometimes in controlling symptoms and stabilizing RBC values. Blood transfusions containing plasma (complement) should be avoided, but saline-washed RBCs may be given during crises. Heparin should be used cautiously, since it may accelerate hemolysis, but its use in thrombotic disease appears warranted. Oral iron supplements are useful.

ANEMIAS DUE TO MECHANICAL INJURY

Traumatic Hemolytic Anemias (Microangiopathic Hemolytic Anemias)

RBCs fragment when exposed to excessive shear or turbulence in the circulation. RBC fragments in the peripheral blood provide the diagnosis. They appear as triangles, helmet shapes, etc. Trauma may be (1) external to the vessel, as occurs in march hemoglobinuria or during karate or bongo playing; (2) within the heart, as in calcific aortic stenosis and with faulty aortic valve prostheses; (3) in arterioles, as in malignant hypertension and some malignant tumors; or (4) in end arterioles as in thrombotic thrombocytopenic purpura and disseminated intravascular coagulation **(DIC).** Coagulation factor deficits occur in DIC (see Ch. 95). **Treatment** is directed toward the underlying process. Iron-deficiency anemia occasionally is superimposed on hemolysis as a result of chronic hemosiderinuria, and, when demonstrated, may respond to iron therapy.

Hemolysis Due to Infectious Agents

Infectious agents may produce hemolytic anemia by the direct action of toxins (e.g., from *Clostridium perfringens*, α- or β-hemolytic streptococci, or meningococci), or by invasion and destruction of the RBC by the organism (e.g., *Plasmodia* and *Bartonellae*).

HEMOLYSIS DUE TO INTRINSIC RED CELL DEFECTS

ANEMIAS DUE TO ALTERATIONS OF RED CELL MEMBRANE

Congenital

Congenital erythropoietic porphyria: (See ANOMALIES IN PIGMENT METABOLISM in Ch. 82).

Hereditary elliptocytosis (ovalocytosis): This rare disorder is inherited as an autosomal dominant trait. The RBCs are oval or elliptical in shape. Hemolysis is usually absent or slight, with little or no anemia. Splenomegaly is often present. Splenectomy is required only in patients with anemia or a clinical complex as seen in hereditary spherocytosis. Splenectomy does relieve the hemolysis.

Hereditary spherocytosis (chronic familial icterus; congenital hemolytic jaundice; chronic acholuric jaundice; familial spherocytosis; spherocytic anemia): *An inherited chronic disease characterized by hemolysis of spheroidal RBCs, anemia, jaundice, and splenomegaly.*

Etiology and Pathogenesis

Hereditary spherocytosis results from an inherited abnormality of the RBC membrane, whose precise nature is unknown. Cell membrane lipids are decreased, and the cell membrane surface area is decreased out of proportion to the lipid lack. Structural instability of the membrane to sodium requires the expenditure of excess energy (in the form of ATP) to extrude sodium. The decreased surface area of the cell impairs the flexibility needed to traverse the spleen's microcirculation. RBCs trapped in the spleen are destroyed. The condition is inherited as a simple mendelian dominant trait. There is usually a history of one or more family members with jaundice, anemia, or splenomegaly. However, one or more generations may be skipped because of variations in the degree of penetrance of the gene.

Symptoms and Signs

Symptoms and signs are usually mild. Moderate jaundice and symptoms of anemia are present in severe cases. Aplastic crises due to intercurrent infection may exacerbate the anemia. Splenomegaly is almost invariable and, rarely, may cause abdominal discomfort. Hepatomegaly may be present, and cholelithiasis is common. Congenital skeletal abnormalities, such as tower-shaped skull and polydactylism, are seen occasionally.

Laboratory Findings

The anemia varies greatly in degree. The RBC count is usually between 3 and 4 million, but during an aplastic crisis it may fall to < 1 million. The Hb level drops proportionately with the cell count. Since RBCs are spheroidal and the MCV is normal, the mean corpuscular diameter is somewhat below normal, and the cells resemble microspherocytes. Reticulocytosis of 15 to 30% and leukocytosis are common.

The osmotic fragility of RBCs is characteristically increased, but in mild cases it may be normal unless sterile defibrinated blood is first incubated at 37 C (98.6 F) for 24 h. Coombs' test is negative. Glucose can correct an increased autohemolysis.

Prognosis and Treatment

Splenectomy, the only treatment, is indicated in patients under age 45 (especially when anemia exists), episodes of jaundice or biliary colic occur, or if the patient has had episodes of erythroblastopenia (aplastic crisis). At surgery a gallbladder with stones or evidence of disease should be removed. After splenectomy, symptoms usually abate, the RBC count rises, and the reticulocyte count returns to normal; since spherocytosis persists, the osmotic fragility of the blood is still increased, but the patient is improved without the removal moiety (spleen) for these abnormal cells.

Acquired

Stomatocytosis: *Condition of RBCs in which a mouth-like or slit-like pattern replaces the normal central zone of pallor.* These cells are associated with both congenital and acquired hemolytic anemia.

The rare congenital form is best characterized and can be used to describe some of the aspects of this anemia in the acquired form; it has autosomal inheritance. The RBC membrane is considered very "leaky" with hyperpermeability to monovalent cations; movement of divalent cations and anions is normal. Circulating RBCs (20 to 30%) are stomatocytic; osmotic fragility is increased, as is autohemolysis with inconstant correction with glucose. Splenectomy results in amelioration of the anemia in some.

Acquired stomatocytosis with hemolytic anemia occurs primarily with recent excessive alcoholism. Stomatocytes in the peripheral blood and the accelerated RBC destruction disappear within 2 wk of alcohol withdrawal.

Anemia due to hypophosphatemia: RBC pliability depends upon intracellular ATP, calcium, and magnesium levels. Since red cell ATP content is related to the serum phosphorus concentration, hypophosphatemia (serum levels < 0.5 mg/dl) results in erythrocyte ATP depletion; this in turn causes RBC membrane rigidity, and hemolysis occurs.

Severe hypophosphatemia may occur in alcoholic withdrawal states, diabetes mellitus, the recovery (diuretic) phase after severe burns, hyperalimentation, severe respiratory alkalosis, or in uremic patients on dialysis being treated with antacids.

The metabolic sequelae of hypophosphatemia are complex and include red cell ATP and 2,3-DPG depletion, a shift in the O_2 dissociation curve to the left, decreased glucose utilization, and lactate production. The resultant rigid, nonyielding RBCs are susceptible to injury in the capillary circulatory bed, leading to a hemolytic anemia with membrane injury and microspherocytosis.

Since these changes are prevented or reversed if cellular ATP is maintained with phosphate supplements, therapy should be directed toward protection against hypophosphatemia in the potential clinical setting and phosphate administration when depletion is recognized.

ANEMIAS DUE TO ABNORMALITIES OF RED CELL METABOLISM (Hereditary Enzyme Deficiencies)

Glucose is the prime energy source for the RBC. Following its entry into the RBC, glucose is converted to lactate either by anaerobic glycolysis (the Embden-Meyerhof pathway) or via the hexose monophosphate shunt. Hemolytic anemias may result from hereditary deficiencies in the enzyme systems involved in these pathways of glucose metabolism.

Embden-Meyerhof Defects

Embden-Meyerhof pathway defects are relatively rare and share the following characteristics: the trait is autosomal recessive, and hemolytic anemia occurs only in homozygotes; spherocytes are absent, but small numbers of crenated spheres may be present; hemolysis and anemia persist after splenectomy, though there may be some improvement. The most common form is that of pyruvate kinase deficiency due to a deficient or defective enzyme. Deficiencies in virtually every enzyme reaction are associated with a congenital hemolytic anemia. The exact mechanism of RBC destruction is unknown. In general, assay of ATP and diphosphoglycerate help identify presence of a metabolic defect and assist in localizing the sites in the pathway for further biochemical characterization.

Hexose Monophosphate Shunt Defects

The only important defect in this pathway is that due to glucose-6-phosphate dehydrogenase deficiency. In some cases this is due to a genetic abnormality of the enzyme, a form of genetic polymorphism. Clinically, the commonest is that of the drug-sensitive type.

Glucose-6-phosphate dehydrogenase (G6PD) deficiency—drug-sensitive variety: This X-linked disorder (see also in Ch. 241) is fully expressed in males and homozygous females and variably expressed in heterozygous females. It occurs in about 10% of American black males and fewer black females. It is also seen in low frequency among people from the Mediterranean basin; e.g., Italians, Greeks, Arabs, and Sephardic Jews.

In affected blacks and most affected whites, hemolysis occurs in older RBCs after exposure to drugs or other substances that produce peroxide and cause oxidation of Hb and RBC membranes. These include primaquine, aspirin, sulfonamides, nitrofurans, phenacetin, naphthalene, some vitamin K derivatives, and, in some whites, fava beans. Acute viral and bacterial infections and diabetic acidosis also may precipitate hemolysis. Anemia, jaundice, and reticulocytosis develop. Heinz bodies may be seen early during the hemolytic episode, but they do not persist in patients with spleens, since they are removed by the spleen. Often the best diagnostic clue is the presence of **"bite cells"** in the peripheral blood. These are RBCs which appear to have had one or more bites (1 μm in size) taken from the cell periphery, possibly as a result of Heinz body removal by the spleen. Since older cells are selectively destroyed, in most episodes hemolysis is self-limited, affecting < 25% of the RBC mass in blacks. However, in whites, the deficiency is more severe, and profound hemolysis may lead to a sufficient intravascular component with hemoglobinuria and acute renal failure. Whether the patient will develop a compensated hemolytic state or lethal hemolysis if the offending drug is continued depends on the degree of G6PD deficiency in the patient and the oxidant potential of the drug. Chronic congenital hemolysis in the absence of drugs occurs in some whites.

A large number of screening tests for G6PD are available. Following hemolysis, false-negative results may be obtained due to the absence of older, more deficient RBCs and the presence of reticulocytes rich in G6PD. Specific enzyme assays are the best diagnostic test. Affected patients should be advised to eliminate drugs or substances that initiate this deficiency.

ANEMIAS DUE TO DEFECTIVE HEMOGLOBIN SYNTHESIS (Hemoglobinopathies)

Genetic abnormalities of the Hb molecule shown by changes in chemical characteristics, electrophoretic mobility, or physical properties.

The normal adult Hb molecule (Hb A) consists of 2 pairs of polypeptide chains designated α and β. Fetal Hb (Hb F) is present at birth, gradually decreases in the first months of life, and makes up < 2% of total Hb in adults. In Hb F, γ chains are substituted for β chains. In certain disorders of Hb synthesis and in aplastic and myeloproliferative states, Hb F may be increased. Normal blood also contains up to 2.5% of Hb A_2, which is composed of α chains and δ chains.

The types of chains and the chemical structure of individual polypeptides in the chains are controlled genetically. Genetic defects may result in Hb molecules with abnormal physical or chemical properties, some of which may result in anemia. Such anemias are severe in homozygotes and mild in heterozygous carriers. Some individuals may be heterozygous for 2 such abnormalities and show an anemia with characteristics of both traits.

The abnormal Hbs are distinguished by their electrophoretic mobility and have been designated by letters. The first to be discovered was sickle cell Hb (Hb S). The designations since then have followed alphabetical sequence in order of discovery; thus, C, D, E, G, H, etc. Structurally different Hbs with the same electrophoretic mobility are named also by the city in which they were discovered (e.g., Hb C_{Harlem}, Hb $S_{Memphis}$). The important hemoglobinopathies in the USA are those due to Hb S and Hb C and the thalassemias. (For a discussion of these disorders, as well as Hb S–C and Hb S–Beta Thalassemia, see Vol. II, Ch. 25)

---

93. BLOOD TRANSFUSION

The procedure of transferring human blood or a component of blood from a donor to a recipient.

Blood is a living tissue; transfusion of blood or its cellular components is a form of transplantation. About 11 to 12 million transfusions of blood and components are given yearly in the USA, and the number is steadily increasing. The decision to transfuse is a *clinical* judgment that requires weighing the possible benefits and known hazards with alternative treatments. A transfusion that is not specifically indicated is contraindicated. Clinical use of blood and components is discussed below.

Collection and Storage of Blood

In the USA, regulations for collecting, storing, and transporting blood and its components have been established by the FDA, and sometimes also by state or local health authorities. The American National Red Cross and the American Association of Blood Banks also have standards affecting their respective systems. The screening of a donor includes interviewing him, testing for Hb, and taking his temperature, pulse rate, and BP. **Causes for disqualification** are history of (1) hepatitis, (2) heart disease, (3) cancer, other than mild treatable forms, such as small skin cancers, (4) severe asthma, (5) bleeding disorder, or (6) convulsions. **Temporary deferments** are for (1) malaria, (2) exposure to malaria, (3) exposure to hepatitis, (4) pregnancy, (5) major surgery, (6) hypertension, (7) hypotension, and (8) anemia. Some of these criteria protect would-be donors from possible ill effects of donation; others protect the recipient. Donation is limited to once every 2 mo.

Paid donation is discouraged because of abuses inherent in the "skid row" blood banks in big cities, because blood from such banks has 5 to 10 times the usual rate of hepatitis infectivity, and because of a desire to encourage voluntary donation and thus broaden the donor base.

The standard donation is 450 ml, taken into a plastic bag containing either Citrate Phosphate Dextrose **(CPD)** or adenine-supplemented CPD (CPDA-1). CPD blood may be stored for 21 days, CPDA-1 blood for 35 days. Heparin is a poor preservative but is occasionally used, mostly for pediatric heart surgery or exchange transfusion. Stored whole blood differs considerably from circulating blood. Changes that occur in blood during refrigerated storage are collectively referred to as the "storage lesion." Some changes (see TABLES 93–1, 93–2, and 93–3) may affect certain recipients.

Before use, blood must be tested for classification and suitability. This includes ABO and Rh typing (see below), antibody screening, STS, and a test for hepatitis B surface antigen (HBsAg). The container label and the federally required Circular of Information give the results of these tests and important information and cautions and should be consulted by physicians using blood transfusions.

When conditions permit, the safest blood for transfusion is the patient's own: **autologous transfusion.** With appropriate precautions, several units of blood can be collected in the few weeks preceding elective surgery, and can then be used for blood replacement during or after surgery. The collection, storage, and issue of autologous blood are necessarily done in a blood bank, with special precautions for protection of the donor-patient. The interested physician should consult the local hospital or community blood bank for information.

Blood Components

The various components of blood can be separated, concentrated, and stored individually; replacement should be restricted to those items definitely needed by the patient.

Anticoagulants, used for whole blood storage and designed to protect RBCs, are not optimal for other components. Labile components are best stored after separation from whole blood. The demand for components such as platelets, antihemophilic factor **(AHF)**, and fresh plasma for fractionation is so high that blood banks must separate fresh components from a majority of blood donations. To do this and continue to supply whole blood ad lib wastes donors' RBCs, which are a by-product of component separation. Whole blood is now considered more of a raw material than a transfusion medium.

For anything other than simple RBC transfusion, consulting the blood bank physician before writing orders provides optimal choices and service. TABLE 93–4 shows some characteristics of blood and components as ordinarily prepared by the blood bank, not including purified manufactured derivatives that are essentially pharmaceutical rather than blood bank items. Clinical indications for individual components are discussed below (amounts must always be individualized).

TABLE 93–1. WHOLE BLOOD: STORAGE IN CPD*

Weeks in storage	0	1	2	3
RBC survival at 24 h after transfusion (%)	100	98	85	80
2,3-diphosphoglycerate (% of initial value)	100	99	80	44
pH (at 37 C)	7.20	7.00	6.89	6.84
Plasma K (mEq/L)	3.9	11.9	17.2	21.0
Plasma Hgb (mg/dl)	1.7	7.8	12.5	19.1

* Ranges of statistical variation have been omitted to make the table easier to read.

Modified from "Blood Storage and Shipment," in *Technical Manual of the American Association of Blood Banks,* ed 7, p. 55, edited by W.V. Miller. Copyright 1977 by American Association of Blood Banks. Used with permission of American Association of Blood Banks.

TABLE 93-2. RED BLOOD CELLS: STORAGE IN CPDA-1
(HEMATOCRIT 80%)*

Weeks in storage:	0	1	2	3	4	5
RBC survival at 24 h after transfusion (%; 75% Hct)	100†				83	78
2,3-diphosphoglycerate (% of initial value)‡	100	83	37	14	9	8
pH (at 37 C)	7.04	6.92	6.8	6.65	6.58	6.55
Percent hemolysis	0.025	0.037	0.072	0.141	0.245	0.336
Plasma K (mEq/L)	4.4	59.1	77.2	88.4	95.6	102.5
Plasma NH_3 (mg/dl)	1.29	6.32	9.76	12.6	16.0	20

* Ranges of statistical variation have been omitted to make the table easier to read.
† Actually, slightly less than 100%.
‡ Initial value represents 4 h of storage.
Data in part from G. Moroff and D. Dende, American Red Cross Blood Services Laboratories, Bethesda, MD, and in part from Fenwal Laboratories, Deerfield, IL. Used with permission.

Red blood cells (RBCs) are transfused to replace Hb or O_2 carrying capacity, including blood lost at surgery and in priming extracorporeal circuits. When volume expansion is required, other fluids can be used concurrently or separately (see SHOCK in Ch. 24).

Frozen-thawed RBCs are indicated mainly for patients who have leukocyte antibodies and repeated febrile transfusion reactions and for patients with multiple blood group antibodies or antibodies to high frequency antigens. The high cost of freezing and thawing RBCs precludes their general use.

Leukocyte-poor RBCs, prepared by inverted centrifugation, can be used for patients who have repeated febrile reactions.

Washed RBCs (by continuous-flow washing) are free of almost all traces of plasma and are suitable for patients who have severe reactions to plasma (e.g., severe allergies or IgA immunization). Modified washing is suitable for patients with congestive heart failure and hypervolemia, or for pediatric heart surgery to avoid citrate.

Whole blood, which is less available because of the demand for plasma, components, and fractions, is used for rapid massive blood loss and exchange transfusions. Whole blood may be necessary if a component is unavailable; conversely, RBCs and other fluids or components can be used instead of whole blood. **Heparinized whole blood,** nearly out of use, is requested for some cases of pediatric heart surgery, primarily to eliminate citrate. Frozen-thawed RBCs or RBCs subjected to a single saline wash may be substituted. Heparinized blood has also been used in exchange transfusions for adults with fulminant hepatitis and for babies with severe hemolytic disease.

Platelet concentrates are used for severe thrombocytopenia (platelet count < 10,000/cu mm) or for a bleeding tendency related to less severe thrombocytopenia (e.g., counts between 10,000 and 50,000/cu mm). They are sometimes necessary for surgical patients who tend to bleed following massive transfusion or prolonged periods on extracorporeal circulation. Since a single fresh platelet concentrate in an adult usually causes a rise of about 12,000 in the platelet count, 6 to 8 concentrates are usually needed. A purpuric patient often shows no rise in count because the transfused platelets are immediately consumed.

TABLE 93-3. WHOLE BLOOD: STORAGE IN CPDA-1*

Weeks in storage	0	5
RBC survival at 24 h after transfusion (%)	100†	82
pH	7.2	6.78
Plasma K (mEq/L)	3.54	26.9
Plasma Hgb (mg/dl)	5.0	34

* Ranges of statistical variation have been omitted to make the table easier to read.
† Actually, slightly less than 100%.
Data in part from G. Moroff and D. Dende, American Red Cross Blood Services Laboratories, Bethesda, MD, and in part from Fenwal Laboratories, Deerfield, IL. Used with permission.

TABLE 93–4. BLOOD COMPONENTS AS PREPARED FROM CPD* OR CPDA-1* WHOLE BLOOD

Component	Storage Period	Storage Temperature (C)	Hct (%)**	Vol/unit (ml)**	Remarks
RBCs*	21 days 35 days***	4 to 6	70	300	
Frozen glycerolized RBCs	2 or more yr	−85 (high glyc.) −190 (low glyc.)	n.a.* n.a.	n.a. n.a.	There are several different freeze-thaw protocols having somewhat different characteristics
Thawed deglycerolized RBCs	24 h	4 to 6	70 to 90	200 to 300	
Leukocyte-poor or washed RBCs	21 days	4 to 6	70 to 90	200 to 230	
WB*	21 days 35 days***	4 to 6	40	513	
WB, heparinized	48 h	4 to 6	40 to 45	477	Deteriorates during 2nd 24 h
Platelet concentrate	3 days 3 days	4 to 6 20 to 24	n.a. n.a.	25 to 30 30 to 50	Best given fresh Best given fresh. Must be agitated continuously during storage
Cryoprecipitated AHF*	1 yr	below −18	0	10	Contains (/unit) about 100 u. AHF and 250 mg fibrinogen
Fresh frozen plasma	1 yr	below −18	0	220	Contains all clotting factors except platelets, but unconcentrated
Granulocytes	24 h	4 to 6 (Probably best)	Depends on technic	Depends on technic	Several technics, giving concentrates of varying characteristics

* CPD = citrate phosphate dextrose solution; CPDA-1 = adenine-supplemented CPD; RBCs = red blood cells; WB = whole blood; AHF = antihemophilic factor; n.a. = not applicable.
** Approximate.
*** Storage in CPDA-1.

Cryoprecipitated antihemophilic factor (AHF, factor VIII) is a concentrate prepared by rapid freezing and slow thawing of fresh plasma. It is used mostly for hemophiliacs, in a dosage depending on the patient's size and degree of AHF deficiency. Cryoprecipitate may also be used in von Willebrand's disease (see HEREDITARY COAGULATION DISORDERS in Vol. II, Ch. 25). Each concentrate usually contains about 100 u. AHF plus about 250 mg **fibrinogen** and can also be used as a source of the latter. Fibrinogen concentrates are not commercially available.

Fresh frozen plasma is an unconcentrated source of all clotting factors except platelets. It can be used to correct a bleeding tendency of unknown cause, or one associated with liver failure. It can also supplement RBCs when whole blood is unavailable for exchange transfusion.

Granulocyte transfusion, still somewhat experimental, is used increasingly in hematology-oncology centers in conjunction with chemotherapy for cancer or leukemia when sepsis occurs during a period of bone marrow depression.

"Fresh" blood or its components are required in few conditions. See TABLE 93–5 for definitions of "fresh" and suitable component alternatives to fit special clinical situations.

Transfusion Technic

CAUTION: *Before starting any transfusion, the label and the cross-match report should be checked to make sure that the blood is indeed for the patient concerned, that it is compatible, and that the component is correct.*

An 18-gauge needle, or larger, is desirable. Smaller needles may have to be used in young people, but hemolysis may occur if excess pressure is necessary. A Y blood-administration set with a filter should be used, with the RBCs attached to one limb and isotonic saline to the other. Since most transfusions are RBCs, which are more viscous than whole blood, 50 to 100 ml of saline are allowed to run into the RBCs before starting. *No IV solution other than isotonic saline should be allowed into the blood bag or in the same tubing with blood, since many solutions exert deleterious effects;* e.g., D/W causes clumping and decreased survival of RBCs; Ringer's solution causes clotting. Transfusion of a single unit of RBCs should not take > 2 h.

Close observation is important during the first 15 min, since most severe reactions will be evident by then. The patient should be kept warm and well covered to prevent chills that might otherwise be interpreted as a reaction. Elective transfusions at night should be discouraged, since observation of the patient is more difficult and his sleep is disturbed.

If any untoward reaction appears to be related to transfusion (see COMPLICATIONS OF TRANSFUSION, below), the transfusion should be stopped and the blood bank notified so that an investigation can begin. *That unit should not be restarted.* Unless the clinical situation is urgent, it is best to delay further transfusions until the cause of the reaction is known.

TABLE 93–5. USE OF "FRESH" BLOOD, AND REASONABLE ALTERNATIVES

Clinical Indication	Realistic Definition of "Fresh" Blood (Assuming CPD RBCs or WB)*	Reasonable Substitutes
Bleeding due to massive blood replacement	< 12 h	Platelet concentrates plus RBCs**
Open-heart surgery, before and during extracorporeal circulation	Preferably < 1 wk	Bank or frozen-thawed RBCs plus volume expanders
Open-heart surgery, oozing after extracorporeal circulation	< 12 h	Platelet concentrates plus bank RBCs
Optimal RBC survival and function	< 1 wk	RBCs stored < 1 wk, or frozen-thawed RBCs
Exchange transfusion	< 1 wk	Bank or frozen-thawed RBCs plus fresh plasma
Liver failure	< 1 wk	Bank or frozen-thawed RBCs plus fresh plasma
Chronic renal disease	< 1 wk	Frozen-thawed or leukocyte-poor RBCs

* CPD = citrate phosphate dextrose solution; RBCs = red blood cells; WB = whole blood.

** Some patients may also need fresh plasma and occasionally fibrinogen or cryoprecipitated antihemophilic factor (AHF).

Modified from D. W. Huestis, "Fresh Blood: Fact and Fancy," in *A Seminar on Current Technical Topics.* Copyright 1974 by the American Association of Blood Banks. Used with permission of the Association and the author.

Divided transfusions (one half one day, one half the next) should be avoided, since this increases the hazard of bacterial growth. When incipient heart failure or hypervolemia is a concern, washed RBCs should be used and a whole unit given in the usual way. Otherwise, to prevent overload, some of the patient's own blood may have to be removed as RBCs are given. For small pediatric transfusions, the blood bank can provide blood or RBCs in multiple interconnected bags which can be subdivided with safety.

IMMUNOHEMATOLOGY

General Principles

Clotted blood is optimal for determining antigens on the RBCs and antibodies in the serum. Blood from a skin puncture may be added directly to isotonic saline for RBC typing. Washed, resuspended RBCs from anticoagulated blood (citrate, oxalate, or EDTA) may also be used. Cells are tested against antisera, and serum against test RBCs of known type, and the presence or absence of agglutination or hemolysis is recorded. Scrupulous attention to both technical and clerical details is vital to avoid errors that may have catastrophic consequences. Reagent manufacturers' instructions should be followed.

ABO and Rh Typing

The four ABO blood groups are determined by testing for the presence or absence of A and B antigens on the RBCs using Anti-A and Anti-B reagents (forward or cell typing), and by testing for Anti-A and Anti-B in the serum using reagents A and B RBCs (serum or reverse typing). A confirmatory cell typing with anti-A,B is also advised. See TABLE 93–6 for the test results seen in each of the four groups. Both cell typing and serum typing are done routinely, because the serum and cell grouping occasionally disagree. When this occurs, the true group must be identified by testing with additional reagents before proceeding with a transfusion. Cell typing is done in test tubes or on slides. Reverse typing should be done by a tube technic because, with the less sensitive slide method, weakly agglutinating Anti-A and Anti-B may lead to misclassification.

As a rule, blood selected for transfusion must be of the same ABO type as the recipient. In urgent situations, type O RBCs may be used for patients of other blood types, or *either* A or B RBCs may be used for AB recipients (*not* both together).

Rh typing should be done routinely whenever ABO typing is done. The test determines whether the Rh factor $Rh_o(D)$ is present (Rh-positive) or absent (Rh-negative) in the RBCs.

Rh$_o$ Variant (D^u) Test

Occasionally, RBCs that have a weakly reacting Rh factor, called Rh$_o$ Variant (D^u), will react negatively in the Rh typing test but will be agglutinated by Anti-Rh$_o$(D) if the more sensitive indirect antiglobulin method is used. If an apparently Rh-negative blood specimen is from a donor or a pregnant woman or her mate, the test for Rh$_o$ Variant (D^u) should always be done. If the Rh-negative blood specimen is from a prospective recipient of a transfusion, the Rh$_o$ Variant (D^u) test need not be done. Persons positive for D^u are considered Rh-positive.

Except for life-threatening emergencies when Rh-negative blood may not be available, Rh-negative patients should always receive Rh-negative blood. Rh-positive patients may receive either Rh-positive or Rh-negative blood.

Screening for Unexpected Antibodies

Routine screening for unexpected RBC antibodies is done on each blood specimen submitted for blood grouping; i.e., blood from donors, recipients, and prenatal patients. Unexpected antibodies are specific for RBC blood group antigens other than A and B, such as Rh$_o$(D), Kell (K), Duffy (Fy^a), and hr'(c). Early detection of such antibodies is important because they can cause hemolytic disease of the newborn and serious transfusion reactions, and they greatly complicate and delay the cross-matching and procurement of compatible blood. Serum is screened for the presence of such an

TABLE 93–6. CHARACTERISTICS AND REACTIONS
OF THE FOUR ABO BLOOD TYPES

ABO type	Red Cells				Serum		
	Antigens present	Reactions with reagents			Antibody present	Reactions with reagents	
		Anti-A	Anti-B	Anti-A, B		A Cells	B Cells
O	Neither	−	−	−	Anti-A & -B	+	+
A	A	+	−	+	Anti-B	−	+
B	B	−	+	+	Anti-A	+	−
AB	A&B	+	+	+	Neither	−	−

antibody by multiple agglutination tests including the sensitive indirect antiglobulin technic, using Group O reagent human RBCs. This reagent is a pool of carefully selected Group O Rh-positive and Rh-negative RBCs that are jointly positive for most important RBC antigens.

Antibody Identification

Once an unexpected antibody is demonstrated by screening, its identity should be determined by testing the serum against a panel of Group O reagent RBCs of known antigenic composition. Further studies such as antibody elution and absorption and subtyping of the patient's RBCs may be required. Knowing the identity of an irregular RBC antibody is helpful for future transfusion therapy or for prognosis and management of hemolytic disease of the newborn if such an antibody is found in the serum of a pregnant woman.

Antibody Titration

When an irregular RBC antibody, especially of Rh specificity, is identified in the serum of a pregnant woman, it should be titrated to estimate its strength, even though there is poor correlation between the maternal antibody titer and the severity of hemolytic disease in the incompatible fetus. A significant rise in antibody titer means that the fetus carries the antigen and may be affected. In such cases, repeated spectrophotometric examination of the amniotic fluid for bilirubin is the only way to monitor directly the condition of the fetus.

Antiglobulin Testing

The **direct antiglobulin (Coombs') test** detects antibodies that coat the patient's RBCs. Washed RBCs are treated with Antihuman Serum and observed for agglutination. The test is done on the cord blood of babies of Rh-negative mothers, or of any babies suspected of having hemolytic disease of the newborn caused by maternal antibody. This test is also used to investigate anemias. If positive, it suggests an autoimmune hemolytic anemia that may be spontaneous or indicative of underlying lymphoma or SLE.

The **indirect antiglobulin test** aids in the recognition of an antibody in the serum and is done by in vitro incubation of normal RBCs with the unknown serum. The test RBCs are then washed in saline and Antihuman Serum is added; agglutination indicates the presence of an antibody (adsorbed from the unknown serum) coating the cells. This part of the routine for cross-match and antibody detection is sometimes positive in autoimmune hemolytic anemias.

Cross-Match Testing

After determining the ABO and Rh type and doing antibody screening on both prospective recipient and donor bloods, cross-matching tests must be done to ensure that the recipient's serum does not contain antibodies that will react with the transfused RBCs. Cross-matching procedures are designed to detect IgG as well as IgM antibodies. A high-protein procedure or enzyme-modified RBCs may be used, but the indirect antiglobulin test is essential in all cases.

Even if the antibody screening test on the patient's serum is negative, an incompatibility may still be found on cross-match, since the donor RBCs may have an antigen not present in the reagent RBCs used for screening, or may have an antigen in a more reactive form. If the recipient has a positive screening test, his antibody should be identified and prospective donor blood should be pretested with the corresponding reagent antiserum, if it is available and if there is time, to select blood donor units negative for the RBC antigen concerned. In an emergency, units compatible by cross-match may be transfused before such identification and donor testing have been completed.

As a rule, the cross-match must be compatible before a transfusion is given. The few exceptions usually concern patients with autoantibodies.

Donor whole blood with an irregular antibody is not usually used for transfusion, but it is suitable for partial use as frozen-thawed or washed RBCs. Antibodies active only at room temperature or below can be disregarded in donor blood. A "minor" cross-match, testing donor serum against recipient's RBCs, can be done, but most authorities consider it superfluous if a proper antibody screening test is done.

Rh Immune Globulin

$Rh_o(D)$ immune globulin must be given to every Rh-negative mother immediately after every abortion or delivery (live or stillborn) unless the baby is $Rh_o(D)$- and D^u-negative, or if the mother's serum already contains Anti-$Rh_o(D)$.

Preparatory testing is done on dual specimens: (1) **Cord blood** is analyzed for ABO and Rh type, including Rh_o Variant (D^u); and a direct antiglobulin test is done. (2) **Maternal blood** drawn immediately postpartum is analyzed for ABO group and Rh type, including Rh_o Variant (D^u), and antibody screening and identification are done. An apparent maternal D^u-positive result may indicate a fetomaternal bleed and should be interpreted with caution.

Genotyping of Mates

The mate of every Rh-negative woman should be Rh-typed. If he is also Rh-negative, Rh hemolytic disease in the newborn is most unlikely, although the possibility of other antigens' causing the disease should be borne in mind. If he is Rh-positive, his zygosity for the Rh factor (Rh genotype) should be determined for purposes of genetic counseling, for estimating prognosis, and for planning management if maternal anti-Rh appears during a pregnancy. The probable zygosity is determined by testing the mate's RBCs with the common Rh reagents, anti-$Rh_o(D)$, anti-rh'(C), anti-rh"(E), anti-hr'(c), and anti-hr'''(e), and evaluating the results statistically. *If the mate of an Rh-sensitized woman is homozygous Rh-positive, every fetus will be affected with Rh hemolytic disease*; if he is heterozygous, there is a 50% chance that each fetus will be Rh-negative and therefore free from hemolytic disease.

COMPLICATIONS OF TRANSFUSION

Reactions that accompany or follow IV administration of blood or blood components. The more serious reactions occur during the transfusion.

HEMOLYTIC REACTIONS

Reactions accompanied by hemolysis of the recipient's or the donor's RBCs—usually the latter—during or following the administration of solutions, plasma, blood, or blood components. The most severe reaction occurs when donor RBCs are hemolyzed by antibody in the recipient's plasma.

Etiology

Hemolysis can result from blood group incompatibility, incompatible plasma or serum, hemolyzed or fragile RBCs (e.g., by overwarming stored blood or contact with inappropriate IV solutions), injections of distilled water or nonisotonic solutions, or instillation of water into the bladder following transurethral prostatic resection.

Incompatibility is the most frequent cause of hemolysis despite advances in blood grouping and cross-matching. Human error (e.g., mislabeling or confusing samples or blood containers) is usually responsible. Poor laboratory technic, including inadequate cross-matching or incorrect identification of the ABO group or Rh type of both donor and recipient, is less common.

Except in an emergency, Rh-negative recipients should receive only Rh-negative blood. Routine typing for other Rh factors (e.g., hr'[c]) is unnecessary. Recipients who have formed any blood group antibody must *always* receive blood negative for the antigen in question.

Antibodies against blood group antigens other than ABO or Rh may occur naturally or may be acquired as a result of transfusion or pregnancy. They can cause a hemolytic transfusion reaction or fetal erythroblastosis. The most important of these are anti-Kell (K) and anti-Duffy (Fyª). Although cross-matching will detect almost all such antibodies, an occasional patient will have a hemolytic reaction despite negative pretransfusion tests.

Group O whole blood, the plasma of which contains Anti-A and Anti-B of the hemolytic or IgG (incomplete) form, may be dangerous when given in emergencies to a recipient with another blood group. Tests to determine hemolytic or incomplete Anti-A and Anti-B are unreliable. The plasma containing most of the antibody should be removed first. Adding specific A and B substances to Group O blood is *not* recommended, since the dangerous IgG antibodies are not neutralized and the material itself may cause anaphylactic reactions.

Symptoms, Signs, and Diagnosis

Hemolytic reactions vary in severity depending on the degree of incompatibility, the amount of blood given, the rate of administration, and the integrity of the kidney, liver, and heart. Onset is usually acute and may occur during or immediately following a blood transfusion; rarely, later. The patient complains of discomfort and anxiety, or may have no symptoms. He may have difficulty in breathing, precordial oppression, a bursting sensation in the head, flushing of the face, and severe pain in the neck, the chest, and especially the lumbar area. Evidence of shock may appear, with a rapid feeble pulse, cold clammy skin, dyspnea, fall in BP, nausea, and vomiting. This acute phase usually develops within 1 h. Free Hb may be found in the plasma and urine, followed by an elevated serum bilirubin and clinical jaundice.

After the acute phase, one of several courses may follow: (1) no further symptoms; (2) temporary oliguria with mild nitrogen retention, then complete recovery; (3) more persistent oliguria, then possibly anuria and uremia, with death in 5 to 14 days. Prolonged oliguria is a poor prognostic sign. When recovery occurs, it is usually marked by diuresis with elimination of retained nitrogenous wastes.

Hemolytic reactions may occur under general anesthesia, when most of the symptoms are masked. The only evidence may be uncontrollable bleeding at the site of incision and from mucous membranes, caused by an associated disseminated intravascular coagulation syndrome.

An important quick aid to diagnosis is to take a blood sample from the patient immediately, centrifuge it, and examine it visually for serum Hb. Significant hemolysis will be clearly visible as a pink to dark red color.

For medicolegal reasons, pretransfusion specimens of both the donor's and the patient's blood should be retyped and again cross-matched. Post-transfusion samples from patient and donor blood should also be retyped and cross-matched again to check on any possible technical or clerical errors or mislabeling of the initial samples.

Prognosis

This depends primarily on the amount of blood given, the degree of incompatibility, and the clinical condition of the patient. Shock at the time of the reaction is a grave prognostic sign. Diuresis is usually a happy sign. Significant permanent kidney damage is unusual.

Prophylaxis

Hemolytic reactions may be avoided by meticulous identification and indelible labeling of patient blood samples intended for cross-matching, and by equally careful identification of donor blood and of the recipient at the time of transfusion. Also important are proper storage of blood; avoidance of warming of blood; allowing 15 min to give the first 50 ml, with close observation for untoward reactions; and careful and complete laboratory procedures to detect incompatibilities. Serious sequelae may be avoided by prompt interruption of the transfusion at the onset of symptoms and by adequate treatment.

Treatment

The transfusion should be stopped. Immediate manifestations are treated symptomatically. Blankets may be used to relieve chills. To establish osmotic diuresis, an infusion of 20 gm of mannitol (e.g., 100 ml of 20% solution) should be started at once and continued at a rate of 10 to 15 ml/min until 1000 ml have been given.

If diuresis ensues, the mannitol infusion should be continued to a maximum of 100 gm/day, or volume may be maintained with other IV fluids until hemoglobinemia and hemoglobinuria have cleared. If no urine appears, the patient should be treated for acute renal failure (see Ch. 145).

FEBRILE REACTIONS

Reactions consisting of chills, fever with a rise of at least 1 C, and sometimes headache and back pain, rarely progressing to cyanosis and shock.

In some patients, after many transfusions or pregnancies, leukocyte antibodies appear in response to the antigens of transfused or fetal WBCs. These antibodies may react with the WBCs in succeeding transfusions to produce a reaction. When symptoms occur repeatedly with the use of otherwise compatible blood, further transfusions should utilize leukocyte-poor or frozen-thawed RBCs. Rarely, febrile reactions can be caused by bacterial pyrogens in solutions or tubing, but these have been almost completely eliminated by the use of disposable infusion sets.

ALLERGIC REACTIONS

Reactions due to hypersensitivity of the patient to an unknown component in the donor's blood are common, usually due to allergens in the donor plasma, or, less often, to antibodies from an allergic donor. Immunized IgA-deficient patients may react violently (anaphylaxis) to IgA in donor plasma.

Symptoms and Signs

Allergic reactions are usually mild, with urticaria, edema, occasional dizziness, and headache during or immediately after the transfusion. Less frequently, dyspnea, wheezing, and incontinence may be present, indicating a generalized spasm of smooth muscle. Rarely, anaphylactic shock may occur.

Prophylaxis

In a patient with a history of known allergies or an allergic transfusion reaction, an antihistamine may be given immediately before or at the beginning of the transfusion (e.g., diphenhydramine 50 mg orally or IM). *It must never be mixed with the blood.*

Treatment

Stop the transfusion immediately. An antihistamine is usually sufficient in mild cases (e.g., diphenhydramine 50 mg IM). For more severe reactions, epinephrine 0.5 to 1 ml of 1:1000 solution s.c. (or, in extreme emergencies, 0.05 to 0.2 ml diluted and injected slowly IV) should be given. A parenteral corticosteroid (e.g., dexamethasone sodium phosphate, 4 to 20 mg IV) may occasionally be required.

CIRCULATORY OVERLOADING

In heart disease with chronic anemia, when the cardiac musculature and reserve are likely to be deficient, transfusions may raise the venous pressure and cause heart failure, rapid pulse, falling BP, rapid, shallow breathing, pulmonary edema, and cyanosis.

Prophylaxis: When such patients must be transfused, *whole blood is contraindicated.* A rise in venous pressure can be avoided by infusing packed RBCs at a slow-to-moderate rate. The patient should be observed for evidence of increased venous pressure or pulmonary congestion. If possible, direct observation of venous pressure during the course of the infusion is a useful precaution. If packed RBCs cause congestion, or must be given at an unduly slow rate (e.g., > 2 h/u.), it is better to use washed RBCs. Prolonged transfusions pose a hazard of bacterial growth because the blood quickly reaches ambient temperature.

Treatment

The transfusion should be discontinued, and treatment for congestive heart failure should begin immediately (see in discussion of acute pulmonary edema associated with right ventricular failure under CONGESTIVE HEART FAILURE in Ch. 25).

AIR EMBOLISM

Transmission of large amounts of air into the vein is potentially dangerous and can cause foaming of blood in the heart with consequent inefficiency of pumping, leading to heart failure. It is largely a complication of pressure infusion of blood from rigid glass bottles, but can also happen when changing IV sets or by erroneously venting a plastic blood bag.

Prophylaxis consists of guarding attentively against air in tubing with any pressure infusion and when changing IV sets. **Treatment** involves turning the patient on his left side, head down, to allow the air to escape a little at a time from the right atrium.

MICROAGGREGATES

Standard blood transfusion sets include a filter that traps the few visible clots and fibrin shreds present in stored blood units. In proportion to the duration of storage, blood also forms microaggregates—microscopic collections of platelets, leukocytes, and fibrin. These microaggregates can be detected in the lungs after massive transfusions and have been incriminated as a cause of the syndrome of post-traumatic pulmonary insufficiency, though direct evidence is lacking.

This potential hazard can be avoided by the use of special microaggregate filters which remove particles as small as 20 to 40 μ. Their use is advised only for patients likely to receive very large amounts of blood that has been stored $>$ 5 or 6 days. (CAUTION: *Since these special filters may also remove platelets, platelet transfusions should not be passed through them.*)

EFFECTS OF COLD

Rapid transfusion of ice-cold blood can chill the patient's heart and cause arrhythmia or arrest. This can be avoided by the use of an IV set that includes a heat exchange device to warm blood gently during delivery. In no case should blood be warmed above 37 C (98.6 F). Warming devices applied to the blood container itself, such as microwave warmers, are contraindicated because (1) a high incidence of hemolysis occurs, (2) any interruption in transfusion may result in warmed blood remaining connected while bacteria grow, and (3) the blood bank has no way of knowing if an unused unit of blood may have been warmed and rechilled.

MASSIVE TRANSFUSION COMPLICATIONS

When a patient receives large amounts of stored blood in a short time (e.g., $>$ 20 u. in a day), his own blood is in effect washed out and the deleterious effects of storage on donor blood may become important, though such complications rather seldom occur.

Bleeding tendency is manifested by abnormal oozing and continued bleeding from raw and cut surfaces. This is associated with the patient's loss of platelets, and regular stored blood does not contain useful numbers. Since clotting factors other than platelets are seldom involved, platelet concentrates should be given; 4 are usually enough for an adult. If these are unavailable, very freshly collected RBCs usually will be effective (see TABLE 93–5), but they should not be given to patients on extracorporeal circulation until the pump has been discontinued.

Citrate and potassium: Patients with liver failure may be unable to metabolize citrate; those with chronic renal disease may have a problem with potassium. These overrated hazards are reduced by removal of plasma from donor blood. Potassium accumulation is insignificant in blood stored $<$ 1 wk (see TABLE 93–2).

OXYGEN AFFINITY

Older stored blood has an increased affinity for O_2, caused by a decrease in RBC 2,3-diphosphoglycerate **(DPG)**. As a result, it releases O_2 to the tissues abnormally slowly. With the possible exception of exchange transfusions in erythroblastotic babies and some patients with severe cardiac deficiency, little clinical evidence shows that DPG deficiency has a significant effect on the recipient; in fact, it is rapidly restored after transfusion. RBCs collected in CPD and CPDA-1 have adequate DPG during the first 2 wk of storage (see TABLES 93–1 and 93–2).

INVESTIGATION AND REPORTING OF REACTIONS

All transfusion reactions, even those that seem inconsequential, should be investigated and reported in writing. The investigation can be minimal in minor reactions (e.g., allergic), but should be full and complete for any suspected hemolytic reactions. A scheme of investigation is given in TABLE 93–7. The report may omit laboratory details, although the blood bank should keep a permanent record of these, but it should include an interpretation of results as well as recommendations regarding the handling of future transfusion therapy.

TABLE 93–7. SCHEDULE OF INVESTIGATION OF REPORTED TRANSFUSION
REACTIONS

I. **All reported reactions**
   A. Specimens needed:
      1. Pretransfusion blood of recipient
      2. Posttransfusion blood of recipient
   B. Investigation (numbers refer to specimens listed above)
      Check donor and patient identification and crossmatch report
      Repeat ABO and Rh typing (2)
      Direct antiglobulin test (2)
      Examine for visible hemolysis (2); if necessary, compare (2) with (1)

If these procedures reveal no evidence of incompatibility or hemolysis and if there is no additional
information to arouse suspicion, no further investigation is needed. Otherwise, proceed as follows:

II. **If there is evidence of hemolysis or incompatible transfusion***
   A. Specimens needed:
      1. Pretransfusion blood of recipient
      2. Posttransfusion blood of recipient
      3. Pilot samples of donor blood
      4. Blood from container implicated in reaction
      5. Posttransfusion urine
   B. Immunologic investigation
      Repeat ABO, Rh, and direct antiglobulin test (1,3,4)
      Repeat crossmatch (1,2,3,4 if indicated—major; minor only if indicated)
      Repeat antibody screen (1,2,3—special, sensitive technics if necessary)
      Identification of any unexpected antibody or incompatibility
   C. Other procedures as indicated
      Serum haptoglobin (1,2)
      Bacteriologic smear and culture (4)
      Serum urea and bilirubin (1,2)
      Urine hemoglobin (5)
      Urine hemosiderin (5)
      Nonimmune causes of hemolysis

* The procedures and specimens listed are generally applicable. Different approaches may be
needed for particular cases.

From *Practical Blood Transfusion* by D. W. Huestis, J. R. Bove, and S. Busch, ed. 3, 1981. Used with
permission of Little, Brown and Company and the author.

DISEASE TRANSMISSION

Virus hepatitis may follow the infusion of whole blood, plasma, or other products prepared from
human blood, notably fibrinogen. Serum albumin and plasma protein fraction, which have been
heated to 60 C for 10 h during preparation, are, with rare exceptions, noninfectious. Depending on
the geographic area and the methods used for testing, **hepatitis B surface antigen** (HBsAg) is detectable in the blood of 0.05% to 1 or 2% of donors. In pooled human plasma products such as fibrinogen and antihemophilic factor, it is disseminated in accordance with the size of the pool. It is active
in freshly frozen and liquid plasma.

Laboratory tests for HBsAg (required on all donor blood) permit detection of 30 to 60% of carriers;
the remainder are undetectable by present methods. This test will not detect **hepatitis A (infectious)**
or the non-A–non-B virus or viruses that now cause the majority of cases of post-transfusion hepatitis. Since hepatitis is known to be more prevalent in certain population groups (e.g., drug addicts,
commercial blood donors), avoidance of such donors and avoidance of unnecessary transfusions
are important preventive measures.

Bacterial infection: Despite careful preparation, from 2 to 5% of all blood drawn contains a few
bacteria, presumably from the skin of the donor. Most organisms will not grow in blood if it is refrigerated properly (4 to 10 C), but some will, mainly gram-negatives of the coliform or aerogenes
groups. Transfusion of heavily contaminated blood may be fatal. Procedures that allow blood to
reach room temperature (prolonged transfusions or warming blood) may greatly accelerate the
growth of any bacteria, and are potentially hazardous.

Malaria is transmitted easily by infected donor blood. Many donors are unaware that they have
malaria, certain varieties of which may be latent and transmissible for 10 to 15 yr. All prospective
donors must be asked whether they have ever had malaria or have been in a region where malaria is

prevalent. Donors who have had malaria or suppressive antimalarial therapy are disqualified for 3 yr; those who have been exposed to malaria without suppressive therapy should be deferred for 6 mo. Storage does not render blood safe.

Syphilis may be transmitted by fresh blood from a donor with the disease, but the incidence is very rare. Storing the blood for 96 h or more at 4 to 10 C kills the spirochete. An STS is required on all donor blood, but infective donors are often in a seronegative phase.

---

94. POLYCYTHEMIA

POLYCYTHEMIA VERA

A chronic, life-shortening, myeloproliferative disorder involving all bone marrow elements and characterized by an increase in RBC mass (erythrocytosis) and hemoglobin concentration.

Etiology, Incidence, and Pathophysiology

Polycythemia vera is classified with chronic myelocytic leukemia, myelofibrosis, and thrombocythemia as a **myeloproliferative disease.** The average age at onset is 60 yr, but 5% of patients are under 40 at age of onset. More often seen in males and in Jews, the disorder occurs in about 7:million persons.

There is hyperplasia of all bone marrow elements (erythrocytes, megakaryocytes, granulocytes, and fibroblasts). Hypervolemia, increased cardiac output, hyperviscosity, and the resultant impaired blood flow are responsible for most clinical manifestations.

With **myelofibrosis,** a late development, anemia occurs. Erythrokinetic patterns show that the total RBC volume decreases as the result of shortened RBC survival and progressive sequestration of RBCs in the spleen, but are incompletely compensated by increased synthesis of RBCs. As the disease progresses, the central marrow develops fibrosis, but the peripheral marrow (e.g., of the long bones), normally not involved in blood production, shows increased erythropoiesis; extramedullary hematopoiesis in the spleen, liver, and other sites becomes prominent.

Symptoms and Signs

Initial complaints, usually of recent onset (6 to 12 mo), are fatigue, decreased efficiency, difficulty in concentration, headache, drowsiness, forgetfulness, and vertigo. Pruritus is present in 50% of the patients, particularly after a hot bath. Rubor may be seen or patients may have normal skin color with only dusky redness of the mucous membranes, particularly the conjunctivas. Patients are not cyanotic. The retinal veins may be dark red, full, and tortuous. The spleen is usually palpable. Some patients are asymptomatic.

Laboratory Findings

The RBC count ranges from 6 to 10 million/cu mm. Hb levels exceed 18 gm/100 ml in men and 16 gm/100 ml in women. The Hct is above 54% in men and above 49% in women. The WBC count ranges from normal to 20,000/cu mm; basophilia may be present. The platelet count is usually increased. The recognition of absolute polycythemia (either vera or secondary) is based on an increased RBC mass. When measured with ^{51}Cr, the RBC mass exceeds 36 ml/kg in men and 32 ml/kg in women, and is sometimes more than twice normal (normal, 28 to 33 ml/kg in men; 24 to 29 ml/kg in women). Since the normal RBC mass is related to height, weight, and BSA, 20% of the overweight should be added to the ideal weight of obese patients to obtain comparable values on a per kg body weight basis.

Arterial blood gases (Sa_{O2} and P_{O2}) are normal. The leukocyte alkaline phosphatase score is > 100 in most patients (normal, 24 to 100). Elevated histamine levels in blood and urine may generate pruritus and an increased frequency of peptic ulcer. Serum B_{12} levels may exceed 900 pg/ml (normal, 200 to 900 pg/ml). Unsaturated B_{12} binding capacity may exceed 2200 pg/ml (normal, 900 to 1700 pg/ml).

The bone marrow shows hyperplasia of the RBCs, granulocytes, megakaryocytes, and sometimes fibroblasts; in 10% of patients the marrow is normal at the time of initial diagnosis; marrow iron is absent in 95% of patients.

Uric acid metabolism is often increased. Serum uric acid levels may be 3 to 4 times normal (normal, 3 to 7 mg/100 ml). Most patients develop hyperuricemia and hyperuricosuria.

Clinical Course and Complications

If phlebotomy is the only treatment, some degree of iron-deficiency anemia develops, manifested by microcytosis, low serum iron, and high total iron-binding capacity.

Anemia without evidence of iron deficiency is usually an early sign of **myelofibrosis,** which develops in both untreated and treated patients. An enlarged spleen; distortion of the RBCs into ovoid, elliptical, or tear-shaped cells; leukocytosis of 20,000 to 50,000/cu mm with a shift to the left; appearance of giant platelets with or without thrombosis; and presence of reticulin fibers in the bone marrow are characteristic findings. If bone marrow aspiration is impossible, bone marrow biopsy will show fibrosis. Extramedullary hematopoiesis becomes increasingly prominent.

The transition to acute, usually myeloblastic (occasionally erythroblastic), **leukemia** occurs rarely. The incidence is greater in patients treated with ^{32}P or chemotherapy than in those treated by phlebotomy. The blood smear shows many bizarre blast cells. The anemia becomes progressively more severe and the bone marrow shows diffuse infiltration with malignant cells. Death usually occurs in a few weeks.

Although platelets are plentiful, they do not function normally; therefore, thromboses (e.g., CVAs) and hemorrhages (e.g., GI) may develop, especially in untreated patients. The frequency of peptic ulcer is increased. Gouty arthritis occurs in $< 10\%$ of patients, mostly in later stages, and may be accompanied by uric acid kidney stones. Hemorrhage is a frequent surgical complication. If possible, patients should be in hematologic remission before surgery. Blood loss at surgery is replaced by whole blood transfusions.

Patients with polycythemia are medically (though not always legally) acceptable as blood donors. Recipients benefit from the relatively high Hct.

Diagnosis

Polycythemia vera must be considered in any man with a Hct $> 52\%$ and any woman with a Hct $> 49\%$. Other conditions that might raise the Hct should be considered; e.g., the use of diuretics or male hormones, the presence of congestive heart failure, accommodation to living at altitudes above 7000 ft, and smoking.

Minimal criteria for diagnosis are an elevated RBC mass, an Sa_{O_2} above 92%, and an enlarged spleen. Normal carboxyhemoglobins should be present. If the spleen is not enlarged, leukocytosis (especially basophilia) and elevations in the platelet count, leukocyte alkaline phosphatase score, serum vitamin B_{12} level, or B_{12}-binding capacity should be present.

Prognosis

Treatment reduces symptoms and appears to prolong life by reducing the incidence of thrombosis and hemorrhage. Adequately treated patients may remain in complete clinical and hematologic remission for many years, but complications usually develop after 5 to 10 yr. Average survival time with treatment is 13 yr. Death is usually due to myelofibrosis, acute leukemia, or diseases of old age.

Treatment

Phlebotomy is probably the safest therapy; it does not depress marrow function and is not mutagenic. Symptoms of hypervolemia are eliminated, but pruritus and symptoms of hypermetabolism remain. Iron-deficiency anemia usually develops following repeated phlebotomy. Phlebotomy is less effective in patients with high iron absorption rates or greatly elevated platelet counts (> 1.5 million/cu mm), and is inconvenient in patients with poor veins.

Usually, 3 to 6 phlebotomies are required to reduce the Hct to $< 50\%$ and to return the RBC mass to normal. Most patients tolerate a 500-ml phlebotomy 3 times/wk, but elderly patients with advanced arteriosclerosis or cardiac complications should have no more than 250 ml of blood removed at a time. Following the initial series of phlebotomies, the Hct should be maintained at 42 to 47%, if possible. The number of phlebotomies needed depends upon the patient's ability to absorb iron and thereby raise the Hct again. Since 1 pint of blood contains 250 mg of iron, a patient who absorbs 4 mg/day will need a phlebotomy every 2 mo; a patient who absorbs only 1.5 mg/day will need only 2 phlebotomies/yr. The average is 5 phlebotomies/yr.

When phlebotomy is the only therapy, supplemental iron must *not* be given, since it accelerates Hb production. A low-iron diet is impractical, but foods of very high iron content (e.g., clams, oysters, liver, legumes) should be avoided.

Phlebotomy followed by radiophosphorus (^{32}P) produces clinical and hematologic remission in almost all patients. Remissions usually last 18 mo, but vary from 6 mo to several years. Fewer follow-up visits are required and there are no immediate side effects, though about 10% of patients treated with ^{32}P develop acute leukemia, usually not until after > 10 yr of treatment.

Initially, 3 to 5 mCi (or 2.3 mCi/sq m BSA) of ^{32}P are given IV; if given orally, the dose should be increased 25%. The patient is seen at 3- to 4-wk intervals until remission is achieved. Platelets should begin to decrease in 2 wk, reaching a low point in 3 to 5 wk; RBCs usually begin to decrease in 1 mo, reaching a low point 3 to 4 mo after treatment. If there is no decrease in platelets or RBCs within 3 mo of initial treatment, an additional 2 to 3 mCi of ^{32}P are given. A 25% increase in dose is given 6 mo after initial treatment if there is still no remission. Once blood counts return to normal, patients are reexamined every 3 mo. The total initial effective dose is given at one time when relapse occurs.

Chemotherapy is no longer advised because of the risk of developing acute leukemia.

Hyperuricemia requires treatment with allopurinol. Gouty arthritis is treated as for primary gout.

OTHER CAUSES OF POLYCYTHEMIA

Reversible polycythemic values may be caused by smoking $> 1\frac{1}{2}$ packs of cigarettes a day, or inhaling when smoking cigars or a pipe; Hct can exceed 60%. The mechanism is the production of carboxyhemoglobin with an associated left shift of the Hb dissociation curve. This form of polycythe-

TABLE 94-1. CHARACTERISTIC FINDINGS IN SOME OF THE POLYCYTHEMIAS

	Hct	RBC Mass	Plasma Volume	Spleen	Arterial Oxygen	Erythro-poietin Production
Polycythemia vera	↑	↑	N	Enlarged	N	↓
Stress polycythemia	↑	N	↓	N	N	N
Secondary polycythemia (anoxia)	↑	↑	N	N	↓	↑
Secondary polycythemia (tumor)	↑	↑	N	N	N	↑

N = Normal; ↑ = increased; ↓ = decreased.

mia probably accounts for most individuals presenting with moderately elevated Hct values. For characteristic findings in some of the polycythemias, see TABLE 94-1.

In **stress polycythemia (stress erythrocytosis)**, the Hct is persistently elevated to 55 to 60%. Plasma volume, measured with ^{131}I-labeled albumin, is usually decreased to 36 to 41 ml/kg (normal, 44 ml/kg in men; 43 ml/kg in women). The RBC mass, measured with ^{51}Cr, is at the upper limits of normal. Since stress erythrocytosis is not true polycythemia, it does not require therapy.

Erythrocytosis secondary to arterial hypoxemia (secondary polycythemia) may be due to an arteriovenous shunt, pulmonary fibrosis, altitude hypoxia, and the pickwickian syndrome. At rest, Sa_{O_2} may be slightly decreased in polycythemia vera and normal in cardiopulmonary disease or respiratory alkalosis. Measured after exercise, Sa_{O_2} rises in patients with polycythemia vera and decreases in those with secondary polycythemia. After breathing 100% O_2, P_{O_2} values exceed 500 mm Hg in polycythemia vera but are under 400 mm Hg in secondary polycythemia. Sa_{O_2} may be particularly misleading in patients with respiratory alkalosis. Because the pH is above 7.4, the O_2 dissociation curve shifts to the left and Sa_{O_2} may be nearly normal despite depressed Pa_{O_2}. (See TABLE 94-2.) RBC mass is increased in both polycythemia vera and secondary polycythemia.

Tissue hypoxia and erythrocytosis occur in patients with some rare **hemoglobinopathies** associated with high O_2 affinity and a shift to the left in the O_2 dissociation curve. A patient with apparent polycythemia who is very young or has a family history of erythrocytosis should be suspected of having a hemoglobinopathy. The diagnosis can be confirmed by O_2 dissociation curve. Some of these mutant hemoglobins are identifiable on Hb electrophoresis.

Renal cysts and tumors are associated with erythrocytosis in < 5% of patients with an increased RBC mass. Removal of the lesions is curative.

Rarer causes of erythrocytosis include large uterine myomas, cerebellar angioblastoma, and hepatoma. Platelet and WBC counts are not increased and the spleen is not enlarged. The increased production of RBCs is probably due to excessive elaboration of erythropoietin.

TABLE 94-2. ARTERIAL O_2 VALUES IN POLYCYTHEMIA VERA AND HYPOXIA

	Normal		Polycythemia Vera		Hypoxia	
	Mean	Range	Mean	Range	Mean	Range
Sa_{O_2}(%)						
Rest	96	93–97	94	90–96	85	71–92
Exercise	96	92–97	94.5	92–96	77	60–95
Pa_{O_2} (mm Hg)						
Rest	88	67–97	71	64–80	55	43–63
Exercise	88	67–100	75	66–83	44	32–59

95. HEMORRHAGIC DISORDERS

Disorders characterized by a tendency to bleed.

Effective hemostasis requires the combined activity of vascular, platelet, and plasma factors as well as counterbalancing mechanisms to prevent excessive clotting. Defects, deficiencies, or excesses in any of these components can lead to hemorrhagic or thrombotic consequences.

Physiology

The fibrin clot is the end result of a sequence involving vascular, platelet, and coagulation phases. In the **vascular phase,** blood flow is reduced at the site of trauma: (1) by local vasoconstriction (an immediate reaction to injury) and (2) by mechanical pressure on injured vessels from blood extravasated into surrounding tissues.

The **platelet phase:** The platelet's role in hemostasis is critical because it adheres to and plugs the site of injury, releasing factors that augment vasoconstriction and platelet aggregation and initiate clotting via the intrinsic system (see below).

Circulating platelets ordinarily are nonadherent to each other or to normal endothelium, but when the endothelial lining of the vessel is broken, the platelets adhere to exposed subendothelial collagen. Next, membrane phospholipids are converted to arachidonic acid and thence to various prostaglandins, primarily **thromboxane A_2,** the potent vasoconstricting and platelet-aggregating agent. This substance produces platelet release of ADP (which stimulates further aggregation) as well as calcium, serotonin (another vasoconstrictor), and phosphatides (platelet factor 3) that provide a surface for plasma factor interactions. Within several seconds, platelets *adhere, aggregate,* and *release,* providing a firm platelet plug that obstructs further blood loss from a damaged vessel and serves as a meshwork for the fibrin clot (see also Hematologic Effects in Ch. 252).

The **coagulation phase** involves interaction of **coagulation factors** (plasma proteins) in addition to tissue thromboplastin and calcium. The factors are designated by Roman numerals (see TABLE 95-1), although earlier terminology uses fibrinogen, prothrombin, thromboplastin, and calcium for factors I-IV. Several theories account for the conversion of prothrombin to thrombin. One of these, the cascade or waterfall theory, states that the sequence begins when factor XII (Hageman factor) is changed to its active form, XIIa, by contact with foreign surfaces (collagen). In the presence of platelet factor III, activation of the factors XI, VIII, IX, X, and V leads to thrombin formation from prothrombin by the **intrinsic pathway** (see FIG. 95-1). Tissue substances released into the circulation from areas of injury or tissue breakdown outside the bloodstream also initiate thrombin formation. This coagulation sequence is called the **extrinsic pathway.** Both pathways require calcium and factors V and X, and both pathways terminate by activating factor X to factor Xa, which is the major amplification step for thrombin formation. The intrinsic pathway, which also requires factors VIII and IX, is sensitive to the activated forms of XI and XII and to the Fletcher and Fitzgerald factors, which represent kallikrein and high mol wt kininogen. The extrinsic pathway depends upon factor VII and is influenced minimally by contact activation; i.e., factor XII.

Formation of fibrin from fibrinogen is the next step in the coagulation phase. It is a thrombin-dependent reaction, as seen in FIG. 95-2, resulting from the proteolytic action of thrombin, which separates the small A and B peptides from the α, β, and γ double strands of the fibrinogen molecule. These peptides act as an antithrombin or inhibitor of blood coagulation and interfere with thrombin action to limit the size of the clot. Large fragments, the fibrin monomers, combine to form a gel that, in the presence of factor XIII (the fibrin stabilizing factor) and calcium, is transformed into a structured fibrin clot providing a sturdier clot, resistant to dissolution.

Clot retraction, which ensues, is produced by a contractile muscle-like protein (thrombasthenin) contained in platelets. The retracted clot is tough, resilient, and not easily friable when exposed to flowing blood.

The **fibrinolysin system,** responsible for clot resolution, becomes active when coagulation is completed. As seen in FIG. 95-3, circulating profibrinolysin (plasminogen) can be activated to the proteolytic enzyme fibrinolysin (plasmin) by a number of substances derived from tissues, by bacterial products (streptokinase), or by the plasma factor XII (activating prekallikrein, also known as Fletcher factor, to kallikrein) after contact with collagen. Kallikrein appears to be a major activator for this system. Urokinase in the urine may represent an excretory product of the activator. (Concentrates of urokinase as well as streptokinase are used therapeutically in thrombotic disorders to lyse clots.) Interaction of the fibrinolysin enzyme with fibrinogen or fibrin results in the breakdown of these molecules and formation of distinct fragments, designated X and Y, that have antithrombin activity. With further exposure to fibrinolysin, the X and Y fragments are degraded into smaller fragments (D and E) and finally into undesignated small peptides.

Naturally occurring inhibitors of the coagulation system are present in plasma and include **antithromboplastin, antithrombin** (called **antithrombin III**), and **antifibrinolysin,** in addition to less spe-

TABLE 95–1. COAGULANTS AND PROCOAGULANTS*

Factor	Comments
I. Fibrinogen	Precursor of fibrin (polymerized protein) which forms the clot structure.
II. Prothrombin	Precursor of the serine protease thrombin (converts fibrinogen to fibrin). Vitamin K-dependent, formed in the liver, and shares common properties with factors VII, IX, and X.
III. Thromboplastin	A tissue lipoprotein acts with factor VII to convert prothrombin to thrombin.
IV. Calcium	Necessary for prothrombin (and other factors) binding to lipid surfaces (platelet or tissue) prior to thrombin formation.
V. Accelerator globulin (AcG)	Factor Va is the active form. The rapid destruction of the active factor by thrombin does not permit identification of the activity in serum. Accelerates formation of thrombin.
VII. Serum prothrombin conversion accelerator (SPCA, convertin, stable factor)	A plasma and serum factor, part of the prothrombin complex produced in the liver. Vitamin K-dependent. Accelerates prothrombin conversion by interaction with thromboplastin. Adsorbed with $BaSO_4$, decreased by dicumarol, warfarin anticoagulants, remains in serum.
VIII. Antihemophilic globulin (Cofactor I, AHG) (Hemophilia A factor)	A plasma factor interacting with platelet factor III and factor IX to activate X to Xa which initiates prothrombin activation. Labile on standing, destroyed by thrombin, not present in serum, and bound to von Willebrand factor, which acts as a carrier.
IX. Plasma thromboplastin component (PTC, Christmas factor) (Hemophilia B factor)	A plasma and serum factor associated with platelet factor III and factor VIII. Becomes activated IXa and in turn activates VIII to VIIIa and X to Xa, which activates prothrombin. Stable on standing, adsorbed with $BaSO_4$, decreased by warfarin, vitamin K-dependent.
X. Stuart-Prower factor	A plasma and serum factor. Accelerator of prothrombin conversion, adsorbed with $BaSO_4$, decreased by warfarin, vitamin K dependent. (Xa, the active form, amplifies thrombin formation.)
XI. Plasma thromboplastin antecedent (PTA)	A plasma factor which is activated by Hageman factor, an accelerator of thrombin formation. XIa is the active form.
XII. Hageman factor (glass factor)	A plasma factor activated by negatively charged surfaces (glass, kaolin, fatty acids); activates PTA (XI), prekallikrein (plasminogen activator) and high mol wt kininogen and factor X.
XIII. Fibrin stabilizing factor	A plasma factor activated by thrombin to form a transamidase. Produces a strong fibrin clot that is insoluble in urea and resistant to destruction.
Fitzgerald factor (high mol wt kininogen)	Interacts with factor XII. Kinins are vasoactive and influence leukocyte migration.
Fletcher factor (prekallikrein)	Interacts with factor XII and Fitzgerald factor; activates both factors and accelerates thrombin formation through activation of factor XI. Kallikrein activates plasminogen (profibrinolysin).

* The letter (a) designates the active form of the factor.

cific protease inhibitors, α_2 macroglobulin, and α_1 antitrypsin. Antithrombin III, the physiologic circulating inhibitor of thrombin, is present in sufficient quantities to neutralize all thrombin activity that can develop in plasma. Antithrombin III, a **heparin cofactor**, acts with heparin to produce a marked immediate binding of thrombin, in contradistinction to the slow progressive inhibition of thrombin that occurs without heparin. Several other sources of antithrombin activity have been described: (1) the absorption of thrombin onto fibrin, (2) the activity of fibrinogen and fibrin degradation (split) products (see below), (3) the progressive binding of thrombin by α_2 macroglobulin, and (4) the

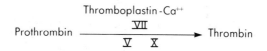

Extrinsic System: (Prothrombin Time)

$$\text{Prothrombin} \xrightarrow[\underline{\text{V}\quad\text{X}}]{\overset{\text{Thromboplastin -Ca}^{++}}{\underline{\text{VII}}}} \text{Thrombin}$$

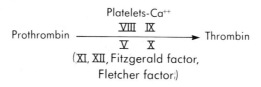

Intrinsic System: (Partial Thromboplastin Time)

$$\text{Prothrombin} \xrightarrow[\underline{\text{V}\quad\text{X}}]{\overset{\text{Platelets-Ca}^{++}}{\underline{\text{VIII}\quad\text{IX}}}} \text{Thrombin}$$
$$(\text{XI, XII, Fitzgerald factor,}$$
$$\text{Fletcher factor})$$

Fig. 95–1.   Thrombin formation.

nonspecific binding by abnormal proteins found in macroglobulinemia, multiple myeloma, etc. The other naturally occurring inhibitors, antithromboplastin, antifibrinolysin, and α_2 glycoprotein have similar capabilities for neutralizing thromboplastin and fibrinolysin respectively.

If the release of thromboplastin and tissue products is gradual and slow—probably a common occurrence *unrelated* to injury—the rate of action of the inhibitors is fast enough to block coagulation and prevent inappropriate clot formation. The inhibitors act slowly, however, when compared with the action of the clotting factors themselves, and as a result of these differential rates, clotting can develop at sites of injury if sufficient platelet lipid or thromboplastin is available. With injury, procoagulant activation is so rapid that the inhibitor system cannot interfere with clot formation, but it is available to neutralize activated clotting factors as they drift from the site of injury.

Laboratory Tests

To evaluate hemostatic disorders, 5 primary screening tests identify vascular, platelet, or plasma coagulation phase abnormalities (see TABLE 95–2). These are the bleeding time, platelet count, clot retraction, prothrombin time, and partial thromboplastin time.

The **bleeding time** indicates the effectiveness of platelet thrombus formation. The Ivy method is preferred, which uses a BP cuff on the upper arm inflated to 40 mm Hg. A stab wound with a lancet or No. 11 scalpel blade is made on the volar aspect of the forearm. The time is recorded and the blood is absorbed on the edge of a piece of filter paper at 30-second intervals until all bleeding has stopped. Normal bleeding time is < 5 min. It is prolonged in severe thrombocytopenia, platelet dysfunction syndromes, vascular defects, and mixed abnormalities such as von Willebrand's disease.

Platelet counts can be estimated by examining a blood smear, prepared immediately from unanticoagulated blood. Platelet clumping and morphology also can be noted. More precise counts are usually performed in the laboratory.

Clot retraction and observation consists of collecting about 5 ml of blood in a tube without anticoagulant. The clot usually starts to separate from the walls of the tube in 30 to 60 min and is usually completely separated in 12 to 24 h. The retracted clot should not change significantly for 72 h.

Since proper clot retraction depends upon normal platelet number and function, clot retraction is delayed, impaired, or absent when platelets are decreased or function abnormally. If a clot forms and

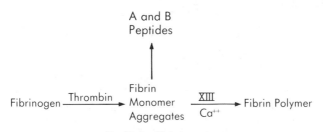

$$\text{Fibrinogen} \xrightarrow{\text{Thrombin}} \overset{\uparrow}{\underset{\text{Aggregates}}{\underset{\text{Monomer}}{\text{Fibrin}}}} \xrightarrow[\text{Ca}^{++}]{\underline{\text{XIII}}} \text{Fibrin Polymer}$$

(A and B Peptides)

Fig. 95–2.   Fibrin formation.

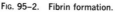

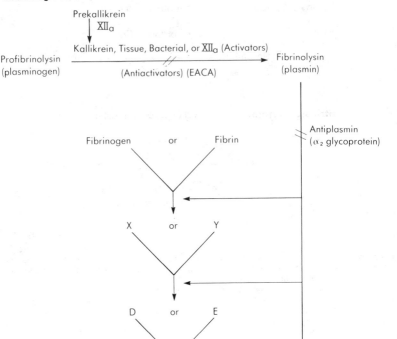

FIG. 95–3. **Fibrinolysin system.**

then becomes fluid, clot lysis has occurred. More elaborate studies for fibrinolysis (euglobulin lysis time, thrombin time, tests for split products of fibrin) should then be considered.

The **partial thromboplastin time (PTT) and prothrombin time (PT)** measure plasma factor activity as indicated in TABLE 95–2. Both procedures require the presence of a substrate, prothrombin (which is activated to thrombin in the assay), and an indicator system in the form of fibrinogen, which is converted to the fibrin clot. If the concentrations of prothrombin and fibrinogen are adequate, the PTT indicates the presence of the hemophilic factors VIII and IX, the contact factors XI and XII, and the Fitzgerald and Fletcher factors, as well as V and X.

The PTT is an excellent screening test for single or multiple coagulation defects. It detects most patients with hemophilia and Christmas disease. Unexplained abnormalities can be clarified by assays of specific coagulation factors and by other tests which are usually performed in a coagulation laboratory. PTT is also used to monitor heparin therapy. The patient's plasma and a normal control plasma are treated with activated partial thromboplastin. The time in seconds that it takes for each to clot is recorded and compared.

The PT requires the presence of factor VII in addition to factors V and X. The time in seconds that it takes for clotting to occur when a small amount of thromboplastin extract is added to plasma is the prothrombin time. This is performed on a control specimen as well as on the patient's specimen. The PT is a valuable screening test for disordered blood coagulation in a variety of acquired conditions (e.g., liver disease, disseminated intravascular coagulation) and is useful for following therapy with coumarin anticoagulants. It should be emphasized that a "minor" prolongation of the PT may signify a major coagulation defect, since certain clotting factors may be greatly reduced without significantly prolonging the PT. Whenever the PT is consistently 4 or more seconds longer than the control time, further investigation is indicated.

Using the PTT and the PT, a factor deficiency can be identified and measured by combining plasma to be tested with plasma having a known deficiency. If the factor is present, the test plasma will correct the known deficient plasma; if absent, it will not. It is possible to obtain a quantitative measurement of each factor by determining the PT or PTT with varying mixtures of test and known

TABLE 95–2. LABORATORY TESTS OF COAGULATION

Coagulation Function or Phase	Test	Comments
Vascular and/or platelet function	Tourniquet test (Rumpel-Leede)	May indicate vascular fragility or thrombocytopenia
	Bleeding time (Ivy)	Requires platelet function (adhesion, aggregation, release, and clot retraction), also small amounts of platelet forms of factor V and fibrinogen
	Platelet count (or estimate)	Quantitation of platelet number
	Clot retraction	Measures thrombasthenin-ATP* activity
	Platelet aggregation	Mechanical procedure to determine platelet response to added ADP**, collagen, and epinephrine. Ristocetin aggregation measures von Willebrand factor activity
	Platelet adhesiveness	Platelet attachment to foreign surface (collagen, glass, etc.) requires von Willebrand factor
	Prothrombin consumption	Measures release of platelet factor III
	Platelet factor IV assay	Measures platelet factor IV (antiheparin factor) released in circulation in conditions with increased platelet turnover
	β–thrombo-globulin assay	Similar to platelet factor IV released from platelets during aggregation and found in circulation when platelet turnover is increased
Plasma factor function	Prothrombin time (PT)	Measures extrinsic system activity (factors I, II, V, VII, and X)
	Partial thromboplastin time (PTT)	Measures intrinsic system activity (factors I, II, V, VIII, IX, X, XI, XII, Fitzgerald, and Fletcher)
	Fibrinogen assay	Measured by the thrombin clotting time procedure
	Specific assays for factors V-XII	Requires depleted plasma or artificial substrate
Fibrinolytic activity	Euglobulin lysis time	Shortened with increased fibrinolytic activity, and prolonged in Fitzgerald and Fletcher factor deficiency
	Chromogenic assay	Measures profibrinolysin, fibrinolysin, and activators using a synthetic substrate, commercially available
Antithrombin activity (heparin)	Thrombin clotting time (TCT)	Measures antithrombin activity (heparin) and is affected by decreased antithrombin III
	Heparin cofactor assay	Measures antithrombin III
	Progressive antithrombin	Measures antithrombin III plus α_2 macroglobulin and other nonspecific antithrombins
Fibrin (fdp) and fibrinogen (FDP) degradation products (collectively designated as split products or FSP)	Protamine sulfate assay	Measures fibrin monomer and X fragments to lesser degrees
	Staphylococcal clumping	Measures products of thrombin- or fibrinolysin-induced degradation of fibrin or fibrinogen
	Immune assay	Measures all products of thrombin- or fibrinolysin-induced degradation of fibrin or fibrinogen, including residual fibrinogen
	(Latex clumping)	

* Adenosine triphosphate.
** Adenosine diphosphate.

deficient plasmas comparing values to a reference curve created by using mixtures of normal and deficient plasmas.

The terms **fibrin split products (FSP)** and **fibrin, or fibrinogen, degradation products (fdp or FDP)** are synonyms that refer to any fragment resulting from the enzymatic cleavage of fibrin or fibrinogen by either fibrinolysin or thrombin. They include the fibrin monomer, X, Y, D, and E fragments, and many small peptides. The *laboratory test* designated FSP (fibrin split products) customarily refers to detection of the fibrin monomer produced when thrombin acts on fibrinogen.

Small amounts of fdp/FDP are present in normal serum but fdp/FDP is markedly elevated in the serum of patients with thromboembolic conditions such as myocardial infarction, deep vein thrombosis, pulmonary emboli, and disseminated intravascular coagulation **(DIC)**. Resting levels of fdp/FDP are about 5 μg/ml; levels rise slightly after exercise or stress. The determination may be made by hemagglutination inhibition **(HI)** immunoassay, by the use of sensitized latex particles which agglutinate at concentrations > 2 μg/ml, or by radioimmunoassay **(RIA)**. The blood specimens must be collected in tubes that contain thrombin to enhance clotting and trypsin inhibitor to prevent fibrin degradation in the specimen after collection. The test may also be done on urine and shows increased levels with kidney disease. It may aid in distinguishing renal from bladder infections, the value being normal in the latter.

The presence of increased **fibrinolysin activity** is determined by measuring the lysis time of the euglobulin fraction of blood **(euglobulin lysis time)**. Euglobulin is an amorphous coagulum of various plasma proteins that precipitate from plasma when it is acidified slightly with acetic acid. The euglobulin fraction contains most of the fibrinolysin originally present in the whole plasma, whereas the antifibrinolysin remains in the supernatant. With fibrinolytic activity separated from antifibrinolytic, the former can act quickly to degrade any adjacent proteins, in this case the euglobulin fibrin gel that has entrapped the fibrinolysin. The time required for the euglobulin clot to lyse visibly is called the lysis time, normally about 1½ to 2 h. The test can measure increased fibrinolytic activity (shortened lysis times).

Other tests of blood coagulation of value for specific purposes are listed in TABLE 95-2 by categories in accordance with the function or phase that they test. Further information on the platelet count can be found under CLINICAL HEMATOLOGY in Ch. 230.

VASCULAR DISORDERS

Vascular disorders seldom lead to serious blood loss. The tourniquet test may be positive, but other laboratory tests of hemostasis and blood coagulation usually are normal; diagnosis must often be made from typical clinical findings.

COMMON PURPURA

The most common vascular bleeding disorder, manifested by increased bruising, and representing increased vascular fragility. This inherited condition occurs more frequently in women, particularly following menopause when estrogen levels decrease and thinning of subcutaneous tissue occurs. The result is **simple, or senile, purpura,** which most often affects fatty thigh tissue producing unsightly bruises rather than significant hemorrhage. The bleeding pattern is usually subcutaneous and, occasionally, mucosal. Enhanced surgical or traumatic bleeding also can occur. Vascular fragility can appear transiently as a result of fever, generalized illness, hypothyroidism, or exposure to certain drugs, especially aspirin. The defect is in the small vessels; however, qualitative platelet disorders can produce apparent increased vascular fragility due to the mutually dependent association of platelet and small vessel functions.

Laboratory findings reveal a positive tourniquet test and a normal or slightly prolonged bleeding time. Other coagulation studies are normal. No definitive therapy exists, but brief courses of corticosteroids may assist in reducing surgical or traumatic bleeding, and estrogen may be effective, particularly after menopause.

ALLERGIC PURPURA (Henoch-Schönlein or Anaphylactoid Purpura)

An acute or chronic vasculitis primarily affecting skin, joints, and the GI and renal systems. The process may result from formation of immune complexes of gamma globulin (IgG) that often follow a streptococcal infection and damage the vascular endothelium. Purpura results from the effusion of blood and plasma into subcutaneous, submucous, and subserous surfaces. Skin lesions vary in appearance, but such nonthrombocytopenic purpura usually is associated with erythema or urticaria and, in contrast to other purpuras, the lesions may be pruritic. Fever and malaise often are present, and effusions into the joints or viscera may produce joint pain **(Schönlein's purpura)** or bouts of abdominal pain **(Henoch's purpura).** The latter may mimic acute abdominal conditions. Renal disease occurs in 10% of cases, with kidney failure as the principal cause of mortality. The incidence of progressive renal failure is probably between 10 and 20%. Renal involvement may appear early or late. Hematuria and proteinuria (< 1 gm/day) are common findings with renal involvement, but the development of the nephrotic syndrome portends severe disease. Renal biopsy is useful to define the extent of the process. Typical early lesions are those of focal and segmental proliferative glomerulonephritis, but there may be diffuse glomerular involvement. The finding of crescentic changes in a majority of glomeruli predicts a poor outcome.

Laboratory findings are useful only to exclude other disorders. The **diagnosis** is largely based on recognition of the clinical findings. **Treatment,** except for the elimination of possible allergens, is primarily symptomatic. The use of corticosteroids usually is disappointing. Immunosuppressive therapy (cyclophosphamide) has been used in a few cases with some success. Exchange plasmapheresis represents another approach that may be of benefit in acute situations. Current therapy has not improved the outcome of diffuse disease with renal involvement. However, the disorder often is self-limited with a good prognosis.

HEREDITARY HEMORRHAGIC TELANGIECTASIA (Rendu-Osler-Weber Syndrome)

A vascular anomaly characterized by telangiectatic lesions of the skin and mucosa, inherited as an autosomal dominant trait. Small red-to-violet lesions consist of thin, dilated vessels that blanch on pressure and tend to bleed spontaneously or from trivial trauma; they often can be seen on the lips, oral and nasal mucosa, tongue, and the tips of the fingers and toes. Symptoms result from bleeding and a consequent anemia; in general they progress in severity with advancing age. Bleeding from superficial lesions may be profuse; that from mucosal lesions (epistaxis and GI bleeding) is more common and more serious. Rarely, involvement of visceral vessels may lead to systemic symptoms (e.g., pulmonary arteriovenous fistulas).

Diagnosis depends upon recognizing the characteristic lesions. If they are absent or overlooked, perplexing diagnostic problems may result, such as protracted and recurrent GI bleeding of "unknown" etiology. **Laboratory studies** usually are normal but may disclose evidence of acute hemorrhage or iron-deficiency anemia.

Treatment is nonspecific. However, estrogens administered systemically and corticosteroid nasal sprays (for nasal mucosal bleeding) have been effective. Accessible lesions may be treated with pressure, styptics, and topical hemostatics. Blood transfusions may be needed for acute hemorrhage. Iron therapy is frequently required on a continuous basis to replace iron lost in repeated bleeding.

MISCELLANEOUS VASCULAR PURPURAS

In **scurvy,** hemorrhage may be prominent. Bleeding gums, perifollicular petechiae on the thighs and buttocks, and large intramuscular or internal hemorrhages may occur. Periosteal hemorrhages are characteristic in children. For therapy see VITAMIN C DEFICIENCY in Ch. 78.

Autoerythrocyte sensitization (Gardner-Diamond syndrome) is characterized by spontaneous painful propagating ecchymoses that represent an immune reaction to the patient's erythrocyte stroma; the ecchymoses may be reproduced by injecting 0.1 ml of the patient's erythrocytes intradermally. Psychoneurotic disorders are associated with this condition.

Purpura associated with hypergammaglobulinemia in which vasculitis often is apparent may be related to various collagen disorders or dysproteinemias. Correction of the underlying disease produces improvement. Corticosteroids may be helpful.

PLATELET DISORDERS

Platelet disorders are considered in terms of a deficiency, either of numbers **(thrombocytopenia)** or of function **(thrombocytopathy).**

THROMBOCYTOPENIA

Disorders manifested by thrombocytopenia can be characterized by failure of production, increased destruction, increased utilization, or dilution, as outlined in TABLE 95–3. The **symptoms and signs** of all these conditions include bleeding into the skin (petechiae, ecchymoses) and from the mucosa (epistaxis; GI tract, GU, and vaginal bleeding). Bleeding into the CNS is uncommon as an early sign, while hemarthroses and delayed bleeding, characteristic of plasma factor deficiency, are rare. Splenomegaly, hepatomegaly, and lymphadenopathy usually are not seen unless other disorders are responsible for the thrombocytopenia (Hodgkin's disease, lymphosarcoma, Gaucher's disease, etc.). As a result of bleeding, anemia may develop and produce weakness, fatigue, and signs of congestive heart failure. The clinical course ranges from the appearance of mild obscure petechiae to severe intractable bleeding. Placental transfer of maternal antiplatelet antibodies may cause thrombocytopenia and purpura in the neonate.

Laboratory findings are the same regardless of etiology: a prolonged bleeding time, delayed prothrombin consumption, and deficient clot retraction. However, an accurate platelet count can obviate these tests. Other coagulation assays are normal, unless the thrombocytopenia is associated with another condition such as liver disease or disseminated intravacular coagulation **(DIC).**

Bone marrow aspirate is of value in excluding marrow failure due to a decrease or absence of megakaryocytes. The marrow may demonstrate displacement of megakaryocytes by tumor or fibrosis or diversion of marrow production as seen in leukemia or simply hypoplasia characterized by

TABLE 95-3. CHARACTERISTICS OF THROMBOCYTOPENIC DISORDERS

Production Failure (Megakaryocytopenia)	Increased Destruction (Megakaryocytosis)	Increased Utilization (Megakaryocytosis)	Dilution
Marrow hypoplasia: Idiopathic Irradiation Drugs (antineo- plastic, benzene compounds, chloramphenicol, etc.) Infection (TB, septicemia, etc.)	**Immune:** ITP* Drugs (quinine, quinidine, thiazides, sulfonamides) Post-transfusion (antibodies to platelet antigen Pla-1) Neonatal (maternal antibodies to infant platelet antigen Pla-1 or maternal ITP)	**DIC† syndromes:** Gram-negative septicemia (Schwartzman- Sanorelli reaction) HUS‡ TTP§ Hemangiomas Neoplasms Burn injury Traumatic injuries	**Massive blood replacement or exchange transfusion** (stored blood rapidly becomes platelet- poor)
Marrow displacement: Fibrosis (agnogenic myeloid metaplasia) Neoplasm Lymphoma Granuloma (TB, sarcoid, etc.) **Marrow diversion and dyspoiesis:** Leukemia Folic acid and B_{12} deficiency	**Hypersplenic:** Lymphoma Leukemia Agnogenic myeloid metaplasia Gaucher's disease **Toxic:** Alcohol Snake venom **Mechanical:** Extracorporeal circulation (renal dialysis, open heart procedures)		

* Idiopathic thrombocytopenia purpura.
† Disseminated intravascular coagulation.
‡ Hemolytic-uremic syndrome.
§ Thrombotic thrombocytopenic purpura.

increased marrow fat and a marked decrease in all cellular elements. Some drugs (see TABLE 95-3) and various toxic or infectious agents may cause hypoplasia, although many cases without known drug exposure are classified as idiopathic.

Management of thrombocytopenia caused by marrow damage or failure may require administration of platelet concentrates. Androgens have been advocated in hypoplastic disorders, primarily for stimulating erythropoiesis. Corticosteroids seem to be ineffective in this form of thrombocytopenia.

IDIOPATHIC THROMBOCYTOPENIC PURPURA (ITP) (Purpura Hemorrhagica; Werlhof's Disease)

Thrombocytopenia without a readily apparent exogenous cause or underlying disease is a common presentation of this condition characterized by increased platelet destruction. Although no specific etiology has been identified, occasionally an acute viral infection precedes the symptoms. Current evidence supports an immunologic basis, since most patients have antiplatelet antibodies that are identifiable on the platelet surface. Symptoms, signs, and laboratory findings are as described above under thrombocytopenia. The bone marrow aspirate generally reveals abundant megakaryocytes; most appear inactive or nonproductive.

The disorder occasionally is self-limited, but most adult forms require therapy. About 15% respond to corticosteroids (hydrocortisone 200 mg/day, or its equivalent, prednisone 60 mg/day orally in divided doses for 2 to 4 wk). Splenectomy can achieve a remission in 50 to 60% of those who fail to respond to steroids or who fail to maintain a remission when steroids are discontinued. Immunosuppressive therapy (cyclophosphamide and azathioprine) has been used effectively in some cases refractory to steroids and splenectomy; vincristine also is of value. Platelet concentrates can be administered for control of bleeding until more specific therapy takes effect; the short survival of platelets in this disease, however, limits their usefulness.

OTHER FORMS OF THROMBOCYTOPENIA

Other forms of thrombocytopenia result from increased platelet destruction (see TABLE 95-3). Specific drugs (such as quinine, quinidine, and chlorothiazide) appear to mediate the formation of platelet antibodies. When the drug is stopped, platelet values return to normal, usually within 1 wk. A direct toxic effect may be responsible for the thrombocytopenia of acute alcoholic intoxication. Specific viral disease (measles, infectious mononucleosis, etc.) may cause the nonidiopathic type often seen in the younger age group in which spontaneous remissions can be expected. Collagen disorders such as SLE can produce an immune form of thrombocytopenia similar to ITP. Steroids and splenectomy also are effective in this condition.

Thrombocytopenia due to **hypersplenism** (increased sequestration of platelets in the enlarged spleen) is associated with disorders that produce splenomegaly (see Ch. 100, below). Splenectomy is the only effective measure in these conditions, although transient responses may follow therapy (irradiation, chemotherapy, corticosteroids) that reduces the size of the spleen.

Increased platelet destruction is prominent in the syndrome of **disseminated intravascular coagulation** (see below). This pattern appears in the **hemolytic-uremic syndrome (HUS)**, but is less well-defined in **thrombotic thrombocytopenic purpura (TTP)** where antigen-antibody complex and complement appear to be more prominent. In both HUS and TTP, the erythrocyte survival time is shortened and occasionally the Coombs' test for antiglobulins is positive. HUS and TTP differ primarily in age of onset and in organ systems involved.

HUS occurs more frequently in children < 5 yr old, but can develop in adults. Although HUS in both groups usually follows an infectious illness, it may occur as a complication of pregnancy or following the use of oral contraceptives. Some patients with SLE may have a clinical presentation indistinguishable from either HUS or TTP.

HUS is characterized by acute renal failure, with thrombocytopenia and hemolytic anemia developing 5 to 10 days after the onset of GI or upper respiratory tract symptoms. Pallor, lethargy, and hypertension are common. In children, splenomegaly and hepatomegaly also are common. Classic signs of erythrocyte fragmentation can be seen in the stained blood smear and although fibrin degradation products can be found in the urine and serum, major consumption of clotting factors does not occur. Hematuria, RBC casts, and proteinuria usually are present. The major histologic findings in HUS are in the glomeruli and arterioles. Vascular changes correlate well with the clinical course. When renal dysfunction is mild, only glomerular endothelial cells swell; prolonged oliguria, however, is associated with lesions involving the media of renal arterioles, while large vessel thrombosis produces irreversible renal failure with cortical infarction. In most children, renal function improves within 1 mo, but adults usually develop progressive failure. Although steroids, anticoagulants (heparin), and antiplatelet drugs (dipyridamole) have been advocated, proof of their efficacy is lacking.

TTP shows a predilection for multiple organ involvement, whereas HUS involves the blood and the kidneys primarily. TTP occurs most commonly in young adults, with a higher incidence in women, and produces severe renal involvement in > 50% of cases. Neurologic complications, apparently the result of diffuse vasculitis, are common and frequently cause death. The disease is fulminant and proves fatal in 80% of cases. Renal failure occurs later in TTP than HUS. Although the hematologic findings are similar to those described for HUS, hemorrhagic complications are more common. Most patients are affected by renal involvement resulting in proteinuria, hematuria, and excretion of cellular casts.

The histologic features are similar to those in HUS except that thrombi in renal afferent arterioles are commoner in TTP. Renal arterioles may have a conspicuous proliferation of endothelial cells, while glomeruli may exhibit only endothelial cell swelling or segmental infarction. Tubular and interstitial changes are minimal and variable. Recent studies suggest that a widespread endothelial lesion is primarily responsible producing a pattern of disseminated platelet thrombi. The plasma clotting system is secondarily involved and the appearance of DIC with diminished levels of fibrinogen and factors V and VIII signals a terminal stage of the disorder.

Unlike HUS, TTP is almost universally fatal if untreated. Treatment with corticosteroids, dextran, anticoagulants, and splenectomy has had limited success. Antiplatelet drugs (dipyridamole and aspirin) in large doses (dipyridamole 600 mg or more daily), exchange transfusion and plasma administration (up to 1000 ml/day) have been beneficial in many cases. Plasmapheresis, 5 L exchange/day for as long as 30 days, should be initiated if administration of high-dose dipyridamole is not followed by clinical improvement and a significant increase in circulating platelets within 24 h. Failure of all recommended measures has been observed in > 30% of cases.

ABNORMALITIES OF PLATELET FUNCTION

In some patients the platelets are normal in number but functionally defective; defects are both congenital and acquired. In addition, a variety of common drugs inhibit platelet function. As a result, the bleeding time usually is prolonged. In a patient who provides a history of easy bruising and bleeding after tooth extractions, tonsillectomy, or other surgical procedures, finding of a normal platelet count and a prolonged bleeding time should suggest the possibility of a qualitative platelet defect. Most other routine coagulation screening tests, such as the PT, PTT, and clotting times, will be normal and will help to differentiate these patients from those with defects in the coagulation mechanism. Since platelets play a role in activation of the plasma clotting factors, an abnormal prothrombin consumption assay may be found as a result of defective release of the phospholipid platelet factor III. Special studies (i.e., platelet aggregation) not available in many laboratories may be needed to identify more specifically qualitative defects. Note that von Willebrand's disorder also will present with a similar clinical and laboratory pattern. The deficiency of the factor VIII-associated von Willebrand's factor may not be sufficient to prolong the activated PTT. Quantitative measurement of the von Willebrand factor, assay for factor VIII clotting activity and antigen may be necessary to rule out this possibility.

Therapy

In most congenital disorders, the only known therapy is transfusion of normal platelets to control bleeding episodes. When platelet dysfunction is associated with an acquired disorder, successful treatment of the underlying disease often results in improved platelet function. Drugs known to inhibit platelet function, such as those containing aspirin and anti-inflammatory agents used in the treatment of arthritis, should be avoided when optimum hemostasis is desired. Acetaminophen may be used to provide analgesia, as it does not inhibit platelet function.

HEREDITARY DEFECTS

Thrombasthenia: In this rare disorder, clot retraction is abnormal. The bleeding time is prolonged and the platelets are not aggregated by any concentration of ADP or by most other agents except ristocetin. On direct blood smear (obtained without anticoagulant), the platelets appear isolated without aggregates.

Defects of collagen-induced platelet aggregation: In this group of disorders, aggregation by collagen is abnormal and usually is due to an inability to induce thromboxane formation from membrane phospholipid which affects release of endogenous ADP, calcium, and other platelet substances responsible for platelet aggregation. Unlike the findings in thrombasthenia, aggregation by ADP (added to the platelets) is normal. Two broad types of defects may account for the inability to release ADP. In one, the platelets are deficient in the substances (serotonin, ADP) normally found in the storage granules **(storage-pool disease);** in another, the platelets contain these agents but are unable to release them. These disorders probably are heterogeneous; both familial and isolated cases are described. Acquired abnormalities of this type are common: aspirin and other drugs affect platelet aggregation and release in the same manner. A careful drug history must be obtained before considering a diagnosis of storage pool disorder.

Platelet disorders associated with abnormal platelet morphology: In one congenital disorder— **Bernard-Soulier syndrome**—unusually large platelets (some the size of RBCs) are found that do not adhere to glass or collagen and do not aggregate with ristocetin, but aggregate with other agents; because they lack the glycoprotein binding site, they are unable to bind to von Willebrand factor. Large platelets associated with functional abnormalities also are associated with the **May-Hegglin anomaly,** a thrombocytopenic disorder with abnormal leukocytes, and in the **Chédiak-Higashi** syndrome (see Vol. II, Ch. 25). In the **gray platelet syndrome,** platelets lacking granules have been reported; the platelets, which look like gray cytoplasmic fragments, do not aggregate or release with ADP, collagen, or epinephrine.

Platelet disorders associated with other congenital defects: Abnormal platelet function also has been found in the Wiskott-Aldrich syndrome, in Down's syndrome, and in the **TAR** (thrombocytopenia with absent radius) syndrome.

von Willebrand's disease: Although the prolonged bleeding time in these patients is due to an abnormality in platelet function during the primary arrest of bleeding, the basic defect is a plasma factor deficiency (see discussion in Vol. II, Ch. 25).

ACQUIRED PLATELET DYSFUNCTION

Abnormalities of platelet function are described in a wide variety of clinical disorders. The platelet defect in uremia is attributed to a low mol wt substance that accumulates in uremic blood; the defect usually disappears after dialysis. Other disorders with qualitative defects are cirrhosis, dysproteinemias, scurvy, pernicious anemia, SLE, the myeloproliferative disorders, and leukemia. In many of these disorders, thrombocytopenia also occurs frequently.

Drug-induced platelet defects: Among drugs that may inhibit collagen-induced platelet aggregation are the nonsteroidal anti-inflammatory agents such as aspirin, indomethacin, and phenylbutazone. The inhibitory effects on platelet function obtained by ingesting a single dose (0.3 to 1.5 gm) of aspirin may persist for 4 to 7 days. Aspirin also produces a modest prolongation of the bleeding time in normal subjects and may produce a marked increase in patients who have platelet dysfunction of other forms (e.g., von Willebrand disorder). The deleterious effect of dextran on hemostasis also is attributed to an inhibitory effect on platelet function. Other drugs that may inhibit platelet aggregation include the tricyclic antidepressants, antihistamines, and phenothiazines.

ACQUIRED COAGULATION DISORDERS

DEFICIENCY OF THE VITAMIN K-DEPENDENT COAGULATION FACTORS

A complex coagulation disorder due to a combined deficiency of factors VII, IX, X, and prothrombin. These factors are synthesized in the liver by a process that requires vitamin K; consequently, the combined deficiencies may result from diverse pathologic conditions (see VITAMIN K DEFICIENCY in Ch. 78). In the adult, chronic liver disease or oral anticoagulants such as warfarin and dicumarol, which compete with vitamin K, are frequently responsible for this coagulopathy. Postoperative patients receiving gut-sterilizing antibiotics without vitamin K supplements may develop this problem. In the newborn, a similar hemorrhagic disease may develop as a result of the vitamin K deficiency associated with inadequate vitamin K formation in the sterile gut, of maternal deficiency, and of liver immaturity.

Clinical signs include bleeding into the skin and mucosa, hematemesis, and melena. Bleeding from the umbilical cord and into the scalp are common in the newborn.

Laboratory findings: PTT and PT are prolonged. In liver disease, other hemostatic abnormalities may be present (e.g., increased fibrinolytic activity, thrombocytopenia).

Treatment: Phytonadione (vitamin K_1) orally, IM, or IV (10 to 50 mg in adults, 1 mg in neonates) is effective within 24 h for both vitamin K deficiency and bleeding from an overdose of oral anticoagulants. (CAUTION: *For IV administration, see Ch. 78.*)

To control bleeding before vitamin K takes effect, or for patients with nonobstructive liver disease, replacement therapy with plasma 8 to 10 ml/kg (5 ml/lb) infused in a short period of time followed by supplements of 3 to 5 ml/kg (2 to 3 ml/lb) q 6 h is effective. Commercially available prothrombin complex also is of value although these products may increase risks of thrombosis or viral hepatitis.

DISSEMINATED INTRAVASCULAR COAGULATION (DIC) (Consumption
Coagulopathy; Defibrinogenation Syndrome)

A complex coagulation disorder resulting from widespread activation of the clotting mechanism.

Etiology and Pathophysiology

Activation of the clotting mechanism by tissue and bacterial products introduced directly into the bloodstream can result in extensive fibrin deposition on arterial surfaces with depletion of fibrinogen, prothrombin, factors V and VIII, and platelets, and formation of fibrinogen breakdown products (fibrin monomer and peptides). In addition, the fibrinolytic system is stimulated, resulting in further formation of fibrinogen and fibrin degradation products **(FDP and fdp).**

Essentially, the process represents the conversion of plasma to serum within the circulation. Frequently seen in severe or terminal disease states, it is one of the most serious of the acquired coagulation disorders. It develops when substances entering the circulation accelerate coagulation processes; included are (1) tissue products (thromboplastin) as in abruptio placentae, placenta previa, metastatic carcinoma, or from ischemic tissue following acute injury or shock; (2) bacterial endotoxin in gram-negative sepsis or meningococcemia; (3) lipid substances released from erythrocytes in acute hemolytic disorders, or from platelets in patients with thrombocytosis or thrombocythemia; and (4) factor XII, activated in immune disorders by antigen and antibody complexes.

Symptoms and Signs

Early in the course of the disorder, laboratory findings may be the only abnormality. Profuse bleeding associated with a severe depletion of platelets and fibrinogen is dominant in late stages. Mucosal bleeding with generalized ecchymoses can lead to exsanguination and shock. Renal necrosis resulting from vascular thrombi represents one of the major risks of thrombosis during periods of DIC, especially in the presence of shock, and is indicated by oliguria or renal shutdown and increasing levels of creatinine and blood urea nitrogen. Venous thrombosis may develop in other areas as well. Careful observation of many severe, debilitating diseases and infections often provide evidence of DIC, although most cases do not proceed to a severe stage. Occasionally, a chronic persistent form develops (as with vascular disorders, aortic aneurysm, giant hemangioma) with mild to moderate hemorrhagic complications resulting from platelet destruction which initiates DIC. This chronic form also may occur in cases of disseminated malignancy or obstetric patients with retained placental remnants. In both of these latter situations, necrosis of tissue with thromboplastin release into the circulation maintains the DIC until the necrotic tissue is removed or destroyed.

Laboratory Findings

Laboratory findings vary depending upon the inciting agent and the stage of the disorder. Tissue products, thromboplastins, tend to affect plasma clotting factors initially, while septic conditions with endotoxin release induce a rapid decrease in platelets. Very early in the thromboplastin release disorders, modest thrombocytopenia may develop, and the PT and PTT actually may be shorter than normal as a result of the activation of factors V, VII, VIII, IX, and X. Factors V and VIII function briefly in the active form before being destroyed by the evolving thrombin. Fibrinogen levels often increase in infection to levels of two to three times normal, so that initially values may appear within the normal range despite increased fibrinogen destruction. As the disorder proceeds, thrombin destroys factors V and VIII, and the PTT and PT are prolonged because of these deficiencies as well as the depletion of fibrinogen. The platelet count declines to levels of 10,000 or less. Fibrinogen levels eventually may drop to less than 50 mg/100 ml. FDP can be identified in the circulation and, although present laboratory procedures vary in sensitivity, a positive test supports the diagnosis. RBC changes (**microangiopathic hemolytic anemia**) are more common in the subacute and chronic varieties.

Diagnosis

Overt DIC is suspected when bleeding occurs in clinical settings known to predispose; e.g., complicated pregnancy, postoperative infection, chemotherapy for cancer. It is confirmed by laboratory studies, as described above. Occult DIC is best anticipated with prospective monitoring of fibrinogen, platelets, FDP, and blood cultures.

Treatment

Supportive therapy with treatment of the underlying disease is the most effective approach. The principal treatment of overt DIC is that of the etiologic condition (e.g., evacuation of the uterus, treatment of gram-negative sepsis). If the patient bleeds as a result of a DIC-induced coagulation deficiency, replacement therapy is necessary initially to control bleeding; e.g., the administration of platelet concentrates and sometimes plasma as well. (Note that platelet concentrates also contain factor V and VIII activities.) *If thrombosis is present (particularly if renal dysfunction has developed) and hemostasis has been accomplished*, anticoagulant therapy can be considered, using heparin either continuously or by IV bolus q 6 h. Anticoagulants should not be employed in the patient with a head injury or if CNS bleeding or thrombosis is suspected. The dose of heparin should be low: 300 u./kg/day and gradually increased to 500 to 800 u./kg/24 h; i.e., as necessary depending on improvement in platelet count and fibrinogen level. The higher heparin dosage may be required as a result of depletion of antithrombin III (heparin cofactor) activity that commonly occurs in this condition and reduces the effectiveness of heparin. In some instances, additional antithrombin III may be necessary. Once the activation of the clotting mechanism is interrupted, platelets, fibrinogen, and other factors increase and the fibrin degradation products disappear from the circulation. Heparin will not affect the underlying cause of the disorder, however, and seldom influences survival. (Note that heparin does not interfere with the effect of endotoxin on platelets.)

PRIMARY FIBRINOLYSIS

Rarely, fibrinolysins are activated in the general circulation by release of tissue kinases following major trauma or surgery, or from neoplasms of the prostate or pancreas. The resulting widespread hemorrhage resembles that seen in plasma factor depletion (as opposed to the mucosal and skin pattern of thrombocytopenia). This disorder must be considered when fibrinogen depletion develops, but it is far less frequent than DIC, with which it may be confused. Laboratory studies are similar to those of DIC in that PT and PTT are prolonged by the lack of fibrinogen, and fibrinogen degradation products are increased. However, if present, thrombocytopenia is not marked, and factors V and VIII are decreased to only a moderate degree. Fibrinolytic activity is pronounced (euglobulin lysis time). In testing, addition of fibrinogen or normal plasma to the patient's plasma may be necessary to provide sufficient fibrinogen substrate to detect increased fibrinolysin activity in the euglobulin fraction. **Treatment** with ε-aminocaproic acid (1 to 2 gm/h IV) can block fibrinolysin activation and restore hemostasis.

ABNORMAL INHIBITORS OF COAGULATION (The Circulating Anticoagulants)

Endogenous substances that inhibit blood coagulation. In some cases, inhibitory substances appear to be antibodies against specific coagulation factors, most commonly factor VIII. They produce a clinical and laboratory picture identical to that of factor VIII deficiency. Sometimes the inhibitor is powerful enough to bind factor VIII in other deficient plasma substrates and give the appearance of factor IX deficiency in addition to VIII. Such inhibitors may develop in patients with hereditary factor VIII or IX (hemophilia A or B) deficiency, and they are described in pregnancy and following drug reactions (penicillin). Immunosuppressive drugs and plasmapheresis have been employed with limited success. Some concentrates of the prothrombin complex used to treat hemophilia B contain active factors X and VII and have controlled bleeding in these cases. A dose of 30 to 75 factor VIII correction units has been recommended (see treatment for hemophilia in Vol. II, Ch. 25).

Other inhibitors described are most frequently antithrombins that develop in some cases of liver disease, SLE, or primary macroglobulinemia. The fibrinogen degradation products from thrombin or fibrinolysin action also can act as weak antithrombins. Mild factor V and factor VII inhibitors also have been described; several are associated with dysproteinemias, but others are idiopathic.

Laboratory findings in the presence of a strong antithrombin are similar to those seen with heparin. An increase in thrombin clotting time **(TCT)** occurs as well as an increase in all clotting time assays, PT, and PTT. However, protamine sulfate does not correct the abnormal assays as it does when heparin is present. Antithromboplastin also develops in some of the dysproteinemias and SLE; it produces a prolongation of the PT only. Factor V inhibitors prolong both the PT and PTT, while factor VII inhibitors prolong the PT only. Many inhibitors interfere with coagulation nonspecifically and may alter all clotting time assays.

Therapy is nonspecific for these conditions; however, chronic plasmapheresis, particularly in patients with macroglobulinemia, reduces the level of abnormal protein to a point where interference with coagulation mechanisms is reduced. In some cases immune suppressive therapy (cyclophosphamide) is successful.

96. LEUKOPENIA

GRANULOCYTOPENIA

(Neutropenia; Agranulocytosis; Agranulocytic Angina)

An acute or chronic reduction in peripheral blood granulocytes resulting in increased susceptibility to bacterial infection in proportion to the severity and duration of the granulocytopenia.

Etiology

Impaired granulocyte production, accelerated destruction or utilization, or combinations of these may result in granulocytopenia with concomitant reduction in the large reserve pool of bone marrow neutrophils.

Chronic granulocytopenia due to **diminished granulocyte production** may be associated with a rare hereditary disorder (e.g., infantile genetic agranulocytosis, familial neutropenia, cyclic neutropenia, pancreatic insufficiency neutropenia) or with a congenital one (e.g., alymphocytosis, dysglobulinemia, thymic alymphoplasia). Whether acute or chronic, reduced granulopoiesis most frequently occurs in association with acquired systemic problems (e.g., myelophthisis due to bone marrow neoplasm, starvation, drug toxicity, irradiation).

The most common cause of acute agranulocytosis is pharmacologic (dose-related) impairment of granulocyte production. Frequently involved are many of the alkylating agents, chemotherapeutic antimetabolites, phenothiazine derivatives, dibenzazepine compounds, antithyroid drugs, sulfonamides, antihistamines, and anticonvulsants. Synthetic penicillins, chloramphenicol, benzene, nitrous oxide, and arsenic also have been incriminated. Their granulopoietic effects vary widely in individuals. Less common are idiosyncratic (non–dose-related) forms of drug-induced depression of granulocyte production that may be either acute (e.g., cinchona alkaloids, indomethacin, procainamide, phenylbutazone, nitrofurantoin, sulfonamides, antithyroid compounds, thiazides) or chronic (e.g., benzene, chloramphenicol, gold salts, phenylbutazone).

Some drugs (e.g., cytarabine, phenytoin, methotrexate, pyrimethamine) may produce granulocytopenia as a consequence of **excessive** (intramedullary) **destruction** of granulocyte precursors. Rarely, acute agranulocytosis due to excessive (intramedullary and extramedullary) granulocyte destruction is caused by the presence of a drug-induced leukocyte antibody (e.g., aminopyrine, dipyrone, phenylbutazone, meralluride, sulfapyridine, gold salts). Most disease-associated granulocytopenia is due to accelerated neutrophil destruction through a variety of mechanisms. This may occur in association with excessive leukophagocytosis (histiocytic medullary reticulosis, lymphoma), systemic infection (e.g., viral, protozoal, severe bacterial sepsis), various forms of hypersplenism (e.g., Felty's syndrome, congestive splenomegaly), collagen disease, intrinsic granulocyte defects (e.g., Chédiak-Higashi syndrome), and, rarely, leukocyte isoantibody (e.g., neonatal immunization neutropenia). Complement-mediated acute reversible neutropenia sometimes occurs during hemodialysis.

The drugs in the USA with the highest absolute risk of granulocytopenia induction, exclusive of the cancer chemotherapeutic agents, are the phenothiazines, antithyroid compounds, sulfonamides, and phenylbutazone in about that order. The greatest relative risk, however, probably is with phenylbutazone.

Pathology and Pathogenesis

Diminished neutrophil production usually involves injury to granulocyte-committed stem cells or blockade of metabolic steps in granulocyte precursors resulting in partial or complete absence of granulocyte proliferation in the marrow. In contrast, increased granulocyte destruction is associated with compensatory increased bone marrow granulocyte production. The marrow usually is hypercellular with a preponderance of myeloid precursors.

In all types of granulocytopenia, leukocyte phagocytic and bactericidal functions are reduced. The risk of bacterial infection is slight when the granulocyte count is in the 1000 to 1500/cu mm range, moderate from 500 to 1000/cu mm, and greatly increased below 500/cu mm. Virtually all patients with granulocyte counts of 500/cu mm or less for a few weeks or more will develop serious bacterial infection. Successful bacterial invasion and proliferation, however, depend upon such additional factors as (1) the number of monocytes, (2) the number of reserve granulocytes in storage, (3) alterations in immunoglobulins, complement, and reticuloendothelial function, and (4) duration of granulocytopenia.

Symptoms and Signs

Clinical manifestations depend upon the type, severity, and duration of associated bacterial infection. Painful buccal or pharyngeal mucosal ulcers associated with dysphagia may herald the onset of **acute granulocytopenia**. The initial symptoms may often be fever, chills, weakness, or extreme prostration due to bacterial sepsis. Untreated, the disease can progress rapidly to bacterial shock and death. **Chronic granulocytopenia** may have a similar acute onset, but frequently the disease progresses slowly with a series of multiple focal infections that commonly involve the skin, perirectal region, and bronchopulmonary system. Some patients may develop either recurrent aphthous stomatitis or cyclic infections.

Although granulocyte counts usually rise to a normal range in 7 to 21 days following cessation of an offending drug or an acute illness, the severe forms of metabolic-induced depression may last for weeks, and certain idiopathic reactions persist for months or years. Severe granulocytopenia of $>$ 3 to 4 wk duration is usually fatal.

Diagnosis

Granulocytopenia is suspected whenever any of the aforementioned signs or symptoms are present, especially in patients using high-risk drugs. The diagnosis is established when the granulocyte count (total WBC $\times$ % granulocytes) is $<$ 1500/cu mm after the 1st mo of life. The total leukocyte count usually is in the range of 300 to 3000/cu mm with a disproportionate reduction in the percent of neutrophils. In pure granulocytopenia the other formed elements of the blood are within the normal range.

Bone marrow examinations help define the type of granulocytopenia. Reduction in marrow myeloid precursors is compatible with diminished granulopoiesis. Normal or increased numbers of marrow myeloid precursors with left shift are most consistent with increased intramedullary or peripheral granulocyte destruction or early marrow recovery.

In chronic forms of granulocytopenia, ancillary diagnostic tests are required to rule out functional hypersplenism (e.g., liver-spleen scan, RBC survival, liver function tests, barium swallow), rheumatoid or collagen disorder (e.g., SLE test, antinuclear factor), dysproteinemia (e.g., immunoelectrophoresis, quantitative immunoglobulins), infection (e.g., blood cultures, viral antibody studies), or leukocyte antibody (e.g., leukoagglutination test).

Treatment

Patients with **acute granulocytopenia** should be considered to have a potentially reversible, acute, acquired disease until proved otherwise. Any possible offending agents (drugs, occupational exposure, etc.) must be identified and eliminated. Patients with fever, other signs of sepsis, or total granulocytes $<$ 1000/cu mm should be hospitalized in a separate room with reverse isolation technics (see BARRIERS in Ch. 7), and thoroughly evaluated to determine the focus of infection. Patients with severe granulocytopenia may lack the requisite cells to localize an infection. Blood, nose, throat, sputum, and urine cultures should be obtained at frequent intervals.

Antimicrobial therapy is not routinely administered, but is given whenever there is (1) a significant fever spike, (2) persistent fever of 38.3 C (101 F) or more, (3) shock, (4) a significant focus of local infection, or (5) a positive blood culture. Initial antimicrobial therapy must be designed to cover a wide range of gram-negative (especially *Escherichia coli*, *Pseudomonas*, *Klebsiella*, and *Proteus*) or gram-positive (especially *Staphylococcus aureus*) organisms. Combination antimicrobial therapy with an aminoglycoside such as gentamicin or tobramycin 1.5 to 1.7 mg/kg IM q 8 h plus a penicillinase-resistant penicillin such as cephalothin 40 to 60 mg/kg IV q 6 h, oxacillin 1 to 2 gm IV q 4 h or carbenicillin 100 mg/kg IV q 4 h is recommended as the initial form of therapy for adults (see ANTIMICROBIAL CHEMOTHERAPY in Ch. 246). Appropriate antibiotics for the types of infection identified should be continued at maintenance dose levels up to 7 to 10 days following defervescence. Extended antibiotic treatment predisposes to the development of renal complications and superinfection with resistant bacteria and fungae. Infection and fever usually ebb with the return of 1000 to 1500 granulocytes/cu mm in the peripheral blood.

There is no certain method to stimulate bone marrow myeloid recovery, but encouraging results have been reported in adults following the daily administration of lithium carbonate 300 mg orally t.i.d. for several weeks. Corticosteroids may be used in the management of bacterial shock, but are not recommended to treat acute granulocytopenia, since they may mask bacterial infections and may impede the migration of granulocytes into tissues. Androgenic steroid therapy results for acute agranulocytosis have been disappointing. Human γ-globulin in doses initially of 1.2 ml/kg IM followed by 0.6 ml/kg IM q 3 to 4 wk should be given to patients with hypogammaglobulinemia. Severely neutropenic patients with antibiotic-resistant sepsis may benefit from repeated daily infusions of massive numbers of leukocytes from compatible normal donors, but this procedure is costly and not without risk and therefore is not recommended for routine use. The value of antimicrobial drug sterilization of the GI tract and the maintenance of agranulocytic patients in sterile environments during cancer chemotherapy remains uncertain.

Saline or hydrogen peroxide gargles every few hours or anesthetic lozenges (benzocaine 15 mg q 3 to 4 h) may relieve the discomfort associated with oropharyngeal ulcerations. Oral thrush (see Ch. 208) is treated with nystatin mouthwashes (400,000 to 600,000 u. q.i.d.). Semi-solid or liquid diet may be necessary during acute mucositis.

Chronic granulocytopenic patients are hospitalized only during acute episodes of infection; therapy is similar to that for patients with acute granulocytopenia. Patients should be taught to recognize the early symptoms and signs of acute infection and to seek immediate medical attention. Those patients who take low-dose oral antibiotics on a rotating basis must be monitored for the emergence of resistant bacterial strains and infections with opportunistic organisms (fungi, pneumocystis, cytomegalovirus, etc.). Therapy directed at improving the number of neutrophils depends on the type of granulocytopenia. Patients with decreased granulopoiesis may be tried on a course of lithium carbonate 300 mg orally t.i.d. (for adults) for a period of at least 3 to 5 wk. If this form of therapy is unsuccessful, adult patients may be given oxymetholone 1 to 2 mg/kg/day orally combined with a small dose of prednisone 10 to 20 mg/day orally for 2 to 3 mo. Patients with primary and secondary hypersplenic forms of granulocytopenia who have had repeated infections usually will respond well to splenectomy. Improvement with splenectomy also usually occurs in some patients with SLE, cyclic neutropenia, and certain forms of marrow dysplasia either with or without splenomegaly.

LYMPHOCYTOPENIA

(Lymphopenia; Alymphocytosis) (See also Ch. 17 and Vol. II, Ch. 25)

An acute or chronic reduction in peripheral blood lymphocytes due to anomalous development of the lymphoreticular system, acquired illness-induced suppression of lymphopoiesis, or increased loss or destruction of body lymphocytes.

Etiology

Chronic impairment of lymphocyte production in several rare primary immunologic deficiency disorders may be severe (e.g., Swiss-type agammaglobulinemia, thymic alymphoplasia, DiGeorge syndrome, Wiskott-Aldrich syndrome), or slight to moderate (e.g., Bruton-type agammaglobulinemia, thymoma, ataxia telangiectasia). Acute or chronic impairment of production also may occur with a variety of acquired conditions (e.g., acute agranulocytosis, aplastic anemia, phenytoin administration, sarcoidosis, renal failure, SLE, leukemia, carcinomatosis, Hodgkin's disease, lymphosarcoma, multiple myeloma).

Lymphocytopenia due to excessive destruction may occur acutely (e.g., stress, corticosteroid or alkylating agent administration, radiation exposure, episodic lymphopenia) or chronically (Cushing's syndrome).

Excessive loss of lymphocytes may result from thoracic duct leakage, abnormalities of intestinal lymphatic drainage, intestinal lymphangiectasia, or severe right heart failure.

Pathology and Pathogenesis

Most patients with thymus-mediated (T cell) immunologic deficiency disorders have underdeveloped central areas in lymph nodes, severe lymphocytopenia involving the larger lymphocytes, and altered cell-mediated immunity. Those with the B cell type are deficient in peripheral zone lymph node development and plasma cells, have modest lymphocytopenia involving the smaller lymphocytes, and demonstrate impairment of humoral antibody responses. The lymphocytopenia usually is permanent or progressive. The lymphocytopenia of most acquired disorders is due to malignant transformation of lymphocytes, tumor disruption of lymphopoiesis, or stem cell failure. Drug-, hormone-, or radiation-induced lympholysis also will result in depletion of tissue lymphocytes. Excessive loss of lymphocytes due to increased external leakage, however, may result in lymphocytopenia associated with hyperplasia of lymphopoietic tissue.

Chronic lymphocytopenia may be associated with reduced serum immunoglobulins, abnormal delayed hypersensitivity responses, or poor lymphocyte transformation. These changes may result in increased susceptibility to bacterial, viral, mycotic, and parasitic infections as well as the development of autoimmune disorders, malignant tumors, and delayed or absent homograft rejection.

Symptoms and Signs

Lymphocytopenia per se causes no symptoms, but the clinical manifestations of any associated illnesses may be present. Chronic tissue lymphocyte depletion frequently is manifested by a reduction in size of lymph nodes, spleen, and tonsils. Lymph node tumor invasion or chronic loss of lymphocytes may result in lymphadenopathy.

Diagnosis

Lymphocytopenia is present when the absolute blood lymphocytes (total WBC $\times$ % lymphocytes) are < 1500/cu mm in adults and < 3000/cu mm in children. The clinical picture, bone marrow and lymph node pathology, and immunologic characteristics usually will define etiology. Immunologic deficiency disorders are discussed in Ch. 17 and Vol. II, Ch. 25.

Treatment

Lymphocytopenia in some of the primary immunologic deficiency disorders has been corrected in a few patients following bone marrow transplantation. Some acquired forms of lymphocytopenia are potentially correctable following remission in the underlying illness or removal of the offending agent. The usual antibiotic therapy of certain infections may be further improved through the use of pooled γ-globulin or specific hyperimmune serum. Corticosteroids, alkylating agents, and ionizing radiation may be very useful in the therapy of certain autoimmune and lymphoproliferative disorders despite their lympholytic effects.

97. LEUKEMIA

Generalized neoplastic disorders of the blood-forming tissues, primarily those of the leukocytic series.

Etiology and Pathogenesis

Some forms of leukemia in cats, chickens, mice, and rats are due to viruses; a similar cause in man is unverified. Exposure to environmental factors, such as irradiation and certain chemicals (especially benzene), may be etiologic factors.

The pathogenesis of the leukemias is becoming clearer. Leukemogenesis occurs in pluripotent hematopoietic stem cells. Cellular kinetic studies indicate that leukemic cells accumulate because of a defect in normal maturation and differentiation. Immature cells retain the ability to proliferate and survive longer than mature cells. Excessive numbers accumulate, presumably first in their tissues of origin (e.g., granulocytes in the bone marrow, lymphocytes in lymph nodes) and then throughout the body. This accumulation leads to organ enlargement (e.g., hepatomegaly, splenomegaly, lymphadenopathy, marrow hypercellularity) and to aberrations in organ functions. The anemia and thrombocytopenia commonly seen in leukemia result from growth inhibition of normal stem cells by leukemic cells, probably mediated by humoral or direct cellular mechanisms. Leukemias involving mature cell types tend to be chronic more often than those involving immature forms.

Classification

Any type of blood cell or its precursor may be involved in the neoplastic process. However, nearly all cases of leukemia are of the following types: **acute lymphoblastic leukemia (ALL),** primarily a disease of children; **acute myeloblastic leukemia (AML)** and **acute monoblastic leukemia (AMOL)** or **myelomonoblastic (AMMOL),** seen at any age but especially in adult life; **chronic lymphocytic leukemia (CLL),** primarily a disease of late life, after age 50; **chronic granulocytic leukemia (CGL),** seen primarily in adults aged 20 to 50.

Acute lymphoblastic leukemia in children and adults has been subclassified by cell surface markers into null or T-cell subtypes. The enzyme terminal deoxynucleotidyl transferase has been associated with pre–T-cell leukemia. Some investigators have reported that T-cell ALL has a worse prognosis than null cell ALL, though this is not a universal finding. A recent classification for both acute lymphoblastic leukemia and acute nonlymphoblastic leukemia (AML, AMOL, and AMMOL) has been reported by a French-American-British (FAB) cooperative study group. This is the FAB classification which classifies acute lymphoblastic leukemia into the L-1, L-2, or L-3 variety by morphologic appearance; the acute nonlymphoblastic leukemias ($>$ 50% blasts in the marrow) are subclassified into the M-1, M-2, M-3, M-4, M-5, and M-6 categories, depending upon the type and percentage of immature cells seen. The leukemias with $<$ 50% blasts are listed as myelodysplastic diseases and are subclassified into refractory anemia with excess blasts or chronic myelomonocytic leukemias.

Leukemias in which other cell types predominate (e.g., eosinophils, basophils, reticulum cells, plasma cells, a variety of poorly identified stem cells, promyelocytes, and erythroleukemia) are rare and will not be considered here.

In many cases of acute leukemia, the peripheral blood leukocyte concentration is normal or even less than normal, but generally the marrow is hypercellular. A **leukemoid reaction,** or blood picture resembling CGL, may appear with some infections (e.g., whooping cough, infectious mononucleosis, tuberculosis) or in non-neoplastic blood dyscrasias and advanced cancer.

While leukemia is usually not difficult to diagnose, certain preleukemic states and poorly defined leukemic variants may be difficult to classify. Features helpful in diagnosing the common forms of leukemia are shown in TABLE 97–1.

Treatment and Prognosis

Therapy can arrest the pathologic process in most cases. The abnormal accumulation of leukocytes may diminish and complete remissions may be gained.

In recent years, dramatic improvement has marked prognosis of the acute leukemias. Improvements in therapy induce higher rates of remission and longer survival. Variations depend upon the specific type of acute leukemia (discussed below). No significant improvement in survival has occurred in the chronic leukemias in recent years.

Although specific therapy (see below) varies with the morphologic type of the disease, certain principles apply to all forms of leukemia. Mass destruction of cells by x-ray and antileukemic drugs liberates large amounts of the nucleic acid metabolite, uric acid, that is relatively insoluble in acid urine and may precipitate in the renal tubules and collecting ducts. Attention to hydration, ensuring a urine output of at least 1500 ml/day, and maintaining an alkaline urine will prevent this complication. In addition, the drug allopurinol, a potent xanthine oxidase inhibitor, blocks the conversion of xanthine to uric acid and thus minimizes hyperuricemia. However, allopurinol also interferes with the degradation of purine analog 6-mercaptopurine **(6MP),** used in therapy; *if the two drugs are used together, the dose of the antileukemic purine analog must be reduced by about 75%.* 6-Thioguanine **(TG),** a purine analog similar to 6MP, does not utilize the xanthine oxidase pathway for degradation,

TABLE 97-1. FINDINGS AT DIAGNOSIS IN THE FOUR MOST COMMON TYPES OF LEUKEMIA

	Acute Lymphoblastic	Acute Myeloblastic	Chronic Granulocytic	Chronic Lymphocytic
Peak age incidence	Childhood	Any age	Young adulthood	Middle and old age
Leukocyte concentration	H* in 50%; N* or L* in 50%	H in 60%; N or L in 40%	H in 100%	H in 98% N or L in 2%
Differential WBC count	Many lymphoblasts	Many myeloblasts	Entire myeloid series	Small lymphocytes
Anemia	In > 90%, severe	In > 90%, severe	In 80%, but mild	In about 50%, mild
Platelets	L in > 80%	L in > 90%	H in 60%; L in 10%	L in 20–30%
Lymphadenopathy	Commonly seen	Occasionally seen	Infrequently seen	Commonly seen
Splenomegaly	60%	50%	Usual and severe	Usual and moderate
Other features	50% CNS occurrence after 1 yr	Rare CNS occurrence	Leukocyte alkaline phosphatase low; Ph1** chromosome positive in 85%	Occasional hemolytic anemia and hypogammaglobulinemia

* L = low; N = normal; H = high.
** Ph1 = Philadelphia.

so no dose reduction is necessary when used with allopurinol. Generally, TG can be used interchangeably with 6MP, but TG in combination with cytarabine (Ara-C) has a greater additive action than 6MP.

Packed RBCs or platelet transfusions should be given for severe anemia (Hb < 8 gm) or thrombocytopenia (platelet count < 30,000/cu mm). Granulocyte transfusions are available for patients who have a transient drug-induced neutropenia and systemic infection. The risk of transfusion reactions and hepatitis is always present. Ideally, transfusion should be with blood products obtained from histocompatible (HLA-matched) single donors.

Antibiotics are used when there is clinical evidence of infection, but only after suitable cultures and diagnostic procedures have been initiated. Prophylactic antibiotic therapy is not recommended, as it often results in infection with resistant organisms (see Ch. 6).

THE ACUTE LEUKEMIAS

(Acute Lymphoblastic Leukemia [ALL]; Acute Myeloblastic or Granulocytic Leukemia [AML or AGL]; Acute Monoblastic Leukemia [AMOL]; Acute Myelomonoblastic Leukemia [AMMOL])

Rapidly progressive forms of leukemia characterized by replacement of normal bone marrow by primitive or blast cells of the blood-forming series. Classification into cell type—ALL as opposed to AML and other forms—is important in treatment and prognosis.

Incidence

ALL is predominantly a disease of childhood. While most patients are under 10, a significant number are teenagers, and a few adults are up to and past 40. **AML** (or **AGL**) occurs at all ages, with a somewhat higher proportion of adults. Patients with **AMOL** or **AMMOL** are often included in this group, since prognosis is similar and therapy is the same.

Pathology

Primitive WBCs in the bone marrow accumulate rapidly and invade many tissues, including liver, spleen, lymph nodes, and CNS. These cells may be early representatives of the myeloid or lymphoid series, but in many instances recognition is difficult. Such leukemias accordingly are classified as **stem cell leukemias.** Bone marrow involvement results in severe anemia and thrombocytopenia with marked bleeding tendencies. Leukocytes in the peripheral blood are predominantly blast forms; the WBC count may be depressed, normal, or elevated.

Symptoms and Signs

Acute leukemia frequently presents as an apparent infectious process with an abrupt onset and high fever. Joint pains may lead to a diagnosis of acute rheumatic fever. Thrombocytopenia may cause petechiae and ecchymoses, as well as bleeding from mouth, nose, kidneys, and bowel. Moderate enlargement of liver, spleen, and lymph nodes is frequent but not invariable. The disease may also have an insidious onset associated with progressive weakness and pallor.

Laboratory Findings and Diagnosis

The total WBC count is not elevated consistently, and leukopenia is often found. Blast forms, usually in the peripheral blood smear, indicate the diagnosis in many cases, but bone marrow aspiration should always confirm it. This typically shows an extreme and uniform accumulation of blast cells, with decreased or absent erythroid and granulocytic elements and megakaryocytes.

Prognosis

The average untreated patient survives about 4 to 6 mo from clinical onset; some die within a few days. Some chemotherapeutic agents produce hematologic and clinical improvement, thus prolonging life for several months, a year, or even longer. Eradicating CNS involvement is more difficult. Death usually occurs from hemorrhage or secondary infection in both ALL and AML.

Prognosis is generally worse for patients presenting with peripheral blood counts of over 100,000 cells/cu mm in both acute lymphoblastic and nonlymphoblastic leukemias. Age as a prognostic factor is an unresolved point. Some investigators feel that patients over 60 do not respond as well as those under 60; others feel that patients between 60 and 75 and in good physical condition will do as well as those under 60. Children with acute lymphoblastic leukemia of the L-1 morphology have a better prognosis in terms of response and survival than the L-2 or L-3 varieties. The prognostic value of null versus T cells is still controversial.

ALL: Survival in children has increased as new agents and combinations thereof achieve remissions in > 90% of cases. Remissions last 5 yr in > 50% of responders. The use of intensive cytotoxic chemotherapy subsequent to remission induction succeeds in prolonging remissions and survival. On a regimen using drugs generally available (see below), median survival is 36 mo. Patients living past 36 mo have the possibility of being cured.

AML, AMOL, AMMOL: Remissions are achieved in 70 to 85% of cases with drugs and treatment programs that are generally available. In patients who respond, survival is usually longer than 1 yr; in those who do not respond, it is 3 to 4 mo. Responders have a 25 to 40% probability of living 3 yr and longer.

Treatment (See also ANTITUMOR DRUGS in Ch. 250)

Survival in acute leukemia depends upon achieving a complete remission. Treatment can accomplish this goal in > 90% of ALL patients and 70 to 80% of AML patients. Each newly diagnosed patient must be given this chance for remission. Since concepts of both antileukemic therapy and supportive therapy are constantly revised and improved, a physician caring for patients with acute leukemia should be knowledgeable and capable of providing contemporary management, and should see enough patients to be able to provide results comparable to those generally achieved. Ideally, patients should be treated at specialized medical centers.

The major difference in treatment of ALL compared to AML (and AMOL or AMMOL) is that the former responds to a wider variety of drugs, some of which are not particularly myelosuppressive. In AML, treatment usually results in significant myelosuppression; thus, patients often get clinically worse before they improve. The period of myelosuppression prior to marrow recovery requires meticulous anticipatory and supportive care.

ALL: Remission induction can be achieved with daily oral prednisone and weekly IV vincristine and an anthracycline in > 90% of children and 85% of adults. Remissions can be maintained with intermittent methotrexate therapy given biweekly either IV or orally. Cyclophosphamide and 6MP may be used together with methotrexate maintenance.

Other treatment schemes utilizing induction with vincristine, prednisone, and anthracyclines, then intensive therapy with multiple cytotoxic agents in combination (daunorubicin or hydroxydaunorubicin, Ara-C, TG, cyclophosphamide, BCNU [carmustine], hydroxyurea, and methotrexate) offer high induction rates and also remission durations of > 3 yr for most patients. The treatment regimens with cytotoxic drugs generally continue for 3 yr. After cessation of chemotherapy, the relapse rate is about 15%, most occurring within the first year.

Leukemic infiltration of the CNS occurs increasingly with the prolongation of life resulting from current therapy. This is usually suggested by headache, increasing irritability, and apathy, which often occur when the patient is otherwise in good remission, because chemotherapeutic agents do not cross the blood-brain barrier. The diagnosis is confirmed by blurred optic discs and the presence of leukemic cells in the CSF. Intrathecal injection of methotrexate (6.25 mg/m^2) or Ara-C (30 mg/m^2) twice weekly is usually effective in controlling symptoms. An Omaya reservoir with its catheter implanted into the cerebral ventricle is also an effective method to administer intracerebral chemotherapy. Whole-brain irradiation to 2400 R may be used with intrathecal or intracerebral chemotherapy.

Prophylactic CNS therapy during or immediately after remission induction prevents leukemic infiltration of the CNS and prolongs survival. The optimal prophylactic treatment modality and regimen are not established, but it appears that intrathecal methotrexate with or without radiation of 2400 R to the cranial vault is indicated.

AML, AMOL, AMMOL: Single cytotoxic agents, such as 6MP or methotrexate, resulted in short remissions in < 20% of cases. Ara-C and 6TG increased remission rates to 50% with a slight prolongation of remission duration from 4 to 10 mo. Currently, the most effective combination of agents for induction is Ara-C at 100 to 200 mg/m²/24 h given as a continuous IV infusion for 5 to 7 days, and daunorubicin 45 mg/m² IV for the first 3 days. The induction rate is > 70% regardless of age. The duration of remission is > 1 yr, with about 30% of patients living 3 yr. Various maintenance programs are evolving, usually with treatment for about 15 mo.

No prophylactic CNS therapy is indicated, since involvement of the CNS is relatively low even with longer survival.

AMOL, AMMOL, and the various stem cell leukemias usually run a course similar to that of AML and are best treated with the same regimen.

CHRONIC GRANULOCYTIC LEUKEMIA

(Chronic Myeloid, Chronic Myelocytic, or Chronic Myelogenous Leukemia; CML; CGL)

Abnormal accumulation of the granulocytic elements of the blood, usually progressing slowly and responsive to treatment during the major period of the disease. The disease, slightly more prevalent in males, occurs at any age but chiefly in the 30s and 40s.

Pathology

CGL is characterized by excessive accumulation of leukocytes, principally in the bone marrow, spleen, liver, and blood. As the disease progresses, leukemic cells may infiltrate other organ systems (e.g., intestinal tract, kidneys, lungs, gonads, lymph nodes). The major cell types are granulocytes of all types in all stages of maturation, but with young forms (metamyelocytes, myelocytes, promyelocytes, and myeloblasts—normally seen only in the bone marrow) very much in evidence in the blood and other tissues.

Symptoms and Signs

Patients often show nonspecific symptoms such as fatigue, weakness, anorexia, or weight loss, or are diagnosed from blood studies for other reasons (e.g., elective surgery). When the patient is first seen, the spleen is usually moderately enlarged, which may result in vague epigastric distress or heaviness. Minor lymphadenopathy occurs occasionally, but is much less evident than in CLL. Hemostasis is rarely impaired until late, after "blastic transformation" develops, or after therapy and/or the evolution of the disease lead to thrombocytopenia. In patients who develop thrombocytosis (platelets > 1000 × 10³/cu mm), hemostatic problems may be secondary to inadequate platelet function.

Laboratory Findings

Characteristic early findings are an elevated WBC count (15,000 to 500,000 or higher) with a shift to the left, mild or no anemia, and normal or often elevated platelet count. The blood smear shows young granulocytes normally seen only in the marrow (metamyelocytes and younger). The absolute number of lymphocytes and monocytes may be normal, but all granulocytic forms are usually increased in number, and basophils are often prominent. A few nucleated erythrocytes may also be present. The bone marrow is very cellular. The leukocyte alkaline phosphatase score is regularly low. Hemostatic tests are usually normal except in some patients with thrombocytosis. The serum uric acid may be elevated. Chromosome analysis of bone marrow or peripheral blood shows the Philadelphia (Ph¹) chromosome (translocation of portion of long arm of chromosome 22 to 9) in > 80% of typical CML and is diagnostic. CML without the Ph¹ chromosome tends to be more acute.

Late in the disease, anemia and thrombocytopenia become more evident. They may signal beginning resistance to therapy and the downhill course frequently associated with "**blastic transformation**" (over 50% blasts and promyelocytes in the marrow with associated anemia and thrombocytopenia).

Diagnosis

CGL should be considered in patients with an elevation in blood granulocyte concentration when the more usual explanations of infection and inflammation seem unlikely. The differential diagnosis includes myelofibrosis, polycythemia vera, other causes of leukocytosis (e.g., inflammation or infection), and leukemoid reactions secondary to cancer or disseminated infection (e.g., tuberculosis). The presence of splenomegaly, the characteristic blood picture, bone marrow aspirate, the leukocyte alkaline phosphatase test, and the presence of the Ph¹ chromosome help in differentiation.

Prognosis

The course is invariably progressive and ultimately fatal. Average survival time is 3 to 4 yr from clinical onset; about 20% of patients survive longer than 5 yr; 2% longer than 10 yr. During most of the disease, treatment may maintain the patient in almost normal health and activity without prolonging survival time appreciably. "**Blast transformation**" eventually occurs, when the patient responds less to antileukemic treatment; he usually succumbs within 4 to 6 mo to infection or bleeding.

Ph¹-negative CGL: A form of CGL, without the Ph¹ chromosome, occasionally seen in children and adults, commonly includes lymphadenopathy, skin lesions, and thrombocytopenia. It tends to run a rapid downhill course.

Treatment

Choice of therapy depends upon the experience of the physician, ease of administration, and convenience to the patient. Successful therapy results in symptomatic improvement by decreasing the proliferation of leukemic cells, manifested in the peripheral blood by a fall in the WBC count to normal levels, a decrease in number of immature leukocytes, a rise in Hb, and a reduction of the splenomegaly. Maximum improvement usually coincides with maintenance of the WBC count at normal levels. Because the aim of therapy is palliation, asymptomatic patients should not be treated, despite moderately elevated leukocyte counts; the benefits of therapy in such patients are questionable. Since patients often begin to have symptoms, and the risk of leukostasis in the brain and lung increases when the leukocyte count rises to over 50,000, this level is a reasonable indication for cytoreductive therapy.

Antineoplastic drugs: Busulfan, generally regarded as the most satisfactory drug, is well tolerated and can be given orally. The usual beginning adult dose is 4 to 6 mg/day orally, but adjustments must be made, since total dosage producing a satisfactory remission varies considerably from patient to patient. The simplest and probably most effective regimen is to continue oral busulfan until the WBC count returns to normal, and then to stop therapy until it begins to rise. Some evidence suggests that intermittent treatment until the WBC count falls into the high-normal range results in longer remissions.

The rate of fall of the WBC count in a given patient on a constant dose of this drug is generally predictable and may be determined by plotting **WBC count** on the vertical axis of a semilogarithmic graph against **time** on the horizontal axis. After several points on the curve have been determined, one can approximate how long therapy must continue before counts will be normal, and adjust return visits accordingly.

Some physicians use continuous low-dose (1 to 2 mg/day) maintenance therapy during remissions, but no evidence shows that doing so will prolong survival or the duration of remissions. For this reason, and since patients derive a psychologic boost from treatment-free periods, most hematologists prefer a regimen of intermittent treatment. Also, long-continued or excessive busulfan therapy may cause hyperpigmentation, splenomegaly with bone marrow aplasia, or pulmonary fibrosis—sufficient reason to limit total dosage to that actually needed to control symptoms.

Hydroxyurea is also useful. Unlike busulfan, it has a shorter duration of action with no known cumulative toxicity. However, the drug has to be given in almost a continuous fashion because of its short duration of action. Patients can be started on hydroxyurea at doses of 20 to 40 mg/kg orally in a single daily dose. Blood counts should be monitored weekly and the dose of hydroxyurea adjusted accordingly. Like busulfan, the rate of fall and maintenance schedule is generally predictable after a while.

Other drugs: Alkylating agents such as melphalan and thiotepa are reported as useful in lowering the marked thrombocytosis in patients with end-stage CGL. Folic acid antagonists, benzene, and the fluorinated pyrimidines are *not recommended.*

Splenic irradiation has been largely relegated to a secondary role, since the response and convenience to busulfan and hydroxyurea is so good. Splenic irradiation does not improve survival, but refractory cases of CGL or terminal phase patients with marked splenomegaly may obtain significant relief and transient lowering of the WBC count. The initial radiation dose should be low (25 or 50 R) to avoid a rapid and severe drop in the WBC count. The dose should be increased cautiously, following the peripheral WBC count closely.

Local irradiation may also relieve leukemic infiltration in skin, lymph nodes, and mucosa.

Treatment of the terminal phase: Blastic transformation is the terminal event for 70 to 90% of CGL patients. The remainder enter a refractory or accelerated phase of CGL that is unresponsive to drugs. In both cases, patients develop anemia, thrombocytopenia, hepatosplenomegaly, occasional lymphadenopathy, and, rarely, thrombocytosis. The peripheral WBC count progressively rises with increased numbers of eosinophils or basophils and some blasts in accelerated cases, and predominantly blasts in the blastic transformation phase. There is no known effective chemotherapy program for the terminal phase of CGL.

About 10 to 15% of blastic transformations may be lymphoblastic with elevated surface terminal transferase activity rather than the expected myeloblastic transformation. Treatment of lymphoblastic transformation with intensive multiple drug programs has resulted in remissions.

CHRONIC LYMPHOCYTIC LEUKEMIA

(Chronic Lymphatic Leukemia; CLL)

Abnormal accumulation of the lymphocytic elements of the lymph nodes and lymphoid tissues, with infiltration of the bone marrow and replacement of the normal hematopoietic elements. The disease, almost three times more common in males, occurs chiefly from age 50 to 70, but may occur at any age.

Pathology

Accumulation of lymphocytes probably begins in the lymph nodes, then involves other lymphoid tissues. The liver and spleen are moderately enlarged because of lymphocytic infiltration. The bone marrow may be almost completely infiltrated by lymphocytes, eventually resulting in anemia, agranulocytosis, and thrombocytopenia. Hemolytic anemia in varying degrees of severity is not uncommon. Some cases may begin with lymph node enlargement and marrow involvement without significant changes in the circulating blood; but, as the disease progresses, lymphocytes appear in the peripheral blood.

It is established that most CLL cases are B-cell types, although some are T-cell CLL (frequently associated with cutaneous involvement at presentation).

Symptoms and Signs

Onset is insidious, with increasing weakness, fatigue, anorexia, and lymphadenopathy. In about 25% of patients, the disease is discovered from a routine blood count. Patients usually show generalized lymphadenopathy, slight to moderate enlargement of liver and spleen, and mild pallor. Skin lesions may result from leukemic infiltration. A few patients show minor hemorrhagic manifestations. Hypogammaglobulinemia and a diminished resistance to infection are common in late stages. Autoimmune hemolytic anemias occur occasionally.

Laboratory Findings

Moderate anemia and reduction in platelets is present in about 50% of patients at diagnosis. The WBC count is usually elevated (up to 1,000,000), with 80 to 90% of cells being small lymphocytes. Lymphocytes predominate in the bone marrow; the granulocytic and erythrocytic series and the megakaryocytes may be reduced correspondingly.

Diagnosis

CLL should be suspected when patients with chronic weakness and debility have generalized lymphadenopathy, hepatosplenomegaly, or unusual generalized skin lesions. Diagnosis is ordinarily made by examination of the peripheral blood, but bone marrow aspirations should confirm it. The histologic appearance of lymph nodes is similar to that seen in malignant lymphoma. However, surface immunofluorescence studies have shown that B cells in CLL have weak reactivity in contrast to the more intense patterns seen in malignant lymphoma with "spillover" leukemia. Additionally, B cells in CLL form rosettes with mouse red cells, while B cells from malignant lymphomas generally do not. Other causes of lymphocytosis (e.g., pertussis, infectious mononucleosis) should be considered, but these can be differentiated by history, physical findings, and absence of anemia and bone marrow infiltration.

Clinical staging of patients (Rai Staging System) provides prognostic and comparative measures during therapeutic trials: Stage 0—peripheral blood absolute lymphocytosis > 15,000 cells/cu mm; Stage I—lymphocytosis and lymphadenopathy; Stage II—Stage I plus hepatosplenomegaly; Stage III—Stage II plus anemia; Stage IV—Stage III plus thrombocytopenia.

Prognosis

The disease is progressive, but some patients may be asymptomatic for many years and treatment may induce lengthy remission. Ultimately, the disorder becomes more active, with progressive involvement of the bone marrow leading to severe anemia and thrombocytopenia. The usual cause of death is intercurrent infection. Average survival time with treatment is many years after onset of symptoms. Patients with Stage III or IV have significantly shorter survivals than those with Stage I or II.

Treatment

No therapy is indicated until active progression is evident. Overtreatment is probably more dangerous than undertreatment. Various therapeutic modalities destroy most abnormal leukemic tissue but will not regularly improve anemia, neutropenia, and thrombocytopenia. The usual cause of death is infection, often with associated hypogammaglobulinemia, and no known therapy predictably improves this.

X-ray therapy may be given to the node-bearing areas and to the liver and spleen, generally for symptomatic palliation. Excessive irradiation may markedly depress hematopoiesis and precipitate anemia, thrombocytopenia, and bleeding.

Antineoplastic drugs: Chlorambucil is the drug most commonly used. The leukemic process may be unusually sensitive to treatment; the starting dose is 6 mg/day orally, adjusted as necessary. When a satisfactory response occurs, the drug should be stopped temporarily, since continuous treatment may result in severe bone marrow depression. As the disease enters the thrombocytopenic and anemic phase, further treatment may be hazardous and greater caution is indicated. However, some investigators report significant response in some patients with Stage III or IV CLL.

Methotrexate and 6MP may be harmful and generally *should not be used*. Investigative treatment plans utilizing a combination of alkylating agents, e.g., vincristine and prednisone, have been shown to induce complete marrow remission in 10 to 15% of cases.

Corticosteroid therapy may produce remarkable temporary improvement: a reduction in size of enlarged lymph nodes, liver, and spleen; possibly a rise in Hb level; and a decrease in bleeding tendency. Initially, the lymphocyte count may rise before falling on continued treatment. Corticosteroids are the initial drug of choice in management of acquired hemolytic anemia or thrombocytopenia sometimes present in CLL. The usual dosage of prednisone, the preferred corticosteroid agent, varies from 10 to 100 mg/day orally in 4 divided doses, the larger doses being used in acute situations. If a patient does not respond to 100 mg/day of prednisone, larger doses rarely prove effective. After a response, the dosage is decreased to a maintenance level (often 15 to 25 mg/day).

Adjuvants: Blood component transfusions are given as indicated. Problems of bleeding and infection are comparable to those present in the other leukemias and are handled similarly.

98. LYMPHOMA

A heterogeneous group of neoplasms arising in the reticuloendothelial and lymphatic systems. The major types are Hodgkin's disease and non-Hodgkin's lymphoma. Rarer forms include Burkitt's lymphoma and mycosis fungoides.

HODGKIN'S DISEASE

A chronic disease with lymphoreticular proliferation of unknown cause that may present in localized or disseminated form. Its extent should be definitively evaluated and staged (see below), since effective treatment is based upon such staging.

Incidence and Etiology

Annually in the USA, 5000 to 6000 new cases of Hodgkin's disease are diagnosed. The male-to-female ratio is 1.4:1. The disease is rare under age 10; however, a binodal age distribution exists with one peak at ages 15 to 34 and another after age 54. Epidemiologic studies find no evidence of horizontal spread. Hodgkin's disease resembles a low-grade graft-versus-host reaction. Recent evidence of tumor-associated antigens in Hodgkin's tissue is consistent with this interpretation. A number of infectious agents, including viruses, are postulated as causes.

Pathology

Diagnosis depends upon identification of large multinucleated reticulum cells **(Reed-Sternberg cells)** in lymph node tissue or other sites. Hodgkin's infiltrates are heterogeneous and consist of abnormal reticulum cells, histiocytes, lymphocytes, monocytes, plasma cells, and eosinophils. The four histopathologic classifications are (1) **lymphocyte predominance**—few Reed-Sternberg cells and many lymphocytes; (2) **mixed cellularity**—a moderate number of Reed-Sternberg cells with a mixed infiltrate; (3) **nodular sclerosis**—generally similar to mixed cellularity except that dense fibrous tissue, which shows a characteristic birefringence with polarized light, surrounds nodules of Hodgkin's tissue; and (4) **lymphocyte depletion**—few lymphocytes, numerous Reed-Sternberg cells, and extensive fibrosis or abnormal reticulum cell infiltrate.

Symptoms and Signs

Most patients present with cervical and mediastinal adenopathy but without systemic complaints. Despite apparent localized or regional disease (clinical stage), further studies are needed to define accurately the pathologic stage (see below). The following discussion considers the range of possible symptoms and signs, which usually do not all occur in the same patient.

A variety of symptoms and signs develop as the disease spreads through the reticuloendothelial system. Its rate of progress varies greatly from a relatively slow or quiescent condition (lymphocyte predominance or, occasionally, in the nodular sclerosis type) to an aggressive process (mixed cellularity or lymphocyte depletion type). An intermediate or moderately progressive clinical pattern is also recognized (nodular sclerosis or mixed cellularity). Intense pruritus may occur early; fever, night sweats, and weight loss occur frequently when internal nodes (bulky mediastinal or retroperitoneal), viscera (liver), or bone marrow are involved. The **Pel-Ebstein fever** pattern—a few days of high fever regularly alternating with a few days to several weeks of normal or subnormal temperature—occasionally is seen. An unexplained symptom is immediate pain in diseased areas after drinking alcoholic beverages.

Bone involvement may produce pain with vertebral osteoblastic lesions ("ivory" vertebra) and, rarely, osteolytic lesions with compression fracture. Pancytopenia is occasionally due to bone marrow invasion, usually by lymphocyte-depleted types. Epidural invasion that compresses the spinal cord may result in paraplegia. Horner's syndrome and laryngeal paralysis may result from pressure on the cervical sympathetic and recurrent laryngeal nerves, respectively. Neuralgic pains follow nerve root compression. Intracranial lesions may occur rarely.

Intra- or extrahepatic bile duct obstruction by tumor masses produces jaundice. Congestion and edema of the face and neck can result from pressure on the superior vena cava (superior vena cava or superior mediastinal syndrome). Leg edema may follow lymphatic obstruction in the pelvis or groin. Tracheobronchial compression can cause severe dyspnea and wheezing. Infiltration of the lung parenchyma may simulate lobar consolidation or bronchopneumonia and may result in cavitation or lung abscess. Ureteral compression from pelvic lymph nodes may interfere with urinary flow and cause secondary renal damage.

Most patients have a slowly progressive defect in delayed or cell-mediated immunity (T-cell function) that contributes in advanced disease to common bacterial and unusual fungal, viral, and protozoal infections (see Ch. 6). Humoral immunity (antibody production) or B-cell function is depressed in far-advanced disease. Evidence of cachexia is present. Patients frequently die from sepsis.

Laboratory Findings

A slight to moderate polymorphonuclear leukocytosis may be present. Lymphocytopenia may occur early and become pronounced with advancing disease. Eosinophilia is present in about 20% of patients, and thrombocytosis may be observed. Anemia, often hypochromic and microcytic, usually develops with advanced disease. In the latter setting, defective iron reutilization is characterized by low serum iron, low iron-binding capacity, and increased bone marrow iron. Hypersplenism may appear, but mainly in patients with marked splenomegaly. Elevation of serum alkaline phosphatase usually indicates bone marrow or liver involvement, or both. Increases in leukocyte alkaline phosphatase, serum haptoglobin, ESR, and serum copper usually reflect active disease.

Diagnosis

The symptom complex of lymph node enlargement (especially cervical) and mediastinal adenopathy, with or without fever, night sweats, and weight loss highly suggests Hodgkin's disease, but the diagnosis can be proved only by biopsy and demonstration of Reed-Sternberg cells in a characteristic histologic setting. In the absence of lymphadenopathy, the diagnosis can sometimes be established by biopsy of bone marrow, liver, or other parenchymal tissue.

The differential diagnosis of Hodgkin's disease from lymphadenopathy due to infectious mononucleosis, toxoplasmosis, cytomegalic inclusion disease, leukemia, or non-Hodgkin's lymphoma (see below) may be difficult. The clinical picture can also be simulated by bronchogenic carcinoma, sarcoidosis, and tuberculosis, and by various diseases with splenomegaly as their outstanding feature (see Ch. 100).

Staging of Hodgkin's Disease

It is essential at the time of diagnosis to document completely the extent of the disease, since the application of curative radiotherapy, chemotherapy, or both depends upon such staging. The disease is localized (Stage I or II) initially in 50% of patients. The Ann Arbor staging system is generally used:

Stage I: Disease limited to one anatomic lymph node region.

Stage II: Disease involving two or more anatomic lymph node regions on the same side of the diaphragm.

Stage III: Disease on both sides of the diaphragm involving lymph nodes or spleen.

Stage IV: Extranodal involvement, such as bone marrow, lung, or liver.

Subclassification E: Extranodal involvement adjacent to an involved lymph node. For example, a patient with cervical nodes and hilar adenopathy with adjacent lung infiltration is classified as Stage IIE, not Stage IV.

These stages are also significantly modified by the presence **(B)** or the absence **(A)** of constitutional symptoms (weight loss, fever, or night sweats).

A variety of procedures provide the data needed to stage these patients appropriately. Noninvasive procedures of value include ultrasound and computerized tomographic scans of the abdomen and pelvis, and, in selected cases, gallium body scans and bone scans. Bipedal lymphangiograms should be performed in patients with nodal disease. Since clinical and lymphangiographic studies attempting to detect disease below the diaphragm are falsely positive or negative in 25 to 33% of patients, laparotomy including splenectomy, biopsy of mesenteric and retroperitoneal lymph nodes (especially those enlarged on lymphangiograms), and core biopsy of the bone marrow and liver should be considered in the majority of patients who do not have unequivocal Stage IIIB or IV disease.

Treatment

Curative chemotherapy and radiotherapy are available for most patients. With nodal disease, 3500 to 4000 rads of radiotherapy in 3 to 4 wk can eradicate Hodgkin's tissue within the treated field 95% of the time. However, irradiation of adjacent uninvolved nodes (extended field or total nodal therapy) is standard practice since the disease spreads by lymphatic contiguity in about ⅔ of patients. Patients with subclassification E may respond to radiotherapy as well as patients with a comparable degree of lymph node involvement only. The following treatment is based upon surgically staged patients.

Stage I and IIA disease can be treated with radiotherapy alone to an upper mantle (all lymph-node–bearing areas above the diaphragm) and at least the upper periaortic lymph nodes. Such treatment is curative in approximately 90% of patients.

For **Stage IIB** disease, and IIIA disease due mainly to splenic involvement, extended field and total nodal radiotherapy (upper mantle, periaortic, and inverted "Y") respectively are probably most effective and are curative for about 60% of patients. Patients with Stage IIIA with extensive retroperitoneal nodal involvement may benefit from combination chemotherapy after radiotherapy (current studies are comparing this approach with the use of chemotherapy alone).

Since radiotherapy alone may not cure **Stage IIIB** Hodgkin's disease, either combination chemotherapy alone or such therapy combined with radiotherapy is needed.

In extranodal Hodgkin's disease **(Stage IVA and B)**, combination chemotherapy, particularly with mechlorethamine, vincristine, procarbazine, and prednisone ("MOPP" program), has produced a complete remission in 70 to 80% of patients, with > 50% remaining disease-free and probably cured at 5 to 10 yr. Such multiagent chemotherapy programs (as well as others utilizing a variety of other effective agents) represent a major advance over single-agent chemotherapy. Other effective agents include vinblastine, doxorubicin, bleomycin, dacarbazine (dimethylimidazolecarboxamide), nitrosoureas, and streptozocin.

NON-HODGKIN'S LYMPHOMA
(Malignant Lymphomas; Lymphosarcoma and Reticulum Cell Sarcoma)

A heterogeneous group of diseases, consisting of neoplastic proliferation of lymphoid cells that usually disseminate throughout the body. The terms lymphosarcoma and reticulum cell sarcoma have been replaced by newer terms (see below). Their courses vary from rapidly fatal to very indolent and initially well tolerated. A leukemia-like picture may develop in up to 50% of children and about 20% of adults with some types of non-Hodgkin's lymphoma.

Incidence and Etiology
Non-Hodgkin's lymphoma occurs more frequently than Hodgkin's disease. Each year in the USA, 7000 or 8000 new cases are diagnosed. It occurs in all age groups, the incidence increasing with age. Its cause is unknown, although, as with the leukemias, there is substantial experimental evidence for a viral etiology.

Pathology
Classification systems, although complex and transitional, offer reasonable means to distinguish subgroups with different prognoses and provide guidelines for management. In general, longer survival is related to a follicular or nodular nodal architecture and smaller lymphoid cell size; larger cell types or undifferentiated cells are usually diffuse and have a poorer prognosis.

The Rappaport classification for the histopathology of non-Hodgkin's lymphoma is based on the degree of differentiation of the tumor and on the presence or absence of nodularity. Large immature cells are designated as "histiocytes" and smaller ones as "lymphocytes" or "undifferentiated cells." Non-Hodgkin's lymphoma is classified as (1) malignant lymphoma, undifferentiated Burkitt's type or non-Burkitt's (pleomorphic type); (2) malignant lymphoma, histiocytic; (3) malignant lymphoma, mixed lymphocytic-histiocytic; (4) malignant lymphoma, lymphocytic (well differentiated or poorly differentiated); or (5) malignant lymphoma, lymphoblastic. All classes are further divided into nodular or diffuse except for (1) and (5), which occur only in a diffuse pattern. Nodular involvement includes cases in which fibrous strands separate the lymphoma infiltrate into nodules.

The Lukes and Collins classification is based upon the cell of origin and divides non-Hodgkin's lymphoma into **T-cell** (thymus-derived) types that include immunoblastic sarcoma and convoluted cell lymphoma (similar to lymphoblastic lymphoma), or **B-cell** (bone marrow-derived) types that include well-differentiated lymphocytic, plasmacytic, follicular center cell (small and large cleaved and non-cleaved cell type) lymphomas, and a B-cell immunoblastic sarcoma. A third category includes rare cases of "true" **histiocytic (or monocyte) origin,** while a fourth category includes **unclassifiable cases.**

Symptoms and Signs
While a variety of clinical manifestations exist, many patients present with asymptomatic adenopathy involving cervical or inguinal regions, or both. Enlarged lymph nodes are rubbery and discrete and later become matted. Local disease is apparent in some patients, but the majority have multiple areas of involvement. Various patterns of disease follow. The tonsils are occasional sites of involvement. Mediastinal and retroperitoneal lymphadenopathy may cause pressure symptoms on various organs. Extranodal sites may dominate the clinical picture; e.g., gastric involvement can simulate GI carcinoma, and intestinal lymphoma may cause a malabsorption syndrome. The skin and bones are initially involved in 15% of patients with histiocytic lymphoma and 7% of patients with lymphocytic lymphoma. Histiocytic lymphoma may rarely remain localized to bone. When extensive abdominal or thoracic disease is present, about 33% of patients develop chylous ascites or pleural effusion respectively due to lymphatic obstruction. Weight loss, fever, night sweats, and asthenia indicate disseminated disease.

Anemia is initially present in about 33% of patients and eventually develops in most. It may be due to bleeding from GI involvement or low platelet levels, hemolysis due to hypersplenism or Coombs-positive hemolytic anemia, bone marrow infiltration by lymphoma, or marrow suppression by drugs or irradiation. A leukemic phase develops in 20 to 40% of lymphocytic lymphomas and 10% of histiocytic lymphomas. Hypogammaglobulinemia due to progressive decrease in immunoglobulin production occurs in 15% of patients and may predispose to serious bacterial infection.

In children, non-Hodgkin's lymphoma may be of the undifferentiated, diffuse histiocytic or lymphoblastic type. These childhood lymphomas present different problems and require different management approaches than those seen in adults. The lymphoblastic type represents a variation of acute lymphoblastic leukemia (T-cell type) since both have a predilection for marrow, peripheral blood, skin, and CNS involvement, and patients frequently present with mediastinal adenopathy (Sternberg sarcoma) and superior vena cava syndrome. Nodular histologies are rarely seen in children.

Diagnosis

Non-Hodgkin's lymphomas must be differentiated from Hodgkin's disease, acute and chronic leukemia, infectious mononucleosis, TB (especially primary TB with hilar adenopathy and tuberculous adenitis), and other causes of lymphadenopathy, including pseudolymphoma due to phenytoin. Diagnosis can be made only by histologic study of excised tissue. Destruction of normal lymph node architecture and invasion of the capsule and adjacent fat by characteristic neoplastic cells are the usual histologic criteria. Immunologic studies to determine B, T, or other cell of origin will identify specific subtypes and help to define prognosis, and may be of value in management decisions (see below).

Staging and Prognosis

Localized non-Hodgkin's lymphoma does occur, but the disease is disseminated in about 90% of nodular histology and 70% of diffuse histology cases when first recognized. Staging procedures, similar to those for Hodgkin's disease, are of value except that laparotomy and splenectomy are rarely required. Lymphangiogram and CT scans of the abdomen are often helpful for staging and sequential comparison.

Initially, constitutional symptoms tend to be less common in non-Hodgkin's lymphoma than in Hodgkin's disease and do not per se alter prognosis. Organ infiltration is more widespread, and the bone marrow and peripheral blood may be involved. Bone marrow biopsy is useful to determine marrow involvement and should be done in most patients.

The prognosis and response to treatment are significantly influenced by histopathology and surface marker studies. Favorable prognostic types include nodular histologies and well-differentiated lymphocytic types that are usually B-cell lymphomas. Unfavorable prognostic groups include T-cell or lymphoblastic lymphomas, diffuse, poorly differentiated lymphocytic, histiocytic, and undifferentiated types (including Burkitt's lymphoma).

Treatment

After clinical and limited pathologic staging, localized lymphoma (Stage I or II) with "favorable" prognostic cell types may be cured by radiotherapy. Localized "unfavorable" prognostic types can be irradiated and about half of Stage I cases will be cured. Chemotherapy with or without radiotherapy is used with Stage II disease. Therapy of disseminated disease (Stage III or IV) of the "favorable" prognostic type is variable, including radiotherapy or chemotherapy. In some instances, when there are no symptoms and tumor growth is indolent, no initial treatment is indicated. Unfortunately, over a 2- to 6-yr period, most patients develop slowly progressive disease that is resistant to most treatment programs.

Advanced "unfavorable" prognostic types may respond dramatically to multiagent chemotherapy and as many as 50% will have long-term remissions and perhaps be cured. Effective agents include cyclophosphamide, vincristine, prednisone, doxorubicin, procarbazine, methotrexate, and bleomycin. Complete remission in 50 to 70% of patients with diffuse histiocytic lymphoma can be achieved by current combination chemotherapy programs, with prolonged disease-free survival in 30 to 40% of all patients. Thus, use of new intensive chemotherapy programs results in improved prognoses in some patients, even with "unfavorable" prognosis histology. Current regimens rarely result in cure of advanced "favorable" prognosis histology, although survival may be prolonged.

Patients with lymphoblastic lymphoma of T-cell type are managed in similar fashion to those with acute childhood T-cell lymphocytic leukemia with intensive chemotherapy regimens including prophylactic treatment of the CNS. Results are encouraging, with an estimated 50% cure rate.

BURKITT'S LYMPHOMA

A highly undifferentiated B-cell lymphoma that tends to involve sites other than the lymph nodes and reticuloendothelial system.

Burkitt's lymphoma, unlike other lymphomas, has a specific geographic distribution. Rare in the USA, it is most common in Central Africa, where its distribution appears to be determined by climatic factors, suggesting an unidentified insect vector and an infectious agent. Strong evidence, not yet verified, points to the herpes-like Epstein-Barr virus (see also INFECTIOUS MONONUCLEOSIS in Vol. II, Ch. 27).

Staging and Treatment

Stages A and B indicate single or multiple extra-abdominal sites. Stage C is defined by intra-abdominal disease including kidneys or gonads. Stage D disease is similar to C but with involvement of extra-abdominal sites including bone marrow or CNS. Prognosis is improved when bulk abdominal tumor can be resected.

Intermittent intensive chemotherapy (high doses of cyclophosphamide alone or lower doses combined with methotrexate and vincristine) produces long-term disease-free survival in 70 to 80% of patients with Stage A or B disease and in 30 to 40% of patients with Stage C and D disease.

MYCOSIS FUNGOIDES

An uncommon chronic T-cell lymphoma primarily affecting the skin and occasionally internal organs.

The disease is rare compared to Hodgkin's disease, and, unlike most other lymphomas, is insidious in onset. It may appear as a chronic, pruritic rash that is difficult to diagnose. Initially plaquelike, it may spread to involve most of the skin, become nodular, and eventually have systemic involvement. Lesions may become ulcerated. Pathologic diagnosis is delayed because sufficient quantities of lymphoma cells appear in the skin lesions only very gradually. Most patients are over age 50 by the time of diagnosis. From then until death, even without treatment, the time span is much longer than for the other lymphomas. Average life expectancy is about 7 to 10 yr after diagnosis. In some cases, a leukemic phase called **Sézary's syndrome** is characterized by small T lymphocytes with cerebriform nuclei in the peripheral blood.

Electron beam radiotherapy, in which most of the energy is absorbed in the first 5 to 10 mm of tissue, and topical nitrogen mustard have proved highly effective in controlling the disease. Plaques may also be treated with sunlight and topical steroids. Systemic treatment with alkylating agents and folic acid antagonists produces transient tumor regression.

---

99. PLASMA CELL DYSCRASIAS

(PCDs; Monoclonal Gammopathy)

A group of clinically and biochemically diverse disorders characterized by the disproportionate proliferation of one clone of cells normally engaged in immunoglobulin synthesis, and the presence of a structurally and electrophoretically homogeneous (monoclonal) immunoglobulin or polypeptide subunit in serum or urine. The disorders vary from asymptomatic and apparently stable conditions to progressive, overtly neoplastic disorders such as multiple myeloma. The classification of plasma cell dyscrasias appears in TABLE 99-1. Both clinical and immunochemical criteria must be used to diagnose these disorders.

The cause of PCDs is unknown. Most monoclonal immunoglobulins (M-components) synthesized by plasma cells are not qualitatively abnormal; rather, they appear to be normal products of a single clone that has undergone intense proliferation. Some of these M-proteins show antibody activity, most frequently directed toward autoantigens and bacterial antigens. Serum levels of normal immunoglobulins are commonly reduced.

The normal structural features of immunoglobulin molecules and the development of the major immunoglobulin classes are outlined in Ch. 16. Normal plasma cell production of immunoglobulins is heterogeneous, with individual clones of plasma cells producing the different immunoglobulins (IgG, IgM, IgA, IgD, or IgE). Each plasma cell clone secretes only one class of heavy chain (γ, μ, α, δ, or ε) and one class of light chain (κ or λ) at any one time in its lifespan. A slight excess of light chains is normally produced, and small amounts of free polyclonal κ and λ chains (up to 50 mg/24 h) are excreted in the urine of normal subjects.

A disproportionate proliferation of one clone results in a corresponding increase in the serum level of its secreted molecular product. This monoclonal immunoglobulin protein (the M-component) is readily detected by finding a tall symmetric spike with α_2, β, or γ mobility on cellulose acetate electrophoresis of serum or urine, but immunoelectrophoresis is required to identify the heavy and light chain class of the protein. The magnitude of M-component is related to the number of cells in the body producing that component; thus these proteins are valuable markers in diagnosing and managing patients with PCDs.

Most commonly, serum M-components are found in patients with malignant PCD (multiple myeloma, Waldenström's macroglobulinemia, primary systemic amyloidosis, or the various heavy chain diseases). Serum M-components are also found in a few asymptomatic, apparently healthy persons; the incidence is age-related—1% of persons over age 25 and 4% of those over age 70. Although many asymptomatic cases remain unchanged for years and are therefore seemingly benign, others represent incipient or **"premyeloma"** fortuitously discovered on routine serum protein electrophoresis. It is impossible to predict the course in any individual patient, and clinically symptomatic myeloma may not evolve for as long as 20 yr. The designation **plasma cell dyscrasia of unknown significance (PCDUS)** is therefore preferred for asymptomatic individuals with monoclonal serum components. Patients with PCDUS usually have low serum levels of M-components ($<$ 2.5 gm/dl) that are stable with time, and show mild marrow plasmacytosis, normal levels of serum immunoglobulins, and no lytic bone lesions or Bence Jones proteinuria. PCDUS also occurs in association with a variety of other diseases (TABLE 99–1). No treatment for the PCD is recommended; patients should be observed for change in status at 4- to 6-mo intervals.

TABLE 99-1. CLASSIFICATION OF PLASMA CELL DYSCRASIAS (PCDs)

	Disorder	Comments and Examples
Malignant (PCDs) Symptomatic, progressive	Multiple myeloma	IgG, IgA, light chains (Bence Jones) only, IgD, IgE, nonsecretory
	Waldenström's macroglobulinemia	IgM
	Primary systemic amyloidosis	Usually light chains (Bence Jones) only, but occasionally intact immunoglobulin molecules (IgG, IgA, IgM)
	Heavy chain diseases	IgG heavy chain (γ-chain) disease IgA heavy chain (α-chain) disease IgM heavy chain (μ-chain) disease IgD heavy chain (δ-chain) disease
Plasma cell dyscrasias of unknown significance (PCDUS) Asymptomatic, most nonprogressive	Associated with lymphoreticular neoplasms	Leukemia, lymphoma
	Associated with nonlymphoreticular neoplasms	Especially carcinomas of the colon, biliary tree, and breast
	Associated with chronic inflammatory conditions	Especially chronic cholecystitis
	Associated with various other disorders	Lichen myxedematosus, diabetes mellitus, thyrotoxicosis, pernicious anemia, chronic obstructive lung disease, Gaucher's disease, etc.
	In apparently healthy individuals; age-related incidence	

MULTIPLE MYELOMA

(Plasma Cell Myeloma; Myelomatosis)

A progressive and ultimately fatal neoplastic disease characterized by marrow plasma cell tumors and overproduction of an intact monoclonal immunoglobulin (IgG, IgA, IgD, or IgE) or **Bence Jones protein** *(free monoclonal κ or λ chains) only, and often associated with numerous osteolytic lesions, hypercalcemia, anemia, renal damage, and increased susceptibility to bacterial infections.* The impaired normal immunoglobulin production observed in multiple myeloma may be due to the presence of a monocyte or macrophage which prevents the maturation of normal B cells into polyclonal immunoglobulin-secreting plasma cells. Persons over the age of 40 are most commonly affected.

Pathology

The pelvis, spine, ribs, and skull are most frequently involved. Skeletal x-rays may show diffuse osteoporosis or discrete osteolytic lesions due to replacement by expanding plasma cell tumors or a factor (osteoclast-activating factor) secreted by the malignant plasma cells. Usually multiple, the osteolytic lesions occasionally occur as a solitary intramedullary mass. Extraosseous plasmacytomas are unusual, but diffuse plasma cell infiltrates may occur in any organ. Extensive cast formation in the renal tubules, atrophy of tubular epithelial cells, and interstitial fibrosis may result in renal failure **(myeloma kidney).** Amyloid deposits (see in Ch. 83) occur in 10% of myeloma patients and are especially likely in those with Bence Jones proteinuria.

The plasma cell tumors produce IgG in 50 to 55% of myeloma patients and IgA in about 20%; 40% of these IgG and IgA patients also have Bence Jones proteinuria. About 25% of patients have "light chain" myeloma; their plasma cells secrete *only* free monoclonal light chains (κ or λ Bence Jones protein). The light chain subgroup tends to have a higher incidence of lytic bone lesions, hypercalcemia, renal failure, and amyloidosis than do other myeloma patients. IgD myeloma accounts for about 1% of cases; serum levels are often relatively low, and heavy Bence Jones proteinuria (80 to 90% type λ) is characteristic. Only a few cases of IgE myeloma have been reported. Nonsecretory myeloma (no identifiable M-component in serum or urine) is very rare.

Symptoms and Signs

Persistent unexplained skeletal pain (especially in the back or thorax), renal failure, or recurrent bacterial infections, especially pneumococcal pneumonias, are the commonest presenting symptoms. Anemia with weakness and fatigue predominates in some patients, and a few have manifestations of the hyperviscosity syndrome (see in MACROGLOBULINEMIA, below). Pathologic fractures and vertebral collapse are common; the latter may lead to spinal cord compression and paraplegia. Lymphadenopathy and hepatosplenomegaly are unusual.

Diagnosis

Physical examination usually is not helpful unless bone pain or pallor is present. Laboratory findings include a normocytic normochromic anemia with rouleau formation evident on peripheral smear. The WBC and platelet counts usually are normal. The ESR is often markedly elevated (> 100 mm/h, Westergren), and BUN, serum creatinine, and serum uric acid are frequently elevated. Hypercalcemia occurs in about 1/3 of patients.

Proteinuria is common because of excess synthesis and secretion of free monoclonal light chains (Bence Jones protein). Significant albuminuria does not occur in myeloma; this finding suggests the presence of coexisting amyloidosis. A quantitative 24-h urinary protein determination is best for detecting significant proteinuria. Chemical paper strip tests of urine do *not* reliably detect Bence Jones protein, and the heat test is often misleading, but sulfosalicylic acid and toluene sulfonic acid are useful screening tests. Serum protein electrophoresis will show a tall, narrow, homogeneous M-spike in 75% of cases; the mobility of the spike may lie anywhere from the α_2 to the slow γ region. The remaining 25% of patients synthesize free monoclonal light chains (Bence Jones protein) only, and their serum electrophoretic patterns usually disclose hypogammaglobulinemia without a monoclonal spike. However, in essentially all patients with light chain myeloma, a homogeneous M-spike is demonstrable on protein electrophoresis of concentrated urine. Immunoelectrophoresis employing monospecific antiserum identifies the immunoglobulin class of the monoclonal spike in either serum or urine.

X-ray of the bones may show typical punched-out lytic lesions or diffuse osteoporosis. The bone marrow usually contains increased numbers of plasma cells at various stages of maturation; rarely is the number of plasma cells normal. The morphology of the plasma cells does not correlate with the class of immunoglobulin synthesized. Although sheets and clusters of plasma cells are diagnostic of marrow tumors, myeloma is a patchy disease and often only modest nonspecific plasmacytosis is observed.

Prognosis

The disease is progressive, but optimal management improves both the quality and duration of life. Life expectancy is related to the extent of disease at diagnosis, adequacy of supportive measures, and response to chemotherapy. About 60% of treated patients show objective improvement; the median survival for responding patients is 2 to 3 yr. High levels of M-protein in serum or urine, diffuse bone lesions, hypercalcemia, pancytopenia, and renal failure are unfavorable signs.

Treatment

General measures: Maintenance of ambulation is vital. Analgesics and palliative doses of radiotherapy (1000 to 2000 rads) to localized areas of symptomatic bone involvement relieve pain significantly. Adequate hydration is also essential. *(Dehydration before an IVP may precipitate acute oliguric renal failure in patients with Bence Jones proteinuria.)* Even patients with prolonged heavy Bence Jones proteinuria (10 to 30 gm/day or even more) may have no evidence of severe renal functional impairment if they are well hydrated (urine output > 1500 ml/day). Prednisone 60 to 80 mg/day orally is useful for hypercalcemia, and allopurinol 100 mg orally t.i.d. controls hyperuricemia. Antibiotics are indicated for active bacterial infection, and although prophylactic antibiotics are not recommended, monthly doses of gamma globulin may be helpful if bacterial infections recur. Transfusion of packed RBCs is indicated for severe anemia.

Chemotherapy: Objective improvement (as documented by a 50% or greater reduction in serum or urine M-component) usually follows the use of oral alkylating agents (melphalan or cyclophosphamide). Median survival may be extended three- to sevenfold. Melphalan may be given intermittently (0.25 mg/kg/day for 4 days every 6 wk) or continuously (6 to 10 mg/day for 8 to 10 days followed by 2 mg/day for maintenance). Prednisone given intermittently (1 mg/kg/day for 4 days every 6 wk) may improve the response to melphalan. Cyclophosphamide (200 mg/day for 5 to 7 days, then 50 to 100 mg/day for maintenance) appears to be equally effective. Because leukopenia and thrombocytopenia develop with these agents, dosage must be titrated in each patient. WBC levels of 2500/cu mm and platelet counts $> 90,000$/cu mm are usually safe. Various multiple drug regimens are being assessed for nonresponding or relapsing patients; occasional responses have been reported.

MACROGLOBULINEMIA

(Primary or Waldenström's Macroglobulinemia)

A plasma cell dyscrasia involving cells that normally synthesize IgM. Macroglobulinemia, a clinical entity distinct from myeloma and other PCDs, resembles a lymphomatous disease. Many of its clinical manifestations are directly due to the large amount of high mol wt macroglobulin circulating in the plasma. Some of these monoclonal IgM proteins are antibodies directed to autologous IgG (rheumatoid factors) or to the I red cell antigen (cold agglutinins). Cryoglobulinemia may be identified. The cause is unknown.

Small monoclonal IgM components are found in the sera of about 5% of patients with diffuse non-Hodgkin lymphoma; this circumstance has been termed "**macroglobulinemic lymphoma.**"

Symptoms and Signs

The patient is usually elderly, with symptoms of the **hyperviscosity syndrome:** fatigue, weakness, skin and mucosal bleeding, visual disturbances, headache, and a variety of other changing neurologic manifestations. When cardiopulmonary abnormalities predominate, they are associated with an increased plasma volume that also contributes to circulatory impairment. A history of cold sensitivity or Raynaud's phenomenon may be associated with the presence of a cryoglobulin or cold agglutinin. Recurrent bacterial infections are a major problem in some patients. Examination may disclose modest generalized lymphadenopathy, purpura, hepatosplenomegaly, and "sausaging" of the retinal veins (see Diagnosis, below). Amyloidosis occurs in 5% of patients.

Laboratory Findings

Moderate anemia with profound rouleau formation and a very high ESR are characteristic. Leukopenia, relative lymphocytosis, and thrombocytopenia occasionally occur. Cryoglobulins, rheumatoid factor, or cold agglutinins may be present; in the last instance the direct Coombs' test usually is positive. A variety of coagulation abnormalities may be present. Results of routine blood studies may be spurious if a cryoprotein is present or if viscosity is markedly increased. Relative serum viscosity is usually > 4.0 (normal 1.4 to 1.8) in patients with the hyperviscosity syndrome.

Diagnosis

A typical M-spike on serum protein electrophoresis that proves to be IgM by immunoelectrophoresis establishes the diagnosis. Immunoelectrophoretic studies of concentrated urine frequently demonstrate a monoclonal light chain (usually κ), but gross Bence Jones proteinuria is unusual. X-rays of bones may show osteoporosis, but lytic lesions are rare. The marrow shows a variable increase in plasma cells, lymphocytes, and intermediate forms (plasmacytoid lymphocytes). Lymph node biopsy is frequently interpreted as diffuse well-differentiated lymphocytic lymphoma. The **hyperviscosity syndrome** can be diagnosed by the findings of marked retinal venous engorgement and localized narrowing that gives the veins a sausage-like appearance. Retinal hemorrhages, exudates, microaneurysms, and papilledema indicate far-advanced stages.

Prognosis and Treatment

The course is variable but tends to be more benign than in myeloma. Many patients survive for > 5 yr. If hyperviscosity is present, initial management consists of reducing the serum viscosity by plasmapheresis which effectively and rapidly reverses the bleeding and neurologic abnormalities caused by the high IgM levels. Repeated plasmaphereses can be employed to control viscosity.

Long-term chemotherapy with oral alkylating agents is effective in most patients. Chlorambucil (2 to 6 mg/day) is the treatment of choice. Melphalan and cyclophosphamide, given as for multiple myeloma, are alternative agents.

PRIMARY SYSTEMIC AMYLOIDOSIS

(See Ch. 83)

HEAVY CHAIN DISEASES

Neoplastic plasma cell dyscrasias characterized by overproduction of homogeneous γ, α, μ, or δ immunoglobulin heavy chains. Some of these proteins are fragments of the normal heavy chain counterparts and may result from structural mutations.

IgG Heavy Chain (γ-chain) Disease

Approximately 40 cases have been reported, primarily in elderly men. Clinically they resemble malignant lymphoma; fever, anemia, and recurrent infections are common, and lymphadenopathy and hepatosplenomegaly are usual. Palatal edema is present in about 1/3 of patients. Bone marrow and lymph node histopathology is variable. Lytic lesions are absent in x-rays of bones. Diagnosis is based on electrophoretic and immunoelectrophoretic demonstration of free homogeneous heavy chain fragments of IgG in serum and urine. Half the patients have monoclonal serum components (often appearing broad and heterogeneous) in excess of 1 gm/dl, and half have proteinuria > 1 gm/day. Bence Jones protein is absent. The course is variable—from a few months to > 5 yr. Death usually results from infection or malignancy. Chemotherapy with alkylating agents or corticosteroids is ineffective.

IgA Heavy Chain (α-chain) Disease (Mediterranean Lymphoma)

This is the most common heavy chain disease and appears in young people. Most patients live in the Middle East; the disease is very rare in the Western Hemisphere. The clinical findings are uniform; almost all patients present with diffuse abdominal lymphoma and malabsorption syndrome. The abdominal nodes and lamina propria of the GI tract are massively infiltrated with lymphocytes, plasma cells, and reticulum cells—often accompanied by villous atrophy. The marrow, liver, and spleen are usually not involved. No osteolytic lesions are seen on x-ray. A discrete M-spike may not appear on routine serum protein electrophoresis. The diagnosis is based on the finding of an α-chain–related protein lacking light chains. Because it is often difficult to demonstrate light chains in IgA myeloma proteins, chemical methods are usually necessary to document their absence. The abnormal protein is not always present in concentrated urine. The course is usually progressive but remissions have been reported following use of radiotherapy, corticosteroids, cyclophosphamide, and antibiotics. A very rare pulmonary form of the disease has been reported.

IgM Heavy Chain (μ-chain) Disease

This very rare heavy chain disorder is clinically similar to chronic lymphocytic leukemia. Visceral organs (spleen, liver, abdominal lymph nodes) are primarily involved, with little peripheral lymphadenopathy. Vacuolated plasma cells are present in the bone marrow. Bence Jones proteinuria, pathologic fractures, and amyloidosis may occur. Routine serum protein electrophoresis shows hypogammaglobulinemia. The diagnosis is made by finding a rapidly migrating serum component that reacts with antiserum to μ chains but not with antiserum to light chains. Free IgM heavy chains are rarely found in the urine. Treatment is as described for chronic lymphocytic leukemia in Ch. 97, above.

IgD Heavy Chain (δ-chain) Disease

A single case has been reported recently. The patient was an elderly man with a clinical picture similar to multiple myeloma. Marked marrow plasmacytosis and osteolytic lesions in the skull were present. A small M-component was evident on serum protein electrophoresis which reacted with a monospecific anti-IgD antiserum, but not with other antisera of heavy or light chain specificity. Proteinuria was absent. Death occurred from renal failure.

100. THE SPLEEN

Analysis of the structure and function of the spleen reveals that it is actually comprised of two organs—an immune one, the **"white pulp,"** consisting of periarterial lymphatic sheaths and germinal centers, and a reticuloendothelial one, the **"red pulp,"** consisting of phagocytic macrophages and granulocytes lining vascular spaces (the cords and sinusoids).

The functions of the white pulp include (1) generation of humoral antibodies to circulating antigens; on occasion inappropriate autoantibodies to circulating blood elements are synthesized, as in immune thrombocytopenic purpura **(ITP)** or Coombs-positive, immune hemolytic anemias; (2) production of a leukocyte-modulating hormone, **"tuftsin"**; this protein nonspecifically increases neutrophil phagocytosis and chemotaxis, and its absence in the congenitally asplenic or splenectomized individual may be partly responsible for the increased susceptibility to infection seen in such patients; and (3) production and maturation of B and T lymphocytes and plasma cells as in other lymphoid organs.

Functions of the red pulp include (1) removal of unwanted particulate matter such as bacteria or senescent blood elements; e.g., in immune cytopenias (ITP, Coombs-positive hemolytic anemias, and in some neutropenias), rosette formation and phagocytosis of antibody-coated cells by red pulp macrophages underlie their destruction; (2) a reservoir function for blood elements; leukocytes and platelets especially can be released to the circulation from the human spleen by epinephrine; (3) a culling and pitting function which removes inclusion bodies such as Heinz bodies, Howell-Jolly bodies, and whole nuclei from RBCs; after splenectomy, circulating nucleated RBCs or cells with pieces of nuclei (Howell-Jolly bodies) are commonly encountered, reflecting loss of this function; and (4) a hematopoietic function: under abnormal conditions the spleen may replace bone marrow as a blood-forming organ. Normally hematopoiesis occurs in spleens only during fetal life; with marrow damage, as by fibrosis or scarring (myelofibrosis), hematopoietic stem cells may repopulate the adult spleen and liver **(myeloid metaplasia).**

HYPERSPLENISM

Various disorders in which blood cytopenia is associated with splenomegaly. The cardinal features of the syndrome are (1) splenomegaly; (2) a reduction of one or more blood cell elements, resulting in anemia, leukopenia, thrombocytopenia, or any combination thereof in association with hyperplasia of the marrow precursors of the deficient cell type; and (3) correction of the cytopenias by splenectomy.

Etiology

Abnormalities of the spleen are almost always secondary to primary disorders elsewhere; the many causes of hypersplenism are summarized in TABLE 100–1. Lymphoproliferative, myeloproliferative, and connective tissue diseases are the most commonly encountered causes in temperate climates, while infectious diseases such as malaria and kala-azar predominate in the tropics. Unsuspected hepatic cirrhosis or portal or splenic vein thrombosis resulting in congestive splenomegaly is uniformly distributed and a frequent cause of "idiopathic" splenomegaly.

Pathogenesis

Although sporadic data have suggested that splenic humors may exist which depress hematopoiesis, hypersequestration of blood in large spleens is generally considered the predominant mechanism for cytopenia in hypersplenism. The following evidence favors this conclusion: (1) Major decreases in leukocyte and platelet counts occur in splenic venous (compared to arterial) blood. (2) Inordinate and progressive accumulation of ^{51}Cr-labeled RBCs or platelets occurs in enlarged spleens, indicating preferential trapping of these cells. (3) Typical hypersplenism can be induced in animals injected with poorly metabolizable polymers such as methylcellulose. Storage of these substances leads to splenomegaly, pancytopenia, and splenic accumulation of ^{51}Cr-labeled RBCs associated with increased marrow Hb synthesis. (4) Viable spleen transplants placed in diffusion chambers in the peritoneal cavity of splenectomized animals have no effect on blood cell counts, arguing against the existence of splenic humors. (5) Administration of epinephrine to laboratory animals leads to splenic shrinkage and concomitant elevations of peripheral leukocyte and platelet counts; this response is greatly enhanced in hypersplenic humans, suggesting that excessively sequestered blood elements are released by the drug.

The fact that splenomegaly occurs in most chronic hemolytic anemias suggests that spleen growth may be stimulated by an increase in its "work load"—in this case, the work of trapping and destroy-

TABLE 100–1. ETIOLOGIES OF SECONDARY HYPERSPLENISM

Disease Category	Disease
Lympho- and myeloproliferative diseases	Lymphomas—including Hodgkin's disease
	Leukemias—especially chronic lymphocytic and chronic myelocytic
	Polycythemia vera
	Myelofibrosis with myeloid metaplasia
Inflammatory diseases	Acute infections—including infectious mononucleosis, infectious hepatitis, subacute bacterial endocarditis, psittacosis
	Chronic infections—including miliary TB, malaria, brucellosis, kala-azar, syphilis
	Sarcoidosis
	Amyloidosis
	Connective tissue diseases—including SLE and Felty's syndrome
Reticuloendothelioses	Lipoid—including Gaucher's, Niemann-Pick, and Schüller-Christian diseases
	Nonlipoid—Letterer-Siwe disease
Chronic, usually congenital, hemolytic anemias	Red cell shape abnormalities—including hereditary spherocytosis, hereditary elliptocytosis
	Hemoglobinopathies—including thalassemias, sickle Hb variants (e.g., Hb S-C disease), congenital Heinz body hemolytic anemias
	Red cell enzymopathies—e.g., pyruvic kinase deficiency
Congestive splenomegaly	Cirrhosis of the liver
	External compression or thrombosis of portal or splenic veins
Splenic cysts	Usually due to resolution of previous intrasplenic hematoma

Modified from *Hematology,* by W. J. Williams et al. Copyright 1976 by McGraw-Hill, Inc. Used with permission of McGraw-Hill Book Company.

ing abnormal RBCs. The commonly observed vicious spiral of hemolysis in many chronic hemolytic states (e.g., hereditary spherocytosis and thalassemia) may reflect this "work hypertrophy," and splenectomy may be of marked clinical benefit in such cases. In addition, splenic tissue, when stimulated to become hyperplastic by chronic hemolysis, may not be discriminating in its hyperfunction; thus thrombocytopenia and leukopenia are common features of many chronic hemolytic diseases. Similarly, common transient and nonspecific blood cytopenias are observed in patients with acute splenomegaly provoked by circulating microorganisms. Such infections are diverse and include subacute bacterial endocarditis, miliary tuberculosis, infectious hepatitis, psittacosis, and infectious mononucleosis.

Symptoms and Signs

Most of the presenting symptoms and signs may be those of the underlying disease. Besides palpable splenomegaly, the following may be encountered: (1) Left upper quadrant abdominal pain associated with splenic friction rubs indicates splenic infarction, a common concomitant of marked splenomegaly. (2) Epigastric and splenic bruits secondary to inordinate blood return from massively enlarged spleens may presage bleeding esophageal varices. (3) Early feeding satiety may be caused by encroachment on the stomach by the enlarged spleen. (4) Purpura and manifestations of mucosal bleeding may occur, although total platelet mass (the circulating pool plus that sequestered in the enlarged spleen) may be normal. Even though the excessive splenic pool can be mobilized by epinephrine, mild hemorrhagic diatheses may be seen in patients with severe depressions of platelet counts. Significant prolongation of bleeding time may be found, but severe hemorrhage is rare; its occurrence suggests additive effects of an underlying primary disease such as leukemia.

Diagnostic Approach to Splenomegaly

The sequence of diagnostic procedures is generally determined by formulation of the data from the history and physical examination.

1. Peripheral blood smear. (a) Excessive basophils, eosinophils, or nucleated or tear-drop RBCs suggest myeloproliferative disorders. (b) Lymphocytosis may occur in lymphoproliferative disorders. (c) Abnormality in RBC shape may suggest hereditary spherocytosis or a hemoglobinopathy (e.g., Hb S or C, or thalassemia).

2. Special blood chemistries. (a) **Serum electrophoresis:** monoclonal gammopathy or decreased immunoglobulins suggest lymphoproliferative disorders or amyloidosis; diffuse hypergammaglobulinemia may be noted in chronic infections (e.g., malaria, kala-azar, brucellosis, tuberculosis) or in cirrhosis with Banti's syndrome, sarcoidosis, and collagen vascular diseases. (b) **Uric acid:** Elevations occur in myeloproliferative disorders and less frequently in lymphoproliferative disorders. (c) **Leukocyte alkaline phosphatase** and **serum vitamin B_{12}:** elevated in myeloproliferative disorders. (d) **Liver function tests:** Diffusely abnormal in Banti's syndrome associated with cirrhosis; a solitary elevation of **serum alkaline phosphatase** suggests hepatic infiltration as in myeloproliferative and lymphoproliferative disorders and miliary tuberculosis.

3. Bone marrow examination. (a) General cellular hyperplasia with peripheral cytopenia is found in all hypersplenism syndromes. (b) Lymphocyte infiltration is found in lymphoproliferative disorders. (c) Hyperplasia of myeloid elements suggests myeloproliferative disorders. (d) Blast cell increase is found in leukemias. (e) Fibrosis occurs in myeloid metaplasia. (f) Periodic acid-Schiff staining clumps are present in amyloidosis. (g) Lipid-laden macrophages occur in Gaucher's and related storage disease.

4. ^{51}Cr-labeled RBC and platelet survival and splenic uptake studies are useful in assessing the degree of hypersequestration of these elements for splenectomy decision. The studies may be performed with epinephrine infusion to document hypersequestration of leukocytes and platelets in hypersplenic conditions—an excessive rise in these elements in the post-infusion circulation documents this phenomenon.

5. Splenic scan with technetium-labeled colloid (see also p. 1225). Patchy uptake is found in infiltrative diseases. Solitary defects suggest infarct or splenic cyst (which commonly follows trauma and resolution of an intrasplenic hematoma).

6. ^{59}Fe kinetics with splenic scanning. Early uptake of label (within 24 h) is observed in myeloid metaplasia.

7. Esophagogram and splenic venography. Varices and dilated splenic (or portal) veins suggest congestive splenomegaly (Banti's syndrome or splenic vein thrombosis).

8. Lymphangiography. Abnormal abdominal nodes occur in lymphoproliferative disorders.
Some of these diagnostic clues are summarized in TABLE 100–2.

Treatment of Splenic Disorders

Most patients with splenomegaly require therapy of the underlying disease, not splenectomy. Since asplenic individuals have increased susceptibility to serious systemic infections with encapsulated bacteria (*H. influenzae*, pneumococci, etc.), **indications for splenectomy or irradiation** should be strict, and include: (1) hemolytic syndromes in which the shortened survival of intrinsically abnormal RBCs is further curtailed by the additive effect of splenomegaly, as in hereditary spherocytosis and thalassemia; (2) severe pancytopenia associated with enormous splenic enlargement (up to 30

TABLE 100-2. HELPFUL CLINICAL FEATURES IN EVALUATING
COMMON SPLENIC DISORDERS

Disease	Spleen Size	Bone Marrow Findings	Blood Smear Findings	Special Studies
Myeloproliferative disorders: polycythemia vera (PV); myeloid metaplasia (MM); chronic myelogenous leukemia (CML)	Moderate (PV); massive (MM & CML)	Hyperplastic (PV & CML); fibrotic (MM)	↑*All blood cells (PV); pancytopenia (MM); ↑blasts (CML)	^{59}Fe splenic accumulation (MM); leukocyte alkaline phosphatase—↑(PV & MM), ↓*(CML)
Lymphoproliferative disorders	Moderate	Lymphoid infiltration; Reed-Sternberg cells (Hodgkin's Disease); amyloid deposits	↑Lymphs (chronic lymphocytic leukemia)	Abnormal serum immuno-globulins
Lipid-storage diseases (e.g., Gaucher's)	Massive	Lipid-filled macrophages	Pancytopenia (if hypersplenism is severe)	Enzyme studies for glycolipid metabolic defects

* ↑=increased; ↓=decreased.

times normal has been recorded in lipid-storage diseases); (3) vascular accidents involving the spleen—either chronic infarctions or bleeding esophageal varices associated with excessive splenic venous return; (4) mechanical encroachment on other abdominal organs (e.g., stomach with early satiety or left kidney with calyceal obstruction); and (5) intolerable hemorrhagic tendency, if definitely related to hypersplenic thrombocytopenia.

SOME SPECIFIC SPLENOMEGALIC SYNDROMES

Myeloproliferative disorders: In polycythemia vera, myelofibrosis with myeloid metaplasia, myelogenous leukemia, and essential thrombocythemia (collectively referred to as "myeloproliferative syndrome") the spleen becomes enlarged, particularly with myelofibrosis in which bone marrow is obliterated and the spleen assumes an increasing hematopoietic function. Splenomegaly may be massive, and if it is associated with infarcts, esophageal varices, or early satiety, splenectomy may be beneficial.

Lymphoproliferative disorders: The spleen is enlarged in chronic lymphocytic leukemia and the lymphomas (including Hodgkin's disease); see Chs. 97 and 98, above. Splenomegaly is usually associated with lymphadenopathy, immunoglobulin abnormalities, and lymphocyte dysfunction (e.g., anergy). Finding invasion of bone marrow by lymphoid elements is helpful in diagnosis.

Lipid-storage diseases: Glucocerebroside (in **Gaucher's disease)** or sphingomyelin (in **Niemann-Pick disease)** may accumulate in splenic reticuloendothelial cells, leading to spleen enlargement. In Gaucher's disease hypersplenism may be the only significant problem; splenectomy may be beneficial, although glycolipid accumulation in liver and bones may worsen after surgery. The finding of typical lipid-laden macrophages in bone marrow preparations frequently aids the diagnosis, and the specific glycolipid metabolic error can be diagnosed by leukocyte incubation studies. (See also ANOMALIES IN LIPID METABOLISM in Ch. 82.)

Collagen vascular disorders: In both SLE and RA, splenomegaly and leukopenia may coexist. In the latter, termed **Felty's syndrome,** leukopenia may be severe and associated with frequent infections. The pathogenesis of splenomegaly in this syndrome is unknown, and splenectomy is only beneficial in about 50% of cases. Splenic amyloidosis should also be considered in RA with splenomegaly.

Congestive splenomegaly (Banti's syndrome): Chronically increased splenic venous pressure may result from hepatic cirrhosis, portal or splenic vein thrombosis, or certain malformations of the portal venous vasculature. Associated bleeding from esophageal varices may be worsened by the superimposed thrombocytopenia induced by splenomegaly. Splenic venography, which may demonstrate or exclude extrahepatic portal obstruction, aids in diagnosis. Depending on etiology, surgical shunting procedures for venous obstructions or medical management of cirrhosis will be appropriate.

SPLENIC DEFICIENCY DISORDERS

(See SPLENIC DEFICIENCY SYNDROMES in Vol. II, Ch. 25)

§10. MUSCULOSKELETAL AND CONNECTIVE TISSUE DISORDERS

101. INTRODUCTION

In less than 2 generations, the broad field of arthritis, rheumatic disorders, and connective tissue diseases has reached maturity. The 7th Edition of THE MERCK MANUAL, published in 1940, contained 2 main categories of the commonest types of arthritis: atrophic or inflammatory arthritis (later called rheumatoid arthritis **[RA]**), and hypertrophic arthritis or degenerative joint disease (later identified as osteoarthritis **[OA]**); and a few other entities in general medicine such as gout and a bacterially incited arthritis. In this edition, the number of specifically identifiable conditions exceeds 100, including several new syndromes recently recognized, notably Lyme disease, eosinophilic fasciitis, and polymyalgia rheumatica.

The recognition of more syndromes has been accompanied by the introduction of new, highly effective drugs. Fifty years ago, colchicine for gouty arthritis and salicylates for arthritis generally completed the list of available drugs in the field except for 3 minor agents discussed below. In the late 1940s, interest in antiarthritic drugs increased with the discovery of corticosteroids and probenecid. Cortisone was initially recommended for management of RA, while probenecid, designed as a drug to inhibit penicillin excretion during its use in a variety of infectious diseases, was serendipitously found to have excellent uricosuric properties. It soon proved to be highly valuable in treating primary and secondary intercritical gout. Later, phenylbutazone and indomethacin emerged as improved aspirin substitutes, nonsteroidal anti-inflammatory drugs **(NSAID)**, useful in a number of arthritic conditions including acute gouty arthritis and acute chondrocalcinosis. Other NSAID drugs followed, e.g., naproxen, tolmetin, fenoprofen, ibuprofen, and sulindac, each selectively helpful in cases of RA and OA and other nonspecific symptoms associated with musculoskeletal disorders.

Meanwhile, 3 agents that enjoyed varying degrees of approbation in the 1930s were rediscovered and reintroduced into clinical medicine. Gold salts, which had been promoted in Europe and discounted in the USA, found new friends on both continents. And the onetime helpful bee or snake venom evolved in the 1970s as the venom of the fiery ant. Chloroquine was another drug that found acceptance by some rheumatologists. Currently it has some advocates in treating systemic lupus erythematosus **(SLE)**.

During the past 20 yr, the corticosteroids have lost favor for treating RA, except for intra-articular injection, while their value in relatively large doses has been accepted as highly desirable in treating fulminating symptoms of acute dermatomyositis, progressive systemic sclerosis, periarteritis nodosa, SLE, polymyalgia rheumatica, eosinophilic fasciitis, and a number of other conditions only remotely related to arthritis. Furthermore, with progress in the clinical recognition of the unusual connective tissue diseases came the association and probably pathogenic significance of many immunologic features, leading to treatment with immunosuppressive or cytotoxic drugs. Such agents include cyclophosphamide, azathioprine, methotrexate, and D-penicillamine. Also, methotrexate was found to be especially helpful in some patients with psoriatic arthritis. Recently, levamisole has been recommended, especially in RA, because of its immunostimulative (rather than immunosuppressive) properties.

Also, a xanthine oxidase inhibitor, allopurinol, has been used in treating intercritical gout, while patients with Paget's disease respond selectively to calcitonin, mythramycin, or diphosphonates. There are no specific drugs for treating Sjögren's syndrome, Reiter's syndrome, sarcoidosis, hemochromatosis, ochronosis, and Lyme disease.

The management of joint disease, regardless of diagnosis, usually involves specific or nonspecific drugs plus one of a variety of medical-surgical procedures that contribute in varying degrees to alleviation of joint, tendon, and muscle distress. These include such supportive measures as rest, heat, splinting, exercise, active or passive motion, elastic supports, massage, traction, hydrotherapy, canes, crutches, walkers, ultrasound, psychotherapy, acupuncture, and reconstructive orthopedic surgery, particularly of the hips and digits but also of some shoulders, elbows, or knees.

Much is yet to be learned and better therapies are needed, but the advances of the past 40 yr are impressive and warrant optimism.

102. APPROACH TO THE PATIENT WITH JOINT DISEASE

A complete history and physical examination, necessary for the diagnosis of joint disease and correct interpretation of physical changes (laboratory and x-ray data are usually only of supplementary help), are important also because joint symptoms may be part of a systemic disease. Even mildly inflammatory or noninflammatory arthritis may be the first indication of SLE, acute rheumatic fever, or hypertrophic pulmonary osteoarthropathy due to bronchogenic carcinoma. Conditions easily misinterpreted as arthritis by the patient include phlebitis, arteriosclerosis obliterans, cellulitis, edema, neuropathy, vascular compression syndromes, the stiffness of Parkinson's disease, periarticular stress fractures, myositis, and fibromyositis.

Extra-articular findings can be significant (e.g., tophi in gout, nodules in RA, and pustular rash in gonococcemia). Coexisting periarticular disease also may facilitate diagnosis. For example, tendinitis commonly coexists with gonococcal arthritis, RA, and other systemic diseases; popliteal cysts due to knee arthritis cause local popliteal pain, venous compression, or rupture into the calf; prominent tenderness of bones adjacent to joints and joint effusions occur in sickle cell disease and hypertrophic pulmonary osteoarthropathy.

TABLE 102–1 contains a classification of rheumatic diseases. Many times, the arthritis is transient and does not fulfill the criteria for any of these diseases, or it resolves without diagnosis. A final diagnosis should not be forced. A tentative diagnosis is made for treatment, with other possibilities kept in mind. A systemic disease should be considered in all atypical and undiagnosed conditions.

Certain problems require immediate attention and prompt treatment. Hemorrhagic fluid suggests fracture or malignancy. Intensely inflammatory effusions suggest pyogenic infection requiring immediate antibiotic therapy and aspiration drainage to prevent joint destruction.

Physical Examination of the Musculoskeletal System

A sequence of **inspection, palpation,** and **determination of the range of motion** of each involved joint area is followed. In most cases, this determines the presence of joint disease and establishes whether the joint, the adjacent structures, or both are involved. Involved joints should be compared with their uninvolved opposites or with those of the examiner. Information is recorded objectively and quantitatively, e.g., by using a numbered grading system and by measuring the range of motion in degrees.

Joint motion, generally painful in joint disease, may not be in periarticular, bone, or soft tissue disease. **Swelling** is an important finding. All swollen joints should be palpated. The examiner should then ballotte the joint to (1) elicit the presence of fluid; (2) differentiate between simple effusion, synovial thickening, and capsule or bony enlargement; and (3) determine whether the swelling is confined to the joint or is periarticular. Tenderness or swelling at only one joint margin may actually be arising in adjacent ligaments, tendons, or bursae; findings from several approaches to the joint substantiate articular involvement. **Increased heat** over the joint should be noted and carefully localized. **Crepitus** may arise from intra-articular structures or from tendons; the crepitus-producing motions should be determined. At the knee, for example, crepitus may arise from patellofemoral "grinding" or from femorotibial motion. **Monarthritis** always suggests infection, crystal-induced arthritis, or tumor.

Small joints, such as the acromioclavicular joint near the shoulder, the tibiofibular joint at the knee, the radioulnar joint, and the lateral epicondyle (the site of tennis elbow), can be the source of pain initially believed to be in the major joint.

The hand: The main differential features of **osteoarthritis** and **rheumatoid arthritis** are outlined in TABLE 102–2. In **psoriatic arthritis,** the distal interphalangeal joints **(DIP)** are commonly affected, psoriasis often is evident around the adjacent nail, and other joint involvement is more asymmetric than in RA. In **Reiter's syndrome,** synovial, periarticular, and periosteal changes are present in a few DIP, proximal interphalangeal **(PIP),** or metacarpophalangeal **(MCP)** joints, and there is asymmetric finger joint involvement. Asymmetric and DIP joint involvement also occur in **gout,** in which irregular peri- or extra-articular tophaceous deposits occur, some of which can be seen under the skin as cream-colored spots. Changes in the hand are more generalized in the **shoulder-hand syndrome** (reflex dystrophy), with diffuse edema and mottled, mildly cyanotic skin. In **progressive systemic sclerosis,** the skin is thickened, flexion contractures often develop, and the history is positive for Raynaud's phenomenon. Findings in **hypertrophic pulmonary osteoarthropathy** include clubbing of the fingertips and bony tenderness of the distal radius and ulna due to underlying periostitis. Joint synovitis similar to that seen in RA occurs in **SLE** and, less often, in **dermatomyositis,** though arthralgias and sore painful hands lacking demonstrable pathologic joint changes are more typical of both these disorders. Finger deformities resembling RA can occur in SLE but are due to soft tissue disease, not advanced erosive arthritis. Raynaud's phenomenon is often present in SLE, and erythema may be found over the extensor joint surfaces in dermatomyositis.

The elbow: Synovial swelling and thickening due to joint disease is sought in the lateral area between the radial head and olecranon, where it produces a bulge. Fluid or thickening in the olecranon bursa, rheumatoid nodules, and epitrochlear nodes should also be sought. Full 180° extension of the joint should be attempted. Though full extension is possible with nonarthritic or extra-articular lesions, its loss is an early change in **arthritis.** In **tennis elbow,** sharply localized pain is elicited by firm pressure over the lateral epicondyle.

The shoulder: Limitation of motion, weakness, pain, and disturbed mobility can be screened for by having the patient raise both arms above his head. Muscle atrophy and neurologic changes should be sought. Though swelling is not common, a bulge in the anterior or lateral superior area of the

TABLE 102–1. CLASSIFICATION OF THE RHEUMATIC DISEASES

I. **Polyarthritis of unknown etiology**
   A. Rheumatoid arthritis
   B. Juvenile rheumatoid arthritis
   C. Ankylosing spondylitis
   D. Psoriatic arthritis
   E. Reiter's syndrome
   F. Palindromic rheumatism
   G. Adult-onset Still's disease
   H. Others

II. **"Connective tissue" disorders (acquired)**
   A. Systemic lupus erythematosus
   B. Progressive systemic sclerosis (scleroderma)
   C. Polymyositis and dermatomyositis
   D. Mixed connective tissue disease
   E. Eosinophilic fasciitis
   F. Necrotizing arteritis and other forms of vasculitis
      1. Polyarteritis nodosa
      2. Hypersensitivity angiitis
      3. Wegener's granulomatosis
      4. Takayasu's (pulseless) disease
      5. Goodpasture's syndrome
      6. Henoch-Schönlein purpura
      7. Cogan's syndrome
      8. Giant cell arteritis (including polymyalgia rheumatica)
   G. Amyloidosis
   H. Others
      (See also Rheumatoid arthritis, I, A; Sjögren's syndrome, VI, I)

III. **Acute rheumatic fever**

IV. **Degenerative joint disease (osteoarthritis, osteoarthrosis)**
   A. Primary
   B. Secondary

V. **Nonarticular rheumatism**
   A. Fibrositis
   B. Intervertebral disk and low back syndromes
   C. Tendinitis and peritendinitis (bursitis, tenosynovitis)
   D. Fasciitis
   E. Carpal tunnel syndrome
   F. Jaccoud's syndrome
   G. Others
      (See also Shoulder-hand syndrome, VIII, C)

VI. **Disorders with which arthritis is frequently associated**
   A. Sarcoidosis
   B. Relapsing polychondritis
   C. Henoch-Schönlein purpura
   D. Ulcerative colitis
   E. Regional enteritis
   F. Whipple's disease
   G. *Yersinia enterocolitica* infection
   H. Intestinal bypass surgery
   I. Sjögren's syndrome
   J. Familial Mediterranean fever
   K. Others
      (See also Psoriatic arthritis, I, D)

(Continued)

TABLE 102–1. CLASSIFICATION OF THE RHEUMATIC DISEASES *(Cont'd)*

VII.   Associated with known infectious agents
   A.   Bacterial
       1.   *Gonococcus*
       2.   *Meningococcus*
       3.   *Pneumococcus*
       4.   *Streptococcus*
       5.   *Staphylococcus*
       6.   *Salmonella*
       7.   *Brucella*
       8.   *Streptobacillus moniliformis* (Haverhill fever)
       9.   *Mycobacterium tuberculosis*
      10.   *Treponema pallidum* (syphilis)
      11.   *Treponema pertenue* (yaws)
      12.   Others
            (See also Acute rheumatic fever, III)
   B.   Rickettsial
   C.   Viral
       1.   Rubella
       2.   Mumps
       3.   Viral hepatitis
       4.   Others
   D.   Fungal
   E.   Parasitic
   F.   Mycoplasmal

VIII.   Traumatic and/or neurogenic disorders
   A.   Traumatic arthritis (the result of direct trauma)
   B.   Neurogenic (neuropathic) arthropathy (Charcot's joints)
       1.   Syphilis (tabes dorsalis)
       2.   Diabetes mellitus (diabetic neuropathy)
       3.   Syringomyelia
       4.   Myelomeningocele
       5.   Congenital insensitivity to pain (including familial dysautonomia)
       6.   Others
   C.   Shoulder-hand syndrome
   D.   Mechanical derangement of joints
   E.   Others
        (See also Degenerative joint disease, IV; Carpal tunnel syndrome, V, E)

IX.   Associated with known or strongly suspected biochemical or endocrine abnormalities
   A.   Gout
   B.   Chondrocalcinosis (pseudogout)
   C.   Apatite crystal disease
   D.   Alkaptonuria (ochronosis)
   E.   Hemophilia
   F.   Sickle cell disease and other hemoglobinopathies
   G.   Agammaglobulinemia (hypogammaglobulinemia)
   H.   Gaucher's disease
   I.   Hyperparathyroidism
   J.   Acromegaly
   K.   Thyroid acropachy
   L.   Hypothyroidism
   M.   Scurvy (hypovitaminosis C)
   N.   Hyperlipoproteinemia Type II (xanthoma tuberosum and tendinosum) and Type IV
   O.   Fabry's disease (angiokeratoma corporis diffusum or glycolipid lipidosis)
   P.   Hemochromatosis
   Q.   Wilson's disease
   R.   Others
        (See also Inherited and congenital disorders, XII)

TABLE 102–1. CLASSIFICATION OF THE RHEUMATIC DISEASES *(Cont'd)*

X. Neoplasms

    A. Synovioma
    B. Primary juxta-articular bone tumors
    C. Metastatic malignant tumors
    D. Leukemia
    E. Multiple myeloma
    F. Benign tumors of articular tissue
    G. Others
       (See also Hypertrophic pulmonary osteoarthropathy, XIII, I)

XI. Allergy and drug reactions

    A. Arthritis due to specific allergens (e.g., serum sickness)
    B. Arthritis due to drugs
    C. Others
       (See also Systemic lupus erythematosus, II, A, for drug-induced lupus-like syndromes,
       e.g., hydralazine and procainamide syndromes; Hypersensitivity angiitis, II, F, 2)

XII. Inherited and congenital disorders

    A. Marfan syndrome
    B. Homocystinuria
    C. Ehlers-Danlos syndrome
    D. Osteogenesis imperfecta
    E. Pseudoxanthoma elasticum
    F. Cutis laxa
    G. Mucopolysaccharidoses (including Hurler's syndrome)
    H. Arthrogryposis multiplex congenita
    I. Hypermobility syndromes
    J. Myositis (or fibrodysplasia) ossificans progressiva
    K. Tumoral calcinosis
    L. Werner's syndrome
    M. Congenital dysplasia of the hip
    N. Arthro-onychodysplasia
    O. Arthro-ophthalmopathy
    P. Others
       (See also Arthropathy associated with known biochemical or endocrine abnormalities, IX)

XIII. Miscellaneous disorders

    A. Pigmented villous synovitis and tenosynovitis
    B. Behçet's syndrome
    C. Erythema nodosum
    D. Relapsing panniculitis (Weber-Christian disease)
    E. Avascular necrosis of bone
    F. Juvenile osteochondritis
    G. Osteochondritis dissecans
    H. Erythema multiforme (Stevens-Johnson syndrome)
    I. Hypertrophic pulmonary osteoarthropathy
    J. Multicentric reticulohistiocytosis
    K. Disseminated lipogranulomatosis (Farber's disease)
    L. Familial lipochrome pigmentary arthritis
    M. Tietze's syndrome
    N. Thrombotic thrombocytopenic purpura
    O. Pancreatitis or pancreatic carcinoma
    P. Steroid-crystal–induced synovitis
    Q. Polymyalgia rheumatica
    R. Intermittent hydrarthrosis
    S. Subacute bacterial endocarditis
    T. Others

TABLE 102–2. THE HAND IN RHEUMATOID ARTHRITIS AND
IN OSTEOARTHRITIS

Criteria	Rheumatoid Arthritis	Osteoarthritis
Character of swelling	Synovial, capsular, "soft tissue;" bony only in late stages	Bony with irregular spurs; occasional soft cysts
Tenderness.	Usual	None or minimal except during occasional acute onset
Distal interphalangeal (DIP) involvement	Not usual, except thumb	Characteristic
Proximal interphalangeal (PIP) involvement	Characteristic	Frequent
Metacarpophalangeal (MCP) involvement	Characteristic	Rare, except thumb
Wrist involvement.	Usual or common	Never, except base of thumb

Modified from P. J. Bilka, *Bulletin on the Rheumatic Diseases,* Vol. 20, pp. 596–599, March 1970. Used with permission of The Arthritis Foundation and the author.

shoulder is occasionally present in **RA** as a result of forward dissection of glenohumeral synovitis. Careful palpation of the relaxed shoulder may allow one to identify inflammation of bursae or tendons, a common condition occurring primarily in the subacromial area or the long head of the biceps tendon. Exact localization may permit aspiration and injection of a corticosteroid-xylocaine solution for relief of acute **tendinitis.**

The foot and ankle: Since weight bearing may elucidate certain abnormalities, part of the examination should be performed with the patient standing. In the normal ankle joint, 15° dorsiflexion and 40° plantar flexion are possible. Swelling just below and in front of the malleoli is characteristic of synovial or intra-articular disease. In **RA,** palpation of tender, rubbery swelling below, in front of, and behind the malleoli demonstrates synovitis of the ankle joint. Ankle edema, which is associated with normal ankle joint subastragalar motion, can be differentiated from true joint swelling by its diffuse, superficial, pitting, and nontender character. Metatarsophalangeal joints are very commonly swollen and tender in RA. Interphalangeal synovitis, not common in the feet in RA, may indicate **Reiter's syndrome, psoriatic arthritis,** or **gout.** In **gout,** the first metatarsophalangeal or bunion joint is most commonly affected. Diffuse erythema is striking in an acute attack of gout.

The knee: Such gross deformities as swelling (e.g., popliteal cysts), quadriceps muscle atrophy, and joint instability may be more obvious when the patient stands and walks. Careful palpation of the knee, especially noting the presence of joint fluid, synovial thickening, and local tenderness, helps detect arthritis. Tender extra-articular bursae and true intra-articular disturbances should be differentiated.

Detection of small knee effusions is a common problem in joint evaluation and is best done using the "bulge sign." The knee is extended and the leg is slightly externally rotated while the patient is supine with muscles relaxed. The medial aspect of the knee is stroked to express any fluid away from this area. The examiner places one hand on the suprapatellar pouch and then strokes or presses gently on the lateral aspect of the knee, creating a fluid wave or bulge visible medially.

Full 180° extension of the knee should be attempted to detect knee flexion contractures. With **meniscus tears** or **collateral ligament injuries,** forceful lateral or medial bending while extending the leg produces pain by compressing the meniscus and simultaneously stretching the opposite collateral ligament. The joint line can be located by medial and lateral palpation while slowly flexing and extending the knee. A displaced meniscus is painful on firm pressure; a collateral ligament injury is tender in a longitudinal direction. The intactness of the cruciate ligaments can be determined by grasping the leg with the knee flexed at 90° (best done with the patient sitting on a table edge with his legs dangling) and estimating the amount of posterior-anterior movement (which should be minimal). The patella should be tested for free, painless motion. To gauge excess mobility of the joint, especially lateral instability, the thigh is firmly fixed and an attempt is made to rock the relaxed, almost extended, knee from side to side.

The hip: A limp is common in patients with significant hip **arthritis.** It may be due to pain, shortening of the leg, flexion contracture, or muscle weakness. Though these gross abnormalities are not always obvious early in the course, some loss of internal rotation, flexion, extension, or abduction can usually be demonstrated. One hand should be placed on the patient's iliac crest to detect pelvic movement that might be mistaken for hip movement. Tenderness over the femoral greater trochanter indicates local **bursitis** rather than arthritis.

The vertebral column: Cervical and lumbar motion should be measured. Inability to reverse the normal lumbar lordosis on flexion occurs in **degenerative arthritis.** Limited flexion is characteristic of **ankylosing spondylitis.** The effect of movement on pain should be noted. Pain and limitation can be due to soft tissue disease as well as to arthritis. Palpation and firm percussion over each vertebra and sacroiliac joint may elicit superficial or deep bone tenderness that should be distinguished from muscle spasm. Localized bone pain suggests such disorders as **osteomyelitis, leukemia, primary or metastatic cancer, compression fracture,** or **herniated disk.** The examiner should note psychogenic ("touch-me-not") reactions. Chest expansion should be measured, as it is typically impaired in **ankylosing spondylitis.**

Diagnostic Studies

Laboratory studies are useful in diagnosing the specific type of arthritis present. Specific tests are discussed in the chapters for each disease. An elevated Westergren sedimentation rate suggests inflammatory disease. Serum uric acid levels are elevated by low doses of aspirin, by diuretics, other drugs, diet, or alcohol, which lower urate clearance, and in gout. Latex fixation tests for rheumatoid factor are often highly positive in RA and may also be positive in cirrhosis, sarcoidosis, SBE, TB, and other diseases. Antinuclear factors may be positive in RA, Sjögren's syndrome, progressive systemic sclerosis, SLE, and other diseases. Serum CPK and SGOT are also elevated in peripheral muscle disease, including certain forms of muscular dystrophy, crush injury, and gangrene of muscle, and in dermatomyositis.

X-rays are important in the initial evaluation of relatively localized unexplained complaints to detect possible primary or metastatic tumors, osteomyelitis, bone infarctions, periarticular calcifications, or other changes in deep structures that may escape physical examination. They are also especially useful in examination of the spine.

Other studies useful in selected patients include needle or surgical synovial biopsy, arthroscopy, arthrography, bone and marrow scans, electromyography, nerve conduction times, thermography, and muscle biopsy. Evaluation of synovial fluid is discussed below.

Differentiating Inflammatory and Noninflammatory Joint Disease

Inflammatory and noninflammatory processes must be differentiated once joint involvement has been established. Among the typical local signs of inflammation, increased heat and erythema are most helpful in this differentiation. Erythema should not be expected over the chronically inflamed joints in RA. Fever and an elevated ESR tend to occur with severe inflammatory arthritis, but may also be due to an inflammatory process elsewhere in the body. Soft tissue swelling tends to favor an inflammatory process, but aspiration of any effusion is essential to determine its nature. Routes of aspiration are the same as those shown for joint injection in Fig. 103–1 under Rheumatoid Arthritis in Ch. 103. An outline for performing arthrocentesis is shown in Table 102–3. Preparation for handling the fluid obtained is critical so that the studies most pertinent for each patient can be properly performed. Not all tests need to be done on each fluid.

Table 102–3. An Outline for Performing Arthrocentesis

Find the effusion.

Mark the site for entry.

Scrub with soap, paint with tincture of iodine, and rinse with alcohol.

Anesthetize the skin by spraying it with ethyl chloride or by infiltrating the skin and subcutaneous tissue with 1% lidocaine.

Aspirate with a 20-gauge needle.

Record the volume, viscosity, color, and clarity of the synovial fluid.

If infection is considered a possibility, immediately place 0.5 ml of the synovial fluid in a sterile tube for routine cultures, in an anaerobic tube for anaerobes, and if gonorrhea is suspected, plate at bedside onto Thayer-Martin medium.

Place 0.5 ml of the synovial fluid in a heparinized tube for a leukocyte count. *Use a 0.3% (hypotonic) saline solution as diluent for the WBC.*

Prepare smears for Wright's and Gram stains.

Prepare a wet smear of fluid to look for crystals and inclusions by placing a drop of synovial fluid on a slide (using a flamed loop) and covering with a cover slip, the edges of which are promptly sealed with clear nail polish to delay drying.

Place the remainder of the fluid in a tube for chemical studies (e.g., glucose in a fluoride tube).

Freeze at -70 C for complement.

Draw fasting serum to compare synovial fluid and serum complement and glucose content.

TABLE 102–4. CLASSIFICATION OF SYNOVIAL EFFUSIONS

	Normal	Noninflammatory	Inflammatory	Septic
Gross examination:				
Viscosity	High	High	Low	Variable
Color	Colorless	Yellow	Yellow	Variable
Clarity*	Transparent	Transparent	Translucent	Opaque
Routine laboratory examination:				
WBC**	< 200/cu mm	200 to 2,000/cu mm	2,000 to 100,000/cu mm	> 100,000/cu mm
PMNs**	< 25%	< 25%	> 50%	> 75%
Culture	Negative	Negative	Negative	Often positive
Glucose (AM fasting)	≅ to simultaneously drawn blood	≅ to simultaneously drawn blood	< 25 mg/100 ml lower than simultaneously drawn blood	> 25 mg/100 ml lower than simultaneously drawn blood

* Extremely cloudy or opaque effusions can also be produced by crystals, tissue fragments, amyloid, or "rice bodies," as well as by leukocytes.

** WBC and % PMNs (polymorphonuclear leukocytes) in septic arthritis will be less if organism is less virulent or partially treated.

Modified from R. A. Gatter and D. J. McCarty, "Synovianalysis," in *Rheumatism,* Vol. 20, pp. 2–6, Jan. 1964. Used with permission.

Synovial fluid measurements that allow classification are shown in TABLE 102–4. These differentiate most effusions as normal or "noninflammatory," inflammatory, and septic arthritis. Effusions can also be hemorrhagic. Each type of effusion suggests certain joint diseases, as shown in TABLE 102–5.

Microscopic examination of a wet synovial fluid smear for crystals (even a few drops of fluid or washings from a joint can be used for culture or examination of crystals), using polarized light, is essential for diagnosis of gout. By placing an inexpensive polarizer over the light source and another between the specimen and the examiner's eye, crystals with a shiny white birefringence will be visible. Compensated polarized light is provided by inserting a first-order red plate, as in commercially available microscopes. One can also reproduce the effects of a compensator by placing 2 strips of clear adhesive tape on a glass slide and placing this slide over the lower polarizer. Sodium

TABLE 102–5. DIFFERENTIAL DIAGNOSIS BASED ON SYNOVIAL FLUID CLASSIFICATION (PARTIAL LISTING)

Noninflammatory	Inflammatory	Septic	Hemorrhagic
Degenerative joint disease	Rheumatoid disease	Bacterial infections	Trauma with or without fracture
Trauma	Reiter's syndrome		Villous pigmented synovitis
Osteochondritis dissecans	Psoriatic arthritis		
Neurogenic (neuropathic) arthropathy	Ankylosing spondylitis		Synovioma
Sickle cell disease	Ulcerative colitis		Neurogenic (neuropathic) arthropathy
Osteochondromatosis	Regional enteritis		
Subsiding or early inflammation	Acute crystal synovitis (gout and pseudogout)		Hemangioma
Hypertrophic pulmonary osteoarthropathy	Partially treated or less virulent bacterial infections		Hemophilia
Ehlers-Danlos syndrome			Anticoagulant treatment
Amyloidosis			Scurvy
	Systemic lupus erythematosus		
	Rheumatic fever		
	Progressive systemic sclerosis		

Modified from R. A. Gatter and D. J. McCarty, "Synovianalysis," in *Rheumatism,* Vol. 20, pp. 2–6, Jan. 1964. Used with permission.

urate crystals then appear strongly *negatively* birefringent, i.e., yellow parallel to the axis marked on the compensator (or the long axis of the slide); calcium pyrophosphate dihydrate **(CPPD)** crystals appear weakly *positively* birefringent, i.e., blue in the direction that urates are yellow. Sodium urate crystals tend to be needle- or rod-shaped; CPPD crystals are rhomboid or rod-shaped. Cholesterol, recently injected intra-articular corticosteroids, oxalate anticoagulants, fibrils from lens paper, and dirt also appear crystalline or as birefringent objects and may be confused with the crystals. Clumps of apatite crystals are not birefringent with polarized light but appear as shiny, slightly irregular "coinlike" particles.

LE cells formed in vivo, marrow spicules (due to fracture), brown cartilage fragments (due to ochronosis), Gram stains or acid-fast stains showing specific organisms, Congo-red–staining amyloid fragments, sickled erythrocytes (due to sickle-cell hemoglobinopathies), or iron in large mononuclear synovial cells on Prussian blue stain (due to hemochromatosis or villous pigmented synovitis) may also be found in the synovial fluid, yielding a specific diagnosis.

Comparing synovial fluid and serum complement levels may be helpful. The synovial fluid complement tends to be < 30% of the serum complement level in RA, but is often higher in gout, Reiter's syndrome, and infectious arthritis. Synovial fluid complement levels will be low in normal and noninflammatory effusions in which little protein is present. Measurements of rheumatoid factor in synovial fluid can give misleading false-positive or false-negative results.

103. ARTHRITIS; RELATED DISORDERS

RHEUMATOID ARTHRITIS (RA)

A chronic syndrome characterized by nonspecific, usually symmetric inflammation of the peripheral joints, potentially resulting in progressive destruction of articular and periarticular structures; generalized manifestations may also be present.

Etiology and Incidence

Etiology is unknown. The immunologic changes (see also in Ch. 19, AUTOIMMUNE DISORDERS) may be initiated by multiple factors. About 1% of all populations are affected, women 2 to 3 times more commonly than men. Onset may be at any age, but most often occurs between 25 and 50.

Pathology

In chronically affected joints, the normally delicate synovial membrane develops many villous folds and thickens because of increased numbers and size of synovial lining cells and colonization by lymphocytes and plasma cells. The colonizing cells, initially perivenular but later forming lymphoid follicles with germinal centers, synthesize rheumatoid factor **(RF)** and other immunoglobulins. Fibrosis and necrosis are also present. These findings are typical but not diagnostic. Hyperplastic synovial tissue (pannus) may erode cartilage, subchondral bone, articular capsule, and ligaments. Polymorphonuclear leukocytes are not prominent in the synovium, but often predominate in the synovial fluid.

The **rheumatoid nodule,** usually found subcutaneously at sites subject to trauma, is the most characteristic pathologic lesion. It is a nonspecific necrobiotic granuloma consisting of a central necrotic area surrounded by "palisaded" mononuclear cells with their long axes radiating from the center, all enveloped by lymphocytes and plasma cells. Nodules and vasculitis have been found at necropsy in many visceral organs in severe cases of RA, but are clinically significant in only a few cases.

ADULT RHEUMATOID ARTHRITIS

Symptoms and Signs

Onset may be abrupt, with simultaneous inflammation in multiple joints, or (more frequently) insidious, with progressive joint involvement. Tenderness in nearly all "active" (inflamed) joints is the most sensitive physical sign. Synovial thickening, the most specific physical finding, eventually occurs in most active joints. Symmetric involvement of small hand joints (especially the proximal interphalangeal and metacarpophalangeal), feet, wrists, elbows, and ankles is typical, but initial manifestations may occur in any joint. Stiffness lasting more than 30 min on arising in the morning or after prolonged inactivity is common; early afternoon fatigue and malaise also occur. Deformities may develop rapidly, particularly flexion contractures. Ulnar deviation of the fingers with slippage of the extensor tendons off the metacarpophalangeal joints is typical.

Subcutaneous rheumatoid nodules, though not usually an early manifestation, can be a major aid in diagnosis; they should be biopsied to differentiate gouty tophi and amyloid and other nodules. Visceral nodules, vasculitis causing leg ulcers or mononeuritis multiplex, pleural or pericardial effusions, and Sjögren's syndrome or episcleritis are other extra-articular manifestations. Fever may be present and is usually low-grade, except in the adult-onset Still's disease, a variant of RA.

Laboratory and X-ray Findings

A normochromic or slightly hypochromic, normocytic anemia, typical of other chronic diseases, is found in 80% of cases; the Hb is usually > 10 gm/100 ml, but may rarely be as low as 8 gm/100 ml. Superimposed iron deficiency or other causes of anemia should be sought if the Hb is < 10 gm/100 ml. Neutropenia is found in 2% of cases, often with splenomegaly **(Felty's syndrome)**. Mild hyper-gammaglobulinemia and thrombocytosis may be present.

The ESR is elevated in 90% of cases. Antibodies to altered γ-globulin, the so-called **rheumatoid factors (RF)**, as detected by agglutination tests (such as the latex fixation test) that show IgM RF are found in about 70% of cases. Though RF are not specific for RA and are found in many diseases (including granulomatous diseases, chronic liver disease, and subacute bacterial endocarditis), a high RF titer provides helpful confirmation when the typical clinical syndrome is present. The **latex** and **bentonite tests**, utilizing human IgG adsorbed to particulate carriers such as latex or bentonite, are less specific but more sensitive than the sensitized sheep cell test using animal (rabbit) IgG. A latex slide test can be used for screening, but if positive, should be followed by a tube dilution test for a titer. In most laboratories, a latex fixation tube dilution titer of 1:160 is considered the lowest positive value for a diagnosis of RA. A high RF titer indicates a poor prognosis and is often associated with progressive disease, nodules, vasculitis, and pulmonary involvement. The titer can be influenced by treatment or spontaneous improvement and often falls as inflammatory joint activity decreases.

The synovial fluid, always abnormal during active joint inflammation, is cloudy and sterile, has reduced viscosity, and contains 3000 to 50,000 WBCs/cu mm. Polymorphonuclear cells typically predominate, but more than 1/2 of the cells may be lymphocytes and other mononuclear cells in very early or subsiding inflammation. Leukocyte cytoplasmic inclusions may be seen on a wet smear, but are also present in other inflammatory effusions. Synovial fluid complement is often $< 30\%$ of the serum level. Crystals are absent, excluding gout and pseudogout.

Radiologically, only soft tissue swelling is seen in the first year of the disease. Subsequently, periarticular osteoporosis, joint space (articular cartilage) narrowing, and subchondral erosions may be present. The rate of radiologic deterioration, like the rate of clinical deterioration, is highly variable.

Differential Diagnosis

The American Rheumatism Association has established criteria for the diagnosis of "possible," "probable," "definite," and "classic" RA (see TABLE 103–1). While primarily intended as a communication aid for those in clinical research, these criteria can serve as a guide to clinical diagnosis. Almost any other disease that causes arthritis must be ruled out by exclusion. These exclusions should be considered relative, since 2 diseases causing arthritis can occasionally coexist.

RA shares many features of other collagen vascular diseases, particularly SLE, but the latter can usually be distinguished by the characteristic skin lesions on light-exposed areas, temporal-frontal hair loss, oral and nasal mucosal lesions, joint fluid with a high viscosity and a WBC count often < 2000/cu mm (predominantly mononuclear cells), positive anti-DNA antibodies, renal disease, and low serum complement. LE cells, positive antinuclear factors, and visceral organ involvement are found in about 5% of otherwise typical RA patients, giving rise to the term "overlap syndrome." Some of these cases may represent severe RA; others have associated SLE or other collagen disease. Polyarteritis, progressive systemic sclerosis, and dermato(poly)myositis may also have features that resemble RA.

Sarcoidosis, amyloidosis, Whipple's disease, and other systemic diseases may also involve joints; biopsy of appropriate tissues often differentiates these conditions. Acute rheumatic fever is differentiated by a migratory pattern of joint involvement, changing cardiac murmurs, chorea, erythema marginatum, and evidence of antecedent streptococcal infection (culture or changing antistreptolysin-O **[ASO]** titer). Infectious arthritis is usually monarticular or asymmetric. Diagnosis depends on identification of the causative agent. It should be remembered, however, that infection can be superimposed on a joint affected by RA. Gonococcal arthritis usually presents as a migratory arthritis involving tendons around the wrist and ankle and finally settling in 1 or 2 joints. Reiter's syndrome is characterized by asymmetric involvement of the heel, spine, sacroiliac joint, and large joints of the leg and by urethritis, conjunctivitis, iritis, painless buccal ulcers, and balanitis circinata or keratoderma blenorrhagica on the soles and elsewhere. Serum and joint fluid complement levels are elevated. Psoriatic arthritis tends to be asymmetric and is not usually associated with RF, but differentiation may be difficult in the absence of characteristic nail or skin lesions. Ankylosing spondylitis may be differentiated by its predilection for males, spinal and axial distribution of joint involvement, absence of subcutaneous nodules, and negative RF test. Gout may be mon- or polyarticular with complete recovery between acute attacks early in the disease. Typical negatively birefringent sodium urate crystals are present in the synovial effusion and can be seen by compensated polarized light. Hyperuricemia does not establish gout as the diagnosis. Response to colchicine is highly suggestive of gout, but other diseases may also subside with colchicine, or spontaneously. Chondrocalcinosis may produce mon- or polyarticular acute or chronic arthritis, but the presence of weakly positively birefringent calcium pyrophosphate dihydrate crystals in joint fluid and x-ray evidence of articular cartilage calcification differentiate this condition. A common variant of osteoarthritis involves the proximal and distal interphalangeal joints, first carpometacarpal and first metatarsopha-

TABLE 103-1. DIAGNOSTIC CRITERIA FOR RHEUMATOID ARTHRITIS

A. Classic Rheumatoid Arthritis
This diagnosis requires 7 of the following criteria. In criteria 1 through 5 the joint signs or symptoms must be continuous for at least 6 wk.
1. Morning stiffness.
2. Pain on motion or tenderness in at least 1 joint (observed by a physician).
3. Swelling (soft tissue thickening or fluid, not bony overgrowth alone) in at least 1 joint (observed by a physician).
4. Swelling (observed by a physician) of at least 1 other joint (any interval free of joint symptoms between the 2 joint involvements may not be more than 3 mo).
5. Symmetric joint swelling (observed by a physician) with simultaneous involvement of the same joint on both sides of the body (bilateral involvement of proximal interphalangeal, metacarpophalangeal, or metatarsophalangeal joints is acceptable without absolute symmetry). Terminal phalangeal joint involvement will not satisfy this criterion.
6. Subcutaneous nodules (observed by a physician) over bony prominences, on extensor surfaces, or in juxta-articular regions.
7. X-ray changes typical of rheumatoid arthritis (which must include at least bony decalcification localized to or greatest around the involved joints and not just degenerative changes). Degenerative changes do not exclude patients from any group classified as rheumatoid arthritis.
8. Positive agglutination test—demonstration of the rheumatoid factor by any method which, in 2 laboratories, has been positive in not > 5% of normal controls.
9. Poor mucin precipitate from synovial fluid (with shreds and cloudy solution). An inflammatory synovial effusion with > 2000 WBC/cu mm and no crystals can be substituted for this criterion.
10. Characteristic histologic changes in synovial membrane with 3 or more of the following: marked villous hypertrophy; proliferation of superficial synovial cells; marked infiltration of chronic inflammatory cells (lymphocytes or plasma cells predominating), with tendency to form "lymphoid nodules"; deposition of compact fibrin either on surface or interstitially; foci of cell necrosis.
11. Characteristic histologic changes in nodules showing granulomatous foci with central zones of cell necrosis, surrounded by a palisade of proliferated mononuclear cells, peripheral fibrosis, and chronic inflammatory cell infiltration.

B. Definite Rheumatoid Arthritis
This diagnosis requires 5 of the above criteria. In criteria 1 through 5 the joint signs or symptoms must be continuous for at least 6 wk

C. Probable Rheumatoid Arthritis
This diagnosis requires 3 of the above criteria. In at least 1 of criteria 1 through 5 the joint signs or symptoms must be continuous for at least 6 wk.

D. Possible Rheumatoid Arthritis
This diagnosis requires 2 of the following criteria and total duration of joint symptoms must be at least 3 wk.
1. Morning stiffness.
2. Tenderness or pain on motion (observed by a physician) with history of recurrence or persistence for 3 wk.
3. History or observation of joint swelling.
4. Subcutaneous nodules (observed by a physician).
5. Elevated ESR or C-reactive protein.
6. Iritis (of dubious value as a criterion except in the case of juvenile rheumatoid arthritis).

Modified from *Bulletin on Rheumatic Diseases*, Vol. 9, No. 4, pp. 175–176, December 1958, and *Primer on the Rheumatic Diseases*, JAMA, Vol. 224, p. 799, April 30, 1973. Copyright 1973, American Medical Association. Used with permission of JAMA and The Arthritis Foundation.

langeal joints, knees, and spine **(Kellgren's syndrome, erosive osteoarthritis).** Symmetry of involvement, prominent joint swelling with signs of inflammation, joint instability, and subchondral erosions on x-ray may prove confusing; the absence of RF, rheumatoid nodules, and systemic involvement, and the characteristic osteoarthritis pattern of joint involvement permit differentiation from RA.

Treatment
As many as 75% of patients improve with conservative treatment during the first year of disease; 5 to 10% are eventually disabled despite full treatment.

Rest and nutrition: Complete bed rest is occasionally indicated for a short period during the most active painful stage of severe disease. Although symptoms and signs often subside with little other treatment, they will probably recur unless anti-inflammatory drugs are given. In less severe cases, regular rest periods should be prescribed and carefully explained. Splints provide local joint rest. An ordinary nutritious diet is sufficient. Food and diet quackery is common and should be discouraged.

Salicylates are relatively safe, inexpensive, analgesic, and anti-inflammatory, and are the corner-stone of drug therapy in RA. Aspirin (acetylsalicylic acid) is prescribed **in writing.** Dosage is begun with 0.6 to 1.0 gm (2 to 3 five-grain tablets) in 4 divided doses with meals and a bedtime snack. Dosage is then adjusted upward until achieving a maximally effective or mildly toxic dose (e.g., tinnitus, diminished hearing). The final dose may vary from 3 to 7.5 gm (about 10 to 25 five-grain tablets). The average dose is 4.5 gm (14 tablets) per day; 3 tablets are given with each of 3 meals and 5 at bedtime. Antacids between meals can be taken for mild GI symptoms without discontinuing the aspirin. Enteric-coated and buffered tablets offer some advantage in patients with concomitant peptic ulcer or hiatus hernia. Sustained-release tablets provide longer relief for some patients and may be given at bedtime. Patients awakened at night by severe pain may take a dose at 2 or 3 AM. Salicylates such as choline salicylate, salsalate, and choline magnesium salicylate seem to have better GI tolerance than aspirin and do not impair platelet adhesiveness, but are not as effective anti-inflammatory agents.

Indomethacin, one of the nonsteroidal anti-inflammatory agents with analgesic and antipyretic activity, is an effective nonsteroidal agent in some patients with RA. The nonsteroidal agents should be considered for patients who do not tolerate or are unsuccessful with aspirin. Initially, 25 mg is given orally t.i.d. with food or immediately after meals. If the response is inadequate, the daily dosage is increased by 25 mg at daily to weekly intervals depending on disease severity until the response is satisfactory or a dosage of 150 to 200 mg/day has been reached. After the acute phase of the disease is controlled, it is often possible to reduce the dosage gradually to a maintenance level of 75 to 100 mg/day.

The most frequent adverse reactions are headache, dizziness, lightheadedness, and GI disturbances (e.g., nausea, anorexia, vomiting, epigastric distress, abdominal pain, diarrhea). GI effects may be minimized by giving the drug immediately after meals or with food. The drug should be **stopped** if GI bleeding occurs. Indomethacin **should not be given** to patients with active peptic ulcer, gastritis, or ulcerative colitis, and should be used with caution if there is a history of these disorders. Fluid retention occurs occasionally. CNS effects are often transient and disappear with continued treatment or after dosage reduction; occasionally, they are of such severity that therapy must be discontinued. Patients just beginning treatment with the drug or showing significant CNS symptoms should not operate automotive equipment or engage in hazardous occupations.

Other nonsteroidal anti-inflammatory drugs are also available for patients who do not tolerate sufficient aspirin to obtain a good effect. Only one agent is usually given at a time. Ibuprofen 400 mg q.i.d. to 800 mg t.i.d. can be given; the larger dose is usually needed. Naproxen often requires only a 250-mg tablet b.i.d.; a total of 750 mg/day may be used. Fenoprofen is given 300 to 600 mg q.i.d.; daily dose should not exceed 3200 mg. Tolmetin is usually initiated with 400 mg t.i.d.; the maximum recommended daily dose is 1800 mg. Sulindac is given 200 mg b.i.d. Meclofenamate is given 200 to 400 mg/day. Though initially felt to be less of a GI irritant than aspirin, these nonsteroidal agents can produce gastric symptoms and GI bleeding. Other possible side effects include CNS symptoms, edema, and decreased platelet adhesiveness. These nonsteroidal anti-inflammatory drugs should be considered aspirin alternatives; however, patients allergic to aspirin may also have allergic reactions to the other nonsteroidal agents. There is no suggestion that they have the potential for remission that gold compounds do. If aspirin and nonsteroidal agents do not seem to be having definite benefit after 3 to 4 mo of treatment, addition of one of the low-acting agents such as gold, penicillamine, or hydroxychloroquine should be considered.

Gold compounds are usually given in addition to salicylates if aspirin or 1 or 2 other nonsteroidal agents do not provide sufficient relief. Gold is effective only against active joint inflammation and is not usually helpful in advanced RA with pronounced joint destruction and minimal residual inflammation. It is not analgesic but can produce remission and is the drug of choice after aspirin. Gold may also decrease the formation of new bony erosions. Gold sodium thiomalate or gold thioglucose (aurothioglucose) can be used. Gold is given IM at weekly intervals: 10 mg the first week, 25 mg the second, and 50 mg/wk thereafter until a total of 1 gm has been given or significant improvement is apparent. When maximum improvement is achieved, dosage is gradually decreased to 50 mg every 2 to 4 wk. Relapse usually occurs in 3 to 6 mo if no further gold is given following remission. Remissions often can be sustained with prolonged maintenance administration of 25 to 50 mg every 3 to 4 wk.

Gold compounds are **contraindicated** in patients with hepatic or renal disease, blood dyscrasia, or acute SLE. **Before receiving** gold, the patient should have a urinalysis, Hct, total and differential WBC count, and an estimate of the number of platelets on the smear, with a count if they seem scarce. These tests should be repeated before each injection during the first month and every 1 to 2 wk thereafter. Toxic reactions are due to sensitivity to the compound or its vehicle, or to heavy metal toxicity; they include pruritus, dermatitis, stomatitis, vague GI discomfort, albuminuria with or without a nephrotic syndrome, hematuria, agranulocytosis, thrombocytopenic purpura, and aplastic anemia. Other rare side effects include diarrhea, hepatitis, and pneumonitis. Gold should be **discontinued** when any of these manifestations appear. If hematopoietic toxicity develops, gold should be **stopped** and corticosteroids begun, preferably in the hospital. Eosinophilia $> 5\%$ and pruritus may precede appearance of a rash and are possible danger signals. Dermatitis is usually pruritic and ranges in severity from a single eczematous patch to generalized and fatal exfoliation. Minor toxic manifestations (e.g., mild pruritus or minor rash) may be eliminated by temporarily withholding gold therapy, then resuming it cautiously. However, if toxic symptoms progress, gold should be withheld and the patient given a corticosteroid. Corticosteroid dosage should be quantitated to the severity of symptoms; a topical corticosteroid or oral prednisone 15 to 20 mg/day in divided doses is given for mild gold dermatitis; larger doses may be needed for hematologic complications. A gold chelating agent, dimercaprol 2.5 mg/kg body wt may be given IM up to 4 to 6 times/day for the first 2 days and then b.i.d. for 5 to 7 days after a *severe* gold reaction. In severe toxic reactions, D-penicillamine can also be given orally 250 mg q.i.d. as a gold chelator until toxicity has subsided. A transient "**nitritoid reaction**" with flushing, tachycardia, and faintness can occur several minutes after injections of gold sodium thiomalate. This occurs more often if the gold is not stored in the dark. If these reactions occur, aurothioglucose can be used, as this does not seem to cause them.

D-**Penicillamine** given orally has a beneficial effect similar to that of gold and may be used in some cases if gold fails or produces toxicity in patients with active RA. Suggested doses start at 250 mg/day for 30 to 90 days; the dose is then increased to 500 mg/day for another 30 to 90 days and, if definite improvement does not occur, may be increased to 750 mg/day for 60 days. When the patient starts to respond, further increases should *not* be made. Benefit usually is not expected until the dose is up to 500 mg/day. The dose should be kept to the minimally effective level. Before therapy and every 2 to 3 wk during treatment, platelets must be checked and urinalysis and CBC performed. This drug can cause marrow suppression, proteinuria, nephrosis, rash, a foul taste, or other serious toxic effects (including myasthenia gravis, pemphigus, Goodpasture's syndrome, polymyositis, or a lupuslike syndrome), all of which require discontinuation. Fatalities due to D-penicillamine have been reported. *It must be monitored carefully*, and should be given by, or with guidance from, one experienced with the drug.

Hydroxychloroquine occasionally controls symptoms of mild to moderate active RA. Toxic effects are usually mild and include generally reversible corneal opacity. However, irreversible retinal degeneration has been reported. Ophthalmologic evaluation with testing of visual fields using a red test object is required before and every 3 to 6 mo during treatment. An initial dose of 200 mg is given orally b.i.d. with breakfast and the evening meal; therapy is continued at that dosage for 3 mo. The drug should be discontinued if the patient fails to improve after 3 mo. If definite improvement is achieved, the dosage is decreased to 200 mg/day and continued as long as effective. Frequent eye examinations must be continued.

Corticosteroids are the most dramatically effective short-term anti-inflammatory drugs. RA, however, is usually active for years, and clinical benefit from corticosteroids frequently diminishes with time. They do not prevent the progression of joint destruction. Furthermore, when the disease is active, severe rebound phenomena follow their withdrawal. Because of their side effects, corticosteroids should be given only after careful and usually prolonged evaluation of less potentially hazardous drugs. Corticosteroids suppress clinical manifestations and may be used to maintain joint function and allow continued performance of customary duties, but the patient should be cautioned about complications occurring with long-term use. Dosage should not exceed 7.5 mg of prednisone/day except for patients with severe systemic manifestations of RA such as vasculitis, pleurisy, or pericarditis. Large "loading doses" followed by rapid dosage reduction are **not recommended.** Alternate-day therapy is **not recommended,** since RA is usually too symptomatically active the days corticosteroids are not given. Contraindications to the use of corticosteroids include peptic ulcer, hypertension, untreated infections, diabetes mellitus, and glaucoma. A PPD should be performed before corticosteroid therapy is begun.

Intra-articular injections of corticosteroid esters may temporarily help to control local synovitis in 1 or 2 particularly painful joints. Triamcinolone hexacetonide may suppress inflammation for the longest period; prednisolone tertiary-butylacetate also is effective. The 21-phosphate preparations of prednisolone or dexamethasone are **not recommended,** because of rapid clearance from the joint and very short duration of action. Overuse of the recently injected, less painful joint may accelerate joint destruction. Since corticosteroid esters are crystalline, local inflammation transiently increases within a few hours in about 2% of injections.

Technic of intra-articular injection: Before attempting paracentesis of a joint, the physician should be familiar with its anatomic features. The optimum approach is on the extensor surface where the synovial pouch is closest to the skin and remote from major nerves, arteries, or veins. (For recommended sites for injecting selected joints, see FIG. 103–1.)

Aseptic technic must be observed. Ethyl chloride spray may produce local skin analgesia. The aspirating needle (seldom more than 20 gauge) is quickly inserted through the skin, subcutaneous tissue, joint capsule, and synovial membrane. Synovial fluid should be aspirated for analysis and to relieve joint distention. If there is no evidence of infection, the aspirating syringe is detached, and the needle remains in place. A small syringe containing the corticosteroid is attached and the drug is

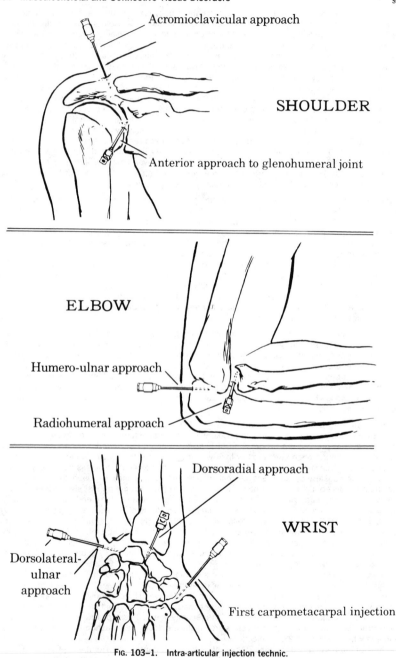

Fig. 103–1. Intra-articular injection technic.

injected into the joint cavity. Doses vary with joint size. The injection site is then covered with a small sterile dressing. Individual joints should not be injected more than 2 to 3 times/yr.

Immunosuppressive drugs such as cyclophosphamide, methotrexate, and azathioprine are used only experimentally in RA. They can suppress inflammation and may allow reduction of corticosteroid doses. Major side effects occur with these drugs, however, including bone marrow suppression

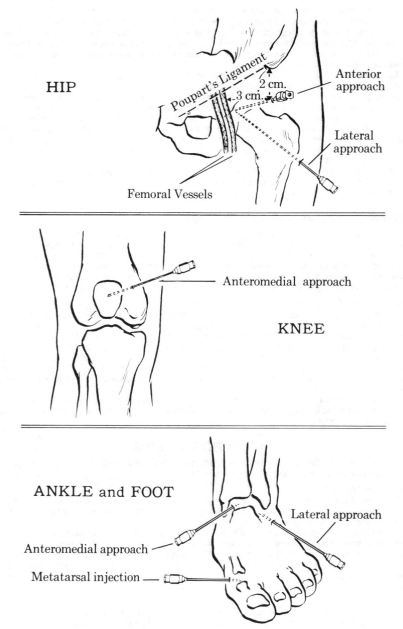

FIG. 103-1.   Intra-articular injection technic. (Cont'd)

and increased risk of malignancy following long-term use. Patients should be fully informed of these potential side effects.

Exercise, physiotherapy, and surgery: Flexion contractures can be prevented and muscle strength restored most successfully after the inflammation is suppressed. Joint splinting reduces local inflammation and may relieve symptoms. Before the acute inflammatory process is controlled, passive exercise to prevent contracture is given carefully and within the limits of pain. Active exercise to restore muscle mass and preserve the normal range of joint motion is desirable as inflammation subsides, but should not be fatiguing. Self-help devices have enabled many patients with severe debilitating RA to perform activities essential to daily living. Orthopedic shoes, modified to fit individual needs, are frequently helpful; metatarsal bars placed posteriorly to painful metatarsophalangeal joints decrease the pain of weight bearing.

Established flexion contractures may require intensive exercise, serial splinting, or orthopedic measures. Though synovectomy provides only temporary relief of inflammation, it may be used in key joints to help preserve joint function if anti-inflammatory drugs have been unsuccessful. Arthroplasty with prosthetic replacement of joint parts is indicated if the degree of joint damage severely limits function. Total hip replacement is the most consistently successful of available prosthetic procedures. Total knee replacement is somewhat less successful but useful. Prosthetic hips and knees cannot be expected to tolerate resumption of activities such as vigorous athletics. Excision of subluxated painful metatarsophalangeal joints may greatly aid ambulation. Surgical procedures must always be considered in terms of the total disease. Deformed hands and arms limit crutch use during rehabilitation; seriously affected knees and feet prevent full benefit from hip surgery. Reasonable objectives for the patient must be determined and function must be considered before appearance. Surgery may be undertaken while the disease is active.

JUVENILE RHEUMATOID ARTHRITIS (Still's Disease)

RA in children is similar in many respects to the adult type. The disease tends to affect the larger joints, resulting in interference with growth and development. Micrognathia due to impaired mandible growth may be seen. Rash, fever, iritis, splenomegaly, and generalized lymphadenopathy are frequently present, at times preceding appearance of the arthritis. Pericarditis and pleural effusion may also be present. The RF is usually absent. Antinuclear antibodies are present in some children. Prognosis is more favorable than in the adult; complete remissions occur in up to 75% of patients.

Treatment

Therapy is generally similar to that for adults except that hydroxychloroquine is not used. Aspirin is well tolerated and effective in large doses (90 to 130 mg/kg/day); salicylate levels should be checked with the higher doses. Systemic corticosteroids can usually be avoided except with severe systemic disease. Growth retardation is an additional hazard of using corticosteroids in children. Intra-articular corticosteroids can be given if the dose is adjusted to the smaller size of the joints. Gold salts can be given to children who do not respond to aspirin. Dosage is built up gradually with precautions, as in adults. Gold dosage must be adjusted to the body weight; 1 mg/kg/mo is considered a maintenance dose.

Passive and active exercises and splints usually prevent flexion contractures. Ophthalmologic examinations should be given semiannually to detect possible uveitis, even in quiescent cases, before eye damage occurs.

PSORIATIC ARTHRITIS

A rheumatoid-like arthritis associated with psoriasis of the skin or nails and a negative RA serology; HLA-B27 antigen is present in most patients.

Symptoms and Signs

Psoriasis of the nails or skin may precede or follow joint involvement. Patients with seronegative inflammatory polyarthritis should be examined for unrecognized or minimal psoriasis. The distal interphalangeal joints (fingers and toes) are especially affected. Asymmetric involvement of large and small joints, including the sacroiliacs and the spine, is common. Rheumatoid nodules are not present. Exacerbations and remissions of joint and skin symptoms may coincide. Arthritic remissions tend to be more frequent, rapid, and complete than in RA, but progression to chronic arthritis and severe crippling may occur. X-ray findings include distal interphalangeal involvement, resorption of terminal phalanges (sausage toes), arthritis mutilans, and extensive destruction and dislocation of large and small joints.

Treatment

Treatment is similar to that for RA, but with significant differences. Antimalarials are **contraindicated.** Toxic reactions to gold salts appear more frequently. Triamcinolone is the preferred corticosteroid. Folic acid antagonists and immunosuppressive agents, especially methotrexate (CAUTION: *Highly toxic*), used under rigidly controlled conditions, have relieved psoriatic lesions and joint symptoms. Treatment of psoriasis is discussed in Ch. 195.

ANKYLOSING SPONDYLITIS

(Marie-Strümpell Disease)

A chronic progressive form of arthritis distinguished by inflammation and eventual ankylosis of a number of joints, primarily involving the spine and paraspinal structures. Calcification and eventual ossification of the anulus fibrosus of the intervertebral disks and adjacent connective tissue are characteristic. The sacroiliac and apophyseal vertebral joints and the paravertebral soft tissues are usually involved in fully developed cases.

Etiology

The disease usually begins in patients aged 10 to 30 and is uncommon after age 30. Susceptibility is higher in men (> 90% of those afflicted), in male relatives, and in persons born with the histocompatibility antigen HLA-B27, who are 300 times more likely to develop the disease than those without the antigen.

Symptoms and Signs

Onset usually is insidious with episodes of low back aching, especially in the sacroiliac and lumbar regions. Pain may occur in a sciatic nerve distribution pattern. There often is well-defined morning back stiffness. Symptoms become progressively worse, spreading from the low back frequently into the mid back and occasionally the neck. In later stages peripheral joints may be affected, especially large joints such as the hips and shoulders (about ⅓ of cases) and, less frequently, the knees and other more peripheral joints. Fatigue, weight loss, mild anemia, and muscle stiffness may occur in severe disease. Iritis (< 25% of cases) and involvement of the heart (< 10% of cases), including cardiac arrhythmias or aortic insufficiency, may develop in longstanding disease.

Sacroiliac joint involvement usually is seen on x-ray at the first examination. Findings may be limited to tenderness on palpation of those joints or on fist percussion of the low back. The normal lumbar concave curve may be flattened because of muscle spasm and involvement of adjacent spinal joints. Normal expansion of the spine does not occur during flexion of the back, and some decreased joint mobility is evident when the patient bends forward, sometimes as if he had a board in his back. This is due to muscle spasm early in the course and to bony ankylosis or bridging later. The costovertebral joints may also be involved, causing diminution of chest expansion and a decrease in vital capacity. Neck movements may be mildly or seriously limited. Ankylosis of the entire spine (resulting in an erect "poker spine") or dorsal kyphosis may develop from forward flexion of the thoracic spine in advanced disease.

Laboratory and X-ray Findings

Laboratory abnormalities are minimal. The ESR may be elevated in 40% of the patients and there may be a mild hypochromic anemia. Although HLA-B27 usually is present (90+%), not all persons possessing this antigen develop spondylitis.

X-ray features are characteristic. In the usually early sacroiliac joint changes, there is blurring of the bony margins with some erosion, especially on the iliac side of the joint; patchy sclerosis is present bilaterally. These joints become fused and obliterated after several years. Similar changes may occur in the symphysis pubis, the vertebral apophyseal joints, and the other joints mentioned above. Calcification of the anterior and lateral spinal ligaments eventually occurs, with generalized demineralization and squaring of the bodies of the vertebrae because of filling in with bone or calcification of the front or anterior aspects of the vertebrae. The "bamboo spine," as seen by x-ray, is a late feature. Bony growths (syndesmophytes) may weld the vertebrae about their disks in late stages. These are found especially on the lateral sides of the vertebrae.

Prognosis

Treatment does not modify progression of the disease, which smolders and progresses slowly for 10 to 20 yr, then either partially or completely remits. Disease may be confined to the sacroiliac or lumbar joints, or may involve the entire spine and other joints and organs.

Treatment

Posture-maintaining exercises should be performed as soon as the diagnosis is made, to retain as much appropriate upright posture as possible. Exercises should stress back movements, straightening of the thoracic spine, deep-bending exercises, and as full a range of motion of the spine in all directions as possible. Flexion postures should not be maintained for long periods of time. To avoid flexion of the neck and upper back, the patient should sleep supine on a firm mattress and use only a small pillow or none at all. The pectoral muscles should be stretched and the upper back straightened by locking the fingers behind the head and pushing the elbows as far back as possible. Hot baths or packs can be applied before exercising to attain a better range of motion. The patient should have ample rest each day and avoid exhaustion.

An analgesic may help relieve pain, permitting better sleep and increasing the ability to exercise. A nonsteroidal anti-inflammatory agent such as indomethacin 25 mg 3 to 5 times/day or one of the newer nonsteroidal anti-inflammatory agents may be tried. Aspirin is less satisfactory but may be helpful in some patients. Narcotics and systemic corticosteroids should be **avoided**. X-ray therapy to the back is **contraindicated**.

If the above measures are followed, surgical procedures to straighten the spine will be needed only rarely. A back brace may help but is usually uncomfortable and unnecessary.

SJÖGREN'S SYNDROME (SS)

A chronic, systemic inflammatory disorder of unknown etiology, characterized by dryness of the mouth, eyes, and other mucous membranes and frequently associated with rheumatic disorders sharing certain autoimmune characteristics (e.g., RA, scleroderma, and SLE) and in which lympho-

cyte infiltration into affected tissues is seen. The relative risk of lymphoma occurring in SS patients is about 44 times that expected in the general population. These patients are also at increased risk for Waldenström's macroglobulinemia. An association has been found between SS and HLA-Dw3 antigen in patients with primary SS (those without associated connective tissue disease). The syndrome occurs most often in women over age 40; prevalence is about 1 in 2000 persons.

Pathophysiology, Symptoms, and Signs

In some, SS affects only the eyes or mouth **(primary SS; sicca complex; sicca syndrome)**; in others, almost every body system may be involved at various times.

Ocular symptoms occur when atrophy of the secretory epithelium of the lacrimal glands causes desiccation of the cornea and conjunctiva **(keratoconjunctivitis sicca,** discussed in Ch. 178). In advanced cases, the cornea is severely damaged and epithelial strands hang from the corneal surface **(keratitis filiformis)**

One third of SS patients develop **enlarged parotid glands** that are usually firm, smooth, fluctuating in size, and mildly tender. Chronic salivary gland enlargement is rarely painful. Ductal alterations in the parotid gland are characterized by intraductal cellular proliferation leading to narrowing of the lumen and eventual formation of compact cellular structures termed epimyoepithelial islands. When salivary glands atrophy, saliva diminishes, and the resulting extreme dryness of the mouth and lips **(xerostomia)** causes difficulty in chewing and swallowing and promotes calculi formation in the salivary ducts. Tooth decay greatly increases because healthy dentition requires saliva. Taste and smell faculties may be lost.

Similarly, desiccation may also be found in the skin and in mucous membranes of the nose, throat, larynx, bronchi, vulva, and vagina. Alopecia may occur. Dryness of the respiratory tract causes a high frequency of lung infections leading, in some, to fatal pneumonia.

Other manifestations: GI effects are associated with mucosal or submucosal atrophy and diffuse infiltration by plasma cells and lymphocytes. Chronic hepatobiliary disease is often associated with SS, as is pancreatitis (not surprisingly, since exocrine pancreatic tissue is similar to that of salivary glands). Fibrinous pericarditis is the commonest cardiovascular feature. Sensory neuropathy is common, especially of the 2nd and 3rd divisions of the 5th cranial nerve. Approximately 20% of SS patients have renal tubular acidosis; in many, decreased renal concentrating ability is demonstrated. Although glomerulonephritis is unusual, interstitial nephritis is frequent. Patients who have had parotid enlargement, splenomegaly, and lymphadenopathy may develop pseudolymphoma or malignant lymphoma.

Diagnosis and Prognosis

Clinically, one suspects SS when complaints suggest dryness of the eyes and mouth; the addition of joint inflammation completes the classic triad. Arthritis occurs in about 1/3 of patients and is similar in distribution to that seen in RA; however, joint symptoms in SS tend to be milder and rarely lead to destruction. Some patients with undiagnosed SS who have rheumatic symptoms may not complain spontaneously of sicca complex; SS is then defined by laboratory evaluation.

When bilateral parotid enlargement occurs in conditions such as hyperlipoproteinemia, malnutrition, cirrhosis, or diabetes mellitus, the glands are soft and puffy, in contrast to the firm glands of SS; oral dryness is absent.

Diagnostic procedures and laboratory findings: The **Schirmer test** measures the quantity of tears secreted in 5 min in response to irritation from a filter paper strip placed under a lower eyelid. A young person normally moistens 15 mm of the paper strip. Since hypolacrimation occurs with aging, 1/3 of normal elderly persons may wet only 10 mm in 5 min. Most persons with SS moisten < 5 mm, although about 15% of test results are false-positive and 15% false-negative. **Ocular staining** with a drop of rose bengal solution into the eye is highly specific. In SS, the portion of the eye filling the palpebral aperture takes up the dye, and red triangles with their bases toward the limbus are seen. **Tear breakup time, tear lysozyme concentration,** and **slit-lamp examination** are also useful.

Salivary glands are evaluated by **salivary flow, sialography,** and **salivary scintiscan.**

One of the most characteristic features of SS is the remarkable immunologic reactivity detected in blood serum; most patients have elevated levels of antibodies against γ-globulin, nuclear protein, and many tissue constituents. Precipitating antibodies to nuclear antigens (identified by immunodiffusion analysis), termed SS-A and SS-B antibodies, are highly specific for SS. Rheumatoid factor is present in > 70% of cases; the LE cell preparation is positive in 15 to 20%. The VDRL test is negative. ESR is elevated in 70% of patients. One third of patients have anemia; 1/4, leukopenia and eosinophilia. Urinalysis may show proteinuria, reflecting interstitial nephritis.

Biopsy of the readily accessible labial salivary glands confirms the diagnosis when foci of lymphocytes and plasma cells associated with atrophy of acinar tissue are seen.

Prognosis in SS is often related to the associated connective tissue disorder, although death may also result from pulmonary infection and, rarely, renal failure or lymphoma.

Prophylaxis and Treatment

Ocular symptoms require diligent care; see KERATOCONJUNCTIVITIS SICCA in Ch. 178.

Management of oral complications is aimed at avoiding the desiccation that promotes ductal calculi and rampant dental caries, e.g., by sipping fluids throughout the day and chewing sugarless gum. Drugs that decrease salivary secretion, such as decongestants and antihistamines, should be avoided. Fastidious oral hygiene and regular dental supervision are advised. Any calculi must be promptly removed, preserving viable salivary tissue. The temporary pain of suddenly enlarged salivary glands is best treated only with analgesics.

Connective tissue involvement is usually mild and chronic; therefore, steroids and immunosuppressive agents are indicated only occasionally, e.g., in a patient with severe vasculitis or visceral involvement. Irradiation and drugs that increase the risk of lymphoproliferative disorders and infections should be avoided.

LYME DISEASE

(LD; Lyme Arthritis)

A tick-transmitted inflammatory disorder best recognized clinically by an early skin lesion, erythema chronicum migrans **(ECM)**, *that may be followed weeks to months later by neurologic, cardiac, or joint abnormalities.*

Etiology, Epidemiology, and Pathophysiology

The illness is caused by a newly discovered spirochete transmitted by the minute tick *Ixodes dammini*. The disease was recognized in 1975 because of close geographic clustering of cases in the small community of Lyme, Connecticut. It has since appeared elsewhere in foci along the northeastern coast of the USA from Massachusetts to Maryland, in Wisconsin, and in California and Oregon. Onset usually is in the summer and early fall and occurs at any age and in either sex, although most patients are children and young adults living in heavily wooded areas.

The *I. dammini* spirochete has been cultured from the blood, skin (ECM), and spinal fluid of LD patients and is thus probably either injected into the skin or bloodstream in tick saliva, or deposited in fecal material on the skin. After an incubation period of 3 to 32 days, the organism migrates outward in the skin (ECM), is spread in lymph (regional adenopathy), or is disseminated in blood to organs or other skin sites. Currently it is not known whether the organism is still present when arthritis is active.

LD is associated with characteristic immune findings. Over 85% of patients with subsequent arthritis have, in the prearticular (ECM) phase, serum cryoglobulins containing IgM (reflecting high serum IgM levels), compared to < 15% of patients without subsequent arthritis. Besides having prognostic value, these differences may represent different ways of responding to an immune stimulus, and may be determined genetically. It appears that patients have an increased frequency of the B cell alloantigen HLA-DRw2 but not of HLA-B27 (as in the spondyloarthropathies).

More direct evidence for circulating immune complexes (e.g., abnormal C1q-binding activity) is found in sera of most patients with ECM. These complexes tend to persist in the circulation of patients who develop neurologic or cardiac abnormalities. By the time arthritis appears, immune complexes are no longer evident in most sera but are found systematically in synovial fluid, and in higher titer than in concomitant sera.

Synovial membrane from affected joints may be indistinguishable from that of RA (see above). Findings include villous hypertrophy, vascular congestion, and colonization with lymphocytes and plasma cells that may resemble early lymphoid follicles and, as in RA, are presumably capable of producing antibody locally. Pannus formation and erosion of cartilage and bone may occur.

The histology of ECM resembles that of an insect bite—epidermal and dermal involvement at the center (which is often indurated), dermal in the periphery. All layers of the epidermis are heavily infiltrated with mononuclear cells around blood vessels and skin appendages. At the center there is edema of the papillary dermis, and intra- and extracellular edema and a thickened keratin layer in the epidermis.

Symptoms, Signs, and Course

ECM begins as a red macule or papule, usually on the proximal portion of an extremity or on the trunk (especially the thigh, buttock, or axilla), that expands, often with central clearing, to a diameter as large as 50 cm. About 25% of patients report having been bitten at that site by a minute tick 3 to 32 days before onset of ECM. The lesion, which may be inapparent to the patient, is often hot to touch. Soon after onset, nearly half the patients develop multiple, usually smaller, lesions without indurated centers. ECM generally lasts for a few weeks; evanescent lesions may appear during resolution. Former skin lesions may reappear faintly, sometimes before recurrent attacks of arthritis. Mucosal lesions do not occur.

The most common symptoms accompanying ECM (or preceding it by a few days) are malaise and fatigue, chills and fever, headache, and stiff neck. Less common are backache, myalgias, nausea and vomiting, sore throat, lymphadenopathy, and splenomegaly. Symptoms characteristically are intermittent and changing, but malaise and fatigue may linger for weeks.

Arthritis occurs in about half of patients with ECM within weeks to months of the onset of ECM; the interval has been as long as 2 yr. Early in the illness, migratory polyarthritis without joint swelling may occur; later, longer attacks of swelling and pain in several large joints, especially knees, typically recur for several years. The knees commonly are much more swollen than painful, often hot, rarely red. Baker's cysts may form and rupture. Those symptoms accompanying ECM, especially malaise, fatigue, and low-grade fever, may also precede or accompany recurrent attacks of arthritis. About 10% of patients develop chronic (unremittent for 6 mo or more) knee involvement.

Frank neurologic abnormalities develop in about 15% of patients within weeks to months of ECM (often before arthritis occurs), commonly last for months, and usually resolve completely. They include lymphocytic meningitis (about 100 cells/cu mm) or meningoencephalitis, chorea, cerebellar ataxia, cranial neuritis (including bilateral Bell's palsy), motor and sensory radiculoneuritis, mononeuritis multiplex, and myelitis. Myocardial abnormalities occur in about 8% of patients within weeks of ECM. They include fluctuating degrees of atrioventricular block (first degree, Wenckebach, or 3rd degree) and, less commonly, myopericarditis with reduced left ventricular ejection fractions and cardiomegaly.

Laboratory and X-ray Findings

Recovery of the *I. dammini* spirochete from blood, ECM, or CSF is so far rare, difficult, and slow (weeks). Specific anti-spirochetal antibodies in significant titer—first IgM, then IgG—appear within weeks of ECM. IgG titers are higher later in the illness when arthritis is present.

Cryoprecipitates and circulating immune complexes are often seen early in the illness (see Pathophysiology, above). The ESR may be elevated when patients feel ill; the Hct, WBC, and differential counts are usually normal. Rheumatoid and antinuclear factors are rarely present. Serum complement components either are normal or elevated during active disease (but see Pathophysiology, above). The urinalysis and serum creatinine are usually normal; SGOT and LDH levels may be slightly abnormal when ECM is present.

Synovial fluid findings vary, but typically show about 25,000 white cells/cu mm (range, 500 to 110,000), mostly granulocytes; about 5 gm/dl of protein; and C3 and C4 levels usually > ⅓ those of serum.

Radiologic findings usually are limited to soft tissue swelling, but a few patients have had erosion of cartilage and bone.

Differential Diagnosis

In children, LD must be distinguished primarily from juvenile RA; in adults, from Reiter's syndrome and atypical RA. The distinguishing features of LD described above may occur in any combination. Important negative findings include absence (usually) of morning stiffness, subcutaneous nodules, iridocyclitis, mucosal lesions, rheumatoid factor, and antinuclear antibodies. Acute rheumatic fever is considered in the occasional patient with migratory polyarthritis and either an increased P-R interval or chorea (as a manifestation of meningoencephalitis). However, patients with LD rarely have heart murmurs or evidence of a preceding streptococcal infection. Spondyloarthropathies with peripheral joint involvement can be distinguished from LD by the lack of axial involvement in the latter.

Treatment

For adults, the drug of choice for early LD is tetracycline 250 mg q.i.d. for at least 10 days and for up to 20 days if symptoms persist or recur. Second choice is penicillin V 500 mg q.i.d., and third choice is erythromycin 250 mg q.i.d., in each instance for 10 to 20 days. In children, penicillin V is recommended rather than tetracycline. For neurologic abnormalities, penicillin G 20 million u./day IV in divided doses is now recommended. It is not yet clear whether antibiotic therapy is helpful later in the illness when arthritis is active. Aspirin (90 mg/kg [1.5 grains/kg] in children) or other nonsteroidal anti-inflammatory agents often relieve arthritis (rarely dramatically) but do not appear to prevent recurrences and are therefore unnecessary during remissions. For tense knee joints due to effusions, crutches are helpful; aspiration of fluid and injection of a corticosteroid may be beneficial. If the patient has marked functional limitation, synovectomy may be performed for chronic knee effusions (6 mo or more despite therapy), but spontaneous remission can occur after more than a year of continuous knee involvement.

INFECTIOUS ARTHRITIS

Arthritis resulting from infection of the synovial tissues with pyogenic bacteria or other infectious agents.

Etiology and Pathogenesis

Any pathogenic microbe may infect a joint. Bacteria are most often the etiologic agents, typically producing an acute arthritis. In young children, the predominating pathogens are staphylococci, *Hemophilus influenzae*, and gram-negative bacilli. Older children and adults are most commonly infected with gonococci, staphylococci, streptococci, or pneumococci. Acute arthritis at any age may be associated with rubella, mumps, or hepatitis B virus infections. Chronic arthritis may be caused by *Mycobacterium tuberculosis* and other mycobacteria or fungi such as *Sporothrix schenckii*, *Coccidioides immitis*, and *Histoplasma capsulatum*.

Microbes usually reach the joint hematogenously; however, direct inoculation of bacteria or fungi into the joint may occur during surgery or drug injection, or secondary to trauma. Patients with RA and chronically inflamed joints are particularly susceptible to bacterial arthritis.

Symptoms and Signs

An infant with septic arthritis is irritable and has a fever. Examination usually reveals failure to move a limb spontaneously, tenderness, or pain with passive motion of the involved joint. Older children and adults complain of acute joint pain and stiffness; on examination, the joint is warm,

TABLE 103-2. INITIAL ANTIMICROBIAL PROGRAMS RECOMMENDED FOR ACUTE BACTERIAL ARTHRITIS

Gram Stain	Antimicrobial
Gram-positive cocci	Nafcillin 50 mg/kg q 6 h IV
Gram-negative cocci	Penicillin G 75,000 u./kg q 6 h IV
Gram-negative bacilli.	Gentamicin 1.5 mg/kg q 8 h IM plus Ampicillin 50 mg/kg q 6 h IV
No organism present Gonococcal infection suspected. . . Other bacterial possibilities	Penicillin as above Nafcillin and gentamicin as above

tender, and swollen, with evidence of effusion. Other signs of infection, such as fever, chills, or leukocytosis, are usually present. Patients receiving anti-inflammatory drugs, however, may show remarkably little systemic or local response. A history of recent urethritis, salpingitis, or hemorrhagic vesicular skin lesions suggests gonococcal arthritis (see under GONORRHEA in Ch. 162).

Mycobacterial and fungal arthritides are typically chronic and monarticular.

Diagnosis

The diagnosis requires a high index of suspicion, particularly in patients with underlying chronic joint disease. *Even the remotest possibility that a joint might be septic demands aspiration of synovial fluid from the involved joint and a search for the infecting organism by Gram stain and culture.* Cultures should also be taken from other likely sources of infection, such as blood, sputum, and abscesses. The etiologic agent may not grow in the early stages of gonococcal arthritis or if antimicrobial therapy is begun before joint aspiration. In these patients, the diagnosis may be supported by the following joint fluid characteristics: WBC count $> 10,000$; $> 90\%$ polymorphonuclear leukocytes; synovial fluid/blood glucose ratio < 0.5; poor mucin clot; and absence of uric acid or calcium pyrophosphate dihydrate crystals.

Mycobacterial and fungal agents should be considered in any case of chronic monarticular arthritis. These agents are difficult to isolate from synovial fluids, and successful diagnosis often depends on their demonstration by microscopic examination and culture of synovial biopsy tissue.

Treatment

Acute bacterial arthritis may destroy the joint if not promptly treated. Successful therapy depends on early and appropriate antibiotic use, which may have to be started before isolating the infecting organism and evaluating its antimicrobial sensitivity pattern. The appropriate antimicrobial (see TABLE 103-2) should be given parenterally, since absorption of oral antimicrobials may be inadequate. Intra-articular antimicrobials may cause synovitis and are rarely indicated. Treatment should be continued for at least 2 wk after all symptoms and signs of inflammation have disappeared. The joint should be aspirated and cultured daily or more often to confirm sterilization of the joint fluid and to remove accumulated pus. If a clinical response and sterilization of the joint fluid are not apparent after 48 h of therapy, the choice and dose of antimicrobials should be adjusted until bactericidal activity of the joint fluid against the infecting organism can be demonstrated at a dilution of 1:8 or greater. Surgical drainage is indicated when needle aspiration of the joint is difficult, as in hip infections, or if the infection is not controlled after 48 h. Splinting is useful for pain relief during the acute stage. Physical therapy is indicated during convalescence to assure optimal return of function.

Antimicrobial therapy for mycobacterial or fungal arthritis is the same as for other serious infections with these agents (see appropriate chapters in this volume, §1). Viral arthritis is usually self-limited and responds to symptomatic therapy.

REITER'S SYNDROME

Arthritis associated with nonbacterial urethritis and conjunctivitis, usually seen in adult males following recent sexual exposure; it may also follow an acute attack of unexplained diarrhea (dysentery). Most patients carry the histocompatibility antigen HLA-B27. The syndrome seems to be a response to infection with shigella or infectious agents transmitted venereally (e.g., chlamydia) in a genetically susceptible host.

Symptoms, Signs, and Course

Typically, nonbacterial urethritis develops 7 to 14 days following sexual exposure, and low-grade fever, conjunctivitis, and arthritis develop over the next few weeks. The urethritis is less painful and productive of purulent discharge than that seen with acute gonorrhea, and may be associated with hemorrhagic cystitis or prostatitis. The conjunctivitis is usually mild, but complications of keratitis and anterior uveitis may occur. The arthritis is asymmetric and polyarticular and generally occurs in the larger joints of the lower extremities and the toes. Small, painless superficial ulcers are commonly seen on the oral mucosa, tongue, and glans penis (balanitis circinata). Many patients also develop hyperkeratotic skin lesions of the palms and soles and around the nails (keratoderma blennorrhagica).

The initial illness typically resolves in 3 to 4 mo, but 50% of patients experience transient recurrences of arthritis or the full syndrome over a period of several years. Joint deformity, ankylosis, sacroiliitis, and spondylitis may occur in the few patients who develop chronic illness.

Diagnosis

Diagnosis requires demonstration of the triad of urethritis, conjunctivitis, and arthritis, and is aided by findings such as the typical skin lesions and the development of plantar fasciitis or Achilles tendinitis. Since the various manifestations may occur at different times, diagnosis may require several months. Positive gonococcal cultures and a rapid response to penicillin therapy differentiate the typical acute case in a sexually active young male from gonococcal arthritis. In patients who develop the chronic form of Reiter's syndrome, the arthritis and skin lesions may resemble those characteristic of psoriatic arthritis, ankylosing spondylitis, or Behçet's syndrome; some rheumatologists classify these very similar entities (often HLA-B27 positive) as **"seronegative spondyloarthritis."**

Prognosis and Treatment

Only a few patients are disabled by chronic or persistent disease. Treatment is nonspecific, with anti-inflammatory agents such as aspirin or indomethacin in doses simlar to those used for RA (see above), or phenylbutazone 100 mg orally q.i.d. Physical therapy is helpful during the recovery phase. Corticosteroids have not been of value. Methotrexate or the folic acid antagonists may lead to symptomatic improvement in patients with severe illness; however, because of their toxicity, they are not warranted in that majority of patients whose illness is self-limited. Tetracycline 500 mg orally q.i.d. may control the urethritis.

BEHÇET'S SYNDROME

A multisystem inflammatory disorder that may include mucocutaneous, genital, ocular, articular, vascular, CNS, and GI involvement. Etiology is unknown; however, histopathologic vasculitic changes are common to all involved organs. Autoimmune and viral causes and an HLA-related immunogenetic predisposition have been suggested. The syndrome generally begins in the 3rd decade and occurs twice as often in men as in women. Although uncommon in the USA, Behçet's syndrome must be considered frequently in differential diagnosis.

Symptoms and Signs

The first manifestations usually are painful oral ulcers resembling those of aphthous stomatitis. Similar ulcers occur on the penis and scrotum, where they are painful, or on the vulva and vagina, where they may be asymptomatic. Other symptoms follow in days to years. The most common ocular lesion is a relapsing iridocyclitis with hypopyon. The posterior segment may also be involved, with choroiditis, retinal vasculitis, and papillitis. Various skin lesions occur in 80% of cases: papules, pustules, vesicles, and folliculitis. Particularly suggestive are erythema-nodosum–like lesions and inflammatory reactions to minor trauma, e.g., needle punctures. A relatively mild, self-limiting, and nondestructive arthritis involving the knees and other large joints occurs in 50% of patients. Recurrent superficial or deep migratory thrombophlebitis develops in 25% of patients and may lead to vena caval obstruction. Arterial damage may cause aneurysms or thrombosis. CNS involvement (18% of cases) may present as chronic meningoencephalitis, benign intracerebral hypertension, or life-threatening brainstem and spinal cord lesions. GI manifestations vary from nonspecific abdominal discomfort to a syndrome resembling ulcerative colitis.

Diagnosis

Diagnosis is clinical, and detection of manifestations may require months. Differential diagnosis includes Reiter's syndrome, Stevens-Johnson syndrome, SLE, ulcerative colitis, and ankylosing spondylitis. Behçet's syndrome has no specific findings that exclude all alternative possibilities, but is often distinguished by the relapsing course and multiple organ involvement.

Laboratory abnormalities are nonspecific but characteristic of inflammatory disease (elevated ESR and α_2- and γ-globulins, and mild leukocytosis). Numerous immunologic abnormalities may be detected, including the presence of autoantibodies to affected tissues and circulating immune complexes.

Prognosis and Treatment

The syndrome is generally benign, but with periods of remission and relapse extending over several decades. Blindness, vena caval obstruction, and paralysis may complicate the course; the occasional fatalities are usually associated with neurologic, vascular, and GI involvement. Symptomatic therapy of the various manifestations is reasonably successful. Needle punctures should be avoided when possible, since they provoke inflammatory skin lesions. Topical corticosteroids may provide temporary symptomatic relief for ocular and oral disease. However, topical or systemic corticosteroids do not alter the frequency of relapses. Occasional patients with severe uveitis or CNS involvement will respond to high doses of systemic corticosteroids (prednisone 60 to 80 mg/day). Immunosuppressive drugs such as cyclophosphamide and azathioprine have been used with some success in patients with severe disease.

OSTEOARTHRITIS

(OA; Degenerative Joint Disease; DJD)

The most common form of arthritis, characterized by degenerative loss of articular cartilage, subchondral bony sclerosis, and cartilage and bone proliferation at the joint margins with subsequent osteophyte formation. Secondary synovial tissue inflammation is common.

Etiology and Incidence

The cause is unknown, but genetic, metabolic, endocrine, biomechanical, and hydrolytic enzyme factors have been suggested. Biomechanical stresses may lead to chondrocyte damage and proteolytic enzyme release resulting in articular cartilage degeneration. OA develops when cartilage repair does not keep pace with degeneration. OA also may be secondary to chronic trauma or underlying joint disease. Under age 45, prevalence is greater in men; over age 45, in women.

Pathology

Grossly, the cartilage becomes yellow-white and soft. Fibrillation, pitting, and ulcers are found in superficial cartilage layers. Marginal osteophytes form. Histologically, fissuring and fibrillation are prominent. Degenerating chondrocytes and reactive clonal chondrocyte proliferation are present. Subchondral bone is thickened; cyst formation occurs. Synovitis is mild to moderate.

Symptoms and Signs

Onset usually is gradual and localized to one or a few joints. Pain, generally the earliest symptom, is greatest after exercise. Stiffness (fibrositis) commonly follows inactivity but is usually of short duration (less than 15 to 30 min). Joint motion is limited in severe cases. Tenderness and crepitus or grating are present. Joint enlargement is present, caused by proliferative reactions in cartilage and bone and by secondary chronic synovial inflammation. Acute flares of synovitis may occur secondary to calcium apatite or calcium pyrophosphate crystal deposition disease. Deformity and subluxation are late findings. Constitutional symptoms and extra-articular manifestations are absent.

The specific clinical picture varies with the joints involved. Enlargement of the terminal interphalangeal joints (**Heberden's nodes**) is common; painful gelatinous cysts may also be present. Women are affected by this form of the disease 10 times as often as men. Similar deformities may develop at the proximal interphalangeal joints. Disease of the first carpometacarpal joint causes pain and limitation of use of the thumb. Knee involvement produces pain, swelling, and instability. OA of the hip causes local pain and a limp; pain may be present at the knee due to referral along the obturator nerve. Spinal OA is common; severe degenerative changes may occur without symptoms. Osteoarthritic changes are most common in the midcervical and lower lumbar areas of maximal spinal motion (see NERVE ROOT DISORDERS in Ch. 130). Compression of contiguous neurologic structures by large osteophytes or a degenerated disk may cause severe radicular pain. Vascular insufficiency syndromes may follow compromise of cervical vascular structures.

Erosive inflammatory osteoarthritis, a clinical variant of OA, involves the terminal and proximal interphalangeal joints of the hands. Painful synovitis is followed by joint deformity and ankylosis. X-rays show bony erosions, osteophytes, and evidence of fusion. **Diffuse idiopathic skeletal hyperostosis (DISH, ankylosing hyperostosis)**, another OA variant, is characterized by a flowing ligamentous ossification along the anterior aspect of the spine. Osteophytes may be present, but disk height is characteristically preserved. Peripheral joints reveal irregular new bone formation and ligamentous calcification.

Laboratory Findings

The ESR may be normal or slightly accelerated. Anemia and leukocytosis are absent. Rheumatoid factor studies are negative. Synovial fluid analysis (see TABLES 102–4 and 102–5 in Ch. 102) reveals minimal abnormalities: the fluid is transparent, viscosity is good, mucin clot formation with glacial acetic acid is normal, and slight increases in cell count are noted. Narrowing of the joint space, osteophyte formation, bone cysts, and subchondral bony sclerosis are present on x-ray.

Differential Diagnosis

Polyarticular RA is usually easily differentiated. Psoriatic arthritis, Reiter's syndrome, and arthritis associated with ulcerative colitis commonly involve the terminal interphalangeal joints, but these disorders may be excluded by their associated findings in other involved systems. In chondrocalcinosis, cartilage calcification and joint fluid crystals are present. Neurologic symptoms of spinal OA may simulate primary neurologic disorders.

Prognosis and Treatment

OA is usually benign, and the overall outlook is favorable. Hip, knee, or spinal involvement, however, may be disabling.

Reassurance is important, and management goals should be outlined. Rest of involved joints is advisable. Canes, crutches, or walkers protect weight-bearing joints in severe cases. Weight reduction should be encouraged in obese patients. Heat relieves pain and muscle spasm; hot packs, electric pads, or warm soaks for 15 to 30 min b.i.d. are usually effective. Isometric exercises maintain muscle tone and build power (isotonic exercises help maintain motion but may damage joints). Exercises, b.i.d. to t.i.d., should begin with a few repetitions each time and progress to 10 or 15.

Drug therapy also may be required. Aspirin 650 to 975 mg (10 to 15 grains) orally q.i.d. is preferred. Analgesics (acetaminophen 650 mg t.i.d., propoxyphene hydrochloride 65 mg q.i.d., or ethoheptazine citrate 75 mg q.i.d.) may be helpful on an as-needed basis. Acetaminophen overuse may cause liver damage. Narcotic agents such as codeine or pentazocine hydrochloride are rarely indicated. Newer nonsteroidal anti-inflammatory agents can be used, including indomethacin 75 to 150 mg/day in divided doses; ibuprofen 1200 to 2400 mg/day in divided doses; fenoprofen 1200 to 3200 mg/day; naproxen 500 to 750 mg/day; tolmetin 200 to 400 mg q.i.d.; sulindac 150 to 200 mg b.i.d.; and meclofenamate 200 to 400 mg/day. Adverse reactions include GI intolerance, peptic ulceration, rash, dizziness, and leukopenia. Amblyopia has been described with ibuprofen. Phenylbutazone, less attractive with the availability of these less toxic nonsteroidal agents, may be given in acute symptomatic cases. An initial dose of 100 mg q.i.d. is gradually reduced and finally discontinued after 1 wk. Chronic symptoms may respond to continued long-term phenylbutazone (100 mg b.i.d. or less), but side reactions may contraindicate its use. Systemic corticosteroids are **contraindicated**. Intra-articular corticosteroids may produce significant relief for variable periods (see RHEUMATOID ARTHRITIS, above), but since degenerative changes may actually be accelerated, injections are best limited to treatment of acute inflammatory flares precipitated by trauma or joint overuse. Muscle relaxants (diazepam 2 to 5 mg t.i.d.) may be helpful.

Traction and a properly fitted cervical collar or lumbodorsal corset may relieve cervical and lumbodorsal spinal symptoms. Transcutaneous nerve stimulation **(TNS)**, a modality that delivers an electric current through the skin to a peripheral nerve, may help relieve pain, especially in spinal disease. Symptomatic relief attributed to traditional acupuncture does not exceed that seen with placebo.

Joint debridement, resection, osteotomy, fusion, arthroplasty, or prosthetic joint replacement may be necessary if conservative measures fail and joint changes are advanced. Total hip replacement relieves pain and markedly improves joint function. Durability considerations generally limit hip replacement to older patients with moderate to severe disease. Total knee replacement is less successful but should be considered if the knee is severely damaged. Decompression laminectomy and fusion may be indicated for severe neurologic changes secondary to cervical or lumbar spinal disease (see NERVE ROOT DISORDERS in Ch. 130).

NEUROGENIC ARTHROPATHY

(Neuropathic Arthropathy; Charcot's Joints)

A destructive arthropathy of joints, with impaired pain perception or position sense.

Etiology

Loss of the sensation of deep pain or of proprioception affects the joint's normal protective reflexes, often allowing trauma (especially repeated minor episodes) and small periarticular fractures to pass unrecognized. For conditions associated with Charcot's joints, see TABLE 103–3. Intra-articular deposition of calcium pyrophosphate dihydrate crystals and the consequent inflammatory reaction may accelerate joint destruction due to other conditions. Local joint infection may play a causative role in some cases associated with leprosy and diabetes mellitus. Muscle hypotonia, ligamentous laxity, and distention of the joint capsule by an effusion are contributory factors tending to accelerate disease progression.

TABLE 103–3. CONDITIONS UNDERLYING NEUROGENIC ARTHROPATHY

Diabetes mellitus	Impaired pain sensitivity due to use of:
	Intra-articular and systemic corticosteroids
Tabes dorsalis	Phenylbutazone
Syringomyelia	Indomethacin
	Excessive amounts of ethyl alcohol
Spina bifida with meningomyelocele (in children)	Congenital insensitivity to pain
Leprosy	Familial-hereditary neuropathies:
	Peroneal muscular atrophy (Charcot-Marie-Tooth disease)
Tumors and injuries of the peripheral nerves and spinal cord	Hereditary sensory neuropathy
	Hypertrophic interstitial neuropathy (Déjérine-Sottas disease)
Subacute combined degeneration of the spinal cord	Familial dysautonomia (Riley-Day syndrome)
	Hypertrophic neuropathy associated with gigantism
Amyloid neuropathy	

Clinical Features

In its early stages, the condition is often confused with osteoarthritis (OA). Some pain, a prominent—often hemorrhagic—effusion, and subluxation and instability of the joint are usually present. Acute joint dislocation sometimes occurs at this stage. Neurogenic arthropathy progresses much more rapidly than OA. Although there may be a long delay from onset of the neurologic condition to onset of arthropathy, once the arthropathy starts it may be rapidly progressive and lead to complete disorganization of the joint in a few months.

In a fully developed Charcot joint, hypertrophic or destructive changes may predominate, or findings may be mixed. Pain is often absent or less severe than would be expected from the degree of joint destruction, but may be severe if the disease has progressed rapidly and there are periarticular fractures or tense hematomas. The joint is swollen from bony overgrowth and massive synovial effusion. Deformity results from fracture with displacement, or dislocation following destruction of articular surfaces, ligamentous laxity, and muscular hypotonia. Fractures and bony metaplasia will cause many loose bodies (pieces of cartilage or bone) to slough into the joint, producing a coarse, grating, often audible crepitus that is usually more unpleasant for the observer than for the patient. The joint may feel like "a bag of bones."

Though most joints can be involved, the knee is affected as often as the sum of all other joints. Distribution depends largely on the underlying disease. Thus, in tabes dorsalis and diabetes mellitus, the lower limbs are affected (knee and hip in tabes; foot in diabetes). In syringomyelia, the upper limb joints are most commonly affected, especially the elbow and shoulder. Frequently, only one joint is affected; usually not more than 2 or 3 (except for the small joints of the feet), in an asymmetric distribution.

The diagnosis should be considered in a patient with an appropriate neurologic disorder who develops a destructive but relatively painless arthropathy. A lapse of several years from the onset of the underlying neurologic condition to the onset of the arthropathy is usual.

X-ray Findings

X-rays show a swollen joint with synovial effusion and subluxation of the articular surfaces. Sclerosis of the bone ends, usually present, may be absent in advanced destructive disease. The bones are deformed, and there is usually evidence of new bone formation adjacent to the cortex starting within the joint capsule and often extending well up the shaft of a long bone. Calcification and ossification occur in the soft tissues, on rare occasions leading to bony bridging across the joint. However, this may be transient, and even extensive soft-tissue calcification may disappear on a subsequent radiograph. Large, bizarrely shaped osteophytes are seen at the joint margins; these may break off to form the numerous intra-articular loose bodies that characterize this condition. Radiologic evidence of spinal involvement (the characteristic "parrot's beak" osteophytes) is frequently found in the absence of any clinical suggestion of disease at this site.

Prophylaxis and Treatment

Prevention of onset of arthropathy is important in a patient at risk (e.g., with severe tabes). Early diagnosis and immobilization of an often painless fracture may stop evolution of the neuroarthropathy. An unstable joint should be protected by splints, special boots, or calipers. Arthrodesis using internal fixation, a compression technic, and an adequate bone graft may be successful in a grossly disorganized joint. Successful treatment of the underlying neurologic condition may slow progression of the arthropathy and, if joint destruction is still in the early stages, reverse the process.

GOUT

A recurrent acute arthritis of peripheral joints which results from deposition, in and about the joints and tendons, of crystals of monosodium urate from supersaturated hyperuricemic body fluids; it may become chronic and deforming. Not all hyperuricemic persons develop gout. The greater the degree and duration of hyperuricemia, the greater the chance of crystal deposition and of acute attacks of gout.

Pathophysiology

Most gouty patients are hyperuricemic. Normal ranges for serum urate levels depend on the method used for its determination. The upper limit in most men is < 7 mg/100 ml of serum. The mean serum urate of women is about 1 mg/100 ml lower until after menopause, at which time it may approach that of men. This difference correlates with the clinical observation that only 5% of gouty patients are women, most of them postmenopausal.

Limited solubility of uric acid and its salts in biologic fluids accounts for the major pathologic features characteristic of gout. Monosodium urate crystals are deposited in and about the joints and tendons and in the tubules or the interstitial tissue of the renal parenchyma. An inflammatory reaction to the deposits of monosodium urate causes the acute attack of gout; continued accretion of the crystals produces the characteristic gouty tophi responsible for erosive joint damage and chronic disability. In the urinary tract, because of the lower pH of urine, free uric acid is precipitated to form calculi with an incidence 1000 times that of the general population. Less than 5% of patients with gout develop slowly progressive renal dysfunction causing death.

Hyperuricemia may be caused by various underlying abnormalities of purine metabolism, both genetic and acquired. Excessive purine synthesis is the most common; diminished renal clearance of uric acid, the other major factor. Medical disorders associated with hyperuricemia and gout include proliferative hematopoietic diseases, psoriasis, myxedema, hypo- and hyperparathyroidism, hypertension, myocardial infarction, advanced primary renal diseases, obesity, and several hereditary diseases (including Down's syndrome and glycogen storage disease, Type I). A rare but well-defined example is sex-linked uricaciduria with a deficiency of the enzyme hypoxanthine-guanine phosphoribosyltransferase. It is associated with markedly excessive uric acid production, a tendency to develop uric acid kidney stones, and severe gouty arthritis and nephropathy at an early age. A spectrum of clinical neurologic symptoms may be present, which correlate with the severity of the enzyme deficiency (the **Lesch-Nyhan syndrome**—with choreoathetosis, spasticity, and mental retardation—is the extreme example). Acute gouty arthritis may thus be the presenting symptom of another underlying metabolic disorder. Hyperuricemia and gouty arthritis also can develop secondary to chronic lead poisoning or diuretic therapy (usually with thiazides).

Symptoms and Signs

Acute gouty arthritis usually appears without warning. It may be precipitated by minor trauma (as from ill-fitting shoes), overindulgence in food or alcohol, surgery, fatigue, emotional stress, infection, or administration of penicillin, insulin, or mercurial diuretics. Acute mon- or polyarticular pain, often of nocturnal onset, is usually the first symptom. The pain becomes progressively more severe each hour and is often described as throbbing, crushing, or excruciating. Examination shows signs of an acute inflammatory response resembling an acute infection, with swelling, warmth, redness, and exquisite tenderness. The overlying skin is tense, hot, shiny, and dusky red or purplish in color. The metatarsophalangeal joint of the great toe is involved most frequently, but the instep, ankle, knee, wrist, and elbow also are common sites. Initially, only a single joint may be affected; in later attacks, several can be affected simultaneously or sequentially. Systemic reactions may include fever, tachycardia, chills, malaise, and leukocytosis.

The first few attacks usually last only a few days, but later untreated attacks may persist for weeks. Local symptoms and signs eventually regress and joint function returns to normal. Asymptomatic intervals between acute bouts of gouty arthritis vary considerably, but tend to become shorter as the disease progresses. Without prophylaxis, several attacks may occur each year.

Chronic gout can be prevented, or its symptoms markedly reduced, by prophylactic therapy. Without it, tophaceous deposits appear in and about the joints and tendons, and symptom-free intervals progressively decrease. Chronic joint symptoms develop, in addition to the superimposed recurrent acute attacks, as permanent erosive joint deformity appears. Limitation of motion often involves multiple joints of the hands, feet, or both; rarely, the shoulder, sacroiliac, sternoclavicular joints, or the cervical spine are involved. Urate deposits are common in the walls of bursae and tendon sheaths. Enlarging tophi on the hands and feet may erupt and discharge chalky urate crystals.

Diagnosis

The clinical features of acute gouty arthritis are so distinctive that a tentative diagnosis usually can be made by history and examination. An elevated serum urate content ($>$ 7 mg/100 ml) supports the diagnosis but is not specific, since other conditions may cause hyperuricemia. Demonstration in tissue or synovial fluid of needle-shaped urate crystals that are free in the fluid or engulfed by phagocytes, and a therapeutic response to colchicine within 12 to 48 h are pathognomonic for gout. The crystals may be identified in the light microscope and are *negatively* birefringent when viewed under crossed polarizing filters attached to a microscope. These findings are particularly helpful in establishing the diagnosis in atypical gout.

Radiologic examination of the peripheral joints in a well-developed case shows punched-out lesions in subchondral bone, commonly in the first metatarsophalangeal joint. The urate deposits must grow to about 5 mm in diameter before becoming visible on x-ray. Such lesions are not specific or diagnostic, since similar lesions may be seen in a variety of joint diseases.

In patients with chondrocalcinosis (see below), the acute synovitis is due to *positively* birefringent calcium pyrophosphate dihydrate crystals of various shapes; in addition, radiopaque calcium deposits are present in articular cartilage (particularly the knee), and the clinical course is milder than in gout. An acutely septic joint may be confused with an acute gouty joint, but the absence of regional lymphadenopathy in gout and the serum uric acid content help differentiate. Microscopic examination and culture of the synovial fluid provide proof by demonstrating either urate crystals or bacteria. Acute rheumatic fever with joint involvement and polyarticular rheumatism may simulate gout in young persons. In RA, joint involvement tends to be symmetric; the duration of a single acute attack is longer and the onset more gradual than in acute gout. Heberden's nodes of osteoarthritis may resemble gouty tophi but are seldom associated with acute symptoms.

Prognosis

Current therapy permits virtually all patients to live a full and productive life without serious disability, if the diagnosis is made early and permanent medical supervision and prophylactic medication accepted by the patient. For those with advanced disease, some reconstitution of joint structure can be achieved. Tophi can be resolved, joint function improved, and any renal dysfunction arrested. Gout is more severe in patients whose clinical symptoms first appear before age 30. Almost 10 to 20% of patients with gout develop urolithiasis. Possible complications include obstruction and infection, with secondary tubulointerstitial disease. Untreated progressive renal dysfunction, usually related to coexisting hypertension, diabetes, or some other cause of nephropathy, leads to further impairment in the removal of urate from the body, accelerating the pathologic process in the joints. It is also the greatest threat to life.

Treatment

Objectives are (1) termination of the acute attack with an anti-inflammatory drug, (2) prevention of recurrent acute attacks by daily use of colchicine, and (3) prevention of further deposition of monosodium urate crystals in tophi and resolution of existing tophi (achieved by lowering the urate concentration in body fluids that bathe the deposits). A preventive maintenance program should aim at averting both the disability resulting from erosion of bone and joint cartilage and the renal damage. Specific treatment depends on the stage and severity of the disease.

Acute attack: Colchicine is still the preferred drug in the first few attacks, particularly when the diagnosis is in doubt. The response usually is dramatic. Joint pains generally begin to subside after 12 h of treatment and are gone within 36 to 48 h. The dose of colchicine is 1.0 mg orally q 2 h until a response is obtained or until diarrhea or vomiting results. Severe episodes may require from 4 to 7 mg (average, 5). Because of the toxic effects of colchicine overdosage, not more than 7 mg should be taken in 48 h for a given attack. When treatment causes diarrhea, paregoric 5 ml orally q 2 to 4 h is helpful.

Nonsteroidal anti-inflammatory agents are effective in acute attacks of established gout. They are especially useful for patients intolerant of colchicine. Daily doses for 2 or 3 days are usually taken with food: indomethacin 100 mg t.i.d., ibuprofen 400 mg t.i.d., naproxen 250 mg t.i.d., or phenylbutazone 200 mg q.i.d.

Treatment with drugs that lower the serum urate concentration should be deferred until acute symptoms have subsided.

Corticosteroids can produce rapid and complete remission but generally are used only when other drugs are contraindicated. In an effusion of the knee, withdrawal of fluid followed by instillation of prednisolone tebutate 25 mg usually brings relief.

In addition to specific therapy, rest, abundant fluid intake to combat dehydration and decrease urate precipitation in the kidneys, and a soft diet are indicated. To control the pain, codeine 30 to 60 mg or meperidine 50 to 100 mg orally q 4 h may be needed.

Intercritical period: The frequency of acute attacks is reduced by daily prophylactic use of colchicine 0.6 mg orally b.i.d. to q.i.d. (depending on tolerance). An extra 1 or 2 mg of colchicine taken at the first suggestion of an attack will abort most.

Colchicine does not retard the progressive joint damage produced by tophi. It can be prevented, however, and many tophaceous deposits resolved, by lowering the serum urate concentration to the normal range and maintaining it there indefinitely, either by increasing uric acid excretion with a uricosuric drug, or by blocking uric acid production with allopurinol, or, in tophaceous gout, by using both drugs daily. Such anti-hyperuricemic therapy is indicated for gouty patients with tophaceous deposits, a serum urate concentration consistently > 9 mg/100 ml, persistent joint symptoms despite only a modest increase in serum urate, or impaired renal function.

Control of hyperuricemia should be started in conjunction with daily colchicine treatment during a quiescent phase, because all such therapy is associated with an increased tendency to develop acute attacks during the first few weeks or months of treatment. Periodic determination of serum urate concentration is a helpful guide to drug effectiveness; the dosage and selection of a drug should be adjusted to achieve a significant reduction in serum urate concentration. Resolution of susceptible tophi may take months or years.

In uricosuric therapy, either 0.5-gm tablets of probenecid or 100-mg tablets of sulfinpyrazone are given orally; the dose is adjusted to maintain a serum urate concentration in the normal range. The starting dose should be 1/2 tablet b.i.d., gradually increasing the dosage over 10 days to up to 4 tablets/day. Sulfinpyrazone has a greater uricosuric effect than does probenecid, but is more toxic. Salicylates antagonize the uricosuric effect of either drug and should be **avoided.** Acetaminophen provides a comparable analgesic effect without interfering with the uricosuric action.

Inhibition of uric acid synthesis by allopurinol, 200 to 600 mg/day in divided doses, also controls serum urate concentration. In addition to blocking the enzyme (xanthine oxidase) responsible for uric acid formation, it corrects excessive purine synthesis. It is especially helpful in managing patients who repeatedly pass uric acid calculi or who have severe renal dysfunction. Established calculi may be dissolved by allopurinol. Adverse effects of allopurinol include mild GI distress, skin rash, and drowsiness.

Adjuncts to treatment: A high fluid intake of at least 3 L/day is desirable for all gouty patients and especially those who are chronic uric acid stone formers. Alkalinization of the urine with sodium bicarbonate or trisodium citrate 5 gm t.i.d. is recommended also. Drugs are so effective in lowering the serum urate concentration that rigid restriction of the purine content of the diet usually is unnecessary. Weight reduction in obese patients should be undertaken during a quiescent phase of the disease.

Surgical correction of severely damaged joints or removal of tophi to relieve tendon entrapment or for cosmetic reasons should be deferred until the disease and the serum urate concentration have been controlled medically. Large tophi should be removed surgically; all others except those walled off by extensive fibrosis should resolve under adequate prophylactic therapy.

Idiopathic Hyperuricemia

There are no hard data regarding specific treatment of non-gouty asymptomatic hyperuricemia. Until this deficiency is corrected, it is suggested that either probenecid, sulfinpyrazone, or allopurinol be given daily to those patients under age 40 with a persistent hyperuricemia of 12 mg/100 ml or greater, whose urinary excretion in a 24-hour sample is < 1000 mg. Any person with a similarly high persistent hyperuricemia and a urinary excretion of uric acid > 1000 mg/day should receive allopurinol daily.

CHONDROCALCINOSIS

(Pseudogout; Calcium Pyrophosphate Dihydrate [CPPD] Crystal Deposition Disease)

A specific joint disease with intermittent attacks of acute arthritis and x-ray evidence of calcinosis of the articular cartilage.

Etiology and Incidence

The cause is unknown. Its frequent association with other conditions such as osteoarthritis, diabetes mellitus, hyperparathyroidism, gout, and hemochromatosis suggests that the deposits of CPPD in the cartilage are secondary to degenerative changes in the joints. The disease appears in maturity. Both sexes are affected equally. A familial pattern of incidence has been observed in several countries. The incidence of asymptomatic calcinosis of the cartilage in persons over age 50 is appreciable.

Symptoms and Signs

Acute or subacute attacks of arthritis **(pseudogout)** occur, usually in the peripheral joints. Such attacks sometimes follow the pattern of uric acid gout but are less severe. There may be complete freedom between attacks, or distress may persist, with low-grade symptoms similar to RA. These patterns tend to persist for life. Asymptomatic calcinosis has been observed by x-ray in the intervertebral cartilages and in the symphysis pubis.

Diagnosis

Identifying large or small CPPD crystals in a drop of synovial fluid is diagnostic (see Differentiating Inflammatory and Noninflammatory Joint Disease in Ch. 102). Crystals may be seen engulfed in leukocytes or floating free. They are weakly *positively* birefringent in contrast to the strongly *negatively* birefringent urate crystals. The x-ray finding of linear calcification in the articular cartilage supports the diagnosis.

Prognosis and Treatment

The prognosis usually is excellent. Chondrocalcinosis (per se) does not progress into chronic deforming arthritis. Colchicine usually is ineffective, although the disease resembles acute gouty arthritis. An acute synovial effusion should be drained, the fluid inspected for crystals, and hydrocortisone 25 mg instilled into the joint. Indomethacin 75 to 150 mg daily is helpful during the acute attack.

---

104. COLLAGEN VASCULAR DISEASES

VASCULITIS

Inflammation of blood vessels, which is often segmental and may be generalized or localized, constituting the basic mechanism of the production of lesions in a variety of rheumatic diseases and syndromes.

A large number of diseases are characterized by or strongly associated with vasculitis. These include the collagen vascular diseases, described in detail below. (Also, the rheumatoid nodule and other lesions of the rheumatic diseases appear to have central foci of vasculitis as their pathogenetic mechanism.) Much of SLE pathophysiology can be ascribed to vasculitis with or without secondary vascular occlusion. The polymyositis or dermatomyositis of childhood frequently includes an element of vasculitis not only in the obvious muscular target organs but also at extramuscular and extracutaneous sites. Even the bland-appearing and extensive intimal proliferation of small arteries typifying progressive systemic sclerosis is believed to be a postinflammatory event. Several other syndromes dominated by serious vasculitis are adequately characterized so as to permit diagnosable clinical profiles. Examples of these include polyarteritis nodosa, Wegener's granulomatosis, and other diseases which follow a less predictable course.

Pathology

Vasculitis may follow a large variety of pathogenetic mechanisms, but the spectrum of histologic abnormalities is limited. Inflammation of a blood vessel may be acute or chronic, with the predominant inflammatory cell being either polymorphonuclear leukocytes in the acute lesions or lymphocytes in the chronic lesions. Moreover, the inflammatory process is often segmental, so that major portions of the vascular tree may be normal yet contain scattered focal areas of intense inflammation. At the affected sites, variable degrees of cellular infiltration and necrosis or scarring within one or more layers of the vessel wall are seen. Thus, the inflammatory process may be most intense within the media or the adventitia, with or without an intimal or periadventitial fibrous scar reaction. Inflammation within the media of a muscular artery tends to destroy the internal elastic lamina. Inflammation at any point in the vessel wall tends to resolve by fibrosis and intimal hypertrophy. On occasion, certain distinguishing histologic events are seen, such as the development of numerous giant cells, or patchy areas of fibrinoid necrosis where complete sections of the vessel wall have undergone inflammatory destruction and liquefaction. Wherever inflammation of a vessel wall is seen, secondary occlusion of the lumen due to intimal hypertrophy and/or intraluminal thrombus formation may be expected. In addition, once the integrity of the vessel wall is breached, RBCs and fibrin may leak into the surrounding perivascular connective tissue.

Any type and size of vessel may be involved in an inflammatory response—arteries, arterioles, veins, venules, or capillaries. However, most of the versatile and variable pathophysiology resulting from vasculitis can be ascribed to arterial inflammation with the potential for total or partial vascular occlusion and subsequent tissue necrosis. Although the primary inflammatory process of a blood vessel is invariably a segmental or focal event, biopsy of even clinically involved tissue may not always provide definitive histologic evidence of vasculitis. However, the intimal and periadventitial fibrous response to a focus of intense vessel wall inflammation frequently extends up and down the vessel from the primary insult, so that the histologic appearance of intimal hyperplasia and fibrosis or perivasculitis would imply the presence of an adjacent area of vasculitis.

Classification

In categorizing the numerous vasculitic disorders, classification according to the size of the predominant vessel involved is most useful. This often reflects the depth of the lesions beginning from the integument and working viscerally. Thus, predominant inflammation of a postcapillary venule with neutrophilic infiltration leads to the typical histologic appearance of leukocytoblastic angiitis manifesting clinically as palpable purpura, and best typified by **Henoch-Schönlein syndrome** or *Pseudomonas* **septicemia.** The vascular inflammation of the deep dermal panniculus, mediated mainly by septal perivascular lymphocytes and presenting clinically as tender, deep, indurated red bumps on the arms and legs, is typical of **erythema nodosum.** Inflammation of medium-sized muscular arteries with the histologic features of a pleomorphic transmural infiltrate, fibrinoid necrosis, destruction of the internal elastic lamina, and postinflammatory aneurysm formation is exemplified by **polyarteritis nodosa.** When a similar type of process is largely confined to the extracranial carotid tree and is associated with a lymphocytic infiltrate and the formation of giant cells clustered around the luminal aspect of the disrupted elastic lamina, severe headaches are induced and **giant-cell arteritis** is recognized. Finally, when inflammation of the largest central vessels such as the aorta and its branches is evident, mainly mediated by adventitial and/or medial lymphocytic infiltration and fibrous scarring with a tendency to postinflammatory stenosis, the loss of major pulses may become clinically evident and **Takayasu's arteritis** is recognized.

DISCOID LUPUS ERYTHEMATOSUS

(DLE; Cutaneous LE; Chronic Discoid LE)

A chronic and recurrent disorder primarily affecting the skin and characterized by sharply circumscribed macules and plaques displaying erythema, follicular plugging, scales, telangiectasia, and atrophy. There are 2 varieties: one with lesions above the chin, the other with or without facial involvement but with lesions on the rest of the body.

Etiology, Incidence, and Course

The cause is unknown. Exposure to sunlight frequently precedes the initial appearance of lesions (50% of patients have a history of photosensitivity). The disease is more common in females, appearing most often during their 30s.

Active lesions may persist or recur for years. Initially, they are erythematous, round, scaling papules 5 to 10 mm in diameter, with follicular plugging. They appear most frequently on the malar prominences, bridge of the nose, scalp, external auditory canals, and the remainder of the pinnae. The lesions may be generalized over the upper portion of the trunk and extensor surfaces of the extremities. Mucous membrane involvement is unusual, though the lips and oral mucosa are occasionally involved. The lesions of untreated DLE gradually extend peripherally, while the center atrophies. The residual scars are noncontractile. A "carpet tack" invagination of the scales into the dilated follicles may be seen in heavily scaled lesions. Alopecia of the scalp may be permanent. Leukopenia and mild and transitory systemic manifestations, such as arthralgias, are common.

Patients with extensive skin lesions are more likely to have internal manifestations suggestive of SLE. Though the disease is limited to the skin in 90% of patients with typical DLE, approximately 10% eventually develop varying degrees of systemic manifestations; approximately 5% develop SLE even when an initial study does not suggest systemic disease.

Differential Diagnosis

Systemic lupus erythematosus **(SLE)** must be excluded. *Since the cutaneous lesions of DLE and SLE may be identical, a patient presenting with typical discoid lesions must be evaluated to determine whether systemic involvement is present.* Skin biopsy will not differentiate these 2 types. A medical history and physical examination are required. Occurrence in a patient younger than age 30 suggests the possibility of an early cutaneous manifestation of SLE. Diagnostic studies should include biopsy from the active margin of the lesion, CBC, ESR, LE cell preparation, test for antinuclear factor, and renal function studies.

The discoid lesions of cutaneous LE are differentiated from those of rosacea by the absence of pustules and the presence of atrophy. The lesions of seborrheic dermatitis are never atrophic and frequently involve the nasolabial area, which is rarely affected by DLE. Polymorphous light sensitivity must also be differentiated; ordinary lesions caused by photosensitivity are not atrophic and usually disappear when direct sunlight is avoided. Lymphoma or plaques of sarcoidosis may also mimic DLE clinically. When the lips and oral mucosa are involved, lichen planus and leukoplakia must be ruled out.

Treatment

Early treatment is advisable, before atrophy is permanent. Excessive exposure to sunlight (or ultraviolet light) should be avoided. In the majority of cases, exposure of 5 to 10 min is innocuous. If a longer period is anticipated, a sunscreen preparation should be applied, e.g., a combination of methyl anthranilate and titanium dioxide, or a liquid preparation with aminobenzoic acid.

It is usually possible to effect involution of small lesions by applying topical corticosteroid ointments or creams t.i.d. to q.i.d. (e.g., triamcinolone acetonide 0.1% or 0.5%, fluocinolone 0.025% or 0.2%, flurandrenolide 0.05%, betamethasone valerate 0.1%, or betamethasone dipropionate 0.05%). The latter may be most effective. Plastic tape coated with flurandrenolide is frequently helpful in resistant lesions. Individual recalcitrant plaques may respond to intradermal injection of 0.1% suspension of triamcinolone acetonide, but secondary atrophy frequently follows.

Systemic antimalarial therapy is indicated for extensive and resistant lesions. Hydroxychloroquine is suggested as the drug of choice rather than chloroquine because the side effect of retinopathy is rare. Adults weighing more than 45.4 kg (100 lb) are given 200 mg b.i.d. orally until involution occurs; the medication is then tapered slowly. Maintenance therapy may be required to prevent significant relapses. The patient must be evaluated by an ophthalmologist before, and at 4-mo intervals during, hydroxychloroquine treatment. Chloroquine 250 mg/day orally may be given if hydroxychloroquine is poorly tolerated. Quinacrine 100 mg/day orally is effective and does not damage the retina; however, it produces a significant yellow stain and in rare instances may cause aplastic anemia. For patients with extensive resistant lesions, quinacrine may be combined with either hydroxychloroquine or chloroquine in the dosages given above.

Some patients with recalcitrant widespread lesions may require systemic corticosteroid therapy (e.g., prednisone 5 to 10 mg/day orally for weeks to months, or longer) in addition to antimalarial and local treatment.

SYSTEMIC LUPUS ERYTHEMATOSUS

(SLE; Disseminated LE)

An inflammatory connective tissue disorder of unknown etiology occurring predominantly in young women, but also in children and older adults; 90% of cases occur in women. Fibrinoid necrosis and bodies of altered nuclear material **("hematoxylin bodies")** may be found in the tissues of any organ. Antinuclear antibodies, including the LE cell factor, are present in the serum of most patients. The presence of these antibodies not only facilitates recognition of the disease in its milder forms, but also supports the favored hypothesis that SLE is an "autoimmune" disorder. The pathogenetic mechanisms of autoimmune reactions are discussed in Ch. 19.

Pathology, Symptoms, and Signs

The clinical findings vary with the acuteness of the process and the distribution of the lesions. SLE may begin abruptly with fever, simulating acute infection, or may develop insidiously over months or years with only episodes of fever and malaise. Manifestations referable to any organ system may appear. As many as 90% of patients complain of articular symptoms ranging from intermittent arthralgias to acute polyarthritis, some for months or years before other manifestations appear, and are usually assumed to have RA.

The characteristic malar "butterfly" erythema is one of several cutaneous lesions that may occur; others include the discoid lesions described above under DLE, and erythematous, firm, maculopapular lesions of the face, exposed areas of the neck, upper chest, and back, and other light-exposed areas. Confluent lesions may become markedly edematous. Blistering and ulceration are rare, though ulcers on the mucous membrane (particularly the central portion of the hard palate near the junction of the hard and soft palate, the buccal and gum mucosa, and the anterior nasal septum) are common. Generalized alopecia is frequent during active phases of the disease. Mottled erythema of the sides of the palms with extension onto the fingers, periungual erythema with edema, and macular reddish-purple lesions on the volar surfaces of the fingers may also occur. Purpura may develop secondary to thrombocytopenia or necrotizing angiitis of small vessels. Photosensitivity occurs in

40% of patients. Following longstanding disease, joint deformity is common, particularly ulnar deviation of the fingers and subluxation of the proximal interphalangeal joints, without x-ray evidence of erosion (Jaccoud's arthritis).

Recurrent pleurisy, with or without effusion, is frequent. Bacterial or viral pneumonia is common, but lupus pneumonitis is rare. Pericarditis is often present. Atypical verrucous endocarditis (Libman-Sacks syndrome) and pericarditis are not usually associated with cardiac dysfunction. The endocarditis usually appears on the mitral and aortic valves and occasionally on the tricuspid, primarily producing a systolic and occasionally a diastolic murmur. The endocarditis is usually apparent at autopsy, occurring in as many as 1/3 of cases. Diffuse myocarditis may produce congestive heart failure.

Generalized adenopathy is frequent, particularly in children, young adults, and blacks. Splenomegaly occurs in 10% of patients. Histologically, the spleen may show periarterial fibrosis ("onion-skin" lesion). Involvement of the CNS causes personality changes, epilepsy, psychoses, and organic brain syndrome.

Renal involvement occurs in the majority of patients and may pursue a benign and asymptomatic, or a relentlessly progressive, fatal course. A nephritic or nephrotic syndrome may result. The histopathology of the renal lesion varies from a focal, usually benign, glomerulitis to a diffuse, usually fatal, membranoproliferative glomerulonephritis. **Kidney biopsy** is unnecessary unless the diagnosis is uncertain. Although the findings on biopsy are of academic interest, there is usually a good response to treatment regardless of the findings. Biopsy may be helpful late in the course of renal disease to determine whether another course of medical therapy is indicated or whether dialysis and transplantation should be considered.

Laboratory Findings

Both the "hematoxylin bodies" in tissue lesions and the LE cell factor in the serum reflect the presence of abnormal immunoglobulins behaving like antibodies to nucleoprotein. The **LE cell factor**, one of several autoantibodies reacting with nuclear constitutents, transforms nuclei into homogeneous globular bodies that are phagocytized by intact granulocytes to form typical LE cells (LE cell phenomenon). A positive LE cell test is most closely correlated with SLE, but it is not pathognomonic. Failure to demonstrate LE cells does not exclude the diagnosis, since only 70 to 90% of patients with SLE exhibit a positive LE cell test at some time during the disease. Fluorescent technics for detecting **antinuclear antibodies (ANA)** are more sensitive but less specific for SLE than is the LE cell test. The most specific but least sensitive test is the titer of Sm antibodies.

Multiple serum protein abnormalities occur. Since the immunoglobulins are usually elevated in active SLE, hyperglobulinemia and positive cephalin flocculation tests are common. Rheumatoid factor, a false-positive STS, circulating anticoagulants, a positive Coombs' test, and cryoglobulins may be found in additon to ANA. The serum complement level is markedly depressed in active disease, especially when a diffuse proliferative glomerular lesion is present. The nephrotic serum protein pattern may predominate in patients with advanced renal disease.

A moderate normochromic, normocytic anemia is found in the majority of patients; rarely, an acute hemolytic crisis is observed. Leukopenia with a normal differential count is common. Thrombocytopenia may be severe and symptomatic. The ESR is elevated almost uniformly during active disease.

Urinalysis may be repeatedly normal despite early renal involvement confirmed by biopsy. Kidney damage can become evident at any time, even when other features of SLE are absent. Urinalyses should be repeated at 4- to 6-mo intervals while monitoring patients in apparent remission. Abacterial pyuria, hematuria, and a slight increase in proteinuria are the initial signs of nephropathy. Proteinuria increases as the disease progresses, and red cell casts, granular casts, and oval fat bodies appear. Urinalysis may show some improvement following adequate treatment of advanced disease, but a return to normal cannot be expected with a badly scarred kidney even though renal function is restored.

Diagnosis

Recognition of SLE is obvious when a young woman has a febrile disease with an erythematous skin rash, polyarthritis, evidence of renal disease, intermittent pleuritic pain, leukopenia, and hyperglobulinemia with LE cells. SLE may be difficult to differentiate from other connective tissue (collagen vascular) disorders in its early stages. It may be mistaken for RA or rheumatic fever if arthritic symptoms predominate. Some cases are mistakenly diagnosed for years as idiopathic thrombocytopenic purpura until other manifestations of SLE appear. Epilepsy or psychoses may be initial findings. Meticulous evaluation and long-term observation may be required before the diagnosis is established. Patients with discoid lesions must be critically evaluated to determine whether they have discoid or systemic LE. Histologic changes in the spleen and kidney are strongly suggestive of the diagnosis.

A detailed medication history should be obtained when the disease is suspected. Numerous drugs may have a causative role, including procainamide, hydralazine, methyldopa, and chlorpromazine.

The American Rheumatism Association has proposed criteria helpful in confirming the diagnosis. A minimum of 4 of the following manifestations must be present serially or simultaneously during any interval: (1) facial erythema (butterfly rash); (2) DLE; (3) Raynaud's phenomenon; (4) alopecia; (5) photosensitivity; (6) oral or nasopharyngeal ulceration; (7) arthritis without deformity; (8) LE cells; (9) chronic false-positive STS; (10) proteinuria > 3.5 gm/24 h; (11) cellular casts; (12) pleuritis, pericarditis, or both; (13) psychosis, convulsions, or both; (14) leukopenia ($<$ 4000/cu mm), thrombocyto-penia ($<$ 100,000/cu mm), hemolytic anemia, or any combination of the 3.

Mixed connective tissue disease (MCTD) is a syndrome with clinical features of SLE overlapping with those of progressive systemic sclerosis **(PSS)** and dermatomyositis. The disorder is discussed in this chapter, below.

Prognosis

This varies widely, depending on the organs involved and the intensity of the inflammatory reaction. Patients with nephritis or myocarditis have a poorer prognosis than those with inflammation limited to serous membranes, joints, and skin. The course of SLE is commonly chronic and relapsing, often with long periods (years) of remission. Rarely, the disease pursues an acute, fulminant course, ending fatally within a few weeks. After diagnosis, mortality averages approximately 5%/yr.

Treatment

When drug-induced SLE produces clinical symptoms, discontinuing the drug will result in symptom reversal within several weeks. Management of idiopathic SLE must be individualized, depending on the location and severity of the disease. To simplify the concept of therapy, SLE should be classified as "mild" or "severe." Mild disease is characterized by fever, arthritis, pleurisy, small pleural and pericardial effusions, pericarditis, or rash; severe life-threatening disease, by hemolytic anemia, thrombocytopenic purpura, massive pleural and pericardial involvement, significant renal damage, acute vasculitis of the extremities or GI tract, or CNS involvement. Treatment depends on the current clinical condition. The course is totally unpredictable. The following drugs and dosages are for adults, unless otherwise specified.

Mild disease should be treated first with salicylates in doses increased to toxicity. If joint pain or fever is not adequately controlled, indomethacin up to 200 mg/day should also be given. Alternatively, ibuprofen 1600 to 3200 mg/day is helpful for patients with gastritis or ulcer history. Other nonsteroidal anti-inflammatory agents may also be useful.

If rash or mucous membrane lesions are present, or if the disease is mild but inadequately controlled by the formerly mentioned drugs, one of the following antimalarials may be added: hydroxychloroquine 200 mg orally b.i.d. (for adults weighing more than 45.4 kg [100 lb]), chloroquine 250 mg/day orally (for adults weighing more than 45.4 kg), quinacrine 100 mg/day orally. For children, the dose is adjusted on a weight basis. Combinations of quinacrine and one of the other 2 agents are often used. Ophthalmologic evaluation is needed every 4 mo as long as hydroxychloroquine or chloroquine is being given. Prednisone 2.5 to 5 mg/day orally may be added to the prior regimen if polyarthritis and myalgia are not controlled. Corticosteroid dosage should be increased by approximately 20% every 1 to 2 wk, but in order to lessen toxicity and withdrawal difficulties, doses should not be larger than necessary for moderate relief.

Severe disease requires immediate corticosteroid therapy, the mainstay of treatment. The other previously mentioned anti-inflammatory agents are not used in acutely ill patients because they are not as effective as corticosteroids. Prednisone is given before meals twice daily to febrile patients and once daily to others. Alternate-day treatment is satisfactory for patients with hematologic and renal complications. The suggested doses are for adults, but children may require almost as much. **Prednisone dosages** for specific manifestations are as follows:

Hemolytic anemia—60 to 80 mg/day. The dose is increased to 100 to 120 mg/day if there is no clinical and laboratory improvement within several days or a week.

Thrombocytopenic purpura—80 mg/day. Platelets may not rise for 4 to 6 wk.

Severe polyserositis—40 to 60 mg/day. Response begins within days.

Renal damage—50 to 60 mg/day or 100 to 120 mg every other day. Improvement does not usually occur for 4 to 12 wk and may not be evident until corticosteroid dosage is reduced. The initial course of therapy should be with corticosteroids alone. If prompt relapse of nephropathy occurs following withdrawal, combined experimental use of high-dose steroids and cytotoxic agents such as cyclophosphamide or chlorambucil can be tried. Azathioprine is of doubtful value in managing any form of SLE. Nitrogen mustard is helpful in half the steroid-resistant cases when a 2nd course of treatment fails.

Acute vasculitis—40 to 100 mg/day. Response usually appears within a few days, but gangrene of the extremities improves over several weeks.

Acute CNS injury, such as psychosis—50 to 100 mg q 12 h for several days. If there is no improvement, hydrocortisone is given parenterally as described just below. For patients with severe CNS damage (i.e., coma, status epilepticus, transverse myelitis), treatment is begun with parenteral hydrocortisone 250 to 500 mg given IM or IV q 12 h; the dose of hydrocortisone is doubled every 24 to 48 h until 3000 mg is being given daily. This level is maintained for several days up to 4 wk, until the patient develops cushingoid features. The dose is then tapered by decrements of about 20% every 4 days until a maintenance level is established. The risk of infection is great with such large doses.

In both mild and severe disease, after the inflammatory process is controlled, the minimal dose of corticosteroids and other agents necessary to suppress tissue inflammation must be determined. This is usually done by decreasing the dose by 10% at intervals varying with how fast clinical improvement occurs. For example, if fever and arthritis are the initial active manifestations, the dose is reduced at weekly intervals; if thrombocytopenia or renal disease (both of which respond more slowly to initiation of therapy) are problems, reductions are made every 2 to 4 wk. Rebound (temporary flare) and relapse tend to occur in the system with the most recent exacerbation. Response to therapy is measured by relief of symptoms and signs, rise in Hct, or improvement in other laboratory tests. A return of low serum complement toward normal may or may not occur with treatment. Should serum complement levels rise with therapy and fall when corticosteroids are reduced, the corticosteroid must be tapered more slowly, and the patient observed for relapse. The dose should not be kept elevated to maintain serum complement or anti-DNA antibody at normal levels when there is an adequate clinical response, because of the complications that occur with high corticosteroid doses. Since positive ANA and LE cell tests and elevated ESR may persist despite clinical remission, these parameters should not be used as guides to therapy.

General medical management is also important. Intercurrent infection, often complicating the disease and easily mistaken for some of its manifestations, should be treated vigorously. The usual measures to combat heart failure and renal insufficiency must be taken in addition to using anti-inflammatory agents. Close medical supervision is imperative during surgical procedures and pregnancy. Elimination of emotional stress, physical fatigue, any implicated drugs, and excessive sun exposure, and avoidance of such sensitizing agents as nonessential medication may inhibit exacerbations of SLE.

PROGRESSIVE SYSTEMIC SCLEROSIS
(PSS; Scleroderma)

A chronic disease of unknown cause, characterized by diffuse fibrosis, degenerative changes, and vascular abnormalities in the skin (scleroderma), articular structures, and internal organs (especially the esophagus, intestinal tract, thyroid, lung, heart, and kidney). The disease varies in severity and progression, its features ranging from generalized cutaneous thickening (PSS with diffuse scleroderma) with rapidly progressive and often fatal visceral involvement, to a form distinguished by restricted skin involvement (often just the fingers and face) and prolonged passage of time, often several decades, before full manifestation of characteristic internal manifestations (**CREST syndrome:** Calcinosis, Raynaud's phenomenon, Esophageal dysfunction, Sclerodactyly, Telangiectasia). In addition, overlap syndromes exist, e.g., **sclerodermatomyositis** *(muscle weakness indistinguishable from polymyositis),* and **mixed connective tissue disease (MCTD)**—discussed separately below.

PSS is about 4 times more common in women than men, and is comparatively rare in children.

Symptoms, Signs, and Diagnosis

The most common **initial complaints** are Raynaud's phenomenon and insidious swelling of the acral portions of the extremities with gradual thickening of the skin of the fingers. Polyarthralgia is also a prominent early symptom. GI disturbances (e..g, heartburn and dysphagia) or respiratory complaints are occasionally the first manifestation of the disease.

Induration of the skin is symmetric and may be confined to the fingers (sclerodactyly) and distal portions of the upper extremities, or affect most or all of the body. As the disease progresses, the skin becomes taut, shiny, and hyperpigmented; the face becomes masklike; telangiectases appear on the fingers, face, lips, and tongue. Subcutaneous calcifications develop (calcinosis circumscripta), usually on the fingertips and over bony eminences. Biopsy of indurated skin shows an increase in compact collagen fibers in the reticular dermis, epidermal thinning, loss of rete pegs, and atrophy of dermal appendages. There may be variably large accumulations of lymphocytes in the dermis and subcutis (which may also be the seat of extensive fibrosis); these cells have been identified as T-dependent lymphocytes.

Friction rubs develop over the **joints** (particularly the knees), tendon sheaths (tendinitis), and large bursae, because of fibrin deposition on synovial surfaces. Flexion contractures of the fingers, wrists, and elbows result from fibrosis of the synovium and periarticular structures. Trophic ulcers are common, especially on the fingertips and overlying the finger joints.

Esophageal dysfunction is the most frequent visceral disturbance and eventually occurs in the majority of patients. Dysphagia, acid reflux due to lower esophageal sphincter incompetence, and peptic esophagitis with possible ulceration and stricture are common. Hypomotility of the **small intestine** may be associated with malabsorption resulting from anaerobic bacterial overgrowth. Pneumatosis cystoides intestinalis may occur following degeneration of the muscularis mucosa and entry of air into the submucosa of the intestinal wall. Characteristic large-mouthed sacculations develop in the **colon** and **ileum** because of atrophy of the smooth muscle of these segments. **Biliary** cirrhosis has occurred in individuals with the CREST syndrome.

Fibrosis of the **lungs,** with exertional dyspnea its most prominent symptom, is associated early with an impairment in gas exchange. Pleurisy and pericarditis with effusion may occur. Pulmonary hypertension may develop as a result of longstanding interstitial and peribronchial fibrosis or intimal hyperplasia of small pulmonary arteries; the latter is associated with the CREST syndrome. **Cardiac** arrhythmias, conduction disturbances, and other ECG abnormalities are common. Cardiac failure may develop and tends to be chronic and to respond poorly to digitalis.

Severe renal disease may develop as a consequence of intimal hyperplasia of interlobular and arcuate arteries and is a major cause of death in PSS. This is usually heralded by the abrupt onset of accelerated or malignant hypertension that, if untreated, is soon followed by rapidly progressive and irreversible renal insufficiency.

Rheumatoid factor tests are positive in ⅓ of PSS patients; serum antinuclear and/or antinucleolar antibodies are present in 90% or more of cases. An antibody that reacts with centromeric protein is found in the serum of a high proportion of patients with the CREST syndrome (anti-centromere antibody).

In MCTD (see in this chapter, below), scleroderma and other evidence of PSS such as Raynaud's phenomenon and esophageal dysfunction occur in association with clinical and serologic features of SLE, polymyositis, and/or RA. Patients with this syndrome have extremely high titers of a serum antibody that reacts with nuclear ribonucleoprotein.

Localized forms of scleroderma occur as circumscribed patches (morphea) or linear sclerosis of the integument and immediately subjacent tissues without systemic involvement; antinuclear antibodies are often found in the latter condition.

Prognosis

The course of PSS is variable and unpredictable. It is often only slowly progressive. Most if not all patients eventually show evidence of visceral involvement. Prognosis is poor if cardiac, pulmonary, or renal manifestations are present at diagnosis. However, the disease may remain limited in extent and nonprogressive for long periods of time in patients with the CREST syndrome; other visceral changes (including pulmonary hypertension due to vascular disease of the lung, and a peculiar form of biliary cirrhosis) eventually develop, but the course of this form of PSS is often remarkably benign.

Treatment

Corticosteroids may be helpful in patients with disabling myositis or MCTD. Recent studies indicate that prolonged administration (1.5+ yr) of D-penicillamine (0.5 to 1.0 gm/day) leads to a reduction in skin thickening and the rate of new visceral involvement. Colchicine and various immunosuppressive agents are also under trial in PSS. Vasodilators may induce temporary and limited improvement in Raynaud's phenomenon, but are often ineffective. Reflux esophagitis is relieved by frequent small feedings, antacids, and cimetidine (300 mg q.i.d.—30 min before meals and at bedtime), and by having the patient sleep with the head of the bed elevated. Esophageal strictures may require periodic dilation; successful correction of gastroesophageal reflux by gastroplasty has been reported. Tetracycline 1 gm/day orally, or another broad-spectrum antibiotic, suppresses intestinal flora and may alleviate symptoms of intestinal malabsorption. Physiotherapy may be helpful in preserving muscle strength but is ineffective in preventing joint contractures.

For kidney disease in PSS, therapy with currently available vasodilators (minoxidil), β-adrenoceptor blockers, and agents inhibiting formation of angiotensin (e.g., captopril) is usually effective in permitting control of hypertension and preventing renal function deterioration. In the past, bilateral nephrectomy was done in an effort to control BP. When treatment is unsuccessful in preventing end-stage renal disease, dialysis and transplantation can be used, although the mortality is still high.

EOSINOPHILIC FASCIITIS (EF)

Diffuse fasciitis with skin swelling and induration, transient eosinophilia, and elevated ESR and IgG. Newly described and of unknown etiology, the syndrome probably represents another variant of autoimmune connective tissue disease. Of the fewer than 100 cases reported in the USA, most have been men in the middle decades of life.

Symptoms and signs: The first signs are induration of the skin and soft tissues, creating a characteristic orange-peel configuration, that is most evident over the anterior (volar) surfaces of the arms and legs. In some, the face and the trunk also may be involved, with changes closely resembling scleroderma. The symptoms usually appear insidiously, with gradual restriction of movement of arms and legs. Strenuous physical activity often precipitates symptoms in those who previously led a sedentary life. Contractures appear, apparently secondary to induration and thickening of the fascia, and are most common in hands, wrists, elbows, and shoulders. Raynaud's phenomenon and systemic involvement, such as pulmonary fibrosis and delayed esophageal motility, usually are absent. Aplastic anemia, thrombocytopenia, Sjögren's syndrome, and cardiac abnormalities have been reported in single cases.

Laboratory studies show an elevated ESR. The serum globulins and blood eosinophils may be increased in concentration; immunofluorescent studies may be positive. Antinuclear antibodies and rheumatoid factor are absent. The **diagnosis** is confirmed by a biopsy of affected skin and fascia deep enough to include adjacent muscle fibers. The dermis may show cellular infiltration. The subdermal fascia is markedly thickened, with collagenous hypertrophy. Marked cellular infiltrates within the fascia include histiocytes, plasma cells, lymphocytes, and in some cases, eosinophils. **Differential diagnosis** includes localized scleroderma or morphea, or the early stages of PSS.

Treatment: Most patients respond to high initial doses of prednisone, 40 to 60 mg/day, with rapid reduction to 5 to 10 mg/day. The long-term outcome is unknown. Some patients experience spontaneous remission. Recurrences have been described in others after 1 or more years of daily prednisone.

POLYMYOSITIS; DERMATOMYOSITIS

*A systemic connective tissue disease characterized by inflammatory and degenerative changes in the muscles—**polymyositis** (and frequently also in the skin—**dermatomyositis**), leading to symmetric weakness and some degree of muscle atrophy, principally of the limb girdles.* Certain clinical findings are shared with progressive systemic sclerosis **(PSS)** or, less frequently, SLE or vasculitis.

Classification of the several types of myositis includes primary idiopathic polymyositis; childhood dermatomyositis (or polymyositis); primary idiopathic dermatomyositis in adults; dermatomyositis (or polymyositis) associated with malignant neoplasms; polymyositis or dermatomyositis associated with various connective tissue disease overlap syndromes, including sclerodermatomyositis and mixed connective tissue disease.

Etiology and Incidence

The etiology is unknown. The disease may be caused by an autoimmune reaction; deposits of IgM, IgG, and the 3rd component of complement have been found in the blood vessel walls of skeletal muscle (with particularly high frequency in childhood dermatomyositis). Recent studies have provided even stronger evidence that a cell-mediated immune reaction to muscle plays a role in pathogenesis. Viruses may participate, since picornavirus-like structures have been found in muscle cells, and tubular inclusions resembling paramyxovirus nucleocapsid have been identified by electron microscopy in myocytes and endothelial cells of vessels in the skin and muscle. The association of a malignant tumor and dermatomyositis suggests that the neoplasm may incite myositis as the result of an autoimmune reaction directed against a common antigen in muscle and tumor.

The disease is not rare; it is less common than SLE or PSS, but more frequent than polyarteritis nodosa. The female:male ratio is 2:1. The disease may appear at any time from infancy through age 80, most commonly from age 40 to 60, or, in children, from age 5 to 15.

Pathology

Microscopic examination of the skin may show epidermal atrophy, basal cell liquefaction and degeneration, vascular dilation, and lymphocytic infiltration of the dermis. Structural changes in affected muscle vary greatly. The most frequent abnormalities consist of necrosis; phagocytosis; regenerative activity reflected by basophilia, large vesicular nuclei, and prominent nucleoli; atrophy and degeneration of both type I and II fibers, especially in a perifascicular distribution; internal migration of nuclei; vacuolation; fiber-size variation; and a lymphocytic infiltrate, often most prominent in a perivascular location. There is an increase in endomysial and later perimysial connective tissue. In childhood dermatomyositis there may be widespread ulceration and infarction in the GI tract related to necrotizing arteritis. There is intimal proliferation and thrombosis of small arteries and veins.

Symptoms and Signs

Onset may be acute or insidious. An acute infection may precede or incite the initial symptoms, which consist of proximal muscle weakness, polymyalgia, rash, polyarthralgias, Raynaud's phenomenon, dysphagia, and constitutional complaints, most notably fever and weight loss. The **muscle weakness** may appear suddenly and progress over weeks to months. The patient may have difficulty raising the arms above the shoulders, climbing steps, or arising from a sitting position, and may be unable to raise the head from the pillow after lying down. Patients may become wheelchair- or bedridden because of weakness of pelvic and shoulder girdle muscle groups. The flexors of the neck may be severely affected. Weakness of the laryngeal musculature is responsible for dysphonia. Involvement of the striated muscle of the pharynx and upper portion of the esophagus leads to dysphagia and regurgitation. A diminution in peristaltic activity and dilatation of the lower esophagus and small intestine may be indistinguishable from that found in PSS. (It may be argued that the diagnosis in patients with such GI changes who are described as having minimal or mild scleroderma may in fact be PSS with CREST syndrome—see above.) The muscles of the hands, feet, and face escape involvement. Contractures of limbs may develop late in the chronic stage.

The **cutaneous eruption,** which tends to be dusky and erythematous, may have an SLE-like butterfly distribution on the face. Periorbital edema with a heliotrope hue is pathognomonic. The skin rash may be slightly elevated and smooth or scaly, and may appear on the forehead, V of the neck and shoulders, chest and back, forearms and lower legs, elbows and knees, medial malleoli, and dorsum of the proximal interphalangeal and metacarpophalangeal joints. The base and sides of the fingernails may be hyperemic. The skin lesions frequently fade completely but may be followed by brownish pigmentation, atrophy, scarring, or vitiligo. Muscular pain, tenderness, and induration tend to be associated with the rash. The skin changes suggest scleroderma in a few patients. Subcutaneous calcification may occur, particularly in childhood dermatomyositis; this is similar in distribution to that encountered in PSS, but tends to be more extensive **(calcinosis universalis),** particularly in untreated or undertreated disease.

Polyarthralgia, accompanied at times by swelling, joint effusions, and other evidence of nondeforming arthritis, occurs in approximately 1/3 of patients. These rheumatic complaints tend to be mild and respond well to corticosteroids. Raynaud's phenomenon occurs, with particularly high frequency in those patients in whom polymyositis coexists with other connective tissue disorders.

Visceral involvement (with the exception of the pharynx and esophagus) is relatively uncommon in polymyositis compared to the high frequency of internal changes in other connective tissue diseases, such as SLE and PSS. Interstitial pneumonitis (manifested by dyspnea and cough) occurs and may precede myositis and dominate the clinical picture. Cardiac involvement, detected chiefly in the ECG (arrhythmias, conduction disturbances abnormal systolic time intervals), has been reported with increasing frequency. Acute renal failure as a consequence of severe rhabdomyolysis with myoglobinuria (crush syndrome) has been reported. Sjögren's syndrome occurs in some patients. Abdominal symptoms, commoner in children, may be associated with hematemesis or melena from GI ulcerations that may progress to perforation and require surgical intervention.

An associated malignancy, usually a carcinoma, occurs in approximately 15% of men (and a smaller proportion of women) over age 50. There is no characteristic type or site.

Laboratory Findings

Laboratory studies are helpful but nonspecific. The ESR is elevated. Antinuclear antibodies and LE cells are found in a few patients, most often those with evidence of other connective tissue disease. The muscle enzymes, especially the transaminases, creatine phosphokinase (CPK), and aldolase, usually show elevated serum levels; of these, the most sensitive and useful is CPK. Periodic enzyme determinations are helpful in monitoring treatment: elevated levels decrease with effective therapy. However, these enzymes may be normal despite active disease in patients with chronic myositis and widespread muscle atrophy.

Increased titers of antibodies to *Toxoplasma gondii* are significantly frequent and suggest that polymyositis may in some cases be associated with recent active toxoplasma infection.

Diagnosis

Five major criteria are useful in diagnosing polymyositis/dermatomyositis: proximal muscle weakness; a characteristic skin rash; elevated muscle enzymes in the serum; a characteristic triad of electromyographic abnormalities; muscle biopsy changes. Electromyography usually shows (1) spontaneous fibrillations and positive sharp potentials, with increased insertional irritability; (2) polyphasic short potentials during voluntary contraction; and (3) bizarre, repetitive, high-frequency discharges during mechanical stimulation. The preferred sites for muscle biopsy are the muscles that show electrical abnormalities, usually the deltoid and quadriceps femoris, but on the opposite extremities in order to avoid sites previously explored.

Any affected adult should be studied for a possible malignancy.

Prognosis

This is better in children than in adults, but is critical in those with an associated malignancy. Relatively satisfactory and long remissions, even apparent recovery, have been reported, especially in children. Death in adults follows severe and progressive muscle weakness, dysphagia, malnutrition, aspiration pneumonia, or respiratory failure with superimposed pulmonary infection. Polymyositis tends to be more severe and resistant to treatment in those individuals with evidence of cardiac involvement. Death in children usually is a result of vasculitis of the bowel.

Treatment

Corticosteroids are widely accepted as the drugs of choice in the initial treatment of polymyositis/dermatomyositis. For acute disease, prednisone is given in divided doses of 40 to 60 mg or more/day, together with antacids and potassium supplements. Serial measurements of muscle enzyme activity in serum provide the best guide of the effectiveness of therapy. Reduction of these enzymes toward or to normal values is noted in a majority of patients in 4 to 6 wk. This is followed by an improvement in muscle strength. Once the enzyme levels have returned to normal, the dose of prednisone is reduced slowly; if muscle enzymes rise, the dose is increased. In most cases of adult polymyositis, prolonged maintenance therapy with prednisone (10 to 15 mg/day) is necessary indefinitely. In childhood dermatomyositis, it may be possible to discontinue prednisone after a year or more, with apparent remission. Immunosuppressive agents, including methotrexate, cyclophosphamide, chlorambucil, and azathioprine have been beneficial in patients who fail to respond to corticosteroids alone. Some patients have received methotrexate for 5 yr or longer for the control of this disease.

POLYMYALGIA RHEUMATICA

(See also TEMPORAL ARTERITIS in Ch. 28)

Pain and stiffness in proximal muscle groups without permanent weakness or atrophy. The syndrome is well defined and relatively common, occurring in those > 50 yr. The female-to-male ratio is 4:1. Pathogenesis is unknown.

Symptoms and Signs

Onset may be sudden or gradual; pain and stiffness may appear symmetrically in the neck, back, or shoulder or pelvic girdle muscles. Morning stiffness is marked, with some patients finding it difficult to get out of bed. Fever, anorexia, malaise, weight loss, and apathy may be present. In spite of the severe pain, examination of the muscles is essentially negative. A markedly high ESR with values over 100 mm/h may be diagnostic. A nonhemolytic anemia with Hct as low as 30% may be present.

Diagnosis

Differentiation from RA is made by the absence of demonstrable synovitis on physical examination, and by a negative RF; from an adenosine diphosphate disorder, by muscle biopsy and normal enzyme levels; from osteoarthritis, by the rapid ESR; and from multiple myeloma, by a normal protein electrophoresis and bone marrow. A number of patients have an associated **temporal arteritis.** *Irreversible blindness with headache may develop rapidly.* Joint scintigrams with ⁹⁹ᵐtechnetium as pertechnetate have shown evidence of synovitis. Biopsy of an asymptomatic temporal artery may show the typical changes of giant cell arteritis.

Treatment

The disease responds so well to corticosteroids that a therapeutic trial also has diagnostic value. Treatment should be started immediately on diagnosis, with prednisone 30 mg/day orally, which is reduced promptly as symptoms subside. Prednisone at 5 to 10 mg/day should be continued as long as symptoms persist; in some, this may be required for many months. Salicylates, indomethacin, gold, and other nonsteroidal anti-inflammatory drugs have been used in patients without temporal arteritis, but if that disease is probable, doses of prednisone, at least 60 mg/day for 1 mo or longer, should be taken while under joint supervision with an ophthalmologist.

POLYARTERITIS

(Polyarteritis Nodosa; Periarteritis Nodosa)

A disease characterized by segmental inflammation and necrosis of medium-sized muscular arteries, with secondary ischemia of the tissue supplied by the affected vessels.

Etiology and Incidence

Though polyarteritis has been ascribed to a hypersensitivity reaction, the cause has not been definitely established; the variety of clinical and pathologic features of the disease suggests multiple pathogenic mechanisms. Arterial lesions like those found in spontaneously occurring polyarteritis are seen in hyperimmunized human volunteers, in animals with experimental serum sickness, and in patients developing allergic reactions. Drugs (e.g., sulfonamides, penicillin, iodide, thiouracil, bismuth, thiazides, guanethidine, methamphetamine) and vaccines, bacterial infections (e.g., with streptococci or staphylococci), and viral infections (e.g., serum hepatitis, influenza) have been associated with onset of the disease. In a majority of patients, however, no predisposing antigen can be incriminated.

Onset usually is between ages 40 and 50, but has been reported in patients of every age group. The disease is 3 times commoner in men than in women.

Pathology

Segmental, necrotizing inflammation of media and adventitia characterizes the lesion. The pathologic process most commonly occurs at points of vessel bifurcation, beginning in the media and extending into the intima and adventitia of medium-sized arteries, often disrupting the internal elastic lamellae. Lesions can usually be seen in all stages of development and healing. Early lesions contain polymorphonuclear leukocytes and occasionally eosinophils; later lesions contain lymphocytes and plasma cells. Immunoglobulin, complement components, and fibrinogen are deposited in the lesions, although their significance is unclear. Intimal proliferation with secondary thrombosis and occlusion leads to organ and tissue infarction. Weakening of the muscular vessel wall may cause small aneurysms and arterial dissection. Healing can result in nodular fibrosis of the adventitia. Renal, hepatic, cardiac, and GI involvement are most frequent, though any organ may be involved. Renal lesions are of 2 distinct types: large-vessel (in which the renal lesion is a tubular infarction, and renal failure is uncommon) and microvascular, including the glomerular afferent arterioles (in which the lesion is diffuse, and renal failure is common and occurs early in the course). Half of all patients with massive hepatic infarction have polyarteritis.

Several syndromes associated with polyarteritis have been separated from typical polyarteritis nodosa on the basis of pathogenic or clinical differences: hypersensitivity angiitis; Cogan's syndrome (where the disease begins as interstitial keratitis and inner ear infarction); pure mesenteric polyarteritis (recognized in IV methamphetamine addicts); Kawasaki's disease (mucocutaneous lymph node syndrome in infants and children complicated by coronary arteritis); and necrotizing arteritis associated with hepatitis B infection (either acute hepatitis or chronic active liver disease). The interrelationships of polyarteritis nodosa and these various forms of arteritis are unclear.

Symptoms and Signs

Polyarteritis manifestations are protean; many other diseases may be mimicked. The course may be that of an acute and prolonged febrile illness, or may be subacute with fatal termination after several months; or it may be insidious and present as a chronic debilitating disease. Symptoms are determined largely by the location and severity of the arteritis and by the extent of secondary circulatory impairment, and may be referable to virtually any organ system or combination thereof.

The most common initial complaints are fever (85%), abdominal pain (65%), symptoms related to peripheral neuropathy, often a mononeuritis multiplex (50%), weakness (45%), weight loss (45%), and asthma (20%). Hypertension (60%), edema (50%), and oliguria and uremia (15%) may be present in the 75% of patients with renal involvement; proteinemia and hematuria are early manifestations. Diffuse or localized abdominal pain, nausea, vomiting, and bloody diarrhea may lead to a mistaken diagnosis of an acute surgical abdomen. Acute ischemia of the gallbladder or intestines may lead to perforation with secondary peritonitis. Hemorrhage from the GI tract or into the retroperitoneal space may also occur. Precordial pain occurs in 25% of patients, though ECG evidence indicates coronary disease in 45%. CNS disease produces headache (30%), convulsions (10%), and organic psychosis. Myalgias and arthralgias are common, but frank arthritis is rare. Dermal lesions, including subcutaneous nodules and irregular areas of skin necrosis, are seen in 20% of patients.

Laboratory Findings

Leukocytosis of 20,000 to 40,000 (80% of patients), proteinuria (60%), and microscopic hematuria (40%) are the most frequent abnormalities. Eosinophilia, either transient or permanent, is unusual but may be present in patients with an extended clinical course or with pulmonary involvement or asthmatic attacks. Thrombocytosis, an elevated ESR, and anemia due to blood loss or renal failure are usual. Hypoalbuminemia and elevated serum immunoglobulins are frequently found, but autoantibodies, though often encountered in other collagen vascular diseases, are rarely present.

Diagnosis

Polyarteritis should be considered as a possible diagnosis when unexplained fever, abdominal pain, renal failure, or hypertension is present, or when a case simulating nephritis or a cardiac disorder is accompanied by eosinophilia or by unexplained symptoms such as arthralgia, muscle tenderness or weakness, subcutaneous nodules, purpuric skin rashes, pain in the abdomen or extremities, or rapidly developing hypertension. The diagnosis is usually suggested by a confusing combination of clinical and laboratory features, especially when other causes of a febrile, multisystem illness have been excluded. A systemic illness associated with peripheral, usually multiple, neuritis involving major nerve trunks (e.g., radial, peroneal, sciatic) in a bilaterally asymmetric or symmetric fashion **(mononeuritis multiplex)** is also highly suggestive of polyarteritis. Any of the above clinical profiles become particularly suggestive of polyarteritis nodosa when seen in a previously healthy middle-aged male.

Since there are no specific serologic tests for polyarteritis, definite diagnosis depends on demonstration of necrotizing arteritis by **biopsy of typical lesions.** Biopsies of skin, subcutaneous tissue, sural nerve and/or muscle should be obtained when clinically involved by an acute inflammatory reaction. Biopsy may be negative, however, because of the focal nature of the disease. Electromyography and nerve conduction studies may be helpful in selecting the site of muscle or nerve biopsy in the absence of clinical findings. The gastrocnemius muscle should *not* be biopsied unless it is the only symptomatic muscle, because of the risk of postoperative venous thrombosis. Testicular biopsy has been advocated because of the frequency of microscopic lesions at this site, but should be *avoided* if there are other accessible sites of suspected involvement. Renal biopsy in patients with evidence of nephritis and liver biopsy in patients with grossly abnormal liver function tests may be appropriate if other sites fail to provide diagnostic material. Blind biopsy of clinically uninvolved tissue is, however, usually futile. Selective angiography may demonstrate small aneurysms in the renal, hepatic, and celiac vessels, and may be considered diagnostic, even in the absence of a firm tissue diagnosis. A diagnosis of polyarteritis nodosa is hardly credible without a clear demonstration of the tissue lesion or angiographic display of the typical aneurysms on medium-sized vessels.

Prognosis

Whether acute or chronic, the untreated disease is usually fatal, often terminating in failure of the heart, kidneys, or other vital organs, or in GI catastrophes or ruptured aneurysm. Without therapy, only 1/3 of patients survive for 1 yr; 88% are dead within 5 yr. Glomerulonephritis with renal failure occasionally responds to therapy, but anuria and hypertension are ominous findings; renal failure is the cause of death in 65% of patients.

Treatment

Therapy must be vigorous and many-faceted. The offending antigen, including drugs, must be sought and avoided. **Corticosteroids** in high dosage (e.g., prednisone 60 mg/day in divided doses) may prevent progression of the disease and appear to induce a partial or near-complete remission in about 30% of patients. Because long-term therapy is necessary, corticosteroid side effects, including hypertension and hypercalciuria (which may accelerate preexisting renal damage), often intervene, and the already present serious risk of supervening infection is enhanced. (See the discussion of corticosteroids in Ch. 251.) Efforts should be made to reduce the daily dose commensurate with evidence of improvement, e.g., reduction of fever, fall in ESR, improvement in cardiac and renal function, improvement in nerve conduction velocity, disappearance of cutaneous lesions, and lessening of pain. Some of the manifestations of long-term hyperadrenocorticism can be minimized by eventually giving corticosteroids in a single morning dose every other day. Though such a regimen may be adequate as maintenance therapy, it is rarely successful in the early stages of treatment.

Immunosuppressive drugs, either alone or initially with corticosteroids, are widely used empirically with some success when corticosteroids alone are inadequate. Cyclophosphamide 2 to 3 mg/kg body weight may be given to patients who do not respond to corticosteroids during the first few weeks of therapy or for whom prohibitively high doses of corticosteroids appear to be necessary to maintain disease control (by these criteria, the majority of patients would qualify). The drug dose should be adjusted to maintain the peripheral blood white cell count between 2,000 and 3500/cu mm. The physician must be aware of the additional risks these drugs impose. Patients must be carefully observed for signs of microbial infections, which must be promptly treated.

Antihypertensive therapy, careful fluid management, attention to renal impairment, digitalization, and other measures based on specific problems are also important. Surgical intervention is required if GI involvement leads to intussusception or mesenteric artery thrombosis and bowel or viscous infarction.

WEGENER'S GRANULOMATOSIS

An uncommon disease that begins as a localized granulomatous inflammation of upper and lower respiratory tract mucosa and usually progresses into generalized necrotizing granulomatous vasculitis and glomerulonephritis.

Etiology and Incidence

The etiology is unknown. Though the disease resembles an infectious process, no causative agent has been isolated. Because of the characteristic histologic tissue changes, hypersensitivity has been postulated as the basis for the disease. Men are affected about twice as often as women. Disease can occur at any age.

Pathology

Biopsy of the inflamed and granular material in the nose and nasopharynx discloses granulomatous tissue containing epithelioid cells, Langhans' cells, and foreign-body giant cells. Pulmonary and skin biopsies show inflammatory perivascular exudate and fibrin deposition in small arteries, capillaries, and venules. Renal biopsy shows a focal and segmental glomerulonephritis of varying degrees of severity, occasionally with necrotizing vasculitis. Immunohistochemical studies of the kidney biopsy show extensive deposits of fibrin within blood vessels and glomeruli. Fibrin deposition in glomeruli suggests a partial activation of a clotting factor (Hageman factor). Immune complexes precipitated by C1q have been found and shown to disappear on therapy with cyclophosphamide and prednisone. Dense subepithelial deposits of material suggestive of immune complex are detectable by electron microscopy on the epithelial side of the basement membrane. Immunofluorescence has shown scattered deposits of complement and IgG in some cases.

Symptoms, Signs, and Laboratory Findings

Onset may be insidious or acute. Presenting complaints are usually referable to the upper respiratory tract and include severe rhinorrhea, paranasal sinusitis, nasal mucosal ulcerations (with consequent secondary bacterial infection), serous or purulent otitis media with hearing loss, cough, hemoptysis, and pleuritis. The patient usually presents with a granulomatous process of the nose often mistaken for chronic sinusitis. The nasal mucous membrane has a red, raised granular appearance and is friable and bleeds easily. Other initial symptoms include fever, malaise, anorexia, weight loss, migratory polyarthropathy, skin lesions, and ocular manifestations with nasolacrimal duct obstruction and proptosis. Chondritis of the ear, myocardial infarction caused by the vasculitis of this disease, and aseptic meningitis and nonhealing granuloma of the CNS may occur.

After a few weeks or months, a disseminated vascular phase characteristically develops and is associated with necrotizing inflammatory skin lesions, pulmonary lesions with cavitation, diffuse vasculitis, and focal glomerulitis that may progress to generalized glomerulonephritis with subsequent hypertension and uremia. Renal disease is the hallmark of generalized disease; urinalysis shows proteinuria, hematuria, and RBC casts. Functional renal impairment is inevitable without immediate appropriate therapy. Occasionally, the disease is limited to pulmonary involvement.

Serum complement levels are normal or elevated. The ESR is elevated. Leukocytosis is present. Antinuclear antibodies and LE cells are not found.

Diagnosis

Diagnosis is established by the characteristic clinical and pathologic findings. Renal biopsy is important in diagnosis, in determining the extent of renal involvement, and in early detection of renal dissemination. Clusters of densely packed atypical cells may be found in the sputum of patients with pulmonary involvement. Differential diagnosis includes polyarteritis, the vascular renal phase of SBE, rapidly or slowly progressive glomerulonephritis, SLE, and midline malignant reticulosis. RA may be simulated for as long as a year before diagnosis becomes apparent. Polyarteritis is ruled out by biopsy of the skin lesions and by different pathologic localization of the vascular lesions. Eosinophilia, not a feature of Wegener's granulomatosis, is often present in polyarteritis; nasal and pulmonary granulomatous inflammation is absent. Characteristic blood cultures and changing cardiac murmurs are present in SBE. In SLE, antinuclear antibodies and LE cells are present in the serum, and the serum complement level is depressed. Vasculitic granulomatous inflammation is absent in midline malignant reticulosis.

Course, Prognosis, and Treatment

The complete syndrome usually progresses rapidly to renal failure once the diffuse vascular phase begins. Patients with the limited form of the disease may have only nasal and pulmonary lesions with little or no systemic involvement. Pulmonary manifestations may improve or may worsen spontaneously.

Early diagnosis and **treatment** are important in view of the potential success of chemotherapy with cytotoxic drugs. The prognosis for this once uniformly fatal disease has been improved by treatment with immunosuppressive cytotoxic agents. Cyclophosphamide (1 to 2 mg/kg/day) is the drug of choice, though azathioprine (2 mg/kg/day) and chlorambucil (0.1 to 0.15 mg/kg/day) have also been used. Duration of therapy depends on the patient's clinical response. Leukocyte counts are monitored. Dosages are reduced gradually to the lowest effective one to prevent severe leukopenia. Attempts should be made to discontinue therapy if disease activity has been absent for 1 yr. Renal disease relapse is carefully sought when tapering the dosage or discontinuing the drug. Long-term, complete remissions can be achieved with therapy, even with advanced disease. Kidney transplantation has been successful for renal failure. Corticosteroids can be used intermittently for nonrenal symptoms in conjunction with the above agents.

MIXED CONNECTIVE TISSUE DISEASE (MCTD)

A rheumatic disease syndrome characterized by overlapping clinical features similar to those of systemic lupus erythematosus (SLE), scleroderma, and polymyositis, and by very high titers of circulating antinuclear antibody to a nuclear ribonucleoprotein (RNP) antigen.

Etiology, Pathogenesis, and Prevalence

The etiology is unknown, but certain findings suggest that immune injury may be involved in the pathogenesis: (1) marked hypergammaglobulinemia; (2) persistence of extremely high titers of RNP antibody; (3) mild to moderate hypocomplementemia in 25%; (4) circulating immune complexes during active disease; (5) specific deposition of IgG, IgM, or complement within the walls of blood vessels or muscle fibers and along the glomerular basement membrane; (6) recent reports that RNP antibodies may penetrate live human mononuclear cells through Fc receptors, and that suppressor T cell function may be abnormal in active disease; and (7) chronic inflammatory infiltration by lymphocytes and plasma cells in various tissues.

Recent findings that HLA-D–related antigen DRw1 and B lymphocyte antigen(s) recognized by serum Ia 505 are increased in MCTD support the hypothesis that it is a unique disease syndrome with a genetic background different from that of normal individuals and of patients with SLE. Generally lower levels of circulating immune complexes, infrequency of high levels of antibodies to native DNA, infrequency of progressive glomerulonephritis, and usually normal reticuloendothelial system Fc receptor clearance of circulating immune complexes further distinguish MCTD from SLE.

Prevalence is unknown; MCTD appears to be seen more commonly than polymyositis and less frequently than SLE. Approximately 80% of patients are female. The age range in published series is from 5 to 80 yr with a mean of 37 yr.

Symptoms, Signs, and Pathology

The **typical clinical syndrome** is characterized by Raynaud's phenomenon, polyarthralgia or arthritis, swollen hands, inflammatory proximal myopathy, esophageal hypomotility, and pulmonary disease. Raynaud's phenomenon may precede other disease manifestations by years, and frequently the initial findings suggest early SLE, scleroderma, polymyositis, or RA. Whatever the initial presentation, there is a tendency for more limited disease to progress and become more widespread and for transitions in the clinical pattern to occur over time.

The most frequent **skin finding** is swelling of the hands resulting in a sausage appearance of the fingers. Diffuse scleroderma-like changes and ischemic necrosis or ulceration of the fingertips, common in scleroderma, are much less frequent in MCTD. Other skin findings include lupus-like rashes, erythematous patches over the knuckles, violaceous discoloration of the eyelids, diffuse nonscarring alopecia, and squared telangiectasia over the hands and face.

Almost all patients have **polyarthralgias**, and ³/₄ have frank **arthritis**. Often the arthritis is nondeforming, but erosive changes and deformities may be present, suggesting RA. **Proximal muscle weakness** with or without tenderness is common. Electromyograms are typical of **inflammatory myopathy**, and muscle biopsies show degeneration of muscle fibers and interstitial and perivascular infiltrates of lymphocytes and plasma cells.

Esophageal abnormalities including decreased lower sphincter pressure, decreased amplitude of peristalsis in the distal ²/₃, and a decrease in upper sphincter pressure occur in 80%, including 70% of asymptomatic patients. **Pulmonary involvement** also occurs in about 80%, and significant abnormalities of diffusing capacity may develop before the disease is clinically apparent. Chest x-rays may show pleuritis and/or diffuse interstitial infiltrates. In some patients, pulmonary involvement becomes the predominant clinical problem, leading to exertional dyspnea and/or pulmonary hypertension. Lung biopsies have revealed interstitial mononuclear infiltrates, fibrosis, and vascular intimal proliferation and medial hypertrophy severe enough in some cases to cause vascular obliteration.

Pericarditis is the most frequent cardiac finding. **Myocarditis** may also be present, leading to congestive heart failure; aortic insufficiency is a less frequent finding. **Renal disease** occurs in only about 10% of patients and often is rather mild. However, kidney involvement occasionally becomes a major clinical problem, and patients have died with progressive renal failure. Renal biopsies usually show mesangial hypercellularity, focal glomerulitis, and membranous glomerulonephritis, while membranoproliferative glomerulonephritis and proliferative vascular lesions are much less frequently seen. Serious **neurologic abnormalities** including organic mental syndrome, aseptic meningitis, seizures, multiple peripheral neuropathies, and cerebral infarction or hemorrhage occur in only about 10% of patients. A trigeminal sensory neuropathy appears to be seen much more frequently in MCTD than in other rheumatic diseases.

Other findings which may be present in patients with MCTD include Sjögren's syndrome, Hashimoto's thyroiditis, fever, lymphadenopathy (often of massive proportions), splenomegaly, hepatomegaly, intestinal involvement similar to that seen in scleroderma, and persistent hoarseness.

Laboratory Findings

Almost all patients with MCTD have high titers (often > 1:1000) of fluorescent antinuclear antibodies **(ANA),** which produce a speckled pattern. Antibodies to extractable nuclear antigen **(ENA)** are usually detected at very high titers (> 1:100,000) by hemagglutination. The ANA and hemagglutination reactions are typically eliminated by digestion with ribonuclease **(RNase),** since the ENA component to which antibodies are directed in MCTD is an RNase-sensitive nuclear ribonucleoprotein **(RNP)** antigen. By immunodiffusion it can be confirmed that antibody to RNP is present, while antibody to the RNase-resistant Sm component of ENA is usually absent.

Antibodies to native DNA and LE cells are infrequent in MCTD. Rheumatoid agglutinins are frequently positive and titers are often high. The ESR is frequently elevated, and 75% of patients have diffuse hypergammaglobulinemia often ranging from 2 to 5 gm/dl. Levels of serum complement are slightly to moderately reduced in only about 25% of patients. Serum levels of creatinine phosphokinase and aldolase are usually elevated when active myositis is present.

Moderate anemia and leukopenia occur in 30 to 40% of patients with MCTD. Clinically significant Coombs-positive hemolytic anemia and thrombocytopenia are uncommon. However, in one report of childhood MCTD severe thrombocytopenia was more common, and 2 children required splenectomy because they were only partially responsive to corticosteroids. Hematuria, casts, and proteinuria are detected on urinalysis when glomerulonephritis occurs.

Diagnosis

MCTD should be considered when additional overlapping features are present in patients appearing to have SLE, scleroderma, polymyositis, RA, juvenile RA, Sjögren's syndrome, vasculitis, idiopathic thrombocytopenic purpura, lymphoma, or "viral pericarditis." MCTD may occasionally present as a fever of unknown origin. Since the characteristic serologic finding of high titers of antibody to RNP only is much more frequently associated with MCTD than with other rheumatic diseases, detection of RNP antibody permits a presumptive diagnosis early in the evolution of the disease when clinical manifestations are limited. If RNP antibody is detected at a high titer, a thorough evaluation of the muscle, esophageal, and pulmonary systems (especially diffusing capacity) will frequently reveal abnormalities even when the patients are asymptomatic with respect to these systems.

Prognosis

In a recent report of over 300 patients with MCTD whose mean duration of disease was 7 yr, only 7% had died, suggesting a rather good prognosis. Causes of death have included pulmonary disease, renal failure, myocardial infarction, colonic perforation, disseminated infection, and cerebral hemorrhage. Sustained remissions for several years on little or no maintenance corticosteroid therapy have now been observed in some patients. However, pulmonary hypertension and proliferative vascular lesions, which usually develop insidiously, represent serious complications for some. Recent studies using in vivo widefield nailfold microscopy have revealed severe capillary abnormalities characteristic of scleroderma in patients who subsequently developed pulmonary hypertension.

Treatment

General medical management and drug therapy in MCTD are similar to the approach used in SLE. Most patients are responsive to corticosteroids, particularly if treated early in the course of the disease. Mild disease is often controlled by salicylates, nonsteroidal anti-inflammatory drugs, antimalarials, or very low doses of corticosteroids. Severe major organ involvement usually requires larger doses of corticosteroids, an initial dose of 1 mg/kg of prednisone often being used. Even in patients whose disease is very progressive and widespread, more prolonged high-dose corticosteroid therapy, sometimes in combination with cytotoxic drugs, may be associated with clinical improvement. However, with disease of longer duration resulting in greater functional impairment, the response may not be so complete, and drug toxicity may contribute to serious and sometimes fatal complications. In general the scleroderma-like features of MCTD are the least likely to respond to treatment.

---

105. BURSITIS

Acute or chronic inflammation of a bursa. Bursae are found where tendons pass over bony prominences. If destroyed, they re-form when motion is regained. Deep bursae may communicate with joints. Most bursitis occurs in the shoulder (subacromial bursitis, supraspinatus tendinitis, and bicipital tendinitis), but other common forms exist: olecranon (miner's elbow), pre- or suprapatellar (housemaid's knee), retrocalcaneal (Achilles), iliopectineal (iliopsoas), ischial (tailor's or weaver's bottom), trochanteric, and first metatarsal head (bunion). The **etiology** of most bursitis is unknown, though it may be caused by trauma, acute or chronic infection, inflammatory arthritis, gout, or RA. It is rarely caused by pyogenic or tuberculous organisms.

Symptoms and Signs

Subacromial bursitis presents with localized pain and tenderness and with immobility in all ranges but particularly in rotation. It is differentiated from **supraspinatus tendinitis,** in which rotation usually is normal, with a painful abduction arc at 40°, and from **bicipital tendinitis,** in which the tenderness is over the bicipital groove of the humerus and the local pain is aggravated by resisted flexion of the elbow joint. Bursitis may be acute or chronic.

Acute bursitis is characterized by pain, localized tenderness, and limitation of motion. The bursal wall secretes a serous effusion when inflamed. Swelling and redness are frequently present if the bursa is superficial (e.g., prepatellar, olecranon).

Chronic bursitis may follow previous attacks of bursitis or repeated trauma or foci of infection. Acute symptoms may develop following unusual exercise or effort. The bursal wall is thickened, with degeneration of the endothelial lining. The bursa eventually may develop adhesions, villi formation, tags, calcareous deposits, and conspicuous muscle atrophy. Pain, swelling, tenderness, muscle weakness, and limitation of motion vary. Subdeltoid calcific deposits may be demonstrated radiographically. Attacks may last from a few days to several weeks, with multiple recurrences. In gout, crystal deposits are present in the olecranon and prepatellar bursae.

Diagnosis

Periarticular tendons or muscle tears, osteomyelitis, TB, and cellulitis must be ruled out. Pathologic processes may simultaneously involve a communicating bursa and joint.

Treatment

For acute bursitis, high doses of nonsteroidal anti-inflammatory agents (e.g., indomethacin, ibuprofen, or naproxen) accompanied by analgesics may be helpful. If not, intrabursal injection of hydrocortisone 20 to 40 mg following infiltration with 1% procaine is the treatment of choice. Phenylbutazone (300 mg for 2 to 3 days, followed by 100 mg for 10 days) is also effective. Systemic corticosteroids (prednisone 15 to 30 mg/day or equivalent for 3 days) have been used. Rest and splinting are only moderately effective. Early active movement inhibits development of limiting adhesions; voluntary movement should be increased as pain subsides. Pendulum exercises are particularly helpful for the shoulder joint.

Chronic bursitis is treated as for acute bursitis, except that splinting and rest are even less likely to be helpful. Surgical removal or large-needle aspiration of radiologically demonstrated calcium may be necessary if corticosteroid injections are not helpful. Disabling adhesions may require physical therapy. Manipulation under anesthesia does not improve the long-term results. Muscle atrophy should be corrected by exercises.

106. TENDINITIS AND TENOSYNOVITIS

Inflammation of the lining of the tendon sheath (tenosynovitis) and of the enclosed tendon (tendinitis) usually occur simultaneously. The synovial-lined tendon sheath usually is the site of maximum inflammation, but the inflammatory response may involve the enclosed tendon (e.g., as a result of a calcium deposit).

Etiology

The etiology is unknown. The tendon sheaths may be involved in systemic diseases (most commonly RA, progressive systemic sclerosis, gout, Reiter's syndrome, and amyloidosis) and when blood cholesterol levels are elevated (hyperlipoproteinemia, Type II). Extreme or repeated trauma, strain, or excessive (unaccustomed) exercise may also be causative. The most common sites of inflammation are the shoulder capsule and associated tendons, flexor carpi ulnaris, flexor digitorum, hip capsule and associated tendons, hamstrings, and Achilles tendons.

Symptoms and Signs

The involved tendon sheaths may be visibly swollen because of fluid accumulation and inflammation, or may remain dry but irregularly contoured, causing friction rubs felt on movement of the tendon in its sheath or heard with a stethoscope. Localized tenderness of variable severity is present; it may be severe and associated with disabling pain on movement. Calcium deposition in the tendon and its sheath may be seen by x-ray as calcific tendinitis.

Treatment

Symptomatic relief is provided by rest of the part, application of heat or cold (whichever benefits the patient), analgesic agents locally, and nonsteroidal anti-inflammatory agents systemically, locally, or both. Anti-inflammatory drugs consist of full doses of aspirin (650 mg [10 grains] 10 to 15 times/day), or indomethacin (25 mg 4 or 5 times/day) or phenylbutazone (100 mg t.i.d.). Colchicine may be helpful (see GOUT in Ch. 103 for dosage regimens) if urate deposits are responsible. Controlled exercise several times daily (becoming progressively more vigorous with tolerance) is indicated, especially to prevent "frozen shoulder."

Injection into the tendon and tendon sheath of a corticosteroid such as prednisolone or hydrocortisone, 10 to 30 mg depending on severity and site, may be helpful. Following infiltration with 1% procaine or lidocaine, a 25-gauge needle with bevel down is thrust into the tendon substance with moderate pressure on the plunger. The needle is withdrawn slowly with pressure maintained; as it reaches the space between tendon and sheath, resistance is suddenly released, whereupon the tendon sheath will be evident and felt to balloon as the injectate enters the synovial space. The injection is made blindly at the site of maximum tenderness if the specific inflammation site cannot be identified. Reexamination of a less inflamed site 3 or 4 days later often discloses the specific lesion, and a second injection can be made with greater precision.

Injections and symptomatic therapy may be required every 2 or 3 wk for 1 or 2 mo for complete resolution. Surgical exploration and removal of inflamed or calcific deposits, followed by graded physical therapy, usually is curative in persistent cases.

TENNIS ELBOW
(Lateral Humeral Epicondylitis)

A strain of the lateral forearm muscles (extensor wad) near their origin on the lateral epicondyle of the humerus. It is caused by repetitive strenuous supination of the wrist against resistance, as in manual screwdriving, or by violent extension of the wrist with the hand pronated, as in tennis. It can be disabling. The disorder must be differentiated from that involving the radiohumeral joint.

Symptoms and Signs

Pain over the lateral epicondyle of the humerus may be severe and radiate to the outer side of the arm and forearm. It is aggravated by dorsiflexion and supination of the wrist against resistance. Point tenderness is present just distal to the lateral epicondyle. Weakness of the dorsiflexed wrist may be pronounced. X-rays are negative. Infiltrating the area around the lateral epicondyle with 1 to 2 ml of 1% procaine relieves symptoms and signs and establishes the diagnosis in doubtful cases.

Treatment

In mild cases, avoiding the pain-producing movement results in gradual improvement. A 4-inch strap worn tightly around the forearm just distal to the elbow transfers the origin of the affected muscles and splints the sprained area, relieving symptoms in 1 to 3 wk. To prevent recurrences, the strap should be worn during the aggravating activity. Hydrocortisone 20 to 40 mg may be injected into the tender soft tissues following infiltration of 1 to 2 ml of 1% procaine, if strapping is unsuccessful. Surgical release of part of the origin of the extensor muscles from the lateral epicondyle is indicated and usually successful if symptoms repeatedly recur or are not alleviated after 3 or 4 injections.

DUPUYTREN'S CONTRACTURE

Contracture of the palmar fascia due to fibrous proliferation, resulting in flexion deformities and loss of function of the fingers.

Etiology and Incidence

The etiology is unknown. The familial incidence is > 50%; men are more often affected than women. The incidence increases progressively after age 40 and is higher in chronic invalids, alcoholics, epileptics, and patients with pulmonary TB and diabetes mellitus. It may appear as a late sequel to the shoulder-hand syndrome following myocardial infarction. Usually it appears spontaneously and without any associated condition, except for liver disease, alcoholism, etc.

Symptoms, Signs, and Diagnosis

One or both hands may be affected; the right hand is more frequently affected when involvement is unilateral. The ring finger is involved most often, followed in order by the little, middle, and index fingers. **Diagnosis** is by inspection and palpation. Initially, a small painless plaque or nodule develops in the palmar fascia and eventually extends into a longitudinal cordlike band. The skin adheres to the fascia and becomes puckered; flexion contracture of the fingers gradually follows. Nodules may be palpated under the skin pucker or over the dorsum of the joints. Extension of the affected fingers is impossible when the wrist is flexed and, in advanced cases, in any position. When the shoulder-hand syndrome is involved, the hands may resemble those affected by scleroderma or Raynaud's disease. The disorder progresses at a variable and unpredictable rate. The fibrosis may not advance for months or years and may remain confined within the distal palmar crease. The process is benign.

Treatment

Local corticosteroid injection into the affected tendon sheaths, analgesics, and physiotherapy are ineffective. Advanced flexion contractures usually require surgery. Subcutaneous fasciotomy, limited fasciectomy, or radical fasciectomy is performed according to the extent of the deformity. The more radical the procedure, the longer the convalescence. Whirlpool baths, passive and active exercises, and posterior extension splints may be helpful postoperatively. Recurrence is possible. Amputation of a finger has been indicated for severe deformity.

107. FIBROMYOSITIS

A group of common nonspecific illnesses characterized by pain, tenderness, and stiffness of joints, muscles, joint capsules, and adjacent structures.

The term **myalgia** indicates simple muscular pain, in contrast to **myositis,** which is due to inflammation of the muscle tissues. **Fibrositis** is a similar inflammation of the fibrous connective tissue components of muscles, joints, tendons, ligaments, and other "white" connective tissues. Various combinations of these conditions may occur together as "simple rheumatism." Any of the fibromuscular tissues may be involved, but those of the low back **(lumbago),** neck **(torticollis),** shoulders, thorax **(pleurodynia),** and thighs **(aches and "charleyhorses")** are especially affected. There is no specific histologic entity.

Etiology

The conditions may be induced or intensified by trauma, exposure to dampness or cold, and occasionally by a systemic, usually rheumatic, disorder. A virus infection or sometimes toxemia from a remote bacterial infection may be causative. Some cases may be of psychogenic or psychophysiologic origin; symptoms can be exacerbated by environmental or emotional stress.

Symptoms, Signs, and Diagnosis

Onset of pain frequently is sudden and the pain is aggravated by movement. Tenderness may be present, sometimes localized in a few small "trigger" zones or nodules. There may be local muscle spasm, though it cannot be regularly demonstrated by electromyography. Fever is not characteristic and only occurs when there is a provoking systemic condition. Diagnosis is by exclusion of other systemic diseases (e.g., early onset of RA, polymyositis, polymyalgia rheumatica, or other connective tissue disease), and (most difficult of all) of psychogenic muscle pain and spasm.

Prognosis and Treatment

Fibromyositis may disappear spontaneously within a few days or weeks, but may become chronic or recur at frequent intervals. Relief may be obtained from such simple measures as rest, local applications of heat, gentle massage, and aspirin 650 mg orally q 3 to 4 h. Trigger nodules or areas of focal tenderness may be injected with 1% procaine or lidocaine solution, 0.5 to 1 ml alone or in combination with a 2.5% hydrocortisone acetate suspension.

108. SPASMODIC TORTICOLLIS
(Wryneck)

Tonic or intermittent spasm of the neck muscles, causing rotation and tilting of the head.

Etiology

Etiology varies and often cannot be defined, but underlying psychologic disturbance, basal ganglia disease, CNS infections, or tumors in the bones or soft tissues of the neck may occasionally be implicated.

Symptoms, Signs, and Course

Onset may occur at any age, but most frequently between the 3rd and 6th decades; it may be sudden or (more likely) gradual. Both sexes are equally affected. Intermittent or continuous painful spasms of the sternomastoid, trapezius, and other neck muscles usually occur unilaterally and cause turning and tilting of the head. Sternomastoid muscle contraction causes rotation of the head to the opposite side and flexion of the neck to the same side. The condition varies from being one of mild or occasional episodes to one that is difficult to treat, may recur often or persist for life, and may result in minimal movement and postural deformity.

Diagnosis

Onset in the 4th and 5th decades precludes congenital torticollis. Pathologic processes in the neck itself must be ruled out by examination of the cervical region and by x-rays of the cervical spine. A history of encephalitis or evidence of extrapyramidal disease may be present. Electromyographic, neurologic, and psychologic studies are usually negative.

Prognosis and Treatment

Prognosis is good for correctable local causes; neurologic and psychiatric processes are more difficult to treat. The spasm can sometimes be temporarily inhibited by applying slight tactile pressure to the same side of the jaw as the head rotation. In general, however, medical remedies are useless. Relapses after thalamic surgical procedures and anterior cervical rhizotomy are common. Psychiatric treatment is indicated if there is clear evidence of an emotional problem; prognosis is best if onset is directly related to exogenous stress.

---

109. NECK, SHOULDER, AND UPPER LIMB PAIN

Pain in these regions is common and may be due to a single pathologic process or combined, extraordinarily diverse ones. The head, neck, shoulders, and upper limbs are all highly mobile and regularly involved in very complex movements that also often require heavy weight-bearing or the use of great force. Soft tissues (nerves, blood vessels, muscles, ligaments, and capsules) of this region are compressed into tight compartments, increasing their susceptibility to stress.

Pathologic processes producing symptoms may be local (e.g., inflammation of a joint, a capsule, or adjacent ligaments, muscles, or nerves), may be distant and cause radiation along the course of neurovascular bundles or brachialgia beginning anywhere from the spinal cord to the end of the extremity, or may be referred pain from diseased intrathoracic or upper abdominal organs. Symptoms also include paresthesias, muscle weakness, and reflex and sensory losses. Accordingly, diagnostic considerations involve good clinical evaluation that, in turn, requires an understanding of inflammatory processes such as the arthritides of either the shoulder or acromioclavicular joints, bursitis (e.g., subacromial), tendinitis (e.g., supraspinatus syndrome, epicondylitis of the elbow), synovitis, capsulitis, fibromyositis, vascular and neurologic disorders (the latter being further subdivided into those originating in the spinal cord, nerve roots, or peripheral nerves from cervical disk protrusion, cervical spondylosis, etc.), and a wide variety of intrathoracic and some abdominal processes that can refer pain to these areas. Discussions can be found under these designations elsewhere in this volume.

---

110. LOW BACK PAIN AND SCIATICA

Low back pain is felt in the low lumbar, lumbosacral, or sacroiliac region. It is often accompanied by *sciatica*, pain radiating down one or both buttocks and/or legs in the distribution of the sciatic nerve.

Etiology

Most low back pain is related to degenerative joint disease of the lumbosacral area resulting from shear in the lumbosacral junction caused by man's upright posture. The incidence of this condition increases with age, reaching 50% in persons > 60 yr. Low back pain may also be caused by (1) a ruptured intervertebral disk with subsequent herniation of the nucleus pulposus into the spinal canal, causing inflammatory or direct mechanical nerve root pressure; (2) fracture, infection, or tumor involving the back, pelvis, or retroperitoneum, or traumatic ligament rupture or paraspinous muscle tear; (3) commonly occurring, mild congenital defects of the low lumbar and upper sacral spine (e.g., spina bifida occulta, abnormal intervertebral facets, sacralization of L-5 transverse processes); (4) bilateral loss of substance in the pars interarticularis and subsequent slipping forward of a vertebra upon the one below (spondylolisthesis); and (5) back strain due to stretching of the abdominal muscles by obesity or pregnancy.

Any type of back pain may be simulated on the basis of psychosocial problems and conflicts; these factors regularly alter the patient's perception and reporting of structurally mediated pain, as well as the resultant degree of disability and response to therapy.

Symptoms, Signs, and Diagnosis

Differential diagnosis may be difficult. It begins with **careful definition of the character and precise location of the pain,** which may be *localized* (felt at the site of pathology and associated with tenderness), as in fibrositis; *diffuse* (arising from deeper-lying tissue), e.g., lumbago; *radicular*, as in sciatica (see below); or *referred* (due to spinal or visceral disease that shares the same spinal segment distribution as the site where the pain is perceived), e.g., osteomyelitis. **Mechanisms that intensify the pain** are also important diagnostically: Limitation of back motion because of pain and tenderness of the paravertebral muscles is common in all conditions, but increased pain following Valsalva's maneuver (straining, coughing, or sneezing), limitation of straight-leg raising, loss of reflexes, and sensory change are more characteristic of conditions affecting spinal nerve roots and the sciatic nerve.

Sciatica usually accompanies low back pain, but may be more severe and may occur alone. It is most commonly caused by peripheral nerve root compression from intervertebral disk protrusion or intraspinal tumor; less often, from infection. Compression may be within the intervertebral foramen by tumor or bony irregularities such as spondylolisthesis or osteoarthritis. The nerves can also be compressed outside the spinal cord, in the pelvis or buttock. Toxic inflammation (e.g., due to alcoholism, diabetic neuritis) is a rare cause. Such processes are confirmed by the presence of sensory and/or motor deficits, findings that are discussed further under NERVE ROOT DISORDERS in Ch. 130.

Spinal stenosis is *an uncommon form of sciatica that mimics vascular disease by simulating intermittent claudication.* It involves the sciatic nerve roots and is manifested by pain in the buttocks, thighs, or calves on walking, running, or climbing stairs. Evaluation will not reveal the anticipated vascular insufficiency. The disorder occurs in middle-aged or elderly patients and results from a narrowed spinal canal space due to osteoarthrosis, Paget's disease, or spondylolisthesis with edema of the cauda equina. Severity of the pain is relieved by rest (although paresthesias may continue) and by performing decompression laminectomies at several levels. This type of claudication can be differentiated from vascular intermittent claudication by the presence of a neurologic deficit and by the pain persisting for hours after resting and not coming on rapidly when exercise is begun. Obviously, the pulses are normal with good skin nutrition.

Congenital bony defects, degenerative disease, or **bony instability** may be demonstrated by x-rays, including oblique films showing the intervertebral facet joints. **Ruptured disk** (see in Ch. 130), **ligamentous sprain,** and **muscle tear** are suggested by sudden onset. Symptoms usually begin within 24 h after heavy lifting. Localized tenderness over a particular area is significant and suggests a process in the back itself rather than in the pelvis or retroperitoneal area. Examination by CT scan is proving valuable in outlining axial spatial deformations. **Fracture** and **fracture dislocation** are ruled out by the history, nature of the trauma, and x-rays. **Chronic arthritis** and **underlying skeletal defects** such as spondylolisthesis are suggested by gradual onset of low back pain; onset in adolescence is highly suggestive of the latter. **Intrapelvic** and **retroperitoneal conditions** may be suggested by the presence of associated symptoms and by the absence of localizing signs in the back, other than limitation of motion due to pain. **Tumors** and **infections** are more difficult to diagnose and may mimic a ruptured disk. A space-occupying tumor is frequently diagnosed by myelography. CSF examination does not always differentiate ruptured disk from tumor, since spinal fluid protein may be elevated in both conditions. CSF examination is indispensable in the diagnosis of spinal meningitis and other infections.

In **psychogenic pain,** a history of trivial trauma commonly is followed by disproportionately severe, disabling pain and no evidence of injury or significant, appropriate underlying disease. Additionally, predisposing anxiety or depression usually is present, with persistence of these affects not fully explained on the basis of the low back pain. While any organic disorder may be mimicked, carefully obtained descriptions of the pain and findings on examination tend to be vague or inconsistent with any known neuroanatomic pathways or disease process. In many cases, an organic disorder reasonably accounts for the symptoms, but psychogenic factors become evident when symptoms and disability persist or worsen after the signs of injury or disease have cleared. Monetary considerations, such as worker's compensation or other insurance, rarely cause the problem but commonly facilitate its perpetuation. **Malingering** is less common than psychogenic pain and is difficult to prove. When suspected, it can only be established by garnering evidence that the patient is faking. Such evidence is best acquired by someone other than the physician.

Prognosis and Treatment

Recovery from a single attack of low back pain is common, but attacks may recur or symptoms may become chronic in all conditions.

Acute low back pain is treated first by relieving muscle spasm with bed rest in a comfortable position, local heat, oral analgesics (aspirin up to a total of 3.6 gm [55 grains] on the first day, codeine up to 60 mg q 4 h, or meperidine up to 100 mg q 4 h), and muscle relaxants (methocarbamol 1 to 2 gm orally q.i.d. for 48 to 72 h; for maintenance, 1 gm q.i.d.; carisoprodol 350 mg t.i.d. to q.i.d.; meprobamate 400 mg t.i.d. to q.i.d.; or diazepam 10 mg t.i.d.). Traction, although useful in relieving muscle spasm, is not usually necessary, since bed rest is equally effective. Manipulation is helpful if the pain is due to muscle spasm alone; it may aggravate an arthritic joint or further rupture a disk.

Patients with ligamentous muscle strain may walk wearing lumbosacral corsets after the initial muscle spasm has subsided. When symptoms permit, abdominal muscle-strengthening exercises and lumbosacral flexion exercises (maneuvers that lessen lumbar lordosis and increase intra-abdominal pressure) are indicated to strengthen the supporting structures of the back and prevent the condition from becoming chronic or recurrent.

Chronic low back pain treatment is directed toward alleviating the cause. Analgesics may relieve pain; narcotics should be **avoided.** Intervertebral joint arthritis may respond to proper bracing and abdominal muscle-strengthening exercises. Lumbosacral flexion exercises may increase symptoms.

Obese patients with longstanding ligamentous or muscle injury or postpartum women with stretched abdominal muscles may benefit from wearing a corset to splint the affected muscles until their strength is regained through exercises. Significant weight loss may be required first. Spinal fusion is indicated if there is instability or severe, well-localized arthritic changes in 1 or 2 interspaces.

Managing psychosocial factors may be quite simple or very difficult. Such factors must be identified as etiologic or complicating issues early in the illness. When the key problems are acute anxiety or trauma, prompt and firm reassurance following a careful history and examination often will suffice. Otherwise, the most important management principles involve what *not* to do. The physician should not behave indecisively or in an accusatory manner; he should not delay appropriate studies (e.g., x-rays, ESR, electromyography) or demanding procedures (e.g., myelography, laminectomy); prescriptions should not be given for narcotics. It is best to be thorough, kind, and firm, providing support by permitting the patient to talk about his concerns, offering nonaddictive medications and physical therapy, and patiently awaiting improvement. If improvement does not occur in a reasonable period, the problem should be privately discussed with a psychiatric colleague in consideration of referral.

111. OSTEITIS DEFORMANS

(Paget's Disease)

A slowly progressive bone disorder characterized by an initial osteolytic phase usually followed by an osteoblastic phase, with resulting abnormal histologic patterns and gross deformity.

Etiology and Incidence

The etiology is unknown. Though a familial incidence has been observed, the specific genetic pattern is unclear. X-ray studies show that about 3% of persons over age 40 have Paget's disease; the incidence increases to about 10% of persons in their 80s. Men are more frequently affected than women. The disease appears to be more common in parts of Europe, England, Australia, and New Zealand; it is rare in Scandinavia, Africa, Japan, India, and South America. Recent studies have demonstrated the presence of viral particles in the pagetic bone.

Pathophysiology

The disease can be divided into 2 histologic phases. The initial phase is osteolytic and primarily involves bone resorption. At this time, x-rays show a characteristic expanding V-shaped osteolytic lesion, particularly in the tibia. An osteoblastic phase follows, during which new bone is formed. Both types of activity frequently occur simultaneously in adjacent sections of a bone. The architecture of the new bone is greatly distorted; bone formation is often bizarre, patternless, and characteristically mosaic.

Symptoms and Signs

Onset is frequently insidious. The disease is usually discovered in an asymptomatic patient when routine blood chemistry studies show an elevated alkaline phosphatase, or when x-rays are obtained for other reasons. Although any bone can be involved, the most commonly affected bones, in order, are the pelvis, femur, skull, tibia, vertebrae, clavicle, and humerus. The patient may seek medical attention for a bony deformity such as bowing of the tibia or femur, enlargement of the skull (changing hat size), shortened stature, or progressive kyphosis, or for severe aching in the affected bones. Occasionally, hypervascularity may cause a sensation of increased heat in the region. Encroachment of neural foramina may lead to neurologic symptoms such as deafness, or spinal cord compression accompanied by paresis or paraplegia. Since the lesions are highly vascular and act as arteriovenous shunts, high output cardiac failure may occur with severe involvement.

Diagnosis

Although any of the symptoms and signs discussed above may be suggestive, the diagnosis is usually based on **x-ray findings.** Increased density, abnormal architecture, cortical thickening, bowing, and overgrowth are evident in the bone. The long bones may show evidence of pseudofractures in the tibia and femur; the outer plate of the skull characteristically appears fuzzy after a prolonged period of osteoporosis circumscripta cranii. **Laboratory studies** further confirm the diagnosis, usually revealing elevated serum alkaline phosphatase and increased urinary excretion of hydroxyproline. Radionuclide bone scans using agents such as technetium-labeled diphosphonate show increased uptake at the site of active lesions. Serum calcium and phosphorus levels are usually normal. Paget's disease may be confused with hyperparathyroidism, bone metastasis from prostatic or breast carcinoma, multiple myeloma, and fibrous dysplasia.

Prognosis

The course is usually slowly progressive. Some patients have localized disease with few or no symptoms for many years. Deformities may develop from bowing of the bones or involvement of adjacent joints. Pathologic fractures of the femur or tibia may occur. Sarcomatous degeneration occurs in about 1% of patients. Spinal cord compression occurs in patients with lumbar spine involvement. Severe pelvic disease is frequently accompanied by acetabular protrusion.

Treatment

Localized asymptomatic lesions require no treatment, but should be monitored. Several agents produce a decrease in bone resorption and levels of serum alkaline phosphatase and urinary hydroxyproline. Calcitonin (50 to 100 MRC u./day subcutaneously) reduces alkaline phosphatase levels, decreases cardiac output, and decreases bone turnover by inhibiting bone resorption. Mithramycin (15 to 25 µg/kg/day IV for 10 days) has been shown to have similar effects in reducing alkaline phosphatase. It is *a cytotoxic drug* frequently used for testicular tumors. Use of oral etidronate disodium (5 to 10 mg/kg/day for 6 mo and then intermittently as needed) has resulted in reduction of urinary hydroxyproline and serum alkaline phosphatase levels, improvement in isotopic bone scans, relief of bone pain, and decrease in cardiac output.

112. OSTEOPOROSIS

An absolute decrease in bone tissue mass; the remaining bone is morphologically normal. The greater proportional loss of trabecular than of compact bone accounts for the primary complications of the disease, i.e., crush fractures of the vertebrae (which consist primarily of trabecular bone) and fractures of the neck of the femur and distal end of the radius (which consist of both cortical and trabecular bone).

Etiology and Incidence

Primary osteoporosis is associated with increased bone resorption; bone formation appears to be normal, though some believe defective bone formation may be involved. The etiology probably is multifactorial. Primary osteoporosis is much more common in women than in men (though it is rare in premenopausal women), in older than in middle-aged individuals, and in whites than in blacks. Failure to develop sufficient bone mass during young adult life, accentuation of age-related bone loss, increased sensitivity to endogenous parathyroid hormone, defective intestinal calcium absorption, and menopause are potentially important factors. **Secondary osteoporosis** may be produced by a number of medical disorders, most commonly hypercortisonism, hypogonadism, multiple myeloma, and subtotal gastrectomy.

Symptoms, Signs, and Diagnosis

Patients with uncomplicated osteoporosis may remain asymptomatic or may have aching pain in the bones, particularly the back. **Crush fractures** of the vertebrae are characteristically associated with minimal or no trauma and usually occur in weight-bearing vertebrae (T-8 and below). The resulting pain is acute, does not usually radiate, is aggravated by weight bearing, may be associated with local tenderness, and generally subsides in a few days or weeks. Patients with multiple compression fractures may develop dorsal kyphosis and exaggerated cervical lordosis, and often complain of a chronic, dull, aching pain particularly prominent in the lower thoracic and lumbar area. Hip and Colles' fractures, when they occur in the elderly, are most commonly due to preexisting osteoporosis.

Serum calcium, phosphorus, and alkaline phosphatase levels, protein electrophoresis, and ESR are normal in primary osteoporosis. Abnormal biochemical findings suggest secondary osteoporosis and should prompt a search for the cause.

On **x-ray examination,** the vertebrae show decreased radiodensity due to loss of trabecular structure. Reliance on subjective impressions of bone density may be misleading, however. The loss of horizontally oriented trabeculae results in increased prominence of the cortical endplates and of the remaining vertically oriented, weight-bearing trabeculae of the vertebrae. Anterior wedging in the thoracic region and ballooning of the vertebral interspaces in the lumbar area are characteristic of vertebral fractures. Although the cortices of long bones may be thin because of excessive endosteal absorption, the periosteal surface remains smooth (in contrast to what occurs in hyperparathyroidism). **Osteomalacia** may be radiologically confused with osteoporosis, but can be distinguished by abnormal serum biochemical findings and by bone biopsy. Corticosteroid-induced osteoporosis is likely to produce radiolucency of the skull, rib fractures, and exuberant callus formation.

Treatment

Treatment is supportive and empiric. Severe acute back pain due to a recent vertebral crush fracture should be treated with an orthopedic support, analgesics, and (when muscle spasm is prominent) heat and massage. Patients with longstanding osteoporosis may develop chronic backache due to abnormal stress from previous vertebral compressions on the muscles and ligaments attached to the spine. This pain may be relieved by an orthopedic garment or, more physiologically, by hyperextension exercises to strengthen flabby paravertebral muscles. Protecting the spinal column by avoiding heavy lifting or accidental falls is critical.

Treatment with diet and drugs is empiric, since the cause of the disease is unknown. At least 2 glasses of milk/day and a small daily supplement (1000 u.) of vitamin D are helpful. Oral calcium supplements and sex hormones decrease bone resorption and arrest or decrease progression of the disease, but these effects may be partly negated by secondary decrease in bone formation after long-term treatment. Large doses of calcium are well tolerated. For milder disease, calcium carbonate tablets 600 mg 4 to 6 times/day (equivalent to 1 to 1.5 gm of calcium/day) are given. Serum and urine calcium values should be determined after 1 mo of therapy and then semiannually while the patient is taking calcium. Patients with more severe disease should be given sex hormones in addition to calcium supplements. Women are given an estrogen such as conjugated equine estrogen 0.625 to 1.25 mg/day (omitting 5 consecutive days of each month to prevent uterine endometrial hyperplasia) or a synthetic anabolic hormone such as oxandrolone 5 mg/day. Estrogen administration produces withdrawal menstrual bleeding in about half the postmenopausal women thus treated and may increase the risk of uterine cancer. Synthetic anabolic hormones produce mild virilization and increased SGOT or plasma lipid levels in about ¼ of treated postmenopausal women. Osteoporotic men are given testosterone enanthate 200 mg IM every 2 or 3 wk. In older men, this may exacerbate symptoms of prostatic hypertrophy or stimulate growth of occult prostatic cancer. Although combined therapy with sodium fluoride 50 mg/day and supplementary calcium also appears to stimulate bone formation, the long-term safety and efficacy of this form of therapy have not been determined.

113. OSTEOMYELITIS

An infection of the bone and bone marrow. Osteomyelitis usually is caused by *Staphylococcus aureus*; however, a variety of gram-positive and -negative bacteria, acid-fast bacilli, fungi, and rickettsias can also be the cause.

Pathology

Infection may reach the bone hematogenously, directly (as in a compound fracture or other trauma), or by extension from an adjacent infection. The hematogenous origin, more common in children, generally is secondary to an acute local infection (e.g., a furuncle, otitis media, pneumonia), and only one organism usually is isolated (e.g., *S. aureus*, gram-negative organisms). In overwhelming bloodstream invasions, there may be a true pyemia with multiple abscesses throughout the body, the osteomyelitis being only a part of the general infection. Often a recent contusion or local bone injury acts as a point of decreased resistance. In children, the metaphyseal areas of the long bones and vertebrae are most often affected; in adults, the pelvis and vertebrae.

Bone marrow is the first tissue involved, usually near the end of the shaft if it is in a long bone. Local necrosis of tissue soon spreads. If the center of infection is near the surface, the exudate may break through and form a subperiosteal abscess. This may spread along the surface of the shaft while the infection is extending along the marrow cavity. The entire shaft can become involved, with complete necrosis; or spread may be arrested at any point. In osteomyelitis secondary to a contiguous focus of infection, i.e., a direct infection of bone by spread from a nearby infected focus (e.g., soft tissue infections following trauma or surgery, infected sinuses or teeth), mixed infections with gram-positive and -negative organisms are found. The femur and tibia are most commonly involved. Osteomyelitis associated with vascular insufficiency is seen in patients with severe atherosclerosis and diabetes mellitus. Again, mixed infections with gram-positive and -negative organisms usually are seen.

The periosteum, which separates from the dead bone, soon commences to lay down a tube of new bone around the old shaft (**involucrum**). Through it, openings (**cloacae**) develop, and sinuses, through which pus escapes, communicate with the surface. The necrotic bone becomes separated from the surrounding living bone, to form a **sequestrum.**

If the infection is near a joint, the joint may become inflamed, with swelling of the synovial membrane and an increase in joint fluid, but with no bacteria present. However, the infection may penetrate into a joint, especially one that partially surrounds the bone, as the hip joint surrounds the neck of the femur. A purulent exudate forms in the joint cavity and the articular cartilage may be destroyed.

In the **chronic stage,** a deep-seated infection appears around the sequestra in the depths of the bone. This is subject to periodic exacerbations, probably caused by obstruction to drainage from intermittent closure of the sinuses. Small sequestra may be extruded through the sinuses.

Symptoms, Signs, and Diagnosis

Characteristically, acute hematogenous osteomyelitis begins with sudden pain in the affected bone and a sharp rise in temperature. In children, this is often preceded for several days by the symptoms and signs of sepsis; in adults, few constitutional features may be present, the first symptoms and signs being those of bone involvement. There is tenderness over the bone, and movement is painful and involuntarily restricted. Later, swelling appears over the bone and, often, in an adjacent joint. Acute osteomyelitis may be confused initially with poliomyelitis, rheumatic fever, myositis, sprains, and fractures, all of which cause local tenderness, pain, and limitation of motion.

Leukocytosis is almost always present. The ESR is elevated. Blood cultures are occasionally positive. If fluctuation is present over the bone or if there is an effusion in the neighboring joint, the fluid should be aspirated and the causative organism identified in smears and cultures. A presumptive clinical diagnosis is often necessary, because x-rays may not give evidence of bone involvement until the infection has been present for some time. Osteomyelitis resulting from direct extension from an infected wound, subcutaneous abscess, or compound fracture may be difficult to detect clinically until the infection has become well established and chronic. With the clinical availability of radionuclide scanning technics, technetium and gallium isotope scans are positive as early as 72 h after the onset of symptoms of osteomyelitis and can be helpful in early diagnosis. However, acute trauma, tumor, synovitis, arthritis, and inflammation can all give positive radionuclide scans; therefore, a positive scan must be interpreted with the clinical picture. Tuberculous and fungal osteomyelitis are distinguished from acute hematogenous osteomyelitis by an insidious and chronic course. Tuberculous involvement of the vertebral column **(Pott's disease)** causes pathologic fractures and angular kyphosis of the spine.

Prognosis

Many of the infections that are precursors of osteomyelitis are overcome so promptly and effectively with antimicrobial therapy that bone infection is prevented. When acute osteomyelitis develops, it usually is controlled if treatment is started promptly. Chronic osteomyelitis has a poorer prognosis, but is less common.

Treatment

Acute osteomyelitis: Most important is the administration of an effective antibiotic as soon as osteomyelitis is suspected, without waiting for any x-ray or laboratory evidence other than a blood count. If treatment is delayed until necrosis of bone has taken place, the antimicrobial cannot reach the dead bone to combat the infection.

Since acute hematogenous osteomyelitis is caused by *S. aureus* in 75 to 80% of patients, and since the penicillinase-resistant penicillins such as methicillin, oxacillin, and nafcillin are effective against most staphylococci, one of these may be given initially, even before the causative organism is identified. Penicillin G may be used, if the organism is susceptible. A patient who is allergic to penicillin may be given a cephalosporin, erythromycin, or clindamycin. (For usual dosages, see in ANTIBIOTICS in Ch. 246.) The choice of an antibiotic for osteomyelitis caused by gram-negative bacteria, tubercle bacilli, fungi, or rickettsias should be determined by cultures and susceptibility studies.

Antibiotics should be continued for 8 to 12 wk after all local signs of swelling and tenderness have subsided, with close clinical and x-ray surveillance after treatment. The affected bone should be immobilized by plaster or traction until all evidence of active infection has disappeared, after which early motion is desirable.

If an abscess has formed, it should be evacuated and its contents cultured to identify the organism and determine its sensitivity to antibiotics. The appropriate antibiotic should then be instilled in the cavity daily, in addition to being given systemically. If the patient has been taking antibiotics and has evidence of persistent osteomyelitis from which no bacteria have been recovered, cultures should be placed on appropriate hypertonic media in an effort to recover cell-wall–deficient forms. Joints from which an organism is cultured should also be treated by daily aspiration or incision and drainage, and by systemic administration of the appropriate antibiotic until the inflammation subsides and the joint fluid becomes clear.

Later, if an abscess forms beneath the cortex of the bone, a window should be made in the cortex to drain the abscess. Treatment of suppurative arthritis requires surgical judgment. Some joint infections subside after simple daily aspiration and the administration of appropriate antibiotics IV. However, hyaline articular cartilage is destroyed so rapidly by the enzymes in pus that it may be advisable to incise and drain early—a much less harmful decision in some cases than the consequences of delaying this procedure.

Chronic osteomyelitis: The basic principles in the treatment of the now rarer chronic case are wide surgical exposure ("saucerization"), removal of dead bone (sequestrum), immobilization, and the use of an appropriate antibiotic to prevent the spread of infection and to sterilize the remaining viable bone. (NOTE: *Antibiotic therapy is not a substitute for removal of all infected dead bone.*)

In both acute and chronic osteomyelitis, the organism's sensitivity to the antibiotic should be tested periodically, since resistance may develop during treatment.

---

114.   NEOPLASMS OF BONES AND JOINTS

Any persistent or progressive pain of the trunk or extremities, particularly if associated with a mass, must be considered to be due to a bone tumor until proved otherwise. Even distress after trauma must be investigated to exclude bone neoplasms, which are often discovered in such investigation. The most common problem in diagnosing and treating bone tumors is failure to suspect their presence. Symptomatic treatment of joint or extremity pain without pretreatment diagnostic x-rays can lead to tragedy. Hence, it is imperative to suspect a tumor and obtain x-rays in 2 planes before proceeding with biopsy and specific treatment.

Host-tumor immunologic factors play a role in the clinical course of malignant lesions. Both humoral and cellular expressions of immunoincompetence in patients with sarcomas have been reported. A correlation has been shown between the degree of general depression of immunologic responsiveness and the subsequent clinical progression of disease. However, the routine use of immunologic monitoring remains experimental, and its clinical usefulness unknown.

Sophisticated approaches to adjunctive chemotherapy are being utilized in a number of experimental clinical trials; their efficacy is unproved.

Diagnosis

X-rays: Certain roentgenographic signs help to distinguish benign from malignant lesions, but none are infallible. X-rays help primarily in determining the tumor's location. For example, Ewing's tumor commonly appears first in the shaft of the long bone, while osteogenic sarcoma usually appears in the metaphysis toward the end of a long bone. Giant-cell tumor usually affects the epiphyseal end of a long bone. An aneurysmal bone cyst may be seen in any bone, but is usually located in the metaphyseal portion of a long bone.

The **patient's age** is helpful. In children, primary bone tumors prevail; metastatic tumors are rare. In adults, the incidence of metastatic bone tumors is about 20 times that of primary malignant tumors.

A **general medical examination** is required once a bone lesion has been discovered and a neoplasm is suspected. Stereo films and at least one lateral projection of the lung fields should be performed to rule out pulmonary metastatic involvement. Skeletal surveys and radioisotopic bone scans should be performed in a search for multicentric or metastatic lesions.

Biopsy is essential to the diagnosis and should be performed after the general medical evaluation is completed. Histopathologic diagnosis of bone tumors is difficult and requires an adequate amount of tissue from a representative portion of the tumor. Blind needle aspiration biopsy should be reserved for large, easily accessible lesions when only metastatic confirmation is required, or, occasionally, for investigation of a vertebral lesion. Open incisional biopsy is preferred because wrong diagnoses are frequent if only a few cells are obtained. The pathologist should be given pertinent details of the clinical history and of the x-rays. Since almost all bone tumors have soft portions that can be sectioned and examined for immediate diagnosis by fresh-frozen technic, and since these portions are usually the best material for diagnosis, an immediate, accurate, definitive diagnosis is possible in more than 90% of bone tumors. Facilities should be available to proceed immediately with appropriate definitive treatment of malignant tumors that are best treated by ablative surgery, which can then be carried out under the same anesthetic as for the biopsy.

BENIGN TUMORS

Osteochondromas (osteocartilaginous exostoses) are the most common benign bone tumors, occur most often in persons aged 10 to 20, and may be singular or multiple. Each osteochondroma is covered by a cartilaginous cap. A strong familial tendency to multiple osteochondromas may exist. Secondary malignant chondrosarcoma (see below) appears in > 10% of multiple osteochondromas.

Benign chondromas are located centrally within a bone (i.e., within the marrow cavity). They most commonly occur in persons aged 10 to 30. On x-ray, they may appear as lytic lesions with areas of stippled calcification.

Chondroblastoma is a rare benign neoplasm arising in an epiphysis. It is most common in persons aged 10 to 20.

Chondromyxofibromas occur before age 30. Their x-ray appearance (usually eccentric, sharply circumscribed, lytic, and located near the end of long bones) suggests the diagnosis.

Osteoid osteoma is a benign lesion which may occur in any bone, but is most common in long bones. The characteristic appearance on x-ray is a small radiolucent zone surrounded by a large sclerotic zone. Technetium-99 bone scans are valuable in helping to identify and localize this lesion. Pain relieved by small doses of aspirin is a classic feature. Treatment is surgical; relief is obtained only if the small radiolucent zone is located and removed.

A giant form of this lesion, **benign osteoblastoma,** occurs in persons aged 10 to 30 and is usually located at the end of a long bone or in the spine. These lesions develop slowly; the central nidus is usually large. Pain is the cardinal symptom. Surgical excision is recommended.

Giant-cell tumor occurs most commonly in the 20s and 30s. The lesions occur in the epiphyses of long bones and produce a lytic appearance on x-ray. They may erode the parent bone and produce soft tissue extensions. Treatment for small lesions usually consists of complete exteriorization, excision by curettage, and bone grafting. For larger lesions, complete excision of the lesion may be necessary. Giant-cell tumor is notorious for its tendency to recur, which may make surgical management difficult. A sarcoma eventually develops and complicates the course in < 10% of cases.

Fibromatous lesions may affect the long bones. The nature of these lesions can be ascertained only by biopsy. Not true neoplastic growths, the lesions probably result from faulty ossification. Many of them regress spontaneously without treatment.

PRIMARY MALIGNANT TUMORS

Osteogenic sarcoma (osteosarcoma), except for myeloma, is the most common primary bone tumor. It is highly malignant with a tendency to metastasize to the lungs. These tumors are most common in persons aged 10 to 20, though they can occur at any age. About half the lesions are located in the region of the knee, though they may be found in any bone. Pain and a mass are the usual symptoms. The x-ray findings vary greatly, with no characteristic appearance, and the tumor may be predominantly sclerotic or lytic. Accurate diagnosis rests on pathologic examination of representative biopsy tissue.

Formerly, the survival rate was low (5-yr survival, about 20%). Today > 50% of patients survive for 5 yr or longer. It is unclear whether the recent improved prognosis is due to adjunctive chemotherapy or to unidentified factors. Currently, a number of clinical trials are testing the efficacy of various adjunctive treatments. Amputation remains the treatment of choice for most lesions; however, limb salvage procedures are being used in select cases in experimental clinical trials.

Fibrosarcomas have the same general characteristics as osteogenic sarcomas, above, and pose the same problems.

Malignant fibrous histiocytoma, a recently described entity, behaves clinically in a manner similar to osteosarcoma and fibrosarcoma. Treatment is the same as for osteosarcoma.

Chondrosarcomas, malignant tumors of cartilage, are clinically, therapeutically, and prognostically unlike osteogenic sarcomas. They develop in more than 10% of patients with multiple benign osteochondromas. However, 90% of chondrosarcomas are primary, arising de novo without an osteochondroma or any prior benign cartilaginous lesion. Diagnosis can be made only by biopsy. Many chondrosarcomas can be graded histologically. Grade 1 lesions are slow-growing and have a good prognosis for cure. Grade 4 lesions (at the opposite end of the spectrum) grow more rapidly and are much more likely to metastasize. Regardless of grade, the outstanding feature of these tumors is their ability to "seed" or implant in surrounding soft tissues.

Treatment is surgical. Because of the potential to seed, the biopsy wound should be closed and ablative surgery carried out meticulously. Care must be taken to avoid entry into the tumor and spillage of tumor cells into the soft tissues of the wound, since recurrence is inevitable if this happens. Total resection when possible is the treatment of choice, with maintenance of the integrity and usefulness of the part. If surgery is performed without spilling the tumor contents into the wound, the cure rate is 50% or more, depending on the grade of the tumor. When surgical ablation and maintenance of function are impossible, amputation is obligatory. Neither radiation nor chemotherapy is effective in either primary or adjunctive treatment.

Mesenchymal chondrosarcoma is a rare but histologically distinct type of chondrosarcoma. It has a great potential for metastasizing; the cure rate is low.

Ewing's tumor (Ewing's sarcoma) is a radiosensitive round-cell bone tumor. Males are affected more frequently than females. Ewing's tumor appears at a younger age than any other primary malignant bone tumor. The peak incidence is between ages 10 and 20. Most of the tumors develop in the extremities, but any bone may be involved. Microscopically, the lesion consists of solidly packed, small round cells. Pain and swelling are the most common symptoms. Ewing's tumor tends to be extensive, sometimes involving the entire shaft of a long bone. Generally, more of the bone is pathologically involved than is apparent from the x-rays. Lytic destruction is the most common finding, but there may be multiple layers of subperiosteal reactive new bone formation, giving the onionskin appearance once considered a classic diagnostic sign. Since many other malignant bone tumors produce an identical appearance, diagnosis depends on biopsy.

Amputation is only indicated for huge lesions, for pathologic fractures, and for lesions in the distal lower extremity of young, growing children. Resection may be considered for lesions in expendable bones such as the ribs. Radiation therapy is indicated for most primary lesions. Several multiple drug chemotherapy programs have shown an improved overall survival. Since this is a rare tumor, most clinical trials report only small series of patients; hence, no one drug regimen is preferred.

Malignant lymphoma of bone is a small round-cell tumor that affects adults, most commonly persons in their 40s and 50s. It may arise in any bone. While the lesion may be referred to as reticulum cell sarcoma, a mixture of reticulum cells, lymphoblasts, and lymphocytes is common in these neoplasms. When malignant lymphoma is responsible for an osseous lesion, one of 3 clinical conditions may be found: (1) The malignant lymphoma may be primary in bone, without evidence of disease elsewhere. (2) In addition to the bone lesion, similar disease may be found in other osseous or soft tissue sites. (3) A patient with known soft tissue lymphomatous disease may have metastatic spread into any bone.

Pain and local swelling are the usual symptoms. On x-ray, bone destruction is predominant. Depending on the stage, the involved bone may be mottled or patchy, or, in more advanced disease, the entire outline of the affected bone may be lost. Pathologic fracture is common.

When malignant lymphoma is primary in bone and no disease is present elsewhere, the prognosis is better than in any other primary malignant bone tumor; the 5-yr survival rate is at least 50%. The tumors are radiosensitive. Amputation is not indicated except when function is lost because of pathologic fracture or extensive soft tissue involvement. Combination radiation and chemotherapy is as effective in achieving cure as amputation or other extensive ablative surgery.

Multiple myeloma (see also Ch. 99) is a tumor of hematopoietic derivation and is the most common bone neoplasm. The neoplastic process is regularly multicentric and often involves the bone marrow so diffusely that bone marrow aspiration usually is diagnostic. Patients with myeloma have predominantly hematologic problems. Only rarely is any form of surgical intervention, except biopsy, indicated.

Malignant giant-cell tumor is rare; even its existence is controversial. The lesion usually is located at the extreme end of a long bone. The classic features of malignant destruction (predominantly lytic; cortical destruction; soft tissue extension; pathologic fracture) are seen on x-ray. To be sure of diagnosis, zones of typical benign giant-cell tumor must be demonstrated in a malignant neoplasm or in previous tissue obtained from the neoplasm. A sarcoma that develops in a previously benign giant-cell tumor is characteristically radioresistant. The same prinicples of treatment apply as in osteogenic sarcoma, above. Ablative surgery, notably amputation, is the treatment of choice; the cure rate is low.

Many other types of primary malignant bone tumors exist, most of them so rare as to be medical curiosities. **Chordoma** develops from the remnants of the primitive notochord. It has a predilection for the ends of the spinal column and usually is located in the sacrum or near the base of the skull. Pain is a virtually constant feature of a chordoma located in the sacrococcygeal region. When the chordoma is located in the base of the occipital region, the symptoms may be referred to any of the cranial nerves, but symptoms resulting from involvement of the nerves to the eye are most common. The duration of symptoms varies from months to several years. A chordoma is seen on x-ray as an expansile, destructive bone lesion that may be associated with a soft tissue mass. Hematogenous metastasis is rare. Local recurrence is more troublesome than metastatic spread. Chordomas located in the spheno-occipital region are usually inaccessible to surgery, but may respond to radiation therapy. Those located in the sacrococcygeal region may be managed successfully by radical en bloc excision.

CONDITIONS THAT COMMONLY SIMULATE PRIMARY TUMORS OF BONE

Many non-neoplastic conditions of bone may simulate bone tumors, either clinically or radiologically. **Heterotopic ossification (myositis ossificans)** or **exuberant callus** after fracture may be mistakenly interpreted as malignant neoplasms; histopathologic tissue examination differentiates the conditions.

Simple **unicameral bone cysts** occur in the long bones in children. Most come to the clinician's attention when pathologic fracture occurs. Small ones heal and may obliterate themselves in the process of fracture healing. Larger ones may require evacuation and bone grafting.

Fibrous dysplasia is a cystic bone lesion probably resulting from an anomaly in bone development. The lesion may appear in one or several bones. When several bones are involved and cutaneous pigmentation and endocrine abnormalities are present, the condition is called **Albright's syndrome.** On x-ray, the lesions appear cystic and may be extensive and deforming. The lesions commonly stop growing at puberty. Spontaneous malignant degeneration is rare. Treatment should be conservative, though deformity secondary to disease in the long bones may require surgical correction.

Aneurysmal bone cyst is a cystic bone lesion of unknown cause that usually appears before age 20. The cyst may occur in the metaphyseal region of the long bones, but almost any bone may be affected. Pain and swelling occur. The lesion may be present for a few weeks to a few years. It tends to increase slowly in size until therapy is begun. The appearance on x-ray is often characteristic; the rarefied area is usually well circumscribed, eccentric, and associated with soft tissue extension produced by periosteal bulging. Periosteal new bone formation tends to delimit the periphery of the tumor. Surgical removal of the entire lesion, or as much of it as possible, is the most successful treatment. Complete regresssion after incomplete removal sometimes occurs. Radiation therapy for aneurysmal bone cysts should be used cautiously, since postirradiation sarcomas occasionally occur. Radiation is the treatment of choice in surgically inaccessible vertebral lesions that are compressing the spinal cord.

Histiocytosis X (Letterer-Siwe disease, Hand-Schüller-Christian syndrome, eosinophilic granuloma) occurs as solitary or multiple osseous lesions. It is a disease of the reticuloendothelial system. The lesions usually are well defined on x-ray. When the lesion is solitary with periosteal new bone formation, the x-ray may suggest a malignant bone tumor; accurate diagnosis depends on biopsy. When only one or a few osseous lesions are present, local radiation therapy is effective in producing a cure. The prognosis is ominous, however, in patients < 3 yr old or at any age with more than 8 bones involved, and particularly in those with hemorrhagic manifestations and enlarged spleens.

More extensive involvement, particularly skull lesions, may occur, and extreme widespread involvement may produce fulminating, rapidly fatal disease with death usually the result of respiratory or cardiac failure. (See also Histiocytosis X in Ch. 43.)

MALIGNANT METASTATIC LESIONS

Any cancer, regardless of the primary site, may metastasize to bone. Metastases from carcinomas are the most common malignant tumors affecting the skeleton. Any bone may be involved, but metastatic osseous lesions distal to the knees and elbows are uncommon. *Tumors that most frequently metastasize to bone arise in the breast, lung, prostate, kidney, and thyroid.* Any patient being treated for cancer or known to have had cancer and presenting with skeletal complaints should undergo a thorough examination to exclude the possibility of metastatic osseous lesions. Roentgenographic skeletal surveys should be made as indicated. Whole-body bone scintigrams, using technetium polyphosphates or another suitable isotope, occasionally demonstrate the metastatic lesions before they are obvious on x-ray. The origin may be obscure, but the pathologist, describing the appearance of the tissue, may be able to give clues as to the location of the primary tumor. Pain, swelling, and skeletal disability representing a metastatic focus of carcinoma occasionally occur before a primary tumor is suspected.

Treatment of metastatic osseous lesions and of the primary disease depends on the type of tissue involved and the organ of origin. Radiation combined with selected chemotherapeutic or hormonal agents is the most common modality. The availability of increasingly effective treatment for most carcinomas makes proper treatment of skeletal metastasis more important. Even when the metastatic osseous focus has grown so that pathologic fracture is imminent or present, surgical technics can be used to avoid amputation. Frequently, when the primary disease has been controlled and only a single osseous metastasis remains, excision combined with radiation, chemotherapy, or both may be curative.

---

115. COMMON FOOT DISORDERS

EXAMINATION OF THE FOOT AND ANKLE

Diagnosis and management of the patient's complaint depend on a working knowledge of foot anatomy, to determine the structures involved, i.e., tendon, nerve, ligament, or bone, and whether the problem is articular or extra-articular. If more than one site is involved, the patient should be asked to indicate the location of greatest discomfort and grade the amount of pain elicited by palpation at each site. Certain areas of the foot are normally tender to palpation, e.g., the sinus tarsi and the distal aspect of the ball between the metatarsals.

Once the problem is localized, its cause is considered: whether it is a local process, the result of trauma or an abnormality in foot structure or function, or a sign of systemic disease.

Examination of the ankle region: To check for tenderness or edema, the skin is first examined by moving it side to side and distally to proximally over the ankle. The skin is compressed, using the fingers of both hands to determine if the problem rests in the skin. Below the skin, the sensory branches of the superficial peroneal nerve can be visualized and palpated by plantar flexing and inverting the foot. Tapping these nerves may elicit pain, discomfort, or tingling **(Tinel sign)**; they are commonly tender following trauma to the foot and ankle. At this level, anterior and lateral to the medial malleolus, the great saphenous vein should be observed for signs of injury, and palpated to determine if it is tender. Below this level, the extensor tendons are then examined by placing the patient's foot at a right angle with the forefoot twisted out in abduction and asking the patient to hold the foot in that position while the examiner plantar flexes it against resistance. This maneuver accentuates the slips of the long extensor tendons. Each slip should be examined individually and palpated for signs of tenderness, pain, or swelling. The anterior tibial tendon can be similarly examined by dorsiflexing and inverting the foot as counter-resistance is applied. **Tenosynovitis** may occur, due to overuse, infection, or collagen disease, e.g., RA.

The ankle joint is then examined by deep palpation medial and lateral to the extensor digitorum longus tendon. Tenderness at the anterior lateral aspect of the ankle joint between the lateral malleolus and talus is common following inversion sprains of the anterior talofibular ligament. A small nodular swelling (sometimes referred to as a meniscoid body) over the anterior talofibular mortise may result from impingement of the ligament in the mortise following ankle sprain. Swelling below and anterior to the lateral malleolus suggests effusion from the ankle joint. Such effusions are found in patients with intra-articular disease, e.g., trauma causing osteoarthritis, ball and socket ankle joints due to abnormal frontal motion in the ankle, or ankle diastasis. Swelling over the anterior talofibular mortise may also be caused by juxta-malleolar lipoma, commonly found in menopausal women. These swellings are usually larger, bilateral, and symmetric, and may be painful because of entrapment of the intermediate dorsal cutaneous branch of the superficial peroneal nerve. Swelling of the entire ankle as opposed to these localized swellings usually represents either venous disease, lymphedema, or the edema of congestive heart failure. Edema tends to accumulate at the ankle because of shoe compression. Swelling behind one or both malleoli, usually painful, suggests tenosynovitis.

The heel should be examined with the foot at a right angle to the leg. Pain, as described by the patient or elicited by palpation on examination, can usually be localized, thus aiding in the diagnosis. In the discussion below, disorders will be described in groups based on such localization. Deep, firm palpation to the center of the heel will elicit pain in patients with biomechanical abnormalities, fascial problems, and heel spur syndromes. Pain at the medial and lateral margins of the heel in children is a common symptom of epiphysitis of the calcaneus (Sever's disease). Pain anterior to the Achilles tendon at the retromalleolar space may suggest bursitis (retromalleolar bursitis, Albert's disease). Pain posterior to the tendo Achilles may result from an enlarged posterior-superior aspect of the calcaneus (Haglund's deformity), a common finding in children and adults whose subtalar joint functions in an inverted position, associated with painful adventitious bursae between the tendon and the skin. Tenderness at the calcaneal insertion of the Achilles tendon may be a sign of an overuse syndrome in athletes or a tight heel chord secondary to abnormal foot structure and function.

Occasionally, the heel will be the location of certain inflammatory arthropathies (e.g., ankylosing spondylitis, Reiter's syndrome), and the heel is second only to the first metatarsophalangeal joint for the occurrence of gouty arthritis. RA commonly is the cause of heel pain resulting from inflammatory erosion at the posterior aspect of the calcaneus. These arthropathies can usually be distinguished from local causes of heel pain by the presence of moderate to severe heat and swelling; they are discussed elsewhere in this volume.

HEEL PAIN

PAIN ON THE PLANTAR SURFACE OF THE HEEL

Strain at the Periosteal Attachment of the Plantar Fascia and the Flexor Digitorum Brevis

The plantar structures of the foot and those of its inner side are subjected to a great strain on weight bearing; excessive strain results in overstretching and other adverse sequelae. Principally involved are the plantar fascia and the flexor digitorum brevis muscle, as well as the muscles controlling the inner sides of the foot and their ligaments and supporting fascial bands. Injuries to the periosteal attachments of these ligaments and the plantar fascia may ensue, resulting in the formation of exostoses where the periosteum is injured (see Calcaneal Spur Syndrome, below).

The strain may be due to obesity or a vocation demanding standing or walking for many hours on hard-surfaced floors. Restricted flexion of the foot caused by shortened calf muscles as a result of prolonged wearing of high-heeled shoes or of abnormal foot structure or function is a common factor. The sudden change from high-heeled shoes in the winter and spring to heelless summer tennis shoes is a common cause. Joggers who run on their toes are more susceptible to strain than those who land on their heels.

Symptoms occur along the course of the intrinsic musculature of the foot and inner border of the plantar fascia. Pain usually is bilateral, but the degree of strain and discomfort on each side varies greatly. Patients often complain of feeling that their foot is "breaking apart."

Diagnosis: The plantar fascia is examined by flexing the foot on the leg to its maximum while *firmly* palpating the inner border of the plantar fascia at its origin at the calcaneus and along its course to the first metatarsal. Rubbing the thumb along the inner border of the plantar fascia when the foot is maximally flexed on the leg also causes a great deal of pain and discomfort.

Treatment begins with rest and other measures to reduce stretching of the fascia. Strapping and padding beneath the arch are indicated. Specific treatment depends on identifying the cause of the strained plantar fascia. Where limitation of dorsiflexion by shortened calf muscles is responsible for the strain, the shortened muscles could be stretched, if possible, to increase ankle flexion. Until an increase in the range of flexion is obtained, the shortened calf muscles must be accommodated by wearing a heel somewhat higher than that found in the common walking shoe or by placing one or more felt cushions in a low-heeled shoe. Either a temporary felt pad arch support or a more permanent orthosis fitted especially for the patient's foot is also needed. When the condition is caused by long hours of standing or walking or abnormal biomechanical function, referral for biomechanical evaluation and construction of an orthosis is required.

Calcaneal Spur Syndrome

The spur is a bony exostosis that originates at the inner weight-bearing tuberosity of the calcaneus and extends forward horizontally in the direction of the plantar fascia. It results from strain that injures the periosteal attachment to the heel bone of the plantar fascia. Spurs usually are present bilaterally and are more or less uniform in shape. They are commonly found in individuals who exhibit limited ankle joint flexion caused by contracted heel chords.

Calcaneal spurs do not always cause symptoms. Even when there is pain in the heel and a spur is present, the spur is not necessarily the cause of the pain. Asymptomatic spurs commonly are discovered incidentally in an x-ray taken for other reasons. A spur may be present for many years without causing symptoms, but pain can develop suddenly as a result of movement producing obliquely downward pressure on the tissues and cutaneous nerves in the area. Pain is experienced only on weight bearing or directly applied digital pressure. It is most pronounced just anterior to the inner weight-bearing tuberosity of the calcaneus but can radiate to other parts of the heel and sometimes forward to the foot. Inferior calcaneal bursitis with accompanying mild heat and swelling may also be seen. While physical examination may demonstrate pain in the central portion of the heel, this may represent only a strain in the plantar fascia. In a few subjects with a very thin fat pad, the spur may be palpated. An x-ray is the only certain means of demonstrating a spur.

Treatment: Symptoms can be controlled with a corticosteroid/lidocaine injection (1 ml of triamcinolone acetonide [10 mg/ml] with 1.5 ml of 2% lidocaine with epinephrine) given perpendicular to the medial border of the heel pointing toward the painful trigger point located at the central portion of the heel. Strapping is recommended to alleviate tension along the plantar fascia as well as orthotic devices to control abnormal elongation of the foot causing strain along the plantar fascia. Biomechanical evaluation of the patient's locomotion is recommended to determine the extent to which it may be a factor in the cause of plantar fascial strain.

Displacement of the Calcaneal Fat Pad

The calcaneus and soft tissue structures, i.e., calcaneal nerves and blood vessels, are protected during the contact phase of gait by a thick, soft tissue buffer composed of fat known loosely as the heel pad. In normal individuals, this heel pad is evenly distributed medially and laterally around the heel. In individuals whose rearfoot functions in excessive inversion, the fat pad has a tendency to be displaced medially; in individuals whose rearfoot functions move in an everted position, the fat pad tends to be displaced laterally. When this displacement occurs, the calcaneus and its surrounding soft tissues no longer are protected and become easily traumatized, causing heel pain.

Diagnosis: The heel should be examined with the patient prone. Under normal conditions the heel pad should be distributed evenly around the heel. In fat pad displacement the pad appears more prominent at the margin aspects of the heel, medially or laterally.

Treatment consists of soft tissue supplements to the shoe to cushion the heel—heel cushions, sponge rubber, or lamb's wool. If these fail to give relief, an orthosis with a hollow heel cup should be used, preferably constructed to transfer weight from the heel to a spot slightly more towards the middle of the foot.

PAIN LOCATED AT THE MARGINS OF THE HEEL

Epiphysitis of the Calcaneus (Sever's Disease)

A painful condition of the heel affecting children. The calcaneus is the only bone in the tarsus that develops from 2 centers of ossification: one from the body of the calcaneus and one from its epiphysis, which later forms the posterior part of this bone. Ossification of the body of the calcaneus begins at birth. Ossification of the epiphysis usually does not begin before the 8th yr. At the age of 16 and sometimes somewhat later, complete ossification with union of the body and the epiphysis of this bone usually has taken place. Between the ages of 8 and 16, before bony union has been effected, the 2 parts of the bone are connected by cartilage. Excessive strain on the epiphysis by jumping or other athletic activities sometimes results in breaking the cartilaginous union between the 2 bones or fibers of the tendinous insertion at the epiphysis. Children who are unable to dorsiflex their foot normally are more prone to this condition. Heat and swelling occasionally are present. The disorder may take several months to become asymptomatic, with healing taking place by fibrous or fibrocartilage replacement.

Diagnosis is based on the age of the patient, a history of athletic involvement, and the typical location of pain along the margins of the growth centers. X-rays are not helpful. Other causes of heel pain in children, such as RA, should be ruled out.

Treatment is often disappointing. Heel pads placed within the shoe are used to alleviate the pull of the Achilles tendon on the heel. Immobilization of the foot in a plaster cast is sometimes effective. Reassurance is important to the patient and the parents.

PAIN LOCATED CHIEFLY AT OR ENTIRELY ABOVE THE POSTERIOR PART OF THE HEEL

Haglund's Deformity (Posterior Tendo Achilles Bursitis)

Immediately above the insertion of the Achilles tendon, posterior to the heel, a bursa develops over the posterior superior lateral aspect of the calcaneus between the tendon and the skin. The bursa develops as a result of variations in heel position and function. This problem is seen mostly in young women but can occur in men. The heel then tends to function in an inverted position throughout the gait cycle, thereby placing excessive soft tissue compression between the posterior lateral aspect of the calcaneus and the counter of the shoe. In these cases the posterior lateral aspect of the calcaneus becomes prominent and can be easily palpated. It is often mistaken for an exostosis.

Symptoms and Signs: In early stages only a small erythematous, slightly indurated tender area may be seen at the posterior superior aspect of the heel, and in this stage, patients often are seen placing bandaids over the area to reduce shoe counter pressure. When the inflamed bursa enlarges, it appears as a painful red lump over the tendon. Sometimes swelling extends to both sides of the tendon depending upon the type of shoe gear the patient wears. In chronic cases, the bursa becomes permanently fibrotic.

Treatment consists of heel raises made of foam rubber or felt to elevate the heel, which eliminates pressure from the counter of the shoe. In addition, stretching of the counter of the shoe or opening the seam in the back of the shoe will relieve inflammation in a small percentage of the cases. Padding placed around the bursa often relieves pressure to the area. Infiltration of a soluble corticosteroid with a local anesthetic is effective in reducing inflammation. Orthotic devices constructed for the shoes are also indicated to control abnormal heel motion. When conservative therapy is ineffective, surgical excision of the posterior lateral aspect of the calcaneus may be indicated.

PAIN AT THE RETROCALCANEAL SPACE

Fracture of the Posterior Lateral Tubercle of the Talus

The fracture develops as a result of a plantar flexion injury in which forces are applied to the talar tubercle by the posterior inferior lip of the tibia. Toe walkers who have elongated lateral talar tubercles (Stieda's processes) seem more prone to this injury. Occasionally, this tubercle may be connected by a cartilaginous bar to the talus, representing a separating center for ossification known as an ostrigonum. This separation often is mistaken for a fractured tubercle on x-ray. At times, fracture of this cartilage juncture occurs, usually as a result of a sudden jump on the ball of the foot or toes in such sports as basketball and tennis. Similarly, the trauma can occur by stepping backward off a chair with force.

Symptoms, Signs, and Diagnosis: Pain and swelling located behind the ankle (at the retrocalcaneal space, between the Achilles tendon and the calcaneus), as well as difficulty in walking downhill or downstairs, is common. Persistent swelling may be present with no obvious history of an injury. Heat may or may not be present depending upon the chronicity of the injury; if present, it is mild. Plantar flexing the foot on the leg will reduplicate the patient's pain, and at times dorsiflexing the hallux is said also to do the same, although this maneuver is questionable. Lateral x-rays of the ankle are necessary to confirm the diagnosis. Bilateral x-rays are ordered to rule out an ostrigonum.

Treatment: Immobilization in a plaster cast for 4 to 6 wk is indicated. If pain persists and soft tissue inflammation is present, infiltrations of corticosteroid/anesthetic combinations may be effective. If conservative therapy is ineffective, surgical excision of the lateral tubercle is indicated.

Anterior Achilles Bursitis (Albert's Disease)

Inflammation of the bursa that lies between the Achilles tendon and the calcaneus at a point of attachment of the former to the bone occurs as a result of trauma and in association with inflammatory arthritis (usually RA). When the bursitis is caused by trauma, its onset is rapid; when caused by systemic disease, it usually develops gradually. Any condition associated with increased strain of the tendo Achilles can be responsible. Other factors, such as a rigid or high shoe counter, may also be causes. Inflammatory changes in this bursa may cause erosive changes in the calcaneus.

Symptoms, Signs, and Diagnosis: Pain, swelling, and heat in the retrocalcaneal space and difficulty walking or wearing shoes are common symptoms. Initially, the swelling is localized just anterior to the tendo Achilles but in time extends both medially and laterally. Swelling and heat contiguous to the tendo Achilles with pain located primarily within the soft tissue differentiates this condition from a fractured posterior lateral tubercle. X-rays should be ordered to rule out fracture or rheumatoid erosive calcaneal changes.

Treatment: Intrabursal injection of a soluble corticosteroid with lidocaine (1 ml of dexamethasone phosphate [4 mg/ml] with 1/2 ml of 2% lidocaine with epinephrine) is effective in relieving symptoms. Warm compresses may also help.

DISORDERS ASSOCIATED WITH METATARSALGIA

Metatarsalgia is a general term used to describe *pain over the ball of the foot*, usually the result of injury to the interdigital nerves or as a result of trauma to the metatarsal-phalangeal articulations. The most common cause of metatarsalgia is **Morton's neuroma** and variations thereof, such as neuralgia involving the interdigital nerves, and malalignment of the metatarsal-phalangeal articulations; the latter are seen more commonly in individuals who exhibit rigidity and stiffness of the forefoot.

Interdigital Nerves (Morton's Neuroma)

The interdigital nerves of the foot travel beneath and between the metatarsals extending distally over the ball of the foot to innervate the toes. The 3rd plantar interdigital nerve is composed of a branch of the medial and lateral plantar nerves. It is at this site that neuroma formation usually occurs, although it is not uncommon for neuromas or neuralgia to develop at other interdigital nerves. Neuroma formation is more often unilateral than bilateral, being more common in women than in men.

Symptoms and Signs: In early stages, patients may only complain of a mild ache or discomfort in the area of the head of the 4th metatarsal. Occasionally, a burning sensation or tingling may be experienced. These symptoms are more pronounced with one type of shoe than with others. As the condition progresses, these sensations become more specific, often causing constant burning that radiates to the tips of the toes. Patients often complain of symptoms with all forms of shoe gear and commonly feel as if a marble or a pebble were inside the ball of the foot.

Diagnosis is established by eliciting the characteristic history and by palpation of the interdigital space plantarly. Pressure is exerted with the thumb between the heads of the 3rd and 4th metatarsals. Patients with neuroma often complain and wince with pain when this maneuver is performed.

Treatment: Lidocaine is often effective, yielding lasting results in cases of simple neuralgia. Otherwise, perineural infiltrations of long-acting corticosteroids with a local anesthetic (e.g., $1/8$ to $1/4$ ml of triamcinolone acetonide [40 mg/ml] with 1 ml of 2% lidocaine with epinephrine) is often quite effective. Injection is at a $45°$ angle with the foot into the interspace at the level of dorsal aspect of the metatarsal-phalangeal joints. Injections may have to be repeated on 2 or 3 occasions. Concomitant use of foot orthoses is helpful. When conservative therapy is ineffective, surgical excision of the neuroma often yields complete relief.

Atrophy of the Plantar Metatarsal Fat Pad

With advancing age, the normal plantar fat pad becomes atrophic and no longer protects pressure-sensitive joints, nerves, and tendons; arteriosclerosis obliterans plays a major role. Trauma to the joint capsule of the metatarsal-phalangeal joints and to the interdigital nerves of the ball of the foot causes pain and burning.

Diagnosis is established by palpation of the metatarsal-phalangeal articulations in order to elicit joint pain and direct compression between the metatarsal heads plantarally to elicit involvement of the interdigital nerves. In addition, atrophy of subcutaneous tissue is always present. This disorder must be differentiated from diabetic neuropathy and ischemia. Diabetic neuropathy tends to more commonly involve the dorsal aspect of the feet and legs. The symptoms of both diabetic neuropathy and ischemic pain are more commonly perceived at night.

Treatment consists of fabricating and prescribing soft tissue supplements for the shoe utilizing foam rubber of various new thermoplastic materials to replace the atrophic fat pad.

Metatarsal-Phalangeal Articulation Pain (Lesser Toes)

Pain involving the metatarsal-phalangeal joint is a common occurrence. This symptom is almost entirely due to malalignment of the joint surfaces, causing subluxations and capsular and synovial impingement with eventual destruction of joint cartilage (degenerative joint disease). Such subluxations are seen in patients who have hammer toe deformities, cavus or highly arched feet, excessive eversion of the subtalar joint (rolling-in of the ankles [pronation]), and hallux valgus deformity (**bunion**). As a result of an overriding hallux, patients with bunion usually also have traumatic subluxations and pain in their second metatarsal-phalangeal articulations. Painful subluxation of the metatarsal phalangeal articulation can also be caused by collagen diseases such as RA.

Diagnosis: The absence of significant heat and swelling over the joint generally rules out collagen disorders, but a rheumatic disease work-up is helpful. Joint pain can be differentiated from neuralgia or neuroma of the interdigital nerves by the absence of such symptoms as burning, numbness, and tingling. In addition, palpation of the joint and moving it through its range of motion usually reveals tenderness of the dorsal as well as plantar aspect of the joint; in neuralgia, symptoms are usually limited to the plantar surface.

Treatment should correct the initiating cause. When excess subtalar eversion (rolling-in of the ankles) is present, a device to control this motion should be fabricated for the shoes. In patients with highly arched feet or hammer toe deformities, the cause should be sought; a weak anterior tibial muscle, tight heel chord, neurologic disease such as Friedreich's ataxia, Charcot-Marie-Tooth disease, or post-stroke toe contractures should be ruled out. Orthotics should be prescribed to redistribute and relieve pressure from the affected articulations. Injections of local anesthetics with or without soluble corticosteroids may have to be given weekly for 2 to 3 wk, but may yield dramatic results lasting for a few months.

Hallux Rigidus (Degenerative Joint Disease of the First Metatarsal-Phalangeal Joint)

Osteoarthritis of the first metatarsal-phalangeal joint is an extremely common occurrence. Most often it is the result of variations in position of the 1st metatarsal due to excessive rolling-in of the ankles (pronation), lateral deviation of the hallux (hallux valgus), dorsiflexion of the 1st metatarsal (metatarsal elevatus), or increased length or medial deviation of the first metatarsal. Occasionally, trauma will be a factor.

Symptoms and Signs: Initially, the only sign may be slight swelling of the joint due to capsular thickening. The joint is tender to the touch, and shoes irritate the condition further. As the condition worsens, pain increases and exostosis formation begins to limit joint motion; the patient no longer bends the joint during walking. Motion now appears to be taking place at the distal interphalangeal joint and an accentuated skin crease is observable at this joint. Although increased heat in the area usually is not present, it may develop late in this disorder, as a result of secondary impingement of the synovial membrane.

Diagnosis is established by observing an enlarged 1st metatarsal-phalangeal joint with limitation of its motion, pain on palpation of the joint capsule (particularly at its lateral aspect), and resulting increased dorsiflexion of the distal phalanx. Dorso-plantar x-rays will reveal spurs laterally, and lateral x-rays may show a dorsal exostosis extending from the metatarsal head in advanced cases.

Treatment: Initially, the aim of treatment is to increase joint motion using passive exercises and toe traction. Relief of pain with lidocaine infiltrations (1.5 ml of a 2% solution with epinephrine) periarticularly will decrease muscle spasm, thereby increasing motion. Early biomechanical control of the foot will restore proper position and function of the metatarsal. In cases recalcitrant to conservative therapy, limitation of motion may be advised to decrease pain and is accomplished by prescribing a foot orthosis with a Morton's extension; a steel splint extending from the end of the toe to the heel between the inner and outer sole or a metatarsal bar may also be prescribed. Surgery may be indicated.

DISORDERS OF THE NERVES OF THE FOOT AND ANKLE

Intermediate Dorsal Cutaneous Nerve

The intermediate dorsal cutaneous nerve has the rare distinction of being visible and palpable in a living foot by simply plantar flexing and inverting the foot. The nerve appears as a band-like structure extending from about 5 cm above the ankle-crossing anterior and medial to the lateral melleolus, losing prominence over the midtarsal area. Because it is so superficial, it is prone to direct trauma.

Symptoms and Signs: Pain is the usual presenting symptom and a history of trauma may be elicited, most commonly inversion sprains. Commonly, there is diffuse, nonspecific pain over the dorsal lateral aspect of the foot and/or ankle. When asked to localize the source of the pain, the patient often rubs his ankle or foot in a semicircular fashion, unable to pinpoint the pain precisely. While paresthesias may be present, frank sensory loss does not usually occur. Patients having neuropathy from ankle sprain generally continue to have pain during treatment while in short leg casts, and after cast removal. Sometimes casts are reapplied because additional immobilization of a sprained ankle is erroneously thought to be necessary.

Diagnosis is suggested by a recalcitrant pain syndrome of the anterior-lateral aspects of the foot and ankle, particularly if palpation and percussion of the nerve reproduces the patient's pain pattern. Confirmation by sensory nerve conduction testing is rarely indicated.

Treatment: Perineural infiltration of local anesthetics (1.5 ml of 2% lidocaine with epinephrine) usually yields dramatic and permanent relief.

Medial Dorsal Cutaneous Nerve Syndrome

The superficial peroneal nerve divides approximately 10.5 cm above the ankle into medial and intermediate dorsal cutaneous nerves. The medial dorsal cutaneous nerve innervates the medial aspect of the great toes in the adjacent sides of the 2nd and 3rd. The nerve can be seen in most patients by plantar flexing and inverting the foot. When it cannot be seen it can be palpated.

Symptoms and Signs: Because the nerve is so superficial it becomes accessible to external trauma, which commonly occurs during sleep. When patients sleep "coffin" style (with one foot placed upon the dorsal aspect of the other, putting direct pressure on the medial dorsal cutaneous nerve) they often complain of numbness of the big toe upon arising in the morning. Patients undergoing foot surgery for correction of bunion deformities often develop numbness and paresthesias along the medial aspect of the great toe as a result of surgical trauma to the medial dorsal cutaneous nerve or postoperative tissue fibrosis surrounding the nerve at the level of the first metatarsal phalangeal joint. Athletes participating in soccer will occasionally damage this nerve.

Diagnosis: By plantar flexing and inverting the foot, the medial dorsal cutaneous nerve often becomes prominent. Palpation or tapping of the nerve will in many instances reduplicate the patient's pain pattern (Tinel's sign). Confirmation may be possible by performing nerve conduction velocities.

Treatment in cases of fibrous entrapment consists of local infiltrations of long-acting corticosteroids, (e.g., 1/4 ml of triamcinolone acetonide [40 mg/ml] with 1 ml of 2% lidocaine with epinephrine) injected perineurally. Padding of the shoe or foot at the adjacent margins of the nerve helps prevent continued trauma.

Posterior Tibial Nerve Neuralgia

At the level of the ankle the posterior tibial nerve passes through a fibroosseous canal within the laciniate ligament. At its exit it terminates into medial and lateral plantar nerves. **Tarsal tunnel syndrome** refers to compression of the nerve within this fibro-osseous canal, but this diagnosis has been loosely used to label neuralgia of the posterior tibial nerve due to varied causes. Synovitis of the flexor tendons of the ankle caused by either abnormal foot function or inflammatory arthritis may on occasion cause secondary pressure neuralgia of the posterior tibial nerve. Occasionally, phlebitis of the communicating veins of the ankle and, in a small percentage of cases, abnormal foot structure and function associated with excessive subtalar eversion may cause the condition.

Symptoms and Signs: Patients complain of pain, usually of a burning and tingling quality, in and around the ankle and often extending to the toes. Difficulty in standing, walking, and wearing various types of shoes may be present. The pain is worse during ambulation and is relieved by rest.

Diagnosis: Tapping the posterior tibial nerve at a site of compression or injury will often produce distal tingling (Tinel's sign). Palpating the nerve may also elicit the patient's syndrome. These objective signs along with the classic complaints of burning pain and tingling in and around the ankle will suggest the possibility of posterior tibial neuralgia. When there is swelling in the area of the nerve, attempts should be made to determine its cause, e.g., rheumatic disease, phlebitis, or fracture. Electrodiagnostic testing often will confirm the diagnosis and should be performed in all patients undergoing foot surgery for decompression.

Treatment: When there is no true compression of the posterior tibial nerve within the fibro-osseous canal, local infiltration of insoluble corticosteroids (1/4 ml of triamcinolone acetonide [40 mg/ml] with 2 ml of 1% lidocaine with epinephrine) may be effective. Strapping the foot in neutral position or slight inversion or constructing an orthotic device for the shoe that keeps the foot in an inverted position will reduce tension on the nerve. Surgery should be reserved for those cases that are recalcitrant to conservative therapy.

ANKLE SPRAINS

Classification

Ankle sprains can be classified according to the extent of soft tissue damage.

Grade 1: Mild or minimal sprain with no actual ligamentous tear. Mild tenderness with some swelling may be present.

Grade 2: Moderate sprain consisting of incomplete or partial rupture with obvious swelling, ecchymosis, and difficulty in ambulation.

Grade 3: A complete tear of a ligament with swelling, hemorrhage, ankle instability, and inability to ambulate.

Pathogenesis and Etiology

The ankle is supported laterally by 3 ligaments: the anterior talofibular, fibulocalcaneal ligament, and posterior talofibular ligament. In an ankle sprain episode, the anterior talofibular ligament is usually ruptured first. Only after this ligament is ruptured can the calcaneofibular ligament divide. The posterior talofibular ligament rarely ruptures. Therefore, if the anterior talofibular ligament is intact, one can surmise that the fibulocalcaneal ligament is also intact; conversely, if the anterior talofibular ligament is ruptured, examination for concomitant rupture of the lateral fibulocalcaneal ligament must be sought. In a study of 321 ligamentous injuries of the ankle, 64% of cases injured the anterior talofibular ligament alone and 17% also injured the lateral fibulocalcaneal ligament.

Predisposing influences leading to ankle sprain may be present. Individuals with ligamentous laxity who display extensive ranges of subtalar inversion are often more prone to inversion episodes. Prophylactic control of rear foot motion in these patients using functional foot orthoses appears indicated. The peroneals are responsible for normal subtalar joint eversion. Occasional weakness of the peroneals occurs in individuals with lumbar disk disease involving L-5/S-1 nerve root or other causes of peripheral neuropathy involving the peroneal nerve. These persons are candidates for sprained ankles. Forefoot valgus, a condition in which the forefoot tends to function in an everted manner during the gait cycle, causing the subtalar joint to compensate by inversion, may be a predisposing factor in ankle sprain. Some individuals inherit a tendency to develop inverted subtalar joints (subtalar varus) and are predisposed to ankle sprain.

Examination

Examination of foot structure and function is required to rule out predisposing influences as described above. Then, topographic examination will determine the site of the ligamentous injury. This is accomplished by simple palpation of the ligaments around the lateral ankle. Classification of the ankle sprain usually can be made clinically. A useful test to determine anterior talofibular rupture is known as the **Drawer sign:** The anterior talofibular ligament prevents the talus from subluxing anteriorly on the tibia. When this ligament is ruptured, anterior displacement of the talus becomes possible. The patient is asked to sit on the side of a table with his legs dangling. With the left hand of the examiner placed in front of the patient's lower leg, the right hand grasps the patient's heel posteriorly and attempts to move the talus anteriorly.

Stress x-rays of the ankle may help to determine the extent of ligamentous injury. Mortise views of the ankle consisting of an anteroposterior x-ray taken with 15° internal rotation are ordered. Both ankles are inverted to maximum (local anesthesia may be indicated) and the degree of lateral tilt of the talus is noted. If a talar tilt difference of 5° or more can be demonstrated, functional impairment should be considered. If the difference is > 10°, symptoms increase significantly and an unstable ankle often results.

Arthrography of the ankle helps to determine the exact site and extent of ligamentous injury. This procedure offers few complications but is indicated only when surgical correction of a ruptured ligament is contemplated. To be useful, the technic must be performed within the first few days of trauma, since further delay technically nullifies the procedure.

Treatment

Grade 1: Strapping and elastic bandages, tape, or Unna boot immobilization; elevation, followed by gentle exercise and ambulation.

Grade 2: Below-knee walking cast immobilization for 3 wk.

Grade 3: Cast immobilization or surgery. The role of surgery is controversial because the extreme fragmentation of ligaments makes surgical repair difficult. Some surgeons will cast solitary anterior talofibular ruptures but recommend surgical repair if the fibulocalcaneal ligament also is torn.

Sequelae of Inversion Ankle Sprains

Meniscoid body: As a result of Grade 2 or 3 injuries of the anterior talofibular ligament, impingement of the ligament can occur between the lateral malleolus and talus. Since this ligament is capsular, its lining is synovial and impingement causes persistent synovitis culminating in time with permanent induration and fibrotic swelling. Further immobilization is of little value, but infiltration of insoluble corticosteroids (1/4 ml of triamcinolone acetonide [40 mg/ml] with 3/4 ml of 2% lidocaine with epinephrine) between the talus and the lateral malleolus often yields dramatic and lasting improvement. Surgery is rarely indicated.

Neuralgia of the intermediate dorsal cutaneous nerve, a sensory branch of the superficial peroneal nerve, crosses over the anterior talofibular ligament and is often injured as a result of inversion sprains. Tapping the nerve will often elicit a Tinel sign, and treatment utilizing local anesthetic nerve blocks often yields gratifying results. (See Intermediate Dorsal Cutaneous Nerve, above).

Peroneal tenosynovitis: Chronic swelling below the lateral malleolus resulting from tenosynovitis of the peroneal tendons is seen in individuals who tend to compensate for painful inversion sprains by chronically everting their subtalar joint while walking. In a small percentage of cases, dislocated peroneal tendons resulting from severe ankle sprains may also cause swelling and tenderness.

Sudeck's post-traumatic reflex dystrophy: *Painful swelling of the foot associated with spotty osteoporosis* may result from angiospasms secondary to ankle sprain. The edema often confuses the clinician, and it is sometimes viewed as swelling resulting from a ligamentous injury. Characteristically, in Sudeck's dystrophy the pain appears out of proportion to the clinical findings; multiple trigger points of pain moving from one site to another associated with spotty osteoporosis help characterize the condition.

Sinus tarsi syndrome, *a persistent pain at the sinus tarsi following ankle sprains:* The pathogenesis is unclear. Partial rupture of the interosseous talocalcaneal ligament or stem of the inferior cruciate ligament of the ankle may be implicated. Diagnosis should be reserved for patients who complain of persistent pain in the sinus tarsi and who exhibit pain on palpation. Since the sinus tarsi is normally tender, both ankles should be examined. Since the anterior talofibular ligament is tender near the sinus tarsi, patients with persistent pain over the anterior talofibular mortise are often misdiagnosed as having sinus tarsi pain. **Treatment** consists of infiltration of 1/4 ml of triamcinolone acetonide [40 mg/ml] with 3/4 ml of 2% lidocaine with epinephrine into the sinus tarsi.

§11. NEUROLOGIC DISORDERS

116. THE NEUROLOGIC EXAMINATION

The neurologic history and examination give rapid, accurate information about the condition of the brain, spinal cord, nerves, and muscles. A well-directed, knowledgeable clinical approach to the patient is not only feasible but can sometimes be lifesaving. The patient's mental activity and behavior are functions of the brain, and appraisal of these higher integrative functions is as important a part of the neurologic examination as examination of station and gait, cranial nerves, motor functions, reflexes, and the state of the various special and somatic sensations. Today's precise chemical tests and laboratory procedures may be helpful, but a well-taken history and careful neurologic examination can still provide 90% of the diagnoses in neurology.

Intracranial disorders (increased intracranial pressure, brain tumor, cerebrovascular disease, meningitis), spinal cord diseases (compressive lesions, intrinsic disease), peripheral nerve disorders (mononeuritis, polyneuritis), and myopathies—each presents with a typical cluster of clinical manifestations. Symptoms and signs of these disorders are discussed in the appropriate chapters elsewhere in this section. Evaluation of the unconscious patient is discussed in Ch. 118.

In the **history,** since different disorders can affect the same area of the nervous system producing similar effects, attention should be given to the mode and temporal sequence of onset and course, symptom by symptom, as well as to the overall disorder. Also, many neurologic disorders result in behavioral changes, pain, or disturbances of sensation that are only apparent to the patient (e.g., headache) and have no abnormalities on examination. Both the patient and the physician must have a mutual understanding of the terms that are being used. For example, some patients will use the word "numbness" in different ways and may be expressing concepts such as weakness, incoordination, or clumsiness instead of the loss of sensation. Similarly, terms such as weakness, dizziness, fainting, unsteadiness, and others should be clarified. A neurologic disease may disturb consciousness, memory, and thinking, so it is often necessary to get historical details from those who know the patient. Social factors, geography, recent travel, work, and home environment—all may give useful clues (e.g., exposure to toxins or infectious agents). A thorough **systems review** is important, since many generalized diseases are accompanied by neurologic manifestations. Since many CNS disorders are hereditary, the **family history** is also important.

The examination described here is intended as a thorough initial screening. The history and initial findings will indicate those areas requiring further detailed study. *An organized and systematic approach is essential;* it expedites the examination, helps to avoid omissions, and saves the patient repeated postural changes. The examination may be divided into a series of tests on different systems: (1) **mental status examination and language assessment,** (2) **cranial nerves,** (3) **reflexes,** (4) **motor function,** (5) **sensory function,** (6) **cerebellar function including coordination, station, and gait,** and (7) **cerebrovascular.** Negative as well as positive findings should be recorded as a basis for future comparisons.

The mental status is evaluated during history-taking and after. In most instances the ability of the patient to give an adequate history in proper temporal sequence and to answer questions properly is testimony to preserved intellectual function. The same observation holds for **language assessment.** Inconsistencies and inaccuracies while giving the history may in themselves be significant signs. **Attention, memory,** and **clarity of thought** are further tested by questions on personal and general knowledge (the former verified by another person), by questions on **orientation** in time and place, and by having the patient perform simple calculations (serially subtracting 7, beginning at 100; solving a problem in making change; or 5-min recall of 3 objects). Memory disorders are essentially problems with getting information in, keeping it, and getting the information out. When a memory deficit is apparent, the observer should note whether it applies to all, recent, or remote details.

Language and speech function may be further evaluated by observing the patient's spontaneous conversation for hesitancy or circumlocutions to avoid forgotten words, and by his ability to follow simple spoken and written commands, e.g., to rapidly identify familiar objects and their use, to write a dictated sentence, and to read aloud and explain what he has read. Problems with these simple tasks may indicate that further special tests for **aphasia** are needed. If defects in higher cortical function are suspected on the basis of mental status examination or language assessment, other simple tests can help localize the lesion. Identification of small objects in the hand, e.g., keys or coins, and testing of 2-point discrimination will elicit disturbances of **cortical sensory function.** Copying simple line drawings will give information about the ability to appreciate **spatial relationships.** Performance following simple verbal commands such as taking a match out of a matchbook and lighting it, will provide information about the ability to carry out sequences of movements or **practic function.** Right-left orientation can be checked by simple tests such as asking the patient to place the right hand on the left ear and similar maneuvers.

The patient's **attitude** toward his presenting symptoms as well as his **insight** into his current problems should be investigated; defects in these areas may be due to an emotional disorder, a cognitive deficit, or anosognosia.

Gait, posture, and **balance** may be observed as the examination begins. The patient's normal walking gait is noted for associated movements, the length of the stride, the width of the base with which the patient walks, whether or not there are any extraneous movements, and the proper sequence of movements. The walking patient may give evidence of weakness or spastic disorders of the trunk or legs. A high-stepped gait suggests leg or ankle weakness; a waddling gait, weakness of the pelvic girdle muscles. Difficulty in walking on the toes or heels suggests mild weakness. Diminished arm-swing on one side may indicate a mild hemiparesis or the early stage of Parkinson's disease. Disorders of balance may cause a grossly ataxic gait or, in less severe cases, inability to stand on one leg, or to walk heel-to-toe. Inability to stand with feet together and eyes closed **(Romberg's sign)** indicates posterior column disturbance. **Tandem walking,** i.e., having the patient walk a straight line with one foot placed in front of the other, is an excellent test for balance, and patients with either posterior column disease or cerebellar disease cannot perform this properly. **Abnormal involuntary movements** (the abrupt jerking of chorea; the slow writhing of athetosis or dystonia; a rest or intention tremor) should be noted.

Cranial nerve function is best examined in a sequence that follows the numerical order of the cranial nerves, with certain exceptions. **The 1st cranial nerve (olfactory nerve)** is tested by having the patient identify materials with characteristic odors, e.g., coffee, soap, tobacco, and cloves. Each nostril may be tested separately while occluding the other to give information about the ipsilateral olfactory nerve. (NOTE: The usual complaint in olfactory nerve disturbance is not inability to smell, but disturbance in the sense of taste.)

The **2nd, 3rd, 4th, and 6th cranial nerves** are part of the visual system, which is considered separately under NEURO-OPHTHALMOLOGIC EXAMINATION, below.

The **5th cranial nerve (trigeminal)** has sensory and motor functions. Sensation is tested on the face in all 3 of the nerve's major divisions. Both pin and light touch are tested above the eye, between the eye and the mouth, and below the mouth to the angle of the jaw. **Corneal reflex** testing is extremely useful because there is objective evidence of a sensory response. The cornea is touched lightly, and the resulting blink reflex mediated by the 7th nerve is noted. Motor function of the 5th nerve is tested by palpating the masseter muscles while the mouth is held tightly closed, and noting any deviation of the jaw when the mouth is opened. The jaw tends to deviate to the side of the muscles innervated by the damaged 5th nerve motor portion.

The **7th cranial nerve (facial nerve)** is the major nerve for facial expression. The following are noted and compared on the 2 sides: the ability to wrinkle the forehead, close the eyes tightly, elevate the corners of the mouth, puff out the cheeks, and tense the anterior muscles of the neck as in a grimace. The 7th nerve is part of the efferent portion of the corneal reflex. Sensory testing may also be done, as it supplies taste to the anterior $2/3$ of the tongue. Distinctive-tasting substances are placed on one side of the tongue. The patient must describe the taste before withdrawing the tongue, as the substance will immediately diffuse to the opposite side.

The **8th cranial nerve** has auditory and vestibular portions. Tests to evaluate each function are described in Ch. 164.

Separating out the functions in the **9th (glossopharyngeal)** and **10th (vagus) nerves** is difficult, as many of the motor functions arise from the same nucleus in the brainstem. Elevation of the palate should be noted; it deviates away from the paralyzed side. Gag reflex can be checked by touching the posterior pharyngeal wall on either side of the midline. Comparison of the 2 sides is necessary, as many people have an inactive gag reflex normally. Hoarseness of the voice may indicate some paralysis of the vocal cords, and, if suspected, they should be visualized.

The **11th nerve (spinal accessory)** innervates the sternocleidomastoid muscle and the upper border of the trapezius muscle. Interruption of this nerve can be ascertained by having the patient turn his head to either side while being actively resisted by the examiner's hand. The sternocleidomastoid turns the head to the opposite side; weakness can be picked up by the loss of this movement and by flabbiness on direct palpation of the muscle. With 11th nerve deficit, weakness of the upper border of the trapezius muscle causes the shoulder to droop on the affected side and some weakness on attempting to shrug the shoulder.

The **12th cranial nerve (hypoglossus)** supplies the musculature of the tongue. If it is interrupted, the tongue atrophies on that side and, on protrusion, the tongue deviates to the affected side. Early bilateral involvement may be difficult to ascertain, as there is no deviation of the tongue and mild atrophy may not be apparent.

Deep tendon (muscle stretch) reflex testing gives information about the afferent nerve, the synaptic connections within the spinal cord, and the motor nerves, in addition to information about the descending motor pathways. The principal muscle stretch reflexes with their spinal segments are biceps (C5–6), radial (C6–7), triceps (C7-8), quadriceps (L2–4), and ankle jerk (S1–2). Asymmetry of stretch reflexes as well as bilateral absence or hyperresponse should be noted. Reflexes should not be considered absent unless one cannot elicit them with reinforcement (e.g., in testing the patellar reflex, the patient vigorously locks his hands together and pulls just before the tendon is percussed).

Lesions of the anterior horn cell on out to the muscle decrease muscle stretch reflexes. Central lesions above the anterior horn cell increase the reflexes. **Superficial reflexes** usually tested are the abdominal and cremasteric reflexes. These are diminished with central lesions. The plantar response is an important reflex to test the integrity of the pyramidal tract. Structural or functional disturbance of the pyramidal tract results in the **Babinski response**—extension of the great toe and fanning of the other toes. **Clonus** is the rhythmic, jerking, rapid alternating muscle contraction and relaxation detected by sudden, passive tendon stretching, and can most easily be elicited at the knee and ankle. Patellar clonus may be evoked by sharply pushing the patella towards the foot; ankle clonus by sudden passive dorsiflexion of the foot. Clonus that persists while a sustained stretch is applied suggests damage to pyramidal pathways. **Reflexes that indicate diffuse cortical disease** are the snout reflex, sucking reflex, and grasp reflex.

Muscle tone is determined by noting resistance during passive flexion and extension. Initial resistance followed by relaxation is seen in upper motor neuron disease, lack of tone in lower motor neuron disease, and increased tone or rigidity throughout the movement is seen in Parkinson's disease and some other disorders of the basal ganglia.

Examination of the motor system is described further below in Approach to the Patient with Muscle Weakness.

Sensory testing is difficult for the patient and the examiner. A full explanation should be given to the patient so that he or she understands the purpose and how to respond. If there is a specific complaint of sensory disturbance or a defect is demonstrated, more exhaustive sensory testing can be carried out.

With the patient's eyes closed, testing begins with a bilateral pinprick survey of the face, neck, arms, trunk, and legs (asking the patient when he feels the stimulus, as well as whether the 2 stimuli feel the same, so as not to suggest the answer), in order to find differences between the 2 sides, a level below which sensation is lost, and areas of hypesthesia or anesthesia.

The examination is continued with **bilateral tests of joint position and postural sense** (by having the patient say whether the terminal phalanges of fingers, then toes, are being moved upwards or down—very small movements can normally be identified, and if even large movements cause confusion, the other joints should be tested, progressing proximally) and of **vibration** (using a 128-cycle tuning fork, applied to the ankle and wrist bones for a quick check, then elsewhere if the vibrations are not felt). **Light touch** may be tested with a cotton ball or the examiner's finger; **heat** and **cold** with water in test tubes. Questions about **paresthesias** are appropriate here, since these commonly accompany distortion of cutaneous sensory function. **Stereognosis,** which involves central interpretation as well as peripheral sensation, may also be tested at this time by having the patient identify objects placed first in each hand, then in both hands simultaneously.

With abnormalities of cutaneous sensation, one should distinguish the patterns created by lesions of particular nerve roots or of single or multiple peripheral nerves (glove-stocking distribution), or by central disorders involving the brain (hemisensory pattern) or spinal cord (level lesion). Repeating the sensory examination on several occasions helps establish a consistent pattern of sensory disturbance. One should map altered areas in detail, proceeding from insensitive to normal zones (for

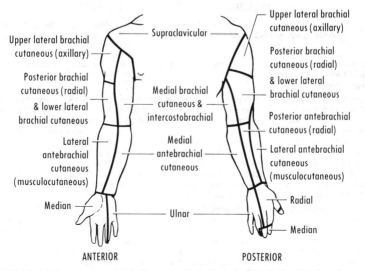

Fig. 116–1a. **Cutaneous nerve distribution: upper limb.** (Redrawn from E. Gardner, D. J. Gray, and R. O'Rahilly, *Anatomy,* ed. 4, 1975. Copyright 1975 by W. B. Saunders Company. Used with permission.)

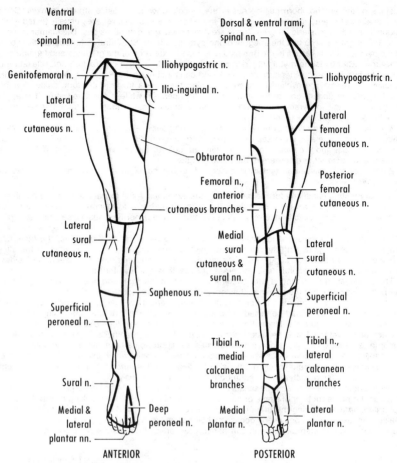

Fig. 116–1b. **Cutaneous nerve distribution: lower limb.** (Redrawn from E. Gardner, D. J. Gray, and R. O'Rahilly, *Anatomy*, ed. 4, 1975. Copyright 1975 by W. B. Saunders Company. Used with permission.)

more accurate boundary determinations), and carefully record the results; a knowledge of the peripheral nerve distributions (Figs. 116–1a and 116–1b), segmental dermatomes (Fig. 116–2), and central sensory pathways is essential.

Coordination of movements depends on the integrity of the motor, sensory, and cerebellar systems. It is checked by having the patient put his index finger to his nose with his eyes open, then closed. Inaccurate placing both times suggests cerebellar disease; if correct only with the eyes open, kinesthetic sensory loss is the likely cause. Fine coordination can be checked by having the patient undo and do up buttons, or open and close a safety pin. Rapidly alternating movements of the hands and feet, with sudden changes in speed and direction, will also test coordination. Defects may be due to cerebellar disease or to pyramidal tract disturbances. With the patient supine and his eyes first open, then closed, leg coordination is evaluated by the toe-finger and heel-knee test (the patient touches the examiner's finger with his toe, then his own opposite knee with his heel) and by the heel-shin test (the patient runs his heel up and down the opposite shin).

Cerebrovascular assessment: Palpation of the carotid arteries is often not useful, and vigorous palpation may indeed be dangerous. Auscultation of the carotid arteries is a much better test for stenotic lesions. The bell of the stethoscope is applied stepwise along the length of the carotid arteries in the neck. Also, the supraclavicular arteries are auscultated. Stenotic lesions will often produce a high-pitched bruit. These should be traced down the neck to be certain that the bruit is not emanating from the heart. Auscultation over the orbit and the cranium may reveal a bruit, usually caused by arteriovenous malformations, more rarely by a carotid-cavernous sinus fistula or a tumor. In children, bruits have much less significance. Occasionally, with occlusion of the carotid artery in

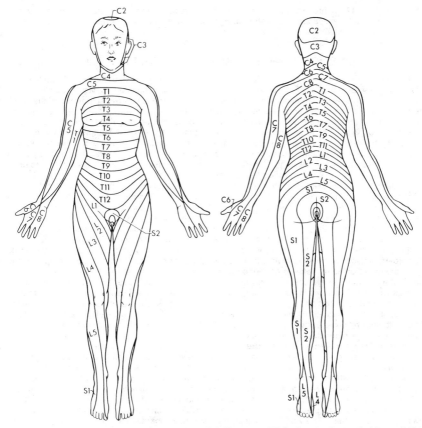

FIG. 116–2.   The dermatomes. (Redrawn from J. J. Keegan and F. D. Garrett, *Anatomical Record* Vol. 102, pp. 409–437, Sept.–Dec. 1948. Used with permission of The Wistar Institute.)

the neck, collateral circulation may be established from the external carotid system to the internal system, resulting in exaggerated pulsations of certain small external arteries over the face. These arteries are the supraorbital just above the midportion of the orbit, the trochlear between the internal canthus of the eye and the base of the nose, and the angular in the region of the nasolabial fold. In a patient with spinal cord disease, auscultation should be done over the affected area, as rarely there may be bruit over a vascular malformation.

The **general physical examination** may provide etiologic clues to a neurologic disorder. A stiff neck may indicate meningeal irritation. A distended bladder may have a neurogenic cause. Skin lesions may indicate neurocutaneous disorders, dermatomyositis, meningococcal meningitis, or SLE. A red, smooth tongue suggests pernicious anemia. Exterior abnormalities of the skull or spine may indicate associated brain or cord disease. Adenopathy or masses in the neck, abdomen, pelvis, or rectum may suggest a metastatic tumor. A heart murmur with cerebrovascular disease suggests SBE.

The history and physical examination are complemented by **laboratory aids,** which should generally progress from the harmless to the more hazardous: for cerebral disorders, CT scan, EEG, and chest and skull x-rays, followed if needed by cerebral arteriography or pneumoencephalography (echoencephalography or radioactive brain scan will seldom be of additional use if CT scanning is available); for peripheral nerve and myoneural disorders, serum enzyme determinations (SGOT, CPK, lactic dehydrogenase isoenzymes), electromyography (EMG), and muscle biopsy; for spinal cord disease, lumbar puncture, manometric testing, and myelography.

Lumbar puncture (see Ch. 117) in patients with intracranial disease is controversial, since it is essential in the diagnosis of many disorders, but its effect on CSF pressure in the presence of intracranial mass lesions may cause potentially fatal shifts in the brain tissues. Papilledema alone does not necessarily contraindicate a spinal puncture, but calls for judicious caution. CSF examination (see Ch. 117 for procedure) may be omitted if physical or laboratory signs of an intracranial mass are present (e.g., papilledema *and* focal signs; evidence on CT scan, brain scan, echoencephalograms, or skull films).

NEURO-OPHTHALMOLOGIC EXAMINATION

Examination of the visual system gives information about many parts of the nervous system. For example, assessment of the function of the optic nerve, chiasm, optic tracts, visual radiations, and visual cortex provides information about lesions occurring in the anterior-posterior axis of the brain. By checking ocular movements and pupillary action, lesions can be located along the superior-inferior axis in the brainstem and in the cerebellum. Information may be gained about the function of the 2nd through the 8th cranial nerves, and data about the intactness of the autonomic system in the brain, the brainstem, spinal cord, and peripheral autonomic nerves. Also, proper funduscopic examination provides information about intracranial pressure, the presence of various neurologic and systemic diseases, and knowledge of the cerebrovascular system. Most of the testing can be done easily and does not require specialized equipment.

Visual acuity is checked in each eye with a standard wall chart or convenient hand-held chart. Each eye is tested individually. From a neurologic standpoint, it is important to ascertain the best possible vision; the patient's glasses should therefore be used. If there is a refractive error and no correction is available, the patient may read through a pinhole in a card, which will minimize the refractive problem. If the vision cannot be quantitated by these means, some statement of acuity should be noted, such as the ability to count fingers at a certain distance or the ability to distinguish light. The baseline should be established, as there may be sudden changes in visual acuity in some disorders, particularly those involving the vascular system or compressive lesions of the optic nerve.

Assessment of visual fields is performed by confrontation examination. The examiner faces the patient who, with one eye covered, fixes his gaze on the examiner's eye. The examiner then slowly brings wiggling fingers from the periphery into each of the 4 visual quadrants; the patient reports when the finger first becomes visible. This gross test will miss subtle visual field defects. It is best to use smaller targets, such as red or blue match heads. If this is done carefully, even the normal physiologic blind spots can be detected. If defects are picked up, careful mapping of the visual fields with quantitative perimetric studies should be done.

Extraocular eye movements are checked by having the patient fix on the physician's finger, which is moved to the extreme gaze horizontally, upward, downward, and then in diagonal directions to either side. The extent of the movements should be noted in all these directions of gaze. The patient should be asked whether or not he sees double. With minimal nerve or muscle involvement, often the defect is not apparent by external observation, but does result in diplopia for the patient. If diplopia is reported in one direction, the eyes are individually occluded, and the patient is asked which of the 2 images disappears, the peripheral one or the near one. The following 2 rules apply to ascertain the weak muscle or affected nerve: (1) the objects increase their separation when moving in the direction of the affected movement; and (2) the image seen with the defectively moving eye is always the most peripheral. For example, if moving the finger horizontally to the patient's left results in an increasing separation of the fingers, then one must conclude that either the left lateral rectus or the right medial rectus is involved. If, on occluding the left eye, the most peripheral image disappears, one can conclude that the fault is with the left lateral rectus. Also, the patient will tend to turn or tilt his head in the direction of the faulty eye movement so that diplopia is minimized.

In checking the eye movements, observations also can be made about the presence of **nystagmus.** Nystagmus on extreme lateral gaze which fatigues quickly is usually physiologic. If it is sustained, then it should be described in regard to the direction of fast and slow component, and to its character as regular, irregular, rotatory, or some other descriptive term. Also, the degree of involvement of either eye should be noted.

Pupillary size, equality, and regularity should be noted, as well as **pupillary reactions to light and accommodation.** The "swinging flashlight test" should be used routinely in order to detect an afferent lesion of the optic nerve. The lighted flashlight is swung slowly from one eye to the other, noting the pupillary light response. Normally, the pupils should react by constriction promptly and equally on both sides. If there is an afferent lesion of one optic nerve, then there is a paradoxic dilation of that pupil as the light is brought to that side. This occurs because escape from the consensual light reflex is still progressing and the direct light reflex in the presence of even a very slight optic nerve lesion is not great enough to overcome it; hence, the paradoxic dilation.

The presence or absence of **ptosis** should be noted and quantitated by measuring the distance of the palpebral fissures. In oculosympathetic paresis **(Horner's syndrome)** one pupil is small and minor degrees of ptosis may be noted.

The presence or absence of **exophthalmos** can be ascertained by inspecting the eyes from above by looking down on the head. Information about the 5th and 7th nerve is learned from checking the **corneal response,** and noting the ability to blink the eyes. Often, the first sign of 7th-nerve involvement is a decrease in blinking on the affected side.

Opticokinetic nystagmus (so-called "railroad nystagmus") is a nystagmus induced by the passage of patterned vision in front of the eye, providing a useful test. Various types of tapes are made for this purpose but, essentially, they have a regular sequence pattern, such as black and white stripes. A standard tape measure is passed in front of the patient's field of vision with instruction to the patient to count the numbers as they move rapidly in front. This can be passed from left to right, right to left, and repeated in the vertical direction. Patients with field defects, for example, will have decreased opticokinetic nystagmus when the tape is moving from the affected to the intact visual field. It is also helpful to rule in or out hysterical blindness.

Neuro-ophthalmologic tests in checking brainstem function in a patient with depressed responsivity are valuable and simple. Instillation of 5 ml ice water into the ear canal should elicit forced deviation of the eyes conjugately to the same side. This implies that the nerve pathway from the labyrinth through the brainstem to the nuclei controlling those eye movements, and the peripheral mechanism responsible for those eye movements, are intact. Similarly, rapid turning of the head will result in a lag of eye movement as if the gaze were fixed. This is followed by a slow drift back to central fixation. This is known as the **"doll's eye" response,** and implies intact brainstem mechanisms, if present.

Funduscopic examination should include observations of the optic nerve, blood vessels, and appearance of the retina to detect papilledema, optic atrophy, vascular disease, retinitis, or other disorders. Papilledema usually implies an increase in intracranial pressure and shows up as blurring and disappearance of the disk margins, elevation of the nerve head, absence of pulsation of retinal vessels, and, occasionally, hemorrhages and exudates. It is important to survey the retinal vessels in cases of stroke, as often small emboli can be picked up in the vessels. Other characteristic findings in various disorders are included in specific disease sections of this volume.

APPROACH TO THE PATIENT WITH MUSCLE WEAKNESS

Weakness is a common complaint of many disorders, ranging from muscle to psychiatric disorders. The exact complaint of the patient must be characterized, since weakness may mean different things to the patient, including fatigue, clumsiness, or numbness. The exact location, the time of occurrence, precipitating and ameliorating factors, and associated symptoms and signs are important. Examination of muscles is only part of the neurologic examination which, in turn, is only a part of the general examination. Isolated muscle testing without a complete examination will lead to grave diagnostic and therapeutic errors.

Synthesizing data from the history, physical examination, and pertinent laboratory tests should differentiate between upper and lower motor neuron disease. In the latter disease, the location of the disorder can be localized at the anterior horn cell, peripheral nerve, neuromuscular junction, or within the muscle itself. To make these distinctions, knowledge about associated sensory findings, muscle tone, cerebellar function, and tendon reflexes is necessary (see above). Specific examination of muscles includes observation, palpation, and strength testing. TABLES 116–1 and 116–2 summarize some of the main differentiating elements.

Observation of muscles provides information about the presence or absence of atrophy, hypertrophy, and extraneous movements. While the patient is seated, and with the extremities in the resting position, the muscles are examined for bulk, contour, and fasciculation. **Atrophy** is evident by decreased muscle bulk, but with large or concealed muscles this may not be obvious until quite advanced. When the atrophy is bilateral, it may not be obvious when comparing one side with the other; in older people, some loss of muscle bulk is common. **Hypertrophy** occurs when one muscle works harder substituting for another, or there may be **pseudohypertrophy** when muscle tissue is replaced by excessive fibrous tissue or some storage material. The commonest extraneous movements are **fasciculations,** *brief, fine, irregular twitches of the muscle visible under the skin.* Fasciculations usually indicate disease of the lower motor neuron, but can sometimes occur in normals, particularly in the calf muscles of older people. **Myotonia** is the decreased relaxation of muscle following a sustained contraction or direct percussion of the muscle itself. It is particularly seen in myotonic dystrophy and may cause a disability due, for example, to inability to relax and quickly open the closed hand.

Palpation of muscle may reveal atrophy, the presence of fasciculations, tenderness, or an abnormal consistency.

Assessment of strength is essential to establish weakness, localize it, and quantitate it for subsequent changes. The patient extends his arms, and next his legs, to be inspected for weakness (a weak limb will soon begin to sag) and for tremor or other involuntary movements. Strength of specific

TABLE 116–1. MUSCLE WEAKNESS: UPPER VS. LOWER NEURON DISEASE

	Upper Motor Neuron Disease (UMN)	Lower Motor Neuron Disease (LMN)
Reflexes	Hyperactive	Diminished or absent
Atrophy	Absent	Present
Fasciculations	Absent	Present
Tone	Increased	Decreased or absent

TABLE 116-2. MUSCLE WEAKNESS: NEUROGENIC VS. MYOGENIC

Neurogenic Weakness	Myogenic Weakness
Wasting out of proportion to weakness	Weakness out of proportion to wasting
Fasciculations	No fasciculations
Reflexes often absent with minimal weakness (amyotrophic lateral sclerosis is an exception)	Reflexes often present with severe weakness
May have sensory changes	No sensory changes

muscle groups may be tested against resistance. Pain in a muscle or involved joint may preclude an active contraction, which complicates testing. Hysterical weakness or malingering may be difficult to evaluate, but usually there is a "giveaway" reaction in which resistance to movement may be quite normal, but the subject suddenly gives way. The absence of atrophy and the presence of normal reflexes also help in these diagnoses.

Grading muscle strength is done in a number of ways. One of the most universal grading systems is: 0 = no movement; 1 = flicker or trace of contraction; 2 = active movement when gravity is eliminated; 3 = active movement against gravity; 4 = active movement against gravity and resistance; and 5 = normal power. While this system has some exactness, it frequently tells little about the functional capacity of the patient. Often, functional testing gives a better picture of the disability. This can be accomplished by having the patient perform various maneuvers and noting any deficiencies. Arising from a squatting position or stepping onto a chair gives good indication of proximal leg strength; standing on the heels, then the toes, tests distal strength. Hand grip strength should also be noted. A patient with quadriceps weakness has to push off with the arms to get out of a chair. Some patients with weakness of the shoulder girdle swing their bodies to move the arms passively to other positions. Patients with weakness about the pelvic girdle characteristically arise from the supine position by first turning prone, then kneeling and slowly pushing themselves erect by standing bent forward and using the arms to climb up the thighs.

117. DIAGNOSTIC PROCEDURES

CT Scan (see in Ch. 225)

Echoencephalography

This procedure was one of the earliest applications of diagnostic ultrasonography and was first proved to be practical in 1954 using A-mode technics. In the adult, ultrasonography in A mode is used very little except to detect midline shift or ventricular size on a screening basis. Attenuation by the skull and the echo reverberations within the skull prevent its use for displaying an anatomic picture of intracranial structures. CT scanning is the method of choice for brain imaging in adults. In contrast, in children < 2 yr where attenuation by the skull is negligible, ultrasonography is most effective in displaying the ventricular system and intracranial anatomy. Under age 2, tissue patterns for specific ultrasonic scans can be done rapidly, usually without need for anesthesia (required for CT scanning).

Other diagnostic applications of ultrasonography in the head include the study of intracranial pulsations, their distribution patterns, and their contours. Some investigators believe that the slope of the pulsatile wave pattern can be correlated with rate of blood flow in a specific area.

Radionuclide Imaging (see also Ch. 227)

Radionuclide scanning provides substantially less information than CT scanning, and its use has declined proportionately where CT instruments are available. When CT cannot be obtained, radionuclide imaging gives about an 80 to 85% rate of accuracy in detecting intracranial masses. The effectiveness of the procedure depends on injury to the capillary membranes of the blood-brain barrier, through which radioactive molecules injected into the bloodstream "leak" and concentrate in abnormal sites. The findings on scanning may direct angiographic studies to a particular part of the brain and are sometimes useful in postoperative situations when CT is unavailable and repetitive radiocontrast studies are impractical.

Neoplasms, including meningioma, glioblastoma multiforme, and metastatic lesions from breast and lung, are readily and accurately detected. The more differentiated tumors are detectable at a lower frequency. Certain low-grade, less common astrocytomas may not be detected. Lesions < 2 cm in diameter and posterior fossa tumors are not usually detected. Pituitary tumors and craniopharyngiomas must be large enough to invade the brain before they are detectable. Abscesses and granulomas are rarely missed by brain scan.

In cases of head trauma, isotope scanning is decidedly inferior to CT scanning, but if the latter is unavailable, has about a 70% accuracy in detecting hematomas, contusions or, occasionally, severe cerebral edema.

Radionuclide scanning is of less diagnostic assistance in the diagnosis of cerebral vascular disease, especially in identifying arteriovenous (A-V) malformations.

CSF kinetics and distribution of isotope over the convexities after intrathecal injections of indium 111 DTPA has been evaluated by isotope scanning in efforts to diagnose surgically treatable hydrocephalus. Unfortunately, correlation between scan results and clinical postoperative outcome has been only moderately good. Variations of this technic have been used to evaluate shunt patency postoperatively.

Cerebral Angiography

With the advent of accurate CT scanning technics, cerebral angiography has increasingly become a supplementary technic, relied upon especially for identifying the site and nature of cerebral vascular lesions and to gain information about the vascularity and possible nature of intracranial neoplasms.

Catheterization of the femoral, axillary, or brachial artery with flexible catheters that can be threaded into the carotid or vertebral arteries has generally replaced percutaneous puncture of the cerebral vessels in the neck. The technic minimizes trauma to atherosclerotic vessels. An intimate knowledge of the cerebral vasculature is necessary for interpretation. Angiography (1) provides information on thrombotic lesions of both cervical and intracranial vessels and almost always precedes consideration of direct surgical approach, such as carotid endarterectomy; (2) may establish the site and source of bleeding in subarachnoid hemorrhage (e.g., intracranial aneurysm, A-V malformation, or vascular tumor); (3) supplies information about blood supply and pattern in intracranial neoplasms.

Most angiograms are performed with local anesthesia at the injection or insertion site. Mild sedation with a barbiturate or diazepam is useful. The cooperation of the patient is necessary to prevent unnecessary movement and for positioning. The injection of the radiopaque material is usually accompanied by a burning sensation in the head, and the patient should be warned of this. The procedure has a relatively low incidence of complications in experienced hands. However, transient and even permanent neurologic deficits can result in as many as 2 to 3% of patients, so that the procedure should generally be reserved for those in whom surgery is contemplated or in whom the diagnosis is not established. A previous history of sensitivity to contrast material requires special preparations or even avoiding the procedure.

Myelography

Myelography demonstrates both intrinsic and extrinsic spinal cord lesions and, less commonly, intracranial lesions or those at the craniocervical junction. A radiopaque material (e.g., iophendylate, metrizamide) or, less commonly, a gas is introduced into the subarachnoid space via a lumbar puncture. With the patient on a tilt table, the material is maneuvered to the suspected area under fluoroscopic control. Appropriate spot films are taken for later viewing and study. Non–water-soluble radiopaque materials are usually removed by aspiration after the study; newer soluble agents need not be removed. Newer technics combine metrizamide injection with cranial or spinal CT scanning to clarify the nature of difficult-to-diagnose lesions.

Myelography is particularly useful to diagnose tumors of or adjacent to the spinal cord, diseases of the intervertebral disk spaces, and spondylytic lesions of the vertebral column. Contraindications to myelography are the same as those for spinal puncture (see below). The procedure of myelography may worsen the effects of a complete spinal canal block. In such instances the patient's neurologic status must be closely watched; occasionally emergency decompressive surgery is necessary.

Electroencephalography (EEG)

The EEG records the electrical activity of the brain's cellular and nerve tract activity, which may be altered by numerous structural and functional changes. Electrical activity in either 8 or 16 locations or pairs of locations is recorded simultaneously by scalp electrodes, usually small metal disks connected by wires to an amplifier. The resultant wave form is recorded in ink on a moving paper strip. Electrode placement is important to assure that similar areas on both sides of the scalp be recorded and that the placement be similar on repeated examinations and for different patients. For example, the International 10–20 System refers to 10 and 20% of distances either along the sagittal line between the nasion and inion, or along the circumference, and in intermediate locations. Uniform lettering and numbering is used, as shown in FIGS. 117–1a and 117–1b.

Recording is done with the patient relaxed and his eyes closed, and reports describe the wave forms recorded. The predominant normal adult wave form is the α rhythm (8 to 13 cycles/second), most prominent in the occipital region. Other wave frequencies are designated as δ (1 to 4 cycles/second), θ (5 to 8), and β ($>$ 13). Generally, it is desirable to record during a relaxed, drowsy, and sleep period and also a period of 3 min of hyperventilation and photic stimulation at various frequencies. Since a variety of natural and unnatural states affect the EEG, knowledge of the patient's clinical condition and responsiveness (e.g., sleeping, comatose, alert) is necessary. For patients who have seizures in sleep, some portion of the recording should be taken during sleep; patients suspected of having temporal lobe seizures may require recording from the medial aspect of

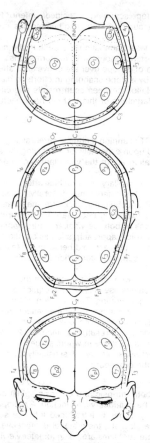

FIG. 117–1a. **Standard electrode placement: Frontal, superior, and posterior views.** (Redrawn from "Appendix: The Ten–Twenty Electrode System of the International Federation" in *Electroencephalography and Clinical Neurophysiology* 10:374, 1958. Used with permission of Elsevier/North Holland Biomedical Press, Amsterdam.)

the temporal lobe by means of nasopharyngeal electrodes in order to demonstrate an abnormality. In certain instances "activation" procedures are used to bring out abnormal patterns. Some of these (e.g., hyperventilation, stroboscopic light stimulation) are easily accomplished. Others, such as sleep deprivation, require planning prior to the test.

The EEG is particularly useful in diagnosing seizure disorders (any patient with a transient disturbance in responsiveness is a candidate). The EEG may provide supplementary information in diagnosing or following the course of patients with metabolic disturbances accompanied by altered mentation, as well as various structural disorders, such as hemorrhage, tumor, degenerative, and infectious diseases. The EEG provides confirmatory information in the diagnosis of brain death and one should probably always have evidence of an isoelectric tracing before making such a diagnosis as an antecedent to organ transplantation. This latter admonition is dependent on local statutes, some states accepting "brain death" while others do not.

Measurement of Cortical Evoked Responses

This is a special application of the EEG in which stimulation of a sensory system (e.g., visual, auditory, somatosensory) activates the nerve tracts linking the receptor and cortical sensory area, resulting in a cortical potential. Ordinarily, these potentials are small and masked by other activity. However, when a series of stimuli are given (usually ≥ 50) and the recordings are superimposed, they summate into a detectable wave form. This can be done electronically to display the stimulus and the following wave form.

Sensory responses of any type are difficult to quantify clinically, as the patient is the observer and reporter. Sensory evoked responses eliminate the subjective factors. However, the requesting physi-

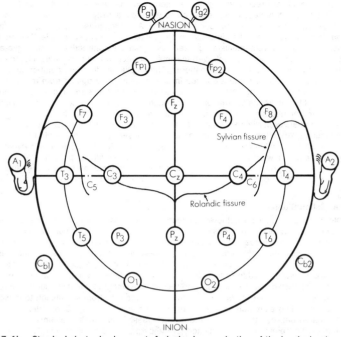

Fig. 117–1b. **Standard electrode placement: A single plane projection of the head,** showing all standard positions and the location of the Rolandic and Sylvian fissures. The outer circle was drawn at the level of the nasion and inion. The inner circle represents the temporal line of electrodes. This diagram provides a useful stamp for the indication of electrode placements in routine recording. (Redrawn from "Appendix: The Ten–Twenty Electrode System of the International Federation" in *Electroencephalography and Clinical Neurophysiology* 10:374, 1958. Used with permission of Elsevier/North Holland Biomedical Press, Amsterdam.)

cian must indicate the clinical condition and explain what information is desired. This technic, rapidly expanding in clinical use, is improving diagnostic capability in neurologic diseases that affect sensory systems.

The method has been most often used to evaluate **visual evoked responses (VER)**. The patient fixes on a point, and a visual stimulus, usually a rapid alternating checkerboard pattern, is used for the stimulus. Recording is done with EEG scalp electrodes over the occipital or visual cortex area. The display provides the time interval between the stimulus and the response, and the wave form. In certain diseases (e.g., cryptic or past retrobulbar neuritis) in which little abnormality can be detected by other means, stimulation evokes an unusually long conduction time along the optic pathways.

Auditory evoked responses (AER) are more complex, and reflect the complicated auditory conducting system with its many synapses and tracts. Since this system is distributed along the brainstem, AER are useful in detecting abnormalities in the brainstem, an area that generally eludes other diagnostic means. The evoked response method has also been applied to somatosensory systems, to identify lesions at various levels in the CNS.

Electromyography (EMG)

EMG records the electrical potentials of a muscle with electrodes, usually consisting of a fine wire within a 24-gauge hollow needle. The electrical activity is amplified and displayed on a cathode ray oscilloscope, and a permanent record is obtained by photographing the display or by recording on a magnetic tape. Usually a parallel output is fed into a loudspeaker. Some pain accompanies insertion of the needle, and the patient must be so informed.

The technic is useful in detecting 3 classes of disease: disease involving the lower motor neuron from the anterior horn cell to the neuromuscular junction, defects in transmission at the neuromuscular junction, and primary muscle disease. It also provides an evaluation following nerve damage. The electromyographer must be supplied with exact clinical information so that the EMG examination can be directed appropriately. Judgments regarding the extent of nerve and muscle involvement can then be made: e.g., whether it is generalized or localized; if localized, the distribution of affected muscle groups may indicate segmental, root, plexus, or nerve involvement.

Electrical potentials are recorded during the insertion of the needle, with the muscle at rest, and during contraction of the muscle. Normally, some electrical activity occurs when the needle is inserted. Repetitive discharges may be seen in myotonia. A relaxed muscle is electrically silent. Fibrillation and fasciculations may be detected in the relaxed denervated muscle. During voluntary contraction, muscle action potentials are present. With minimal contraction, often single-action potentials can be detected and analyzed. With maximal contraction in a normal muscle, the individual potentials fuse to form an "interference pattern." The amplitude, duration, number, and configuration of the muscle action potential are noted in differentiating neurogenic from myogenic involvement, an often useful role of EMG. In myogenic weakness, the size of the action potential is decreased, with little decrease in number. In neurogenic weakness, the action potential size usually is normal, but the numbers are decreased. Typical patterns are illustrated in Fig. 117–2.

Following complete or partial nerve damage, it is essential to know the sequence of changes in the innervated muscle. At first the only change noted is the absence or decrease of muscle contraction noted on the EMG. Fibrillation potentials begin to appear with the insertion or movement of the recording needle after a week or so. In 2 to 4 wk, spontaneous fibrillation potentials appear. Sequential examinations may show a decrease of fibrillations as reinnervation takes place, and the emergence of low amplitude, often polyphasic, action potentials which gradually develop more normal patterns.

Nerve Stimulation Studies

Valuable information can be gathered by recording an electric shock stimulus of a peripheral nerve and muscle contraction response. Both motor and sensory nerves can be tested. The physician performing the test needs full clinical information about the location and nature of the illness and often must devise innovative technics to fit special circumstances. Nerve stimulation testing may be uncomfortable; the nature and necessity of the test must be fully explained to the patient.

Motor nerve testing: A surface-stimulating electrode is placed over the appropriate nerve and either a needle or surface electrode is used to record. Movement of the stimulating electrode along the nerve determines the site of nerve injury; measuring the time from stimulation to muscle activation from 2 stimulating sites determines the nerve conduction velocity. Conduction velocities can also be compared between the affected and normal sides. Similar measurements may be made for **sensory nerves.** These methods are depicted for the carpal tunnel syndrome in Fig. 117–3.

When weakness is due to muscle disease, nerve conduction velocities remain normal. In disease affecting peripheral nerves, conduction is often slow, and the response patterns may show a dispersion of the potentials due to unequal involvement of the nerve axons. Observation of muscle action

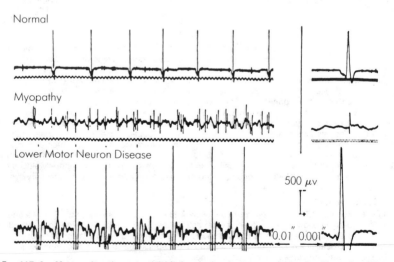

Fig. 117–2. **Motor unit action potentials during weak voluntary contraction** (m. biceps brachii) in a normal person, in progressive muscular dystrophy (myopathy), and in amyotrophic lateral sclerosis (lower motor neuron disease). Action potentials on the left are recorded with a slow time base (time signal is 100 cycles/second). Action potentials on the right are recorded with a more rapid time base (time signal is 1,000 cycles/second). (Redrawn from Mayo Clinic: *Clinical Examinations in Neurology*, ed. 4, 1976, p. 312. Copyright 1976 by W. B. Saunders Company. Used with permission of W. B. Saunders Company and the Mayo Foundation.)

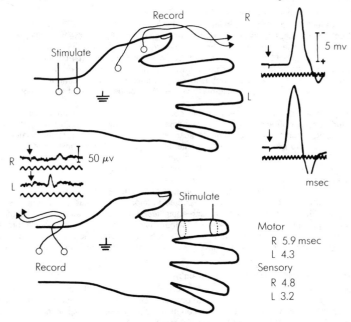

Fig. 117–3.   **Latency of muscle and nerve action potentials in right carpal tunnel syndrome.** Nerve action potentials evoked by stimulation of digital nerves in index finger are detected by surface electrodes over median nerve at wrist. The action potentials of thenar muscles evoked by stimulation of the median nerve at the wrist are recorded by surface electrodes over belly and tendon of abductor pollicis brevis. Latency of both responses (to start of muscle action potential and to peak of nerve action potential) is prolonged on the right side. (Redrawn from Mayo Clinic: *Clinical Examinations in Neurology*, ed. 4, 1976, p. 324. Copyright 1976 by W. B. Saunders Company. Used with permission of W. B. Saunders Company and the Mayo Foundation.)

potentials during repetitive stimulation of a nerve is used to study the fatigability of the muscle in diseases of the neuromuscular junction. In myasthenia gravis, for example, the action potential shows a progressive decremental response.

Electronystagmography (ENG)

The degree and direction of nystagmus can be quantitated with ENG, using the retinal/corneal (negative/positive) voltage differences in the eye, which acts as a dipole. The direction of this dipole can be measured with standard EEG electrodes placed on either side of the eye in the direction of the eye movement. The potential is amplified and recorded with a pen writer. Various means to elicit the nystagmus can be applied, e.g., caloric testing and position changes. Medications such as diazepam that suppress eye movement must be discontinued many hours prior to the test.

Detection of Visual Field Defects

Major defects in the visual fields may be detected by confrontation in the neurologic examination (see Ch. 116). If a defect is detected, its more exact delineation is required. The site of a lesion from the retina back to the visual cortex can be determined and serial observations used to follow the progression or resolution of lesions. Two methods are used: perimetry, which records the total extent of the visual field, and tangent screen, which records the central visual field from the point of fixation out to 30°.

In **perimetric testing,** the subject fixes on a central point, and a white test object is moved out along an arc. Each eye is tested separately. The point at which the object disappears is noted, and then the object is brought back into the seeing field; this is recorded. The arc is then rotated and another meridian is checked. The process usually is repeated at 30° or lesser intervals to define the defect. Test objects of varying sizes are used. The data are presented on a chart of concentric circles with radii at 30° intervals.

Tangent screen testing is done with a flat surface, usually black, on a wall 1 m from the subject. A wand with the test object at the tip is moved out along meridians from the central fixation point to 30°. Test objects of varying sizes and colors can be used to outline the field and any scotomas. The density of a defect is determined by comparing the defect obtained with varying-sized test objects. The information is presented similarly to that of perimetry.

Noninvasive Measurement of Extracranial Arterial Disease

Noninvasive technics can be divided into 2 categories:

1. **Indirect technics** that assess the functional hemodynamics distal to the bifurcation of the common carotid artery. These include ophthalmodynamometry, oculopneumoplethysmography, thermography, and directional Doppler flow studies. **Oculoplethysmography (OPG)** is the most useful of the indirect tests in detecting carotid lesions that cause a reduction in blood flow to the ipsilateral orbit when compared to flow in the opposite eye. Nonstenotic lesions cannot be identified and bilateral stenotic lesions may give false-negative results. Occlusion cannot be distinguished from stenosis.

2. **Direct technics** that outline the anatomic configurations of the extracranial carotid arteries. These include Doppler ultrasonic scanning, real-time B-scan imaging, and phonoangiography.

Direct imaging technics, such as B-mode scanning, that can demonstrate the anatomy of the carotid bifurcation are promising new developments. Small ulcerated lesions that do not compromise blood flow distally can be imaged. Obese patients and those with anatomic variations pose difficulties for this technic. Calcifications in the arterial wall may give false-positive images, while a fresh occluding thrombus may give a false-negative result.

Improvements in these technics and development of additional procedures such as computer-enhanced IV contrast angiography may be expected to improve the reliability of noninvasive tests.

Noninvasive studies are most useful as screening tests to evaluate patients with asymptomatic carotid bruits, patients with puzzling symptoms that may or may not be due to cerebrovascular disease, and to follow patients after carotid endarterectomy to detect recurrence or progression of disease. Arteriography remains the definitive diagnostic test for patients with symptomatic cerebrovascular disease.

Cerebrospinal Fluid (CSF) Collection and Examination

Lumbar puncture is performed most often to obtain a CSF specimen for diagnostic study (see TABLE 117–1); it is used also to administer radiopaque material or to give medications intrathecally. Possible **contraindications** include local infection near the puncture site, papilledema (or other signs of increased CSF pressure), and coagulation disorders.

The patient lies on his side at the edge of a firm bed or table with knees drawn up and head bent forward to put the spine in hyperflexion (see FIG. 117–4). The usual site for lumbar puncture is the midline between the 3rd and 4th (or 4th and 5th) lumbar vertebrae; palpation will locate the depression between the vertebrae. The area should be cleansed with an antiseptic and locally anesthetized, first by hypodermic and then by deep injection.

The lumbar puncture needle (3 to 3½ in., 20- to 22-gauge) is inserted through the skin in the midline between the vertebrae, perpendicular to the surface of the back, and directed slightly upward toward the patient's head. If it impinges on bone, it should be withdrawn and aimed in a slightly different direction. The bevel of the needle should face laterally so as to separate the fibers of the ligaments and the dura without tearing them. When the needle penetrates the dura and enters the spinal canal, a slight easing of resistance can be felt. The stylet of the needle is then withdrawn, and drops of CSF will appear. With the needle in place, the CSF pressure is read on a manometer before and after removing fluid.

A procedure now seldom employed is the **Queckenstedt test,** designed to determine the presence or absence of hydrostatic block. Bilateral pressure is exerted on the jugular veins, hampering the egress of blood from the cranium and thereby increasing intracranial pressure. This, in turn, increases the pressure within the spinal canal rostral to the needle if there is no obstruction. Generally speaking, the Queckenstedt test gives little information that cannot better be obtained by other technics and *should not be performed when increased intracranial pressure or a spinal block is suspected,* since the increased pressure may produce cerebral or cerebellar herniation with serious consequences.

The amount of CSF withdrawn is equal to the volume of fluid to be introduced or is sufficient for the laboratory investigation planned. Drugs to be injected should first be warmed to body temperature and should be injected slowly. The removed CSF may be used as a diluent.

At the end of the procedure, the needle is withdrawn quickly and the puncture site covered with sterile gauze and adhesive tape.

Gross examination: Normal CSF is clear and colorless and does not coagulate. Haziness appears when 300 to 600 cells/cu mm are present. More than 600 cells/cu mm results in a turbid or purulent fluid. Bloody fluid that does not coagulate on standing and has a uniform appearance in all test tubes is seen with bleeding into the subarachnoid space. Fluid that is at first bloody but clears on continued collection is the result of trauma due to faulty technic. Xanthochromic (yellow- or amber-tinged) fluid is obtained whenever blood has been present for > 4 h or when bile pigment is present. The fluid may appear faintly yellow when the protein content is > 100 mg/100 ml. Clots, either coarse or in the form of delicate webs, indicate the presence of fibrinogen and fibrin ferment. Coarse clots commonly form in fluids with a "high" WBC count. Web formation is common in tuberculous meningitis. (For differential diagnoses, see TABLE 117–1.)

TABLE 117-1. CSF ABNORMALITIES IN VARIOUS CONDITIONS*

	Pressure	Cells/cu mm	Predominant Cell Type	Glucose	Protein
Normal	100–200 mm	0–3	L	50–100 mg/100 ml	20–45 mg/100 ml
Acute bacterial meningitis	↑	500–5000	PMN	↓	About 100 mg/100 ml
Subacute meningitis (tuberculous, cryptococcal, sarcoid, leukemic, carcinoma)	N or ↑	100–700	L	↓	↑
Viral infections	N or ↑	100–2000	L	N	N or ↑
Brain abscess or tumor	N or ↑	0–1000	L	N	↑
Lead encephalopathy	↑	0–500	L	N	↑
Meningismus	N or ↑	N	L	N	N or ↓
Acute syphilitic meningitis	N or ↑	25–2000	L	N	↑
Paretic neurosyphilis	N or ↑	15–2000	L	N	↑
Guillain-Barré syndrome	N	0–100	L	N	>100 mg/100 ml
Cerebral hemorrhage	↑	Bloody	RBCs	N	↑
Cerebral thrombosis	N or ↑	0–100	L	N	N or ↑
Cord tumor	N	0–50	L	N	N or ↑

* N = normal; ↑ = increased; ↓ = decreased; PMN = polymorphonuclear; L = lymphocyte; RBCs = red blood cells.

NOTE: Figures given for pressure, cell count, and protein are approximations; exceptions are not infrequent. Similarly, PMNs may predominate in conditions usually characterized by lymphocyte response, especially early in the course of viral infections or tuberculous meningitis. Alterations in glucose are less variable and more reliable.

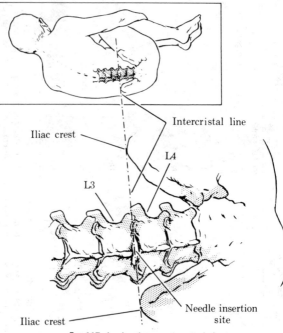

FIG. 117–4.   Lumbar puncture technic.

Protein: The fluid is analyzed quantitatively for protein using standard laboratory assays. Special examinations for γ-globulin percentage (should be < 15%), oligoclonal banding, and the presence of myelin basic protein may be helpful in diagnosing demyelinating diseases. Such special tests should be ordered in advance and sufficient fluid obtained for their determination. CSF protein contents > 50 mg/dl are abnormal.

Sugar: Normally, CSF sugar is above 50 mg/dl. Sugar values below this level should be checked against blood sugar to rule out the presence of hypoglycemia as a cause. The analytic method is the same as that used on blood.

The microscopic examination should be performed promptly after collection. For the cell count, the CSF may be unstained or polychrome methylene blue may be used. If the fluid is crystal clear, each side of the hemocytometer counting chamber is filled. The number of cells found in 9 squares approximates the number of cells/cu mm. When the fluid is not clear, the stain should be used. This solution colors WBCs blue and RBCs yellow. Stain is drawn to the 1 mark in a WBC pipette, which is then filled to the 11 mark with CSF. The counting chamber is filled and the number of cells in the entire WBC and RBC areas (9 sq mm) is counted. The cells/cu mm equal the number of cells in 9 sq mm divided by 9 and multipled by 11 to correct for chamber depth and stain dilution.

A differential count should also be made. The specimen is centrifuged and the sediment smeared on a slide with a wire loop. The specimen is dried and treated with Wright's stain. The types of cells found are reported as percent of the total cell count. Should the WBC count be < 30/cu mm, a rough estimation is made of the WBC count from the preparation in the counting chamber.

If infection is suspected, additional slides should be made from the centrifuged CSF specimen and stained with appropriate stains for bacteria (Gram stain and methylene blue), for TB (acid-fast stain), and for cryptococcus (India ink). For such special stains the sediment from at least 10 ml of fluid should be taken and specially prepared slides should be used for best results.

Spinal fluid cultures: The CSF should be cultured immediately (unless TB is the *only* consideration, in which case the specimen may be incubated overnight in the original sterile test tube). Cultures should be placed on chocolate and blood agar and incubated anaerobically. In addition, special media or animal inoculation may be required for accurate identification.

118. COMMON NEUROLOGIC MANIFESTATIONS

FOCAL DISORDERS OF HIGHER NERVOUS FUNCTION

Disorders of the higher (integrative) mental processes, characterized by specific symptoms and signs, and caused by lesions at specific sites in the cerebral cortex, either defined or presumed.

The patient's mental activity, cognitive processes, emotional responses, and behavior—all activities of the brain—are as much an expression of nervous system activity as are motor functions, reflexes, cranial nerve function, and the various special and somatic sensations. While the appraisal of many higher nervous functions often lies within the domain of psychiatry, the neurophysiologic origin of these processes bears reemphasizing.

The higher mental processes may be deranged diffusely or focally. Diffuse disorders (e.g., delirium, dementia) are discussed in Ch. 119. In addition to the focal disorders discussed in this chapter, focal manifestations that are typically associated with epilepsy, cerebrovascular disorders, and certain intracranial neoplasms are also described in Chs. 120, 122, and 125, respectively.

APHASIA

A defect or loss of language function, in which the comprehension or expression of words (or nonverbal equivalents of words) is impaired as a result of injury to the language centers in the cerebral cortex.

Language function resides predominantly in the left hemisphere of most persons, including the left-handed; more specifically, in the posterosuperior temporal lobe, the adjacent parietal lobe, the inferolateral frontal lobe, and the deep connections between those regions. Damage to any part of this roughly triangular area (e.g., by infarct or tumor) will interfere with some aspect of language function, resulting in an **aphasia**.

Lesions that impinge on the posterosuperior temporal gyrus and the adjacent angular gyrus of the temporal lobe disrupt the neural connections that receive and integrate linguistic information coming to the brain, producing a **receptive**, or **sensory**, **aphasia**. With large lesions in this area, the patient cannot understand *any* sensory information having to do with language, be it auditory, visual, or tactile. Smaller injuries selectively interfere with comprehension of some more specific form of symbolic information; for example, with the ability to read **(dyslexia, alexia, word blindness)**.

Injury to the inferior frontal gyrus just anterior to the facial and lingual areas of the motor cortex **(Broca's area)** produces an **expressive**, or **motor**, **aphasia** in which the patient's comprehension and ability to conceptualize are relatively preserved, but his ability to form language and express himself is impaired. Usually, the impairment affects both speech **(dysphasia)** and writing **(agraphia, dysgraphia)**. **Anomia**, the inability to name objects, may be receptive or expressive. In dysarthria, the inability to articulate words properly is not an aphasia, but a motor disorder.

Brain lesions large enough to damage language function significantly will seldom produce pure defects; thus an isolated receptive or expressive aphasia is rare.

APRAXIA

Inability to execute purposeful learned motor acts, despite the physical ability and willingness to do so. Typically, the patient is unable to follow a motor command even though he understands it and is physically able to execute the individual component movements. The defect is apparently a lesion in the neural pathways that retain the memory of learned patterns of movement, so that the patient cannot conceptualize the necessary movement patterns or translate them into purposive action. Apraxia is common in many metabolic and structural diseases that involve the brain diffusely, particularly those that seem to impair frontal lobe function. Selective apraxias with loss of specific movements (e.g., **constructional apraxia**, an inability to draw or build simple constructions; or an apraxia for getting dressed) may occur in dementia or, occasionally, with parietal lobe lesions.

FOCAL CORTICAL SENSORY DISORDERS

The discriminative aspects of sensation—recognition, localization, and interpretation of sensory stimuli—depend on functional mechanisms in the parietal sensory cortex. All higher sensory recognition requires that the common peripheral sensory pathways be intact as well as cortical sensory discrimination, however, so that central disorders must be differentiated from peripheral neural interruptions by testing peripheral sensation.

The inability to recognize sensory stimuli, or to appreciate their import **(agnosia)** may be visual, tactile, or auditory. **Astereognosis**, the inability to identify the shape, size, weight, and texture of objects, results from lesions in the post-central gyrus.

When **2-point discrimination** is impaired peripherally, the patient cannot distinguish 2 points < 5 mm apart on the fingertips (normal: 2 to 3 mm); with a cortical lesion the patient cannot consistently distinguish 2 points from one.

Disturbances in the **perception of spatial relationships** may occur with parietal lobe lesions. Lesions in the posterior parts of the right parietal lobe usually lead to altered awareness of the body image, with neglect or denial of the contralateral side of the body **(anosognosia)**, accompanied at times by unawareness of external objects on the same side. The patient may deny that there is anything wrong with him, or may acknowledge his disability but disregard it. Anosognosia is commonly seen with a left hemiplegia, and presents special problems for those caring for a stroke patient. **Finger agnosia**, difficulty in identifying the fingers, is seen commonly with diffuse dementias or parietal lesions of the left hemisphere. Disturbed spatial perception may also play a role in some apraxias (see above) that result from left parietal lobe lesions.

AMNESIC SYNDROMES

(See Ch. 119)

IMPAIRED CONSCIOUSNESS

A fully alert state with intact mentation requires a fully intact interaction between the mechanisms governing the cognitive functions of the cerebral hemispheres and the arousal mechanisms of the reticular activating system, a part of the **reticular formation**, the extensive network of nuclei and interconnecting fibers found throughout much of the diencephalon, midbrain, pons, and medulla. The **reticular activating system** is a functional, not a morphologic, unit located along the central core of the diencephalon and upper brainstem. It receives afferent impulses from many somatic, visceral, auditory, and visual sensory pathways, and relays the impulses to the thalamic reticular nucleus which in turn activates areas widely distributed throughout the cerebral cortex.

Impairment of consciousness may be brief or prolonged, mild or profound. Brief unconsciousness occurs with **syncope** (see in Ch. 24); with a convulsive seizure it may last somewhat longer, and in concussion may last up to 24 h. Prolonged unconsciousness usually results from severe intracranial or metabolic disorders. **Obtundation** is *reduced alertness*, usually combined with hypersomnia. **Stupor** is *unresponsiveness from which the patient can be aroused only briefly and only by vigorous and repeated stimulation*. **Coma** is *unarousable unresponsiveness;* in deep coma, even primitive avoidance reflexes may be absent.

Hypersomnia (excessively long or deep sleep from which the patient can be awakened only by energetic stimulation), and **delirium** and **confusional states**—see Ch. 119, below (patients are disoriented for place or time, are confused in their interpretation of sensory stimuli, may have hallucinations [predominantly visual], have a short attention span, and are often drowsy or agitated)—are also states of impaired consciousness.

Etiology

A clouded or depressed state of consciousness implies dysfunction of the cerebral hemispheres, the upper brainstem, or both areas. **Lesions in supratentorial structures** may extensively damage both hemispheres or may produce so much brain swelling that the hemispheres compress the diencephalic activating system and may even squeeze it through the tentorium (transtentorial herniation—see under INTRACRANIAL NEOPLASMS in Ch. 125), causing brainstem damage. **Primary subtentorial (brainstem or cerebellar) lesions** may compress or directly damage the reticular activating system anywhere between the level of the mid-pons and (by upward pressure) the diencephalon. **Metabolic or infectious diseases** may depress hemispheric and brainstem function by a change in blood composition or a direct toxic effect. Impaired consciousness may also be due to **reduced blood flow** (as in syncope or infarction) or a **change in electrical activity** (as in epilepsy). Either inadequate blood flow or a chemical change may alter the electrical activity. **Concussion** and **psychologic disturbances** impair consciousness without detectable structural changes in the brain. TABLE 118–1 lists the major disorders that produce unconsciousness.

Diagnosis

The cause of unconsciousness is often not immediately evident, and diagnosis requires an orderly approach. The airway must be patent and BP supported before a detailed history or examination is undertaken. Observers or relatives should be questioned about the mode of onset or injury; ingestion of drugs, alcohol, or other toxic substances; infections, convulsions, headache, and previous illnesses (e.g., diabetes mellitus, nephritis, heart disease, hypertension). The patient may be wearing a tag or carrying a diagnostic card in his wallet. Police can help in locating relatives or associates. Containers suspected of having held food, alcohol, drugs, or poisons should be examined and saved (for chemical analysis and as possible legal evidence). Signs of hemorrhage, incontinence, and cranial trauma should be sought. The patient's age may be significant: epilepsy and systemic infection are frequently responsible in those under 40; cardiovascular disease (especially stroke), metabolic disorders (diabetes mellitus, hypoglycemia), and uremia are more common after 40.

TABLE 118–1. THE MOST FREQUENT CAUSES OF IMPAIRED
CONSCIOUSNESS

Supratentorial mass lesions
Epidural hematoma
Subdural hematoma
Cerebral infarct or hemorrhage
Brain tumor
Brain abscess

Subtentorial lesions
Brainstem infarct
Brainstem tumor
Brainstem hemorrhage
Cerebellar hemorrhage
Brainstem trauma

Diffuse and metabolic cerebral disorders
Trauma (concussion; cerebral lacerations or contusions)
Anoxia or ischemia (syncope; cardiac arrhythmia; pulmonary infarct; shock; pulmonary
    insufficiency; carbon monoxide poisoning; collagen vascular disease)
Epilepsy
Postictal states (following epileptic seizure)
Infection (meningitis; encephalitis)
Subarachnoid hemorrhage
Exogenous toxins (ethyl alcohol; barbiturates; glutethimide; morphine; heroin; methyl alcohol;
    hypothermia)
Endogenous toxins and deficiencies (uremia; hepatic coma; diabetic acidosis; hypoglycemia;
    hyponatremia)
Psychomotor status epilepticus

Psychiatric disorders
Malingering
Hysteria
Catatonia

Adapted from *The Diagnosis of Stupor and Coma,* ed. 3, by F. Plum and J. B. Posner. Copyright
1980 by F. A. Davis Company. Used with permission.

Physical examination should note (1) **rectal temperature;** (2) **skin:** color, evidence of trauma or
hypodermic injections (narcotics, insulin), rashes, petechiae; (3) **scalp:** contusions or lacerations;
(4) **eyes:** pupil size and reaction to light, ocular palsy, corneal reflex, oculocephalic reflex ("doll's
eye" response to head rotation), fundic signs of papilledema, vascular sclerosis, or diabetic or uremic retinitis; (5) **ENT:** escape of CSF or blood, scarred or bitten tongue, breath odor (alcohol, acetone, paraldehyde, bitter almonds [cyanide]); (6) **respiration pattern:** hyperventilation; Cheyne-
Stokes (periodic) breathing; (7) **cardiovascular signs:** apical rate and rhythm, character of the pulse,
BP in both arms, signs of cardiac decompensation, sclerosis in peripheral vessels, cyanosis or clubbing of the fingers and toes; (8) **abdomen:** spasm, rigidity; (9) **neurologic signs:** paresis, stiff neck,
reflexes, muscular twitching, convulsions.

The neurologic appraisal provides the key to whether the disease is supratentorial, subtentorial, or
metabolic. **Breathing** is Cheyne-Stokes (periodic) with hemispheric disease and irregularly irregular
with pontomedullary disease; hyper- or hypoventilation occurs with metabolic disease. The **pupils**
are small and reactive to light with hypothalamic and pontine disease or narcotic poisoning, fixed in
midposition with midbrain damage or severe glutethimide overdosage, light-reactive with metabolic
disorders, dilated with anoxia or 3rd nerve compression, and normally reactive with hemispheric
disease or psychogenic unresponsiveness. **Oculovestibular responses** to caloric stimulation show
bilateral tonic conjugate deviation with hemispheric depression, are absent or dysconjugate with
brainstem impairment, and are normal with psychogenic unresponsiveness. **Motor responses** to
painful stimuli are hemiplegic with hemispheric lesions. Decerebrate rigidity (neck, back, and limbs
extended; jaws clenched) occurs with diencephalic-midbrain dysfunction; flaccidity, with pontomedullary brainstem dysfunction. Symmetric motor abnormalities, often including asterixis or a multifocal
myoclonus, occur with metabolic diseases, and motor signs and reflexes are normal with psychogenic unresponsiveness.

Characteristically, neurologic signs and symptoms in supratentorial mass lesions first indicate
involvement of one cerebral hemisphere. Then, because of enlargement of the mass and consequent

shifts in brain tissues as a result of pressure changes, signs show progressive rostral-caudal deterioration indicating involvement first of the diencephalon and finally of the brainstem (see Complications in Ch. 123). With unconsciousness from a primary brainstem lesion, pupillary and oculomotor signs are abnormal from the start.

Laboratory studies: In coma of unknown cause, and where hypoglycemia is possible, the first step is to **draw blood** for glucose determination and then to give 50 ml hypertonic glucose IV. Other blood determinations should include Hct, respiratory gases, WBC, BUN, sodium, potassium, bicarbonate, chloride, alcohol, and bromide content, and spectroscopy for sulfhemoglobin and methemoglobin. **Urine** should be collected by catheterization and examined for sugar, acetone, albumin, and sedative drugs. **Gastric lavage** is required for diagnosis and treatment in suspected poisoning, with care to avoid esophageal or gastric perforation if the poison may have been corrosive (see also Ch. 258). For patients in deep coma, endotracheal intubation should precede lavage, to prevent pulmonary aspiration. **Skull x-rays** are frequently necessary, but must be deferred in shock. **Carotid arteriography** or **CT scanning** to exclude subdural or epidural hematoma may be indicated. In urgent cases, **lumbar puncture** to detect infection should be performed as soon as possible if no diagnosis is established, unless increased intracranial pressure from an expanding lesion is suspected.

The principal diagnostic points for some of the more common causes of unconsciousness are as follows (further details are discussed in the appropriate chapters elsewhere in this volume).

Acute alcoholism: Alcoholic breath; patient usually stuporous, not comatose, responding to noxious stimuli; face and conjunctivas hyperemic; temperature normal or subnormal; pupils moderately dilated, equal, and reactive to light; respirations deep and noisy, not stertorous; blood alcohol > 200 mg/100 ml.

Cranial trauma: Onset of coma sudden or gradual; often local evidence or history of injury, perhaps with bleeding from ear, nose, or throat; temperature normal or elevated; pupils usually unequal and sluggish or inactive; respirations variable, often slow or irregular; pulse variable, rapid initially and then slow; BP variable; reflexes frequently altered, often with incontinence and evidence of paralysis; CSF possibly bloody and under increased pressure; possible fracture lines or pineal displacement on skull x-rays.

Stroke: Patient usually over 40, with cardiovascular disease or hypertension; onset sudden; face flushed or cyanotic, often asymmetric; temperature, pulse, and respirations variable; pupils usually unequal and inactive; BP often elevated; focal neurologic signs common, including hemiplegia; CSF often bloody or xanthochromic with increased pressure.

Epilepsy: History of previous "fits"; onset sudden and convulsive; incontinence common; temperature, pulse, and respirations usually normal, but possibly elevated after repeated convulsions; pupils reactive; tongue bitten or scarred from previous attacks.

Diabetic acidosis: Onset gradual; skin dry, face flushed; breath odor fruity; temperature often subnormal; eyeballs may be soft; air hunger (hyperventilation); glucosuria, ketonuria, hyperglycemia; decreased CO_2 combining power.

Hypoglycemia: Onset possibly acute, with convulsions, but usually preceded by lightheadedness, sweating, nausea, vomiting, pallor, palpitations, headache, abdominal pain, hunger; skin moist and pale; hypothermia; pupils reactive; deep reflexes exaggerated; positive Babinski sign; hypoglycemia during attack.

Syncope: Onset sudden, often associated with emotional crisis or heart block; coma seldom deep or prolonged; pallor; pulse slow at onset, later rapid and weak.

Barbiturate or glutethimide poisoning: Appearance often of deep sleep. Skin sometimes cyanotic; hypothermia; pupils variable according to degree of poisoning—fixed small in severe cases of barbiturate poisoning, in midposition with glutethimide; respirations shallow and slow; muscles usually flaccid; reflexes sluggish or absent.

Treatment

Immediate findings may call for **emergency measures:** control of hemorrhage, cardiopulmonary resuscitation, airway maintenance (by intubation or tracheostomy), treatment of shock, O_2 administration (for the hypoxia that complicates all unconsciousness), catheterization, fluid or electrolyte replacement, and chemotherapy. Temperature, pulse, respirations, and BP should be checked at frequent intervals. If the diagnosis is not immediately evident, glucose infusion may be started once blood has been drawn for blood sugar determination. Nothing should be given by mouth because of the danger of aspiration. Stimulants should be avoided. Morphine depresses respiration and is therefore *contraindicated*. Parenteral feeding and prevention of decubitus ulcers are essential in protracted unconsciousness.

Cerebral Death

Modern methods of resuscitation and support of BP and respiration have created new problems in defining death. If, for 12 h, there has been no spontaneous respiration despite apneic oxygenation for 3 to 5 min, no other voluntary movement, no cranial reflexes (pupillary reflexes, corneal reflex, oculovestibular reflex, jaw reflex, gag reflex), no response to noxious stimuli, and a flat EEG reading at maximal gain, coma may be considered irreversible. *These criteria apply only when drug intoxication can be completely ruled out.*

PAIN

Pain, the most common symptom for which patients seek help, can reflect either physical or emotional discomfort. **Physical pain** is a result of tissue injury, and arises from stimulation of pain endings in somatic or visceral structures. The pain-conducting fibers synapse with neurons in the dorsal gray horn of the spinal cord; the pain impulse then travels up the contralateral spinothalamic tract to synapses in the midbrain and thalamus, and from the latter to the sensory cortex.

Somatic pain tends to be localized, often follows dermatomal or spinal segmental (myotomal) patterns, is described in familiar terms, and is rarely continuous except in certain easily identified acute or subacute tissue-damaging lesions. **Visceral pain** is poorly localized and often spreads from the injured organ to other visceral regions or to somatic dermatomes with a common spinal afferent pathway **(referred pain).** Visceral pain may be more difficult for the patient to describe and is often more disturbing than somatic pain.

Some **"psychogenic"** pains arise from chronic muscle tension; others represent an excessive preoccupation with minor somatic sensation. Some complaints of pain originate in the patient's imagination. Psychogenic pains most frequently involve the head, the abdomen, or the low back and may be described vaguely or in colorful terms but generally are difficult to reconcile with neuroanatomic pathways or physiologic mechanisms. They often occur in "pain-prone" persons with a long history of nonorganic suffering. The suffering may be severe despite apparent good health, and it may be continuous, defying most analgesics.

Pain of thalamic origin ("central pain") is uncommon but may be seen with thalamic lesions. It is characterized by severe, often continuous and burning pain on the contralateral side, which may be greatly accentuated by even a light touch. Since it is frequently accompanied by emotional disturbance and may not respond to analgesics, it may be mistaken for psychogenic pain.

Tolerance to discomfort varies widely, and the medical and emotional history is often helpful in evaluating a complaint of pain. Pain of recent onset deserves careful attention, particularly in an adult not previously subject to repeated pain. On the other hand, excessive medical attention to spurious complaints or to pain that is based on an underlying emotional depression can reinforce invalidism in physically healthy patients.

Treatment

Management of the cause is the prime consideration, but when this fails to relieve pain or while the cause is being sought, symptomatic therapy is indicated (see also Chs. 247 and 249). Rest of the painful part, heat, cold, change in position, or counterirritants may suffice. Analgesics that act by peripheral sensory nerve depression are preferred; thus, localized pain due to burns or surface inflammation may be treated with 1% dibucaine or 5% benzocaine ointment.

The *mildest effective agent* should be used for central analgesia. (NOTE: Doses given here are average adult doses.) Mild pain usually responds to an oral salicylate (e.g., aspirin 300 to 600 mg [5 to 10 grains] q 2 to 3 h), to acetaminophen 325 to 650 mg q 4 h, to a salicylate with small doses of codeine [15 to 30 mg q 4 h]), or to propoxyphene 65 mg t.i.d. or q.i.d. More severe pain may require oral or s.c. codeine 30 mg q 3 to 4 h; hydromorphone 2 to 3 mg q 4 to 6 h; meperidine 25 to 150 mg q 4 h; methadone 2.5 to 10 mg q 3 to 6 h; or morphine 10 to 15 mg q 4 h. Analgesics are additive and often best used together. For rapid relief of severe pain, morphine 2 to 4 mg can be injected slowly IV. Effectiveness of analgesics may be enhanced by mild sedatives such as pentobarbital 50 mg orally. Sedatives alone can control mild pain, but their continued use is habit-forming. Trigeminal neuralgia and the lightning pains of tabes dorsalis are often relieved by the anticonvulsant carbamazepine 200 mg orally 3 to 5 times/day. Acupuncture and cutaneous stimulation sometimes relieve pain of a musculoskeletal origin, but results are unpredictable.

Chronic pain is physically and psychologically debilitating and represents a special problem for the physician and patient. Every effort must be taken to determine the degree to which the pain reflects chronic anxiety or depression. Analgesics generally have little effect in such circumstances and may be habit-forming. **Intractable pain** (e.g., in trigeminal neuralgia, cancer, or [rarely] other destructive diseases) may sometimes be relieved by surgical interruption of afferent sensory pathways. Cordotomy, cutting the ascending spinothalamic pathways in the spinal cord, is the most widely employed surgical procedure. Its greatest benefit is in cancer patients with pain from a clearly unilateral, spinal, or extremity source. With other chronic pain, success is unpredictable, and adverse effects are not easily reversed. In conditions such as cancer, risking addiction is preferable to permitting chronic unrelieved suffering. Severe intractable pain from cancer or organic disease of the nervous system can sometimes be alleviated with a psychotropic drug alone (e.g., amitriptyline 75 mg, or fluphenazine 1 to 3 mg, daily), but in general these agents are best used in combinations with appropriate analgesics, at least in the initial stages of development. (See also NARCOTICS AND NARCOTIC ANTAGONISTS in Ch. 247.)

HEADACHE
(Cephalalgia)

Etiology and Pathogenesis

Headache is a common manifestation of acute systemic or intracranial infection, intracranial tumor, head injuries, severe hypertension, cerebral hypoxia, and many diseases of the eye, nose, throat, teeth, and ear. However, such conditions account for only a few patients who consult a physician because of headache. The remainder usually suffer from muscle tension headache, migraine, or head pain for which no structural cause can be found.

The first task when a patient complains of headache is to determine precisely what hurts. Headaches may result from stimulation or traction of, or pressure on, any of the pain-sensitive structures of the head: all tissues covering the cranium; the 5th, 9th, and 10th cranial nerves and the upper cervical nerves; the large intracranial venous sinuses; the large arteries at the base of the brain and the large dural arteries; and the dura mater at the base of the skull. Dilation or contraction of blood vessel walls stimulates nerve endings, causing headache.

Diagnosis

TABLE 118–2 gives salient features of the history, physical findings, and special studies in conditions commonly associated with headache. The frequency, duration, nature, location, and severity of the headache help to identify the cause. Infrequent headaches can usually be related to acute causes such as fatigue, fever, or alcohol ingestion. The cause of chronic or recurrent headaches is often difficult to diagnose. Headache of recent origin especially requires careful attention. Useful tests include blood count, blood serology, BUN, CSF examination, skull and sinus x-rays, visual tests (acuity, visual fields, refraction), echoencephalography, and an EEG. CT or cerebral angiography is occasionally indicated when abnormal neurologic signs are present or the headache is of recent origin.

Recurrent headaches associated with disease of intra- or extracranial structures are characterized by remissions lasting hours or days. Headaches from brain tumors or other intracranial lesions are usually of recent origin. They tend to be intermittently persistent for several hours each day, and may be precipitated or relieved by change of posture. The headache at first may be localized in the region of the tumor, but it tends to become generalized as intracranial pressure increases.

Headache associated with emotional tension tends to be chronic or continuous, and commonly arises in the occipital or bifrontal region and spreads over the entire head. It is described usually as a pressure sensation or as a viselike constriction of the skull. Febrile illnesses, arterial hypertension, and migraine usually cause throbbing pain in any part of the head.

Treatment

Besides attention to the cause, symptomatic analgesic therapy is usually indicated. Many headaches are trivial, of short duration, and require no further treatment. Management of chronic psychogenic, post-traumatic, or migrainous headaches is a common and more difficult problem. Both psychotherapy and pharmacotherapy are necessary.

Psychotherapy need not be extensive in most cases. An understanding, reassuring physician who accepts the pain as real, not imaginary, helps greatly. The patient should be seen at frequent, regular intervals and encouraged to discuss his emotional difficulties. The physician should reassure the patient that no organic lesion is present and explain the emotional basis of the headache. Environmental readjustments, removal of irritants and stresses, and reeducation may help.

The **pharmacotherapy** of chronic headache includes a variety of drugs. Those used for migraine are discussed under that topic below. In psychogenic and post-traumatic headache, analgesics are most effective. Aspirin 300 to 600 mg orally q 4 h may be given alone, with acetaminophen 325 mg and caffeine, or with phenobarbital. Many physicians empirically supplement analgesia with tranquilizers (e.g., diazepam 2 to 5 mg orally q.i.d.). Continued use of a mild sedative such as phenobarbital 15 to 30 mg orally once or twice/day is sometimes adequate. The value of drug therapy depends not only on the particular medication, but on concomitant psychotherapy and the quality of the associated doctor-patient relationship.

MIGRAINE

A paroxysmal disorder characterized by recurrent attacks of headache, with or without associated visual and GI disturbances.

Etiology and Incidence

The cause is unknown, but evidence suggests a functional disturbance of cranial circulation. Prodromal symptoms (e.g., flashes of light, hemianopia, paresthesias) are probably due to intracerebral vasoconstriction, and the head pain to dilation of scalp arteries. Migraine may occur at any age but usually begins between ages 10 and 30, more often in women than in men. Remission after age 50 is not uncommon. A family history is obtained in > 50% of cases.

Symptoms and Signs

Headache may be preceded by a short period of depression, irritability, restlessness, or anorexia, and in some patients by scintillating scotomas, visual field defects, paresthesias, or (rarely) hemipa-

TABLE 118-2. DIFFERENTIAL DIAGNOSIS OF HEADACHE

Cause	Typical History	Physical & Neurologic Findings	Special Studies Indicated
ORGANIC DISEASE: **A. Intracranial (increased pressure)** 1. Expanding lesions Brain tumor	Headache: mild to severe, localized or generalized, intermittent. Slowly progressive weakness on one side, convulsions, visual changes, aphasia, vomiting, mental changes	Papilledema, visual field changes, aphasia, paralysis, mental changes	Skull & chest x-rays, EEG, lumbar puncture (unless signs of intracranial pressure are present), or arteriogram. CT scan often diagnostic
Brain abscess	As above; history of ear disease, sinusitis, bronchiectasis, lung abscess, rheumatic or congenital heart disease	As above; evidence of local or distant infective focus; temperature need not be elevated, pulse may be slow	As above; cultures from infection site, CSF, and blood
Subdural hematoma	As above; history of trauma, fluctuating changes in consciousness	As above; signs of recent head injury	As above for non-infective lesions
2. Meningeal irritation Meningitis, acute	Headache: recent, severe, generalized, constant, radiates down neck. Malaise, fever, with vomiting. Preceding sore throat or respiratory infection	Patient usually acutely ill; may be confused, irrational, excited; may have stiff neck, positive Kernig's sign	Blood culture, lumbar puncture, smear & culture of CSF
Meningitis, chronic Syphilis Tuberculosis Cryptococcosis	Headache: dull to severe, generalized or over vertex. Moderate fever. History of syphilis or tuberculosis	Signs of meningeal irritation less marked than in acute form; cranial nerve palsies, delirium or confusion	Lumbar puncture with smear & culture of CSF; CSF protein, blood counts, & sugar; chest x-ray. Blood & spinal fluid STS
Subarachnoid hemorrhage	Headache: sudden onset, severe & constant. Prodromal pain in & about one eye; ptosis	Patient drowsy or comatose; stiff neck, positive Kernig's sign, bilateral Babinski's sign, third nerve paralysis; elevated BP	Lumbar puncture, arteriogram
B. Cranial (changes in skull) 1. Metastatic neoplasms	Headache localized; symptoms of primary cancer elsewhere; often neurologic symptoms	Scalp mass; cranial nerve signs; evidence of primary lesion or metastases elsewhere	X-ray of skull & other bones

(Continued)

TABLE 118–2. DIFFERENTIAL DIAGNOSIS OF HEADACHE *(Cont'd)*

Cause	Typical History	Physical & Neurologic Findings	Special Studies Indicated
ORGANIC DISEASE: *(Cont'd)* **B. Cranial (changes in skull)** *(Cont'd)* 2. Paget's disease	Headache: mild, burning, intermittent or constant, localized or generalized. History of increasing size of skull; pain in back, limbs	Skull tender; suggestive configuration of skull; evidence of compression of brain & cranial nerves	Skull x-ray, serum alkaline phosphatase
C. Involvement of sensory nerves of scalp	Headache: radiates along course of nerve. Pain of herpes zoster may be constant	Nerve may be tender on pressure, occasionally cutaneous hyperalgesia along distribution of nerve; vesicles or scars in herpes	
D. Vascular disturbances 1. Migraine	Headache: usually generalized, but may be unilateral, throbbing, beginning in & about eye, spreading to involve one or both sides; accompanied by anorexia, nausea, & vomiting. Similar periodic attacks over extended period. Family history frequently positive. Prodromata: changes in mood, anorexia, scintillating scotomas, occasionally hemiparesis	Examination negative between attacks; some cases may disclose transient neurologic findings during an attack	Skull x-ray, brain scan, EEG to rule out organic disease. Trial with a vasoconstrictor (dihydroergotamine or methysergide)
2. Toxic states; infections; alcoholism; uremia; lead, arsenic, morphine, carbon monoxide poisoning; encephalitides	Headache: moderate, generalized, pulsating, constant. History of exposure to toxins, or of other symptoms produced by causative agent	Other signs produced by causative agent	Studies applicable to the agent suspected; lumbar puncture, blood & urine studies
3. Hypertension	Headache: throbbing, paroxysmal, occipital or vertex. History of cardiovascular or renal disease	Elevated BP, retinal changes, cardiac findings, edema	Blood chemistry, renal studies
4. "Cluster" headaches (histamine headache)	Headache: paroxysmal, abrupt, severe, unilateral, involving eye, temple, neck, and face. Symptoms of vasodilation on same side as pain, edema below eye, rhinorrhea, lacrimation. Periods of remission	Evidence of facial vasodilation, pupillary constriction, tenderness on pressure of external & common carotid arteries, injection of conjunctiva, flushing of side of face	Therapeutic trial of methysergide or vasoconstrictor drugs. Corticosteroid trial. Indomethacin

E. Extracranial		
1. Lesions of eye (eyestrain, iritis, glaucoma)	Headache: frontal or supraorbital, moderate or severe pain, frequently worse after use of eyes. Pain in eye	Changes in appearance of iris; increased intraocular tension; errors of refraction	Ophthalmic examination
2. Lesions of middle ear (otitis media, mastoiditis)	Headache: temporal or aural, unilateral, intermittent, stabbing sensations. Feeling of fullness in ear, increasing deafness, tinnitus, otorrhea, general malaise with fever & acute illness	Acutely ill; tender over mastoid; red, congested, or retracted drum on affected side. Fever. Signs of meningeal irritation in children	Otoscopic examination, mastoid x-ray
3. Lesions of nasal sinuses	Headache: frontal, dull or severe, usually worse in morning, improved in afternoon; worse in cold, damp weather. History of preceding URI, pain in one part of face. Purulent nasal discharge	Evidence of nasal obstruction, swollen mucous membranes, tenderness on percussion over affected sinus	X-ray of sinuses, transillumination
4. Lesions of oral cavity (teeth, tongue, pharynx)	Headache: bilateral or unilateral, variable in intensity, periodic. Pain in mouth, jaw, or throat	Lesion in oral cavity. Tenderness on tapping affected teeth or pain on syringing with ice water	Dental evaluation, including x-ray study
POST-TRAUMATIC	Headache: localized to site of injury or generalized, variable in intensity, frequency, duration. Made worse by emotional disturbances. Vertigo, worse on change of position. History of trauma, irritability, insomnia, inability to concentrate, inability to tolerate alcohol	Usually normal physical and neurologic examination	Skull x-ray, EEG, lumbar puncture, thorough psychologic study
PSYCHOGENIC:		
1. Conversion hysteria, anxiety states	Headache: frequently bizarre, bitemporal, constant, generalized, vise-like pain over vertex, made worse by emotional disturbance	Appearance may be bland or apprehensive. Tachycardia, elevated systolic pressure, moist palms, hyperactive reflexes. Examination often normal	Studies to rule out organic disease. Evaluation of psychologic factors and personality
2. Muscle tension	Headache: intermittent, moderate, fronto-occipital or general, feeling of tightness or stiffness	Muscles may be tender, otherwise normal	As above

resis. These symptoms may disappear shortly before the headache appears or may merge with it. Pain is either unilateral or generalized. Symptoms usually follow a pattern in each patient, except that unilateral headaches may not always be on the same side. The patient may have attacks daily or only once in several months.

Untreated attacks may last for hours or days. Nausea, vomiting, and photophobia are common. The extremities are cold and cyanosed, and the patient is irritable and seeks seclusion. The scalp arteries are prominent, and their amplitude of pulsation is increased. Intracranial vascular malformations are a rare cause of migrainous headaches; other major manifestations are seizures, cranial bruits, signs of a mass lesion, or subarachnoid hemorrhage.

Diagnosis

This is based on the symptom patterns described above in a patient who shows no evidence of intracranial pathologic changes. The diagnosis is more probable with a family history of migraine or if visual prodromata occur.

Prophylaxis

Various nonspecific medical and surgical procedures have been recommended for decreasing the frequency of attacks; their effectiveness depends largely on the patient's confidence in, and the enthusiasm of, the physician. The most effective prophylaxis is supportive psychotherapy. Methysergide 4 to 8 mg/day orally is effective but can cause retroperitoneal fibrosis and should not be used for periods > 3 mo at a time, with rest periods in between. It is **contraindicated** in pregnancy or in occlusive vascular disease.

Propranolol 10 to 20 mg orally 3 to 4 times/day has received a few successful trials in migraine prophylaxis but has only limited usefulness. Some patients are now being helped with biofeedback approaches in which they are ostensibly taught to control vascular tone; the long-term effect is uncertain.

Treatment of the Acute Attack

Aspirin or codeine may alleviate mild attacks. In severe attacks, only ergot derivatives and codeine or stronger analgesics offer relief and usually only if taken before the headache has lasted 2 h. Immediately after onset, ergotamine tartrate 0.5 mg s.c. or 0.25 mg IV can be given, repeated once in 1 h if necessary (the IV route is more likely to cause emesis). Alternatively, dihydroergotamine 1 mg s.c., IM, or IV is given, repeated in 1 or 2 h if needed.

Much larger doses of oral ergot preparations are required. Oral ergotamine tartrate and caffeine preparations are sometimes more effective and require a smaller total dose of ergot (2 mg, then 1 mg q 30 min if necessary to a maximum of 9 mg ergotamine). The drugs may be given by rectal suppository if nausea precludes oral administration.

VERTIGO

(Dizziness)

A disturbance in which the individual has a subjective impression of movement in space (subjective vertigo) or of objects moving around him (objective vertigo), usually with a loss of equilibrium.

Etiology

True vertigo, as distinguished from faintness, lightheadedness, or other forms of "dizziness," results from a disturbance somewhere in the equilibratory apparatus: vestibule; semicircular canals; 8th nerve; vestibular nuclei in the brainstem and their temporal lobe connections; and eyes. These structures may be affected by any of a large variety of disorders: (1) **otogenic:** Ménière's syndrome, myringitis, otitis media, acute vestibular neuronitis, herpes zoster oticus, labyrinthitis, middle ear or labyrinthine tumors, petrositis, otosclerosis, obstructed external auditory canal or eustachian tube; (2) **toxic:** alcohol, streptomycin, opiates; (3) **psychogenic:** hysteria; (4) **environmental:** motion sickness; (5) **ocular:** diplopia; (6) **circulatory:** transient vertebrobasilar ischemic attacks; (7) **neurologic:** multiple sclerosis, skull fracture, temporal lobe seizures, encephalitis; (8) **neoplastic:** tumors of the pons, cerebellopontine angle, or 8th nerve; (9) **hematogenic:** leukemia involving the labyrinth. Stimulation of proprioceptors in muscles, joints, and tendons may induce a sense of dysequilibrium, but this is not true vertigo.

Diagnosis

Nystagmus, past-pointing, inability to walk a straight line, and persistent deviation to one side when walking all indicate a disturbance of the labyrinthine vestibular apparatus or its CNS connections. Determining whether the vertigo is **peripheral** (arising from the labyrinth or vestibular nerve) or **central** (arising from the vestibular nuclei or their higher connections) is the first step in establishing the cause (see also Nystagmus in Ch. 173).

Peripheral nystagmus is conjugate, horizontal, or horizontal-rotary, maximal towards the affected labyrinth, and has its fast component away from the side of the lesion. Central nystagmus can be horizontal or vertical, characteristically has its fast component in the direction of gaze to either side, and may be pendular or unequal in the 2 eyes. Upgaze or downgaze nystagmus always arises from central abnormalities.

Paroxysmal, episodic, or severe attacks of vertigo separated by normal interludes indicate a peripheral vertigo. Persistent vertigo or dysequilibrium accompanied by nystagmus and gait disturbance usually indicates CNS disease. Vertical or rotary nystagmus also indicates a central lesion. Unilateral deafness and tinnitus indicate cochlear nerve involvement and are therefore reliable indicators of a peripheral nerve lesion. Labyrinthine disease produces more intense symptoms than does involvement of vestibular nuclei. Headache is more common with central lesions, and other findings such as double vision, slurred speech, incoordination of an extremity, or unilateral weakness are unlikely with peripheral lesions.

Vestibular function tests (see in Ch. 164) are important—absence of the caloric response indicates a dead labyrinth. Audiograms may differentiate between cochlear and neural hearing loss. Special studies of the vestibular apparatus and CNS are often necessary. Skull x-rays with special views and tomography of the petrous pyramids, CSF examination, and EEG help to exclude pathologic CNS changes. CT scan or cerebral angiography may be indicated.

Sudden, episodic attacks of vertigo, tinnitus, and progressive deafness, accompanied by nausea and vomiting and persisting for minutes to hours, are characteristic of **Ménière's syndrome.** Vertigo persisting for days or weeks may be due to **vestibular neuronitis.** This diagnosis is made from the nonrecurrent nature of the attack, preservation of hearing, and absence of any neurologic signs except nystagmus and equilibratory disturbance. In patients with **postural hypotension** who become vertiginous on changing from recumbent to upright position, examination before and after this shift in posture demonstrates the exaggerated fall in BP. However, vertigo with sudden change in body or head position—e.g., on rising from a recumbent posture, or on rolling over in bed **(postural** or **positional vertigo)**—is more often due to labyrinthine disturbance, as occurs after skull fracture. Vertigo that occurs on sudden turning or extending of the head may occasionally be due to **vertebral artery insufficiency** or **tumors of the floor of the 4th ventricle;** occasionally, especially in the elderly, it occurs as an isolated, idiopathic disorder **(benign positional vertigo;** see also in Ch. 167), perhaps related to degeneration changes in the ampullae of the semicircular canals.

True vertigo is not a symptom of psychoneurosis, but giddiness and fear of losing one's balance while walking may be symptoms of an anxiety neurosis or depression. Diagnosis is established by absence of objective findings, by negative laboratory tests, and by psychologic evaluation.

Treatment

Treatment depends on determining and eliminating the cause. Treatment of Ménière's syndrome and other otogenic causes of vertigo is discussed in Ch. 167. CNS disorders causing vertigo—posterior fossa tumors, cerebellar disorders, and multiple sclerosis—are discussed elsewhere in this section.

Symptomatic relief may be obtained by bed rest and dimenhydrinate 50 to 100 mg orally q 4 to 6 h, perphenazine 4 to 8 mg orally or 5 mg IM t.i.d., or meclizine 25 mg orally t.i.d. All these drugs are moderately effective against both intermittent and continuous vertigo in ambulatory patients.

HICCUP

(Hiccough; Singultus)

Repeated involuntary spasmodic contractions of the diaphragm, followed by sudden closure of the glottis, which checks the inflow of air and produces the characteristic sounds.

Etiology

The condition, which is more common in men, follows irritation of afferent or efferent nerves or of medullary centers controlling the muscles of respiration, particularly the diaphragm. The cause of transient episodes may never become apparent, but with prolonged or recurrent attacks the cause can usually be determined. Afferent nerves may be stimulated by swallowing hot or irritating substances. Hiccups accompanying diaphragmatic pleurisy, pneumonia, uremia, or alcoholism are not infrequent. Abdominal causes include disorders of the stomach and esophagus, bowel diseases, pancreatitis, pregnancy, bladder irritation, hepatic metastases, or hepatitis. Thoracic and mediastinal lesions or surgery may be responsible. Posterior fossa tumors or infarcts may stimulate centers in the medulla oblongata. Persistent hiccups occasionally may result from psychogenic causes.

Treatment

High blood CO_2 inhibits hiccups; low CO_2 accentuates them. Numerous simple measures may be tried: increasing Pa_{CO_2} by a series of breath-holdings or by rebreathing into a paper bag (CAUTION: *Not a plastic bag, as it may cling to the nostrils*); drinking a glass of water rapidly; swallowing dry bread or crushed ice; inducing vomiting; traction on the tongue; pressure on the eyeballs; or ethyl chloride spray to the epigastrium. Carotid sinus compression (massage) may be tried with proper precautions (see PAROXYSMAL SUPRAVENTRICULAR TACHYCARDIA in CARDIAC ARRHYTHMIAS, Ch. 25). Strong digital pressure may be applied over the phrenic nerves behind the sternoclavicular joints.

If these measures fail, an often successful method is to introduce a plastic or rubber suction catheter through the nose to a distance of 3 or 4 in. and, with a to-and-fro movement, to stimulate the pharynx in the sensitive area behind the uvula and opposite the second cervical vertebra.

Other maneuvers include gastric lavage, galvanic stimulation of the phrenic nerve, or esophageal dilation with a small bougie. Gastric overdistention can be relieved by continuous suction. Inhalation of 5% CO_2 in O_2 is of value, particularly in postoperative patients. In diaphragmatic pleurisy, tight adhesive support of the lower chest may help. The list of drugs for control of persistent hiccup includes phenobarbital, scopolamine, amphetamine, prochlorperazine, chlorpromazine, and narcotics.

When simpler methods fail, the phrenic nerve may be blocked by small amounts of 0.5% procaine solution, caution being taken to avoid respiratory depression and pneumothorax. Even bilateral phrenicotomy does not cure all cases.

---

119. NEUROPSYCHIATRIC SYNDROMES IN ORGANIC CEREBRAL DISEASE

(Organic Brain Syndrome)

Psychologic or cognitive disorders caused by or associated with impaired cerebral tissue function.

Toxic-metabolic, inflammatory, and structural brain disorders may produce symptoms simulating functional neurotic or psychotic syndromes, which may be the presenting or predominant feature of the disorder. These neuropsychiatric syndromes manifest themselves in one or more of these spheres: disorders of (1) attention, arousal and consciousness, and motivation; (2) perception (internal and external, ideational and physical); (3) mood and affect; (4) intellectual function; and (5) personality.

The neurotic or psychotic syndromes that occur with brain involvement due to metabolic disease (e.g., vitamin B_{12} deficiency) or a secondary metabolic disorder (e.g., secondary to carcinoma of the pancreas) may be the earliest manifestations of the underlying disorder. In psychiatric appraisal, diagnosis is facilitated by evidence of change from premorbid psychologic status, by careful mental status assessment, and by a high index of suspicion. In addition to information obtained during a general psychiatric examination, mental status testing should focus on attention, language function (fluency, comprehension, repetition, quality of language and speech output), memory (old, well-learned information, recent events, new information), and specific intellectual functions (reading, writing, mathematics, and copying of 2- and 3-dimensional figures). An EEG and CT scanning are appropriate initial screening procedures in suspicious cases. Cerebral arteriography or brain scan should be reserved for cases with a peculiar presentation or frank organic features.

Any neurotic syndrome or personality disorder may occur in the course of a cerebral disease, but conversion symptoms are the most common. Such symptoms appearing for the first time in middle or late life are particularly suggestive, and the possibility of organic disease should be considered in such cases unless the patient has just suffered clear-cut precipitating psychosocial stress.

Any brain disorder may present as a psychotic syndrome, but drugs, cerebral tumors, temporal lobe epilepsy, multiple sclerosis, vitamin B_{12} deficiency, head injury, infarctions, and degenerative disease are the commonest organic causes of psychosis. The entire range of psychotic disorders can occur in the context of cerebral disease. Schizophrenic states due to excessive consumption of amphetamines, alcohol (alcoholic hallucinosis), or other toxic compounds are frequently misdiagnosed as primary schizophrenic illnesses. General paresis (dementia paralytica) is a great mimic of psychosis, although it is less common now. In those conditions that are progressive, unmistakable organic features eventually appear, and dementia supervenes unless the underlying condition is treatable.

Depressive states often follow influenza, typhoid, infectious hepatitis, or childbirth or may be associated with medications such as antihypertensive drugs, notably reserpine. Sometimes gross **euphoria** may follow the administration of corticosteroids or ACTH.

Neuropsychiatric syndromes associated with organic disease are conveniently grouped as follows: (1) delirious states, (2) dementia, (3) the amnesic syndromes, (4) the frontal lobe syndrome, and (5) seizure disorders.

DELIRIUM AND CONFUSIONAL STATES

Syndromes (often reversible) most commonly found in either toxic or inflammatory conditions affecting the brain diffusely or multifocally. They are characterized by fluctuating disturbances of attention, perception, intellectual function, and affect.

Etiology and Incidence

Delirium, a disorder marked by irritability, fear, visual hallucinations, and sometimes a complete loss of contact with the environment, may occur at any age. **Confusional states,** milder clinical states, are more common in the elderly and in patients with preexisting brain disease. In susceptible individuals, confusional states can occur after sudden or unexpected environmental changes.

Delirium may occur with a wide range of clinical conditions, broadly falling into 2 groups: **metabolic disorders** and **structural lesions.** Clouding of consciousness implies disturbance of function of the reticular activating system, and because of its polysynaptic nature, this region of the brainstem and diencephalon is susceptible to the action of many abnormal metabolites and toxins. Thus, a severe and potentially fatal delirious reaction may occur when chronically ingested alcohol, sedatives, or anesthetic agents are suddenly withdrawn; less severe delirious reactions can accompany febrile conditions, liver or renal failure, acute intermittent porphyria, myxedema, or either hypo- or hyperglycemia, or occur in association with thiamine or nicotinic acid deficiencies or in the course of cardiac failure.

Structural lesions can lead to delirious states. These include meningitis and encephalitis; cerebral neoplasms when multiple or causing an intracranial pressure rise and shift; cerebral abscess; large subdural hematomas; head injury; or cerebral infarct or bleeding. The brain is displaced, and there is stretching and spasm of the perforating branches originating from the basilar, superior cerebellar, posterior communicating, and posterior cerebral arteries that supply the central region of the brainstem and diencephalon, including the reticular activating system. Necessarily, this interference with blood supply also leads to disturbed cerebral cortical function.

Symptoms and Signs

Most cases of delirium begin fairly suddenly. The cardinal feature is clouding of consciousness, but this sign must be inferred from its resulting clinical features. Since new memory traces are formed with difficulty, if at all, recent memory is impaired. Disorientation results from a lack of appreciation of time, perhaps location, and in severe cases, person. Confusion is shown in difficulty with intellectual tasks, in speech, and in behavior, which may become purposeless and childish. The severity of the findings may vary from patient to patient, and in the same patient from time to time. One delirious patient may have only a fuzzy feeling and some slowness in thinking; another may be detached from his environment or border on coma. Increased or decreased motor activity is common.

The delirious patient becomes inattentive and distractable and has difficulty in comprehension. Remaining in touch with reality is difficult, since perceptions and imaginings are no longer clearly distinguished; illusions and hallucinations appear, most frequently visual though often auditory or tactile. The environment is likely to be misinterpreted, and often frank delusional beliefs emerge. The patient's emotional responses are often blunted or labile, but in many cases overwhelming fear is obvious. Elation or depression is less common, but a depressive tinge to a delirious or clouded state implies a serious suicidal risk. Occasionally, the patient may be excitable, irritable, violent, and paranoid.

The patient's disturbed behavior often can be related to his abnormal affect and paranoid beliefs. Apathy or restlessness is common, but the most serious behavioral problems are the patient's inability to cooperate with the medical staff in treatment (sometimes amounting to outright rejection of treatment) and suicidal behavior, which is most often seen in fearful patients.

Sleep is frequently disturbed and often punctuated by vivid dreams. Partial or complete amnesia for the period of the illness is usual and includes periods in which the patient appeared lucid. Seizures may occur, particularly in delirium following drug withdrawal.

Diagnosis

An arbitrary distinction between delirium and coma is drawn, depending on whether the patient can communicate. If the frankly delirious symptoms of vivid hallucinations, fear, and florid delusions are lacking and only clouding of consciousness is present, delirium may often be difficult to demonstrate at a single interview, but successive examinations will provide a clearer picture. In mild cases, simple tests of memory and orientation may appear normal, but the patient shows considerable affective or behavioral disturbance. Clinical tests of concentration (e.g., serial subtraction) may prove helpful. In some cases (often misdiagnosed as acute schizophrenic illnesses), marked paranoid ideation is directed against the medical and nursing staff. The paranoid symptoms usually settle in a few hours or days. In delirium, the EEG is particularly helpful and shows slowing of the α rhythm and excessive diffuse θ and even δ activity.

Clinical Course and Prognosis

The illness may continue for hours or weeks, but most cases last a few days. The course is often fluctuating, and a patient may be able to answer questions accurately at one time but become totally irrational and out of reach shortly afterwards. Patients tend to be worse in the evenings and at night and in circumstances of sensory deprivation such as isolated private hospital rooms. The prognosis is good if the underlying condition is reversible.

Treatment

The underlying condition must be treated vigorously if possible; the delirious syndrome itself requires ensuring that no harm comes to the patient, that food intake is adequate, and that fluids and electrolytes are well maintained. A quiet, relaxed environment—the opposite of the intensive treatment area—should be provided. Simple, but very important, general measures that help the patient to become reoriented are described in the treatment of Dementia, below. High-potency multiple vitamin preparations have been advised. Quiet delirious reactions usually require little or no pharmacotherapy; medications should be avoided when possible. Restlessness and recalcitrance are best managed using haloperidol 5 to 10 mg 3 to 4 times a day. For agitated deliria, such as occur with delirium tremens, the drug of choice is diazepam given IV slowly in doses of 5 to 10 mg every 15 min until the patient is quiet. The agent can then be given at wider intervals as necessary to keep the patient quiet but not asleep.

Treatment of delirium as a psychiatric emergency is discussed in Ch. 142.

DEMENTIA

A syndrome of progressive, irreversible cerebral dysfunction caused by structural neuropathologic alterations and characterized by predominant cognitive functional loss.

Symptoms and Signs

Dementia is often considered to be dominated by cognitive difficulties, and in many patients the earliest changes do occur in the cognitive field. However, depression, paranoia, anxiety, or any of several other psychologic symptoms may be the predominant presenting feature. Except in rare cases of brainstem involvement, the brain lesions that cause dementia are widespread, involving the cortex, limbic system, and perhaps the white matter of the cerebral hemispheres. Since pathologic changes proceed at different rates in different brain areas and with different diseases, early symptoms differ widely from patient to patient.

The most common clinical picture is of slow disintegration of personality and intellect due to impaired insight and judgment and the loss of affect. Usually, progression of the disease is more painful to the beholder than to the patient. Interests become restricted, outlook becomes rigid, conceptual thinking becomes more difficult, and some poverty of thought becomes apparent. Familiar tasks may be performed well, but acquiring new skills is difficult. Initiative is diminished, and the patient may become distractable. In addition, a global defect eventually develops, involving all aspects of higher cortical function. Along with the cognitive dysfunction, specific disturbances of speech (aphasia), motor activity (apraxia), and recognition of perceptions (agnosia) may be discernible. Memory impairment increases, beginning with problems recalling recent events or finding names; the impairment varies greatly from time to time and often from moment to moment. It can be circumvented at first, but as the defect increases, remote memory is also progressively impaired. Characteristically, orientation becomes impaired at first for time, later for place, and finally for person.

In some patients, cognitive dysfunction is preceded by modifications in their usual behavior and emotional responses. Typically, affect is blunted, but in early stages it may be excessive. Normal personality traits may become exaggerated or caricatured; an obsessive patient may be unbearably pedantic and rigid (organic orderliness), or a sociable extrovert may be facile and inappropriately jocular. The initial affective change may be dominated by irritability, with periods of anger and violence. Depression is common. If the mood change (depression, anxiety, or elation) is sustained, the disorder may be misdiagnosed as a primary affective condition. Affect becomes more and more shallow and evanescent as the condition progresses, and finally gives way to severe blunting, masked perhaps by a fatuous euphoria without depth.

The patient may embark on foolish and ill-judged, perhaps illegal, activities, but he cannot sustain them as his motivation and drive decline. Habits deteriorate, and the patient becomes slovenly, dirty, and eventually incontinent, culminating with the need for total nursing care in later stages of the illness.

Coexisting neurologic features depend on the distribution and nature of the brain lesions, and these in turn on the etiology. They are marked in some syndromes, but in others, such as senile dementia, they are unusual despite the widespread atrophic process.

While dementia tends to run an insidious and progressive course as described above, it is quite common for patients who have subtle, borderline, or mild signs of dementia to become acutely and severely confused and disturbed. This is usually due to a sudden stress, e.g., acute illness of any kind, treatment with medications that affect cerebral metabolism, sudden changes in environment and daily routines, psychosocial stresses (particularly loss of a close relationship with another person). Typically, the stresses are multiple, as when an elderly person fractures a hip, is hospitalized, and has anesthesia, surgery, medications for pain, frequent changes of personnel, and a move to a nursing home. Recognition of these sudden changes and their causes demands a description of the prestress status, because judicious care may result in substantial improvement.

Classification and Etiology

Dementia may result from a wide variety of distinctive pathologic processes.

Alzheimer-type dementia is due to a degenerative process, with a large loss of cells from the cerebral cortex and other brain areas. Clinically, memory loss is the most prominent early symptom. Disturbances of arousal do not occur early in the disease course. The brain shows marked atrophy with wide sulci and dilated ventricles. Senile plaques and neurofibrillary tangles are present. **Alzheimer's presenile** and **senile onset dementias** are similar in both clinical and pathologic features, with the former commonly having its beginning in the 5th and 6th decades and the latter in the 7th and 8th decades, sometimes earlier, rarely later. The dementia usually progresses steadily, becoming well advanced in 2 to 3 yr. **Pick's disease** also presents in the presenile period and shows a similar clinical picture. The primary difference is found pathologically: circumscribed convolutional atrophy affects mainly the frontal and temporal lobes. In general, Pick's disease patients are apt to be more dull and lacking initiative. Patients with either Alzheimer's or Pick's disease may occasionally show mild extrapyramidal signs, with decreased arm swing, masked faces, and bradykinesia, but without tremor. Some cases of dementia occurring in the presenile period are hard to classify and are sometimes labelled **idiopathic,** or **simple presenile dementia.**

Chronic communicating hydrocephalus with "normal" pressure can cause an insidiously developing dementia in mid to late middle age, affecting men more than women. Clinically, such patients are slow and slovenly in contrast to the more alert behavior that characterizes Alzheimer's disease. The gait is unsteady, slow, and shuffling, and many patients have episodes of urinary incontinence. Pathogenesis is based on impeded CSF circulation and absorption. There may have been a previous attack of meningitis, encephalitis, or head injury, and a few cases prove to have tumors, particularly of the midbrain. CT scanning shows large dilated ventricles with little or no cortical atrophy. The CSF pressure is in the upper ranges of normal limits. Some improvement may follow the introduction of a ventriculoatrial shunt.

Multi-infarct dementia is more common in men and begins most frequently in the 7th decade. Small and large cerebral infarcts of varying ages are present. Hypertension is frequently associated but is not an essential precursor. Hypertensive patients are most susceptible to repeated lacunar infarcts. Because the pathologic process involves infarction, the dementia tends to progress in a steplike manner, each step initiated by a period of clouding of consciousness and perhaps the development or aggravation of neurologic signs. In the early stages of the illness, personality and insight tend to be better preserved than in senile dementia. Depressive symptoms are particularly common, and suicide is possible. As the condition advances, neurologic features, especially hemiplegias, are likely, and pseudobulbar palsy, with pathologic laughing and crying, or signs of extrapyramidal dysfunction may develop. Treatment is similar to that of other forms of cerebral ischemic disease (see Ch. 122). Control of hypertension may be especially important.

Infectious dementia has been recognized with increased frequency and is characterized by a relatively acute onset, prominent disturbances in attention, focal and fluctuating neurologic deficits, and rapid progression. **Creutzfeldt-Jakob disease** (subacute spongiform encephalopathy) is discussed under CENTRAL NERVOUS SYSTEM VIRAL DISEASES in Ch. 12. It is a rare form of dementia caused by a slow virus infection and typically runs a 6- to 24-mo course. The progressive dementia is accompanied by ataxia, and extrapyramidal and often pyramidal features. Myoclonic attacks are frequent. The EEG pattern characteristically shows a flat background interrupted by regular brief polyphasic complexes with sharp wave components, although this is not pathognomonic. Brain biopsy is appropriate in **suspected herpes encephalitis** and should be considered in possible cases of **multifocal leukoencephalopathy** or **subacute sclerosing panencephalitis.**

Huntington's disease (see in Ch. 127) is caused by a single autosomal dominant gene with complete penetrance. The symptoms may begin at any age, but in most cases onset is between 35 and 50 yr of age. Personality changes with frequent psychosis, intellectual impairment leading to profound dementia, and abnormal involuntary movements all contribute to this syndrome; any one of these symptom clusters can present initially.

A severe **head injury** may cause sufficient brain damage to result in nonprogressive dementia. With repeated head injury, as in boxers, progressive dementia accompanied by extrapyramidal features **(chronic progressive traumatic encephalopathy)** may develop even though boxing may be abandoned.

Other causes: Dementia may occur with cerebral **tumors** (particularly midline tumors or those involving the corpus callosum), with **subdural hematomas,** in **syphilis** (either as general paresis or as a result of meningovascular disease), and in **alcoholism, myxedema, SLE, vitamin B$_{12}$ deficiency, nicotinic acid deficiency (pellagra),** and **multiple sclerosis.** It may also occur in the course of other degenerative conditions of the CNS, such as **Friedreich's ataxia,** or after **meningitis, encephalitis,** or **poisoning** with lead or carbon monoxide. Dementia may be the presenting feature in a significant number of such cases, and early and accurate diagnosis is necessary if treatment is to be begun while useful brain function remains. Intellectual deterioration with cortical atrophy and ventricular enlargement is found in some individuals who have had schizophrenia for a prolonged period.

Diagnosis

Diagnosis of dementia is a matter of clinical judgment. A neuropsychologic diagnosis of dementia should *not* be accepted if the clinical evaluation is dubious, especially in patients who appear depressed or who may have other primary psychiatric disorders. The results of psychometric tests can only be depended upon when the patient is freely communicative. Muteness or a failure to supply complete answers can result from depression as easily as from dementia. CT studies should also be correlated with the clinical state. Cerebral cortical "atrophy" increases with age in persons with normal mental status, and CT scan provides no reliable indication of intellectual impairment. *Because dementia is sometimes secondary to a treatable condition, adequate investigations must be made unless the etiology is obvious.* These should include a CBC, lumbar puncture, serum vitamin B$_{12}$ level, tests of thyroid function, chest and skull x-rays, CT scan, EEG, and serologic tests for syphilis.

Differentiating dementia from delirium is seldom difficult. The delirious patient usually has a brief history and a more florid illness. By the time a patient with dementia is seen in the clinic, symptoms have typically been present for an extended period of time. An EEG may be helpful in difficult cases, as when a confused patient is seen with no accompanying informant; the EEG disturbance is generally greater in delirium.

Distinguishing dementia from a primary psychiatric disorder may be a more difficult problem. **Pseudodementia,** a reversible disorder if treated, can closely mimic neuropathologically caused disorders. Though most common in depressed elderly individuals, it can occur in patients with schizophrenic or personality disorders. Neuropsychologic testing and CT scanning may not distinguish pseudodemented patients from those who have persistent neuropathologic syndromes. A depressed patient readily creates an illusion of dementia because of apathy, slowness and poverty of thought, poor concentration, and inattention. The risk of misdiagnosis increases with age. Since depression may sometimes be an early symptom of dementia, evident depression may be mistakenly dismissed as a secondary feature. In doubtful cases, the patient should be treated as having a depressive illness. Patients with a primary dementia may also experience depression; antidepressant therapy may prove beneficial.

Chronic barbiturate or bromide intoxication, vitamin deficiency states, and myxedema may mimic dementia.

Treatment

The initial management of acute dementia should always include noting whether a prominent recent worsening has occurred in the patient's mental status. If so, the prior capabilities must be described, since there is reason to try for substantial improvement. This is particularly true when the dementia has suddenly become worse because of stress. Such patients benefit from improvement in a precipitating illness, withdrawal of known toxic drugs, and minimal use of drugs that affect brain metabolism. They require time to adjust to and become familiar with new surroundings, routines, and people.

Quiet, dark private rooms for these patients should be avoided. The room should be reasonably bright and provide sensory stimuli such as a night light and a radio or a television set to assist the patient in remaining oriented and in focusing his attention. Excessive stimuli, however, should be avoided. Familiar people or a familiar supportive family member in attendance, and frequent visits by medical personnel, encourage the patient to relate. Attention should be paid to assisting him in his discrimination of reality and to allaying his anxiety. Explanations should be precise and simple, and nonessential procedures omitted. Orientation to time is helped by using large calendars and clocks and routinizing daily activities; orientation to person, by medical personnel wearing large name tags and repeatedly introducing themselves. *Diligent application of such simple procedures often can lead to marked improvement.*

Patients with dementia should be as much as possible in familiar surroundings with minimal variation in environmental stimuli, yet should be encouraged to continue with performable tasks. Major problems develop when awareness of their difficulties causes them to feel an acute sense of frustration, loss of self-esteem, and, at times, overwhelming anxiety **(catastrophic reaction).** The family should be counseled and should encourage the patient in activities that promote a sense of participation and accomplishment. If catastrophic reactions can be averted, hospitalization or institutionalization may be avoided.

Prognosis

Dementia is regarded generally as an insidious, slowly progressive, untreatable condition. However, onset can be acute, as occurs sometimes in cerebrovascular disease or after meningitis; the disorder may not be progressive, as after a head injury; and in a few cases, treatment may arrest the progress of the condition or even lead to frank recovery. Removal of alcohol in patients with alcoholic dementia can lead to substantial long-term improvement. In depressed, demented individuals, antidepressants can substantially (though transiently) improve function. Therefore, dementia should not be regarded as a hopeless condition to be diagnosed and then ignored. Each case requires careful consideration, and the most appropriate investigations should be selected for each patient.

AMNESIC SYNDROMES

Amnesia can result from either diffuse cerebral impairment or focal lesions, since specific neuroanatomic pathways in the cerebrum take part in the complex, poorly defined processes of memory storage and recall. The pathways underlying memory are found in the **limbic system,** extending along the hippocampal formation of the medial temporal lobes, fornix, and mammillary bodies, to the anterior nuclei of the thalamus, cingulum, septal area, and the orbital surface of the frontal lobes. There is a close connection between the hypothalamic-mammillary area and the brainstem reticular formation (see IMPAIRED CONSCIOUSNESS, in Ch. 118), suggesting a close relationship between reticular formation and limbic system in the memory process. Recent memory and the ability to form new memories are profoundly impaired by bilateral lesions involving the limbic memory route, most often seen in the temporal lobes (from trauma, stroke, herpes simplex encephalitis) or in the mammillary bodies and medial thalamus (from thiamine deficiency, hypothalamic neoplasms, and ischemia).

The **retrograde** and **post-traumatic amnesia** for the periods immediately preceding and following concussion or more severe head trauma also appear to result from an interruption of limbic function, although more diffuse cerebral processes involved in memory storage and recall are probably also affected, as they are in many of the diffuse dementia-producing diseases.

KORSAKOFF'S SYNDROME (Dysmnesic Syndrome)

An amnesic state in which the inability to record new memory traces may lead to confabulation and a seemingly paradoxic situation in which the patient can carry out complex tasks learned before his illness but cannot learn the simplest new skills.

Etiology

The disorder results from damage to the medial aspects of both temporal lobes, notably the hippo-campal gyri and hippocampi; to interference with the pathways of the limbic system; or to damage to the mammillary bodies or dorsal medial nucleus of the thalamus. The hippocampal areas may be affected by bilateral infarction, subarachnoid hemorrhage, head injury, acute necrotic encephalitis (herpes simplex), invasive cerebral tumors, or neurosurgical interference. Mammillary body or me-dial thalamic involvement occurs in chronic alcoholism and is often associated with an initial attack of Wernicke's encephalopathy.

Symptoms and Signs

The typical syndrome occurs only when the pathologic process severely damages the appropriate areas of the brain but not other brain areas. Because the destructive process is seldom discrete or total, the clinical picture is often incomplete or obscured by other features. In "pure" cases, how-ever, the memory defect is highly characteristic. Since memory for new information is affected but memories for distant events are not, the patient's previous experience is available to guide his ac-tions; there may be little apparent intellectual loss. Memory of events since the onset of the illness—and often, for unknown reasons, for a period of weeks or months before it—is severely or totally disturbed. Disorientation in time is inevitable with such a gross defect of memory.

Confabulation is a striking feature that frequently occurs during the early course of the illness in association with the defect in recent memory. It is less apparent in more chronic cases. The bewil-dered patient substitutes imaginary or confused experiences for those he cannot recall. Convincing confabulations may deceive the doctor into seeing the patient's mental state as normal. Since other cognitive functions must be preserved to allow confabulation to develop, this symptom is absent or poorly developed in dementia.

Since the limbic system is concerned also with the experience of emotion, emotional changes usually develop; these include apathy, blandness, or mild euphoria with little or no response to environmental events, including fear-inducing situations. The emotional changes, together with the loss of insight, protect the patient from the distress of his disability.

Prognosis and Treatment

The course of Korsakoff's syndrome reflects its cause. It is often transient and has a good progno-sis in head injury and subarachnoid hemorrhage. In alcoholism, acute necrotic encephalitis, and other conditions where destruction is irreversible, the prognosis is poor and prolonged institutional care may be required. However, improvement may occur for as long as 12 to 24 mo after onset, and one must beware of premature institutionalization. **Treatment** is that of the underlying condition.

TRANSIENT GLOBAL AMNESIA

Attacks of transient global amnesia lasting 6 to 24 h can occur in adult patients of any age, especially men. Pathogenesis is related to ischemia involving midline limbic structures. Migraine may sometimes represent their cause among younger subjects; in older patients, pathogenesis is be-lieved to be similar to the transient ischemic attacks of cerebrovascular disease. Loss of recent memory is severe, and disorientation and confusion last minutes or hours. Nevertheless, recovery is generally complete, with few recurrences.

FRONTAL LOBE SYNDROME

A syndrome in which the range of emotional expression is constricted, inhibition is lessened, and foresight is impaired or lost. There is a fundamental change of personality; intellectual function may be variable, but is usually impaired.

Any pathologic process leading to destruction or interference with the function of the gray matter of both frontal lobes will give rise to the frontal lobe syndrome, but some of the features also occur with lesions restricted to the temporal lobes. Degenerative conditions (see DEMENTIA, above), cere-bral tumors, general paresis, and head injury are the most common causes of frontal lobe destruc-tion.

The patient becomes careless and uncaring, his work unreliable and shoddy. He becomes untrust-worthy and cannot concentrate his thoughts or energies for any length of time on any particular task. A shallow, inappropriate, jocular euphoria is common, though some patients tend to a dispirited and indifferent state of apathy. Habits deteriorate and judgment is impaired, often to the disadvantage of his family. Insight is lost. The patient generally does not complain, although his family does. The frontal lobe syndrome may be the initial presentation in dementia. **Treatment** is that of the underlying condition.

SEIZURE DISORDERS

(See Ch. 120)

POSTCONCUSSIONAL SYNDROME

A syndrome including a wide variety of symptoms such as headaches and complaints of impaired memory, although no defect can be demonstrated objectively.

After a mild head injury, headache, dizziness, difficulty in concentration, depression, apathy, and perhaps anxiety are more common than after severe head injuries. These symptoms can cause a considerable disability. The part played by brain damage is unclear; the postconcussional syndrome is more common in patients with a premorbid neurotic disposition, though recent studies suggest that even mild trauma can cause neuronal damage. It is especially common when compensation for the injury is possible. The results of treatment with drugs or psychotherapy vary, and symptoms commonly persist after compensation claims are settled.

---

120. SEIZURE DISORDERS

(Epilepsy)

Epilepsy: *A recurrent paroxysmal disorder of cerebral function characterized by sudden, brief attacks of altered consciousness, motor activity, sensory phenomena, or inappropriate behavior.* **Convulsive seizures,** the most common form of attacks, begin with loss of consciousness and motor control, and tonic or clonic jerking of all extremities, but any recurrent seizure pattern may be termed epilepsy.

Seizure disorders in the newborn are also discussed in Vol. II, Ch. 21.

Etiology

Epilepsy is classed etiologically as symptomatic or idiopathic, "symptomatic" implying that a probable cause has been identified which at times permits a specific course of therapy. No obvious cause can be found in about 75% of adults and a smaller percentage of children under age 3. Some authorities believe that idiopathic epilepsy is due to a microscopic scar in the brain resulting from birth trauma or other injury, and, indeed, many patients classed during life as idiopathic show evidence of a causative lesion at autopsy. However, it is more likely that unexplained metabolic abnormalities underlie most idiopathic cases.

Idiopathic epilepsy generally begins between ages 2 and 14. Seizures before age 2 are usually related to developmental defects, birth injuries, or a metabolic disease affecting the brain; those beginning after age 25 are usually secondary to cerebral trauma, tumors, or other organic brain disease. Focal diseases of the brain can cause seizures at any age.

Convulsive seizures may be associated with a variety of cerebral or systemic disorders, as a result of a focal or generalized disturbance of cortical function. These include **hyperpyrexia** (acute infection, heat stroke), **CNS infections** (meningitis, encephalitis, brain abscess, neurosyphilis, rabies, tetanus, falciparum malaria, toxoplasmosis, cysticercosis of the brain), **metabolic disturbances** (hypoglycemia, hypoparathyroidism, phenylketonuria), **convulsive or toxic agents** (camphor, pentylenetetrazol, strychnine, picrotoxin, lead, alcohol), **cerebral hypoxia** (Adams-Stokes syndrome, carotid sinus hypersensitivity, anesthesia, carbon monoxide poisoning, breath-holding), **expanding brain lesions** (neoplasm, intracranial hemorrhage, subdural hematoma in infancy), **brain defects** (congenital, developmental), **cerebral edema** (hypertensive encephalopathy, eclampsia), **cerebral trauma** (skull fracture, birth injury), **anaphylaxis** (foreign serum or drug allergy), and **cerebral infarct or hemorrhage.** Convulsions may also occur as a **withdrawal symptom** after chronic use of alcohol, hypnotics, or tranquilizers. **Hysterical patients** occasionally simulate convulsive attacks.

The seizures are only transient in many of these conditions and do not recur once the illness ends. However, convulsions may recur at intervals for years or indefinitely if there is a permanent lesion or scar in the CNS, in which case a diagnosis of epilepsy is made.

Pathogenesis

Convulsive seizures result from an acute focal or generalized disturbance in cerebral function. Though this disturbance can usually be demonstrated by EEG, its cause is not known. Apparently, a small focus of diseased tissue in the cerebrum will discharge abnormally in response to certain endogenous or exogenous stimuli, and spread of the discharge to other portions of the cerebrum results in convulsive phenomena and loss of consciousness. Whether seizures that are generalized from the outset can begin as a diffuse abnormal discharge or must originate focally is not yet known.

Given a sufficient stimulus (e.g., convulsant drugs, hypoxia, hypoglycemia), even the normal brain can discharge in a disorganized fashion and produce a seizure. Seizures may occasionally be precipitated in susceptible persons by exogenous factors (sound, light, cutaneous stimulation).

TABLE 120-1. INTERNATIONAL CLASSIFICATION OF EPILEPTIC SEIZURES

I. Partial seizures (seizures beginning locally)
   A. Partial seizures with elementary symptomatology (generally without impairment of consciousness)
      1. With motor symptoms (includes jacksonian seizures)
      2. With special sensory or somatosensory symptoms
      3. With autonomic symptoms
      4. Compound forms
   B. Partial seizures with complex symptomatology (generally with impairment of consciousness) (temporal lobe or psychomotor seizures)
      1. With impairment of consciousness only
      2. With cognitive symptomatology
      3. With affective symptomatology
      4. With "psychosensory" symptomatology
      5. With "psychomotor" symptomatology (automatisms)
      6. Compound forms
   C. Partial seizures secondarily generalized
II. Generalized seizures (bilaterally symmetrical and without local onset)
      1. Absences (petit mal)
      2. Bilateral massive epileptic myoclonus
      3. Infantile spasms
      4. Clonic seizures
      5. Tonic seizures
      6. Tonic-clonic seizures (grand mal)
      7. Atonic seizures
      8. Akinetic seizures
III. Unilateral seizures (or predominantly)
IV. Unclassified epileptic seizures (due to incomplete data)

Modified from "Clinical and electroencephalographical classification of epileptic seizures," by H. Gastaut, in *Epilepsia* 11:102–113, 1970. Used with permission of Elsevier/North Holland Biomedical Press, Amsterdam, and the author.

Classification and Incidence

Epileptic seizures can be classified according to several different criteria. TABLE 120-1 gives a current internationally agreed-upon classification. **Partial seizures** begin focally with a specific sensory, motor, or psychic aberration that reflects the affected part of the cerebral hemisphere where the seizure originates. TABLE 120-2 gives some of the characteristic manifestations and their sites of origin. Focal manifestations that immediately precede generalized convulsions are called **aura,** and also reflect where the seizure begins. Sometimes a focal lesion of the hemispheres will activate deeper parts of the brain so rapidly that it produces a generalized grand mal seizure before any focal sign appears. **Generalized seizures** usually affect both consciousness and motor function from the outset. The seizure itself is initiated in the deeper part of the brain and frequently has a genetic or metabolic cause.

Epilepsy affects about 2% of the population. Most patients have only 1 type of seizure; about 30% have 2 or more types. About 90% experience grand mal seizures, either alone (60%) or in combination with other seizures (30%). Absence (petit mal) attacks occur in about 25% (4% alone, 21% in combination). Psychomotor attacks occur in 18% (6% alone, 12% in combination).

TABLE 120-2. FOCAL MANIFESTATIONS OF PARTIAL SEIZURES AND SITES OF THE CEREBRAL DYSFUNCTION

Focal Manifestation	Site of Dysfunction
Localized twitching of muscles (jacksonian seizure)	Frontal lobe (motor cortex)
Localized numbness or tingling	Parietal lobe (sensory cortex)
Chewing movements or smacking of lips	Anterior temporal lobe
Olfactory hallucinations	Antero-medial temporal lobe
Visual hallucinations (formed images)	Temporal lobe
Visual hallucinations (flashes of light)	Occipital lobe
Complex automatic behaviorisms	Temporal lobe

Symptoms and Signs

Partial or focal seizures begin with specific motor, sensory, or psychomotor focal phenomena. Common manifestations are given in TABLE 120–2. In **jacksonian seizures,** focal motor symptoms begin in one hand or foot and then "march" up the extremity, or spread similarly from a corner of the mouth. The dysfunction may remain localized or may spread to other parts of the brain, with consequent loss of consciousness and generalized convulsive movements.

Partial seizures with complex symptoms are characterized by a variety of patterns of onset (see TABLE 120–1). In most instances, the patient has a 1- to 2-min loss of contact with the surroundings. The starting patient may stagger, perform automatic purposeless movements, and utter unintelligible sounds. He does not understand what is said and may resist aid. Mental confusion continues for another 1 or 2 min after the attack is apparently over. **Psychomotor attacks** may develop at any age and are usually associated with structural lesions, most often in the temporal lobe. **Status psychomotor epilepsy** may occur, in which affected subjects act in a slow, bewildered, and sometimes confused state for hours or, rarely, days. Diagnosis of such psychomotor fugue states is made by EEG.

Partial seizures of temporal lobe origin rarely are characterized by unprovoked aggressive behavior. If restrained, however, such patients may occasionally lash out at the person restricting their movement. No satisfactory evidence suggests that complex acts of premeditated or unprovoked aggression can ever be attributed to attacks of temporal lobe epilepsy.

Patients with temporal lobe epilepsy experience a significantly higher incidence of interictal psychiatric disorders than do either the normal population or patients with other forms of epilepsy. Selection factors in evaluation make exact figures difficult to be sure of, but some studies show as many as 1/3 of patients with temporal lobe epilepsy having substantial psychopathologic difficulties, with up to 10% showing symptoms of schizophreniform or depressive psychoses. The behavior abnormalities are slightly more frequent among patients with left temporal lobe epileptic foci. Neither anticonvulsant medication nor surgical treatment has shown a predictably favorable effect on these psychiatric disorders.

Generalized seizures can be minor or major in their manifestations. **Absence (petit mal) attacks** are brief generalized seizures manifested by a 10- to 30-second loss of consciousness, with eye or muscle flutterings at a rate of 3/second, and with or without loss of muscle tone. The patient suddenly stops any activity in which he is engaged and resumes it after the attack. Petit mal seizures are genetically determined and occur predominantly in children: they never begin after age 20. The attacks are likely to occur several or many times a day, often when the patient is sitting quietly. They are infrequent during exercise. Petit mal attacks rarely indicate gross brain damage, and many patients are highly intelligent.

Infantile spasms are characterized by sudden flexion of the arms, forward flexion of the trunk, and extension of the legs. The attacks last only a few seconds but may be repeated many times a day. They are restricted to the first 3 yr of life, often to be replaced by other forms of attacks. Brain damage is usually evident.

Tonic-clonic (grand mal) seizures occasionally begin with a sinking or rising sensation in the epigastrium (the **aura**) followed by an outcry; the seizure continues with loss of consciousness; falling; and tonic, then clonic contractions of the muscles of the extremities, trunk, and head. Urinary and fecal incontinence may occur. The attack usually lasts 2 to 5 min. It may be preceded by a prodromal mood change, and may be followed by a **postictal state**, with deep sleep, headache, muscle soreness or, at times, focal motor or sensory phenomena. The attacks may appear at any age.

Akinetic seizures are brief, generalized seizures seen in children. The child falls or pitches to the ground, so that attacks carry the risk of serious trauma.

Epileptic equivalents is a now outmoded term describing certain types of partial seizures that tend to be confined to a single symptom. The disturbances appear in partially treated patients or those subject to more complex seizures and include repetitive auras, paroxysmal attacks of abdominal pair (abdominal epilepsy), or periods of mental cloudiness that may last for several hours. They generally represent fragments of more widespread seizures or the close fusion (i.e., status) of petit mal attacks

In **status epilepticus,** seizures follow one another with no intervening periods of consciousness Grand mal status epilepticus may persist for hours or days, and may be fatal. It may occur spontaneously or result from too rapid withdrawal of anticonvulsants.

Diagnosis

Idiopathic epilepsy must be distinguished from symptomatic epilepsy for proper treatment. Th type of seizure seen in the newborn is not helpful in distinguishing between structural and metaboli causes. In older children and adults, however, focal seizures generally imply a focal structural lesio in the brain, while generalized seizures are more likely to have a metabolic cause.

The history should include an eyewitness account of a typical attack and information on the fre quency of seizures and the longest and shortest intervals between attacks. A history of prior traum (e.g., cranial injury producing unconsciousness, birth trauma), **infection** (e.g., meningitis, encepha tis, pertussis), or **toxic episodes** (e.g., excessive alcohol or drug consumption and its relation seizures) must be sought and evaluated. A family history of convulsions or neurologic disorders significant.

Fever and stiff neck accompanying convulsions of recent onset should suggest meningitis or subarachnoid hemorrhage. Focal cerebral symptoms and signs in association with seizures suggest brain tumor, cerebrovascular disease, or residual traumatic abnormalities. Grand mal seizures, particularly in an adult, always require an extensive diagnostic search for an unsuspected focal lesion.

Appropriate studies include serum glucose and calcium, skull x-rays, and EEG. If these are abnormal, and in all cases of adult-onset seizures, lumbar puncture and CT scan are indicated.

The EEG in grand mal attacks is characterized by sharp spikes with an increased rate of 25 to 30/second. In petit mal, spikes and slow waves appear at the rate of 3/second. Temporal lobe foci (spikes or slow waves) are frequent with psychomotor attacks. The presence of a focal EEG abnormality may aid in the differential diagnosis of brain disease, as may the presence of a characteristic centrencephalic abnormality. Since an EEG taken during a seizure-free interval is normal in about 15% of patients, one normal EEG does not exclude epilepsy. In some cases even repeated EEGs may be normal and the diagnosis of epilepsy as opposed to a behavioral disorder may have to be made on clinical grounds; this is rare, however.

Prognosis

Drug therapy can control grand mal seizures in 50% of cases and greatly reduce the frequency of seizures in another 35%; control petit mal seizures in 40% and reduce the frequency in 35%; control psychomotor attacks in 35% and reduce the frequency in 50%. Newer anticonvulsant agents promise to improve these results even more.

Most patients with epilepsy are normal between attacks, although overuse of anticonvulsants can dull alertness. Progressive mental deterioration is usually related to an accompanying neurologic disease that itself caused the seizures; only rarely do seizures per se impair mental abilities. The outlook is better when no brain lesion is demonstrable. About 70% of noninstitutionalized patients with epilepsy are mentally normal, 20% show a slight reduction in intellect, and 10% have a moderate to pronounced impairment.

Management and Treatment

1. **General principles:** In idiopathic epilepsy, treatment is primarily control of seizures. In symptomatic epilepsy, the associated disease must be treated as well; continued anticonvulsant treatment is usually needed after surgical removal of cerebral lesions.

A normal life should be encouraged. Moderate exercise is recommended; such sports as swimming and horseback riding are permitted with proper safeguards. Movies, dancing, and other social activities should be encouraged. Most state licensing agencies permit driving after seizures have stopped for 1 yr. Alcoholic beverages are **contraindicated.**

Members of the family must be taught a common-sense attitude toward the patient's illness. Instead of overprotection and oversolicitude, sympathetic support should be directed against feelings of inferiority, self-consciousness, and other emotional handicaps, and emphasis should be placed on preventing invalidism. Vocational rehabilitation may help. Institutional care is advisable only for patients with severe mental retardation or with attacks that are frequent, violent, and not controlled by medication.

2. **Management of a convulsion,** whatever its etiology, is limited to preventing injury. A firm but reasonably soft object (e.g., a folded handkerchief) should be inserted between the teeth, but attempts to protect the tongue should not be too vigorous or teeth may be damaged. Clothing about the neck should be loosened, and a pillow may be placed under the head. A responsible fellow worker may be trained to give emergency aid if the patient concurs.

3. **Elimination of causative or precipitating factors:** Physical disorders (e.g., infections and endocrine abnormalities) should be corrected. The first rule in treating seizure disorders is to seek for progressive organic lesions of the brain, such as tumors and abscesses, and, if found, to remove surgically. Cortical scars from trauma, vascular lesions, or birth injuries can sometimes be excised when focal attacks resist medical therapy. After surgical removal of organic lesions, continued medical treatment is usually necessary.

4. **Drug therapy** has undergone substantial advances in recent years, with new and effective drugs available for previously intractable seizure types. Also, the widespread availability of accurate estimations of drug levels has made clinical management more secure and effective.

No single drug controls all types of seizures, and different drugs are required for different patients. Furthermore, some patients may require several drugs. For the newly treated patient with a seizure disorder, the single first drug of choice for the particular type of epilepsy is selected, starting with relatively low doses and increasing over a week or so to the standard therapeutic dose. After about a week at such dosage, **blood levels** are obtained to determine the individual's pharmacokinetic response and, if appropriate, whether the effective therapeutic level has been reached. If seizures continue, the daily drug is increased by small increments as doses rise above the usual. If toxic blood levels or symptoms are encountered, a second anticonvulsant is added slowly, again guarding against toxicity, since interaction between agents can interfere with their rate of metabolic degradation. Once seizures are brought under control, medication should be continued *without interruption* at least 5 seizure-free years.

Many anticonvulsant drugs are available; the most effective for chronic use are given in TABLE 120–3. Therapeutic and toxic blood levels are reasonably well established for phenytoin, phenobar-

TABLE 120–3. DRUGS USED IN EPILEPSY

Drug	Indications	Daily Dose Levels		Blood Level		Toxicity
		Child	Adult	Therapeutic	Toxic	
Phenytoin	Generalized motor, partial motor seizures	5–10 mg/kg	300–500 mg	10–20 μg/ml	>25 μg/ml	Nystagmus, ataxia, dysarthria, lethargy, megaloblastic anemia, gingival hyperplasia Idiosyncratic: rash, exfoliative dermatitis, grand mal convulsions (rare)
Phenobarbital	Generalized motor, partial motor seizures	<4 yr, 5–10 mg/kg	5 yr to adult, 2–5 mg/kg	20–30 μg/ml	>35 μg/ml	Sedation, nystagmus, ataxia, learning difficulties Idiosyncratic: anemia, rash, hyperkinesis
Primidone	Partial complex, generalized motor seizures	10–20 mg/kg Increase slowly	.75–1.5 gm Increase slowly	See phenobarbital. Primidone levels are approximately ¼ phenobarbital levels		See phenobarbital
Carbamazepine	Partial complex, generalized motor seizures	10–20 mg/kg Increase slowly	0.8–1.2 gm Increase slowly	5–9 μg/ml	>12 μg/ml	Nystagmus, diplopia, dysarthria, lethargy, nausea Idiosyncratic: granulocytopenia, thrombocytopenia, liver toxicity
Ethosuximide	Petit mal	<6 yr, 0.5 gm b.i.d. >6 yr, 0.5 gm t.i.d.	0.5 gm q.i.d.	40–100 μg/ml	>100 μg/ml	Nausea, lethargy, dizziness, headache Idiosyncratic: leuco- or pancytopenia, dermatitis, SLE
Trimethadione	Petit mal	<6 yr, 0.3 gm b.i.d. >6 yr, 0.3 gm t.i.d.	0.6 gm t.i.d.	15–25 μg/ml	>25–30 μg/ml	Sedation, nausea Idiosyncratic: hemeralopia, neutropenia, aplastic anemia, dermatitis, SLE

Clonazepam	Petit mal, atypical petit mal, myoclonus, akinetic seizures; infantile spasms	Initial: 0.005–.01 mg/kg t.i.d. Maintenance: 0.03–0.06 mg/kg t.i.d.	Initial: 0.5 mg t.i.d. Maintenance: up to 5–7 mg t.i.d.	5–50 µg/ml (preliminary)	>80 µg/ml	Drowsiness, ataxia, behavorial abnormalities Serious reaction rare, but partial or complete tolerance to beneficial effects usual in 1–6 mo
Valproate	Petit mal, myoclonus, generalized motor, akinetic, partial motor seizures	15–30 mg/kg (Total given in divided doses t.i.d. Start slowly, especially if other drugs are being taken.)	1.0–1.5 gm/day	>50 µg/ml (before A.M. dose)	>100 µg/ml	Nausea and vomiting, transient drowsiness, transient neutropenia

bital, primidone, and ethosuximide, and are given in TABLE 120-3. The table also gives standard dose responses for other anticonvulsants, but it is not presently known if these levels are therapeutically optimal. Estimates of drug concentrations in blood are useful (1) to indicate the particular response to specific drugs (individuals can vary widely); (2) if abnormally high, to warn against toxicity in susceptible individuals; and (3) if abnormally low, to reflect the patient's noncompliance in taking medication. Despite these potential advantages, management must give first attention to the patient's epilepsy. Once the drug response is known, blood levels become substantially less useful to follow than the clinical course.

For **partial (focal) motor** or **generalized motor (grand mal)** seizures, phenytoin is the drug of choice; 300 mg/day orally can be given in divided doses or at bedtime. If seizures continue, doses can be increased cautiously to 500 mg/day with blood level monitoring. Phenobarbital 100 mg/day at bedtime or primidone up to 1.5 gm/day can be added *slowly* to minimize drowsiness. Combinations of phenytoin-phenobarbital often are more effective than either drug alone.

For **partial complex (psychomotor) seizures**, treatment of choice begins with phenytoin or primidone. The latter tends to be particularly effective but is not the first choice because it may cause drowsiness. Carbamazepine appears even more effective, but its hematopoietic effects require close supervision. Clonazepam has produced results superior to valproate, but the drug has not been extensively tested in the USA.

For **absence (petit mal) seizures**, ethosuximide orally is preferred. Valproate and clonazepam orally also are effective, but the latter shows a high incidence of tolerance. Trimethadione 300 mg to 2 gm/day orally in divided doses or acetazolamide 250 mg t.i.d. are reserved for otherwise refractory cases. A ketogenic diet may be helpful but is difficult to maintain.

Akinetic seizures, myoclonic seizures, and infantile spasms all are difficult to treat. Valproate is preferred, followed by clonazepam. Ethosuximide sometimes is successful, as is acetazolamide (in dosages as for petit mal). Phenytoin has only limited effectiveness. For infantile spasms, corticosteroids, given for a total of 8 to 10 wk, are often effective. Prednisone 2 mg/kg orally is given for 4 wk, then reduced to about half this amount for maintenance. ACTH 20 to 60 u./day IM may also be used.

For **status epilepticus**, diazepam 5 to 10 mg (for adults) is given IV, followed by phenobarbital 200 to 400 mg IV; alternatively, diazepam 10 mg IV q 10 to 15 min for up to 1 h may be given, in amounts up to 40 mg/h for adults and 0.3 mg/kg for children. To prevent recurrence, in adults 500 mg to 1 gm of phenytoin may be given IV at a rate of 50 mg/min for the first 500 mg and 100 mg/30 min thereafter. Smaller doses should be used for children, according to weight. Giving the full amount in one successively administered "loading" dose produces better results than do divided doses. Anesthetic doses of pentobarbital (IV or rectally) may be necessary in some refractory cases; hypothermia may be beneficical in others. Intubation and O_2 therapy are desirable to prevent anoxemia.

Acute convulsive seizures from febrile illnesses, ingestion of alcohol or other toxins, or acute metabolic disturbance require emergency therapy, especially for the causative condition as well as for the convulsion. Status epilepticus should be treated at once. If there has been only one seizure, both phenytoin and phenobarbital should be given in full dosages (see TABLE 120-3) for 7 to 10 days. Anticonvulsants are of little value in preventing alcoholic withdrawal seizures.

Whether children with a *single* febrile convulsion should receive long-term anticonvulsant therapy is not settled. There is little evidence to support this approach, although some physicians favor it. It is more conservative to give drugs for a short interval only, unless the EEG is grossly abnormal or seizures recur in the absence of infection. Children with recurrent generalized febrile convulsions should be treated as for grand mal epilepsy.

Undesirable side effects of drug therapy: Phenobarbital frequently causes incapacitating drowsiness and, in < 1% of cases, an allergic scarlatiniform or morbilliform rash. When a rash appears in a patient taking phenobarbital and phenytoin, the latter is more often responsible. In high doses phenytoin may also cause restlessness, nervousness, nystagmus, nausea, vomiting, unsteady gait, dermatitis, hypertrophy of the gums, and confusion. Adenopathy is a rare complication. Megaloblastic anemia (responsive to folic acid) and aplastic anemia have also been reported with the hydantoins. Phenytoin may alter the serum PBI and other thyroid function tests. Tri- and paramethadione may cause a generalized rash, photophobia, blurred vision, leukopenia, and, rarely, severe anemia, agranulocytosis, or nephrosis. Because the methadiones may be teratogenic, another anticonvulsant (e.g., ethosuximide) is indicated in pregnancy.

Patients receiving paramethadione, trimethadione, or mephenytoin should have a CBC once/month for the first year of therapy. If the WBC or RBC counts decrease significantly, these drugs should be **discontinued immediately**. LE cells in the blood may be demonstrated with either para- or trimethadione. Another drug should be substituted if this happens. The blood should be examined for LE cells whenever suggestive symptoms appear.

When an overdose reaction occurs, one reduces the amount of drug until the intoxication subsides. When more serious toxicity appears, the patient is given ipecac syrup or, if obtunded, is lavaged. After emesis or lavage, activated charcoal is administered, followed by a saline cathartic such as magnesium citrate. The suspect drug should be discontinued and a new anticonvulsant promptly substituted.

121.   SLEEP DISORDERS

The physiologic requirement for sleep is self-evident, yet its precise homeostatic contribution is unknown. The 2 types and varying depths of sleep are marked by characteristic changes in eye movements and in the EEG. EEG low-voltage fast activity accompanies one type (rapid-eye-movement **[REM]**) with periods that occur 5 to 6 times during a normal night's sleep and account for 20 to 25% of the total sleep time. The remainder (nonREM **[NREM]**) is characterized by slow waves on the EEG and ranges in depth through 4 stages (1 to 4), with commensurate difficulties in arousal. Some evidence implicates norepinephrine pathways in the brainstem with REM sleep and serotoninergic pathways with slow wave or NREM. Most dreaming occurs during REM and stage 3; most night terrors, sleep walking, and sleep talking in stages 3 and 4. Selective interruption of REM sleep produces hyperactive and emotionally labile behavior in experimental subjects, but this relationship has not been observed under natural circumstances. Although sleep is necessary for survival, individuals vary widely in their requirements, which are influenced by a number of factors including the current emotional state.

Sleep disorders are frequent and include night terrors and nightmares, somnambulism, sleep paralysis, reversals of the sleep rhythm, sleep apnea, insomnia, and narcolepsy. Enuresis is discussed in Ch. 156 and in Behavioral Problems in Vol. II, Ch. 24.

Night terrors, more frequent in children than adults, often are accompanied by sleep walking and may represent hypnagogic phenomena (see Narcolepsy, below) during partial arousal from deep sleep. They tend to be self-limiting in children, but in adults often are associated with psychologic difficulties or alcoholism. Diazepam 2 to 5 mg at bedtime sometimes is preventive.

Nightmares occur frequently, affecting adults and (especially) children. They occur during REM sleep and are more common during fever, with excess fatigue, or after alcohol ingestion. Treatment is directed at the underlying conflicts or disorder.

During **somnambulism,** the patient may sit or walk, or behave in a complex fashion. The eyes usually are open but without evidence of recognition. Patients may mumble repetitiously, and some injure themselves on obstacles or stairs. There is no accompanying dream, and the concurrent EEG looks more like wakefulness than sleep. Treatment is to protect the subject against injury and deal with any underlying disorder.

Sleep paralysis: See Narcolepsy, below.

Reversals of the sleep rhythm usually reflect jet lag or disease or damage to the hypothalamic region of the diencephalon, as occurs following severe head injury or encephalitis. Sedative misuse can sometimes induce such reversals (see Insomnia, below).

Sleep apnea can occur either from airway obstruction (the most frequent cause) or from primary brainstem medullary failure due to neurologic causes of medullary depression such as poliomyelitis, tumors of the posterior fossa, or idiopathic (primary) central hypoventilation. **Obstructive sleep apnea** occurs in obese patients with secondary pulmonary insufficiency **(Pickwickian syndrome).** In such subjects the obesity, perhaps combined with a constitutional defect, leads to pulmonary failure, resulting hypercapnia, and upper airway narrowing. Repeated nocturnal obstruction may cause further respiratory failure and repeated awakenings, and result in a continuous cycle of night and day episodes of sleep, obstructive choking, startled awakening with gasping, and drowsiness. Similar but less pronounced sequences also sometimes occur in nonobese subjects, presumably due to congenital abnormalities of the upper airway. Weight reduction in the obese sometimes is effective, but some patients require tracheostomy. Relief of the obstruction usually reverses the commonly associated pulmonary and systemic hypertension and cardiac arrhythmias.

INSOMNIA

Difficulty in sleeping, or disturbed sleep patterns leaving the perception of insufficient sleep. Insomnia is common, and may be due to several physical and emotional disorders.

With advancing age, the total amount of sleep tends to shorten and sleep becomes more interrupted. These changes may be subjectively distressing and lead to requests for treatment. There is no evidence, however, that such insomnia interferes with health. **Initial insomnia,** *difficulty in falling asleep,* is commonly associated with an emotional disturbance such as anxiety, a phobic state, or depression; other symptoms of the emotional problem will be present.

In **early morning awakening,** the patient falls asleep normally but awakens several hours before his usual time and either cannot fall asleep again or drifts into a restless, unsatisfying sleep. This pattern is sometimes a phenomenon of aging, but is often associated with depression and should be investigated, since tendencies to anxiety, self-reproach, and self-punitive thinking are often magnified in the morning.

An **inverted sleep rhythm** (see also above) may develop, especially in elderly persons, due to inappropriate use of sedatives, often prescribed for insomnia. Patients become drowsy in the morning, sleep or doze much of the day, and have fitful and interrupted sleep at night. If sedation is increased, restlessness and wandering in a clouded or confused state may occur at night. When sedation is withdrawn from a patient who regularly takes heavy doses of hypnotics to control "chronic insomnia," a rebound wakefulness commonly ensues, which the patient interprets as a recurrence of his insomnia.

Diagnosis

Insomnia may be *primary*, i.e., longstanding and with little apparent relationship to immediate somatic or psychic events, or *secondary* to some acquired pain, anxiety, or depression. Insomnia of recent onset is usually due to current dilemmas, e.g., marital strife, problems at work, guilt over sexual conflicts, or concerns about health. If no such personal difficulties or symptoms of an emotional disturbance emerge, a physical cause should be considered. Substantial amounts of alcohol consumed in the evening can lead to withdrawal effects in the early morning so that the patient awakens restless or, if he is severely dependent, fearful and tremulous. Insomnia unresponsive to simple measures often is due to a severe emotional disturbance, especially depression.

Treatment

This depends on the underlying cause. Many patients respond to reassurance that their sleeplessness is a result of normal anxieties or a treatable physical disorder. Providing an opportunity to ventilate anxieties often will ease distress and help to reestablish normal sleep patterns. Elderly patients experiencing a normal change in sleep patterns require reassurance, encouragement to take more exercise during the day, and instruction in relaxation. For insomnia due to emotional disturbance, and in refractory cases due to more common causes, hypnotic medication may be required, especially if the sleeplessness impairs the patient's efficiency and sense of well-being (see also Ch. 247 and TABLE 247–1). Flurazepam 15 to 30 mg at bedtime is the least toxic of the hypnotics. Chloral hydrate 1 to 2 gm is preferred over barbiturates or glutethimide because of the tendency of the latter to induce tolerance and withdrawal symptoms. Patients who awaken because of pain should be given aspirin 325 to 650 mg (5 to 10 grains) at bedtime. Warm milk helps some patients sleep. For insomnia accompanying depression, a tricyclic antidepressant taken about 1 h before bedtime usually suffices (see Ch. 139 and ANTIDEPRESSANTS in Ch. 247).

All hypnotics should be prescribed in limited quantities, and the patient encouraged to do without them as soon as possible. All depressed patients represent the risk of suicide attempts by overdosage with any hypnotic.

NARCOLEPSY

A rare syndrome of recurrent attacks of sleep, sudden loss of muscle tone (cataplexy), sleep paralysis, and hypnagogic phenomena, with a characteristic initial REM sleep pattern. About 10% of narcoleptics show the full tetrad of symptoms.

Etiology and Incidence

The cause is unknown. No pathologic changes are seen in the brain. Symptoms usually begin in adolescents or young adults with no previous illness, and persist throughout life; longevity is unaffected. Narcolepsy is 4 times more common in men than women; some patients give a family history of the disorder.

Symptoms and Signs

The 4 components of the syndrome are as follows:

1. Sleep attacks: Outwardly, normal sleep is resembled except in frequency and untimely occurrence. Physiologically, however, the contrast is significant. In normal persons, NREM sleep precedes REM sleep, and usually lasts about 60 min. In narcolepsy, REM sleep is almost instantaneous, with no preceding NREM phase. This differing pattern is so consistent that it almost defines the disease. The sleep attacks vary from few to many in a single day, and may last minutes or hours. The desire to sleep can be resisted only temporarily, but the patient can be roused from narcoleptic sleep as readily as from normal sleep. Attacks are apt to occur in the monotonous conditions conducive to normal sleep, but may also occur in hazardous circumstances, e.g., while driving. The patient may feel refreshed on awakening, yet fall asleep again in a few minutes. It is debatable whether the total amount of sleep is actually increased; the frequent episodes of sleep during the day make it seem so, but many patients sleep poorly at night and nocturnal sleep may be interrupted by vivid, frightening dreams.

2. Cataplexy: Momentary paralysis occurs in association with sudden emotional reactions, such as mirth, anger, fear, or joy. An element of surprise seems important. Weakness may be confined to the limbs (e.g., the patient may drop the rod when a fish strikes his line) or may cause a limp fall (when the patient laughs heartily or is suddenly angry). These attacks resemble the loss of muscle tone occurring in REM sleep or to a lesser degree in many persons who become "weak with laughter."

3. Sleep paralysis: Occasionally, just when falling asleep or immediately on awakening, the patient wants to move and finds that for a moment he cannot. Although these episodes resemble the motor inhibition that accompanies REM sleep, they also are common in normal children and in some normal adults.

4. Hypnagogic phenomena: Particularly vivid auditory or visual illusions or hallucinations may occur at the onset of sleep and are difficult to distinguish from intense reverie. These are somewhat similar to vivid dreams occurring in normal REM sleep. Hypnagogic phenomena occur commonly in young children and occasionally in adults who do not have narcolepsy or other sleep disorders.

No specific laboratory abnormalities are seen, except that in EEG records during an attack, the low-voltage fast record of REM sleep appears immediately.

Diagnosis

The history of typical sleep attacks is characteristic, and other symptoms of the clinical tetrad should be sought. Occasional patients have sleep attacks only, and also lack the typically prompt appearance of REM sleep; they may be affected by another, yet uncharacterized disorder. Many otherwise normal individuals experience occasional episodes of sleep paralysis or hypnagogic phenomena but recognize them as benign and do not seek medical assistance. Patients with intracranial mass lesions, encephalitis, or metabolic encephalopathy may be hypersomnolent; this, however, is apt to be recent in origin and constant (i.e., not occurring in attacks). The periodic hypersomnia of the **Kleine-Levin syndrome** seen in adolescent boys is accompanied by overeating; the somnolence of the **sleep apnea syndrome,** by obesity, chronic hypercapnia, mild hypoxia, and erythrocytosis. Exhaustion, sleepiness, and neurotic fatigue are differentiated by evaluation of personality, circumstances of sleep, and lack of cataplexy.

Treatment

Stimulant drugs may help; the dosage is regulated according to individual need: ephedrine 25 mg, amphetamine 10 to 20 mg, or dextroamphetamine 5 to 10 mg, orally q 3 to 4 h during the day. Methylphenidate in oral doses of 60 to 120 mg/day may be even more successful. Though directed primarily against sleep attacks, these drugs also seem to lessen the attacks of cataplexy. The recommended doses are tolerated without serious untoward effects. The last dose must be taken early enough to avoid interfering with nocturnal sleep. Imipramine and MAO inhibitors have recently been found useful in treating narcolepsy; *they must not be combined with an amphetamine.*

122.   CEREBROVASCULAR DISEASE

(Stroke; Cerebrovascular Accident; CVA)

Cerebrovascular disease is the commonest cause of neurologic disability in Western countries. Although vascular injury to the brain can occur as part of a number of relatively rare diseases, most cerebrovascular illnesses are secondary to atherosclerotic disease, hypertension, or a combination of both. The major *specific* types of cerebrovascular disease are (1) **cerebral insufficiency** due to transient disturbances of blood flow or, rarely, to hypertensive encephalopathy; (2) **cerebral infarction,** due either to embolism or to thrombosis of the intra- or extracranial arteries; and (3) **cerebral hemorrhage,** which includes hypertensive parenchymal hemorrhage and subarachnoid hemorrhage from congenital aneurysm. The vernacular terms "stroke," "cerebrovascular accident," and "CVA" lack specificity and are commonly applied to the clinical syndromes that accompany either ischemic or hemorrhagic lesions.

Both ischemic and hemorrhagic stroke tend to develop abruptly, with cerebral hemorrhage generally having the most catastrophically acute onset. Symptoms and signs in cerebrovascular disease reflect the area of brain that is damaged and not necessarily the specific artery that is affected. Occlusion of either the middle cerebral artery or internal carotid artery, for example, can produce a similar clinical neurologic abnormality. Nevertheless, cerebral vascular injuries generally conform to fairly specific patterns of arterial supply, and a knowledge of these distributions is important in distinguishing stroke from space-taking lesions such as brain tumor or abscess.

The most important step in accurate diagnosis of cerebral vascular lesions consists of an accurate history. The most important step in treatment consists of identifying patients with potential or impending strokes so that effective measures can be attempted to prevent brain damage.

ISCHEMIC SYNDROMES

Cerebrovascular disorders caused by insufficient cerebral circulation.

Etiology and Pathophysiology

Normally, an adequate blood flow to the brain is ensured by an efficient collateral system: from one carotid to the other; from one vertebral artery to the other and to the carotids via the anastomoses at the circle of Willis; and via collateral circulation at the level of the hemispheres. Congenital anomalies and the vascular changes of atherosclerosis impair these compensatory mechanisms, so that **brain ischemia** and consequent neurologic symptoms can result from an intra- or extracranial interruption in arterial blood flow. Thrombosis or emboli from an atherosclerotic plaque or other causes (e.g., arteritis, rheumatic heart disease) commonly produce the ischemic arterial obstruction. If the blood supply to the ischemic region is promptly restored, the brain tissues recover and symptoms disappear, but if ischemia lasts for more than a few minutes, **infarction** results and neurologic damage is permanent.

Atheroma, which underlies most thromboses, may affect any of the major cerebral arteries. Large atheromas are more commonly **extracranial,** affecting the common carotid and vertebral arteries at their origins, the cervical bifurcation of the internal carotid, the carotid siphon, and the basilar artery just proximal to the origin of the posterior cerebral artery. Occlusions can occur either in these large extracranial arteries or in any of the smaller, intracranial arteries. An occlusion may be partial or complete, and in the extracranial vessels is sometimes bilateral. Whether ischemia and infarction occur depends upon the efficiency of collateral circulation; e.g., a concomitant stenosis of the vertebral arteries, by compromising collateral circulation, may intensify the effects of carotid lesions. **Intracranial thrombosis** may occur in one of the large arteries at the base of the brain, in a deep perforating artery, or in a small cortical branch, but the main trunk of the middle cerebral artery and its branches are the most common sites.

Less frequently, thrombotic occlusion is secondary to **vascular inflammation,** as in a collagen vascular disease, acute or chronic meningitis, or syphilis. Very rarely, **arterial compression** is due to bony vertebral projections (osteophytes). Cerebral thrombosis in young women is rare but quadruples in incidence when oral contraceptives are used.

Cerebral emboli originate in extracranial vessels and usually derive from atheromas in the large arteries supplying the brain, or (in children as well as adults) from thrombi in damaged hearts. The fragments, which may lodge temporarily or permanently in major or minor branches of the cerebral arterial tree, may come from an accumulation of platelets, fibrin, and cholesterol on the surface of ulcerated plaques in atherosclerosis; from vegetations on the heart valves in bacterial, mycotic, or marantic endocarditis; from mural thrombi in atrial fibrillation (particularly in rheumatic heart disease) or following myocardial infarction; or from clots following open-heart surgery. Rarely, cerebral emboli may originate as fat (from fractures of the long bones), air (caisson disease), or venous clots that pass from the right to the left side of the heart through a patent foramen ovale (paradoxical embolus).

Physiologic circulatory insufficiency is a relatively uncommon cause of ischemia and infarction. The diminished perfusion may occur alone or be superimposed on an already existing partial occlusion. Many processes may produce diminished perfusion. Profound anemia, by reducing the O_2-carrying capacity of the blood, and severe polycythemia, by increasing its viscosity, can contribute to cerebral vascular problems. A pronounced, sustained fall in arterial pressure is ordinarily needed in order to cause a severe compromise in regional blood flow, but in the presence of arterial disease or hypertension a lesser fall in BP can cause local ischemia and infarction. Orthostatic hypotension, acute blood loss, myocardial infarction, or, less often, cardiac arrhythmias are common mechanisms producing a fall in BP. A hypersensitivity to carotid sinus compression (e.g., from a sudden turning of the head) usually causes bradycardia and syncope; it is doubtful whether it can cause transient ischemia or an infarction in atherosclerotic patients.

TRANSIENT ISCHEMIC ATTACKS (TIAs)

Focal neurologic abnormalities of sudden onset and brief duration (usually minutes, never more than a few hours) that reflect dysfunction in the distribution of either the internal carotid–middle cerebral or the vertebral-basilar arterial system. The attacks are often recurrent and at times presage a stroke. Most TIAs are due to cerebral emboli arising from plaques or atherosclerotic ulcers involving the carotid or vertebral arteries in the neck. Emboli also may arise from mural thrombi in a diseased heart. The attacks are most common in the middle-aged and elderly. TIAs occasionally can occur in children in whom severe cardiovascular disease produces emboli or greatly increased Hct.

Hypertension, atherosclerosis, heart disease, diabetes mellitus, and polycythemia are predisposing. Some TIAs may be due to a brief reduction in blood flow through stenosed arteries. A rare variation is the **subclavian steal syndrome** (see below), in which a subclavian artery distal to a stenosis "steals" blood from the vertebral artery when exertion requires increased blood to the arm.

Symptoms, Signs, and Course

TIAs appear suddenly, last from 2 or 3 min to 30 min or more (seldom over 1 or 2 h), and then disappear without neurologic residua. Consciousness remains intact throughout the episode.

Symptoms depend on the arterial system affected. **With carotid artery involvement,** symptoms generally are unilateral. Ipsilateral blindness and contralateral hemiparesis, often with paresthesias, is classic, but less complete symptoms are more frequent. Aphasia indicates involvement of the dominant hemisphere. **When the vertebrobasilar system is involved,** symptoms reflect brainstem dysfunction. Confusion, vertigo, binocular blindness or diplopia, and unilateral or, more often, bilateral weakness, and paresthesias of the extremities may be present. "Drop attacks" (falling without loss of consciousness) may result from bilateral leg weakness. Slurred speech (dysarthria) may occur with either carotid or vertebrobasilar involvement.

Patients may have several attacks daily, or only 2 or 3 over several years. The symptoms usually are similar in repeated carotid attacks, but vary somewhat in successive vertebrobasilar attacks. How often TIAs presage a completed stroke is unknown. In some patients, especially those with carotid artery involvement, stroke eventually occurs; in others, TIAs occur shortly before a stroke; in still others, symptoms repeatedly appear without sequelae.

Diagnosis

Differentiation from convulsive seizures, neoplasms, migraine, Ménière's disease or other forms of vertigo, or hyperinsulinism in diabetics is sometimes necessary. Angiography or Doppler sonography can confirm the presence of stenosis and identify the involved artery and is needed to identify potentially operable lesions in the carotid arteries. With associated subclavian artery occlusion, the brachial BP in the affected arm is significantly lower than in the opposite arm.

Treatment

In addition to treating the atherosclerosis, hypertension, or other underlying disorder, vascular surgery or anticoagulants may be indicated. If the obstruction is at the carotid bifurcation or in the prevertebral subclavian artery, endarterectomy or resection and prosthetic replacement of the affected portion of the artery may be beneficial.

If the obstruction is intracranial or vertebrobasilar, or if vertebral and carotid arteries are affected, and if the patient is not hypertensive, therapy is usually with platelet inhibitors or anticoagulants. Surgical anastomosis between the external carotid and middle cerebral artery (EC-MCA bypass) has been attempted in some cases, but results are too preliminary to evaluate. Heparin is used if attacks are of recent origin and occur daily; a warfarin derivative, when attacks are frequent but occur less often. Details on dosage and risks can be found in Ch. 254. For patients with only occasional TIAs, most authorities now give a trial of aspirin therapy before starting anticoagulants. Once started, duration of anticoagulant therapy is difficult to specify. Most authorities continue anticoagulants for 2 to 3 mo in basilar artery involvement, and for 6 to 12 mo in carotid artery involvement; a trial without therapy may then be attempted. Unless specifically contraindicated, therapy with drugs that inhibit platelet aggregation should be continued indefinitely. At present, aspirin 0.3 gm (5 grains) once or twice daily is the agent of choice, especially in males. Relative values of sulfinpyrazone, dipyridamole, or clofibrate have not been established.

STROKE IN EVOLUTION AND COMPLETED STROKE

Stroke in evolution: *The clinical condition manifested by neurologic defects that increase over a 24- to 48-h period, reflecting enlarging infarction or progressive edema, usually in the territory of the middle cerebral artery.*

Completed stroke: *The clinical condition manifested by neurologic deficits of varying severity, usually abrupt in onset and either fatal or showing variable improvement, resulting from infarction of brain tissue due to arteriosclerotic or hypertensive stenosis, thrombosis, or embolism.*

Symptoms, Signs, and Course

In **stroke in evolution,** unilateral neurologic dysfunction (often beginning in one arm) increases painlessly and without headache or fever over several hours or a day or two to involve progressively more of the body ipsilaterally. The progression is usually stepwise, interrupted by periods of stability, but may be continuous. **Acute completed stroke** is by far the more common condition. Symptoms develop rapidly, and typically are maximal within a few minutes. By convention, **completed stroke** also refers to the patient's condition, after either evolving or acute stroke, once symptoms have ceased to progress and are either stable or improving.

In either evolving or acute completed stroke, deficits may worsen and consciousness may become clouded during the next few days because of cerebral edema or, less often, from extension of the infarct. Severe cerebral edema can cause a potentially fatal shift in intracranial structures (transtentorial herniation; see under INTRACRANIAL NEOPLASMS in Ch. 125). However, early improvement in function is common unless severe infarction or edema has occurred. Further improvement is then gradual over days, weeks, or months.

The **specific neurologic symptoms** are determined by the *site* of the brain infarct. The involved artery can often be inferred from the symptom pattern, although the correlation is not exact. Occlusion of several arteries can cause symptoms described under several of the following categories.

The distribution of the **middle cerebral artery** or one of its deep penetrating branches is most commonly involved. Occlusion of the proximal part of the artery, which supplies large portions of the frontal, parietal, and temporal lobe surfaces, results in contralateral hemiplegia, usually severe, with hemianesthesia and a homonymous hemianopia. Aphasia occurs when the dominant hemisphere is affected; apraxia or anosognosia when the nondominant hemisphere is involved. A contralateral hemiplegia of the face, arm, and leg, sometimes with hemianesthesia, also results from occlusion of one of the deep branches, which supply the basal ganglia, internal and external capsules, and thalamus. Motor or sensory impairment may be less severe when terminal branches are involved.

Occlusion of the **internal carotid artery** leads to infarction in the central-lateral portion of the cerebral hemisphere, with symptoms indistinguishable from those of middle cerebral artery occlusion.

Anterior cerebral artery occlusion is uncommon, but affects portions of the frontal and parietal lobes, corpus callosum, and sometimes the caudate nucleus and internal capsule. Contralateral hemiplegia, especially affecting the leg, may be seen. A grasp reflex and urinary incontinence may occur. Bilateral occlusion may cause emotional disturbances with apathy, confusion, and occasional mutism, plus spastic paraplegia.

Posterior cerebral artery occlusion can affect areas in the temporal and occipital lobes, internal capsule, hippocampus, thalamus, mammillary and geniculate bodies, choroid plexus, and upper brainstem. Contralateral homonymous hemianopia, hemisensory loss, spontaneous thalamic pain, or sudden hemiballism may occur; alexia may follow an infarct in the dominant hemisphere.

The vertebrobasilar system supplies the brainstem, cerebellum, and portions of the temporal and occipital lobes. Branch occlusions cause combinations of cerebellar, corticospinal, sensory, and cranial nerve signs. Complete occlusion of the basilar artery usually causes ophthalmoplegia, pupillary abnormalities, bilateral corticospinal signs (tetraparesis or tetraplegia), and changes in consciousness. Pseudobulbar manifestations (dysarthria, dysphagia, emotional instability) occur frequently. The course is often fatal.

Diagnosis

Stroke usually can be diagnosed clinically, especially in a patient over age 50 with hypertension, diabetes mellitus, or signs of atherosclerosis, or in any patient with a known source of emboli. Clinical diagnosis seldom is difficult. In the unusual case, differentiation from a rapidly growing or suddenly symptomatic tumor is aided by a negative skull x-ray or by a CT scan (which is sometimes negative for as much as several days after an acute infarction). Arteriography is limited to patients in whom the diagnosis is in doubt or a remedial vascular obstruction is suspected.

Determining the immediate cause of a stroke may be difficult. Onset during sleep or on arising suggests infarction; onset during exertion, hemorrhage. Headache, coma or stupor, marked hypertension, and convulsive seizures are more likely with hemorrhage.

Diminished carotid artery pulsation and localized vascular bruits and thrills in the neck may be present and suggest the presence of stenosis and plaque formation in an extracranial vessel, while the neurologic symptoms and signs can suggest the artery involved.

A stroke due to a large embolus tends to be an acute completed stroke, sudden in onset, with focal disorders that are maximal within a few minutes. Headache may precede it. Thrombosis is less frequent and is suggested by a slower onset, or a gradual progression of symptoms, as in evolving stroke. However, the distinction is not entirely reliable. Concomitant signs of myocardial infarction, atrial fibrillation, or vegetative heart disease further suggest embolization.

Studies should be done to identify hypertension and to rule out anemia, polycythemia, and infections. Plasma lipids should be determined. A chest x-ray should be taken to search for a primary lung tumor and cardiovascular disorders, and an ECG should be performed.

Laboratory findings are nonspecific. The CSF in all forms of ischemic stroke is usually normal, but leukocytes may be transiently increased to 500/cu mm, sugar may be slightly reduced, and protein may be elevated to 80 mg/100 ml. The CSF is usually clear after an infarct, but bloody, with increased pressure, after intracranial hemorrhage. Red cells may be present due to infarction, but are far fewer than the number seen in hemorrhages. Angiography is sometimes needed to identify the site of arterial occlusion (e.g., when surgery is contemplated). A CT scan helps to differentiate an ischemic stroke from intracerebral hemorrhage, hematoma, or tumor.

Prognosis

During the early days of either evolving or completed stroke, neither progression nor ultimate outcome can be predicted. About 35% of patients die in the hospital; the mortality rate increases with age.

The eventual extent of neurologic recovery depends on the patient's age and general state of health as well as on the site and size of the infarction. Impaired consciousness, mental deterioration, or aphasia all suggest a poor prognosis. Complete recovery is uncommon, but the sooner improvement begins, the better the prognosis. About 50% of patients with moderate or severe hemiplegia, and most of those with lesser deficits, recover functionally by the time of discharge and are ultimately able to care for their basic needs, have a clear sensorium, and can walk adequately, although use of an affected limb may be limited. Any deficit remaining after 6 mo is likely to be permanent, although some patients continue slowly to improve. Recurrence of cerebral infarction is common, and each recurrence is likely to add to the neurologic disability.

Treatment

Immediate care of a comatose patient includes airway maintenance, adequate oxygenation, nasogastric feeding or IV fluids to maintain nutritional and fluid intake, attention to bladder and bowel function, and measures to prevent decubitus ulcers. Corticosteroids have no proved value.

Heart failure, cardiac arrhythmias, severe hypertension, and intercurrent respiratory infection must be treated. IV spasmolytic agents such as sodium nitroprusside are preferable in malignant hypertension. Barbiturates and other sedatives are *contraindicated,* as they increase the risk of respiratory depression and subsequent pneumonitis. Passive movements, particularly of paralyzed limbs, and breathing exercises, if possible, should be begun early.

Heparin (see in Ch. 254) may stabilize symptoms in evolving stroke, but anticoagulants are useless (and possibly dangerous) in acute completed stroke and are *contraindicated* in hypertensive patients because of the increased possibility of hemorrhage into the brain or other organs.

Vascular surgery is not indicated as an emergency measure and is pointless when atheromatous stenosis is widespread, but thromboendarterectomy or resection and prosthetic replacement may sometimes help to prevent recurrent neurologic episodes in patients with partial, isolated carotid occlusion.

Rehabilitation and aftercare: Early and repeated appraisals of the patient's status by physician, physiotherapist, and nursing staff allow a remedial program to be designed. Elaborate programs are probably unnecessary, and the value of speech therapy is unproved. Younger age, limited sensory and motor deficit, intact mental function, and a helpful home environment favorably influence reha-bilitation. Early treatment, continuing encouragement, and orientation toward the outside environ-ment are important. The patient and his relatives and friends must understand the nature of his disabilities and the likelihood that progress will occur but will take time, patience, and perseverance. Mood changes may be the result of the infarct as well as a reaction to the situation; they should be expected, and treated by reassurance and understanding; tranquilizers or antidepressants may be helpful after the patient's condition has stabilized. Occupational and physical therapy should empha-size using affected limbs and achieving proficiency in eating, dressing, toilet functions, and other basic needs. Appliances such as hearing aids and walking frames often are needed; in the living quarters, handbars (e.g., at tub and toilet) and ramps can be of great help (see also Ch. 229).

HYPERTENSIVE ENCEPHALOPATHY

An acute or subacute condition occurring in patients with severe hypertension, and marked by headache, obtundation, confusion or stupor, and convulsions. Modern hypertensive treatment has made the condition rare. Although both ischemic and hemorrhagic stroke are more common in hypertension, hypertensive encephalopathy is an additional, specific cerebral disorder confined to patients with severe hypertension. Often, one finds rapidly changing neurologic abnormalities, in-cluding cortical blindness, hemiparesis, and hemisensory defects. BP always is elevated, usually with diastolic pressures > 110 to 140 mm Hg. Grade 3 or 4 retinopathy usually is present and the CSF pressure commonly is > 200 mm with a CSF protein content usually > 60 mg/100 ml. The patho-genesis is believed to involve either multifocal areas of hypertensive-induced arteriolar spasm or perhaps blood-brain barrier leakage adjacent to an area of loss of vascular autoregulation.

Diagnosis depends on the characteristic clinical picture and the exclusion of other possible ill-nesses. Clinically the picture most resembles uremia, from which it is differentiated by a BUN < 100 mg/100 ml. Other metabolic encephalopathies must also be excluded but are less of a problem, since most are not particularly associated with an elevated BP.

Treatment consists of deliberate (not abrupt) but progressive reduction of BP to more nearly normal ranges by the use of sodium nitroprusside, if other agents fail.

HEMORRHAGIC SYNDROMES

Cerebrovascular disorders caused by bleeding into brain tissue or meningeal spaces.

Intracranial hemorrhage may occur into the brain substance, the epi- or subdural spaces, the subarachnoid space, or a combination of these sites. Epidural and subdural hemorrhage are often the consequence of head trauma, and are discussed in Ch. 123.

INTRACEREBRAL HEMORRHAGE

Etiology and Pathogenesis

Intracerebral hemorrhage usually results from rupture of an arteriosclerotic vessel either long exposed to arterial hypertension or made ischemic by local thrombus formation. Less often, the cause is a congenital aneurysm or other vascular malformation. Mycotic aneurysms, brain infarct, blood dyscrasias, collagen diseases, and other systemic diseases are occasional causes. Hyperten-sive or aneurysmal cerebral hemorrhage is usually large and single; hemorrhages from most other causes are apt to be small and diffusely scattered.

Most severe intracerebral hemorrhages, like infarcts, are located in the region of the basal ganglia, internal capsule, and thalamus, since a branch of the middle cerebral artery is most often involved. CT scanning reveals that smaller and less clinically severe hemorrhages also arise elsewhere in the cerebrum. Hemorrhages in the cerebellum or brainstem are less common.

The hematoma compresses and displaces adjacent brain tissue and, if large, increases intracranial pressure. Pressure from the hematoma and the accompanying edema may cause **transtentorial her-niation** (see under INTRACRANIAL NEOPLASMS in Ch. 125), compressing the brainstem and often causing secondary hemorrhages in the midbrain and pons. If the hemorrhage ruptures into the ventricular system, blood may reach the subarachnoid space.

Symptoms and Signs

Cerebral hemorrhage characteristically begins abruptly with headache, followed by steadily increasing neurologic deficits. Large hemorrhages produce hemiparesis when located in the hemispheres, and symptoms of cerebellar or brainstem dysfunction (conjugate eye deviation or ophthalmoplegia; stertorous breathing, pinpoint pupils, and coma) when located in the posterior fossa. Loss of consciousness is common; it may occur within a few minutes after onset or develop gradually. Nausea, vomiting, delirium, and focal or generalized seizures also are common. Large hemorrhages are fatal within a few days in more than 50% of patients. In those who survive, consciousness returns and neurologic deficits gradually recede as the extravasated blood is resorbed. Some degree of impairment usually remains, including some dysphasia if the dominant hemisphere was affected, but many patients make a reasonable degree of functional recovery.

Smaller hemorrhages cause focal deficits like those seen in ischemic stroke; as with infarcts, the deficits reflect the site of the damage.

Diagnosis and Treatment

It is often difficult clinically to distinguish small cerebral hemorrhages from ischemic stroke. If available, CT scanning is the procedure of choice. Lumbar puncture must be done cautiously, if at all, when patients are unconscious or symptoms are worsening, since the consequent change in CSF pressure may precipitate transtentorial herniation. With large hemorrhages, the CSF is almost always bloody (Hct > 1%) and under increased pressure. Other distinguishing features are given above under diagnosis of ischemic stroke.

Therapy following hemorrhage is similar to that for ischemic stroke (see above), except that anticoagulants are **contraindicated** in hemorrhage. Codeine 60 mg q 4 h may be needed to relieve headache, and diazepam will relieve anxiety. Hypnotic sedatives are contraindicated, as in ischemic stroke. Nausea or vomiting may require IV fluid administration during the first few days. Surgical decompression of large hemorrhages producing brain displacement is sometimes attempted, but results are inconclusive.

SUBARACHNOID HEMORRHAGE

Sudden bleeding into the subarachnoid space.

Etiology and Pathology

Secondary bleeding into the subarachnoid space is most commonly due to head trauma. Spontaneous or primary subarachnoid hemorrhage is usually from a ruptured congenital intracranial aneurysm. Less frequently it may be due to mycotic or arteriosclerotic aneurysm, arteriovenous (A-V) malformation, or hemorrhagic disease. It may occur at any age, but is most common from age 25 to 50.

Hemorrhage from aneurysm usually arises from outpouchings at the bifurcation of an artery at or near the base of the brain, a point where the muscular coat is poorly developed, thus predisposing to aneurysm formation; arteriosclerosis and especially hypertension probably also play a role. Most aneurysms are located along the middle or anterior cerebral arteries or the communicating branches of the circle of Willis.

A secondary increase in intracranial pressure is common after subarachnoid hemorrhage and may last for days or a few weeks. The associated communicating hydrocephalus may contribute to headache or the posthemorrhage delirium.

Symptoms and Signs

Before rupture, most aneurysms are asymptomatic. A few may manifest themselves as a result of pressure on adjacent structures. Ocular palsies, diplopia, squint, and facial pain due to pressure on the 3rd, 4th, 5th, and 6th cranial nerves may be present. Visual loss and a bitemporal field defect signify pressure on the optic chiasm. Pressure on the optic tract produces a homonymous hemianopia.

Following rupture, there usually is acute severe headache, often followed or accompanied by at least brief syncope. Some patients remain in coma, but more often the patient is merely obtunded. The mixture of escaping blood and CSF irritates the meninges and increases intracranial pressure, producing headache, vomiting, dizziness, convulsions, and alterations in pulse and respiratory rates. Stiffness of the neck usually is not present initially unless the cerebellar tonsils are herniated downwards. Within 24 h, however, moderate to marked stiffness of the neck, Kernig's sign, and bilateral Babinski's signs are present. The temperature may be elevated during the first 5 to 10 days, and the patient often continues to have headaches and confusion during this time. Focal signs, generally including hemiplegia, are present in about 25% of cases, as a result of bleeding into the brain substance or associated vasospasm and ischemia. Later, the extravasated clot may act as an intracranial tumor.

Spinal puncture is indicated for diagnosis and at first yields a bloody CSF under increased pressure; after 6 h or more, a xanthochromic supernatant is found. Once active hemorrhage ceases, the CSF gradually clears, and the pressure usually returns to normal in about 3 wk.

Differential Diagnosis

Acute subarachnoid hemorrhage occasionally simulates myocardial infarction because of the associated syncope and neurogenic abnormalities on the ECG. In cases with obvious neurologic signs, subarachnoid hemorrhage must be differentiated from parenchymatous cerebral hemorrhage, bleeding from A-V malformation, cerebral contusion and laceration, subdural hematoma, and sometimes brain tumor with hemorrhage. CT scanning plus cerebral angiography is necessary for differential diagnosis and as a guide to surgical therapy. All 4 cerebral vessels should be inspected, because several aneurysms may be present. Skull x-rays may show calcification in the wall of an aneurysm.

Prognosis

The mortality rate with first hemorrhages is about 35%, and an additional 15% of patients die from a subsequent rupture within a few weeks. A second rupture after 6 mo occurs at a rate of about 5/yr. In general, the prognosis is grave with cerebral aneurysm, better with bleeding from A-V malformations, and best when no lesion is discovered with 4-vessel arteriography, presumably because the bleeding source was small and possibly had collapsed or thrombosed later.

Prophylaxis and Treatment

Underlying vascular disease, blood dyscrasia, cardiac disease, or syphilis should be treated appropriately. Exertion should be *avoided.* Bed rest is mandatory until bleeding has stopped. Fluid balance and nutrition should be maintained, parenterally if necessary. Diazepam may be used for restlessness, and codeine or meperidine 25 to 50 mg parenterally may be required to relieve headaches. Constipation induces straining and should be prevented. Anticoagulants are **contraindicated.**

The desirability of spinal puncture to reduce intracranial pressure depends on the patient's reaction to the initial diagnostic puncture. If he improves, small amounts of CSF may be removed at intervals, in order to slowly reduce the intracranial pressure to normal.

In experienced hands, surgery that succeeds in trapping or obliterating an aneurysm reduces the risk of subsequent fatal bleeding and lowers long-term mortality. Procedures include extirpating or clipping the aneurysm, ligating the proximal carotid artery, inducing thrombosis, or covering the aneurysmal sac with plastic, gauze, or muscle. Surgical mortality is unjustifiably high in patients operated on when in stupor or coma. In less neurologically damaged patients, arteriography and surgical therapy should be carried out as soon as practicable after the initial bleed. Choice of surgical procedure depends on the site of the aneurysm.

Even with surgical treatment, subarachnoid hemorrhage leaves many patients with residual neurologic damage. In a few patients, obtundation, confusion, and delayed motor recovery continue for weeks after subarachnoid hemorrhage, because of a secondary communicating hydrocephalus. Cerebral ventricular shunting is only rarely necessary.

ARTERIOVENOUS (A-V) MALFORMATIONS

Abnormal, tangled collections of dilated blood vessels that result from congenitally malformed vascular structures in which arterial afferents flow directly into venous efferents without the usual resistance of an intervening capillary bed. The result is a progressively enlarging vascular anomaly that can produce neurologic abnormalities either because of its size, because it compresses neural tissue in its interstices, or because it bleeds. The malformations are particularly likely to arise at junction points between cerebral arterial beds and are found most frequently within the cerebral parenchyma in the frontal-parietal region, in the frontal lobe, or in the lateral cerebellum or overlying occipital lobe.

Clinical Syndromes

A-V malformation produces 3 relatively distinct neurologic disorders. Most often, perhaps half the time, they bleed to produce the clinical picture of **parenchymal** or **subarachnoid hemorrhage.** Little or nothing distinctive identifies A-V malformations as the source except that such hemorrhages tend to be less neurologically devastating than those due to hypertensive or congenital aneurysm and they have a high frequency of recurrence over the years. The other 2 syndromes include **focal epilepsy,** with the nature of the focus related to the site of the malformation (see TABLE 120–2 in Ch. 120), and progressive **focal neurologic sensory-motor deficit** due to the enlarging malformation acting as a mass lesion.

Diagnosis and Treatment

Specific diagnosis of A-V malformations is difficult except by laboratory means. Some patients have arterial bruits, detectable on the overlying cranial vault. CT generally outlines malformations exceeding 1.5 cm in diameter, but arteriography is required for definitive diagnosis and to determine if the lesion is operable.

Treatment includes anticonvulsants to control seizures (see Drug Therapy in Ch. 120). Surgical removal can be attempted and, if all the arterial feeders can be identified and ligated, sometimes produces a cure. In most instances, however, the location and size of these lesions precludes satisfactory therapy.

THORACIC OUTLET OBSTRUCTION SYNDROMES

(Neurovascular Compression of the Shoulder Girdle; Scalenus Anticus Syndrome; Cervical Rib Syndrome)

A group of somewhat inconsistent disorders characterized by subjective complaints of pain and paresthesias in the neck, shoulder, arm, and hand, most often distributed medially in the members and sometimes extending into the adjacent anterior chest wall. The condition is commoner in women than men and most frequent between ages 35 and 55. Many patients have minor to moderate degrees of sensory impairment in the C8 to T1 distribution on the painful side, and a few will have prominent vascular-autonomic changes in the hand including cyanosis, swelling and, rarely, Raynaud's phenomenon or distal gangrene. The pathogenesis is believed to be due to compression of the subclavian vessels and, sometimes, the lower or medial trunks of the brachial plexus against a cervical rib, an abnormal 1st thoracic rib, or a putatively abnormal insertion or position of the scalene muscles.

Symptoms, Signs, and Diagnosis

The condition, which is seen clinically less often today than a generation ago, can be suspected by the distribution of symptoms and is supported by the finding of obliteration of the pulse with elevation of the arm and turning of the head to the opposite shoulder **(Adson's maneuver)**. Also helpful are the auscultation of bruits at the clavicle or the apex of the axilla, or the finding of a cervical rib by x-ray. Some patients will show kinking or partial obstruction of axillary arteries or veins on angiography, but these are not incontrovertible evidence of disease.

Treatment

Most patients respond to physical therapy and exercises. Except when obvious cervical ribs can be identified, surgical treatment is best left to the experienced specialist.

SUBCLAVIAN STEAL SYNDROME

An uncommon cerebrovascular symptom complex in which an obstruction in the subclavian artery proximal to the origin of the vertebral artery is envisaged as causing reversed flow down the latter. The putative effect is to divert (steal) blood from the brainstem into the brachial circulation. The symptom complex consists of symptoms of vertebral–basilar insufficiency presumed to be induced or accentuated by muscular activity in the arm served by the obstructed subclavian artery. **Treatment** should be directed at the fundamental vascular disease process. Some surgeons recommend a common carotid-subclavian artery anastomosis to bypass the subclavian obstruction.

---

123.   TRAUMA OF THE HEAD AND SPINE

HEAD INJURY

Head injury causes more deaths and disability than any other neurologic cause in subjects under age 50. Mortality in severe injury approaches 50% and is only little reduced by treatment. Damage results from penetration of the skull or from rapid acceleration or deceleration of the brain, which injures tissue at the point of impact, at its opposite pole **(contrecoup)**, and also diffusely along the frontal and temporal lobes. Nerve tissue, blood vessels, and meninges are sheared, torn, and ruptured, resulting in neural disruption, intra- and extracerebral ischemia or hemorrhage, and cerebral edema. Hemorrhage or edema acts as an expanding intracranial lesion, causing increased intracranial pressure that can lead to fatal herniation of brain tissue through the tentorial opening. Skull fractures may lacerate meningeal arteries or large venous sinuses, producing epidural or subdural hematoma. Infectious organisms may reach the meninges even when a fracture is not clearly evident, especially when it involves the paranasal sinuses (see Ch. 168). Few head injuries occur in isolation, and most cases require simultaneous attention to other seriously traumatized parts of the body.

Symptoms and Signs

Concussion is characterized by post-traumatic loss of consciousness lasting less than 24 h (usually much less), without structural lesions in the brain. Although unconscious, the patient with concussion rarely is deeply unresponsive. Pupillary reactions and other signs of brainstem function are intact; thus, extensor plantar responses may be present, but not hemiplegia or decerebrate postural responses to noxious stimulation (see Motor Responses under IMPAIRED CONSCIOUSNESS, Diagnosis, in Ch. 118). Lumbar puncture reveals a clear CSF.

Cerebral contusion, lacerations, and edema constitute more severe injuries. They are often accompanied by severe surface wounds and by fractures located at the base of the skull or having depressed bone fragments (see also FRACTURES OF THE TEMPORAL BONE in Ch. 167). Respiration is often labored because of pulmonary congestion (or chest trauma). Hemiplegia, decorticate rigidity (arms flexed and adducted; legs and often trunk extended), or decerebrate rigidity (jaws clenched, neck retracted, all limbs extended) is common. Lumbar puncture reveals bloody CSF, usually under increased pressure. Pupils may be unequal. Fixation of the pupils to light and loss of oculovestibular reflexes are ominous prognostic signs. Increased intracranial pressure, particularly when associated with compression or distortion of the brainstem, may produce a rising BP coupled with a slowing of the pulse and respiratory rates.

The cerebral hemispheres and underlying diencephalon are generally more exposed and susceptible to the effects of trauma than is the brainstem. **Signs of primary brainstem injury** (coma; stertorous breathing; pinpoint pupils; quadrispasticity with arms flexed and trunk and legs extended, but without raised intracranial pressure) almost always imply severe injury and carry a poor prognosis.

Since severe head injuries are frequently accompanied by thoracic damage, the neurologic problems created by the injury are often complicated by pulmonary edema (some of which is undoubtedly neurogenic), hypoxia, and an unstable circulation. Damage to the cervical spine, also a common accompaniment, can cause fatal respiratory paralysis or permanent quadriplegia from cord injury; other cord damage can be almost as disastrous.

Immediate Management

Multiple injuries are likely when an accident has caused severe head injury. Therefore, at the accident site, once a clear airway is secured (with an oral or endotracheal tube if possible) and acute bleeding controlled, the accident victim should be moved en bloc, with particular care to avoid displacing the spine or other bones and thereby injuring the spinal cord or blood vessels. Splinting can be confined to supporting the entire body for transport to a medical facility. For care of the victim with possible cord injuries, see below. Morphine and other depressants are **contraindicated**.

In the hospital, once the airway is secured (by tracheostomy when injuries are severe), fluids are started, and internal bleeding and other emergency complications are evaluated and treated, a careful assessment should be made of the state of consciousness, breathing pattern, pupil size and reaction to light, and motor activity in the limbs. These functions, BP, pulse, and temperature should be recorded at least hourly, since any deterioration demands prompt attention. Once the baseline data are obtained, x-rays should be taken and checked, particularly for skull fracture lines that could affect blood vessels, and for associated cervical spine fractures. When extensive injury is obvious, lumbar puncture is unnecessary and may be hazardous, since it can precipitate tentorial herniation. CT scans are valuable for detecting potentially operable intracranial hematomas. If CT is unavailable, cerebral angiograms are indicated when specific complications (e.g., subdural or epidural hematoma) are suspected; radioactive scans and EEG are of little diagnostic help in the immediate post-trauma situation.

Treatment

Patients should be protected against heat loss, fluid depletion, and airway obstruction, and should be monitored closely for signs of deterioration. Patients with concussion should be kept under close supervision for at least 48 h to be certain no complications arise.

Skull fractures, if aligned, require no treatment. Depressed fractures are best handled by a neurosurgeon, and may require emergency management of lacerated blood vessels. Antibiotic prophylaxis is avoided, since it only encourages drug-resistant strains.

To protect against complications, arterial hypoxia should be minimized by partial (40%) oxygenation, combined if necessary with IPPB. Fever should be controlled with cooling blankets. Blood and fluid loss should be replaced promptly. One must prevent hypo- or hyperthermia and be alert for acute renal failure. Anticonvulsants (e.g., phenytoin 1 gm IV in 12 h followed by 300 to 400 mg/day) will protect against seizures. Osmotic diuretics (urea, mannitol, glycerol) given IV reduce brain swelling but should be reserved for deteriorating patients or for preoperative use in patients with hematomas. Corticosteroids are often used for this purpose, but their benefit is questionable.

Restlessness occurring during improvement from coma may require sedation (e.g., with chlorpromazine 50 mg IM or haloperidol 2 to 5 mg IM). When unconsciousness begins to improve within 1 wk, the outlook for reasonable recovery is good.

Complications

Acute subdural or **intracerebral hematomas** are common in severe head injury and, together with severe **brain edema,** are present in most fatal cases. All 3 conditions cause signs of progressive rostral-caudal neurologic deterioration: deepening coma, widening pulse pressure, dilated pupils, spastic hemiplegia with hyper-reflexia, quadrispasticity, pupillary fixation to light, decorticate rigidity, decerebrate rigidity (see Symptoms and Signs, above). Angiograms are usually diagnostic, but bilateral burr holes over the parieto-occipital and temporal regions provide a more rapid and equally effective diagnostic approach.

Epidural hematoma is most often temporal (middle meningeal artery), less often occipital (venous sinus). Symptoms—increasing headache, deterioration of consciousness, motor dysfunction, pupillary changes—develop 24 to 96 h after trauma. An epidural hematoma is uncommon but important, because continued bleeding for longer than 24 h may cause potentially fatal compression of brain tissue. Temporal fracture lines suggest the diagnosis, but may not be present. Angiograms should be made or, preferably, burr holes drilled promptly for diagnosis and evacuation of the clot.

Chronic subdural hematoma is a late complication that may not develop until some weeks after trauma. Although diagnosis in early cases (2 to 4 wk after trauma) may be suggested by a clinical course of delayed neurologic deterioration, diagnosis is usually difficult because of the time lapse between the injury and the onset of symptoms and signs. Most patients are over age 50, and the head injury may have been relatively trivial, even forgotten. Increasing daily headache, fluctuating drowsiness or mental changes, and mild to moderate hemiparesis are typical. Pupillary abnormalities occur in only 10% of patients, and lumbar puncture may be normal in longstanding cases. Brain scans become abnormal in 80% of cases; these or angiograms are diagnostic.

Convalescence after any severe head injury is marked by **amnesia** for the periods both immediately preceding and following loss of consciousness. **Retrograde amnesia** is usually brief; the duration of **post-traumatic amnesia** (measured until the restoration of complete, continuous awareness) gives a good estimate of the extent of brain damage in closed head injuries. Giddiness, attention difficulties, anxiety, and headache **(postconcussional syndrome)** occur for a variable period after concussion, but seldom persist or require more than reassurance unless lawsuits are pending—in which case careful assessment of psychosocial factors is needed.

Objective assessment of residual disability is important after severe head injury, when subjective complaints may be fewer precisely because of the residual effects. Personality changes from frontal lobe damage and memory deficits from temporal lobe damage, unless tested for, may go unnoticed at first, yet cause problems later at work and at home. Focal deficits, including damage to cranial nerves, are more obvious. Anosmia is permanent; other cranial nerve deficits usually recover spontaneously but are sometimes permanent. Hemiparesis and aphasia usually recover well, except in the elderly or after severe cerebral laceration.

Most recovery after severe head injury occurs in the adult within the first 6 mo, with smaller adjustments continuing for perhaps as long as 2 yr. Children fare better, showing both better immediate recoveries from even very severe injuries and continuing improvement for longer periods of time.

Post-traumatic epilepsy, with seizures beginning as late as 24 mo after trauma, follows about 10% of severe closed head injuries and 40% of penetrating head wounds. To reduce the risk, patients with such injuries should receive prophylactic anticonvulsants (e.g., phenytoin 100 mg orally t.i.d.) for up to 3 yr.

The worst complication of severe head injury is that of near-complete damage to forebrain functions with sparing of the brainstem. Such patients are fortunately rare, but may exist in a **chronic vegetative state** for many years if they survive. In general, few patients recover from the vegetative state when it lasts as long as 2 mo after injury.

SPINAL CORD INJURY

Loss of neurologic function after a spinal injury can result briefly from concussion or more lastingly from compression of the spinal cord due to contusion or hemorrhage, as well as permanently from lacerations or transection. In **contusion,** rapid edematous swelling of the cord with a rise in intradural pressure can cause severe dysfunction for several days. This is followed by spontaneous improvement, but some residual disability may remain. **Hemorrhage** is usually confined to the central gray matter **(hematomyelia)** and produces signs of lower motor neuron damage (muscle weakness and wasting, fasciculation, diminished tendon reflexes) that are usually permanent. The motor weakness often is proximal rather than distal and accompanied by selective impairment of pain and temperature sensations. **Extradural, subdural,** or **subarachnoid hemorrhage** can also occur. **Lacerations** or **transection** inevitably leave permanent dysfunction.

Symptoms, Signs, and Diagnosis

An acute transverse cord lesion causes immediate flaccid paralysis and loss of all sensation and reflex activity (including autonomic functions) below the level of injury **(spinal shock).** The flaccid paralysis gradually changes, over hours or days, to spastic paraplegia due to exaggeration of the normal stretch reflexes. Later, if the lumbosacral cord is intact, extensor or flexor muscle spasms appear, and deep tendon reflexes and autonomic reflexes return (see also NEUROGENIC BLADDER in Ch. 156).

Less complete lesions cause partial motor and sensory loss. Voluntary movement becomes disordered. Sensory loss depends on the tracts affected: posture, vibration, and light touch, if the posterior columns; pain, temperature, and light or deep touch, if the spinothalamic tracts. Hemisection of the cord results in ipsilateral spastic paralysis and loss of postural sense, and contralateral loss of pain and thermal sense **(Brown-Séquard's syndrome).**

Clinical clues identify the level of cord damage. (Abbreviations here refer to vertebrae; one must remember that the cord is shorter than the spine, so that as one descends the spine, the cord segments and vertebral levels are increasingly out of alignment.) Lesions above C-5, if serious, cause respiratory paralysis and are often fatal. Lesions at or above C-4 to C-5 cause complete quadriplegia; with a lesion between C-5 and C-6, the arms can abduct and flex. Damage between C-6 and C-7 paralyzes the legs, wrists, and hands but allows shoulder movement and elbow flexion. Transverse lesions above T-1 cause miotic pupils; lesions at C-8 to T-1 cause **Horner's syndrome**

(constricted pupil, ptosis, facial anhidrosis). Lesions between T-11 and T-12 affect the leg muscles above and below the knee; lesions at T-12 to L-1 cause paralysis below the knee. Trauma to the cauda equina causes hypo- or areflexic paresis of the lower extremities and, usually, pain and hyperesthesia in the distribution of the nerve roots. Damage to the 3rd, 4th, and 5th sacral nerve roots or to the conus medullaris at L-1 causes complete loss of bladder and bowel control.

Prognosis

As in the brain, severed or degenerated nerve processes in the cord cannot recover, and damage is permanent, while compressed nerve tissue usually recovers its function. Return of a movement or sensation during the first week after injury heralds a favorable recovery; any dysfunction remaining after 6 mo is likely to be permanent.

Severe cord injury above C-5 is usually fatal. Cauda equina lesions are seldom complete, and motor or sensory loss is therefore likely to be partial, but reflex arcs controlling micturition, sexual activity in men, and bowel function are in the conus medullaris, and if they are destroyed even reflex micturition cannot be established. Damage to the cauda equina anywhere in the lumbar or sacral spine may cause permanent impotence and loss of sphincter control for bladder, bowel, or both, as will any permanent cord injury at a higher level.

Immediate Management

To protect the cord from further damage, any accident victim suspected of having a spinal injury, especially in the cervical region, must be handled with the utmost care. Until the extent of injury is known, all spinal injuries should be treated as potentially unstable. Either flexion or extension of the spine can contuse or transect the cord if an intervertebral disk has ruptured or the spine is fractured. Getting accident victims out of damaged cars can present a risk of quadriplegia or even death from cervical cord damage. The patient should be moved en bloc and should be transported on a firm, flat board or door, with careful padding to stabilize his position without excessive pressure; proper alignment of the spine by traction is critical. Those with thoracic or lumbar spine injuries should be carried prone or supine; those with cervical cord damage are likely to have respiratory difficulties and should be carried prone, with attention to a patent airway and any possible constrictions around the chest.

Treatment

When the spine is stable, injuries are treated by rest until swelling and local pain have subsided. Unstable injuries must be immobilized, until bone and soft tissues have healed, with traction to ensure proper alignment. Surgery with internal fixation is occasionally needed. It is doubtful whether surgical decompression favorably influences traumatic cord injuries, but osmotic diuretics to reduce edema (as with head injuries) may be indicated.

Nursing care includes prevention of urinary infection, moving the paralyzed patient q 2 h (on a Stryker frame when necessary), and other measures to prevent bedsores. Exercises and rehabilitative measures should begin as soon as possible.

---

124. CNS INFECTIONS

MENINGITIS; ENCEPHALITIS

(See also NEONATAL MENINGITIS in Vol. II, Ch. 21)

Meningitis: *Inflammation of the meninges of the brain or spinal cord.* The brain as well as the meninges can be involved; the cerebral manifestations of bacterial invasion are termed **cerebritis;** those of viral agents, **encephalitis.**

Most bacteria cause an acute meningitis, but tuberculous and syphilitic meningitis are subacute. Viral infections cause an acute **aseptic meningitis,** while fungal infections, disseminated malignancies, and chemical reactions to certain intrathecal injections usually cause a subacute aseptic meningitis.

ACUTE BACTERIAL MENINGITIS

Etiology and Causative Organisms

Acute meningitis may be caused by any of several bacteria, all of which induce similar disorders. Data on the relative incidence of causative bacteria are imprecise because the incidence varies with such factors as the patient's age, immune competence, and probability of exposure, but the following order of frequency is a reasonable approximation: (1) *Neisseria meningitidis,* (2) *Hemophilus influenzae,* (3) *Streptococcus (Diplococcus) pneumoniae,* (4) Group A *Streptococcus,* (5) *Escherichia coli* or other gram-negative organisms (chiefly *Pseudomonas*), (6) *Staphylococcus aureus.* Individual cases may show clinical clues to the nature of the organism, as discussed under Diagnosis, below.

Recurrent meningitis, largely a phenomenon of the antibiotic era, occurs in special situations: (1) with communications to the exterior that may be congenital (myelomeningocele, neurenteric cyst, cranial or spinal midline dermal sinus) or post-traumatic (with or without CSF rhinorrhea or otorrhea); (2) with parameningeal foci of infection, as in mastoiditis, sinusitis, brain abscess, subdural empyema, or spinal epidural abscess; (3) in immunologic deficiency states.

Pathology

The purulent exudate may be restricted or may cover the meninges throughout the brain and spinal cord. The amount of fibrin in the CSF may vary also. The brain may be swollen, its convolutions flattened, and its ventricles compressed. Inflammation may extend around the optic and other cranial nerves, causing secondary demyelination. Particularly in pneumococcal and staphylococcal infection, adhesions may obstruct CSF pathways and cause communicating hydrocephalus late in the course or after resolution of the acute infection.

Symptoms and Signs

A prodromal respiratory illness or sore throat often precedes the fever, headache, stiff neck, and vomiting that characterize acute meningitis. Adults may become desperately ill within 24 h; the course can be even shorter in children. In older children and adults, changes in consciousness progress through irritability, confusion, drowsiness, stupor, and coma. Dehydration is common and vascular collapse may lead to shock **(Waterhouse-Friderichsen syndrome)**, especially in meningococcal septicemia. Hemiparesis is uncommon early in the course but may be seen later as a result of cerebral infarction.

Symptoms and signs are less predictable in infants between 3 mo and 2 yr of age. Fever, vomiting, irritability, convulsions, a high-pitched cry, and a bulging or tight fontanel are commonly present; stiff neck may be absent. Since the incidence of meningitis is highest in this age group, any unexplained fever is suspect, warranting close monitoring and, if necessary, lumbar puncture. Recognition of meningitis in a neonate is even more difficult (see NEONATAL MENINGITIS in Vol. II, Ch. 21).

Subdural effusions may develop after several days in infants and young children; typical signs are seizures, persistent fever, or enlarging head size. Subdural taps through the coronal sutures show a high protein content in the subdural fluid.

Diagnosis

The patient's age or the history may give a clue to the causative organism (see also NEONATAL MENINGITIS in Vol. II, Ch. 21). The incidence of pneumococcal and *H. influenzae* meningitis is highest between the ages of 3 mo and 1 yr; both are rare before then, and *H. influenzae* is a common infection until age 10 yr. After the neonatal period, staphylococcal meningitis occurs primarily in individuals with chronic skin, bone, or sinus infections, or following neurosurgical penetration of the subarachnoid space. Only meningococcal meningitis is apt to occur in epidemics, and only in segregated populations (e.g., in military installations or boarding schools), where it may be cultured from asymptomatic carriers.

Bacteria that invade the CNS always come from elsewhere in the body. In most cases, however, meningitis occurs without clinical clues to the origin, which is presumably septicemia after respiratory or nasopharyngeal infection. However, organisms may also reach the meninges by direct extension following otitis (particularly pneumococci or *H. influenzae*), or following head trauma, especially when a fracture (which may not be clearly evident) involves the paranasal sinuses. Congenital communications with the subarachnoid space should be suspected in meningitis due to *E. coli*, staphylococci, or other unusual organisms.

The head, ears, and skin of all patients should be inspected for sources of infection. A petechial or hemorrhagic rash is common in generalized septicemia, especially when meningococcal, and requires prompt investigation. The skin over the entire spine should be inspected for dimples, sinuses, nevi, or tufts of hair, which may indicate a congenital anomaly communicating with the subarachnoid space. The joints may be involved in meningococcal or *H. influenzae* infections.

Abrupt neck flexion in the supine patient results in involuntary flexion of the knees **(Brudzinski's sign)**. Attempts to extend the knee from the flexed-thigh position are met with strong passive resistance **(Kernig's sign)**. Both signs are presumably due to irritation of motor nerve roots passing through inflamed meninges as they are brought under tension. Unilateral or bilateral **Babinski's sign** may be present. Cranial nerve abnormalities (oculomotor or facial nerve palsy, and occasionally deafness) may be seen.

Laboratory Findings: Diagnosis requires lumbar puncture and CSF examination (see TABLE 117–1 and discussion in Ch. 117) to obtain the following information: (1) pressure, (2) appearance of fluid, (3) cell count, including differential and cell type on spun sediment, (4) protein and glucose concentrations, (5) Gram stain of spun sediment (regardless of cell count, since bacteria may be seen before the count increases), and (6) culture. The CSF is almost always under increased pressure and opalescent or cloudy; cell count varies from a few hundred to several thousand/cu mm, and polymorphonuclear cells (PMNs) usually predominate; protein is generally increased; and glucose is almost always < 40 mg/100 ml. Blood and CSF glucose should be determined at the same time, since CSF glucose is ordinarily about 60% of the blood glucose level and a depressed CSF glucose may not be appreciated if blood glucose is elevated. Meningococci can be recognized readily on

Gram stain, but identification of pneumococci, *H. influenzae*, and other organisms on smear may be difficult. CSF culture may be positive when the cell count is normal, or falsely negative when a bacterial infection has been partially treated with antibiotics. Counterimmunophoresis, using CSF, may be useful in the rapid detection of bacterial meningitis. Culture specimens from the nose, throat, blood, and other obviously infected sites should always be taken. Leukocytosis is usually present and serum electrolyte abnormalities are common.

Differential Diagnosis

Viral infections: Differentiation of viral from bacterial CNS infections is often difficult and is based chiefly on CSF findings (see TABLE 117-1 in Ch. 117). Patients with bacterial meningitis who have been partially treated with antibiotics may have CSF findings identical to those seen in viral infection.

Partially treated meningitis: The widespread use of antibiotics to treat minor respiratory infections has made the diagnosis of subsequent bacterial meningitis more difficult, since doses may be sufficient to partially reverse or obscure clinical meningeal symptoms and signs, and the CSF may be more nearly normal, as in a viral infection. This also poses a therapeutic dilemma, as discussed below.

Nonspecific infections in infants: Lumbar puncture should be performed with little hesitation if FUO is present in young children, especially infants, since clinical signs of meningitis are less likely to be present.

Subacute meningitis: The slowly evolving symptoms and the CSF findings usually differentiate subacute meningitis from acute bacterial meningitis. Other diagnostic points are discussed under SUBACUTE MENINGITIS, below.

Meningismus (meningism): All the symptoms and signs of meningitis may occur without demonstrable meningeal infection, but this diagnosis requires that the CSF be normal. Meningismus is especially common in young children with pneumonia or shigella infections.

Lead encephalopathy: The clinical findings may mimic bacterial meningitis although onset is usually less explosive and fever is uncommon. CSF glucose is usually normal. Other symptoms, signs, and tests diagnostic of plumbism are discussed under ACCIDENTS AND POISONING in Vol. II, Ch. 24.

Prognosis

Antibiotics have reduced the fatality rate of acute bacterial meningitis to below 10% in cases recognized early. However, when meningitis is diagnosed late or occurs in neonates or the elderly, it is still frequently fatal. A low WBC count is a bad prognostic sign. Persistent leukopenia, delayed therapy, and development of the Waterhouse-Friderichsen syndrome diminish the chances of survival. Survivors occasionally show signs of cranial nerve damage, evidence of cerebral infarction, recurrent convulsions, or mental retardation. Meningococcal vaccine is used mainly in epidemic areas and closed populations where epidemic spread is feared.

Treatment

1. Initial therapy: If the clinical findings and characteristic CSF abnormalities are diagnostic, specific therapy (see below and TABLE 124-1) should usually be started immediately, as soon as specimens are taken for culture. If the organism cannot be identified positively on smear, a combination of chloramphenicol and penicillin G or chloramphenicol and ampicillin is the treatment of choice (TABLE 124-1). If *Pseudomonas* infection is suspected at any age, ampicillin with gentamicin and carbenicillin, or with amikacin, is given (this combination protects against other, unsuspected agents as well as *Pseudomonas*).

Treatment problems arise when CSF pleocytosis and normal glucose content make it difficult to determine whether viral meningitis, partially treated bacterial infections, or early bacterial meningitis is the diagnosis. Moreover, antibiotics can cause anaphylactic reactions, drug fever, and difficulty in evaluating the response to therapy. It may therefore be advisable, *if the patient's condition permits it,* to withhold antibiotics and examine the CSF in 8 to 12 h, or sooner if his condition deteriorates. If CSF glucose remains normal and no organisms grow on culture, it is best to continue without antibiotics on the assumption that the infection is not bacterial. However, if the patient's condition is serious, and especially if he has already received antibiotics that may hinder the growth of organisms on culture, a bacterial infection must be assumed and treatment begun with ampicillin or another appropriate antibiotic.

2. **Specific therapy:** (For dosages, see TABLE 124-1.) Once the organism is identified, penicillin G may be substituted for ampicillin in infections caused by meningococci, pneumococci, β-hemolytic streptococci, and susceptible staphylococci. Penicillinase-producing staphylococci should be treated with methicillin or nafcillin. For *H. influenzae* infections, ampicillin is still the drug of choice except in cases of ampicillin-resistant *H. influenzae* or in patients allergic to penicillin. In such cases, chloramphenicol should be used. When *Pseudomonas* is identified, gentamicin is given alone if the organism is sensitive. If the sensitivity is not known or is uncertain, gentamicin plus carbenicillin, or amikacin alone, should be used. Two new cephalosporins, cefotaxime and moxalactam, may prove to be more effective against enteric gram-negative bacilli, especially *E. coli, Klebsiella, Enterobacter,* and most strains of *Serratia.* The antibiotics should be continued for at least 1 wk after fever subsides and the CSF returns to normal.

TABLE 124–1. ANTIBIOTIC THERAPY FOR ACUTE BACTERIAL MENINGITIS*

Organism	Antibiotic	*Total* Daily Dose	Frequency of **Fractional** Dosage**
Unknown: Before age 2 mo	Ampicillin with	200 mg/kg IV	q 6 h
	Kanamycin or with	15 mg/kg IM or IV	q 8 h
	Gentamicin	5 mg/kg IV	q 8 h
Unknown: After age 2 mo	Chloramphenicol with	100 mg/kg body wt IV	q 6 h
	Penicillin G or with	200,000 u./kg	q 4 h
	Ampicillin	200 mg/kg IV	q 6 h
Meningococcus	Penicillin G	200,000 u./kg	q 4 h
H. influenzae	Ampicillin or	200–400 mg/kg IV	q 6 h
	Chloramphenicol	100 mg/kg IV	q 6 h
Pneumococcus	Penicillin G	200,000 u./kg	q 4 h
Streptococcus	Ampicillin or	200 mg/kg IV	q 6 h
	Penicillin G	200,000 u./kg IV	q 4 h
Staphylococcus	Methicillin or	100–200 mg/kg IV	q 4 h
	Nafcillin	100 mg/kg IV	q 4 h
E. coli	Kanamycin or	15 mg/kg IM or IV	q 8 h
	Gentamicin	5 mg/kg IV	q 8 h
Pseudomonas	Gentamicin; or	5 mg/kg IV	q 8 h
	Carbenicillin and	400 mg/kg IV	q 6 h
	Gentamicin; or	5 mg/kg IV	q 8 h
	Amikacin	15 mg/kg IV	q 8 h
Proteus	Ampicillin with	200 mg/kg IV	q 6 h
	Kanamycin or with	15 mg/kg IM or IV	q 8 h
	Gentamicin	5 mg/kg IV	q 8 h

* See TABLE 21–6 in NEONATAL INFECTIONS, Vol. II, Ch. 21, for dosages in neonates.

** Though fractional doses are stated, in the treatment of seriously ill patients it is advantageous to give antimicrobials continuously by IV infusion.

3. Supportive therapy: Dehydration and electrolyte disorders require correction (see Ch. 81). Convulsions and status epilepticus are treated appropriately (see Ch. 120, and SEIZURE DISORDERS in Vol. II, Ch. 21). Care should be taken to avoid secondary infections from indwelling venous or urethral catheters.

Vascular collapse and shock **(Waterhouse-Friderichsen syndrome)** should be watched for. Although attributed to adrenal insufficiency, loss of tissue fluid may be equally important, and the value of ACTH and corticosteroids remains controversial. Plasma expanders and BP support with metaraminol or levarterenol are indicated.

If necessary, cerebral edema may be treated with 15% mannitol solution 1 to 2 gm/kg IV, or 30% urea solution 0.5 to 1.5 gm/kg IV, either drug given over 30 min and repeated in 8 to 12 h if necessary. Dexamethasone 4 mg IV, then 2 mg IV q 4 h (for adults), or glycerin (glycerol) 1.5 gm/kg/24 h orally may be used as a nonspecific agent.

In infants with subdural effusion, the fluid usually subsides with repeated daily subdural taps through the sutures. To avoid sudden shifts in the intracranial contents, not more than 20 ml/day of CSF should be removed from one side. If the effusion persists after 3 to 4 wk of taps, surgical exploration is indicated.

ACUTE VIRAL ENCEPHALITIS AND ASEPTIC MENINGITIS

Encephalitis: *An acute inflammatory disease of the brain due to direct viral invasion or to hypersensitivity initiated by a virus or other foreign protein.* **Encephalomyelitis:** *The same disorder affecting spinal cord structures as well as the brain.*

Aseptic meningitis: *A febrile meningeal inflammation characterized by CSF pleocytosis, normal glucose, and an absence of bacteria on examination and culture.*

Etiology and Causative Viruses

Virus infection may cause encephalitis as a primary manifestation or as a secondary complication. Viruses causing primary encephalitis may be epidemic (arbo-, polio-, echo-, and coxsackie viruses) or sporadic (herpes simplex, herpes zoster). Arbovirus encephalitides (St. Louis, Eastern and Western equine, and California) are mosquito-borne and infect man only during warm weather.

Most cases of encephalitis occur as a complication of viral infection and are considered to have an immunologic mechanism. Examples are the encephalitides following measles, chickenpox, rubella, smallpox vaccination, vaccinia, and many other less well defined virus infections. These **parainfectious** or **postinfectious encephalitides** typically develop 5 to 10 days after onset of illness and are characterized by a perivascular demyelination in the brain of patients who succumb; a virus has rarely been isolated from the brain. (The condition is sometimes referred to as **acute disseminated encephalomyelitis** and classified with the primary demyelinating diseases.) In mumps, both primary and postinfectious CNS involvement may occur.

Meningitis with CSF findings of pleocytosis, normal glucose, and no evidence of bacterial organisms (hence, "**aseptic**") may be due not only to viral infections (see also ENTEROVIRAL DISEASES in Vol. II, Ch. 24) but also to other organisms and noninfectious causes (see TABLE 124–2).

Very rarely, encephalitis or other encephalopathies occur as a late consequence of viral infections. The best known of these are **subacute sclerosing panencephalitis (SSPE)**, associated with the measles virus; **kuru,** a "slow virus" infection seen in New Guinea, and **Creutzfeldt-Jakob disease,** a rare dementia of middle age. These nonacute encephalitides are discussed in SLOW VIRUS INFECTIONS in Ch. 12.

Pathology

Cerebral edema is present, and numerous petechial hemorrhages are scattered throughout the hemispheres, brainstem, cerebellum, and occasionally the spinal cord. Direct viral invasion of the brain is likely to be associated with neuron necrosis, and, frequently, with visible inclusion bodies. In para- and postinfectious encephalomyelitis, perivenous demyelinating lesions are characteristic.

Symptoms and Signs

CNS viral infections may take 3 forms: (1) **Asymptomatic:** There may be no symptoms, or fever and malaise may be present with no clinical meningeal manifestations. The CSF, however, may be abnormal, with lymphocytic pleocytosis, and a virus may be isolated from the CSF. (2) **Meningitis:** Fever, headache, vomiting, malaise, and stiff neck and back may be the predominant symptoms. (3) **Encephalitis:** Meningitis may be associated with evidence of cerebral dysfunction (alteration in consciousness, personality change, seizures, paresis) and cranial nerve abnormalities. The distinction

TABLE 124–2. CAUSES OF ASEPTIC MENINGITIS (INCLUDING COMMON ENCEPHALITIDES)

Infectious

Virus: Mumps, echovirus, poliovirus, coxsackievirus, lymphocytic choriomeningitis, herpes simplex, herpes zoster, Eastern and Western equine, St. Louis, infectious hepatitis, infectious mononucleosis

Postinfectious: Measles, rubella, varicella, smallpox, vaccinia

Bacterial: Tuberculosis, syphilis, partially treated bacterial meningitis

Miscellaneous infections: Leptospirosis, toxoplasmosis, torulosis, trichinosis, syphilis, coccidioidomycosis, mycoplasma, lymphogranuloma venereum, cat-scratch disease

Noninfectious

Parameningeal disease: Brain tumor, stroke, multiple sclerosis, abscess, chronic sinusitis or otitis

Reaction to intrathecal injections: Air, serum, antibiotics, iophendylate and other dyes

Poison: Lead

Vaccine reactions: Many, especially rabies, pertussis, smallpox

Meningeal disease: Sarcoidosis, meningeal leukemia, meningeal carcinomatosis

between aseptic meningitis and encephalitis is based on the extent and severity of cerebral dysfunction, independent of signs of meningeal inflammation.

Diagnosis

Viral CNS infections must be differentiated from nonviral and noninfectious causes (see TABLE 124-2), but the major diagnostic problem is differentiation from acute or partially treated bacterial meningitis (see ACUTE BACTERIAL MENINGITIS above, and TABLE 117-1 in Ch. 117). Diagnosis is usually based on the CSF characteristics, including normal glucose and failure to grow bacteria on culture. Even under ideal circumstances, viruses causing aseptic meningitis and encephalitis are identified in fewer than half the cases. Viruses are occasionally isolated directly from the CSF or from other tissues. A precise diagnosis, however, usually requires the use of paired sera documenting a rise in antibodies. Since many forms of encephalitis and aseptic meningitis have important public health implications, serum should be drawn and preserved whenever the diagnosis of encephalitis or aseptic meningitis of uncertain etiology is first suspected. Information regarding more precise viral diagnosis can be obtained from local departments of health.

Although **herpes simplex encephalitis** is clinically similar to other viral encephalitides, repeated seizures occurring early in the course, and localizing signs indicating temporal or frontal lobe involvement, strongly suggest herpes simplex as the cause. The presence of erythrocytes in the CSF following an atraumatic spinal tap also suggests herpes simplex infection. The virus is rarely present in the CSF, and serologic tests are not sufficient to implicate herpes simplex virus, since antibody levels normally fluctuate even in healthy persons. Diagnosis is certain only upon demonstration of the virus (by recovery of the virus or immunologic technics) in cerebral tissue obtained by brain biopsy or at postmortem examination.

Prognosis and Treatment

Even desperately ill patients may recover completely. The mortality rate varies with the etiology, and epidemics with the same virus vary in severity in different years. Permanent cerebral disorders are more likely to occur in infants, but young children continue to show improvement over a longer period than do adults with similar infections.

In herpes simplex encephalitis, early treatment with vidarabine (adenine arabinoside) 15 mg/kg/day IV over a 12-h period reduces mortality from 70 to 28% and also the incidence of sequelae in survivors. However, after onset of coma, the outcome is not significantly altered by this drug. Vidarabine may also be useful in varicella encephalitis. For other forms of viral encephalitis, no effective antiviral agent is yet available.

Supportive therapy is as for acute bacterial meningitis. Fluid balance should be maintained but overhydration avoided.

SUBACUTE MENINGITIS

Meningitis in which the duration of the disease, in the absence of antibiotics, is $>$ 2 wk but $<$ 3 mo.

Etiology

Subacute meningitis may occur with (1) systemic fungal infections; (2) TB; (3) dissemination of malignant cells, as in leukemia, metastatic carcinoma (especially of lung and breast), or primary brain tumors such as gliomas; (4) syphilis; (5) sarcoidosis.

A marked increase in fungal CNS infections has paralleled the decline of TB and accompanied the increase in immunosuppressive therapy. *Cryptococcus* is the most common offender; *Coccidioides*, Mucorales, *Candida*, *Actinomyces*, and *Aspergillus* are encountered occasionally. Cryptococcal meningitis may be a complication of Hodgkin's disease or other lymphomas.

Neoplastic meningitis with diffuse leptomeningeal involvement is a continuing problem in acute lymphoblastic leukemia, especially in leukemic children being treated with antileukemic drugs, which do not cross the blood-brain barrier. Neoplastic meningitis may also occur with gliomas (particularly glioblastoma, ependymoma, or medulloblastoma) or with carcinoma metastatic to the brain. Rarely, the first sign of malignant disease may be a subacute meningeal inflammation.

Symptoms and Signs

These are essentially the same as in acute meningitis, but the illness evolves more slowly—over a period of weeks rather than days. Fever may be minimal. Chronic communicating hydrocephalus may be seen as a complication. In neoplastic meningitis, headache, dementia, and cranial and peripheral nerve palsies are common, and the course is progressive; death occurs within a few weeks or months after the onset of symptoms.

Diagnosis

Because of the slow evolution of cerebral symptoms, the differential diagnosis includes structural lesions such as brain tumors, abscesses, and subdural effusions. Active TB elsewhere in the body or a known malignancy suggests the etiology, but the CSF must be examined to establish a diagnosis unless contraindicated by evidence of increased intracranial pressure from an expanding lesion. The CSF cell count is generally $<$ 1000/cu mm with lymphocytes predominant; glucose is frequently low except in syphilis, and protein may be high. Besides lymphocytic pleocytosis, CSF findings in neoplastic meningitis include low glucose, slightly elevated protein, and, frequently, elevated pressure; at times, tumor cells may be found. Microscopic examination or culture of the CSF is needed to identify malignant cells or a causative organism. Fungi can frequently be identified by examination of a centrifuged sediment; TB can be identified on stained smear. In syphilis, CSF pressure, cell count, and protein resemble findings in other subacute meningitides but the CSF glucose is usually normal; CSF and blood VDRL tests and STS are positive in most patients. Since most causative infections must be treated over a prolonged period with highly specific drugs, precise identification of the organism is essential before therapy is begun.

Treatment

Tuberculous meningitis: See EXTRAPULMONARY TUBERCULOSIS in Ch. 8.

Syphilitic meningitis: See Ch. 162.

Leukemic meningitis: See THE ACUTE LEUKEMIAS in Ch. 97.

Sarcoid meningitis: Prednisone 80 mg/day orally is given for 3 wk, then decreased by 5 mg/day every 3 days.

Actinomyces **meningitis:** The drug of choice is penicillin G, 20 million u./day IM or IV (200,000 u./kg/day for children), given for at least 6 wk. Treatment may be continued for an additional 2 to 3 mo with penicillin V, 1 to 2 million u./day orally (proportionately less for children).

Mycotic meningitis: Amphotericin B is the drug of choice for all fungi and yeasts. Starting at 50 mg/day, amphotericin B is given by slow IV infusion in gradually increasing doses as tolerated. (CAUTION: *Daily dosage should not exceed 1.5 mg/kg for adults and 1 mg/kg for children. See General Therapeutic Principles in Ch. 9 for other information on administration and other precautions.*) A total of 4 to 6 gm is usually given but the optimal total dose is uncertain. Treatment duration need not exceed 10 wk if the blood level of amphotericin B can be maintained at a concentration at least twice that needed to inhibit growth of the fungus in culture. Intrathecal administration is occasionally useful but not without hazard.

BRAIN ABSCESS

An intracerebral encapsulated collection of pus.

Etiology and Pathology

An abscess within the brain is due to extension from a bacterial infection outside the brain. **Direct extension** is from infection of the skull itself (e.g., osteomyelitis, mastoiditis, sinusitis) or infection within the skull (e.g., subdural empyema); an abscess can also result from penetration by a foreign body. **Indirect extension**, via the bloodstream, occurs with bacterial endocarditis, pulmonary infection (e.g., bronchiectasis), and cyanotic congenital heart disease. Occasionally, the primary source of bacterial infection cannot be identified.

The first stage is characterized pathologically by a poorly localized bacterial encephalitis (cerebritis). Subsequently, glia and fibroblasts form a limiting capsule that reduces systemic signs of inflammation. Cerebral edema may be marked at any stage.

Symptoms, Signs, and Diagnosis

Symptoms and signs resemble those seen in brain tumor: headache, nausea and vomiting, papilledema, hemiparesis, ataxia, and convulsions. Evidence of systemic inflammation, such as fever, chills, and leukocytosis, is usually present but may be absent when the abscess is encapsulated. Symptoms have generally been present for a few days to a few weeks at the time of diagnosis.

Signs of brain tumor in association with evidence of infection suggest brain abscess, especially when there has been an antecedent infection that is the probable primary site. CSF findings commonly include increased pressure, mild pleocytosis (average, 135 cells/cu mm), and mild elevation of protein. CSF glucose is not usually decreased, and bacteria can only occasionally be cultured from the CSF. If the abscess is well encapsulated and remote from CSF pathways, the CSF may be normal.

Primary or metastatic brain tumor, subdural effusion, cerebrovascular disease, subacute and chronic meningitis, and degenerative diseases must be excluded.

Treatment

Brain abscess is fatal unless treated. Mixed bacterial infections are common and often include anaerobic organisms that are difficult to culture. When the causative bacteria cannot be identified, treatment should be with ampicillin 200 mg/kg/day IV plus tetracycline 50 mg/kg/day orally, or ampicillin plus chloramphenicol 100 mg/kg/day orally.

Surgical excision or aspiration plus antibiotics is the treatment of choice. Antibiotic treatment should be given for a minimum of 4 to 8 wk, but a cure with antibiotics alone is exceptional and can be expected only with very early diagnosis.

125. CNS NEOPLASMS

INTRACRANIAL NEOPLASMS
(Brain Tumors)

An expanding intracranial lesion may be a neoplasm (metastatic or primary), granuloma, parasitic cyst, hemorrhage (intracerebral, extradural, or subdural), aneurysm, or abscess. This chapter deals primarily with neoplasms arising from intracranial tissues. These growths are common and are frequently misdiagnosed.

Primary intracranial neoplasms are divided into 6 classes: (1) tumors of the skull (osteoma, hemangioma, granuloma, xanthoma, osteitis deformans); (2) tumors of the meninges (meningioma, sarcoma, gliomatosis); (3) tumors of the cranial nerves (glioma of the optic nerve, schwannoma [neurilemoma] of the 8th and 5th cranial nerves); (4) tumors of the supportive tissue (gliomas); (5) tumors of the pituitary or pineal body (pituitary adenoma, pinealoma); and (6) congenital tumors (craniopharyngioma, chordoma, germinoma, teratoma, dermoid cyst, angioma, hemangioblastoma).

Secondary metastases may involve the skull or any intracranial structure.

Pathology and Incidence

CNS changes result both from invasion and destruction by the tumor and from its secondary effects (increased intracranial pressure, cerebral edema, and compression of brain tissue, cranial nerves, and cerebral vessels).

Brain tumors are found in about 2% of routine autopsies. They may occur at any age but are most common in early adult or middle life. **Common primary childhood tumors** are cerebellar astrocytomas and medulloblastomas, ependymomas, gliomas of the brainstem and optic nerve, germinomas (pinealomas), and congenital tumors. The most **common metastatic invaders in childhood** are neuroblastoma (usually epidural) and leukemia (meningeal). **Primary adult tumors** include meningiomas, schwannomas, gliomas of the cerebral hemispheres (particularly the malignant glioblastoma multiforme and more benign astrocytoma and oligodendroglioma). **Metastatic tumors** in adults arise most commonly from bronchogenic carcinoma, adenocarcinoma of the breast, and malignant melanoma. Overall incidence in males and females is about equal, but cerebellar medulloblastoma and glioblastoma multiforme are more common in males; meningioma and schwannoma, in females.

The relative frequency of various types of intracranial tumors is gliomas 45%, pituitary adenomas 15%, meningiomas 15%, schwannomas 7%, congenital tumors 3%, metastatic and other types 15%.

Symptoms and Signs

1. General symptoms and signs result from increased intracranial pressure. This may be due to the space-occupying tumor mass itself or to associated cerebral edema, obstructed flow of CSF (occurring early in 3rd ventricle or posterior fossa tumors), obstructed dural venous sinuses (especially by bony or extradural metastatic tumors), or obstructed CSF absorption mechanisms (as in leukemic or carcinomatous involvement of the meninges). Headache and vomiting result, as may mental symptoms. Papilledema develops in about 25% of patients with brain tumor and may not be an early sign; its absence does not rule out a tumor or elevated intracranial pressure. In young children, elevated intracranial pressure may enlarge the head. The intracranial pressure is usually normal in patients with small tumors of the cerebral hemispheres, pituitary adenomas, or brainstem tumors that do not obstruct the aqueduct of Sylvius. Changes in temperature, pulse or respiratory rate, or BP are unusual except terminally.

Convulsive seizures, either focal or generalized, occur with cerebral hemisphere tumors and may precede other symptoms by months or years. They are more frequent with meningiomas and slowly growing astrocytomas than with malignant gliomas. Focal seizures help to locate the tumor.

Mental symptoms (e.g., drowsiness, lethargy, obtuseness, personality changes, disordered conduct, impaired mental faculties, psychotic episodes) may appear at any time. They are the initial symptoms in 25% of malignant brain tumors.

2. Special (focal) symptoms and signs are due to localized destruction or compression of nervous tissue or to altered endocrine function, and depend on the location of the tumor.

A. Tumors of the Cerebral Hemispheres

Frontal lobe tumors (commonly meningiomas or gliomas) involving the frontal convexity are characterized by progressive hemiplegia, focal or generalized seizures, and mental changes. Expressive aphasia may accompany a tumor of the dominant hemisphere. A tumor at the base of the frontal lobes (particularly meningioma of the olfactory groove) produces ipsilateral anosmia. A tumor on the medial surface of a frontal lobe may cause precipitate urination. Mental changes (especially inattention and loss of motivation) and ataxic gait are common when the tumor spreads across the corpus callosum to both frontal lobes. Meningioma of the tuberculum sellae may compress the optic chiasm, producing a visual field defect similar to that of a pituitary adenoma (see Tumors of the Pituitary and

Suprasellar Region, below). Meningioma of the inner third of the sphenoid ridge may cause exophthalmos and unilateral amblyopia. Meningioma of the outer part of the sphenoid ridge may invade the temporal lobe (see Temporal lobe tumors, below).

Parietal lobe tumors may produce either generalized convulsions or sensory focal seizures. Cutaneous tactile, pain, and temperature senses are unimpaired, but stereognosis and the cortical sensory modalities (position sense, 2-point discrimination) are impaired contralaterally. Contralateral homonymous hemianopia, apraxia, and anosognosia (nonrecognition of bodily defects) may also be present. Denial of illness is characteristic, especially if obtundation is present. Speech disturbances, agraphia, and finger agnosia may occur when the tumor involves the dominant hemisphere.

Temporal lobe tumors, particularly in the nondominant hemisphere, are often relatively "silent" except when they cause convulsive seizures. A tumor deep in the temporal lobe may cause contralateral hemianopia, psychomotor seizures, or convulsive seizures preceded by an olfactory aura or visual hallucinations of complex formed images. Tumors involving the surface of the dominant temporal lobe produce mixed expressive and receptive aphasia or dysphasia, chiefly anomia.

Occipital lobe tumors usually cause a contralateral quadrant defect in the visual field or a hemianopia with sparing of the macula. Associated convulsions may be preceded by an aura of flashing lights, but not formed images.

Subcortical tumors commonly involve the internal capsule and produce contralateral hemiplegia. They may invade any of the lobes of the hemisphere, producing corresponding symptoms. Thalamic invasion produces contralateral cutaneous sensory impairment. Invasion of the basal ganglia usually does not produce parkinsonian symptoms, but athetosis, bizarre tremors, or dystonic postures are occasionally present.

Cranial, extradural, or subdural metastatic tumors, by compressing or invading the underlying cortex, may produce the same localizing signs as those caused by a primary cortical tumor.

As lesions enlarge, brain tissue may be displaced through the fixed intracranial openings, producing various herniation syndromes. Thus, the medial surface of a hemisphere may be forced beneath the falx cerebri. **Transtentorial herniation** occurs with displacement of brain tissue through the tentorial notch. In **central herniation,** there is symmetric bilateral tissue displacement, while **temporal lobe herniation** is an asymmetric displacement of a cone of temporal lobe tissue through the tentorial notch. Both types of herniation compress vital brainstem structures: central herniation leads to coma, mid-position fixed pupils, altered respiration, loss of oculocephalic and oculovestibular reflexes (failure of the eyes to move in response to head rotation or to caloric stimulation, respectively), and bilateral motor paralysis (decerebrate rigidity or flaccidity). Temporal lobe herniation may produce an early 3rd nerve palsy (unilateral dilated fixed pupil and extraocular paralysis) in addition to the central signs. Less commonly, a cerebellar cone may be forced through the foramen magnum, producing respiratory and cardiac arrest.

False localizing signs may accompany prolonged elevated intracranial pressure. They include uni- or bilateral lateral rectus palsy from 6th nerve compression, hemiplegia on the same side as the tumor from compression of the opposite cerebral peduncle against the tentorium, and visual field defect on the same side as the tumor from compromise of the opposite posterior cerebral artery.

B. Tumors of the Pituitary and Suprasellar Region

Pituitary adenomas may present as intrasellar secretory or nonsecretory masses, or masses with extrasellar extension. Secretory adenomas produce hormones that cause specific endocrinopathies. Traditionally, adenomas with particular histologic staining characteristics have been associated with specific endocrinopathies: e.g., **acidophilic** adenoma overproduces growth hormone, leading to gigantism prior to puberty, acromegaly after puberty; **basophilic** adenoma overproduces ACTH, leading to Cushing's syndrome. **Chromophobe** adenomas were thought not to secrete hormones, but are now known to be responsible for most of the endocrinopathies caused by pituitary tumors. The most common endocrine hypersecretion is prolactin, producing amenorrhea and galactorrhea in women and, less frequently, impotence and gynecomastia in men. Many secretory tumors are microadenomas, found only after an endocrine abnormality is discovered (see Ch. 85).

Enlarging pituitary adenomas cause headache. As the tumor grows out of the sella, it compresses the optic chiasm, nerves, or tracts, and the hypothalamus. The common visual field defect is bitemporal hemianopia, but unilateral optic atrophy, contralateral hemianopia, or any combination of the 3 may occur. Hypothalamic compression usually causes diabetes insipidus from injury to the supraoptic-pituitary tract. The tumor may destroy functioning glandular tissue and cause pituitary deficiency. X-rays show a characteristic balloon-shaped appearance of the sella, but microadenomas may only cause laterally placed focal bulging of the sella floor, visible only on tomograms.

Other tumors in the region of the sella turcica (e.g., meningiomas, craniopharyngiomas, metastases, dermoid cysts) or aneurysms may compress the optic chiasm, invade the sella, and produce symptoms similar to those of chromophobic adenoma.

C. Pineal Tumors

Pineal tumors (usually germinomas) occur at any age, but are most common in childhood. Precocious puberty may result, especially in boys. The tumor compresses the aqueduct of Sylvius, causing hydrocephalus, papilledema, and other signs of increased intracranial pressure. The pretectum rostral to the superior colliculi is also compressed, resulting in paralysis of upward gaze, ptosis, and loss of pupillary light and accommodation reflexes.

D. Tumors of the Brainstem

Gliomas of the brainstem are usually astrocytomas. Common symptoms, resulting from destruction of nuclear masses, are unilateral or bilateral paralysis of the 5th, 6th, 7th, and 10th cranial nerves, and paralysis of lateral gaze. Damage to the motor or sensory pathways causes hemiplegia, hemianesthesia, or cerebellar disturbances (ataxia, nystagmus, intention tremor). Increased intracranial pressure appears late in brainstem tumors.

E. Posterior Fossa Tumors

Tumors of the 4th ventricle and cerebellum (usually medulloblastomas, gliomas, ependymomas, or metastases) interfere with CSF circulation, and symptoms of increased intracranial pressure appear early. Ataxic gait, intention tremor, and other signs of cerebellar dysfunction follow.

Cerebellopontine angle tumors, particularly neurilemomas (acoustic neurinomas, schwannomas), are characterized by tinnitus, unilateral hearing impairment, and, sometimes, vertigo. Pressure on the adjacent cranial nerves, brainstem, and cerebellum produces loss of corneal reflex, facial palsy and anesthesia, palatal weakness, signs of cerebellar dysfunction, and, rarely, contralateral hemiplegia or hemianesthesia. Loss of vestibular response to caloric stimulation, enlargement of the porus acusticus as shown by x-ray, and high CSF protein content suggest an acoustic neurilemoma (see also ACOUSTIC NEURINOMA in Ch. 167).

F. Meningeal Neoplasm

Diffuse involvement of the leptomeninges was common in acute lymphoblastic leukemia but is much less so as a result of prophylactic radiation therapy and chemotherapy. Meningeal neoplasm may complicate gliomas (particularly the glioblastomas or medulloblastomas) or metastatic carcinoma of the brain. Symptoms and signs are discussed under SUBACUTE MENINGITIS in Ch. 124.

Diagnosis

A brain tumor should be considered and neurologic consultation requested for patients with slowly progressive signs of focal cerebral dysfunction, focal or generalized convulsions, headaches of recent onset, or other evidence of increased intracranial pressure (e.g., vomiting, papilledema).

Studies should include a complete neurologic examination, testing of visual acuity and visual fields, audiometric tests, a CT scan, and x-rays of the chest (for a source of metastases). Cerebral angiography may be necessary as a preoperative measure, less often for diagnosis.

CSF examination is unnecessary if the diagnosis is obvious but may be useful if the diagnosis or the nature of the lesion is not clear after preliminary studies; it is essential in the diagnosis of chronic or subacute neoplastic meningitis or benign intracranial hypertension (**pseudotumor cerebri**—see below). Lumbar puncture is **contraindicated** in the presence of papilledema if an expanding lesion is suspected, since the sudden pressure change in such instances can precipitate transtentorial herniation.

Treatment

Treatment of brain tumor is surgical excision or irradiation. Firm, encapsulated tumors (e.g., meningiomas, schwannomas) and congenital tumors are not affected by irradiation and should be excised. Infiltrating gliomas cannot be completely extirpated surgically, and partial removal is followed by x-ray therapy. If the tumor is inaccessible, as in the thalamus or brainstem, irradiation is the primary therapy. Pituitary tumors may be removed by trans-sphenoidal microsurgery or craniotomy. They may also be treated by irradiation alone or irradiation after surgery. Surgery is indicated if vision is threatened, but the method of treatment of microadenomas is controversial. Hyperprolactinemia from pituitary adenomas may be effectively treated with bromocriptine 2.5 to 7.5 mg/day orally, but resection or irradiation is necessary to treat the tumor itself. Treatment of leukemic meningitis is discussed in Ch. 97.

Chemotherapy of brain tumors (e.g., with carmustine [BCNU], lomustine [CCNU], or semustine [methyl CCNU]) is playing an increasing role in treatment (see also Ch. 250).

If neurologic or neurosurgical consultation is not readily available, temporary measures may be necessary to relieve increased intracranial pressure and prevent herniation. Mannitol 25 to 100 gm infused IV is given to relieve pressure immediately, and should be accompanied by a corticosteroid (e.g., dexamethasone 16 mg/day orally or parenterally, or prednisone 60 to 80 mg/day orally, in divided doses) to maintain the reduced pressure. Lumbar puncture is **contraindicated** for reduction of intracranial pressure accompanying brain neoplasms.

PSEUDOTUMOR CEREBRI

(Benign Intracranial Hypertension)

A disorder characterized by increased intracranial pressure in the absence of any evidence of intracranial space-occupying lesion, obstruction of the ventricular or subarachnoid pathways, infection, or hypertensive encephalopathy. Etiology in most instances is unknown; the syndrome undoubtedly includes several disorders of different causes. Generally, however, both onset and eventual disappearance are spontaneous. The condition is more common in women between ages 20 and 50, and especially affects those who are overweight. Symptoms consist of headache of varying severity (often mild), papilledema, and the appearance of generally good health. Partial or complete monocular visual loss occurs in about 5% of patients, and is the only serious neurologic sign. On the other hand, the blind spots are frequently enlarged. CT scans generally are normal, or show a somewhat small ventricular system. EEG is normal. The lumbar puncture pressure is elevated, and the fluid is normal. A similar picture can be the result of occlusion of an intracranial venous sinus involving the posterior third of the sagittal sinus or one of the circumflex sinuses; excessive ingestion of Vitamin A or tetracycline; increased intracranial pressure secondary to chronic CO_2 retention and hypoxia; and other less well established abnormalities, including iron-deficiency anemia and hypoparathyroidism. **Treatment** varies according to the cause, but once the diagnosis is made, the syndrome generally has no serious consequences and can be managed symptomatically. However, visual loss, if it occurs, may be permanent regardless of treatment. Pseudotumor recurs in about 10% of cases.

SPINAL CORD NEOPLASMS

Lesions that compress the spinal cord or its roots, arising from the cord parenchyma, roots, meninges, or vertebrae.

Pathology and Incidence

Primary neoplasms of the spinal cord are much less common than intracranial tumors and are rare in childhood or old age. Only about 10% of spinal tumors are intramedullary. Meningiomas and neurofibromas account for about 2/3 of all primary spinal tumors; others include gliomas and sarcomas. Extradural metastatic lesions are not uncommon; they may accompany carcinoma of the lung, breast, prostate, kidney, or thyroid, or lymphoma (Hodgkin's disease, lymphosarcoma, and reticulum cell sarcoma).

Symptoms and Signs

Extramedullary neoplasms: The first symptoms are usually from compression of nerve roots— pain and paresthesias followed by sensory loss, muscular weakness, and wasting along the distribution of the affected roots. Growth of the tumor leads to cord compression, causing progressive spastic weakness and impaired cutaneous and proprioceptive sensation below the level of the lesion. Sphincter control may be affected. Depending on the location and nature of the tumor, cord symptoms may be mild or severe and are often asymmetric. Occlusion of spinal vessels by the tumor may cause myelomalacia with symptoms of cord transection (see SPINAL CORD INJURY in Ch. 123).

Intramedullary neoplasms (gliomas, ependymomas) frequently extend over several spinal segments and clinically may mimic syringomyelia. A tumor localized in one segment may clinically resemble an extramedullary tumor, but pain is usually less prominent and sphincter symptoms occur earlier.

Diagnosis

Spinal neoplasms must be differentiated from other diseases of the spinal cord, e.g., vascular malformations, syphilis, multiple sclerosis, syringomyelia, pernicious anemia, amyotrophic lateral sclerosis, anomalies of the cervical spine and base of the skull, cervical spondylosis, and ruptured intervertebral disk.

X-rays of the spine may show bone destruction, widening of the vertebral pedicles, or distortion of paraspinal tissues. The CSF protein concentration is usually increased and manometric examination shows subarachnoid block. Iophendylate myelography is the definitive diagnostic test for tumors and may provide the first clue that the offending lesion is an arteriovenous malformation; this can then be identified by selective arteriography.

Treatment

Extramedullary compressive growths may be removed surgically; the prognosis depends on the damage already done. For intramedullary and nonexcisable extramedullary tumors, radiotherapy is used, either alone or following surgical decompression. The tumor may be arrested; reversal of the clinical syndrome occurs in about 1/2 of patients. Corticosteroid hormones may reduce spinal cord edema and preserve function.

126. DEMYELINATING DISEASES

The myelin that sheaths many nerve fibers is a complex of lipoprotein layers formed in early life by the oligodendroglia in the CNS and by the Schwann cells peripherally (see also in Ch. 130). The two myelins differ both chemically and immunologically, but serve the same function: to promote transmission of the neural impulse along the axon.

Many congenital metabolic disorders (e.g., phenylketonuria and other aminoacidurias; Tay-Sachs, Niemann-Pick, Gaucher's, and Hurler's diseases; Krabbe's disease and other leukodystrophies) affect the developing myelin sheath. Unless the innate biochemical defect can be corrected or compensated for before this occurs, permanent and often widespread neurologic deficits result.

Demyelination in later life is a feature of many neurologic disorders, since it can occur as a result of neuronal damage as well as damage to the myelin itself, whether the damage is due to local injury, ischemia, toxic agents, or metabolic disorders. Extensive myelin loss is usually followed by axonal degeneration and often by cell body degeneration, and may be irreversible. However, in many instances remyelination occurs; and repair, regeneration, and complete recovery of neural function can take place rapidly—this is often seen, for example, following the segmental demyelination that characterizes many peripheral neuropathies, and may explain the exacerbations and remissions of multiple sclerosis.

Demyelination also occurs as the predominant finding in several disorders of uncertain etiology that have come to be known as the **primary demyelinating diseases**. Of these, **multiple sclerosis (MS)** is the most prominent, and is discussed in detail below. Brief descriptions of the others follow.

Acute disseminated encephalomyelitis (postinfectious encephalitis) is a perivascular CNS demyelination that can occur spontaneously but usually follows a viral infection or inoculation (or, very rarely, a bacterial vaccine), suggesting an immunologic cause. It is discussed under ACUTE VIRAL ENCEPHALITIS in Ch. 124. The "neuroparalytic accidents" and peripheral neuropathies that can follow rabies vaccination with brain tissue preparations, and the Guillain-Barré syndrome (discussed under PERIPHERAL NEUROPATHY in Ch. 130) are similar demyelinating disorders with the same presumed immunologic pathogenesis.

In **optic neuromyelitis,** the demyelination selectively and acutely affects the optic nerves and (usually a short time later) the spinal cord at a thoracic or, less often, a cervical segment. The optic demyelination produces acute visual loss or central scotoma; spinal cord involvement results in the same symptoms and signs as are seen in MS. The syndrome may follow febrile diseases, may occur as a feature of MS, or apparently may occur spontaneously. Early **treatment** with ACTH or corticosteroids to control the assumed inflammation has been used empirically.

Adrenoleukodystrophy (formerly called **Schilder's disease**) is a rare, sex-linked recessive metabolic disorder that occurs in boys and is characterized by adrenal atrophy and widespread, diffuse cerebral demyelination. It produces mental deterioration, corticospinal tract dysfunction, and cortical blindness. There is laboratory evidence of adrenal cortical dysfunction. Death invariably occurs in 1 to 5 yr.

MULTIPLE SCLEROSIS

(MS; Disseminated Sclerosis)

A slowly progressive CNS disease characterized by disseminated patches of demyelination in the brain and spinal cord, resulting in multiple and varied neurologic symptoms and signs, usually with remissions and exacerbations.

Etiology and Incidence

The cause is unknown but an immunologic abnormality is suspected, with few clues that presently indicate a specific mechanism. Postulated etiologies include infection by a slow or latent virus, and myelinolysis by enzymes. IgG is elevated in the CSF of most patients with MS, and elevated titers have been found to a variety of viral agents, including measles. The full significance of these findings as well as variously reported associations with HLA allotypes is presently unclear, and the evidence somewhat conflicting. An increased family incidence suggests that genetic factors may influence susceptibility. Women are affected somewhat more often than men. The disease is more common in temperate climates (1:2000) than in the tropics (1:10,000), but relocation after age 15 does not alter the risk.

Pathology

Plaques, or islands, of demyelination with destruction of oligodendroglia and perivascular inflammation are disseminated through the CNS, primarily in the white matter, with a predilection for the lateral and posterior columns (especially in the cervical and dorsal regions), the optic nerves, and periventricular areas. Tracts in the midbrain, pons, and cerebellum are also affected, and gray matter in both cerebrum and cord may be invaded. Cell bodies and axons are usually preserved, especially in early lesions. Later, axons may be destroyed, especially in the long tracts, and a fibrous gliosis gives the tracts their "sclerotic" appearance. Both early and late lesions may be found simultaneously. Chemical changes in lipid and protein constituents of myelin have been demonstrated in and around the plaques.

Symptoms and Signs

The disease is characterized by various complaints and findings, with remissions and persistently recurring exacerbations. Onset usually is insidious. In most cases, patients present between age 20 and 40 with one or more symptoms, their nature depending on the sites of initial demyelination. Paresthesias in one or more extremities, in the trunk, or on one side of the face; weakness or clumsiness of a leg or a hand; or visual disturbances, such as partial blindness and pain in one eye (**retrobulbar optic neuritis**), diplopia, dimness of vision, or scotomas, are the most frequent presenting symptoms. Other common early symptoms are a fleeting ocular palsy, transient weakness, slight stiffness or unusual fatigability of a limb, minor gait disturbances, difficulties with bladder control, vertigo, or mild emotional disturbances—all evidence of scattered involvement of the CNS and often occurring months or years before the disease is recognized.

Findings on examination are many and varied:

Mental: Apathy, lack of judgment, or inattention may occur. Emotional lability is common and, along with the widespread, mild signs, often leads to the initial impression of hysteria. Euphoria occurs in many patients, but in some a reactive depression is understandably present. Sudden weeping or forced laughter (concomitants of pseudobulbar palsy) indicates that corticobulbar pathways of emotional control are involved. Convulsive seizures may occur. Severe changes such as mania or dementia are uncommon and occur late in the disease. Scanning speech (slow enunciation with a tendency to hesitate at the beginning of a word or syllable) is common in advanced disease, but aphasic symptoms are rare.

Cranial nerves: In addition to the initial optic neuritis, one or more of the following ocular signs are usually present at some time: partial atrophy of the optic nerve with temporal pallor; changes in the visual fields (central scotoma or general narrowing of the fields); transient ophthalmoplegia with diplopia (from involvement of the brainstem tracts connecting the 3rd, 4th, and 6th nerve nuclei). Choked disks are found with optic neuritis, but pupillary changes, Argyll Robertson pupils, or total blindness are rare. Nystagmus, a common finding, may be due to cerebellar or oculomotor damage.

Other evidence of cranial nerve involvement is uncommon, and when present is usually due to brainstem injury in the area of the cranial nerve nuclei. Deafness is rare, but vertigo is not. Numbness on one side of the face, or pain resembling trigeminal neuralgia, is seen occasionally.

Motor: Deep reflexes (e.g., knee and ankle jerks) are generally increased; Babinski's sign and clonus are often present. Superficial reflexes, particularly upper and lower abdominals, are diminished or absent. Often, the patient complains of unilateral symptoms but examination elicits signs of bilateral corticospinal tract involvement. Intention tremor from cerebellar lesions is common, and continued purposeful effort accentuates it. The motion is ataxic: shaky, irregular, tremulous, and ineffective. Static tremor, especially obvious when the head is unsupported, may be seen. Muscular weakness and spasticity from corticospinal damage produce a stumbling, weaving, drunken gait; later, a combination of spasticity and cerebellar ataxia may be totally disabling. The cerebral lesions may result in hemiplegia, sometimes the presenting symptom. Muscular atrophy or painful flexor spasms in response to sensory stimuli (e.g., bedclothes) may appear in late stages.

Charcot's triad—nystagmus, intention tremor, and scanning speech—is a common cerebellar manifestation in advanced disease. Mild dysarthria may result from cerebellar damage, disturbance of cortical control, or injury to the bulbar nuclei.

Sensory: Complete loss of any form of cutaneous sensation is rare, but paresthesias, numbness, and blunting of sensation such as hemianesthesia to pain or disturbances of vibratory or position sense may occur and are often localized, e.g., to the hands or legs. The objective changes are fleeting and are often elicited only with careful testing.

Autonomic: Difficulty in micturition, partial retention of urine, or slight incontinence is common with spinal cord involvement, as are sexual impotence in men and genital anesthesia in women. Bladder and rectal incontinence may occur with severe advanced involvement.

A hot bath may be useful in exposing new signs, but intensification of existing symptoms or signs is nonspecific.

The **CSF** is abnormal in over 80% of cases. Gamma globulin may be $> 13\%$, and cells (lymphocytes) and protein content may be slightly increased, but these findings are not pathognomonic. Oligoclonal bands may be found on agarose electrophoresis of the CSF of up to 90% of patients with MS, but their absence does not rule out the disease.

Course

The course is highly varied and unpredictable and in most patients, remittent. At first, months or years of remission may separate episodes, especially when the disease begins with retrobulbar neuritis, but usually the intervals of freedom grow shorter, and eventually permanent and progressive disablement occurs. Life span probably is not shortened. The average duration of illness probably exceeds 25 yr, but there is great variability. Remissions have lasted longer than 25 yr. Some patients, however, have frequent attacks and are rapidly incapacitated; in a few, particularly when onset is in middle age, the course is progressively and unremittingly downhill; and occasionally the disease is fatal within a year.

Diagnosis

MS is so likely a cause of the above symptoms and signs that the physician risks misdiagnosing a curable disorder. A firm diagnosis rarely can be made during the first attack, although it can be suspected. Later, *a history of remissions and exacerbations and clinical evidence of CNS lesions in more than one area are highly suggestive*, but the diagnosis should only be made after exclusion of all other possibilities. Small cerebral infarctions, syringomyelia, amyotrophic lateral sclerosis, syphilis, pernicious anemia, arthritis of the cervical spine, ruptured intervertebral disk, platybasia, and the hereditary ataxias must all be considered. CNS tumors, abscesses, or other mass lesions, vascular malformations of the brain or spinal cord, and anomalies of the spine or base of the skull must be ruled out by the clinical findings, skull and spinal x-rays, brain scans, and CSF examination. Particular attention should be paid to the area within the foramen magnum, since treatable lesions at the junction of the spinal cord and medulla (e.g., subarachnoid cyst, foramen magnum tumors) can also cause a highly variable and fluctuating spectrum of motor and sensory symptoms.

Treatment

There is no specific therapy. Spontaneous remissions make any treatment difficult to evaluate. However, prednisone 60 mg/day for 5 to 7 days may hasten recovery in acute attacks (e.g., retrobulbar neuritis), especially if given very early in the episode. Long-term corticosteroid therapy and immunosuppressive agents are rarely justified. Intrathecal corticosteroid therapy has no value and may cause secondary arachnoiditis.

The patient should maintain as normal and active a life as possible, but should avoid overwork and fatigue. Massage and passive movement of weakened spastic limbs make patients more comfortable. Muscle training is physically and psychologically beneficial. Encouragement and reassurance are essential; a hopeless outlook should be avoided. Invalidism may be prevented by prompt treatment and in late stages can be postponed by physiotherapy and prompt treatment of infections and urinary difficulties. Decubitus ulcer and urinary tract infections should be prevented in bedridden patients. Several drugs reduce spasticity by inhibiting the spinal cord reflexes (diazepam 15 to 30 mg/day in divided doses, baclofen 70 to 80 mg/day in divided doses). While the short-term toxicity of these agents appears to be minimal (usually lethargy), their long-term effects are largely unknown. Cautious and judicious use is required because reducing spasticity in MS patients often exacerbates weakness, thus further incapacitating the patient.

ACUTE TRANSVERSE MYELITIS

(See under DEMYELINATING CORD DISORDERS in Ch. 129)

127. EXTRAPYRAMIDAL AND CEREBELLAR DISORDERS

The **pyramidal tracts** (named for the pyramid formed where the fibers traverse the medulla) are upper motor neuron pathways that connect the motor cortex with lower motor neurons in the spinal ventral horns via the **corticospinal tracts.** The **extrapyramidal system** (so called because the pathways do not run through the medullary pyramid) is a multisynaptic complex of neurons that interconnect the basal ganglia, thalamic and subthalamic nuclei, red nucleus, and substantia nigra with one another and with parts of the reticular formation, cerebellum, and cerebrum.

The extrapyramidal system is a functional integrative unit, not a morphologic unit as is the pyramidal system. Both pyramidal and extrapyramidal systems work inseparably together in the control of movement and posture, the extrapyramidal system modulating and integrating motor impulses that originate in the cortex.

Chemical mediators (the monoamines dopamine and serotonin; acetylcholine; GABA [gamma amino butyric acid]; perhaps endorphins) play an important role in the extrapyramidal transmission of neural impulses, and much evidence indicates that the pathogenesis of extrapyramidal symptoms often has a significant chemical component.

Pyramidal disorders cause weakness plus spasticity, producing the classic "lengthening and shortening" or **"clasp-knife" phenomenon:** when an affected part is moved passively, it shows a gradual increase in resistance, then a sudden letting go. Deep tendon reflexes are increased also, and Babinski's sign is present.

Extrapyramidal disorders are characterized by involuntary movements (tremors, tics, athetosis, chorea, ballism); impairment of voluntary movement (brady-, hypo-, or akinesia); and changes in muscle tone and posture (dystonia, muscle rigidity, dysequilibrium). Muscular weakness and reflex changes are *not* prominent features.

TREMORS

Involuntary movements in one or more parts of the body produced by successive alternate contractions of opposing muscle groups. Tremors often reflect extrapyramidal or cerebellar disturbance. Transient tremors without particular significance may occur normally with hunger, chilling, physical exertion, or excitement.

Classification

In differentiating tremors, one should note their rate, rhythm, and distribution, and the effect of movement or rest. A rapid (fine) tremor oscillates 8 to 10 times/second, a slow (coarse) tremor 3 to 5 times/second. **Intention tremor** appears during, or is accentuated by, voluntary movement of the affected part and is characteristic of cerebellar disorders. **Rest (passive) tremor** is present when the involved part is more or less at rest but diminishes or disappears with active movements; it is seen in extrapyramidal disorders. **Static tremor** appears during attempts to maintain the position of the affected part without support.

Other involuntary movements may accompany metabolic disorders. **Asterixis** is an arrhythmic hand flapping evoked with the arms outstretched and the wrists dorsiflexed. **Myoclonus** is a sudden, nonrhythmic contraction of one or more muscles or part of a muscle resembling the normal leg or whole-body jerk of light sleep.

Causes of Tremor

1. Organic diseases of the CNS

Benign hereditary tremor (essential tremor): A fine to moderate tremor of the hands, head, and voice may appear during adolescence or later in successive family generations. There are no pathologic findings. Voluntary movement and emotion tend to increase the tremor; alcohol often suppresses it (and therefore may be abused).

Parkinsonism (see in this chapter): The coarse alternating tremor, with 4 to 8 movements/second in several planes, is a prominent symptom. It is most common in the fingers, often progresses to the forearm, head, eyelids, and tongue, is present during rest, and usually disappears or diminishes with movement and during sleep.

Senility: The tremor of old age may be an intention tremor similar to benign essential tremor.

Hepatolenticular degeneration (Wilson's disease; see in Ch. 79): Various types of tremor may be seen, including the coarse multiplane parkinsonian tremor of basal ganglia disease or the intention tremor of cerebellar disease. However, the characteristic (though not pathognomonic) abnormal involuntary movement is a "wing-beating" tremor with violent, rapid flapping movements of the hand or entire arm.

Paresis (dementia paralytica; see Neurosyphilis in Ch. 162): A fine rapid tremor involving the face, tongue, and hands, often increased by voluntary movement, is an early symptom. It is probably due to damage to the frontal lobe and its connections with the brainstem and cerebellum.

Multiple sclerosis (see in Ch. 126): The tremor appears during movement of a limb and disappears at rest, and is evidence of involvement of the cerebellum or its pathways. Occasionally, a static tremor of the head may be present.

Friedreich's ataxia and other heredodegenerative diseases of the cerebellum (see under SPINO-CEREBELLAR DISEASES in Vol. II, Ch. 25): The tremor in hereditary ataxias and related cerebellar disorders resembles that of multiple sclerosis.

2. Toxic states

Intoxication: Alcoholism is the most common toxic state producing a tremor. A rapid coarse tremor of the fingers, tongue, limbs, and head is often most evident in the morning before breakfast, and is abolished or diminished by an alcoholic drink. Alcoholic tremor is most severe during delirium tremens. Persons dependent on morphine and cocaine show a fine tremor of the facial muscles and fingers that is particularly pronounced on drug withdrawal. Tremor is frequently a prominent symptom in poisoning. Chronic mercurial poisoning causes a coarse, fairly slow tremor of the muscles of the face and extremities, usually more marked during movement.

Metabolic encephalopathy: Asterixis is common in hepatic failure but can also occur in uremia and respiratory acidosis. Myoclonus is also seen in metabolic encephalopathies.

3. Endocrinopathy: The tremor of **hyperthyroidism** is fine, regular, and rapid, and usually confined to the outstretched fingers and hands.

4. Tremors associated with functional disease may simulate those of organic CNS disease and make diagnosis difficult. Psychiatric evaluation is helpful. Tremor is a fairly common symptom in both **chronic** and **acute anxiety states.** In the former it resembles that of hyperthyroidism; in the latter, it is coarser and more irregular. **Hysterical neuroses** may cause constant or paroxysmal tremor that may be generalized or limited to an extremity. Frequently fine and rapid, the tremor may also be a coarse irregular shaking intensified by emotion and voluntary movement.

Treatment

Hereditary tremor may be diminished or controlled by sedatives such as phenobarbital 15 to 30 mg or diazepam 2 to 10 mg (if not too sedating), either drug orally t.i.d. or q.i.d. Propranolol 120 to 240 mg/day orally relieves many patients. The tremor of parkinsonism or other basal ganglia disease is decreased by atropine-like drugs and levodopa. The intention tremor of multiple sclerosis and cerebellar disease is not modified by drugs, but muscular reeducation enables patients to move the affected extremity with less tremor—in the arm, for example, by performing movements with the arm held adducted on the chest if possible. Neurosurgically induced lesions in the ventral thalamus may help severely affected patients. Tremors of hyperthyroidism are alleviated by treatment of the disease and may be diminished by reserpine 0.1 to 0.25 mg orally once or twice/day or propranolol 60 to 240 mg/day in divided doses. In other conditions, therapy of tremor is also that of the underlying disease. Thus, the tremor of paresis improves with penicillin therapy. The tremors due to toxins improve with removal of the toxin and general supportive measures; diet and vitamin therapy are also essential in alcoholism. Psychotherapy is recommended in anxiety or hysterical states.

BALLISM; HEMIBALLISM

Violent, flinging limb movements caused by injury in the area of the subthalamic nucleus, usually a small infarct. **Ballism** is bilateral; **hemiballism** is confined to the side contralateral to the injury. The head is sometimes also affected. The repeated violent movements incapacitate and may exhaust the patient. They usually wane after 6 to 8 wk. In **diagnosis,** chorea, drug-induced dyskinesia, and focal seizures must be excluded.

Treatment

Several months of oral therapy with chlorpromazine 50 to 200 mg/day or haloperidol 2 to 10 mg/day suppresses the ballistic movements and speeds the return to normal function. Higher doses are occasionally required.

PARKINSONISM

(Parkinson's Disease; Paralysis Agitans; Shaking Palsy)

A chronic, progressive CNS disorder characterized by slowness and poverty of purposeful movement, muscular rigidity, and tremor.

Parkinson's disease itself is idiopathic, but symptoms resembling parkinsonism may also result from various causes. Drug-induced parkinsonian symptoms caused by the phenothiazines, haloperidol, and reserpine are discussed under Tranquilizers in Ch. 247. Carbon monoxide or manganese poisoning, bilateral infarcts of the basal ganglia, hydrocephalus, tumors near the basal ganglia, and cerebral trauma can also cause the syndrome. Postencephalitic parkinsonism, now rare, commonly followed the 1919–1924 pandemic of encephalitis lethargica.

In idiopathic parkinsonism, there is usually a loss of cells in the substantia nigra, locus ceruleus, and other pigmented neurons, and a decrease of dopamine content in axon terminals of cells projecting from the substantia nigra to the caudate nucleus and putamen. The same cells were involved in encephalitis lethargica.

Symptoms and Signs

Parkinson's disease occurs in the middle-aged and elderly. It is slowly progressive but may not be incapacitating for many years. Onset is insidious, and often begins with tremor in one hand, followed by increasing bradykinesia and rigidity. With full-blown disease, the patient's appearance is characteristic. The facial expression is fixed, with muscles smoothed out and almost immobile; the eyes are unblinking and staring, and the mouth is slightly open, frequently with drooling from the corners. The facial skin is often greasy, with seborrheic scaling. Posture is typically stooped. The characteristic tremor affects the hand most severely, producing the "pill-rolling" movement of fingers and thumb, accompanied by wrist flexion and extension. A passive (rest) tremor, it is relatively slow (4 to 8 seconds), is aggravated by emotional tension (e.g., embarrassment) and fatigue, diminishes or may disappear with voluntary movement, and disappears during sleep. It may remain in one arm or may spread gradually to the other extremities and ultimately to the jaw and neck.

Hypertonia produces a muscular rigidity that involves opposing muscle groups equally and throughout the range of motion, so that, for example, when the elbow is moved passively, the arm typically responds with a series of ratchet-like catches (**"cogwheel rigidity"**) or with a uniform resistance (**"lead-pipe rigidity"**).

All voluntary movements, particularly those carried out by the small muscles, are notably slowed (**bradykinesia**), and spontaneous movement is diminished (**akinesia**). The patient finds it hard to start walking, and may begin with small, hesitant steps and then break into a run in order to prevent falling forward (**festination**). Once in motion, he walks with slow, shuffling steps, the arms flexed, adducted, and unswinging, the trunk bent slightly forward. Walking may stop, with the patient "frozen" and unable to set himself in motion again. When pushed, he may pitch forward or backward (**propulsion** or **retropulsion**). Because of the hypokinesia, micrographia is common, and speech may become almost unintelligible because of its soft pitch and slow cadence, sometimes interrupted by rapid jumbled sounds analogous to the festinating gait.

Rigidity and secondary joint changes often cause cramplike pains in the limbs and spine. Muscle strength may be diminished. Sensation is intact, and reflexes are normal unless muscular rigidity interferes.

Oculogyric crises (prolonged fixation of the eyeballs in one position), bizarre tics, and torticollis are seen in the postencephalitic form; these and other dystonic or choreiform movements may also occur with phenothiazines.

As many as half the patients suffer mild dementia, which becomes severe in a few. Depression is even more common, and may make physical and mental functions difficult to assess.

Diagnosis

Diagnosis is usually easy once the clinical picture is characteristic, but may be difficult in the early stages. Clues are the lack of facial expression, infrequent blinking, the shuffling gait, the hand tremor with associated impairment of rapid finger movements, and the hypertonic muscle resistance to passive movement.

Other forms of tremor must be excluded (see TREMORS, above). Involutional depression and cerebral arteriosclerosis must be differentiated. Intracranial tumors may cause similar hypokinesia, but rarely cause the characteristic alternating tremor and cogwheel rigidity. Wilson's disease, the rigid form of Huntington's chorea, and Farr's disease (calcification of the basal ganglia) should be considered whenever parkinsonian symptoms appear before age 30. Phenothiazine use or toxic exposure must be excluded.

Treatment

Levodopa, the atropine-like or anticholinergic drugs, and amantadine all provide symptomatic treatment but are not curative.

Levodopa (L-dopa), the metabolic precursor of dopamine, is used for replacement therapy since dopamine itself does not cross the blood-brain barrier. Its greatest effect is on bradykinesic symptoms. Early cases respond most favorably; however, bedridden patients may become ambulatory. Levodopa must be given in large doses because much of the drug is metabolized before it reaches its site of action in the brain. It is therefore often given in combination with **carbidopa,** a dopa decarboxylase inhibitor that prevents the systemic metabolism of levodopa until it reaches the brain. The initial dose is carbidopa/levodopa 10/100 mg t.i.d. after meals, with 10/100-mg increments every 4 to 7 (or more) days, depending on toleration. Carbidopa/levodopa must be given in divided doses, with or after meals. The maintenance dose is determined by the response and the bothersome side effects, which are kept to a minimum by increasing and adjusting the dose gradually and carefully. Most patients require 40 to 80/400 to 800 mg/day; some less, some as much as 200/2000 mg/day. Patients who need only 200 to 400 mg of levodopa/day may experience nausea with the 10/100-mg carbidopa/levodopa tablet but not with a 25/100-mg tablet.

When levodopa is used alone, early side effects include anorexia, nausea and vomiting, and orthostatic hypotension. These disappear when carbidopa is used with levodopa. Dystonic, choreiform, or oral-facial movements **(dyskinesias)** may appear with large doses or even with the standard dose after several months to 2 yr of treatment. They are dose-related, and the threshold dose for their occurrence gradually decreases as treatment continues. A desirable mood elevation often occurs with levodopa. Mania, depression, and toxic delirium may rarely be seen, especially in patients with preexisting mental problems, but usually subside with a reduction in dosage. Impairment of postural reflexes and rapid, unpredictable, marked changes in motility (the "on-off effect") are complications of prolonged levodopa therapy in longstanding parkinsonism. Their frequency can be somewhat decreased by keeping the dose of levodopa as low as possible and by giving the medication in small amounts q 1 to 3 h throughout the day.

Drugs that may interfere with the therapeutic action of levodopa include pyridoxine, reserpine, phenothiazines, butyrophenones, thioxanthenes, and probably papaverine and related isoquinolines.

Amantadine is presumed to release dopamine from basal ganglia neurons; it acts synergistically with levodopa. Doses of 200 to 300 mg/day orally are moderately effective in some patients, either alone or in combination with levodopa. Pedal edema, livedo reticularis, and confusion are the chief side effects.

Some physicians prefer to use **atropine-like drugs (anticholinergics)** in advance of levodopa or as a supplement to it in order to keep the levodopa dosage as low as possible. The anticholinergics are given in a small initial dose, increasing until improvement is maximal or untoward effects prevent further increases. For example, trihexyphenidyl 1 mg/day orally is given for a few days, then increased by 1- to 2-mg increments every 7 to 14 days until the optimum dosage (usually 4 to 10 mg/day in divided doses) is determined. Adverse effects due to excess amounts include urinary retention, constipation, delirium, dry mouth, and impaired temperature regulation due to decreased sweating. Antihistamines, commonly diphenhydramine 25 to 100 mg/day orally, can be given to ameliorate parkinsonism through their mild anticholinergic effect and as safe, mild sedatives.

Some **ergot dervatives** (e.g., **bromocriptine**) mimic the effect of dopamine at its receptor and have an antiparkinsonian effect, especially in combination with carbidopa/levodopa. Excess bromocriptine causes nausea, dyskinesia, or toxic delirium.

Most patients with mild parkinsonism are treated initially with atropine-like drugs or amantadine, alone or in combination. If functional disability remains significant despite use of these drugs, levodopa and a dopa decarboxylase inhibitor should be tried (see above) before the illness becomes advanced or severe. Common practice is to continue former medication at regular dosage when levodopa is started. The other drugs may be reduced as levodopa becomes effective. Continuing one or more of them may be beneficial, especially for tremor.

A tricyclic antidepressant (see Ch. 139 and ANTIDEPRESSANTS in Ch. 247) may help depression; monoamine oxidase inhibitors **must not be given with levodopa.**

Cryosurgical destruction of various thalamic nuclei alleviates tremor and rigidity contralaterally, but bradykinesia is not benefited. Since both sides are usually involved and bilateral cryosurgery may cause dementia, mutism, and postural difficulties, most patients are now treated with levodopa.

PROGRESSIVE SUPRANUCLEAR PALSY
(Steele-Richardson-Olszewski Syndrome)

A rare disorder of middle age characterized by progressive external ophthalmoplegia beginning in the vertical plane, parkinsonian-like facies and bradykinesia, spastic-ataxic gait disturbances, progressive neck and trunk rigidity, and **pseudobulbar palsy** *(dysphagia, dysarthria, inappropriate emotion, and intact bulbar reflexes).* Dementia is common. Pathologic examination shows neuronal deterioration in the cerebral cortex and basal ganglia. Patients are usually men. The cause is unknown. The poor voluntary control of vertical gaze, of oral-pharyngeal movement, and of affect is indicative of damage to corticobulbar regulatory centers bilaterally rather than to bulbar structures themselves (hence, "pseudobulbar"). A similar pseudobulbar disorder that may follow multiple small strokes ("**lacunar state**") is differentiated by the history of a stepwise progression of deficits characteristic of strokes.

There is no satisfactory **treatment,** although the extrapyramidal symptoms occasionally improve somewhat with levodopa.

SHY-DRAGER SYNDROME
(See in Orthostatic Hypotension in Ch. 24)

WILSON'S DISEASE
(See Ch. 79)

HUNTINGTON'S CHOREA
(Chronic Progressive, Hereditary, or Degenerative Chorea)

A hereditary disease beginning in adulthood, characterized by choreic movements and mental deterioration.

The disease is transmitted as an autosomal dominant trait. Pathologic findings include gross atrophy of the corpus striatum, with neuronal degeneration in the caudate and other deep nuclei and in the frontal cerebral cortex.

Symptoms and Signs

Onset is insidious; symptoms usually begin between ages 30 and 50. Personality changes (obstinacy, moodiness, lack of interest) and inappropriate behavior may antedate or accompany the involuntary jerky, irregular choreic movements. These usually appear first in the arms, neck, and face, and progress from mild fidgeting to facial grimaces, hesitant speech, torticollis, and irregular trunk movements. The gait is wide-based and prancing. Some patients become euphoric; others, irascible and violent. Paranoia is common. As the disease progresses, walking becomes impossible, swallowing difficult, and dementia profound. A subtype of Huntington's disease has been described, which begins during childhood and causes rigidity and bradykinesia that evolves into chorea.

Tragically, although 1/2 the children of an affected parent are at risk of developing and transmitting the disease, their fate may be unknown until they are well into childbearing age. A provocative levodopa test to detect carriers is of unknown reliability. Therefore, all potential carriers should be urged not to have children. Those who escape the disease themselves do not transmit the trait.

Treatment

The chorea responds to piperazine phenothiazines such as perphenazine (up to 20 mg/day) or fluphenazine (2.5 to 10 mg/day), and to haloperidol (0.5 to 12 mg/day). There is no treatment for the mental decline.

OTHER CHOREIC DISORDERS

SYDENHAM'S CHOREA (See Bacterial Infections in Vol. II, Ch. 24)

CHOREA GRAVIDARUM

Choreiform movements developing during pregnancy. Usually occurring in the first pregnancy and during the first trimester, the disorder is similar to Sydenham's chorea, but not necessarily associated with rheumatic fever. Recurrence in subsequent pregnancies does not indicate progressive disease. **Treatment** is tempered by concern for the developing fetus. Sedation with barbiturates is safest.

A similar disorder can occur in women taking oral contraceptives and is treated by discontinuing the drugs.

TICS

(Habit Spasms)

Brief, repetitive, purposeless, semivoluntary or involuntary contractions of a muscle or functional group of muscles, often of the face, shoulder, or arm. A typical "nervous tic" is a twitching of the corner of the eye or the mouth. Tics typically start around age 6 and regress as the child matures. However, they may persist into adulthood. Tics may at first be voluntarily controlled, but persistent tics become automatic.

Tics associated with encephalitis are presumed to be extrapyramidal in origin. The pathophysiologic basis of ordinary tics is not known. Since they often accompany tension or emotional upset, they are usually attributed to psychologic mechanisms, but even hereditary tremor and established organic disorders such as parkinsonism are known to be worsened by emotional stress.

Gilles de la Tourette's syndrome begins in childhood with single or multiple tics (facial blinking, grimaces, shoulder shrugging, arm movements) which may gradually worsen in extent and severity. Vocal tics such as grunting, sniffing, shouting, and barking noises develop, and, in about half the patients, coprolalia or compulsive swearing occur. Mentation remains normal. Symptoms wax and wane throughout adult life. In contrast with most movement disorders, Tourette tics are suppressed in group settings, and expressed when the patient is alone. Various psychologic mechanisms have been postulated but not substantiated. The dramatic response to haloperidol, a dopamine antagonist, suggests an organic basis. A high frequency of single or multiple tics has been found in relatives of patients with Tourette's syndrome, but there is no clearcut genetic pattern.

Diagnosis

A tic syndrome in a child must be differentiated from Sydenham's chorea, Wilson's disease, and a mass lesion of the cerebellum or basal ganglia. Gilles de la Tourette's syndrome is a clinical diagnosis and can be made with assurance only as the typical course unfolds.

Treatment

Mild childhood or adult tics may respond to phenobarbital, chlordiazepoxide, or diazepam. Gilles de la Tourette's syndrome responds best to haloperidol, starting with 0.5 mg/day orally and gradually increasing by 0.5- to 1-mg increments until the tics are controlled (often requiring 3 to 10 mg/day). Adverse effects (akathisia, parkinsonism, depression) are titrated against tic suppression with the goal of controlling most (not necessarily all) tics at the lowest possible dose. The concomitant use of an anticholinergic such as benztropine 1 to 3 mg/day may limit the adverse effects of haloperidol. Psychotherapy is clearly ineffective as a treatment for the syndrome but may be indicated for secondary emotional problems.

DISORDERS OF THE CEREBELLUM

The cerebellum is an integration center for the control of posture and voluntary movement. It consists of a phylogenetically old midline portion (vermis and flocculonodular lobe) and 2 phylogenetically recent lateral hemispheres. The cerebellum receives input from the many afferent systems concerned with proprioception and movement (muscle spindles, vestibular nuclei, sensory and motor cortex, visual and auditory systems, skin) and projects to efferent motor-coordinating pathways (extrapyramidal system, vestibular nuclei, and cerebral cortex).

The flocculonodular lobes play an important role in the maintenance of equilibrium; the anterior lobe of the hemispheres, in maintaining posture; and the posterior lobe, in adjustments and precision of voluntary movements. Further, some somatotopic mapping has been established: the midline cerebellum is responsible for trunk and lower extremity coordination; the hemispheres are concerned mainly with limb coordination. Thus, childhood medulloblastomas, which involve the cerebellar vermis, characteristically affect the trunk and legs, while lesions in the lateral cerebellar hemispheres (e.g., childhood cerebellar astrocytoma or other tumors, infarcts, the demyelinating plaques of multiple sclerosis) affect the ipsilateral limbs.

The signs of cerebellar disease are (1) ataxia (clumsy, wide-based gait); (2) dysmetria (difficulty in controlling the range of voluntary movement, usually with an overshooting of the intended goal [hypermetria]); (3) intention tremor; (4) dysdiadochokinesia (clumsy, rapid, alternating movements); and (5) hypotonia. Nystagmus often occurs with cerebellar disorders because of associated vestibular involvement; the fast component is maximal toward the side of the lesion. Dysarthria with inappropriate accenting of syllables (scanning speech) is also found.

Cerebellar dysfunction is a component of a number of neurologic disorders. Multiple sclerosis and infarctions are discussed elsewhere in this section. The hereditary spinocerebellar ataxias are discussed in Vol. II, Ch. 25. Other possible causes include the Arnold-Chiari malformation, severe hyperpyrexia, toxic agents (heavy metals, carbon monoxide, phenytoin), repeated head trauma (as in boxing), and hypothyroidism.

ALCOHOLIC–NUTRITIONAL CEREBELLAR DEGENERATION

(Parenchymatous Cerebellar or Cerebellar Cortical Degeneration)

Sudden, severe lower extremity incoordination and imbalance occurring in "binge" drinkers or in persons with severe nutritional deprivation. Necrosis of the anterior superior cerebellar vermis is found pathologically.

Symptoms, Signs, and Diagnosis

Typically, the patient has been on an alcoholic binge and awakens to find that he cannot walk. Less often, symptoms follow nutritional depletion (e.g., from pellagra or a GI disorder). Examination shows severe lower-extremity dysmetria and hypotonia, but intact strength. The stance is wide-based with severe parkinson-like retropulsion and an extensor posture of the legs. Gait is extremely ataxic, if walking is possible.

The condition must be differentiated from cerebellar neoplasms, multiple sclerosis, proprioceptive deficits due to peripheral neuropathy, and bilateral vestibular impairment.

Prognosis and Treatment

Adequate nutrition, abstinence from alcohol, and physical therapy are the only treatment available. Recovery is poor, and several bouts may lead to a step-wise deterioration of gait.

---

128.   CRANIOCERVICAL ABNORMALITIES

Disorders occurring at the juncture of cord and medulla within the foramen magnum, where the neural structures and the vascular supply are multiple and complex. The cervical cord is flexible and therefore liable to intermittent compression. In consequence, several types of lesions at this level can cause symptoms that vary considerably from patient to patient and that may come and go.

Symptoms and Signs

Axons of upper motor neurons in the decussation of the pyramids may be affected, often causing weakness, spasticity, and hyperactive reflexes in one upper and both lower extremities. Lower motor neuron involvement may cause muscular atrophy and weakness in the arms and hands. Involvement of sensory fibers may cause occipital and neck pain; diminished touch, vibration, or position sensation in the limbs may occur, singly or in combination, and may be bilateral, ipsilateral, or contralateral, or even ipsilateral at one level and contralateral at another. A tingling down the back on neck flexion **(Lhermitte's sign)** may occur. Involvement of the median longitudinal fasciculi in the cervical cord may cause nystagmus or an internuclear ophthalmoplegia with horizontal nystagmus on lateral gaze that is maximal in the eye closest to the object of gaze. Downbeat nystagmus (fast component downward) is characteristic of craniocervical junction lesions.

Diagnosis

It is important to identify a treatable cause. The cause is difficult to determine clinically, since the spectrum of variable and intermittent medullary or cervical symptoms can occur with multiple sclerosis, a vascular disorder, a syrinx, subluxation due to RA, a foramen magnum tumor such as a meningioma or chordoma, or another mass lesion. Congenital anomalies of the craniocervical junction may cause symptoms in adulthood and are associated with basilar invagination, which should be sought on plain x-rays of the skull and cervical spine. Vertebral angiography or CT scanning may disclose cerebellar tonsils within the cervical canal in the **Arnold-Chiari malformation.** Myelography with spilling of contrast medium over the rim of the foramen magnum into the cisterna magna and onto the clivus, with the patient both supine and prone, is necessary to rule out a mass lesion in this region.

---

129.   SPINAL CORD DISORDERS

The spinal cord extends caudally from the medulla at the foramen magnum to terminate at the upper lumbar vertebrae. In the **white matter** at the periphery are the ascending and descending tracts of myelinated sensory and motor nerve fibers. The **central H-shaped gray matter** is composed of cell bodies and nonmyelinated fibers. The **anterior (ventral) horns of the H** contain lower motor neuron cells that receive their impulses from the motor cortex via the descending corticospinal tracts; the axons of the anterior horn cells become the efferent fibers of the spinal nerves. The **posterior (dorsal) horns** contain afferent sensory nerve fibers whose cell bodies lie in the dorsal root ganglia. The **gray matter of the cord** also contains many internuncial neurons that carry motor, sensory, or reflex impulses from dorsal to ventral nerve roots, from one side of the cord to the other, and from one level of the cord to another.

The **segments of the cord** are conceptual, not actual, divisions, and correspond approximately to the attachments of the 31 pairs of spinal nerves. In spinal cord disorders, the integrity of individual segments is assessed clinically by examining the reflexes and the sensory and motor responses in the distribution of the segments (see SPINAL CORD INJURY, Symptoms and Signs, in Ch. 123).

SPINAL CORD COMPRESSION

Many diseases affect the spinal cord by mechanical compression, which often presents in a stereotyped fashion and can be treated effectively if caught early.

Acute spinal cord compression usually is traumatic, presenting as flaccid paraplegia or quadriplegia ("spinal shock"— see SPINAL CORD INJURY in Ch. 123).

Subacute cord compression is usually caused by an extramedullary neoplasm (see also SPINAL CORD NEOPLASMS in Ch. 125) or an epidural abscess or hematoma (see below). It is announced by local back pain, with or without a radicular distribution. Reflex changes from corticospinal tract dysfunction (hyper-reflexia, Babinski signs) follow, then weakness (often proximal) of the lower extremities, sensory loss, and loss of sphincter control. The phase of back pain and mild weakness may last hours to days, but the transition to total loss of function caudal to the lesion may take only minutes. Therefore, it is essential to suspect, diagnose, and treat cord compression promptly.

Chronic spinal cord compression is a consequence of bony or cartilaginous protrusions into the spinal canal (e.g., from osteophytes, spondylosis, or a herniated nucleus pulposus; these are discussed in Ch. 130) or of slow-growing extramedullary neoplasms (neurofibroma, meningioma—see SPINAL CORD NEOPLASMS in Ch. 125). It follows the course outlined for subacute compression except that pain may be dull, both motor and sensory abnormalities may evolve at the same time, and spasticity is found in the lower limbs.

Diagnosis is based on the clinical signs—spine tenderness, paraparesis, sensory deficits of the legs and trunk, and corticospinal reflex changes. Spine x-rays may disclose erosion, collapse, fracture, or subluxation at the level of the lesion. A myelogram is necessary to confirm compression of the cord and to fully define the level of the lesion.

Treatment depends on the underlying illness. Management of acute injuries and of conditions causing chronic compression is discussed in the chapters referred to above.

The need for prompt intervention in subacute compression cannot be overemphasized. Many patients, if treated before weakness becomes marked, recover full neurologic function, whereas few do well once paraplegia or autonomic deficits have occurred. Corticosteroids (dexamethasone 100 mg/day for 3 days) are given promptly. If the tissue type of a compressing metastatic neoplasm is known, immediate radiation therapy is as effective as rapid surgical decompression. Immediate surgery is performed if a tissue diagnosis is needed or for epidural hematoma or abscess. Patients having surgery for epidural metastases should receive radiotherapy, starting 5 days postoperation.

SPINAL EPIDURAL ABSCESS AND HEMATOMA

The epidural space in the spinal column is much more easily expanded by a lesion than is the cranial epidural space, typically by an abscess or a hematoma. Spinal epidural **abscess** usually occurs in a patient with an underlying infection, either remote (e.g., a furuncle or dental abscess) or contiguous (e.g., vertebral osteomyelitis, decubitus ulcer, or retroperitoneal abscess). *Staphylococcus aureus* is the commonest causative organism, followed by *Escherichia coli* and mixed anaerobes. Spinal epidural **hematoma** may result from back trauma or may occur during anticoagulant therapy.

Either condition begins with local back pain and tenderness, usually thoracic or lumbar, which is often severe and may radiate in a root distribution. Weakness in a paraplegic or root pattern progresses over hours to days with abscess, but within minutes to several hours with hematoma. Whether sensory or sphincter deficits occur depends on the site and size of the lesion. With an abscess, patients are usually febrile and the CSF has a high protein content and a lymphocytic pleocytosis; x-rays of the spine show osteomyelitic findings in about 1/3 of cases.

Both conditions are **diagnosed** and localized with myelography. If the lumbar epidural space is the suspected site, it is preferable to instill the contrast medium into the subarachnoid space via a cisternal needle puncture to avoid traversing the abscess or hematoma.

Treatment of epidural abscess or hematoma is by prompt surgical decompression and removal. In suspected abscess, cultures of blood and of focal infections should be obtained before surgery, and treatment should be started with a penicillinase-resistant penicillin. Any pus found at operation should be gram-stained and cultured. Patients with suspected hematoma who are taking coumarin anticoagulants should be given vitamin K_1 2.5 to 10 mg s.c.

SYRINGOMYELIA; SYRINGOBULBIA

A fluid-filled neuroglial cavity (syrinx) within the substance of the spinal cord (syringomyelia) or brainstem (syringobulbia). It is a congenital lesion, but for unknown reasons often expands during the teens or young adult years. Usually irregular and longitudinal, the **spinal syrinx** is paramedian and commonly begins in the cervical area, but may extend across or virtually the length of the spinal cord. It may be associated with an additional congenital anomaly such as the Arnold-Chiari malformation (in which cerebellar tissue extends into the spinal canal) or dysraphic syndromes (e.g., encephalocele, myelomeningocele). About 30% of spinal cord tumors have an associated syrinx. **Syringobulbia** usually occurs as a slitlike gap within the lower brainstem that may affect the lower cranial nerves or ascending sensory or descending motor pathways by disruption or compression.

Symptoms and Signs

The **syrinx,** being paramedian, first interrupts fibers crossing from one side of the spinal cord to the other. Since these are predominantly pain and temperature fibers, and usually cervical, the patient may first notice a lack of sensation for noxious stimuli in his fingers (e.g., a painless burn or cut). Other sensory losses follow. A capelike sensory defect over the shoulders and back is common. Impairment of corticospinal tracts leads to spasticity and weakness of the lower extremities. Anterior horn cells may be involved at the level of the syrinx, causing segmental muscular atrophy and fasciculations. **Syringobulbia** may cause vertigo, nystagmus, uni- or bilateral facial sensory impairment, lingual atrophy, dysarthria, dysphagia, and, at times, more distal sensory or motor dysfunction due to medullary compression.

Diagnosis

Syringomyelia must be distinguished from neoplasms and vascular malformations, and an associated parenchymal cord neoplasm must always be sought. The diagnosis is aided by air myelography, which demonstrates expansion and collapse of the cord at the level of the syrinx as the patient changes position. Surgical exploration may be necessary to confirm the diagnosis and to rule out an associated neoplasm.

Treatment

Surgical drainage of the syrinx, plugging of the obex in the 4th ventricle, or section of the spinal cord (and central canal) at the filum terminale have been advocated by some, but benefits are hard to appraise since the course of symptoms and signs in syringomyelia is variable. Radiation therapy has proved useless.

DEMYELINATING CORD DISORDERS

MULTIPLE SCLEROSIS (See in Ch. 126)

ACUTE TRANSVERSE MYELITIS

Inflammation affecting both gray and white matter in one or several adjacent cord segments, causing sudden local back pain followed by symptoms of spinal cord transection that develop over a few hours. Some cases are associated with acute encephalomyelitis, syphilis, viral infections, or demyelinating disease elsewhere in the nervous system, particularly optic neuromyelitis or multiple sclerosis, but usually no cause is found. The deficit is usually severe, with global sensorimotor paraplegia below the level of the lesion, urinary retention, and loss of bowel control. The thoracic area is most often involved, so that abdominal paralysis also occurs. Eventual improvement is only slight, except in cases caused by viral encephalomyelitis or an acute inflammatory edema.

Diagnosis

The condition must be differentiated from anterior spinal artery occlusion and acute cord compression, particularly from an epidural abscess. The CSF may show mononuclear leukocytes and a slightly increased protein content. Myelography may demonstrate swelling of the cord, sometimes even producing a subarachnoid block at the level of the lesion.

Treatment

Corticosteroids (e.g., dexamethasone 100 mg IV initially; then 16 mg IV q 6 h) may be given to decrease inflammation, although the effectiveness is uncertain. Surgical decompression may be indicated if a mass lesion cannot be excluded as the cause.

VASCULAR DISORDERS

The vascular supply of the spinal cord originates superiorly from the vertebral arteries, and in the low thoracic area from a branch of the aorta. Branches of the anterior spinal artery supply the anterior 2/3 of the cord, and branches of the posterior spinal artery supply the posterior 1/3.

INFARCTION

Because the spinal circulation is supplied by 2 or 3 major arterial branches, the cord is especially vulnerable to infarction—with resultant softening **(myelomalacia)**—in the "watershed" area between the connection of these branches, around the 2nd to 4th thoracic segments. Infarction is uncommon, however, and is more often due to vascular compression (from tumors, acute disk compression) or to remote causes (e.g., surgery, dissecting aneurysm) than to intrinsic disease of the spinal arteries.

Symptoms and Signs

Sudden pain in the back and in the distribution of the affected segment is followed by bilateral flaccid weakness and impaired pinprick and temperature sensation below the level of the infarct. The distribution of the anterior spinal artery is usually involved, so that touch, proprioception, and vibration sense are likely to be spared since they are conducted in posterior tracts of the cord. As with all infarcts, the deficit is most marked during the first few days and may partially resolve with time.

Diagnosis and Treatment

Transverse myelitis, cord compression by a tumor or other mass, and demyelinating disease cause similar findings and must be excluded. Treatment is symptomatic, with frequent turning and skin care (see Ch. 199), attention to pulmonary toilet, and physical and occupational therapy. If urinary bladder function is compromised, intermittent catheterization with rigorous attention to antisepsis is preferable to an indwelling catheter (see also Neurogenic Bladder in Ch. 156).

ARTERIOVENOUS (A-V) MALFORMATIONS

Large, tortuous veins predominate in A-V malformations of the cord. The malformations may be small and localized or may involve up to $1/2$ the cord. They may, like a mass lesion, compress or even replace normal parenchymal tissue; or may rupture, causing a focal or generalized hemorrhage. The most common location is on the posterior aspect of the cord at the thoracic level. A cutaneous angioma sometimes overlies the spinal one.

Symptoms, Signs, and Diagnosis

Hemorrhage can provoke sudden pain in the area and loss of neurologic function below the level of the hemorrhage; fever and nuchal rigidity may result from blood in the subarachnoid space. Malformations that compress or infiltrate the cord present much like a spinal cord tumor; syringomyelia, demyelinating disease, and infections produce similar symptoms. Diagnosis is suggested by a "bag of worms" appearance on myelogram (with the needle removed and the patient supine), and confirmed by selective arteriography, injecting thoracic branches of the aorta until the branch that feeds the malformation is found.

Treatment

Surgery, using specialized microtechnics, is indicated if spinal cord function is threatened, but special experience is required. Occlusion of feeder arteries by embolization through an arterial catheter is practiced in a few large medical centers.

COMBINED SYSTEM DISEASE

(Subacute Combined Degeneration of the Spinal Cord)

The neurologic manifestations of pernicious anemia. The hematologic and GI features are discussed in Anemia Due to Vitamin B_{12} Deficiency in Ch. 92.

Pathology

The descriptive names (above), which antedate discovery of vitamin B_{12} deficiency as the cause, refer to the degenerative changes seen in the posterior columns and corticospinal tracts. These changes, which are also seen in the cerebral white matter and peripheral nerves, involve both axons and myelin sheaths; the peripheral nerve abnormality usually precedes the spinal cord changes. There may be degeneration of cortical neurons as well, but neuronal changes are minor in comparison to those in myelinated tracts. Occasionally, the optic nerves are also involved.

Symptoms and Signs

The neurologic symptoms occasionally precede the hematologic abnormalities. Onset is gradual, with peripheral pins-and-needles paresthesias and weakness, progressing to leg stiffness, unsteadiness due to proprioceptive difficulties, lethargy, and fatigue. Delirium or confusion, spastic ataxia, and at times postural hypotension are seen in advanced cases.

Examination in the early stages shows peripheral loss of position and vibration sense in the extremities, accompanied by mild to moderate weakness and reflex loss. Later in the course, spasticity, Babinski responses, more severe loss of proprioceptive and vibratory sensations in the lower extremities, and ataxia emerge. Tactile sensation may be impaired, but involvement of pain and temperature sensations usually is minor. The upper extremities are involved later and less consistently.

Diagnosis and Treatment

These are described in Ch. 92. The condition must be differentiated from compressive cord lesions and multiple sclerosis, as well as from other anemias. Early diagnosis is important, since the neurologic defects become irreversible if allowed to persist for months or years. CAUTION: Folic acid therapy without vitamin B_{12} corrects the hematologic abnormalities, but can aggravate the neurologic manifestations; therefore, it is *contraindicated*.

TABES DORSALIS

(See SYPHILIS in Ch. 162)

130. PERIPHERAL NERVE DISORDERS

The peripheral nervous system comprises the cranial and spinal nerves from their point of exit from the CNS to their terminations in peripheral structures. By convention, the olfactory and optic nerves, though not true nerves but CNS tracts, are also included.

The **cranial nerves** (except for the olfactory, optic, and a part of the spinal accessory) leave the CNS from the brainstem. Their motor nuclei lie deep within the brainstem; their sensory nuclei in ganglia just ouside it. The 31 pairs of **spinal nerves** each emerge from a segment of the spinal cord as an anterior (ventral) motor root and a posterior (dorsal) sensory root. The efferent motor fibers originate as anterior horn cells in the gray matter of the cord; the afferent sensory fibers originate in dorsal root ganglia. The ventral and dorsal roots combine to form the nerve, which exits via an intervertebral foramen. Because the cord is shorter than the spine, the foramina lie progressively farther from the original cord segment, so that in the lumbosacral region the nerve roots from the lower cord segments descend within the spinal column in a near-vertical sheaf (the **cauda equina**).

The spinal nerves anastomose peripherally into the cervical, brachial, and lumbosacral **plexuses** (the intercostal nerves remaining segmental), and then branch into the nerve trunks that terminate (as much as 3 ft distant) in peripheral structures. By convention, the term "**peripheral nerve**" is often used to connote this portion of a spinal nerve, lying peripheral to the roots and plexuses.

The peripheral nerves are bundles of nerve fibers that range in diameter from 0.5 to 22 μm. The larger fibers convey motor or touch and proprioceptive impulses; the smaller fibers convey pain and autonomic impulses. The supporting satellite **Schwann cells** envelop each nerve fiber in a thin cytoplasmic tube, covered by the **neurilemma (sheath of Schwann)**. Within the neurilemma, the Schwann cells further wrap the larger fibers in a multilayered insulating membrane, the **myelin sheath,** which enhances conduction of neural impulses, so that large fibers tend to be fast conductors, and small fibers, slow conductors.

Peripheral nerve dysfunction may result from damage to the nerve fibers, cell body, or myelin sheath. When ischemic or traumatic injury stops the flow of axoplasm down the nerve fiber, the nerve process dies distally **(Wallerian degeneration)**. When metabolic injury to the cell body alters the axoplasmic nutrients, the most distal part of the cell process is affected first, and axonal degeneration ascends proximally, producing the distal-to-central pattern of symptoms characteristic of the metabolic neuropathies. Injury to the myelin sheath, either directly or from Schwann cell or neuronal damage, results in **demyelination** with a consequent slowing of nerve conduction. Each Schwann cell maintains the myelin sheath along one segment of the nerve fiber, so that selective Schwann cell damage results in **segmental demyelination**, a pathologic finding characteristic of many neuropathies.

After a crush injury, nerve fiber regrowth proceeds within the Schwann cell tube at about 1 mm/day. Regrowth may be misdirected, causing **aberrant innervation** (e.g., of fibers in the wrong muscle; of a touch receptor at the wrong site; of a temperature instead of a touch receptor). The myelin sheath can regenerate rapidly, especially after segmental demyelination, with complete recovery of function unless axonal destruction has also occurred.

CRANIAL NERVE DISORDERS

OLFACTORY NERVE DISORDERS (See ANOSMIA in Ch. 168)

OPTIC NERVE DISORDERS (See Ch. 184)

OPHTHALMOPLEGIA (See EXTRAOCULAR MUSCLE PALSIES in Ch. 173)

TRIGEMINAL NEURALGIA (Tic Douloureux)

Bouts of severe brief lancinating pain in the distribution of one or more divisions of the 5th cranial nerve, most often the superior mandibular or maxillary. The cause is unknown, and no pathologic changes can be found. Older patients are usually affected. The pain is often set off by touching a trigger point or by activity such as chewing or brushing the teeth. Pain is intense, and although each bout is brief, successive bouts may incapacitate the patient.

Diagnosis

The history usually is typical and diagnostic. No signs, clinical or pathologic, occur with trigeminal neuralgia, so that finding a sensory abnormality or cranial nerve dysfunction rules out trigeminal neuralgia as the cause of pain. If cranial nerve dysfunction is found, a neoplasm or other lesion impinging on the nerve or its distribution in the brainstem should be sought. Tumors or other lesions usually produce persistent pain and sensory impairment. Post-herpetic pain is diagnosed by the typical antecedent rash, scarring, and its predilection for the ophthalmic division of the 5th nerve. Multiple sclerosis, which sometimes causes typical trigeminal neuralgia, can be distinguished by the typically fluctuating and changing neurologic symptoms. Trigeminal neuropathy may occur in Sjögren's syndrome or RA, but with a sensory deficit that is often perioral and nasal. Migraine and atypical facial pain from other causes can be excluded by their prolonged throbbing or burning pain, in contrast to the brief sharp pains of trigeminal neuralgia.

Treatment

Carbamazepine 200 to 1600 mg/day is generally effective; liver and hematopoietic functions should be monitored. Phenytoin 300 to 600 mg/day also is effective in some cases. Peripheral block or section of the 5th nerve branches is seldom beneficial. Major surgical approaches to treatment at present include the separating away of structures (especially arteries) pressing against the trigeminal root in the posterior fossa (Jennetta procedure) and the placement of electrolytic lesions of the Gasserian ganglion via a percutaneous stereotaxically positioned needle. Occasionally, to relieve intractable pain, surgical section of 5th nerve fibers proximal to the Gasserian ganglion, at the brainstem level, is resorted to.

GLOSSOPHARYNGEAL NEURALGIA

A rare syndrome characterized by recurrent attacks of severe pain in the posterior pharynx, tonsils, back of the tongue, and middle ear. The cause is unknown, and no pathologic changes can be found, except in the rare case due to a tumor in the cerebellopontine angle. Men are affected more commonly than women; the syndrome usually appears after age 40.

Symptoms and Signs

As in trigeminal neuralgia, intermittent attacks of brief, severe, excruciating pain occur paroxysmally, either spontaneously or precipitated by movement (e.g., chewing, swallowing, talking, sneezing). The pain, lasting seconds to a few minutes, usually begins at the base of the tongue and radiates to the ears or down the neck anterolaterally. Occasionally, increased activity of the vagus nerve causes cardiac sinus arrest with syncope. Attacks may be separated by long intervals.

Diagnosis

The location of the pain, precipitation of an attack on swallowing or by touching the tonsils with an applicator, and temporarily eliminating the pain with 0.15% tetracaine applied locally (after which the pain cannot be evoked by stimulation), will distinguish glossopharyngeal neuralgia from trigeminal neuralgia involving the mandibular division. Tonsillar, pharyngeal, and cerebellopontine angle tumors must be ruled out.

Treatment

As in trigeminal neuralgia, carbamazepine is the drug of choice. If ineffective, cocainization of the pharynx may provide temporary relief, and surgery may be necessary. When pain is restricted to the pharynx, the nerve in the neck may be avulsed; it must be sectioned intracranially if pain is widespread.

FACIAL NERVE DISORDERS

Unilateral facial weakness is a common neurologic sign. Of the many disorders that can affect the facial nerve and cause facial weakness, only the commonest, Bell's palsy, is discussed here; other causes are mentioned under diagnosis of that condition.

BELL'S PALSY

Idiopathic unilateral facial paralysis of sudden onset. The cause is unknown, but the mechanism is presumed to involve swelling of the nerve due to immune or viral disease, with ischemia and compression of the facial nerve in the narrow confines of its course through the temporal bone.

Symptoms, Signs, and Course

Pain behind the ear may precede the facial weakness, which develops, sometimes to complete paralysis, within hours. The involved side is flat and expressionless, and patients may complain about the seemingly twisted intact side rather than the involved side. In severe cases the palpebral fissure is wide, and the patient cannot close his eye. Examination may show an area of decreased pinprick sensation along the distribution of Arnold's nerve behind the involved ear. A lesion just proximal to the nerve branches may affect salivation, taste, and lacrimation, and may cause hyperacusis.

Prognosis depends on the extent of nerve damage. Complete recovery within several months invariably follows partial facial paralysis. The results after total paralysis are variable. The likelihood of complete recovery is 90% if the nerve proximal in the face retains normal excitability to supramaximal electrical stimulation, but it is only about 20% if electrical excitability is absent. Misdirected regrowth of nerve fibers may innervate lower facial muscles with periocular fibers and vice versa, resulting in contraction of unexpected muscles on voluntary facial movements **(synkinesia)**, or "crocodile tears" during salivation. Facial muscle contractures may follow chronic weakness.

Diagnosis

The weakness of the entire half of the face distinguishes Bell's palsy from supranuclear lesions (e.g., stroke, cerebral tumor), in which the weakness is mainly below the eye because of the bilateral cerebral innervation of the frontalis muscles. However, Bell's palsy must be differentiated from unilateral facial weakness due to other disorders of the facial nerve or its nucleus, chiefly geniculate herpes **(Ramsay Hunt syndrome)**, middle ear or mastoid infections, fractures of the petrous bone, carcinomatous or leukemic invasion of the nerve, or cerebellopontine angle or glomus jugulare tumors. Since the facial nerve may be involved by any invasive cranial nerve disorder, such as tumor or infection, the other cranial nerves should be tested. Skull x-rays are negative in Bell's palsy but may reveal a fracture line, bony erosion by infection or neoplasm, or internal auditory canal expansion from a cerebellopontine angle tumor.

Treatment

Methylcellulose drops or temporary patching may suffice to protect the exposed eye; tarsorrhaphy may be needed when eye closure weakness is prolonged. Definitive treatment is aimed at decompressing the facial nerve before denervation occurs. Corticosteroids appear to be more successful than surgical unroofing of the facial canal; e.g., prednisone 60 to 80 mg/day orally beginning soon after onset and given for 1 wk, then decreased gradually over the 2nd wk. Faradic stimulation of the nerve and physical therapy are useful only to provoke motion and prevent contractures in paralyzed muscles. Hypoglossal-facial nerve anastomosis may partially restore facial function if none has returned in 6 to 12 mo.

EIGHTH NERVE DISORDERS (See Differentiation of Sensory (Cochlear) and Neural (8th Nerve) Hearing Losses in Ch. 164 and Vertigo in Ch. 118)

NERVE ROOT DISORDERS

(See also Ch. 110)

Etiology

Nerve root dysfunction generally follows pressure upon, or invasion of, the root. A spotty syndrome of nerve root dysfunction may occur when spinal nerve roots are invaded by a metastatic tumor that has spread to the subarachnoid space and involves the meninges and contiguous structures **(neoplastic meningitis**—see Ch. 125 and Subacute Meningitis in Ch. 124). The CSF shows cancer cells, a high protein content, and a decreased sugar content. Nerve roots may also be involved by systemic diseases such as pernicious anemia and tabes dorsalis, producing a profound loss of proprioceptive sensation. Intra- or extradural tumors may invade or compress the spinal roots. Mechanical compression by a herniated disk is discussed below.

Diagnosis

Diseases of the spinal roots present a characteristic radicular syndrome that distinguishes them from other peripheral nerve diseases. **Ventral (motor) root involvement** causes weakness and flaccidity of the muscles supplied by that root. After 6 wk, atrophy and occasionally fasciculations are seen. **Dorsal (sensory) root abnormalities** cause sensory impairment, pain, or both in the dermatome of that root. Deep tendon reflexes are depressed.

Pain is typical of root syndromes and is often precipitated by movement of the spine. Pain from disease of low lumbar and high sacral roots, which form the sciatic nerve, involves the buttock and posterolateral thigh and calf **(sciatica)**. Large lesions in the lumbosacral region involve the many roots of the **cauda equina**, producing bilateral radicular symptoms and signs in the lower extremities as well as impaired sphincter and sexual functions due to involvement of lower sacral roots. **Thoracic root syndromes** produce little motor change, but cause bandlike pain around the thorax or flank. **Cervical root syndromes** cause weakness, atrophy, depressed tendon reflexes, pain, and dermatomal sensory loss in one or both upper extremities. Large cervical or thoracic lesions may involve the spinal cord as well as roots.

Myelography can define soft tissue deformation of the dura mater or nerve root and delineate the level of a disk protrusion or the appearance of an intraspinal space-occupying lesion. The lumbar puncture required for myelography provides information on CSF dynamics, cytology, and biochemistry.

HERNIATED NUCLEUS PULPOSUS (Herniated, Ruptured, or Prolapsed Intervertebral Disk; Disk Syndrome)

Etiology

Cartilaginous disks, consisting of an outer anulus fibrosus and an inner nucleus pulposus, separate the spinal vertebrae. Degenerative changes or trauma may rupture the anulus fibrosus, most commonly in the lumbosacral and cervical areas, and pressure transmitted through the spine forces the nucleus posterolaterally or posteriorly into the extradural space. Symptoms result when the herniated nucleus compresses a nerve root, either within the spinal canal or at the intervertebral foramen. Root compression usually is unilateral but may be bilateral if the herniation is large. Posterior protrusion of a cervical (or, rarely, a thoracic) disk may compress the cervical spinal cord; a lumbar disk may compress the cauda equina, impairing many roots at once.

Symptoms and Signs

Pain in the distribution of the compressed root may begin suddenly and severely, or insidiously. It is worse on movement and may be exacerbated by the Valsalva maneuver (coughing, laughing, straining at stool, etc.), since this transmits pressure to the disk through the subarachnoid space. Paresthesias or numbness in the sensory distribution of the root may occur. Deep tendon reflexes in the root distribution are depressed. With a lumbosacral herniation, straight leg raising, which stretches the roots, may produce back pain; neck flexion is similarly painful with herniated cervical disks. Muscles supplied by the impaired root eventually become weak, wasted, and flaccid and may show fasciculation. Cervical cord compression may cause spastic paraparesis of the lower limbs, and cauda equina compression often results in urine retention or incontinence from loss of sphincter function; *these occurrences signal a situation requiring urgent care and close supervision.*

Diagnosis

Compression of a nerve root may also be caused by an extramedullary spinal tumor such as a meningioma or a neurofibroma of the root itself, by involvement of the vertebrae with metastatic tumor, by spondylosis with protrusion of osteophytes into the intervertebral foramen, or by subluxation of one vertebra upon another (spondylolisthesis); these must all be considered in the differential diagnosis. Plain x-rays may disclose a small intervertebral disk space or may show erosion by tumor or the changes of spondylosis or spondylolisthesis. Electromyography may reveal neuropathic changes within muscles supplied by the affected root. Diagnosis and localization are confirmed by myelography, which is best reserved as a preoperative localizing measure. In cases where diagnosis is in doubt, CT scans of the implicated spinal region are helpful.

Treatment

For a first attack of disk syndrome, 2 wk of conservative therapy should be tried. The treatment of choice is bed rest, supine, on a firm surface. Immobilization by traction may be helpful but does not fully relieve pressure on the nerve. Analgesics and mild sedative tranquilizers such as diazepam 5 to 20 mg orally q.i.d. provide symptomatic relief. A rigid brace or cervical collar may help in immobilization during recovery. Exercises during and after recovery strengthen paraspinal muscles and thereby provide better splinting of the injured disk. The patient should be taught to avoid twisting the spine and to lift with bent knees rather than with bent back. If a disk syndrome does not respond to these measures—e.g., if objective neurologic findings (weakness, atrophy, sensory deficit) remain or grow worse—surgical removal of the disk with fusion of the involved vertebrae or decompression of the involved root should be performed.

Cervical-thoracic herniations that acutely compress the cord, and cauda equina herniations that impair bladder function, require *immediate surgery.*

PLEXUS DISORDERS

Diseases of the **brachial** or **lumbosacral plexuses** cause a mixed motor and sensory disorder of the corresponding limb. The pattern does not fit the distribution of individual roots or nerves. Disorders of the rostral brachial plexus produce disability about the shoulder, and those of the caudal brachial plexus produce dysfunction in the hand. In infants they may be caused by traction during birth; in adults, by invasion of metastatic cancer (typically breast or lung carcinoma in brachial plexus disorders and bowel or genitourinary neoplasms in the lumbosacral plexus).

Acute brachial neuritis occurs mainly in young men, producing supraclavicular pain, weakness and diminished reflexes in the distribution of the brachial plexus, and minor sensory abnormalities. Profound weakness develops within several days to weeks of onset, then regresses over the next few months. The rostral plexus and therefore proximal muscles are involved in 2/3 of cases. The **etiology**

is unknown, although viral or immunologic processes are suspected. **Treatment** with corticosteroids (e.g., prednisone 60 to 80 mg/day orally) is advocated by some.

CERVICAL SYNDROMES (Cervical Musculoskeletal Discomfort; Cervical Radiculopathy; Cervical Spondylosis with Nerve Root or Spinal Cord Compression)

A spectrum of acute and chronic neuromuscular disorders affecting the cervical region, the distribution of the cervical nerve roots, or both. Acute cervical syndromes are common and range in seriousness from nonspecific painful muscle spasms in the posterior neck and occiput to acute painful radiculopathy with sensorimotor defects in the distribution of the C-6 to C-8 nerve roots. Chronic cervical radiculopathy is less prominently painful but can produce weakness, wasting, and discomfort in the upper extremities or, when the spinal cord is compressed, a progressive paraparesis.

Etiology

Trauma and arthritis are frequent causes of cervical muscle pain, although psychogenic muscle tension is the offender perhaps equally as often. The great flexibility of the cervical spine predisposes it to acute injury from sudden deceleration (e.g., "whiplash" injury). When pain lasts more than a few days after such trauma, secondary reactions to the injury must be considered, especially after vehicular accidents when the question of compensation is raised. Other causes of acute stiff neck include athletic injuries, sudden thrusts or pulls on the arms, and falls. Less frequently, nontraumatic inflammation, infections, neoplasms, and metabolic disorders may affect the cervical structures.

Wear and tear of the ligamentous and capsular structures probably cause recurrent low-grade inflammation in almost everyone and, quite commonly, the changes of **osteoarthritis**. Over the years this may become chronic and result in mild scarring and hyperplasia. The consequent thickening of the anterior and posterior walls of the intervertebral canals causes chronic foraminal narrowing, which occasionally may be sufficient to compress and irritate the nerve roots as they traverse the foramina. With continued motion, osteophytes develop at the margins of the joints and cause further narrowing. These osteoarthritic changes are referred to as **cervical spondylosis**. RA and other causes of nontraumatic inflammation also may produce a similar chronic root compression unless ankylosis prevents movement.

Symptoms and Signs

With cervical muscle contraction, pain is the most frequent complaint; not necessarily localized to the neck, it may occur anywhere along the distribution of the neck muscles. Pain most commonly radiates between the shoulder blades and to the tops of the shoulders, with little evidence of a nerve root distribution. In some patients, associated muscle contraction may cause pain radiating into the upper arms or even to the occiput. Neck or shoulder motion, particularly neck extension or tilting, may be limited or may cause pain or "crunching" sounds in the neck muscles; "knots" may be present in the neck muscles. Tenderness of deep muscles and over the spinous processes posteriorly, spasms in the lateral and anterior neck muscles, and localized muscle spasms at sites of referred pain also may be present.

Nerve root involvement may be accompanied by numbness and tingling in the proximal part of the dermatome, and by sensory loss distally. Often there are varying degrees of muscle weakness and wasting, and diminished reflexes along the segmental nerve root distribution. Acute symptoms of this type that involve single roots tend to occur in younger persons, mostly those under 45, and reflect acute intervertebral disk rupture with nerve root compression. Among older persons, when nerve root involvement occurs, it emerges more slowly as part of the chronic degenerative arthritic process of cervical spondylosis. Spinal tumors in both age groups tend to involve several adjacent dermatomes and have a progressive course.

Cervical spondylosis is part of the process of degenerative arthritis and produces proliferative changes that result in narrowing and lipping of the intervertebral spaces and spurs in the articular facets that often protrude into the intervertebral foramina where they compress the nerve roots. Most often the 5th, 6th, and 7th vertebrae are involved with resulting injury to the 6th, 7th, and 8th nerve roots, particularly the 6th and 7th. Symptoms usually begin in middle age or later as mild, often intermittent, neck pain and stiffness, or discomfort and paresthesias in the arm and hand. More severe compression leads to muscular atrophy and sensory deficits in the distribution of the involved roots. Deep tendon reflexes may be diminished or hyperactive, depending on whether the spinal cord is compressed and at what level. Spinal cord compression, caused by protrusion of osteophytes posteriorly from the vertebral bodies into the spinal canal, results in progressive spastic motor weakness of the lower extremities, with increased tendon reflexes and Babinski signs. Vibratory sense in the lower extremities is usually diminished; proprioceptive and touch abnormalities are less common.

X-Ray Findings

With cervical muscle pain, x-ray findings may be normal. With clear signs of nerve root disease or spinal cord involvement, x-ray changes are more prominent, although the degree of abnormality often correlates poorly with physical findings. The films may show small vertebral subluxations (some resulting from ligamentous and capsular instability), rotation of one vertebra upon another, or narrowed disks. Osteophytic formations may be seen at the vertebral margins or at the lateral interbody (Luschka) joints or posterior apophyseal joints, with consequent foraminal narrowing at one or more levels. Evidence of old fractures and other skeletal disorders are sometimes found. Straightening or reversal of the normally forward cervical curve may be seen, but this is diagnostic only of muscle tension.

X-rays may not localize the painful lesion in the neck, since changes may be seen at several interspaces or may be limited to the soft tissues and thus not be visible on routine films. When neurologic dysfunction is prominent or progressive, myelography is best for definition of lesions that compress nerve roots or the spinal cord, such as a herniated disk or tumor.

Diagnosis

The patient's history is helpful, including an account of recent or old injuries or accidents, the patient's activities at the time of onset of symptoms and whether onset was gradual or sudden, and possible aggravating social or emotional factors. The cervical spine may be hyperextended for 1 min or compressed by pressure on the patient's head to reproduce the pain and aid in establishing a diagnosis. In contrast, manual traction with the neck in slight flexion may give symptomatic relief. These manipulations should be performed only after x-rays have ruled out an unstable fracture or subluxation.

Sympathetic nerve deficit, most commonly ipsilateral **Horner's syndrome**, suggests a supraclavicular lesion (e.g., Pancoast's pulmonary superior sulcus tumor). The combination of weakness, atrophy, depressed reflexes, and sensory loss in the distribution of lower cervical roots, and spastic paraparesis with vibratory impairment in the legs, is typical of cervical spondylosis. Space-occupying lesions must be considered and, when suspected, ruled out by myelography. Cervical spondylosis must also be differentiated from herniated disk, combined system disease of pernicious anemia, and amyotrophic lateral sclerosis.

Prognosis

Prognosis depends on the underlying cause and should be guarded following injury. If symptoms rapidly improve and disappear within 6 wk, the residual disability will be minimal; otherwise, chronic intermittent disability of varying degree may be anticipated.

Treatment

Specific therapy depends on the underlying cause. For general management, conservative measures usually are satisfactory; surgery is rarely indicated. The patient must adjust to the limitations of the cervical spine to prevent aggravation and exacerbation of symptoms. Activities requiring repeated or prolonged hyperextension or hyperflexion of the neck should be avoided; a protective collar should be worn during strenuous exercise or heavy lifting. A cervical contour pillow to keep the neck from assuming an extreme position during rest or sleep may provide adequate relief with little or no other treatment.

Heat helps relieve pain and muscle spasm. Analgesics (aspirin 600 mg alone or with up to 65 mg codeine, given orally q 3 h) and muscle relaxants (e.g., diazepam 5 mg orally q.i.d.) are also frequently effective. When symptoms are acute, bed rest for 1 to 2 wk may be necessary. Whether the prolonged use of a cervical collar provides advantages is debatable.

Traction as well as a cervical collar is recommended initially. Cervical traction effectively relieves muscle spasm even when severe nerve root involvement and motor weakness are present. It is usually applied at home for 15 min 3 to 4 times/day, using static weights. The required amount of pull varies according to the individual's size and body type, but is usually between 5 and 15 lb. Neck position during traction is important: the most comfortable straight or mildly flexed position is used; extension should be avoided. The traction is applied through a head halter, with the weight attached on a rope put through a pulley that is placed above and slightly in front of the patient to ensure that the neck is pulled in flexion. The traction should relieve the pain, and relief should begin to last beyond the traction periods within a few days. The frequency of treatments may be decreased as symptoms subside.

If static home traction does not provide relief, intermittent traction using a motorized device in a physical therapy facility is indicated. Hospitalization for further evaluation is indicated if motor weakness progresses or does not rapidly subside. **Surgical decompression** may be indicated to prevent further deterioration when spastic paraparesis due to cervical spondylosis does not respond to conservative measures, keeping in mind that decompression may prevent further disability but will probably not reverse the weakness that is already present.

Isometric exercises and manipulation are rarely effective.

PERIPHERAL NEUROPATHY

(Peripheral Neuritis)

A syndrome of sensory, motor, reflex, and vasomotor symptoms, singly or in any combination, produced by disease of a single nerve (**mononeuropathy, mononeuritis**), *2 or more nerves in separate areas* (**mononeuritis multiplex**), *or many nerves simultaneously* (**polyneuropathy, polyneuritis,**

multiple peripheral neuritis). The lesions, usually degenerative and rarely accompanied by signs of inflammation, may be in the nerve roots or peripheral nerves. The term "neuritis" does not specifically connote nerve inflammation; and the term "neuralgia," which refers to recurrent idiopathic paroxysms of acute pain along the distribution of a nerve (as in trigeminal and glossopharyngeal neuralgia, discussed above), should not be used as a synonym for neuritis.

Etiology

Mechanical stress (compression, direct blows, penetrating injuries, contusions, avulsion resulting from fracture or dislocation of bones) usually causes mononeuritis; sometimes mononeuritis multiplex. Pressure paralysis usually affects superficial nerves (ulnar, radial, peroneal) at bony prominences (e.g., during sound sleep or anesthesia in thin or cachectic persons and frequently in alcoholics) or at narrow canals (e.g., in entrapment neuropathies, such as the median nerve in the carpal tunnel syndrome). Pressure palsies also may result from tumors, bony hyperostosis, casts, crutches, or prolonged cramped postures (e.g., from gardening). Violent muscular activity or forcible overextension of a joint may produce a mechanical neuritis, as may repeated small traumas such as those encountered by engravers through tight gripping of small tools, or by air-hammer operators through excessive vibration. Hemorrhage into a nerve, and exposure to cold or to radiation, may cause neuropathy.

Vascular or collagen vascular conditions (polyarteritis nodosa, atherosclerosis, SLE, scleroderma, sarcoidosis, and RA) usually cause mononeuritis multiplex. **Volkmann's ischemic paralysis** occurs when occlusion of a major artery affects nerves with a common blood supply in one limb.

Microorganisms may cause mononeuritis by direct invasion of the nerve (e.g., in leprosy or TB; the facial nerve in mastoiditis). Polyneuritis with acute febrile diseases may be due to a toxin (diphtheria), direct invasion of multiple nerves (malaria), or a probable autoimmune reaction (virus infections, the Guillain-Barré syndrome); the polyneuritis that sometimes follows immunizations is also probably immunologic (see also Ch. 126 and ACUTE VIRAL ENCEPHALITIS in Ch. 124).

Toxic agents generally cause a polyneuropathy, but sometimes a mononeuropathy. They include emetine, hexobarbital, barbital, chlorobutanol, sulfonamides, phenytoin, nitrofurantoin, the vinca alkaloids, heavy metals, carbon monoxide, triorthocresylphosphate, orthodinitrophenol, many solvents, and other industrial poisons.

Metabolic neuritis, almost always a polyneuropathy, can result from nutritional deficiency (especially of B vitamins)—e.g., in alcoholism, beriberi, pernicious anemia, isoniazid-induced pyridoxine deficiency, malabsorption syndromes, psychoses, and hyperemesis gravidarum. Polyneuropathy also occurs in hypothyroidism, acute porphyria, sarcoidosis, amyloidosis, and in many uremic patients receiving dialysis. Diabetes mellitus causes several forms of neuropathy: a sensorimotor distal polyneuropathy (most common), a vascular mononeuritis multiplex, and an isolated mononeuritis (often of the oculomotor or abducens cranial nerves).

Malignancy (bronchogenic carcinoma, myeloma, lymphoma) may cause polyneuritis by an unknown mechanism as well as by invasion.

For **hereditary neuropathies,** see Vol. II, Ch. 25, and TABLE 25–19 in Vol. II, Ch. 25.

Symptoms, Signs, and Clinical Forms

Mononeuritis, both single and multiplex, is characterized by pain, weakness, and paresthesias in the distribution of the affected nerve. Mononeuritis multiplex is asymmetric, and all the affected nerves may be involved from the outset or progressively. Extensive involvement of many nerves may simulate a polyneuropathy.

Compression and entrapment neuropathies result from mechanical compromise of a nerve. **Ulnar nerve palsy** is caused by trauma to the nerve in the ulnar groove of the elbow by repeated leaning on the elbow or by asymmetric bone growth after a childhood fracture ("tardy ulnar palsy"). There are paresthesias and sensory deficit in the 5th and lateral 4th fingers plus weakness and atrophy of the thumb adductor, 5th finger abductor, and interossei muscles. Severe, chronic ulnar palsy produces a "claw-hand" deformity. The **carpal tunnel syndrome** (see FIG. 117–3 in Ch. 117) results from compression of the median nerve in the volar aspect of the wrist between the longitudinal tendons of forearm muscles that flex the hand and the transverse superficial carpal ligament. This compression produces paresthesias in the radial-palmar aspect of the hand plus pain in the wrist, in the palm, or sometimes proximal to the compression site in the forearm. Sensory deficit in the palmar aspect of the first 3 digits and/or weakness of thumb opposition may follow. The syndrome is relatively common, may be uni- or bilateral, and is seen more often in women. It is associated with the synovial changes of acromegaly, myxedema, and RA, and also with occupations that require repeated forceful wrist flexion. The chief distinction to be made is from C6 root compression due to cervical osteoarthropathy.

Peroneal nerve palsy is caused by compression of the nerve against the lateral aspect of the fibula. It is most common in emaciated nonambulatory patients and in thin people who habitually cross their legs. Weakness of foot dorsiflexion and eversion (foot drop) are present. Occasionally, a sensory deficit is found on the dorsal aspect of the web between the 1st and 2nd metatarsals. **Radial nerve palsy** ("Saturday night palsy") is caused by compression of the nerve against the humerus—e.g., as the arm is draped over the back of a chair during intoxication or deep sleep. Symptoms include weakness of wrist and finger extensors (wrist drop) and occasionally a sensory loss on the dorsal web between 1st and 2nd metatarsals.

The site of local nerve damage can be identified by **Tinel's sign,** a distal paresthesia in the distribution of the nerve that is elicited by percussion over the site of compression. Electrical nerve conduction studies help in localization.

Polyneuropathy is bilaterally symmetric, and all nerves (sensory, motor, vasomotor, or a combination) are involved simultaneously. There are several forms of polyneuropathy. An acute, rapidly progressive form, the Guillain-Barré syndrome, is discussed separately below. The most common form of polyneuropathy is seen with metabolic diseases such as diabetes mellitus or malnutrition. This form develops slowly, often over months or years, and often begins with sensory abnormalities in the lower extremities. Peripheral tingling, numbness, burning pain, or deficiencies in joint proprioception and vibratory sensation are often prominent. Pain is often worse at night and may be aggravated by touching the affected area or by temperature changes. In severe cases, objective signs of sensory loss can be demonstrated, characteristically in stocking-and-glove distribution. The Achilles and other deep tendon reflexes are diminished or absent. Painless ulcers on the digits or Charcot's joints may be seen when sensory loss is profound. Sensory or proprioceptive deficits may lead to gait abnormalities that simulate tabes dorsalis. Weakness and atrophy of distal limb muscles and flaccid tone characterize involvement of motor fibers.

The autonomic nervous system may be additionally or selectively involved, leading to nocturnal diarrhea, bladder and bowel incontinence, impotence, or postural hypotension. Vasomotor symptoms (hyperemia, sweating, and bullae) are more common in partial lesions; complete lesions generally produce pallor, dry skin, and osteoporosis. Trophic changes are common in severe and prolonged cases.

Uncommonly, an exclusively sensory polyneuropathy is seen in carcinoma, especially bronchogenic, which begins with peripheral pains and paresthesias and progresses centrally to a loss of all forms of sensation.

Diagnosis

Neuropathy is a symptom complex rather than a disease entity, and the cause must be sought. The etiology is often suggested during the general assessment. In mononeuropathy, attention should be directed toward a mechanical or traumatic origin, though infectious agents may be responsible. Mononeuritis multiplex usually is due to polyarteritis or diabetes mellitus; sometimes to sarcoidosis, SLE, leprosy (patients from the Caribbean, Asia, or Africa), or brucellosis. Polyneuropathy is most commonly toxic, parainfectious, or metabolic (diabetic, or due to vitamin deficiency in alcoholism). Poliomyelitis, tabes dorsalis, and progressive muscular atrophies and dystrophies must be excluded; arthritis, fibrositis, and dermatomyositis may also simulate neuritis.

Physical examination may show hypertension, weight loss (which reflects an underlying systemic disease), signs of atherosclerosis, infection, anemia, or malignancy. Scars, fractures, and bony callus suggest a traumatic neuritis. There may be weakness, muscle atrophy, hypotonia, hyporeflexia, or sensory impairment, depending on which nerve fibers are affected. These findings are most severe in the distal parts of the extremities in polyneuropathy.

Laboratory findings are often helpful. Examination of the blood may disclose the megaloblasts of pernicious anemia, the stippled RBCs of lead poisoning, or polyarteritic eosinophilia. The urine may show porphyrins, porphobilinogen, heavy metals, or evidence of renal disease. Glucosuria or hyperglycemia may disclose diabetes mellitus. X-rays may show a herniated disk or bone changes due to trauma, malignancy, or osteoarthritis. Thyroid function tests may be indicated. Gastric analysis for free acid, the Schilling test, and serum folate and B_{12} levels will diagnose pernicious anemia.

The CSF is normal in traumatic mononeuritis and often in polyneuropathy, but the protein content may be moderately or greatly increased in diphtheritic and diabetic polyneuropathy and in the Guillain-Barré syndrome. Malignant cells are found, protein content is high, and sugar content is usually low when lymphoma, leukemia, or carcinoma is producing a polyneuropathic syndrome.

Electromyography, nerve conduction velocity tests, and muscle and sural nerve biopsy help to distinguish the weakness of peripheral neuropathy from that of myopathic and motor neuron disorders. Motor nerve conduction is often slowed in peripheral neuropathy (because of demyelination) but not in motor neuron diseases. Slowed conduction may also confirm a suspected entrapment neuropathy. **Muscle biopsy** may sometimes provide specific diagnosis (trichinosis, sarcoidosis, polyarteritis). Special histologic technics may differentiate axonal degeneration from segmental demyelination in sural nerve biopsies.

Prognosis and Treatment

Mild neuritis usually recovers rapidly with treatment, but may recur if the cause is not avoided. Recovery may be incomplete, with sensory, motor, or vasomotor residua and, in severe cases, chronic muscular atrophy as well.

Specific therapy is directed toward the cause by control of diabetes, administration of vitamins, avoiding further mechanical trauma, or surgery for tumors and perhaps for ruptured intervertebral disk. Nerve suture or neurolysis and nerve transplant may be advisable in some traumatic lesions. In peripheral nerve entrapment or compression neuropathy, surgical decompression of the ulnar or median nerves is beneficial; peroneal and radial compression neuropathies are treated by avoiding pressure on the areas. Recovery is slow; physical therapy and splints avoid contractures.

GUILLAIN–BARRÉ SYNDROME (Acute Polyneuropathy; Acute Polyradiculitis; Infectious or Acute Idiopathic Polyneuritis; Landry's Ascending Paralysis; Acute Segmentally Demyelinating Polyradiculoneuropathy)

An acute, rapidly progressive form of polyneuropathy characterized by muscular weakness and mild distal sensory loss that usually begins shortly after a banal infectious disorder, surgery, or an immunization.

Etiology

The many synonyms given to this disorder reflect its variant manifestations and postulated causes. Since it is often para- or postinfectious, it is now presumed to be due to an immunologic attack on peripheral nerves.

Symptoms and Signs

Symptoms begin peripherally, often in the digits, and progress centrally. Although numbness, tingling, and other paresthesias are common and there may be mild distal sensory loss, flaccid muscular weakness predominates, with associated muscle tenderness and diminished tendon reflexes. The weakness often ascends from legs to arms to face. The sphincters usually escape. In severe cases, motor cranial nerves and trunk muscles may be involved and respiration may be impaired. Sympathetic involvement is indicated by hyperhidrosis, edema, a livid skin, and postural hypotension. The respiratory paralysis and autonomic deficits may be life-threatening.

Diagnosis

Because the initial symptoms are subtle and subjective, some patients are erroneously thought to be hysterical. Substances toxic to the neuromuscular junction, such as organic phosphates in insecticides and botulinus toxin in improperly canned food, also cause rapidly progressive weakness, usually with abnormalities of ocular and pharyngeal muscles plus parasympatholytic symptoms (dry mouth, hyperpyrexia). Acute poliomyelitis is differentiated by the GI prodrome and by the presence of lymphocytes in the CSF. The CSF in the Guillain-Barré syndrome shows no cells and has a high protein content (albumino-cytologic dissociation). CSF pressure may also be increased, with an associated blood Pa_{CO_2} increase, as a result of respiratory embarrassment.

Treatment and Prognosis

Severe acute polyneuropathy represents a medical emergency, requiring constant monitoring and vigorous support of vital functions. The airway must be kept clear, and vital capacity should be measured frequently, so that respiration can be assisted if necessary. Fluid intake should be sufficient to maintain a urine volume of at least 1 to 1.5 L/day; serum electrolytes should be monitored to prevent water intoxication. The extremities should be protected from trauma and from pressure of bedclothes. Immobilization may cause ankylosis and is to be avoided. Heat aids in pain relief and permits early physical therapy. Passive full-range joint movement should be started immediately and active exercises begun when acute symptoms subside.

Corticosteroids have been advocated, but best present evidence is that their usage improves the acute signs, but not the eventual outcome. Prednisone in doses of up to 60 to 80 mg/day orally has been effective in improving the course of certain patients with *chronic* polyneuropathy. If so used, the drug should be given in intermittent courses.

Recovery over a period of months is usual if the patient survives the acute episode. Residual defects may require retraining, orthopedic appliances, or corrective surgery.

CAUSALGIA

A syndrome of persistent, severe, diffuse burning pain, almost always in an extremity, triggered by many stimuli, and resulting from partial interruption of sensory nerve fibers, especially of the median nerve. Even contact with air or drying of the skin may be a sufficient stimulus. The excruciating pain is accompanied by vasomotor and dystrophic changes and may cause severe emotional disturbances. Discoloration, hyperhidrosis, and coldness are signs of localized autonomic dysfunction. Vasospasm is often so severe that major pulsations in the involved extremity are greatly reduced. Disuse atrophy of the muscles follows continuous protective immobilization of the extremity.

Treatment

Sympathectomy provides relief in severe cases; paravertebral nerve block with procaine may be adequate in milder cases. Occasionally, local procaine infiltration or warm, wet dressings of methacholine give relief. A combination of amitriptyline 50 to 150 mg/day and fluphenazine 1 to 5 mg/day orally in divided doses may control the pain, as may carbamazepine 100 to 1200 mg/day. The variety of suggested remedies indicates their uncertain efficacy.

NEUROFIBROMATOSIS

(von Recklinghausen's Disease)

A hereditary (autosomal dominant) disorder that produces pigmented spots and tumors of the skin, tumors of peripheral, optic, and acoustic nerves, and subcutaneous and bony deformities.

Symptoms, Signs, and Diagnosis

One third of patients with neurofibromatosis are asymptomatic and are discovered on routine examination. In 1/3 of patients cosmetic problems are the initial complaints. Characteristic skin lesions, apparent at birth or in infancy in > 90% of patients, are medium-brown (café-au-lait) patches distributed most commonly over the trunk, pelvis, and flexor creases of elbows and knees. The presence of 6 or more of these freckle-like lesions with one larger than 1.5 cm is diagnostic of neurofibromatosis. Multiple cutaneous tumors, flesh-colored and of variable size and shape, appear in late childhood. There may be only a few or thousands of these lesions. Subcutaneous nodules or amorphous overgrowth of subcutaneous tissues **(plexiform neuromas)** and underlying bone may produce grotesque deformities, but this happens only rarely. Skeletal anomalies include absence of the greater wing of the sphenoid bone (posterior orbital wall) with consequent pulsating exophthalmos, fibrous dysplasia, subperiosteal bone cysts, vertebral scalloping, scoliosis, and tibial pseudoarthrosis.

The remaining 1/3 of patients present with neurologic problems. **Neurofibromas** (tumors of Schwann cells and nerve fibroblasts), which rarely appear before puberty, can be felt along the course of subcutaneous peripheral nerves. These tumors may involve spinal nerve roots, characteristically growing through an intervertebral foramen to produce intraspinal and extraspinal masses ("dumbbell" tumor). The intraspinal component may cause spinal cord compression. Plexiform neuromas may involve peripheral nerves producing deficits distal to the lesion. Tumors of cranial nerves may produce progressive blindness (optic glioma) or dizziness, ataxia, and deafness (acoustic neuroma). Bilateral acoustic neuromas are characteristic of neurofibromatosis, and gliomas and meningiomas are abnormally frequent. A recent survey of unselected outpatients with neurofibromatosis showed a 40 (male) to 87 (female) times increase in risk for neural tumors vs. the general population.

Treatment

The various deep tumors are treated by appropriate surgical removal or radiation. The underlying cellular disorder is unknown and no general treatment is available. Genetic counseling is advisable.

---

131. MUSCULAR ATROPHIES AND RELATED DISORDERS

The diseases falling under this heading are all characterized by motor dysfunction (usually muscular weakness) due to an abnormality in some part of the **motor unit.** This comprises a single lower motor neuron (an anterior horn cell, its efferent root and peripheral nerve fiber, and its terminal arborization), the motor end-plate at the neuromuscular junction, and the 10 to 600 muscle fibers that the neuron innervates.

It is convenient to classify the disorders according to the part of the motor unit principally affected (see TABLE 131-1). Thus, in the diseases known as **muscular atrophies,** the major defect is a loss of efferent innervation caused by degeneration of either (1) an anterior horn cell (spinal muscular atrophies), or (2) an axon at the level of an anterior efferent root or peripheral nerve. In some of the atrophies, the nuclei of upper motor neurons in the motor cortex or their axons in the brainstem (corticobulbar tracts) or spinal cord (corticospinal tracts) are also involved; in others, cranial nerve motor nuclei in the brainstem (bulbar nuclei) are affected (bulbar palsies).

In the myopathies, the major involvement is at the level of the muscle fibers. By convention, certain hereditary progressive myopathies are known as **muscular dystrophies.** Other myopathies may result from inflammation or from an endocrine or metabolic abnormality. Those that are hereditary are discussed in Vol. II, Ch. 25; other disorders that can cause myopathy or muscular weakness (polymyositis, dermatomyositis, trichinosis, thyroid and adrenal disorders, hypercalcemia, hypophosphatemia) are discussed elsewhere in this volume.

In **myasthenia gravis** and drug-induced **cholinesterase inhibition,** the defect is at the neuromuscular junction.

TABLE 131–1. CLASSIFICATION OF THE MUSCULAR ATROPHIES, DYSTROPHIES, AND RELATED NEUROMUSCULAR DISORDERS

I. Neurogenic Muscular Atrophies
  A. Anterior horn cell degeneration
    1. Amyotrophic lateral sclerosis (including progressive spinal muscular atrophy and progressive bulbar palsy)
    2. Infantile spinal muscular atrophy
    3. Juvenile spinal muscular atrophy
  B. Anterior root and peripheral nerve involvements
    1. Peroneal muscular atrophy
    2. Hypertrophic interstitial neuropathy
    3. Guillain-Barré syndrome (see Ch. 130)
    4. Metabolic neuropathies (see PERIPHERAL NEUROPATHY in Ch. 130)

II. Disorders of Muscle Fibers
  A. Muscular dystrophies
    1. Pseudohypertrophic muscular dystrophy
    2. Limb-girdle muscular dystrophy
    3. Facioscapulohumeral muscular dystrophy
    4. Myotonic muscular dystrophy (see Myotonic Myopathies, below)
    5. Rare forms: distal muscular dystrophy; ocular myopathy; benign juvenile muscular dystrophy
  B. Inflammatory myopathies
    1. Dermatomyositis, polymyositis
    2. Trichinosis
  C. Myotonic myopathies
    1. Myotonia atrophica
    2. Myotonia congenita
  D. Glycogen storage diseases of muscle (McArdle's, Tarui's, and Pompe's diseases)
  E. Familial periodic paralysis
    1. Hypokalemic type
    2. Hyperkalemic type
    3. Normokalemic type
  F. Endocrine myopathies (e.g., in thyroid, parathyroid, adrenal disorders; hypercalcemia; hypophosphatemia)

III. Neuromuscular Junction Disturbance
  A. Myasthenia gravis
  B. Drug-induced cholinesterase inhibition (e.g., from neostigmine, insecticides)

MUSCULAR ATROPHIES

(Motor Neuron Diseases)

Disorders characterized by muscle weakness and wasting due to denervation.

AMYOTROPHIC LATERAL SCLEROSIS; PROGRESSIVE SPINAL MUSCULAR ATROPHY; PROGRESSIVE BULBAR PALSY

Motor neuron disease of unknown etiology characterized by progressive degeneration of corticospinal tracts and anterior horn cells or bulbar efferent neurons. The symptoms and descriptive designation vary according to the part of the nervous system most affected. Onset is generally after age 40, and the incidence is greater in males.

Symptoms and Signs

Amyotrophic lateral sclerosis: Muscular weakness and atrophy begin in the hands and spread to the forearms and legs. Muscle fasciculations are commonly visible. Sensory abnormalities are absent. Spasticity, increased tendon reflexes, and extensor plantar reflexes are characteristic and occasionally may precede evidence of atrophy. Death usually occurs within 2 to 5 yr. Pathologic examination shows degeneration of upper and lower motor neurons, chiefly in the anterior horns and corticospinal tracts.

In the variant known as **progressive spinal muscular atrophy (Aran-Duchenne muscular atrophy),** anterior horn cell involvement outpaces corticospinal involvement, and the condition is more benign.

Muscle wasting and marked weakness begin in the hands, progress to the arms, shoulders, and legs, and are eventually generalized. Fasciculations are readily seen in the limb muscles and sometimes in the tongue. Survival for 20 to 25 yr is possible.

Progressive bulbar palsy (Duchenne's paralysis, labioglossolaryngeal paralysis): In this variant, the muscles innervated by cranial nerves and corticobulbar tracts are predominantly involved, so that chewing, swallowing, and talking are difficult. A pseudobulbar emotional response, with labile and inappropriate emotions, may be seen. Because of the dysphagia the prognosis is particularly poor, and death in 1 to 3 yr (often from respiratory complications) is not uncommon.

Diagnosis

Diagnostic features include the late onset, the progressive and generalized motor involvement, absence of sensory abnormalities, and clinical evidence of upper and lower motor neuron involvement. Electromyography and muscle biopsy can document the lower motor neuron involvement. Late-onset myopathies and atrophies due to cervical spondylosis, ruptured intervertebral disk, spinal cord tumor, syringomyelia, congenital malformations of the cervical spine, and multiple sclerosis must be differentiated.

Treatment

There is no specific treatment. Physiotherapy may help to maintain muscle function. Patients with pharyngeal weakness should be fed with extreme care.

MYASTHENIA GRAVIS

A disease characterized by sporadic muscular fatigability and weakness, occurring chiefly in muscles innervated by cranial nerves, and characteristically improved by cholinesterase-inhibiting drugs.

The causative defect is believed to be located at the neuromuscular junction and to be related to an impairment of acetylcholine's ability to induce muscle contraction. Recent evidence indicates that the primary defect in the disorder consists of an immunologically induced abnormality in the receptor protein neuromuscular junction. The disease may affect patients of any age group, but especially involves (1) adolescents and young adults, females more often than males, and (2) adults over age 40, many of whom show evidence of thymoma. Most **neonatal myasthenia** reflects the passive transfer of antibodies to receptor protein from a myasthenic mother to the fetus. The motor weakness in such instances may be profound but rarely lasts longer than 2 to 3 wk. The myasthenia in the mother may or may not be clinically evident at the time that the newborn is affected. About 5% of myasthenic syndromes occur in more disseminated immunologic disorders and as complications of certain drugs, e.g., D-penicillamine. Thyroid disorders occur more often in myasthenic patients than in the general population. A myasthenia-like syndrome **(Eaton-Lambert syndrome)** may occur in association with small-cell lung carcinoma; the tumor that may be underlying is sometimes not evident for several years.

Symptoms and Signs

Onset can be sudden or insidious; the most common symptoms are ptosis and diplopia, followed by dysphagia, dysarthria, and limb weakness. Respiratory muscle weakness can occur and is dramatic and life-threatening. Symptoms are exaggerated after use of the affected musculature, and may vary in intensity from day to day. Sensation and reflexes are not altered. Spontaneous remission occurs in about 25% of patients.

Muscle weakness in Eaton-Lambert syndrome mainly occurs in the proximal pelvic and shoulder muscles. Unlike myasthenia gravis, ocular and bulbar muscles are usually not involved, and repeated activity seems to increase muscle strength.

Diagnosis

The tendency toward fatigue and increased weakness of involved muscle groups after their continued use is characteristic of myasthenia gravis and usually can be discerned from the history and demonstrated on examination. The fluctuating course and especially the reversal of objective neurologic signs by edrophonium or neostigmine differentiate this disorder from others causing similar muscular weakness and fatigability. Eaton-Lambert syndrome, frequently responsive to anticholinesterase drugs, is differentiated from myasthenia gravis by electromyography; action potential amplitude *increases* after the first (reduced reaction) stimulus.

In testing adults for myasthenia gravis, edrophonium, a very short-acting anticholinesterase, is valuable diagnostically and in determining the need for additional drug therapy. (Details of the edrophonium test are described under CHOLINERGIC DRUGS in Ch. 248.) In doubtful instances, electromyography with repetitive nerve stimulation and recording of muscle action potentials (Jolly test) may be diagnostic. Most patients with active myasthenia will have detectable levels of antiacetylcholine receptor antibodies in the serum. The presence of such antibodies is valuable for diagnosis but does not correlate with fluctuations in the intensity of the disease. For evaluating infants or extremity strength in adults, neostigmine 1.5 mg with atropine 0.6 mg, both IM, is preferable to edrophonium since the pharmacologic effects persist for an hour, allowing time for an adequate examination. In long-standing disease, the usual test agents may not reverse extraocular muscle weakness.

A concurrent thyroid disorder should be excluded once the diagnosis is established. Mediastinal laminagrams to exclude thymoma should be carried out in all adults.

Treatment

Treatment is with cholinesterase inhibitors, thymectomy, and, sometimes, corticosteroids. One or more courses of plasmapheresis have improved patients refractory to other treatment. Thymectomy, which should be considered in all patients except those with only ocular involvement or with myasthenia from drugs or another disease, may cure 30 to 40% of cases.

Neostigmine 15 to 60 mg orally q 3 to 4 h and pyridostigmine 60 to 240 mg orally q 3 to 4 h are the drugs most commonly used. The dose must be carefully adjusted to individual requirements, and mild exacerbations may require an increase in dosage. Long-acting capsules are available for nighttime use by patients with severe dysphagia who would otherwise find it difficult to swallow medication in the morning. For some patients, abdominal cramps and diarrhea are less troublesome with pyridostigmine. Atropine 0.4 to 0.6 mg orally b.i.d. to t.i.d. may be given for GI side effects. When parenteral therapy is necessary (e.g., with dysphagia), neostigmine 0.5 mg IV or 1.5 mg IM may be substituted for 15 mg orally. The cholinergic drugs may not relieve all symptoms, especially extraocular muscle paralysis, in which case ephedrine 25 mg orally t.i.d. or q.i.d. may be tried as an adjunct.

Excessive neostigmine or pyridostigmine dosage causes weakness that cannot be differentiated clinically from myasthenia itself. Patients may also become refractory to the medication. Thus, if a patient who has been doing well should deteriorate, the cause must be determined. Edrophonium IV should be given; if the patient's weakness improves, the maintenance dose has been inadequate. If the weakness worsens, either the dose was too large or the patient's illness is refractory. Patients with respiratory paresis who are unresponsive to medication require complete respiratory support in a respiratory care unit.

Prednisone 100 mg orally every other day provides an alternative approach and frequently induces a remission, but long-term experience with this therapy is lacking.

The Eaton-Lambert syndrome, if weakness is severe, can be treated with guanidine 35 mg/kg. The drug sometimes suppresses bone marrow, and blood counts must be closely monitored.

DRUG-INDUCED NEUROMUSCULAR JUNCTION BLOCK

The cholinergic agents used to treat myasthenia gravis inhibit cholinesterase, the enzyme that breaks down acetylcholine, and hence they prolong the action of acetylcholine and cause persisting depolarization at the neuromuscular junction. Large doses can produce weakness that is clinically similar to myasthenia gravis. Organophosphate insecticides (e.g., parathion) and most nerve gases are also cholinesterase inhibitors and can produce marked miosis, tightness in the chest, bronchial secretion, GI hyperactivity, and a prolonged myasthenia-like weakness and muscular twitching.

Treatment (doses are for adults) is with atropine 2 to 4 mg IV, repeated as often as q 10 to 20 min if necessary to control tracheal, bronchial, and salivary secretions; and for muscular weakness, pralidoxime chloride 1 gm IV, given within not less than 2 min and repeated if necessary in 20 min.

§12. PSYCHIATRIC DISORDERS

132. INTRODUCTION

Psychiatry, a branch of medicine, is responsible for the study, diagnosis, treatment, and prevention of human behavior disorders. Abnormal behavior may be determined or modified by genetic, physicochemical, psychologic, and social factors, and the physician must acquire the information, knowledge, and skill appropriate to his task.

In addition to mastery of objective observation, the psychiatrist must also acquire the knowledge and skills of participant, subjective, and self observation. Skills in objective observation have been his principal heritage from his background in natural science, but as he learns other types of observation, he finds that this differentiation of his role function is necessary for him to understand the relationship to his patient and to his growing capacity for human intimacy. Only then can the general notion of personality and its underlying principles be learned: the genetic and ontogenic factors in growth, development, and decline; recognition of unconscious and preconscious factors as determinants of behavior; the idea that the personality is integral and indivisible; the recognition that man is a social animal and that the emerging stages of the life cycle reflect coordination between the developing individual and his social environment.

Historically, the introduction of rauwolfia and the phenothiazines in the early 1950s contributed to the effective treatment and symptomatic management of many severely psychotic patients, reduced the duration of hospital stays, and increased the percentage of patients discharged from hospitals after acute episodes, making deinstitutionalization possible.

In addition, there were new psychosocial methods of treatment of psychotic patients, leading to the avoidance of seclusion and restraint; the development of large group technics, such as the therapeutic community; upgrading of the education of nonprofessionals; efforts at early discharge; attempts to break down administrative and other barriers between the hospital and the community; involvement of the family in therapy; and reform of the internal social organization within the hospital.

Pharmacologic investigation of the neuroleptic drugs has led to biochemical studies of the neurotransmitters and their possible role in the cause or course of mental illness, including delirium, dementia, and mental deficiency.

There is a movement toward greater precision in diagnosis, greater understanding of genetic factors in psychopathology, greater exactness in the appropriate use of psychoactive drugs, neuroleptics, antidepressants, anxiolytics, and lithium, and more realistic expectations of the benefits of psychotherapy.

Interest has increased in the treatment of psychotic patients, including those who are chronically disabled, with concern as to whether they are cared for properly in the hospital or in the community; and in the important role family physicians can play in their rehabilitation.

There is greater awareness of the patient's membership in his family and in his community and in the reciprocal relations that may enhance health or provoke illness in the patient and family.

In spite of these real advances, understanding of the basic causes of mental illness has yet to be achieved and requires continued and vigorous research in all of the fields relevant to the determinants of abnormal human behavior.

Classification of Mental Disease

In all medical disciplines, classifications of disease are a dynamic process, ever changing to incorporate new knowledge. Access to the brain and technics for measuring and evaluating its functions, particularly mental activities, are still limited; thus, our understanding of the etiology and pathogenesis of mental disorders is scant. Nevertheless, attempts to categorize mental illness for the past half century have attempted to include theoretical concepts of causality, mixed with descriptive criteria. As a result, terminology and definitions of terms have varied widely among different psychiatrists and in different places. Since diagnosis implies prognosis and determines choices of therapy and since commonality of diagnostic categories is essential to research design, the need for revision of psychiatric nomenclature and classification is great.

The American Psychiatric Association started such a revision in 1974 and introduced a new *Diagnostic and Statistical Manual of Mental Disorders*, Third Edition (DSM-III) in March 1980. This new classification attempts to rely entirely on descriptions of symptoms and signs, i.e., what the patient says and does as indicators of how he thinks and feels. In this edition of THE MERCK MANUAL, we have not completely discarded the old terminology, but have attempted to identify new terms together with their predecessors and to reflect the diagnostic criteria in our discussions.

133. THE PSYCHIATRIC INTERVIEW

Although the detail and emphasis in psychiatric and medical interviews differ, the same purposes apply: to establish a therapeutic doctor-patient relationship and obtain information leading to accurate diagnosis and treatment. In psychiatry especially, effective treatment depends on establishing and maintaining a therapeutic relationship, and the technics that foster such a relationship will be effective in eliciting relevant data from the patient. The initial interview is therefore a significant encounter.

Several different levels of data are obtained simultaneously in the psychiatric interview; appreciation of the exquisite richness of such data grows with the physician's increasing experience and sophistication. The data sources include the patient's verbal content (what he says), manner of speaking (how he says it), nonverbal communication (body language) and associated somatic clues, as well as the interviewer's own emotional responses. Obvious but often overlooked sources of important clinical data include dress, posture, gait, facial expression, complexion, weight, and movement. A mental posture of free-floating attention to the entire gestalt of the patient-interviewer interactions is the most effective way to obtain information from all levels. Data at one level will often augment, modify, or even contradict data at another level. Thus, the alert interviewer will note the patient who shifts position or fidgets with his watch while verbally denying that he is concerned about the item of history currently under discussion. Blushing, blanching, perspiration, increase in respiratory rate, and increase in tics or mannerisms are all sensitive indicators of emotional arousal. Often a subtle cue (a shift of gaze or slight change of expression) will suggest covert emotions, fantasies, or impulses. Body language also may communicate more eloquently than words the pain of a deep depression, the terror of acute anxiety, or the eroticism of seductive behavior.

The patient's behavior is determined by the reality of the present situation, his past experiences, his personality, and his outlook on life. Commonly, he will initially have mixed feelings; while he usually acknowledges his need for help and is relieved to share his concern with a potentially helpful professional, he may also be fearful of rejection, criticism, or humiliation. Thus, his perceptions of and reactions to the interviewer contain both rational and irrational elements, and his behavior may appear inconsistent, puzzling, or inappropriate. With psychotic illness or severe organic brain syndrome, these aberrations of perception and behavior may be extreme.

The interviewer may experience diverse emotions during the interview: most commonly, anxiety, sadness, sympathy, indifference, irritability, or resentment. Recognizing these emotions, learning what in the patient's behavior elicited them, and preventing them from disrupting the interview are essential.

Patients are often accompanied by a spouse, relative, or friend. Usually the patient is seen first. Sometimes, however (e.g., when there is an organic problem or language difficulty, or when the patient is aged or a child), seeing the relative first or even both together may be profitable, but permission must be obtained from the patient. The opportunity to interview someone who knows the patient should not be missed, since it will add valuable perspective, but the confidentiality of each source must be respected.

The appropriate interview length cannot be arbitrarily established. With some patients 15 min are ample, as in cases of severe delirium, psychosis, or dementia. Conversely, an hour may be insufficient in a complex case where the patient is articulate and cooperative. The patient's tolerance for fatigue and anxiety and the physician's time limits place constraints on the interview length. However, a too-brief interview may prevent establishment of the relational bond necessary for the patient to communicate openly. At least 30 min usually are required for the psychiatric interview; more often, 45 or 60 min. When time constraints are inflexible, the patient should be assured of further opportunity to complete the assessment. In crisis situations with an acutely agitated patient, or when the patient is otherwise incapable of supplying a complete history, the interview goals must be realistically limited. **Termination of the interview** is usually straightforward, although a loquacious or demanding patient may require firm interruption. The patient's questions should be encouraged and answered truthfully. Overly optimistic reassurance or unjustified guarantees of treatment efficacy should be avoided; the attempt to provide comfort and hope must be tempered with realism.

Obtaining the History

The tone for the entire interview is established within the first few minutes. Therefore, attention to the interview setting and the interviewer's manner will be rewarded by increased effectiveness; e.g., a quiet, comfortable, and private place lends dignity to the encounter and encourages free discussion. The interviewer should communicate professionalism, concern, and willingness to take the necessary time. Thus, the physician greets the patient by name, performs introductions, indicates the purpose of the interview, and inquires regarding the patient's comfort at the moment.

Having set the tone for the interview, the physician then establishes its direction. Needless controversy has existed concerning interviewing technic, with the two extremes represented by an entirely directed, doctor-oriented interview, and a totally open-ended, patient-oriented interview. No technic is uniformly successful under all circumstances, since the time available, the specific purpose of the interview, and the patient's clinical state will require appropriate modifications. The following approach is usually applicable and productive.

Inquiry should begin by asking the patient to identify the problem (in broad outline) for which he is seeking help. Questions such as "What has been the problem that brought you here?" or "Please tell me what has led you to come to see me today" are useful. Comments such as "Um-humm" or "Tell me more about that" at this stage encourage the patient to talk freely, as does repeating with a questioning inflection a key word or phrase spoken by the patient. As the patient talks, clarification is sought of key words such as depression, panic, nervousness, and anxiety, since these terms mean different things to different people. However, premature efforts to determine the exact details and their chronologic order at the very beginning of the interview may inhibit and distract the patient, and actually reduce the information available to the interviewer. In this early phase of the interview, the major focus is to learn what is significant to the patient himself, how he narrates his story, what emotions are manifest, and what nonverbal cues he communicates, as well as areas of vagueness, inconsistency, or confusion. Exceptions to this approach occur in some psychotic and organic states, where it is obvious immediately that the patient needs structure and direction in order to furnish useful information.

Once the patient has related his difficulties in his own words, a more structured approach is used to follow up leads in the original narrative and to open up new areas for discussion. Again, questions should be initially open-ended in order to encourage elaboration by the patient. For each problem area, one must clarify the time and mode of onset and get a detailed description of the symptoms or situations, chronology of events, aggravating and alleviating factors, and associated elements or manifestations. Progressively more directed, specific questions are required to obtain all pertinent information.

Personal and family histories are obtained next, to provide a background against which the illness can be viewed and to find clues to the genesis of the illness and to possible therapeutic approaches. One inquires regarding the patient's marital and family relations; a family history of mental or nervous disorder; the patient's birth, developmental milestones, childhood memories, and home atmosphere; school (academic, social, and behavioral aspects); then sex education and sexual maturation. Work history, social relationships, other interests, and future goals complete this section of the interview. The interviewer must observe evidence of emotional arousal or conflict in the patient during this review and encourage further elaboration in sensitive areas.

The physician's attitude, while attentive, friendly, and encouraging, should retain an appropriate objectivity in relation to the patient and his problem. Total emotional neutrality is neither possible nor desirable, but the physician should be especially aware of feelings of irritability, impatience, or special attraction toward the patient. The temptations to outdo the patient by recounting personal experiences, to moralize about the patient's behavior, to give gratuitous advice, or to provide dogmatic opinions should be resisted. Questions generally should be turned back to the patient ("Well, what do you think yourself?"), although at times it is beneficial to directly answer a patient's question and promptly return the focus of the interview to the patient.

To complete the history, inquiry may need to be directed toward some symptoms merely to establish that the patient does not have them; e.g., direct but sympathetic questions may be needed to establish the presence of hallucinations or suicidal thoughts.

Recording the History

In contrast to the flexibility used in obtaining a history, a particular format should be followed to record the history. The schema below is commonly used (alternatively, the developmental approach is acceptable, starting at birth or with the family history so that the illness is described in the perspective of the patient's life story). (1) **Identifying characteristics:** name, age, sex, race, marital status, occupation, and source of referral. (2) **Presenting problems:** a brief verbatim statement. (3) **History of present illness:** a chronologic account of the current symptoms and behavioral changes together with coincident life events and their relationships. Events are dated as accurately as possible, and symptoms recorded in the patient's own words, with qualifying details. Previous treatments and the responses to them are noted, and the present degree of disability estimated. (4) **Personal history:** birth and infancy (nature of delivery, temperament and habits, ages at passing milestones); childhood (emotional adjustment, neurotic symptoms, physical illnesses, relationships with peers and siblings); education (duration and details of schooling; achievements, attitudes, and adjustment); work record (list of jobs, reasons for changing, achievements, and adjustments); sexual maturation (date of menarche or puberty; growth of sexual interest and practice; courtship, marriage, and children; emotional and sexual compatibility with spouse). (5) **Previous medical history:** physical and psychiatric illnesses. (6) **Personality prior to illness:** social relationships within the home, at work, and in the community; individual and social activities and interests; predominant moods; character traits, strengths and weaknesses, coping style, methods of handling challenge and stress, and temperament; religious and moral standards; ambitions and aspirations; habits, including drinking, drug use, and smoking. (7) **Family history:** details of each parent and sibling in turn in regard to age, health, occupation, personality, and relationship with the patient; familial diseases, including psychiatric illness. If a relative is dead, the date and cause of death are recorded.

Mental Status Examination

The distinction between history and examination is even more blurred in psychiatry than in general medicine. Most (and frequently all) of the mental status examination is carried out while the history is being obtained. It is insulting and pointless to demand from an intelligent, coherent patient the names of the last six heads of state, a recitation of long sequences of numbers, or the interpretation of proverbs and fables. However, when a specific mental status test is *required* to document the patient's mental state, the interviewer tactfully requests cooperation and is not deterred because of possible embarrassment.

The mental state may be recorded under the following headings. (1) **Appearance and behavior:** dress, posture, facial expression, motor activity such as agitation, impulsivity, mannerisms, retardation, relationship to the interviewer. (2) **Stream of talk** (thought processes): poverty or rigidity of thought; pace and progression of speech; whether speech is logical and to the point or confusing and irrelevant; the presence of thought disorder, flight of ideas, obsessional qualification, or distractibility. The stream of talk is recorded verbatim if relevant. (3) **Thought content:** special preoccupations, obsessional ideas, misinterpretations, ideas of reference or influence, delusions, derogatory or grandiose ideas. (4) **Perceptual abnormalities:** auditory, visual, or tactile hallucinations; depersonalization; derealization. (5) **Affect:** happiness, elation, sadness, depression, irritability, anger, suspicion, perplexity, fear, or anxiety; blunting or incongruity of affect; lability or reactivity of mood; appropriateness to context. (6) **Cognitive functions:** (a) Sensorium: level of consciousness; (b) Memory and orientation: immediate recall; memory for recent and remote events; digit span; orientation in time, place, and person; (c) Concentration: serial sevens; months of the year in reverse order; (d) General information: the President, capitals, distances, etc.; (e) Intelligence: compatibility of school and work records with current performance; interpretation of proverbs; general vocabulary. Psychometric testing may be necessary; (f) Insight and judgment, especially in regard to present illness and plans for the future.

Formulation

An essential aspect of the psychiatric evaluation is the formulation, a concise statement of the interviewer's understanding of and plans for the case. It begins with a summary of the relevant data from the history and mental status examination organized in terms of an explanatory hypothesis concerning the patient's condition. This includes an assessment of the patient's personality strengths and vulnerabilities, as well as the identification of antecedent and proximal factors that have contributed to the origin and evolution of the illness. Next, a differential diagnosis is given and necessary further investigations are listed. Then an initial treatment plan is outlined. A statement of prognosis completes the formulation.

---

134.   PSYCHIATRY IN MEDICINE

PSYCHIATRIC CONSIDERATIONS IN THE MEDICAL INTERVIEW

Relating a patient's complaints and disabilities to his personality helps to form a sound clinical judgment about the nature and causes of the disorder.

To form a picture of the individual patient's personality, the physician has to listen attentively and show interest in the patient as a person (see also Ch. 133). A rigid interview conducted hastily and in an emotionally indifferent way will more likely cause the patient to conceal relevant information than help him divulge it. While tracing the history of the presenting illness with open-ended questions that permit the patient to tell his story in his own words, it is important to note comments that describe associated social circumstances and emotional reactions, as well as attitudes toward physicians and medicines.

Attention then should turn to the patient's social background, previous medical and psychiatric history, and adjustment at different stages of his life. Parental characteristics and the family atmosphere during his childhood are important because personality features that influence the way a person will handle illness and adversity are partly determined early in life. The way the patient has handled different family and social roles provides important clues. His schooling, manner of handling puberty and adolescence, stability and effectiveness at work, sexual adaptation, and the pattern of his social life and quality and stability of his marriage provide information valuable in appraising his personality. Use or abuse of alcohol and tobacco, behavior in driving, and any tendencies to antisocial conduct should be tactfully inquired after. The patient's responses to the usual vicissitudes of life—failures, setbacks, losses, and previous illnesses—are important; he may have endured stresses and misfortunes with courage and resilience or his history may suggest a poor capacity for tolerating frustration.

The personality profile that emerges from these inquiries may reveal traits such as narcissism, immaturity, excessive dependency, anxiety, tendencies to deny illness, histrionic behavior—or conscientiousness, modesty, and adaptability. In particular, the history may reveal patterns of repetitive behavior that the patient exhibits under stressful conditions; i.e., whether distress is expressed in somatic symptoms (e.g., headache, abdominal pain) or in psychologic symptoms (e.g., phobic behavior, depression) or whether the expression is in social behavior, such as withdrawal or rebelliousness. With this information the physician can better interpret the patient's complaints, anticipate his reactions to his illness, and plan appropriate therapy.

Observation during the interview also provides valuable data. A patient may be depressed and pessimistic, or cheerful, facile, and prone to deny illness; he may be friendly and warm, or reserved, cold, and suspicious. Nonverbal communication may reveal attitudes and affects denied by the patient's words. For example, a patient who "chokes up" or becomes tearful when discussing a parent's death is revealing that it was a significant loss; the possibility that unresolved grief is still troubling him should occur to the physician. A tear in the eye, overt weeping, or other such manifestations of emotion should be considered as **physical signs** and should be recorded as such in the patient's chart.

Similarly, when a patient denies being angry, anxious, or depressed while his posture, gestures, and facial expression reveal these emotions, further inquiry may reveal stresses and emotionally depressing circumstances possibly related to the evolution of the present illness. However, the physician should be cautious and remember the possibilities of error in such inquiries. Discriminating and experienced judgment is needed to assess whether psychologic conflicts are highly significant, of limited importance, or perhaps merely coincidental to the patient's physical illness.

Referral for a psychiatric opinion: About 10% of patients admitted to a hospital are referred for a psychiatric consultation. Many of these patients have attempted suicide, and a substantial proportion have other conspicuous psychologic disturbances requiring appraisal and treatment. Particularly important are delirium, dementia, and functional psychiatric syndromes due to organic or metabolic brain disorders (see Ch. 119). In or out of the hospital, awareness of each patient's personality and its relation to his somatic complaints will aid in managing all physically ill patients and increase the physician's awareness of psychiatrically ill or disturbed persons. Many of these patients will suffer from complex, difficult, or refractory problems that will require referral to a psychiatrist. An infrequently used, but very helpful, procedure is for the primary care physician to discuss the situation with a psychiatric colleague *before* making a referral. Advice obtained in such an exchange may obviate the need for referral or help to make the referral in the most appropriate manner. When referral is planned, it should be discussed openly and sensitively with the patient.

PSYCHOSOMATIC MEDICINE

(Biopsychosocial Medicine)

Psychologic factors may contribute directly or indirectly to the etiology of some physical disorders; in others, psychiatric symptoms may be a direct expression of a lesion involving neural or endocrine organs. Psychologic symptoms also may occur as a reaction to the physical illness. The use of the term "psychosomatic" to encompass all these possibilities is a diffuse concept, but it draws attention to the ubiquity of emotional disturbances and psychologic interrelationships with somatic disease and disability throughout the entire field of medicine.

In a more limited sense, "psychosomatic" refers to conditions in which psychologic factors have some etiologic importance. Even in these disorders, however, the etiology is always complex and multifactorial, and psychologic factors are *not* the only contributors to the illness. It is useful to consider a *necessary* **biological** component (e.g., the genetic tendency to diabetes mellitus) which, when combined with **psychologic** reactions (e.g., depression) and **social** stress (e.g., loss of a loved person), results in a set of conditions *sufficient* to produce the illness; hence, the term **biopsychosocial**. The stressful environmental events and psychologic reactions may be viewed as triggers or precipitants of illness. These reactions are *nonspecific* and have been noted in association with a wide variety of diseases, such as diabetes mellitus, SLE, leukemia, and multiple sclerosis. Furthermore, the importance of psychologic factors is relative and varies widely in different patients with the same illness (e.g., asthma, in which inheritance and allergy and infection, as well as the patient's personality, interact to varying degrees).

Psychologic factors may influence the development of physical disease in other ways. For example, certain personality types may predispose to the development of particular disorders, exemplified by the apparent relation of coronary artery disease to Type A and Type B personalities. (Type A [coronary-prone] patients are characterized by enhanced aggressiveness and competitive drive, preoccupation with deadlines, a chronic sense of impatience, and a feeling of time urgency. The opposite behavior pattern, type B [coronary-resistant], is more relaxed and less hurried.)

Increasingly, physicians are dealing with disorders that result in chronic disability or that are liable to recurrence, e.g., myocardial infarction, hypertension, cerebrovascular disease, diabetes mellitus, malignancy, RA, and chronic respiratory illness. Psychologic and social stress are entwined with these disorders; however, cause and effect are difficult to disentangle in investigating such associations. Psychosocial pressures contribute to the clinical course of these disorders in interaction with numerous other factors, including the individual's hereditary predisposition, personality features, and the autonomic and endocrine effects that arise in response to individual vicissitudes.

Psychologic Factors as Indirect Etiologic Agents

Although research has recently uncovered some of the most lethal etiologic agents of disease, the knowledge in many cases has proved difficult to apply in practice. Cigarette smoking and overeating are socially sanctioned forms of addiction, and smoking is also encouraged and reinforced by vast and subtle advertising campaigns that link the habit with assertiveness and virility. The roots of dependence on tobacco or excessive eating, as in other addictions, lie in the individual's personality, his reaction to his psychosocial environment, and his susceptibility to stress and to the relief of anxiety and tension provided by the addicting agent. Any attempt to control these conditions is likely to fail unless the individual psychologic determinants are appreciated, sought out through psychologic appraisal, and dealt with effectively.

Similar situations may arise in a variety of illnesses. In diabetes, for example, a patient may become depressed over his endless dependence on insulin injections and careful dietary management, resulting in neglect of his therapy. Unless his needs for independence are dealt with, medical treatment for this type of "brittle diabetes" may be frustrated.

Somatic Symptoms Reflecting Psychic States

Psychosocial stress producing conflict and requiring an adaptive response may appear *disguised in somatic form* with what appear to be symptoms of organic disease. The emotional disturbance is often overlooked or even denied by the patient and sometimes by the doctor. The mechanisms responsible for such symptoms are unclear although they are generally ascribed to tension, acting directly (e.g., increased muscle tension) or through a conversion process.

Conversion is *the unconscious process of transforming psychic conflict and anxiety into a somatic symptom.* The term was traditionally linked to hysterical (histrionic) behavior (see HYSTERICAL NEUROSIS in Ch. 138), but in primary care medicine it should be considered separately, as it occurs in both sexes and all types of patients. This type of symptom formation is seen virtually every day in a busy primary care practice but unfortunately is seldom recognized as such and is poorly understood. As a result, patients may be subjected to multiple, tedious, expensive, and sometimes dangerous investigations in a search for an elusive organic illness.

Virtually any symptom that can be imagined by a patient may become a conversion symptom, and the history usually reveals how the patient "selected" his particular symptom. Commonly, the patient will have **previously experienced the symptom on an organic basis,** e.g., a painful fracture, angina pectoris, or a ruptured lumbar disk. Then, at a time of psychosocial stress, the symptom reappears (or persists following adequate treatment) as a psychogenic symptom. Alternatively, the patient may "borrow" the symptom from another person; e.g., the medical student who imagines his lymph nodes are swollen while caring for a patient with lymphoma, or the person who presents with chest pain after an associate or relative has a myocardial infarction. In each case, the patient has **identified with someone else who had the symptom.** Finally, the symptom may have been unconsciously selected because of its **value as a metaphor** for his psychosocial condition, e.g., the patient with chest pain following rejection by a lover ("broken heart"), or the patient with back pain who feels that his burdens are too difficult to carry. While literally any symptom may be a conversion symptom, *pain* of one sort or another is most common, e.g., atypical facial pain, vague headaches, poorly localized abdominal discomfort and colic, backache or nuchal pain, limb pain that sometimes simulates intermittent claudication, dysuria, dyspareunia, or dysmenorrhea.

Anxiety and **depression** are commonly seen affects caused by psychic stress and may be expressed as symptoms in any of the body systems. No diagnostic difficulties are encountered if several body systems are involved and the patient also describes his personal anguish and apprehension. But if the patient's symptoms are expressed through a single system and he fails to emphasize emotional discomfort, diagnostic problems are created. Such cases are often described as **masked depression,** although in some instances **masked anxiety** would be a more appropriate term. Mental suffering and depressive symptoms such as insomnia, self-disparagement, psychomotor retardation, and a pessimistic outlook are common, but the patient may deny actual depression of mood or attribute it to his alleged physical disorder. Alternatively, the patient may acknowledge the presence of depression (or anxiety), but insist that it is secondary to some elusive physical condition.

Psychologic Reactions to Physical Disease

Patients with differing personalities will respond differently to being ill, and it is wise to keep in mind the psychologic effects of chronic illnesses, the effect of the patient's knowledge or lack of understanding of the diagnosis, and the patient's response to the physician's attitudes and communications. Individual responses to the side effects of drugs are also highly variable.

Many patients with recurrent or chronic physical disorders experience depression that frequently aggravates the disability and sets up a vicious circle. The gradual decline in well-being due to the physical disorder in hypertension, Parkinson's disease, cardiac failure, or RA creates a depressive reaction that in turn lessens the sense of well-being still further. Antidepressive treatment in these cases often promotes improvement.

MUNCHAUSEN'S SYNDROME (Pathologic Malingering; Chronic Fictitious Illness; Hospital Hobos)

Repeated fabrication of illness, usually acute, dramatic, and convincing, by a person who wanders from hospital to hospital for treatment. Many of the disorders in medical textbooks may be closely mimicked; e.g., individual patients have produced the clinical picture of myocardial infarction, hematemesis or hemoptysis, acute abdominal conditions, or a pyrexia of unknown origin. They can reproduce symptoms of cerebral tumor or disseminated sclerosis with uncanny skill. A patient's abdominal wall may be a criss-cross of scars, and a digit or a limb may have been amputated. Pyrexias are often due to self-inflicted abscesses, and the culture, usually *Escherichia coli*, clearly indicates the source of the infecting organism.

In a bizarre variant of the syndrome, a child may be used as a surrogate patient. The parent falsifies history and may injure the child with drugs, add blood or bacterial contaminants to urine specimens, etc.—all in order to simulate disease.

Patients with Munchausen's syndrome initially and sometimes interminably become the responsibility of medical or surgical clinics. Nevertheless, the disorder is primarily a psychiatric problem, is more complex than simple dishonest simulation of symptoms, and is associated with severe emotional difficulties. The patient's personality may show prominent histrionic features, but these individuals are usually quite intelligent, resourceful, and successful in simulating a variety of conditions. Their deceits and simulations are conscious, but the motivations for their forgery of illness and quest for attention are largely unconscious.

Commonly, there is an early history of emotional and physical abuse. Patients appear to have problems with their identity, intense feelings, inadequate impulse control, a deficient sense of reality, brief psychiatric episodes, and unstable interpersonal relationships. The need to be taken care of is at odds with the inability to trust authority figures, who are manipulated and continually provoked or tested. Feelings of guilt and the associated need for punishment and expiation are obvious.

Treatment

In these patients with psychopathology of psychotic proportions encompassed within a characterologic disorder, successful treatment is rare. Acceding to the patients' manipulations will relieve their tension, but their provocations escalate, ultimately surpassing what physicians are willing or able to do. Refusal to meet treatment demands or confrontation results in angry reactions, and the patient generally moves on to another hospital. Psychiatric treatment is usually refused or circumvented, but consultation and follow-up care may be accepted, at least to help resolve a crisis. However, management is generally limited to early recognition of the disorder and avoidance of risky procedures and excessive or unwarranted medication.

---

135. PERSONALITY DISORDERS

Disordered patterns of behavior characterized by relatively fixed and inflexible reactions to stress. The behavior patterns are rigid and stylized, representing the individual's pattern of dealing with other people and external events regardless of the realities that exist. This rigidity, together with lack of insight and resistance to change, is the key to recognition of personality disorders and a source of frustration to those who must live or deal with them.

From childhood and through much of their life span, individuals with personality disorders exhibit characteristic patterns of maladjustment in their social, interpersonal, and work relationships. In the absence of environmental frustration these persons tend to show little anxiety or mental or emotional symptoms, and they feel that their behavior patterns are "normal" and "right." Thus, they rarely seek help because of their own anxiety and discomfort; more often they are referred by their families or by social agencies when the patient's behavior causes trouble for others. Patients may seek help, usually after environmental frustrations, but unlike neurotic persons will view their difficulties as *outside* of themselves.

Personality disorders are of medical and psychiatric importance for 3 reasons: (1) Their externalization of internal conflicts often leads to clashes with others in ways that bring the patient under medical observation. The result is often a maladaptive doctor-patient relationship, with the patient refusing to take appropriate responsibility and the doctor blaming, distrusting, and ultimately rejecting the patient. (2) Persons with severe personality disorders are at high risk of becoming addicted to alcohol or drugs, of behaving in a self-destructive manner, of pursuing sexually deviant lives with which they cannot cope, and of clashing with society and its mores. (3) These individuals are susceptible to breakdown on exposure to stress. The type of personality disorder may or may not determine the kind of psychiatric illness that complicates it; e.g., a person with a hysterical personality may respond to excess emotional stress by hysterical conversion or dissociative symptoms, or a suicidal depression.

Diagnosis of personality disorders *is based upon recognition of typical behavior patterns and the patient's apparent inability to learn from experience.* The maladaptive behavior patterns seen in personality disorders tend to be exaggerations of **mental coping mechanisms** used *unconsciously* at times by most people. Some mechanisms, when used chronically and maladaptively, may result in the diagnosis of a personality disorder: (1) **Dissociation** (neurotic denial) effects temporary but drastic modification of one's personality or one's sense of personal identity. These modifications can include fugues, hysterical conversion reactions, short-term denial of responsibility for one's acts or feelings, trance states, chance-taking, and pharmacologic intoxication to numb unhappiness. (2) **Projection** allows one to attribute one's own *unacknowledged* feelings to others; it leads to prejudice, rejection of intimacy through paranoid suspicion, overvigilance to external danger, and injustice-collecting. (3) **Schizoid fantasy** is a tendency to use imaginary relationships and private belief systems for the purpose of conflict resolution and relief from loneliness. It is associated with eccentricity and global avoidance of interpersonal intimacy. In contrast to the psychotic person, the user of schizoid fantasy who has a personality disorder does not fully believe in or insist on acting out his or her fantasies. Unlike dissociation, the use of fantasy remakes the outer, not the inner, world. (4) **Hypochondriasis** transforms reproach towards others (which may have arisen from bereavement, loneliness, or anger) into unremitting somatic complaints, as an expression of the entrenched belief that some organic disease is present. In contrast to neurotic conversion reaction where distress is muted and the doctor fascinated, in hypochondriasis the patient's distress is exaggerated, he is resistant to logical reassurance and treatment, and the physician feels helpless and resentful. (5) **Turning against the self** allows aggression toward others to be expressed indirectly and ineffectively through passivity. It includes failures and illnesses that affect others more than oneself, and silly, provocative clowning. The mechanism underlies most sadomasochistic relationships. (6) **Acting out** is the direct, often impersonal, behavioral expression of an unconscious wish or impulse in order to avoid being conscious of the affect—painful or pleasurable—that accompanies it. It includes many delinquent, impulsive, and deviant acts that seem motiveless because the actor is unaware of his or her own feelings.

Unlike neurotic defense mechanisms that trouble the user but not the observer, the use of these immature defense mechanisms is like smoking a strong cigar in a crowded elevator—only the outsider objects. Although these mechanisms may not be breached by reason or interpretation, they respond to improved interpersonal relationships and to supportive but forceful confrontation in prolonged psychotherapy or peer encounters.

Diagnostic Groups

The following classification largely reflects the nomenclature suggested in the American Psychiatric Association's *Diagnostic and Statistical Manual of Mental Disorders,* Third Edition **(DSM-III).**

1. Hysterical (histrionic) personalities are conspicuously egocentric. Since winning the esteem and admiration of others is important to them, attention-seeking and theatrical behavior tends to be characteristic. Their emotional immaturity is expressed with an exaggerated, childish, emotional response to any wounding of their vanity. Inconsistencies in behavior arise because the hysterical personality can adopt whatever pattern of conduct will place him or her in a favorable light or boost self-esteem. In our culture this form of personality disorder is noted more often in women but is also seen in men.

A hysteric person's lively manner lends itself to easily established superficial relationships, but these persons are rarely deeply involved emotionally. They may combine provocativeness or sexualization of nonsexual relationships with sexual dysfunction or fears. Their relationships are affected by a seemingly insatiable need for affection, and behind their sexually seductive behavior lies a childlike wish for nonsexual affection and protection; i.e., they tend to be dependent. Promiscuous entanglements with many partners are possible because of the hysteric's lack of real involvement with any of them. The crises that arise from these relationships are managed with manipulative behavior that may include suicidal threats and shrewd exploitation of the other's emotional susceptibilities. Insight fails to develop in hysteric persons because they can easily repress or forget unpleasant or discreditable experiences; responsibility for misfortunes and failures is usually ascribed to others.

2. Antisocial personalities (previously used designations: **psychopathic, sociopathic**) characteristically act out their conflicts and flout normal rules of social order. These individuals are impulsive, irresponsible, amoral, and unable to forego immediate gratification. They cannot form affectionate relationships with others, but their charm and plausibility may be highly developed and skillfully used for their own ends. They tolerate frustration poorly, and opposition is likely to elicit hostility, aggression, or serious violence. Their antisocial behavior shows little foresight and is not associated with remorse or guilt, since these people seem to have a keen capacity for rationalizing and for blaming their behavior on others. Failure and punishment rarely modify their behavior or improve their judgment and foresight. A person with an antisocial personality may attempt suicide if his aggressions are turned inward instead of being directed against others.

This personality type is often associated with a history of alcoholism, drug addiction, sexual deviation, promiscuity, occupational failure, or imprisonment. In our culture men are more often labeled as antisocial and women as hysterical personalities, but the two personality patterns have much in common. In families of patients with both patterns, there may be antisocial male and hysterical female relatives, and in both patterns there is frequently a history of parental strife and severe emotional deprivation in the formative years. Life expectancy is diminished, but among those surviving there is some tendency to stabilization after age 40. The effects of either severe cerebral injury or undiagnosed alcoholism may closely simulate the picture of an antisocial personality. Unless repetitive antisocial behavior is observed before age 15, the diagnosis of antisocial personality must be doubted.

3. Paranoid personalities are characterized by projection of their own hostilities and conflicts onto others. These persons are markedly sensitive to interpersonal relationships and tend to find hostile and malevolent intentions behind trivial, innocent, or even kindly acts by others. Often their suspicious attitudes lead to aggressive feelings or behavior or bring about rejection by others, which seems to justify their original feelings; however, they are unable to see their own roles in this cycle. Their behavior may be designed to prove their adequacy, while their sense of worthiness becomes exaggerated and is accompanied by belittlement of others. In many spheres these persons may be highly efficient and conscientious, although envious and inflexible. They may be litigious, especially when they feel a sense of righteous indignation.

Paranoid tendencies are especially likely to develop among those who feel particularly inferior because of a disfiguring defect such as lameness or a facial deformity that makes them noticeably different from their peers. Likewise, sensory impairment, particularly chronic deafness, has a similar effect since it impairs their capacity for reality testing and thus leads to the misinterpretation of being talked about or laughed at.

4. Obsessive-compulsive personalities are conscientious and have high levels of aspiration, but they also tend to be perfectionistic and are often unable to gain adequate satisfaction from their achievements. They are reliable, dependable, orderly, and methodical, but their inflexibility often makes them incapable of adapting to changed circumstances. They are cautious and weigh all aspects of a problem; consequently, making decisions may be difficult for them. They bear responsibilities seriously but may suffer much anxiety over them. They pay attention to every detail and are therefore in danger of becoming entangled with means and forgetting the main purposes of their tasks. Compulsiveness is in tune with Western cultural standards, and when the disorder is not too marked, these people are often capable of high levels of achievement, especially in the sciences and academic fields where order is desirable. On the other hand, they often feel a sense of isolation and have difficulties with interpersonal relationships, in which their feelings are less under strict control, events are less predictable, and they must rely on others.

5. Cyclothymic personalities (see also Ch. 139) fluctuate in their moods between states of high-spirited buoyancy and states of gloom and pessimism, each sustained for weeks or longer. Characteristically, the rhythmic mood changes are regular and predictable and occur either without external cause or in response to trivial events. In one common variant of this disorder, the mood is predominantly marked by elation, energy, an infectious gaiety, and optimism; the depressive phases are relatively short-lived and unnoticed. In other individuals the depressive phase is the predominant one. It is uncertain whether the cyclothymic personality disorder lies on a continuum with manic-depressive illness or is a different entity. Many gifted and creative individuals have personalities conforming to a cyclothymic pattern. (The diagnosis has been omitted from DSM-III.)

6. Schizoid personalities are introverted and withdrawn, solitary, emotionally cold, and distant. They are most often absorbed with their own thoughts and feelings and are fearful of closeness and intimacy with others. They are reticent, given to daydreaming, and prefer theoretic speculation to practical action. This personality pattern is found in about 40% of schizophrenic patients before they become ill (see also Ch. 140). However, many schizoid people do not develop schizophrenia or other mental disorders.

7. Passive-aggressive personalities are characterized by helplessness, clinging dependency, and procrastination. The apparent passivity is designed to gain attention and affection, to avoid responsibility, or to control or punish others covertly. Passive-aggressive behavior is characterized by obstinacy, inefficiency, and sullenness, often disguised under a superficial compliance. Frequently, individuals with this disorder agree to perform a task and then proceed to subtly undermine its completion with complaints and passive obstructionism. They also may manifest provocativeness and argumentativeness, especially with those in authority. Such behavior usually serves to deny or conceal marked dependency needs. The behavior is maladaptive in that, ironically, it drives others away and prevents the individual from receiving even a normal amount of support. In most cases sadomasochism is seen as a variant of passive-aggressive behavior.

8. Dependent personalities surrender responsibility for major areas of their lives to others and permit the needs of those on whom they are dependent to supersede their own needs. They lack self-confidence, and feel intense discomfort when alone for more than brief periods. The features of this syndrome are commonly seen in other personality disorders and are frequently obscured by the more obvious aspects of them. For example, hysterical behavior patterns are quite striking and may mask severe underlying dependency. Therefore, use of the syndrome as a discrete diagnosis may prove untenable.

9. **Borderline personalities** are unstable in several areas, including interpersonal relationships, behavior, mood, and self-image. To some extent, the borderline personality has features of all the personality disorders listed above. Brief but frank delusions and hallucinatory experiences are common. Unlike the schizoid personality, however, interpersonal relationships are far more dramatic and intense; unlike the antisocial personality, there is more disturbance of formal thought processes, and aggression is more often turned against the self; and unlike the hysterical personality, there is greater expression of overt anger and greater confusion over sexual identity. Borderline personalities are commonly seen in primary care medical practices, where they tend to appear frequently with vague somatic complaints, often do not comply with therapeutic recommendations, and tend to be very frustrating to their physicians.

10. **Avoidant personalities** are usually hypersensitive to rejection, and fear starting relationships without being very sure of uncritical acceptance; there is, however, a strong desire for affection and acceptance. Unlike schizoid personalities, these individuals are openly distressed by their lack of ability to relate comfortably with others.

11. **Schizotypal personalities** display oddities of thinking, perception, communication, and behavior that suggest schizophrenia but are never severe enough to meet the criteria for that disorder (see Ch. 140). These oddities in cognition may be expressed as magical thinking, ideas of reference, and paranoid ideation, and by definition are more marked than those found in schizoid and avoidant personalities.

12. **Narcissistic personalities** have an exaggerated sense of self-importance, are absorbed by fantasies of unlimited success, and exhibitionistically seek constant attention. Extreme swings between overidealization and devaluation characterize the relationships of these persons, who also display marked entitlement, interpersonal exploitiveness, and oversensitivity to failure. The primary care physician is often frustrated by these patients' incessant and frequently urgent demands relating to what he views as minor problems. As in the case of the hypochondriacal patient, the complaints and entitlement of the narcissistic patient may be caused by genuine but assiduously concealed emotional pain and unhappiness. Like the dependent personality, the narcissistic personality is seen so commonly in the other personality disorders that it may prove inappropriate to treat it as an independent disorder.

Some patients with narcissistic personalities are also characterized by a tendency to complain of multiple somatic symptoms, and this group (also referred to under a variety of terms including **hysterical personality disorder, primitive hysterics**, etc.), which may more properly be viewed as having a personality disorder, has been designated in DSM-III as having a neurosis referred to as **somatization disorder (Briquet's syndrome)**. Therefore, this disorder is discussed in Ch. 138.

Treatment

While specific technics of treatment and problems encountered with the various personality disorders may differ, several general concepts can be considered. Motivation for therapy often comes from someone other than the person involved, and the patient often feels that the reasons for therapy are foreign to him or that he is being victimized. The doctor's job is to contain the patient's externalization through setting limits, confrontation, and avoiding his own tendency to become overinvolved—first to rescue and then to condemn. The temptation of both doctor and patient to hope that drugs will relieve the patient's distress must be recognized and rejected. Over the long term, the anxiety and depression of personality disorders are rarely abolished by pharmacotherapy, while drug abuse and suicide attempts are common complications of prescribing drugs to these individuals.

Commonly, therapeutic gains are made only in the setting of a long-term relationship with another person, who must be flexible, reassuring, and usually more active than passive. Patients need to be confronted with the way their behavior affects other people. Frequently, limits on behavior need to be set and reality issues dealt with. In many cases the family should be involved, since group pressure seems to be effective. Group and family treatment, group living situations, therapeutic social clubs, milieu hospital therapy—all can be valuable in treatment. The patient's self-esteem must be supported while his maladaptive modes of behavior are confronted. It is also important that those undertaking treatment be aware of the difficulties and avoid the disappointment, annoyance, and moral judgments that tend to creep in. The middle years tend to bring maturation for those with personality disorders, and this process can sometimes be given a helping hand.

136. DRUG DEPENDENCE

(Substance Use Disorders; Drug Addiction; Drug Abuse; Drug Habituation)

A single definition for drug dependence is neither desirable nor possible. The term **drug dependence of a specific type** emphasizes that different drugs have different effects, including the type and hazard of the dependence they produce. **Addiction** refers to a style of living that includes drug dependence, generally both physical and psychologic, but mainly connotes continuing use and overwhelming involvement with a drug. Addiction additionally implies the risk of harm and the need to stop drug use, whether the addict understands and agrees or not.

Drug abuse is definable only in terms of societal disapproval and involves different types of behavior: (1) experimental and recreational use of drugs; (2) use of psychoactive drugs to relieve problems or symptoms; (3) use of drugs at first for the above reasons but development later of dependence and continuation at least partially to prevent the discomfort of withdrawal.

Recreational drug use has increasingly become a part of our culture, although in general not sanctioned by society and often illegal. Users who apparently do not suffer harm tend toward episodic use involving relatively small doses, precluding clinical toxicity and the development of tolerance and physical dependence. The drugs used are often "natural," i.e., close to plant origin and containing a mixture of compounds, and are not isolated psychoactive chemicals, e.g., crude opium, alcoholic beverages, marijuana products, coffee and other caffeine-containing beverages, hallucinogenic mushrooms, and coca leaf. The drugs are most often taken orally or are inhaled. The use of active potent compounds administered by injection is seldom easily controllable. Recreational use is also often accompanied by ritualization with a set of observed rules and is seldom practiced alone. Most drugs used in this fashion are psychostimulants or hallucinogens used to obtain the "high" rather than to relieve psychic distress; depressant agents are seldom used in this controlled manner.

Two general aspects are common to most types of drug dependence: (1) **Psychologic dependence** involves feelings of satisfaction and a drive to repeated or continuous administration of the drug to produce pleasure or avoid discomfort. This mental state is a powerful factor involved in chronic use of psychotropic drugs, and with some drugs psychologic dependence may be the only factor involved in intense craving and compulsive use. (2) **Physical dependence** is defined as a state of adaptation to a drug accompanied by the development of tolerance and manifested by a withdrawal or abstinence syndrome. **Tolerance** is defined as the need to increase the dose progressively in order to produce the effect originally achieved by smaller amounts. Physical dependence and tolerance do not accompany all forms of drug dependence. A **withdrawal syndrome** is characterized by unpleasant physiologic changes that occur when the drug is discontinued abruptly or when its effect is counteracted by a specific antagonist.

Drugs that produce dependence act on the CNS and have one or more of the following effects: reduced anxiety and tension; elation or other mood changes seen as pleasurable by the user; feelings of increased mental and physical ability; altered sensory perception; and changes in behavior. These drugs may be divided into (1) those causing chiefly psychic dependence and (2) those causing both psychic and physical dependence. Important drugs in the first category are cocaine, marijuana, amphetamine, bromides, and the hallucinogens, such as lysergic acid diethylamide (LSD), mescaline, and psilocybin. A major stereotyped abstinence syndrome does not follow withdrawal of these drugs, but some cause tolerance; and in some cases reactions following withdrawal resemble an abstinence syndrome (e.g., depression and lethargy following withdrawal of cocaine or amphetamine; characteristic changes in the EEG with amphetamine). TABLE 136–1 lists some commonly used psychoactive drugs and their potential for various types of dependence.

In the USA, the Comprehensive Drug Abuse Prevention and Control Act of 1970 (Public Law 91–513) and subsequent changes require the drug industry to maintain physical security and strict record-keeping over certain types of drugs, and divide controlled substances into 5 schedules (or classes) on the basis of their potential for abuse, accepted medical use, and accepted safety under medical supervision. Substances included in Schedule I are those with a high potential for abuse, no accepted medical use, and a lack of accepted safety. Those in Schedules II through V decrease in potential for abuse. Placing a drug into one of these schedules determines the nature of control that must be exercised. Prescriptions for drugs in all these schedules must bear the physician's Federal Drug Enforcement Administration (DEA) license number. (See also Refills in Ch. 244.)

Etiology

The development of drug dependence is complex and unclear. At least 3 components require consideration: the addictive drugs, predisposing conditions, and the personality of the user. The psychology of the individual and drug availability determine the choice of addicting drug and the pattern and frequency of use.

Drug dependence is partly related to cultural patterns and socioeconomic classes, and the progression from experimentation to occasional use and the development of tolerance and physical dependence are poorly understood processes. Factors leading to increased use and habituation or addiction appear to include peer or group pressure and emotional distress that is symptomatically relieved by specific drug effects. Factors involved in the mechanisms leading to drug abuse include hypophoria, low self-esteem, social alienation, and environmental stress, particularly if accompanied by feelings of impotence to effect change or to accomplish goals. The medical profession may contribute to harmful psychoactive drug use inadvertently through overzealous drug application to the problems of living and through failure to prevent the obtaining of drugs from multiple doctors. Advertising in mass media may contribute to social expectations that drugs can relieve distress or gratify needs.

Pharmacologic factors: Persons who become addicted or dependent have no known biochemical, drug dispositional, or physiologic responsiveness differences from those who do not, although many efforts have been made to find such differences. After 2 to 3 days of treatment with full doses

TABLE 136–1. COMMONLY USED SUBSTANCES WITH POTENTIAL FOR DEPENDENCE

Drug	Physical Dependence	Psychologic Dependence	Tolerance
CNS Depressants			
Opiates	+ + + +	+ + + +	+ + + +
Synthetic narcotics	+ + + +	+ + + +	+ + + +
Barbiturates	+ + +	+ + +	+ +
Glutethimide	+ + +	+ + +	+ +
Methyprylon	+ + +	+ + +	+ +
Ethchlorvynol	+ + +	+ + +	+ +
Methaqualone	+ + +	+ + +	+ +
Alcohol	+ + +	+ + +	+ +
Minor Tranquilizers			
Meprobamate	+ + +	+ + +	+
Benzodiazepines	+	+ + +	+
Stimulants			
Amphetamine	?	+ + +	+ + + +
Methamphetamine	?	+ + +	+ + + +
Cocaine	0	+ + +	0
Hallucinogens			
LSD	0	+ +	+ +
Mescaline, peyote	0	+ +	+
Marijuana			
(low-dose Δ-9 THC)	0	+ +	0
(high-dose Δ-9 THC)	0	+ +	?

Abbreviations: LSD, Lysergic acid diethylamide; THC, tetrahydrocannabinol; 0, no effect; +, slight, to + + + +, marked, effect.

of a narcotic analgesic, some physical dependence may exist. Such patients have a mild withdrawal syndrome, scarcely noted, or described as a case of influenza; they do not become addicted. Even patients with chronic pain problems requiring long-term administration usually are not addicts, although they may experience some problems with tolerance and physical dependence. Some substances have a high potential for physiologic dependence and are more prone to abuse even when used in a social or recreational setting. Pharmacologic effects are important, but not exclusive, factors in the development of drug dependence.

Personality factors: The "addictive personality" has been described variously by behavioral scientists, but there is little scientific evidence that characteristic personality factors exist. Some have concluded that addicts are basically escapists, persons who cannot face confronting realities and who run away. Others have described addicts as schizoid individuals who are fearful, withdrawn, and depressed, and who have a history of frequent suicide attempts and numerous self-inflicted injuries. Addicts have also been described as basically dependent and grasping in their relations and frequently exhibiting overt and unconscious rage and immature sexuality. These descriptions may have a genesis in the describer's attitudes.

Abuse of prescription drugs may occur in persons with an advanced education and professional status. Before developing the drug dependence, they did not demonstrate the pleasure-oriented, irresponsible behavior usually prejudicially attributed to addicts. Sometimes the patient justifies the use of medication because of a crisis, job pressure, or family catastrophe that produces temporary anxiety or depression. Most of these patients abuse alcohol or another drug at the same time and may have repeated hospital admissions for overdose, adverse reactions, or withdrawal problems.

DEPENDENCE ON ALCOHOL

The development of characteristic deviant behaviors associated with prolonged consumption of excessive amounts of alcohol. Alcoholism is a chronic illness of undetermined etiology with an insidious onset, showing recognizable symptoms and signs proportionate to its severity.

The discussion of alcoholism needs 2 separate foci. Consumption of large amounts of ethyl alcohol is usually accompanied by significant clinical toxicity and tissue damage, the hazards of physical dependence, and a dangerous abstinence syndrome. Additionally, the term alcoholism is applied to the social impairment occurring in the lives of addicted individuals and their families. Usually, the 2 foci are recognized simultaneously, but occasionally one predominates to the apparent exclusion of the other.

An **alcoholic** is identified by severe dependence or addiction and a cumulative pattern of behaviors associated with drinking. (1) Frequent intoxication is obvious and destructive; it interferes with the individual's ability to socialize and to work. Drunkenness may lead to (2) marriage failure and eventually, after work absenteeism becomes intolerable, to (3) being fired. Alcoholics may (4) seek medical treatment for their drinking. They may (5) suffer physical injury, (6) be apprehended for driving while intoxicated, or (7) be arrested by the police for drunkenness. Eventually, they may (8) be hospitalized for delirium tremens or cirrhosis of the liver. Women alcoholics have been in general more likely to drink alone, and less likely to experience some of the social stigmata.

The frequency and severity of these 8 symptoms and the age at which they occur are accepted as defining alcoholism. The earlier in life these behaviors are evident, the more crippling is the disorder.

Incidence of alcoholism among women, children, adolescents, and college students is increasing. The male:female ratio is now approximately 4:1. It is generally assumed that 75% of American adults drink alcoholic beverages, and 1 in 10 will experience some problem with alcoholism.

Etiology

The etiology is unknown. Psychologic hypotheses have noted the frequent incidence of certain personality traits, including (1) schizoid qualities (isolation, loneliness, shyness), (2) depression, (3) dependency, (4) hostile and self-destructive impulsivity, and (5) sexual immaturity. Families of alcoholics tend to have a higher incidence of alcoholism. Genetic or biochemical defects leading to alcoholism are suspected but have not been clearly demonstrated, although a higher incidence of alcoholism has been reported in biological children of alcoholics, as compared to adoptive children. Societal factors affect patterns of drinking and consequent behavior, the attitudes transmitted through the culture or child rearing. Alcoholics frequently have histories of broken homes and disturbed relationships with parents.

Physiology and Pathology

Alcohol is absorbed into the blood, principally from the small intestine. It accumulates in the blood because absorption is more rapid than oxidation and elimination. Depression of the CNS is a principal effect of alcohol: a blood alcohol level of 50 mg/100 ml produces sedation or tranquility; 50 to 150 mg/100 ml, lack of coordination; 150 to 200 mg/100 ml, intoxication (delirium); and 300 to 400 mg/100 ml, unconsciousness. (For symptoms of unconsciousness due to acute alcoholism, see Ch. 118.) Blood levels > 500 mg/100 ml may be fatal. The legal driving level is 100 mg/100 ml or less in most states, and intoxication is often defined as a blood level of 150 mg/100 ml. From 5 to 10% of ingested alcohol is excreted unchanged in urine, sweat, and expired air; the remainder is oxidized to CO_2 and water at a rate of 5 to 10 ml/h (of absolute alcohol), each ml furnishing about 7 kcal.

The most common forms of specific organ damage seen in alcoholics are cirrhosis of the liver, peripheral neuropathy, brain damage, and cardiomyopathy. Gastritis is common and pancreatitis may also develop. Alcohol seems to have a direct hepatotoxic effect, although inadequate nutrition secondary to heavy alcohol intake may exacerbate this effect. Irreversible impairment of liver function occurs in some alcoholics; this may prevent adequate glycogen storage and promote a tendency to hypoglycemia from inability to mobilize glucose. Symptomatic hypoglycemia may result from the absence of adequate food intake. (See also discussions of alcoholic ketoacidosis and hypoglycemia in Ch. 90.) Both the direct action of alcohol and the accompanying nutritional deficiencies (particularly of thiamine) are considered responsible for the frequent peripheral nerve degeneration and brain changes. Alcoholic cardiomyopathy may develop after approximately 10 yr of heavy alcohol abuse and is attributed to a direct toxic effect of alcohol on the heart muscle, independent of nutritional deficiencies. It is manifested clinically as cardiomegaly and congestive heart failure and pathologically usually as diffuse myocardial fibrosis and hypertrophy with glycoprotein infiltration. In addition, thiamine deficiency associated with alcohol abuse can produce a cardiomyopathy ("beriberi heart disease") in which high output failure is prominent, and cardiac conductive disturbances can occur related to electrolyte imbalance. Gastritis in alcoholics may be related to the effect of alcohol on gastric secretions, which are increased in volume and acidity while the pepsin content remains low.

Tolerance, Physical Dependence, and Abstinence Syndromes

Patients who drink large amounts of alcohol repetitively become somewhat **tolerant** to its effects, a phenomenon also noted with other CNS depressants (opiates, barbiturates, meprobamate, etc.); later doses do not have the same intoxicating effect as earlier ones. This tolerance is not based primarily on changes in drug disposition or metabolism but is caused by adaptational changes of CNS cells (cellular or pharmacodynamic tolerance). Those tolerant to alcohol may have incredibly high blood alcohol concentrations; a few have survived concentrations of > 700 mg/100 ml. Even so, the tolerance is incomplete and individuals can always manifest some degree of intoxication and impairment with a high enough dose. In fact, in tolerance animals, the *lethal* dose increases minimally. The **physical dependence** accompanying tolerance is profound, and withdrawal produces a series of adverse effects that may lead to death. Individuals tolerant to alcohol are cross-tolerant to many other CNS depressants (barbiturates, nonbarbiturate hypnotics, and benzodiazepines).

Alcohol withdrawal syndrome: A continuum of symptoms and signs accompanies alcohol withdrawal, usually beginning 12 to 48 h after cessation of intake. The mild withdrawal syndrome includes tremor, weakness, sweating, hyperreflexia, and GI symptoms. Some patients may suffer generalized grand mal seizures, usually not more than 2 in short succession ("**alcoholic epilepsy**" or "**rum fits**").

Alcoholic hallucinosis follows prolonged excessive use of alcohol. The symptoms are auditory illusions and hallucinations, usually of a paranoid nature and frequently accusatory and threatening; the patient is usually apprehensive and may be terrified. The condition resembles schizophrenia, but there is usually no thought disorder and the history is not typical of schizophrenia. The symptoms do not resemble the delirious state of an acute organic brain syndrome as much as do delirium tremens or the other pathologic reactions associated with withdrawal. Consciousness remains clear, and the signs of autonomic lability seen in delirium tremens are usually absent. When the syndrome occurs, it usually precedes delirium tremens. The hallucinosis is usually transient and responds to treatment with moderately large doses of phenothiazines. Chlorpromazine or thioridazine 100 to 300 mg q.i.d. is recommended. Recovery usually occurs in 1 to 3 wk; recurrence is likely if the patient resumes drinking.

Delirium tremens (the severe withdrawal syndrome) begins with anxiety attacks, increasing confusion, poor sleep, marked sweating, and a profound depression. Autonomic lability, evidenced by diaphoresis and increased pulse rate and temperature, accompanies the delirium and parallels its progress. Mild delirium is usually accompanied by marked diaphoresis, a pulse rate of 100 to 120/min, and a temperature of 37.2 to 37.8 C (99 to 100 F). Marked delirium, with gross disorientation and cognitive disruption, is associated with marked restlessness, a pulse greater than 120/min, and temperature over 37.8 C (100 F).

Initially, fleeting hallucinations and nocturnal illusions that arouse fear and restlessness may occur. Typical of these delirious, confused, and disoriented states is a return to a habitual activity—e.g., the patient frequently imagines that he is back at work and attempts to perform some related activity. Visual hallucinations involving animals are frequent and often incite terror. The patient is suggestible to all sensory stimuli and particularly to objects seen in dim light. Vestibular disturbances may cause him to believe that the floor is moving, walls are falling, or the room is rotating. As the delirium progresses, a persistent coarse tremor of the hand at rest develops, sometimes extending to the head and trunk. Marked ataxia is present; care must be taken to prevent self-injury. Symptoms vary among patients but are usually the same with each recurrence for a particular patient.

Temperature may be elevated during the withdrawal of any addictive agent, but elevated temperature in alcohol withdrawal is a poor prognostic sign. The mortality of delirium tremens may be as high as 15%. However, the course is usually self-limited, terminating in a long sleep. The acute period persists from 2 to 10 days but can be more prolonged in severe withdrawal syndromes. Delirium tremens should begin to clear within 12 to 24 h, and if there is no evidence of marked improvement within this interval, other conditions such as subdural hematoma, a systemic disorder, or other disturbances of mentation should be suspected.

Patients with **cirrhosis and impending hepatic coma** become dull, lethargic, and stuporous and develop a "flapping" tremor of the extended arms (**asterixis**). The apprehension, panic, and restlessness seen in delirium tremens are absent. These patients are extremely ill and require immediate medical intervention. (See also PORTAL-SYSTEMIC ENCEPHALOPATHY, in Ch. 64.)

Korsakoff's syndrome (see also Ch. 119) is characterized by a gross disturbance in the patient's recent memory. He may confabulate to conceal the defects in his retention. For example, if a patient who has been hospitalized for a week is asked what he has done the previous day, he may happily describe having gone shopping, having lunch, and attending a football game. If the question is repeated immediately, he may give another equally interesting account that has no bearing on the first. This disorder is attributed to the patient's excessive intake of alcohol, to his being chronically malnourished, and to a diet deficient in the B vitamins, particularly thiamine. Korsakoff's syndrome may begin insidiously, or it may suddenly follow bouts of delirium tremens. Unlike the delirious patient, an alcoholic with this disorder is comfortable, rather cheerful, and generally noncomprehending. The prognosis is poor because the patient usually cannot alter his previous pattern of excessive alcohol intake; the outcome is graver if **Wernicke's encephalopathy** also develops. Usual symptoms of Wernicke's encephalopathy include ocular palsy, impaired mentation, ataxia, and polyneuropathy. *Vitamin therapy should be started urgently.* These patients should be given large doses of B-complex vitamins orally and 50 mg of thiamine daily parenterally until a normal dietary intake is possible.

Pathologic intoxication is a rare syndrome characterized by repetitive and automatic movements and the occurrences of extreme excitement with aggressive, uncontrolled irrational behavior after ingesting a relatively small amount of alcohol. The episode may last for minutes or hours and is followed by a prolonged sleep with amnesia for the event upon awakening.

Treatment

Medical evaluation is needed initially to detect any intercurrent illness that might complicate withdrawal and to rule out any CNS symptoms from injury that might mimic or be masked by the withdrawal syndrome. It is especially important to differentiate delirium tremens from the mental changes found in acute hepatic insufficiency, because of the difference in management.

Delirious patients are extremely suggestible and respond well to reassurance. They should not be restrained. Fluid balance must be maintained and large doses of vitamin C and B-complex vitamins, particularly thiamine, given promptly. A dehydrated alcoholic patient should be given 1000 ml of 5% dextrose in physiologic saline solution followed by 1000 ml of 10% dextrose in distilled water.

Some drugs frequently used to treat alcohol withdrawal are similar to alcohol in pharmacologic effects. In fact, the most useful agents are apparently those to which alcohol induces cross-tolerance. All patients entering withdrawal are candidates for CNS-depressant drugs, but not all need them. Nondrug "detoxification" can be utilized in many individuals if proper attention is paid to psychologic support, reassurance, and a nonthreatening approach and environment. Unfortunately, most of these are not readily available in a general hospital or emergency room venue.

Paraldehyde, once a mainstay of therapy, has been largely abandoned because of its unpleasant smell and because a few unexplained instances of sudden death have followed its use. It may be used in initial doses of 10 ml orally, if the patient will accept it. This dose has been repeated as often as q 4 h in the severely agitated patient. Similarly, **rapidly acting barbiturates** (pentobarbital and secobarbital) are seldom used today, but phenobarbital is quite useful. However, benzodiazepines have become the mainstay of therapy. **Chlordiazepoxide** is recommended in most situations in initial 50- to 100-mg oral doses which may need repetition q 3 h. **Diazepam** is a useful alternative. Isolated seizures need no specific therapy, and repeated seizures will respond to 1- to 3-mg doses of IV diazepam. **Phenothiazines** are not recommended, since they may not control severe delirium tremens and since they lower the seizure threshold. The routine administration of **phenytoin** is not necessary. Outpatient therapy with phenytoin is almost always a waste of time and drug, because these seizures only occur under the stress of alcohol withdrawal, and withdrawing (or heavily drinking) patients do not take their antiseizure medication.

The first treatment phase consists of acute withdrawal of alcohol. The delirious state that may accompany withdrawal and its management has been described above. After correction of any nutritional deficiencies associated with excessive alcohol intake, the patient's behavior must be changed to stop drunkenness. Maintaining sobriety once it has been established is difficult because the patient has fixed patterns of nonsobriety. The patient should be warned that after a few weeks, when he has recovered from his last bout, he is likely to find some excuse to take a drink. He should also be told that he may be able to drink in a controlled manner for a few days or, rarely, even for a few weeks, but with depressing regularity he will repeat the pattern and again drink without control.

Various types of psychotherapy have been recommended for alcoholism, but a general rule is that group processes are superior to one-on-one processes. Some feel that newer behavioral technics may hold promise. Aversive therapy using electric shock or inducing nausea and vomiting with disulfiram, emetine, or apomorphine has been used. If benzodiazepines were used judiciously, they would be effective substitutes for alcohol. Unfortunately, many patients will utilize them as they did alcohol. Unlike most people who take these drugs, alcoholics may achieve intoxication and even physical dependence and withdrawal with diazepam or chlordiazepoxide.

Alcoholics Anonymous (AA): No other approach has benefited so many alcoholics as effectively as the help they have offered themselves through AA. The patient must find an AA group in which he is comfortable, preferably one where he has common interests with the other members in addition to his alcohol problem; e.g., in some metropolitan areas there are AA groups of physicians and dentists. These groups provide the patient with nondrinking friends who are always available as well as an area in which to socialize—away from the tavern. The patient also hears others, more expert than he, confess before the group every rationalization the patient has ever thought up privately to justify his own drinking. Finally, the help he gives to other alcoholics may afford him the self-esteem and confidence formerly found only in alcohol.

Disulfiram therapy: Disulfiram interferes with the metabolism of acetaldehyde (an intermediary product in the oxidation of alcohol) so that acetaldehyde accumulates, producing toxic symptoms and great discomfort. Drinking alcohol within 12 h after taking disulfiram produces facial flushing in 5 to 15 min, then intense vasodilation of the face and neck with suffusion of the conjunctivae, throbbing headache, tachycardia, hyperpnea, and sweating. Nausea and vomiting follow in 30 to 60 min and may be so intense as to lead to hypotension, dizziness, and sometimes fainting and collapse. The reaction lasts 1 to 3 h. Discomfort is so intense that few patients will risk taking alcohol as long as they are taking disulfiram. The patient should also avoid medications containing alcohol (e.g., tinctures, elixirs, some OTC liquid cough/cold preparations, which contain as much as 25% ethanol).

Disulfiram may be given on an outpatient basis after the patient has been free of alcohol for 4 or 5 days. The initial dose is 0.5 gm orally once/day for 1 to 3 wk. The maintenance dose is adjusted individually; 0.25 to 0.5 gm once/day is usually adequate, but some patients may require more. Both patient and relatives should be warned that the effects of disulfiram may persist for 3 to 7 days following the last dose. In Great Britain and some other European countries, disulfiram is available for use as a subcutaneous implant, obviating the need to take daily oral doses in long-term management. The patient must want to be helped, must cooperate, and should be seen periodically by the physician to encourage his continuing to take disulfiram.

Disulfiram therapy is **contraindicated** in pregnancy and in decompensated cardiac patients. Few studies convincingly indicate a general utility of the drug, and many patients are noncompliant. However, when patients succeed they are often users of disulfiram, and the lack of proof should not interfere with its availability to patients and therapists.

DEPENDENCE OF THE OPIATE TYPE

The characteristics of dependence of the opiate type are a strong psychic dependence manifested as an overpowering compulsion to continue taking the drug, the development of tolerance so that the dosage must be continually increased in order to obtain the initial effect, and physical dependence that increases in intensity with increased dosage and duration of use. The physical dependence necessitates continued administration of the same opiate or a related drug to prevent withdrawal symptoms and signs. Withdrawal of the drug or administration of an antagonist precipitates a characteristic and self-limited abstinence syndrome.

Tolerance and physical dependence on the opiates and synthetic narcotics develop rapidly; therapeutic doses taken regularly over a 2- to 3-day period can lead to some tolerance and dependence, and the user may show symptoms of withdrawal when the drug is discontinued. Narcotic drugs often induce cross-tolerance. Abusers may substitute one for another. With increased use of methadone in detoxification and maintenance programs, illicitly obtained methadone has become an additional substance for abuse. People who have developed tolerance may show few signs of drug use and function normally in their usual activities. Tolerance to the various effects of these drugs frequently develops unevenly; for example, a meperidine user may tolerate large doses but show many of the stimulant and atropine-like side effects. Heroin users may become completely tolerant to the euphoric and lethal effects but will still have constricted pupils and constipation.

Symptoms and Signs

Acute intoxication with opiates is characterized by euphoria, flushing, itching of the skin, miosis, drowsiness, decreased respiratory rate and depth, hypotension, bradycardia, and decreased body temperature.

The **withdrawal syndrome** from an opiate generally includes symptoms and signs opposite to the drug's pharmacologic effects (e.g., CNS hyperactivity). The severity of the withdrawal syndrome increases with the size of the opiate dose and the duration of dependence. Symptoms begin to appear as early as 4 to 6 h after withdrawal and reach a peak within 36 to 72 h for heroin. The initial anxiety and craving for the drug are followed by other symptoms increasing in severity and intensity. A reliable early sign of abstinence is an increased resting respiratory rate, > 16/min, usually accompanied by yawning, perspiration, lacrimation, and rhinorrhea. Other symptoms include mydriasis, piloerection ("gooseflesh"), tremors, "muscle-twitching," hot and cold flashes, aching muscles, and anorexia. The withdrawal syndrome in persons who have been taking methadone develops more slowly and is overtly less severe than heroin withdrawal, although users may perceive it as worse.

Complications

Many but not all complications of heroin addiction are related to unsanitary administration of the drug. The more frequent complications include pulmonary problems, hepatitis, arthritic conditions, immunologic alterations, and neurologic disorders. The effect of heroin addiction on pregnancy (see below) merits special mention.

Pulmonary problems: Pulmonary conditions found in narcotic addicts include aspiration pneumonitis, pneumonia, lung abscess, septic pulmonary emboli, atelectasis, and pulmonary fibrosis from talc granulomatosis. Chronic heroin addiction results in a decreased vital capacity and a mildly to moderately decreased pulmonary diffusion capacity. These effects are distinct from the unusual pulmonary edema that may be associated with overdose. In addition, many addicts smoke one or more packages of cigarettes/day. As a result, the addict is particularly susceptible to a variety of pulmonary infections.

Liver disturbance: Heroin addicts have a higher incidence of viral hepatitis, both Type A and Type B. The combination of viral hepatitis and the frequently high alcohol intake may account for a high incidence of liver dysfunction.

Musculoskeletal conditions: The most common problem is osteomyelitis (particularly lumbar vertebral), probably due to hematogenous spread of organisms from unsterile injections. Infectious spondylitis and sacroileitis have been reported. **Myositis ossificans ("drug abuser's elbow")** is extraosseous metaplasia of muscle damaged by inept needle manipulation; injury to the brachialis muscle is followed by replacement of the muscle bundle by a calcific mass.

Immunologic abnormalities: Hypergammaglobulinemia, involving both IgG and IgM, may be detected in up to 90% of addicts. A number of serologic tests have been found to be positive in heroin addicts (see TABLE 136-2). The reason for the immunologic changes is unknown, but they may reflect repeated antigenic stimulation, either from infections or from the daily parenteral injection of foreign substances. This altered immune state in heroin addicts may lead to such problems as splenomegaly, arthritis and arthralgia, lymphadenopathy, nephritis, and false-positive VDRL results.

Neurologic disorders that occur in heroin addicts are usually noninfectious complications of coma and cerebral anoxia. Additionally, toxic amblyopia (apparently due to quinine contamination of heroin), transverse myelitis, and a variety of mono- and polyneuropathies have been described. Recently, Guillain-Barré syndrome has been reported. Cerebral complications include those secondary to bacterial endocarditis (bacterial meningitis, mycotic aneurysm, brain abscess, and subdural and epidural abscesses), acute cerebral falciparum malaria, and the cerebral complications of viral hepa-

TABLE 136–2. PERCENTAGE FREQUENCY OF POSITIVE SEROLOGIC TESTS
IN HEROIN ADDICTS ENTERING TREATMENT

Serologic Tests	Frequency (%)
VDRL	15–30
Latex fixation	20
Tests for mononucleosis	10
C-reactive protein	20–30
Serum hepatitis	5–10
Lymphogranuloma venereum	20
Typhoid, O and H	15–25
Paratyphoid, A and B	10–30
Proteus OX-19	15–25
Q fever	5–15
Brucella	10–25
Coombs	5

titis and tetanus. Some neurologic complications are thought to be due to allergic responses to the heroin-adulterant mixture.

Other complications include superficial cutaneous abscesses, cellulitis, lymphangitis, lymphadenitis, and phlebitis from contaminated needles. Many heroin addicts begin with subcutaneous injections ("skin popping"). They may return to this mode when extensive scarring makes their veins no longer accessible. As addicts become more desperate, cutaneous ulcers in unlikely sites may be found. Contaminated needles and inoculum may also lead to bacterial endocarditis.

Pregnancy and opiate addiction: Problems of the heroin-addicted mother are transferred to the fetus; because heroin and methadone freely cross the placental barrier, the fetus readily becomes drug-dependent. Pregnant addicts seen early enough should be encouraged to enter a methadone maintenance program. Obviously, such plans should include the obstetrician and pediatrician who will treat the dependent infant. Pregnant women withdrawn from heroin or methadone late in the 3rd trimester of pregnancy risk the precipitation of labor. Pregnant women seen at or near term may be stabilized on methadone. The infants of dependent mothers may present with tremors, a high-pitched cry, jitters, convulsions, and tachypnea. For a discussion of problems of the neonate, including the **fetal alcohol syndrome,** see METABOLIC CONDITIONS in Vol. II, Ch. 21.

Treatment

The clinical management of narcotics addicts is extremely difficult. Physicians treating narcotic drug addicts should be fully aware of the federal, state, and local regulations concerning the treatment of addicts. Few physicians have had formal training or experience in the difficulties encountered in dealing with narcotics addicts and their companions and families, as well as the attitudes of society (including law enforcement officers, other physicians, and allied health personnel) toward the treatment of such individuals. The physician should be aware of locally available resources and usually should refer narcotics addicts to specialized treatment centers and not attempt to care for them in an office. If there are no specialized centers, close supervision of the patient with frequent contacts and close work with the patient's family and friends are necessary.

In order to legally use a narcotic drug in treating an addict, the existence of a physiologic heroin dependence must be established. This is a difficult diagnosis, since many individuals seeking treatment have minimal physical opiate dependence; this high incidence of psychologic heroin dependence has occurred because recently only low-grade heroin has been available and most addicts have not maintained a high enough level of heroin use to produce physiologic dependence. The following are helpful in assessing physiologic dependence: (1) a history of 3 or more narcotic injections/day, (2) the presence of fresh needle marks, (3) the presence of narcotic in a properly obtained urine specimen, and (4) observation of withdrawal symptoms and signs.

Management of acute intoxication (overdose): Naloxone (0.4 to 0.8 mg) given IV is the drug of choice, since it possesses no respiratory depressant properties. If the patient's unconsciousness is due to a narcotic, dramatic recovery occurs immediately following the administration of this antagonist. Since some patients become agitated, delirious, and combative as they recover from their comatose state, secure physical restraints may be required and should be applied before the narcotic antagonist is given. All patients treated for narcotic overdose should be hospitalized and observed for at least 24 h, since the action of the opiate antagonist is relatively short and respiratory depression may recur within several hours (especially with methadone). Pulmonary edema that may be severe enough to cause death from hypoxia is usually not responsive to naloxone and has an unclear relationship to overdosage.

The opiate withdrawal syndrome is self-limited, and although severely discomforting is not life-threatening. A patient admitted for withdrawal should be told that he will probably experience some unpleasant symptoms and should be reassured that they will not be allowed to progress to a dangerous level but that the medication he receives will be based on some objective physical signs of withdrawal. The patient's drug-seeking behavior usually begins with the first symptoms of withdrawal, and hospital personnel must always be alert to the possibility that he will try to obtain illicit supplies of drugs. Visitors may have to be restricted. Many patients with withdrawal symptoms have other medical problems that must be diagnosed and treated. Opiate users may have mixed addictions, and although providing appropriate withdrawal measures for each drug is theoretically feasible, for practical purposes this is not required.

Currently, **methadone substitution** is the preferred method of opiate withdrawal. Methadone is given orally in the smallest amount that will prevent severe signs of withdrawal but not necessarily all signs. Close observation of the patient is important, since his subjective symptoms are unreliable. Many of the symptoms of withdrawal can be mimicked by anxiety states. Generally, 20 mg/day of methadone will block the symptoms of severe withdrawal in almost all addicts. Higher doses should be given only on direct observations of the physical signs of withdrawal, since addicts are notoriously unreliable in reporting the size of their habits. Doses of 25 to 45 mg can produce unconsciousness if the person has not developed tolerance for heroin or methadone. Once a suppressing dose has been established, it should be reduced progressively *by not more than 20% each day.* Patients commonly become emotionally upset and frequently request additional medication. Chloral hydrate 500 to 1000 mg may be given orally for several nights to improve sleep. The acute manifestations of withdrawal usually subside within 7 to 10 days, but patients often complain of weakness, insomnia, and a severe pervasive anxiety for several months. Minor metabolic and physiologic effects of withdrawal may persist for up to 6 mo. It is appropriate to treat heroin withdrawal with oral methadone, but the usual low-grade level of dependence can be treated with propoxyphene napsylate or even benzodiazepines, which are not cross-tolerant to opiates.

It is now well documented that the central α-adrenergic drug **clonidine** can halt essentially all signs of opiate withdrawal. This probably relates to diminution of central adrenergic outflow secondary to stimulation of central α receptors (the same mechanism by which clonidine lowers BP). This theory supports the importance of central adrenergic discharge in the evolution of the opiate withdrawal syndrome. Clonidine is not a benign drug. In addition to causing hypotension and drowsiness, its withdrawal may precipitate restlessness, insomnia, irritability, tachycardia, and headache. Its general utility in treating opiate withdrawal awaits further study.

Recently a narcotic antagonist, **buprenorphine,** has provoked some interest. Unlike other antagonists used in treating opiate dependence, it has some agonist effects and users may find a tempering of withdrawal. Early studies indicate that the drug provokes little physical dependence itself. If this proves true the drug could be valuable both in detoxification and long-term treatment of opiate dependence.

Withdrawal from methadone: The abstinence syndrome induced by methadone is similar to that of heroin, but its onset is more gradual and delayed, beginning 36 to 72 h after discontinuing the drug. Deep muscle aches and "bone pains" are frequent complaints. Because the abstinence syndrome begins gradually, methadone addicts may be initially observed on admission. A urine sample should be obtained to document the methadone habit, and methadone provided as symptoms develop. Methadone withdrawal for individuals coming from methadone maintenance programs may be particularly difficult, since the addict's dose of methadone may be as high as 100 mg/day. In general, ambulatory detoxification should be begun by reducing the dose to 60 mg/day or less over several weeks before attempting complete detoxification.

Treatment of chronic opiate dependence: No consensus exists regarding long-term treatment of opiate-dependent users. Despite fiscal withdrawal, thousands of American opiate addicts are still in methadone maintenance programs. It was hoped that large enough doses of oral methadone in treating addicts (chiefly heroin) would enable them to move to socially productive lives because their supply problems would be met. Additionally, the methadone would block any effects of injected heroin and alleviate user's "drug hunger." For some, the plan has worked. For others, methadone just adds another drug problem to their alcohol use, intermittent heroin use, and desperate lives. Additionally, the widespread availability of methadone has established its role as an important drug of abuse in the culture.

Experiments with L-acetyl α-methadol (LAAM), a longer-acting synthetic opiate, give hope of help to some addicts and of removing the problem of expensive daily client visits or take-home medication which insures some diversion.

The therapeutic community concept emerged nearly 25 yr ago in response to the heroin problem. Synanon, Daytop Village, and Phoenix House pioneered this non-drug treatment in residential centers, and the movement has grown. The communal, relatively long-term (usually 15-mo) residential setting would, it was hoped, by training, education, and redirection help users achieve new lives. Like methadone maintenance, this mode has helped, indeed transformed, some. How well it works, how widely it may be applied, and how much funding the greater society will give remain unanswered questions.

DEPENDENCE OF THE BARBITURATE TYPE

Barbiturates and alcohol are strikingly similar in their syndromes of dependence, withdrawal, and chronic intoxication. The characteristics of drug dependence of the barbiturate/alcohol type are psychic dependence that may lead to periodic, as often as continuous, abuse, and a physical dependence that can be detected only after consumption of amounts considerably above the usual therapeutic or socially acceptable levels. When intake is reduced below a critical level, a self-limited abstinence syndrome ensues. Symptoms of withdrawal from barbiturates and other sedative-hypnotics can be suppressed completely with a barbiturate. Tolerance to barbiturates develops irregularly and incompletely so that considerable behavioral disturbances and psychotoxicity persist, depending on the pharmacodynamic effects of the drug. Some mutual but incomplete cross-tolerance exists between alcohol and the barbiturates as well as the nonbarbiturate sedative-hypnotics, including benzodiazepines.

Symptoms and Signs

Drug effects: In general, those dependent on sedatives and hypnotics, including barbiturates and benzodiazepines, prefer the rapid-onset drugs, e.g., secobarbital and pentobarbital. The signs of progressive sedative intoxication are depression of superficial skin reflexes, fine lateral-gaze nystagmus, slightly decreased alertness with coarser or rapid nystagmus, ataxia and slurred speech, and a positive Romberg's sign. With progression there is nystagmus on forward gaze, somnolence, marked ataxia with falling, confusion, deep sleep, small pupils, respiratory depression, and ultimately death. Patients on large doses of depressants frequently have difficulty thinking and show slowness of speech and comprehension with some dysarthria, poor memory, faulty judgment, narrowed attention span, and emotional lability. In general, the combination of slow thought, slurred speech, and bruises on the extremities from falling may suggest dependence on depressants.

Withdrawal effects: In susceptible patients, psychologic dependence on the drug may develop rapidly and, after only a few weeks, attempts to discontinue the drug exacerbate any initial insomnia and result in restlessness, disturbing dreams, frequent awakening, and feelings of tension in the early morning. The extent of physical dependence is related to the barbiturate dose and the length of time that it has been taken; for example, pentobarbital 200 mg/day may be ingested for many months without significant tolerance developing; 300 mg/day may induce an abstinence syndrome on terminating medication if ingested for more than 3 mo; and 500 to 600 mg/day may provoke an abstinence syndrome after 1 mo. Large doses of barbiturates (4 to 10 times the usual hypnotic dose) taken for 1 mo or more will probably induce some form of abstinence syndrome.

An abrupt withdrawal syndrome from large doses of barbiturates or tranquilizers produces a severe, frightening, and potentially life-threatening illness essentially similar to delirium tremens. Withdrawal from barbiturates carries a significant mortality rate and should always be undertaken in the hospital. Once the withdrawal syndrome has begun, reversing it is difficult, but with a careful schedule the symptoms can be minimized. The reestablishment of CNS stability requires about 30 days. Occasionally, after even properly managed withdrawal over 1 to 2 wk, a seizure may occur in the following 2 wk. Within the first 12 to 20 h after the withdrawal of a short-acting barbiturate, the patient becomes increasingly restless, tremulous, and weak. By the 2nd day, the tremulousness becomes more prominent, the deep tendon reflexes may be increased, and the patient becomes weaker. During the 2nd and 3rd days, convulsions occur in 75% of all patients taking 800 mg/day or more. The convulsions may progress to status epilepticus and death. From the 2nd to the 5th day, the untreated abstinence syndrome includes delirium, insomnia, confusion, and frightening visual and auditory hallucinations. Hyperpyrexia and dehydration often occur. With longer-acting barbiturates, symptoms may not begin for > 24 h, do not reach a peak for 5 to 7 days, and may last as long as 10 to 14 days.

It is now clearly established that a withdrawal syndrome similar to the barbiturate syndrome, although seldom as severe, may occur with benzodiazepines, particularly diazepam. Almost all patients so described have been heavy users of alcohol. The syndrome with these agents may be very long in development because of a long persistence of the drugs in the body. There are now a few reports of withdrawal syndromes from diazepam in patients who have taken relatively low doses (30 to 50 mg/day).

Treatment

The procedure for treating dependence on depressants, particularly barbiturates, is to reintoxicate the patient and then withdraw the drug on a strict schedule, being alert for signs of marked withdrawal. Before beginning withdrawal from barbiturates, one can evaluate sedative tolerance with a test dose of pentobarbital 200 mg orally given to the nonintoxicated, fasting patient; 1 to 2 h later this test dose produces drowsiness or sleep with response to arousal in individuals with no tolerance to pentobarbital. Patients with intermediate levels of tolerance may show some impairment, while patients tolerant to 900 mg or more show no signs of intoxication. If the 200-mg dose has no effect, the tolerance level can be determined by repeating the test q 3 to 4 h with a larger dose. Severe anxiety or agitation may increase the patient's tolerance. Once the 24-h dose to which the patient is tolerant has been ascertained, that dose of pentobarbital is usually given q.i.d. for 2 or 3 days to stabilize the patient, and is then decreased by 10%/day.

Alternatively, phenobarbital can be used: it does not produce the "high" of the more rapidly acting drugs, its action is prolonged so that it provides smoother sedation, and it is the anticonvulsant of choice. Shorter-acting barbiturates or other sedative-hypnotics or minor tranquilizers can be replaced by a dose of phenobarbital equivalent to ⅓ the average daily dose of the drug on which the patient has become dependent (see Table 136–3). Phenobarbital is given orally q.i.d., and the initial phenobarbital dose is reduced by 30 mg/day until the patient is drug-free. For example, if the patient has been taking secobarbital 1000 mg/day, the stabilizing dose of phenobarbital is 300 mg/day or 75 mg q 6 h. Since the initial daily dose must be estimated from the patient's history, there is obviously a large margin of error, and the patient must be observed closely for the first 72 h. If he remains agitated or anxious, the dosage should be increased; if he is drowsy, dysarthric, or has nystagmus, the dosage should be decreased. While patients are being detoxified, other sedatives and psychotropic medications should be avoided. However, if the patient is also taking antidepressant medications, especially the tricyclics, the antidepressant should not be abruptly discontinued but should be reduced over 3 to 4 days.

DEPENDENCE OF THE CANNABIS (MARIJUANA) TYPE

Drug dependence of the cannabis type arises from chronic or periodic administration of cannabis or cannabis substances. Its characteristics include some psychologic dependence because of the desired subjective effects but no physical dependence so that there is no abstinence syndrome when the drug is discontinued. The use of this agent on an episodic but continuous basis may be carried out without evidence of social or psychic dysfunction. In many users the term dependence with its obvious connotations probably is misapplied.

Use of this drug is widespread. In the USA it is commonly used in the form of cigarettes made from the dried plant, *Cannabis sativa*, or as hashish, the pressed resin of the plant. Recently, synthetic Δ-9 tetrahydrocannabinol (THC), an active constituent of marijuana, has become available for research; despite claims of dealers and users, it does not appear on the street.

Cannabis produces a dreamy state of consciousness in which ideas seem disconnected, uncontrollable, and freely flowing. Time, color, and spatial perceptions are distorted and enhanced. In general, there is a feeling of well-being, exaltation, excitement, and inner joyousness that has been termed a "high." Many of the psychologic effects seem to be related to the setting in which the drug is taken. An occasional panic reaction has occured, particularly in naive users, but these have become unusual as the culture has gained increasing familiarity with the drug. Communicative and motor abilities are decreased during the use of these drugs. Difficulty in depth perception and altered sense of timing, both of which are particularly hazardous during automobile driving, have been demonstrated. There are now several published reports of the exacerbation of schizophrenic symptoms by marijuana even in patients being treated with antipsychotic medication (e.g., chlorpromazine).

Metabolic products of marijuana are retained in the tissues for as long as 8 days. Lowered testosterone levels have been reported, although the biologic significance of this is uncertain.

In recent years, critics of marijuana use have become prominent and have enlisted much scientific data in support. A counter-reform movement opposed to decriminalization and the easy acceptance

Table 136–3. DOSES OF SOME COMMON SEDATIVES AND TRANQUILIZERS THAT HAVE PRODUCED PHYSICAL DEPENDENCE

Drug	Doses Producing Dependence (mg/day)	Time Necessary to Produce Dependence (days)	Dosage Equivalent to 30 mg Phenobarbital (mg)
Secobarbital	500– 600	30	100
Pentobarbital ("yellow jackets")......	500– 600	30	100
Amobarbital ("blues")	500– 600	30	100
Amobarbital-secobarbital combination ("rainbows")...................	500– 600	30	100
Glutethimide....................	1250–1500	60	500
Methyprylon....................	1200–1500	60	300
Ethchlorvynol	1500–2000	60	500
Meprobamate...................	2000–2400	60	400
Chlordiazepoxide	200– 300	60	25
Diazepam	60– 100*	40	10
Methaqualone...................	1800–2400	30	300
Chloral hydrate.................	2000–2500	30	500

* See also discussion of withdrawal effects, above.

of the drug in American society has emerged. Many of the claims regarding severe biologic impact are still uncertain, but some other points are not. The content of THC in American marijuana has increased. Much material is more potent than that used in the past and users now take more drugs at an earlier age. The emerging literature may answer questions as to higher dose toxicity; but the politics of marijuana use will remain controversial for a long time.

DEPENDENCE OF THE COCAINE TYPE

Cocaine is the prototype of a stimulant drug that in high doses produces euphoric excitement and, occasionally, hallucinatory experiences. These properties are highly esteemed by experienced drug users and lead to some degree of psychic dependence. Cocaine is probably the best example of a drug to which neither tolerance nor physical dependence develops, but to which psychic dependence develops that can lead to addiction. Since physical dependence does not occur, there is no abstinence syndrome when the drug is withdrawn. The tendency to continue taking the drug is strong. The effects differ strikingly with different modes of use. When injected or inhaled, cocaine produces a condition of hyperstimulation, alertness, euphoria, and feelings of great power. The excitation and "high" are similar to that produced by injection of high doses of amphetamine. Since cocaine is a very short-acting drug, heavy users may resort to injecting it IV q 10 or 15 min. With this repetition, toxic effects such as tachycardia, hypertension, mydriasis, muscle-twitching, formication ("cocaine bugs"), miniaturized visual hallucinations, sleeplessness, and extreme nervousness appear. Hallucinations and paranoid delusions may develop, as well as violent behavior; the individual may be dangerous at this time. The action of the drug, however, is sufficiently brief to prevent sustained aggressive activity. The pupils are maximally dilated, and elevations of heart rate, BP, and respiration result from the drug's sympathomimetic effect. An **overdose** of cocaine produces tremors, convulsions with a temporal lobe seizure pattern, and delirium. Death may be due to a cardiovascular collapse or respiratory failure. These severe toxic effects occur in the compulsive heavy user, who often has a history of heroin use. Probably a majority of users are episodic recreational users who voluntarily curtail their use, or find that the drug's high cost mandates episodic use.

Two recent developments should be mentioned. The smoking of "free-base" cocaine has become popular. This necessitates the conversion of the hydrochloride salt to the more combustible form. A flame is held to the converted material and the smoke inhaled. The speed of onset is shortened and the intensity of the high is magnified. Because the extraction utilizes flammable solvents, there have been a few serious explosions and burns.

Procaine when snorted produces local sensations not unlike cocaine and may even produce some "high." Powdered procaine is widely used to cut cocaine and is occasionally mixed with mannitol or lactose and sold as cocaine. It is widely sold by mail-order suppliers and is sometimes called "synthetic cocaine."

Treatment of acute cocaine intoxication is generally unnecessary because of the extremely short action of the drug. If an overdose requires intervention, IV barbiturates or diazepam may be used. However, the respiratory depression that accompanies cocaine poisoning can be worsened with large doses of sedatives. Anticonvulsants do not effectively prevent convulsions in cocaine overdose. Discontinuing the chronic and sustained use of cocaine requires considerable assistance, and the depression that may occur requires close supervision and treatment.

DEPENDENCE OF THE AMPHETAMINE TYPE

Because amphetamine and drugs with similar pharmacologic properties can elevate mood and induce a feeling of well-being, they are widely used as stimulants and anorexiants. Little physical dependence is created, and the withdrawal syndrome, if one exists, is not severe. Withdrawal is followed by a state of mental and physical depression and fatigue. Qualitatively, the psychologic effects are similar to those produced by cocaine; the psychologic dependence is variable. Unlike cocaine and most other CNS stimulants, amphetamine induces **tolerance.** Tolerance to amphetamine develops slowly, but a progressive increase in dosage can occur and permits the eventual ingestion or injection of amounts several hundredfold greater than the original therapeutic dose. The tolerance to various effects develops unequally, so that nervousness and sleeplessness persist and psychotoxic effects, such as hallucinations and delusions, may occur. However, even massive doses are rarely fatal. Chronic drug users have reportedly injected as much as 15,000 mg of amphetamine in 24 h without observable acute illness. For neophytes, however, rapid injection of 120 mg **may be fatal,** although some individuals have survived 400 to 500 mg.

Abusers of amphetamine are prone to accidents because of the excitation and grandiosity produced and the accompanying excessive fatigue of sleeplessness. IV administration may lead to serious antisocial behavior and can precipitate a schizophrenic episode. Adverse reactions to continued high doses of methamphetamine include (1) anxiety reactions during which the person is fearful and tremulous and concerned about his physical well-being; (2) an amphetamine psychosis in which the person misinterprets others' actions, hallucinates, and becomes unrealistically suspicious; (3) an exhaustion syndrome, involving an intense feeling of fatigue and need for sleep, after the stimulation phase; and (4) a prolonged depression during which suicide is a possibility.

A **paranoid psychosis** almost inevitably results from long-term use of high doses IV but can also result from large oral doses. This psychosis may rarely be precipitated either by a single large dose or by chronic moderate doses. Typical features of the amphetamine psychosis include feelings of persecution, delusions of reference, and feelings of omnipotence. Those who use high doses IV usually accept that they will sooner or later experience paranoia and are often able to cope with it. Nevertheless, when drug use becomes very intense, or toward the end of a long run, even well-practiced intellectual awareness may fail, and the user may respond to a delusional system. Recovery from even prolonged amphetamine psychosis is usual. The slow but complete recovery of users who have become thoroughly disorganized and paranoid is a striking phenomenon. The more florid symptoms fade within a few days or weeks, although some confusion and memory loss and some delusional ideas may commonly persist for months. There is significant sale of fake amphetamine, and many users now consume large amounts of caffeine in concert with phenylephrine, phenylpropanolamine, or pseudoephedrine.

Treatment

Symptomatically, other than general fatigue, sleepiness, and depression, there are no **withdrawal phenomena.** However, EEG changes are seen that fulfill physiologic criteria for dependence. Abrupt discontinuance of amphetamine is not without complications; withdrawal can uncover an underlying depression, or it may precipitate a depressive reaction, often with a suicidal potential. In many persons whose amphetamine intake masks chronic fatigue, withdrawal is followed by 2 or 3 days of intense tiredness or sleepiness. Patients recovering from an amphetamine psychosis may demonstrate severe anxiety and extreme restlessness. Therefore, withdrawal should generally be undertaken in a drug-free environment where hospital and nursing facilities are available.

The acute agitated psychotic state with paranoid delusions and auditory and visual hallucinations responds remarkably to phenothiazines; chlorpromazine 25 to 50 mg IM rapidly reverses the toxic psychotic conditions but may produce severe postural hypotension. Haloperidol 2.5 to 5 mg IM has been used effectively, since it rarely produces hypotension, but it greatly increases the risk of an alarming acute extrapyramidal motor reaction. Usually, reassurance and a quiet, nonthreatening environment will permit the patient to recover. Acidification of the urine with ammonium chloride 500 mg orally q 4 h will aid in amphetamine excretion.

DEPENDENCE OF THE HALLUCINOGEN TYPE

Hallucinogens include lysergic acid diethylamide (LSD), psilocybin, mescaline, peyote, 2,5-dimethoxy-4-methylamphetamine (DOM, "STP"), 5-methoxy-3,4-methylenedioxyamphetamine (MMDA), and other substituted amphetamines. Generally, other than LSD, the listed hallucinogen exotica are not available on the street, despite the beliefs of dealers and users. These substances induce a state of excitation of the CNS and central autonomic hyperactivity, manifested as changes in mood (usually euphoric, sometimes depressive) and perception. True hallucinations apparently rarely occur. Psychic dependence on hallucinogens varies greatly but is usually not intense. No evidence of physical dependence can be detected when the drugs are abruptly withdrawn. A high degree of tolerance to LSD develops and disappears rapidly. Individuals tolerant to any of these drugs are cross-tolerant to the others. The chief dangers to the individual are the psychologic effects and impairment of judgment, which can lead to dangerous decision-making or accidents.

Responses to the hallucinogens depend on several factors, including the individual's expectations, the setting, and his ability to cope with the perceptual distortions. Untoward reactions to LSD apparently have become rare. Adverse reactions to hallucinogens appear as anxiety attacks, extreme apprehensiveness, or panic states. Most often, these reactions quickly subside with appropriate management in a secure setting. However, some individuals (especially after using LSD) remain disturbed and may even show a **persistent psychotic state.** It is unclear whether the drug use has precipitated or uncovered a preexisting psychotic potential or whether this can occur in previously stable individuals.

Some persons, especially among those who are chronic or repeated users of hallucinogenic drugs and particularly with the use of LSD, may experience drug effects after they have discontinued use of the drug. Referred to as **"flashbacks,"** these episodes most commonly consist of visual distortions but can include distortions of virtually any sensation (including perceptions of time, space, or self-image) or hallucinations. Such episodes can be precipitated by use of marijuana, alcohol, or barbiturates, by stress or fatigue, or they may occur without apparent reason. The mechanisms that produce flashbacks are not known, but they tend to subside over a period of 6 mo to a year.

Treatment

Reassurance that the bizarre thoughts, visions, and sounds are due to the drug and not to a "nervous breakdown" will usually suffice in acute adverse reactions to hallucinogens. **Phenothiazines must be used with extreme caution,** because of the danger of hypotension, particularly if phencyclidine (see below) has been ingested. Short-acting barbiturates or minor tranquilizers such as chlordiazepoxide or diazepam may help reduce overwhelming anxiety.

For heavy users of hallucinogens, withdrawal of the drug is the simplest part of treatment; some may need psychiatric treatment for associated problems. Frequent contact and establishing a helpful relationship with a physician can be beneficial. Maintaining the patient's social functioning (e.g., school or work performance) may be more realistic than aiming for complete abstinence.

Persistent psychotic states or other psychologic disorders will require appropriate psychiatric care. Flashbacks may be transient and may not be unduly distressing to the patient, requiring no special treatment. However, they may be associated with anxiety and depression and may require therapy similar to that of the acute adverse reactions.

DEPENDENCE ON PHENCYCLIDINE (PCP)

PCP has emerged as an important drug of abuse. It is not easily classified and should be considered separately from the hallucinogenic drugs. It has a bewildering number of effects in the CNS, and its neuropharmacology is only poorly understood.

PCP was tested as an anesthetic agent in humans in the late 1950s because of an ability to isolate humans from noxious sensory input (dissociative anesthesia). It was withdrawn because individuals often experienced severe anxiety, delusional states, or frank psychosis postoperatively. Clinical testing stopped in 1962 and PCP appeared as a street drug in 1967. Initially sold deceptively as "THC," in recent years it has established its own market. Although once available as a veterinary anesthetic, essentially all street material results from illegal synthesis, not difficult to perform. Occasionally injected or ingested, it is most frequently sprinkled on smoking material (parsley, mint leaves, tobacco, marijuana), combusted, and inhaled. In recent years, much random violence and crime has been attributed to users of this drug, although as with past drug horror stories, this is not often well documented. There is some evidence that the number of emergency room visits caused by the drug has begun to decline, but PCP is one of the most dangerous agents to appear in American recreational drug use circles.

A giddy euphoria usually occurs with lower doses, often followed by bursts of anxiety or mood lability. Effects of higher doses include a withdrawn catatonic state, ataxia, dysarthria, muscular hypertonicity, and myoclonic jerks. Rotatory nystagmus is often helpful in making the diagnosis. Cardiovascular status is usually unaffected. At very high doses, coma, convulsions, severe hypertension, and death may occur, although fatalities are unusual. Prolonged psychotic states have apparently followed use.

In treatment, diazepam is often helpful, and is mandatory when seizure activity is present. Some clinicians feel that haloperidol is useful. There have been reports of hypotension when chlorpromazine was used. Diazoxide may be used when severe hypertension is present. PCP is highly lipid-soluble and may have a prolonged biologic persistence. It or its metabolites may remain in the CNS for lengthy periods. The basic character of the drug leads to surprisingly high secretion into the stomach, and prolonged gastric lavage has recovered large amounts. Lavage must be accompanied by acidification with ammonium chloride (or other agents) because this maneuver results in dramatic ionic trapping in the stomach and urine. Anecdotally, street users may resort to cranberry juice to hasten urinary excretion.

DEPENDENCE ON VOLATILE SOLVENTS

Use of industrial solvents and aerosol sprays to achieve a state of intoxication continues to be an endemic problem among juveniles. These volatile solvents (e.g., aliphatic and aromatic hydrocarbons, chlorinated hydrocarbons, ketones, acetates) along with ether, chloroform, and alcohol produce temporary stimulation before depression of the CNS occurs. Partial tolerance to the fumes develops with daily use, as does psychologic dependence, but an abstinence syndrome does not occur.

Acute symptoms of dizziness, slurred speech, unsteady gait, and drowsiness are seen early. Impulsiveness, excitement, and irritability may occur. As the CNS becomes more deeply affected, illusions, hallucinations, and delusions develop. The user experiences a euphoric dreamy "high," culminating in a short period of "sleep." Delirium with confusion, psychomotor clumsiness, emotional lability, and impairment of thinking are seen. The intoxicated state may last from minutes to an hour or more.

Complications may result from the effect of the solvent or from other toxic ingredients such as lead in gasoline. A syndrome of hepatic and renal failure may result from carbon tetrachloride. Injuries to brain, liver, kidney, and bone marrow occur and may be the effects of heavy exposure or hypersensitivity. Death occurs from respiratory arrest, cardiac arrhythmias, or asphyxia due to occlusion of the airway.

Treatment of solvent-dependent children is difficult, and relapse is frequent. Intensive attempts to improve the patient's self-esteem and status in family, school, and society may be helpful.

DEPENDENCE ON VOLATILE NITRITES

Reinhalation of amyl nitrite ("poppers") to alter consciousness and enhance sexual pleasure has emerged in recent years. This use has been particularly prominent in urban male homosexual society. When amyl nitrite was returned to the prescription drug category, entrepreneurs began to market other nitrites (butyl, isobutyl) under a variety of tradenames, e.g., "Locker Room," "Rush," and others. At this time there is little evidence that the products have significant hazard, although they produce a predictable nitrite vasodilating effect with brief hypotension, dizziness, and flushing, followed by reflex tachycardia.

137. PSYCHOSEXUAL DISORDERS

Accepted norms of sexual behavior and attitudes vary greatly within and among different cultures. **Masturbation,** once widely regarded as a perversion and a cause of mental disease, is now recognized as a normal sexual activity throughout life. It is considered a symptom only when it suggests an inhibition of partner-oriented behavior. Its cumulative incidence is approximately 97% in males and 80% in females. While masturbation per se causes no harm, guilt over masturbation created by disapproving and punitive attitudes may create considerable distress and damage the capacity for sexual performance.

The Kinsey report revealed that about 5% of the population are preferentially **homosexual** for their entire lives. Several countries have passed laws permitting homosexual relationships between consenting adults. The American Psychiatric Association has officially ruled that homosexuality should no longer be considered a psychiatric disease, but this concept is in dispute. Provision is made, however, for the treatment of homosexuals whose desires create such distress that they are motivated to reduce their homosexual arousal and to increase their capacity for heterosexual arousal.

Frequent sexual activity with many partners, often one-time-only encounters, is an indication of diminished capacity for pair-bonding. **Extramarital sexuality** is discouraged by most cultures, but **premarital coitus** is accepted as normal by most. In the USA over 80% of both men and women have intercourse prior to marriage. This is in keeping with a recent shift in developed countries toward more freedom of sexual expression. **Dysfunction of arousal and orgasm** in the male and female is discussed in Vol. II, Ch. 9. **Illegitimacy** arouses disapproval and causes social disadvantage in many countries, while in others a high proportion of children are born out of wedlock and are not ostracized. Although illegitimacy is well tolerated in some cultures, illegitimate children reared by a single parent or handed over to surrogates who cannot form a close emotional bond with the child in the formative years in some instances may be less likely to mature normally and may be at increased risk of developing emotional disorders or frank mental illness. The data are inconclusive on **children** (not illegitimate) **raised by a single, divorced parent.** Many parents remarry; others have a variety of support systems, e.g., grandparents.

Individuals whose sexual practices include small amounts of **fetishism** and **sadomasochism** generally have normal love relationships. Such tendencies may excite anxiety and distress but call for reassurance rather than therapy. However, if sexual drives are absorbed entirely in submission to flagellation, are vented only on articles of clothing, or are expressed wholly in **exhibitionism** or **voyeurism,** the individual's capacity for establishing love relationships is stunted, and other aspects of his personal and emotional adjustment suffer.

Doctors can offer sensitive and disciplined advice on sexual matters, and should not miss opportunities for helpful intervention by overestimating the influence of cultural diversity. The strength of the sexual drive, the needs of individuals, and the frequency of sexual contact are subject to great variation.

Etiology and Incidence

Etiology is complex and includes a variety of factors whose relative importance varies from case to case. Inherited or subtle constitutional factors probably play a part. The important role of fetal androgens in preparing the brain for later sexual activity suggests that interference with this process may render a person vulnerable to damaging environmental influences occurring during childhood psychosexual development. Parental attitude toward sexual behavior is important. A forbidding puritanical rejection of physical sexuality engenders guilt and shame and inhibits the capacity for enjoying sex.

In forming a secure **sexual identity (sense of maleness or femaleness)** and **gender identity (sense of masculinity or femininity**—see below) the character of the parents' emotional bond and the relationship that each of them has with the child is important. The parent of the same sex must be a person with whom the child can identify. The opposite-sex parent must engender enough love and trust so that the child later feels comfortable with members of the opposite sex. Relations with parents may be damaged by excessive emotional distance, by punitive behaviors, or by seductiveness and exploitation. The child has to feel accepted and lovable. Children exposed to hostility, rejection, and cruelty are liable to sexual maladjustment. (Establishing the individual's confidence that he is capable and worthy of being loved for himself is one of the goals of therapy.)

These potentially damaging parent-child relationships can lead to disorders of gender identity such as transsexualism, to one of the paraphilias, to homosexuality, or to dysfunctions in sexual performance. Another outcome can be a **dissociation of sexual behavior,** so that emotional bonds can be formed with others from the individual's own social class or intellectual circle, but physical sexual relationships are possible only with those considered as inferiors, such as prostitutes, with whom the individual has no affinity and no emotional ties. In these maladjustments the sexual act is associated with guilt and anxiety, and other outlets are found in relationships or practices in which sexual emotions are not aroused.

Sexual deviation is far more common among men than women, and this unequal distribution has been found in most cultures studied. Since reproductive competence in the female is of decisive importance for the species, and less so in the male, biologic reasons for the unequal distribution may exist. Developmentally, males must transfer their infantile identification with their mothers to their fathers during the preschool or oedipal period, from about the age of 3 to about 6, whereas females need not pass through this process of changing identification. The need to "disidentify" during a critical period of psychosexual development creates greater vulnerabilities for the male, hence the enormous preponderance of males affected by the paraphilias.

The pattern of erotic arousal is fairly well developed before puberty; therefore, if something goes awry, the causes for gender or paraphiliac disorders should be sought in the prepubertal years. Three general factors are present: (1) anxiety interferes with normal psychosexual development; (2) a displacement to another pattern of arousal allows the person to avoid the standard pattern of erotic arousal while retaining the capacity for sexual pleasure; and (3) the pattern of sexual arousal often has both symbolic and conditioning facets (e.g., the fetish "chosen" symbolizes the object of arousal but may have developed by an accidental association of the fetish with sexual curiosity, desire, and excitement). Whether *all* transsexual or homosexual development is created by these psychodynamic processes is still controversial; for many, it is true.

GENDER IDENTITY DISORDERS

Disorders due to feelings of discomfort and inappropriateness about one's anatomic sex. When there is confusion in sex-labeling and rearing, children will become confused about their gender identity. However, even the presence of ambiguous genitalia will not affect the child's gender identity if sex-labeling and rearing are unambiguous.

TRANSSEXUALISM

A transsexual believes that he is the victim of a biologic accident, cruelly imprisoned within a body incompatible with his real sexual identity. Most are men who consider themselves to have feminine gender identity and regard their genitalia and masculine features with repugnance. Their primary objective in seeking psychiatric help is not to obtain psychologic treatment but to secure surgery that will give them as close an approximation as possible to a female body. The diagnosis is made only if the disturbance has been continuous (not limited to periods of stress) for at least 2 yr, is not symptomatic of another mental disorder such as schizophrenia, and is not associated with genital ambiguity or genetic abnormality.

In true **male transsexuals** the condition begins in early childhood with indulgence in girls' games, fantasies of being female, repugnance at the physical changes that attend puberty, and thereafter a quest for a feminine gender identity. Many transsexuals are adept at acquiring the skills that enable them to adopt a feminine gender identity. Some patients are satisfied with being given help to achieve a more feminine appearance, together with employment and an identity card that enables them to work and live in society as women. Others are not content with changing their social identity but can be helped to achieve a more stable adjustment with small doses of feminizing hormones. Many transsexuals request feminizing operations in spite of the sacrifices entailed. The decision for surgery sometimes raises grave social and ethical problems. Since some follow-up studies have provided evidence that *some* true transsexuals achieve more happy and productive lives with the aid of surgery, it is justified in carefully selected men. After surgery, the patients need assistance with movement, gesture, and voice production. Some homosexual men, usually with serious personality problems, request reallocation surgery. The results in these patients are unsatisfactory from both a medical and social viewpoint.

Female transsexuals increasingly present in medical and psychiatric practice. Nearly all those who seek treatment are the dominant members in lesbian partnerships. The patient asks for mastectomy, hysterectomy, and oophorectomy and also wants androgenic hormones to alter her voice and promote a more masculine appearance. She may ask for an artificial phallus to be fashioned by plastic surgery. Stable and effective personalities whose social adaptation in most spheres of their lives has been successful may sometimes be helped to achieve greater satisfaction through limited surgical help, but heroic surgery should be avoided.

GENDER IDENTITY DISORDER OF CHILDHOOD

DSM-III (*Diagnostic and Statistical Manual of Mental Disorders* of the American Psychiatric Association, Third Edition) describes the essential features of this disorder as a persistent feeling of discomfort and inappropriateness in a child about his or her anatomic sex and a desire to be, or a conviction that he or she is, of the opposite sex. This disorder is apparently rare, and the clinician must be careful to differentiate between the child with this disorder and the much more frequent rejection of stereotypical sex-role behavior (e.g., tomboyishness in girls or sissyish behavior in boys). The children with a gender identity disorder have a profound disturbance of the normal sense of maleness or femaleness, and will strongly and persistently state a desire to be of the other sex, or will insist that they are. (Individuals who develop transsexualism have evidenced gender identity problems as children.)

Girls regularly have male peer groups and are avidly interested in sports and rough-and-tumble play; they are disinterested in playing with female-type dolls or in playing house. Boys invariably are preoccupied with female stereotypical activities such as dressing in girls' or women's clothes, or have a compelling desire to participate in the girls' games. They choose toys and games that are most usually favored by girls, and frequently demonstrate gestures and actions usually regarded as feminine. They encounter considerable male peer-group teasing and rejection.

Of the boys who cross-dress, 75% begin prior to their 4th birthday. Doll-playing begins during the same period. Social ostracism and conflict become significant at about age 7 or 8. The age of onset in females is also early, but a majority give up this pattern in late childhood or adolescence. A minority of the girls remain identified as males, and some of these develop a homosexual arousal pattern. A smaller number from each sex may later develop transsexualism. The condition may be reversible with long-term psychotherapy and family therapy; the data are not yet conclusive.

Intersexuality

Confusion over gender identity may arise if the child is born with ambiguous genitalia. These children are sometimes called **hermaphrodites,** although most are **pseudohermaphrodites.** Male pseudohermaphrodites have testicular tissue; females have ovarian tissue. In true hermaphrodites, both testicular and ovarian tissues coexist.

The sex of rearing should be determined by the probable course of development at adolescence. If corrective surgery is recommended, it should be carried out very early, whenever possible prior to 18 mo of age. Intersex states are discussed in more detail in Vol. II, Ch. 25.

PARAPHILIAS

DSM-III defines these disorders as *gross impairment in the capacity for affectionate sexual activity between adult human partners.* The paraphilias are far more common in males than females. They usually require long-term psychotherapy, with the individual's motivation not coerced, e.g., by court order. Group therapy for some sex offenders is helpful. Anti-androgen treatment for pedophiliacs, rapists, and lust murderers may be helpful.

FETISHISM

The essential feature of fetishism is the use of nonliving objects as the preferred exclusive method of producing sexual excitement. When a man achieves gratification by sexual stimulation caused by his wearing some feminine garment, usually an article of underclothing, the diagnosis of transvestism rather than fetishism should be made. The fetish may replace sexual activity with a partner or may be integrated into sexual behavior with a partner. When the latter occurs, the fetish is required for erotic arousal. Commonly used fetishes are female undergarments, shoes, and boots—less commonly, parts of the human body such as hair or nails. Minor fetishistic behavior incorporated into heterosexual behavior cannot be regarded as aberrant. When the fetishistic arousal pattern is more intense, it generates serious problems in the relationship. When the fetish becomes the sole object of sexual desire, normal sexual relations are avoided.

TRANSVESTISM

Dressing by men in the clothes of the opposite sex. Usually the transvestite achieves a certain amount of sexual excitement, and public display may give much satisfaction. Despite their deviation, many transvestites manage to have reasonably happy marriages. When their wives are cooperative, men have intercourse in feminine attire. When their wives are not cooperative, anxiety, depression, guilt, and shame associated with the desire to cross-dress are common. Unless there is marital conflict, few transvestites seek treatment.

ZOOPHILIA

Sexual excitement produced by the act or fantasy of engaging in sexual activity with animals as the preferred or exclusive method. DSM-III states that the animal may be the object of intercourse or may be trained to sexually excite the human partner by licking or rubbing. The animal is preferred even when other forms of sexual outlet are available. Shame, guilt, and social isolation with depression, anxiety, and loneliness may result from the intense and persistent desire to engage in this extremely rare form of sexual activity.

PEDOPHILIA

As described by DSM-III, *a preference for repetitive sexual activity with prepubertal children.* Arbitrarily, the age difference between the adult with this disorder and the child victim is set at 10 yr or more. Twice as many pedophiliacs prefer opposite-sex children to same-sex children. Heterosexually oriented males tend to prefer girls 8 to 10 yr; in most cases, the adult is known to the child. Looking or touching seems to be more prevalent than genital contact. With homosexually oriented males, the age of the preferred partner is 10 to 13 yr, and casual acquaintanceship is higher than in the heterosexually oriented group. Adults who have no sexual preference prefer children under the age of 8.

Sexual offenses against children constitute a significant proportion of reported criminal sexual acts. The recidivism rate for homosexual pedophilia is second only to exhibitionism, and ranges from 13 to 28% of those apprehended—roughly twice the rate of heterosexual pedophilia.

EXHIBITIONISM

As described by DSM-III, *repetitive acts of genital exposure to an unsuspecting stranger for the purpose of producing sexual excitement.* It is rare that further sexual contact is sought. About 1/3 of apprehended male sex offenders are exhibitionists. These persons have the highest recidivism rate of all sex offenders; about 20% get rearrested. The victim is usually a female adult or child. Most exhibitionists are married, but the marriage is often troubled by poor sexual adjustment, including frequent psychosexual dysfunction. A very few cases of exhibitionism in women have been reported.

VOYEURISM

Voyeurs become sexually aroused by looking at unsuspecting women who are naked, in the act of disrobing, or engaging in sexual activity. The essential feature of this condition is a repetitive seeking-out of these situations. Orgasm usually produced by masturbation may occur during the voyeuristic activity. The voyeur does not initiate further sexual contact. The disorder has to be differentiated from normal sexual curiosity occurring between people who know each other.

SEXUAL MASOCHISM

Intentional participation in an activity in which the individual is physically harmed or the individual's life is threatened in order to produce sexual excitement, or if the preferred or exclusive mode of producing sexual excitement is to be humiliated, bound, beaten, or otherwise made to suffer. Masochistic fantasy without masochistic behavior is an insufficient basis for the diagnosis of sexual masochism. Fantasies are fairly frequent, whereas masochistic behavior is relatively uncommon. A potentially dangerous form of masochism entails various forms of physical self-constraint and partial asphyxiation, which can lead to accidental death. These have been reported only for men.

SEXUAL SADISM

The inflicting of physical or psychologic suffering on the sexual partner as a method of stimulating sexual excitement and orgasm. Generally there are insistent and persistent fantasies in which sexual excitement is produced as a result of suffering inflicted on the partner, but the fantasies alone without behavior are an insufficient basis for the diagnosis. The partner may or may not be consenting, but even if consenting, the diagnosis is warranted if bodily injury is extensive or mortal. Sadism has to be differentiated from minor manifestations of aggression in normal sexual activity. There is a spectrum of intensity with regard to sexual sadism. DSM-III states that at the more extreme end are individuals who require that the sexual partner must suffer in order for sexual excitement to occur; such individuals may brutally rape or torture victims. At the most extreme part of the spectrum are lust murderers, in whom sexual excitement is produced by the death of the victim. The act of rape is essentially aggressive, not sexual, and most rapists are not motivated by sexually sadistic impulses. Approximately 1 rapist in 4 experiences enhanced sexual excitement by sadistic fantasies or behavior.

HOMOSEXUALITY

A transient stage of homosexual conduct in puberty and adolescence is common (1/3 of male adolescents), but almost all persons who experience this, even those who engage in some form of physical contact, later become exclusively heterosexual in their preferences. Approximately 5% of males are exclusively homosexual during their entire lives. A majority report some heterosexual contact that was soon abandoned after initial experiences. Perhaps 33% of male homosexuals and a larger percentage of female homosexuals **(lesbians)** are capable of heterosexual performance and even pleasure, even though they are preferentially homosexual. About 20% of homosexual men and 33% of homosexual women marry, but their heterosexual marriages are unstable.

Preferential or exclusive homosexuality has to be distinguished from **situational (facultative) homosexuality,** frequently exhibited by men and women confined for long periods with members of their own sex, as on board ship or in prison. Usual sexual behavior is resumed on release from such environments.

Sexual acts between homosexuals consist mostly of expressions of tenderness, fondling, caressing, and kissing. Orgasm is achieved through mutual masturbation, fellatio (taking the penis in the mouth), or anal intercourse. It is uncommon for one partner to adopt an exclusively active or passive role, and most homosexuals participate in the relationship in a variety of ways.

Between 15 to 20% of homosexuals are capable of long-lasting partnerships. Casual, shallow contacts with strangers are more frequent; 28% of male homosexuals report having more than 1000 partners. Because of this promiscuity, sexually transmitted diseases are frequent. Only 5% of homosexuals posture effeminately; most homosexuals are repelled by such behavior. Many homosexuals are emotionally stable, conducting normal lives and considering themselves happy, but the prevalence of depression, psychosomatic illness, and suicide seems higher among homosexuals than in the general population. Emotional disturbance increases with advancing years. Unless they have formed "close-coupled" relationships, many homosexuals suffer increasing isolation and rejection as they advance to middle or late life and are rejected by the homosexual culture, which highly values youth and physical attractiveness.

Female homosexuals are more capable than male homosexuals of "close-coupled" relationships, and engage in casual sexual contacts far less frequently than their male counterparts. Psychiatric illnesses are also less common among lesbians than among male homosexuals. Whether this is intrinsic or due to more favorable societal reactions, or is a result of a combination of the 2 is not clear.

Etiology

Etiology is not known. Some psychiatrists ascribe the condition to failure of identification with the parent of the same sex and a close-binding seductive relationship with the parent of the opposite sex; however, many children raised in such environments do not exhibit homosexual behavior. The constitutional factors involving hormonal programming of the brain during fetal life may be a significant factor, but this is still a speculative hypothesis.

Treatment and Prognosis

Unless the homosexual wishes to change his sexual orientation, treatment for homosexuality is not indicated. If there is, however, a sustained pattern of homosexual arousal that is a persistent source of distress, the diagnosis is **ego-dystonic homosexuality**, and treatment is warranted. Some homosexuals enter treatment for alleviation of distress caused by problems in their relationships or employment, and develop a motivation for change, but most have no wish to do so. Treatment is possible only if motivation for change is high. The prognosis for change is better if there is a history of heterosexual behavior and fantasies. Otherwise, limited goals must be set in treatment. Help in overcoming crises or mitigating emotional distress, and simple psychotherapy to assist the individual in achieving a realistic, satisfying adjustment to his social predicament are all that is needed in most cases. The best methods of therapy for those homosexuals who are strongly motivated to change draw on both behavior therapy technics and psychotherapy, including group therapy. The advice of specialists should be sought before even raising questions about treatment aimed at altering fundamental attitudes in any particular case. Endocrine treatments are valueless.

138.　THE NEUROSES

Disorders in which specific, usually ego-alien, and distressing neurotic symptoms occur, i.e., anxieties, phobias, obsessions, compulsions, and hysterical conversion and dissociative phenomena.

The neuroses comprise one of the 3 major categories of nonorganic psychiatric disorders, which also include the psychoses and personality (or character) disorders. Neurotic illness is not usually characterized by the major alterations in mental function and severe disturbances in cognitive and perceptual processes (e.g., delusions, hallucinations) seen in the psychoses; also, the capacity to distinguish between fantasy and reality (reality testing) remains generally intact in neurotic illness, in contrast to its partial or complete absence in the psychoses. The significant aberrations in behavior patterns and personal relationships seen in the personality disorders also may occur in neurotic individuals.

ANXIETY NEUROSIS

(Anxiety Disorder; Anxiety Reaction)

A neurotic disorder characterized by chronic, unrealistic anxiety often punctuated by acute attacks of anxiety or panic. Anxiety neurosis afflicts 5% of the population, is characteristically a disorder of young adults, and affects women twice as often as men.

Etiology

Both psychologic and physiologic factors cause anxiety neurosis, and there also is evidence of a genetic influence.

Psychologic factors: Emotional stress often precipitates anxiety (e.g., threatened or actual changes in personal relationships). The precipitant is not so obvious when inner emotional drives (sexual, aggressive, or dependency needs) are a source of conflict, because psychologic defenses keep them from the individual's conscious awareness. The drives are aroused by environmental events to which the person is especially sensitized, and anxiety represents the individual's fear of losing control of these drives and of his resulting actions.

Physiologically, anxiety is associated with autonomic nervous system discharge (fight or flight reaction) set in motion by the arousal of frightening inner impulses and emotions. The resulting bodily sensations (see below) are mediated by limbic system discharges (in which catecholamine metabolism plays a central role) and their peripheral effects on the neurohumoral processes of the autonomic nervous system.

Clinical Features

Anxiety is a symptom in all psychiatric disorders, but it occurs alone or as the primary symptom in anxiety neurosis. **Acute anxiety attacks (panic)** form the cardinal feature of anxiety neurosis and are among the most painful life experiences. They may occur repetitively over a period of time and are self-limited, generally lasting a few minutes to an hour or 2. The patient experiences a subjective sense of terror that arises for no evident reason, and a haunting dread of some nameless, imminent catastrophe, temporarily preventing rational thinking. Of the somatic symptoms integral to anxiety, the most common are cardiorespiratory, with tachycardia, palpitations, occasional premature beats, and precordial pain usually described as sharp or sticking in quality. Trembling, visible as a fine tremor of the outstretched hands, sweating, complaints of "butterflies in the stomach," and generalized motor weakness and dizziness are common; nausea and occasionally diarrhea occur. The patient may notice a feeling of unreality and loss of contact with people and objects in his environment. A sense of air hunger leading to hyperventilation often is experienced. This can result in a secondary respiratory alkalosis, and varying degrees of muscular stiffness in the extremities and a feeling of pins and needles or numbness around the mouth and in the fingers and toes— **hyperventilation syndrome** (see Respiratory Alkalosis in Ch. 81 and the discussion of psychogenic dyspnea in Ch. 29). These secondary symptoms compound the patient's anxiety and add to his frequent conviction that he is about to lose consciousness or die.

Chronic anxiety: Symptoms are similiar to those of acute anxiety attacks, but are less intense and of longer duration, lasting days, weeks, or months. The patient is aware of a generalized tension and apprehension, a tendency to startle easily, an uneasiness and nervousness at work or with people, a vague, nagging uncertainty about the future that may be accompanied by chronic fatigue, headaches, insomnia, and a variety of subacute autonomic symptoms. Although the syndrome is not completely disabling, the patient is chronically uncomfortable in his daily activities and personal relationships, and often finds his capacity for effective work compromised by chronic fatigue and difficulties in concentration.

Diagnosis

Because of the cardiac manifestations, anxiety attacks may be mistaken for myocardial infarction. Similarly, the autonomic symptoms secondary to a pheochromocytoma and the hyperarousal resulting from Graves' disease may imitate the clinical picture of anxiety neurosis. Appropriate physical and laboratory examinations usually establish the proper diagnosis.

Course and Prognosis

Mild anxiety tends to be chronic, punctuated by acute anxiety attacks of varying frequency and intensity. Roughly 1/3 of patients recover, with men having a better prognosis than women. Anxiety symptoms often become less severe and troublesome with middle age.

Treatment

Psychologic measures: Insight psychotherapy (in patients properly selected by the criterion of psychologic-mindedness), aimed at uncovering the unconscious conflicts, may bring about psychologic changes that lead to increased self-knowledge and tolerance of internal drives. **Supportive psychotherapy** may reduce symptoms through reassurance and the relationship with an understanding, sympathetic physician. **Relaxation technics** permit some voluntary control over autonomic functions that diminish hyperactivity. **Meditation** is a specific and often effective form of relaxation. In individuals with a capacity for entering hypnotic trance, **hypnosis** can potentiate the effects of the relaxation technics.

Pharmacologic measures: Medications that lower responsiveness to stress are helpful. Minor tranquilizers such as chlordiazepoxide (5 to 10 mg 3 to 4 times/day orally) or diazepam (2 to 5 mg 3 to 4 times/day orally) are often effective in controlling the symptoms of chronic or anticipatory anxiety (see Agoraphobia, below). Furthermore, recent clinical studies indicate the often dramatic relief from panic attacks to be obtained with therapeutic doses of tricyclic antidepressant medication (imipramine) or monoamine oxidase (MAO) inhibitors (phenelzine). Medications generally should be used along with, not as a substitute for, appropriate psychotherapy.

PHOBIC NEUROSIS

(Phobic Disorder; Phobic Reaction)

A neurotic disorder characterized by the presence of irrational or exaggerated fears of objects, situations, or bodily functions not inherently dangerous or the appropriate source of the anxiety. Anxiety, both acute and chronic, is a prominent feature, but unlike the free-floating anxiety of anxiety neurosis, it is bound to and associated with exposure to specific environmental stimuli. Phobic disorders affect less than 1% of the population, comprise about 5% of neuroses found in patients > 18 yr, and occur more frequently in women.

Etiology

Etiology is in many respects similar to that of neurotic anxiety in general; i.e., phobias appear to be associated with an increased family history of anxiety disorders, and the anxiety itself is a fearful reaction to the threatened emergence of forbidden, unconscious drives, a reaction that is expressed in excessive activity of the autonomic nervous system. However, a further set of psychologic mechanisms **(projection, displacement)** focuses the anxiety on specific external objects or situations, which then come to represent the underlying, original source of the anxiety. The shifting and binding of the anxiety to the external secondary symbol enables the individual to utilize the further defensive maneuver of **avoidance** of the object in order to control arousal of the painful anxiety. Choice of the phobic symbol is often determined by a chance exposure to the object at a time when the anxiety over a threatening inner impulse first appeared. The phobic object, in other words, becomes a conditioned stimulus, and the phobic neurosis is, in effect, a learned response.

Clinical Features

The very thought of the phobic object is sufficient to induce anxiety, and as the patient comes closer in reality to the phobic stimulus, the anxiety mounts to an intensity reaching a state of panic. As a result, the patient protects himself from experiencing the anxiety by avoiding the phobic stimulus, which often leads to a disabling constriction in his daily life and capacity for normal functioning. In some phobic individuals, **counterphobic behavior** develops (*the active seeking out of exposure to phobic, often dangerous situations, e.g., the individual with a fear of heights who becomes an alpine rock climber*).

Agoraphobia (*a fear of open, public places or of situations where crowds are to be found*) is the commonest (60%) of the phobic disorders. The individual's activities are severely restricted; in the extreme he cannot leave the security of his home. Agoraphobia often begins with the sudden onset of a panic attack in some public place; subsequently, anticipatory anxiety that the attack will recur causes the individual to remain at home to avoid a reemergence of the painful affect. Frequently, the agoraphobic patient can face the phobic situation without undue discomfort if in the company of someone with whom he has a close relationship— the so-called **obligatory companion.**

Phobias of objects (simple phobias) are commonly seen as transitory phenomena during early childhood (e.g., fear of the darkness or of animals). Adults also may develop specific, localized neurotic fears of a variety of objects. If the objects are uncommon or easily avoided, no serious disability results. However, great inconvenience may occur, e.g., in a businessman with a phobia of planes whose work requires frequent air travel.

Phobias of function (social phobias), in which anxiety is aroused by the presence of others, are less common than the other types. Most frequent manifestations are a fear of blushing (erythrophobia), which causes the victim to shun social situations, or a fear of eating, which leads to an avoidance of dining in public places.

Diagnosis

The sudden outbreak of severe phobias may herald the onset of a schizophrenic psychosis or occasionally may be seen in patients with a chronic schizophrenic disorder. The course of the latter illness and the presence of thought disorder and other psychotic features (hallucinations, delusions) suggest a psychosis. Phobic patients sometimes become depressed because of their failure to overcome their phobic avoidance, but this is secondary to the phobic neurosis itself and disappears when the phobia is resolved.

Course and Prognosis

The phobic disorder usually begins in early adulthood and has a chronic course of exacerbations and remissions. Agoraphobia is not only severely disabling but is the least likely of the phobic disorders to manifest significant remissions. Spontaneous remission of phobic neurosis is less likely in patients steadily symptomatic for over a year.

Treatment

Psychotherapy: Insight psychotherapy may be effective. However, despite significant changes in the patient's psychologic functioning and structure, the phobic symptoms may persist and require more active technics focused specifically on bringing about their removal, e.g., **behavior therapy.** These technics decondition the patient to the phobic stimulus by requiring him to confront the stimulus while using relaxation technics (including hypnosis) to combat the anxiety aroused by the stimulus (reciprocal inhibition). **Flooding** is an extreme behavioral procedure that requires the patient to experience prolonged intense anxiety from a direct, continued exposure to the phobic stimulus.

Pharmacotherapy: Minor tranquilizers (see in Ch. 247) are helpful in reducing the intensity of the anticipatory anxiety; the patient is better able to face the phobic stimulus and work toward complete desensitization. Furthermore, the eruption of panic attacks often is completely prevented with therapeutic doses of tricyclic antidepressive medication (imipramine) or MAO inhibitors (phenelzine).

OBSESSIVE-COMPULSIVE NEUROSIS

(Obsessive-Compulsive Disorder; Obsessional Neurosis)

A neurotic disorder characterized by the presence of recurrent ideas and fantasies (obsessions) and repetitive impulses or actions (compulsions) that the patient recognizes as morbid and toward which he feels a strong inner resistance.

Anxiety is a central feature, but in contrast to the phobias (where the patient is anxious in the face of external dangers of which he perceives himself to be the passive victim), the anxiety arises in response to internally derived thoughts and urges that the patient fears he may actively carry out despite his wishes not to. Obsessive-compulsive patients comprise less than 5% of those with neurotic disorders, and about 0.05% of the population at large. The neurosis affects men and women equally and tends to be found in individuals from upper socioeconomic levels and with higher intelligence.

Etiology

There is some evidence of a higher incidence in the families of obsessive-compulsive patients than in control populations.

Psychodynamic theory: The obsession is the ideational component of an underlying, forbidden impulse, most commonly aggressive in quality, that emerges into consciousness. Through the defense mechanism of **isolation,** the affective component of the drive is separated from the ideational content, so that the individual experiences only an insistent thought, unaccompanied by any awareness of a wish to realize the idea or that it stems from a hidden impulse. Despite the defense of isolation, the idea is too close to the forbidden drive. Therefore, the idea becomes the source of anxiety and motivates the further defensive maneuver of **undoing,** in the form of a secondary magical compulsive act.

Learning theory: An originally neutral thought becomes capable of arousing anxiety through its association with an unconditioned anxiety-provoking stimulus. When a subsequent action reduces that anxiety, the act becomes fixed as a compulsive ritual and a stable, but nonadaptive, learned psychologic structure is created.

Clinical Features

Obsessions: Ideas, words, and images, usually disconnected and unrelated to what the individual is doing, force themselves on his attention with a power and insistence that he cannot resist. They are often colored by an aggressive, sexual, or scatologic quality that the individual perceives as totally alien to himself as a person. The patient frequently is convinced that he has done something harmful or antisocial, and feels considerable concern and anxiety. Despite this, he recognizes that the ideas are untrue and nonsensical while at the same time spending considerable energy trying to resist them and banish them from his consciousness. His efforts may be momentarily successful; but inevitably the ideas return again moments later, and the struggle is renewed.

Compulsions and compulsive acts: A compulsion has the same autonomous characteristics as an obsession, but rather than being merely an idea or image, it is an overwhelming urge to do something aggressive, disgraceful, or obscene. As with the obsessions, the patient experiences anxiety, recognizes the absurdity of the impulse, and resists putting it into action. Not infrequently, however, he does in fact act on the compulsive urge and indulges in a repetitive behavioral pattern in the form of compulsive acts or rituals. These are often found to be secondary to a primary obsessional idea and serve the function of combating or neutralizing its harmful qualities. A young man, for example, had the insistent thought every time he turned off an electric light: "My father will die." (Obsession.) To quell the anxiety associated with that thought, he would feel compelled to touch the light switch again and say to himself, "I take back that thought." (Compulsion.) The quality of **magical thinking** characterizes both obsessions and compulsions. Neither has anything to do with the real, physical world of cause and effect—a fact of which the patient is aware.

Diagnosis

The often bizarre quality of obsessive-compulsive ideas and rituals may at times resemble the similar bizarreness of schizophrenic thinking, but in the obsessional patient reality testing is intact.

Course and Prognosis

Onset of symptoms occurs during early adolescence in 10 to 15% of patients. The disorder tends to run a chronic, remitting course, with symptomatic periods generally lasting < 1 yr before a remission brings relief. With treatment, about 25% of patients improve markedly; the rest are partially improved or unchanged. Prognosis is better for those patients who begin treatment early.

Treatment

Properly selected patients may respond to **insight psychotherapy** with disappearance of symptoms, but in many patients the symptoms are stubbornly resistant. **Supportive therapy,** with an emphasis on reassurance and encouragement to activity, may provide sufficient relief to enable patients to perform daily activities fairly comfortably. **Behavioral technics,** especially those aimed at **flooding** the patient with anxiety by forcibly preventing him from carrying out compulsive rituals, have been reported to be successful, but are still experimental.

No drugs have a specific effect on the symptoms. However, when depression is present, its successful treatment with antidepressant medication may also relieve the obsessional symptoms.

HYSTERICAL NEUROSIS

(Conversion Reaction; Conversion Disorder; Dissociative Reaction; Dissociative Disorder)

A neurotic disorder characterized by a wide variety of somatic and mental symptoms resulting from dissociation, typically beginning during adolescence or early adulthood and occurring more commonly in women than men. Since the concept of hysteria as a disease is over 2000 yr old, its limits as a disorder have become blurred by a variety of definitions. This chapter restricts discussion to those phenomena classified as **conversion and dissociative disorders of consciousness,** which have a common basis in the mental phenomenon of dissociation.

Etiology

The concept of **dissociation,** *a process whereby specific internal mental contents (memories, ideas, feelings, perceptions) are lost to conscious awareness and become unavailable to voluntary recall,* is central to an understanding of the genesis of hysterical symptoms. Though unconscious, these mental contents can be recovered under special circumstances (e.g., in dreams or a hypnotic trance). Furthermore, they are able to affect the individual's awareness and behavior in a variety of ways. For example, the dissociation and loss from consciousness of memories of motor patterns lead to paralysis; the emergence of a fragment of a dissociated visual memory may produce an ego-alien visual hallucination; the emergence of a complex of mental associations forming a dissociated personality may effect a complete change in the individual's behavior. All phenomena of conversion and dissociative hysteria may be viewed as the effects of either the dissociation itself or of the eruption into consciousness of portions of the dissociated mental contents of varying degrees of complexity. Proneness to dissociation may in part be genetic.

Two factors concerning dissociation should be noted: (1) It is closely correlated with hypnotizability, and individuals prone to spontaneous dissociation rate high on hypnotizability scales. (2) It works as a psychologic defense; i.e., it provides a mechanism for banishing anxiety-provoking, painful, unpleasant mental contents from consciousness. However, the individual becomes subject to the unconscious substitution of hysterical symptoms.

Clinical Features

Conversion symptoms: Almost any organ disease symptom can be simulated on an hysterical basis, e.g., symptoms mimicking the illness of a deceased relative. A variety of **sensorimotor symptoms** have been considered to be specific to and characteristic of hysterical neurosis. (Conversion symptoms are also commonly seen in nonpsychiatric practice in patients who do *not* have classical hysterical neurosis; see in PSYCHOSOMATIC MEDICINE, Ch.134.) Weakness and paralysis of muscular groups are common; spasms and abnormal movements, less frequent. The motor disturbances are usually accompanied by altered sensibility, especially those involving touch, pain, temperature, and position sense. Especially characteristic are the "glove" and "stocking" distribution of the motor and sensory disturbances when these affect the limbs; i.e., the distribution is determined by the body-image concept of a functional arm and leg rather than the dermatome innervation of the area affected. Another common distribution is complete hemianesthesia, which extends exactly to the midline of the body fore and aft. Less frequently, special senses and functions may be affected, such as in hysterical blindness, deafness, and aphonia; both visual and auditory hallucinations may occur.

Dissociative phenomena: A variety of altered states of consciousness may result from the dissociative process. In **somnambulism** (see also Ch. 121), the patient appears to be out of contact with his environment, is seemingly unresponsive to external stimuli, and in many cases appears to be living out a vivid, hallucinated drama, often the memory of some past emotionally traumatic event. In **amnesia,** the commonest form of dissociative hysteria, the patient typically has a complete loss of memory for all past events covering a period of several hours to several weeks. **Anterograde amnesia** may occur, wherein the amnesia covers the memory of events as they are experienced, the patient forgetting continuously from moment to moment what he has just been thinking, feeling, and doing. For a discussion of amnesia as a functional syndrome in organic cerebral disease, see Ch. 119.

Far less common but more dramatic and eye-catching are the conditions of fugue states and multiple personalities. Central to both is a loss of personal identity. Typically, in a **fugue state** the individual suddenly loses all recollection of his past life and any awareness of who he is. He disappears from his usual haunts, leaving family and job, and traveling far from home, begins new work with a new identity, quite unaware of any change in his existence or life. Suddenly after a matter of days to weeks, he "comes to." Totally amnesic for the period of the fugue, he recaptures his former identity and, greatly distressed, wonders how he came to be in such strange surroundings. In the **multiple personality** a similar sudden change of identity occurs without, however, any wandering from home and with a frequent, unpredictable alternation between personalities. Most commonly 2 such personalities exist: the primary, or A personality, often afflicted with disabling neurotic symptoms and with no awareness of the existence of the B, or secondary personality. The latter, on the contrary, is fully aware of all the thoughts and activities of A, and whereas A is chronically depressed and sick, B is healthy, vivacious, and scornful of the restricted life and personality that characterize A's existence.

Diagnosis

The sensorimotor symptoms of hysteria are distinguished from neurologic disease by the absence of pathologic neurologic signs, by recognition of precipitating psychosocial stress and conflict, and by the specific characteristics of the distribution of hysterical motor and sensory disturbances. Dissociative disorders of consciousness are differentiated from those caused by gross brain disease by the absence of positive indications of the latter (e.g., EEG changes, abnormal CT scan, pathognomonic changes in tests of cognitive functions). When the hysterical symptoms imitate those of medical diseases, the diagnosis is often more difficult. It is best established by the absence of findings pointing to disorders in organ functions and by the positive stigmas of hysteria, such as high hypnotizability, a previous history of clear-cut conversion or dissociative symptoms, and evidence that the symptoms represent a symbolic expression and resolution of psychologic conflicts.

Course and Prognosis

The paucity of studies on the natural history of hysteria precludes definite statements about its course and prognosis. Clinical experience suggests that it is a chronic illness. While patients may recover from specific symptoms, these are frequently replaced by others, especially during periods of emotional tension and stress, as a result of the propensity for dissociation.

Treatment

Psychoanalytic treatment, once thought to be specific for hysterical symptoms, is effective in a small number of hysterical patients who are capable of using the insights gained by psychoanalytic exploration. For others, family therapy, environmental manipulation (e.g., job changes, homemaking assistance), reassurance, and a supportive physician relationship may be helpful. Hypnosis can remove specific symptoms, but a substitute symptom often arises. However, in patients with amnesia, hypnosis can be an effective tool to bring repressed ideas and feelings into consciousness, enabling the patient to face and resolve them more directly as the first step in the therapeutic process. Continued psychotherapeutic work is necessary to help the patient come to a more healthy and adaptive resolution of his problem.

SOMATIZATION DISORDER

(Briquet's Syndrome)

A neurotic illness characterized by the presence of multiple somatic symptoms, including those seen in classical conversion hysteria. Patients usually consult a physician other than a psychiatrist. Formerly considered a form of hysteria and viewed by many as a hysterical personality disorder (see NARCISSISTIC PERSONALITIES in Ch. 135), somatization disorder has recently been allocated a diagnosis of its own as a neurosis in DSM-III on the basis of phenomenologic clinical research. The disorder begins in adolescence or early adulthood, occurs predominantly in women (1 to 2% of the female population), and tends to be associated with sociopathy and alcoholism in male relatives.

Etiology

Etiology is not known, although the disorder often runs in families, and it is clear that the narcissistic personality structure of these patients (i.e., their marked dependency needs and exaggerated rage when frustrated) is involved in their somatic complaints. The symptoms are a somatized message expressing a desperate plea for help and attention, and their intensity and persistence reflect the extreme degree of the wish to be cared for in every aspect of the patient's life.

Clinical Features

Central to the disorder is the presence of multiple, vague somatic complaints that may be referable to any part of the body but most commonly take the form of headaches, nausea and vomiting, abdominal pain, bowel difficulties, dysmenorrhea, fatigue, syncope, dyspareunia, and sexual frigidity. Anxiety and depression are common accompaniments. The somatization appears to be part of a personality disorder, which has other characteristics. In their relationship with the doctor and others, patients are seen to be dramatic and emotional in presenting their complaints, and may be openly seductive and exhibitionistic. As the relationship develops, a marked, insatiable dependency emerges. Patients increasingly demand help and emotional support, may exhibit outbursts of rage when they feel that their needs are not gratified, and often attempt to manipulate others by threatening or attempting suicide. Often dissatisfied with their care, they go from doctor to doctor.

Diagnosis

Somatization disorder is distinguished from anxiety neurosis, hysterical neurosis, and depression by the predominance, multiplicity, and persistence of somatic complaints, the absence of the biologic signs and symptoms characterizing endogenous depression, and the gestural, manipulative nature of the suicidal behavior. The most difficult challenge lies in assessing the presence or absence of physical disease. Since such patients may develop concurrent physical illnesses, appropriate physical and laboratory examinations should be carried out during the initial clinical evaluation or whenever a significant shift occurs in the symptomatic picture.

Course and Prognosis

The disorder tends to run a fluctuating but chronic course. Complete relief of symptoms is rare, and unnecessary examinations and medical and surgical procedures may add to the patient's complaints or dysfunction. In some patients, depression becomes more prominent after many years, the frequent references and gestures relating to suicide become more ominous, and suicide may be carried out.

Treatment

Treatment usually is extraordinarily difficult, requiring tact and patience. The physician must walk a narrow clinical line between avoiding unnecessary diagnostic procedures and being alert to the possibility of developing physical disease. Medications do not help significantly, and attempts to provide insight with specific psychotherapeutic technics usually fail. The patient needs a calm, firm, supporting relationship with a physician who provides reassurance and sets effective, appropriate limits to the patient's histrionically exaggerated behavior and demands.

HYPOCHONDRIACAL NEUROSIS

(Hypochondriasis; Atypical Somatiform Disorder)

A neurotic disorder characterized by a preoccupation with bodily functions and a morbid fear that one is suffering from serious disease. The peak incidence of onset is in the 30s in men, the 40s in women.

Etiology

Etiology is unknown, but some clinical evidence suggests that hypochondriasis, like somatization disorder, is related to a narcissistic character organization marked by excessive concern with self and with the gratification of dependency needs.

Clinical Features

The hypochondriacal patient complains of symptoms in a wide variety of body parts, most commonly in the abdominal viscera, chest, head, and neck. The specific symptom may be based on a heightened awareness of bodily sensation (heartbeat, peristaltic action) or minor disorders of function such as mild, localized pain or discomfort. The complaints often are described in minute, specific detail with respect to location, quality, and duration, but follow no pattern recognizable as organic dysfunction, and are usually not associated with abnormal physical findings. Although the symptoms described by the patient may be odd or bizarre, in *hypochondriasis*, as contrasted with hypochondriacal symptoms seen in psychotic disorders, they are not delusional in quality, and the patient exhibits no other signs of psychosis.

Diagnosis

Although hypochondriasis shares with somatization disorder a central complaint of somatic symptoms, the disorders differ in that hypochondriacal neurosis begins at a later age and the somatic complaints of the hypochondriac are richly detailed and sharply localized. Hypochondriacal symptoms are frequently associated with endogenous depressions, are then usually delusional in quality, and disappear when the affective disorder is relieved.

Course, Prognosis, and Treatment

The course is chronic, fluctuating in some, steady in others. Only a very small proportion of patients (perhaps 5%) recover permanently. The presence of hypochondriacal complaints in association with depression presages a poor prognosis for recovery from the basic affective illness.

Hypochondriasis is notoriously resistant to all forms of treatment, and all such measures are only palliative. Patients may gain some relief from a sympathetic, supportive relationship with a physician, and it is often helpful to work with the patient's family, giving them an awareness of the nature and course of the disorder so that they can provide a supportive home environment.

139. AFFECTIVE DISORDERS

Psychiatric conditions in which a disturbance of affect or mood is either a primary determinant of the psychopathologic state or constitutes its core manifestation. **Anxiety**, **depression**, and **elation** are the 3 affects most commonly elaborated into clinical disorders, but by convention the designation of affective or mood disorder is usually limited to conditions characterized by morbid depression or elevation of mood.

Affective disorders, especially the depressive forms, are heterogeneous and common in both psychiatry and general medicine settings. Thus, depression can occur in the context of, or secondary to, a large number of nonaffective psychiatric and medical conditions, as well as part of the primary mood disorders of unipolar and bipolar illness.

Classification

Normal moods (sadness, grief, and elation) are part of the fabric of everyday life and should be differentiated from the morbid moods of affective disorder.

The term **"the blues"** (*sadness, or normal depression*) refers to a universal human response to separation, disappointment, and loss; the response may actually be adaptive by permitting withdrawal from frustrating situations to conserve inner resources for subsequent use. Transient irritable and depressive periods also occur as reactions to certain holidays or significant anniversaries, as well as during the premenstrual phase and the first week postpartum. Although such **holiday blues, anniversary reactions, premenstrual depressions,** and **maternity blues** are not in themselves psychopathologic, those predisposed to affective illness may break down during such times.

Grief (*bereavement reaction*), the prototype of **reactive depression,** also manifests itself with such anxiety symptoms as initial insomnia, agitation, and autonomic nervous system hyperactivity. These reactions occur in response to significant separations and losses, e.g., death, marital separation, romantic disappointment, financial reverses, leaving familiar environments, forced emigration. Bereavement and loss seem not to cause depressive illness, but provide vulnerable periods for those predisposed to affective disorder.

Elation, although not studied systematically, is popularly linked to success and achievement. However, "paradoxical depressions" also may follow such positive events, presumably because of the increased responsibilities associated with them. Elation is sometimes conceptualized psychodynamically as a defense against depression or as a denial of the pain of loss, e.g., the rare form of bereavement reaction where hyperactivitiy and even elation may completely replace the expected grief. The concept of "flight into health" is invoked to explain the lucid and energetic periods of brief duration encountered in very sick terminal patients or in those who need to take definitive action in the face of unusual life duress. Whether such reactions form the prelude to clinical mania in predisposed individuals is speculative.

Morbid affective states (affective disorders) occur when sadness, grief, or elevated moods are so intense that they do not respond to simple reassurance and continue autonomously well beyond the expected impact of a stressful life event; the morbid mood may also arise "endogenously," i.e., without apparent life stress. In addition to mood change, certain psychologic symptoms and somatic signs (see TABLE 139–3) are ordinarily necessary for the diagnosis of an affective disorder. Different subtypes of affective disorder are distinguished by whether these signs and symptoms cluster into discrete full syndromal episodes (episodic or major affective disorders) or pursue a course of low-grade intermittent chronicity (chronic affective disorders). Each subtype is further divided on the basis of polarity, i.e., presence or absence of elevated moods, and severity (see TABLE 139–1).

Major (episodic) affective disorders consist of the primary mood disorders of **unipolar (depression only)** and **bipolar (manic-depressive)** conditions; the severest (melancholic and psychotic) manifestations are commonly seen in these subgroups. Half of all unipolar depressions occur just once in a lifetime, with complete recovery usually within months; the remainder are recurrent, with variable intervening periods (usually many years) of freedom from episodes. Manic-depressive illness has a bipolar course, with both depressive and elevated periods, and is therefore almost always recurrent. The circular and predominantly depressive forms outnumber the predominantly manic forms, which comprise not $> 15\%$.

Chronic affective disorders usually occur on an attenuated or subsyndromal plane of severity, pursue an irregularly intermittent course (often lifelong), and occur in the setting of significant personality disturbance. **Cyclothymia** is *an alternating pattern between depressive (gloomy, pessimistic, worrisome, and preoccupied with personal inadequacy) and hyperthymic (cheerful, vigorous, optimistic, and overconfident) traits;* it is best viewed as a spectrum of affective temperaments that imperceptibly merge with manic-depressive illness, to which it is genetically linked. Of the **chronic depressive disorders,** only a small percent are the **dysthymic disorders** proper (*attenuated subclinical forms of major depression*); these temperamental dysthymias may form the adolescent or even childhood precursors of adult major depressive episodes, or constitute the residua of partially remit-

TABLE 139–1. CLINICAL SUBTYPES OF AFFECTIVE DISORDERS

Major (or Episodic)	Chronic
Bipolar affective disorder	Cyclothymia
Unipolar depression	Chronic depression
	Dysthymia
	Characterologic neurotic depression
	Atypical depression

Modified from *Diagnostic and Statistical Manual of Mental Disorders,* Third Edition (DSM-III), American Psychiatric Association, Washington, D.C., APA, 1980.

ted unipolar episodes. The characterologically based **neurotic depressions** and **atypical depressions** represent the most common types of chronic depression.

Incidence and Epidemiology

About 1 in 4 individuals suffers some form of affective disturbance during a lifetime. However, the lifetime risk for clinically significant mood disorders is probably not more than 15% (12% in men and 18% in women) for depressions and 1% for manic-depressive illness; the rates are more skewed in the direction of women for the milder forms of depression, and nearly even in manic-depression. Affective illness has a positive correlation with age, largely contributed by depressive disorders, which peak in the 40s to 60s; bipolar disorders usually begin in the teens, 20s, and 30s. As the most prevalent psychiatric condition, depression is estimated to vary from about 25% in public mental institutions to almost 40% in outpatient psychiatric clinics, reaching 50% in private psychiatric facilities, and up to 70% of all psychiatric diagnoses in nonpsychiatric medical practice. However, the suggestion that depression is such an integral part of the human condition that few people will escape it is not warranted. Although sadness and transient depressive affect are universal human experiences, depressive illness is limited to those individuals with a special vulnerability.

Culture, social class, and race have not been conclusively shown to make significant differential contributions to the overall rates of affective illness. However, sociocultural factors are known to modify the clinical manifestations; e.g., somatic complaints, worry, tension, and irritability are more common in the lower socioeconomic classes; guilty ruminations and self-reproach are more characteristic of depressions in Anglo-Saxon cultures; and in some Mediterranean and African countries, as well as in American blacks, mania tends to manifest itself more floridly.

Etiology and Pathogenesis

The syndromes of depression and mania—analogous to many medical conditions, such as congestive heart failure—represent the final common pathways of various processes.

Secondary affective states are chronologically superimposed on preexisting nonaffective disorders and are often, but not always, understandable developments from them—somatically (see TABLE 139-2), psychologically, or via both mechanisms. Some, such as myxedema depression and steroid euphoria, are largely attributable to physiochemical factors and can be considered **symptomatic affective disorders**. Others, such as the chronic depressive states that accompany seriously debilitating cardiopulmonary or neurologic diseases, are explained in terms of the limitations that the

TABLE 139-2. COMMON CAUSES OF SYMPTOMATIC DEPRESSIONS AND ELATIONS

Type of Cause	Depressions	Elations
Pharmacologic	Steroidal contraceptives Reserpine α-Methyldopa Physostigmine Alcohol Sedative-hypnotics Amphetamine withdrawal	Corticosteroids Levodopa Amphetamines Methylphenidate Cocaine Monoamine oxidase inhibitors Tricyclic antidepressants
Infectious	Influenza Viral hepatitis Infectious mononucleosis TB General paresis (tertiary syphilis)	Influenza St. Louis encephalitis Q fever General paresis (tertiary syphilis)
Endocrine	Myxedema Cushing's disease Addison's disease	Thyrotoxicosis
Collagen	SLE RA	SLE Rheumatic chorea
Neurologic	Multiple sclerosis Parkinson's disease Sleep apnea Cerebral tumors Dementing diseases in early stages	Multiple sclerosis Diencephalic and 3rd ventricle tumors
Nutritional	Pellagra Vitamin B_{12} deficiency	
Neoplastic	Cancer of the head of the pancreas	

underlying condition imposes on the lifestyle of the individual. More commonly, however, both orders of causes are operative, e.g., in the schizophrenics' depression which could stem from high doses of depressant neuroleptics, as well as from the profound sense of demoralization imposed by a malignant mental disorder; or in the depressive psychosis of Cushing's disease, where the changes in body image in a female afflicted with acne, hirsutism, obesity, striae, etc., are as relevant as the endocrine impact on the brain. Excessive endogenous production of corticosteroids results in depression, while those exogenously administered cause euphoria; fortunately, corticosteroids are usually given to very sick individuals where some degree of flight into health is both expected and desirable.

In the affective states associated with nonaffective disorders, incomplete syndromes of depression and mania are common, as well as atypical mixtures with paranoia, anxiety, delirium, or dementia. When a full-blown affective syndrome develops in the setting of a medical condition, etiologic factors important in the primary mood disorders are probably operative. For instance, the so-called "reserpine depression" is most commonly a pseudodepression; it is partly attributable to the sedative side effects of the drug and is fully reversible upon its discontinuation. The less frequently occurring irreversible reserpine depressions are seen predominantly in predisposed individuals with family or personal history of affective disorder. This example highlights the arbitrary nature of the primary-secondary distinction and suggests a continuum of pathogenesis for all affective states. However, in clinical practice the dichotomy is useful to facilitate therapy aimed at reversible underlying causes.

Primary affective syndromes arise in the absence of factors listed for secondary affective states. The exact pathogenetic mechanisms are unclear, but an interaction between several contributory causes is most likely.

Heredity is a major predisposing factor in primary mood disorders, although sporadic (nonfamilial) forms also exist. Unipolar depressions are hypothesized to be transmitted polygenically, and bipolar disorders by single dominant genes (either X-linked or autosomal). Alternatively, unipolar and bipolar disorders may lie on a polygenic continuum of severity. The exact mechanisms are uncertain, but the metabolic end results appear to reflect abnormalities in biogenic amine neurotransmitters of the limbic-diencephalic system; norepinephrine, dopamine, and serotonin have been implicated singly or in combination. Despite 15 yr of research, no direct evidence exists for biogenic amine abnormality in affective disorders. However, 2 recent findings in depressive illness—shortened rapid-eye-movement **(REM)** latency and steroidal overproduction resistant to dexamethasone suppression—strongly suggest, albeit indirectly, such an abnormality.

While genetic factors clearly underlie bipolar disorders, what triggers the onset of manic episodes is not fully understood. As compared with depressive illness, the role of psychologic factors is less established here. The switch from depression to mania is often heralded by total insomnia for 1 to 3 days (and experimentally induced by total sleep or REM deprivation).

Stressful life events (especially separations) commonly precede affective episodes, predominantly the unipolar forms. However, such events may represent the prodromal manifestations of an affective episode rather than its cause; e.g., affectively ill persons often alienate their loved ones.

Any **personality type** can develop clinical depression, but the more recurrent unipolar forms are associated with obsessionalism and passive-dependence. The rigid obsessional character is liable to break down when significant departures from routine are imposed by stressful life events, while the passive-dependent character lacks the requisite skills to adjust to such events. The personality structure in bipolar illness tends to be less "neurotic," with 1/3 to 1/2 arising from cyclothymia.

Childhood loss of a parent does not place one at higher risk for affective illness, but such persons tend to have their first depressions at an earlier age, more often pursue an intermittently chronic course, and attempt suicide more often. Unsubstituted childhood loss appears to prevent the development of adult coping skills and thereby contributes to the genesis of neurotic personality traits such as passive-dependent helplessness.

The higher vulnerability of women to depression is customarily traced to their presumed greater passive-dependence and helplessness in controlling their destiny in male-oriented societies. However, biologic vulnerabilities are at least as relevant: women have two X chromosomes (important in bipolar illness, if dominant X-linkage is involved), are more susceptible to marginal hypothyroidism, use depressionogenic steroidal contraceptives, undergo premenstrual and postpartum endocrine changes, and compared to men, have higher levels of monoamine oxidase (the enzyme that degrades the neurotransmitters considered important for mood).

Symptoms, Signs, and Diagnosis

In the **depressive syndrome** (see TABLE 139–3), the mood typically is depressed, irritable, or anxious, or a combination thereof. However, in **masked depressions,** consciously experienced depression may be paradoxically absent. Instead, the patient complains of being somatically ill and may even wear a defensive mask of smiling **(smiling depression).** Others complain of various aches and pains, fears of calamity to themselves or their loved ones, and fears of going insane. Finally, in some the morbid affect is of such depth that tears dry up; here, a return of the ability to cry is usually a sign of improvement. It is in such severe depressions that morbid states of depersonalization and derealization occur, with loss of the capacity to experience usual emotions, and a feeling that the world has become colorless, lifeless, and dead.

TABLE 139–3. CLINICAL MANIFESTATIONS OF DEPRESSIVE AND MANIC STATES

	Depressive Syndrome	Manic Syndrome
Mood	Depressed, irritable, or anxious (the patient may, however, smile or deny subjective mood change)	Elated, irritable, or hostile
	Crying spells (the patient may, however, complain of inability to cry or to experience emotions)	Momentary tearfulness (as part of mixed state)
Associated psychologic manifestations	Lack of self-confidence; low self-esteem; self-reproach	Inflated self-esteem; boasting; grandiosity
	Poor concentration; indecisiveness	Racing thoughts; clang associations (new thoughts triggered by word sounds rather than meaning); distractibility
	Reduction in gratification; loss of interest in usual activities; loss of attachments; social withdrawal Negative expectations; hopelessness; helplessness; increased dependency	Heightened interest in new activities, people, creative pursuits; increased involvement with people (who are often alienated because of the patient's intrusive and meddlesome behavior); buying sprees; sexual indiscretions; foolish business investments
	Recurrent thoughts of death and suicide	
Somatic manifestations	Diurnal variations in mood and activity (typically worse in the AM)	
	Psychomotor retardation; fatigue Pain; agitation	Psychomotor acceleration; eutonia (increased sense of physical well-being)
	Anorexia and weight loss, or weight gain	Possible weight loss from increased activity and inattention to proper dietary habits
	Insomnia, or hypersomnia Menstrual irregularities; amenorrhea	Decreased need for sleep
	Anhedonia; loss of sexual desire	Increased sexual desire
Psychotic symptoms	Delusions of worthlessness and sinfulness	Gradiose delusions of exceptional talent
	Delusions of reference and persecution	Delusions of assistance; delusions of reference and persecution
	Delusions of ill health (nilhilistic, somatic, or hypochondriacal)	Delusions of exceptional mental and physical fitness
	Delusions of poverty	Delusions of wealth, aristocratic ancestry, or other grandiose identity
	Depressive hallucinations in the auditory, visual, and (rarely) olfactory spheres	Fleeting auditory or visual hallucinations

The morbid mood is accompanied by preoccupation with guilt, self-denigrating ideas, decreased ability to concentrate, indecisiveness, diminished interest in usual activities, social withdrawal, helplessness and hopelessness, and recurrent thoughts of death and suicide.

The mood change and the associated psychologic manifestations occur in most clinical subtypes of depression. However, it is in full-fledged **melancholia** (literally, "black-humored" depression) that somatic manifestations dominate the clinical picture. The greater the number of such somatic signs and symptoms, the greater the chance that somatic therapies will be beneficial. This is to be expected, since the somatic manifestations listed in TABLE 139–3 are indicative of limbic-diencephalic dysfunction. It is in such melancholic depression that REM latency is shortened at sleep onset, and elevated steroidal output (sometimes to the level seen in diencephalic Cushing's disease) exhibits early escape from dexamethasone suppression. Furthermore, there is often diurnal variation of mood and activity, with a nadir in the morning. Psychomotor retardation or slowing of thinking, speech, and general activity may progress to **depressive stupor,** where all voluntary activities come to a standstill; others exhibit psychomotor agitation, with restlessness, wringing of the hands, and pressure of speech. Some patients, especially bipolar depressives, tend to be hypersomnolent, while many unipolar depressives typically complain of insomnia, with difficulty falling asleep, multiple arousals, or early morning awakening. Anorexia and weight loss are sometimes serious enough to lead to emaciation and secondary disturbances in electrolyte balance; overeating and weight gain are somewhat less common and more characteristic of milder depressions. There is often loss of sexual desire, with impotence; amenorrhea can also occur. The sexual difficulties may reflect a more generalized loss of ability to experience pleasure (anhedonia). An important feature of depressions of melancholic depth is their **autonomous course.** Even when precipitated by environmental stress, they assume independence from the stress and follow an unrelenting, uninterrupted course, showing little response to psychologic support and reassurance. Whether melancholia is qualitatively different from other types of depression is an unresolved clinical problem; nevertheless, the distinction among them is important, because melancholia requires vigorous somatic therapy.

Psychotic manifestations are present in 15% of depressions, most commonly in melancholia. Patients have delusions of having committed unpardonable sins or crimes; hallucinatory voices accuse them of various misdeeds or condemn them to death. The rare hallucinations of vision take the form of coffins or deceased relatives. Because of feelings of insecurity and worthlessness, patients believe themselves to be observed, watched, and persecuted. Others think they have lost all their fortunes; that their children will consequently starve; that they harbor incurable and "shameful" diseases, like cancer and venereal disease; and that they are contaminating other people. An occasional patient may, rarely, kill family members to "save" them from future misfortune, and then commit suicide.

Dysthymia proper is not easily distinguished clinically from the heterogeneous group of **chronic depressions.** Absence of understandable psychologic factors for the depressive disposition and the presence of positive family history for affective illness may help establish that some forms of low-grade depressions of intermittent chronicity are genetically attenuated major affective disorders. Chronic depression is sometimes the sequel of one or several incompletely remitted episodes of unipolar depression; such chronicity is not uncommon in elderly individuals, and tends to be associated with debilitating somatic disorders, multiple interpersonal losses, and chronic marital conflicts of an irreconcilable nature. These depressions merge imperceptibly with the characterologically based **neurotic depressions,** manifested by chronic low self-esteem, exquisite sensitivity to separation from loved objects, prominent character pathology with passive-dependent or histrionic traits, low threshold for alcohol and sedative-hypnotics, and a repetitive tendency to dysphoric mood and manipulative suicidal gestures; the mood is typically reactive to environmental support. Related to neurotic depressions are the **atypical depressions,** characterized by evening worsening of mood and symptoms of somatic and phobic anxiety with agoraphobic coloring.

The manic psychotic syndrome (see TABLE 139-3) is customarily distinguished from nonpsychotic forms of morbid elation **(hypomania).** In the full-blown manic psychosis, the mood typically is one of elation, but irritability and frank hostility with cantankerousness are not uncommon. The morbid mood colors patients' entire experience and behavior to such an extent that they believe they are in their best mental state. Their lack of insight and inordinate capacity for activity lead to a dangerously explosive psychotic state, in which the patient is impatient, intrusive, and meddlesome, and responds with aggressive irritability when crossed. Interpersonal friction results and may lead to secondary paranoid delusional interpretations of being persecuted. Psychomotor acceleration is experienced as racing thoughts and is manifested by flight of ideas, which in the extreme is difficult to distinguish from the loose associations of the schizophrenic. Attention is quite distractible, with the patient constantly shifting from one theme, one endeavor, to another. Thoughts and activities are expansive and may progress into frank delusional grandiosity, i.e., false convictions of personal wealth, power, inventiveness, and genius, or temporary assumption of a grandiose identity. Patients may believe they are being assisted or persecuted by external agents. Fleeting auditory and visual hallucinations are sometimes present, occur at the height of mania, and are usually understandably linked with the morbid mood. The need for sleep is decreased. Manic persons are inexhaustibly, excessively, and impulsively involved in various activities without recognizing the social dangers involved. In the extreme, activity is so frenzied that any understandable link between mood and behavior is lost (a kind of senseless agitation known as **delirious mania**) this counterpart of depressive stupor is rare today.

Mixed states are *labile mixtures between depressive and manic manifestations or rapid alternation from one to the other,* and occur in $1/3$ to $1/2$ of manic-depressives at one time or another. The most common examples include momentary switches into tearfulness and suicidal ideation, observed at the height of mania, or racing thoughts in the context of a depressive state. Less commonly, the entire affective episode is a mixed state, with dysphorically elevated mood, insomnia, psychomotor agitation, racing thoughts, suicidal ideation, grandiosity, persecutory delusions, auditory hallucinations, etc. Alcohol and sedative-hypnotic abuse often contribute to such full-fledged mixed states.

In **cyclothymia**, the clinical manifestations are similar to those described for manic-depressive illness, but are attenuated. Most typically, there are brief cycles (usually days) of alternating retarded depression and elevated periods or labile irritability. In another form, depressive features predominate; the bipolar tendency is shown by the ease with which elation or irritability is elicited by the administration of tricyclic antidepressants. In a form rarely seen clinically, elevated periods predominate, with occasional periods of irritability. Although a relationship seems to exist between these milder cyclothymic manifestations of manic-depressive illness and social and creative success, it is important to recognize cyclothymic disorders because their affective nature is often masked by serious interpersonal and social problems, such as repeated marital failure or romantic breakups, episodic promiscuous behavior, uneven work and school record, geographic instability and dilettantism, and an episodic pattern of alcohol and drug abuse. A family history for frank bipolar psychosis is a useful clue to diagnosis.

Differential Diagnosis

The most common diagnostic error equates affective psychosis with **schizophrenia** or **schizoaffective disorder.** The differential diagnosis between affective and schizophrenic psychoses (TABLE 139–4) is important clinically because of the relative specificity of lithium for treating affective illness (and the potential for neurotoxicity in schizophrenia), and because affectively ill individuals should be protected from the unnecessary risk of tardive dyskinesia. No pathognomonic differentiating features exist, and diagnosis must be based on the overall clinical picture, family history, course, and associated features. Not only mood-congruous psychotic features occur in affective illness; mood-incongruous delusions or hallucinations are sometimes secondarily superimposed on the basic mood disorder because of the concomitant presence of alcoholic hallucinosis, sedative-hypnotic withdrawal, psychedelic-induced psychosis, or other systemic or brain disease mimicking schizophrenia. In a remitting illness with mixed affective and schizophrenic features, a schizoaffective diagnosis should not be made unless such complicating factors are excluded. When in doubt, because of the better prognosis of affective disorder, therapeutic trial with a thymoleptic drug (an antidepressant or lithium carbonate) is indicated.

Therapeutic trial with thymoleptics is also justified in elderly individuals to clarify the differential diagnosis between **early dementia** (which often presents with affective change) and **pseudodemented depression.** In the latter, psychomotor retardation, decreased concentration, and memory impairment contribute to the appearance of dementiform clinical features. Because of the better prognosis of depressive illness, it should be preferentially diagnosed, especially when past episodes have occurred or when family history is suggestive. Reversible neurologic or systemic diseases may, however, coexist with or contribute to an unmistakable depressive disorder.

The dual and related concepts of **masked depression** and **affective equivalents** are often invoked to explain certain disorders with prominent somatic symptoms or behavioral disturbance with mini-

TABLE 139–4. DIFFERENTIATION OF AFFECTIVE AND SCHIZOPHRENIC PSYCHOSES

Validating Criteria	Affective Psychosis	Schizophrenic Psychosis
Age	Any	Rarely begins after 40
Premorbid personality	Extroverted, dysthymic, cyclothymic, or compulsive	Often introverted, or schizotypal
Onset	Usually abrupt	Usually insidious
Affect	Usually "infectious"	Rigid, blunted, or inappropriate
Thought processes	Usually intelligible: slowed down or accelerated	Typically difficult to follow (loose associations)
Delusions and hallucinations	Usually mood-congruous, but occasionally Schneiderian in form	Typically idiosyncratic, bizarre, and involving multiple areas of the patient's life; commonly Schneiderian in form
Family history	Affective disorder; alcoholism	Schizophrenia
Course	Usually remitting or periodic; personality preserved	Usually nonremitting; personality often deteriorated
Biologic criteria (for depressive disorders)	Shortened REM latency; abnormal dexamethasone suppression test (DST)*	Normal results with these tests

*Serum cortisol $\geq$ 5 μg/dl at either 4 PM or 11 PM following overnight 11 PM 1–mg dexamethasone (Carroll et al standardization).

Adapted from H.S. Akiskal and V.R. Puzantian, *Psychiatric Clinics of North America* Vol. 2, No. 3, pp. 419–439, 1979. Used with permission.

mal or absent mood change. These include antisocial acting out (especially in children and adolescents), substance use disorders, pain, hypochondriasis, anxiety states, and psychophysiologic disorders. In the absence of clear-cut affective symptoms, the diagnosis of an affective disorder is not recommended unless past episodes of affective illness have occurred, the condition is periodic, and the family history is positive for affective illness. Therapeutic trial with a thymoleptic drug, sometimes justified in such cases on empirical grounds, may assist in differential diagnosis if unequivocal response occurs.

Depressive disorders are uncommon before adolescence, at which time they often herald the onset of manic-depressive illness. The basic manifestations of **childhood depressive illness** (see also Vol. II, Ch. 26) are not different from adults; they are simply manifested in areas of typical concern to children and parents, such as school work and play. In the presence of standard "adult" signs and symptoms of depression, the diagnosis of affective disorder should be made in preference to adjustment reactions or neurotic and behavior disorders; the latter are often given exaggerated prominence in child psychiatry. Conversely, when affective symptoms are lacking, hyperactivity and behavioral disturbances should not be considered affective equivalents unless validating criteria as outlined above are present. It must be remembered that affective disorders do occur in mentally retarded children (and adults), in whom somatic symptoms and behavioral disturbances are especially likely to mask the basic affective disorder.

Alcohol is more likely to be sought by the manic, rather than the depressed, patient in an attempt at self-treatment; thus, unipolar depression is less often a cause of alcoholism and drug abuse than has been thought. Affective symptoms, especially depression, of a transient or intermittent nature (due to pharmacologic or social causes) that often accompany **substance use disorders** should not be confused with major affective disorders that most typically have a sustained duration of several months. Differentiation from intermittently chronic affective disorders such as cyclothymia is more problematic. The diagnosis of primary alcoholism, other substance use disorders, and antisocial personality should be preferentially considered in individuals with prominent alcohol and drug histories. However, episodic substance abuse, especially that of alcohol (dipsomania), or onset after age 40, favors the diagnosis of primary affective disorder with secondary substance abuse.

Neurotic symptoms such as anxiety, phobias, and obsessions are common in primary depressive disorders; they disappear when the affective episode remits. In primary neurotic syndromes, on the other hand, there are usually irregular exacerbations and remissions of the neurotic symptoms beginning with early adulthood. Nevertheless, such conditions as periodic obsessional or anxiety states making their first appearance after age 40 are often due to primary mood disorder. The differentiation between neurotic and affective disorders is more problematic when mild symptoms common to both groups of illnesses coexist. Such conditions, variously diagnosed as **mixed anxiety-depression, neurotic depression,** or **atypical depression** usually pursue chronically intermittent courses. Some authorities consider them as the neurotic end of an affective spectrum. Despite symptomatologic overlap, however, primary affective and primary neurotic syndromes are distinct in genetic backgrounds and, to some extent, in treatment response.

Treatment of Major (Episodic) Affective Disorders

Depressive illness as a single unipolar episode:

1. **Medical or neurologic causes should be excluded,** especially after age 40.

2. **Hospitalization:** Persistent suicidal ideation (particularly when family support is lacking), stupor, agitated-deluded depression, and physical debilitation require hospitalization and, often, electroconvulsive therapy **(ECT)**; the response to 4 to 8 treatments in such cases is usually dramatic and may be lifesaving. A 2- to 4-wk course with neuroleptics (e.g., thioridazine up to 400 mg/day orally given in 2 to 3 divided doses, or thiothixene up to 40 mg/day orally or IM given in 2 to 3 divided doses) represents an alternative in agitated psychotic patients. Continuation therapy with a tricyclic antidepressant usually prevents relapse in ECT- or neuroleptic-treated patients.

3. **Most depressions are handled on an outpatient basis.** Pharmacotherapy is the treatment of choice for depressions of melancholic depth; nonmelancholic depressions are treated either with drugs or psychotherapy or, preferably, by combining the two. Initially, the patient is seen on a weekly or biweekly basis to provide support and monitor progress. Since most patients are embarrassed and demoralized by the implications of having a mental disorder, especially one that seriously diminishes the capacity for work, it is extremely important to tell the patient, his family, and his employer (when appropriate) that depression is a self-limiting medical illness with a generally good prognosis; an explanation also may be given in terms of our current understanding of the biochemical basis of depression.

4. **Guidelines for drug therapy** (see also ANTIDEPRESSANTS in Ch. 247). The family history of response to a specific monoamine oxidase inhibitor **(MAOI)** or a **tricyclic antidepressant** guides drug choice. Otherwise, because of ease of administration, it is best to begin with a tricyclic. Although different tricyclics are considered to be equally effective in the average case of depression, certain practical, pharmacodynamic, and theoretical considerations provide reasonable guidelines in their choice. For instance, it is convenient to treat the agitated insomniac patient with a sedating tricyclic (amitriptyline, doxepin, or trimipramine), the retarded insomniac patient with a less sedating tricyclic (imipramine or nortriptyline), and the hypersomnic retarded patient with nonsedating tricyclics (desipramine or maprotiline). For patients with cardiac disease, doxepin may offer relatively low cardio-

toxicity. For many patients who should stay alert with the least amount of dry mouth, desipramine is a suitable drug. For other patients with concurrent GI disorders (except in esophageal hiatus hernia), amitriptyline is desirable because of its anticholinergic potency; amitriptyline also helps the depressed patient with concurrent pain and insomnia (not an uncommon combination) while decreasing the need for analgesic medication.

In view of the 2-type biochemical hypothesis of depression, the patient who fails to respond to an adequate trial of a serotonergic tricyclic should receive a trial with a noradrenergic tricyclic, and vice versa. Generally, the more sedating tricyclics are serotonergic, and the least sedating ones are noradrenergic. Except for protriptyline (10 to 60 mg/day) and nortriptyline (50 to 150 mg/day), the range of therapeutic doses for tricyclics given by mouth is 75 to 300 mg/day in most Western countries (somewhat lower in certain African and Mediterranean countries); ordinarily, an average of 150 mg/day will suffice, but some may need up to 300 mg/day for remission. Individual and population differences in the pharmacokinetic handling of the tricyclics are the most likely explanation. Giving the entire dose at bedtime renders hypnotics unnecessary, minimizes side effects during daytime, and improves compliance. The dosage is usually raised by units of 50 to 75 mg/wk until therapeutic response is seen in approximately 2 to 3 wk (it can be as early as 7 days or as late as 4 to 5 wk); within 1 to 2 mo following response, a downward adjustment of dosage is attempted, to be maintained at 50 to 150 mg/day for 6 to 9 mo or the natural duration of an episode. Abrupt withdrawal should be avoided to prevent cholinergic rebound, e.g., nightmares, nausea, colic, etc.

The indications and dosage range of the tricyclics for preadolescent depressions are not established; in the rare melancholic child, conservative doses and increments are best, as is true with the elderly (about half the adult dose). Seizures and behavioral symptoms due to toxicity (excitement, confusion, hallucinations, or oversedation) are especially likely to occur in elderly individuals with organic brain disease.

The most troublesome, though generally benign, **side effects of the tricyclics** include sedation, dry mouth, tremor, postural dizziness, blurred vision, sweating, constipation, and urinary hesitancy. During the first 10 to 15 days when the patient is largely reaping side effects and little therapeutic benefit, he should be informed that these are expected effects, that they are the prelude to therapeutic response, and that they will abate with time. The most serious but fortunately rare undesirable effects are precipitation of angle-closure glaucoma, cardiac arrhythmias, and myocardial infarction; patients with such potential should be excluded from tricyclic therapy by appropriate ophthalmologic and cardiologic consultation.

Where anxiety is prominent, a benzodiazepine tranquilizer such as chlordiazepoxide 5 to 25 mg orally b.i.d. or t.i.d. or lorazepam 1 to 2 mg orally b.i.d. or t.i.d. can be added for 2 to 3 wk to the tricyclic regimen. Although neuroleptics alone, such as thioridazine 25 to 100 mg orally b.i.d. or t.i.d., are also advocated for anxious depressions, it is best to reserve them for refractory cases in order not to expose the patient to unnecessary risk for tardive dyskinesia. The MAOI phenelzine is another alternative (see under Chronic Affective Disorders, below).

ECT or a potent MAOI such as tranylcypromine 10 to 30 mg orally b.i.d. may be given for those who are poor risks with tricyclics, cannot tolerate them, or fail to improve on full courses of 2 different tricyclics for 4 to 5 wk each (after dosage adjustment suggested by plasma drug levels). Plasma tricyclic levels are most useful in determining causes of inadequate clinical response on standard oral doses, or when pronounced side effects occur on small doses, or when anticipated side effects might be dangerous because of heart disease or old age.

Especially when combined with a MAOI, the serotonin precursor L-tryptophan 6 to 8 gm/day orally has been advocated for **refractory depressions** on an experimental basis; L-tryptophan and a tricyclic are similarly combined. In 8% of depressions (usually women, detected by augmented thyroid-stimulating hormone [TSH] response to thyrotropin-releasing hormone [TRH] stimulation) significant potentiation of tricyclic antidepressant activity is provided by tri-iodothyronine 25 to 50 μg/day orally. A lithium-tricyclic combination may prove beneficial in cases where an eventual bipolar course is suspected (young, postpartum, hypersomnic-retarded depression with bipolar family history). After a 10-day period of a tertiary amine tricyclic such as amitriptyline 75 to 100 mg orally, the addition of gradually increasing doses of phenelzine 30 to 60 mg/day orally in divided doses is probably safe, and might help refractory cases; but the addition, in reverse order, of a tricyclic on a MAOI may result in hypertensive crisis. All of these unorthodox approaches to refractory cases are best reserved to specialized affective disorder units or clinics.

5. Brief individual psychotherapy may improve coping skills once the acute melancholic phase is over in a few weeks. Couples' therapy may help resolve conjugal conflicts. Elaborate long-term psychotherapy is unnecessary except in the presence of significant personality disturbance.

Recurrent depressions occurring on an infrequent basis can be treated as outlined above for a single episode. However, unipolar illness recurring at intervals shorter than 2 yr should be indefinitely maintained on tricyclics, the dosage periodically adjusted with respect to mood level and side effects. Family history for bipolar illness is often positive in depressions with high episode frequency **(unipolar II disorder),** and patients must be observed for the occurrence of hypomania. As expected, maintenance lithium carbonate (see below) is equally effective in such cases. Relapses, nevertheless, are not uncommon with maintenance chemotherapy; supportive psychotherapy may therefore assist in boosting morale, improving coping skills, and identifying early manifestations of relapse.

Manic-depressive illness. Many bipolar patients with recurrent depressions experience pleasant elevation of mood, usually at the tail end of a depression **(bipolar II disorder)**, but do not report it unless specifically questioned. In the absence of documented history for hypomanic or manic episodes, the **depressive phase** of bipolar illness is not easily distinguishable from unipolar depression (see TABLE 139–5). Tricyclics may overcorrect the mood in a hypomanic direction, giving a clue to the bipolar nature of the illness; such pharmacologic hypomania is also seen with ECT and MAOIs, and probably all centrally acting sympathomimetic drugs. Lithium has a modest acute antidepressant effect in the depressive phase of bipolar illness, and can be given alone or in conjunction with a tricyclic.

Manic psychosis often presents as a social emergency and is preferably managed on an inpatient basis; hypomania usually can be managed on an outpatient basis. After lithium work-up (CBC, urinalysis, thyroid status, serum electrolytes, creatinine, and BUN), lithium carbonate is started 300 mg orally b.i.d. or t.i.d. and increased over a 7- to 10-day period until a serum level of 0.8 to 1.4 mEq/L is reached. Acutely manic patients have high tolerance for lithium and preferentially retain it during the first 10 days, while excreting sodium; regular diet is recommended. Teenagers who enjoy excellent glomerular function need higher doses of lithium to achieve the same level of equilibrium in the serum, while the reverse is true for elderly patients. Because lithium's onset of action has a 4- to 10-day latency period, it is sometimes initially necessary to also administer haloperidol 5 to 10 mg IM as needed (up to 80 mg/day) or another suitable neuroleptic until the manic psychosis is under control. In psychotic, extremely hyperactive patients with precarious food and fluid intake, it is preferable to give neuroleptics and supportive care for a few days before initiating lithium. Mixed states of manic-depressive illness are also best treated with a neuroleptic-lithium combination. In all combination therapies, the neuroleptic can usually be discontinued in a few weeks. Lithium therapy for an isolated manic episode should continue for at least 6 mo; but most manias occur as part of recurrent bipolar illness.

Recurrent bipolar illness with frequent episodes is best treated with indefinite maintenance on lithium, with serum level of 0.6 to 1.0 mEq/L, usually achieved with three to five 300-mg capsules/day. Tricyclics (50 to 300 mg/day) or MAOIs can be added separately when needed, especially during the first 2 yr of maintenance therapy, to control depressive swings; and thioridazine (50 to 400 mg/day) or other suitable neuroleptics for hypomanic swings or mixed states.

Patients may complain of being overcontrolled, of being less alert, and less creative; therefore, considerable psychotherapeutic skills are needed to assure compliance to maintenance doses of lithium, as well as interventions with the patient's spouse or family to abate interpersonal crises secondary to mercurial moods. Actual decrease in creativity is relatively uncommon, as lithium generally offers the opportunity for more "even" periods devoted to interpersonal, scholastic, professional, and artistic pursuits. Individual psychotherapy may assist patients to cope better with their living problems and adjust to their new self-identities. In the noncompliant, cantankerous manic patient, it is customary to give a depot phenothiazine such as fluphenazine decanoate 12.5 to 50 mg IM every 3 to 4 wk; because of the risks for tardive dyskinesia, lithium should be substituted as soon

TABLE 139–5. COMPARISON OF BIPOLAR AND UNIPOLAR DEPRESSIONS

Validating Criteria	Bipolar Depression	Unipolar Depression
Basic personality	Extroverted, cyclothymic, or compulsive	Compulsive or passive-dependent
Age of onset (mean)	30s	40s
Sex ratio	Equal	Women > men
Postpartum episodes	More common	Less common
Onset of episode	Often abrupt	Abrupt or insidious
Psychomotor activity	Retardation > agitation	Agitation > retardation
Sleep	Hypersomnia > insomnia	Insomnia > hypersomnia
Number of episodes	Numerous	Fewer
Duration of episode	Shorter	3 to 9 mo
Family history	Bipolar and unipolar illness; alcoholism?	Unipolar illness; alcholism
Tricyclic antidepressants	Hypomania induction	Hypomania induction uncommon
Lithium	Modest antidepressant effect in acute phase	Usually ineffective in acute phase

Adapted from H.S. Akiskal and W.T. McKinney, Jr., *Archives of General Psychiatry* Vol. 32, pp. 285–305, March 1975. Copyright 1975 by the American Medical Association. Used with permission.

as feasible. In bipolar patients with mood-incongruous psychotic features beyond the usual boundaries of a "pure" affective disorder, intermittent courses of such neuroleptics are often necessary as well.

The **most common acute benign side effects of lithium** consist of tremor, fasciculation, nausea, diarrhea, polyuria, polydipsia, and weight gain (partly attributed to high-calorie beverages). These are usually transient and often respond to a slight decrease in dosage (and use of diet soft drinks). Empirically, some clinicians advocate short courses of propranolol 10 mg orally t.i.d. or q.i.d. for incapacitating tremor. **Toxic effects** are initially manifested by gross tremor, increased deep tendon reflexes, persistent headache, vomiting, and mental confusion, and may progress to stupor, seizures, and cardiac arrhythmias. Apart from overdoses, lithium toxicity is more likely in patients with renal disease with decreased creatinine clearance and with sodium loss that may result from excessive sweating, diarrhea, or diuretics; none of these represent absolute contraindications to lithium, but may dictate assessment of baseline renal function (e.g., creatinine clearance), lower doses, dietary sodium supplementation, and frequent serum lithium determinations, and follow-up of renal function tests. It is likewise desirable to obtain baseline EEG in neurologic, and baseline ECG in cardiac, disease, and to follow progress with frequent serum lithium determinations. Otherwise, in healthy subjects with relatively stable mood, quarterly serum checks are usually sufficient. The more common **chronic side effects** of lithium include mild leukocytosis (of no functional significance), hypothyroidism (successfully managed with thyroid supplementation), acne (tetracycline given if needed), nephrogenic diabetes insipidus (may respond to reduction of dosage or temporary interruption of lithium therapy). Individuals with past history of parenchymal kidney disease may be at some risk for structural damage to the distal tubule; therefore, serum lithium levels generally should be maintained at the lowest level compatible with freedom from incapacitating mood swings.

Treatment of Chronic Affective Disorders

For **dysthymia,** a vigorous trial of a noradrenergic tricyclic such as desipramine up to 300 mg/day or lithium carbonate may help. The value of tricyclics or lithium is not established in the other types of chronic depression. Thus, **secondary chronic depressions** that often accompany incapacitating nonaffective diseases are best handled with various combinations of supportive, group, and family therapies. However, where insomnia, anxiety, or pain (due to demonstrable organic pathology or psychologic factors, or both) is prominent, a sedating tricyclic such as doxepin can be adjunctively given, in the 50- to 150-mg range. Characterologic **neurotic depressions,** although traditionally the domain of psychodynamically oriented psychotherapy, are being increasingly treated by behavioral and cognitive technics. Sedating tricyclics can also be given adjunctively for their tranquilizing or hypnotic properties; minor tranquilizers are generally best avoided. Trial with a MAOI is worthwhile if these approaches fail. The **atypical depressions** respond favorably to maintenance treatment with MAOIs, notably phenelzine, beginning with 15 mg b.i.d. or t.i.d. The dose can be raised by 15 mg/wk until a ceiling of 60 to 75 mg/day is reached. Response may occur as early as a few days or as late as 8 wk. Treatment should continue for 12 mo or longer. Side effects include dry mouth, constipation, nausea, edema, weight gain, and postural hypertension. **To avert paradoxical hypertensive crises,** the patient should be instructed to avoid sympathomimetic drugs, reserpine, and meperidine, as well as tyramine– or ʟ-dopa–containing beers and wine, or foods with such content (fava beans, yeast, canned figs, raisins, yogurt, cheese, sour cream, soy sauce, pickled herring, caviar, liver, and meat prepared with tenderizer).

Cyclothymia can be treated very much like recurrent bipolar illness, with considerable psychotherapeutic attention paid these persons' stormy interpersonal relations. The decision to give a lithium trial depends on the functional impairment produced by the unpredictable mood swings.

Complications

Social consequences. Frequent episodes of bipolar illness, often due to inadequate treatment or lack of compliance with maintenance chemotherapy, result in uneven productivity, dilettantism, bankruptcy, ruined careers, and repeated marital breakdown. Furthermore, all types of recurrent chronic affective disorders may poison family life and rob children of optimal parenting. Early recognition and comprehensive approaches (i.e., psychotherapeutic, sociotherapeutic, and pharmacotherapeutic) to the treatment of recurrent affective disorders minimize such complications.

Secondary alcoholism and sedative-hypnotic abuse, the latter often iatrogenically facilitated, are common risks in inadequately treated or unrecognized recurrent affective disorders. Recognition of affective disorders and their pharmacologic management is important for primary care physicians; minor tranquilizers and sedative-hypnotics are of little value as primary treatment for affective disorders.

Modest increase in mortality from cardiovascular causes occurs in bipolar illness, is not accounted for by cardiotoxicity from lithium and tricyclics, and tends to involve nonaffective first-degree biologic relatives as well. The reasons for this are obscure.

Suicide, the most serious risk, causes 15 to 20% of deaths in untreated affective illness, and tends to occur within 4 to 5 yr from the first clinical episode. The recovery phase from depression (when psychomotor activity is returning to normal but the mood is still dark) is a major risk period, as are the premenstrual phase and personally significant anniversaries. Other risk factors and management of suicidal patients are discussed in Ch. 141.

140.   SCHIZOPHRENIC DISORDERS

(See also Vol. II, Ch. 26)

The schizophrenic disorders, as defined by **DSM-III** (the American Psychiatric Association's *Diagnostic and Statistical Manual*, Third Edition), are *mental disorders with a tendency toward chronicity which impairs functioning and which is characterized by psychotic symptoms involving disturbances of thinking, feeling, and behavior.* Six specific criteria for the diagnosis include (1) certain psychotic symptoms, delusions, hallucinations, formal thought disorder; (2) deterioration from a previous level of functioning; (3) continuous signs of the illness for at least 6 mo; (4) a tendency towards onset before age 45; (5) not due to affective disorders; and (6) not due to organic mental disorder or mental retardation.

The DSM-III definition eliminates several entities included in the DSM-II concept. Syndromes which look like schizophrenia but which last < 6 mo are called **schizophreniform.** Psychotic syndromes of < 2 wk duration which follow a significant psychosocial stressor are now called **brief reactive psychoses.** Borderline or latent schizophrenia and simple schizophrenia are now diagnosed **borderline** or **schizotypal personality disorders.** Late onset of schizophrenia-like syndromes, e.g., the involutional paraphrenias, are diagnosed **paranoid disorder** or **atypical psychosis.** Organic mental disorder or mental retardation and affective disorder are specifically excluded.

The exclusion of affective disorder is complicated and problematic, but in the final draft of DSM-III, the category of **schizoaffective** (see below) was significantly narrowed. Most patients with mixtures of schizophrenic and affective symptoms are now to be diagnosed schizophrenia or affective disorder.

The DSM-III codes for subtypes of schizophrenia essentially remain the standard subtypes, i.e., **disorganized (hebephrenic), catatonic, paranoid, undifferentiated,** and **residual.** DSM-III also allows for the classification for the course of the illness, namely, **subchronic** (< 2 yr), **chronic** (> 2 yr), **subchronic with acute exacerbation, chronic with acute exacerbation,** and **in remission.**

Incidence and Etiology

Schizophrenia has a worldwide distribution. Using a relatively narrow concept of the disorder, studies of European and Asian populations have found the lifetime prevalence from 0.2% to almost 1%. However, in the USA and USSR, higher rates have been found although the criteria used are very much broader. Schizophrenia most commonly becomes manifest in late adolescence or early adult life, although paranoid schizophrenia typically has a later onset. Even with available forms of treatment, schizophrenic patients occupy about ½ the hospital beds of mentally ill and mentally retarded patients, and about ¼ of all available hospital beds. The high prevalence of schizophrenia in lower socioeconomic classes has been mainly attributed to social disorganization and consequent stresses, but there is evidence that this association arises partly because some patients in a prepsychotic phase drift down the social scale.

Most cases of schizophrenia are now thought to be caused by a complex interaction between inherited and environmental factors. Approximately 10% of relatives of schizophrenics will be recognized as schizophrenic. A genetic predisposition is probably necessary if schizophrenia is to occur at all, but the overt manifestations of illness seem to be decided partly by stressful life experiences, such as faulty patterns of upbringing and disturbed relationships. Those who develop schizophrenia in middle age or later often are unmarried, widowed, or deaf.

Although no specific type of premorbid personality is seen in all cases, many patients who develop schizophrenia show such traits as sensitivity, shyness and unsociability, lack of affect, and paranoid attitudes. Difficulty in personal relationships and social isolation inevitably result. The term **schizoid personality** is used to describe persons with defective capacity to form social relationships; the term **schizotypal personality** is being introduced to describe those who, in addition to their deficiencies in social relations, show oddities of thinking, perception, communication, and behavior which are not severe enough to meet the criteria for schizophrenia. Schizoid and schizotypal personalities are discussed in Ch. 135.

Clinical Manifestations and Diagnosis

Even in cases with acute onset (commonly of the catatonic or paranoid subtypes) and with an apparent relationship to stressful events in the environment, careful history taking often will reveal a prodromal period of weeks or months of increasing withdrawal and disorganization of the previous level of functioning. During the active phase, characteristic symptoms involve psychologic processes (content of thought, language, perception, affect), volition, motor behavior, sense of self, and relationship to the external world. A residual phase often follows the active phase and may be similar to the prodromal phase, but at times with persistent delusional beliefs and with emotional blunting. In order to distinguish schizophrenic disorders from short-term reversible illnesses, DSM-III requires that schizophrenia be diagnosed only when continuous signs have lasted for at least 6 mo during the person's life, and that this period include an active phase of psychotic symptoms with or without a prodromal or residual phase. However, in many patients the deterioration is so gradual that it is difficult to trace back to a specific time when illness supervened in the schizoid personality. In the early stages of schizophrenia, the patient may become increasingly uneasily aware that his psychologic integrity is impaired. He may worry over his lack of concentration or fear that he is going insane. His personal identity may be threatened by doubts of his sexual gender. He may symbolize his awareness of illness in terms of an internal battle between good and evil or project his feeling of internal dissolution onto the environment as fantasies of the annihilation of the world by some holocaust.

Thought disorder: Clear, goal-directed thinking becomes increasingly difficult, as shown in a diffuseness or woolliness and circumstantiality of speech. Sudden and incomprehensible changes of subject and obvious flaws in reasoning occur because distraction by fringe associations and the patient's private symbolism determines his thinking as much as does normal logic. "I have always believed in the good of mankind but I know I am not a woman because I have an Adam's apple" seems nonsensical. However, the patient who said this suffered doubts about his sexual identity and believed that a battle for good and evil was raging within him; his implicit identification of women with evil, the switch from mankind to woman (presumably because of the syllable "man"), the search for reassurance by choosing a minor sexual difference because of its symbolism, and the condensation of the themes illustrate the schizophrenic disturbance of thinking. Some schizophrenics report a stoppage of thinking **(thought block)** or may claim that their thoughts are broadcast or shared with other people; delusional interpretations of these experiences (see below) lead to the belief that their minds are being controlled by external agencies. Thinking may be impoverished in many schizophrenic patients who have been ill for a long time.

Emotional (affective) changes: Blunting and inappropriateness (incongruity) of affect are the most characteristic emotional changes and are obvious and not easily overlooked in severe cases. Minor blunting and incongruity may be difficult to evaluate, since their assessment is subjective and therefore unreliable. Any mood disturbance—depression, excitement, anxiety, elation—may occur, and perplexity is not uncommon in acute schizophrenia.

Perceptual disorders: Auditory hallucinations are the most common, but hallucinations of sight, touch (including sexual sensations), smell, and taste may occur. The auditory hallucinations range from whistling, humming, or machinery sounds to an indirect muttering of voices or clear complex conversations. Auditory hallucinations can occur in many disorders, but certain types, especially hallucinations of a running commentary on the patient's actions or of voices talking about the patient, strongly suggest a diagnosis of schizophrenia.

Delusions: Delusions of persecution are frequent, as well as those involving hypochondriacal or religious ideas, jealousy, and sexual problems (particularly homosexuality). Delusions of grandeur are common in schizophrenia but are also often found in other disorders, such as in the manic phase of manic-depressive psychosis. Delusional interpretations of strange experiences such as thought blocking or broadcasting and depersonalization may lead the patient to believe that telepathy is occurring, that a mechanical device is recording his thoughts and conversation, or that he is under the control of an external agency. The patient suddenly may develop a delusional system that explains in a flash a whole succession of preceding puzzling events that he viewed with ill-defined suspicion, perplexity, or an inexplicable feeling of menace. This type of delusion, almost invariably diagnostic of schizophrenia, may convince the patient of his special significance—that he is the Messiah or the innocent victim in the center of a conspiracy—or provide immovably strong explanations for previous experiences. The delusional system may seem illuminating to the patient but is baffling and incomprehensible to others.

Catatonic symptoms: Disturbances of movement range from gross overactivity and excitement to marked retardation and even stupor with mutism. Posturing may occur, and the patient may take up a bizarre position (crucifix, or head raised several inches from the pillow) for prolonged periods. Extreme negativism or automatic obedience is sometimes seen. Mannerisms such as a mincing gait, grimaces, or overemphasis of normal movements are more common. Chemotherapy and improved individual management have made severe catatonic symptoms increasingly rare.

Violent behavior: Although threats of violence and even minor aggressive outbursts are common in acute schizophrenic states and relapses, dangerous behavior occurring when the patient obeys commanding voices or attacks his persecutors is uncommon. Occasionally, grotesque violence, with self-mutilation (often of sexual parts) or murderous attacks, may occur. Matricide, the rarest form of murder, is most often perpetrated by schizophrenics. Petty crimes may be committed by a "down and out" chronic schizophrenic patient. The risk of suicide is increased in all stages of schizophrenic illness.

In addition to violent behavior associated with the psychotic state (including organic brain disease), there are persons with personality disorders, including the schizoid or schizotypal types, who become severely isolated, depressed, and paranoid and who may seek resolution of their difficulties in an act of aggression (e.g., physical attack, murder, assassination) against someone whom they perceive as a single source of their abject state. The victim is usually someone in an authoritarian position (e.g., a parent, teacher, popular idol, or prominent political leader), or a sweetheart, spouse, or child. In their tormented thinking, they appear to seek recognition, love, and honor for their "heroic" act, but at the same time they seem to expect and welcome death as punishment and escape.

Nonspecific symptoms: Withdrawal from external reality and failure to coordinate drive are frequent findings. There may be abnormality of psychomotor activity with rocking, pacing, peculiar motor response, or immobility. The patient may often appear perplexed, eccentrically groomed or dressed, and disheveled. Poverty of speech is common and ritualistic behavior associated with magical thinking often occurs. The patient may be depressed and exhibit anxiety, anger, or a mixture of these. There may be ideas of reference and hypochondriacal concerns. Rarely, during a period of excitement, a patient may be found to be confused or disoriented, but usually there is no significant disturbance in the sensorium.

Differential diagnosis: Altered states of consciousness are rare in schizophrenia. However, when this occurs and is accompanied by a clustering of schizophrenic symptoms, the symptoms may indicate an organic cerebral etiology caused by toxic (drug, metabolic, infection) or other organic factors. The organic delusional symptoms associated with amphetamines, cocaine, and phencyclidine should be considered particularly. Paranoid disorders are usually distinguished from schizophrenia by the absence of prominent hallucinations, incoherence, or bizarre delusions.

DSM-III asserts that affective symptoms are consistent with the diagnosis of schizophrenia and that schizophrenic symptoms are consistent with the diagnosis of affective disorders. The distinction for syndromes with both kinds of symptoms rests upon course. The diagnosis of **schizoaffective disorder** should be made whenever the clinician is unable to make a differential diagnosis between schizophrenia and affective disorders. The diagnosis of schizoaffective is to be used when there is an episode of affective illness in which preoccupation with mood-incongruent delusions or hallucinations (persecutory delusions, bizarre delusions) dominates the clinical picture and when affective symptoms are no longer present. DSM-III's use of the diagnoses of **schizophreniform syndromes, brief reactive psychoses,** and **borderline** or **schizotypal personality disorders** are described in the introduction to this chapter.

Classification and Course

DSM-III has classified the course as subchronic (< 2 yr), chronic (> 2 yr), subchronic with acute exacerbation, chronic with acute exacerbation, and in remission. In the past, schizophrenia was divided into 2 distinct patterns of onset. The first **(reactive)** is the development of illness in a person who has shown satisfactory social functioning but who often possesses an anxious and insecure temperament. This type of illness is frequently precipitated by a traumatic event and has a rapid onset. Patients with the second pattern **(process type)** have a history of poor social functioning, have few friends, and show occasional bizarre habits. They are described as isolated, shy, and withdrawn (schizoid). There is no distinct precipitating event; the illness begins with a gradual downhill course into withdrawal and isolation.

Certain symptoms commonly cluster together but no clear demarcation exists between subtypes of schizophrenia, and individual patients may shift from one to another in successive episodes or even in the same illness. The term **undifferentiated** is used when the episode is characterized by prominent psychotic symptoms not classifiable in any specific subtype, or meeting the criteria for more than one. Currently, those subtypes of schizophrenia without overt psychotic symptoms, i.e., latent, borderline, or simple schizophrenia, are to be diagnosed as borderline or schizotypal personality disorders. The emphasis in **hebephrenia (disorganized type)** is on silliness and incongruity of affect and thought disorder with increasing autism. Delusions, hallucinations, and other minor catatonic symptoms (e.g., mannerisms) are often present, and the personality is severely disorganized. In **catatonia,** movement disorders predominate, with increasing motor agitation or retardation and gross posturing. Autism is extreme. **Paranoid schizophrenia** includes delusions of persecution or grandeur, thought disorder, and hallucinations, but there is less personality disintegration than in other subtypes. In **chronic schizophrenia** all subtypes tend to a clinical picture where blunting of emotion and drive, and incoherence or poverty of thought are the dominant features. Delusions, hallucinations, passivity, and catatonic symptoms all may persist, usually with diminished intensity. The diagnostic criteria for **residual type** include a history of at least one previous episode of schizophrenia with chronic psychotic symptoms, a clinical picture without any prominent psychotic symptoms but continuing evidence of the illness, such as blunted affect, social withdrawal, and poverty of thought.

Prognosis

Schizophrenia is not necessarily a chronic disorder. About 30% of patients recover completely, and most of the remainder show some improvement. The florid symptoms can nearly always be controlled, but blunting of emotion and drive may remain intractable. Although even minor defects may impair personal relationships and work efficiency, partial remission is compatible with a reasonable life adjustment. With treatment, an active psychosis commonly is controlled within 4 to 8 wk, but residual defects of varying severity may persist for weeks or months before further improvement. Relapse is common unless adequate follow-up and medication intake are maintained. Acute exacerbations requiring therapeutic intervention often occur; residual impairment usually increases between episodes. A favorable prognosis is associated with good premorbid personality with adequate social function, the presence of precipitating events, abrupt onset, onset late in life, a clinical picture that includes confusion or perplexity, or a family history of affective disorder.

Treatment

The mainstays of treatment are chemotherapy, the development of a therapeutic relationship with a skilled counselor, social support, and graded rehabilitation and retraining. For a first illness or an acute relapse, hospitalization, even if it must be compulsory, is usually indicated to stabilize the patient on a suitable chemotherapeutic regimen; to ensure the physical safety of the patient or other persons; to prevent damage to finances, work prospects, or personal relationships; and to relieve the family. Although most states have enacted legal restrictions insisting that hospitalization take place only on the basis of the patient's being dangerous to himself or to others, the prevailing practice remains dependent on the psychiatrist's clinical judgment of the necessity for hospitalization. However, since schizophrenic patients are readily susceptible to institutionalism and since family ties are loosened by prolonged separation, hospitalization for more than a few months is harmful unless the severity of the illness makes it essential or it is part of an active rehabilitation program.

Chemotherapy: (See also under TRANQUILIZERS in Ch. 247.) A highly disturbed or distressed patient can be given haloperidol 5 to 10 mg IM q 4 to 6 h for a 24-h period. Even larger doses administered within a short period of time are used to treat acutely agitated and excited patients, e.g., haloperidol 5 to 10 mg every hour for 3 to 4 times. Oral chlorpromazine 200 to 1000 mg/day or thioridazine 200 to 800 mg/day is given initially or after the parenteral drugs. Since hypotension may develop with both parenteral and oral drugs, prophylactic antiparkinsonian drugs (trihexyphenidyl HCl, procyclidine HCl) often were prescribed earlier to prevent extrapyramidal complications such as dystonia, parkinsonism, and akathisia. However, cumulative experience has led to avoidance of these drugs, particularly with patients receiving thioridazine. Antiparkinsonian drugs are prescribed now only when extrapyramidal symptoms become manifest or if the risk of extrapyramidal symptomatology is great. The prophylactic use of antiparkinsonian drugs is indicated when the medical risk of certain complications, e.g., respiratory distress, is present, or when patients have reacted adversely to neuroleptic medication in the past. Usually these are given for a short period of time, perhaps < 10 days, but in some instances with continuing parkinsonism, the use may be extended to as long as 3 mo. The clinical efficiency and side effects of the butyrophenones, thioxanthenes, dihydroindolones, and dibenzoxazepines are the same as those of the phenothiazines. (For adverse effects of phenothiazine administration, including tardive dyskinesia, see TRANQUILIZERS in Ch. 247.) The full dosages of antipsychotic medication given to younger patients are liable to cause marked side effects in older patients and are rarely required by them. These drugs in the elderly should be given in gradually increasing dosages and established at a level appropriate to each individual.

Many schizophrenic patients will not continue to take oral antipsychotic medication. Long-acting depot injections of fluphenazine enanthate or decanoate are, therefore, often preferred for maintenance treatment, and they reduce the risk of relapse. Depot fluphenazine is given IM or s.c. in 25- to 37.5-mg doses every 2, 3, or 4 wk from the onset of treatment. Depot fluphenazine therapy requires backup facilities. Recently, special medication clinics have been established, and nurses have been trained to give defaulting patients their injections at home.

With rapid and complete recovery from an acute episode in a patient with a nonschizoid personality, drug treatment need not be continued for more than 3 to 6 mo after recovery. In more serious forms of illness, drugs should be continued for 2 to 3 yr, and some patients may require antipsychotic medication indefinitely. A general rule of thumb of maintenance medication is to continue the patient at 1/3 to 1/5 of the dosage he has required during the acute phase of his psychosis. The maintenance phase should be continued for 3 to 6 mo after discharge and tapered slowly for a trial period. Periods of stress (family discord, job difficulties, emotional losses, physical illness) may require reinstitution of medication. Every attempt should be made to permit the patient to have respite from continuous drug administration, i.e., a "drug holiday," which may consist of no medication over a weekend or for longer periods of a week or a month. Obviously, these measures require vigilance and awareness of symptom recurrence. Depressive periods due to personal problems or a primary affective swing are not uncommon in otherwise well-controlled schizophrenics and require appropriate counseling and perhaps the prescribing of an antidepressant drug such as amitriptyline or imipramine 75 to 150 mg daily in divided doses.

Electroconvulsive therapy (ECT): In catatonic patients or those with severe depression, elation, or excitement, ECT accelerates the response to antipsychotic drugs; 4 to 10 treatments may be required.

Psychotherapy, counseling, and social management: Working with the patient and his family helps to alleviate distress and problems of work and personal relationships, to establish patterns of readjustment, and to uncover and work out stresses precipitating schizophrenic episodes. Depth or analytic psychotherapy is not indicated, but establishing a therapeutic relationship with frequent discussions and the therapist's patient concern and interest, is essential. In the initial stages (except rarely when there is no alternative) the therapist should not argue or flatly deny the reality of the patient's psychotic beliefs. Agreeing with the patient, on the other hand, risks compounding and reinforcing such beliefs. A neutral attitude may be achieved by focusing discussions on problems (including the patient's distress) to which the beliefs have given rise. With increasing insight, simple interpretation of certain ideas may be discussed.

Occupational therapy and graded social involvement should be arranged. For those who are more disabled, a comprehensive structured rehabilitation program including employment retraining may be planned. The needs of the family should be considered, and a trained social worker may be helpful.

Primary in the care of chronic schizophrenics is careful control of environmental pressure. Overstimulation (in the form of high expectancies, high emotional involvement with relatives, or excessive work loads) can cause either a florid exacerbation of symptoms or autistic withdrawal. Understimulation reinforces passivity, dependency, and the tendency to autism. Understimulation may occur in the home, particularly with overprotective parents, and in the hospital (institutionalism). In evaluating the handicaps of a chronic schizophrenic patient, it is good practice to assume, in order to avoid therapeutic nihilism, that secondary handicaps from over- or understimulation are present and outweigh the primary defects of the illness. Individual psychotherapy combined with appropriate family and milieu therapy helps foster direct, forthright, and less stressful communication between the patient and his world.

PARANOID DISORDERS

States of heightened self-awareness with a marked tendency to self-reference and projection of the patient's own ideas to others. In common usage "paranoid" implies persecutory ideas or attitudes held by the patient.

Paranoid states range imperceptibly from a circumscribed delusional system with no loss of affect or associative processes, to the more complete disorganization seen in paranoid schizophrenia. This is reflected in inadequate affective responses, increasingly disorganized associations, and symbolization and projection of mental material as hallucinations.

Etiology, Symptoms, and Signs

The personality that spawns a paranoid illness reflects a need to shield sensitive portions of inner life, a hunger for recognition, and the fears and guilt feelings these conflicts and strivings evoke. Sexual conflicts, often unconscious, may be operative, and homosexual tendencies are often noted. The paranoid patient characteristically has a tense and expectant affective state that stimulates his attention; he sees connections where none exist and at times rationalizes his concepts into an extensive delusional system.

Brief paranoid states: These states, which are often of a psychotic intensity, are reactive illnesses in persons whose personalities are characterized by sensitivity, insecurity, inferiority, and suspiciousness. Isolation from social contact and physical problems (e.g., deafness) are often exacerbating factors, and alcoholism is commonly involved. In acute and chronic brain syndromes, the impaired comprehension and dulling of consciousness favor paranoid interpretations and delusions. Usually, these disorders are of < 6 mo duration. The onset generally is quite sudden, and the condition rarely becomes chronic.

Paranoid psychosis: Typically in these illnesses, highly elaborated delusional systems gradually develop without hallucinations, disorganization of thinking, or other characteristic schizophrenic symptoms. A few patients, however, eventually progress into frank schizophrenic illness. In one form of paranoid psychosis, core symptoms center on some minor or imagined physical defect. The patient delusionally misinterprets facial expressions or overheard scraps of conversation to confirm his beliefs that he is discriminated against because of this defect. In other patients, a trivial or illusory asymmetry of face or enlargement of the nose is the focus for a paranoid system. Such patients may trail from specialist to specialist incessantly demanding plastic surgery. Real or imagined slights or injustices may lead to never-ending litigation, or religious fanaticism may insidiously progress to grandiose but encapsulated messianic beliefs.

In one dangerous form of paranoid psychosis, delusional sexual jealousy is the central theme. Jealousy has a complex psychopathology, and morbid jealousy **(Othello syndrome)** occurs in a variety of conditions, including paranoid states. A primary depression may underlie the illness. The patient's anguish over delusions of his spouse's infidelity is readily converted to rage. The patient may unceasingly make accusations, spy upon or follow his spouse, examine undergarments for seminal stains, and misinterpret simple actions, such as the way a curtain is drawn, as a message to the lover. He may demand confession constantly and assert that forgiveness will ensue. Physical assault is a real danger.

A persecutory delusional system may develop as a result of a close relationship with another person who already has a disorder with persecutory delusions. This type of induction psychosis is a result of sharing the delusions of the dominant person. In the past this disorder has been termed "**folie à deux.**" In rare instances more than 2 persons may be involved. The prognosis for what is now called **shared paranoid disorder** is a function of the emotional strength of the person in whom the psychosis has been induced.

Clinical Course and Prognosis

The history may show that, as a child, the patient needed special appreciation, was moody, resented school and parental discipline, could not form good play adjustments, and was suspicious. While growing up, the rigidity and tendency to pride may have increased, as well as the patient's sensitivity to others' attitudes toward him. Before the psychosis becomes manifest, prodromal symptoms may occur. The patient may have reacted to numerous situations with wounded and bitter pride. He analyzes his moods and sensations, may become hypochondriacal, is reserved, and withdraws in disdain from discussing his problems. Gradually, the idea may be born that his failures have been due to the enmity of others, and he sees new and hidden significance in commonplace events, leading to the belief that people deliberately slight him and that his situation is endangered. He experiences vague fears, becomes increasingly resentful, and defends his suspicions vigorously. Hallucinations may or may not occur.

Patients with classic paranoia or reactions closely approximating it probably never recover; however, they do not necessarily deteriorate and may not require hospitalization. If their conduct remains within bounds, society may view them as "cranks." However, some patients who at first appear to be suffering from circumscribed paranoid psychoses are later recognized to be schizophrenic.

Diagnosis

In contrast to mania, paranoid ideas are more sustained and are supported by a less changeable affect than manic vacillations. The mental operations are exaggerations of normal mechanisms, and differentiating patients with paranoid psychoses from nonpsychotic patients with extremely paranoid embittered personalities can be difficult. A patient is psychotic if the reaction is continuous, if his beliefs cannot be corrected, if they tend to spread, and if they are completely illogical and cause major functional impairment. These reactions can be classified as approximating either the paranoid or the schizophrenic pole by evaluating the degree of disturbance in the individual's contacts with reality; the more the repressed material comes into consciousness as hallucinations and the more archaic the form of adjustment, the nearer the reaction approaches schizophrenia.

The rapid development of a paranoid illness, particularly in a previously well-adjusted personality, should lead to a very careful clinical assessment and investigations to exclude an underlying organic disorder due to systemic illness (e.g., hypothyroidism), brain disease (e.g., neurosyphilis), or drug toxicity (e.g., amphetamines).

Treatment

Whether the patient should be hospitalized is determined by his potential danger to himself and to others. If delusions are directed against specific persons, confinement probably is necessary; the greater the expressed hatred, the more imperative is commitment. (See also the discussion of commitment under treatment of schizophrenia, above.) Establishing a relationship with the therapist is a vital step; psychotherapy then will alleviate distress and often modify behavior, even though essential delusional thinking is unaltered. In dealing with paranoid patients, honesty and truthfulness are necessary. The patient's concerns should be discussed, and the therapist should try to express an understanding of the patient's point of view, without agreeing with his delusions or belittling or strongly contradicting them. Often the patient will follow reasonable suggestions and greatly modify his behavior. The physician may become the patient's one confidant and can help him by being tolerant and combining a philosophic detachment with sympathetic humility, discretion, understanding, warmth, and a sense of humor about his own possible ineptness as well as the patient's peccadilloes. Thus, at least temporary serenity may be achieved by helping the paranoid patient to achieve a calmer environmental adjustment. The physician also can aid in unraveling family problems or irritating work situations.

Phenothiazines and other neuroleptic drugs, as described above for schizophrenia, are helpful and often minimize symptoms, though complete remission is uncommon even after prolonged drug treatment. In morbid jealousy, phenothiazines are most effective when onset was not insidious. However, it is difficult to persuade patients with this illness to undergo prolonged treatment.

---

141.   SUICIDAL BEHAVIOR

(See also Vol. II, Ch. 26)

Suicidal behavior includes both accomplished and attempted suicide. An **attempted suicide** is a suicidal act that was not fatal, possibly because the self-destructive intention was slight, vague, or ambiguous. Most persons who attempt suicide are ambivalent about their wish to die, and the attempt may result from a strong wish to live and a need to communicate a plea for help. When suicide plans and actions appear grossly unlikely to succeed, they are often termed **suicide gestures** and are predominantly communicative in nature. However, a suicide gesture should not be dismissed lightly; it is an important cry for help and requires thorough evaluation and treatment aimed at relief of misery and prevention of further attempts, especially since 1 in 10 of those persons who attempt suicide finally takes his or her life. **Accomplished suicides** differ in many respects from attempted suicides; the differences are discussed below. However, the distinction is not absolute, since attempted suicides also include acts by persons whose determination to die is thwarted only because they are discovered early and resuscitated effectively, and since a suicide attempt may be fatal by miscalculation.

The discussion in this chapter is based on the above categorization. However, a distinction can also be made between **direct destructive behavior** (which usually includes 3 distinctly different groups of phenomena: suicidal thoughts, suicide attempts, and suicides) and **indirect self-destructive behavior** (characterized by taking a life-threatening risk without an intention of dying, generally repeatedly, and often unconsciously in such a way that the consequences are likely to be destructive to the individual before long). This latter behavior covers a wide variety of phenomena, e.g., excessive drinking and drug use, heavy smoking, overeating, neglect of one's health, self-mutilation, polysurgical addiction, hunger strikes, criminal behavior, and deviant traffic behavior.

Incidence

Statistics on suicide are based mainly on verdicts recorded on death certificates and at inquests, and they underestimate the true incidence. Even so, suicide ranks among the first 10 causes of death for adults in urban communities, and accounts for 10% of deaths between the ages of 25 and 34 and for 1/3 of deaths among university students. It is the third-ranking cause of death among adolescents (see also Vol. II, Ch. 26). Of the approximately 200,000 suicide attempts in the USA each year, 10% are successful. More than 70% of successful suicides are over 40 yr of age, and the incidence rises sharply above 60 yr, particularly for men. About 2/3 of attempted suicides, however, are under the age of 40.

Attempted suicides account for about 1/5 of emergency medical admissions and for 1/10 of all medical admissions. Women make 2 to 3 times as many suicide attempts as men, but men are generally more successful in their attempts. Adolescent single girls are overrepresented among attempted suicides, and the incidence is also high among single men in their 30s. Several studies have found a higher incidence of suicides among the families of patients who have attempted suicide.

For both sexes, marriage (particularly when it is a secure relationship) is associated with a significantly low suicide rate; suicide attempts are higher among those alone because of separation, divorce, or death.

The suicide rate among blacks is lower than among whites, but suicide among black women has increased 80% in the last 20 yr. Among American Indians the suicide rate has risen in recent years, and in some tribes it is 5 times the national average.

A number of suicides take place in prisons, particularly by young men who have not committed violent crimes. Hanging is the usual method, and the suicide is most likely to occur during the first week of incarceration. Hunger strikes accompanied by suicidal declarations, particularly among political prisoners, are reported from time to time. Here, the intention to manipulate attitudes and behavior of others is at its most obvious. Self-injury and death are means to an end rather than goals. Group suicides, whether in large numbers or only involving two, as in lovers or spouse suicides, represent extreme forms of identification with others. When in large groups, they tend to occur in highly emotive settings that overcome the strong drive to self-preservation.

Professional persons, including lawyers, dentists, military men, and physicians, have higher than average suicide rates. The physician rate is largely due to female physicians, whose annual rate of suicide is 4 times that of a matched general population. Furthermore, it has been calculated that no fewer than 65% of American women physicians suffer from a primary affective disorder, a finding that correlates highly with the increased suicide rate. As for the suicide method, there is a high incidence of overdosage with drugs among both male and female physicians (as compared with the general population), possibly because of easy access and knowledge as to what constitutes a fatal dose. Of the medical specialties, the highest rate is among psychiatrists.

Suicide is less frequent among practicing members of most religious groups (particularly Roman Catholics), who are generally prohibited by their doctrines from taking their lives and are provided with close social bonds protecting against acts of self-destruction. The low rates that have been reported from Catholic countries are only in part due to a tendency of coroners to avoid verdicts of suicide; i.e., there would appear to be an actually reduced rate of suicide. However, religious affiliation and strong religious beliefs do not necessarily prevent impetuous, unpremeditated suicidal actions that occur in settings of frustration, anger, and despair.

About 1 in 5 suicides leaves a suicide note; notes are more common among elderly suicides and successful suicides. In attempted suicides, a note indicates premeditation and a serious risk of repeated attempts and later, successful suicide. The notes often refer to personal relationships and events that will follow the patient's death. They frequently contain delusional ideas of guilt or paranoia and may be evidence of serious mental illness.

Methods Employed in Suicidal Acts

The choice of methods is determined both by cultural factors and the availability of the agent. The method used may also reflect the seriousness of intention, since some (such as jumping from heights) make survival virtually impossible, whereas others (e.g., drug ingestion) provide a chance of being rescued. However, the use of a method that proves not to be fatal does not necessarily imply that the intention is less serious. The use of bizarre suicide methods suggests an underlying psychosis.

Drug ingestion is the most frequent method used in suicide attempts; barbiturates are less frequently used, as they are prescribed more cautiously in view of their tendency to cause dependence.

The use of psychotropic drugs has increased over recent years, but salicylates, which used to account for > 20% of cases, now only account for about half of these, with acetaminophen (a safer analgesic from the point of view of causing gastric irritation) being prescribed more often. The toxicity of salicylates and acetaminophen often constitutes a serious threat to life.

About 20% of all attempted suicides use 2 or more methods or a combination of drugs. The risk of a fatal outcome is increased, particularly when a combination of drugs with serious interactions is used, and multiple drug ingestion makes it important to determine blood levels of all the possibilities when a patient is seen.

Violent methods such as shooting and hanging (uncommon among attempted suicides) are largely used by men, but the number of women using such means is increasing.

Etiology

The psychologic mechanisms leading to suicidal behavior resemble those frequently implicated in other forms of self-destruction such as alcoholism, reckless driving, self-mutilation, and violent antisocial acts. Suicide is often the final act in a course of self-destructive behavior. Traumatic childhood experiences, particularly the distresses of a broken home or parental deprivation, are significantly more common among persons with a tendency to self-destructive behavior, perhaps because these persons are more likely to have serious difficulties establishing secure, meaningful relationships.

Suicide usually results from multiple and complex motivations. The principal causative factors (see also TABLE 141–1) include **mental disorders** (primarily depression), **social factors** (disappointment and loss), **personality abnormalities** (impulsivity and aggression), and **physical illnesses**. Some or all of these factors may contribute to the crisis that results in the suicidal act; often one factor (commonly a disruption in important relationships) is the final straw. In many suicides an aggressive component is evident; when its distressing impact is considered, the act appears to be directed at other, significant persons. Homicide followed by suicide provides clear evidence of aggression, as does the high incidence of suicide among prisoners serving terms for violent crimes.

Depression causes over half of all attempted suicides, and although endogenous depression may be involved, in most cases the depression is reactive or neurotic. Marital disharmony, broken and unhappy love affairs, disputes with parents among the young, and recent bereavements (particularly among the elderly) may precipitate the depression. Depression associated with physical illness may precipitate a suicide attempt, but **physical disability**, particularly if chronic or painful, is more commonly associated with accomplished suicide. Physical illness in the elderly, particularly serious, chronic, and painful illness, plays an important role in about 20% of suicides.

Among **schizophrenic** patients, accomplished suicide sometimes occurs and in chronic schizophrenia may result from the phases of depression these patients are prone to. The suicide method is usually bizarre and often violent. Attempted suicide is uncommon; it may be the first gross sign of psychiatric disturbance, occurring in the early stages of the illness, possibly when the patient becomes aware of the disorganization of his thought and volitional processes.

Alcohol predisposes to suicidal acts by aggravating the intensity of any depressive mood swing and by lowering self-control. About 1/3 of patients who attempt suicide will have consumed alcohol before the act, and about half of these will have been intoxicated at the time. Since alcoholism itself, particularly "binge alcoholism," often causes deep feelings of remorse in the intervening periods, alcoholic patients are particularly suicide-prone even when sober. In one follow-up study of alcoholics, 1 in 10 patients committed suicide. Improved treatment facilities for alcoholics would probably reduce the suicide rate.

Organic brain disease, particularly arteriosclerotic dementia, may be characterized by emotional lability, and serious violent acts of self-injury may occur during a deep but transient depressive mood swing. Consciousness is usually impaired during the act, and the patient may only have a vague recollection of the event. **Epileptic** patients, especially those with temporal lobe epilepsy, frequently

TABLE 141–1. HIGH SUICIDE RISK FACTORS

Personal and Social Factors	Clinical Features and Symptoms
Male sex	Depressive illness, especially at onset or towards end of illness
Above the age of 55	
Recent divorce or widowhood	Marked motor agitation and restlessness
Social isolation with real or imagined unsympathetic attitude of relatives	Feelings of guilt and inadequacy
	Severe hypochondriacal preoccupations: delusion or near-delusional combination of physical disease, e.g., cancer, heart disease, or sexually transmitted disease
History of suicide in family, or of affective disorder	
Unemployment	Alcoholic or drug abuse
Previous suicidal attempt	Physical illness, especially if chronic, painful, or disabling

suffer brief but profound episodes of depression. These mood disturbances, as well as the availability of drugs prescribed for their condition, put epileptic patients at a greater than normal risk of suicidal behavior.

Individuals with **personality disorders** are prone to attempted suicide, especially emotionally immature persons with a psychopathic personality, who tolerate little frustration and react to stress impetuously with violence and aggression. A history of excessive alcohol consumption, drug abuse, or criminal behavior is found sometimes. The large number of attempted suicides among separated or divorced persons may reflect an inability to form mature, lasting relationships as well as reflecting loneliness and depression; the precipitants in such cases are the stresses that inevitably result from the dissolution of even troubled relationships and the burdens of establishing new associations and life styles. Another important aspect in attempted suicide is the element of "Russian roulette," in which the person decides to let fate determine the outcome. Some unstable persons find a source of excitement in this aspect of such perilous activities as reckless driving, dangerous sports, and other forms of toying with death.

Prevention of Suicide

Any suicide act or threat must be taken seriously. Although some suicides are a surprise and shock even to close relatives and associates, in most cases clear warnings are given, generally to relatives, friends, medical personnel, or volunteers in lay organizations offering a 24-h service to those in distress. These emergency suicide prevention centers attempt to identify the potentially suicidal person, keep him in conversation, evaluate the risk, and offer him help with his immediate problems, usually calling upon others (family, physician, police) for urgent assistance in the crisis and trying to guide the suicidal person to appropriate facilities for follow-up assistance. However, despite this logical approach to helping potentially suicidal individuals, no hard data indicate that it does reduce suicide incidence.

The average physician encounters 6 or more potential suicides in his office each year. More than half of suicides have consulted their physicians within a few months, and at least 20% have been under psychiatric care during the preceding year. Since depressive illness is a major cause of suicide, its recognition and treatment are the most important contributions a physician can make to suicide prevention. Each depressed patient should be questioned carefully about any thoughts of suicide. The fear is baseless that such inquiry, even in a tactful and sympathetic form, may implant the idea of self-destruction in the patient. The questioning will aid the physician in obtaining a clearer picture of the depth of the patient's depression and will encourage constructive discussion and convey to the patient the physician's awareness of his deep despair.

Features indicating a possibly high risk of suicide in a depressed patient (see also TABLE 141–1): (1) **Age and sex**—men over 50 are at the highest risk. (2) **Clinical features**—marked feelings of guilt, self-denigration, or nihilistic delusions; marked anxiety and motor restlessness; delusional or near-delusional hypochondriacal preoccupations with physical illnesses such as cancer or sexually transmitted disease; a history of previous suicide attempts or a family history of suicide; addiction to alcohol or drugs; painful, disabling, or serious physical illness, especially in patients who have previously enjoyed good health; use of drugs, such as reserpine, that can cause severe depression. (3) **Social factors**—marital status (widowed, divorced, or separated); real or self-imposed social isolation; unemployment or financial difficulties, particularly if causing a drastic fall in the patient's economic status.

The treatment of depression is outlined in Ch. 139. The risk of suicide is increased early in the treatment of depression, when retardation and indecisiveness are ameliorated but a depressed mood and feelings of gloom still persist. Early results of treatment may, therefore, enable the patient to set about self-destruction effectively in a state of only partially lifted depression. Psychotropic drugs must be prescribed carefully and in controlled amounts. Hypnotics used to treat insomnia in depressed patients are especially dangerous; insomnia may be a symptom of depression, and to treat it with drugs without treating the underlying depression is not only ineffective but highly dangerous.

For **dealing with an acute suicide threat** (e.g., a patient who calls and declares that he is going to take a lethal dose of barbiturates or the person who threatens to jump from a height), only general advice can be given. In these situations the desire to die is ambivalent and often transient, and the physician or other person to whom the patient appeals for help must ally himself with the desire to live. The person threatening suicide is in an immediate crisis, and the physician should offer hope that it can be resolved. Emergency psychologic aid may be provided by (1) establishing a relationship and open communication with the patient; (2) reminding him of his identity (i.e., using his name repeatedly) and helping him identify the problem that has brought on the crisis; (3) offering constructive help with the problem and encouraging the patient to constructive action; (4) involving the patient's family and friends, reminding the patient that others care for him and want to help.

If a patient calls to say that he has already committed a suicidal act (e.g., taken a drug or turned on the gas) or is in the process, his address should be obtained, if possible, and someone else should contact the police at once to trace the call and rescue the patient. He should be kept talking on the telephone until the police arrive.

A comprehensive follow-up service providing adequate psychiatric and social after-care is, at present, the best means of reducing further suicide attempts and accomplished suicide. Since many successful suicides have a previous history of suicidal attempts, a psychiatric assessment is important for *all* patients as soon as feasible after a suicide attempt. This defines the problems that contributed to the act and permits appropriate treatment to be planned.

Management of Attempted Suicide

Many attempted suicides are admitted to a hospital emergency ward in a comatose state. The usual management of a comatose patient is discussed in Ch. 118. When it is certain that the patient has ingested an overdose of a hypnotic, sedative, or tranquilizer, it is important to (1) remove the poison from the patient, attempting to prevent absorption and expedite excretion; (2) institute symptomatic treatment to keep the patient alive; and (3) administer any known antidote if the specific drug ingested can be firmly identified (see Ch. 258). Every case of life-threatening self-injury should be hospitalized both to treat the physical injury and for psychiatric assessment. Most patients are well enough to be discharged as soon as the physical injury is treated, but all should be offered follow-up care.

In the psychiatric assessment made immediately after a suicide attempt, the patient may deny any problems. Not uncommonly, the severe depression that led to the suicidal act is followed by a short-lived mood elevation, a cathartic effect probably responsible for the finding that further suicide attempts are rare immediately after the initial attempt. Nevertheless, the risk of later, successful suicide is high unless the patient's problems are resolved. The patient needs a secure, strong source of help, which begins when the physician provides sympathetic attention and clear indications of his concern and commitment as well as his understanding of the patient's troubled feelings.

The duration of hospital stay and the kind of treatment required vary. Patients with psychotic illness, organic brain disease, or epilepsy, and some with severe depression whose crisis situation has not resolved, should be admitted to a psychiatric unit for continued supervision until their underlying problems are resolved or they can cope with the problems. The role of the patient's family physician after a suicide attempt is central. If he is not in charge of the case, he should be kept fully informed and given specific suggestions for follow-up care.

Impact of Suicide on Others

Any suicidal act has a potentially destructive impact on other associated persons. The successful suicide, especially, leaves his physician, family, and friends with strong feelings, which include guilt, shame, and remorse at not having prevented the latest attempt, as well as anger, directed toward the suicide or others. However, the physician must realize that neither he nor the patient's family are omniscient or omnipotent and that the patient's eventual successful suicide was ultimately not preventable. The physician should also recognize that he has the remaining important task of helping the suicide's family and friends deal with their guilt feelings and sorrow.

---

142. PSYCHIATRIC EMERGENCIES

An emergency may be created as much by circumstances as by an event. Behavior that excites comment and action in a public place may be tolerated in the home and regarded as hardly worthy of comment in a psychiatric ward. For the purposes of this chapter the circumstances are those of a general practitioner's office, an emergency ward, or a medical ward.

Obtaining a good history in an emergency may be impossible, and accounts given by excited relatives or bystanders can be biased or colored by personal involvement in the dramatic and unusual situation. At times, attention to the emotional concerns and needs of family is essential. In some emergencies diagnosis is critical to decision-making, but in others a symptom such as excitement or aggression constitutes the emergency, and diagnosis may have to await its control.

Panic; Anxiety Attacks (see also in Ch. 138)

In battle and in periods of civil catastrophe, anxiety is a normal state, but individuals who are subjected to particularly severe stress or who are perhaps especially vulnerable may be incapacitated by terror. They may manifest tremors or dissociative symptoms and bizarre or dangerous behavior. Sedation is valuable, and a tactical withdrawal from the stressful situation for a few days is helpful. Prolonged withdrawal, however, is associated with a considerable risk of chronicity.

In less stressful times, attacks of acute anxiety occur in susceptible patients; a phobic anxiety state commonly underlies those attacks. Many anxiety attacks are so brief that the acute phase is over before the patient can reach a doctor. In most cases the anxiety is generalized, but diagnostic problems can arise if various body systems are affected to different degrees, so that cardiovascular manifestations are prominent in one patient and GI symptoms in another. If overbreathing (hyperventilation) is the salient feature, the patient may complain of dizziness, lose consciousness, or show signs of tetany.

In everyday circumstances it may be difficult to determine what precipitated an anxiety attack, and advice to separate the patient from the anxiety-provoking situation is often gratuitous. Reassurance is sometimes sufficient to allay the patient's distress, and reassuring any relatives and bystanders is helpful. If mild sedation is required, the benzodiazepines (e.g., diazepam 5 to 10 mg or oxazepam 15 to 30 mg orally repeated as necessary) are usually effective. In more disturbed patients diazepam 10 mg may be given IM or even IV. Major tranquilizers have no advantage over the benzodiazepines in these circumstances. It has been suggested that small maintenance doses of tricyclic or monoamine oxidase inhibitor (MAOI) antidepressants may prevent the occurrence of phobic anxiety states. Hyperventilation will usually stop if the patient's attention is drawn to it, and he is given quiet and supportive reassurance (see also RESPIRATORY ALKALOSIS in Ch. 81).

Delirium (see also Ch. 119)

Delirious patients are a common problem in medical and surgical wards. Acute delirium may be due to ingestion of drugs such as LSD or marijuana; overdose of prescribed medication; alcohol, barbiturate, or other drug withdrawal; electrolyte imbalance; metabolic disorders; or seizures. It may also occur as an idiosyncratic reaction to a normal dose of medicine and is not uncommonly seen in situations of intense stress, such as cardiac care units.

Difficulties arise when a confused patient with impaired comprehension passively interferes with his medical treatment, or when a patient who becomes paranoid or deluded and begins to hallucinate becomes actively uncooperative and threatens or attacks the nursing staff or dismantles therapeutic equipment. Some patients become elated and overcheerful and disturb the ward by shouting and singing. Others become panic-stricken and may injure themselves in attempts to escape from imaginary persecutors.

Treatment of the cause of the delirium and general measures to make the patient comfortable and keep him safe are needed along with good nursing care. Often a major tranquilizer or diazepam orally or parenterally must be given urgently; the pharmacologic treatment is similar to that of an excited patient (see below).

Acute Memory Disturbances

Although disturbances of memory are most commonly organic (see Ch. 119), memory loss that presents as an emergency is usually hysterical (see in Ch. 138). Patients with massive dissociation can no longer recall their identity or events of their past; language and knowledge of social customs generally survive. In hysterical pseudodementia, of which the Ganser state is one example, cognitive functions are more profoundly dissociated, and regressive behavior results. In many of these patients a traumatic and often "shameful" event precedes the onset of the dissociation. The patient's memory may return with quiet and persistent interviewing, but hypnosis or abreactive drugs such as amobarbital sodium IV (200 mg slowly infused usually is adequate) may be indicated. Other hysterical symptoms (e.g., loss of vision, deafness, muteness, or paralyses) may require similar treatment.

Transient global amnesia (see in Ch. 119) creates similar difficulties and may be mistaken for hysterical amnesia. Remote memory is unaffected. There is no treatment for an attack of transient global amnesia; memory is recovered spontaneously in a few hours.

Dementia rarely presents as an emergency but may create one. A solitary patient who has been quietly deteriorating for months or years may be found in a state of indescribable squalor and neglect or may be brought to a doctor's office or emergency ward with no history and no informant.

Stupor (see also IMPAIRED CONSCIOUSNESS in Ch. 118)

Unconsciousness is always an emergency, and in some psychiatric disorders the degree of withdrawal is so substantial that a noncommunicative and unresponsive patient appears unconscious. This condition may occur in catatonic schizophrenia, in severe depressive illness, and in hysteria. If a history is available from a friend or relative, earlier characteristic symptoms may indicate the diagnosis, but great care must be taken to ensure that organic causes are not overlooked. Amobarbital sodium IV (200 mg slowly infused usually is adequate) is useful diagnostically in distinguishing hysterical, catatonic, and organic states; may relieve hysterical stupors; and often leads to a temporary remission in catatonic stupor. Both catatonic and depressive stupor respond to ECT.

Excitement, Anger, and Aggression

Although excitement, anger, and their physical concomitant, aggression, occur in a wide range of psychiatric disorders (schizophrenia, mania, psychopathy, and, rarely, in temporal lobe lesions including epilepsy and delirium), the precise diagnosis may be academic in the face of a disturbed and violent patient. Calm words may not stem the patient's wrath, but meeting his anger with further anger will only aggravate the situation.

An attempt to persuade the patient to take medication should be considered, i.e., diazepam 5 to 40 mg or haloperidol 5 to 10 mg orally. However, in most cases a parenteral route will be necessary, despite the patient's verbal and physical objections. This raises medico-legal problems, and physicians should be familiar with laws and regulations that apply in their locations to the management (including commitment) of acutely disturbed patients. Consultation with a psychiatrist or appropriate judicial authority will help protect the patient and the physician. Once the decision to give an injection has been made, adequate forces should be mustered; in the case of a muscular young male wielding an ax, several policemen may be regarded as indispensable. Once the patient has been secured, a major neuroleptic such as haloperidol 5 mg should be injected without unnecessary finesse into the nearest available muscle in a struggling patient. However, even in these circumstances the routes of major nerves must be remembered and respected. If the injection is not effective, it may be repeated hourly as necessary.

Suicide (see Ch. 141, above)

§13. RENAL AND UROLOGIC DISORDERS

143. RENAL STRUCTURE AND FUNCTION

The kidneys control the volume, composition, and pressure of body fluids by regulating the excretion of water and solutes. Through hormonal mechanisms they also influence hydroxylation of vitamin D to its biologically active form, red cell production, and BP. Urine is formed in the kidneys as an aqueous solution containing metabolic waste products, foreign substances, and water-soluble constituents of the body in quantities depending upon homeostatic needs.

Anatomy

The kidneys are bilateral, retroperitoneal structures, each consisting of an outer cortex and an inner medulla. The medulla is arranged into several cone-shaped or pyramidal projections separated from each other by sections of cortex called renal columns. The bases of the pyramids face the cortex of the kidney, while the apices (papillae) point toward the hilus and project into the renal pelvis (FIG. 143–1). The cortex contains glomeruli and tubules; the medulla, tubules only.

The kidneys possess numerous blood vessels and, because of their low vascular resistance, receive approximately 1200 ml of blood or 25% of the cardiac output each minute. The major resistance to blood flow occurs in the glomerular capillary bed and is produced by a relatively high resistance in the afferent and efferent arterioles. However, changes in renal arterial pressure produce proportional variations in the afferent arteriolar resistance, which tends to preserve a constant renal blood flow **(RBF)** and glomerular capillary pressure, i.e., **autoregulation.** In addition to autoregulation, the renal circulation is controlled by extrinsic factors such as sympathetic nerves, hormones (epinephrine, angiotensin, prostaglandins, and bradykinin), and the composition of the blood.

The Nephron

The basic functional unit of the kidney is the nephron, a long tubular structure made up of successive segments of diverse structure and transport functions. It includes (1) a **renal corpuscle** (Bowman's capsule and the glomerulus, a tuft of capillaries), (2) a **proximal tubule** (convoluted and straight portion), (3) a hairpin loop **(Henle's loop),** (4) a **distal tubule** (straight portion, macula densa, and convoluted portion), and (5) a **collecting duct system.** Each human kidney contains about one million nephrons; 85% are cortical, with short loops of Henle, and 15% are juxtamedullary, with glomeruli near the cortical medullary junction and with long, thin, looping segments (FIG. 143–2).

Glomerular Filtration

The glomerulus acts as an ultrafilter, allowing passage of water, electrolytes, and small organic molecules such as glucose, but not blood cells and large protein molecules. The ultrafiltrate produced by the glomeruli of both kidneys amounts to about 70 ml/min/sq m or 100 L/day/sq m; this rate is termed the **glomerular filtration rate (GFR).** About 99% of the glomerular filtrate is resorbed during passage through the renal tubules, with most of the resorption taking place in the proximal tubules.

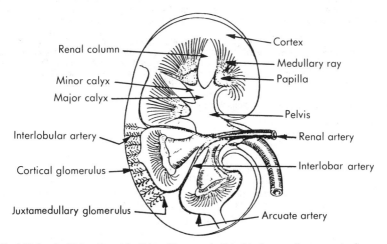

FIG. 143–1. **Sagittal section of the kidney.** The upper half depicts the overall gross anatomic arrangement. The lower half demonstrates the arterial supply. (From *Clinical Nephrology,* ed. 2, by S. Papper. Copyright 1978 by Little, Brown and Company. Used with permission.)

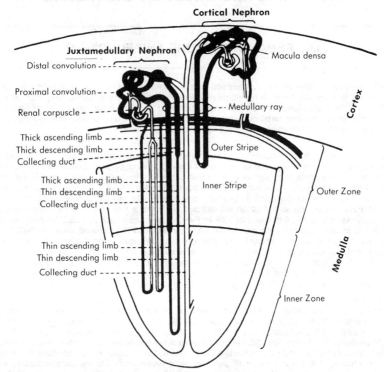

Fig. 143–2. Position of cortico- and juxtamedullary nephrons in the kidney. (From *Histology*, ed. 3, by R. O. Greep and L. Weiss. Copyright © 1973 by McGraw-Hill, Inc. Used with permission of McGraw-Hill Book Company.)

The Concept of "Clearance" and the Measurement of GFR

A principal function of the kidney is to remove or "clear" various solutes from the blood that are not essential to the body, and to conserve those that the body requires. A solute is never totally removed from the blood in any one passage through the kidneys (although sodium *p*-aminohippurate **(PAH)** may have an extraction over 90%); rather, a portion is removed during each sweep of the blood through the renal system. **Clearance** may be defined as *the volume of plasma that is completely cleared of a solute in a unit of time* and is usually expressed in ml/min. Stated another way, *the renal clearance of a substance represents the volume of plasma that would have to pass through the nephrons within a given time period to provide the amount of that substance in the urine.* Substances that are rapidly eliminated have a **high clearance;** those eliminated slowly, a **low clearance.**

The following equations illustrate the relationships involved in clearance calculations. "X" is considered as a substance that is cleared completely in one passage and can be used to measure renal plasma clearance. The symbolic relationships are:

U_x = concentration of "x" in urine
P_x = concentration of "x" in plasma
V = volume of urine excreted/min
Cl_x = renal plasma clearance of "x"
U_xV = rate of urine excretion of "x"
Cl_xP_x = rate of "x" removed or "cleared" by kidneys

When the concentration of substance "x" in the body fluids is in a steady state, the amount leaving the kidneys equals that cleared from the blood. Symbolically, this may be stated as:

$$U_xV = Cl_xP_x$$

or

$$Cl_x = \frac{U_xV}{P_x}$$

Thus, from the urinary excretion rate and the plasma concentration of "x," one can compute its renal clearance. For example, if 550 mg/min of "x" are being excreted, the same amount has entered the nephrons. If the plasma concentration during these steady-state conditions is 1 mg/ml, then 550 ml/min of plasma were virtually cleared of this substance by the kidney:

$$Cl_x = \frac{U_xV}{P_x} = \frac{550 \text{ mg/min}}{1 \text{ mg/ml}} = 550 \text{ ml/min}$$

If a substance does not undergo tubular transport after passing through the glomerulus—i.e., if it is neither resorbed nor secreted within the renal tubule—then its clearance will be a measure of GFR. Because the measurement of GFR is useful in understanding normal function and in treatment of patients with renal disease, it is desirable to have a convenient and quantitative method of its estimation. A substance that is ideally suited for such measurements is **inulin.** It is a fructose polymer with an average size of about 5000 daltons. When given IV it is freely filtered by the glomeruli and passes through the renal tubules undisturbed. The normal GFR for average young adults is about 125 ml/min.

A comparison of the renal clearance of any solute with that of inulin will give information concerning transport of that solute by the renal tubules. For example, a substance that (like inulin) is not protein-bound and is freely filtrable, but which has a lower clearance than inulin, has undergone net tubular resorption; a substance with a clearance greater than inulin, in addition to being filtered by the glomerulus, has had portions secreted by tubular cells. Certain organic substances like PAH are rapidly secreted by tubular cells and are almost entirely removed from the blood perfusing the kidneys in a single circulation. Thus, these substances are useful in determinations of **effective renal plasma flow (ERPF).**

The clearance of endogenous creatinine is often used clinically as an estimate of GFR. Unfortunately, since some creatinine is secreted by the tubules, a true measure of GFR is not obtained. Despite this, the **creatinine clearance** is convenient and adequate for most clinical purposes (see also DIAGNOSTIC PROCEDURES in Ch. 144). If the urinary excretion of creatinine is constant, then the creatinine clearance and its plasma concentration are inversely proportional.

$$Cl_{creat} \, P_{creat} = U_{creat}V$$

$$\begin{array}{c} \text{creatinine removed} \\ \text{from plasma} \end{array} = \begin{array}{c} \text{creatinine excreted} \\ \text{in urine} \end{array}$$

or

$$Cl_{creat} = \frac{U_{creat}V}{P_{creat}}$$

One can thus determine changes in renal function (GFR estimates) through single measurements of plasma creatinine. For example, a patient with an initial creatinine clearance of 100 ml/min and a creatinine plasma concentration of 1 mg/100 ml (0.01 mg/ml) has a urinary excretion rate of creatinine of 1 mg/min or 1.4 gm/day. If the serum creatinine concentration rises to 5 mg/100 ml (0.05 mg/ml) and the total urinary excretion of creatinine remains constant, then the creatinine clearance is $1/5$ the previous value or 20 ml/min.

In the first instance:

$$Cl_{creat} = \frac{U_{creat}V}{P_{creat}} = \frac{1 \text{ mg/min}}{1 \text{ mg/100 ml}} = 100 \text{ ml/min}$$

In the second instance:

$$Cl_{creat} = \frac{U_{creat}V}{P_{creat}} = \frac{1 \text{ mg/min}}{5 \text{ mg/100 ml}} = 20 \text{ ml/min}$$

Thus, one could assume that the number of functioning nephrons in the kidneys has significantly decreased. Similar relationships would exist with the blood concentration of urea, but that is more affected by protein in the diet than is creatinine, which is derived from muscle creatine.

Tubular Function

Transport or movement of solutes and water across tubular cells is one of the principal activities of the renal tubules. Transport is termed **resorption** when it proceeds from the tubular lumen to the interstitial fluid, and **secretion** when it proceeds in the reverse direction. Many solutes are transported in both directions simultaneously, but one direction usually dominates and the resultant is termed **net transport.**

Transport is energy-dependent. Tubular transport is classified according to the energy source used in the transfer process: **active transport** is the movement of a substance against a gradient of electric potential or chemical concentration; **passive transport** or **diffusion** is the migration of a substance down an electrochemical gradient, which is usually generated by the active transport of another solute.

The activity of the tubules may be appreciated by comparing the rates at which substances are filtered into the nephrons with the rates at which they are excreted in the urine (TABLE 143–1). The tubules are largely occupied with conservation of water and essential solutes and the elimination of certain waste products.

TABLE 143-1. FILTRATION AND RESORPTION IN THE NEPHRONS

Substance	Amount Filtered Daily*	Amount in Urine Daily*	Net Tubular Resorption*
Water	180 L	1.5 L	99%
Sodium	26,000 mEq	150 mEq	99%
Potassium	810 mEq	100 mEq	88%
Glucose	1000 mM	nil	100%
Amino acids	65 gm	2 gm	98%
Urea	-1280 mM	500 mM	60%

* These values are approximate.

Fine adjustments of water and solute excretion take place in the distal tubule (convolutions and collecting ducts). Transport in the distal tubule differs from that in the proximal tubule in the former's capacity to resorb and secrete against large gradients. Furthermore, it is the only segment of the nephron that responds to both antidiuretic hormone (ADH) and aldosterone. ADH enhances water resorption, while aldosterone enhances the transport capacity for sodium resorption with reciprocal potassium and hydrogen ion secretion. By being distal, the sodium and water resorption in the collecting duct cannot be reversed by a subsequent segment of the nephron, and thus is the final determinant of urine composition.

Tubular Resorption

Glucose resorption illustrates an active-transport–limited system wherein, at normal plasma glucose levels and GFR, the glucose is completely resorbed and its clearance or excretion is nil. The mechanisms involved permit transporting a fixed amount of glucose in a unit of time (transport maximum or T_m) across the tubular cells. If the filtered glucose load (plasma glucose $\times$ GFR) exceeds the T_m, glucose begins to appear in the urine. The higher the plasma glucose concentration, the greater the amount of glucose filtered, compared to that resorbed. Thus, when the glucose Tm is exceeded, the glucose clearance approaches the GFR as the plasma glucose concentration increases.

Although glucose is the best prototype for illustration, amino acids and other inorganic and organic compounds undergo transport-limited resorption. Phosphate resorption capacity is modulated by parathyroid hormone. The control of other transport processes is generally unknown. Natriuretic hormone may influence sodium transport.

Urea resorption. Urea, like water, is resorbed passively throughout the nephron. Because of passive resorption, the excretion of urea is variable and depends upon urine concentration and flow. About 1/3 of filtered urea is resorbed in man when the urine is copious and dilute, while 80% may be resorbed during dehydration when urine flow is low and the urine concentrated.

Sodium (Na) resorption. Enough resorption of Na and water occurs on passage through the proximal tubules to cause a 60 to 80% reduction in glomerular filtrate volume. Peritubular capillaries and proximal tubular fluid remain isosmotic with arterial plasma throughout proximal tubular resorption (osmotic gradients between them are not seen). Since most of the osmotic activity of water within the proximal tubules is due to Na and its associated anions (chloride and bicarbonate), it follows that Na and water are simultaneously resorbed, and their ratio is set by plasma osmolality. Water resorption seems to be passive and coupled to active Na resorption.

Unlike threshold-limited transport, proximal tubular resorption of Na is not saturable but seems to exhibit gradient-limited characteristics. This is evident when large quantities of nonresorbed solutes (e.g., glucose or mannitol) are present in the proximal tubular lumen. Their presence decreases the resorption of Na and water from the lumen, producing a large volume of urine. This obligate retention of Na and water in the presence of large amounts of unresorbed solutes is the basic mechanism of osmotic diuresis.

The distal nephron is the final arbiter of Na elimination, since it is there that Na can be resorbed against large gradients and there, too, that aldosterone enhances the transport capacity (see Tubular Function, above).

The interrelationship between the filtration and resorption of Na is a central factor in the renal regulation of Na. Under a variety of circumstances, the fraction of filtered Na resorbed in the proximal segment is relatively constant despite acute changes in GFR, a concept termed glomerulotubular balance. This balance is neither perfect nor constant. If the GFR is chronically reduced, the resorption of Na will decrease proportionally more than the decrease in filtration so that Na excretion equals dietary intake. Thus, renal control of Na balance resides not in regulation of filtration but in tubular resorption of Na. Nonetheless, the contribution of acute changes in GFR cannot be ignored, as small changes can produce relatively large variations in the absolute rate of Na excretion before adjustment in tubular resorption occurs.

The physiologic factors that bring about changes in the rate of tubular resorption of sodium are not well understood, but are influenced by certain extrarenal and intrarenal factors (FIG. 143-3). For a discussion of regulation of water and sodium homeostasis see Ch. 81.

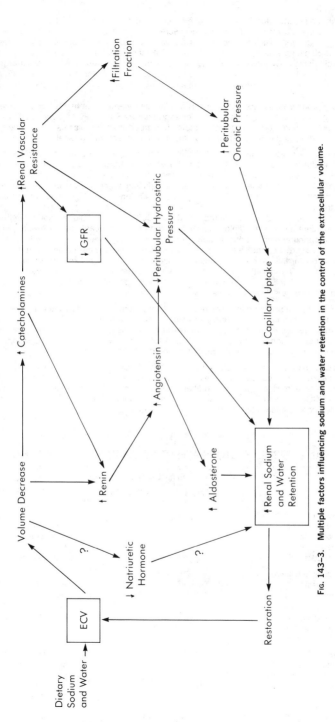

FIG. 143-3.   Multiple factors influencing sodium and water retention in the control of the extracellular volume.

Tubular Secretion

Although tubular transport is mainly concerned with returning the bulk of the glomerular filtrate to the plasma, some plasma solutes are actively secreted into the tubular lumen and excreted. A renal clearance greater than GFR is evidence of tubular secretion. Exogenous organic bases such as thiamine or quinidine and organic acids such as PAH and penicillin are rapidly excreted once they enter the circulation. They are filtered and also actively secreted into the urine. Most organic acids compete with each other for secretion, as do most organic bases (competition between acids and bases is rare). This explains why probenecid, an organic acid, interferes with the secretion of penicillin.

Secretory processes also exhibit transport maximums. Therefore, at high plasma concentrations, filtration may become the dominant mode of excretion. PAH is so avidly secreted that at plasma levels far below saturation it is almost completely cleared from the plasma in a single circulation through the kidney and has, therefore, been found useful in estimating renal blood flow.

Potassium (K) excretion. The usual adult daily diet contains 50 to 100 mEq of K. Small quantities of K are lost in the feces and perspiration, but the kidney is the dominant organ of K excretion and regulation. Studies of renal clearance have demonstrated that K excretion is not closely linked to the filtered load of K. For example, with severe renal insufficiency, the K excretory rate may exceed the quantity filtered by the glomeruli. This also occurs with functional decreases in filtration such as vasoconstriction.

Since approximately 90% of the filtered K and 60 to 80% of tubular fluid is resorbed in the proximal tubule, K concentration in this fluid is lower than the plasma concentration. However, in the distal tubule the K concentration is considerably greater than in plasma, even on a low K intake. Thus, K undergoes net secretion, and renal conservation of K is relatively poor compared to Na resorption, where distal tubular fluid to plasma Na concentration ratios can be below 0.01. Whereas urinary Na concentration may be nil with a marked stimulus for Na conservation, the urinary K concentration rarely is $<$ 5 to 10 mEq/L, even with severe and prolonged K deprivation. The factors affecting potassium secretion are listed in TABLE 143–2.

Hydrogen ion (proton) excretion. The net quantity of protons excreted by the kidney is small (50 to 100 mEq/day) compared to that excreted by the lungs via carbonic acid (15,000 mEq/day). Therefore, *disturbances in pulmonary function can result in acidosis within minutes, while several days are required to produce the same degree of change following cessation of renal function.* The renal regulation of acid-base balance is discussed in Ch. 81.

Bicarbonate (HCO_3^-) resorption. Ordinarily, the rate of HCO_3^- resorption is adjusted to maintain a constant plasma HCO_3^- concentration of about 25 mEq/L. HCO_3^- resorption resembles a threshold-limited mechanism in which increases in filtered load above the threshold level lead to excretion of the excess HCO_3^- in the urine. However, no true threshold for HCO_3^- is demonstrable, and the rate of resorption can be altered by several important factors (see Ch. 81).

TABLE 143–2. FACTORS AFFECTING POTASSIUM SECRETION*

	Renal Change		Steady-State Potassium Balance
	Days 1-2	Days 3+	
Acid-base			
Respiratory alkalosis	↑	0	No change
Metabolic alkalosis	↑↑↑	↑↑↑	Severe depletion
Respiratory acidosis	↓	↑	Minimal depletion
Metabolic acidosis	↓	↑↑	Moderate depletion
Fluid-electrolyte balance			
Sodium loading	↑	↑	Minimal depletion
Sodium deprivation	↓	0	No change
Potassium loading	↑	↑↑	Minimal excess
Potassium deprivation	↓↓	↓	Moderate depletion
Water loading	0	0	No change
Drugs			
Acetazolamide	↑↑↑	0	Minimal depletion
Thiazide, furosemide	↑↑	↑	Minimal depletion
Mannitol or urea diuresis	↑	↑	Minimal depletion
Aldosterone	↑↑	↑↑	Moderate depletion
Spironolactone	↓	↓	Minimal excess
Triamterene	↓	↓	Minimal excess

* ↑=increase; ↓=decrease; 0=no change.

It might be assumed that resorption of HCO_3^- occurs passively as the result of active Na transport. Such passive resorption would require that the tubule be permeable to HCO_3^-. However, although the tubule is quite permeable to Cl^-, it is relatively impermeable to HCO_3^-. Thus, the resorption of bicarbonate must be an active process. A model of a widely held concept of HCO_3^- resorption is shown in Fig. 143-4. About 4,000 mEq of HCO_3^- are filtered daily by the glomeruli in healthy adults. If this HCO_3^- were not resorbed, it would be equivalent to adding > 4 L of 1 N acid to the body. Thus, the resorption of HCO_3^- is a normal conservation process, and essentially none appears in the urine. Carbonic anhydrase within the tubular cell catalyzes the hydration of carbon dioxide (CO_2) to carbonic acid, which dissociates into H^+ and HCO_3^-. The HCO_3^- generated by this reaction moves passively out of the cell and into the peritubular fluid. The remaining H^+ is secreted into the tubular fluid and reacts with filtered HCO_3^- in the tubular lumen, reforming carbonic acid and then CO_2 and water. The CO_2 formed in the tubular lumen diffuses back into the cell, thus completing the cycle. Carbonic anhydrase inhibitors interfere with this sequence by impairing the hydration reaction and thus the generation of H^+ and HCO_3^- from CO_2 and water in the cell; they also inhibit HCO_3^- transport across the peritubular membrane. Both actions limit HCO_3^- resorption and H^+ secretion. Inhibition must be virtually complete to produce diuresis, which in turn is limited by the metabolic acidosis produced. Inhibition plus HCO_3^- repletion has been used to alkalinize the urine and increase urate solubility in diseases where urate uropathy is likely.

H^+ may also react with certain salts such as phosphate to form acid salts, or with NH_3 to form NH_4^+. In this instance, new HCO_3^- is generated and returned to the ECF via the renal veins to restore that which was decomposed by reaction with inorganic and organic acids produced by cellular metabolism. On a quantitative basis, the protons involved in HCO_3^- resorption greatly exceed those that generate new HCO_3^-.

Ammonium excretion. Ammonia (NH_3) is formed in the tubular cells from amino acid precursors, principally glutamine. It carries no electrical charge, is lipid-soluble, penetrates cell membranes readily, and diffuses easily throughout the kidney. It reacts with hydrogen ions, forming ammonium ions (NH_4^+) which are highly soluble in water and do not readily penetrate cell membranes. The difference in membrane penetrability between NH_3 and ammonium ions is referred to as **nonionic diffusion** and best explains why NH_4^+ excretion varies with urine pH. Differences in pH between collecting duct fluid and renal venous blood determine the distribution of ammonium ions between these compartments and thus regulate the proportion leaving the kidney. The lower the urine pH, the more NH_4^+ appears in the urine (Fig. 143-5).

NH_4^+ excretion is also influenced by the production rate of NH_3. Changes in systemic acid-base balance regulate the rate of NH_3 formation from glutamine, with metabolic acidosis stimulating NH_3 production and alkalosis inhibiting it. This alteration in NH_3 formation and, hence, in NH_4^+ excretion in response to acid-base disturbances represents one of the most important mechanisms by which the kidney can adjust hydrogen ion excretion in response to changing rates of hydrogen ion production.

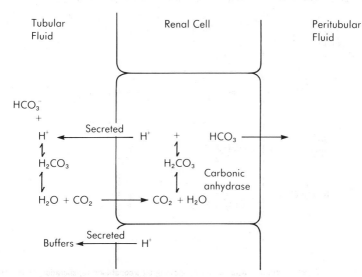

FIG. 143-4. **Bicarbonate resorption model.** (From *The Urinary System,* by W. H. Chapman et al. Copyright 1973 by W. B. Saunders Company. Used with permission.)

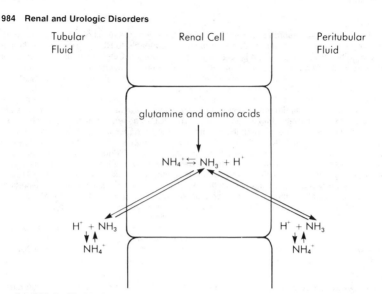

Tubular   Renal Cell   Peritubular
Fluid   Fluid

FIG. 143-5. **Model of ammonium excretion.** (From *The Urinary System,* by W. H. Chapman et al. Copyright 1973 by W. B. Saunders Company. Used with permission.)

Titratable acid. Hydrogen ions secreted into the tubular fluid are buffered by anions of weak acids in addition to NH_3. At the normal pH of urine, phosphate is the major buffer that contributes to the formation of titratable acid. When urine pH is between 4.5 and 5, creatinine and urate also buffer hydrogen ions in significant amounts and contribute to the titratable acid (FIG. 143-6).

Concentration and dilution of urine. Variation in urine osmolality is dependent on 3 physiologic features: (1) varying permeabilities to water in the loop of Henle and collecting tubular segments, (2) active resorption of sodium chloride from luminal fluid, and (3) the unique structural arrangements of the vasa recta, Henle's loop, and the collecting ducts to produce a countercurrent multiplier and exchanger system. Only the juxtamedullary nephrons are involved in the countercurrent operations that concentrate the urine. The other nephrons produce a dilute urine because of the unique characteristics of their tubular cells in the thick segment of the ascending limb, where transport of NaCl occurs *without* passive diffusion of water, thus creating a hypotonic tubular fluid.

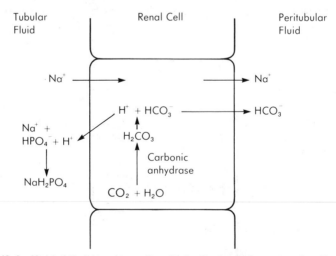

Tubular   Renal Cell   Peritubular
Fluid   Fluid

FIG. 143-6. **Model of titratable acid excretion, showing bicarbonate ion regeneration.** (From *The Urinary System,* by W. H. Chapman et al. Copyright 1973 by W. B. Saunders Company. Used with permission.)

The countercurrent multiplier mechanism. The ability of the kidney to concentrate urine depends on the spatial arrangement of the juxtamedullary nephrons (FIG. 143–7). An osmotic gradient exists between the corticomedullary junction and the papilla. As the glomerular filtrate proceeds through the proximal tubule, resorption of solutes and water greatly reduces filtrate volume while keeping osmolality constant. In a juxtamedullary nephron, however, upon entering the descending limb of Henle's loop, the filtrate begins to increase in osmolality until, at the tip of the loop, or the region of the papilla, tubular fluid osmolality is about 4 times that of plasma. During passage through the ascending limb, this fluid undergoes a reversal in osmolality. As it proceeds through the thick segment of the ascending limb, a net decrease in osmolality (dilution) occurs because of the resorption of NaCl, so that fluid entering the distal convoluted tubule is hypotonic to plasma and cortical interstitial fluid.

Medullary hypertonicity results, apparently from the interstitial accumulation of solutes, primarily NaCl and urea. The driving force for solute accumulation is probably provided by an electrogenic chloride pump in the thick ascending limb of Henle's loop. The active extrusion of NaCl by the thick ascending limb into the medullary interstitium produces a progressive concentration (almost entirely by water abstraction) of the fluid flowing along the descending limb. Thus, fluid entering the ascending thin limb has a higher NaCl concentration and a lower urea concentration than in the medullary interstitium. These chemical differences between lumen and interstitium, coupled with the fact that the thin ascending limb is more permeable to NaCl than to urea, further assist in fluid dilution. As fluid moves up the water-impermeable ascending thin limb, passive NaCl efflux from lumen to interstitium exceeds passive urea influx from interstitium to tubular fluid, producing progressive dilution of ascending fluid and, concomitantly, urea cycling from the medullary collecting ducts through the interstitium to ascending thin limbs. Finally, the process begins again with active NaCl transport from the thick ascending limb. These changes occur regardless of the volume and concentration of the final urine and are not influenced by ADH.

The distal convoluted tubule is water-impermeable, both in the presence and absence of ADH. However, water moves passively across the cortical and medullary collecting tubules just as in the proximal tubule, but water permeability of these segments is variable, unlike that of the proximal tubule. Permeability of the collecting ducts to water varies with the circulating level of ADH. These segments are relatively water-impermeable in the absence of ADH, and increase their water permeability tenfold in the presence of ADH. When high titers of ADH are present, hypotonic fluid entering the cortical collecting ducts rapidly loses water until it becomes iso-osmolar with the surrounding cortical interstitium. As this fluid flows through the collecting ducts, it continues to lose water to the hypertonic medullary interstitium and emerges from the papillae hypertonic to cortical or arterial plasma.

Countercurrent exchange: The anatomic arrangement of the vasa recta facilitates its function as a countercurrent exchanger and assures maintenance of a hypertonic interstitium. As the vasa recta blood descends in the capillary loop, it approaches osmotic equilibrium with the surrounding hypertonic environment, with the passive diffusion of NaCl and other solutes (mainly urea) into the capil-

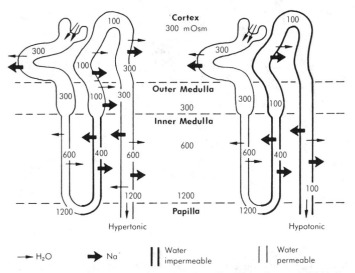

FIG. 143–7. Schema of countercurrent mechanism. (From *The Urinary System*, by W. H. Chapman et al. Copyright 1973 by W. B. Saunders Company. Used with permission.)

lary lumen while water diffuses out. As the blood doubles back on itself and ascends to the corticomedullary junction, these solutes return to the interstitium while water diffuses in. Thus, the countercurrent vascular loops serve as a source of O_2 and other nutrients but tend to minimize the loss of solutes from, and the addition of water to, the medulla. The hypertonic medullary gradient would be rapidly dissipated if blood were flowing in one direction only. This mechanism may also concentrate drugs in the medulla, such as acetaminophen.

The diluting mechanism. From a structural-functional viewpoint, 2 important considerations exist for the development of a hypotonic urine: (1) solute must be removed from the urine without the concomitant diffusion of water, and (2) the tubular area distal to the diluting site must remain relatively water-impermeable.

The process of dilution begins in the thick segment of the ascending limb where NaCl is removed from the tubular fluid without passive diffusion of water. Under all conditions of hydration, urine entering and traversing the distal convoluted tubule is always hypotonic. When the ADH titer is low, the collecting ducts are impermeable to water, and urine traversing these segments remains hypotonic. The exact dilution of the final urine also depends on the amount of Na resorbed by the distal tubule without concomitant water resorption. The most dilute urines are produced by water-loaded and Na-depleted individuals.

RENAL HORMONAL FUNCTIONS

The kidney plays an integral role in many endocrine functions, being a target organ for some hormones (e.g., ADH, aldosterone), affecting intermediary metabolism of others (e.g., converting vitamin D to its most active metabolite [1,25-dihydroxycholecalciferol] and degrading insulin), and actively secreting hormones. Some of these renal-endocrine relations are discussed elsewhere in this volume and in Vol. II; in this chapter, the renin-angiotensin-aldosterone system, erythropoietin, and the kallikrein-kinin system are reviewed.

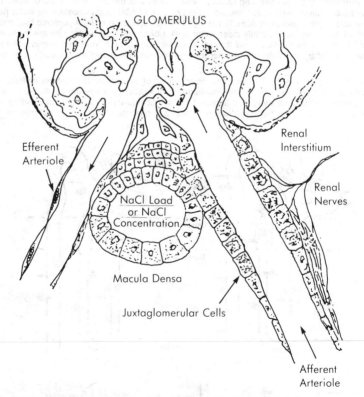

GLOMERULUS

Efferent Arteriole

Renal Interstitium

Renal Nerves

NaCl Load or NaCl Concentration

Macula Densa

Juxtaglomerular Cells

Afferent Arteriole

Fig. 143–8. **Diagram of the juxtaglomerular apparatus.** (Modified from J. O. Davis: "What Signals the Kidney to Release Renin?" *Circulation Research*, Vol. 28, pp. 301–306, Mar. 1971. Used with permission of the American Heart Association, Inc., and the author.)

Renin-angiotensin-aldosterone system. The juxtaglomerular apparatus **(JGA)** is involved in volume and pressure regulations. Renin, a proteolytic enzyme, is formed in the granules of the JGA cells (Fig. 143–8) and catalyzes the conversion of angiotensinogen (a plasma protein) to angiotensin I (Fig. 143–9). This inactive product is cleaved by a converting enzyme, mainly in the lung but also in the kidney and brain, to angiotensin II, which then stimulates the release of aldosterone. The des-Asp heptapeptide, or angiotensin III, is also found in the circulation and is as active as angiotensin II in stimulating aldosterone release but has much less pressor activity.

The secretion of renin is controlled by at least 4 mechanisms that are not mutually exclusive: (1) a renal vascular receptor that apparently responds to changes in tension in the afferent arteriole wall; (2) a macula densa receptor that appears to detect changes in the rate of delivery or concentration of sodium chloride in the distal tubule; (3) a negative feedback effect of circulating angiotensin on renin secretion; and (4) the CNS, that stimulates renin secretion via the renal nerve, the adrenal medulla (catecholamine release), and the posterior pituitary (vasopressin release). A simplified schema for the operation of the renin-angiotensin-aldosterone system is given in Fig. 143–10. In general, factors that block β-adrenoceptors or produce an increase in the circulating blood volume and pressure cause renal afferent arteriolar vasoconstriction, and inhibit renin release. Contrarily, a decrease in the extracellular compartment or β-adrenoceptor stimulation causes renal vasodilatation, resulting in renin release.

Erythropoietin production apparently is responsive to a renal oxygen sensor that detects tissue oxygen deprivation (see Fig. 143–11). For example, increased erythropoietin output has been demonstrated experimentally by a reduction in renal blood flow, in vitro perfusion of isolated kidneys with hypoxic blood, increased renal pressure through ureteral obstruction or large intrarenal cysts, and microinfarction of the kidney. It seems probable that erythropoietin production and oxygen sensing take place in the same cells, but it is unclear whether these cells are located in the cortex or medulla.

Patients with end-stage renal disease as well as anephric patients have a low (5 to 10% of normal) rate of erythrocyte production. (See also Anemia of Renal Disease, p. 713.) Such production is provided by nonrenal synthesis of erythropoietin which appears also to be responsive to tissue hypoxia. Hepatocytes or Kupffer cells are suspected as the site of nonrenal production.

Erythrocytosis from inappropriate secretion of erythropoietin is not uncommon. Renal neoplasms and benign tumors, polycystic kidney disease, solitary renal cysts, and hydronephrosis are renal disorders commonly associated with erythrocytosis. It is felt that the high levels of erythropoietin occasionally seen with these disorders are produced by partially compressed and hypoxic normal renal tissue. The secretion of an erythropoietin-like material has also been reported in a number of

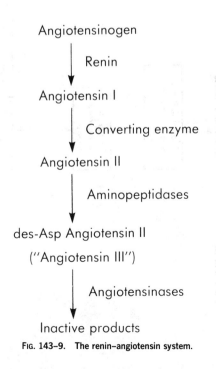

Fig. 143–9. The renin–angiotensin system.

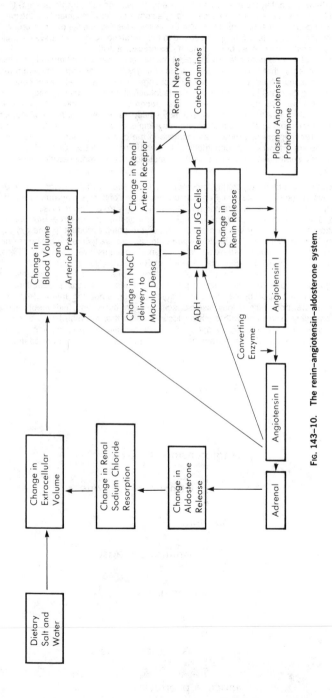

Fig. 143-10. The renin–angiotensin–aldosterone system.

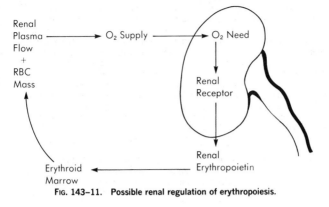

FIG. 143–11. Possible renal regulation of erythropoiesis.

patients with other neoplasms, such as hepatomas and cerebellar hemangiomas. In such cases, it is likely that the erythropoietin production is directly from the neoplastic tissue.

The prostaglandins (see Ch. 252)

Kallikrein-kinin system. The enzyme kallikrein, present mainly in the renal cortex and seen in the urine, may have significance as a local hormone through the local production of the end metabolite bradykinin, a vasodilator peptide. Current evidence suggests that this system is an important part of an intrarenal hormonal regulatory complex which also includes the renin-angiotensin-aldosterone system and prostaglandins. Abnormalities of this system may be involved in certain forms of hypertension, kidney disease, and fluid and electrolyte disorders.

144. CLINICAL EVALUATION OF GENITOURINARY DISORDERS

Symptoms of GU disorders may be nonspecific, but careful acquisition and analysis of data from the history, physical examination, and appropriate laboratory studies should provide accurate diagnosis.

A family history of renal disease in an adult may suggest polycystic disease or, if associated with ear and eye disorders, may indicate hereditary nephropathy. A history of recent infectious diseases involving the skin, respiratory tract, or endocardium is helpful in evaluating possible causes of glomerulonephritis. A specific history of renal disease, trauma to the urinary system, stones, or prior urinary system surgery is important, as is a previous history of hypertension or a systemic disease known to affect the kidney (e.g., diabetes mellitus, SLE). The clinical approach to such data is discussed here; specific disorders are discussed separately in the following chapters.

SYMPTOMS AND SIGNS

Fever, weight loss, and malaise are common. The presence of fever together with symptoms of urinary tract infection is helpful in evaluating the site of the infection. Simple acute cystitis is an afebrile disease, whereas acute pyelonephritis or prostatitis usually produces high fever. Occasionally, renal carcinoma is associated with fever. Weight loss is to be expected in the advanced stages of cancer but it may also be noticed when renal insufficiency from any cause supervenes.

Changes in Micturition

Most people void about 4 to 6 times/day, mostly in the daytime. **Frequency** (*frequent micturition*), unassociated with an increase in urine volume, is a symptom of diminution in bladder effective filling capacity. Infection, foreign bodies, stones, or tumor, causing injury to the bladder mucosa or underlying structures and leading to inflammatory infiltration and edema, resulting in mild stretching of the bladder and a loss of bladder elasticity, produce a functional decrease, pain, and a compelling **urgency** to urinate. Involuntary urination may even occur, if voiding is not immediate. Voidings are usually small in volume and the desire to urinate may be felt as almost constant **urinary tenesmus** until the irritative process resolves. **Dysuria** (*painful urination*) suggests irritation or inflammation in the bladder neck or urethra, usually due to bacterial infection. Persistent symptoms in the absence of such infection require careful evaluation of the bladder and urethra. **Nocturia** (*voiding during the night*) is an abnormal, but nonspecific, symptom, which may reflect early renal disease with a decrease in concentrating capacity but is commonly associated with cardiac and hepatic failure without evidence of intrinsic urinary system disease. Nocturia may also occur without disease, e.g., as a result of excessive fluid intake in the late evening. **Enuresis** *(bed-wetting at night)* is physiologic during the first 2 or 3 yr of life but becomes an increasing problem after that age. It may be produced by delayed neuromuscular maturation of the lower urinary tract, or it may indicate organic disease, e.g., infection or distal urethral stenosis in girls, posterior urethral valves in boys, or neurogenic bladder. (See also Ch. 156 and BEHAVIORAL PROBLEMS in Vol. II, Ch. 24.)

Hesitancy, straining, and **decrease in force and caliber of the urinary stream** are common symptoms of obstructions distal to the bladder. In men, these are most commonly associated with prostatic obstruction, less often with urethral stricture. Similar symptoms in a male child suggest posterior urethral valves, congenital urethral stricture, or meatal stenosis. In women these symptoms suggest meatal stenosis.

Incontinence *(a loss of urine without warning)* is associated with exstrophy of the bladder, epispadias, vesicovaginal fistula, ectopic ureteral orifices, congenital or acquired neurogenic bladder dysfunction, as well as injuries sustained during prostatectomy or childbirth. In women, incontinence with mild physical stress such as coughing, laughing, running, or lifting is commonly associated with a cystocele. Loss of urine due to bladder outlet obstruction or a flaccid bladder may produce **overflow incontinence** when the intravesicular pressure exceeds outlet resistance. Residual urine is always present with overflow incontinence.

Pneumaturia *(the passage of gas in the urine)*, a rare symptom, usually indicates a fistula between the urinary tract and the bowel. This may be a complication of diverticulitis, with abscess formation, enterocolitis, carcinoma of the colon, or vesicovaginal fistula. Rarely, pneumaturia may be due to gas formation from bacteriuria alone. **Chyluria** is *lymph in urine produced by rupture of a lymph vessel or filariasis*. **Milky urine** may be caused by precipitated phosphates in an alkaline urine. **Brick dust urine** usually is produced by precipitated urates in an acid urine.

Changes in Urinary Output

Normally, adults void between 700 and 2000 ml daily. Impairment in renal concentrating capacity may occur with many forms of renal disease and may cause **polyuria** *(a daily urine volume > 2500 ml)*. **Oliguria** *(< 500 ml/day)* tends to be an acute condition that may be due to decreased renal perfusion (prerenal factors), ureteral or bladder outlet obstruction (postrenal factors), or primary renal disease. **Anuria** *(< 100 ml/day)* is usually associated with uremia and may signal acute renal failure or the end stage of chronic progressive renal insufficiency. Since anuria can also be due to urinary obstruction that may be reversible, this possibility must be ruled out when acute anuria occurs.

Changes in the Appearance of Urine

Urine may be clear during water diuresis or may be a deep yellow color due to the presence of chromogens, such as urobilin, when maximally concentrated. If excretion of food pigments (usually red in color) or drugs (brown, black, blue, green, or red) can be excluded, colors other than yellow suggest the presence of disease such as hematuria, hemoglobinuria, myoglobinuria, pyuria, porphyria, or melanoma. Urine frequently appears cloudy, suggesting pyuria due to a urinary tract inflammation, but this is more commonly due to precipitated amorphous phosphate salts in an alkaline urine. Microscopy of the urine sediment and chemical analysis of the urine usually identify the cause.

Hematuria *(blood in the urine)* can produce red to brown discoloration depending on the amount of blood present and the acidity of the urine. Slight hematuria may cause no discoloration and may only be detected by chemical testing or microscopic examination. When hematuria is noted, the presence or absence of pain related to the urinary system is important. Hematuria without pain is usually due to renal, vesical, or prostatic disease. In the absence of RBC casts (which indicate glomerulonephritis), silent hematuria may be caused by bladder or kidney tumor. Such tumors usually bleed intermittently, and complacency must not occur if the bleeding stops spontaneously. Other causes of asymptomatic hematuria include stones, polycystic disease, renal cysts, sickle cell disease, hydronephrosis, and benign prostatic hyperplasia. When discomfort such as renal colic accompanies hematuria, a ureteral stone is suggested, although a clot from renal bleeding could cause the same type of pain. Hematuria with dysuria is also associated with bladder infections or lithiasis.

Pain (see also renal colic in Ch. 158)

Pain related to renal disease is usually in the flank or back between the 12th rib and the iliac crest, with occasional radiation to the epigastrium. Stretching of the pain-sensitive renal capsule is the probable cause and may occur in any condition producing parenchymatous swelling, such as acute glomerulonephritis, pyelonephritis, or acute ureteral obstruction. There is often marked tenderness over the kidney in the costovertebral angle formed by the 12th rib and the lumbar spine. Inflammation or distention of the renal pelvis or ureter causes pain in the flank and hypochondrium, with radiation into the ipsilateral iliac fossa and often into the upper thigh, testicle, or labium. The pain is intermittent but does not completely remit between waves of colic.

The most common cause of **bladder pain** is bacterial cystitis, and the discomfort is commonly suprapubic and referred to the distal urethra during urination. Acute urinary retention causes agonizing pain in the suprapubic area, but chronic urinary retention due to bladder neck obstruction or neurogenic bladder usually causes little discomfort.

Prostatic disease generally is painless, but with prostatitis a vague discomfort or fullness in the perineal or rectal area may be noted. On the other hand, **testicular pain** due to trauma or infection is usually severe and felt locally.

Edema

Edema usually represents excessive water and sodium in the extracellular space due to abnormal renal excretion, but it may be caused by cardiac, hepatic, or renal disease. Initially, the problem is evident only by an increase in weight, but later, edema becomes overt. Edema associated with renal disease may be noted first as facial puffiness rather than swelling in dependent or lower parts of the body, but this characteristic is neither essential nor specific. If fluid retention continues, **anasarca** (*generalized edema*) with fluid transudates (effusions) in the pleural and peritoneal cavities may be seen; it is most frequently associated with continuous, heavy proteinuria (the nephrotic syndrome).

Hematospermia

Less than 2% of urologic referrals are due to bloody semen. Most patients have repeated episodes of hematospermia, although some experience it just once. It is usually idiopathic but may be associated with prolonged sexual abstinence, frequent coitus, interrupted coitus, and bleeding disorders. Many urologists ascribe the symptoms to seminal vesiculopathy as a result of some unidentified infection or vascular congestion. The disorder is benign and rarely associated with malignancy or serious infection. It is always useful, however, to evaluate such patients for prostatic infection or urethral strictures. Because the etiology is unknown in most cases, treatment is largely empirical. Some urologists advocate a 5- to 7-day trial of tetracycline 250 mg q.i.d. followed by gentle massage. In the absence of overt urologic disease, patients should be reassured that the problem is not serious or progressive.

Nonspecific Symptoms and Signs

Most patients with progressive decompensation of the urinary system are asymptomatic early in the process. However, when sufficient renal function is lost (GFR < 10% of normal), disturbances of multiple organ systems occur producing symptoms ascribable to **uremia.** Weight loss, weakness, fatigue, dyspnea, anorexia, nausea and vomiting, itching, failure to grow, tetany, peripheral neuropathy, pericarditis, and convulsions are the usual symptoms and signs. Most of these can be ameliorated or reversed by dialysis or renal transplantation and good nutrition.

Hypertension in childhood is commonly secondary to renal disease (vascular occlusion, glomerulonephritis); progressive renal failure in children and adults usually produces hypertension. However, not more than 5% of adult hypertension is due to renovascular causes (with major renal artery or segmental artery obstruction and demonstrable increased renin secretion from the obstructed side).

The skin may show pallor, suggesting anemia, commonly associated with renal disease; excoriations may be present, suggesting pruritus; and infections, e.g., carbuncles or cellulitis, may be due to glomerulonephritis. Occasionally, skin lesions from vasculitis or endocarditis are present, suggesting a possible cause of renal disease.

Examination of the **optic fundi** helps to evaluate vascular disease and may reveal hemorrhages, exudates, and papilledema. The **mouth** may reveal stomatitis or an ammoniacal odor, while a look at the **face, abdomen,** or **extremities** may indicate edema. The finding by palpation of enlarged **kidneys, bladder,** or **prostate** is an important clue.

DIAGNOSTIC PROCEDURES

Hypoproliferative anemia may be a clue to renal failure in an otherwise asymptomatic patient, but many other causes (such as neoplasia and systemic inflammatory diseases) must be excluded. Likewise, polycythemia may occur in renal cell carcinoma or polycystic disease, but more common causes should be considered first.

Serum chemistries are often abnormal when renal dysfunction is present, but the changes are nonspecific and may be produced by variations in renal blood flow **(RBF)** as well as by parenchymatous renal disease. Hypernatremia, for instance, is most frequently due to lack of adequate water intake in an obtunded patient but can also be produced by excessive water loss from a renal concentrating defect due to tubulointerstitial disease (e.g., nephrogenic diabetes insipidus, hypercalcemic or potassium depletion nephropathy). As another example, the serum bicarbonate may be reduced as a consequence of metabolic acidosis due to renal disease, but other causes such as lactic acidosis or ketoacidosis must be excluded. The most specific serum chemical determination for the diagnosis of renal dysfunction is the serum creatinine (see Measurement of Renal Function, below).

Urinalysis

The urinalysis is the best guide to intrinsic GU disease. It includes a qualitative evaluation for the presence of protein, glucose, ketones, blood, and nitrites; determination of the urinary pH; and microscopic examination of the sediment. The solute concentration of urine should be measured by either refractometry (sp gr) or osmometry (osmolarity).

Proteinuria (see also in NEPHROTIC SYNDROME, Ch. 148): Commercially available dipsticks permit simple and rapid testing. The dipstick technic is sensitive to as little as 5 to 20 mg/dl of albumin, the predominant protein in most renal diseases, but is less sensitive to globulins and mucoproteins and may be negative in the presence of Bence Jones proteins (found in multiple myeloma or a related lymphoproliferative disorder). Electrophoresis, immunoelectrophoresis, and radioimmunoassays are also available to separate or quantitate various urinary proteins.

The major mechanisms producing proteinuria are (1) elevated plasma concentrations of normal or abnormal proteins ("overflow" proteinuria such as lysozymuria in myelomonocytic leukemia or Bence-Jones proteinuria in multiple myeloma); (2) increased tubular cell secretion (Tamm-Horsfall proteinuria); (3) decreased tubular resorption of normal filtered proteins; and (4) an increase of filtered proteins caused by altered glomerular capillary permeability.

In most adults with proteinuria, the abnormality is first observed as an "isolated" finding during a routine physical examination in an asymptomatic subject who appears healthy and exhibits no evidence of systemic or renal disease. Daily total protein excretion is usually < 1 gm (urine protein/creatinine ratio < 0.1). Different qualitative patterns of proteinuria have been described although the correlation of these patterns with long-term prognosis is not well established. Two types of classification have been used, one based on body posture and the other without regard to body posture. In the first approach, repetitive tests identify proteinuria as "**constant**" if it is present during recumbency and quiet upright ambulation, and "**orthostatic**" when it is present only in the upright position. Using the 2nd scheme, the pattern is "**intermittent**" if proteinuria comes and goes, and "**persistent**" if proteinuria is found in all urine samples examined. The exact significance of intermittent or orthostatic proteinuria is not clear; most patients do not show any deterioration of renal function and in about 50% the proteinuria ceases after several years. However, the presence of constant or persistent proteinuria is more serious. Although the course is indolent in the absence of other indicators of renal disease, such as microscopic hematuria, most patients continue to demonstrate proteinuria over a course of many years; many develop an abnormal urine sediment and hypertension, and a few progress to renal failure.

When proteinuria is constant or persistent, quantitative measurements of protein excretion are useful for diagnosis and to follow the clinical progress of patients. These are accomplished by measuring the total protein voided in a 10- to 24-h period; normally, < 150 mg/day of protein are excreted. Alternatively, a random sample of urine is used to relate the amount of protein present to its creatinine content. Normally, the protein/creatinine ratio is < 0.1. Heavy proteinuria (> 2 gm/sq m/day or a protein/creatinine ratio > 2) is usually found in patients with glomerulopathy producing the nephrotic syndrome. Proteinuria is usually minimal, intermittent, or absent in diseases primarily involving the tubulointerstitial area (e.g., pyelonephritis, analgesic nephropathy, benign nephrosclerosis, nephropathies of hypercalcemia and potassium depletion).

Exercise proteinuria is sometimes seen in joggers, marathon runners, and boxers. It is accompanied by elevation of catecholamines and there may be associated hemoglobinuria, hematuria, or even myeloglobinuria.

Glucosuria: Testing by dipstick is both specific and very sensitive, detecting as little as 100 mg/dl of glucose. Methods that depend on Benedict's reagent (the reduction of dilute alkaline copper solution) are useful, but are nonspecific and also measure other reducing substances such as lactose, levulose, pentose, galactose, ascorbic acid, and many commonly prescribed drugs. The most common cause of glucosuria is hyperglycemia with normal renal glucose transport. However, if glucosuria persists with normal blood glucose concentrations, renal tubular dysfunction should be considered.

Ketonuria: The dipstick reagent is much more sensitive to acetoacetic acid than to acetone. It does not react with β-hydroxybutyric acid. In most instances ketonuria is nonspecific, and acetoacetic acid, acetone, and β-hydroxybutyric acid are all excreted in the urine. Consequently, a test that principally determines one of these 3 compounds is generally satisfactory for the diagnosis of ketonuria. Ketonuria offers clues to the causes of metabolic acidosis. It is present in starvation, uncontrolled diabetes mellitus, and occasionally in ethanol intoxication. It is not specific for intrinsic urinary system disease.

Hematuria: The dipstick reagent is sensitive to free Hb and myoglobin. A positive test in the absence of RBCs on microscopic examination suggests the presence of hemoglobinuria or myoglobinuria—an important clue to etiology in the patient with acute renal failure.

Nitrituria is determined by a dipstick test that uses the conversion of nitrate (derived from dietary metabolites) to nitrite by the action of certain bacteria in the urine. If nitrite is present, a pink color forms. Normally no detectable nitrite is present. When there is significant bacteriuria, the test will be positive in 80% of cases where the urine has incubated for at least 4 h in the bladder. Thus, a positive test is a reliable index of significant bacteriuria. However, a negative test should never be interpreted as indicating the absence of bacteriuria. There are at least 4 reasons for a negative test when bacteriuria is present: (1) insufficient bladder incubation time for conversion of nitrate to nitrite; (2) low urinary excretion of nitrate; (3) some urinary pathogens do not contain enzymes to convert nitrate to nitrite; and (4) bacterial enzymes may reduce nitrates all the way to nitrogen.

Urine pH: The dipstick is impregnated with various dyes that respond with different color changes to a pH in the range of 5 to 9. Although this test is routinely done, it neither identifies nor excludes patients with urinary system disease. However, it is often useful to aid in identifying various crystals that may be found in urine on microscopy. Specific pH testing of urine with a pH meter is critical in the diagnosis of the "distal" type of renal tubular acidosis where the diagnosis is suggested by a urine pH greater than 5.5 following an acid load. Patients with other types of renal disease can usually vary urinary pH in a relatively normal manner even though the quantitative capacity to excrete titratable acid and ammonia may be reduced.

Urine solute concentration: The total concentration of solutes in urine (**osmolarity**) is best determined by an osmometer. However, for most clinical purposes, the measurement of urinary sp gr or its refractive index may suffice because of the correlation between these measures and urinary osmolarity. The customary hydrometer (urinometer) has been superseded by the more accurate refractometer, which is calibrated in terms of sp gr as well as refractive index. Readings are easy and rapid and only a few drops of urine are needed. Although the correlation is not a linear one, it is satisfactory for clinical applications except when large amounts of glucose or high mol wt solutes such as protein or organic iodides (radiographic contrast chemicals) are present. In these situations sp gr and refractometry give abnormally high values in contrast to the lower osmolarity values.

Normal urine osmolarity varies between 50 to 1200 mOsm/L depending on the circulating titer of ADH and the rate of urinary solute excretion. Although the loss of urinary concentrating capacity is a sensitive test of renal dysfunction, the measurement of urine osmolarity (or sp gr) in a randomly voided urine is only helpful when it is > 700 mOsm/L (sp gr 1.020), as it excludes significant tubulo-interstitial disease. Osmolarity values less than this may be normal or abnormal depending on the prior state of hydration. Proper use of this test as a measure of renal function is described under Measurement of Renal Function, below.

Urinary sediment examination: Normal urine contains a small number of cells and other formed elements shed from the whole length of the urinary system. With disease, these cells are increased and may help to localize the site and type of injury. Particulate elements in urine can be separated and concentrated by forcing urine through a membrane filter; the residue on the filter requires special staining technics for proper microscopic visualization but does provide a permanent record. More commonly, 10 to 15 ml of freshly voided urine are centrifuged for 5 min at a slow speed (1500 rpm), and the supernatant decanted. The sediment residue at the bottom of the centrifuge tube is best visualized in a hemacytometer chamber, but an ordinary glass slide and coverslip will suffice. Using reduced light with the low-power objective, several fields are scanned to detect casts and cells. Then the light is increased, and with the high-power objective, specific cells and casts are identified. A semiquantitative estimation of the numbers of these formed elements is made by a per–high- or low-power field count (e.g., 10 to 15 WBC/high-power field **[hpf]**).

A **classification of urinary formed elements** is listed in TABLE 144-1. Voided urine in women contains genital tract cells as well. It is uncommon to observe more than one leukocyte, erythrocyte, or epithelial cell/hpf (400X) in a normal male, or more than 4 leukocytes/hpf in a normal female. An increased number of cells suggests urinary system disease. Excessive numbers of RBCs may indicate infection, tumor, stones, or inflammation. Excessive leukocytes may indicate infection or other inflammatory diseases. The finding of occasional bacteria in a centrifuged urine sediment is not necessarily evidence of a significant urinary tract infection. However, the finding of bacteria in an uncentrifuged *fresh* urine sample is commonly associated with urine cultures of > 10^5 organisms/ml of voided urine and suggests a urinary tract infection rather than contamination.

The finding of **casts** (*cylindrical masses of mucoprotein in which cellular elements, protein, or fat droplets may be entrapped*) in urine sediment is most important in distinguishing primary renal disease from diseases of the lower tract. The types of casts possible and the diseases with which they are associated are noted in TABLE 144-2. **RBC casts are virtually pathognomonic of glomerulonephritis** (exceptions are rare). Although **WBC casts** suggest pyelonephritis, they are specific only for the presence of tubulointerstitial inflammation and are also common in certain stages of proliferative glomerulonephritis. On the other hand, the rare **bacterial cast** is pathognomonic of bacterial pyelonephritis. **Renal cells with fat inclusions** are common with various types of tubulointerstitial disease; however, a large number of such cells and fatty casts are rarely present except when the nephrotic syndrome exists. Lastly, the finding of **waxy** and **broad casts,** which are formed in the most distal

TABLE 144-1. URINARY FORMED ELEMENTS

Cells from Blood	Cells from GU System	Foreign Cells	Crystals
Erythrocyte	Epithelial	Bacterial	Oxalate
Leukocyte	Renal tubular	Fungal	Phosphate
Plasma	Transitional	Parasitic	Urate
	Squamous	Neoplastic	Drug
	Sperm		

Modified from W. H. Chapman et al, *The Urinary System,* p. 236. Copyright 1973 by W. B. Saunders Company. Used with permission.

TABLE 144–2. URINARY CASTS

Type	Description	Significance
Plain cast		
Hyaline	Mucoprotein matrix secreted by tubules	Nonspecific; present in normal urine but increased numbers when urine flow is low
Waxy	Matrix contains serum proteins. Formed in distal nephron	Present in advanced renal failure
Casts with inclusions		
RBC	Protein matrix variably filled with red cells. Often have red-orange appearance	Present in proliferative glomerulo-nephritis. (Rarely, may also be found with cortical necrosis and occasionally with acute tubular injury.)
Epithelial cell	Protein matrix variably filled with tubular cells	Found with acute tubular injury, glomerulonephritis, and nephrotic syndrome
WBC	Protein matrix variably filled with leukocytes	Found with proliferative glomerulo-nephritis and interstitial nephritis
Granular	Tubular protein droplets in hyaline cast	Present with any form of nephritis causing tubular injury
Fatty	Free fat droplets or tubular cells with fat droplets in a protein matrix	Found with any form of nephritis but most abundant with nephrotic syndrome and Fabry's disease
Mixed	Hyaline cast with various cells such as red, white, and tubular	Usually found in proliferative glomerulonephritis
Miscellaneous.	Crystals or bacteria	Bacterial cast pathognomonic of bacterial pyelonephritis
Pseudocasts	Composed of clumped urates, leukocytes, bacteria, artifacts	Important not to confuse with true cast

parts of the nephron, suggests diffuse, widespread nephron involvement with tubular dilatation of residual nephrons and is thus common in far-advanced renal failure.

Although a thorough examination of fresh, unstained, properly prepared urine sediment will usually reveal to the expert all of the important diagnostic elements present, a **stained urine sediment** may speed and enhance recognition of certain morphologically similar elements in urine such as renal tubular cells and leukocytes. Special stains such as Sudan III will also clarify the presence of free and cellular fat globules. TABLE 144–3 contains a list of some of the commonly used supravital stains and their characteristics.

TABLE 144–3. URINARY SEDIMENT STAINS

Stain	Characteristics
Benzidine or orthotolidine	Used to identify hemoglobin; can distinguish yeast from RBC or pigmented casts from hemoglobin casts
Gram	Used to differentiate between gram-positive (purple) and gram-negative (red) bacteria
Papanicolaou	Useful in identifying malignant cells, cellular inclusion bodies in measles, and intranuclear inclusions in cytomegalic disease
Prescott-Brodie	Peroxidase stain plus eosin stains WBC blue-gray to black and other cells pink-red
Sternheimer-Malbin	A crystal violet and safranin stain that identifies white cells (granular motility or "glitter" cells)
Sudan III	A red, fat-soluble azo dye in 70% alcohol that stains fat pink-red
Wright	A mixture of eosin and methylene blue that is useful in identifying various types of leukocytes

Urine cultures. Collection of specimens (see also LOWER URINARY TRACT AND MALE GENITAL TRACT INFECTIONS in Ch. 151): To diagnose urinary tract infection, one must obtain a sample that reflects bladder urine without undue contamination from other sources. This can be accomplished directly by a urethral catheter or suprapubic needle aspiration of the bladder. However, noninvasive technics using clean-voided urine collections and quantitative culture methods can give adequate information without the hazards of instrumentation in most patients. Culture of a clean-voided specimen in women is representative of bladder urine about 80% of the time; this increases to 90% when 2 consecutive specimens are positive, and to 100% when 3 consecutive specimens are positive and all demonstrate the same organism. In the adult male, a single clean-voided specimen is diagnostic provided that he is circumcised or has retracted the foreskin and cleansed the glans.

The first voided urine specimen following sleep is the best, because bacterial counts will be highest at this time from a long period of incubation in the bladder. Specimens obtained at other times of the day or in patients who are forcing fluids may have a colony count less than the usually accepted 10^5/ml. Specimens that cannot be examined and cultured within 1 h after voiding must be refrigerated. Multiplication of contaminating organisms in urine left standing at room temperature will invalidate the results of both microscopic examination and urine culture.

Localization of infection (see also Ch. 151): Bacteriuria can occur from infection in any part of the urinary tract as well as certain parts of the reproductive system. Most patients, however, appear to have only bladder bacteriuria without evidence of tissue invasion. In the absence of urinary tract obstruction, such cases readily respond to appropriate antimicrobial treatment, and localization studies are not indicated. However, in the patient who has frequent relapsing infections, localization may help to uncover the cause and lead to different therapeutic management.

Localization studies may be divided into several types as shown in TABLE 144–4. Ureteral catheterization and bladder washout technics have become the standards for distinguishing lower from upper tract infections. These methods are based on the hypothesis that bacteria coming from the ureters suggest renal infection. Actually, such localization studies do not prove the existence of renal infection, since renal tissue is not sampled. The bladder washout method is probably the most benign localization procedure, since it avoids cystoscopy and ureteral catheterization.

For localization of lower urinary tract infections in men, the voided urine and expressed prostatic secretions are partitioned into segments: the first voided 5 to 10 ml; the midstream portion; the secretions expressed by prostatic massage; and the first voided 5 to 10 ml immediately after prostatic massage.

In women, the presence of antibody-coated bacteria in the urine correlates closely with renal bacteriuria as determined by the bladder washout method. Apparently antibody-coated bacteria appear in the urine only when tissue invasion has occurred which elicits a local antibody response. These antibodies then react with the surface antigens of the bacteria. The presence of antibody coating the bacteria can then be detected by fluorescein-conjugated immunoglobulins raised against human antibodies in an animal. Although these immunoglobulins are present in the urine of patients with cystitis, they do not react with bacteria in urine. This further supports the hypothesis that coating a bacteria with antibody occurs only in infected tissue. As with all localization tests that depend on indirect evidence, the antibody-coated bacteria may not be specific. Nonspecific fluorescence may be observed with certain organisms such as *Candida*. In men, the test is often positive in bacterial prostatitis as well as pyelonephritis.

Measurement of Renal Function

Renal function tests are useful in evaluating the severity of kidney disease and in following its progress. These can be divided into specific aspects of nephron function such as glomerular filtration, blood flow, and tubular transport, all of which are discussed in detail in Ch. 143, above. TABLE 144–5 provides a summary of tests that have been found useful.

In clinical practice, the GFR is adequately estimated from the endogenous creatinine clearance. The normal value for men is between 140 to 200 L/day (70 ± 14 ml/min/sq m) and for women, 120 to 180 L/day (60 ± 10 ml/min/sq m). Plasma concentration of creatinine varies inversely with the

TABLE 144–4. USEFUL METHODS FOR LOCALIZING URINARY TRACT INFECTION

Methods	Comments
Clinical	Distinct features of pyelonephritis, perinephric abscess, cystitis, prostatitis, urethritis
Urinalysis	Bacterial cast pathognomonic of pyelonephritis; WBC cast suggests nonspecific tubulointerstitial inflammation; tissue may indicate papillary necrosis
Differential culture	Controlled voidings plus prostatic secretions or semen; bladder washout methods or ureteral catheterization to distinguish upper from lower tract infection
Antibody-coated bacteria	Indicate bacterial invasions of tissues (kidney, prostate)

TABLE 144-5. RENAL FUNCTION TESTS

Nephron Function	Specific Test	Clinical Test
Glomerular filtration	Clearance of inulin ^{125}I-Iothalamate ^{169}Yb-DTPA ^{51}Cr-EDTA	Creatinine clearance Plasma creatinine Plasma urea
Renal plasma flow	Clearance of PAH ^{125}I-Hippuran	PSP excretion
Proximal tubular transport	T_m glucose (reabsorption) T_m PAH (secretion)	Plasma phosphate, urate Urinary amino acids
Distal tubular transport	Maximal urine/plasma osmolarity Acidifying capacity (urine pH, TA, NH_4^+)	Maximal urinary osmolarity Acid and bicarbonate loading

DTPA = Diethylenetriaminepentoacetic acid; EDTA = Ethylenediaminetetraacetic acid; PAH = Para-aminohippurate; PSP = Phenolsulfonphthalein; T_m = Transport maximum; TA = Titratable acid.

Modified from W. H. Chapman et al, *The Urinary System*, p. 239. Copyright 1973 by W. B. Saunders Company. Used with permission.

GFR and is therefore a useful index of the GFR if production (related to muscle mass, age) and metabolism (increased in uremia) are considered. The upper limit of plasma creatinine concentration in men with normal GFR is 1.2 mg/dl; in women, 1 mg/dl. A formula useful for estimation of the GFR from the plasma creatinine concentration is:

$$C_{creat} = \frac{(140 - age\ [yr])\ (body\ wt\ [kg])}{(72)\ (serum\ creat\ [mg/dl])}$$

Creatinine clearance is not useful for detecting early kidney damage due to hypertrophy of residual glomeruli. After loss of 50 to 75% of the normal glomerular filtration surface, a decrease in creatinine clearance is clearly detectable. Thus, a normal creatinine clearance cannot exclude the presence of mild renal disease (see Ch. 143). Because of clinical convenience, **serum creatinine** measurements are used as an index of renal function. This is possible because creatinine production and excretion are reasonably constant in the absence of muscle disease. In contrast to the serum creatinine, the **blood urea nitrogen (BUN)** is unsuitable as a single measure of renal function (the blood concentration is influenced by variations in urine flow rate as well as the production and metabolism of urea). The BUN/creatinine ratio is often used to differentiate prerenal, renal, or post-renal (obstructive) azotemia. A ratio > 15 is abnormal and suggests prerenal or postrenal azotemia. The BUN/creatinine ratio is also elevated whenever urea production is increased by diet or steroid therapy, with some neoplasms and antibiotics, and with excessive protein catabolism as seen in infections and uncontrolled diabetes mellitus. The causes of prerenal azotemia include shock, dehydration, and massive GI hemorrhage. The BUN/creatinine ratio is normal with renal azotemia. A low ratio is found in pregnancy, overhydration, severe liver disease, and malnutrition.

Measurement of the **renal plasma flow** is no more useful clinically than the GFR and is considerably more difficult and costly. However, tests of **renal concentrating ability** are simple and diagnostically helpful. A loss of concentrating capacity in the presence of adequate ADH stimulation is associated with tubulointerstitial disease (edema, infiltrate, fibrosis) except when nephrogenic diabetes insipidus is present. The loss of concentrating ability is frequently present long before a depression of GFR is measurable.

Renal concentration capacity is best tested by 2 procedures: (1) water deprivation for a period of 12 to 14 h, and (2) the response to exogenous vasopressin. After the patient has fasted for 12 to 14 h overnight, the osmolarity of the initial morning urine and subsequent hourly samples is measured. When there is < 30 mOsm/L difference in consecutive hourly measurements, the maximum concentration capacity has been reached with water deprivation. The 5 u. of aqueous vasopressin s.c. are given, and the urine osmolarity is measured after another hour. The results of this type of testing are noted in FIG. 144-1. (CAUTION: *In persons with renal failure, water deprivation may be harmful and is usually not useful in diagnosis; the concentrating capacity is always abnormal when the GFR is significantly reduced.*) A lack of response to either water deprivation or exogenous vasopressin suggests an intrinsic renal concentrating defect that may be due to one or more of the following: **functional tubular impairment**, which may be congenital (e.g., nephrogenic diabetes insipidus [DI] or Fanconi's syndrome) or acquired (e.g., osmotic diuresis, certain diuretics [furosemide, ethacrynic acid], potassium deficiency, or hypercalcemia). Otherwise, one considers **tubulointerstitial disease**, as seen in sickle cell disease, toxic nephritis, pyelonephritis, nephrosclerosis, or any renal disease severe enough to produce azotemia.

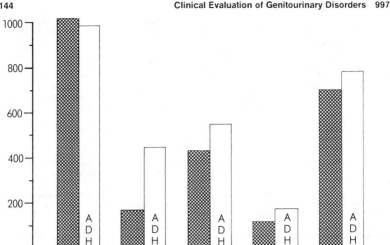

FIG. 144-1.   **Maximum urinary osmolarities after water deprivation** (shaded bars) **vs. urinary osmolarity after administration of exogenous vasopressin** (open bars). (Data taken from "Recognition of partial defects in antidiuretic hormone secretion," by M. Miller et al, *Annals of Internal Medicine* Vol. 73, No. 5, pp. 721–729, November 1970. Used with permission of The American College of Physicians and the authors.)

Additional special tests of renal tubular function usually require research laboratories and are reserved for patients with specific problems. However, tests that measure plasma phosphate and urate, urinary amino acids, and urine pH are readily available and may prove useful in screening specific clinical problems.

Radionuclide, Radiographic, and Ultrasound Procedures

Radionuclide procedures (see Ch. 227)

Radiographic procedures: A **plain x-ray of the abdomen** (kidney, ureter, bladder [KUB]) is performed first to demonstrate the size and location of the kidneys. Since GI and GU diseases tend to mimic each other, the x-ray may be helpful in differential diagnosis. However, the renal outline can be obscured by bowel content, lack of perinephritic fat, or a perinephric hematoma or abscess. This difficulty may be overcome by tomography. Congenital absence of a kidney may be suggested. If both kidneys are unusually large, polycystic kidney disease, multiple myeloma, lymphoma, amyloid disease, or hydronephrosis may be present. If both are small, the end stage of a sclerosing disease such as glomerulonephritis, tubulointerstitial nephritis, or nephrosclerosis must be considered. Unilateral enlargement should suggest renal tumor, cyst, or hydronephrosis, whereas a small kidney on one side is compatible with congenital hypoplasia, atrophic pyelonephritis, or an ischemic kidney. Normally, the left kidney is 0.5 cm longer than its mate.

In 90% of cases, the right kidney is lower than the left because of displacement by the liver. The long axes of the kidneys are oblique to the spine and tend to parallel the borders of the psoas muscles. If both kidneys are parallel to the spine, the possibility of horseshoe kidneys should be considered. If only one kidney is displaced, a tumor or cyst may be present.

Because an x-ray film is two-dimensional, a positive diagnosis of a stone in the urinary tract is practically impossible except in the instance of a staghorn calculus. However, suspicious opaque bodies may be noted in the region of the adrenal, kidney, ureter, bladder, or prostate. Oblique and lateral films, as well as visualization of the urinary tract with radiopaque fluids, are necessary in order to place the calcification specifically within these organs.

Excretory urography (commonly called IVP) is used to visualize the kidney and lower urinary tract. Studies are done by an IV infusion of a triiodinated benzoic acid derivative. The iodine molecule provides radiopacity, while the benzoic acid molecule is rapidly filtered by the kidney. After IV injection of a contrast agent, the drug becomes concentrated in the renal tubules within the first 5 min, providing a nephrogram. Tomography of the kidney should be done routinely at this stage to show renal outlines that may otherwise be obscured by overlying gas or bowel content. In addition, cysts can frequently be differentiated from solid neoplasms. Later, the contrast agent appears in the collecting system, outlining the renal pelvis, the ureters, and finally the bladder. This ability to visualize the urinary system is dependent on adequate renal function and, to some degree, on the absence of an osmotic or water diuresis, which would dilute the contrast agent. Therefore, the best radiograms are obtained in patients with a normal GFR who have been water-restricted or given ADH. It is usually difficult to obtain an adequate study in patients with a BUN > 70 mg/dl or a plasma creatinine > 7 mg/dl, but occasionally delayed films (up to 24 h) are satisfactory in excluding obstructive uropathy. Excretory urography is indicated when disease of the urinary tract is suspected. This test may be useful in investigating cysts and tumors of the kidneys (space-occupying lesions), infections of the kidney (distortion of the calyces), hydronephrosis, vesicoureteral reflux, hypertension, and lithiasis. If renal injury is suspected, excretory urography will confirm that the contralateral uninjured kidney is normal, and will provide functional information about the injured kidney. Finally, excretory urograms are indispensable in infants, particularly males, for whom cystoscopy may be unduly traumatic.

(CAUTION: *Acute renal failure is occasionally [incidence < 0.5%] seen following radiocontrast procedures. The mechanism is unknown, but concomitant risk factors include prior renal insufficiency, diabetes mellitus, advanced age, dehydration, and multiple myeloma. When contrast studies need to be done in high-risk patients, adequate hydration and a reduction in contrast dosage may prevent this problem.*)

In the **retrograde pyelogram,** radiopaque agents similar to those used in excretory urography are introduced directly into the urinary tract following cystoscopy and catheterization of the ureter. The technic provides more intense opacification of the collecting and voiding system when the excretory urogram has been unsuccessful owing to poor renal function. Retrograde evaluation may also be indicated to assess the degree of ureteral obstruction or when the patient is allergic to IV radiopaque chemicals. Retrograde pyelography is useful for detailed examination of the pelvicalyceal collecting system, ureters, and urinary bladder. Its disadvantages are (1) potential infection; (2) distortion of the calyces by overdistention; (3) backflow phenomena that obscure detail; (4) acute ureteral edema and obstruction of secondary stenosis and stricture formation; (5) potential rupture of the renal pelvis and ureters; (6) the need for anesthesia.

The cystogram is obtained as a part of the excretory urogram but may be unsatisfactory owing to poor opacification or incomplete filling. Controlled bladder filling utilizing a catheter **(retrograde cystogram)** is then necessary for adequate visualization. Retrograde cystograms are advisable for study of neurogenic bladder, bladder rupture, or recurrent urinary tract infections. Such causes as vesicoureteral reflux or vesical fistulas can be diagnosed by this technic or by radionuclide bladder scan.

The male urethra may be examined by the retrograde injection of a contrast agent, although the information needed is frequently seen in a voiding film after an excretory urogram. When the retrograde urethral injection is combined with this cystography, the combined procedure is called **retrograde urethrocystography.**

Computed tomography (CT) is more expensive than ultrasound and excretory urography and in general offers few advantages. CT scans are most useful in evaluating renal mass lesions or determining the etiology of a retroperitoneal mass distorting the normal urinary tract (e.g., an enlarged abdominal lymph node). Renal cysts are of low density on CT scanning, and following an IV injection of contrast material there is no enhancement. Rather, the cyst stands out as a prominent "lucency" against the contrast-containing parenchyma. Renal carcinoma, on the other hand, generally is isodense on the unenhanced scan and with enhancement may show an increased density due to hypervascularity of the lesion. Contrast enhancement often helps demonstrate necrotic areas within the mass. It is often possible to determine by CT scan the extent of extrarenal involvement by tumor.

When bladder carcinoma is suspected or known, CT after sequential intravesical air and contrast agent is the best current noninvasive technic for evaluating the extent of these lesions.

Angiography: Renal arteriography and aortography are particularly useful for outlining the renal arterial and venous systems, especially in relation to renovascular hypertension and renal neoplasia. Technics include the translumbar method, in which percutaneous needle puncture of the aorta is performed, and the retrograde method, in which a catheter is introduced through a peripheral artery and extended to the desired level in the aortic lumen. The retrograde method is safest and simplest and provides superior arteriograms. The translumbar method is only used in older patients with aortoiliac occlusive disease, for whom the transfemoral method is contraindicated, or in those few in whom a catheter cannot be passed. To enhance the films obtained during angiography, subtraction studies often give additional information, particularly when bowel content obscures essential parts of the renal angiogram.

Renal angiography is indicated when it is necessary to determine the anatomy of the renal arteries, demonstrate the relationship of the vascular supply to lesions of the parenchyma, or obtain information concerning differential renal function. Examples of such situations include the following: (1) suspected renal hypertension; (2) possible renal or suprarenal masses; (3) congenital renal anomalies of structure, position, or vascular supply; (4) persistent unilateral renal bleeding in the presence of a normal excretory urogram; (5) a poorly functioning kidney of relatively recent onset when the retrograde pyelogram is normal or if retrograde ureteral catheterization is technically unsuccessful; (6) a suspected aberrant artery in the presence of hydronephrosis with ureteropelvic obstruction; and (7) cases of contemplated partial nephrectomy, heminephrectomy, or transplant donors in which accurate knowledge of the blood supply before operation is necessary. Contraindications to angiography are mainly those of a markedly atherosclerotic aorta. Complications include injury to the cannulated vessels and neighboring organs, reactions to the contrast agent, and bleeding.

Abdominal cavography: Visualization of the inferior vena cava for diagnostic purposes is usually done by percutaneous puncture of the femoral vein. Complications of this procedure have been few and are limited to those of extravasation of blood and the contrast agent in the area of injection. Renal vein catheterization provides samples for renal vein renin assays, for diagnosing renal vein thrombosis, and in evaluating the extent of malignant renal neoplasms.

Ultrasound, a noninvasive, innocuous technic, is advantageous in that visualization does not depend on function. Nevertheless, some functional information can be inferred, especially in the fetus, in whom the kidneys can be identified with certainty after about 20 wk gestation, permitting measurement of urine production rate by serial estimations of the bladder volume. For neonates, ultrasound is a first-choice technic for investigating abdominal masses, since the procedure is atraumatic and results are highly accurate.

The kidney can be effectively outlined and the caliceal-pelvic echo pattern critically examined by scanning in the posterior and lateral positions. Ultrasound has proved particularly effective in diagnosing polycystic kidney disease, differentiating between renal cysts and tumors, detecting hydronephrosis and perirenal fluid collections or intrarenal hemorrhage, estimating renal size, and locating the optimal site for percutaneous renal biopsy or nephrostomy. It is the preferred diagnostic method in a uremic patient when uptake of contrast agent or isotope is impaired. It is effective in evaluating renal transplantation for sudden changes in kidney size; in detecting obstruction, lymphocele, or perirenal hemorrhage; and in detecting retroperitoneal pathology such as tumor, lymphadenopathy, or hemorrhage.

The urine-filled bladder is readily outlined by ultrasound. Normally, bladder wall contour changes depend on the amount of urine present. Absence of normal contour changes or distortion of bladder position indicates pelvic or bladder wall pathology. Although bladder tumors may be observed with ultrasound, CT is a superior evaluation technic.

Although ultrasound is not frequently used for this purpose, it permits urine volume in the bladder to be calculated to within about 10% of the catheterized amount. Thus the amount of residual urine in the bladder after voiding can be determined without catheterization.

Morphologic Procedures

Renal biopsy is performed for 4 reasons: (1) to help establish a histologic diagnosis; (2) to help estimate prognosis and the potential reversibility or progression of the renal lesion; (3) to estimate the value of therapeutic modalities; and (4) to determine the natural history of renal diseases. The only absolute contraindication to a biopsy is an uncontrollable bleeding disorder. The biopsy of a solitary kidney is a relative contraindication to be weighed against the need for information. Biopsies of a single, functioning, transplanted kidney are done frequently to diagnose and study possible graft rejections. Conditions associated with an increased morbidity following biopsy are deemed relative contraindications; these include renal tumors, large renal cysts, hydronephrosis, perinephric abscesses, severe reduction in blood or plasma volume, severe hypertension, and advanced renal failure with symptoms of uremia.

There are 2 biopsy technics, **open** and **percutaneous;** the percutaneous technic is most common. The open surgical method is rarely necessary—only when the percutaneous method has been unsuccessful or when direct visual control of the biopsy is critical. For the percutaneous technic the patient is sedated, and the kidney is visualized by radiographic or ultrasonic technics. With the patient in the prone position, and following local anesthesia of the overlying skin and muscles of the back, the biopsy needle is inserted and tissue is obtained for light, electron, and immunofluorescent microscopy.

Urine cytology is useful in screening for possible urinary tract neoplasia in high-risk populations such as industrial dye workers and patients with painless hematuria from nonrenal causes, and in following patients after resection of bladder tumors. The 2nd voided morning urine sample is best, since the exfoliated cells in the initial morning specimen often show extensive deterioration. The initial morning sample may be rendered as useful as the 2nd by giving the patient 1 gm of ascorbic acid the night before; this pretreatment may retard the natural cellular changes in an overnight bladder urine specimen. Abnormal cytology is seen in 70 to 85% of patients with known urinary tract epithelial neoplasia, but inflammatory or reactive hyperplastic lesions of the urinary tract may produce falsely positive results. Falsely negative examinations are usually associated with neoplasia having a low-grade histologic appearance. Diagnostic accuracy may be increased by instrumental brushing prior to urinary cytology collections.

---

145. RENAL FAILURE

ACUTE RENAL FAILURE (ARF)

*The clinical conditions associated with rapid, steadily increasing **azotemia**, with or without oliguria (< 500 ml daily).*

Etiology and Classification

The causes of ARF can be grouped into 3 diagnostic categories: **prerenal** (inadequate renal perfusion), **postrenal** (obstruction), and **renal.** Major causes of acute renal failure are noted in TABLE 145–1. Prerenal and postrenal causes are potentially reversible if diagnosed and treated early, and

TABLE 145-1. MAJOR CAUSES OF ACUTE RENAL FAILURE

Prerenal	Postrenal	Renal
Fluid and electrolyte depletion Hemorrhage Septicemia Cardiac failure Liver failure Heatstroke (myoglobinuria ± fluid/elect depletion) Burns (fluid/elect depletion + myoglobinuria and hemoglobinuria)	Prostatism Bladder, pelvic, or retroperitoneal tumors Calculi	Acute tubular injury (ischemia, toxins, hemoglobinuria, myoglobinuria, heatstroke, burns) Acute glomerulonephritis Arterial or venous obstruction Acute tubulointerstitial nephritis (drug reaction, pyelonephritis, papillary necrosis) Intrarenal precipitation (hypercalcemia, urates, myeloma protein)

some of the causes of primary renal injury that result in acute vascular and tubulointerstitial nephropathy are also treatable, such as malignant hypertension, vasculitis, bacterial infections, drug reactions, and metabolic disorders (e.g., hypercalcemia or hyperuricemia).

Pathophysiology

Prerenal azotemia is caused by inadequate renal perfusion due to extracellular volume depletion, cardiac or hepatic failure, or sepsis. Oliguria occurs as a result of reduced GFR and enhanced sodium and water resorption, normal responses to an inadequate circulating blood volume.

Intrinsic renal causes of ARF are multifactorial, with the most common being prolonged renal ischemia or a nephrotoxin. In experimental studies the factors that initiate and those that maintain ARF may differ. At least 3 mechanisms appear responsible for oligura: (1) a marked decrease in GFR due to renal cortical ischemia and/or a marked change in glomerular membrane permeability; (2) tubular obstruction from cellular and interstitial swelling and/or blockage from cellular debris; and (3) diffusion of glomerular filtrate across injured tubular epithelium. These factors are interdependent but all are not necessarily present in every patient; moreover, they vary in importance from patient to patient, and even in the same patient from time to time. The importance of all these factors in producing acute renal failure points up the inadequacy of the previously popular term **"acute tubular necrosis"** as a description of the basic abnormality. The tubular lesions are variable, but edema and inflammation of the interstitial tissue are always present. While the general structural integrity of the vessels appears normal, the glomerular epithelial cells are usually swollen when viewed with scanning electron microscopy.

Postrenal azotemia is usually associated with glomerular and tubular dysfunction, and the urinary changes may mimic those in patients with primary renal injury.

Symptoms, Signs, and Diagnosis

Initially, diagnostic focus rests on the exclusion of immediately reversible prerenal or postrenal factors. Extracellular volume depletion, cardiac and liver failure, and vasodilation from sepsis may be the principal factors causing renal hypoperfusion and prerenal azotemia. Correction of the underlying hemodynamic abnormality with abatement of ARF is conclusive evidence.

In the absence of prerenal factors, obstructive causes are excluded. Bladder outlet obstruction is probably the commonest cause of sudden, and often total, cessation of urinary output. A history of voiding difficulty or urinary stream reduction is particularly important in infants and older men. An enlarged kidney or palpable bladder is suggestive. Rectal and vaginal examinations are done when obstructive uropathy is suspected.

A history of intrinsic renal disease is often absent, but edema, the nephrotic syndrome, or signs of arteritis in the skin and retina may suggest glomerulonephritis. A history of hemoptysis may suggest Wegener's granulomatosis, Goodpasture's syndrome, skin rash, polyarteritis, or SLE. A history of drug ingestion and a maculopapular or purpuric skin rash may suggest drug allergy and tubulointerstitial nephritis. Primary vascular causes of ARF may be present without symptoms or signs. Bilateral renal artery occlusion may cause a bruit or flank pain but is usually asymptomatic. In infants, bilateral renal vein thrombosis usually results in enlarged, tender kidneys.

Laboratory findings: Oliguria or **anuria** suggests ARF or end-stage renal failure. However, a daily urine output of 1 to 2.5 L is frequently seen in ARF. Anuria suggests obstruction or intrinsic renal disease.

The **urinary sediment** may give valuable etiologic clues. In prerenal azotemia the sediment is usually unremarkable. This may also be true with obstructive uropathy, although white and red cells are not infrequently seen, as well as casts (granular and tubular cells). With primary renal injury, the sediment characteristically contains tubular cells, tubular cell casts, and many brown pigmented granular casts. Urinary eosinophils suggest an allergic tubulointerstitial nephritis; red cell casts suggest vasculitis or glomerulonephritis.

TABLE 145-2. DIAGNOSTIC INDEXES IN ACUTE RENAL FAILURE

	Prerenal	Postrenal	ARF	AGN*
U/P osmt	> 1.5	1 to 1.5	1 to 1.5	1 to 1.5
Urine sodium, mEq/L	< 20	> 40	> 40	< 30
U_{cr}‡/S_{cr}§	> 30	< 25	< 25	> 30
Renal failure index**	< 1	> 2	> 2	< 1

    * Acute glomerulonephritis
    † Urine to plasma osmolarity ratio
    ‡ Urine creatinine concentration
    § Serum creatinine concentration
    ** Urine sodium, mEq/L/urine to serum creatinine ratio
    Adapted from T. R. Miller et al, "Urinary Diagnostic Indices in Acute Renal Failure," *Annals of Internal Medicine* Vol. 89, No. 1, pp. 47–50, July 1978. Used with permission of the American College of Physicians and the author.

A progressive daily rise in the serum creatinine is diagnostic of ARF. However, urinary and serum chemical analyses permit the use of indexes early in the course of ARF, which may help to distinguish the various etiologies (see TABLE 145-2). Although the urine to plasma osmolarity ratio, urine sodium concentration, and urine creatinine to serum creatinine ratio are discriminating in most patients, the most discriminating index is the "renal failure index," which is < 1 in prerenal azotemia or acute glomerulonephritis and > 2 in patients with postrenal or other renal causes of ARF.

Characteristic laboratory findings in ARF are those of progressive azotemia, acidosis, hyperkalemia, and hyponatremia. A modest daily rise in serum creatinine (1 mg/dl) and urea nitrogen (< 15 mg/dl) usually occurs. Acidosis is ordinarily moderate, with a CO_2 content between 15 and 20 mEq/L. Serum potassium concentration increases slowly. However, when catabolism is markedly accelerated by trauma, sepsis, surgery, or steroids, the serum urea nitrogen may rise at the rate of 30 mg/dl/day and the serum potassium by 1 mEq/L/day. Hyponatremia is usually moderate (serum sodium 125 to 135 mEq/L) and is related to a surplus of body water. The hematologic picture is that of a normochromic, normocytic anemia of moderate severity. Hct usually ranges from 25 to 30%.

In evaluating suspected postrenal azotemia, a postvoiding urethral catheterization helps assess bladder outlet obstruction. Urolithiasis as a cause of obstructive azotemia is not usually missed, as it is rarely silent, and simultaneous blockage of both ureters is unlikely. An x-ray of the abdomen can detect 90% of urinary tract calculi that are radiopaque. Ultrasound and radionuclide scans are also used in assessing possible upper tract obstruction and may obviate the need for retrograde ureteral catheterization. Excretory urography should be cautiously used in this setting, as it occasionally may cause or worsen ARF.

Three phases, prodromal, oliguric, and postoliguric, are typical of ARF from acute tubular injury. The prodromal phase varies in duration depending on causative factors such as the amount of toxin ingested or the duration and severity of hypotension. During the **oliguric phase**, urine output typically varies between 50 to 400 ml/day. However, a considerable number of patients are never oliguric and have a lower mortality, morbidity, and need for dialysis. Although the average oliguric period is about 10 to 14 days, it may persist for only 1 to 2 days or for as long as 6 to 8 wk. During this phase, the serum creatinine typically increases by 1 to 2 mg/dl daily and the urea nitrogen by 10 to 15 mg/dl. However, the serum urea nitrogen levels may be misleading as an early index of renal function because elevated values are frequently associated with increased protein catabolism due to surgery, trauma, burns, transfusion reactions, and GI or internal bleeding.

The **postoliguric phase** is associated with a gradual return of urine output to normal levels; however, serum creatinine and urea levels may not fall until several days later. Tubular dysfunction may persist and is manifested during this time by sodium wasting, polyuria (*which may be massive*) unresponsive to vasopressin, or hyperchloremic metabolic acidosis.

Prognosis

Except in fulminant ARF, death should not result from the renal failure and its immediate complications (e.g., hyperkalemia, uremia, bleeding diathesis). However, the survival rate (approximately 50%) is not apparently improving, perhaps because more profoundly ill patients are treated than in the past and because of the intrinsic mortality of associated conditions such as sepsis, pulmonary failure, major wounds, burns, surgical complications, and consumption coagulopathy.

Prophylaxis and Treatment

ARF often can be prevented by proper maintenance of normal fluid balance, blood volume, and BP during and after major surgery; by adequate infusions to maintain normal plasma volume in patients with severe burns; and by prompt transfusion in hemorrhagic hypotension. When a vasopressor agent is required, dopamine at an IV rate of 1 to 10 µg/kg/min may augment renal blood flow and urine output and prevent some cases of ARF. When intravascular hemolysis or rhabdomyolysis is detected, mannitol or furosemide should be given until pigment has disappeared from the urine. In incipient ARF, furosemide 2 to 3 mg/kg IV combined with mannitol 0.5 to 1 gm/kg IV or dopamine 0.5 to 3 μg/kg/min IV may reestablish normal urine flow or convert oliguric to nonoliguric ARF, but evidence of their beneficial effects otherwise is inconclusive except when they are given prophylactically in certain high-risk patients (e.g., those undergoing aortic or open-heart surgery).

Dehydration should be avoided in the patient requiring cholecystography or the patient with renal insufficiency requiring urography, particularly those with multiple myeloma. Urography should be avoided in the patient with diabetic nephropathy because of the high incidence of renal deterioration. Severe hyperuricemia ($>$ 10 mg/dl) should be treated with allopurinol before radiographic contrast studies. To prevent intrarenal tubular blockade with urates during cytolytic therapy in patients with neoplastic disease, prior treatment with allopurinol should be considered along with alkalinizing the urine (oral sodium bicarbonate and/or acetazolamide) and increasing urine flow with increased oral fluids.

The conservative management of established ARF without dialysis requires meticulous limitation of the intake of all substances requiring renal excretion, and is only advocated when dialysis facilities are not readily available. Water intake should be restricted to a volume equal to urine output and measured extrarenal losses plus an allowance of about 500 ml/day for insensible loss. Daily weight determination serves as a check on fluid intake, since any weight gain must be attributed to excess fluid. Sodium and potassium intake are eliminated. Dosage of certain medications that are principally eliminated by the kidney (e.g., digitalis and some antibiotics) must be modified. To prevent negative nitrogen balance, oral or IV administration of essential amino acids in addition to glucose has been advocated; the risks of such treatment include fluid overload, hyperosmolarity, and, when IV therapy is used, infection.

An indwelling bladder catheter should be used with extreme caution and only when necessary. In the postoliguric phase, careful attention to fluid and electrolyte balance is mandatory to prevent extracellular volume, osmolar, acid-base, and potassium disturbances that may be serious or even lethal.

Since patients with advanced azotemia may deteriorate in an unpredictable manner, it is desirable to start dialysis (see Ch. 146, below) as soon as possible after the diagnosis is established. The use of dialysis allows more aggressive nutrition and may improve prognosis.

CHRONIC RENAL FAILURE

The clinical condition resulting from a multitude of pathologic processes that lead to derangement and insufficiency of renal excretory and regulatory function (uremia).

Etiology and Classification

Chronic renal failure may result from any cause of renal dysfunction of sufficient magnitude. The functional effects of chronic renal failure can be grouped into 3 stages: **diminished renal reserve, renal insufficiency (failure),** and **uremia.** The concept of renal functional adaptation explains the observation that a loss of 75% of renal tissue only produces a fall in GFR to 50% of normal. With diminished renal reserve there is a measurable loss of renal function, but homeostasis is preserved at the expense of some hormonal adaptations such as secondary hyperparathyroidism and intrarenal changes in glomerulotubular balance. At the stage of renal insufficiency, there is slight retention of nitrogenous compounds **(azotemia),** reflected in elevated plasma urea nitrogen and creatinine. With further renal dysfunction, fluid and electrolyte balance is disturbed, azotemia increases, and systemic manifestations **(uremia)** occur. This is usually seen with a GFR $<$ 6 ml/min/sq m.

Symptoms and Signs

Patients with just diminished renal reserve are asymptomatic, and renal dysfunction can only be detected by careful testing. A patient with renal insufficiency may have only vague symptoms despite the elevated BUN and creatinine; nocturia is noted at this stage, principally due to a failure to concentrate the urine during the night. Lassitude, fatigue, and decreased mental acuity are often the first manifestations of uremia. Neuromuscular features include coarse muscular twitches, peripheral neuropathies with sensory and motor phenomena, muscle cramps, and convulsions (usually the result of hypertensive encephalopathy). GI manifestations (anorexia, nausea, vomiting, stomatitis, an unpleasant taste in the mouth) are almost uniformly present. In advanced disease, GI ulceration and bleeding are common. Malnutrition leading to generalized tissue wasting is a prominent feature of chronic uremia. The skin may develop a yellow-brown discoloration, and, occasionally, urea from sweat may crystallize on the skin as **uremic frost.** Pruritus is an especially uncomfortable feature of chronic uremia in some patients. Hypertension is often present in advanced renal insufficiency and is usually related to hypervolemia and, in an occasional case, to elevated serum angiotensin levels. Hypertension and renal retention of sodium and water may lead to congestive heart failure. Pericarditis, usually seen in chronic uremia, may occur in acute, potentially reversible, uremia.

Laboratory Findings

Characteristic findings are those of nitrogen retention, acidosis, and anemia. Urea and creatinine are elevated. Plasma sodium concentrations may be normal or reduced. Acidosis ordinarily is moderate, with CO_2 content between 15 and 20 mEq/L. Hypocalcemia and hyperphosphatemia are found regularly. The serum potassium is normal or only moderately elevated ($<$ 6.5 mEq/L). Urinary volume is often relatively fixed between 1 and 4 L/day and does not respond to variations in water intake. Urinary osmolarity is usually fixed close to that of plasma (300 to 320 mOsm/L). The findings on urinalysis depend on the nature of the underlying disease, but broad (especially waxy) casts are often prominent in advanced renal insufficiency of any cause. The hematologic picture (see also Ch. 92) is that of a normochromic, normocytic anemia of moderate severity. Hct usually ranges from 20 to 30%.

Prognosis

The outcome depends on the nature of the underlying disorder and superimposed complications. The latter may cause acute reductions in renal function that are reversible with therapy. However, progression of underlying chronic renal disease is generally not susceptible to specific treatment, and oliguria, progressive hyperkalemia, and pericarditis are often manifestations of a preterminal state. Even in these situations, if no other major organ failure exists, dialysis or transplantation will improve the outlook.

Treatment

Factors aggravating or producing kidney failure (e.g., salt and water depletion, nephrotoxins, congestive heart failure, infection, hypercalcemia, obstruction) must be treated specifically. When it has been established that uremia is the result of a progressive and untreatable disorder, conservative management will often prolong useful, comfortable life until dialysis or transplantation is required. General principles of conservative management follow.

Meticulous attention to dietary management as renal failure progresses from moderate to end-stage disease is important. Because anorexia is an early symptom of uremia, an attempt should be made to evaluate caloric intake. An increase in caloric intake should be coupled with a reduction in the total content of **dietary protein** (see TABLE 145–3). Endogenous protein catabolism is minimized by providing sufficient carbohydrate and fat to meet energy requirements and prevent ketosis. Disappearance or reduction in the severity of anorexia and nausea is a benefit of reduced dietary protein. An intake of 0.6 gm/kg of a mixed protein diet, which includes some low-quality protein to add variety, greatly improves patient acceptance. To this basic protein allowance should be added the equivalent of daily urinary protein loss. Though life is not prolonged, many uremic symptoms (fatigue, nausea, vomiting, twitching, confusion) are markedly improved and the immediate need for dialysis or transplantation may be deferred for a short time.

Hypertriglyceridemia is commonly observed in uremia. Since reduction of carbohydrate intake and a proportional increase in protein is not possible in uremia, clofibrate has been used successfully. Because this drug is eliminated in large part by the kidney, the customary dose must be reduced to 500 mg 3 times/wk. A reduction in **vitamin intake** often accompanies the dietary reductions in uremia; patients should take a multi-vitamin preparation containing water-soluble vitamins. There is no demonstrated need for administration of vitamins A or E.

TABLE 145–3. SAMPLE MODIFIED GIOVANNETTI DIET (18-20 GM PROTEIN)*

Breakfast	Lunch	Dinner
1/2 cup cranberry juice 1/2 cup cream of rice, unsalted 2 slices toast, low-protein 4 tsp butter 2 tsp honey 1/4 cup milk 2 tsp sugar 1 cup tea	1 egg, soft-cooked 1/2 cup cooked carrots 1/2 cup rice 6 slices cucumber on 1 leaf lettuce 2 slices bread, low-protein 6 tsp butter 1 tbsp grape jelly 2 low-protein cookies 1 cup Kool-Aid	Special fruit plate: 2 peach halves and 2 pineapple slices on lettuce 2 slices bread, low-protein 4 tsp butter 1 tbsp grape jelly 1/2 cup milk
Midmorning Nourishment	*Midafternoon Nourishment*	*Evening Nourishment*
2 slices low-protein rusk 4 tsp butter Cinnamon and 2 tsp sugar	6 pieces low-protein caramels 1 cup lemonade with sugar	2 low-protein cookies 6 oz 7-Up

Approximate Composition:

Protein	20 gm	Sodium	1417 mg
Fat	95 gm	Potassium	888 mg
Carbohydrate	456 gm	Kilocalories	2760

* This diet provides 18 to 20 gm of high-quality protein primarily in the form of 1 egg and 6 oz of milk. Protein of low biologic value (vegetables, grains) can be added to give more variety and increase daily intake to 0.6 gm/kg. Caloric intake should be as high as possible. Foods are cooked without salt, and fluid is drained from the food when served.

Water intake should be controlled by thirst or prescription to maintain a serum sodium concentration of 135 to 145 mEq/L; when forced or restricted, water intake may exceed limited renal concentrating and diluting capacities. Sodium intake should be unrestricted, unless contraindicated by edema or hypertension. Potassium intake is closely related to protein and fruit ingestion and does not typically require adjustments. Occasionally supplementation may be required for the hypokalemia associated with renal tubular dysfunction or vigorous diuretic therapy. Except for hyporeninemic-hypoaldosteronism or spironolactone therapy, hyperkalemia is infrequent until end-stage renal failure, or in severe metabolic acidosis or with potassium loads (GI bleeding, excessive oral intake). Mild hyperkalemia ($<$ 6 mEq/L) can be treated by reduction in protein intake and correction of metabolic acidosis. Severe hyperkalemia ($>$ 7 mEq/L) is an indication for starting dialysis, but a cation-exchange resin such as sodium polystyrene sulfonate 50 gm in a 10 or 20% glucose solution as a retention enema for 30 to 60 min, or 20 to 50 gm in 100 ml of a 20% sorbitol solution q.i.d. orally, may be useful if dialysis is not immediately contemplated. The benefits of cation-exchange resins are relatively slow—30 to 60 min when used rectally and 1 to 2 h when taken orally. Activity need not be restricted, as fatigue and lassitude usually keep it within acceptable limits.

Mild acidosis requires no therapy. However, when the plasma CO_2 content is below 15 mM/L, alkali therapy may help to reduce such symptoms as anorexia, lassitude, and dyspnea. Alkali therapy consists of sodium bicarbonate (initial dose is 1 gm t.i.d.) or sodium citrate (initial dose is a 10% solution, 1 tsp t.i.d.). Doses are increased gradually until the CO_2 is about 20 mEq/L and symptoms are relieved, or until evidence of sodium overloading prevents further therapy.

Hypocalcemia and hyperphosphatemia, although asymptomatic, are associated with osteodystrophy (osteitis fibrosa or osteomalacia). The bone disease is related to secondary hyperparathyroidism and a disturbance of vitamin D metabolism. Medical management includes phosphate-binding compounds (aluminum hydroxide gels or aluminum carbonate), calcium carbonate orally, and judicious doses of calcitriol 0.25 to 1 μg/day. The effect of therapy is monitored by frequent measurements of plasma calcium, phosphate, and alkaline phosphatase. Hypocalcemia may cause tetany during alkali therapy, especially if alkalinization has been rapid; in such cases, calcium gluconate IV may be needed.

The anemia of uremia responds only to transfusion, which should not be undertaken unless anemia is severe (Hct $<$ 18%) or symptomatic. Transfusions should be given slowly, and packed RBCs should be used to avoid circulatory overloading. It is always appropriate to check for and treat other sources of anemia, particularly nutritional deficiencies such as iron, folate, and cyanocobalamin.

Congestive heart failure, most commonly due to fluid retention by the kidney, responds to sodium restriction. If myocardial damage is present, digitalis may be necessary, but it must be remembered that the distribution volume and excretion rate of digoxin are reduced in renal failure. Diuretics such as furosemide and bumetanide (the latter drug not yet available in the USA) are usually effective even when renal function is markedly reduced. Moderate or severe hypertension should be treated by careful reduction of BP to avoid the deleterious effect of persistent hypertension on renal function. Patients who fail to respond to moderate reduction in sodium intake (100 mEq/day) need further dietary sodium restriction and diuretic therapy (furosemide 80 to 240 mg b.i.d. or bumetanide 1 to 5 mg b.i.d.). Adjunctive doses of hydrochlorothiazide 50 mg b.i.d. or metolazone 5 to 10 mg/day may be carefully added to high-dose furosemide or bumetanide therapy if hypertension or edema is not controlled. If careful reduction of the extracellular volume does not control BP, then conventional hypertensive drugs are added. Vasodilators (hydralazine, prazosin, minoxidil) or β-adrenoceptor blockers are preferred.

When the limits of effectiveness of conventional therapy have been reached, long-term dialysis or transplantation should be considered. When chronic dialysis is used to treat irreversible uremia, anemia and hypertension may still persist and require transfusions and restriction of fluid and salt intake, respectively. Occasionally, peripheral neuropathy may progress and become disabling despite frequent dialysis. Fatigue and lassitude may be major problems in the days just prior to each dialysis.

146. THERAPEUTIC PROCEDURES

When disease causes kidney failure, or otherwise compromises the ability of the kidneys to remove toxic materials from the blood and maintain fluid, electrolyte, and acid-base balance, therapeutic modalities such as dialysis, hemoperfusion, hemofiltration (discussed below), and transplantation (see Ch. 20) may be used. These measures may be required urgently in acute renal failure, as in certain types of poisoning or acute renal ischemia, or when a patient with progressive renal disease decompensates. Management of the patient with end-stage renal failure involves cooperation between the nephrologist, psychiatrist and/or social worker, nursing staff familiar with dialysis and transplantation, dietitian, and frequently the transplant surgeon or coordinator. Assessment of the patient should begin when it is clear that he has progressive, irreversible renal disease, but before the actual need for dialysis or transplantation is present. Patients can then (1) have their psychosocial strengths and weaknesses assessed in a noncrisis atmosphere; (2) be informed concerning and participate in the choice of therapy; and (3) have a vascular access created early to allow time for maturation. The choice of therapeutic modality is individualized, taking into consideration the trade-offs inherent in each, the patient's psychosocial resources and desires, and the medical resources of the community.

Dialysis patients require special dietary care and medications (discussed below) and awareness and support regarding the psychosocial aspects of dialysis (see PSYCHOSOCIAL ASPECTS OF CHRONIC DIALYSIS, below).

Generally, patients eat a protein-restricted diet containing 1 to 1.2 gm of protein/kg ideal body weight/day. This diet generally emphasizes, but is not limited to, high biologic value proteins, and is limited to 2 gm of sodium and 2 gm of potassium. Limitation of phosphorus intake may also be required. Daily fluid intake is limited to 500 to 1000 ml plus measured urinary output, and must be monitored by weight gain.

The following medications are commonly prescribed: Vitamin B complex, folic acid 1 mg/day, vitamin C 500 mg, ferrous sulfate 300 mg t.i.d., calcium carbonate (1 to 2 gm elemental calcium), an anabolic steroid (e.g., nandrolone decanoate or testosterone enanthate). Aluminum hydroxide gel is given before meals in sufficient doses to maintain the predialysis serum phosphate within normal limits. In approximately 80% of patients, hypertension can be controlled simply by achieving dry weight through ultrafiltration during dialysis. In the remaining 20%, propranolol, hydralazine, prazosin, clonidine, or methyldopa may be required. In resistant cases, a combination of the above agents plus minoxidil is frequently necessary. Impairment in renal excretion must be considered whenever any drug is given to these patients. Digoxin and aminoglycoside antibiotic doses are always reduced.

DIALYSIS

The process of separating elements in a solution by diffusion across a semipermeable membrane. The patient's own peritoneum or a machine using a synthetic semipermeable membrane such as cellophane may be used—**peritoneal dialysis** and **hemodialysis,** respectively.

Five types of maintenance dialysis programs are available for management of chronic renal failure: home hemodialysis, home peritoneal dialysis, self-care (performed in-center by the patient, with limited supervision) and passive-care dialysis, and continuous ambulatory peritoneal dialysis **(CAPD).** Home dialysis generally is the least expensive and promotes the greatest patient independence. About 50% of patients are suitable candidates for home dialysis. A dialyzing partner is generally required for hemodialysis, but seldom for peritoneal dialysis. Training for patient and partner takes 3 to 8 wk.

Indications for Peritoneal Dialysis and Hemodialysis

Indications for the 2 types of dialysis are similar and will be considered together. Generally, both forms are effective. Exceptions for which peritoneal dialysis is less desired are those patients who have diminished peritoneal membrane (e.g., heat stroke, systemic sclerosis) or those in whom transport is insufficient to most clinical needs (e.g., life-threatening hyperkalemia and catabolic states). Hemodialysis is less desired in the face of bleeding (e.g., thrombocytopenia).

Acute renal failure presents the following pathophysiologic problems correctable by dialysis: (a) retention of nitrogenous solutes (urea, creatinine, uric acid); (b) overexpansion of extracellular fluid **(ECF)** volume; (c) hyperkalemia; and (d) metabolic acidosis. The decision to dialyze a patient is a complex clinical judgment that cannot be made solely on the basis of laboratory determinations. Dialysis is often necessary in patients with the combination of prolonged oliguria (over 14 days), increasing acidosis, and congestive heart failure. Since patients with uremia from acute renal failure may deteriorate rapidly and die, dialysis is often begun early in the course of the disease.

Although many patients can survive **acute drug intoxication** if prompt and proper respiratory and cardiovascular support is given, dialysis can be very effective in the treatment of many specific drug poisonings (see TABLE 258–2 in Ch. 258). The decision to institute dialysis depends on the clinical and biochemical characteristics of the poisoning, including the severity of coma, whether a potentially lethal dose was ingested, whether an impaired route of excretion may make autodetoxification unlikely, and whether the poison can be metabolized to a more toxic form (e.g., oxidation of ethylene glycol to oxalic acid). The hazards of prolonged coma and the relationship between toxicity and blood concentration are important factors in the clinical assessment. Furthermore, the risk of compromised ventilatory support during transit must be considered before moving a patient to a medical center with an artificial kidney.

Patients with **stable chronic renal failure** may not require dialysis. However, if an intercurrent illness such as gastroenteritis, congestive heart failure, sepsis, or lactic acidosis produces acute metabolic or circulatory decompensation, the patient's condition may suddenly deteriorate. Congestive heart failure may be difficult to correct in these patients because response to diuretics is poor. Likewise, they may not tolerate the sodium load produced when metabolic acidosis is corrected with sodium bicarbonate. Dialysis corrects the metabolic acidosis without expanding the ECF volume, which it can actually reduce by ultrafiltration.

In **chronic renal failure,** periodic maintenance dialysis is usually needed when the GFR falls to < 5 to 8 ml/min. Intractable nausea and vomiting, uremic encephalopathy and neuropathy, pericarditis, and pleuritis are urgent indications for dialysis. Many centers prefer to begin dialysis when the patient can no longer perform his usual activities. Dialysis may be employed as the sole form of therapy for chronic renal failure or may be used to support renal transplantation.

PERITONEAL DIALYSIS (Peritoneal Lavage)

Technic

Peritoneal dialysis requires inserting a sterile plastic catheter into one of the pelvic gutters and irrigating the peritoneum with sterile solutions. The bladder is emptied first. If the patient cannot void, a single sterile catheterization is performed. The patient is initially given 50 mg meperidine IM, and the abdomen is shaved and prepared aseptically as for laparotomy. The operator wears a mask, cap, and gloves. Intradermal and subcutaneous infiltration with 1% procaine or lidocaine at the site of introduction of the catheter provides local anesthesia. A small stab wound is made in the midline, 1/3 of the way from the umbilicus to the symphysis pubis. Sites of previous surgery should be **avoided** because of the increased bleeding tendency of scar tissue, and because adhesions may have fixed a viscus to the site. If the midline is not suitable, a lateral approach may be used. The patient should tense his abdomen as when moving his bowels, while a catheter with a pointed obturator is advanced with firm pressure. A "pop" will be felt when it pierces the parietal peritoneum. The obturator is immediately withdrawn to prevent possible laceration of the viscera. The catheter is then "walked" along the anterior peritoneum towards either of the lower quadrants. When sufficiently advanced, it is rotated so that the tip lies posteriorly in the pelvic gutter. The patient may feel a sudden urge to defecate if the catheter tip touches the rectum. Some physicians instill 1 L of peritoneal dialysate through a 13-gauge needle to facilitate the puncture and catheter placement. Others prefer to perform paracentesis with a gallbladder trocar. The peritoneal catheter is threaded through the trocar after the stylet has been removed, or the trocar may be used to direct the catheter into the proper quadrant. Upon placement, 1 L of solution is infused rapidly and allowed to drain immediately to test the adequacy of drainage. A purse-string suture is placed in the skin around the puncture site to minimize leakage, a sterile dressing is applied, and the catheter is taped in place and connected to a sterile closed infusion-drainage system.

The **irrigation schedule** is usually organized into inflow, dwell, and outflow periods. Inflow of 2 L of solution is usually accomplished within 5 to 10 min. The fluid is allowed to remain in the abdomen for a 30-min dwell period and is then drained by gravity into a sterile closed system over 15 to 20 min. Thus a single 2-L exchange requires about 1 h. Shortening the dwell time enhances the removal of small molecules such as urea, but increases the amount of dialysis solution needed. Duration of treatment varies from 24 to 72 h, depending on clinical indications. If the dialysate is not completely drained within 20 min, the next infusion should be started rather than wait for complete drainage. The slight residual volume that results does not significantly interfere with clearance. Repeated failure to recover instilled fluid requires repositioning of the catheter.

Automated peritoneal dialysis systems and development of the "permanent" silastic catheter (Tenckhoff) have made chronic intermittent peritoneal dialysis a suitable technic for use in chronic renal failure. This equipment prepares sterile dialysate from tap water and concentrate, infusing it into and draining it from the peritoneal cavity on a prearranged schedule. With this technology the incidence of peritonitis has been greatly reduced.

Continuous ambulatory peritoneal dialysis (CAPD) differs from manual peritoneal dialysis in that dwell times are generally 4 to 8 h; the technic is employed continuously 24 h/day, 7 days/wk, rather than intermittently; and the peritoneal dialysate must be supplied in collapsible plastic containers. Because it is continuous, greater clearances are achieved. Four 2-L exchanges/day generally suffice for adequate control of uremia. Clinical experience to date indicates that patients generally feel better and have greater dietary lattitude with this technic. Since it does not require elaborate machinery, it is relatively easy to learn and allows the patient much greater mobility. Its principal drawbacks are frequent episodes of peritonitis, a tendency toward backache, and excessive weight gain due to absorbed glucose from the solution. Moderate hypertriglyceridemia is common. Occasional patients reach levels of > 1000 mg/dl. Recent developments in tubing design promise to substantially reduce the incidence of peritonitis.

Dialysis Solutions

The composition of a typical commercially available peritoneal dialysis solution is listed in TABLE 146–1. It mimics electrolyte composition of interstitial fluid but differs in that acetate or lactate replaces bicarbonate and the solution is potassium-free. Glucose, which is absorbed from the peritoneum relatively slowly, can be used as an osmotic force to balance the oncotic pressure in the plasma and to produce ultrafiltration in higher concentrations. Solutions with 1.5% glucose are used when the ECF volume is not to be changed. Solutions with 4.25% (or, rarely, 7%) glucose produce ultrafiltration at rates up to 1 L/h. These hypertonic solutions also have been used intermittently to enhance clearances. All peritoneal dialysis solutions are prewarmed to 37 C to promote efficient diffusion and prevent cooling of the patient.

Potassium chloride injection is frequently added to each exchange to regulate the amount of potassium removed. The serum potassium concentration usually approaches that of the dialysis solution after 48 h of treatment, except in patients with a high endogenous potassium production

TABLE 146-1. COMPOSITION OF TYPICAL DIALYSATE

		Peritoneal Dialysis (Sterile)	Hemodialysis (Nonsterile)
Glucose	mg/100ml	1500–4250	200
Sodium	mEq/L	140	135
Chloride	mEq/L	100.5	106
Potassium	mEq/L	*	2
Acetate	mEq/L	45	35
Calcium	mEq/L	4	3.5
Magnesium	mEq/L	1.5	1.0

* Added as indicated.

(hypercatabolic states, severe metabolic acidosis, or rhabdomyolysis), for whom potassium-free dialysate is indicated. For chronic renal failure, most physicians use potassium-free dialysate. Other measures, such as oral or rectal administration of ion-exchange resins or vigorous treatment of acidosis with bicarbonate, may control serum potassium more effectively.

Heparin sodium 1000 u. is added to each 2-L exchange to prevent fibrin formation around the catheter tip. Antibiotics are not used routinely but are reserved for specific peritoneal infections.

Results

Inflow and outflow volumes must be measured accurately to determine ultrafiltration. In many euvolemic patients, peritoneal dialysate containing 1.5% glucose will produce significant ultrafiltration. If no ultrafiltration is desired, this net volume should be replaced IV with 5% dextrose in 0.45% sodium chloride solution or equivalent oral fluid and electrolyte intake.

Urea clearance with peritoneal dialysis varies between 15 and 27 ml/min, depending on dwell time. Usually 48 exchanges in 48 h will reduce BUN to 50% and plasma creatinine to 60% of the predialysis values. This is equivalent to a 6-h treatment with coil hemodialysis.

Complications

Bleeding during peritoneal dialysis is usually from the subcutaneous tissues around the puncture site and can be controlled easily with an additional deep purse-string suture around the catheter. If the drainage fluid is cloudy, **peritonitis** should be suspected and may be confirmed by Gram stain and culture of the fluid. It can be treated by adding appropriate antibiotics to the dialyzing solution. Dialysis need not be discontinued prematurely. Entrance of air into the peritoneum may cause local pain or poor fluid drainage. Other complications include **perforation of viscus, hydrothorax, atelectasis, protein loss, hyperosmolar coma, hypernatremia,** and **hypotension.**

Contraindications

Recent surgery for abdominal vascular prosthesis is the most serious contraindication. Focal peritonitis, fecal fistula, and extensive abdominal adhesions are relative contraindications. Peritoneal dialysis is less effective than hemodialysis in acute life-threatening hyperkalemia.

HEMODIALYSIS

A hemodialysis system, "kidney machine," has 3 essential components: a tubing system for conducting blood from the patient to the membrane unit; a membrane unit where blood and dialysate come into contact with opposite surfaces of the cellophane membrane and dialysis takes place; and a dialysate supply system.

Access to the circulation for hemodialysis is generally obtained with an arteriovenous shunt or fistula. An **arteriovenous shunt** (FIG. 146-1a) consists of Teflon® vessel tips inserted into the radial artery and cephalic vein (or other accessible vessels in an upper or lower extremity). These vessel tips are linked by a silicone rubber cannula or tube external to the skin. Two sections of the cannula are joined by a connecting piece of Teflon and are separated at the connector for dialysis. After each dialysis session, the cannula loop is rejoined with a new Teflon connector. Subcutaneous **arteriovenous fistulas** (FIG. 146-1b) avoid the recurrent infections and clotting associated with shunts. The radial artery is anastomosed to the cephalic vein in an end-to-end, end-to-side, or side-to-side fashion. The forearm veins dilate, eventually arterialize, and are suitable for repeated puncture.

Dialysis Membrane Units

There are 3 types of membrane units: coil dialyzers, parallel sheet (plate) dialyzers, and hollow fiber dialyzers. In **coil dialyzers** (FIG. 146-2), tight concentric coils of cellophane tubing are separated by screening or mesh spacers. Blood is pumped through the inside of the tubing, and dialysate circulates through the coil outside. Ultrafiltration is accomplished by partially obstructing the outflow of blood from the coil with a screw clamp, thus increasing the blood pressure within the coil.

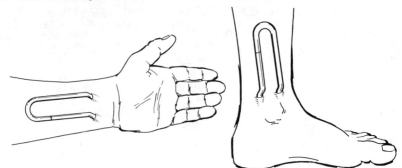

FIG. 146-1a.   Arteriovenous shunts.

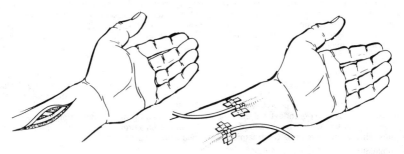

FIG. 146-1b.   Subcutaneous arteriovenous fistulas.

Parallel sheet dialyzers (plate-type dialyzer, FIG. 146-3) consist of parallel sheets of cellophane sealed at the edges between grooved polypropylene membrane supports. Blood passes one way between the sheets, while dialysate passes in the opposite direction outside of the membranes. The arterial-venous pressure gradient is sufficient to circulate the blood through the membranes without a pump. Ultrafiltration is achieved by applying a negative pressure to the dialysate.

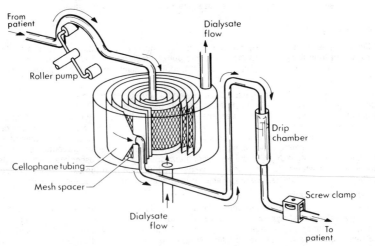

FIG. 146-2.   Coil-type dialyzer.

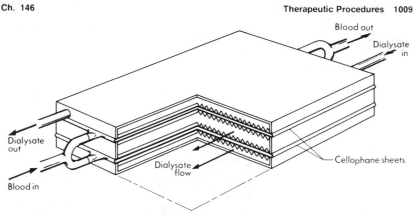

Fig. 146-3. Plate-type dialyzer.

Hollow fiber dialyzers (Fig. 146-4) consist of a bundle of hollow cellulose fibers 200 μm in diameter, through which the blood passes. Dialysate is circulated around the outside of these fibers in a countercurrent fashion. This dialyzer is compact and efficient because of the high ratio of surface area to blood volume. Blood flow resistance is low as in a parallel sheet dialyzer; thus, these units do not need a blood pump when operating from an arteriovenous shunt.

Dialysis Solutions

The composition of the dialysate used in hemodialysis depends on clinical requirements. It is prepared by diluting a concentrated solution with water. In some areas water must be treated by deionization, water softeners, or reverse osmosis to make it suitable for hemodialysis. The typical diluted electrolyte composition is listed in Table 146-1. Unlike peritoneal dialysate, this solution is not sterile. The accuracy of the dilution is checked by measuring the conductivity, osmolality, or the chloride content. Two types of systems can be used to deliver dialysate to the membrane units. In a **batch system,** 120 L of dialysate is prepared at one time from the concentrate. Some machines require only 5.5 L of dialysate because a sorbent cartridge is used to regenerate dialysate. In **proportioning systems,** dialysate is prepared by continuously diluting concentrate in a 1:35 ratio in an inline system. Batch systems are usually used with coil dialyzers, but parallel flow and hollow fiber dialyzers work best with proportioning systems.

Technic

The patient's blood is heparinized during hemodialysis, producing a whole-blood clotting time > 30 min. This is required to prevent clotting in the extracorporeal circuit. In patients with recent surgery or concurrent bleeding, regional heparinization (limited to the extracorporeal circuit) is accomplished by matched infusions of heparin into the blood before it enters the dialyzer and protamine into the blood before it re-enters the body.

A typical acute hemodialysis treatment takes 4 to 6 h. It reduces the BUN and creatinine by approximately 50%, and corrects metabolic acidosis and hyperkalemia. Most patients receiving chronic maintenance hemodialysis require 4- to 8-h treatments 3 times/wk to maintain a state of well-being. Technical complications of hemodialysis include hypotension due to excessive ultrafiltration, hemorrhage due to systemic heparinization or accidental blood line separation, hypokalemia, air embolism, pyrogenic reactions, hemolysis due to improper dialysate preparation, and seizures due to osmotic dysequilibrium.

HEMOPERFUSION, HEMOFILTRATION, AND HEMODIAFILTRATION

In **hemoperfusion** (*perfusion of blood through a sorbent device instead of a hemodialyzer*), the sorbents employed are either activated charcoal or resin beads. This technic is particularly useful in the treatment of drug overdose, especially where the drug involved is poorly soluble in water, and has also been used to treat liver failure and as an adjunct in treating uremia. While these sorbents are effective in removing solutes such as potassium, creatinine, and uric acid from uremic blood, urea removal remains a clinical problem. Aside from its use in drug intoxication, hemoperfusion is primarily a research technic.

Hemofiltration and **hemodiafiltration,** similar technics used in uremia, differ from hemodialysis in that they use *convective transport of solute through ultrafiltration across the membrane rather than diffusion.* The theoretical rationale is that convective transport is a more effective means of removing larger mol wt solutes (500 to 5000 daltons) from the blood than diffuse transport. The principal

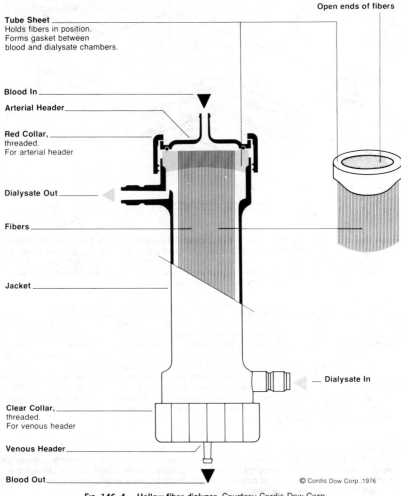

Open ends of fibers

Tube Sheet
Holds fibers in position.
Forms gasket between
blood and dialysate chambers.

Blood In

Arterial Header

Red Collar,
threaded.
For arterial header

Dialysate Out

Fibers

Jacket

Dialysate In

Clear Collar,
threaded.
For venous header

Venous Header

Blood Out   © Cordis Dow Corp.,1976

FIG. 146–4.   Hollow fiber dialyzer. Courtesy Cordis Dow Corp.

clinical advantage is better control of hypertension. Although this technic is very expensive, it can sustain the life of uremic patients as the sole form of therapy.

Hemofiltration has also been used with ordinary dialyzers to enhance fluid removal, generally being employed for periods up to 1 h at the beginning of dialysis. Symptoms of dysequilibrium, cramps, and hypotension are less frequent than with ultrafiltration during dialysis because hemofiltration does not produce the serum hypotonicity usually associated with hemodialysis. Because removal of small molecules (e.g., urea and creatinine) is less effective during hemofiltration, the price paid is a slight lengthening of the treatment time required to produce equivalent small-molecule clearances.

ALTERED NEUROLOGIC AND MENTAL STATES IN DIALYSIS PATIENTS

The symptoms and signs of **acute uremic encephalopathy** (see Ch. 145) are generally reversed rapidly by dialysis, although in rare cases restoration to the premorbid state may take 2 wk. However, sensitive psychologic tests can demonstrate differences in function before and after dialysis in otherwise stable patients. Furthermore, patients on chronic dialysis therapy may develop a variety of neurologic and psychiatric disorders which affect their mental functioning. Since hemodialysis patients are regularly anticoagulated, problems such as **subdural hematoma** and **intracerebral hemor-**

rhage may develop. Disequilibrium associated with osmotic shifts produced by hemodialysis may produce **seizures.** Because of enhanced atherosclerosis in renal failure, **thrombotic strokes** may occur.

A peculiar neurologic syndrome, **dialysis dementia,** is characterized by progressive dementia, dyspraxia, facial grimaces, myoclonic seizures, and characteristic EEG. This disorder may be associated with high brain aluminum concentrations. The exact source of the aluminum is controversial, but high aluminum concentrations in tap water have been found in areas where epidemics of this condition have occurred. Another source of aluminum may be the aluminum-containing antacids prescribed to control phosphorus balance. Secondary hyperparathyroidism also may be pathogenetic.

Besides organic brain syndromes, dialysis patients are also subject to a wide range of **functional disorders,** from schizophrenia and manic depression to maladaptive coping behavior. The differential diagnostic approach used to separate these disorders is the same as that used for patients who do not have kidney failure. A careful neurologic and psychiatric evaluation is always warranted before assuming the disorder is functional or attempting symptomatic relief.

PSYCHOSOCIAL ASPECTS OF CHRONIC DIALYSIS

The chronic dialysis patient depends on a machine for his life. Medical, social, and emotional complications make the patient and family constantly vulnerable to crises. How patients, families, and staff cope with these pressures affects not only adjustment but also patient survival. In general, psychosocial problems are reduced by dialysis programs that encouage patient independence and resumption of former life interests as much as possible.

Psychosocial Stresses of Chronic Dialysis

Losses or threatened losses in every area of the patient's life abound; **loss of independence** is major among these. The patient is dependent on the medical team to manage the illness and treatment; dialyses, often scheduled at the discretion of others, influence the patient's work and leisure activities; regular employment may be precluded, and usual family roles and responsibilities are often modified, creating tension and feelings of guilt and inadequacy; community help is often necessary for high treatment costs, medications, special diets, and transportation.

Also stressful are **losses and changes in body function,** including loss of urination and of physical energy; loss or change in sexual function; changed appearance due to access surgery, needle marks, bone disease, neuropathy, myopathy, or other signs of physical deterioration; and ultimately, the threat of loss of life.

Chronic dialysis has a major psychosocial **impact on the patient's family,** particularly in home dialysis when a family member is the treatment partner; but in any setting, patient dependence and reduced work capacity and physical abilities may cause role reversals in the family. The marital relationship is especially vulnerable.

Reactions of Patients and Familiies

Favorable prognostic indicators for long-term adjustment to dialysis include those premorbid personalities and life adjustments which demonstrate the patient's adaptability, independence and self-control, tolerance to frustration, and optimistic perception of life. An emotionally stable and encouraging family also fosters adjustment. A consistently supportive approach from the medical team towards patient and family and their inclusion as key participants are essential. Age, sex, education, and other socioeconomic factors seem to be less important. Persons of many different personality types can adjust quite comfortably to dialysis. The availability of both passive-care and self-care treatment options gives the treatment team more flexibility in designing programs around individual personality types and needs.

Coping reactions among dialysis patients range from full rehabilitation to suicide. Stages of adjustment may include a "honeymoon" period at dialysis onset experienced by persons who are physically much improved, optimistic, and euphoric; a period of depression, disillusionment, and discouragement, when the long-term reality of the illness and treatment sets in; and finally, the beginning of long-term adaptation, characterized by the individual's premorbid personality and coping skills.

Specific coping reactions include **denial,** particularly useful in helping a patient to avoid the reality of his dependence on a machine and his life-threatening situation. Thus, the patient is not overwhelmed and can resume life activities. However, if denial is excessive, the patient may reject the need for treatment and die. Lack of denial may result in severe anxiety or depression or permit the situation to become overwhelming and lead to psychosis or suicide.

Increased dependence or independence is a common coping reaction. Dependent personalities may more easily accept their circumstances, but excessive dependence can create extreme demands on others and impede rehabilitation. Patients may accept the sick role too well and be unable to relinquish it. Independence as a coping reaction may create adjustment problems to the machine and the sick role initially, and may lead to rejection of advice and treatment. However, ultimately it can favor social rehabilitation and patient responsibility, reducing the burden on family members.

Depression, a normal response to loss, may be especially pronounced. **Guilt, hostility, and ambivalence** are seen in patients who view the machine as both miracle and monster. They may feel both grateful and resentful toward those on whom they depend, and may be ambivalent about the very desire to live.

Some dialysis patients **act out** their feelings, e.g., by noncompliance with diet and medication or arriving late or not at all for dialysis. The staff or the home dialysis partner may become the target for the patient's anger. However, many patients express their feelings and direct their energy in productive ways. They may return to work, resume former interests, or become "lay counselors" to fellow dialysis patients. Self-care and home dialysis help the patient regain a sense of control and independence by making him largely responsible for his own treatment, able to integrate it into his life more flexibly.

Coping reactions in patients' families are similar. Denial can be functional or can interfere with emotional support to the patient. Depression, resentment, guilt, ambivalence, and psychosomatic and behavioral problems are manifested by family members. However, families can provide very important support to their ill members and can also develop a network of mutual support with other dialysis families.

Special Demands on the Medical Team

The medical team is intensely involved with patients whom they see gradually deteriorate rather than get well. Strong emotional attachments are inevitable. Staff, like patients, sometimes cope by using denial, but it is generally an unsatisfactory reaction. Denying the seriousness of the patient's illness and his limitations may lead to unrealistic staff expectations. The resulting feelings of guilt in the patient and resentment in the staff impede meeting realistic rehabilitation goals. Realistically appropriate staff attitudes promote the patient's desire to live, self-esteem, and rehabilitation.

KIDNEY TRANSPLANTATION

(See in Ch. 20)

---

147. IMMUNOLOGICALLY MEDIATED RENAL DISEASE

(Immune Renal Disease; IRD)

The majority of glomerular and many tubulointerstitial renal diseases are mediated by host immune mechanisms. In some instances, the kidney itself participates as the antigenic stimulus for destructive immune injury (e.g., renal allograft rejection). Alternatively, the kidney may act as the antigenic target for cross-reactive antibody-mediated damage (e.g., anti–glomerular-basement-membrane **[anti-GBM]** disease), or as an unwitting bystander involved when complexes of a variety of immune components are deposited within the kidney.

The critical roles played by host immune mechanisms in mediating many renal diseases were demonstrated by examining renal tissue specimens using light, immunofluorescence, and electron microscopy in concert with specifically designed reagents to identify and localize host immune components. The presence and pattern of host immune reactants such as antibody, complement, immune complexes, or sensitized lymphoid cells, as well as the detection of alterations in immune components in blood and urine, have provided the diagnostic and prognostic clues to understanding IRD.

Related discussions of immune mechanisms are in Chs. 16 and 18.

Pathogenesis

Although IRD may result from a wide range of host immune responses, Type III immune injury will be discussed first, since the deposition of immune complexes appears to be the commonest underlying mechanism.

Type III immune complex (I-C) renal diseases *result from deposition of antigen-antibody-complement complexes in the mesangium, interstitium, or glomerular capillary wall of the kidney.* The type and location of antibody identified in renal biopsy sections is regarded as the "fingerprint" of the underlying immune mechanism. Immune complexes are classically deposited in a **"lumpy-bumpy" pattern** as demonstrated by immunofluorescence and electron microscopic study of renal tissue sections. In I-C renal diseases, circulating I-C may also be demonstrated in the blood.

The underlying mechanisms of I-C renal diseases have been determined by analogy to experimental IRD produced in laboratory animals by administration of foreign proteins. The foreign protein stimulates production of specific antibody; the antibody combines with the protein to form circulating I-C. At first, resulting I-C are small and remain in circulation. As antibody production increases, the size of the circulating I-C increases, favoring localization in the mesangium or glomerular capillary wall. This is the most vulnerable phase for the kidney. As I-C become larger, they are preferentially removed by reticuloendothelial organs of the body (spleen, liver, and lymphatics), minimizing localization in the kidney.

Once localized within the kidney, I-C produce renal tissue damage in patients with Type III IRD by activation of the complement (C) system. On exposure to I-C, the series of proteins known as C combine to form immune reactants capable of mediating injury. (See also THE COMPLEMENT SYSTEM, Ch. 16.) An example of one such immune reactant is chemotactic factor, which causes polymorpho-nuclear leukocytes (PMNs) and other phagocytic cells to localize in the area of immune injury. These phagocytic cells release their intracellular enzymes (lysozymes), which are capable of causing tissue damage. Once completely activated through C9, complement is capable of causing direct tissue destruction.

A wide variety of antigens have been associated with I-C in mediating the development of Type III IRD (see TABLE 147–1). For convenience, these antigens can be categorized as self or foreign. **Self antigens** are best exemplified by the IRD of SLE, where the host's own nuclear proteins constitute the antigens of the circulating I-C. Tumor antigens and renal tubular antigens may also provide self-antigen for I-C development leading to IRD. **Foreign** (or **exogenous**) **antigens** include a host of bacterial, viral, and parasitic antigens as well as foreign protein antigens and drugs. In some in-stances of Type III IRD, the antigen may be demonstrated in deposits or eluted from renal tissues (e.g., the treponeme in syphilis or the hepatitis-associated antigen in hepatitis-associated postinfec-tive glomerulonephritis). More commonly, however, the involved antigen cannot be identified or recovered.

Deposition of I-C in the glomerular capillary wall, predominantly in subepithelial sites, underlies the pathogenesis of Type III immune glomerular diseases; however, the precise mechanism whereby I-C localize in these sites is unclear. A variety of factors appear to influence or favor such localization, including release of vasoactive substances to enhance vascular permeability, and the size, shape, and antigen:antibody ratio of the complexes. Nevertheless, none of these factors provides a com-plete explanation for I-C deposition. A possible explanation is offered by demonstration of the pres-ence of 2 forms of normally occurring binding sites for host immune reactants; one for the 3rd component of complement (C3) on the glomerular epithelial cell, and another for the Fc fragment of IgG in the renal interstitium. Hypothetically (see FIG. 147–1), I-C containing antigen-antibody and C3 may fix to subepithelial C3 binding sites after passing through the endothelial cells of the capillary wall. Their passage to the C3 binding site may be affected by release of vasoactive amines as well as the structure of the I-C molecule. In tubulointerstitial Type III IRD, localization of IgG-containing I-C may result from attachment to interstitial Fc binding sites.

Type II (cytotoxic antibody-mediated) IRD results from the fixation of cytotoxic antibody to kidney tissue, with subsequent activation of the C sequence and the propagation of immune inflammatory injury. Although not as common as Type III IRD, Type II is the most clearly understood form. For example, **anti-GBM disease** or **hyperacute renal allograft** rejection results from the fixation of an antibody layer to affected areas of the kidney. Often, the cytotoxic antibody can be detected in the plasma. In contrast to the "lumpy-bumpy" pattern of antibody deposition in Type III IRD, antibody in cytotoxic IRD is deposited in a smooth, linear fashion. In Type II IRD, the cytotoxic antibody is directed against kidney antigens resulting in tissue injury by local activation of C. As in Type III IRD, the antigens within the kidney may be self (the GBM, as in Goodpasture's disease) or foreign (histo-compatibility antigens, as in hyperacute renal graft rejection). (See TABLE 147–2.)

TABLE 147–1. ANTIGENS ASSOCIATED WITH IMMUNE COMPLEXES IN DISEASES ASSOCIATED WITH TYPE III IMMUNE RENAL INJURY

Antigen	Examples	Disease
Foreign		
Bacterial	β-Hemolytic streptococcus	Streptococcal pharyngitis
	Staphylococcus	Furunculosis
Viral	Varicella	Chickenpox
	Hepatitis B-associated antigen	Viral hepatitis
Parasitic	Malaria	Malaria
	Treponeme	Syphilis
	Toxoplasma	Toxoplasmosis
Foreign Protein	Serum	Serum sickness
Drugs	Heroin	Drug addiction
Self		
Nuclear	DNA, RNA	SLE
Tumor	CEA	Carcinoma

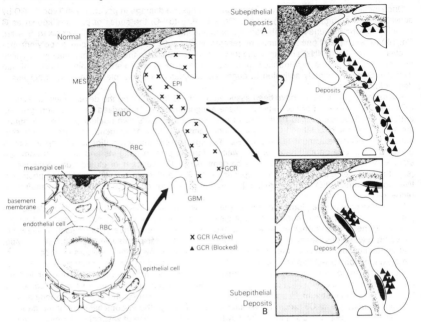

FIG. 147–1. Hypothesis to explain the development of subepithelial immune deposits as a result of binding of immune complexes to complement (C3) receptors on the visceral epithelial cell. Immune complexes composed of antigen, antibody, and C3 circulate to the kidney, migrate through the capillary wall, and come in contact with active glomerular complement receptors (GCR) on epithelial cells (EPI). The deposits are bound to the active GCR and accumulate to form larger deposits, thereby occupying available GCR binding sites.

Type IV (cell-mediated) IRD is characterized by the infiltration of mononuclear cells that have become sensitized to antigens within the kidney. Sensitized lymphocytes may cause tissue injury either directly or by releasing soluble products (lymphokines) that have the capacity to support local inflammation and release tissue-destructive intracellular enzymes. Although not completely proved, **chronic glomerulonephritis (GN)** may represent an example of cell-mediated sensitization to self-renal antigens, stimulated by exposure to cross-reactive streptococcal cell wall antigens. Sensitization to foreign renal antigens is exemplified by **chronic renal allograft rejection.**

Type I (immediate hypersensitivity) IRD: Type I immune reactions are caused by immediate hypersensitivity and are mediated by the action of IgE on basophils and mast cells after contact with specific antigen. As one of their mechanisms of action, these vasoactive substances trigger platelet-mediated coagulation, thrombosis, and fibrin deposition. Participation of IgE-mediated mechanisms in IRD has not been definitively established, but a number of renal diseases are associated with IgE deposition as shown by immunofluorescence, e.g., **minimal change nephropathy** and **malignant hypertension.**

In immunologic inflammatory reactions mediated by IgE on contact with specific antigen, antibody is capable of releasing a number of humoral substances into the area of inflammation. Histamine, one of these substances which is stored in mast cells and basophil granules, causes smooth muscle contraction of small blood vessels and increased permeability of capillaries. Another substance is platelet-aggregating factor (PAF), which can be shown experimentally to result in the aggregation of platelets and the release of histamine into the area of inflammation. Other substances include slow reactive substance of anaphylaxis (SRS-A), bradykinin, and prostaglandins. All these substances are capable of causing contraction of smooth muscles and propagation of IgE-mediated inflammation.

Direct complement-mediated IRD: Complement-mediated damage to the kidneys may also result from direct activation of complement through the alternative pathway (see also THE COMPLEMENT SYSTEM, Ch. 16). This type of renal injury is characterized predominantly by the deposition of C3 and another serum protein called properdin in the mesangium and glomerular capillary wall. Early components of complement and immunoglobulin are not demonstrable using immunofluorescence techniques. Alternative pathway activation of the C system results when properdin cleaves C3, using as cofactors C3 proactivator, C3 proactivator convertase, and native C3 in the presence of magnesium

TABLE 147-2. PATTERNS OF IMMUNOLOGICALLY MEDIATED RENAL DISEASES

Type of Immune Response	Associated Renal Disease	Antigen	Pattern of Deposition of Immune Components		
			Ig	Complement	Fibrin
Type I (Anaphylactic)	1. Minimal change disease (?)	(?)	Focal mesangial IgE (?)	—	—
Type II (Cytotoxic)	1. Anti-GBM disease	GBM[1]	Linear along GBM	Linear along GBM (sometimes absent)	Extracapillary
	2. Anti-TBM disease	TBM[2]	Linear along TBM	Linear along TBM	—
	3. Hyperacute rejection	HLA[3]	Diffuse vascular	—	Diffuse cortical vascular
Type III (Immune complex)	1. Immune complex GN, (e.g., poststreptococcal, serum sickness, hepatitis B, SLE)	Variety of exogenous & endogenous[4]	"Lumpy-bumpy" in capillary wall or interstitium	"Lumpy-bumpy" in capillary wall or interstitium	Minimal
Type IV (Cell-mediated)	1. Chronic renal allograft rejection	HLA	Diffuse granular	Diffuse granular	Vascular
	2. Chronic GN	Renal	Variable	Variable	Vascular
Direct complement activation (alternative pathway)	1. Membranoproliferative GN	(?)	Often none, occasional IgG in mesangium	C3, subendothelial or intramembranous	Rare

1-Glomerular basement membrane.
2-Tubular basement membrane.
3-Histocompatibility antigens.
4-See Table 147-1.

Modified from J. A. Bellanti, *Immunology II*, p. 601, 1978. Copyright 1978 by W. B. Saunders Company. Used with permission.

ions. While all these compounds are constituents of normal serum, activation normally proceeds at a controlled rate without resulting in renal deposition of activated C3. The exact mechanism whereby alternative pathway activation becomes disordered, with resultant renal C3 deposition, is not clear. About half the patients who develop membranoproliferative GN have a serum protein capable of direct cleavage of C3 to active C3b. This molecule, called **C3 Nephritic Factor**, is a heat-stable 7S γ-globulin of 150,000 mol wt that is not immunoglobulin. C3b may then deposit in the phagocytic mesangium of the kidney or in C3b binding sites within the capillary wall and result in local immune inflammatory injury.

Direct C activation results in IRD characterized by proliferation of cellular elements within the renal corpuscle and increase in the thickness of the capillary wall. These changes in renal biopsy sections are described as **membranoproliferative GN**, of which 2 forms have been described. In Type I disease, deposited immune components are found mostly in the mesangium and subendothelial sites. In Type II disease, the deposits are found intramembranously within the capillary wall. Although both forms appear to result from alternative pathway C3 activation, the subendothelial variety may be associated with I-C alternative pathway activation, while Type II disease is more commonly associated with the presence of C3 Nephritic Factor in the serum.

Diagnostic Features of IRD

Renal biopsy: Although analyses of blood and urine usually are performed first, renal biopsy material ultimately provides the definitive data for the diagnosis of IRD. Consideration of the normal structure and the basic pathologic changes that are possible provides an understanding of IRD. The renal corpuscle consists of cells and extracellular material **(ECM)**. Possible cellular changes are an increase in number (hyperplasia), a decrease in number (atrophy), necrosis, and exudation (infiltration by neutrophils). The possible ECM changes are an increase in amount of material (sclerosis or scarring) or the accumulation of foreign protein deposits. All of every glomerulus **(diffuse change)**, all of a few glomeruli **(focal change)**, or part of a few glomeruli **(local change)** may be involved (see TABLE 147–3).

The biopsy specimen is usually examined by light, immunofluorescence, and electron microscopy. Light microscopic examination of the biopsy reveals the morphologic changes, e.g., cellular proliferation, membrane thickening, sclerosis, and hyalinization. Since various immune mechanisms may result in similar morphologic alterations, immunofluorescence microscopy is utilized to reveal the type and location of immune components deposited. Electron microscopic examination of the kidney specimen may be used to provide further clarification of the location of deposits.

Type III IRD are associated with deposits of antigen, antibody, complement, or a combination of these immune reactants throughout the capillary wall or in the renal interstitium in a "**lumpy**" **distribution**. **Linear deposition** of IgG or IgM and C3 along the subendothelial surface suggests Type II IRD. Type I IRD is associated with the **deposition of IgE**. Direct complement-mediated IRD may be associated with **deposition of IgG or IgM in the mesangium**. In Type IV IRD, there may be no immunoglobulin deposited.

The **type and pattern of C deposition** help in diagnosing and distinguishing IRD. Complement deposition usually follows the pattern of immunoglobulin deposition. However, the presence of C3 deposition in the absence of immunoglobulin, Clq, or C4 deposition suggests alternative pathway activation and membranoproliferative GN.

Urine examination: In many instances, the precise diagnosis of IRD can be made by careful examination of the urine. The urine in IRD nearly always contains abundant amounts of protein and

TABLE 147–3. RENAL PARENCHYMAL TISSUES AND THEIR RESPONSES TO IMMUNE INJURY

Renal Parenchymal Tissue	Response
Glomerulus	PMN,* mononuclear cell infiltration; sclerosis
Glomerular capillary endothelial cell	Hyperplasia
Glomerular basement membrane	Thickening
Mesangial cell	Hyperplasia
Glomerular visceral epithelial cell	Hyperplasia
Epithelial cell of Bowman's capsule	Hyperplasia (crescent formation)
Interstitium	Cellular infiltration; fibrosis
Tubular epithelial cells	Swelling, necrosis
Interstitial macrophages	Hyperplasia

* Polymorphonuclear

Modified from J. A. Bellanti, *Immunology II*, p. 600, 1978. Copyright 1978 by W. B. Saunders Company. Used with permission.

lipid-laden macrophages (the **Maltese crosses** seen by polarized light microscopy). Thus, nephrotic syndrome (see in Ch. 148) is present in virtually all forms of IRD. The excretion of excess protein into the urine appears to result from loss of the ability of the glomerular capillary wall to retain large mol wt proteins or to repel negatively charged albumin molecules. The latter may be the consequence of immune injury altering the normal negative charges on the epithelial cell surface. While the nephrotic syndrome may be observed in nonimmune renal diseases such as diabetes, the presence of ne-phrotic-range proteinuria suggests an underlying immune mechanism.

RBCs, WBCs, and cellular casts may also be found in the urine. Injury resulting in necrosis, as in acute Type II injury of anti-GBM disease, results in significant hematuria. Forms of Type III injury (e.g., postinfective glomerulonephritides) are associated with hematuria and RBC casts. SLE, with active renal disease, is associated with hematuria, lymphocyturia, RBC casts, epithelial cell casts (the "**telescopic urine**" of SLE nephritis), and some other collagen vascular diseases. Membranous, membranoproliferative, focal sclerosing, and minimal-change glomerulonephritides are associated with nephrotic syndrome but usually otherwise benign urinary sediments.

Serologic analyses: In Type II IRD, cytotoxic antibodies may be present in the circulation (e.g., anti-GBM or anti-kidney antibodies). Circulating antinuclear antibodies may be seen in SLE, or circulating I-C in a variety of Type III IRD.

Alterations in levels of C proteins often are significant in differentiating IRD. In instances where alternative pathway C activation predominates, early components of C (Clq and C4) are *not* depressed, since C consumption occurs via direct activation of C3 (e.g., membranoproliferative GN and frequently in poststreptococcal GN **[PSGN]**). In classical pathway activation (as in SLE), early components of C are depressed. The presence of C3 Nephritic Factor with depressed C3 but normal Clq and C4 virtually establishes the diagnosis of membranoproliferative GN with alternative pathway C activation.

Other helpful serologic analyses include rising titers of antibodies to streptococcal antigens in PSGN. Other postinfective glomerulonephritides can be diagnosed by serologic studies such as a positive test for syphilis, the presence of hepatitis-associated antigen, or rising antibody titers to a variety of infective organisms.

Course and Prognosis

These are highly variable and depend on the underlying pathogenetic mechanisms. The clinical courses of IRD can be grouped into general categories: (1) acute onset, (2) acute onset with rapid progression, (3) slowly progressive, and (4) nephrotic syndrome (see Ch. 148).

Treatment

Although the immunologic mechanisms underlying many renal diseases are now understood, treatment in most instances is either nonspecific or unavailable. The principles of therapy involve modulation of the host's immune mechanism by means of antigen, antibody, or I-C removal; immuno-suppression; and/or administration of anti-inflammatory and in some cases anticoagulation agents (see TABLE 147-4). If the antigenic stimulus cannot be removed, the goal is to reduce the antigen load and create antibody excess to favor reticuloendothelial removal of I-C. A few diseases are particularly responsive to corticosteroid therapy (e.g., minimal change disease). Azathioprine may provide additional benefit in transplant rejection and SLE. Cyclophosphamide appears to be helpful in Wegener's granulomatosis.

In Type II renal diseases, reduction of cytotoxic antibody levels is difficult, since the stimulating antigen remains present. Therefore, nephrectomy may be lifesaving in some instances. Therapeutic benefit has been achieved by plasmapheresis in anti-GBM disease, acute allograft rejection, and SLE. Additionally, in Type II disease associated with fibrin deposition, epithelial cell crescent forma-tion, and thrombosis, anticoagulation has met with some success. Unfortunately, the majority of IRD remain resistant to therapy.

TABLE 147-4. TREATMENT OF IMMUNE RENAL DISEASE

Type of IRD	Treatment
Minimal change nephropathy	Corticosteroids
SLE	Corticosteroids, azathioprine, plasmapheresis (?)
Membranous GN	Corticosteroids
Rapidly progressive GN (Anti-GBM disease)	Anticoagulants, plasmapheresis, nephrectomy (?)
Wegener's granulomatosis	Cyclophosphamide
Acute renal allograft rejection	Corticosteroids, ALS,* plasmapheresis
Chronic allograft rejection	Corticosteroids, azathioprine, ALS
Allergic interstitial nephritis	Corticosteroids

* Antilymphocyte serum.

148. THE GLOMERULAR DISEASES

A group of diverse conditions including, but not limited to, glomerulonephritis, in which the disease process appears mainly to affect the glomerulus. Due to the limited number of ways that a tissue can respond to injury and that these injuries can be expressed as symptoms and signs, there are structural, functional, and clinical similarities within the group. Clear-cut differentiation may be impossible.

Consideration of the normal glomerular structure and the basic pathologic changes that are possible provides an understanding of glomerular disease. The glomerulus consists of cells and extracellular material **(ECM)**. The possible cellular changes are an increase in number (hyperplasia), a decrease in number (atrophy), necrosis, and inflammatory cell infiltration. The possible ECM changes are an increase in amount of material (sclerosis or scarring) or the accumulation of foreign protein deposits. All of every glomerulus **(diffuse** change), all of a few glomeruli **(focal** change), or part of a few glomeruli **(local** change) may be involved (see TABLE 147–3).

Glomerular damage is associated with changes in glomerular capillary permeability, with the appearance of proteinuria and various components of the blood such as RBCs and WBCs. Occasionally at this stage abnormalities also can be detected in tubular function, because of inflammatory changes in the interstitial area. When present, these interstitial changes produce a reduction in urinary concentrating capacity and ammonium excretion. Such functional abnormalities may be caused by a disturbance in normal peritubular fluid and solute exchange in the distal nephron. Because there is some inherent capacity for glomerular hypertrophy, such defects in tubular function usually occur before reductions in GFR are noted. However, with further glomerular derangement, the total filtration surface is reduced, GFR falls, and azotemia occurs.

The clinical presentation of these various glomerulopathies can be grouped into 5 general categories: (1) acute onset, (2) acute onset with rapid progression, (3) slowly progressive, (4) nephrotic syndrome, and (5) systemic disease.

GLOMERULAR DISEASE OF ACUTE ONSET

(Acute Glomerulonephritis; PSGN; Postinfectious Glomerulonephritis)

A disease characterized pathologically by diffuse inflammatory changes in the glomeruli and clinically by the abrupt onset of proteinuria, hematuria, and, usually, RBC casts.

Etiology and Pathophysiology

The classic example of glomerular disease of acute onset is post-streptococcal glomerulonephritis **(PSGN)**. Strong evidence exists that this is an immune complex disease in which streptococcal antigens provoke an antibody response, and the subsequent antigen-antibody complexes in the circulation are deposited in the glomerular capillary walls. These complexes activate the complement pathway with the liberation of chemotactic factors causing polymorpholeukocytic infiltration. The release of lysosomal enzymes from neutrophils and the direct effect of the complement system lead to damage of the capillary wall including the glomerular basal lamina **(GBL)**. PSGN may occur during epidemics of streptococcal infection, or sporadically. The streptococcal infection is most often in the respiratory tract (pharyngitis, sinusitis, tonsillitis), but infections at other sites (skin and middle ear) may also precede nephritis. Cultures show no evidence of streptococcal infection of the kidneys in acute nephritis.

Certain other forms of postinfectious glomerulonephritis are also felt to produce injury via immune complexes. The glomerulopathy associated with bacterial endocarditis, infected ventriculoatrial shunts (established to relieve hydrocephalus), varicella, infectious hepatitis (HBsAg-positive), syphilis, and malaria are considered to be examples of immune complex diseases. The latter three may cause a sclerosing lesion and excessive proteinuria (the **nephrotic syndrome**) rather than acute glomerular disease, possibly because of chronic but low-level antigenemia.

Pathology

The lesion is mainly confined to the glomeruli, which characteristically are enlarged and hypercellular. Initially, there are large numbers of neutrophils and/or eosinophils; later, there are relatively large numbers of mononuclear cells. Epithelial cell hyperplasia is a common early and transient feature after onset of the clinical syndrome, and cellular crescents may be seen in a few glomeruli. True synechiae (bridges of basement membrane between the capillary loops and Bowman's basement membrane) rarely form. Endothelial cells increase in number, and the usual fenestration of the endothelial cell cytoplasm is often not apparent. The mesangial regions are often greatly expanded by increased cells and edema. Neutrophils, dead cells, cell debris, and deposits of electron-dense material are often seen within the confines of the mesangium. The deposits presumably represent circulating or in-situ–formed antigen-antibody complexes.

The peripheral GBL is most remarkable because of the large numbers of deposits on its epithelial aspect. Experimental evidence suggests that such deposits are formed in situ. The foot processes of the epithelial cells are invariably fused over the deposits. Deposits within the substance of the GBL are principally found near or over mesangial regions. By fluorescence microscopy, deposits of IgG and C3 globulins can be seen distributed irregularly over the peripheral capillary loops and in the mesangium, appearing as discrete, well-outlined specks of irregular size and shape in a subepithelial position. They are best described as diffuse, irregular deposits.

Symptoms, Signs, and Diagnosis

Though PSGN is most common in children after age 3 and in young adults, it is not rare even in older individuals. A latent period of from 5 days to 6 wk occurs between the streptococcal infection and the onset of nephritis. Edema, oliguria, dark urine due to the presence of blood, and (if the fluid retention is severe enough) hypervolemia, headaches, and visual disturbances secondary to hypertension may be the presenting complaints of PSGN. History of a sore throat, impetigo, or better yet, culture-proven streptococcal infection 1 to 6 wk prior to onset of these symptoms and elevated serum titers of antistreptococcal antibodies are especially helpful in documenting PSGN. The course is not stereotyped. For many patients, the first clue to PSGN is the incidental discovery of gross or microscopic hematuria. Transient renal insufficiency is frequently seen. For an unfortunate few, the disease presents with anuria, severe hypervolemia, hyperkalemia, and the possibility of death in the initial phase. For the majority, the symptoms and signs gradually abate over some days.

Other forms of postinfectious glomerulonephritis generally are easier to diagnose than PSGN, for they usually have a much shorter lag period or are present when the infectious process is active and apparent. However, the nephritis of subacute bacterial endocarditis (SBE) can present a diagnostic enigma, since a wide spectrum of renal involvement is possible, from mild hematuria, a histologic glomerulitis, and no demonstrable renal functional impairment, to significant renal functional impairment representing a diffuse proliferative and exudative lesion with tubulointerstitial involvement. The primary disease is often difficult to detect, and the systemic manifestations often mimic other diseases such as SLE or polyarteritis. Indeed, since some microorganisms may be difficult to grow and routine blood cultures may be sterile in this syndrome, patients have been treated with corticosteroids, rather than antibiotics, with disastrous results.

Laboratory Findings

The urine may be scanty, brown, smoky, or frankly bloody. From 0.5 to 2 gm/sq m/day of protein may be excreted. The urinary sediment contains RBCs, WBCs, and renal tubular cells; casts containing RBCs and Hb are characteristic but WBC casts and granular (protein droplets) casts are also common. **The RBC cast is pathognomonic of glomerulitis from any etiology,** but when found with the previously described clinical picture, is strongly suggestive of glomerular disease of acute onset.

The antibody titer against the causal infectious agent rises in most patients within 1 to 2 wk. Serum complement levels (C3, C4, and total hemolytic activity) are usually diminished during the active phase of the disease. Cryoglobulinemia is usually present and persists for several months, whereas circulating immune complexes are detectable for only a few weeks. Ultrasound or radiologic evaluation is helpful in distinguishing the acute disease from an exacerbation of chronic disease. In acute glomerular disease the kidneys are usually of normal size or slightly enlarged; with chronic disease the kidneys are usually small. Renal function can be estimated by changes in the serum creatinine concentration or directly by creatinine clearance measurements. Although renal function usually returns to normal over a matter of 1 to 3 mo, proteinuria may persist for 6 mo to 1 yr, and microscopic hematuria for several years. Urine sediment changes may recur transiently following minor respiratory infections.

Clinical Course and Prognosis

Patients with immune complex glomerular disease of acute onset have a good prognosis if the initial renal damage is not severe (marked decline in GFR, nephrotic syndrome, many crescents) and the source of antigenemia can be effectively removed. In children with PSGN, renal cellular proliferation disappears within a period of weeks, but the severity of the inflammatory response varies widely, and residual sclerosis occurs frequently. The majority of children (85 to 95%) retain or regain normal renal function. Progression to late renal failure is uncommon, although abnormal urinary findings (proteinuria, hematuria) may exist for many years. When progression does occur in the course of PSGN, extensive extracapillary proliferation (crescent formation) and necrosis are usually prominent.

PSGN in adults is not as benign, and progression, or at least persistence of the prior damage, is noted by an abnormal urinalysis in up to 50% of cases. Healing is characterized by scarring. Thus, the prognosis depends on the patient's age and the state of the renal lesion when the inflammatory stimulus is removed.

Postinfectious glomerulonephritis secondary to an infected ventriculo-atrial shunt (from cerebral ventricle to the atrium, to relieve hydrocephalus) has a good prognosis when the infection (usually *Staphylococcus epidermidis [albus]*) can be eradicated, but this often requires removal of the shunt together with appropriate antibiotic therapy. In SBE, as with the other forms of postinfectious nephritis, removal of the source of the antigen will usually (70 to 80%) cause resolution of the renal injury if extensive damage (crescents, necrosis) has not occurred prior to effective antimicrobial therapy.

Treatment

No specific treatment is known for glomerular disease of acute onset. If a bacterial infection is still present when nephritis is discovered, it should be treated with an appropriate antimicrobial drug. If azotemia and metabolic acidosis are present, dietary protein is restricted. Sodium intake is restricted only when circulatory overload, edema, or severe hypertension is present. Diuretics such as the thiazides or furosemide may also help in the management of the expanded extracellular fluid volume producing these findings. Hypertensive encephalopathy may require parenteral therapy with antihypertensive agents (hydralazine, diazoxide, nitroprusside).

RAPIDLY PROGRESSIVE GLOMERULAR DISEASE

(RPGN; Subacute Glomerulonephritis)

A syndrome characterized pathologically by extracapillary proliferation in most glomeruli and clinically by fulminant renal failure associated with proteinuria, hematuria, and RBC casts.

Etiology

In most instances, etiology is unknown; the pathophysiologic mechanisms are varied (see TABLE 148-1). Fortunately, RPGN is uncommon. The syndrome occurs as part of a multisystem disease in about 40% of cases. This chapter discusses RPGN with primary renal involvement, most of which is idiopathic; about 30% appears to be caused by antibody directed against the GBL, and a small amount by immune complex disease.

The initiating events leading to autoimmunity directed against the GBL are unknown. Antibodies to the GBL are present in the blood and can be demonstrated by the immunofluorescence technic on the GBL. In certain patients, a circulating antibody is present that cross-reacts with pulmonary alveolar basement membrane, leading to a pulmonary-renal complex called **Goodpasture's syndrome** (see Ch. 42).

Pathology

The typical picture is marked proliferation of glomerular epithelial cells to form a cellular mass (crescent) filling Bowman's space. The glomerular tuft is collapsed and usually appears to be hypocellular. Neutrophils in large numbers may be seen between epithelial cells. Necrosis within the tuft or involving the crescent is not common but may be the most prominent abnormality. In such patients, a careful search for histologic evidence of a vasculitis is important.

Interstitial edema is often a striking early finding. Most often it is diffuse and associated with infiltration of diverse types of inflammatory cells. Infiltration by mononuclear leukocytes between tubular cells is seen when interstitial infiltration is extensive. Later, the interstitium is diffusely fibrotic and the number of inflammatory cells decreases. The initial tubular changes include vacuole and hyaline droplet formation. RBC and hyaline casts in distal tubules are not prominent features. Atrophy and basal lamina thickening occur as the disease progresses.

A linear deposition of IgG (usually associated with the C3 complement component) along the GBL is the most marked abnormality seen by fluorescence microscopy, but this pattern is not constant or specific. Diffuse, irregular deposits of IgG and C3 are found in patients with severe immune complex disease. Such cases often have proliferation of intraglomerular cells as well as crescents.

Symptoms, Signs, and Diagnosis

The clinical presentation may be similar to that of acute, but nonprogressive, disease. However, the onset is usually more insidious with weakness, fatigue, and malaise as the most prominent symptoms; nausea, anorexia, and vomiting are also common. A few patients have a preceding history of proteinuria, hematuria, or hypertension. About 50% of the patients have edema and a history of an acute, febrile, influenza-like illness within 1 mo of the onset of renal failure. This is generally followed by severe oliguria, and most patients are azotemic when initially seen. Hypertension is uncommon and rarely severe.

Clinical findings and laboratory data usually indicate the diagnosis. Renal biopsy may help in differential diagnosis and in defining potentially reversible lesions that may also present with acute renal failure.

Laboratory Findings

Azotemia of varying degrees is typical. Hematuria is always present and is often macroscopic. RBC casts are always found, and a "telescopic" sediment (RBC, WBC, granular, waxy, and broad casts) is common. Anemia, sometimes severe, is a constant finding. Leukocytosis is not infrequent.

Serologic findings may help distinguish an anti-GBL antibody nephritis from severe immune complex disease. Immune complex disease is suggested by rising titers of antibodies to streptococci,

TABLE 148-1. CAUSES OF RAPIDLY PROGRESSIVE GLOMERULONEPHRITIS

Primary Renal Disease	Multisystem Disease
Idiopathic	Henoch-Schönlein purpura
Immune complex disease	Polyarteritis nodosa
Anti-GBL nephritis	Wegener's granulomatosis
	SLE

circulating immune complexes, or cryoglobulinemia. Hypocomplementemia is uncommon in anti-GBL antibody nephritis while common in immune complex disease. A serum assay for circulating anti-GBL antibodies is helpful when positive, but unfortunately is not readily available. The initial ultrasound or radiographic examination may show enlarged kidneys. As the disease persists, however, they become progressively smaller.

Prognosis

Although the entire course of the disease may occur over a period of several months, it is common for many patients to present in the terminal stages of renal failure. Without dialysis, death with total and irreversible anuria is common within a few weeks. The prognosis depends on preceding factors. If PSGN, lupus, or periarteritis nodosa is the cause, renal function may improve with appropriate therapy. However, with idiopathic RPGN, only an occasional case has a spontaneous remission. Patients who ultimately recover normal renal function have histologic changes, principally in the glomeruli, which consist primarily of hypercellularity with little or no sclerosis within the glomerular tuft or the epithelial cells; the interstitium shows minimal fibrosis.

Treatment

A renal biopsy early in the course of suspected RPGN is useful to establish diagnosis, estimate prognosis, and plan management. Serologic tests and a check for possible infectious disease should be done. Where severe crescentic disease is found on biopsy ($>$ 75% of glomeruli) without extensive glomerular obsolescence, tubulointerstitial lesions, multisystem or infectious disease, and a GFR $>$ 6 ml/min/sq m, a trial of heparin 500 u./kg/day IV for 5 days, azothioprine or cyclophosphamide 1 mg/kg/day orally, and intermittent prednisone 2 mg/kg orally every other day for 1 mo is reasonable. Alternatively, plasmapheresis may be safer and more effective when high titers of anti-GBL antibodies are present or in the case of fulminant immune complex disease. However, none of these treatment regimens have been tested or compared by randomized prospective trials for efficacy. Such therapy can only be expected to be effective in the early phase of the disease.

For those patients with more severe disease, maintenance dialysis should be offered and aggressive drug treatment withheld. Only renal transplantation can resolve the therapeutic problem, but even here, there is a risk that the transplant may be compromised by the development of the original disease in the donor kidney. The certainty and extent of this risk, however, are not clearly established, even when anti-GBL antibodies are present.

SLOWLY PROGRESSIVE GLOMERULAR DISEASE

(Chronic Glomerulonephritis)

A syndrome associated with several diseases of different etiologies, characterized pathologically by diffuse sclerosis of glomeruli and clinically by proteinuria, cylindruria, hematuria, usually hypertension, and slow, progressive loss of renal function. The incidence in the general population is unknown. Incidence in autopsy series is 0.5 to 1%. Because of its slow, progressive nature, it is asymptomatic for years longer than it is symptomatic. Therefore, the majority of these patients are undetected.

Etiology

Etiology is diverse. In a recent series of patients with end-stage renal disease who had bilateral nephrectomy, a primary glomerular disease could be identified in about 50% of patients. Histologic changes suggesting focal and segmental sclerosis were present in 28%, nonspecific glomerulonephritis in 28%, membranoproliferative or lobular glomerulonephritis in 25%, extensive crescentic disease in 15%, and severe membranous nephropathy in 4%. Only nonspecific glomerulonephritis is discussed here. In most of these patients the nephrotic syndrome develops (see below) during the progression to renal failure.

A history of previous acute glomerular disease is uncommon. Serologic studies implicating preceding streptococcal infections are unconvincing. Although immunoglobulins and complement can be histologically demonstrated in a variable distribution in the glomeruli, this is, at best, indirect evidence of immune etiology. Furthermore, searches for an infectious, toxic, or metabolic etiology have thus far been fruitless. Intrarenal coagulation has been implicated based on the findings of fibrinopeptides from activation of the coagulation system in the urine, blood, and, occasionally, the renal parenchyma. However, it is not known whether their presence is causal or secondary to the injury.

Pathology

The amount of ECM (usually mesangial matrix) is increased without significant hypercellularity. In many areas this is the result of collapsed capillary loops as well as an actual increase in mesangial matrix and GBL. Organized glomerular synechiae are often present and may involve up to 50% of the glomerular architecture. Deposits of immunoglobulins by fluorescence microscopy are inconstant and may be absent.

Depending on the stage of the disease, the interstitium is variably affected, but it often appears to be involved early and extensively by infiltration and fibrosis. In such areas, tubular atrophy is also present. The vascular lesion is nonspecific, mimics nephrosclerotic changes, and may be the result of hypertension.

Irreversible and progressive renal disease is suggested by the presence of severe and diffuse glomerular sclerosis, synechiae in a number of glomeruli, interstitial disease out of proportion to the degree of glomerular change present, and a marked increase in ECM.

Symptoms and Signs

The insidious nature of the disease makes it difficult to accurately date its onset. At one end of the clinical spectrum, it may be discovered during a routine medical examination at a time when the patient is asymptomatic and renal function is normal except for proteinuria and, possibly, hematuria. At the other extreme, the patient may present with uremic symptoms (nausea, vomiting, dyspnea, pruritus, easy fatigability) due to end-stage renal disease. During the course of chronic glomerulonephritis, gross hematuria is rare, but the illness may present with recurrent episodes of gross hematuria and proteinuria, possibly representing progressive Berger's disease (or other types of idiopathic renal hematuria), flareups of a slowly progressive illness, or separate, unrelated episodes of acute glomerulonephritis. Dependent edema may occur, usually with moderate renal failure, as a manifestation of the nephrotic syndrome. Hypertension is common, may be of any degree of severity, and usually accompanies renal insufficiency but occasionally may be prominent before azotemia is significant.

Laboratory Findings

Proteinuria is a consistent finding. Hematuria and RBC casts are frequently present but may be absent in some patients with established disease. Finely and coarsely granular tubular cell and hyaline casts are usually present in moderate numbers in the urinary sediment, depending on the severity of the injury. Waxy and broad casts only appear when there is significant interstitial scarring and tubular atrophy with dilation. When 50% or more of the functioning renal mass is destroyed, the BUN and creatinine become progressively elevated and the biochemical findings of uremia appear.

Diagnosis

In the early stages of the disease, **renal biopsy** may be helpful in distinguishing between (1) idiopathic recurrent hematuria, (2) nonglomerular disease (tubulointerstitial disease), or (3) slowly progressive glomerular disease. Clinical presentations of many renal diseases may be identical, and renal biopsy is the most reliable method of differentiation. It is most helpful during the early stages of the syndrome, before there is significant renal functional impairment, and is rarely indicated in the advanced stages of the disease. When the kidneys are shrunken and scarred, little specific etiologic information can be learned from histologic examination.

Treatment

Although many forms of therapy have been attempted, none has proved conclusively effective in preventing progression. Blood pressure control by sodium restriction and antihypertensive drugs as needed is felt to be useful. The management of uremic symptoms is discussed in Ch. 145.

IDIOPATHIC RECURRENT RENAL HEMATURIA

A disorder with the clinical findings of recurrent episodes of macroscopic hematuria, mild proteinuria, a variety of glomerular changes, and slow or no progression to renal failure.

Based on renal biopsy findings, 2 groups are currently recognized. **Mesangial IgA nephropathy (Berger's Disease)** was first described as a distinct clinical pathologic entity and separated from other causes of idiopathic renal hematuria on the basis of an immunofluorescent study of renal biopsies. The distinguishing feature was a granular deposition of IgA principally involving the glomerular mesangium in a generalized and diffuse fashion. It is important to note, however, that the glomerular IgA deposits are not specific for Berger's disease and may occur in other conditions such as Schönlein-Henoch purpura, SLE nephritis, and in association with chronic liver disease. In the second type, histologically, a spectrum of abnormalities ranging from minimal changes to mild diffuse proliferative glomerulonephritis has been described. The most commonly encountered lesion is a focal and segmental proliferative glomerulonephritis.

Symptoms and Signs

Approximately 50% of patients with recurrent renal hematuria demonstrate prominent mesangial IgA deposits. The initial presentation of both types of idiopathic hematuria occurs during childhood or in young adults. The syndrome is described most often as occurring 1 to 2 days after an episode of a febrile upper respiratory illness, thus mimicking PSGN, except that the onset of hematuria is coincident with the febrile illness. In Berger's disease, males are affected twice as frequently as females, but the sex ratio is equal with non-IgG idiopathic hematuria. There is no evidence of a systemic disease. Mild proteinuria (< 1 gm/day) is typical but occasional patients will develop the nephrotic syndrome. Microscopic hematuria is always present but RBC casts are noted infrequently. The serum creatinine and serum complement levels are usually normal, and hypertension is unusual at the time of diagnosis. Loin pain may accompany the hematuria, although the symptom is more common in those patients with idiopathic renal hematuria who do not demonstrate mesangial IgA deposits.

Patients with recurrent hematuria and a positive family history should be suspected of having hereditary nephritis and receive careful auditory and ocular examination.

Course and Treatment

The long-term outlook for patients with idiopathic hematuria *without* mesangial IgA deposition appears to be benign. Frequently, a spontaneous remission of hematuria occurs and renal function is well preserved in most patients. However, IgA nephropathy usually progresses slowly and most patients develop renal insufficiency over a period of several decades. Persistent heavy proteinuria, reduced GFR, and diffuse proliferative glomerulonephritis are unfavorable prognostic findings. When uremia occurs, treatment is similar to that of other renal diseases. Renal transplantation has been successful although some patients demonstrate immunologic evidence of recurrence.

NEPHROTIC SYNDROME (NS)

A predictable complex that follows a severe and prolonged increase in glomerular permeability for protein; the major features are edema, hyponatruria, hypoalbuminemia, lipiduria, and hyperlipemia, all of variable relative severity.

Incidence

New cases of NS in children average 2:100,000/yr in the USA and United Kingdom. An adult survey yielded 3:1,000,000/yr of new cases. The literature contains conflicting reports of the percentages of lipoid nephrosis (minimal change-nil disease [foot process "fusion" is the only morphologic change]) in various series and age groups, but the variations depend on patient selection and referral patterns, local incidence of focal glomerulosclerosis, and geographic prevalence of predisposing diseases (e.g., schistosomiasis in Egypt, malaria in Nigeria and Uganda). There is a predilection for males in the young and more equal sex distribution in older patients. NS has been seen at all ages.

Etiology

NS may be due to pure lipoid nephrosis, primary glomerular disease (e.g., the immune complex nephritides), focal segmental and mesangial diseases, a vast array of systemic diseases (e.g., SLE, diabetes, myeloma, and amyloid), neoplasms such as Hodgkin's and lymphomas, infections like malaria and syphilis, nephroallergens, nephrotoxins, and renal transplants. Familial nephrotic syndromes occur. Congenital NS (Finnish type) is an hereditary and autosomal recessive disorder, usually leading to death or to dialysis within 1 yr. A simplified classification of causes of NS is presented in TABLE 148–2; the disorders touch almost every branch of medicine.

Pathology

The lesion depends on the cause. Lipoid nephrosis shows only endothelial edema and "fusion," or effacement, of foot processes of the epithelial podocytes proportionate to proteinuria. Vacuoles, lysozymes, and increased organelles may also be seen. Mesangial hypercellularity occurs in about 5%. Focal segmental sclerosis (hyalinosis) may be superimposed on the lesions of lipoid nephrosis and begins in the juxtamedullary glomeruli. It is easily missed by inexperienced pathologists and correlates with poor response to steroids and a less favorable prognosis. Global sclerosis leads to obsolete glomeruli. Proliferation may be focal or diffuse in the NS associated with acute poststreptococcal, Schönlein-Henoch's rapidly progressive, Goodpasture's, and other forms of glomerulonephritides. Most of the other etiologies of NS have distinctive lesions: e.g., diabetic nephropathy shows intercapillary glomerulosclerosis, diffuse or nodular; amyloid has a fibrillar infiltrate that is diagnostic on electronmicroscopy and on polarizing microscopy with Congo red; sickle cell nephropathy shows a microangiopathy.

Immune complexes are seen as dense deposits in membranous glomerulonephritis with intermembranous deposits and interjection of basement membrane to form spikes. Deposits are subendothelial, intramembranous, or subepithelial in the glomerulonephritis of SLE. Whenever immune complexes are deposited, immunofluorescent staining is positive for complement and for IgG, IgA, and IgM in varying proportions. In human glomeruli only, a complement receptor has been identified on the epithelial podocyte. The number of receptor sites per glomerulus in vitro is reduced in proportion to the density of the in vivo complement staining.

Tubules show granularity and vacuoles or changes associated with proteinuria and deficits in concentrating ability. A variety of tubular syndromes have been associated with such changes, especially in myeloma.

Symptoms and Signs

At presentation, proteinuria usually exceeds 2 gm/sq m/day or 3.5 gm/day for an average adult, but the onset of NS can be so subtle that it cannot be dated. Anorexia, weakness, malaise, puffy eyelids, retinal sheen, abdominal pain, wasting of muscles, and edema leading to ascites and anasarca are found with varying frequencies.

Localized edema may bring the patient to varied subspecialists for such complaints as pleural effusion, pericardial fullness, scrotal edema, hydrarthrosis, ascites, or laryngeal edema; abdominal pain in the mesentery may be seen in children. Most often, edema is mobile—detected in eyelids in the morning and in the ankles after standing. It is also identified by parallel white lines in fingernail beds. It accumulates primarily by Starling forces, i.e., depending on the relationship between hydrostatic and oncotic pressure in capillaries and interstitium. Fluid retention is increased by activation of the renin-angiotensin-aldosterone system and increased fractional reabsorption of sodium.

TABLE 148–2. CAUSES OF THE NEPHROTIC SYNDROME

Glomerular disease	Minimal change Idiopathic membranous Proliferative Lobular
Metabolic	Diffuse and nodular diabetic glomerulosclerosis Amyloidosis Multiple myeloma Myxedema
Systemic diseases **Immunogenic disease**	SLE Periarteritis Goodpasture's syndrome Dermatomyositis Central pontine myelinolysis Takayasu's disease Erythema multiforme
Circulatory diseases	Sickle cell anemia Spherocytosis Renal artery stenosis Renal vein thrombosis Pulmonary artery thrombosis Inferior vena cava stenosis or thrombosis Constrictive pericarditis Congestive heart failure Tricuspid valvular insufficiency Pheochromocytoma
Nephrotoxins	Organic mercurial diuretics Ammoniated mercury ointment Inorganic mercury Bismuth Gold
Allergens and drugs	Pollen Bee stings Poison oak, poison ivy, and "purified" rhus toxin Trimethadione and paramethadione Insect repellents Snake bites Probenecid Penicillamine Miscellaneous allergens and serum therapy, e.g., wool, "cold pills," globulin and poliomyelitis vaccine
Diseases due to infection	Cytomegalic inclusion disease Syphilis Malaria Typhus Chronic jejunoileitis Tuberculosis Subacute bacterial endocarditis Herpes zoster "Shunt" nephritis (staphylococcus) Miscellaneous bacteremia
Congenital nephrotic syndrome	
Hereditofamilial nephritis	
Miscellaneous causes	Pregnancy Transplantation Cyclic recurrence Intestinal lymphangiectasis

Modified from *Diseases of the Kidney,* ed. 2, 1971, p. 504, edited by M. B. Strauss and L. G. Welt. Copyright 1971. Used by permission of Little, Brown and Company.

Orthostatic hypotension and even shock may be seen in children. Adults may be hypo-, normo-, or hypertensive, as their renin-aldosterone system is stimulated. It is important to examine carefully the degree of muscle wasting, which can easily be masked by edema. Oliguria and even acute renal failure may be seen, due to hypovolemia and diminished perfusion; occasionally, acute tubular necrosis supervenes.

Complications: A wide variety of severe metabolic sequential syndromes may be seen in prolonged NS in children and with membranous GN in both children and adults. These include nutritional deficiencies, including protein malnutrition resembling kwashiorkor, brittle hair and nails, alopecia, stunted growth and dwarfism, demineralization of bone, glucosuria, hyperaminoaciduria of varying types, potassium depletion syndromes, myopathy, decreased total calcium, tetany, and hypometabolism. Peritonitis and an increase of opportunistic infections are also seen. Coagulation disorders, together with decreased fibrinolytic activity and episodic hypovolemia, constitute a serious thrombotic risk. Notable is the relationship between membranous NS and renal vein thrombosis.

Laboratory Findings

Foamy urine has been noticed by patients since the time of Hippocrates ("bubbles on the surface of the urine"). Initial urinalyses may show poor concentration, proteinuria, and hyaline, granular, fatty, and epithelial cell casts. (The granules contain aggregated droplets of serum protein in the outer matrix as Tamm-Horsfall protein.) Anisotropic crystals or double refractile fat bodies are seen on polarized microscopy and may be present in casts. Oval fat bodies and fatty granules in casts are best demonstrated with Sudan stain. White cells are prominent in exudative diseases and SLE. Amyloid fibrils may be seen on electron microscopy.

Microcytic anemia may be present because of urinary loss of siderophyllin. **Coagulation disorders** are common, with a decrease of factors IX and XII due to their urinary loss and an increase of factor VIII, fibrinogen, and platelets.

Lipiduria is determined by Sudan staining of casts containing lipid granules, identifying macrophages containing lipid (oval fat bodies), and by finding anisotropic crystals on polarized microscopy (double refractile fat bodies).

Hyperlipemia may be detected visually by observing lactescent sera. Such patients have lipoprotein lipase deficiency transiently correctable by heparin or a problem in conversion of high- to low-density lipoprotein. In the laboratory, it is documented by elevations of total cholesterol, triglycerides, free and esterified cholesterol, and phosphatides. Unesterified fatty acids are normal. Lipid levels may exceed 10-fold normal in severely hypoalbuminemic patients.

Hypoalbuminemia is detected by chemical measurement or by quantitative electrophoresis. Albumin is often < 2.5 gm/100 ml and in children it is sometimes < 1 gm/100 ml. Values down to 0.2 gm/100 ml have been recorded. Alpha and γ-globulin are usually low as are ceruloplasmin, transferrin, ASO protein, and other immune globulins.

Diagnosis

Diagnosis of NS is based on the clinical features and laboratory findings described above, *but characterization of the cause depends on renal biopsy.* **Proteinuria** is the cardinal finding and must be present to make the diagnosis. The only other common medical conditions that produce *consistent* proteinuria in the nephrotic range are (a) severe right-sided congestive failure (e.g., constrictive pericarditis, tricuspid disease, primary pulmonary hypertension), (b) necrotizing arteriolitis of accelerated (malignant) hypertension, and (c) myeloma. Other causes of proteinuria are discussed in Ch. 144. Patients with the nephrotic syndrome in association with other renal syndromes nearly always have renal insufficiency at the time of onset or develop it early in the course. Thus, heavy proteinuria in the nephritic patient occurs when the disease is far advanced and is, therefore, an ominous sign. In contrast, patients with primary nephrotic syndrome have heavy proteinuria and its biochemical consequences as the main clinical problem; renal failure rarely is a presenting finding. However, renal insufficiency may occur in the primary nephrotic syndrome after a long course of illness.

Urine sodium concentration falls precipitously, and < 1 mEq Na/ml of urine is often seen in the accumulation phase of the nephrotic edema. **Urine K** is usually high, and the Na/K ratio is > 1. Aldosterone secretion and secretion rates are elevated. Nephrotic patients excrete a salt load poorly, and a defect in the response of natriuretic hormone to saline infusion has been postulated.

Prognosis

Prognosis varies with specific etiology; see the discussions in THE GLOMERULAR DISEASES, above, in Ch. 147, and in the chapters on specific systemic diseases. It is generally favorable in the steroid-responsive disorders and in the immunosuppressed frequent relapsers (see Treatment, below). Many of the diseases (e.g., membranous NS) have spontaneous remissions in a significant fraction even after 5 to 7 yr. Prognosis may be altered drastically by infections or by thromboses in cerebral, pulmonary, peripheral, or renal veins. Focal sclerosis, global sclerosis, and mesangiocapillary proliferative disease are associated with poor response to therapy and a guarded prognosis, but modern dialysis technics and transplantation have altered traditional mortality statistics.

Treatment

Supportive: Major features are moderate salt restriction, moderately high protein diets (> 1 gm/kg), graded exercise, and sparing, judicious use of thiazide and loop diuretics to control symptomatic edema. Slow infusions of albumin can be used in hypovolemia. Anabolic hormones occasionally are useful. Hypertension should be treated appropriately, usually with β-blockade or antirenin drugs. Infections (especially bacteriuria, endocarditis, and peritonitis) are life-threatening and should be treated promptly. Anticoagulants may be used in thrombotic events. Nutritional guidance is essential. Sunlight, routine immunization, nephroallergens, insect bites, and potentially nephrotoxic drugs may have to be avoided in hypersensitive subjects. Counseling is important to avoid the "deprived sibling" syndrome when a nephrotic child dominates parental energies. Psychiatric advice is often necessary because of cosmetic effects of disease, corticosteroids, etc.

Anti-lesion: Effective agents include corticosteroids, ACTH, nitrogen mustards, azathioprine, cyclophosphamide, chlorambucil, and indomethacin. Lipoid nephrosis, SLE, and early membranous and limited proliferative disorders have shown some responses, especially lipoid nephrosis without segmental sclerosis. Colchicine produces favorable results in some cases of amyloid NS associated with familial Mediterranean fever (see Ch. 14).

Renal biopsy *is indicated in most cases of adult nephrotic syndrome for rational choice of therapy or prognosis.* After biopsy, in those conditions where a corticosteroid trial is indicated, prednisolone should be given 60 mg/sq m/day or 2 mg/kg/day in children and 1 to 1.5 mg/kg/day in adults for a minimum of 21 days. The patient should then be classified according to the therapeutic classification outline in TABLE 148–3. Class 0, I, and II responders should be tapered gradually and taken off corticosteroids. Class III and IV responders should be converted to 80- to 100-mg prednisolone on alternate days for an additional 4 to 6 wk. These patients should then be tapered off corticosteroids and carefully observed for relapse.

Some patients who respond to corticosteroids have frequent relapses but may respond more favorably to the combination of prednisolone 40 mg/day and cyclophosphamide 1.5 to 2 mg/kg/day for 60 days in a single course. Favorable responses are the rule with this regimen when patients are carefully selected and defined as having lipoid nephrosis with selective proteinuria, are steroid-responsive and steroid-dependent, and are frequent relapsers. However, gonadal toxicity is a serious consideration, especially in prepubertal adolescence. Hemorrhagic cystitis has been noted, but usually at higher cumulative doses. Toxicity is minimized by strictly limiting the dose of cyclophosphamide therapy.

Therapy combining low doses of prednisolone, azathioprine, and cyclophosphamide has been tried in resistant cases of SLE. Immunosuppressives and heparin followed by dicumarol have been used in severe proliferative diseases with deteriorating function. Indomethacin may decrease proteinuria, but is sometimes associated with a fall in GFR. Captopril, an angiotensin-converting enzyme inhibitor sometimes used to treat high renin states, may worsen proteinuria and the NS. It is adversely associated with membrane deposits similar to those seen with penicillamine therapy.

Careful desensitization may reverse NS associated with nephroallergens such as poison oak or ivy and insect antigens. Removal of nephrotoxins such as gold, mercury, penicillamine, and trimethadione may be followed by remission.

Removal of an infectious antigen by specific therapy may also cure the NS, e.g., staphylococcus and *Streptococcus viridans* endocarditis, malaria, syphilis, schistosomiasis, and "shunt" nephritis.

Intractable massive proteinuria with potentially fatal protein malnutrition has been treated with unilateral nephrectomy, bilateral nephrectomy, "medical" nephrectomy with mercury, and therapeu-

TABLE 148–3. THERAPEUTIC CLASSIFICATION OF THE NEPHROTIC SYNDROME—STEROID TRIAL

Groups of Responders	Type of Response	Grade of Response
IV	Complete therapeutic remission[1]	Good
III	Substantial but less than complete remission[2]	Good
II	Quantitative lessening of proteinuria[3]	Intermediate
I	No remission of proteinuria[4]	Poor
0	No response or death	

[1] Clearing all features of the nephrotic syndrome (e.g., reduction of proteinuria to < 90 mg/day, restoration of serum albumin to normal, loss of all signs and symptoms).

[2] Marked decrease in proteinuria (e.g., to < 2 gm/day), increase in serum albumin nearly to normal levels (e.g., > 3.0 gm/100 ml), decrease in hypercholesterolemia (e.g., to < 300 mg/100 ml), and a loss of nephrotic signs and symptoms.

[3] Lessening from 10 to 6 gm/day, but not below the "nephrotic range." Serum albumin concentration does not rise to normal; many clinical features of the nephrotic syndrome, including edema, may show improvement.

[4] No significant change in proteinuria, serum proteins, or lipids.

Modified from *Diseases of the Kidney,* ed. 2, 1971, p. 581, edited by M. B. Strauss and L. G. Welt. Copyright 1971. Used by permission of Little, Brown and Company.

tic renal infarction by injecting thrombosing agents to produce arterial occlusion. Except for unilateral nephrectomy, these procedures are followed by transplantation or dialysis. The mercury technic seems to have the lowest extrarenal morbidity.

Congenital nephrosis is rarely compatible with life beyond 1 yr, but a few patients have been supported nutritionally to the stage of renal failure and then managed with dialysis or transplantation. Many lesions, notably focal segmental sclerosis, SLE, and some forms of immune deposit nephritis may later recur in the transplanted kidney.

149. TUBULOINTERSTITIAL DISEASE

Tubulointerstitial abnormalities occur in all renal diseases, and most are discussed in The Manual in different chapters according to the etiology of the disorders (e.g., bacterial pyelonephritis in Ch. 151; transplant rejection in Ch. 20; toxic nephropathy in Ch. 150; tubulointerstitial nephropathy caused by radiation damage in Ch. 218; and tubulointerstitial disease in malignancy in Ch. 161). This chapter deals with selective circumstances in which tubulointerstitial involvement predominates, producing syndromes that may be due to diverse causes.

ACUTE NONINFECTIVE TUBULOINTERSTITIAL NEPHRITIS

A syndrome of acute renal failure most commonly due to drug hypersensitivity affecting tubules and interstitial tissue.

Etiology

This uncommon disorder previously was often associated with severe systemic infections. With the advent of antimicrobial agents, the dominant cause is a reaction to drugs. Among the most commonly incriminated drugs are methicillin, sulfonamides, anticonvulsants, penicillin, ampicillin, rifampin, diuretics, phenindione, and nonsteroidal anti-inflammatory agents.

Pathology

Glomeruli are usually normal. The earliest finding is interstitial edema typically followed by interstitial infiltration with lymphocytes, plasma cells, eosinophils, and small numbers of polymorphonuclear leukocytes. Tubular epithelium varies from necrotic to normal. The disorder is believed to be immunologic, but immunoglobulins and drug antigens have been found in the tubulointerstitial area in only a few cases. Histologic changes usually are reversible if the cause is recognized and removed; however, some severe cases progress to fibrosis and renal failure.

Symptoms and Signs

The initial presentation may be that of acute renal failure with or without oliguria. Helpful clinical clues include a history of exposure to appropriate drugs and signs of hypersensitivity such as fever, skin rash, eosinophilia, and eosinophiluria. The urine also usually contains protein, RBCs, and other WBCs. Hematuria at times may be macroscopic. The kidneys usually are large because of interstitial edema, and avidly take up radioactive gallium. The interval between exposure to drugs and development of renal involvement varies between 5 days and 5 wk.

Clinical Course, Prognosis, and Treatment

If severe prolonged oliguria is present, patients are treated for acute renal failure. Patients usually recover renal function on withdrawal of the offending drug, but some irreversible cases have been reported. Corticosteroid therapy (e.g., prednisone 1 mg/kg once a day for 3 days followed by decreasing doses over the next 7 to 10 days) may be of value in accelerating recovery of function.

CHRONIC TUBULOINTERSTITIAL NEPHROPATHY

This term includes *all those chronic kidney disorders in which generalized or localized changes in the tubulointerstitial area predominate over glomerular or vascular lesions.* Since some tubulointerstitial changes are associated with all renal diseases, this distinction may be difficult. Furthermore, more than one condition associated with tubulointerstitial inflammation (e.g., diabetes mellitus and urinary tract infection) may be present in a patient. Current data suggest that $1/3$ to $1/2$ of chronic renal failure cases develop as a result of chronic tubulointerstitial nephropathy.

The conditions commonly associated with tubulointerstitial inflammation are listed in Table 149-1. General features of tubulointerstitial nephropathy are discussed here; specific disorders are discussed separately in The Manual.

TABLE 149–1. FACTORS AND CONDITIONS ASSOCIATED WITH CHRONIC
TUBULOINTERSTITIAL NEPHROPATHY

Obstructive uropathies (including reflux nephropathy)
Bacterial pyelonephritis
Immunologic reactions
Transplant rejections
Reactions associated with glomerulonephritis
Sjögren's syndrome
Nephrotoxins
Analgesic nephropathy
Heavy metal poisoning (cadmium, lead)
Metabolic diseases
Gout
Nephrocalcinosis
Oxalosis
Cystinosis
Inherited and congenital disorders
Polycystic disease
Medullary cystic disease
Hereditary nephritis
Sickle cell disease
Malignancy
Radiation nephritis
Balkan nephritis
Idiopathic

Pathology

Although the causes and pathologic changes are variable, certain features are consistent. Grossly, the kidneys are small and atrophic. Toxins, metabolic diseases, inherited disorders, and Balkan nephritis as causes of tubulointerstitial nephritis produce symmetric and bilateral disease, but with other causes renal scarring may be unequal and involve only one kidney. With the exception of pyelonephritis or obstructive uropathy, the pelvic structures may not be affected. However, many disorders (e.g., analgesic abuse, obstructive uropathy, diabetes mellitus) may be associated with renal papillary damage and calyceal dilation with widening of the calyces and an overlying cortical scar. Histologically, glomeruli vary from normality to complete destruction. Tubules may be absent or atrophied. Tubular lumina vary considerably in diameter, but may show marked dilation with homogeneous casts producing a thyroidlike appearance. The interstitium contains varying degrees of inflammatory cells and fibrosis. Nonscarred areas appear reasonably normal.

Symptoms and Signs

Certain clinical features are common to all types of tubulointerstitial nephropathy. Generally, symptoms indicating progression of renal disease are absent, and edema, excessive proteinuria, and gross hematuria are not present in the early stages. Hypertension is a common finding. Patients often present with symptoms of end-stage renal disease or are discovered to have significant abnormalities on being examined for other medical problems.

Three renal syndromes, although not specific for tubulointerstitial nephropathy, may represent the initial clinical manifestations: (1) polyuria, (2) renal tubular acidosis, and (3) inability to conserve sodium. These functional defects result from a loss of tubulointerstitial function out of proportion to interference with renal blood flow and glomerular filtration. These changes occur more often in tubulointerstitial disease than in glomerulonephritis, but even in such cases, a proportionate loss of glomerular and tubulointerstitial function (as in other forms of renal disease) is more usually seen.

ENDEMIC TUBULOINTERSTITIAL NEPHRITIS OF THE BALKANS

In certain well-defined regions of the Balkans, a chronic nephropathy with the histologic characteristics of tubulointerstitial nephritis has been described. The exact cause of the condition is unknown although an environmental toxin is suspected. Although it is endemic, the disease is not familial and there are no associated hearing or ocular defects. The onset is never acute. The disease is discovered on routine examination by the presence of proteinuria or with the findings of chronic renal insufficiency. Special clinical features are the absence of edema, the rarity of hypertension, and the presence of severe anemia. The condition deteriorates rapidly, with chronic end-stage disease appearing within 5 yr after the first signs of the disease. Malignant tumors of the urinary system are found in 30 to 40% of affected patients.

150. NEPHROTOXIC DISORDERS
(Toxic Nephropathy)

Any functional or morphologic change in the kidney produced by a drug or a chemical or biologic agent which is ingested, injected, inhaled, or absorbed. By extension, the concept applies to normal ions circulating in abnormal concentrations (e.g., hypokalemic, hyperkalemic, hypomagnesemic, and hyperuricemic nephropathy).

The kidney has many unique features which render it susceptible to toxicity and its discovery. Its various functions can be measured quantitatively with accuracy, and subtle effects detected early (see Ch. 143). Its effluent (urine) can easily be measured by physical, chemical, microscopic, bacteriologic, and immunologic methods (see Ch. 144). Its affluent (blood) is the core of biochemistry. The kidney has the highest blood supply/gm of any tissue in the body (about 3.5 ml/gm/min vs. about 0.07 ml/gm/min for most organs except the lung). Circulating agents are thus delivered at 50 times the "usual" rate for tissues. The kidney has the largest endothelial surface area/gm, with 2 complete capillary beds in series. The first bed (glomerulus) has the highest hydrostatic pressure and greatest filtration fraction. Solute leaving the circulation is 100 times the mean of most organs. The kidney, therefore, gets a disproportionate sample of absorbed agents.

Physiologic reduction of glomerular filtrate to form concentrated urine may expose the luminal surfaces of cells to as much as 300 times the plasma concentration of *filtered* molecules or 1000 or more times the plasma concentration of those agents undergoing *tubular secretion.* The surface area exposed is astronomical because of a fine brush border on proximal tubular cells. A countercurrent flow mechanism acts like a heat exchanger to increase concentration of both urine and the interstitial fluid of the medulla. No other tissue fluid in the body is exposed to such concentrations, which may range to 4 times plasma concentration. Tubular transport separates drugs from *protein binding,* a common protective device for other cells. Transcellular transport uniquely exposes the interior of the cell and its organelles to newly encountered chemicals. Binding sites (e.g., SH groups) may facilitate *entry* but retard *exit* (e.g., heavy metals). The kidney has the highest O_2 consumption/gm and glucose production/gm, and is, therefore, vulnerable to poisons affecting *cell energetics.* As the leading site of *immune complex deposition,* it is uniquely susceptible to *immunologic* injury. It may also be active in the recognition of antigen. The human epithelial cell podocyte is the prime site of a complex receptor.

Etiology
TABLE 150-1 lists most of the clinically important drugs and chemicals known to produce nephrotoxicity. Most of these are directly toxic to cells by known or unknown cytotoxic mechanisms. Other

TABLE 150-1. COMMON NEPHROTOXIC AGENTS

Heavy metals	Lead, mercury, cadmium, uranium, gold, copper, arsenic, iron, thallium
Antibiotics	Aminoglycosides, polypeptides, amphotericin, bacitracin, rifampin, sulfonamides, co-trimoxazole, cephaloridine, methicillin
Analgesics	Aspirin, phenacetin, acetaminophen, all nonsteroidal anti-inflammatory drugs
Solvents	Methanol, glycols, carbon tetrachloride, trichloroethylene, miscellaneous hydrocarbons
Oxalosis-inducing agents	Oxalic acid, methoxyflurane, ethylene glycol, antirust agents
Anticancer drugs	Cis-platinum, nitrosoureas (CCNU, BCNU, methyl CCNU), adriamycin, daunorubicin, *Corynebacterium parvum,* immunotherapy
Diagnostic agents	Bunamiodyl, iodides, all contrast agents
Herbicides and pesticides	Paraquat, cyanide, dioxin, diphenyl
Botanicals and biologicals	Mushrooms (e.g., *Amanita phalloides*—severe muscarine poisoning), snake and spider venoms, insect bites, aflatoxins
Methemoglobin formers	See TABLE 150-3
Immune complex inducers	Penicillamine, captopril, levamisole, gold salts
Antiepileptics	Trimethadione and paramethadione
Unknown	(Balkan nephropathy)

TABLE 150–2. EXAMPLES OF AGENTS CAUSING NEPHROTOXICITY INDIRECTLY

Agent	Mechanism
Ethylene glycol, methoxyflurane	Via oxalic acid
Phencyclidine (PCP) and amphetamines	Via rhabdomyolysis
Methysergide	Via retroperitoneal fibrosis
Ergot alkaloids	Via severe arteriolar constriction
Heroin	Via lead, staphylococcus and fungal toxin, or other contaminants of illicit use
Chemotherapy of hematopoietic neoplasms and uricosuric drugs	Via obstruction with uric acid crystals—intra- or extra-renal
Vitamin D + milk + alkali + vitamin D analog	Nephrocalcinosis and lithiasis
Diphenyl and some pesticides	Via cysts and dysplasia
Mushroom and colchicine poisoning	Via diarrhea and fluid loss
Aniline, p-phenetidine, and a host of drugs, foods and industrial agents*	Via methemoglobin formation
Phenacetin and oxidant drugs	Only in G6PD-deficient patients

* See TABLE 150-3.

agents can produce renal injury by indirect mechanisms—often not apparent from a knowledge of the biochemistry of the agent. A partial list of such agents is presented in TABLE 150-2. Many agents are nephrotoxic via methemoglobin formation; a list is in TABLE 150-3. A diagrammatic mapping of the effects of some antibiotics on varied portions of the nephron is presented in FIG. 150-1.

In patients with pretreatment renal disease, one should be particularly alert to drugs which depend on the kidney as a major pathway for elimination. TABLE 150-4 provides a partial list. In renal failure

TABLE 150–3. AGENTS INDUCING METHEMOGLOBIN PRODUCTION

Medical Intoxications	Industrial Intoxications	Food Intoxications
Nitrates	Nitrites	Nitrites
Ammonium nitrate	Chlorides	Brines
Bismuth	Potassium ferricyanide	Confusion between nitrite
subnitrate	Aniline and derivatives	and sodium chloride
Nitrites	Trichlorocarbanilide	Nitrates
Potassium chloride	p-nitroaniline	Contaminated water
Potassium	Phenylhydrazine	Spinach, carrots
permanganate	Toluidine and xylidine	Sodium nitrate
Phenacetin	Nitro- and dinitrobenzene	Nitrobenzene (bakery goods)
Acetanilide	Mono- and dinitrophenol	Essence of mirbane
Phenylhydrazine	Dinitro-4,6-ortho-cresol	
Local anesthetics	Nitrogenous derivatives of toluene	
Benzocaine	Nitroglycerin	
Prilocaine	Nitrocellulose	
PAS	Naphthalene and derivatives	
Dinitrophenol	p-dichlorobenzene	
Polyphenols	Polyphenols	
Resorcinol		
Pyrogallol		
Phenazopyridine		
Sulfones		
Sulfonamides*		
Primaquine*		
Methylene blue		

* Use caution in treatment with methylene blue (risk of hemolysis). This intoxication often reveals a latent red cell enzyme defect.

From *Nephrology*, edited by J. Hamburger, J. Crosnier, and J. P. Grunfeld. Copyright 1979 by John Wiley & Sons. Used with permission.

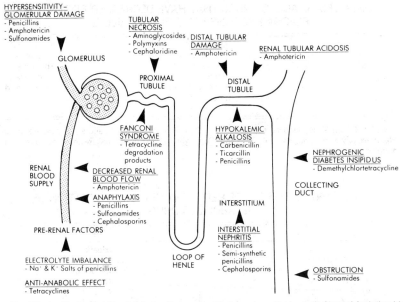

Fig. 150–1. **Nephrotoxicity of antimicrobial agents.** (Redrawn from Nephrotoxic Sites of Antimicrobial Agents, by G. B. Appel and H. C. Neu, in *The New England Journal of Medicine* Vol. 296, No. 12, March 24, 1977, p. 665. Reprinted by permission of *The New England Journal of Medicine*.)

there are significant changes in protein binding of acidic drugs. Protein binding not only is a major determinant of pharmacokinetics but also of cell toxicity in many organs. TABLE 150–5 offers a partial list of acidic drugs with decreased protein binding. Renal failure also affects drug oxidation and reduction; glucuronide, sulfate, and glycine conjugation; acetylation; and hydrolysis. A list of such interactions is given in TABLE 150–6.

Only a few nephrotoxins can be discussed here in greater detail. In hospitals, by far the leading cause of nephrotoxic renal failure (about 25% of all acute renal failure) is **antibiotics**, with aminoglycosides leading the list. Streptomycin, kanamycin, neomycin, gentamicin, tobramycin, amikacin, and

TABLE 150–4. SOME DRUGS FOR WHICH THE KIDNEY IS A MAJOR
PATHWAY OF ELIMINATION

Amikacin	Cycloserine	Neomycin
Ampicillin	Digoxin	Penicillins
Carbenicillin	Ethambutol	Procainamide
Cefamandole	Flucytosine	Streptomycin
Cefazolin	Gentamicin	Sulfinpyrazone
Cefoxitin	Kanamycin	Tetracycline
Cephalexin	Lithium	Ticarcillin
Cephalothin	Methotrexate	Tobramycin
Cimetidine	Methyldopa	Vancomycin
Colistin	Nadolol	

Modified from M. Reidenberg and D. Drayer, "Drug Therapy in Renal Failure," *Annual Review of Pharmacology and Toxicology* Vol. 20, 1980. Copyright © 1980 by Annual Reviews Inc. Used with permission.

TABLE 150–5. ACIDIC DRUGS THAT HAVE DECREASED BINDING TO PLASMA PROTEINS FROM RENAL FAILURE

Benzylpenicillin	Methyl red	Sulfonamides
Clofibrate	Pentobarbital	Thiopental
Congo red	Phenobarbital	Thyroxine
Diazoxide	Phenol red	Tryptophan
Dicloxacillin	Phenylbutazone	Valproic acid
Fluorescein	Phenytoin	Warfarin
Methyl orange	Salicylate	

Modified from M. Reidenberg and D. Drayer, "Drug Therapy in Renal Failure," *Annual Review of Pharmacology and Toxicology* Vol. 20, 1980. Copyright © 1980 by Annual Reviews Inc. Used with permission.

TABLE 150–6. EFFECTS OF RENAL FAILURE ON ELIMINATION OF METABOLIZED DRUGS

Drug	Effect
	Oxidation
Antipyrine	Normal or rapid
Digitoxin	Normal or rapid
Histamine	Normal
Lidocaine	Normal
Meperidine	Normal
Pentobarbital	Normal
Phenacetin	Normal
Phenobarbital	Normal
Phenytoin	Rapid
Propranolol	Normal or rapid
Quinidine	Normal or slow
Tolbutamide	Normal
Xylitol	Normal
	Reduction
Cortisol	Slow
	Synthesis
	(Glucuronide Conjugation)
Acetaminophen	Normal
Chloramphenicol	Normal
Lorazepam	Normal
	(Sulfate Conjugation)
Acetaminophen	Normal
Methyldopa	Normal
	(Acetylation)
PAS	Slow
Isoniazid	Normal or slow
Sulfisoxazole	Slow
	(Glycine Conjugation)
Salicylate	Normal
	Hydrolysis
	(Peptides)
Glucagon	Slow
Insulin	Slow
	(Esters)
Cephalothin	Slow
Clindamycin phosphate	Slow
Procaine	Slow

Modified from M. Reidenberg and D. Drayer, "Drug Therapy in Renal Failure," *Annual Review of Pharmacology and Toxicology* Vol. 20, 1980. Copyright © 1980 by Annual Reviews Inc. Used with permission.

sisomicin are all nephrotoxic. They accumulate in proximal tubular cells, induce cytosegrosomes with amyloid bodies, increase urinary enzymes and protein, decrease creatinine clearance and, unless severe, usually result in **nonoliguric renal failure.** Aminoglycosides appear to be synergistic in toxicity with cephaloridine, cephalothin, and methicillin. Because of accumulation, toxicity may be delayed or may occur early in a repeat course of therapy. Polypeptides such as colistin and polymyxin are directly and predictably nephrotoxic, as are bacitracin and the fungicide amphotericin B. Reported colistin cases have usually occurred in the range of 6 to 28 mg/kg/day. Outdated tetracycline may produce a Fanconi-like syndrome.

Allergy is involved in the acute tubulointerstitial nephritis (**TIN**) of the penicillins (especially methicillin), rifampin, sulfonamides, or combinations of trimethoprim and sulfamethoxazole. Diagnosis of acute TIN is suggested by fever, eosinophilia, elevated IgE, and positive gallium imaging of the kidneys; it is confirmed by renal biopsy.

All radiographic contrast agents are to some extent nephrotoxic. Their incidence of renal toxicity is higher when given intra-arterially. Predisposing risk factors are hypoperfusion, dehydration, existing renal insufficiency, age > 60, solitary kidney, diabetes, melanoma, hyperuricemia, congestive heart failure, and multiple exposures at close intervals.

Analgesic nephropathy accounts for 2.7% of patients in one USA dialysis series and upwards of 20% in Australia, South Africa, and elsewhere. Analgesics account for 1/5 of self-poisoning in the United Kingdom. All anti-inflammatory analgesics are nephrotoxic, including aspirin, phenacetin, acetaminophen, phenylbutazone, oxyphenbutazone, indomethacin, ibuprofen, alclofenac, mefenamic acid, flufenamic acid, N-phenylanthranilic acid, fenoprofen, sulindac, and naproxen. Mixed analgesic nephropathy may occur after a cumulative dose of 1 to 2 kg. The patients are usually prone to self-medication and have anemia, gastric upset or peptic ulcer, urinary infections, papillary necrosis, chronic TIN, hypertension, pigmented liver, and an increased risk of pelvic epithelioma and bladder cancer.

Most **heavy metals** accumulate in segments of the proximal nephron because of transport or binding sites such as SH groups. Toxic effects of lead are seen from pica, industrial exposure, contaminated water, wine or alcohol, mining or inhalation of smoke, or leaded gasoline. Tetraethyl lead goes through intact skin and lungs. **Chronic lead syndrome** includes shrunken kidneys, uremia, hypertension, anemia with basophilic stippling, encephalopathy, peripheral neuropathy, and Fanconi syndrome. More acutely, lead colic may occur. Mercury, bismuth, and thallium nephrotoxicity seem to be decreasing, but cadmium, copper, gold, uranium, arsenic, and iron are still prevalent—the latter associated with proximal myopathy in hemochromatosis and in other forms of iron overload, such as dialysis patients with multiple transfusions.

Solvent nephrotoxicity occurs mainly from inhaled hydrocarbons (Goodpasture's syndrome), methanol, glycols, and halogenated compounds such as carbon tetrachloride and trichloroethylene. Halogenated anesthetics (e.g., methoxyflurane) have also been implicated.

It appears that the chemists of the industrial revolution have far surpassed the toxicologists and clinicians. Drugs inducing immune complex disease in the kidney, proteinuria, and many features of nephrotic syndrome include D-penicillamine, captopril (an angiotensin-converting enzyme inhibitor used in therapy of hypertension), levamisole, and gold salts used by injection for RA.

Diagnosis

Diagnosis of toxic nephropathy requires a detective's mentality. In addition to a broad knowledge of drugs and toxicology, the clinician must be alert to the psychologic profiles associated with possible suicide or homicide, and to the patient's possible exposures to toxic agents at work, during recreation, from his environment, from his hobby, from his food and water. Has he had radiation exposure > 2000 rads, or multiple doses of contrast materials, or does he have risk factors such as dehydration with a single dose of contrast material? Does he have contact with unusual hydrocarbons such as are found in pesticides, paint or stripping agents, solvents, cleaners, or fertilizers? Is he exposed to unregulated foods or alcohol (e.g., lead in moonshine) or street drugs with their contaminants (e.g., glue sniffing)? Does he self-medicate inordinately (analgesics, laxatives, diuretics, ointments)? Does he "borrow" prescription drugs from others? Does he live downstream from a pollution source or drink well water from a contaminated aquifer? (There are 400 industrial-waste, deep injection wells in 22 states.) What is his allergic history and his family history of immunologic disease?

Treatment

Treatment guides are found elsewhere in the discussions of syndromes produced by the particular toxic agent (e.g., acute and chronic renal failure, nephrotic syndrome, tubular acidosis, interstitial nephritis, and in the section on poisoning).

General measures include withdrawal of the offending agent, induction of emesis, enhancing of excretion (e.g., chelates, diuretics) while function remains, and by direct removal from the bloodstream via the most efficient method (usually hemodialysis with large-surface dialyzer, hemoperfusion over charcoal or resins, plasmapheresis, or sorbopheresis).

151. INFECTIONS OF THE KIDNEY, URINARY TRACT, AND MALE GENITAL TRACT

ACUTE BACTERIAL PYELONEPHRITIS
(Acute Infective Tubulointerstitial Nephritis)

An acute, patchy, often bilateral, pyogenic infection of the kidney. Clinically, renal pelvic infection cannot be distinguished from parenchymal infection, and both pelvis and parenchyma are usually affected. Acute infective tubulointerstitial nephritis is a more descriptive term. (**Chronic bacterial pyelonephritis** is discussed separately below).

Etiology
Infections usually occur by the ascending route after entering the urethral meatus. Obstruction (strictures, calculi, tumors, prostatic hypertrophy, neurogenic bladder) predisposes to infection. The role of obstruction, whether anatomic or physiologic (e.g., neurogenic bladder), in predisposing to infection cannot be overemphasized; obstruction causes stasis, stasis invites bacterial invasion, and infection is established. Controversially, some believe that adults with diabetes mellitus may have a higher frequency of symptomatic bacteriuria than nondiabetics, perhaps due both to more frequent urinary instrumentation and a greater susceptibility to tissue invasion. Pyelonephritis is especially likely in females in their childhood or during pregnancy, and after urethral catheterization or instrumentation, but is uncommon in males free from urinary tract abnormalities. *Escherichia coli* is the most common bacterium and accounts for about 85% of uncomplicated infections, followed by *Klebsiella, Proteus,* and *Enterobacter. Pseudomonas,* staphylococci, and Group D streptococci account for 5 to 10% of the remainder. Hematogenous spread to the kidney may occur from any systemic infection but is commonest with staphylococcal bacteremia that produces cortical and perinephric abscesses. Patients subjected to instrumentation or indwelling catheters, who become infected while in the hospital, who are on chronic antimicrobial therapy, or those being treated with corticosteroids or immunosuppressive drugs are particularly likely to colonize with unusual organisms, such as *Serratia, Acinetobacter,* and *Candida.*

Pathology
The kidney is usually enlarged. The parenchyma shows extensive destruction of tissue by the acute inflammatory process, particularly in the cortex. Arteries, arterioles, and glomeruli show considerable resistance to infection. Polymorphonuclear leukocytes are present in large numbers in the interstitial tissue and in the lumina of many tubules, particularly collecting ducts. Chronic inflammatory cells appear within a few days, and medullary abscesses and acute necrosis of papillary tissue may be found. The pelvic and calyceal epithelia show acute inflammation. An important feature of the kidney with acute pyelonephritis is the patchy nature of the disease. Discrete wedge-shaped areas of involvement with no spread of infection outside them are a striking feature.

Symptoms and Signs
Typically, the onset is rapid and characterized by chills, fever, flank pain, nausea, and vomiting. Bladder irritation from infected urine may result in frequency and urgency. Physical examination will sometimes show some abdominal rigidity, which must be distinguished from that produced by intraperitoneal disease. If rigidity is absent or slight, a tender, enlarged kidney may sometimes be palpable. Costovertebral tenderness is generally present on the infected side. In children, symptoms are often slight and less characteristic.

Diagnosis
Diagnosis is suggested by urinary symptoms (frequency and dysuria) associated with signs of sepsis and renal inflammation (chills, fever, costovertebral tenderness); the laboratory provides confirmation. Urine should be collected aseptically (a midstream voiding in the male, a "clean-catch" in the female) for culture and microscopic examination. On urinalysis, the pH may be alkaline due to urea-splitting organisms, proteinuria is minimal (< 1 gm/day), bacteria are found in fresh uncentrifuged urine, and RBCs and WBCs are usually seen. WBC casts, when seen, are pathognomonic of renal inflammation (also seen in glomerulonephritis or noninfective tubulointerstitial nephritis) but may be difficult to separate from renal tubular cell casts unless special stains are used. Bacteria are usually evident on Gram stain of the unspun urine. Culture usually shows $> 100,000$ organisms/ml. Urinary bacteria are usually (60%) coated with antibody—a good indication of tissue invasion. However, antibody-coated bacteria cannot be used to specifically localize the site of infection, as positive tests are seen in cystitis (9%), acute hemorrhagic cystitis (67%), and prostatitis (67%). Males, patients with renal colic, and those who do not respond promptly to treatment require further urologic investigation. Excretory urograms may disclose calculi, anomalies, deformities, or obstructive lesions (see also Diagnostic Procedures in Ch. 144).

Treatment

Antimicrobial therapy should be instituted as soon as the diagnosis has been established and urine has been sent to the laboratory for culture and sensitivity tests. Treatment should be continued for a minimum of 10 to 14 days and in some instances for 4 wk. Urine cultures should be repeated during therapy and after its completion. If obstruction is present, surgery may be required. (For specific treatment, see in Lower Urinary Tract and Male Genital Tract Infections, below.)

CHRONIC BACTERIAL PYELONEPHRITIS
(Chronic Infective Tubulointerstitial Nephritis)

A chronic, patchy, often bilateral, pyogenic infection of the kidney that produces atrophy and calyceal deformity with overlying parenchymal scarring. The disorder causes end-stage renal failure in about 10 to 15% of patients who are treated by dialysis or transplantation. The term pyelonephritis should not be used to describe any tubulointerstitial nephropathy without documented urinary tract infection **(UTI)**. Despite chronic renal bacteriuria, progressive renal failure is infrequent except when associated with obstructive uropathy.

Pathology

The histologic picture is not specific and is similar to that seen with other diseases producing chronic tubulointerstitial nephropathy. The most specific change is a parenchymal scar associated with retraction of the adjacent papilla. Perhaps some initial insult (bacterial or other) produces papillary damage followed by focal tubulointerstitial atrophy, dilated calyces, and overlying cortical sclerosis.

Symptoms, Signs, and Diagnosis

Clinical clues, such as fever and flank or abdominal pain, are often vague and inconsistent. A history of UTI and recurrent acute pyelonephritis is helpful but infrequently obtained except in children with vesicoureteral reflux. A history of recurrent UTI and a typical pattern of renal dysfunction occasionally occurs and strongly suggests the diagnosis. An abnormal urogram showing a dilated calyceal system with an overlying scar is almost diagnostic alone, although a high degree of vesicoureteral reflux without bacteriuria can produce similar findings. Frequently, obstructive uropathy (strictures, stones, reflux, myoneurogenic disease, etc.) is present. In these patients, a positive urine culture does *not* distinguish the site of infection. To differentiate upper from lower tract disease, localization studies, checking for antibody-coated bacteria in women, and using bladder washout with neomycin-fibrinolytic enzyme solutions are helpful. The purpose of these studies is to find the patients who have kidney involvement, so as to predict the probable development of serious renal disease in particular patients and to select the optimal plan for long-term patient management. However, all these efforts at localizing the site of infection are necessarily indirect and usually confirm that which was evident by clinical observation. While localization technics have obvious value in research projects, it is only in the rare patient that they help in the management of UTI.

Proteinuria is absent, minimal, or intermittent until scarring of the kidneys is far advanced. Even then, proteinuria is usually < 1 gm/sq m/day. Urinary sediment tends to be scanty, but renal epithelial cells, granular casts and, occasionally, WBC casts are found. Renal function studies may disclose defects in concentrating ability, and hyperchloremic acidosis before azotemia is found.

Clinical Course and Prognosis

The course is extremely variable, but typically the disease progresses extremely slowly, with patients having adequate renal function for 20 yr or more after the onset. Two important factors influence the outcome of the disorder: (1) recurrent pyelonephritis, and (2) the type of urinary obstruction. Frequent exacerbations of acute pyelonephritis, even though controlled, usually produce some further deterioration of renal structure and function. Continued obstruction acts both by predisposing to or perpetuating renal infection, and by increasing the pelvic pressure, which damages the kidney directly.

Treatment

The most important therapeutic measures are the elimination of obstruction and eradication of urinary bacteria. Where obstruction cannot be eliminated and recurrent infections are common, long-term antimicrobial therapy with drugs such as nitrofurantoin or trimethoprim-sulfamethoxazole (see Lower Urinary Tract and Male Genital Tract Infections, below) are useful. The use of methenamine salts should be avoided because they are not effective in suppressing renal bacterial infections. In the absence of demonstrable obstruction or renal dysfunction, it has not been clearly established that covert renal bacteriuria is deleterious. Therefore, repeated courses of antimicrobials or suppressive therapy are probably not indicated. If uremia or hypertension develops, the principles of treatment are as outlined in the chapters dealing with these subjects.

LOWER URINARY TRACT AND MALE GENITAL TRACT INFECTIONS

Bacterial infections of the lower urinary tract are very common. They occur about 10 times more frequently in the female than in the male, except in the neonatal period when frequency is equal in both sexes. During infancy, the organisms enter the GU system most often by hematogenous or lymphatic spread. In older children and in adults, the main route of infection is an ascending one (from the vagina-urethra-bladder). Antibacterial therapy and surgical procedures have markedly improved the prognosis for most GU tract infections.

While urinary tract obstruction does not in itself cause UTI, its presence often predisposes to infection and makes infection much more difficult to clear with medical therapy. Urologic investigation is therefore mandatory in all but the simplest of UTIs, to detect obstructive uropathy, urinary calculi, congenital anatomic defects, or other abnormalities that may complicate or perpetuate the infection.

BACTERIAL INFECTIONS

The majority of UTIs are caused by gram-negative bacteria. The most common gram-negative organisms are *Escherichia coli* (up to 85% of uncomplicated UTIs), followed by *Klebsiella* species, *Proteus* species, *Enterobacter (Aerobacter) aerogenes*, and *Pseudomonas aeruginosa*. Occasionally, gram-positive pathogens may be involved, including *Staphylococcus epidermidis (albus)*, *S. aureus*, enterococci (*Streptococcus faecalis*), α-hemolytic streptococci, and β-hemolytic streptococci. Infection of the GU system by *Mycobacterium tuberculosis*, always a secondary manifestation of tuberculous disease in another site, is now uncommon. TB is discussed in Ch. 8.

GENERAL CONSIDERATIONS

Symptoms and Signs

Urethritis in men usually presents with a urethral discharge that is purulent (in cases due to *Neisseria gonorrhoeae*) or whitish-mucoid (in cases of nonspecific type). The etiology of the nonspecific or nongonococcal urethritis may be due to infection with *Chlamydia trachomatis* or *Ureaplasma urealyticum*. The man usually experiences burning on urination, urgency and frequency of urination, and inflammation of the urinary meatus. Women who have acute urethritis often have symptoms that are similar to those of acute bladder infections.

Acute cystitis classically presents with burning on urination or painful urination, urinary urgency and frequency, suprapubic and often low back pain, and nocturia. Gross hematuria may also occur, particularly in women. Many women with frequency and dysuria do not have bacteriuria, and symptoms usually resolve. Such symptoms may be caused by infections with gonococci, *Chlamydia*, or viruses, or be secondary to vaginitis.

High back pain or loin pain, chills, fever, nausea and vomiting, and other signs of general toxicity usually imply a kidney infection, such as **acute pyelonephritis, renal abscess,** or **perirenal abscess.**

Acute bacterial prostatitis: See under SPECIFIC CLINICAL FEATURES, below.

Diagnosis

In normal men and women the bladder urine is sterile. The urethral flora normally is either sterile or contains small numbers of gram-postive organisms (*S. epidermidis [albus]*, *Streptococcus* species, diphtheroids, or lactobacilli). External vaginal cultures show a similar normal flora. The presence of gram-negative organisms in either the urethral culture of men or women or in vaginal cultures of women is usually abnormal, and may precede cystitis. (See also the discussion of urine cultures in Ch. 144.)

A clean-catch midstream urine specimen is the most commonly used specific diagnostic study and must be obtained scrupulously for culture and antimicrobial-sensitivity tests when an infection is suspected. Quantitative urine cultures are generally available and markedly reduce the need for specimens obtained by more complex procedures. The presence of >100,000 organisms/ml in a carefully collected clean-voided urine specimen is presumptive evidence of a UTI. The presence of 3 or more species of bacteria in large numbers strongly suggests that the urine was contaminated during collection or was improperly stored (e.g., kept at room temperature for an extended period) prior to culture, unless collected from a patient on chronic long-term catheter drainage.

The most accurate means of establishing the diagnosis of UTI is quantitative culture of the urine obtained by means of suprapubic needle aspiration of the bladder. A clean-voided midstream urine culture suffices in men to establish the diagnosis of UTI. In women the 2nd most accurate way to diagnose UTI is a urine culture obtained by bladder catheterization. Although urethral flora may be pushed into the bladder during catheterization, studies have shown that a bacterial colony count of >1000 colonies/ml in a carefully collected catheterized specimen usually means that a bladder infection is present. Urinary infections rarely occur following bladder catheterization if careful, meticulous sterile technic is used.

In women, lower-tract localization cultures differentiate vaginal, urethral, and bladder infections. The patient is well hydrated to assure a full bladder. The lithotomy position is used. An external vaginal culture is obtained without preliminary skin preparation by swabbing the vaginal introitus with a sterile cotton-tipped applicator and then placing this cotton tip in 5 ml of saline or standard transport broth. With the nurse holding the patient's labia apart, the patient voids while on the table and the first 5 to 10 ml of urine are collected for a urethral culture. The patient then voids about 200 ml and a midstream sample is obtained by the nurse for a bladder culture. When the bacterial colony count of the vaginal culture significantly exceeds those of the urethral and midstream cultures, the diagnosis is vaginitis; when the urethral culture count exceeds the other cultures, the diagnosis is urethritis; when the midstream culture reveals a bacterial count of 100,000/ml, the diagnosis of a bladder or kidney infection is established.

In men, lower-tract localization cultures sort out urethral, bladder, and prostatic infections. The patient is well hydrated to assure a full bladder, and the foreskin is fully retracted to prevent washings from the prepuce from contaminating the specimen. The glans penis is cleansed with an antiseptic solution. The patient voids, and the first voided 10 ml of urine are collected for a urethral culture. The patient next voids about 200 ml, and a midstream aliquot is obtained for a bladder specimen. The patient then bends forward and continues to retract the foreskin. The physician massages the prostate gland and collects drops of expressed prostatic fluid for prostatic culture. The patient voids again, and the physician collects the first voided 10 ml of urine immediately following prostatic massage (prostatic culture). The specimens are refrigerated immediately, cultured, and the quantitative bacterial colony counts of the 4 specimens are compared. When the bacterial count of the urethral specimen significantly exceeds the other specimens, the diagnosis of bacterial urethritis is established. When the bacterial colony counts of the prostatic specimens significantly exceed those of the urethral and bladder specimens, the diagnosis of bacterial prostatitis is established. If the bacterial count of the midstream urine culture is 100,000/ml or greater, the diagnosis of a bladder or kidney infection is established. In the latter case the patient should be treated with a suitable antibacterial agent, and the localization cultures should be repeated in 4 to 5 days. If the patient has bacterial prostatitis, even though the urine will be sterilized by the antibacterial agent, the prostatic fluid cultures may still grow the pathogenic organism, and the diagnosis of bacterial prostatitis is established.

The normal centrifuged midstream or catheterized urine specimen should not contain > 5 WBCs/high-power field; more than this amount constitutes definite pyuria. Similarly, more than 2 RBCs/high-power field is considered abnormal and warrants further investigation. When the urine sample contains $> 100,000$ bacteria/ml, bacteria are usually readily seen on a wet-mount of the unspun sediment. A finding of > 20 bacteria/field of urine sediment, or a Gram stain of uncentrifuged urine demonstrating bacteria in every field, has an 85% correlation with significant bacteriuria ($>100,000$ organisms/ml) by quantitative culture. There is, however, no substitute for quantitative urine culture of carefully prepared samples in making the diagnosis of GU tract infection, and judging the sensitivity of the bacteria to specific antibiotics.

Because congenital anomalies, obstructive uropathy, urolithiasis, or other abnormalities may complicate UTI, an excretory urogram (IVP) with a post-evacuation film should be done as an important part of the evaluation. This is of special value if pyelonephritis is suspected, and to determine residual urine volume without catheterization in the male. It is usually of little value for uncomplicated cystitis in the female. Retrograde pyelography is rarely indicated. Voiding cystourethrograms are important to evaluate the possibilities of vesicoureteral reflux, particularly in children, and may identify urethral strictures or valves as well. Retrograde urethrography is useful in both men and women to evaluate the possibilities of urethral strictures, diverticula, or fistulas.

Cystoscopy may be helpful when a UTI fails to respond readily to therapy. Cystoscopy and ureteral catheterization permit collection of differential urine specimens from the bladder and kidneys to localize the site of infection.

Treatment

Obstructive uropathy, anatomic abnormalities, and neuropathic GU tract lesions may require correction by surgical means. Catheter drainage of an obstructed urinary tract aids in prompt control of UTI. On occasion, as with renal cortical abscess or perinephric abscess, surgical drainage is necessary. Instrumentation of the lower urinary tract in the presence of infected urine should be deferred, if possible, until the urine is sterilized with appropriate antimicrobial therapy to avoid bacteremia with septic shock, especially in the male.

Before antimicrobial treatment, uncomplicated and complicated (structural or neurologic abnormalities, foreign bodies) UTI should be distinguished. For an initial course of therapy of uncomplicated infections, sulfonamides, tetracycline, ampicillin or amoxicillin, trimethoprim, or trimethoprim/sulfamethoxazole are usually adequate (see TABLE 151-1). (Dosages, where indicated, are for the average adult with normal renal function. Dosages of most agents must be altered in states of decreased renal function). Therapy for 7 to 10 days is customary, although 1 to 3 days may be adequate for most initial infections. Post-treatment follow-up is desirable to ascertain cure and rule out asymptomatic bacteriuria.

The treatment of recurrent uncomplicated infections is slightly more complex. Recurrent infections can be relapses or reinfections. Sensitivity tests are highly desirable to guide antimicrobial selection. Most recurrences are a reinfection with a new organism and can be treated in the manner of an initial acute uncomplicated infection. Recurrence within a few weeks of successful treatment may be caused by a relapse—reemergence of a partially suppressed organism. It is often caused by an inadequate course of therapy, urologic abnormalities, or renal infection. For relapses, tetracycline, ampicillin or amoxicillin, an oral cephalosporin, nalidixic or oxolinic acid, trimethoprim/sulfamethoxazole, and nitrofurantoin should be considered. The latter 2 agents are particularly useful for

TABLE 151–1. ANTIMICROBIAL DRUG DOSAGE FOR URINARY TRACT INFECTION

Drug	Adults		Children		Dosing Interval (hr)
	Oral Daily Dose	Parenteral Daily Dose	Oral Daily Dose	Parenteral Daily Dose	
Amikacin		15 mg/kg		15 mg/kg	8–12
Amoxicillin	750–1500 mg		40 mg/kg		8
Ampicillin	1–2 gm		100 mg/kg		6
Carbenicillin	8 tablets*	6–12 gm		50–200 mg/kg	6
Cefazolin		1.5–3 gm		25–50 mg/kg	6–8
Cefadroxil	0.5–1 gm		Not recommended		12
Cephalexin	1–2 gm		25–50 mg/kg		6
Cephalothin		2–4 gm		40–80 mg/kg	4–6
Cephapirin		2–4 gm		40–80 mg/kg	6
Cephradine	2 gm		25–50 mg/kg		6–12
Cefamandole		1.5–6 gm		50–100 mg/kg	4–8
Cefoxitin		3–4 gm		80–160 mg/kg	6–8 / 4–6 (children)
Gentamicin		3–5 mg/kg		3–5 mg/kg	8–12
Kanamycin		15 mg/kg		15 mg/kg	8–12
Methenamine hippurate	2 gm		75 mg/kg		12
Methenamine mandelate	4 gm		75 mg/kg		6
Nalidixic acid	2–4 gm		Not recommended		6
Nitrofurantoin	200–400 mg		5–7 mg/kg		6
Oxolinic acid	1.5 gm		Not recommended		12
Sulfonamides	2–4 gm		150 mg/kg		6
Tetracyclines	1–2 gm		25–50 mg/kg		6
Ticarcillin		4–12 gm		50–100 mg/kg	6
Tobramycin		3–5 mg/kg		3–5 mg/kg	8–12
Trimethoprim	200 mg		Not recommended		12
Trimethoprim/ sulfamethoxazole	320/1600 mg		Not recommended		12

* Each tablet provides 382 mg of carbenicillin.

recurrences because the development of bacterial resistance is minimized. Therapy of relapses may occasionally require higher doses and 4 to 6 wk of treatment.

If frequent recurrences occur despite a course of prolonged treatment, then prophylactic, suppressive therapy with a single dose daily is usually effective. If the infecting organism is sensitive to nitrofurantoin or trimethoprim/sulfamethoxazole, these are good choices. Sulfonamides alone should be avoided for prophylaxis. Methenamine salts may be effective if the urine pH remains acidic and the urine is sterile prior to prophylaxis. Other useful agents include oral cephalosporins and nalidixic or oxolinic acids, but the frequent occurrence of resistant organisms during treatment necessitates periodic urine cultures. Three to 6 mo of prophylaxis are usually adequate. Recurrences should be watched for and treated with an appropriate agent and another course of prophylaxis.

Patients with **complicated infections** will respond to antimicrobial agents for only a few days unless the urologic abnormality can be corrected. Therefore, treatment should be reserved for acute episodes of tissue invasion in order to avoid the occurrence of highly resistant organisms. Aminoglycoside (gentamicin, tobramycin, amikacin) therapy of acute episodes of complicated infections is started after urine cultures because resistance to other antimicrobial agents is common. After initial treatment, sensitivity studies may indicate a less toxic agent can be substituted for the aminoglycoside for the 7- to 10-day course of treatment. When frequent septic recurrences occur, suppression of bacteriuria may be successful with nitrofurantoin, trimethoprim/sulfamethoxazole, or methena-mine salts.

Symptomatic therapy: A variety of preparations are used for relief of UTI symptoms (especially frequency, urgency, and dysuria). These drugs include the anticholinergic agents (atropine, hyoscy-amine, flavoxate, propantheline, or oxybutynin), which produce an antispasmodic effect on the smooth muscle of the urinary tract; and a topical urinary analgesic (phenazopyridine). These drugs may be used *in conjunction with specific antibacterial drug therapy* for 1 or 2 days only in the early stages of treatment when symptomatic relief for the patient is highly desirable, or for treating symp-toms when cultures are negative.

Specific Clinical Features

Kidney: See in discussions of acute and chronic pyelonephritis, above.

Ureter: Ureteritis generally accompanies pyelonephritis and may accompany cystitis. Chronic ure-teral infection may lead to decreased ureteral peristalsis and ureteral dilation with urinary stasis. One peculiar manifestation of chronic ureteritis is **ureteritis cystica,** the development of submucosal blebs that produce negative filling defects in the ureterogram.

Bladder: Most cases of **cystitis in women** are due to ascending infection from the vagina through the urethra, and often occur after sexual intercourse. Those women who develop recurrent UTIs differ from normal women in that they tend to carry large numbers of abnormal organisms for long periods of time on their vaginal vestibules. These pathogenic vaginal bacteria may find their way through the urethra and into the bladder and cause the next bladder infection. Thus the cause of recurrent UTIs in women appears to be a lack of some form of local defense mechanism that allows the colonization of these bacteria on the vaginal vestibule. These women may also have decreased cervicovaginal antibody to enterobacteria.

Cystitis in men generally results from ascending infection of the urethra or prostate or occurs secondary to urethral instrumentation. The most common cause of relapsing bladder infection in men is chronic bacterial prostatitis. Although the bladder urine can readily be sterilized with an appropriate antibacterial agent, most antibacterial agents do not diffuse from plasma into prostatic fluid. Therefore, when drug therapy is stopped, the prostatic pathogen eventually reinfects the blad-der urine.

Recurrent cystitis in both men and women that is associated with passage of air in the urine, especially when changing or multiple organisms are involved, usually implies a vesicoenteric fistula. Recurrent cystitis in women is sometimes secondary to a small and otherwise essentially asympto-matic vesicovaginal fistula.

Hemorrhagic cystitis is an acute bacterial cystitis that presents with gross hematuria, frequency, urgency, and dysuria. **Cystitis cystica** and **vesicular cystitis** are usually secondary to chronic infec-tions with mucosal and submucosal cystic changes similar to those seen in ureteritis cystica (see above). **Cystitis emphysematosa** is due to infection with gas-forming bacilli involving the submuco-sal layer of the bladder wall and is characterized by symptoms of infection plus pneumaturia. **Cystitis glandularis** is associated with chronic infections and exhibits characteristic histologic changes of encysted epithelialized spaces beneath the mucosal lining of the bladder.

Chronic covert bacteriuria (*significant bacteriuria detected by the screening of apparently healthy populations.* The term is preferred to the older one, **asymptomatic bacteriuria**). The prevalence of covert bacteriuria is about 1.2% in school girls and increases with age and sexual activity. Except during pregnancy, when therapy is indicated to prevent acute bacterial pyelonephritis, the proper management of covert bacteriuria in the patient without obstruction is controversial. A common plan is to treat with a 7- to 10-day course of an appropriate oral antimicrobial for each recurrent infection. If recurrence occurs after 2 or 3 short courses of treatment, urologic studies should be done; if no correctable lesion is found, a 6-wk course can be tried. Documenting a sterile urine by culture during prolonged therapy is important. If covert bacteriuria again recurs, 2 choices are possible: treatment of symptomatic episodes only, or prophylaxis with bedtime doses of nitrofurantoin or trimethoprim-sulfamethoxazole for several months.

Covert bacteriuria is rare in the male and should always prompt a thorough search for obstruction, prostatitis, or a hematogenous source.

Urinary infection and chronic renal failure: Most dialysis and transplantation units have found that chronic pyelonephritis accounts for only 10 to 15% of patients with chronic renal failure. Most urinary infections occur in the bladder only, but even chronic renal bacteriuria rarely progresses to chronic renal failure. When end-stage renal disease does occur, associated anatomic or physiologic obstruc-tion is usually present.

Prostate and seminal vesicles: Acute bacterial prostatitis is an acute infection of the prostate gland characterized by chills, high fever, urinary frequency and urgency, perineal and low back pain, varying degrees of symptoms of obstruction to voiding, dysuria or burning on urination, nocturia, and often arthralgia and myalgia. Gross hematuria sometimes accompanies acute prostatitis. The prostate gland is tender, focally or diffusely swollen and indurated, and usually warm to the palpating finger in the rectum. Culture of the expressed prostatic secretions usually yields large numbers of the bacterial pathogen. Enteric, gram-negative organisms are the most common cause of infection.

However, because of the danger of bacteremia, the physician should *not* massage an acutely in-flamed prostate gland until adequate blood levels of an appropriate antibacterial agent have been established. Since acute cystitis usually soon accompanies acute prostatitis, the bacterial pathogen can usually be identified by culture of the voided bladder urine.

Hospitalization with bed rest, analgesics, and hydration is usually required. If sepsis is suspected, ampicillin or amoxicillin should be given for 7 to 10 days. To prevent the development of chronic bacterial prostatitis, trimethoprim/sulfamethoxazole therapy is recommended for 30 days. In patients allergic to penicillin, an alternative treatment until testing of antibacterial susceptibility of the patho-gen is completed is an aminoglycoside. Should complete urinary retention occur, bladder drainage by punch suprapubic cystostomy is preferred over a urethral catheter (which may lead to bacter-emia).

The spectrum of symptoms in **chronic bacterial prostatitis** is variable. The hallmark of chronic bacterial prostatitis is relapsing UTI due to the same pathogen as in the prostatic secretions. Some patients are essentially asymptomatic except for bacilluria that relapses between courses of antimi-crobial therapy. Most patients, however, experience low back and perineal pain, urinary urgency and frequency, and painful urination. Infections involving the scrotal contents produce intense localizing discomfort, swelling, erythema, and severe tenderness to palpation. Rectal palpation of the prostate usually discloses no specific findings, but the prostate may be moderately tender and irregularly indurated or boggy. Secretions may be copious and numerous. WBCs, often in large clumps, may be identified, but the presence of large numbers of WBCs and lipid-laden macrophages (oval fat bodies) does not distinguish between bacterial prostatitis and nonbacterial prostatitis. The only accurate way of making the diagnosis of chronic bacterial prostatitis by laboratory means is with lower-tract local-ization cultures of the urethra, bladder, and prostatic secretions (see in GENERAL CONSIDERATIONS, above).

Chronic nonbacterial prostatitis is even more common than is bacterial prostatitis. The symptoms of this condition simulate those of chronic bacterial prostatitis; likewise, these patients usually show an increase in the number of WBCs and oval fat bodies in their expressed prostatic secretions. However, these patients rarely have a history of UTI, and lower-tract localization cultures fail to reveal a pathogenic organism.

The cause of nonbacterial prostatitis is unknown; thus, the condition is difficult to treat effectively. Antimicrobial agents do not relieve symptoms. Hot sitz baths and anticholinergic drugs provide some symptomatic relief. Some patients improve symptomatically with periodic prostatic massage, espe-cially for congestive prostatitis.

Seminal vesiculitis, an infection of the seminal vesicles, is an uncommon condition and is impos-sible to prove by culture technics. It may be the cause of blood in the ejaculate.

Urethra: The urethra may be the site of acute and chronic infections. The bulbous and pendulous portions of the male urethra and the entire female urethra are richly invested with periurethral glands. Organisms gaining access to the urethra may colonize these glands and produce acute and chronic infection.

Gonorrheal urethritis is a very common form of urethritis in men (see in Ch. 162). Inadequately treated gonococcal urethritis can cause urethral strictures. Urethral stricture predisposes to proxi-mal urethritis, occasionally with development of a periurethral abscess. Urethral diverticula may follow and serve as foci of continuing infection because of urinary stasis. Periurethral abscess may penetrate to and perforate the perineum or scrotum, and a urethral fistula may result. Although gonococcal urethritis may occur in women, the primary sites of infection are the vagina, cervix, and reproductive organs.

Nongonococcal urethritis (nonspecific urethritis—see in Ch. 162) in men is the commonest form of urethritis, exceeding gonococcal urethritis in incidence. *Chlamydia trachomatis, Ureaplasma ure-alyticum,* and other yet unknown agents cause this infection. These organisms are usually sensitive to the tetracyclines (500 mg q.i.d. for 10 to 14 days). The sexual partner should be treated concomi-tantly.

Scrotal contents: Acute bacterial epididymitis usually is a complication of bacterial urethritis or prostatitis and may be unilateral or bilateral. Torsion of the testis (see in Vol. II, Ch. 21, CONGENITAL ANOMALIES) must also be considered as an important differential diagnosis in patients under age 30 yr. The condition is characterized by fever and pain in the scrotum. Physical examination reveals swelling, induration, and marked tenderness of a portion or all of the affected epididymis and at times, the adjacent testis. The infecting organism can usually be identified by culture of the urine, or expressed prostatic secretions. In men < 35 yr, most cases are due to the sexually transmitted pathogens *Neisseria gonorrhoeae* or *C. trachomatis.* Most of these men have demonstrable urethri-tis. In men over 35, most cases are due to coliform gram-negative bacilli. These men have pyuria, infected urine, and urologic abnormalities or recent urologic procedures. Treatment consists of bed rest, scrotal elevation, scrotal ice packs, analgesics, and antimicrobial therapy. In men < 35 yr, tetracycline 500 mg orally q.i.d. for 10 to 14 days is given. Older patients may require gentamicin 5 mg/kg IM or IV in 3 divided doses daily until the identity of the infecting organism is known. Then treatment with an appropriate, less toxic, antimicrobial is given for 15 days. Post-treatment cultures are important to establish adequate treatment. Unless abscess formation occurs, surgical drainage is usually not required. When the inflammation involves the vas deferens, vasitis ensues; when the entire spermatic cord structures are also involved, the diagnosis is funiculitis. **Recurrent bacterial epididymitis** secondary to a chronic urethritis or prostatitis that cannot be cured can usually be prevented by means of vasoligation (vasectomy). Occasionally, **chronic epididymitis** requires an epididymectomy for relief of symptoms. Patients who must continuously wear an indwelling urethral catheter are prone to develop recurrent epididymitis and epididymo-orchitis. Prophylactic bilateral vasectomy should be considered, since most cases result from retrograde infection via the vasa. Placement of a suprapubic cystostomy or institution of a self-catheterization regimen may be useful adjuncts.

Nonbacterial epididymitis and epididymo-orchitis are of unknown etiology but are not rare. They may occur secondary to a retrograde extravasation. Urinalysis is often normal, and urine and prostatic fluid cultures are negative. The symptoms simulate those of bacterial epididymitis and treatment is similar, except that antimicrobial therapy may not be effective. Nerve block of the spermatic cord with a local anesthetic solution can provide marked symptomatic relief.

SEXUALLY TRANSMITTED DISEASES (See Ch. 162 and in Vol. II, Ch. 5)

PARASITIC DISEASES

Parasitic diseases such as schistosomiasis (bilharziasis), malaria, filariasis (*Wuchereria bancrofti*), *Trichomonas vaginalis*, *Entamoeba histolytica*, and *Echinococcus granulosus* affect large numbers of people and are frequent causes of renal and lower urinary tract disease. Parasitic infections are often chronic or recurrent and it is not surprising that immunologic types of renal disease have been described. In Africa the most common type of childhood renal disease is the nephrotic syndrome associated with quartan malaria and a variety of glomerulopathic changes. Similarly, glomerulopathies are commonly associated with schistosomiasis, especially *Schistosoma mansoni* and *S. japonicum*. However, *S. haematobium* infestations are associated with obstructive uropathy, hydronephrosis, and pyelonephritis—a common cause of end-stage renal disease along the Nile river. Chronic cystitis is another frequent complication of schistosomiasis and frequently results in carcinoma of the bladder.

Filariasis involves the lymphatic system, with obstruction leading to chyluria and chronic elephantiasis which may involve the scrotum and legs. **Echinococcosis** is transmitted by the tapeworm ova and leads to hydatid cysts that most often involve the liver but involve the kidney in a significant number of cases. *Trichomonas vaginalis* is a common cause of vaginitis in women but can lead to urethritis and prostatitis in men. Treatment is discussed in Vol. II, Ch. 5. Transmission is by coitus, and the sexual partner should be treated at the same time to prevent reinfection. **Amebiasis** usually affects the GI tract, but may involve the kidney, bladder, and male or female genitalia, usually by blood-borne spread. Treatment is discussed in Ch. 13.

FUNGAL DISEASES

A few mycotic diseases occasionally affect the GU system. *Candida* species are the most frequent fungal agents colonizing or infecting the urine. Multiple antibiotic therapy, antineoplastic drugs, steroids, and chronic catheterization are predisposing factors. Urinary tract infections with *Candida* species may respond to flucytosine orally 50 to 150 mg/kg/day in divided doses q 6 h for 7 to 10 days, but emergence of resistant organisms is a frequent complication. Renal infections may require systemic therapy with amphotericin B. Cystitis will usually respond to bladder instillations of amphotericin B over a 6- to 10-day period. **Actinomycosis** rarely may involve the kidney or prostate; in the prostate it causes a chronic prostatitis resembling that seen in TB. It is diagnosed by finding branching mycelia or sulfur granules with gram-positive filamentous borders in the expressed prostatic secretions. Penicillin or a tetracycline is recommended for therapy. **Blastomycosis,** a rare cause of prostatic, scrotal, and kidney infections, is diagnosed by demonstration of round, budding, yeastlike cells. Treatment is with amphotericin B (0.25 to 1 mg/kg/day IV) or hydroxystilbamidine 225 mg/day IV over 1 to 2 h; duration of therapy varies from 6 wk to 3 mo depending on the infection's severity. Rarely, **coccidioidomycosis** produces a granulomatous reaction in the prostate that resembles granulomatous prostatitis, which is a vascular or allergic phenomenon, not an infection.

INTERSTITIAL CYSTITIS (Hunner's Ulcer)

Interstitial cystitis is probably not an infectious disease, but is included here because of the clinical manifestations of bladder inflammation and irritation. This entity may be related to the collagen diseases, may be an autoimmune disease, may be an allergic manifestation, or may be secondary to an infectious agent not yet identified. Radiation therapy and treatment with such drugs as cyclophosphamide can cause severe cystitis. Histologically, the bladder wall shows a unifocal or multifocal inflammatory infiltration with mucosal ulceration and scarring that ultimately results in contraction of the smooth muscle, diminished urinary capacity, and symptoms of frequent, painful urination and hematuria. Typically, middle-aged women are affected.

No single form of therapy is universally successful. Typical therapy has been repeated dilation and distention of the bladder under anesthesia and sometimes electrofulguration of the ulcerative lesions. Treatment with anticholinergic drugs such as propantheline bromide 15 mg q.i.d. or oxybutynin chloride 5 mg 2 to 3 times/day offers some relief. Bladder instillations of dimethyl sulfoxide (DMSO) are also being used with some success to relieve symptoms. Rarely, augmentation cystoplasty using ileum or sigmoid may be undertaken to increase bladder capacity, and occasionally the disease process may be so severe as to demand cystectomy with urinary diversion by ileal or colon conduit, ureterosigmoidostomy, or other methods. Carcinoma in situ of the urinary bladder can often mimic the symptoms of interstitial cystitis and must always be ruled out in such cases by means of repeated urinary cytology and bladder biopsy.

---

152. VASCULAR DISEASE

VASCULAR DISEASES OF ACUTE ONSET

Excluding vasculitis, 5 types of acute vascular disease produce renal syndromes: (1) malignant nephroangiosclerosis, (2) infarction from occlusion of major renal vessels, (3) atheromatous embolization, (4) renal cortical necrosis, and (5) renal vein thrombosis.

MALIGNANT NEPHROANGIOSCLEROSIS (Malignant Nephrosclerosis; Malignant Hypertension)

Renal arteriolar necrosis associated with hypertension and rapidly progressive renal failure. Most cases of malignant nephroangiosclerosis appear as accelerated cardiovascular disease in the course of idiopathic hypertension, especially in untreated cases. Although 1% of patients with idiopathic hypertension have been reported to develop this complication, the incidence is apparently decreasing. However, about 20% of patients with this condition may have renovascular hypertension. The peak incidence in men occurs during their 40s and 50s; in women, about a decade earlier.

Pathology
The size of the kidneys varies greatly and presumably depends on the length of the clinical course and the presence of preexisting disease. The most striking glomerular change is fibrinoid necrosis in the capillary tuft. Proliferation of intraglomerular cells as well as epithelial crescents may be present. The most important change, the hallmark of malignant hypertension, is fibrinoid necrosis of arterioles. Interlobular arteries usually show considerable intimal thickening by a fine concentric layering of collagen, often causing a virtual obliteration of the vascular lumen.

Symptoms and Signs
Patients present with symptoms representing varying degrees of involvement of the brain, the heart, and the kidneys. Headaches, blurring of vision, and varying degrees of obtundation are usually present at some time during the disease.

On physical examination, neuroretinopathy (hemorrhages, exudates, and often papilledema) is present. The heart is enlarged, with evidence of left ventricular hypertrophy. Findings of congestive heart failure may also be present. Neurologically, patients vary from those slightly obtunded to those with coma due to cerebral hemorrhage.

Varying degrees of renal insufficiency are present. The urinary findings include proteinuria (occasionally in the nephrotic range) and microscopic hematuria. An occasional red cell cast may be found but the numbers are small, except with those renal syndromes associated with proliferative glomerulonephritis. Granular casts are common, and if renal failure is far advanced, broad and waxy casts may be seen. Hematologic abnormalities are common and include coagulopathies as well as hemolysis. Extremely high levels of renin and aldosterone are typical.

Diagnosis
Diagnosis is based on the finding of a persistent diastolic BP > 120 mm Hg and of neuroretinopathy, along with the other clinical features of cardiac and renal involvement described above.

Prognosis and Treatment
Untreated patients die in a relatively short period of time—about 50% by 6 mo, and most of the remainder within 1 yr. Death usually results from uremia (40%), cerebral atherothrombotic infarction (40%), or myocardial infarction (15%). Although some patients have spontaneous remissions, aggressive lowering of BP (see ARTERIAL HYPERTENSION in Ch. 24) and management of renal failure significantly reduce the mortality and morbidity. With therapy, fewer patients die, especially from renal failure and cerebrovascular disease, but the proportion developing myocardial infarction increases. Patients without significant renal failure improve most, and if hypertension can be reduced satisfactorily with dietary and drug therapy, most patients will be alive after 3 to 5 yr. Even patients with progressive renal insufficiency can be kept alive by dialysis and have occasionally shown improvement in renal function, permitting dialysis to be discontinued.

RENAL INFARCTION

A localized area of ischemic necrosis.

Renal infarction is caused by either arterial or venous occlusion. Occlusion of the renal artery is most frequently due to embolism, arteriosclerotic narrowing, and trauma. **Therapeutic infarction** via selective catheterization is occasionally used for renal tumors and massive proteinuria or severe uncontrollable hypertension in end-stage renal disease. **"Medical" nephrectomy** with nephrotoxic doses of mercaptomerin also is used where advanced renal failure exists and the patient is a potential dialysis or transplantation candidate.

Symptoms and Signs

Small occlusions of the renal artery frequently occur without any urinary or systemic findings. Typically, however, a steady aching flank pain develops that is localized to the affected renal area. Fever, nausea, and vomiting may occur. When infarction is a result of arterial occlusion, the kidney is small and not palpable. However, with thrombosis of the renal veins, the kidney is usually tender and enlarged enough to be easily palpated. Hypertension occurs infrequently after infarction; if it occurs, it usually is transient. Leukocytosis, proteinuria, and microscopic hematuria are typically present. Gross hematuria is extremely rare. Serum and urine enzymes such as lactic dehydrogenase, alkaline phosphatase, and glutamic oxalacetic transaminase are frequently elevated early in the disease.

Diagnosis

When renal infarction is suspected, excretory urography is indicated. During the first 2 wk after a large renal infarction, excretion of contrast medium or radionuclide on the involved side is diminished or absent. Because impaired excretion could also be due to obstruction of the ureter, retrograde urography is frequently indicated as the next diagnostic step. A combination of history (atrial fibrillation, recent myocardial infarction or trauma, past embolic episodes), symptoms and signs, virtual absence of excretory function on the involved side, and a normal collecting system is strong evidence for renal infarction. Arteriography is definitive, but is done only if a surgical attempt to relieve the obstruction is being considered. The extent of functional return may be evaluated by repeated excretory urograms or radionuclide scanning at intervals of 1 mo.

Treatment

Although surgical embolectomy may cause reversal of renal dysfunction even up to 6 wk after embolization, conservative medical therapy with anticoagulants is usually indicated, especially in those with serious cardiac disease or unilateral infarction. The recent reports of dislodgments of renal emboli with a Fogarty catheter suggest that this procedure may be more effective and safer than previous medical and surgical procedures.

ATHEROEMBOLIC RENAL DISEASE

A clinical syndrome involving either rapid deterioration of renal function or a more slowly progressive renal failure, depending on the amount of atheromatous material obstructing the renal arteries. The syndrome may occur spontaneously or subsequent to vascular surgery or arteriography. In patients with severe erosive disease of the aorta, the frequency of atheroembolic renal disease is approximately 15 to 30%; in patients with mild atherosclerosis, peripheral embolism has an incidence of only 1%. Embolization to the kidneys occurs most commonly in elderly patients and increases in incidence with age.

Symptoms, Signs, and Diagnosis

Atheroemboli to the kidney should be suspected in patients > 60 yr of age with renal failure of unknown etiology, especially if they have signs of advanced arteriosclerosis. The precise time of embolism is difficult to determine in patients with spontaneous atheroembolism, unlike in those with atheroembolism following arteriography. Most patients with spontaneous atheroembolism are azotemic when first seen, and progressive renal failure subsequently develops.

Most patients with this disorder and renal failure are hypertensive. In those known to be previously normotensive, a substantial rise in BP occurs with the onset of atheroembolism. Embolism of other abdominal organs such as the pancreas and the intestinal tract commonly occur. Signs of peripheral embolism such as livedo reticularis, painful muscle nodules, or overt gangrene strongly suggest the diagnosis but are not often present. When embolism is widespread, however, this syndrome has been confused with polyarteritis because of the multiplicity of organ involvement. Embolization to the retina can cause sudden blindness, and the bright yellow crystalline plaques can be seen lodged at bifurcations of arterioles on fundoscopic examination.

There are no distinctive laboratory or urinary sediment abnormalities. Diagnosis is confirmed only by renal biopsy.

Prognosis and Treatment

No treatment reverses the renal failure. Patients with atheroembolic renal disease and advanced renal insufficiency do not regain normal renal function even transiently. Surgical experience involving severe atheromatous disease of the aorta has shown that careful technic can minimize the likelihood of atheroembolism of the renal arteries.

RENAL CORTICAL NECROSIS

A rare form of arterial infarction characterized by necrosis of cortical tissues with sparing of the medulla.

Renal cortical necrosis can occur at any age; about 10% occurs in infancy and childhood. Over 50% of reported cases are associated with abruptio placentae; the next most common association is bacterial sepsis. Other predisposing conditions are nephrotoxins, renal ischemia, intravascular coagulation, and hyperacute renal allograft rejection. In children, infections, dehydration, shock, and hemolysis are associated. Suggested causes include vasospasm, activation of the clotting mechanism, endotoxin, immunologic injury, and direct endothelial cell injury. The lesion closely resembles the animal experimental forms of generalized Schwartzmann reaction.

Symptoms, Signs, and Diagnosis

Distinguishing this form of acute renal failure from many others may be difficult, but cortical necrosis should be considered when abrupt anuria occurs in any of the clinical settings noted above, and when gross hematuria and flank pain are present. Fever and leukocytosis are common even in the absence of sepsis. The urine contains much protein and RBCs; WBCs and casts (RBC, renal cell, and broad) are frequently seen. If measured early enough, serum LDH and SGOT levels are elevated. In the early stages, mild hypertension, or even hypotension, is common. However, in surviving patients who regain some residual renal function, accelerated or malignant hypertension is typical.

Although a biopsy showing patchy or diffuse cortical necrosis is the only means of confident diagnosis, renal radiograms are also useful. Serial radiograms initially show enlarged kidneys; renal size then diminishes and may be reduced to about 50% of normal in 6 to 8 wk. At this stage, calcification appears, often linear, and especially marked at the corticomedullary junction. The diagnosis can only be firmly established from the typical histologic findings obtained by biopsy, which shows focal or patchy cortical necrosis.

Treatment

Management does not differ from other forms of acute renal failure, although more problems may be encountered because of the prolonged anuria and the precipitating causes. All appropriate means, including maintenance dialysis, are used to allow recovery of any residual function. A few patients after several months may regain enough function to discontinue maintenance dialysis. For the majority, however, chronic dialysis or renal transplantation is the usual solution.

RENAL VEIN THROMBOSIS

Etiology and Incidence

Conditions associated with renal vein thrombosis are (1) retroperitoneal disease (abscess, pancreatitis, tumor, trauma); (2) thromboembolic disease; (3) extracellular volume depletion (mostly in infants); and (4) various nephropathies (amyloidosis, SLE, diabetes mellitus, polyarteritis nodosa, membranous). The frequency is difficult to determine because, aside from the acute forms usually seen in children, most cases induce only mild symptoms that often go unnoticed. Acute thrombosis usually produces hemorrhagic infarction. Partially occlusive, slowly progressive thrombosis is more common in adults. It is associated with nephrotic syndrome even in unilateral thrombosis.

Diagnosis

Clinically, 2 different pictures are seen. With children, loin pain, fever, hematuria, oliguria, edema, leukocytosis, and renal failure are found. In adults, the diagnosis is usually considered only in the presence of the nephrotic syndrome. (Whether the thrombosis is a primary cause of the nephrotic syndrome or is secondary to the hypercoagulable state associated with the nephrotic syndrome is still debated.) Commonly, the onset of the syndrome is gradual with the appearance of proteinuria and a deterioration of GFR. If the disease is acute, x-rays may show an enlarged kidney; slowly progressive thrombosis produces an atrophic kidney. Excretory urography shows absence of excretion of contrast medium. Cavography or selective renal phlebography may show thrombosis manifested by filling defects or a filling of collateral veins.

Prognosis and Treatment

Death due to renal vein thrombosis is rare and is usually related to complications such as pulmonary embolism or the primary condition producing the thrombosis. The effect on renal function is variable, depending on whether one or both kidneys are involved, on the development of collateral circulation or recanalization of the thrombus, and on the prior state of kidney function. These multiple factors influence the natural course of the disease and render evaluation of any treatment difficult. However, surgery is rarely used and nephrectomy is performed only in certain cases of total infarction or for reasons related to the primary disease. Thrombolytic therapy with streptokinase or urokinase has been infrequently tried and is unproved. Anticoagulant therapy is usually associated with improvement of renal function, is particularly useful in preventing pulmonary embolism, and improves patient survival.

SLOWLY PROGRESSIVE VASCULAR DISEASE

Arteriosclerosis is a phenomenon of aging that is accentuated by hypertension. In the kidney, the lesion is usually described as **benign nephrosclerosis** although a more accurate description would be **nephroangiosclerosis**. The vascular lesions are quite distinct from those associated with malignant hypertension, where fibrinoid necrosis of the arteries is the hallmark of the vascular damage. Arteriosclerotic disease is discussed under ARTERIOSCLEROSIS; ATHEROSCLEROSIS in Ch. 24. See also HYPERTENSION in Ch. 24.

RENOVASCULAR HYPERTENSION

(See HYPERTENSION in Ch. 24)

153. RENAL DISEASE ASSOCIATED WITH SYSTEMIC AND METABOLIC SYNDROMES

Renal disease may be prominently involved in many systemic disorders. These include the collagen vascular diseases (e.g., SLE, progressive systemic sclerosis, polyarteritis, Wegener's granulomatosis); hemorrhagic disorders (e.g., the hemolytic-uremic syndrome, thrombotic thrombocytopenic purpura, Henoch-Schönlein purpura); plasma cell dyscrasias (e.g., multiple myeloma); anemia (e.g., sickle cell disease); liver disease (see Ch. 64); pregnancy (see Vol. II, Ch. 18); and endocrine and metabolic disorders (e.g., diabetes mellitus and amyloidosis). Changes in the concentrations of various electrolytes and body fluids may have profound effects on renal function, especially seen in the presence of hypophosphatemia, hypercalcemia, potassium depletion, and gout. The renal abnormalities involved in the above disorders are included in their discussions elsewhere in this volume and in Vol. II.

ANOMALIES IN KIDNEY TRANSPORT

CYSTINURIA

An inherited defect of the renal tubules in which resorption of the amino acid cystine is impaired, urinary excretion is increased, and cystine calculi often form in the urinary tract.

Cystinuria is inherited as an autosomal recessive trait. Heterozygotes may excrete increased quantities of cystine in the urine, but seldom enough to result in stone formation.

Pathophysiology

The diminished renal tubular resorption of cystine increases its concentration in the urine. Cystine is poorly soluble in acid urine; when its concentration exceeds its solubility, precipitation in the urinary tract results, both as crystals and stones.

Renal tubular resorption of dibasic amino acids (lysine, ornithine, and arginine) is also impaired, although these amino acids have an alternative transport system separate from that shared with cystine. Since the dibasic amino acids are more soluble in urine than is cystine, their increased excretion does not result in precipitation. Absorption of cystine and the dibasic amino acids is decreased in the small intestine as well as in the renal tubule. Several patterns of impaired intestinal absorption of these amino acids have been described.

Clinical Features and Diagnosis

Radiopaque cystine stones form in the renal pelvis or bladder. Staghorn calculi are common. Symptoms usually appear between ages 10 and 30, and renal colic is the commonest presenting complaint. Urinary tract infection and renal failure due to obstruction may develop. In longtime survivors, end-stage renal disease is the rule.

Cystine may occur in the urine as yellow-brown hexagonal crystals. The presence of excessive cystine in the urine may be detected by the nitroprusside cyanide test. The diagnosis is confirmed by chromatography or electrophoresis.

Treatment

The concentration of cystine in the urine can be reduced by increasing urine volume. Fluid intake must be sufficient to provide a urine flow rate of 2 ml/min, especially at night when the pH of the urine drops. Alkalinization of the urine to pH > 7.5 with sodium bicarbonate 15 to 30 gm/day orally in divided doses, and acetazolamide 250 mg orally at bedtime, will increase the solubility of cystine significantly. D-Penicillamine 250 mg/day orally initially and gradually increased to 1 to 2 gm/day may be effective when high fluid intake and alkalinization do not reduce stone formation. It reduces cystine excretion by forming the more soluble disulfide, cysteine-penicillamine. *Toxicity of penicillamine limits its usefulness.* About half of all patients treated develop some toxic manifestation, including fever, rash, arthralgias, and, less commonly, nephrotic syndrome, pancytopenia, or an SLE-like reaction.

RENAL TUBULAR ACIDOSIS (RTA)

Impaired ability to secrete hydrogen ions in the distal nephron or to resorb bicarbonate ions proximally, leading to chronic metabolic acidosis which, in the distal form, may be accompanied by potassium depletion and by rickets or osteomalacia.

Distal RTA (Type I) usually is a sporadic disorder, but familial cases occur either in association with another genetic disease or rarely as an isolated autosomal dominant disease. Sporadic cases may develop as a **primary** disease, nearly always in women, or **secondary** to a predisposing cause such as an autoimmune disease with hypergammaglobulinemia (especially Sjögren's syndrome), amphotericin B or lithium therapy, renal transplantation, nephrocalcinosis, or renal medullary cystic disease.

Proximal RTA (Type II) accompanies several inherited diseases, including Fanconi's syndrome, hereditary fructose intolerance, Wilson's disease, and Lowe's syndrome. It also occurs in multiple myeloma, in chronic hypocalcemia with secondary hyperparathyroidism, after renal transplantation, and following treatment with certain drugs, including acetazolamide, sulfonamides, outdated tetracycline, and streptozocin.

Type IV RTA, in which the major defect is diminished renal ammonia production, occurs chiefly in association with selective hypoaldosteronism (hyporeninism).

Pathophysiology and Clinical Features

Tubular resorption and secretion is discussed in Ch. 143. In distal (classic, Type I) RTA the ability to secrete hydrogen ions against a concentration gradient in the distal tubule is impaired so that urine pH does not fall below about 6. In proximal (Type II) RTA, the capacity of the proximal tubule to resorb bicarbonate ion (HCO_3^-) is diminished so that at normal levels of plasma HCO_3^-, increased amounts of HCO_3^- reach the distal tubule and are excreted in the urine. At low levels of plasma HCO_3^- the proximal tubule resorbs enough of the filtered HCO_3^- to allow urinary acidification to occur.

With either Type I or Type II, chronic metabolic acidosis develops. In the distal form this results in 2 other major alterations in homeostasis: potassium wasting in the urine, and continued mobilization of bone calcium with hypercalciuria. Potassium depletion induced by chronic metabolic acidosis causes muscle weakness, hyporeflexia, and paralysis. The continued loss of bone calcium results in rickets and osteomalacia. In the presence of alkaline urine, it also results in calcium precipitation; stone formation, which may be seen on x-ray, may cause renal colic and nephrocalcinosis. Renal parenchymal damage and chronic renal failure may develop eventually. In hereditary types, nephrocalcinosis has been seen by age 6.

Diagnosis

Low plasma HCO_3^- and low blood pH with a normal level of undetermined anions are present. Distal RTA is confirmed by an **acid load test:** Ammonium chloride 100 mg/kg orally normally reduces urine pH to < 5.2 within 3 to 6 h. In distal tubular acidosis, urine pH remains > 6.

A **bicarbonate titration test** helps to identify proximal RTA. Sodium bicarbonate is slowly infused in order to raise plasma HCO_3^-. In proximal tubular acidosis HCO_3^- will appear in the urine before plasma HCO_3^- reaches the normal range.

Treatment

Bicarbonate administration relieves the symptoms and prevents or stabilizes renal failure and bone disease. In distal tubular acidosis, sodium bicarbonate 80 to 200 mg/kg/day (1 to 3 mEq/kg/day) orally in divided doses will eliminate the acidosis. In the proximal form, doses of 800 mg/kg/day or more may be necessary. **Shohl's solution** (140 gm citric acid and 90 gm sodium citrate dihydrate made up to 1 L with water), 50 to 100 ml/day in divided doses, can be substituted for sodium bicarbonate solution and may be better tolerated. Potassium supplements may be required in selected cases after alkalinization.

The acidosis accompanying the syndrome of hyporeninemia and hypoaldosteronism is usually mild. When necessary, it can be treated with sodium bicarbonate as described for distal RTA, above.

FANCONI'S SYNDROME

An acquired or inherited disorder, often associated with cystinosis, with characteristic abnormalities of renal proximal tubular function including glucosuria, phosphaturia, aminoaciduria, and bicarbonate wasting.

Occurrence and Genetics

As an inherited trait, Fanconi's syndrome usually accompanies another genetic disorder, particularly cystinosis. (See TABLE 82–3 in Ch. 82.) When associated with cystinosis, it is an autosomal recessive disease. Heterozygotes may show cystine accumulation in cells but lack other clinical and laboratory manifestations. Fanconi's syndrome may also accompany Wilson's disease, hereditary fructose intolerance, galactosemia, glycogen storage disease, Lowe's syndrome, and tyrosinemia.

Acquired Fanconi's syndrome may be caused by 6-mercaptopurine or outdated tetracycline, renal transplantation, multiple myeloma, amyloidosis, and intoxication with heavy metals or other chemical agents.

Pathophysiology and Clinical Features

A variety of defects of proximal tubular function occur, including impaired resorption of glucose, phosphate, amino acids, bicarbonate, uric acid, water, potassium, and sodium. The aminoaciduria is generalized and, unlike the case in cystinuria, increased cystine excretion is only a minor component. The basic abnormality underlying these diverse changes is unknown. The chief clinical features (proximal tubular acidosis, hypophosphatemic rickets, hypokalemia, polyuria, and polydipsia) usually appear in infancy in hereditary Fanconi's syndrome.

In the **nephropathic form associated with cystinosis,** failure to thrive and growth retardation are common. The retinas show patchy depigmentation. Interstitial nephritis develops, leading to progressive renal failure that may be fatal before adolescence.

Diagnosis and Treatment

Diagnosis is made by demonstrating the abnormalities of renal function, particularly glucosuria, phosphaturia, and aminoaciduria. In cystinosis, slit-lamp examination may show cystine crystals in the cornea.

There is no specific treatment. Acidosis may be improved by giving sodium bicarbonate or Shohl's solution, as in renal tubular acidosis. For treatment of hypophosphatemic rickets, see below. Potassium depletion may require replacement therapy. Renal transplantation has been successful in renal failure; however, when cystinosis is the underlying disease, progressive damage may continue in other organs and eventually end in death.

HYPOPHOSPHATEMIC RICKETS (Vitamin D-Resistant Rickets)

A familial or, rarely, acquired disorder characterized by impaired resorption of phosphate in the proximal renal tubules with consequent hypophosphatemia, defective intestinal absorption of calcium, and rickets or osteomalacia that is unresponsive to vitamin D.

Familial hypophosphatemic rickets is inherited as an X-linked dominant trait. Affected females have less severe bone disease than males and may show only hypophosphatemia. Sporadic acquired cases sometimes are associated with benign tumors.

Pathophysiology and Clinical Features

The 2 major physiologic abnormalities in hypophosphatemic rickets are decreased proximal tubular resorption of phosphate and decreased intestinal calcium absorption. The cause and effect relationship, if any, between these 2 abnormalities is controversial, as is their relationship to the abnormal vitamin D metabolism that is also present. Intestinal phosphate absorption is also impaired. Parathyroid hormone and vitamin D levels are normal.

The disease is manifested as a spectrum of abnormalities from hypophosphatemia alone to severe rickets or osteomalacia with bowing of the legs and other bone deformities, pseudofractures, bone pain, and short stature. Blood phosphate levels are depressed, calcium is normal, and alkaline phosphatase often is elevated. Bony outgrowth at muscle attachments may limit motion. The rickets of the spine or pelvis seen in vitamin D deficiency is rarely found. Craniostenosis and convulsions may be present in children. The age of onset is usually < 1 yr.

Hypophosphatemic rickets must be distinguished from **vitamin D-dependent rickets,** an autosomal recessive disorder with similar clinical features except that hypocalcemia is present, hypophosphatemia is mild or absent, tetany and convulsions are common, and rickets of spine and pelvis are frequent (see also Ch. 78).

Treatment

Treatment consists of oral phosphate 1 to 3 gm/day as neutral phosphate solutions, plus vitamin D or dihydrotachysterol. Treatment is begun with 10,000 to 25,000 u./day of vitamin D, and the dose is increased in 4 to 6 wk until alkaline phosphatase decreases or bone healing occurs. Treatment with vitamin D must be monitored to prevent hypercalcemia, which may cause renal damage or have other harmful effects. Vitamin D alone decreases alkaline phosphatase but does not influence the growth pattern, serum phosphate, or tubular resorption of phosphate. Phosphate alone improves intestinal calcium resorption as well as the hypophosphatemia, and initiates bone healing, but this last is not sustained unless vitamin D is also given. Recent evidence suggests that long-term calcitriol (0.25 to 1 μg/day) plus phosphate supplementation may result in better bone mineralization than occurs with vitamin D plus phosphate. In cases of adult onset, a few patients have improved dramatically after removal of a benign fibrosing hemangiosarcoma.

RENAL GLUCOSURIA (Renal Glycosuria)

Excretion of glucose in the urine in the presence of normal or low blood glucose levels.

Renal glucosuria may be associated with many renal tubular defects involving aminoaciduria and renal tubular acidosis. When it occurs as an isolated finding with otherwise normal renal function, it is usually inherited as an autosomal dominant trait; occasionally it is a recessive trait. The active transport system for glucose in the proximal tubules is discussed in Ch. 143. The maximum rate at which glucose can be resorbed (normally 320 mg/min) is termed the **transport maximum (T_m)** for glucose. In Type A renal glucosuria, the T_m for glucose is reduced and sugar escapes in the urine. In

Type B the T_m is normal, but the renal threshold is reduced so that glucose appears in the urine at a lower than normal plasma concentration. Combined forms of the disease occur. Intestinal glucose transport is normal except in the rare glucose-galactose malabsorption (see CARBOHYDRATE INTOLERANCE in Ch. 56).

Renal glucosuria is asymptomatic and without serious sequelae. A few patients eventually develop diabetes mellitus, which should be ruled out by establishing the diagnosis of glucosuria. **Diagnosis** is made by demonstrating glucose in the urine after an overnight fast in a patient having normal glucose tolerance. Glucosuria should be demonstrated by a specific test for glucose, such as the glucose oxidase test, to distinguish it from other abnormalities wherein reducing substances are found in the urine. No treatment is necessary.

NEPHROGENIC DIABETES INSIPIDUS (DI)

A disease in which renal function is normal except for an inability to concentrate the urine due to lack of response of the renal tubules to antidiuretic hormone.

Nephrogenic DI occurs as an X-linked, probably recessive, disease. Affected males are completely unresponsive to **antidiuretic hormone (ADH, vasopressin).** Heterozygous females show normal or slightly impaired responsiveness to ADH.

Concentration of the urine in normal individuals is the consequence of secretion of ADH by the posterior pituitary in response to changes in the osmolality of the plasma and increased water resorption in response to ADH by the distal convoluted tubule and collecting duct. These parts of the nephron are normally impermeable to water in the absence of ADH, resulting in high flow rates of dilute urine. ADH increases the permeability of the distal tubule and collecting duct to water, allowing it to be passively resorbed along the medullary concentration gradient created by the countercurrent mechanism.

In nephrogenic DI, the formation and secretion of ADH by the posterior pituitary are normal but the nephron is unresponsive to the hormone. The consequences are polydipsia, polyuria, and hypotonic urine, the same features as are seen in pituitary DI, from which the disease must be distinguished. Usually the disease appears soon after birth. Since the infant cannot communicate its thirst, severe water depletion may result, with hypernatremia, fever, vomiting, and convulsions. *Brain damage with permanent mental retardation may occur if the cause of the symptoms is not recognized.* Urine osmolality is usually 50 to 100 mOsm/L but may rise to 280 mOsm/L during a solute diuresis. Other evidence of abnormal tubular function is lacking, and the GFR is normal.

A **nephrogenic DI syndrome** may be seen in disorders preferentially affecting the medulla or distal nephrons, resulting in impaired ability to concentrate the urine and apparent insensitivity to ADH: medullary and polycystic disease; sickle cell nephropathy; release of obstructing periureteral fibrosis; medullary pyelonephritis; hypokalemic, hypercalcemic, and hypomagnesemic nephropathies; the nephrotic syndrome; and myeloma. Certain nephrotoxins, especially aminoglycosides and lithium, also are causes.

Treatment of nephrogenic DI consists of ensuring that the patient has an adequate free water intake. As long as the patient can increase his water intake in response to thirst, serious sequelae seldom occur, but polyuria and polydipsia may be nuisances. Thiazide diuretics may be helpful.

HARTNUP DISEASE

A rare disease due to abnormal absorption and excretion of tryptophan and other amino acids, characterized clinically by rash and CNS abnormalities.

Hartnup disease is inherited as an autosomal recessive trait. Consanguinity is common. Heterozygotes are normal. Small intestine absorption of tryptophan, phenylalanine, methionine, and other monoaminomonocarboxylic amino acids is abnormal. Accumulation of unabsorbed amino acids in the GI tract increases their metabolism by bacterial flora. Some tryptophan degradation products including indoles, kynurenine, and serotonin are absorbed by the bowel and appear in the urine. Renal amino acid resorption is also defective, causing a generalized aminoaciduria involving all neutral amino acids except proline and hydroxyproline. Conversion of tryptophan to niacinamide is also defective.

Clinical signs are due to niacinamide deficiency and resemble those of pellagra, particularly the rash on parts of the body exposed to the sun. Neurologic manifestations include cerebellar ataxia and psychologic abnormalities. Mental retardation, short stature, headache, and collapsing or fainting are common. Symptoms may be precipitated by sunlight, fever, drugs, or other stresses. Poor nutritional intake nearly always precedes appearance of symptoms. The eventual prognosis is good and the frequency of attacks usually diminishes with age.

Diagnosis is made by demonstrating the characteristic amino acid excretion pattern in the urine. Presence of indoles and other tryptophan degradation products in the urine provides supplementary evidence of the disease. **Treatment:** Attacks can be prevented by maintaining good nutrition and supplementing the diet with niacinamide or niacin.

FAMILIAL IMINOGLYCINURIA

An autosomal recessive benign defect in the renal tubular resorption of imino acids and glycine. Homozygotes excrete abnormal amounts of imino acids (proline and hydroxyproline) and glycine; heterozygotes have glycinuria only. Plasma levels of amino acids are normal. Intestinal absorption of proline may be impaired. Iminoaciduria is normal in the newborn.

BARTTER'S SYNDROME

A combination of fluid, electrolyte, and hormonal abnormalities characterized by renal potassium and sodium wasting, hypokalemia, hyperaldosteronism, hyperreninemia, and normal BP. The syndrome usually appears in childhood, either as a sporadic or a familial disorder.

Etiology, Pathophysiology, and Clinical Features

Bartter's syndrome results from a complex disturbance of renal electrolyte handling. The underlying renal tubular disorder (or disorders) has not been defined. The proximal tubule, the ascending thick limb of the loop of Henle, and the distal nephron have all been suggested as possible sites of transport defects which might be etiologic. Both potassium and sodium wasting occur, each contributing to the stimulation of renin release, which is accompanied by hyperplasia of cells of the juxtaglomerular apparatus. Elevated levels of aldosterone are present. Potassium depletion is not eliminated by correction of the hyperaldosteronism. Sodium wasting results in a chronically low plasma volume, which is reflected by a normal BP despite high levels of renin and angiotensin, and by an impaired pressor response to angiotensin infusion. Metabolic alkalosis often is present.

Excretion of prostaglandins and kallikrein in the urine is increased. Inhibition of prostaglandin synthesis results in correction of most of the abnormalities, but potasisum depletion is only partially eliminated.

Affected children have poor growth rates and appear malnourished. Muscle weakness, polydipsia, polyuria, and mental retardation may be present.

Diagnosis and Treatment

Bartter's syndrome is distinguished from other diseases associated with hyperaldosteronism by the absence of hypertension (as in primary hyperaldosteronism) and edema (as in secondary aldosteronism). When the features of the disease are first seen in adults, vomiting or surreptitious diuretic abuse must be explicitly eliminated as causes.

Potassium supplementation plus spironolactone, triamterene, propranolol, or indomethacin will correct most features, but no drug completely eliminates potassium wasting. Indomethacin 1 to 2 mg/kg/day usually maintains plasma potassium level close to the lower limit of normal.

---

154. INHERITED AND CONGENITAL DISORDERS

CYSTIC DISORDERS

The cystic disorders of the kidney represent types of dysplastic malformations. There may be single or multiple cysts varying in size from less than 1 cm to over 10 cm in diameter. Some disorders are congenital, some are acquired, and sometimes a distinction cannot be made. The major groups are (1) polycystic disease (adult and infantile types), (2) cystic dysplasias (multicystic and focal types), (3) cortical cysts (single and multiple types), (4) medullary cystic disorders (medullary cystic disease complex, medullary sponge kidney), and (5) miscellaneous (inflammatory, neoplastic, extraparenchymal types).

POLYCYSTIC RENAL DISEASES

Inherited kidney disorders characterized by many bilateral cysts which cause enlargement of the total renal size, while reducing, by compression, the functioning renal tissue. The disease usually is classified by the pattern of inheritance. Two types are recognized: the **adult form,** an autosomal dominant disorder that progresses to renal insufficiency in middle age; an **infantile form,** a rare autosomal recessive disease that produces renal failure in childhood. The adult type usually develops clinical symptoms after the 2nd decade, although it has been described in a fetus from an affected patient and in several neonates. The incidence of the adult type is lower than 1:1000 persons by age 80 (by which time an individual with the dominant gene has a 100% chance of affliction). About 5% of patients with end-stage renal disease have this disorder. Mechanisms for the development of polycystic disease and progressive enlargement of the cysts are not known. The cysts are dilated nephrons and collecting ducts. The cysts of glomerular origin may end blindly in the cortex, while those of tubular origin communicate proximally with the glomerulus and distally with the renal pelvis.

Clinical Features

The infantile form of polycystic disease is much rarer than the adult form and usually leads to a very early death. Since adult polycystic disease is slowly progressive over many years, it is often asymptomatic initially but may be discovered by ultrasonography in childhood. Clinical onset is in early or middle adult life, although occasionally the disease may not be discovered until later and may be found only at autopsy. Symptoms are usually related to effects of the cysts, such as lumbar discomfort or pain, hematuria, infection, and colic, or may be related to a loss of renal function with uremic symptoms. Chronic infection frequently is superimposed and contributes to the progressive loss of renal function. In about ⅓ of cases, cysts are present in the liver but are of no functional significance. There is also a high associated incidence of intracranial aneurysms. Hypertension is common; about 50% of the patients have this finding at the time of diagnosis.

Though over 50% of patients become uremic within 10 yr of onset of symptoms, the course is quite variable and many will go for more than 20 yr before end-stage renal failure occurs. In the absence of dialysis or transplantation, death is usually due to uremia or the complications of hypertensive cardiovascular disease, and occurs at an average age of 50. About 10% of patients die of intracranial hemorrhage from rupture of aneurysms.

Diagnosis

In advanced cases, when the kidneys are grossly enlarged and palpable, the diagnosis is obvious. The urine shows mild proteinuria and varying degrees of hematuria, but RBC casts are infrequent. Pyuria is common even in the absence of bacterial infection. Episodically, the urine is grossly bloody, apparently because of hemorrhage from a ruptured cyst or a dislodged calculus. The excretory urogram is characteristic, with large kidneys showing irregular outlines because of the many cysts. The calyces, infundibula, and pelvis are compressed and elongated by cysts, giving what is referred to as a "spidery" appearance. Renal and hepatic sonograms and radionuclide scans show a typical "moth-eaten" appearance due to the cysts that displace functional tissue. Polycystic kidney disease, with its progressive azotemia, is distinguished from solitary or multiple cysts of the kidney which do not distort a sufficient portion of the renal parenchyma to cause uremia. The distinction is made on clinical grounds and by ultrasound, excretory urography, or radionuclide scanning.

Treatment

Management of urinary infections and secondary hypertension may prolong life considerably. Genetic counseling is recommended. When uremia supervenes, its management is the same as in other renal diseases (see Ch. 145, above). With dialysis, patients with polycystic kidney disease have more normal Hcts than any other group of patients. Transplantation is feasible, but the use of parental and sibling donors may be impractical in view of the familial characteristics of the disease.

MEDULLARY CYSTIC DISEASE (Familial Juvenile Nephronophthisis)

A diffuse nephropathy, either genetic or congenital in origin, usually seen in children or young adults and characterized by the insidious onset of uremia.

The commonly described variants and their incidence are juvenile nephronophthisis, 50%; adult-onset medullary cystic disease, 18%; and renal-retinal dysplasia, 17%. Isolated cases (with no family history) comprise 15%. A family history is common, and a recessive pattern of transmission is suggested. In a few families the renal disease has been accompanied by pigmentary retinal degradation. The adult-onset variety is less common and shows a dominant pattern of transmission.

Clinical Features and Diagnosis

Symptoms usually begin in the first 2 decades of life, although the disease has been observed as late as the 60s. Polyuria due to a vasopressin-resistant renal concentrating defect is often the earliest symptom. Urinary sodium wastage is frequently present and commonly is severe enough to require a sodium intake of several hundred mEq/day to prevent extracellular volume depletion. Acidosis with or without relative hyperchloremia is often seen. Unexplained uremia is a good early clue in some cases. Retarded growth and evidence of bone disease are common in children. In many patients these problems develop slowly over a period of years and are so well compensated that they are not recognized as abnormal until significant uremic symptoms appear.

Laboratory findings are similar to those in patients with chronic renal failure. Proteinuria is minimal or absent and the urinary sediment is not remarkable. Excretory urography demonstrates only small kidneys, but ultrasound and arteriography may reveal medullary cysts.

Course and Treatment

Progression of the disease is variable and depends on the degree of renal dysfunction when the patient is first seen. As a rule, the disease progresses slowly but inexorably. When uremia supervenes, its management is the same as in other renal diseases (see Ch. 145, above). These patients may do very well with transplantation; menses may be restored and growth resumed.

MEDULLARY SPONGE KIDNEY

Tubular ectasia or dysplasia resulting in congenital cystic dilation of the collecting tubules. This disorder is unrelated to medullary cystic disease. Sponge kidney leads to urinary stasis and nephrocalcinosis.

More common in males, the condition is usually asymptomatic unless the complications of calculus colic, hematuria, or infections supervene. **Diagnosis** is by urography, which shows a pyramidal pattern of calcium deposition and urographic evidence of pyramidal cavities filled with contrast material, giving the appearance of a "bouquet of flowers." Sonography usually is not helpful because the cysts are small and are located deep in the medulla. The lesion may be confused with TB, medullary necrosis, and nephrocalcinosis of other etiologies. If uncomplicated, the condition has an excellent prognosis. **Treatment** is given only for complications. Usually, noncalcinotic forms are asymptomatic and need no therapy. Although nephrocalcinosis may be progressive, no specific medical treatment is effective. However, thiazides (e.g., trichlormethiazide 2 to 4 mg orally daily), high fluid intake, and a low calcium diet may inhibit stone formation and reduce obstructive complications. Infections are treated in the usual manner. Surgery is indicated only when obstruction occurs.

HEREDITARY CHRONIC NEPHROPATHIES

Many of the genetically transmitted renal disorders produce functional or structural abnormalities, or both. Those involving mainly tubular transport defects (see Ch. 153) or metabolic defects with renal involvement as in Fabry's disease (see LIPIDOSES in Ch. 82) are discussed elsewhere. The hereditary, noncystic nephropathies discussed in this section are hereditary nephritis and the nail-patella syndrome.

HEREDITARY NEPHRITIS (Alport's Syndrome)

A familial disorder characterized by hematuria, renal functional impairment, nerve deafness, and, on occasion, ocular abnormalities.

Most evidence supports an autosomal dominant inheritance; however, males are more commonly and severely afflicted but father fewer affected sons than daughters. Thus, transmission is most often through females. The disorder is structurally characterized by abnormal basal lamina production involving both glomeruli and tubules. Histologic changes are initially seen in the glomeruli, with mesangial cell proliferation and multilamination of the basal lamina. Later, similar basal lamina abnormalities are found in the tubules along with interstitial fibrosis and tubular atrophy.

Symptoms and Signs

The onset of the disease may be similar to that of acute glomerulonephritis, but many patients are asymptomatic and the disease is detected by finding hematuria. The urine may contain small amounts of protein, WBCs, and casts of various types. The nephrotic syndrome occurs rarely. Afflicted females are usually asymptomatic and have little functional impairment, while most males with the disease develop evidence of renal insufficiency between ages 20 and 30. Nerve deafness is frequently present, usually perceived in the higher frequencies and more commonly found among affected males than females. Some individuals with a family history may have nerve deafness alone without renal disease; such persons are capable of transmitting the renal disease to a subsequent generation. Eye lesions occur less frequently than acoustic ones; they include cataracts, anterior lenticonus, spherophakia, and nystagmus.

Treatment

Treatment is only indicated when uremia occurs; its management is the same as in other renal diseases. Successful transplants have been done using kidneys from cadavers or living, related adult females with hematuria but no sign of progression. Genetic counseling is indicated.

NAIL-PATELLA SYNDROME (Osteo-onychodysplasia)

A familial disorder of mesenchymal tissue characterized by abnormalities of bone, joints, fingernails, and kidneys.

Inheritance occurs as an autosomal dominant trait linked to the ABO blood group locus. The most common skeletal dysplasia is unilateral or bilateral hypoplasia or absence of the patella, subluxation of the radial heads at the elbows, and bilateral accessory iliac horns. The fingernails are either absent or hypoplastic with pitting and ridges. Ocular abnormalities have occurred but deafness is not found. The renal lesion is characterized by abnormal lamina production. Histologic changes initially show endothelial and visceral epithelial proliferation and irregular areas of rarefaction in the glomerular basal lamina. Later, thickening of the glomerular basement membrane and mesangial sclerosis occur.

Symptoms and Signs

Renal dysfunction occurs in about ½ of patients with this disorder and is manifest by proteinuria and, rarely, hematuria. Proteinuria is usually minimal but occasionally may reach nephrotic syndrome ranges. The disease is diagnosed by the typical clinical and radiographic findings and can be further confirmed by renal biopsy. About ⅓ of patients with renal involvement will slowly progress to renal failure.

Treatment

Genetic counseling is indicated. Management of progressive renal failure is the same as in other renal diseases. Successful transplants have been done without evidence of recurrence of the disease in the renal graft.

CONGENITAL ANOMALIES

(See Vol. II, Ch. 21)

---

155. OBSTRUCTIVE UROPATHIES

Urine flow may be obstructed at any point from the renal infundibula to the external urethral meatus. The consequences include increased intraluminal pressure, urinary stasis, infection, stone formation, and renal failure. Presenting symptoms depend on the obstruction level and acuteness of onset. Infection may cause irritative symptoms, i.e., difficult urination or dysuria, hematuria, and localized or generalized pain.

HYDRONEPHROSIS

Dilatation of the renal pelvis and, usually, of the infundibula and calyces beyond the normal capacity of 3 to 10 ml.

Etiology

Primary hydronephrosis without ureteral dilatation results from obstruction at the ureteropelvic junction: intrinsic stricture, high insertion of the ureter into the renal pelvis, a defect in continuity of smooth muscle at the ureteropelvic junction, kinking of the junction from nephroptosis, or extrinsic compression by fibrous bands or an aberrant artery or vein or from a renal pelvis stone or tumor. **Secondary hydronephrosis** results from obstruction distal to the ureteropelvic junction or occurs as a result of vesicoureteral reflux: ureteral stones or tumors, extrinsic ureteral compression by primary or metastatic tumor, myoneurogenic disease of the ureter or bladder, fibrosis secondary to surgery or radiation, retroperitoneal fibrosis, ureterocele, congenital or acquired vesicoureteral reflux, malignancies of the bladder or other pelvic viscera, bladder outlet obstruction due to prostatic enlargement or carcinoma, or urethral obstruction such as stricture, congenital valves, or meatal stenosis. The hydronephrosis occasionally seen in pregnancy is due to mechanical factors and the effects of progestational hormones. It is usually transient, though some dilatation may persist following delivery. Occasionally, a severe urinary tract infection may induce temporary atony of the urinary tract with hydronephrosis.

Pathology

Chronic dilatation of the renal pelvis causes muscular atony, fibrosis, and loss of peristaltic activity. Since urine is normally excreted at extremely low pressure (estimated at < 10 cm of water pressure), prolonged and severe hydronephrosis will ultimately result in pressure atrophy of the renal parenchyma, which affects the collecting tubules initially, and then the proximal tubules and glomeruli, with gradual loss of renal function.

Symptoms and Signs

Acute hydronephrosis is usually manifested by colicky pain, while chronically progressive hydronephrosis may be asymptomatic or attended by intercurrent attacks of dull, aching flank discomfort. A flank mass may be palpable, particularly in massive hydronephrosis of infancy and childhood. Intermittent hydronephrosis due to nephroptosis or acute overdistention of the renal pelvis **(Dietl's crisis)** generally produces excruciating pain. Hematuria may be seen in 10% of patients with hydronephrosis. Urinary infection with pyuria, fever, and localized discomfort is a fairly common finding. Calculi may result from stasis, and azotemia may occur when both kidneys are involved. Unexplained, vague GI symptoms may be due to hydronephrosis, and are often seen in children with congenital ureteropelvic obstruction.

Diagnosis

Urologic investigation (see also discussions of urinary system evaluation procedures in Ch. 144) begins with an excretory urogram (IVP) performed by standard technic or by infusion. Cystourethrograms may show lower tract obstruction, neurogenic disorders, or vesicoureteral reflux. Cystoscopy and retrograde pyelography may confirm and delineate the anatomic deformity. Following instillation of contrast material and removal of the ureteral catheter, the normal renal pelvis will empty contrast material in 5 to 10 min. Delayed emptying by a hydronephrotic kidney confirms a functional or anatomic abnormality, unless dehydration (which prolongs the emptying time) is a factor. Assessment of the degree of hydronephrosis as well as the comparative delay in emptying time, by either IVP or the retrograde technic, may be enhanced by establishing diuresis with a suitable diuretic before the contrast material is injected. A kidney that is nonfunctioning by delayed films on pyelography may be investigated by radioisotope scan to identify functional renal parenchyma. Hydronephrosis is usually well documented by noninvasive ultrasound studies, and this method is particularly useful in children.

Treatment

Intensive treatment of urinary infections and management of renal failure are imperative. Surgery for primary hydronephrosis should be undertaken promptly if renal function is compromised, infection persists, or pain is significant. Temporary nephrostomy drainage may be needed in severe obstruction, infection, or stones. The percutaneous technic may be used, if indicated. Secondary hydronephrosis may be corrected by attention to the cause, e.g., relief of lower tract obstructive uropathies. Catheter drainage or urinary diversion by a variety of technics is often helpful.

Prognosis

Surgical correction of primary hydronephrosis, either unilateral or bilateral, may be successful in most cases when infection can be controlled, renal function has been preserved, and calculous disease has not supervened. The prognosis is more guarded in secondary hydronephrosis. Surgery must eliminate stasis or reflux, infection must be treated, and normal intraluminal pressure gradients must be preserved to ensure stabilization of renal function.

URETERAL OBSTRUCTION

Ureteral strictures may be congenital or due to trauma, infection, surgery, or external radiation. Ureteral segments lacking myoneural continuity cause proximal ureterectasis and hydronephrosis. Primary resection and reanastomosis of the ureter may afford adequate relief of obstruction and hydronephrosis due to strictures or atonic segments. **Retroperitoneal fibrosis** may be idiopathic or secondary to a variety of drugs, primarily methysergide. Management involves dissection and mobilization of the ureters with intraperitoneal transplantation to avoid recurrence of obstruction. **Ureteral obstruction at the ureterovesical junction** may result from the trauma of stone passage or extraction, hypertrophy of the bladder wall in neurogenic diseases, defects in continuity of ureteral muscle, bladder outlet obstruction, or occasional congenital strictures. Vesicoureteral reimplantation is generally the surgical procedure of choice. Ureteral obstruction by calculi is very common and may result in chronic hydronephrosis.

BENIGN PROSTATIC HYPERPLASIA

(BPH; Benign Prostatic Hypertrophy)

Benign adenomatous hyperplasia of the paraurethral prostate gland commonly seen in men over age 50, causing variable degrees of bladder outlet obstruction. The etiology is unknown but may involve alterations in hormonal balance associated with aging.

Pathology

Multiple fibroadenomatous nodules occur in the paraurethral region of the prostate gland, probably originating within the paraurethral glands themselves rather than in the true fibromuscular prostate **(surgical capsule),** which is displaced laterally by progressive growth of the hyperplastic nodules. The hyperplastic process may involve the lateral walls of the prostate **(lateral lobe hyperplasia)** or may include tissue at the inferior margin of the vesical neck **(middle lobe hyperplasia).** Histologically, the tissue is glandular with varying amounts of fibrous stroma interposed. Secondary infection may induce chronic prostatitis. As the lumen of the prostatic urethra is compromised, there is progressive obstruction to the outflow of urine with hypertrophy of the bladder detrusor, trabeculation, cellule formation, and diverticula. Incomplete bladder emptying causes stasis and infection with secondary inflammatory changes in the bladder and the upper urinary tract. Prolonged obstruction, even though incomplete, may produce hydronephrosis and compromise renal function. Urinary stasis may predispose to calculus formation.

Symptoms and Signs

Symptoms of bladder outlet obstruction may include progressive urinary frequency, urgency, and nocturia as a result of incomplete emptying and rapid refilling of the bladder. Hesitancy and intermittency with decreased size and force of the urinary stream occur. Sensations of incomplete emptying, terminal dribbling, almost continuous overflow incontinence, or complete urinary retention may ensue. Rectal examination may be misleading; a prostate that is small by rectal examination may be sufficiently enlarged to cause urethral obstruction. Congestion of superficial veins of the prostatic urethra and trigone may cause hematuria secondary to rupture while the patient is straining to void. Burning on urination and chills and fever indicate urinary infection. Episodes of acute complete urinary retention may follow prolonged attempts to retain urine, immobilization, exposure to cold, anesthetic agents, anticholinergic and sympathomimetic drugs, or the ingestion of alcohol. The distended urinary bladder may be palpable or percussible on physical examination. Prolonged urinary retention, partial or complete, may result in progressive renal failure and azotemia.

Diagnosis

BPH with bladder outlet obstruction is suspected on the basis of the symptoms and signs. Rectal examination usually discloses an enlarged gland with a rubbery consistency and, frequently, loss of the median furrow. An indurated and tender prostate suggests prostatitis, while a stony, hard nodular prostate usually indicates carcinoma or, occasionally, prostatic calculi. An excretory urogram may disclose upward displacement of the terminal portions of the ureters **(fishhooking)** and a defect at the base of the bladder compatible with prostatic enlargement. The postvoiding cystogram provides information regarding residual urine. Catheterization after voiding provides a measurement of residual urine and permits preliminary drainage to stabilize renal function and afford adequate control of urinary infection. Cystoscopy permits estimation of the size of the gland and the appropriate surgical approach, plus an opportunity to differentiate between contracture of the vesical neck, chronic prostatitis, and other obstructive phenomena. Instrumentation should be avoided until there is a commitment to definitive therapy, since manipulation may induce increased obstruction, trauma, and infection.

Treatment

When urinary infection or azotemia accompanies bladder outlet obstruction, initial therapy should be medical, directed toward stabilizing renal function, discontinuing anticholinergic and sympathomimetic drugs, and eradicating infection. Catheter drainage, either urethral or suprapubic, may be desirable in advanced bladder outlet obstruction. Definitive therapy is surgical. Transurethral resection of the prostate (TURP) is the preferred operative procedure and has the advantage of patient acceptance, since no incision is required and the procedure is associated with low morbidity and mortality. Larger benign prostates may be managed by open surgery using the suprapubic or retropubic approach that permits enucleation of the adenomatous tissue from within the surgical capsule. All surgical methods require postoperative catheter drainage for a few days. The prognosis is excellent and the patient usually maintains preoperative sexual potency.

URETHRAL OBSTRUCTION

Obstruction in the male may result from benign prostatic hyperplasia, prostatic carcinoma, or chronic prostatitis with contracture of the vesical neck or urethral valves. In either sex, congenital and acquired urethral strictures and meatal stenosis may be present, while urethral stenosis (Lyon's ring) may occur in females. Differentiation of the causes requires urologic investigation, which may include cystourethrography and cystourethroscopy. **Treatment** is usually surgical.

156. MYONEUROGENIC DISORDERS

The urinary tract is subject to congenital and acquired disorders of smooth muscle and innervation that result in inadequate urinary control, urinary stasis, infection, calculi, and renal damage. These complications of the underlying myoneurogenic disorders can be life-threatening and require careful evaluation and meticulous attention to management.

NEUROGENIC BLADDER

Vesical dysfunction resulting from congenital abnormality, injury, or disease process of the brain, spinal cord, or local nerve supply to the urinary bladder and its outlet.

Classification

Because of the complexity and variability of neurogenic bladder, clinical classification is unsatisfactory. However, the distinction between the **hypotonic** (flaccid) and the **spastic** (contracted) neurogenic bladder is important in treatment. Congenital spinal cord defects generally result in a hypotonic neurogenic bladder, while acquired disease processes exhibit slowly progressive signs of either hypotonia or hypertonia. Neurogenic bladder following acute spinal cord injury presents as a flaccid hypotonic bladder persisting for days, weeks, or months (shock phase) before permanent spasticity or flaccidity is established.

Etiology

Normal urinary control and voiding are the result of complex interactions of smooth muscle, voluntary muscle, cerebral inhibition, and the autonomic nervous system. Congenital neurogenic bladder may result from myelomeningocele, filum terminale syndrome, or other lesions of the spinal cord, including the cauda equina. The most common acquired cause of severe neurogenic bladder dysfunction is spinal cord injury resulting in paraplegia or quadriplegia, the result of transverse myelitis or transection of the cord. Disease processes that result in neurogenic bladder—either hypotonic or hypertonic—include syphilis, diabetes mellitus, brain or spinal cord tumors, ruptured intervertebral disk, and the demyelinating or degenerative diseases such as multiple sclerosis and amyotrophic lateral sclerosis.

Symptoms and Signs

Neurogenic bladder may cause partial or complete urinary retention, incontinence, or frequent urination. In the chronic phase, with inadequate emptying, urinary infection is common. Urinary calculi result from immobilization, with increased urinary calcium excretion, urinary stasis with crystallization, and superimposed urinary infection. In acute spinal cord injuries, the "**shock bladder**" is atonic and distended and may exhibit continuous overflow dribbling. With lower spinal cord (sacral and lumbar) lesions, the bladder becomes flaccid within a few weeks. Upper cord lesions (thoracic and cervical) produce an automatic or spastic reflex bladder that may empty spontaneously or as the result of somatic stimuli; the effectiveness of emptying depends on urethral resistance. Contracture of the vesical neck is common, particularly in spastic neurogenic bladder, and vesicoureteral reflux with renal damage may follow any type of congenital or acquired neurogenic bladder. Associated sphincter dyssynergia may also be present.

Diagnostic Evaluation

Serial pyelography, cystography, and urethrography demonstrate urinary calculi and help to assess the anatomic patterns and progressions seen in neurogenic bladder. Cystourethroscopic evaluation determines the degree of bladder outlet obstruction. Serial cystometrograms at 2-wk intervals during the recovery phase of flaccid paralysis provide an index of detrusor functional capacity and hence an indication of rehabilitation prospects. Also helpful are urodynamic assessment of voiding flow rates, sphincter electromyograms, and urethral pressure profile studies.

Treatment

In flaccid paralysis of the bladder following acute spinal cord injury, continuous catheter drainage or periodic intermittent catheterization (see BLADDER CARE in Ch. 228) should be established immediately to prevent overdistention with consequent infection and damage to the detrusor muscle.

Ultimately, a decision must be reached regarding long-term management. Patients who establish an automatic or reflex bladder may be managed by condom catheter drainage. Persistent residual urine and contracture of the vesical neck may require transurethral resection in the male or female on one or more occasions, or incision of the external sphincter (sphincterotomy) in the male, to minimize outlet resistance and to maximize emptying. Electrical stimulation of the bladder, the sacral nerves, or the spinal cord may help but remains experimental.

Continuous urethral catheter drainage may be required in some instances and is tolerated better in the female. In the male, the continuing presence of the catheter predisposes to urethritis, periurethritis, abscess formation, and urethral fistula. Intermittent catheterization, preferably done by the patient, is used when feasible. Permanent urinary diversion is occasionally appropriate in some patients with congenital or acquired neurogenic bladder dysfunction, especially those in whom flaccidity persists and reflux occurs (increasing the risk of upper tract damage), or when spasticity or quadriplegia prevents the use of satisfactory continuous or intermittent drainage. Permanent upper tract diversion is best accomplished by ileal or colon conduit. Ureterosigmoidostomy is not favored, because most patients with neurogenic bladder also lose rectal sphincter control. Permanent suprapubic cystostomy affords adequate control in some patients, and cutaneous vesicostomy with an external appliance and no indwelling catheter may be a convenient method of urinary control in patients with no upper tract damage. Cutaneous intubated ureterostomies and nephrostomies are not advisable, since the inlying catheters increase the chances for stone formation and infection.

Continued monitoring of renal function, control of urinary infection, high fluid intake, early ambulation, frequent change of position, and dietary calcium restriction to inhibit stone formation are essential, with or without attendant urinary diversion or catheter drainage. Though total recovery in any form of neurogenic bladder is uncommon, rehabilitation may be excellent with vigorous and appropriate therapeutic measures. Artificial sphincter devices may be surgically inserted to control urinary continence in selected patients.

MEGACYSTIS SYNDROME

The syndrome of megacystis ("large bladder") is poorly understood. It is often seen in girls with large, thin-walled, smooth bladders without evidence of outlet obstruction. The presenting symptoms are related to urinary tract infections. Vesicoureteral reflux is common. IVP with the bladder empty may disclose normal-appearing upper tracts, while cystourethrograms may exhibit reflux with massive dilation of the upper tracts. Rehabilitation by ureteral reimplantation and reduction cystoplasty may be effective, although some patients benefit from intermittent catheterization or require urinary diversion, generally by the ileal or colon conduit method.

URETERAL DYSFUNCTION

Abnormalities of ureteral smooth muscle or ureteral nerve supply may cause ureteral dilation, segmental or total, with demonstrable obstruction. **Megaloureter** is the term applied to severe ureteral dilation, unilateral or bilateral, in which obstruction and reflux are not evident. Ureteral dilation and relative atony may develop above a segmental defect in peristaltic transmission due to failure of smooth muscle continuity or of nerve impulse propagation (adynamic segment). **Treatment** is surgical; prognosis depends on the neuromuscular integrity of the proximal ureter.

ENURESIS

Involuntary and consistent episodic wetting during sleep by a child over age 5 or 6 is abnormal: most children achieve urinary control by age 3, 88% by age 4½, and 93% by age 7½. Enuresis is more common in boys than in girls and is often familial. It may be associated with passive-aggressiveness, dependency, sleepwalking, antisocial behavior, sibling rivalry, and speech disorders (see also BEHAVIOR PROBLEMS in Vol. II, Ch. 24).

Etiology

Persistent enuresis may be due to underlying organic causes, or may be functional or psychogenic. It may be associated with deep sleep—enuretic children sleep soundly and are unusually unresponsive to stimuli. EEG studies have shown that functional enuresis occurs during slow-wave (non–rapid-eye-movement [NREM]) sleep and not during dream (rapid-eye-movement [REM]) sleep.

The commonest anatomic causes are phimosis, meatal stricture and meatitis, urethral stricture, urethral valves, and contracture of the vesical neck. In obstructive uropathies, the bladder detrusor responds by hypertrophy, trabeculation, and increased irritability, predisposing to spontaneous and uninhibited contraction during sleep. Nonobstructive uropathies such as urethritis, trigonitis and cystitis, juvenile diabetes, pinworms, epilepsy, and spina bifida may also cause enuresis. Some children have an idiopathic diminished bladder capacity.

Diagnosis

Urologic evaluation is indicated in enuretic children over age 6, particularly when there are no apparent emotional, familial, or social problems that would predispose to episodic wetting. Enuresis must be distinguished from partial or total incontinence due to neurogenic bladder, vesical fistula, epispadias or other urethral abnormality, or ureteral ectopia with continuous urinary leakage. Definitive studies include IVP and voiding cystourethrography. Instrumentation should be reserved for patients with abnormalities demonstrated by radiologic studies. Psychiatric evaluation may be helpful when psychosocial causes are suspected.

Treatment and Prognosis

Nonsurgical management is discussed in BEHAVIORAL PROBLEMS in Vol. II, Ch. 24. Surgical correction of obstructive uropathies usually results in complete alleviation of bed-wetting within a few weeks or months. Associated urinary infections should be treated simultaneously.

---

157.   URINARY INCONTINENCE

The involuntary loss of urine during the day or night. **Enuresis** or bed-wetting is *the involuntary loss of urine during periods of sleep* (see Ch. 156, above, and BEHAVIORAL PROBLEMS in Vol. II, Ch. 24).

Types

Urge incontinence may occur alone or in conjunction with varying degrees of stress incontinence, and is characterized principally by involuntary loss of urine preceded by an urgent desire to void. In the absence of urinary tract infection, the most common causes of this type of incontinence are idiopathic; uninhibited neurogenic bladder dysfunction; spina bifida occulta; multiple sclerosis; bladder calculi, neoplasms, or TB; and interstitial cystitis. Therapy is directed toward correction of the underlying cause. Cases of the adult idiopathic variety are best treated with anticholinergic drugs, such as propantheline 15 mg or oxybutynin 5 mg orally q.i.d. The dosage should be adjusted to the individual patient's needs.

Stress incontinence (partial incompetence of the urinary sphincter) is the involuntary loss of urine on coughing, straining, sneezing, lifting, or any maneuver that suddenly increases intra-abdominal pressure. This form of urinary incontinence is seen occasionally in men following prostatectomy or trauma to the membranous urethra or bladder neck. It is the most common cause of involuntary loss of urine seen in women. It may be caused by shortening of the urethra and loss of the normal posterior urethrovesical angle resulting from pelvic relaxation (cystocele) that characteristically occurs with aging or multiparity. Diagnosis is established by history, pelvic examination, and the demonstration of loss of urine with coughing, which may be stopped by finger elevation of the paraurethral vaginal tissues at the bladder neck (the Marshall-Marchetti test). Mild cases may respond to a series of exercises of the pubococcygeus muscles (Kegel's exercises—see in Vol. II, Ch. 9) or to sympathomimetic drug therapy, which increases proximal urethral resistance. More severe cases require surgical correction by anterior vesicourethropexy or vaginal repair.

Urinary retention with overflow incontinence (paradoxical incontinence) occurs when the bladder becomes acutely or chronically overdistended and the intravesical pressure increases, eventually overcoming urinary sphincter resistance. Urine then dribbles from the urethra, and the patient may be unable to initiate or maintain a good urinary stream. Examination of the abdomen reveals the distended bladder. The bladder's inability to empty may result from obstruction to urine outflow or from impaired detrusor contraction. In children, the most common causes of obstructive uropathy of the lower urinary tract include urethral meatal stenosis, urethral strictures, urethral valves, and, rarely, bladder neck contracture. In adults the most common causes of bladder outlet obstruction include vesical neck contracture, benign prostatic hyperplasia, carcinoma of the prostate, and urethral stricture. Myelomeningocele, spina bifida occulta, tumors, and injury to the sacral spinal cord may be associated with a bladder that lacks motor impulses, impairing voiding contraction.

Ectopic ureter in female patients characteristically presents a history of lifelong, constant leakage of urine day and night despite voiding normal amounts of urine at regular intervals throughout the day. The ectopic ureteral orifice may be located near the bladder neck, in the urethra, or within the vagina. Diagnosis is facilitated by careful inspection of the vagina and vaginal vestibule, cystoscopy, excretory urography, and voiding cystourethrography. Surgical correction is necessary for cure.

In the male, the ectopic ureter drains proximal to the external sphincter and does not produce urinary incontinence.

Total incompetence of the urinary sphincter is characterized by a constant involuntary dripping of urine from the urethra day and night without bladder distention as determined by physical examination of the abdomen or measurement of residual urine. In children, congenital failure of the urethra to close properly (e.g., epispadias) results in this form of incontinence. In women, the most common cause is trauma to the vesical neck and urethra. In men, the most common cause is surgical trauma to the vesical neck and membranous urethra. Postprostatectomy incontinence, particularly following radical prostatectomy for cancer, is a result of damage to the urinary sphincter mechanism. Various surgical procedures have been devised to treat this form of urinary incontinence, including the application of artificial sphincters.

Various forms of **neurogenic bladder dysfunction** (see Ch. 156, above) may be the underlying cause of urinary incontinence. Therapy varies with the specific type of dysfunction present, as determined by history, physical examination, and urodynamic studies.

Urinary fistulas in women are a cause of involuntary loss of urine from the urethra or vagina. Such fistulas are usually secondary to operative trauma, neoplasms, automobile accidents, traumatic delivery, or gunshot wounds, where a tract becomes established and conducts urine from the ureter, bladder, or urethra into the vagina. The common symptom is the involuntary loss of urine from the vagina. The amount of urine that is lost varies with the size and location of the fistula. The leaking may be constant or intermittent and may or may not be associated with voiding. Diagnosis can usually be established by excretory urography, voiding cystourethrography, and urethrocystoscopy. Inspection of the vagina following filling of the bladder with indigo carmine solution helps identify whether the fistulous opening is from the urethra, bladder, or ureter. Therapy consists of surgical excision of the fistulous tract.

Psychogenic incontinence is occasionally seen in children and even in adults who have underlying emotional disturbances. Diagnosis can only be established after all other causes of incontinence have been ruled out. Treatment consists of anticholinergic drugs and psychotherapy.

Mixed types of incontinence are occasionally seen. A child may have incontinence secondary to both an uninhibited neurogenic bladder dysfunction and psychogenic incontinence, or an adult male may have both overflow incontinence due to prostatic obstruction, and neurogenic bladder dysfunction secondary to diabetic neuropathy or cerebrovascular insufficiency. A complete urodynamic evaluation, including excretory urography, voiding cystourethrography, retrograde urethrography, cystoscopy, cystometrograms, and a careful neurologic examination may be required to detect these mixed forms. Therapy is directed toward identifying and treating the specific types of incontinence present.

158. URINARY CALCULI

Urinary calculi **(stones)** may occur anywhere in the urinary tract and are common causes of pain, obstruction, and secondary infection.

Incidence and Pathogenesis

Approximately 1 in every 1000 adults is hospitalized annually in the USA because of urinary stones. They are found in about 1% of all autopsies. The incidence varies geographically (stone belts) and in time (stone epidemics). The pathogenesis is related to (1) factors increasing the urine concentration of stone crystalloids and (2) factors favoring stone formation at normal urinary concentrations. The first group includes reduction in urine volume (dehydration) and an increased rate of excretion of stone constituents: calcium, oxalate, urate, cystine, xanthine, or, rarely, phosphate. The second group of factors is less well understood but includes urinary stasis (time for crystallization), pH changes, foreign bodies (including other stones), and reduction of normal protective substances.

Calculi vary in size from microscopic crystalline foci to stones several cm in diameter. A large stone, such as a staghorn calculus, may be shaped by and virtually fill an entire renal calyceal system. Stones consist of masses of crystals in a protein matrix that gives cohesion and structure. Their composition may vary with geographic location and age group and is often mixed. In adults in the USA approximately 90% of stones contain calcium, and 65% oxalate; 5% are predominantly urate, and 2 to 3% are cystine. The incidence of magnesium ammonium phosphate stones parallels that of urea-splitting bacterial infections and hence elevated urine pH. Certain types of stones may have characteristic appearances, but the composition should always be determined by analysis.

Symptoms and Signs

Many calculi are "silent." Back pain or **renal colic** may occur when calculi obstruct one or more calyces, the renal pelvis, or the ureter; stones in the bladder may cause suprapubic pain. Typical symptoms of renal colic include excruciating intermittent pain, usually originating in the flank or kidney area and radiating across the abdomen along the course of the ureter, frequently into the region of the genitalia and inner side of the thigh. GI symptoms (nausea, vomiting, abdominal distention, the clinical picture of ileus) may obscure the urinary origin. Chills, fever, hematuria, and frequency of urination are common, particularly as a calculus passes down the ureter. The affected kidney may transiently become nonfunctioning in acute renal colic due to ureteral calculus, even for some time after the stone has been spontaneously passed.

Laboratory Findings

Urinalysis: The urine may be normal despite multiple calculi. Macroscopic or microscopic hematuria is common. Pyuria with or without bacteria may be seen. Various crystalline substances may be identified in the sediment, but the stone's composition should be determined by chemical analysis. The only exception is the presence of the typical benzene-ring crystals of cystine in a concentrated, acidified specimen, which strongly suggests cystinuria.

Roentgenography: Most urinary calculi are demonstrable on x-ray. Only pure uric acid calculi, rare xanthine calculi, and some "matrix stones" (composed largely of protein matrix) are radiolucent. Pyramidal calcium deposits within the renal parenchyma are diagnostic of **nephrocalcinosis** and suggest renal tubular acidosis, sarcoidosis, Cushing's disease, hyperparathyroidism, or the milk-alkali syndrome. Retrograde or intravenous urography may show opaque or nonopaque calculi, as well as the extent and degree of obstruction.

Diagnosis

The symptoms of colic, together with flank or costovertebral angle tenderness, increased sensitivity in the lumbar and groin areas, or complaints of pain in the genitalia with no obvious localized lesions suggest renal colic from stones. Diagnosis is supported by urinalysis and x-ray findings. IVP should be done to evaluate extent of obstruction and to detect radiolucent stones. Differential diagnosis includes appendicitis, cholecystitis, peptic ulcer, and pancreatitis.

Treatment

Many small solitary calculi, uncomplicated by obstruction or infection, require no specific therapy. Eradication of infection should be attempted; if impossible, chronic suppressive therapy may be necessary. Symptoms of colic may be relieved by narcotics (morphine 10 to 15 mg or meperidine 100 mg IM q 3 to 4 h), but antispasmodics are unsatisfactory. Obstructing stones should be removed surgically if they do not pass spontaneously. Calculi impacted in the renal pelvis or ureter may require surgery, particularly when associated with infection. Calculi < 1 cm in diameter in the lower ureter may be approached endoscopically; cystoscopic basket extraction is successful when the calculus is not impacted in an edematous ureter. Uric acid calculi in the upper or lower urinary tract occasionally may be dissolved by prolonged alkalinization of the urine, but chemical dissolution of other calculi is not possible.

Prophylaxis

Knowledge of pathogenesis is required to plan prophylaxis, beginning with recovery and analysis of the stone, preferably by crystallographic technics. A **cystine stone** is diagnostic of cystinuria, which is discussed under ANOMALIES IN KIDNEY TRANSPORT in Ch. 153. A **magnesium ammonium phosphate stone** indicates urinary tract infection. **Abnormalities of calcium metabolism** are most frequently found. Hyperparathyroidism is associated with approximately 5% of calcium stones. Urinary calcium excretion on a low-calcium diet (no dairy products) should be determined for 2 days to see if hypercalciuria (> 3.5 to 4 mg calcium/kg/24 h) is present. If so, hyperparathyroidism, sarcoidosis, vitamin D intoxication, hyperthyroidism, renal tubular acidosis, multiple myeloma, metastatic cancer, and idiopathic hypercalciuria must be considered (see HYPERCALCEMIA in Ch. 81).

Idiopathic hypercalciuria is the most frequent abnormality found with recurrent calcium stones, occurring in about 40% of such patients. Prophylaxis is best carried out in such patients by forcing fluids (especially at night when physiologic concentration of the urine normally occurs) and with hydrochlorothiazide 50 mg b.i.d. This diuretic reduces urinary calcium in normal subjects and patients with idiopathic hypercalciuria. Orthophosphate treatment (in amounts equivalent to 1 gm of phosphorus daily) may also reduce urine calcium and stone recurrence but is not recommended for patients with calcium phosphate stones.

Calcium oxalate stones are rarely due to excess oxalate excretion (> 60 mg/24 h), but this occurs in 4 conditions: pyridoxine deficiency, primary hyperoxaluria Type I (glycolic aciduria), primary hyperoxaluria Type II (glyceric aciduria), and enteric hyperoxaluria. Pyridoxine deficiency responds to vitamin replacement therapy. Both types of primary hyperoxaluria are genetic disorders and are best treated with pyridoxine (100 to 200 mg/day), magnesium oxide (200 mg/day), and forced fluids. Patients with small bowel disease not infrequently absorb excessive oxalate from the diet (over 10%), and a low-oxalate diet is the best approach to treatment of this syndrome.

Uric acid stones occur in association with excessive uric acid excretion (usually in primary or secondary gout) or increased urine acidity. Urate solubility is markedly increased as the pH rises from 5 to 7 (more than 20-fold) because of the shift from free uric acid to sodium urate. Forcing fluids and maintaining urinary pH above 6 with sodium bicarbonate or citrate is usually prophylactic. Allopurinol 200 to 400 mg daily orally may be needed to reduce urate synthesis.

No abnormality is found to account for stones in at least half the patients studied. There may be some defect in formation and excretion of protective substances in the urine, but current methods for identifying and measuring these substances are inadequate. If the calculus is small and solitary and if no abnormality is found, high fluid intake may suffice. If stones recur in the absence of a detectable metabolic abnormality, the program described above for idiopathic hypercalciuria is most likely to help.

159.   MALE GENITAL LESIONS

Abnormalities of the external male genitalia (penis, scrotal, and scrotal contents) are psychologically disturbing and sometimes life-threatening for the patient. A careful, gentle examination and correct diagnosis are mandatory.

PENILE LESIONS

Bacterial and yeast infections beneath the foreskin of the uncircumcised male are common causes of balanoposthitis (generalized inflammation of the glans penis and foreskin), discussed in Ch. 162. Such inflammation predisposes to meatal stricture, phimosis, paraphimosis, and cancer.

Erythroplasia of Queyrat, a premalignant lesion, is a well-circumscribed area of reddish, velvety pigmentation, usually on the glans or at the corona. Biopsy should be considered, and treatment consists of topical application of 5% fluorouracil cream.

Balanitis xerotica obliterans, the result of chronic inflammation, is an indurated, blanched area near the tip of the glans, surrounding the meatus and often causing constriction. Local antibacterial and anti-inflammatory agents may be used, and meatotomy may be required in some instances.

Chancre, the primary lesion of syphilis, is discussed in Ch. 162.

Genital warts (condylomata acuminata) are discussed in Vol. II, Ch. 5.

Paget's and Bowen's diseases are rare skin cancers that may appear on the penis. Other rare penile lesions include diphtheria, TB, mycotic disease of the penis, and herpes zoster. Herpes simplex is more common.

Carcinoma is discussed in Ch. 161.

PRIAPISM

Painful, persistent, and abnormal penile erection, unaccompanied by sexual desire or excitation.

The mechanisms of priapism are poorly understood, but probably involve a complexity of vascular and neurologic abnormalities. Pelvic vascular thrombosis is most often incriminated. It may be secondary to prolonged sexual activity; leukemia, sickle cell disease or trait, or other blood dyscrasias; pelvic hematoma or neoplasm; cerebrospinal disease such as syphilis or tumor; or infection and inflammation of the male genitalia such as prostatitis, urethritis, or cystitis, especially if complicated by a bladder calculus. The corpora cavernosa are rarely thrombosed completely, usually containing only thick, dark venous blood of motor oil consistency. The corpus spongiosum and glans penis are not involved.

Treatment is difficult and frequently unsuccessful. Neurologic priapism may be alleviated by continuous caudal or spinal anesthesia. Estrogens are ineffective, and anticoagulants are effective only in the earliest stages. The corpora may be decompressed by introduction of large-bore needles (12- or 16-gauge) with evacuation and irrigation, though tumescence usually recurs. Creation of a fistula between the glans and corpus cavernosum has proved successful and can be done with a biopsy needle. Semipermanent diversion by means of a saphenous vein shunt from one or both corpora or a cavernoso-spongiosum shunt may result in detumescence for a period of time sufficient to permit reestablishment of normal pelvic circulation. Underlying causes should be treated. **Prognosis** for recovery of sexual function is poor unless treatment is prompt and effective.

PEYRONIE'S DISEASE

Dysplasia of the cavernous sheaths consisting of a fibrous thickening and contracture of the investing fascia of the corpora not unlike Dupuytren's contracture. The cause is unknown. The disease occurs in adult males. The contracture usually results in deviation of the erect penis to the involved side, occasionally causes painful erections, and frequently prevents intromission. Later, the fibrotic process may extend into the corpus cavernosum, compromising tumescence distally.

Treatment is varied and results unpredictable. Resolution may occur spontaneously over many months. Surgical removal of the plaque and replacement with a patch graft may be successful or result in further scarring and exaggeration of the defect. High-potency corticosteroid local injections (dexamethasone 2 to 4 mg once or twice/wk) may be effective; oral corticosteroids have not been. Local ultrasonic treatment has proved beneficial in relieving symptoms in some cases. An asymptomatic plaque does not warrant treatment.

SCROTAL MASSES

Scrotal masses may be due to trauma, inflammatory conditions involving the scrotal wall or contents, neoplasms of the testis or testicular appendages, or mechanical abnormalities involving the scrotal contents or adjacent structures.

Epididymo-orchitis (inflammation of the epididymis and testis) may be a complication of urinary infection with prostatitis or urethritis, a sequel to gonorrhea, a complication of prostatic surgery, or a result of infection secondary to an indwelling catheter. Gram-negative bacteria and *Chlamydia trachomatis* are the organisms usually involved. Tuberculous epididymitis, syphilitic gummas, and the mycotic diseases (actinomycosis, blastomycosis) are rare today. **Treatment** consists of bed rest, scrotal support (adhesive bridge), ice bags, and systemic antibacterials. Scrotal abscesses tend to drain spontaneously and incision is rarely necessary.

Acute **mumps orchitis** is discussed in Vol. II, Ch. 24.

Urethral stricture and **diverticulum** may be accompanied by abscess formation and extravasation of urine into the scrotum and perineum. Urinary diversion by suprapubic cystotomy, incision and drainage, and antibiotics are indicated. Persistent strictures are definitely treated with open or endoscopic surgery.

Hydrocele is a common intrinsic scrotal mass. It results from excessive accumulation of normal fluid within the tunica vaginalis due to overproduction (inflammation of the testis and its appendages) or diminished resorption (lymphatic or venous obstruction in the cord or retroperitoneal space). Congenital hydrocele communicates with the abdominal cavity through a patent processus vaginalis, a potential hernia space, but may resolve spontaneously following neonatal obliteration of the communication. **Treatment** of persistent hydrocele is surgical. Aspiration is only a temporary measure and may introduce secondary infection. **Hematocele** is usually secondary to trauma and is an accumulation of blood within the tunica vaginalis. Unlike hydrocele, it does not transilluminate. **Treatment** is surgical, if the hematocele is large and does not absorb with conservative management.

Inguinal hernia, direct or indirect, may extend into the scrotal compartment. Hernia must be differentiated from hydrocele or hematocele. In the former, the examiner cannot palpate the cord above the mass, while with a hydrocele and hematocele, normal cord structures are usually palpable above the mass. Surgical repair of inguinal hernia is recommended because of the probability of progression and the possibilities of incarceration and strangulation.

Spermatocele (spermatic cyst) occurs adjacent to the epididymis and usually contains sperm. It may be difficult to differentiate from hydrocele, since each will transilluminate and is cystic and painless. Spermatoceles occur at the upper pole of the testis adjacent to the epididymis and may suggest the presence of a "third testis." Surgical excision is indicated if it becomes large and symptomatic.

Testicular torsion: See Vol. II, Ch. 21, in MANAGEMENT OF THE NORMAL NEWBORN and in CONGENITAL ANOMALIES.

Testis tumors: See Ch. 161.

Varicocele is a collection of large veins and usually occurs in the left scrotum and feels like a "bag of worms." It is present in the upright position and should drain in the supine position. Surgical correction may be necessary in treating infertility, and is indicated if the varicocele is symptomatic.

Lymphedema of the scrotum may result from abdominal venous compression, an intra-abdominal tumor, cirrhosis with ascites, filariasis, or Milroy's disease (idiopathic lymphedema). **Treatment** is with a scrotal suspensory, though resection and scrotoplasty may be necessary.

160. GENITOURINARY TRAUMA

Trauma to the GU tract may be caused by penetrating or perforating wounds, blunt crushing injuries, surgery, instrumentation, or irradiation. Hematuria, oliguria, pain, and anuria are the principal manifestations. Localized tenderness, swelling, and ecchymosis may be present; shock may develop. Prompt diagnosis and treatment may be lifesaving and are essential to preserve renal function.

Kidney

Blunt external force is the usual cause of traumatic injury to the kidneys. Penetrating or perforating injuries may result from gunshot or stab wounds. Damage varies widely: contusion may cause massive hematuria without anatomic defect; laceration may be capsular and/or parenchymal; fragmentation or "shattered kidney" may cause massive bleeding and extravasation of urine; laceration or complete disruption of the renal pedicle (artery or vein) may cause shock and sudden death. Infusion pyelography (**IVP**) with tomography usually establishes a diagnosis. Retrograde pyelography is seldom required. Arteriography should be used when there is nonvisualization on IVP or when a major injury is suspected.

Therapy begins with whole blood or blood substitutes to prevent or control shock. Maintenance of BP and establishment of urinary flow also facilitate accurate radiographic diagnosis. Conservative management with bed rest will suffice in many cases. However, severe injuries resulting in uncontrolled bleeding or excessive urine extravasation may require surgical intervention or arterial embolization under radiologic control. **Prognosis** is good with prompt diagnosis and appropriate management. Renal hypertension may be a late consequence of renal injury with segmental ischemia or infarction and subsequent scarring, or may be due to perinephric fibrosis.

Ureter

Most ureteral injuries are the result of pelvic surgery (radical urologic, gynecologic, or colonic procedures) and are frequently unrecognized until oliguria, pain, fever, anuria, or a fistula appears. Ureteral injury from external trauma is uncommon. Blunt injuries, particularly with extreme hyperextension of the trunk, may cause avulsion of the ureter at the renal pelvis or at the pelvic brim. Diagnostic measures should include IVP with tomography and, in some instances, retrograde pyelography. Percutaneous nephrostomy with antegrade pyelography may be valuable for diagnosis and therapy.

Treatment: Prompt recognition of anuria caused by suture ligation of the ureter may result in satisfactory surgical correction. Postsurgical obstruction or urinary fistula may require temporary urinary diversion (nephrostomy, proximal ureterostomy) or primary repair (ureteroureterostomy, ureteroneocystostomy, or transureteroureterostomy). Ureteral catheterization and prolonged ureteral catheter stenting (3 to 6 wk) may dilate a stricture or allow a fistula to close.

Bladder

Traumatic rupture of the overdistended bladder is common with crushing external trauma as may occur in automobile accidents, and is usually associated with pelvic fracture. Rupture may be intra- or extraperitoneal. Oliguria, hematuria, or anuria may be the principal presenting signs. Diagnosis may be established by cystography with sterile contrast materials, which will also identify extravasation of urine. Displacement of the bladder as noted radiographically may or may not indicate rupture, since extravesical bleeding into the paravesical space may cause massive distortion (a "tear-drop bladder" configuration due to extrinsic compression).

Treatment for minor lacerations may only require catheter drainage for 7 to 10 days. With more severe injuries, treatment usually consists of prompt exploration, repair of lacerations, and establishment of urinary drainage, preferably with both suprapubic and urethral catheters.

Urethra

Common causes of urethral injury include pelvic fracture with shearing tears (usually at the prostatomembranous junction), perineal straddle injuries, and traumatic urethral instrumentation. Anuria with suprapubic, scrotal, or perineal extravasation of fluid may be presenting signs. Diagnosis is established by retrograde urethrogram. Cystourethrography defines the location and extent of injury.

Treatment: Most urethral injuries require surgical repair. Suprapubic bladder catheter drainage should be established, and in many instances, urethral surgery may be deferred and done electively. Urethral stricture at the site of injury is a frequent long-term complication, demanding subsequent urethral dilation, internal urethrotomy, or secondary surgical repair. Impotence is a possible complication of severe proximal urethral injury in males.

External Male Genitalia

While penetrating and perforating injuries of the penis or scrotum and its contents may occur, the severe injuries are from crushing blows and avulsion of the skin or the genitalia. Avulsion injuries can occur among industrial and farm workers, when clothing is caught in machinery. Penile injuries may occur secondary to a variety of devices such as penile rings and vacuum cleaner attachments or excessive trauma during intercourse, masturbation, or fellatio.

Treatment: Avulsed skin should be conserved, cooled, and reapplied as quickly as possible. Debridement should be conservative. Skin grafting may be necessary. When the entire scrotum is avulsed, the testes may be buried under the skin of the thigh or the lower abdomen, if possible, in hope of retaining spermatogenesis and hormonal function. Complete traumatic avulsion of the penis is uncommon. Gunshot wounds and other penetrating injuries require debridement and drainage. Hematomas and hematoceles may result from external trauma to the scrotum and are usually managed conservatively.

161. NEOPLASMS

GU neoplasms occur at any age. Gross or microscopic **hematuria** is an important diagnostic sign.

KIDNEY

TUBULOINTERSTITIAL DISEASE IN MALIGNANCY

Renal parenchyma may be invaded by proliferative malignant cells in leukemia and lymphosarcoma. The cortex is involved more than the medulla. These changes are found in about half the patients with generalized lymphosarcoma and a third of those with malignant lymphomas. The kidneys are enlarged, often asymmetrically. Excretory urography reveals elongation and narrowing of the calyces due to this diffuse infiltration. Other factors may cause renal enlargement in a patient with diffuse malignant disease, since neoplastic infiltration is present at autopsy in only 50% of such patients. Despite the extensive interstitial involvement, functional changes are few. Proteinuria is absent or insignificant and there is rarely a rise in the blood urea or creatinine concentration unless some other complication occurs, such as uric acid nephropathy, hypercalcemia, or bacterial infiltration.

CARCINOMA OF THE KIDNEY (Hypernephroma)

Carcinoma of the kidney accounts for 1 to 2% of adult cancers, with 2/3 of cases occurring in males.

Symptoms, Signs, and Diagnosis

Hematuria is the most common presenting sign, followed by flank pain, palpable mass, and FUO. Hypertension (due to segmental ischemia or pedicle compression) and polycythemia (secondary to increased erythropoietin activity) are also seen in some cases.

Pyelography confirms the presence of a mass, and renal angiography is usually diagnostic, showing neovascularization. Nephrotomography, ultrasonography, cyst puncture, and abdominal CT scan are useful aids in evaluating renal masses.

Prognosis and Treatment

Radical nephrectomy with regional node dissection offers the best chance for cure. Removal of the primary tumor may rarely cause regression of metastatic lesions.

The overall 5-yr survival rate in adult nephrocarcinoma is about 45%. Hormonal factors may cause the greater survival rate of females over males. However, therapy with progestational agents and either cortisone derivatives or testosterone has been disappointing.

RENAL PELVIS AND URETER

Malignancies of the renal pelvis and ureter are histologically similar (usually transitional cell in character, but occasionally squamous cell). Hematuria is the principal presenting sign, and colicky pain may accompany obstruction. Diagnosis is established by finding a negative filling defect on IVP or retrograde pyelography. Cytology may be helpful. **Treatment** usually is radical nephroureterectomy, including a cuff of bladder. Occasionally, local excision of a ureteral lesion is indicated (e.g., decreased renal function, solitary kidney). Prognosis in operable lesions is good. Periodic follow-up cystoscopies are indicated, since tumors tend to recur in the urinary bladder and may be treated by transurethral resection.

URINARY BLADDER

Etiology and Incidence

Known urinary carcinogens include β-naphthylamine, p-aminodiphenyl (aniline dyes), certain chemical intermediates in the manufacture of rubber, tryptophan metabolites, and, possibly, excretory products of tobacco tars. Chronic irritation (as in schistosomiasis) predisposes to bladder cancer, and residual urine is thought to play a role. The incidence of bladder malignancies in men vs. women is about 3:1.

Pathology

Transitional carcinoma is most common, often beginning as a papillary growth and proceeding to invasion and loss of differentiation with widespread metastases. Squamous cell carcinoma may represent a metaplastic form of transitional cell tumor, is highly invasive, and offers a poorer prognosis. Adenocarcinoma of the bladder is rarer and may be primary or represent spread from a bowel carcinoma.

Symptoms, Signs, and Diagnosis

Hematuria, pyuria, dysuria, burning, and frequency are the most common presenting symptoms. Pain occurs with invasion, infection, or fixation. A suprapubic mass may be palpable later on bimanual examination. Microhematuria may be the earliest sign of bladder carcinoma.

Filling defects of the bladder by cystogram or in the cystographic phase of the IVP suggest vesical neoplasm. Urinary cytologies are frequently positive for tumor cells. Diagnosis is by cystoscopy and transurethral resectional biopsy. Bimanual examination under anesthesia aids in staging the disease. Pelvic CT scan and ultrasound may also be of value in staging.

Prognosis and Treatment

Malignancies that are superficial or invade only the most superficial portion of the bladder musculature respond to endoscopic therapy, but recurrence at the same or another site in the bladder is relatively common. Deeply invasive lesions of the bladder musculature respond poorly. Bladder malignancies that have metastasized are incurable, though cystectomy and urinary diversion may prolong life and be palliative.

Superficial and early lesions may be treated effectively by transurethral resection. Tumors that invade the bladder wall in depth should be treated by partial, total, or radical cystectomy, the latter methods necessitating concomitant urinary diversion. Preoperative irradiation may be effective in retarding tumor growth. Combined use of radiation therapy and surgery yields the best results. Chemotherapy is not effective except for certain selected superficial papillary growths, which may be treated by repeated bladder instillations of thiotepa (60 mg in 60 ml of distilled water weekly for 6 wk, courses repeated as needed). Other chemotherapeutic drugs have also been used topically with varying degrees of success in decreasing the incidence of recurrence (bleomycin, ethoglucid, doxorubicin).

PROSTATE

Adenocarcinoma of the prostate accounts for the majority of malignancies in men over age 65. The etiology is unknown. Sarcoma of the prostate is rare; it may occur in children. Undifferentiated prostatic carcinoma, squamous cell carcinoma, and ductal transitional carcinoma of the prostate probably represent variants of adult adenocarcinoma and are less responsive to the usual measures of control.

Pathology

The usual prostatic malignancy is glandular, not unlike the histologic configuration of normal prostate. Frequent mitoses, stromal invasion, and involvement of perineural lymphatics constitute the principal histologic criteria of diagnosis.

Symptoms and Signs

Prostatic carcinoma is generally slowly progressive and may cause no symptoms. Late in the course of the disease, symptoms of bladder outlet obstruction, ureteral obstruction, hematuria, and pyuria may appear. Metastases to the pelvis and lumbar spine may cause bone pain. Stony hard induration or a nodule of the prostate suggests prostatic malignancy and must be distinguished from granulomatous prostatitis, prostatic TB, prostatic calculi, and other more unusual prostatic diseases. The firm and nodular irregular prostate is pathognomonic of prostatic carcinoma and later exhibits extension of induration and fixation of the gland to the rectum and the lateral pelvic walls.

Diagnosis

Prostatic carcinoma must be suspected on the basis of rectal findings. A solitary firm prostatic nodule should be biopsied. The more extensive processes may be defined by needle biopsy, either transrectally or transperineally. An **elevated serum acid phosphatase** indicates local extension or metastases. Other diseases causing elevation of this enzyme are benign prostatic hyperplasia (slight elevation following vigorous prostatic massage), multiple myeloma, Gaucher's disease, and hemolytic anemia. Denaturation with tartrate permits the separation of prostatic phosphatase from that originating elsewhere, and this fractionation is available for discrimination. Copper, fluoride, formaldehyde, oxalates, tartrates, androgens, clofibrate, and improper sample storage may cause spurious changes in acid phosphatase levels. Radioactive immunoassay methods for determination of prostatic acid phosphatase may give added information regarding the detection of localized prostatic carcinoma as well as later stages of the disease. The level declines after successful treatment and rises again with recurrence.

Prostatic carcinoma usually produces osteoblastic bony metastases, and their radiographic demonstration in the presence of a stony hard prostate is diagnostic. Aspiration of bone marrow and demonstration of prostatic cellular configuration in metastatic cells confirm a diagnosis of advanced disease.

Prognosis

Ten-year cure rates approaching 65% occur with localized prostatic carcinoma amenable to radical prostatectomy or radiation therapy. Prostatic malignancies not amenable to radical surgery or radiation therapy may respond to adequate hormonal control and/or orchiectomy for 10 yr or more. This is particularly true in older men and when the carcinoma is well differentiated. The presence of obvious metastases at the time of initial diagnosis obviously worsens the prognosis, but therapy may yield significant long-term palliation without cure.

Treatment

Early and localized prostatic carcinoma may be cured by radical perineal or retropubic prostatectomy or radiation therapy. Extensive local disease or metastases may preclude surgical cure, in which case diagnostic confirmation should be followed by hormonal control, irradiation, or both. The treatment of choice is estrogen (diethylstilbestrol 1 mg/day orally; high estrogen doses may predispose to thrombosis or other vascular complications. High-dose, short-term therapy with IV diethylstilbestrol diphosphate may yield dramatic symptomatic relief. Bilateral orchiectomy may be useful for advanced disease early or after estrogen failure. Irradiation may provide prompt relief of pain from bony metastases refractory to other treatment and also may be effective in controlling local disease.

URETHRA

Carcinoma of the urethra is rare. It occurs in both males and females and may be squamous or transitional cell, or occasionally adenocarcinoma. Hematuria and a local mass are the presenting symptoms. Obstructive symptoms are rare. Friable and bleeding masses presenting at the external urethral meatus in the female must be suspect. Differentiation between carcinoma of the urethra, urethral prolapse, and urethral caruncle may require excisional biopsy. Irradiation and radical surgery are equally effective, although the prognosis remains poor.

PENIS

Carcinoma of the penis is more common in uncircumcised males who practice poor local hygiene. The usual lesion, arising in the region of the corona or beneath the foreskin, is epidermoid, extending locally and metastasizing relatively late. Metastases are via the penile lymphatics to the superficial and deep inguinal nodes, often necessitating total or partial penectomy with associated inguinal lymphadenectomy. Penile carcinomas are refractory to radiation, and chemotherapy is ineffective. Partial penectomy may be curative in early lesions, with a penile stump that is satisfactory for urination and sexual activity.

TESTIS

The origin and nature of scrotal masses must be accurately determined, since most growths arising in or from the testis are malignant, while extratesticular scrotal masses are usually benign.

Etiology and Incidence

Etiology is unknown. Testicular tumors account for the majority of solid malignancies in males under 30. Cryptorchid testes are affected by malignancy about 20 times as often as descended testes. This appears to be true even if the cryptorchid testis has been brought down surgically.

Pathology

Most malignant testicular tumors arise from the primordial germ cell and are classified as seminoma, teratoma, embryonal carcinoma, teratocarcinoma, and choriocarcinoma, in order of increasing malignancy. Functional interstitial cell carcinomas of the testis are rare. Tumors arising in the testicular appendages and the cord are usually benign fibromas, fibroadenomas, adenomatoid tumors, and lipomas, although sarcomas occasionally may occur.

Symptoms and Signs

The usual presenting sign in testicular tumor is a scrotal mass, progressively increasing in size and sometimes associated with pain. Many patients relate the mass to minor trauma, indicating the time when the mass was first discovered. Hemorrhage into a rapidly expanding tumor may produce exquisite local pain and tenderness. A firm or cystic scrotal mass arising from the testis is cause for immediate clinical suspicion of testicular tumor.

Diagnosis

The principal diagnostic tool is surgical inguinal exploration, exposing and clamping the cord through an inguinal incision before mobilization of the tumor. Diagnostic studies should include chest x-ray and IVP for direct or indirect evidence of metastases, as well as urinary gonadotropin determination. A positive Aschheim-Zondek or other pregnancy test may be associated with the more active testicular tumors, particularly choriocarcinoma, and may serve as a prognostic indicator following surgery. Radioimmunoassays of α-fetoprotein and the β subunit of human chorionic gonadotropin are reliable markers indicating the presence of tumor and are valuable in follow-up of patients with proven testicular tumors, especially of the nonseminomatous types. Pedal lymphangiography and abdominal CT scans are important in the staging process.

Prognosis

This depends on the histology and extent of the malignancy. Five-year survival rates > 80% are seen with seminomas localized to the testis or even metastatic to the retroperineum. The 5-yr survival rate with highly malignant choriocarcinomas is virtually nil. Other tumors range between these extremes.

Treatment

Inguinal orchiectomy must be performed. Transabdominal retroperitoneal lymph node dissection is recommended for terato- and embryonal carcinoma. Irradiation may be effective, particularly in seminoma, using 3000 to 5000 R to the abdominal and mediastinal lymphatics as well as the left supraclavicular area. Chemotherapy with cisplatin in combination with other agents may cause regression and control of metastatic, nonseminomatous testicular tumors but is highly toxic. Local excision of benign extratesticular solid tumors is satisfactory treatment.

§14. SEXUALLY RELATED DISORDERS

162. SEXUALLY TRANSMITTED DISEASE (STD)
(See also Vol. II, Ch. 5)

The most common communicable diseases in the world, STDs have steadily increased in incidence for the past 2 decades. In that time, diseases such as nonspecific urethritis (discussed in this chapter), trichomoniasis, chlamydial infections, genital candidiasis, genital and anorectal herpes and warts (discussed in Vol. II, Ch. 5), scabies, pediculosis pubis, molluscum contagiosum (see Chs. 192 and 193 in this volume), and other conditions that may be transmitted sexually have been more prevalent than the 5 historically defined venereal diseases—syphilis, gonorrhea, chancroid, lymphogranuloma venereum, and granuloma inguinale. However, because the former group is not consistently reported, incidence figures are not available. For gonorrhea, it is estimated that over 250 million persons are infected annually worldwide, and close to 3 million in the USA. For syphilis, annual worldwide incidence is estimated at 50 million persons, with 400,000 in the USA annually needing treatment. Some enteric infections, including salmonellosis, giardiasis, amebiasis, shigellosis, and typhoid, as well as cytomegalovirus infection, also appear to be sexually transmitted.

A medical paradox exists in that STD incidence has risen despite the progress made in diagnosis and treatment, which renders patients noninfectious rapidly and cures the majority. Factors responsible include changes in sexual behavior, e.g., the widespread use of contraceptive pills and devices and the greater variety of sexual practices, including orogenital and anorectal contact; the emergence of strains of organisms less sensitive to antibiotics; the symptomless carriers of infecting agents; a highly mobile population; a high incidence of sexual activity and infection in homosexual men; ignorance of the facts by doctors and the public; and reticence.

STD control depends on good facilities for diagnosis and treatment, tracing of all sexual contacts of the patients, thorough surveillance of those who have received treatment to ensure that they have been cured, educated awareness by doctors, nurses, and the public, and development of methods for producing artificial immunity and protection against infection.

GONORRHEA

An acute infectious disease of the epithelium of the urethra, cervix, and rectum, which may involve other areas of the body and may give rise to bacteremia, resulting in metastatic complications.

Etiology and Epidemiology

The causative organism is the gonococcus *Neisseria gonorrhoeae*, which can be demonstrated from discharges (by direct smear or after culture) as pairs or clumps of gram-negative, kidney-shaped diplococci, often intracellular, and with their mutually adjacent surfaces slightly concave.

The disease usually is spread by sexual contact. Women are frequently symptomless carriers of the organisms for weeks or months and are often identified through tracing of sexual contacts. Symptomless infection is also common in homosexual men, especially in the oropharynx and rectum, and is being found more frequently in the urethras of both hetero- and homosexual men.

Gonorrhea occurs in the vagina of prepubertal girls, most of whom get the infections from their infected parents.

Symptoms and Signs

In men, the incubation period is from 2 to 14 days. The onset usually consists of a tingling sensation in the urethra followed a few hours later by dysuria and a purulent discharge. Frequency and urgency of micturition develop as the disease spreads to the posterior urethra. Examination shows a purulent, yellowish-green urethral discharge; the lips of the meatus may be red and swollen.

In women, symptoms usually begin within 7 to 21 days after infection. Symptoms generally are mild, but in a few women the onset may be severe, with dysuria, frequency, and vaginal discharge. The vagina, cervix, and reproductive organs are the sites most frequently infected; the urethra, Skene's ducts, Bartholin's glands, and rectum, less frequently. The cervix may be reddened and friable, with a mucopurulent or purulent discharge. Pus may be expressed from the urethra on pressure against the symphysis pubis or from Skene's ducts or Bartholin's glands. Salpingitis is a common complication (see Vol. II, Ch. 4).

In either sex, rectal gonorrhea is common. It usually is symptomless, but perianal discomfort and a rectal discharge may occur. If rectal infection is severe, perianal excoriation may be present and proctoscopy may show mucopus on the rectal wall. **Gonococcal pharyngitis** from orogenital contact is being recognized more frequently. Although there are often no symptoms or signs, some patients may complain of a sore throat and discomfort on swallowing, and the pharynx and tonsillar area may be red, sometimes with a mucopurulent exudate and occasionally with edema of the uvula and faucial pillars.

In female infants and little girls, edema of the vulva with a purulent vaginal discharge may be accompanied by proctitis. The child may complain of soreness or dysuria and the parents may notice staining of the underclothes. Gonococci can be isolated from the discharge.

Diagnosis

A gram-stained smear of urethral discharge allows rapid identification of the gonococcus in most men. However, the cervical Gram stain is only about 60% reliable in women. Identification of the gonococcus by culture of exudate specimens should always be done for women and for men with negative urethral Gram stains. Cultures should be performed in both sexes when symptoms of rectal or pharyngeal infection are present, as Gram stains are *unreliable*. Exudates from the urethra, cervix, rectum, and other infected sites are inoculated onto a suitable medium (e.g., Modified Thayer-Martin medium) and incubated at 35 to 36 C for 48 h in an atmosphere containing 3 to 10% carbon dioxide (a candle jar may be used). Some colonies become visible after 24 h, but most appear after 48 h. The colonies are small, circular, transparent, and usually 1 to 4 mm in diameter, with umbilicated centers and crenated margins. Complete identification depends on characteristic appearance on Gram stain, on the oxidase test, in which positive colonies turn purple and later black on exposure to 1% di- or tetramethyl-*p*-phenylenediamine HCl, and on fermentation reactions. *N. gonorrhoeae* is oxidase-positive, and ferments dextrose (glucose) but not maltose or sucrose. The meningococcus (*N. meningitidis*) is also oxidase-positive, and ferments dextrose and maltose but not sucrose. Nonpathogenic *Neisseria* species ferment either 3 or more carbohydrates, or none.

If adequate laboratory facilities are not immediately available, the specimen may be inoculated onto a transport medium for transfer to a laboratory. Containers with suitable media and self-contained carbon dioxide supply are commercially available. For successful growth of gonococci, the specimens must be subcultured within 48 h, preferably within 24 h. Reliable immunofluorescent or serologic tests for gonococci are not yet available for routine clinical use.

Complications

In men, postgonococcal nonspecific urethritis is the most common complication. The discharge returns 7 to 14 days after treatment and may be due to the presence of other organisms such as *Chlamydia trachomatis*, which were simultaneously acquired with gonorrhea but which have longer incubation periods and which also do not respond to penicillin. **Epididymitis** (see Ch. 151), another important complication, is usually unilateral; if bilateral, sterility may result. Infection descends from the posterior urethra along the vas deferens to the lower pole of the epididymis. The testicle is painful, and the epididymis and spermatic cord become hot, tender, and swollen. A secondary hydrocele may follow. Abscesses of Tyson's and Littré's glands, periurethral abscesses, infection of Cowper's glands and the prostate, urethral stricture, and infection of the seminal vesicles are less common complications.

In women, salpingitis is the most important clinical problem (see Vol. II, Ch. 4).

In either sex, disseminated gonococcal infection with bacteremia may occur, but more commonly in women. The disease presents with a mild febrile illness, malaise, flitting joint pains, and scanty pustular and petechial skin lesions toward the periphery of the limbs. The genital infection may be symptomless, but bacteriologic tests of the genital secretions demonstrate gonococci. The organism can sometimes be grown from the bloodstream or joint fluid and can be demonstrated in the pus from skin lesions, using immunofluorescent technics. Bacteremia has serious potential sequelae; pericarditis, endocarditis, meningitis, and perihepatitis occasionally occur and can be fatal.

Gonococcal arthritis also is more frequent in women than in men. Genital manifestations may be minimal or absent. The onset is acute, with fever, severe pain, and limitation of movement (usually in a single joint). The joint is swollen and tender, and the overlying skin is hot and red. Synovial fluid is increased, and aspiration produces thick pus from which gonococci can be isolated, stained, and cultured. Early destruction of the articular surfaces of the joint occurs, and serious damage may result if the condition is not promptly treated.

Ocular infections may occur in the newborn (see under NEONATAL INFECTIONS in Vol. II, Ch. 21) or in adults (see Ch. 178).

Treatment

The Center for Disease Control now considers 3 treatment regimens to be coequal: (1) aqueous procaine penicillin G 4.8 million u. IM (divided, at 2 sites) plus probenecid 1 gm orally given simultaneously; (2) ampicillin 3.5 gm or amoxicillin 3.0 gm orally given simultaneously with probenecid 1 gm; and (3) tetracycline 500 mg orally q.i.d. for 5 days. Patients with uncertain reliability should be given one of the single-dose regimens. With suspected rectal infection, the penicillin regimen is preferred, and with suspected pharyngeal infection, ampicillin should be *avoided*. Patients who fail therapy or who have possible penicillin-resistant gonorrhea should be given spectinomycin 2 gm IM. Penicillin-allergic patients should be given spectinomycin or tetracycline (unless possibly pregnant).

Blood for serologic tests for syphilis **(STS)** should always be obtained before treatment is started, and the patient should be carefully examined to exclude other STDs. STS should be repeated 3 mo after treatment is concluded.

The infectious nature of gonorrhea should be explained to the patient, who should abstain from sexual activity until cure is confirmed. Men should also be advised not to squeeze the penis in a search for urethral discharges. All sexual contacts of the patient should be traced, examined, and given treatment.

One week after treatment, to confirm that the patient is cured and no longer infectious, specimens from the infected sites should be tested and cultured for gonorrhea. Ideally, a second test for cure should be performed 2 wk later and STS carried out 3 mo after treatment. Many recurrent infections are due to reinfection. However, penicillin-resistant gonococci are occurring in the USA, many imported from Southeast Asia. In patients who fail therapy and deny reexposure, tests for penicillin resistance are indicated.

For treatment of specific complications, see appropriate chapters elsewhere in THE MANUAL.

NONSPECIFIC SEXUALLY TRANSMITTED INFECTION

(NSI; Nongonococcal Urethritis [NGU]; Nonspecific Urethritis [NSU])

Etiology and Incidence

As the nonspecific sexually transmitted causes of cervicitis and urethritis in women, urethritis in men, and proctitis and pharyngitis in both become identified, the terms widely used to describe these infections, nonspecific urethritis (NSU) or nongonococcal urethritis (NGU), are increasingly narrow and inapt. Nonspecific sexually transmitted infection **(NSI)**, although not a reportable disease, may be the most common sexually transmitted disease in the USA, more prevalent than gonorrhea. The probable causal agents include *Chlamydia trachomatis* (thought to be responsible for about 50% of cases) and, probably, *Ureaplasma urealyticum*.

Symptoms and Signs

In men, symptoms of urethritis generally appear between 7 and 28 days after intercourse, usually with mild dysuria and discomfort in the urethra and a mucopurulent discharge. Although the discharge may be slight and the symptoms mild, they are frequently more marked early in the morning when the lips of the meatus often are stuck together with dried secretions. On examination the meatus may be red, with evidence of the dried secretions. Occasionally the onset is more acute, with dysuria, frequency, and a copious purulent discharge; hematuria may be present.

Proctitis and pharyngitis may develop following rectal and orogenital contact.

The majority of **women** are asymptomatic, although vaginal discharge, mild dysuria, frequency, pelvic pain, and dyspareunia, as well as proctitis and pharyngitis, may occur. Cervicitis, sometimes with minute follicles, and urethritis with mucopurulent secretion may be seen.

Diagnosis

Diagnosis is based on bacteriologic examination, and the exclusion of gonorrhea, trichomoniasis, candidiasis, and other causes of discharge. **In men,** Gram-stained slides of the urethral discharge will show a large number of polymorphonuclear leukocytes and some epithelial cells, but no pathogenic organisms. Cultures for gonococci, *Trichomonas*, and *Candida* will be negative. Examination of first-void urine will show an excess of pus cells but few or no organisms. If the diagnosis is in doubt, examination is made early in the morning after the urine has been held for 8 h or more. If infection is present, usually enough material for laboratory examination will be available from the urethra to confirm the diagnosis. *C. trachomatis* can be grown on culture from nearly half the cases. **In women,** Gram stain of a purulent cervical discharge will often show many leukocytes, but urethral Gram stains have not proved reliable.

See also PROCTITIS in Vol. II, Ch. 5.

Complications

In men, local complications include epididymitis, cystitis, prostatitis, and urethral stricture; in women, bartholinitis, cysts of Bartholin's glands, and salpingitis. A serious systemic complication is Reiter's syndrome, consisting of nonspecific urethritis, polyarthritis, and conjunctivitis or uveitis (see in Ch. 103).

Chlamydial ophthalmia neonatorum is increasingly being diagnosed in infants born to women with chlamydial cervicitis (see under NEONATAL INFECTIONS in Vol. II, Ch. 21).

Treatment

Uncomplicated infections are treated with tetracycline 500 mg orally q 6 h for 7 to 14 days. Patients who relapse or develop complications require longer courses (tetracycline 500 mg orally q 6 h for 21 to 28 days) and bed rest. **In pregnant women** with NSI, erythromycin (at the same dosage) should be substituted for tetracycline. Cysts of Bartholin's glands may require aspiration or surgical removal. About 20% of the patients have one or more relapses on follow-up and require retreatment. They often become anxious and depressed, and should be assured that they will eventually be cured.

Penicillin is *ineffective*. If appropriate treatment is not given, the signs and symptoms usually subside within 4 wk in about 60 to 70% of patients, but may recur, often with complications, in the ensuing months or years. Patients with complications usually benefit from bed rest and a longer course of antibiotics.

Patients should be advised to abstain from sexual intercourse until cured. The sexual partners should be examined and treated. All treated persons should be followed for 3 mo with regular clinical examinations, bacteriologic tests, and urine tests. STS should be done before treatment and after 3 mo.

SYPHILIS
(Lues)

A contagious systemic disease caused by the spirochete Treponema pallidum, *characterized by periods of active florid manifestations and by years of symptomless latency.* It can affect any tissue or vascular organ of the body and be passed from mother to fetus (congenital syphilis—see Vol. II, Ch. 5).

Classification (see TABLE 162–1)

ACQUIRED SYPHILIS

Etiology and Pathology

T. pallidum is a delicate spiral organism about 0.25 μm wide and from 5 to 20 μm long. It can be examined under a darkfield microscope or identified by fluorescent technics (see under Diagnosis, below). It does not grow on artifical media and cannot survive for long outside the human body, but it may be kept viable for many hours on special media or by subfreezing temperatures.

In acquired syphilis, *T. pallidum* enters the body through the mucous membranes or abrasions of the skin. Within hours the organisms reach the regional lymph nodes and rapidly disseminate throughout the body. The host tissues react by a perivascular infiltration of lymphocytes, plasma cells, and, later, fibroblasts, resulting in swelling and proliferation of the endothelium of the smaller blood vessels, leading to **endarteritis obliterans.** Healing occurs with scar tissue formation. In late syphilis, tissue hypersensitivity to *T. pallidum* leads to gummatous ulcerations and necrosis. Inflammatory changes are replaced by degenerative processes, especially in the cardiovascular and central nervous systems.

The CNS is invaded early in the infection, and during the secondary stage of the disease more than 30% of patients have an abnormal CSF (see TABLE 117–1 in Ch. 117). During the first 5 to 10 yr after infection, the disease principally involves the meninges and blood vessels, resulting in **meningovascular neurosyphilis;** later in the course of the disease the parenchyma of the brain and spinal cord are damaged, and degenerative changes lead to **parenchymatous neurosyphilis.** Involvement of the cerebral cortex and overlying meninges results in **general paresis.** Degenerative changes in the posterior columns and root ganglia of the spinal cord result in **tabes dorsalis.**

For **aortitis,** see SYPHILIS OF THE CARDIOVASCULAR SYSTEM in Ch. 24.

Epidemiology

Infection is usually transmitted by sexual contact, including orogenital and anorectal, and occasionally by kissing or close bodily contact. Promiscuous homosexual men are at the greatest risk. Untreated patients with primary or secondary syphilis having active lesions are the most infectious, and the risks of contagion are greatest during the first 2 yr (when treponemes are widely disseminated throughout the body), after which they gradually decline. Early latent syphilis is potentially infectious, but not late latent syphilis. Tertiary syphilis is not contagious. Infection with syphilis does not confer any lasting immunity against subsequent reinfection, particularly if antisyphilitic treatment is given early in the course of the disease.

TABLE 162–1. CLASSIFICATION OF SYPHILIS

Acquired	Congenital
Early infectious syphilis	**Early congenital syphilis** (symptomatic)
Primary stage	
Chancre; regional lymphadenopathy	The overt disease seen in infants up to age 2
Secondary stage	
Immediately follows primary stage	**Late congenital syphilis** (symptomatic)
Characterized by varied dermatologic lesions that mimic several disorders (e.g., skin rashes, erosions of mucous membranes, alopecia)	The stigmas seen in later life (e.g., Hutchinson's teeth, scars of interstitial keratitis, bony abnormalities)
Latent stage (asymptomatic; may persist indefinitely or be followed by late stage, below)	
Early latent syphilis (infection < 2 yr* duration; infectious lesions may recur)	(Congenital syphilis can also exist in a permanently latent, or asymptomatic, state.)
Late latent syphilis (infection > 2 yr* duration)	
Late or **tertiary** stage (symptomatic; not contagious)	
Benign tertiary (late benign) syphilis	
Cardiovascular syphilis	
Neurosyphilis	

* For reporting purposes, the division is sometimes made on a 4-yr, rather than a 2-yr, basis.

Symptoms, Signs, and Course

The incubation period of syphilis can vary from 1 to 13 wk, but is usually from 3 to 4 wk. The disease differs clinically with each patient.

Primary syphilis: The primary lesion or **chancre** generally appears within 4 wk of infection and heals within 4 to 8 wk in untreated patients. At the site of inoculation, it develops as a red papule that soon erodes, forming a painless ulcer. It is usually single, occasionally multiple, and has an indurated, hard base. It does not bleed but when abraded exudes a clear serum containing numerous *T. pallida*. A red areola may surround it. The regional lymphatic nodes become painlessly enlarged and are rubbery, discrete, indolent, and nontender on palpation. Primary chancres occur on the penis, anus, and rectum in men; the vulva, cervix, and perineum in women. Chancres may also be found on the lips, tongue, buccal mucosa, tonsils, or fingers, and rarely on other parts of the body.

Secondary syphilis: Cutaneous rashes usually appear within 6 to 12 wk after infection and are most florid after 3 to 4 mo. (About 25% of patients have a healing primary chancre.) The lesions may be transitory or may persist for months. In untreated patients they frequently heal but fresh ones may appear within weeks or months. Over 80% of patients have mucocutaneous lesions, 50% have generalized enlargement of the lymph nodes, and about 10% have lesions of the eyes, bones and joints, meninges, liver, and spleen. Mild constitutional symptoms of malaise, headache, anorexia, nausea, aching pains in the bones, and fatigability are often present, as well as fever, anemia, jaundice, albuminuria, and neck stiffness. At this stage a small number of patients develop acute syphilitic meningitis, with headache, neck stiffness, cranial nerve lesions, deafness, and occasional papilledema.

Syphilitic skin rashes may imitate a variety of dermatologic conditions (see Diagnosis, below). Usually they are symmetric and more marked on the flexor and volar surfaces of the body. They generally occur in crops, and papules may be found with macules, pustules, or squamous lesions. The individual spots are pigmented in black persons and pinkish or pale red in whites, are round and tend to become confluent and indurated, and generally do not itch. They eventually heal, usually without leaving a scar, but in some patients there may be areas of residual hyper- or depigmentation.

Frequently, there is a generalized, nontender, rubbery, discrete enlargement of the lymph nodes affecting the cervical, suboccipital, epitrochlear, axillary, and inguinal groups. The liver and spleen may be palpable in some patients. The surface of the mucous membranes frequently becomes eroded, forming mucous patches that are circular and often grayish-white with a red areola. These patches occur mostly in the mouth; on the palate, pharynx, larynx, glans penis, or vulva; or in the anal canal and rectum. Papules developing at the mucocutaneous junctions and in moist areas of the skin become hypertrophic, flattened, and dull pink or gray in color. They are termed **condylomata lata**, and are extremely infectious. The hair often falls out in patches, leaving a "moth-eaten" appearance. Some patients develop uveitis, meningitis, periostitis, or jaundice.

Latent syphilis: In early latent syphilis, infectious mucocutaneous relapses may occur during the first year, but after 2 yr the development of further contagious lesions is rare, and the patient appears normal. The latent stage may last for a few years or for the rest of the patient's life. In untreated cases, about ⅓ of those infected will develop late or tertiary syphilis. This may not occur for many years after the initial infection.

Late or **tertiary syphilis:** The clinical description of the lesions of late syphilis may be divided into (1) benign tertiary syphilis of the skin, bone, and viscera, (2) cardiovascular syphilis, and (3) neurosyphilis.

Lesions of **benign tertiary syphilis** usually develop within 3 to 10 yr of infection. The typical lesion is a **gumma** (a chronic granulomatous reaction). It is frequently localized but there may be diffuse gummatous infiltration of an organ or tissue. With localized lesions, an area of central necrosis is surrounded by granulation tissue. Gummas are indolent and increase in size slowly, gradually heal, and leave scars. Gummatous lesions may develop in the skin, where they result in nodular, ulcerative, or squamous skin eruptions. If they are subcutaneous, they result in punched-out ulcers with sloughing, washed-leather–appearing bases, which heal leaving typical tissue-paper scars. Often they occur in submucous tissue, especially of the palate, nasal septum, pharynx, and larynx, leading to tissue destruction with perforation of the palate or septum. They are most commonly found on the leg just below the knee, the upper trunk, the face, and the scalp, but may occur almost anywhere in the body, including the stomach, lung, liver, testicle, and choroid of the eye.

Diffuse gummatous infiltration affects the tongue, leading to chronic interstitial glossitis with leukoplakia and deep fissure formation. Carcinoma is a common sequel. A similar condition found in the testicle causes painless swelling with loss of testicular sensation.

Benign tertiary syphilis of the bones results in either periostitis with bone formation or osteitis with destructive lesions. The patient complains of a deep, boring pain, characteristically worse at night. A lump or swelling may be noticed if the area involved is superficial.

Cardiovascular syphilis is a serious manifestation of tertiary syphilis, usually appearing between 10 to 25 yr after the initial infection. (See in Ch. 24.)

Neurosyphilis develops in about 10 to 12% of untreated syphilitics. **Asymptomatic neurosyphilis** generally precedes symptomatic neurosyphilis and is found in about 15% of those originally diagnosed as having latent syphilis, in 12% of those with cardiovascular syphilis, and in 5% of those with benign tertiary syphilis. In asymptomatic neurosyphilis abnormalities may be present in the CSF (see Diagnosis, below).

Meningovascular neurosyphilis: When the cerebral cortex is principally involved, headache, dizziness, poor concentration, lassitude, insomnia, neck stiffness, and blurred vision occur. Mental confusion, epileptiform attacks, papilledema, aphasia, and mono- or hemiplegia may also be present. Cranial nerve palsies and pupillary abnormalities occur with basal meningitis. The **Argyll Robertson pupil,** which generally occurs only in neurosyphilis, is a small irregular pupil that reacts normally to accommodation but not to light.

When the spinal cord is involved there may be bulbar symptoms, weakness and wasting of the muscles of the shoulder girdle and arms, a slowly progressive spastic paraplegia with bladder symptoms, and in rare cases, a transverse myelitis with sudden flaccid paraplegia and loss of sphincter control.

Parenchymatous neurosyphilis: General paresis or **dementia paralytica** generally affects patients in their 40s or 50s. The onset usually is insidious and manifested by behavior changes. It also may present with convulsions or epileptic attacks, and there may be aphasia or a transient hemiparesis. Changes in the patient include irritability, difficulty in concentrating, memory deterioration, and defective judgment. Headaches and insomnia are associated with fatigue and lethargy. The patient's appearance becomes shabby, unkempt, and dirty; emotional instability leads to frequent weeping and temper tantrums; neurasthenia, depression, and delusions of grandeur with lack of insight may be present.

The physical signs include tremors of the mouth, tongue, outstretched hands, and whole body; pupillary abnormalities; dysarthria; brisk tendon reflexes; and, in some cases, extensor plantar responses. The handwriting usually is shaky and illegible. Signs of posterior column involvement accompany taboparesis. The lesions of **tabes dorsalis (locomotor ataxia)** result in pain, ataxia, sensory changes, and loss of tendon reflexes. Onset is slow and insidious. The first and most characteristic symptom usually is an intense, stabbing pain (lightning pain), that occurs in crops and recurs at irregular intervals, generally striking the legs. Later, unsteadiness of gait develops that is worse in the dark, and the patient may walk on a broad base with the feet wide apart. There may be a feeling of walking on foam rubber, with hyperesthesia and paresthesia. Loss of bladder sensation leads to retention of urine, with eventual incontinence. The urine often becomes infected. Impotence is common.

The majority of patients with tabes dorsalis are thin and have a characteristic sad-looking, tabetic facies. Argyll Robertson pupils usually are present and there may be primary optic atrophy. Examination of the lower limbs discloses hypotonia, diminished or absent tendon reflexes, impaired vibration and joint position sense, ataxia in the heel-shin test, and absence of deep pain sensation. **Romberg's sign** is positive and there is ataxia on walking. The bladder is frequently palpable.

Visceral crises appear as paroxysms of pain in various organs, the most common being gastric crises with vomiting. Rectal, bladder, and laryngeal crises also occur. **Trophic lesions** may develop in the later stages of the disease, and trophic ulcers may develop on the soles of the feet, penetrating deeply and involving the underlying bone. **Charcot's arthropathy,** a painless disorganization of a joint, with bony swelling and an abnormal range of movement, is a common manifestation.

Diagnosis

Diagnostic studies for syphilis should include a clinical history, a thorough physical examination, serologic tests, darkfield examination of fluids from lesions, CSF tests, radiologic examination, and investigations of all personal contacts where relevant.

Darkfield examination: In darkfield microscopy, light is directed obliquely through the slide in such a manner that the rays striking any organisms on the slide cause them to appear as bright objects against a dark background. The external morphology and motility of spirochetes present in exudates and tissue fluids from primary and secondary lesions may thus be observed and identified. Experience and skill are needed in taking the specimens and identifying the organism by its white appearance, regular coils, corkscrew rotation, watchspring movements, and angulation. The organism must be distinguished from other treponemes and spirochetes, many of which are not pathogenic.

Serologic tests for syphilis (STS): Two principal types aid in the diagnosis of syphilis and other treponemal diseases: (1) nonspecific screening or standard nontreponemal tests using lipoid antigens and testing for syphilitic reagin, and (2) specific or treponemal tests for antitreponemal antibodies.

The screening tests most frequently used are the **Venereal Disease Research Laboratory (VDRL)** and the **rapid plasma reagin (RPR)** tests. Specific tests include the **fluorescent treponemal antibody-absorption (FTA-ABS)** test, the *Treponema pallidum* **hemagglutination assay (TPHA),** and the *T. pallidum* **immobilization (TPI)** test.

The **VDRL test** is a flocculation test for syphilis in which reagin in the patient's serum reacts visibly with cardiolipin, the antigen. A number of conditions (e.g., acute infectious hepatitis) can increase serum reagin and produce a reactive VDRL test. Results are reported as reactive, weakly reactive, borderline, or nonreactive. Reactive and weakly reactive sera are considered positive for syphilitic antibodies. All reactive and weakly reactive VDRL tests should be confirmed using the more specific **FTA-ABS test,** which uses the Nichols strain of *T. pallidum* as the antigen.

The screening tests are easy to perform and inexpensive, but they lack the specificity of the treponemal tests and sometimes give biologic false-positive (BFP) results. A BFP reaction may be a clue to the presence of autoimmune or collagen vascular disorders, viral infection, or any condition with alterations in the globulin system. STS, carried out periodically, provide valuable information about the activity of the disease and the effects of treatment, but will not give positive results until 3 to 6 wk after the initial infection. Since the chancre usually develops before this, an early negative STS cannot rule out syphilis. If the screening tests are positive but the diagnosis is still uncertain, the more specific treponemal tests are performed. The FTA-ABS test, the most sensitive STS, usually becomes positive when the infection has been established 3 to 4 wk. In patients with undiagnosed genital lesions, the serologic tests should be repeated at 2-wk intervals for the first 6 wk and then monthly for 2 mo before the diagnosis of syphilis can be excluded.

CSF examination: Before treatment is given in all but the early infectious cases, examination of the CSF is essential to exclude neurosyphilis and to establish the diagnosis. The cell count, total protein, colloidal gold, and serologic tests are usually performed.

The diagnosis of primary syphilis depends on demonstrating the presence of *T. pallidum* in exudates taken from the chancre by darkfield microscopy. If the initial results are negative, the examinations should be repeated daily for at least 3 days. Aspirates from lymph node punctures may enable *T. pallidum* to be demonstrated in some cases, especially where topical antiseptics or antibiotics have been used.

The differential diagnosis of genital ulceration includes herpes genitalis, chancroid, lymphogranuloma venereum, scabies, mucous patches of secondary syphilis, erosive balanitis, Behçet's disease, gummatous ulceration, epithelioma, granuloma inguinale, tuberculous ulceration, and trauma. All genital ulcers should be considered syphilitic until proved otherwise. Because the possibility of syphilis is frequently overlooked by the physician, extragenital chancres are often misdiagnosed.

Diagnosis of secondary syphilis: Cutaneous eruptions and mucosal lesions should be considered syphilitic in origin if they are associated with generalized lymphadenopathy. The diagnosis is established by demonstrating the presence of *T. pallidum* on darkfield examination, and by positive STS. These are reactive in 99% of cases, often with a high titer.

A common error in differential diagnosis is to misdiagnose secondary syphilis for the following: a drug eruption, pityriasis rosea, rubella, infectious mononucleosis, erythema multiforme, pityriasis rubra pilaris, or fungal infections. Condylomata lata may be mistaken for warts, hemorrhoids, or pemphigus vegetans; scalp lesions for ringworm or alopecia areata; and mucous patches for a wide variety of other conditions. Syphilis can mimic most skin diseases and should be considered when evaluating skin and mucosal lesions, wherever its incidence is high.

The diagnosis of latent syphilis is made by excluding the other forms of syphilis. Patients should be suspected of latent syphilis who have persistently positive tests (including specific tests such as the FTA-ABS test, and the TPI test) without any clinical evidence of active syphilitic lesions. Their CSF tests are normal (as well as their heart and aorta) on radiologic examination. Latent acquired syphilis must be differentiated from latent congenital syphilis, latent yaws, other treponemal diseases found in patients from tropical areas, and BFP reactions.

Tertiary syphilis: Many patients give no history of primary or secondary manifestations, and it must be presumed that they were asymptomatic during the early stages, the manifestations were trivial or ignored, or the diagnosis was missed.

Benign tertiary syphilis: The history and physical signs should suggest the value of STS, which will be positive in most cases. Differentiation from other granulomatous conditions may be difficult, and biopsy may be helpful.

Cardiovascular syphilis: Symptoms and signs are sometimes so typical that a clinical diagnosis can easily be made. However, it may be confirmed by radiologic examination, ECG, and STS (see SYPHILIS OF THE CARDIOVASCULAR SYSTEM in Ch. 24). The CSF should be examined, as neurosyphilis and cardiovascular syphilis often occur concurrently.

Asymptomatic neurosyphilis: The CSF usually shows an elevated cell count, increased protein, and positive STS. In paresis, STS and the CSF are always positive. Additionally, the CSF will show an elevated cell count of 7 to 100 lymphocytes, increased protein, and a first-zone colloidal gold reaction. In tabes dorsalis the FTA-ABS tests are usually positive, but the serologic screening tests may be negative in 50% of cases. The CSF usually shows an increased cell count, a raised protein, weakly positive STS, and a midzone colloidal gold reaction. In many advanced cases the CSF may be normal.

Treatment

In primary and secondary syphilis, all the implications should be explained to the patient. All sexual contacts of the past 3 mo (in cases of primary syphilis) and those up to 1 yr (in cases of secondary syphilis) should be examined, treated, and informed that they may be contagious and should not have any form of sexual relations until examinations and tests show that they are no longer infectious, often a matter of several months.

Penicillin is the antibiotic of choice for all stages of syphilis, and a serum level of 0.03 IU/ml for 6 to 8 days is required to produce cure in early infectious syphilis. Benzathine penicillin G 2.4 million u. IM will produce a satisfactory blood level for 2 wk (1.2 million u. is usually given in each buttock). Many physicians give a 2nd injection of 2.4 million u. 10 to 14 days later to ensure an adequate blood level. Alternatively, aqueous procaine penicillin G 600,000 u./day IM for 10 days may be given. For penicillin-sensitive patients, erythromycin 500 mg orally q 6 h for 15 days or tetracycline (at the same dosage) may be used.

Patients with **early and late latent syphilis** should be treated with penicillin to prevent the subsequent development of tertiary manifestations. Benzathine penicillin G at a total dosage of 7.2 to 9.6 million u. may be given as single injections of 2.4 million u. IM once/wk for 3 or 4 wk. Alternatively, aqueous procaine penicillin G 600,000 u./day IM for 14 days may be given. Those sensitive to penicillin may be treated with erythromycin 500 mg q 6 h for 15 days. **Benign tertiary syphilis** is treated in the same way as latent syphilis, above; however, for those who cannot tolerate penicillin and are treated with erythromycin, it is advisable to give a second course of erythromycin at the same dosage 3 mo later.

Cardiovascular syphilis: Patients should be advised to avoid heavy lifting and strenuous exertion. Treatment of the syphilitic infection is the same as for latent syphilis, above, but procaine penicillin G usually is given for a total of 21 days. For treatment of the cardiovascular complications, see in Ch. 24.

Neurosyphilis: Penicillin is given as in latent syphilis, above, but procaine penicillin G should be given for a total of 21 days. Treatment of asymptomatic neurosyphilis prevents the development of symptomatic neurosyphilis. Chlorpromazine 25 or 50 mg orally or IM is effective in controlling restless patients with paresis, and analgesics should be used freely for tabetic patients with lightning pains. Carbamazepine 200 mg orally t.i.d. or q.i.d. is sometimes effective in controlling the pains.

Over 50% of the patients with early infectious syphilis, especially those with secondary syphilis, will have a **Herxheimer reaction** within 6 to 12 h after the initial treatment. It is manifested by general malaise, fever, headache, sweating, rigors, and a temporary exacerbation of the syphilitic lesions. It usually subsides within 1 or 2 h and is not dangerous to the patient apart from the anxiety it may produce. However, patients with general paresis or those with a high CSF cell count are likely to develop a Herxheimer reaction that occasionally causes serious disorders, such as a hemiplegia or monoplegia. The Herxheimer reaction should be explained to the patient before treatment is started. Administration of prednisone 5 mg orally q 6 h for 24 h before starting the penicillin and during the first 2 days of penicillin therapy reduces the risk of an unfavorable outcome should a reaction occur.

Surveillance

The importance of tests to confirm a permanent cure should be explained to the patient before treatment. Examinations and quantitative STS should be made monthly for 6 mo and every 3 mo thereafter for an additional 18 mo in **primary and secondary syphilis.** Following successful treatment, lesions heal rapidly and serologic titers fall, the reagin tests usually becoming negative within 9 to 12 mo. The specific tests, such as the FTA-ABS and the TPHA, usually remain positive for years or even for the rest of the patient's life. The CSF should be examined after 1 yr of surveillance. If the VDRL remains positive for more than 1 yr or if the titer starts to rise, re-treatment should be considered. Relapse is uncommon but occasionally occurs about the 6th to 9th mo. It may be clinical or serologic, or may involve the nervous system; it requires re-treatment with double the original dose of antibiotic. If all the clinical and serologic examinations remain satisfactory for 2 yr after treatment, the patient can be reassured that cure is complete and permanent and he need not return.

Patients with **latent syphilis** should be kept under surveillance at intervals of 3 mo for the first 2 to 3 yr, and those with persistently positive serologic tests should be seen annually indefinitely. The prognosis is excellent. Patients with **benign tertiary syphilis** should be examined at regular intervals after treatment, and those with **cardiovascular syphilis** should be followed throughout their lives.

In **asymptomatic neurosyphilis,** the CSF should be examined at 6-mo intervals until it has been normal for 2 yr; if the CSF is abnormal, it should be examined at 3-mo intervals until it is normal, and then annually for 2 yr more. Tabes dorsalis tends to progress despite treatment, and a careful watch should be kept for urinary tract infections.

BALANOPOSTHITIS; BALANITIS

Inflammation of the glans penis and the prepuce.

Etiology

Balanoposthitis (balanitis when in the circumcised) may be caused by complications of gonorrhea, trichomoniasis, candidiasis, Reiter's syndrome, and manifestations of secondary syphilis. Other causes include fixed drug eruptions, contact dermatitis, psoriasis, lichen planus, seborrheic dermatitis, lichen sclerosus et atrophicus, and erythroplasia of Queyrat. In many cases no cause can be found. Balanoposthitis is often associated with a tight prepuce. The subpreputial secretions become infected with anaerobic bacteria or Vincent's organisms, resulting in inflammation and tissue destruction. Diabetes mellitus predisposes to balanoposthitis.

Symptoms and Signs

Soreness, irritation, and a subpreputial discharge often occur 2 or 3 days after sexual intercourse. Phimosis (constriction of the foreskin) due to edema of the surface of the glans penis and prepuce may be present. Both may be eroded with superficial ulcerations. The inguinal lymphatic nodes may be tender and enlarged.

Diagnosis

Common STDs should be excluded, STS performed, and the urine tested for glucose. Smears and cultures of material from the inflamed surface should be taken.

Treatment

The appropriate treatment should be given if a specific cause is found. Saline washes should be carried out several times daily if no cause can be found. Subpreputial irrigations should be given if there is true phimosis. Oral sulfonamides, which will not mask incubating syphilis, should be given if there is significant secondary infection. Circumcision should be considered in patients with persistent phimosis once the inflammation has resolved.

163. THE MEDICAL EXAMINATION OF THE RAPE VICTIM

Rape may be defined as *illegal sexual penetration of any body orifice without consent*. Reported cases of female victims in the USA total 50,000/yr; estimates of unreported rape range from 2 to 10 times that number. Approximately 90% of rapists attack victims of the same race; 50% are known to their victims and are often members of the extended family. This is particularly important for preteen and teenage victims and has implications for follow-up and child abuse prevention. Most rapes are planned (not the result of sudden impulse), and over half the attacks involve a weapon, usually a knife. Approximately 50% of female rape victims show signs of physical trauma; over 10% require medical attention.

Although rape is usually thought of in the context of the female victim, a growing number of rape victims are males who are not necessarily part of a prison or homosexual community. The male victim is more likely to have physical trauma than the female, to have been victimized by several assailants, and to be more unwilling to report the crime. For both males and females, however, the assault is the sexual expression of aggression, anger, or need for power. It is a violent, much more than a sexual, act. A few cases of female rapes of males have been reported in the last several years.

Evaluation Procedures

Although provision of medical care and psychologic support for the rape victim is the first concern, the patient is a victim of a crime, and forensic medicine requires certain special details of medical evaluation and record-keeping. TABLE 163–1 may serve as a guide for examination procedures and the medical record, to be adapted according to local requirements. Such a record is sometimes admissible in court and aids recall if testimony is required later. The record should never, unless subpoenaed, be released without written consent of the patient.

Wherever possible, the patient should be treated in a rape treatment center, which should be separate from routine emergency-room care and staffed by trained, concerned support personnel.

History and physical examination: A brief account of the attack by the patient will indicate areas for medical investigation and treatment. However, recounting the events is often frightening for the patient, and a complete history may have to be deferred until more immediate needs have been met. The reasons for the questions asked and for the examination procedure are not always clear to patients; e.g., it may need to be explained that knowledge of the last menstrual period, or the use of a contraceptive, will help determine the risk of pregnancy, or that information concerning the time of the last previous coitus is important in establishing validity of sperm testing.

Since the patient has been through an experience to which he or she did not consent, enlisting the patient's cooperation in the examination is important. Female rape victims may feel anxiety at being examined by a male physician. For this reason, and also for the purpose of corroborating the procedures, it is essential that a female nurse or volunteer be present during the examination.

The evidence collected during the examination, and all laboratory specimens, are placed in individual packages and carefully labeled, dated, and sealed. Receipts should be obtained upon delivery to the laboratory or police.

Psychologic assessment: Rape presents both psychologic and social problems for the victims, who must handle their own feelings as well as face the often judgmental reactions of friends, family, and officials. Long-range effects of rape include aversion to sex, anxiety, phobias, suspiciousness, and depression.

Primary reactions are fear and anger, although patients' outward responses range from talkativeness, tenseness, crying, and trembling to dispassion, quiescence, and smiling. The latter responses are rarely an indication that the patient is unconcerned; they may be avoidance reactions or may occur in patients who have coping styles that require control of emotion or who are physically exhausted. The anger felt by many victims may be displaced onto hospital personnel, who should be aware of this and not troubled by it.

Guilt feelings occur when the patient feels, generally irrationally, that somehow he or she provoked or should have prevented the attack, or feels that the attack was a punishment for some imagined wrongdoing.

The physician's report may include a brief account of the attack in the patient's words and a statement of the physician's clinical determination as to injuries and sexual activity. It is not necessary to state whether rape occurred, since that is a legal determination, but one should record a diagnosis including all probable or possible physical and psychologic problems.

Treatment

Mild sedation may be necessary. Most physical trauma is minor and is treated conservatively. More severe injuries may require surgical repair.

Psychologic trauma: An unhurried, nonjudgmental, listening attitude by the examiner is therapeutic. *Since the full psychologic impact cannot be ascertained at the first examination, follow-up visits must be scheduled.* If the patient's acute reactions do not subside or if long-range psychologic problems seem likely, psychiatric referral is indicated.

Prophylaxis for sexually transmitted disease: If it is suspected that the assailant had gonorrhea or syphilis, the patient is immediately given probenecid 1 gm orally followed by procaine penicillin G and benzathine penicillin G 4.8 million u. IM in divided doses at 2 sites. Penicillin-allergic patients should be given (for gonorrhea) tetracycline hydrochloride 0.5 gm orally q.i.d. for 5 days; for syphilis, the dosage is for 15 consecutive days.

TABLE 163–1. EXAMINATION FOR ALLEGED RAPE

Name of patient: Date of examination:
    Address: Time:
    Phone: Location:
    Age:
    Sex:
Name of guardian, if patient is under age:
    Address:
    Phone:
Name of person accompanying patient to hospital:
    Address:
    Phone:
Name of police officer, badge number, and department:

HISTORY
    Circumstances of attack
        Date and time:
        Location (familiar to patient?):
        Assailant(s):
            Number:
            Name(s), if known:
            Description(s):
            Weapon:
        Type of sexual contact (vaginal, oral, rectal):
            Condom used?
        Activities of patient after attack
            Douche: Medication:
            Bath: Other:
            Clothing change:
    Last menstrual period:
    Date of previous coitus and time, if recent:
    Contraceptive history (oral, IUD, etc.):

PHYSICAL EXAMINATION
    General trauma (extragenital)
        Head: Chest: Arms:
        Face: Abdomen: Legs:
        Throat: Back: Other:
    Genital trauma
        Perineum: Vulva: Cervix:
        Hymen: Vagina: Anus:
    Foreign material on body (stains, hair, dirt, twigs, etc.):
    Evidence of alcohol or other drugs:
    Evidence of existing pregnancy:

PSYCHOLOGIC ASSESSMENT
    Patient's emotional or mental state:

(Continued)

TABLE 163–1. EXAMINATION FOR ALLEGED RAPE *(Cont'd)*

LABORATORY FINDINGS

Clothing:　Note condition (damaged, stained, foreign material adhering)
　　　　　　Provide small samples, including unstained sample, or give clothing to police or
　　　　　　　laboratory

Hair samples:　Loose hairs adhering to patient or clothing
　　　　　　　Semen-encrusted pubic hair
　　　　　　　Clipped pubic hair of victim—at least ten (for comparison)

Other specimens, as indicated by the history or physical examination:

	Tests	*From*	*To determine*
Semen	Papanicolaou	Vagina	Sperm motility, nonmotility
	Saline suspension*	Cervix	Sperm morphology
	Acid phosphatase†	Rectum	Presence of A, B, or H blood
	Other (e.g., bacterial cultures)	Mouth	group substances‡
		Thighs	Gonorrhea
		Other	

Baseline VDRL and gonorrhea cultures
Blood　　　　　　　　　　　　　　　　　　　　　　　Blood group
　(including dried samples on patient's　　　　　　Presence of drugs, alcohol
　　body and clothing)　　　　　　　　　　　　　　Pregnancy

Urine　　　　　　　　　　　　　　　　　　　　　　Presence of drugs, alcohol
　　　　　　　　　　　　　　　　　　　　　　　　　Pregnancy

TREATMENT

REFERRAL

PHYSICIAN'S CLINICAL COMMENTS
　Signed:　　　　　　　　　　　　　　　　　　　MD State License No:

WITNESS TO EXAMINATION
　Signed:

DISPOSITION OF EVIDENCE
　Delivered by:　　　　　　　　　　　　　　　Date:　　　Time:
　Received by:　　　　　　　　　　　　　　　Date:　　　Time:

* Should be performed by examining physician if time factor permits discovery of motile sperm.
† A useful test, since no sperm will be found if the assailant had a vasectomy, is oligospermic, or used a condom. If test cannot be performed immediately, specimen should be placed in a freezer.
‡ In 80% of cases, blood group substances are found in semen.

Adapted from I. Root, W. Ogden, and W. Scott, "The Medical Investigation of Alleged Rape," *The Western Journal of Medicine* Vol. 120, No. 4, pp. 329–333, April 1974. Copyright 1974 by the California Medical Association. Used with permission.

Pregnancy: Factors determining the possibility of a pregnancy include the patient's menstrual cycle phase and whether or not contraceptives were used. HCG tests make such determinations easier. If pregnancy seems possible, diethylstilbestrol **(DES)** 25 mg orally b.i.d. for 5 days is started within 24 to 48 h, but should be accompanied by antiemetic medication (prochlorperazine 10 mg q.i.d. orally for 5 days). The patient should be told of other possible side effects from DES, such as abdominal pain or vaginal spotting. Other estrogens also may be given. If it is suspected that the patient is already pregnant, estrogens should not be given until this possibility is evaluated. The patient's attitude toward abortion should be explored.

Additional considerations include: (1) Provision of privacy for examination and consultation. (2) Provision of cleansing facilities and toilet. Many patients will want to wash (some will have been urinated on or have been raped out of doors); some will want to use a mouthwash. (3) Provision of money or transportation to get home. (4) If a rape crisis team operates in the area, referral can provide helpful medical, psychologic, and legal support to the victim.

Follow-up should include tests for gonorrhea, syphilis, and pregnancy within 6 wk. If pregnancy occurs, consideration should be given to its termination. A further test for syphilis should be done at 6 mo. (See also discussion of follow-up in psychologic trauma, above.)

164. CLINICAL EVALUATION OF COMPLAINTS REFERABLE TO THE EARS

A thorough history should be taken and a physical examination performed with emphasis on the ear, nose, and nasopharynx, and on transillumination of the paranasal sinuses. In addition, the teeth, tongue, tonsils, hypopharynx, larynx, salivary glands, and temporomandibular joints should be examined, since pain and discomfort may be referred from them to the ears. Radiography of the temporal bone is usually indicated in trauma to the ear, possible basal skull fracture, perforation of the tympanic membrane, hearing loss, vertigo, facial paralysis, and otalgia of obscure origin.

CLINICAL MEASUREMENT OF HEARING

Hearing loss due to a lesion in the external auditory canal or the middle ear is called **conductive**, while hearing loss due to a lesion in the inner ear or the 8th nerve is called **sensorineural**. Conductive and sensorineural hearing loss can be differentiated by comparing the threshold of hearing by air conduction with that by bone conduction (see also DIFFERENTIATION OF SENSORY [COCHLEAR] AND NEURAL [8TH NERVE] HEARING LOSSES, below).

Hearing by air conduction is tested by presenting an acoustic stimulus, in air, to the ear. A hearing loss or elevation of the threshold demonstrated in this way can be caused by a defect in any part of the hearing apparatus—external auditory canal, middle ear, inner ear, 8th nerve, or central auditory pathways.

Hearing by bone conduction is tested by placing a sounding source (e.g., tuning fork) in contact with the head. This causes vibration throughout the skull, including the walls of the bony cochlea, and stimulates the inner ear directly. Because sensitivity of the cochlea is clinically unaffected by outer and middle ear pathology, hearing by bone conduction bypasses the external and middle ear and tests the integrity of the inner ear, 8th nerve, and central pathways.

If the air conduction threshold is elevated and the bone conduction threshold is normal, the hearing loss is *conductive*. If both air and bone conduction thresholds are elevated equally, the hearing loss is *sensorineural*. Occasionally, a **composite** or **mixed** loss of hearing occurs, with both conductive and sensorineural components. Under these circumstances, both bone and air conduction thresholds are elevated, the air conduction more than the bone.

The Weber and Rinne tuning fork tests are used to differentiate a conductive from a sensorineural hearing loss. The **Weber tuning fork test** is performed by placing the stem of a vibrating tuning fork on the midline of the head and having the patient indicate in which ear the tone is heard. The patient with a unilateral *conductive* hearing loss hears the tone louder in the affected ear, for reasons that are unclear. By contrast, the patient with a unilateral *sensorineural* loss hears the tone in the unaffected ear, because the tuning fork stimulates both inner ears equally and the patient perceives the stimulus with the more sensitive, unaffected end organ and nerve.

The **Rinne tuning fork test** compares hearing ability by air conduction with that by bone conduction. The tines of a vibrating tuning fork are held near the pinna (air conduction) and then the stem of the vibrating tuning fork is placed in contact with the mastoid process (bone conduction) and the patient is asked to indicate which stimulus is louder. Normally the stimulus is heard longer and louder by air conduction than by bone conduction; e.g., 40 seconds by air conduction and 20 seconds by bone conduction (AC>BC). With a conductive hearing loss, this ratio is reversed; the bone conduction stimulus will be perceived longer and louder than the air conduction stimulus (BC>AC). With a sensorineural hearing loss, both air and bone conduction perception are reduced, but the ratio remains the same (AC>BC).

The **audiometer** is used to quantitate hearing loss. With this electronic device, acoustic stimuli of specific frequencies are delivered at specific intensities in order to determine the patient's hearing threshold for each frequency. The hearing for each ear is measured from 125 or 250 to 8000 Hz by air conduction (using earphones) and by bone conduction (using an oscillator in contact with the head). Hearing loss is measured in decibels (**db**), which equal 10 times the logarithm of the ratio of the acoustic power of a stimulus required to achieve hearing threshold in a patient to the acoustic power required to achieve threshold in a normal individual. Test results are plotted on a graph called an audiogram (FIG. 164–1). If intense tones are presented to one ear, they may be heard in the other ear. The Rinne tuning fork test and audiometry require the use of masking for accurate results.

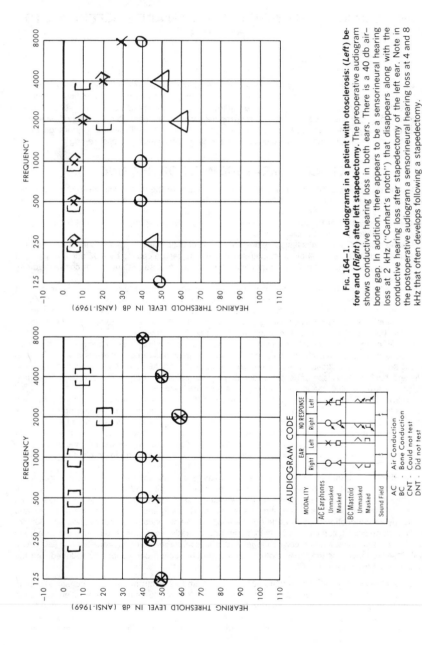

Fig. 164–1.   Audiograms in a patient with otosclerosis: (*Left*) before and (*Right*) after left stapedectomy. The preoperative audiogram shows conductive hearing loss in both ears. There is a 40 db air–bone gap. In addition, there appears to be a sensorineural hearing loss at 2 kHz ("Carhart's notch") that disappears along with the conductive hearing loss after stapedectomy of the left ear. Note in the postoperative audiogram a sensorineural hearing loss at 4 and 8 kHz that often develops following a stapedectomy.

Masking is the presentation of sound (usually noise) to the ear not being tested so that the responses are based on hearing in the ear being tested.

Speech audiometry: The **speech reception threshold (SRT),** the intensity at which speech is recognized as a meaningful symbol, is determined by presenting a list of spondee words (2 syllables equally accented, such as *railroad, staircase, baseball*) at specific intensities, noting the intensity at which the patient repeats 50% of the words correctly. The SRT usually approximates the average hearing levels at the speech frequencies of 500, 1000, and 2000 Hz.

The ability to discriminate the various speech sounds or phonemes is determined by presenting a list of 50 phonetically balanced words, containing the phonemes in the same relative frequency as in conversational English, at an intensity of 40 db above the SRT. The percentage of words correctly repeated by the patient is the **discrimination score,** normally 90 to 100%. The discrimination score remains in the normal range in conductive hearing losses, but is reduced in sensorineural hearing losses because analysis of the speech sounds by the inner ear and 8th nerve is impaired. Discrimination tends to be poorer in neural than in sensory hearing losses.

The impedance of the middle ear to acoustical energy can be measured by **tympanometry** without voluntary participation by the patient, requiring only that the patient remain quiet during the test; a sounding source and microphone sealed in the external auditory canal can measure the acoustical energy absorbed (passing through) or reflected by the middle ear. In conductive hearing loss, the middle ear absorbs relatively less sound and reflects relatively more sound. Normally the greatest compliance of the middle ear occurs with a pressure in the external auditory canal equal to atmospheric pressure. Increasing or decreasing the pressure in the external auditory canal demonstrates various patterns of compliance. With a relatively negative pressure in the middle ear, as in eustachian tube obstruction and middle ear effusion, maximal compliance occurs with a negative pressure in the external auditory canal. With discontinuity of the ossicular chain, as in necrosis or dislocation of the long process of the incus, no point of maximal compliance can be obtained. With fixation of the ossicular chain, as in stapedial footplate ankylosis in otosclerosis, compliance may remain normal or may be reduced. Tympanometry has been used to screen children for middle ear effusions (serous or secretory otitis media), to provide diagnostic clues, and to confirm the type of lesion in patients with conductive hearing losses.

This technic can detect changes in compliance produced by reflex contraction of the stapedius muscle; the reflex is initiated by presenting to the same or opposite ear a tone approximately 80 db above the hearing threshold. The presence or absence of the reflex is important in the topographical diagnosis of facial nerve paralysis. The reflex adapts or decays in neural hearing losses, and presence or absence of reflex adaptation or decay, especially below 2000 Hz, aids in differential diagnosis of sensory and neural hearing losses. The reflex can also confirm voluntary threshold responses.

When the patient cannot or will not respond voluntarily to acoustic stimuli, measuring the cochlear microphonic response and action potentials of the 8th nerve **(electrocochleography)** and evoked responses from the brainstem and auditory cortex **(evoked response audiometry)** to acoustic stimuli has been useful in evaluating infants and children suspected of having profound hearing loss (see also CLINICAL MEASUREMENT OF HEARING IN CHILDREN in Vol. II, Ch. 24 and SCREENING PROCEDURES in Vol. II, Ch. 23), individuals suspected of feigning or exaggerating a hearing loss (psychogenic hypacusis), and patients with sensorineural hearing loss of obscure etiology. Seven sequential wave forms have been identified that occur in the 8th nerve and central auditory pathways in response to acoustic stimuli. Lesions of the 8th nerve and brainstem auditory pathways result in changes in the amplitude and latency of the wave forms; these changes in latency of the wave forms are often of diagnostic value. Evoked-response audiometry is used in coma to determine the functional integrity of the brainstem.

DIFFERENTIATION OF SENSORY (COCHLEAR) AND NEURAL (8TH NERVE) HEARING LOSSES

The term *sensorineural* indicates that it is not certain whether the loss of hearing is due to a lesion in the inner ear or in the 8th nerve. The differentiation between sensory (cochlear) and neural (8th nerve) hearing loss is clinically important. **Sensory hearing losses** result from end-organ lesions (acoustic trauma, viral endolymphatic labyrinthitis, ototoxic drugs, Ménière's disease) that usually represent no threat to life. On the other hand, **neural hearing losses** are frequently due to cerebellopontine angle tumors, and these 8th nerve lesions are potentially fatal.

Sensory and neural hearing losses may be differentiated on the basis of tests for recruitment, sensitivity to small increments in intensity, and pathologic adaptation, including stapedial reflex decay as discussed above.

Recruitment (abnormal increase in the perception of loudness or the ability to hear loud sounds normally despite a hearing loss) is absent in neural hearing losses and present in sensory hearing losses. Recruitment can be demonstrated by having the patient compare the loudness of sounds in the affected ear with the loudness of sounds in the normal ear. In sensory hearing losses, the sensation of loudness in the affected ear increases more with each increment in intensity than it does in the normal ear. In neural hearing losses, the sensation of loudness in the affected ear increases less with each increment in intensity than it does in the normal ear (decruitment).

Sensitivity to small increments in intensity can be demonstrated by presenting a continuous tone of 20 db above the hearing threshold and increasing the intensity by 1 db briefly and intermittently. The percentage of small increments that the patient can detect yields the **short increment sensitivity index (SISI)**. A high SISI (80 to 100%) is characteristic of sensory hearing losses, while a patient with a neural lesion, like a person with normal hearing, cannot detect such small changes in intensity.

Pathologic adaptation is demonstrated when a patient cannot continue to perceive a constant tone above the threshold of hearing **(tone decay)**. The tone decay test for pathologic adaptation is mildly abnormal in sensory lesions and severely abnormal in neural lesions.

Several of these phenomena may be demonstrated with the **Békésy automatic audiometer**, in which the intensity of the stimulus can be controlled by the patient. The patient is instructed to depress a button when he hears the stimulus, which causes the intensity of the stimulus to decrease. When the stimulus is no longer audible, the patient releases the button, and the intensity begins to increase. In this way the patient traces back and forth across his threshold of hearing. Over the course of a 5-min period, the frequency of the test tone may be gradually increased from 100 to 10,000 Hz. If pathologic adaptation is present, it can be demonstrated by decay of the response to a continuous presentation of the test stimulus. The decay of the response can be reduced or eliminated by interrupting the tone for 0.5 second every second. Testing with continuous and interrupted tone presentations yields 5 patterns of tracings. In the Type I pattern, the continuous and interrupted tracings are superimposed. This pattern is found in normal hearing and in conductive hearing losses. In the Type II pattern, the 2 tracings are superimposed up to 1000 Hz. Above this frequency, the continuous tracing separates by about 20 db from the interrupted tracing, and in the higher frequencies the excursions of the continuous tracings become smaller. This pattern is characteristic of sensory hearing losses, as in Ménière's disease, and indicates mild pathologic adaptation. In the Type III pattern, the continuous tracing separates sharply from the interrupted tracing at a lower frequency, and the excursions of the continuous tracing do not become smaller. This pattern is characteristic of neural lesions, such as acoustic neurinomas, and indicates severe pathologic adaptation. In the Type IV pattern, the continuous tracing separates from the interrupted tracing at all frequencies, and the excursions of the continuous tracing may or may not become smaller. This pattern is indicative of active cochlear lesions (such as a recent attack of Ménière's disease) or of early neural lesions. In the Type V pattern, the continuous and interrupted tracings are separated but the apparent threshold of the interrupted tracing is greater than the continuous tracing. This pattern occurs in psychogenic or feigned hearing loss.

Patients with complaints referable to one cranial nerve, such as the 8th cranial nerve, deserve thorough neurologic evaluation. Emphasis has been placed in this discussion on thorough evaluation of the auditory division of the 8th nerve and its end organ. Further evaluation of the patient should include vestibular testing (see below) and may require lumbar puncture, polytomography of the internal auditory canals, CT of the head, and posterior fossa myelography.

TINNITUS

The perception of sound in the absence of an acoustic stimulus. Tinnitus, a subjective experience of the patient, is distinguished from **bruit,** noise that may be heard by the examiner and often by the patient as well.

Tinnitus may be of a buzzing, ringing, roaring, whistling, or hissing quality or may involve more complex sounds that vary over time. Tinnitus may be intermittent or continuous. An associated hearing loss is usually present.

The mechanism involved in the production of tinnitus remains obscure. Tinnitus may occur as a symptom of nearly all ear disorders, including obstruction of the external auditory canal due to cerumen and foreign bodies, infectious processes (external otitis, myringitis, otitis media, labyrinthitis, petrositis, syphilis, meningitis), eustachian tube obstruction, otosclerosis, Ménière's disease, arachnoiditis, cerebellopontine angle tumors, ototoxicity (due to salicylates, quinine and its synthetic analogs, aminoglycoside antibiotics, certain diuretics, carbon monoxide, heavy metals, alcohol, etc.), cardiovascular diseases (hypertension, arteriosclerosis, etc.), anemia, hypothyroidism, hereditary sensorineural hearing loss, noise-induced hearing loss, acoustic trauma (blast injury), and head trauma.

Treatment

The patient's ability to tolerate the tinnitus varies. Treatment should be directed toward the underlying disease, since its amelioration may produce improvement in the tinnitus. Although there is no specific medical or surgical therapy for tinnitus, many patients find relief by playing background music to mask the tinnitus and even go to sleep with the radio playing. Some patients benefit from use of a tinnitus masker, a device that is worn like a hearing aid and that presents a noise more pleasant than the tinnitus.

EARACHE

Pain occurs with infections and neoplasms in the external ear and middle ear or is referred to the ear from remote disease processes. Even mild inflammation in the external auditory canal produces severe pain. Perichondritis of the pinna produces severe pain and tenderness. With eustachian tube obstruction, abrupt changes in middle-ear pressure relative to atmospheric pressure may result in painful retraction of the tympanic membrane. Infection in the middle ear results in painful inflammation of the middle-ear mucous membrane and pain due to increased pressure in the middle ear with bulging of the tympanic membrane. The commonest cause of earache in children, acute otitis media, requires prompt examination by a physician and antibiotic therapy to prevent serious sequelae. In the absence of disease in the ear, the source of referred otalgia should be sought in those areas receiving sensory supply from the cranial nerves that subserve sensation in the external ear and middle ear—i.e., the trigeminal, glossopharyngeal, and vagus nerves. Specifically, the cause of obscure otalgia should be sought in the nose, paranasal sinuses, nasopharynx, teeth, gingiva, temporomandibular joints, mandible, tongue, palatine tonsils, pharynx, hypopharynx, larynx, trachea, and esophagus. Occult neoplasms in these locations often first make their presence known by pain referred to the ear.

Treatment depends on identifying the cause of the pain and providing the therapy appropriate for that disease.

CLINICAL EVALUATION OF THE VESTIBULAR APPARATUS

Patients with vertigo, difficulty with balance, or a sensorineural hearing loss of unknown etiology should have vestibular function tested. Since the results in each ear can be compared, caloric tests are more useful clinically than stimulation with acceleration or deceleration in rotational, torsion swing, and lateral swing tests.

Artificial stimulation of the vestibular apparatus produces nystagmus, past-pointing, falling, and autonomic responses such as sweating, vomiting, hypotension, and bradycardia. **Nystagmus,** the most useful response, can be monitored visually or, more reliably, by recording changes in the corneoretinal potential (electronystagmography). Vestibular nystagmus is a rhythmic movement of the eyes. It has a quick and a slow component and may be rotary, vertical, or horizontal. The direction of the nystagmus is determined by the direction of the quick component because it is easier to see. However, the slow component is the more fundamental response to vestibular stimulation, while the quick component is compensatory. The slow component moves in the direction of the movement of the endolymph. Past-pointing and falling are also in the direction of movement of the endolymph. The hallucination of the movement of the environment is in the direction of endolymphatic flow, and the hallucination of the movement of the subject is in the direction opposite to that of endolymphatic flow.

Caloric stimulation produces convection currents within the endolymph. These currents cause movement of the cupula in the ampulla of the horizontal semicircular canal, which occurs in one direction during cooling and in the opposite direction during warming.

The **Hallpike caloric test,** an accurate and reproducible measure of vestibular sensitivity, is performed with the patient supine and the head elevated 30 degrees to bring the horizontal semicircular canal into a vertical position. Each ear is irrigated with 240 ml of water delivered in 40 seconds, first at 30 C (86 F) and then at 44 C (110 F). The resulting nystagmus is monitored with the patient gazing straight ahead. Irrigation of the ear with cool water produces nystagmus to the opposite side; warm water produces nystagmus to the same side. A mnemonic device is COWS (cold to the opposite and warm to the same).

The duration of the nystagmus, the velocity of the slow component, or the frequency of the nystagmus may be measured. **Canal paresis,** a unilateral reduction or absence of sensitivity, and **directional preponderance,** a relative exaggeration of the nystagmic response in one direction, can be demonstrated. Various combinations of canal paresis and directional preponderance may coexist. The presence of canal paresis, directional preponderance, or combinations of the two signal an organic lesion—end organ, 8th nerve, brainstem, or cerebellar—but do not necessarily indicate on which side the lesion is. Occasionally, an important differential point rests on the caloric examination. Acoustic neurinomas frequently show canal paresis or complete lack of response on the side of the tumor. A normal response to caloric stimulation casts serious doubt on the diagnosis of an acoustic neurinoma.

165.   EXTERNAL EAR

OBSTRUCTIONS
(See Vol. II, Ch. 25)

EXTERNAL OTITIS
(See Vol. II, Ch. 24)

PERICHONDRITIS

Trauma, insect bites, and incision of superficial infections of the pinna may initiate perichondritis, which causes an accumulation of pus between the cartilage and the perichondrium that cuts off the blood supply to the cartilage, with consequent avascular necrosis. Septic necrosis also plays a role. The infection tends to be indolent, long-lasting, and destructive. Perichondritis is often caused by a gram-negative rod. **Treatment:** Wide incision for drainage is followed by a dressing to reapproximate the blood supply to the cartilage. Systemic antibiotic therapy is indicated and should be guided by culture and sensitivity studies.

AURAL ECZEMATOID DERMATITIS

Eczema, characterized by itching, redness, discharge, desquamation, and even fissuring leading to secondary infection, frequently involves the pinna and ear canal. Recurrences are common. **Treatment:** Dilute aluminum acetate solution (Burow's solution) is applied as often as required. Itching and inflammation can be reduced with topical corticosteroids.

TRAUMA

Hematoma

A subperichondrial hematoma may result from blunt trauma to the pinna. The external ear becomes a shapeless, reddish-purple mass when blood collects between the perichondrium and the cartilage. Since the perichondrium carries the blood supply to the cartilage, avascular necrosis of the cartilage may occur. The "cauliflower ear" characteristic of wrestlers and boxers is the consequence of an organized and calcified hematoma. **Treatment:** The clot must be evacuated through an incision, and the skin and perichondrium are reapproximated to the cartilage with suction drainage or with splints of cotton soaked in benzoin, forming a dressing to keep the cartilage and its blood supply in close approximation.

Lacerations

For lacerations of the external ear that penetrate the cartilage and the skin on both sides, the skin margins are sutured, the cartilage is splinted externally with benzoin-impregnated cotton, and a protective dressing is applied. Sutures should not extend into the cartilage.

Fractures

Forceful blows to the mandible may be transmitted to the anterior wall of the ear canal (posterior wall of the glenoid fossa). Displaced fragments from fractures of the anterior wall of the canal may cause stenosis of the canal and must be excised, under general anesthesia.

TUMORS

Sebaceous cysts, osteomas, and keloids may arise in and occlude the ear canal and cause retention of cerumen and a conductive hearing loss. Excision is the treatment of choice.

Ceruminomas arise in the outer third of the external auditory canal. Although these tumors appear benign histologically, they behave in a malignant manner and should be excised widely.

Basal cell and squamous cell carcinomas frequently develop on the external ear following regular exposure to the sun. Early lesions can be successfully treated with cautery and curettage or irradiation. More advanced lesions require surgical excision of V-shaped wedges or larger amounts of the external ear. Invasion of cartilage makes irradiation therapy less effective and surgery the preferred treatment. Basal cell and squamous cell carcinomas may also arise in or secondarily invade the external auditory canal. Persistent inflammation in chronic otitis media may predispose the development of squamous cell carcinoma. Extensive resection is indicated. En bloc resection of the external auditory canal with sparing of the facial nerve is performed when lesions are limited to the canal and have not invaded the middle ear.

166.   TYMPANIC MEMBRANE AND MIDDLE EAR

(See Vol. II, Ch. 24 for INFECTIOUS MYRINGITIS; ACUTE OTITIS MEDIA; SECRETORY OTITIS MEDIA; ACUTE MASTOIDITIS; and CHRONIC OTITIS MEDIA)

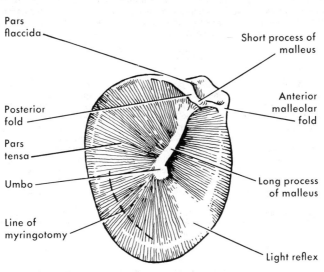

FIG. 166–1.   The tympanic membrane (right ear).

General Considerations

The patient with a middle ear disorder may present with one or more of the following complaints: a feeling of fullness or pressure in the ear; constant or intermittent, mild to excruciating pain; diminished hearing; tinnitus; and vertigo. In acute otitis media, systemic symptoms (e.g., fever) are commonly present in addition. The symptoms may begin with a feeling of fullness and progress serially in additive fashion. Infants and children, especially, may be febrile and present with other prominent systemic manifestations (anorexia, vomiting, diarrhea, lethargy, etc.).

The symptoms may result from infection, trauma, and disturbed pressure relationships secondary to eustachian tube obstruction. In determining the cause, the physician should elicit information about antecedent and associated symptoms (e.g., rhinorrhea, nasal obstruction, sore throat, upper respiratory infection, allergic manifestations; headache or other evidence of meningeal involvement; systemic symptoms). The appearance of the external auditory canal and tympanic membrane often yields diagnostic clues; the nose, nasopharynx, and oropharynx should also be examined for signs of infection and allergy and for evidence of an underlying disorder—e.g., a neoplasm of the nasopharynx.

The function of the middle ear should be evaluated with pneumatic otoscopy, the Weber and Rinne tuning fork tests, tympanometry, and audiometry.

TRAUMA

The tympanic membrane may be punctured and the tympanum penetrated by objects placed in the ear canal (e.g., cotton applicators) or entering the canal accidentally (e.g., twigs on a tree or missiles such as pencils or hot slag). A sudden overpressure, as in an explosion (acoustic trauma), a slap, or swimming and diving accidents, or a sudden negative pressure, as in a kiss over the ear, also can perforate the tympanic membrane. Penetration of the eardrum may cause dislocations of the ossicular chain.

Symptoms and Signs

Traumatic perforation of the tympanic membrane results in sudden severe pain followed by bleeding from the ear. A loss of hearing and tinnitus occur. The loss of hearing is more severe if there has been a disruption of the ossicular chain. Vertigo suggests an associated injury to the inner ear, as occasionally a portion of the stapes or a missile is driven into the inner ear. Purulent otorrhea may begin in 24 to 48 h.

Treatment

Following perforation, oral penicillin G or V 250 mg q 6 h should be given for 7 days to prevent infection. Aseptic technic is used in examining the ear. If necessary, under local anesthesia and microscopic control, the displaced flaps of tympanic membrane may be laid in their original positons to facilitate healing. The ear is kept dry, and topical medication with 0.5% acetic acid, 5 drops t.i.d., though not used prophylactically, may be employed if the ear becomes infected. Spontaneous closure of the perforation is usual; a tympanoplasty is indicated if the perforation does not heal spontaneously within 2 mo. A persistent conductive hearing loss suggests discontinuity of the ossicular chain, and the middle ear should be explored surgically and repaired. Vertigo that persists for hours or longer following the injury indicates penetration of the inner ear and requires an exploratory tympanotomy to repair the damage as soon as possible.

BAROTITIS MEDIA

(Aerotitis)

Damage to the middle ear due to ambient pressure changes. During a sudden increase in ambient pressure, as in descent of an airplane or in deep sea diving (see appropriate chapters in §19), gas must move from the nasopharynx into the middle ear to maintain equal pressure on both sides of the tympanic membrane. If the eustachian tube is not functioning properly, as in URI or allergy, the pressure in the middle ear will be less than the ambient pressure and the relative negative pressure in the middle ear will result in retraction of the tympanic membrane and a transudate of blood in the vessels in the lamina propria of the mucous membrane will form in the middle ear. If the difference in pressure becomes great, ecchymosis and subepithelial hematoma may develop in the mucous membrane of the middle ear and in the tympanic membrane. Very severe pressure differentials cause bleeding into the middle ear and rupture of the tympanic membrane. Pressure differentials between the middle ear and the ambient pressures usually produce severe pain and a conductive hearing loss.

Individuals with acute upper respiratory infections or allergic reactions should be advised not to fly or dive, but if these activities are undertaken, a nasal vasoconstrictor such as phenylephrine 0.25% applied topically 30 min before descent is of prophylactic value.

OTOSCLEROSIS

A disease of the bone of the otic capsule and the most common cause of progressive conductive hearing loss in the adult with a normal tympanic membrane. Histologically, foci of otosclerosis show irregularly arranged, new, immature bone interspersed with numerous vascular channels. These foci enlarge and cause ankylosis of the footplate of the stapes and a consequent conductive hearing loss.

The tendency to otosclerosis is familial. About 10% of adult white populations have foci of otosclerosis, but only about 10% of affected persons develop conductive hearing loss. It becomes clinically evident in the late teenage and early adult years. The fixation of the stapes may progress rapidly during pregnancy.

Treatment is with microsurgical technics: The stapes is removed and replaced by a prosthesis, correcting the hearing loss in most cases. A hearing aid may also improve the hearing of the patient with otosclerosis.

TUMORS

Rarely, the middle ear is the site of origin of squamous cell carcinoma. The persistent otorrhea of chronic otitis media may be a predisposing factor. Radiation therapy and resection of the temporal bone are necessary.

Nonchromaffin paragangliomas (chemodectomas), known as glomus jugulare or glomus tympanicum tumors, arise in the middle ear from glomus bodies in the jugular bulb or the medial wall of the middle ear. They produce a pulsatile red mass in the middle ear. The first symptom is often a tinnitus that is synchronous with the pulse. Hearing loss and, later, vertigo develop. Excision is the treatment of choice. Palliation is achieved with radiation therapy for tumors too large to resect.

---

167.   INNER EAR

For a discussion of the etiology, diagnosis, and treatment of **vertigo**, see also Chs. 118 and 164.

MÉNIÈRE'S DISEASE

A disorder characterized by recurrent prostrating vertigo, sensorineural hearing loss, and tinnitus, associated with generalized dilation of the membranous labyrinth (endolymphatic hydrops).

The etiology of Ménière's disease is unknown, and the pathophysiology is poorly understood. The attacks of vertigo appear suddenly, last from a few to 24 h, and subside gradually. The attacks are associated with nausea and vomiting. The patient may have a recurrent feeling of fullness or pressure in the affected ear. The hearing in the affected ear tends to fluctuate, but over the years the hearing progressively worsens. The tinnitus may be constant or intermittent, and may be worse before, after, or during an attack of vertigo. Although only one ear is usually affected, both ears are involved in 10 to 15% of patients.

In **Lermoyez's variant** of Ménière's disease, hearing loss and tinnitus precede the first attack of vertigo by months or years and the hearing may improve with the onset of the vertigo.

Treatment

Treatment is empirical. A number of operations, including sacculotomy, placement of a stainless steel tack through the footplate of the stapes, endolymphatic-subarachnoid shunt, ultrasonic irradiation, and cryosurgery have been advocated for patients who are disabled by the frequency of vertiginous attacks. Vestibular neurectomy relieves the vertigo and usually the hearing is preserved. A labyrinthectomy can be performed if the vertigo is sufficiently disabling and the hearing has degenerated to a useless level.

Symptomatic relief of the vertigo may be obtained with anticholinergic agents (e.g., atropine 1 to 2 mg or scopolamine 0.6 mg orally or IM q 4 to 6 h) to minimize vagal-mediated GI symptoms, antihistamines (e.g., diphenhydramine, meclizine, or cyclizine 50 mg orally or IM q 6 h) to sedate the vestibular system, or barbiturates (e.g., pentobarbital 100 mg orally or IM q 8 h) for general sedation. Diazepam 2.5 to 5 mg orally or IM q 6 to 8 h is particularly effective in relieving the distress of severe vertigo by sedating the vestibular system.

VESTIBULAR NEURONITIS

A benign disorder characterized by sudden onset of vertigo that is persistent at first and then becomes paroxysmal.

The attacks are frequent at first, gradually become less frequent and less severe, and finally disappear after 18 mo. The disease is thought to be a neuronitis involving the vestibular division of the 8th nerve, and to be viral in origin because of its frequent epidemic occurrence, particularly among adolescents and young adults. There is no associated hearing loss or tinnitus.

The condition is self-limited and may occur as only a single episode. Acute attacks of vertigo may be suppressed symptomatically as in Ménière's disease. With prolonged vomiting, IV fluids and electrolytes may be required for replacement and maintenance.

BENIGN PAROXYSMAL POSITIONAL VERTIGO

(Postural or Positional Vertigo; Cupulolithiasis)

Violent vertigo lasting approximately 30 seconds, induced by certain head positions, and often accompanied by nausea, vomiting, and ataxia.

Etiology

Granular basophilic masses in the cupula of the posterior semicircular canal have been demonstrated. It has been suggested that the cupular deposits represent calcium carbonate derived from the otoliths. Etiologic factors appear to be spontaneous degeneration of the utricular otolithic membranes, labyrinthine concussion, otitis media, ear surgery, and occlusions of the anterior vestibular artery.

Diagnosis

A **provocative test for positional nystagmus** may be performed. The patient is first seated on an examining table, then assumes the supine position with his head dependent over the end of the table and turned so that one ear is undermost. After the position has been assumed, a latent period of several seconds will be followed by vertigo, which is severe, is likely to last for 30 to 40 seconds, and is accompanied by rotary nystagmus. If the left ear is affected, when it is put undermost the nystagmus will be clockwise; if the right ear, the nystagmus is counterclockwise. When the patient sits up, the response recurs, but the nystagmus is rotary in the reverse direction and is milder. The response fatigues, so that with immediate repetition of the test the response will be less strong.

Positional nystagmus may occur with end-organ or CNS lesions. The latency of the response, the severe subjective sensation, the fatigability of the response, the limited duration, and the direction of the rotary nystagmus distinguish benign paroxysmal positional vertigo from a CNS lesion. The positional nystagmus of CNS lesions lacks latency, fatigability, and the severe subjective sensation. The nystagmus may continue as long as the position is maintained. The positional nystagmus of CNS lesions may be vertical or changing in direction and, if rotary, is likely to be perverted (i.e., not in the anticipated direction).

The diagnostic evaluation should include audiometry, electrostagmography, and tomography of the internal auditory canals, to exclude other diagnostic possibilities.

Treatment

There is no effective treatment. The patient is instructed to avoid the provocative positions.

HERPES ZOSTER OTICUS

(Ramsay Hunt Syndrome; Viral Neuronitis and Ganglionitis;
Geniculate Herpes)

Invasion of the 8th nerve ganglia and the geniculate ganglion by the herpes zoster virus, producing severe ear pain, hearing loss, vertigo, and paralysis of the facial nerve. Vesicles can be seen on the pinna and in the external auditory canal in the distribution of the sensory branch of the facial nerve. Other cranial nerves are often involved, and some degree of meningeal inflammation is common. Lymphocytes may be present in the CSF, and the protein content is often increased. Evidence of a mild generalized encephalitis can be found in many patients. The hearing loss may be permanent or there may be partial or complete recovery. The vertigo lasts for days to several weeks. The facial paralysis may be transient or permanent.

Treatment

Corticosteroid therapy is the treatment of choice; e.g., prednisone 15 mg orally q.i.d. for 2 days, then 5 mg orally q.i.d. for 7 to 10 days, followed by gradual tapering of the dose. Pain is relieved with codeine 30 to 60 mg orally q 3 to 4 h as necessary, while the vertigo is effectively suppressed with diazepam 2.5 to 5 mg orally or IM q 4 to 6 h. Decompression of the fallopian canal is indicated when the nerve excitability declines but it only occasionally relieves the facial paralysis.

PURULENT LABYRINTHITIS

(Suppurative Labyrinthitis)

Purulent labyrinthitis may occur secondary to acute otitis media or purulent meningitis. In acute otitis media, the microorganisms may gain access to the inner ear through the oval and round windows; in purulent meningitis, through the cochlear aqueduct. Purulent labyrinthitis is also frequently followed by meningitis as the microorganisms gain access to the subarachnoid space through the cochlear aqueduct.

Purulent labyrinthitis is characterized by severe vertigo and nystagmus. It invariably results in complete hearing loss and, in chronic otitis media and cholesteatoma, is often followed by facial paralysis. **Treatment** includes labyrinthectomy for drainage of the inner ear, radical mastoidectomy, and massive antibiotic therapy.

SUDDEN DEAFNESS

Severe sensorineural hearing loss that usually occurs in only one ear and develops over a period of a few hours or less.

Sudden deafness occurs in about 1:5000 persons every year. Although the sudden onset suggests a vascular etiology (embolism, thrombosis, or hemorrhage) by analogy with vascular accidents in the CNS, the evidence supports a viral etiology in most cases. Sudden deafness tends to occur in children and young and middle-aged adults who have no evidence of vascular disease. The histopathologic findings in the temporal bone in sudden deafness are unlike those seen in the inner ear of animals with experimental vascular occlusion or embolization, but are similar to those seen in human viral infections of the inner ear that result in sudden deafness—e.g., mumps and measles **(viral endolymphatic labyrinthitis).** The viruses of influenza, chickenpox, and mononucleosis and the adenoviruses also produce sudden deafness.

The pathologic findings in individuals with persistent hearing loss due to viral endolymphatic labyrinthitis are similar regardless of the causative virus. The organ of Corti is missing in the basal turn. Individual hair cells tend to be missing. Ganglion cell populations are reduced in the basal turn. The stria vascularis becomes atrophic. The tectorial membrane is often rolled up and ensheathed in a syncytium. Reissner's membrane may be collapsed and adherent to the basilar membrane.

Perilymph fistulas between the inner and middle ears occasionally occur with severe ambient pressure changes and with strenuous activities like weight lifting. Fistulas in the oval or round windows result in a sudden sensorineural hearing loss and vertigo. The patient may experience a popping sound in the affected ear when the fistula occurs.

Symptoms and Signs

The hearing loss is usually profound, but fortunately the hearing returns to normal in most patients and partial recovery occurs in others. Tinnitus and vertigo may be present initially. The vertigo usually subsides in several days. If hearing is going to return, it is likely to do so in 10 to 14 days.

Treatment

Although vasodilators, anticoagulants, low mol wt dextran, corticosteroids, and vitamins have all been advocated, no form of treatment is of proved value. In view of the frequent micropetechiae and extravasation of blood that are characteristic of virus-induced inflammatory reactions, vasodilation and anticoagulation may not be indicated. Furthermore, in an inflammatory reaction the cochlear blood flow is already increased as much as is beneficial. Although corticosteroids have not been proved to be of value, their use appears rational—e.g., prednisone 15 mg orally t.i.d. for 2 days, then

5 mg orally q.i.d. for 5 to 7 days followed by a tapering of dosage. Bed rest also seems advisable.
   Surgical exploration of the middle ear should be carried out for a suspected perilymph fistula, and the fistula should be repaired with an autogenous soft tissue graft.

CONGENITAL SENSORINEURAL HEARING LOSS
(See Vol. II, Ch. 24)

NOISE-INDUCED HEARING LOSS

   Any source of intense noise, such as woodworking equipment, chain saws, gasoline combustion engines, heavy machinery, gunfire, or aircraft, may damage the inner ear. Individuals vary greatly in susceptibility to noise-induced hearing loss, but nearly everyone will lose some hearing if exposed to sufficiently intense noise for a sufficient time. Any noise > 85 db is damaging. The hearing loss is usually accompanied by a high-frequency tinnitus. Loss occurs first at 4 kHz and gradually moves into the lower frequencies with further exposure. In contrast to most sensorineural hearing losses, damage is less at 8 kHz than at 4 kHz. **Prevention** depends on limiting the length of exposure, reducing the noise at its source, and isolating the person from the sound source. Noise may be attenuated by wearing ear protectors, e.g., plastic plugs in the ear canals or glycerine-filled cups over the ears. With severe noise-induced hearing loss, a hearing aid is usually helpful.

PRESBYCUSIS

   The sensorineural hearing loss that occurs as a part of normal aging. It begins after age 20, first affecting the highest frequencies (18 to 20 kHz) and gradually moving into the lower frequencies; it usually begins to affect the 4- to 8-kHz range by age 55 to 65, although there is considerable variation. Some individuals are severely handicapped by age 60 and some are essentially untouched at 90. Men are affected more often and more severely than women. Stiffening of the basilar membrane and deterioration of the hair cells, stria vascularis, ganglion cells, and cochlear nuclei may play a role in pathogenesis, and presbycusis appears to be related in part to noise exposure.
   Speech reading (lip reading); auditory training, making maximum use of nonauditory clues; and amplification with a hearing aid are helpful.

OTOTOXIC DRUGS

   The aminoglycoside antibiotics, salicylates, quinine and its synthetic substitutes, and the diuretics ethacrynic acid and furosemide can be ototoxic. Though affecting both the auditory and vestibular portions of the inner ear, these drugs are particularly toxic to the organ of Corti (cortitoxic). Nearly all ototoxic drugs are eliminated through the kidneys, and renal impairment predisposes to the accumulation of toxic levels. Ototoxic drugs should be avoided in topical medication for the ear in the presence of a perforated tympanic membrane, since ototoxic agents can be absorbed into the inner ear fluids through the secondary tympanic membrane at the oval window.

   Streptomycin damages the vestibular portion of the inner ear more readily than the auditory portion. Vertigo and difficulty with maintaining balance tend to be temporary and eventually completely compensated, but with severe and permanent damage the loss of vestibular sensation may persist, causing difficulty when walking in the dark and Dandy's syndrome (bouncing of the environment with each step). From 4 to 15% of patients receiving 1 gm/day for > 1 wk develop a measurable hearing loss, which usually appears after a short latent period (7 to 10 days) and slowly becomes worse if treatment is continued. Complete, permanent deafness may follow.
   Neomycin has the greatest cortitoxic effect of any antibiotic. With large doses given orally or by colonic irrigation for intestinal sterilization, enough may be absorbed to affect hearing, particularly if GI ulceration or other mucosal lesions are present. Neomycin should not be used for irrigation of wounds or intrapleural or intraperitoneal irrigation because massive amounts of neomycin may be retained and absorbed and cause deafness. **Kanamycin** is close to neomycin in cortitoxic potential.
   Viomycin shows both cochlear and vestibular toxicity. **Vancomycin** causes hearing loss, especially in the presence of renal insufficiency. **Gentamicin** has vestibular toxic properties in man and both vestibular and cochlear toxicity in laboratory animals.
   Ethacrynic acid IV has caused profound and permanent hearing loss in gravely ill patients with renal failure who are given concomitant aminoglycoside antibiotic therapy. Transient hearing loss from **furosemide** has been reported.
   Salicylates produce hearing loss and tinnitus that is usually reversible. **Quinine** and its synthetic substitutes produce a permanent loss of hearing.

   The highest frequencies are usually affected first, and a high-pitched tinnitus or vertigo may develop—though they are not reliable warning symptoms. Ototoxic antibiotics should be **avoided** in pregnancy. Elderly persons and those with a preexisting hearing loss should not be treated with ototoxic drugs if other effective drugs are available. If possible, before treatment is begun with an ototoxic drug (especially an ototoxic antibiotic), the hearing should be measured in order to document a preexisting hearing loss. Hearing should be monitored audiometrically as often as daily while treatment is continued. If renal function is impaired, the dosage of renally eliminated ototoxic drugs should be adjusted so that the blood levels do not exceed those required therapeutically. Serum levels of the agent should be monitored to insure that adequate therapeutic levels have been achieved but not exceeded. Although there is some individual variation in susceptibility, not exceeding the recommended blood level will usually conserve the hearing.

FRACTURES OF THE TEMPORAL BONE

Ecchymosis in the postauricular skin (Battle's sign) suggests a fracture of the temporal bone. Bleeding from the ear following a skull injury is pathognomonic of a temporal bone fracture. The bleeding may be medial to an intact tympanic membrane, may come from the middle ear through a ruptured tympanic membrane, or may come from a fracture line in the ear canal. A hemotympanum gives the eardrum a blue-black color. CSF otorrhea signifies a communication between the middle ear and the subarachnoid space. Fractures longitudinal to the petrous pyramid (80%) extend through the middle ear and rupture the tympanic membrane; they produce facial paralysis in 15% of cases and a profound sensorineural hearing loss in 35%. The middle ear damage may include disruption of the ossicular chain. Transverse fractures (20%) cross the fallopian canal and the cochlea and nearly always produce facial paralysis and a permanent hearing loss. The hearing can be assessed initially with the Weber and Rinne tuning fork tests and subsequently with audiometry. With radiography of the temporal bone, particularly polytomography, the fracture can usually be demonstrated.

Treatment

Antibiotics such as procaine penicillin G 600,000 u. IM q 12 h should be given for 7 to 10 days to prevent meningitis. Persistent facial paralysis requires decompression of the nerve. Ossicular chain disruption is later repaired surgically.

ACOUSTIC NEURINOMA

(Vestibular Schwannoma; Acoustic Neuroma; Eighth Nerve Tumor)

Acoustic neurinomas are derived from Schwann cells. They arise twice as often from the vestibular division of the 8th nerve as from the auditory division and account for approximately 7% of all intracranial tumors.

As the tumor increases in size, it projects from the internal auditory meatus into the cerebellopontine angle and begins to compress the cerebellum and brainstem. The 5th and later the 7th cranial nerves become involved.

Symptoms, Signs, and Diagnosis

A hearing loss and tinnitus are early symptoms. Although the patient complains of dizziness and unsteadiness, true vertigo is not usually present. The sensorineural hearing loss (see Ch. 164) is characterized by greater impairment of speech discrimination than would be expected with a cochlear lesion. Recruitment is absent, and the short increment sensitivity index (SISI) is low. Tone decay is marked. Usually Békésy audiometry shows a Type III or IV pattern. Stapedial reflex decay and increase in the latency of the 5th wave in the brainstem evoked response audiometry provide further evidence of a neural lesion. As a rule, caloric testing demonstrates marked vestibular hypoactivity (canal paresis). Early diagnosis is based on polytomography of the internal auditory meatus, CT, and myelography of the posterior fossa, in addition to the auditory and vestibular findings.

Treatment

Small tumors may be removed with microsurgical technics that allow preservation of the facial nerve, using a middle cranial fossa route to preserve the remaining hearing or a translabyrinthine route if no useful hearing remains. Large tumors are removed by a combined translabyrinthine and occipital approach.

---

168. NOSE AND PARANASAL SINUSES

FRACTURES

The nasal bones are fractured more frequently than are other facial bones. The fracture usually includes the ascending processes of the maxilla and often the septum. The torn mucous membrane results in nosebleed. Soft tissue swelling develops promptly and may obscure the break. Septal hematomas may occur between the perichondrium and the quadrangular cartilage and may become infected; abscess formation leads to avascular and septic necrosis of the cartilage, with a saddle deformity of the nose.

Diagnosis

A fracture should be suspected if blunt injury causes bleeding from the nose. Diagnosis can ordinarily be established by gently palpating the dorsum (bridge) of the nose for deformity, instability, crepitus, and point tenderness, and is confirmed by x-ray. The most common deformity is deviation of the dorsum of the nose in one direction and depression of the nasal bone and ascending process of the maxilla on the other side.

Treatment

Nasal fractures in adults may be reduced under local anesthesia; children require general anesthesia. The fracture is manipulated into a good position by internal and external traction. A blunt elevator is placed under the depressed nasal bone and the depressed bone is lifted anteriorly and laterally while pressure is applied to the other side of the nose, in order to bring the nasal dorsum to the midline. The position of the nose is stabilized by internal packing and external splinting. Septal hematomas must be immediately incised and drained. Septal fractures are difficult to hold in position and often require submucous resection later.

FOREIGN BODIES

(See Vol. II, Ch. 25)

SEPTAL DEVIATION AND PERFORATION

Deviations of the nasal septum from developmental abnormalities or trauma are common but often are asymptomatic and require no treatment. Septal deviation may cause varying degrees of nasal obstruction and predispose the patient to sinusitis (particularly if the deviation obstructs an ostium of a paranasal sinus) and to epistaxis as a result of drying air currents. **Treatment** of symptomatic deviation of the nasal septum is by septoplasty or submucous resection of the septum.

Septal **ulcers** and **perforations** may follow nasal surgery, repeated trauma such as picking the nose, and granulomatous infections such as TB and syphilis. Crusting about the margins and repeated epistaxis may result. Small perforations may whistle. Topically applied bacitracin 500 u./gm in a petrolatum base reduces the crusting. Perforations of the nasal septum may be repaired by using buccal or septal mucous membrane flaps.

EPISTAXIS

(Nosebleed)

Bleeding from the nose occurs secondary to local infections such as vestibulitis, rhinitis, and sinusitis; systemic infections such as scarlet fever, malaria, and typhoid fever; drying of the nasal mucous membrane; trauma (digital, as in picking the nose, and blunt, as in nasal fractures); arteriosclerosis; hypertension; and bleeding tendencies associated with aplastic anemia, leukemia, thrombocytopenia, liver disease, the hereditary coagulopathies, and Osler-Weber-Rendu syndrome (hereditary hemorrhagic telangiectasia—see Ch. 95).

Treatment

Most nasal bleeding occurs from a plexus of vessels in the anteroinferior septum (Kiesselbach's area). **Bleeding may be controlled by pinching the nasal alae together for 5 to 10 min.** If this fails, the bleeding site must be found. The bleeding point may be cauterized; or bleeding can be controlled temporarily by applying pressure over a cotton pledget impregnated with a vasoconstrictor such as phenylephrine 0.25% and a topical anesthetic such as tetracaine 1% until the site is anesthetized. Although electrocautery may be used, silver nitrate in a 75% applicator bead may be used to control bleeding without producing too deep a burn of the mucous membrane.

In epistaxis due to a hemorrhagic disorder, petrolatum gauze is used to apply pressure as atraumatically as possible to the bleeding point; cautery is not used, since the periphery of a cauterized area may begin to bleed. Attention is directed to identifying and correcting the bleeding disorder.

In arteriosclerosis and hypertension, bleeding is likely to be far posterior in the inferior meatus and may be difficult to control. Control requires ligating the internal maxillary artery and its branches or packing the posterior part of the nasal cavity. The arteries may be ligated under microscopic control with a surgical approach through the maxillary sinus. In order to pack the posterior part of the nasal cavity, the choana is obstructed with a postnasal pack made by folding and rolling 4-in. gauze squares into a tight bundle and tying the bundle with 2 strands of heavy silk suture. The ends of one suture are tied to a catheter that has been introduced through the nasal cavity on the side of the bleeding and brought out through the mouth. The catheter is withdrawn from the nose as the pack is placed behind the soft palate into the nasopharynx. The 2nd suture is trimmed below the level of the soft palate so that it can be used to remove the pack. The nasal cavity, particularly the posterior part of the inferior meatus, is firmly packed with petrolatum gauze and the first suture is tied over a roll of gauze at the anterior nares to secure the postnasal pack. The packing remains in place for 4 to 5 days. (Alternatively, the balloon of a Foley catheter may be inflated in the nasopharynx to obstruct the choana.) An antibiotic such as ampicillin 250 mg orally q 6 h is given to prevent sinusitis and otitis media. Postnasal packing lowers the arterial P_{O2}, and supplementary O_2 should be given while the packing is in place.

In Osler-Weber-Rendu syndrome, multiple severe nosebleeds may occur from arteriovenous aneurysms in the mucous membrane and result in profound and persistent anemia that is not easily corrected with administration of iron. A split-thickness skin graft (septal dermoplasty) reduces the episodes of epistaxis and allows the anemia to be corrected.

Severe epistaxis is often associated with liver disease. Blood may have been swallowed in large amounts. It should be eliminated as promptly as possible with enemas and cathartics, and the GI tract sterilized with nonabsorbable antibiotics (e.g., neomycin 1 gm orally q.i.d.) to prevent the breakdown of blood and the absorption of ammonia.

The need for blood replacement is determined by the Hb level, vital signs, and the central venous pressure.

VESTIBULITIS

Infection of the nasal vestibule. **Low-grade infections** and **folliculitis** produce annoying crusts, and bleeding occurs as the crusts come away. Bacitracin ointment 500 u./gm applied topically b.i.d. for 14 days is effective.

Furuncles of the nasal vestibule are usually staphylococcal; they may develop into a spreading cellulitis of the tip of the nose. Systemic antibiotics should be employed along with hot soaks; penicillin G or V is the drug of choice. Furuncles of the central portion of the face should be allowed to drain spontaneously. Incision and drainage increase the risk of retrograde thrombophlebitis and subsequent cavernous sinus thrombosis, and are **contraindicated.**

RHINITIS

The most frequent of the acute upper respiratory infections, characterized by edema and vasodilatation of the nasal mucous membrane, nasal discharge, and obstruction. **Acute rhinitis** is the usual manifestation of a common cold (see in Ch. 12); it may also be caused by streptococcal, pneumococcal, or staphylococcal infections. **Chronic rhinitis** may occur in syphilis, TB, rhinoscleroma, rhinosporidiosis, leishmaniasis, blastomycosis, histoplasmosis, and leprosy, all conditions characterized by granuloma formation and destruction of soft tissue, cartilage, and bone. Rhinoscleroma also causes progressive nasal obstruction from indurated inflammatory tissue in the lamina propria. These conditions produce nasal obstruction, purulent rhinorrhea, and frequent bleeding. Rhinosporidiosis is characterized by bleeding polyps.

Diagnosis and Treatment

Diagnosis and treatment of acute bacterial rhinitis are based on identification of the pathogen and antibiotic sensitivities. The diagnosis in chronic rhinitis is based on demonstration of the causative microorganism by culture or biopsy. Treatment consists of chemotherapy appropriate to the causative agent.

In acute rhinitis, topical vasoconstriction with a sympathomimetic amine (e.g., phenylephrine 0.25%), given for not more than 7 days, provides symptomatic relief. Systemic sympathomimetic amines, such as pseudoephedrine 30 mg orally q 4 to 6 h, may be given for vasoconstriction of the nasal mucous membrane.

ATROPHIC RHINITIS

A chronic rhinitis characterized by an atrophic and sclerotic mucous membrane, abnormal patency of the nasal cavities, crust formation, and foul odor. The mucous membrane changes from ciliated pseudostratified columnar epithelium to stratified squamous epithelium, and the lamina propria is reduced in amount and vascularity. Anosmia results, and epistaxis may be recurrent and severe. The etiology is unknown, although bacterial infection plays a role.

Treatment is directed toward reducing the crusting and eliminating the odor. Topical antibiotics, such as bacitracin 500 u./gm, in a petrolatum base, estrogens topically and systemically, and vitamin therapy may be effective. Occluding or reducing the patency of the nasal cavities, surgically or with a pledget of lamb's wool, decreases the crusting caused by the drying effect of air flowing over the atrophic mucous membrane.

VASOMOTOR RHINITIS

A chronic rhinitis characterized by intermittent vascular engorgement of the nasal mucous membrane, sneezing, and watery rhinorrhea. The turgescent mucous membrane varies from bright red to a purplish hue. The condition is marked by periods of remission and exacerbation. It appears to be aggravated by a dry atmosphere. The etiology is uncertain, and no allergy can be identified.

Treatment is empirical and not always satisfactory. Patients benefit from humidified air; e.g., from a humidified central heating system or a vaporizer in the workroom and bedroom. Systemic sympathomimetic amines—e.g., ephedrine, pseudoephedrine, and phenylpropanolamine 30 mg orally (adult) q 4 to 6 h as necessary—give symptomatic relief but are not recommended for regular long-term use.

Topical vasoconstrictors should be **avoided** because the vasculature of the nasal mucous membrane loses its sensitivity to stimuli—e.g., the humidity and temperature of the inspired air—that result in vasoconstriction. Vasodilatation results, except after application of a strong stimulus, such as a topical sympathomimetic amine.

ALLERGIC RHINITIS

(See Ch. 19)

POLYPS

Allergic rhinitis predisposes to polyp formation; polyps may also occur in acute and chronic infections. Nasal polyps form at the site of massive dependent edema in the lamina propria of the mucous membrane, usually around the ostia of the maxillary sinuses. As a polyp develops, it becomes teardrop-shaped; when mature, it resembles a peeled seedless grape. In acute infections, polyps may regress after the infection resolves. Bleeding polyps occur in rhinosporidiosis.

Treatment: Corticosteroids, such as dexamethasone sodium phosphate as an aerosol (0.1 mg/spray), 2 sprays in each nostril b.i.d. or t.i.d., or methylprednisolone acetate 1 ml of a 20 mg/ml suspension given by injection into the polyp, have reduced or eliminated polyps, but surgical removal is more reliable. Polyps should be removed if they obstruct the airway or promote sinusitis. They tend to recur unless the underlying allergy or infection is controlled. In severe and recurrent cases, ethmoidectomy may be indicated.

WEGENER'S GRANULOMATOSIS

Wegener's granulomatosis, a condition of unknown etiology characterized by granulomas of the nose and lung and glomerulitis of the kidney, is discussed fully in Ch. 104. Most destructive lesions of bone, cartilage, and soft tissue of the nose and paranasal sinuses are ultimately found on thorough biopsy to be malignant tumors such as a lymphoma or carcinoma.

ANOSMIA

Loss of the sense of smell. Although frequently idiopathic, anosmia requires careful evaluation for intranasal and neurologic diseases. Anosmia occurs (1) when intranasal swelling or other obstruction prevents odors from gaining access to the olfactory area; (2) when the olfactory neuroepithelium is destroyed, as in atrophic rhinitis or the chronic rhinitis of granulomatous diseases and neoplasms; and (3) when the olfactory bulbs and tracts or their central connections are destroyed, as by intracranial trauma, infections, or neoplasms.

SINUSITIS

An inflammatory process in the paranasal sinuses due to viral, bacterial, and fungal infections or allergic reactions.

Etiology and Pathogenesis

Acute sinusitis is caused by streptococci, pneumococci, and staphylococci, and is usually precipitated by an acute viral respiratory tract infection. Exacerbations of chronic sinusitis may be caused by a gram-negative rod or anaerobic microorganisms. In about 25% of cases, chronic maxillary sinusitis is secondary to dental infection.

With a URI, the swollen nasal mucous membrane obstructs the ostium of the paranasal sinus, and the O_2 in the sinus is absorbed into the blood vessels in the mucous membrane. The resulting relative negative pressure in the sinus (**vacuum sinusitis**) is painful. If the vacuum is maintained, a transudate from the mucous membrane develops and fills the sinus, where it serves as a medium for bacteria that enter through the ostium or through a spreading cellulitis or thrombophlebitis of the mucous membrane. An outpouring of serum and leukocytes to combat the infection results, and painful positive pressure develops in the obstructed sinus. The mucous membrane becomes hyperemic and edematous.

Symptoms, Signs, and Diagnosis

The symptoms and signs of acute and chronic sinusitis are similar. The area over the involved sinus may be tender and swollen. Maxillary sinusitis causes pain in the maxillary area, toothache, and frontal headache. Frontal sinusitis produces pain in the frontal area and frontal headache. Ethmoid sinusitis causes pain behind and between the eyes, and a frontal headache that is often described as "splitting." Pain from sphenoid sinusitis is less well localized and is referred to the frontal or occipital area. There may be malaise. Fever and chills suggest an extension of the infection beyond the sinuses.

The nasal mucosa is red and turgescent; yellow or green purulent rhinorrhea may be present. The seropurulent or mucopurulent exudate may be seen in the middle meatus in maxillary, anterior ethmoid, and frontal sinusitis, and in the area medial to the middle turbinate in posterior ethmoid and sphenoid sinusitis.

The frontal and maxillary sinuses may be opaque to transillumination, but radiography of the paranasal sinuses more reliably defines the sites and the degree of involvement. Radio-opacity in acute sinusitis may be due to the swollen mucous membrane or a retained exudate. X-rays of the apices of the teeth are required in chronic maxillary sinusitis to exclude a periapical abscess.

Treatment

Improved drainage and control of infection are the aims of therapy in acute sinusitis. Steam inhalation effectively produces nasal vasoconstriction and promotes drainage. Topical vasoconstrictors such as phenylephrine 0.25% spray q 3 h are effective but should be used for a maximum of 7 days; systemic vasoconstrictors such as ephedrine, pseudoephedrine, or phenylpropanolamine 30 mg orally (adults) q 4 to 6 h are less reliably effective.

In both acute and chronic sinusitis, antibiotics should be given for at least 10 to 12 days. In acute sinusitis, penicillin G or V 250 mg orally q 6 h is the initial antibiotic of choice, and erythromycin 250 mg orally q 6 h is the second choice. In exacerbations of chronic sinusitis, a broad-spectrum antibiotic such as ampicillin 250 or 500 mg or tetracycline 250 mg orally q 6 h is better. In chronic sinusitis, prolonged antibiotic therapy for 4 to 6 wk often results in complete resolution. The sensitivities of pathogens isolated from the sinus exudate and the patient's response guide subsequent therapy. Sinusitis not responsive to antibiotic therapy may require operative intervention to improve ventilation and drainage and to remove inspiccated mucopurulent material, epithelial debris, and hypertrophic mucous membrane.

NEOPLASMS

Exophytic papillomas are squamous cell papillomas with a branching, vascular connective tissue stalk with finger-like projections on the surface. In the nasal cavity they often require repeated excision, but have a benign course. **Inverted papillomas** are squamous cell papillomas in which the epithelium is invaginated into the vascular connective tissue stroma. They are invasive and behave in a locally malignant manner; excision must include a large margin of normal tissue.

Other benign tumors that occur in the nasal cavity are fibromas, hemangiomas, and neurofibromas. Fibromas, neurolemmomas, and ossifying fibromas occur in the paranasal sinuses.

Squamous cell carcinoma is the most common malignant tumor in the nose and paranasal sinuses; others are adenoid cystic and mucoepidermoid carcinomas, malignant mixed tumors, adenocarcinomas, lymphomas, fibrosarcomas, osteosarcomas, chondrosarcomas, and melanomas. Hypernephroma is the most common metastatic tumor in the paranasal sinuses. Combined irradiation and radical resection give the best survival rates.

---

169. NASOPHARYNX

ADENOID HYPERTROPHY

(See Vol. II, Ch. 25)

TORNWALDT'S CYST

(Nasopharyngeal Cyst)

A frequently infected cyst found in the midline of the nasopharynx. The cyst lies superficial to the superior constrictor muscle of the pharynx and is covered by the mucous membrane of the nasopharynx. If infected, it may cause persistent purulent drainage with a foul taste and odor, eustachian tube obstruction, and sore throat. Purulent exudate may be seen coming from the opening of the cyst. **Treatment** consists of marsupialization or excision.

NEOPLASMS

JUVENILE ANGIOFIBROMA (See Vol. II, Ch. 25)

NASOPHARYNGEAL CARCINOMA

Squamous cell carcinoma of the nasopharynx occurs in children and young adults, with an unusually high incidence in the Chinese. The first symptom is often nasal or eustachian tube obstruction; the latter may result in middle ear effusion. Purulent bloody rhinorrhea, frank epistaxis, cranial nerve paralysis due to invasion of the parapharyngeal space and cranial cavity by the tumor, and cervical lymphadenopathy due to metastasis are common presenting complaints. **Diagnosis** is by biopsy of the primary nasopharyngeal tumor. Biopsy of the neck metastasis should be avoided until the nasopharynx has been inspected and palpated and any suspicious lesion there has been biopsied. The **treatment** of choice is supervoltage irradiation. The overall 5-yr survival rate is 35%.

170. OROPHARYNX

(See Vol. II, Ch. 24 for PHARYNGITIS; TONSILLITIS; PARAPHARYNGEAL ABSCESS; and RETROPHARYNGEAL ABSCESS. See Vol. II, Ch. 25 for VELOPHARYNGEAL INSUFFICIENCY)

PERITONSILLAR CELLULITIS AND ABSCESS

(Quinsy)

An acute infection located between the tonsil and the superior pharyngeal constrictor muscle. Peritonsillar abscesses are rare in children but common in young adults. Although usually due to a Group A β-hemolytic streptococcus, anaerobic microorganisms such as bacteroides also cause peritonsillar infection. There is severe pain on swallowing; the patient is febrile and toxic, holds his head tilted toward the side of the abscess, and shows marked trismus. The tonsil is displaced medially by the peritonsillar cellulitis and abscess, the soft palate is erythematous and displaced forward, and the uvula is edematous and displaced to the opposite side.

Treatment

Cellulitis without pus formation will respond to penicillin in 24 to 48 h. Initially, penicillin G 1 million u. IV q 4 h is given. If pus is present and does not drain spontaneously, incision and drainage are required. Antibiotic therapy should be continued orally with penicillin G or V 250 mg q 6 h for 12 days. Peritonsillar abscesses tend to recur and tonsillectomy is indicated (usually performed 6 wk after the acute infection has subsided). With antibiotic therapy, the tonsillectomy can be performed at the time of the acute peritonsillar infection.

CARCINOMA OF THE TONSIL

Squamous cell carcinoma of the tonsil is second in frequency only to carcinoma of the larynx among malignancies of the upper respiratory tract. Sore throat is the most common presenting complaint, and pain often radiates to the ear on the same side. A metastatic mass in the neck may be the first symptom. **Treatment** consists of a combination of irradiation and surgery. The 5-yr survival rate approximates 50%.

ZENKER'S (HYPOPHARYNGEAL) DIVERTICULUM

(See in Ch. 50)

171. LARYNX

VOCAL CORD POLYPS

Vocal cord polyps develop from voice abuse, chronic laryngeal allergic manifestations, and chronic inhalation of irritants such as industrial fumes and cigarette smoke. They consist of chronic edema in the lamina propria of the true vocal cord and result in hoarseness and a breathy voice quality. Biopsy of discrete lesions should be done to exclude carcinoma. **Treatment** involves surgical removal of the polyp to restore the voice, and attention to the underlying cause to prevent recurrence, including voice therapy if voice abuse is the cause.

VOCAL CORD NODULES

(Singer's, Teacher's, or Screamer's Nodules)

Vocal cord nodules are caused by chronic voice abuse, such as screaming or shouting, or using an unnaturally low fundamental frequency. The nodules are condensations of hyaline connective tissue in the lamina propria at the junction of the anterior 1/3 and the posterior 2/3 of the free edges of the true vocal cords. Hoarseness and a breathy voice quality result. Carcinoma should be excluded by biopsy. **Treatment** involves surgical removal of the nodules and correction of the underlying voice abuse. Vocal nodules in children usually regress with voice therapy alone.

CONTACT ULCERS

Unilateral or bilateral ulcers of the mucous membrane over the vocal process of the arytenoid cartilage resulting from voice abuse. Mild pain on phonation and swallowing and varying degrees of hoarseness result. Biopsy to exclude carcinoma is important. Prolonged ulceration leads to formation of nonspecific granulomas, which produce varying degrees of hoarseness.

Treatment consists of prolonged voice rest (6 wk minimum) for healing of the ulcers. Patients must recognize the limitations of their voices and learn to adjust their vocal activities to avoid recurrent ulcers. Granulomas tend to recur after surgical removal but respond to extensive voice therapy.

LARYNGITIS

Inflammation of the larynx.

Etiology

Viral and bacterial URIs are the most frequent causes of acute laryngitis. Although viral laryngitis is commoner, β-hemolytic streptococcus and *Streptococcus pneumoniae* are causative microorganisms. It may also occur in the course of bronchitis, pneumonia, influenza, pertussis, measles, and diphtheria. Excessive use of the voice, allergic reactions, and inhalation of irritating substances can cause acute or chronic laryngitis.

Symptoms and Signs

Unnatural change of voice is usually the most prominent symptom. Hoarseness and even aphonia, together with a sensation of tickling, rawness, and a constant urge to clear the throat, may occur. Symptoms vary with the severity of the inflammation. Fever, malaise, dysphagia, and throat pain may occur in the more severe infections; dyspnea may be apparent if laryngeal edema is present. Laryngoscopic examination discloses a mild to marked erythema of the mucous membrane that may also be edematous. If a membrane is present, diphtheria must be suspected (see DIPHTHERIA in Vol. II, Ch. 24).

Treatment

There is no specific treatment for viral laryngitis. Penicillin G 250 mg orally q 6 h for 10 to 12 days is the drug of choice for streptococcal or pneumococcal laryngitis. Treatment of acute or chronic bronchitis may improve the laryngitis. Treatment of chronic bronchitis may require a broader spectrum antibiotic, such as ampicillin 250 or 500 mg or tetracycline 250 mg orally q 6 h for 10 to 14 days. Voice rest and steam inhalations give symptomatic relief and promote resolution of acute laryngitis.

ACUTE LARYNGOTRACHEOBRONCHITIS

(See CROUP and ACUTE EPIGLOTTITIS in Vol. II, Ch. 24)

VOCAL CORD PARALYSIS

Etiology

Vocal cord paralysis may result from lesions at the nucleus ambiguus, its supranuclear tracts, the main trunk of the vagus, or the recurrent laryngeal nerves. Intracranial neoplasms, vascular accidents, and demyelinating diseases cause nucleus ambiguus paralysis. Tumors at the base of the skull and trauma of the neck cause vagus paralysis. Recurrent laryngeal paralysis is caused by neck or thoracic lesions, e.g., aortic aneurysm, mitral stenosis, neoplasms of the thyroid gland, esophagus, lung, and mediastinal structures, or trauma, thyroidectomy, neurotoxins (lead), neurotoxic infections (diphtheria), and viral illness. Vocal cord paralysis is often idiopathic.

Symptoms and Signs

Vocal cord paralysis results in loss of vocal cord abduction, or adduction and abduction; and may affect phonation, respiration, and deglutition; may result in aspiration of food and fluids into the trachea. The paralyzed cord generally lies 2 to 3 mm lateral to the midline, and in recurrent laryngeal nerve paralysis may move with phonation but not on inspiration. In **unilateral vocal cord paralysis**, the voice is hoarse and breathy. There is usually no airway obstruction because the normal cord abducts sufficiently. In **bilateral vocal cord paralysis**, the cords are within 2 to 3 mm of the midline and the voice is of limited intensity but good quality. The airway, however, is inadequate, resulting in stridor and dyspnea on moderate exertion.

Diagnosis

The cause must always be sought. The evaluation may include laryngoscopy, bronchoscopy, and esophagoscopy. Neurologic examination, x-rays of the base of the skull, thyroid gland scan, upper GI series, posteroanterior and lateral chest x-rays, and laminagraphy of the chest are also indicated. Cricoarytenoid arthritis may cause fixation of the cricoarytenoid joint and must be differentiated.

Treatment

In unilateral paralysis, augmenting the paralyzed cord by injection of a Teflon® suspension may allow approximation of the cords for voice improvement and prevention of aspiration. Maintenance of an adequate airway is the problem in bilateral paralysis. Tracheotomy may be needed permanently or during URIs. An arytenoidectomy with lateralization of the true vocal cord will open the glottis and improve the airway but may adversely affect the voice quality.

LARYNGOCELES

Evaginations of the mucous membrane of the laryngeal ventricle. Internal laryngoceles displace and enlarge the false vocal cord and result in hoarseness and airway obstruction. External laryngoceles extend through the thyrohyoid membrane, producing a mass in the neck. Laryngoceles are filled with air and can be expanded by Valsalva's maneuver. They tend to occur in musicians who play wind instruments. They appear on x-ray as smooth, ovoid, radiolucent masses. Laryngoceles may become infected or filled with mucoid fluid. **Treatment** is by excision.

NEOPLASMS

BENIGN

Juvenile papillomas may grow so exuberantly at multiple sites in the larynx that tracheotomy is required to maintain an adequate airway. They are thought to be of viral etiology, and they may appear as early as 1 yr of age and occur in epidemics. **Treatment** is by periodic excision. Recurrence is common. Regression usually occurs spontaneously at puberty.

Other benign laryngeal tumors include hemangiomas, fibromas, chondromas, myxomas, and neurofibromas. They may involve any part of the larynx. Removal restores the voice, the functional integrity of the laryngeal sphincter, and the airway.

MALIGNANT

Squamous cell carcinoma is the most common malignant laryngeal tumor. The incidence is higher in males, heavy drinkers, and heavy smokers. The true vocal cord (particularly the anterior portion), epiglottis, pyriform sinus, and postcricoid area are common sites of origin. Hoarseness is an early symptom and all patients with hoarseness lasting 2 wk should have indirect laryngoscopy. A discrete lesion of the laryngeal mucous membrane should be biopsied at direct laryngoscopy.

Early **treatment** by irradiation or cordectomy results in a 5-yr survival rate of 85 to 95%. Since irradiation usually returns the voice to normal, it is the treatment of choice in early carcinoma. Surgery is necessary in advanced carcinoma with anterior commissure involvement, thyroid cartilage invasion, or impaired vocal cord mobility. Partial laryngectomy, preserving laryngeal phonatory and sphincteric functions, may be possible, but total laryngectomy with radical neck dissection on the side of the lesion is more frequently required. A combination of irradiation and surgery is more successful than surgery alone in advanced supraglottic and hypopharyngeal lesions.

After laryngectomy, rehabilitation requires developing a new voice. The most satisfactory new voice is one that results from training in esophageal speech, a technic that involves taking air into the esophagus either during the negative intrathoracic pressure of inspiration or by swallowing air. The air in the esophagus is gradually eructed through the pharyngoesophageal junction, causing it to vibrate. The pharyngoesophageal junction substitutes for the larynx as the source of sound; the sound is articulated into speech sounds by the pharynx, palate, tongue, teeth, and lips.

Two alternate means of rehabilitation are available: An electrolarynx may be used as the sounding source; this method requires using a hand to hold the device in place while it produces the fundamental sound. In the other method, a tracheoesophageal fistula with a one-way valve is created so that air can be forced into the esophagus during expiration to produce vibration of the pharyngoesophageal segment. This method carries with it the risk of aspiration of fluids and food into the tracheobronchial tree if the tracheoesophageal valve misfunctions.

172. CLINICAL EXAMINATION

Some ocular complaints are nonspecific, so that a complete history and examination of all parts of the eye and its adnexa are necessary to identify the source of the complaint. The patient should be asked about the location and duration of the symptom; the presence and nature of any pain, discharge, or redness; and any change in visual acuity.

Unless chemicals requiring immediate irrigation have splashed into the eye, the first step in ocular evaluation is to record the visual acuity, testing the eyes separately and together, and with and without glasses if the patient wears them. Gross inspection of the glasses will provide an approximation of the degree of ametropia (e.g., nearsightedness, farsightedness, astigmatism). The visual fields and ocular motility may also be determined at this time. The fields can be checked by confrontation examination, as described under assessment of visual fields in NEURO-OPHTHALMOLOGIC EXAMINATION in Ch. 116 and under Detection of Visual Field Defects in Ch. 117.

Under a focal light and magnification (e.g., provided by a headband loupe), systematic examination of the eye should proceed. The eyelids are examined for lesions of the margins and subcutaneous tissues. The area of the lacrimal sacs is palpated and an attempt made to express any contents up through the canaliculi and puncta. The lids are then everted, and the palpebral and bulbar conjunctiva and the fornices are inspected for foreign bodies, signs of inflammation (e.g., follicular hypertrophy, exudate, injection), or other abnormalities.

The cornea should be inspected closely. If pain and photophobia make it difficult for the patient to open his eye, topical anesthesia can be accomplished before examination by instilling 1 drop of 1% proparacaine or tetracaine. Fluorescein staining with sterile, individually packaged fluorescein strips will make corneal abrasions or ulcers more apparent. The strip is moistened with 1 drop of sterile saline and, with the patient's eye turned upward, is touched to the inside of the lower lid for several seconds. The eye is closed for 5 seconds, then examined under good magnification and illumination. Denuded areas will stain green.

The size and shape of the pupils and their reaction to light and accommodation should be noted. Ocular tension and anterior chamber depth should be estimated before dilation, as mydriasis can precipitate an attack of acute glaucoma if the anterior chamber is shallow.

Ophthalmoscopy is aided by dilating the pupil with 1 drop of 0.5% tropicamide or 2.5 or 5% phenylephrine (repeated in 5 to 15 min if necessary); for longer action, 0.5% cyclopentolate or 10% phenylephrine may be used. Atropine is not recommended because of its prolonged action. Ophthalmoscopy will disclose lesions of the cornea, lens, and retina, as well as vitreous opacities and optic

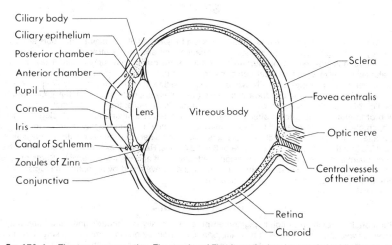

FIG. 172–1. **The eye—cross section.** The **zonules of Zinn** keep the lens suspended, while the muscles of the **ciliary body** serve to focus the lens. The **ciliary epithelium** secretes **aqueous humor,** which fills the **anterior and posterior chambers** and drains primarily via the **canal of Schlemm.** The **iris** regulates the light entering the eye by adjusting the size of its central opening, the **pupil.** The visual image is focused on the **retina,** the **fovea centralis** being the area of sharpest visual acuity. Note that the conjunctiva ends abruptly at the limbus. The cornea is covered with an epithelium that differs in many respects from the conjunctival epithelium.

nerve lesions. The strength of the ophthalmoscope lens required to bring the retina into focus will give an approximate measure of refractive error. The fundus may show changes due to systemic disease (e.g., diabetes mellitus, hypertension).

Other instruments (e.g., slit lamp, gonioscope, tangent screen, perimeter) may be needed for precise diagnosis; their use requires special training. The slit-lamp examination is especially helpful in distinguishing corneal lesions. Though other physicians can care for many diseases of the eye, when in doubt an ophthalmologist should be consulted, especially when the cause of pain or diminished vision is not apparent or when symptoms persist.

173. OCULAR SYMPTOMS AND SIGNS

HEMORRHAGE

Subconjunctival hemorrhages may develop at any age, usually following minor trauma, straining, sneezing, or coughing; rarely, they occur spontaneously. They alarm the patient but are of no pathologic significance, with the rare exception when they are associated with blood dyscrasias. They occur as gross extravasations of blood beneath the conjunctiva and are absorbed spontaneously within 2 wk. Topical corticosteroids, antibiotics, vasoconstrictors, and compresses are of little value in speeding reabsorption; reassurance is adequate therapy.

Vitreous hemorrhages are extravasations of blood into the vitreous and produce a black reflex on ophthalmoscopy. They may occur in such conditions as diabetic retinopathy or hypertension or result from trauma, retinal neovascularization, or retinal tears. In the 3 latter conditions, retinal detachment may ensue. Vitreous hemorrhages tend to absorb slowly, but they may become loosely organized and subsequently form proliferating bands that obscure vision and later contract and detach the retina. Localized bleeding from retinal vessels can sometimes be controlled by photocoagulation with light or laser beams. Periodic evaluation of vascular retinopathies by an ophthalmologist is important, particularly in diabetes mellitus.

Retinal hemorrhages may be flame-shaped in the superficial nerve fiber layer, as in hypertension or venous occlusion, or more localized ("dot and blot") in the deeper layers, as in diabetes mellitus or septic infarctions. Retinal hemorrhages are always significant, reflecting vascular disease that usually is systemic.

SPOTS

(Floaters)

Seeing spots (floaters) before one or both eyes is a frequent adult complaint. The spots are accentuated by bright light, usually are without significance, and are due to vitreous debris derived from the membranous attachment of the vitreous body to the optic nerve and retina. They are more prevalent in highly myopic and older persons and tend to become less noticeable with time. A minute **vitreous hemorrhage** appears as a brown or red spot. **Retinal detachments** usually are preceded by a shower of "sparks" in one quadrant of the field (diagonally opposite the retinal tear), followed by a sensation of a curtain moving across the eye. Spots may be serious; they warrant meticulous examination of the fundus and media after dilation with a short-acting mydriatic or cycloplegic (e.g., 1% cyclopentolate, 1 drop, repeated in 5 to 15 min). Examination is done best by indirect ophthalmoscopy, a technic used by most ophthalmologists. Vitreous floaters can be seen with a high plus lens by looking into the red reflex at a distance of 6 to 12 inches. Repeated examinations are warranted if the complaint continues or worsens, if vision is affected, or if apprehension persists. Spots of recent origin or those accompanied by flashes of light should be evaluated by an ophthalmologist. Disturbance of vision always demands an explanation.

PHOTOPHOBIA

Photophobia, common in lightly pigmented persons, usually is without significance and may be relieved by wearing dark glasses. It is an important, but nondiagnostic, symptom in keratoconjunctivitis, intraocular inflammation, acute glaucoma, and traumatic corneal epithelial abrasions.

PAIN

Ocular pain usually is important and, unless due to an obvious local cause such as a foreign body, acute lid infection, or injury, demands investigation (e.g., for uveitis, especially iridocyclitis, or glaucoma). Sinusitis occasionally causes referred eye pain.

SCOTOMAS

A blind spot in the field of vision is a **negative scotoma.** Frequently it goes unnoticed by the patient unless it involves central vision and interferes significantly with visual acuity. Negative scotomas noticed by the patient usually are due to hemorrhage or choroiditis. A scotoma found in the same visual field area in each eye is most commonly a quadrantic or hemianopic defect due to a lesion in the optic pathways. A **positive scotoma,** perceived as a light spot or scintillating flashes, represents a response to abnormal stimulation of some portion of the visual system; e.g., as in the migraine syndrome.

Examination of the eyes, including the visual fields, always is mandatory to determine the cause of any scotoma. A bilateral scotoma, if not caused by bilateral retinal lesions, demands perimetric examination and neurologic evaluation.

EXOPHTHALMOS

(See Ch. 175)

ERRORS OF REFRACTION

In **emmetropia** no optical defect exists and parallel light rays entering the eye focus clearly on the retina. In **ametropia** an optical defect exists that may be of several varieties: In **hyperopia** (farsightedness), the most common refractive error, the point of focus lies behind the retina, either because the eyeball axis is too short or because the refractive power of the eye is too weak. A convex (plus) lens is used in corrective glasses. In **myopia** (nearsightedness), the image is focused in front of the retina because the axis of the eyeball is too long or the refractive power of the eye is too strong; a concave (minus) corrective lens is used. In **astigmatism,** the refraction is unequal in the different meridians of the eyeball. A cylindric corrective lens (a segment cut from a cylinder) is used that has no refractive power along the vertical axis and is concave or convex along the opposite axis.

Anisometropia, a significant difference between the refractive errors of the two eyes (usually > 2 diopters), is seen occasionally. When the refractive errors are corrected with lenses, image size differences **(aniseikonia)** are produced, which can lead to difficulties in fusion and even to suppression of one of the images.

Presbyopia, a hyperopia for near vision that develops with advancing age, results from a physiologic change in the accommodative mechanism by which the focus of the eye is adjusted for objects at different distances. Beginning in the teens, the lens substance gradually grows less pliable and eventually cannot change shape (accommodate) in response to the action of the ciliary muscles. As a result, the individual becomes unable to focus well for near vision, but usually does not need corrective glasses until he reaches the early to mid-40s.

STRABISMUS

(See Vol. II, Ch. 25)

NYSTAGMUS

Rhythmic oscillation of the eyes in a horizontal, vertical, or rotary direction. **Pendular nystagmus (undulatory** or **oscillating nystagmus)** is seen when vision is poor from birth or from an early age. The eyes move to and fro with roughly the same velocity in both directions. **Jerk nystagmus** is more common. It is characterized by a slow drift, usually away from the direction of gaze, followed by a quick jerk or recovery in the direction of gaze. A motor disorder, it may be congenital or due to a variety of conditions affecting the brain, including ingestion of drugs such as alcohol and barbiturates, palsy of lateral or vertical gaze, disorders of the vestibular apparatus (see Ch. 164) and brainstem and cerebellar dysfunction (see Ch. 127). It is common in multiple sclerosis. The two eyes almost always participate symmetrically in the nystagmus. An exception to this rule is **spasmus nutans,** a poorly understood but usually benign condition of children under age I yr, associated with head bobbing. In adults, asymmetric nystagmus is usually a sign of multiple sclerosis.

Certain acquired types of nystagmus may help to localize a brain disorder—**rotary (rotatory) nystagmus** is usually a sign of vestibular system disease, and **vertical nystagmus** a sign of brainstem disease—but in general, nystagmus indicates unspecified brainstem dysfunction.

Nystagmus may blur a patient's vision, and he may be able to turn his head into a position to avoid this blur, but the ideal treatment is to remove the cause.

EXTRAOCULAR MUSCLE PALSIES

(Ophthalmoplegia)

The oculomotor (3rd cranial) nerve innervates the medial, superior, and inferior rectus and the inferior oblique extraocular muscles, and the pupilloconstrictor and levator palpebrae muscles as well. The superior oblique and lateral rectus muscles are innervated, respectively, by the trochlear and abducens (4th and 6th cranial) nerves. Although all 6 extraocular muscles are involved when the eye moves, 1 or 2 govern each principal direction of movement.

Etiology

The most common causes of acute ophthalmoplegia are neurologic disorders—diabetic neuropathy, pressure from an aneurysm or other space-occupying lesion, brainstem ischemia or other cerebrovascular disorder, trauma to the nerve, infectious or toxic neuritis, multiple sclerosis, and syphilis. Ophthalmoplegia may also result from direct trauma to the extraocular muscles, intrinsic disease of the extraocular muscles (myasthenia gravis), or compression by an orbital mass. It may occur in migraine, temporal arteritis, collagen vascular diseases, trichinosis, or botulism.

The 2 most common known causes of extraocular muscle palsy are diabetes mellitus and aneurysm. Trochlear nerve palsy is often seen after closed head trauma. Abducens nerve palsy is characteristically associated with mastoid bone infections and acute Wernicke's encephalopathy, but is more often due to diabetic neuropathy, pressure from a mass lesion (remote or direct), meningitis, trauma, multiple sclerosis, or syphilis.

Symptoms and Signs

Diplopia of recent onset is the characteristic symptom. It varies in different fields of gaze, depending on the muscles affected. The diplopia becomes greatest in the direction of action of the dysfunctioning muscles. **Oculomotor nerve** damage causes outward deviation of one eye (divergence strabismus) with inability to adduct the eye closer than the midline. Abduction and intorsion are the remaining functions. Lid ptosis and pupillary dilation also occur if the oculomotor lesion is complete. **Trochlear nerve** paralysis causes a vertical deviation with vertical diplopia that is characteristically corrected by tilting the head to one shoulder. **Abducens nerve** paralysis causes one eye to turn in; the eye cannot abduct beyond the midline.

Diagnosis and Treatment

Associated pain and pupillary dilation suggest a structural lesion (most often an aneurysm) pressing on the 3rd nerve; pain also occurs with diabetic neuropathy, but the pupil is usually not dilated. Arteriograms are indicated when aneurysm is suspected.

The direction of the diplopia and the ocular deviations found on examination will usually identify the affected muscles, and hence the nerves presumptively involved, but the cause of the paralysis must always be sought, since **treatment** is to remove or control the cause. Since a metabolic, neurologic, myopathic, or cardiovascular disorder may underlie the palsy, a full medical examination and routine skull x-rays are in order unless the palsy is obviously the result of trauma.

174. INJURIES

Trauma to the eye or adjacent structures requires meticulous examination to determine the extent of injury. The patient's vision, the range of extraocular motion, the location of lid and conjunctival lacerations and of foreign bodies, and the clarity of the ocular media should be carefully determined and recorded in detail for protection of patient, physician, and, in industrial cases, employer.

FOREIGN BODIES

1. **Conjunctival and corneal injuries** by foreign bodies are the most frequent eye injuries. Seemingly minor trauma can be serious if ocular penetration is unrecognized or if secondary infection follows a corneal abrasion.

Treatment: Adequate light, good anesthesia, and proper instruments are essential to ensure minimal trauma when removing embedded foreign bodies. Fluorescein staining (see Ch. 172) renders foreign bodies and abrasions more apparent. An anesthetic (e.g., 2 drops of proparacaine 0.5%) is instilled onto the conjunctiva. Both lids are everted and the entire conjunctiva and cornea inspected with a binocular lens (loupe). Conjunctival foreign bodies are lifted out with a moist sterile cotton applicator. A corneal foreign body that cannot be dislodged by irrigation may be lifted out carefully on the point of a sterile spud or hypodermic needle, under loupe magnification. Unless steel or iron foreign bodies are removed immediately, they leave a "rust ring" on the cornea that also requires removal, under the light and magnification of the slit lamp.

If the foreign body was tiny, only an antibiotic ointment (e.g., erythromycin 0.5% or bacitracin 500 u./gm) should be instilled. If larger, however, treatment is that for any **corneal abrasion:** dilating the pupil with a short-acting cycloplegic (e.g., 1 drop of 1% cyclopentolate); instilling an antibiotic, usually erythromycin or bacitracin; and applying a patch firmly enough to keep the eye closed overnight. Ophthalmic corticosteroid preparations tend to promote the growth of fungi and are **contraindicated.** The corneal epithelium regenerates rapidly; under a patch, large areas will heal within 1 to 3 days. Follow-up examination by an ophthalmologist 1 or 2 days after injury is wise, especially if the foreign body was removed with a needle or spud.

2. Intraocular foreign bodies: A foreign body that has penetrated the eye must be removed by an ophthalmic surgeon, but certain **emergency treatment** should be instituted immediately. The pupil is dilated with 2 drops of 1 to 4% atropine solution. Antimicrobials are indicated, both systemic and topical; e.g., gentamicin ± 2 mg/kg/day (if kidney function is adequate) in combination with methicillin 1 gm IM q 6 h, and gentamicin 0.3% ophthalmic solution 1 drop hourly. Ointment should be avoided if the globe is lacerated. A patch and a metal shield are placed over the eye to avoid inadvertent pressure, which could extrude ocular contents through the penetration site.

LACERATIONS AND CONTUSIONS

During the first 24 h, **lid contusions ("black eye")** should be treated with ice packs to inhibit swelling. The next day, hot compresses may aid absorption of the hematoma. Minor **lid lacerations** may be repaired with fine silk sutures. Lid-margin lacerations are best repaired by an ophthalmic surgeon, since particular care is needed to ensure apposition and avoid a notch in the contour. Major lacerations, especially those involving the lacrimal apparatus, should be repaired by an ophthalmic surgeon.

Trauma to the globe may severely damage internal structures. Hemorrhage into the anterior chamber, laceration of the iris, cataract, dislocated lens, glaucoma, vitreous hemorrhage, orbital-floor fractures, retinal hemorrhage or detachment, and rupture of the eyeball may result. **Emergency treatment** may be needed before care by a specialist. It consists of alleviating pain (e.g., with meperidine 50 mg IM q 3 h), keeping the pupil dilated with 2 drops of 1 to 4% atropine, applying protective dressings (including a metal shield), and combating possible infection with local and systemic antimicrobials as for an intraocular foreign body (see above). One should never forcibly open traumatized lids, as the injury may be aggravated. When a globe laceration is present, topical antibiotics should be given in the form of drops only, to avoid penetration of ointment into the globe. Because of the danger of fungal contamination, corticosteroids are **contraindicated** before open wounds are closed surgically.

Anterior chamber hemorrhage (traumatic hyphema) following blunt injuries is potentially serious and requires attention by an ophthalmologist. It may be followed by recurrent bleeding, glaucoma, and blood-staining of the cornea. The **immediate treatment** is complete bed rest, binocular bandaging, sedation, and, if intraocular pressure rises, a carbonic anhydrase inhibitor (e.g., acetazolamide 250 mg to 1 gm/day orally in divided doses). The non-ophthalmologist should *not* use miotics or mydriatics in these cases. Rarely, recurrent bleeding with secondary glaucoma may require evacuation of the blood by an ophthalmologist.

BURNS

Eyelid burns should be cleansed thoroughly with sterile isotonic saline solution, followed by petrolatum gauze or an antimicrobial ointment (e.g., bacitracin). Sterile pressure dressings are then applied and held by an elastic bandage or stockinet around the head until the surface has healed.

Chemical burns of the **cornea** and **conjunctiva** can be serious and should be treated immediately by copious irrigation with water or other bland fluids. The eye may be anesthetized with 1 drop of 1% proparacaine, if it is available, but irrigation should never be delayed and should be carried out for 5 to 30 min, depending on the estimate of chemical contact. Irrigation until the pH is neutral (as measured with paper indicators) is a reasonable end-point. Pain results from loss of corneal epithelium and chemical iritis, which should be treated by instilling a long-acting cycloplegic (e.g., 1% atropine solution), applying an antibiotic ointment, and patching. Initially, pain may require codeine 30 to 60 mg orally or meperidine 50 mg IM q 4 h. Severe burns require specialized treatment by an ophthalmologist to save vision and prevent major complications such as iridocyclitis, perforation of the globe, and lid deformities. All patients with significant redness of the eye or loss of normal epithelium should be seen by an ophthalmologist within 24 h.

---

175. ORBIT

ORBITAL CELLULITIS

Inflammation of the orbital tissues caused by infection that extends from the nasal sinuses or teeth, by metastatic spread from infections elsewhere, or by the introduction of bacteria via orbital trauma. Symptoms include extreme orbital pain, exophthalmos, impaired mobility of the eye, lid swelling, chemosis, fever, and malaise. Possible complications are loss of vision from optic neuritis, thrombophlebitis of the orbital veins resulting in cavernous sinus thrombosis, panophthalmitis, and spread of the infection to the meninges and brain.

Treatment with appropriate systemic antimicrobials is supplemented by general supportive therapy (including hot applications to localize the infection, bed rest, and fluids). Meperidine 50 mg, or codeine 60 mg with aspirin or acetaminophen, orally q 4 h should be given for pain. Incision and drainage are indicated if suppuration is suspected or if the infection does not respond to antibiotic therapy.

CAVERNOUS SINUS THROMBOSIS

Thrombosis of the cavernous sinus usually results from direct spread of infection along the venous channels draining the orbit and face. It is often secondary to orbital cellulitis or a pyogenic skin infection in the central region of the face; rarely, it is due to metastatic spread from other pyogenic foci. Exophthalmos, papilledema, severe cerebral symptoms (headache, convulsions), and a septic temperature curve are present. The prognosis is grave.

Prompt intensive **treatment** with systemic antibiotics appropriate to the causative organism, intravenous fluids, and bed rest is imperative.

EXOPHTHALMOS

(Proptosis)

Protrusion of one or both eyeballs resulting from orbital inflammation, edema, tumors, or injuries; cavernous sinus thrombosis; or enlargement of the eyeball (as in congenital glaucoma and unilateral high myopia). In hyperthyroidism, edema and lymphoid infiltration of the orbital tissues may cause unilateral or bilateral exophthalmos. Sudden unilateral onset is usually due to hemorrhage or inflammation of the orbit or accessory sinuses. A 2- to 3-wk onset suggests chronic inflammation or orbital pseudotumor (a non-neoplastic cellular infiltration and proliferation); slower onset suggests neoplasm.

An arteriovenous aneurysm involving the internal carotid artery and the cavernous sinus may produce a pulsating exophthalmos with bruit. Post-traumatic onset is probably due to carotid-cavernous fistula, confirmable by auscultation of the globe. Trauma or infection (especially facial) may cause cavernous sinus thrombosis with unilateral exophthalmos and fever. Unilateral high myopia or meningioma may cause unilateral exophthalmos. Thyroid studies should be performed when the cause is not apparent; if normal, the cause must be sought within the orbit by x-ray (including pneumograms, if necessary). The degree of exophthalmos can be followed with the exophthalmometer; if it is progressive, exposure of the globe can lead to corneal drying, ulceration, and infection.

Treatment

Etiology determines therapy. Ligation of the involved common carotid is necessary in arteriovenous aneurysm. The exophthalmos of hyperthyroidism may subside when the hyperthyroidism is controlled, but occasionally it follows a relentless course and requires surgical orbital decompression. Systemic corticosteroids are often beneficial in controlling edema and pseudotumor (e.g., 60 to 80 mg prednisone orally, given daily for 1 wk, then on alternate days for 5 wk, then gradually reduced to the minimal amount needed to control the proptosis). Tumors must be removed.

176.   LACRIMAL APPARATUS

DACRYOSTENOSIS

Stricture of the nasolacrimal duct, often resulting from a congenital abnormality or an infection. Congenital obstruction usually appears between ages 3 and 12 wk as a persistent tearing **(epiphora)** of one eye or, rarely, of both. The later onset and lack of purulent exudate in congenital obstruction differentiate it from neonatal conjunctivitis due to either silver nitrate instillation or bacterial infection. Pressure on the nasolacrimal sac frequently causes a copious reflux of mucus or pus from the punctum. In adults, dacryostenosis with epiphora may result from inflammatory obstruction of the duct due to chronic nasal infection, or from severe or chronic conjunctivitis. Fracture of the nose and facial bones may cause mechanical obstruction. Prolonged blockage usually leads to infection of the lacrimal sac (see DACRYOCYSTITIS below).

Treatment

Congenital dacryostenosis usually resolves spontaneously by age 6 mo. Milking the contents of the lacrimal sac through the nasolacrimal duct with fingertip massage b.i.d. may speed resolution; antibiotic drops may prevent infection. If resolution is not spontaneous, the punctum should be dilated and the nasolacrimal canal probed. Brief general anesthesia usually is necessary in infants. In adults, a local anesthetic such as 0.5% proparacaine is instilled and the punctum is dilated. Isotonic saline is irrigated gently through the nasolacrimal system with a fine, blunt canaliculus needle while the upper punctum is occluded with a punctum dilator. A drop of fluorescein in the saline makes it easily detectable in the nose. If this fails, lacrimal probing may establish patency. Using probes of increasing size followed by irrigation with sterile isotonic saline may be successful in incomplete obstruction. Complete obstruction requires a surgical opening from the tear sac into the nasal passages.

DACRYOCYSTITIS

Infection of the lacrimal sac.

Etiology

Dacryocystitis is usually secondary to obstruction of the nasolacrimal duct. In infants, it is a complication of congenital dacryostenosis; in others, the duct obstruction results from nasal trauma, deviated septum, hypertrophic rhinitis, mucosal polyps, hypertrophied inferior turbinate, or residual congenital dacryostenosis.

Symptoms and Signs

Pain, redness and edema about the lacrimal sac, epiphora, conjunctivitis, blepharitis, fever, and leukocytosis are associated with **acute dacryocystitis;** in **chronic dacryocystitis,** slight swelling of the sac may be the only symptom. On pressure, pus may regurgitate through the punctum. The sac may become distended from retained secretions and form a large mucocele. Recurrent acute inflammations may result in a red, brawny, indurated area over the sac. An abscess, if present, may rupture and form a draining fistula.

Treatment

Acute dacryocystitis is treated by frequent application of hot compresses, incision and drainage if an abscess has formed, procaine penicillin G 1.2 million u. IM followed by penicillin V 250 to 500 mg orally q 6 h and antibiotic ophthalmic preparations to prevent secondary corneal infection. The systemic antibiotic can be changed after results of culture are available. **Chronic dacryocystitis** may be relieved by dilating the nasolacrimal duct with a probe after using a local anesthetic such as 1% proparacaine or tetracaine, or 4% cocaine. Contributory nasal or sinus abnormalities should be treated. If conservative treatment fails, removal of the sac or nasolacrimal intubation or anastomosis may be necessary.

---

177. EYELIDS

LID EDEMA

Allergies (see OTHER ALLERGIC EYE DISEASES in Ch. 19) usually produce marked crinkly lid edema of one or both eyes and may be due to topical agents, such as eyedrops (e.g., atropine or epinephrine), other drugs, or cosmetics. Plant allergens can cause lid edema in atopic individuals. **Trichinosis** produces lid edema that is usually bilateral and resembles the allergic type; the associated fever and other systemic symptoms may not be present initially. An eosinophilia > 10% is characteristic.

In allergic lid edema, removal of the offending cause is often the only treatment needed. Cold compresses over the closed lids may speed resolution; topical corticosteroid creams (e.g., 0.1% triamcinolone) may be needed if swelling persists for more than 24 h.

BLEPHARITIS

Inflammation of the lid margins with redness, thickening, and often the formation of scales and crusts or shallow marginal ulcers.

Etiology

Ulcerative blepharitis is caused by bacterial infection (usually staphylococcal) of the lash follicles and the meibomian glands. The cause of nonulcerative (squamous or seborrheic) blepharitis is often obscure; it may be allergic in origin or associated with seborrhea of the face and scalp.

Symptoms and Signs

A foreign-body sensation is common. Itching, burning, and redness of the lid margins, lid edema, loss of lashes, and conjunctival irritation with lacrimation and photophobia may be present. In ulcerative blepharitis, tenacious adherent crusts appear and leave a bleeding surface when removed. Small pustules develop in the lash follicles and eventually break down to form shallow ulcers. During sleep, the lids become glued together by dried secretions. A history of repeated sties and chalazions is common. In the nonulcerative type, greasy, easily removable scales develop on the lid margins.

Prognosis

Patients should be warned that both types are indolent, recurrent, and stubbornly resistant to treatment. Exacerbations of the nonulcerative type are inconvenient and unsightly, but not destructive. Repeated attacks of the ulcerative type result in loss of eyelashes, scarring of the lids, and occasionally corneal ulceration.

Treatment

Erythromycin or bacitracin ophthalmic ointment should be applied t.i.d. to the lash margins, following 10-min application of warm compresses. Instillation of sulfacetamide-corticosteroid drops is useful in combating secondary conjunctival and corneal irritation or bacterial invasion. Drops may be used during the day, and ointment at night and on arising. Prolonged local treatment with neomycin should be avoided because of possible local allergic reactions. Tonometry is indicated during long-term corticosteroid therapy.

Nonulcerative seborrheic blepharitis also requires attention to the face and scalp (see SEBORRHEIC DERMATITIS in Ch. 189).

HORDEOLUM

(Sty)

An acute localized pyogenic infection of one or more of the glands of Zeis or Moll **(external hordeolum)** *or of the meibomian glands* **(internal hordeolum, meibomian sty).**

Etiology

Staphylococci usually are responsible. Sties often are associated with and secondary to blepharitis. Recurrence is common.

Symptoms and Signs

External hordeolum usually begins with pain, redness, and tenderness of the lid margin followed by a small, round, tender area of induration. Lacrimation, photophobia, and a foreign-body sensation may be present. Though usually localized, edema may be diffuse. A small yellowish spot, indicative of suppuration, appears in the center of the induration ("pointing"). The abscess soon ruptures, with discharge of pus and relief of pain.

Internal hordeolum involving one of the meibomian glands is more severe. Pain, redness, and edema are more localized. Inspection of the conjunctival side of the lid shows a small elevation or yellow area at the site of the affected gland. Later, an abscess forms, pointing on the conjunctival side of the lid; it seldom points through the skin. Spontaneous rupture is rare, and recurrence is common.

Diagnosis

External sties are superficial, well localized, and appear to lie at the base of an eyelash. An internal sty is deeper and can be seen through the conjunctiva. If the hordeolum lies near the inner canthus of the lower lid, it must be differentiated from acute dacryocystitis (see in Ch. 176). Successful lacrimal irrigation rules out dacryocystitis.

Treatment

Suppuration may be aborted in the early stages by topical antimicrobials (e.g., 0.5% erythromycin or 500 u./gm bacitracin ointment t.i.d.). Pointing is hastened by hot compresses applied for 10 min t.i.d. or q.i.d. As soon as suppuration is evidenced by the formation of a central yellow area, the sty should be incised with a sharp, fine-tipped blade and its contents expressed. Antibiotic ophthalmic solutions or ointments (e.g., 10 to 30% sulfacetamide), applied for several days, prevent spread of infection to neighboring structures. Systemic antibiotics are rarely needed.

CHALAZION

Chronic granulomatous enlargement of a meibomian gland from occlusion of its duct, often following inflammation of the gland.

Symptoms and Signs

At onset, a chalazion may be indistinguishable from a sty, with lid edema, swelling, and irritation. After a few days, however, it resolves, leaving a painless, slowly growing, round mass in the lid. The skin can be moved loosely over the swelling, which may be seen in the tarsus of the lid, generally presenting subconjunctivally as a red or gray mass. When the mass is in the lower lid near the inner canthus, chronic dacryocystitis must be ruled out.

Treatment

Most chalazions disappear after a few months, although incision and curettage may be indicated if there is no resolution after 6 wk. Hot compresses and topical antibiotic ointments (e.g., 0.5% erythromycin or bacitracin 500 u./gm) are indicated initially. Systemic antibiotics rarely are necessary.

ENTROPION AND ECTROPION

Inversion of the eyelid **(entropion)** *and* *eversion* **(ectropion)** can result from aging or from scar formation. Entropion causes irritation as the lashes rub against the globe, and may lead to corneal ulceration and scarring. Ectropion is generally the result of tissue relaxation with aging, and leads to poor drainage of tears through the nasolacrimal system. Symptoms may include redness, irritation, and epiphora. Both conditions, if persistent, are best treated surgically.

178.   CONJUNCTIVA

ACUTE CONJUNCTIVITIS

An acute conjunctival inflammation, usually caused by viruses, allergy, or bacteria.

Etiology

Viruses, especially adenoviruses (see under RESPIRATORY VIRAL DISEASES in Ch. 12) and allergies (see ALLERGIC CONJUNCTIVITIS in Ch. 19) are the most common causes in populations with good hygiene. Mixed or unidentifiable pathogens may be present. Conjunctival irritation from wind, dust, smoke, and other types of air pollution often is associated; conjunctivitis may also accompany the common cold, exanthems (especially measles), and corneal irritation due to the intense light of electric arcs, sunlamps, and reflection from snow. Acute hemorrhagic conjunctivitis, associated with infection by enterovirus type 70, has occurred in outbreaks in Africa and Asia (see CONJUNCTIVITIS under ENTEROVIRAL DISEASES in Vol. II, Ch. 24).

Symptoms, Signs, and Diagnosis

TABLE 178–1 indicates prominent symptoms and signs found in acute conjunctivitis. The discharge should be cultured, particularly if it is purulent. Smears should be examined microscopically, stained with Gram's stain to identify bacteria and with Wright's stain to determine the leukocytic response. While cultures can be taken for viral disease, special tissue culture facilities are necessary for growth of the virus.

Lymphoid follicles are present on the undersurface of the lid in viral infection; velvety papillary projections, in allergic disease. The preauricular node should be palpated in all cases; it tends to be enlarged and painful in viral conjunctivitis.

Examination of conjunctival scrapings will rule out inclusion conjunctivitis, trachoma, and vernal conjunctivitis: in the former two, inclusion bodies are present; in the last, eosinophils are present. Retained corneal or conjunctival foreign bodies and corneal abrasion or ulcer may be ruled out by staining the eye with fluorescein (see Ch. 172) and examining it, under magnification, with a good focal light.

The deep ciliary injection of iritis and of acute glaucoma is readily differentiated, since it is due to fine, straight, deep vessels that radiate from the limbus and are immobile when the conjunctiva is moved. The brick-red conjunctival injection of conjunctivitis is composed of coarse, tortuous superficial vessels that move with the conjunctiva; moreover, the conjunctiva blanches when a decongestant (e.g., a drop of phenylephrine 0.125%) is instilled. Other features that distinguish conjunctivitis from acute iritis and acute glaucoma are given in TABLE 181–1 in Ch. 181.

Treatment

After examining the patient, the physician must wash his hands thoroughly and sterilize his instruments to avoid transmitting infection. The patient should be told to use only his own towels. The eyes should be kept free of discharge and not patched. If bacterial infection is suspected, 10% sulfonamide drops and an antibiotic ointment (e.g., 0.5% erythromycin) are applied t.i.d. This treatment can be used for all forms of conjunctivitis; a poor clinical response after 2 or 3 days indicates that an insensitive bacterium is present, or that the cause is viral or allergic. Antibiotic therapy may be modified if necessary when the results of culture and sensitivity studies become available. Corticosteroids should not be used, either separately or with antibiotics, until a causative pathogen is identified or excluded, since herpes simplex virus may be present and may be spread from the conjunctiva to the cornea, with subsequent ulceration and perforation. If allergy is likely on the basis of history and lack of response to antibiotic therapy, topical corticosteroid therapy (e.g., 0.12% prednisolone drops t.i.d.) can be initiated. With long-term use of corticosteroids, intraocular pressure should be monitored and the lens examined periodically for cataracts.

TABLE 178–1. DIFFERENTIATING FEATURES IN CONJUNCTIVITIS

Etiology	Discharge; Cell Type	Lid Swelling	Node Involvement	Itching
Bacterial	purulent; polymorpho-nuclear leukocytes	moderate	no	no
Viral	clear; mononuclear	minimal	yes	no
Allergic	clear, mucoid, ropy; eosinophils	moderate to severe	no	intense

CHRONIC CONJUNCTIVITIS

A chronic inflammation of the conjunctiva characterized by exacerbations and remissions that occur over months or years. The causal agents, when identifiable, are similar to those of acute conjunctivitis; ectropion, entropion, blepharitis, chronic dacryocystitis, and chronic exposure to irritants are also etiologically associated.

Symptoms and Signs

Symptoms are similar to those of acute conjunctivitis but less severe, and include itching, smarting, and a foreign-body sensation; a scant mucoid secretion may be present. The palpebral conjunctiva is reddened, thickened, and velvety. The bulbar conjunctiva may be slightly involved.

Treatment

Irritating factors must be eliminated. Overtreatment may produce drug sensitivity and should be avoided. Prophylactic expression of the meibomian glands with 2 glass rods, after topical anesthesia (e.g., 1 or 2 drops of 0.5% proparacaine), may help. A short course of topical corticosteroid-antibiotic therapy may be soothing and beneficial.

CONJUNCTIVITIS NEONATORUM

(See NEONATAL CONJUNCTIVITIS under NEONATAL INFECTIONS in Vol. II, Ch. 21)

ADULT GONOCOCCAL CONJUNCTIVITIS

A rare, severe, purulent conjunctivitis that occurs in adults as a result of self-inoculation from a gonorrheal genital infection or is acquired from a gonorrheal contact. Usually only one eye is involved. Symptoms similar to those of conjunctivitis neonatorum, but more severe, develop 12 to 48 h after exposure; complications, including corneal ulceration, abscess, perforation, panophthalmitis, and blindness, are common. Treatment involves parenteral antimicrobial therapy and 10 to 30% sulfacetamide drops instilled into the affected eye q 2 h.

TRACHOMA

(Granular Conjunctivitis; Egyptian Ophthalmia)

A chronic conjunctivitis caused by Chlamydia trachomatis *and characterized by progressive exacerbations and remissions, with follicular subconjunctival hyperplasia, corneal vascularization, and cicatrization of the conjunctiva, cornea, and lids.*

Epidemiology

The disease is still endemic in poverty-stricken parts of the dry, hot Mediterranean countries and Far East. It occurs sporadically among American Indians and in mountainous areas of the southern USA. It is most contagious in its early stages and is transmitted by direct contact or, possibly, by handling contaminated articles (e.g., towels, handkerchiefs). The causative organism, a **TRIC** agent (**TR**achoma and **I**nclusion **C**onjunctivitis), is a strain of *Chlamydia trachomatis* and is related to psittacosis and lymphogranuloma venereum (see Ch. 11).

Symptoms and Signs

After an incubation period of about 7 days, conjunctival congestion, eyelid edema, photophobia, and lacrimation gradually appear, usually bilaterally. Small follicles develop in the conjunctiva of the upper lids 7 to 10 days later and gradually increase in size and number for 3 or 4 wk, forming yellow-gray semitransparent "sago-grain" granulations surrounded by inflammatory papillae. Pannus formation begins during this stage, with invasion of the upper half of the cornea by loops of vessels from the limbus. The stage of follicular hypertrophy and pannus formation may last from several months to more than a year, depending on response to therapy. The entire cornea may ultimately be involved, reducing vision. Rarely, the pannus retrogresses completely and corneal transparency is restored without treatment.

Unless adequate treatment is given, the cicatricial stage follows. The follicles and papillae gradually shrink and are replaced by scar tissue that often causes entropion and lacrimal duct obstruction. The corneal epithelium becomes dull and thickened, and lacrimation is decreased. Ulcers form in ischemic areas of the pannus. On healing, the conjunctiva is smooth and grayish-white; the extent of residual corneal opacity and vision loss varies. Secondary bacterial infection is common and contributes to scarring and the chronicity of the disease.

Diagnosis

C. trachomatis can be isolated in culture. In the early stage, the presence of minute granular cytoplasmic inclusion bodies in Giemsa-stained epithelial conjunctival scrapings differentiates trachoma from acute conjunctivitis. Inclusion bodies are also found in inclusion conjunctivitis but the developing clinical picture distinguishes this from trachoma. Palpebral vernal conjunctivitis is similar to trachoma in its follicular hypertrophic stage, but eosinophilia and milky flat-topped papillae are present and inclusion bodies are not found in the scrapings.

Treatment

Tetracycline (or erythromycin) eye ointments, applied b.i.d. or q.i.d. for 4 to 6 wk, are usually effective. A concomitant oral tetracycline is helpful. Lid deformities should be treated surgically.

INCLUSION CONJUNCTIVITIS

(Inclusion Blenorrhea; Swimming Pool Conjunctivitis)

An acute conjunctivitis, known as **inclusion blennorrhea** *in the newborn and* **adult inclusion conjunctivitis** *or* **swimming pool conjunctivitis** *in the adult, caused by* Chlamydia trachomatis, *a TRIC agent* (see TRACHOMA, above). This organism can persist asymptomatically in the cervix for prolonged periods. As a form of ophthalmia neonatorum, inclusion conjunctivitis results from passage through an infected birth canal and occurs in 40 to 50% of the newborns exposed to it. Although most instances of acute inclusion conjunctivitis in adults result from exposure to infected genital secretions, adenovirus acquired in swimming pools has been implicated occasionally.

Symptoms, Signs, and Diagnosis

In the newborn, intense papillary conjunctivitis, lid swelling, chemosis, and mucopurulent discharge develop, usually bilaterally, after a 5- to 14-day incubation period. Epithelial-cell inclusion bodies are present in conjunctival scrapings. Hypertrophied papillae may develop in both conjunctival folds and persist for several months. No corneal damage occurs. The longer incubation time helps to differentiate inclusion blennorrhea from gonococcal ophthalmia neonatorum. In adults, the conjunctivitis is less severe and usually unilateral; the secretion is less profuse but the papillae are larger. Preauricular lymph nodes may be swollen on the side of the involved eye.

Treatment

Tetracycline 1% ophthalmic ointment q.i.d. is specific and should be applied to both eyes in order to prevent bilateral infection. Local application alone is usually curative in 1 wk in the newborn. In adults, oral tetracycline 500 mg q.i.d. for 10 days is also given to cure concomitant genital infection.

VERNAL (ALLERGIC) CONJUNCTIVITIS

A bilateral chronic conjunctivitis, probably allergic in origin, usually recurring in the spring and lasting through the summer. It is most common in males aged 5 to 20. (See also ALLERGIC CONJUNCTIVITIS in Ch. 19).

Symptoms and Signs

Intense itching, lacrimation, photophobia, conjunctival injection, and a tenacious mucoid discharge containing numerous eosinophils are characteristic. Either the palpebral or the bulbar conjunctiva may be affected. In the **palpebral** form, square, hard, flattened, closely packed, pale pink to grayish "cobblestone" granulations are present, chiefly in the upper lids. The uninvolved tarsal conjunctiva is milky white. In the **bulbar (limbic) form,** the circumcorneal conjunctiva becomes hypertrophied and grayish. Occasionally, a small, circumscribed loss of corneal epithelium occurs, causing pain and increased photophobia.

Symptoms usually disappear during the cold months and become milder over the years, but the granulations often persist for life.

Treatment

Frequent applications of a topical corticosteroid are beneficial (e.g., 0.1% dexamethasone drops q 2 h), supplemented if necessary by small oral doses. Dosage should be reduced as soon as possible, with intermittent long-term maintenance therapy of 0.2% prednisolone applied once or twice/day the goal. If topical steroids are used for more than a few weeks, intraocular pressure must be checked routinely. Desensitization to pollens may help some patients.

KERATOCONJUNCTIVITIS SICCA

(Keratitis Sicca; Dry Eyes)

A chronic, bilateral dryness of the conjunctiva and sclera leading to dessication of the ocular surface.

Symptoms and Signs

As an isolated phenomenon or in association with systemic diseases such as rheumatoid arthritis or lupus erythematosus (when it is termed **Sjögren's syndrome**), dryness of the eyes occurs more commonly in adult women. Initial reduction of tear production leads to burning and irritation. This proceeds to photophobia and blepharospasm as the corneal epithelium develops scattered cellular loss, termed superficial keratitis. In its advanced stages, keratinization of the ocular surface occurs, frequently associated with loss of the normal configuration of the conjunctival fornices. In advanced keratoconjunctivitis sicca, ulceration, vascularization, and scarring of the cornea may lead to severe visual disability. Diagnosis is done by evaluating tear production via the use of strips of blotting paper (**Schirmer test**—see in SJÖGREN'S SYNDROME in Ch. 103), with and without topical anesthesia.

Treatment

Frequent use of artificial tears containing methylcellulose or polyvinyl alcohol can be effective. Most cases are treated adequately throughout the patient's life with such supplementation. Intractable cases may respond to the use of soft contact lenses, kept hydrated with frequent applications of saline drops. Occlusion of the nasolacrimal punctum can be tried before eyelid surgery, but in severe cases partial tarsorrhaphy can reduce the loss of tears through evaporation.

EPISCLERITIS

Inflammation of the episcleral tissues, usually localized. A red to purplish tender patch is present just under the conjunctiva; a yellow nodule may also be present. **Treatment** by frequent applications of a topical corticosteroid—e.g., 0.1% dexamethasone drops q 2 h for 5 days, then gradually reduced over 3 wk—is usually rapidly effective.

SCLERITIS

A deep, usually localized, inflammation of the scleral tissues, more purple in appearance than episcleritis. It may be associated with rheumatic disorders. If severe, perforation of the globe and loss of the eye may ensue.

Treatment

Some cases respond to a topical corticosteroid, but careful observation is necessary to forestall increased loss of scleral substance. Systemic corticosteroids may be tried when involvement is quite deep and response to topical therapy is poor, but the prognosis is guarded.

---

179. CORNEA

SUPERFICIAL PUNCTATE KERATITIS

Scattered, fine, punctate loss of epithelium from the corneal surface of one or both eyes. It is often associated with trachoma, staphylococcal blepharitis, conjunctivitis, or a respiratory tract infection. It may be due to a viral infection or may be a reaction to local medication and is commonly the cause of intense pain after exposure to ultraviolet rays (e.g., from welding arcs, sun lamps). Symptoms include photophobia, pain, lacrimation, conjunctival injection, and diminution of vision. An enlarged preauricular node may be present in viral cases. Lesions due to ultraviolet ray exposure do not appear until several hours after the exposure; they last 24 to 48 h, while those secondary to viral or bacterial agents may last for months. Healing is spontaneous and residual vision impairment is rare, regardless of etiology.

Treatment

Topical antimicrobial therapy should be given promptly, particularly if a causative organism can be cultured and identified. For gram-positive organisms, 10 to 30% sulfacetamide drops q 2 h and 0.5% erythromycin or 500 u./gm bacitracin ointment t.i.d. can be used. Gram-negative organisms can be treated with 0.3% gentamicin or 0.5% chloramphenicol drops q 2 h, and bacitracin ointment t.i.d. Dark glasses are useful for photophobia. A systemic analgesic may be needed for control of pain; *topical anesthetics may delay healing and should not be used.* Ultraviolet burns are treated with short-acting cycloplegics, antibiotic ointment, and patching for 24 h. Corticosteroids are not indicated.

CORNEAL ULCER

Local necrosis of corneal tissue due to invasion by microorganisms.

Etiology

A pneumococcal, streptococcal, or staphylococcal infection following trauma or complicating a corneal foreign body is the usual primary cause. Corneal ulcers also occur as complications of herpes simplex keratitis, chronic blepharitis, conjunctivitis (especially bacterial), trachoma, dacryocystitis, gonorrhea, and acute infectious diseases. **Serpent (serpiginous, hypopyon) ulcer** usually is due to pneumococci or *Pseudomonas aeruginosa* and often is associated with chronic lacrimal sac infections. **Indolent ulcers** are considered to be fungal until proved otherwise. Corneal ulcers may also result from disturbances in corneal nutrition secondary to keratomalacia or glaucoma, or corneal exposure due to eyelid injuries or defective closure of the lids **(lagophthalmos).**

Symptoms and Signs

Pain, photophobia, blepharospasm, and lacrimation are present, but may be minimal. The lesion begins as a dull, grayish, circumscribed superficial infiltration and subsequently necroses and suppurates to form an ulcer. This stains green with fluorescein (see Ch. 172 for method) and is readily evident. Considerable ciliary injection is usual, and in long-standing cases blood vessels may grow in from the limbus **(pannus)**. The ulcer may spread to involve the width of the cornea or may penetrate deeply. Serpent ulcer usually begins near the center of the cornea, grows rapidly in size and depth, and may destroy most of the cornea; pus may appear in the anterior chamber **(hypopyon)**.

Ulceration without extensive infiltration may occur in herpes simplex. Fungal ulcerations are densely infiltrated and show occasional discrete islands of infiltrate (satellite lesions) at the periphery.

Complications

The deeper the ulcer, the more severe the symptoms and complications. Ulcers deep enough to involve Bowman's membrane and the substance of the cornea heal with fibrous tissue replacement, causing opaque scarring of the cornea and decreased vision. Iritis, iridocyclitis, corneal perforation with iris prolapse, hypopyon, panophthalmitis, and destruction of the eye may occur with or without treatment. Ulcers caused by fungi are indolent but serious; those caused by *P. aeruginosa* are especially virulent, and those associated with dendritic herpes simplex keratitis may be particularly refractory.

Treatment

Corneal ulcers should be treated only by an ophthalmologist.

HERPES SIMPLEX KERATITIS

Corneal herpes simplex virus infection, with a spectrum of clinical appearances, commonly leading to chronic inflammation, vascularization, scarring, and loss of vision. The initial infection is usually an undistinguished self-limiting conjunctivitis, which may be accompanied by a vesicular blepharitis. Recurrences usually take the form of **dendritic keratitis**, with a characteristic branched lesion of the cornea resembling the veins of a leaf, with knoblike terminals. A foreign-body sensation, lacrimation, photophobia, and conjunctival injection are early symptoms, followed rapidly by corneal hypoesthesia or anesthesia, an important diagnostic sign. Ulceration and permanent scarring of the cornea may result. **Disciform keratitis**, a deep, disc-shaped corneal inflammation with accompanying iritis, frequently follows dendritic keratitis and probably represents an immunologic response to the virus. Rarely, direct invasion of the corneal stroma by herpes simplex virus is seen, and occasionally a recurrent loss of corneal epithelium is seen in patients with herpes simplex virus but without active viral eruption.

Treatment

Idoxuridine **(IDU)**, vidarabine, and trifluridine are specific, though not always effective. The agent, whether an ointment or solution, should be used several times daily. If healing fails to occur after 3 to 5 days, debridement by gentle swabbing with a cotton-tipped applicator is indicated. Topical corticosteroids are **contraindicated** in the early stages of dendritic keratitis, but may be effective in the stromal or uveitic involvement when used with IDU. Atropine 1% instilled t.i.d. is useful in cases with more than epithelial involvement. Cases that fail to heal after 1 wk and those with stromal or uveal involvement require referral to an ophthalmologist.

OPHTHALMIC HERPES ZOSTER

(See also HERPES ZOSTER in Ch. 12)

Involvement of the eyelid or palpebral conjunctiva by herpes zoster is not threatening to the globe. However, when the nasociliary nerve is affected, as indicated by a lesion on the tip of the nose, the cornea invariably becomes involved. Marked lid edema, ciliary and conjunctival injection, corneal infiltration, and pain are all present. Keratitis accompanied by uveitis may be severe, and is followed by scarring. Glaucoma, a common sequel, often develops much later.

Treatment

Unlike herpes simplex, herpes zoster *is* an indication for corticosteroids when the cornea and uveal tract are involved. Topical therapy (e.g., 0.1% dexamethasone, instilled q 2 h initially) is usually adequate. The pupil should be kept dilated with 1% atropine or 0.5 to 1% cyclopentolate solution, 1 drop t.i.d. Intraocular pressure must be monitored.

PHLYCTENULAR KERATOCONJUNCTIVITIS

(Phlyctenular or Eczematous Conjunctivitis)

A conjunctivitis, usually occurring in children, characterized by discrete nodular areas of inflammation (phlyctenules) and resulting from the atopic reaction of a hypersensitive conjunctiva or cornea to an unknown allergen. Proteins of staphylococcal, tuberculous, or other bacterial origin have been implicated. The disease is rare in the USA.

Phlyctenules appear as crops of small yellow-gray nodules at the limbus or on the cornea and bulbar conjunctiva and persist from several days to 1 to 2 wk. They ulcerate, but heal without a scar. When the cornea is affected, blepharospasm, severe tearing, photophobia, and pain may be prominent. Frequent recurrence, especially with secondary infection, may lead to corneal opacity with loss of vision. **Treatment** with a topical corticosteroid-antibiotic combination is valuable in combating the condition and any secondary infection.

INTERSTITIAL KERATITIS
(Parenchymatous Keratitis)

A chronic nonulcerative infiltration of the deep layers of the cornea, with uveal inflammation. It is rare in the USA. Most cases occur in children as a late complication of congenital syphilis. Ultimately, both eyes may be involved. Rarely, acquired syphilis or tuberculosis may cause a unilateral form in adults.

Photophobia, pain, lacrimation, and gradual loss of vision are common. The lesion begins in the deep corneal layers; soon the entire cornea develops a ground-glass appearance, obscuring the iris. New blood vessels grow in from the limbus and produce orange-red areas ("salmon patches"). Iritis, iridocyclitis, and choroiditis are common. The inflammation and neovascularization usually begin to subside after 1 to 2 mo. Some corneal opacity may remain, but vision may be impaired even when the cornea clears completely. An ophthalmologist should be consulted for treatment.

KERATOMALACIA
(Xerotic Keratitis; Xerophthalmia)

A condition associated with vitamin A deficiency and protein-calorie malnutrition, characterized by a hazy, dry cornea that becomes denuded. Corneal ulceration with secondary infection is common. The lacrimal glands and conjunctiva are also affected. Lack of tears causes extreme dryness of the eyes, and foamy Bitot's spots appear on the bulbar conjunctiva. Night blindness may be associated. Further details, including specific therapy, can be found under VITAMIN A DEFICIENCY in Ch. 78. Antibiotic ointments or sulfonamides (e.g., sulfacetamide ophthalmic solution 30% or ointment 10%) are required if secondary infection exists.

KERATOCONUS

A slowly progressive ectasia of the cornea, usually bilateral, beginning between ages 10 and 20. The cone shape that the cornea assumes causes major changes in the refractive power of the eye, necessitating frequent change of spectacles. Contact lenses may provide better visual correction, and should always be tried when eyeglasses are not satisfactory. Surgery may be necessary if the cornea becomes thin or if scarring follows rents in the posterior corneal surface.

BULLOUS KERATOPATHY

A condition caused by excessive fluid accumulation in the cornea, most frequently the result of aging and failure of the posterior corneal endothelium. It is seen occasionally after intraocular operations (e.g., for cataract), where the mechanical stresses further interfere with the process of corneal detumescence.

The fluid-filled bullae on the corneal surface rupture, causing pain and decreased vision. The bullae and swelling of the corneal stroma appear on examination.

Treatment, including the use of dehydrating agents, soft contact lenses, and corneal transplantation, is best carried out by an ophthalmologist.

180.   CATARACT

Developmental or degenerative opacity of the lens. **Developmental cataract** occurs congenitally or during early life from nutritional, toxic, inflammatory, or hereditary metabolic causes (e.g., galactosemia; rubella or other maternal disease early in pregnancy). **Degenerative cataract** is characterized by a gradual loss of lens transparency. The cause may be senile degeneration, x-rays, heat from infrared rays, trauma, systemic disease (e.g., diabetes), uveitis (cataracta complicata), or systemic medications (e.g., corticosteroids).

Symptoms and Signs

The cardinal symptom is a progressive, painless loss of vision. The degree of loss depends on the location and extent of the opacity. When the opacity is in the central lens nucleus (nuclear cataract), myopia develops in the early stages, so that a presbyopic patient may discover that he can read without his glasses ("second sight"). Pain occurs if the cataract swells and produces secondary glaucoma.

Diagnosis

Well-developed cataracts appear as gray opacities in the lens. Ophthalmoscopic examination of the dilated pupil (see Ch. 172) with the instrument held about 1 ft away will usually disclose subtle opacities. Small cataracts stand out as dark defects in the red reflex. A large cataract may obliterate the red reflex. Slit-lamp examination provides more details about the character, location, and extent of the opacity.

Gradual loss of vision beginning in middle age or later is characteristic of glaucoma as well as cataract. Before dilation of the pupils for an ophthalmoscopic examination, increased intraocular tension and a shallow anterior chamber must be ruled out. The vision lost through cataract can be restored surgically, but the deterioration due to glaucoma mistakenly diagnosed as cataract may result in permanent blindness.

Treatment

Frequent refractions and eyeglass prescription changes will help maintain useful vision during cataract development. Occasionally, chronic pupillary dilation (10% phenylephrine) is helpful for small lenticular opacities. Lens extraction is necessary when useful vision is lost; it can be accomplished by removal of the lens intact, or by emulsification followed by irrigation and aspiration. Age is no contraindication to surgery. Corticosteroids must be given topically and systemically when surgery is needed in the presence of uveitis. Refractive correction postoperatively is accomplished by cataract spectacles, contact lenses, or intraoperative implantation of an intraocular prosthetic lens.

---

181. UVEAL TRACT

UVEITIS

Inflammation of the uveal tract (iris, ciliary body, and choroid). Uveitis is anatomically classified as **anterior (iritis, iridocyclitis)** or **posterior (choroiditis, chorioretinitis).** It may be acute, recurrent, or chronic, and granulomatous or nongranulomatous.

ANTERIOR UVEITIS

*Inflammation of the iris **(iritis)** or ciliary body **(cyclitis)** or, more usually, of both **(iridocyclitis).***

Etiology

The causes are varied and seldom identified. Spread of infection from a remote focus, though often blamed, has rarely been verified. Viral infections and hypersensitivity reactions have also been implicated. Granulomatous uveitis may occur with syphilis, tuberculosis, and sarcoidosis, while nongranulomatous uveitis occurs with keratoconjunctivitis, corneal ulcer, episcleritis, ocular trauma, retinal detachment, and some systemic diseases (e.g., ankylosing spondylitis).

Symptoms and Signs

Moderate to severe ocular and periocular pain, photophobia, redness, and lacrimation are common initial symptoms; blurred vision and transient myopia may occur. There is circumcorneal ciliary injection, the surface details of the iris are obscured, and the pupil may be small and irregular. The aqueous humor often appears turbid, fibrin may be seen in the anterior chamber, and inflammatory cells may coalesce to form small, round, pale deposits on the corneal endothelium **(keratic precipitates)**. TABLE 181-1 lists features that distinguish acute anterior uveitis from acute glaucoma and conjunctivitis.

Acute anterior uveitis lasts a few days to several weeks and may recur. Chronic anterior uveitis may last months or years. In severe cases, inflammatory cells and proteinaceous debris gravitate to form a cream-colored meniscus **(hypopyon)** along the lower portion of the anterior chamber, and adhesions develop between the posterior surface of the iris and the lens capsule **(posterior synechiae)**. If synechiae form around the entire pupillary circumference **(total or complete posterior synechia)**, the flow of aqueous between the posterior and anterior chambers is blocked, the iris bulges forward **(iris bombé)**, and an angle-closure glaucoma results *that can be rapidly blinding if unrelieved.* Neglected or chronic anterior uveitis may lead to secondary open-angle glaucoma, corneal disease, or cataract.

Treatment

Mydriasis to prevent development of posterior synechiae, cycloplegia to reduce pain, and suppression of damaging inflammatory activity are the objectives. Therefore, 1% atropine drops 2 to 3 times/day and 0.1% dexamethasone drops, 4 to 6 times/day initially, are instilled. A short-term systemic corticosteroid (e.g., prednisone 25 to 50 mg/day orally) may be required in severe cases; if contraindicated by other medical problems, a depot form of corticosteroid (e.g., methylprednisolone acetate 40 to 80 mg) may be injected under Tenon's capsule, but depot injections of corticosteroids are **contraindicated** in herpetic keratouveitis. Specific therapy is indicated when an underlying cause has been identified.

TABLE 181-1. DIFFERENTIAL DIAGNOSIS OF CERTAIN ACUTE EYE DISORDERS

Acute Iritis	Acute Glaucoma	Acute Conjunctivitis
Pain: moderately severe	Pain: very severe	Pain: burning, but not severe
Vision: moderately decreased	Vision: considerably decreased	Vision: normal
Eyeball tension: usually normal or soft	Eyeball tension: increased	Eyeball tension: unchanged
Lacrimation	Lacrimation	Mucous or mucopurulent discharge
Injection: circumcorneal	Injection: circumcorneal and episcleral	Injection: superficial conjunctival
Cornea: transparent; precipitates may be present on posterior surface	Cornea: appears steamy	Cornea: normal
Anterior chamber: normal depth	Anterior chamber: very shallow	Anterior chamber: normal depth
Iris: dull and swollen	Iris: congested and bulging	Iris: normal
Pupil: small, irregular	Pupil: mid-dilated	Pupil: normal

An ophthalmologist should be consulted. Chronic use of topical corticosteroids may increase ocular tension in predisposed persons ("steroid responders"), may cause lens opacities, and can cause serious ocular disease when bacterial or viral corneal infections (e.g., herpes simplex) are present. Also, response to therapy is best followed by a physician experienced in slit-lamp biomicroscopy.

POSTERIOR UVEITIS

Inflammation of the choroid (choroiditis) and, usually, of the overlying retina (chorioretinitis).

Etiology

Although granulomatous diseases (e.g., toxoplasmosis) are frequently implicated, the cause is often unknown. In children, unilateral chorioretinitis with vitreous membranes may be due to an intraocular parasite.

Symptoms and Signs

Blurred vision, distortion of the size or shape of objects (metamorphopsia), and floating black spots are common presenting symptoms. Ocular pain and lacrimation are less common than in anterior uveitis. Marked reduction in visual acuity may accompany an inflammatory focus in the posterior pole of the eye; peripheral lesions cause little visual deficit. Vitreous haze and opacities and a poorly defined, grayish-yellow or white chorioretinal lesion may be seen through the ophthalmoscope. Punched-out, pigmented, atrophic chorioretinal scars, seen in either eye, usually indicate recurrent uveitis. Complications include exudative retinal detachment, secondary glaucoma, cataract, and endophthalmitis.

Diagnosis

Ophthalmoscopic findings may suggest a specific etiology. Old pigmented geographic chorioretinal scars with an adjacent ("satellite") active focus are common in toxoplasmosis. A central macular lesion associated with a small hemorrhage, peripapillary chorioretinal scarring, and peripheral punched-out atrophic spots is typical of "presumed ocular histoplasmosis." A solitary uniocular inflammatory mass in a young child with a dog or cat at home suggests *Toxocara* infestation.

Skin or serologic tests for tuberculosis, toxoplasmosis, and syphilis; chest x-ray; blood count; and stool examinations of pets for ova and parasites may support a diagnosis.

Treatment

Active chorioretinitis frequently responds to systemic corticosteroid therapy; macular or paramacular involvement demands immediate, vigorous treatment (e.g., with prednisone 50 to 100 mg daily during the acute phase, then on alternate days with decreasing doses until quiescent). The pupil is dilated with 1% cyclopentolate drops or 2% homatropine drops t.i.d. to prevent posterior synechiae and facilitate subsequent examinations. Specific therapy is given when the cause is identified. Since an inflammatory component in the parafoveal "presumed ocular histoplasmosis" lesion is debated, corticosteroids usually are not prescribed. Photocoagulation of the lesion has been helpful in limiting macular damage in some patients.

SYMPATHETIC OPHTHALMIA

A severe bilateral granulomatous uveitis that occurs as a hypersensitivity reaction to uveal pigment following trauma to one eye. The condition usually follows accidental or surgical perforation of the globe or a retained intraocular foreign body. The incidence of this complication is < 0.1%.

Symptoms and Signs

Two weeks to several years after injury or surgery, symptoms of uveal tract irritation (photophobia, lacrimation, transient blurring of vision, neuralgic pain, eye tenderness) develop in both the injured ("exciting") eye and the uninjured ("sympathizing") eye. This is accompanied by ciliary injection, vitreous opacities, keratic precipitates, and other signs of acute uveitis. *Insufficient or delayed treatment can result in phthisis and blindness in both eyes.*

Treatment

Prompt, adequate treatment of a severely injured eye by a specialist is essential; its enucleation before uveal irritation develops in the uninjured eye may be indicated to prevent sympathetic ophthalmia. The injured eye should be enucleated when sightless or when preservation of sight is unlikely, especially if the ciliary body is involved. When there is useful vision in the injured eye, the need for enucleation becomes a difficult decision, since the irritation often subsides without an active sympathetic inflammation.

Purely prophylactic corticosteroid treatment is not recommended. However, at the first signs of uveitis in an injured eye, in which development of sympathetic ophthalmia is suspected, intensive topical and systemic corticosteroid therapy (e.g., 0.1% dexamethasone drops 6 times/day and prednisone orally 80 to 100 mg/day) should be started, then continued as long and as vigorously as necessary to control the disease, 1% atropine being used to keep the pupils well dilated. If this fails, treatment with antimetabolites (e.g. methotrexate, azathioprine, or cyclophosphamide) may be considered. (CAUTION: *These drugs are highly toxic and the patient should be monitored closely during therapy.*)

PANOPHTHALMITIS; ENDOPHTHALMITIS

Panophthalmitis: *A suppurative inflammation involving all three coats of the eye and usually causing its complete destruction.* **Endophthalmitis:** *A similar inflammation restricted to the uveal tract, vitreous body, and retina.* The causative pyogenic organisms may be introduced by trauma, perforating corneal ulcer, metastatic septic embolus, or the extension of orbital cellulitis.

Symptoms and Signs

There is intense eye pain, rapid loss of vision, conjunctival and ciliary injection, chemosis, lid swelling, and rapid spread of pus throughout the interior of the eye. The sclera eventually ruptures and the purulent contents of the eyeball drain, leaving a blind, shrunken globe. Severe constitutional symptoms (fever, headache, vomiting) may be present.

Treatment

Therapy must begin on suspicion of the diagnosis. As soon as possible, specific medications should be selected on the basis of organisms cultured and their sensitivities. Large systemic doses of antibiotics or sulfonamides are indicated. Culture of aspirated intraocular fluids as well as subconjunctival or intraocular administration of antibiotics are sometimes indicated but should be conducted by an ophthalmologist. Concomitant systemic corticosteroid therapy is often of value.

CHOROIDAL MALIGNANT MELANOMA

This is the most common ocular malignancy. It occurs mainly during middle age and is rare in blacks. In the early stages, the melanoma is a slightly convex, slate gray mass with a smooth retinal surface; hemorrhage is rare. As the tumor grows, it may become mushroom-shaped. An overlying secondary nonrhegmatogenous retinal detachment (see in Ch. 182) can mask its presence in advanced cases. **Symptoms** may be absent, but metamorphopsia and decreased visual acuity will be present if the tumor or the retinal detachment involves the macula. Visual field testing will reveal a scotoma caused by the tumor or detachment. Secondary glaucoma may occur.

Diagnosis is aided by indirect ophthalmoscopy, transillumination, fluorescein angiography, and ultrasonography. **Treatment** by enucleation is indicated if distant metastases are not present. If extraocular extension is discovered at surgery, orbital exenteration is necessary. Five-year survival is about 40 to 50%, but metastatic recurrence may appear years later. Some small posterior tumors without retinal detachment may respond to photocoagulation.

182.   RETINA

VASCULAR RETINOPATHIES

Retinal hemorrhage, exudates, edema, ischemia, or infarction due to ocular or systemic vascular disorders.

Arteriosclerotic retinopathy is found in generalized arteriosclerosis and is often secondary to hypertension. The walls of the retinal arterioles become thickened, and the changes are reflected on ophthalmoscopy as a widened arteriolar light reflex. As the sclerosis progresses, one sees indentation of the veins at arteriovenous crossings and an increased difference between the sizes of the venous and arteriolar blood columns. The fine arterioles and veins may become tortuous, and the arteries may appear sheathed. Advanced sclerosis at arteriovenous crossings can cause branch retinal vein occlusion.

Hypertensive retinopathy occurs in chronic essential hypertension, malignant hypertension, and toxemia of pregnancy. The fundi show generalized or focal retinal arteriolar constriction in the early stages. As the disease progresses, superficial flame-shaped hemorrhages and small white or gray foci of retinal ischemia ("cotton-wool spots") develop. Yellow exudates, due to lipid deposition deep in the retina, are seen later, often producing a star-shaped figure around the macula. (See also Hypertension in Ch. 24.) The optic disc becomes congested and edematous in severe hypertension and resembles the choked disc caused by brain tumor (**papilledema;** see in Ch. 184).

Treatment

Arteriosclerotic and hypertensive retinopathies can be managed only by medical control of the primary systemic disorder.

CENTRAL RETINAL ARTERY OCCLUSION

Central retinal artery occlusion produces a painless, sudden, unilateral blindness. The occlusion may be due to embolism (disseminated atherosclerotic plaques, endocarditis, fat emboli [Purtscher's retinopathy], atrial myxoma) or to thrombosis in a sclerotic central artery. Another important cause is cranial arteritis (temporal arteritis; see in Ch. 28). The pupil is semidilated and responds poorly to direct light but constricts briskly when the other eye is illuminated. Ophthalmoscopy discloses a pale, opaque fundus with a bright red fovea ("cherry red spot"). The arteries are attenuated and may appear bloodless; the veins are narrow, with less blood than normal. An embolic obstruction is sometimes visible, and if it is not relieved quickly, retinal infarction occurs and blindness is permanent. If a major branch is occluded rather than the entire artery, fundus abnormalities are limited to that sector of the retina, and a permanent subtotal visual field loss follows unless the occlusion is relieved.

Branch retinal artery occlusion is almost always embolic.

Treatment

Immediate treatment is imperative. Reduction of intraocular tension by intermittent digital massage over the closed eyelids or anterior chamber paracentesis may dislodge an embolus and allow it to enter a smaller branch of the artery, thus reducing the area of retinal ischemia. Inhalation of 5 to 10% CO_2 in O_2 may relieve retinal arterial spasm.

CENTRAL RETINAL VEIN OCCLUSION

Central retinal vein occlusion usually appears in elderly arteriosclerotic patients. Glaucoma, covert diabetes mellitus, hypertension, increased blood viscosity, or an elevated Hct can be predisposing factors. Occlusion in a young person is uncommon; it may be idiopathic or result from retinal phlebitis. Painless visual loss occurs less abruptly than in arterial obstruction. The retinal veins appear distended and tortuous, the fundus is congested and edematous, and numerous retinal hemorrhages appear. These changes are limited to one quadrant if the obstruction involves only a branch of the vein. Neovascularization of the retina or of the iris (**rubeosis iridis)** with secondary glaucoma can occur weeks to months after the occlusion. Fluorescein angiography is essential to determine the state of the circulation. Patients with normal retinal vessel perfusion usually do well; those with poor perfusion are more likely to develop complications.

Treatment

There is no generally accepted medical therapy. Tonometry to detect predisposing glaucoma, a blood-clotting survey, and a glucose tolerance test are worthwhile. Destruction of secondary retinal neovascular overgrowth by photocoagulation may decrease vitreous hemorrhages. Secondary neovascular glaucoma requires panretinal photocoagulation.

DIABETIC RETINOPATHY

This major cause of blindness can be particularly severe in juvenile diabetics but is also frequent in chronic adult-onset diabetes. Although the severity of the metabolic derangement is important, the degree of retinopathy seems more related to the duration of the diabetes than to its stability. Hypertension has a further deleterious effect. The first signs are often venous dilation and small red dots seen ophthalmoscopically in the posterior retinal pole. The dots are caused by single or clustered capillary microaneurysms that can be demonstrated by fluorescein angiography. Dot and blot retinal hemorrhages and deep-lying edema and edema residues may impair macular function. Macular edema is a common cause of visual impairment in diabetics and may best be detected or confirmed by fluorescein angiography. Proliferative retinal neovascularization **(retinitis proliferans)** in the posterior pole occurs in advanced disease; the new vessels may extend into the vitreous cavity with subsequent vitreous hemorrhages, fibrous tissue formation, and secondary retinal detachment.

Treatment

Control of the diabetes and blood pressure is important. Photocoagulation (by xenon arc or argon laser) may reduce the degree of retinal edema and the frequency and severity of hemorrhagic episodes. Some diabetics threatened with blindness have improved after pituitary ablation, but the procedure produces major long-term endocrine deficiencies and candidates must be carefully selected. Vitrectomy may be useful in some cases of longstanding vitreous hemorrhage.

SENILE MACULAR DEGENERATION

Senile macular degeneration is a leading cause of visual diminution in the elderly. There is no sex predilection, but the condition is seen much more commonly in white than in black people. There is no known predisposing, systemic condition and there is some suggestion that the condition may have a hereditary basis. Two different forms of senile macular degeneration can be defined: The first is an **atrophic form** in which there is a pigmentary disturbance in the macular region but no elevated macular scar and little or no hemorrhage or exudation in the region of the macula; the second is called **disciform macular degeneration** and is characterized by the formation of an exudative mound, often with subretinal and intraretinal hemorrhage surrounding the mound. Eventually this exudative mound contracts and leaves a distinct elevated scar at the posterior pole. Both the exudative and the atrophic forms of macular degeneration are generally bilateral and are often preceded by the appearance of multiple drusen in the macular region.

Symptoms, Signs, and Diagnosis

There may be a slow or sudden, painless loss of central visual acuity. Occasionally the first symptom may be visual distortion from one eye, and this can be easily tested with an Amsler Grid. Funduscopy will reveal a pigmentary or hemorrhagic disturbance in the macular region of the involved eye; the contralateral eye almost always shows some evidence of pigmentary disturbance and the presence of drusen in the macula. Fluorescein angiography often demonstrates neovascular membranes beneath the retina, particularly in the disciform variety.

Treatment

No medical therapy is of value in treating senile macular degeneration. Smoking probably should be curtailed. If neovascular nets can be demonstrated by fluorescein angiography and if such nets are not in the immediate area of the fovea, then photocoagulation can be attempted to obliterate the new vessels and perhaps prevent hemorrhage and exudation.

RETINAL DETACHMENT

Separation of the neural retina from the underlying retinal pigment epithelium.

Although detachment may be localized initially, without treatment the entire retina may detach. **Rhegmatogenous detachment** implies a through and through break in the retina and is seen most often in myopia, after cataract surgery, or following ocular trauma. In these cases fluid percolates through the hole from the vitreous into the subretinal space. **Nonrhegmatogenous detachments** can be produced by vitreoretinal traction (e.g., proliferative retinopathy of diabetes or sickle cell disease) or by transudation of fluid into the subretinal space (e.g., severe uveitis, especially in Vogt-Koyanagi-Harada disease, or primary or metastatic choroidal tumors).

Symptoms, Signs, and Diagnosis

Retinal detachment is painless. Premonitory symptoms include dark or irregular vitreous floaters, flashes of light, or blurred vision. As the detachment progresses, the patient notices a curtain or veil in the field of vision. If the macula is involved, central visual acuity fails drastically.

Visual acuity can be measured with the Snellen chart or any reading material. Each eye is tested separately (with glasses, if the patient wears them). Visual fields can be estimated by confrontation testing. Direct ophthalmoscopy may show retinal irregularities and a bullous retinal elevation with darkened blood vessels. Indirect ophthalmoscopy, including scleral depression, may be necessary to detect peripheral breaks and detachment.

If a vitreous hemorrhage obscures the fundus, especially in a myopic, aphakic (post-cataract extraction), or injured eye, retinal detachment should be suspected and ultrasonography performed. The patient should be hospitalized, sedated, and kept in bed with his head elevated. Binocular patching and pupillary dilatation are used until an adequate examination can be carried out.

Any patient with a suspected or established retinal detachment should be seen, on an emergency basis, by an ophthalmologist. Prognosis is best if the condition is treated before macular involvement occurs.

Treatment

Rhegmatogenous detachment is treated by finding the retinal holes and sealing them by diathermy or cryotherapy. The eye may be shortened by scleral "buckling" and by implanting silicone rubber sponges. Fluid may be drained from the subretinal space. Anterior retinal breaks without detachment can be sealed by transconjunctival cryopexy; posterior breaks, by photocoagulation. More than 90% of rhegmatogenous detachments can be reattached surgically.

Nonrhegmatogenous detachments due to vitreoretinal traction may be treatable by intravitreal surgery; transudative detachments due to uveitis may respond to systemic corticosteroid therapy, but occasionally may require antimetabolite therapy. Primary choroidal neoplasms (malignant melanomas) may require enucleation, though radiation and local resection are used occasionally; choroidal hemangiomas respond to localized photocoagulation. Metastatic choroidal neoplasms (the usual primary sites are breast, lung, and GI tract) respond well to radiotherapy, and the eyes should *not* be enucleated.

RETROLENTAL FIBROPLASIA

(Retinopathy of Prematurity)

A bilateral disease characterized by abnormality of the retinal vessels that occurs in premature infants in whom the immature retina was exposed to high postnatal incubation O_2 concentrations. Affected infants usually weigh < 1500 gm at birth. Increased O_2 concentration causes initial retinal vasoconstriction and then vaso-obliteration, especially in the temporal retinal periphery. This may be followed by neovascularization. If severe, fibrovascular invasion of the vitreous and retinal detachment may result. If mild, the abnormal vessels may regress and useful vision is possible. Delayed cicatricial changes occur in some during the lst yr, resulting in dragging of the retinal vessels and macula into a temporal retinal fold. Myopia is a common finding. Other associated problems include glaucoma, retinal detachment (which can occur even in the teens or 20s), and mental retardation.

Prevention and Treatment

Careful monitoring of incubator O_2 is needed to minimize the incidence of this complication of prematurity. The lowest concentration necessary for maintenance should be used. The ocular danger increases with $O_2 > 30\%$. An ophthalmologist should be consulted not only by the neonatologist but also in later years so that long-term complications can be diagnosed and treated. (See also under PREMATURE INFANT in Vol. II, Ch. 21.)

RETINOBLASTOMA

(See Vol. II, Ch. 25)

RETINITIS PIGMENTOSA

(See Vol. I, Ch. 25)

---

183.   GLAUCOMA

A disorder characterized by increased intraocular pressure that may cause impaired vision, ranging from slight loss to absolute blindness. **Primary glaucoma** in adults may be of two types: (1) **chronic open-angle** (wide-angle) or (2) **acute or chronic angle-closure** (closed-angle, narrow-angle, congestive, acute glaucoma attack). **Congenital (infantile) glaucoma** is also primary. **Secondary glaucoma** results from preexisting ocular disease, usually uveitis, intraocular tumor, or an enlarged cataract. Prolonged corticosteroid therapy, especially with topical ophthalmic preparations, can produce an increased pressure, particularly in patients with a predisposition, so-called steroid responders. It may be present after 1 wk, but usually occurs by the 6th to 8th wk of therapy. The increased pressure usually, but not always, subsides with cessation of therapy. Periodic tonometry is advisable during long-term corticosteroid use, to discover early elevated pressure and preclude damage from a severe or prolonged intraocular pressure rise.

TABLE 183-1 lists the salient findings and usual treatment for the most common forms of glaucoma. Rarer forms may occur with associated congenital anomalies (e.g., Sturge-Weber's and Marfan's syndromes) or with vascular or degenerative disorders.

PRIMARY GLAUCOMA

Etiology and Pathogenesis

The causes are unknown. Vasomotor and emotional instability, hyperopia, and especially heredity are among the predisposing factors. The increased intraocular tension is related to an imbalance between production and outflow of the aqueous humor. Obstruction to outflow appears to be mainly responsible for this imbalance. In chronic open-angle glaucoma, the anterior chamber and its anatomic structures appear normal but drainage of the aqueous humor is impeded. In acute and chronic angle-closure (congestive) glaucoma, the anterior chamber is shallow, the filtration angle is narrowed, and the iris may obstruct the trabecular meshwork at the entrance of the canal of Schlemm. Dilation of the pupil may push the root of the iris forward against the angle or may produce pupillary block and thus precipitate an acute attack. Eyes with narrow anterior chamber angles are predisposed to acute angle-closure glaucoma attacks of varying degrees of severity.

CHRONIC OPEN-ANGLE GLAUCOMA

A disorder characterized by a gradual rise in intraocular pressure, causing slowly progressive loss of peripheral vision and, when uncontrolled, late loss of central vision and ultimate blindness. The most prevalent form of glaucoma, it is common after age 30 but may occur in early childhood. It is usually familial. Rarely, it is unilateral.

Diagnosis

Glaucoma should be suspected in any patient, especially if over 40, who requires frequent spectacle lens changes, has mild headaches or vague visual disturbances, sees halos around electric lights, or has impaired dark adaptation. Since glaucoma can be asymptomatic until irreversible damage has occurred, every routine eye examination (and, optimally, every physical examination) in all adult patients should include examination with a tonometer. A single normal reading does not rule out glaucoma, since normal pressure shows diurnal variations of about 3 to 4 mm Hg (and even greater). The pressure rise in early glaucoma may be intermittent. A high-normal pressure reading is an indication for frequent follow-up examinations. In suspected cases, provocative testing is indicated.

Cupping of the optic disk is characteristic but a normal optic disk does not rule out glaucoma, since optic nerve damage develops insidiously and, in some cases, late in the disease. Visual field changes may be subtle, with normal-appearing disks. The earliest changes in the central visual field are a baring of the blind spot and small scotomata above or below fixation, with small and dim visual field targets. Subtle nasal peripheral field defects appear early. The external eye usually appears normal.

Treatment

Most cases can be controlled with eyedrops. Beginning with the weakest available preparations (e.g., 0.5% pilocarpine), the most effective concentration and frequency of administration are determined by trial. Preparations of choice are pilocarpine, timolol maleate, carbachol, and, in aphakic eyes only, potent cholinesterase inhibitors such as isoflurophate (CAUTION: *Patients treated with powerful miotics like demecarium, echothiophate, and isoflurophate may develop cataracts or retinal detachment, which must be looked for periodically during treatment*). Rarely, 2% pilocarpine ointment is used at night to supplement other medication. Carbonic anhydrase inhibitors (e.g., dichlorphenamide 50 to 200 mg/day or acetazolamide 125 to 250 mg q.i.d. orally) are of value when miotics alone do not control abnormal tension but should be used with caution. Epinephrine 0.5 to 2%, 1 drop 1 to 2 times/day, may aid control by reducing aqueous production; recently it has been recommended that for more effective management dipivefrin hydrochloride 0.1% solution used once or twice a day may be substituted for epinephrine. The patient should avoid fatigue, emotional upsets, use of tobacco, and drinking large quantities of fluids. Tonometry and charting of visual fields should be performed semi-annually or more often when indicated. When medication fails to control intraocular tension or visual fields show increasing defects, laser trabeculopexy or filtering surgery to improve aqueous drainage should be considered.

ACUTE ANGLE-CLOSURE GLAUCOMA

A disorder characterized by attacks of suddenly increased intraocular pressure, usually unilateral, with severe pain and loss of vision, caused by acute obstruction of aqueous drainage within the eye.

Symptoms and Signs

Prodromal symptoms occur as transitory episodes of diminished visual acuity, colored halos around lights, and pain in the eye and head. At such times, examination will show a somewhat dilated, poorly reacting pupil and shallow anterior chamber in the affected eye. These episodes may last only a few hours and recur at intervals before a typical prolonged attack of acute angle-closure glaucoma. The acute attack is characterized by rapid loss of sight and sudden onset of severe throbbing pain in the eye; the pain radiates over the sensory distribution of the 5th nerve. *Nausea and vomiting are common and may be mistaken for acute GI disease.* Upper lid edema, lacrimation, circumcorneal injection, chemosis, and a somewhat dilated, fixed pupil may be present. The cornea

TABLE 183–1. CHARACTERISTICS OF

Type of Glaucoma	Age	Iridocorneal Angle	Cornea	Pupil; Iris
Chronic open-angle glaucoma	Rare in children and young adults; incidence rises from age 30 on	Wide open; may show pigment deposits	Not remarkable	Pupil not dilated. Iris may be atrophic late in the course
Angle-closure: acute; glaucoma attack	Any age, but more frequent after age 30	Closed during acute attack; narrow in interim	Cloudy. Microcystic edema of epithelium frequent	Pupil mid-dilated, fixed. Iris appears muddy
Glaucomato-cyclitic crisis (Posner-Schlossman syndrome)	Any age from young adulthood on	Narrow (not closed) or wide open	May be clear with keratic precipitates. Edema may be present	Pupil not dilated or only slightly dilated
Angle-closure: chronic; recurrent glaucoma attack	Any age	Narrow; closable with peripheral anterior synechiae	Usually cloudy during attack, clear between attacks	Pupil usually dilated during attack, normal between attacks
Congenital (infantile) glaucoma	Birth to 1st few mo of life (usually discovered before age 6 mo)	Closed by membrane	Large in diameter, cloudy	Pupil dilated. Iris may show atrophy
Secondary glaucoma	Any age (usually accompanying or following anterior uveitis)	Angle may be blocked by inflammatory debris or pigment	May be cloudy. Microcystic edema may be present	Pupil may be narrow. Iris may appear muddy
Corticosteroid-induced glaucoma	Any age in susceptible individuals ("steroid responders") after prolonged ophthalmic use	Wide open or narrow (not closed)	Usually clear	Pupil reacts; not constricted or dilated

is steamy, the anterior chamber shallow, and the aqueous humor turbid enough to obscure the fundus. Intraocular pressure is increased considerably. (TABLE 181–1 in Ch. 181 lists findings that distinguish acute glaucoma, iritis, and conjunctivitis.) Symptoms usually subside after medical treatment, but may recur. Each acute attack progressively diminishes vision and contracts the visual field. The condition may be bilateral.

Glaucomatocyclitic crisis (Posner-Schlossman syndrome), a recurrent monocular rise in pressure, simulates acute angle-closure glaucoma but is associated with normal anterior chamber depth, keratic precipitates, and other signs of uveitis.

THE COMMON FORMS OF GLAUCOMA

Optic Nerve Head & Visual Field	Intraocular Pressure	Subjective Symptoms	Treatment of Choice
May appear normal or show cupping. Progressive visual field defect if untreated	Elevated slightly (22 to 30 mm Hg) or markedly (30 to 45 mm Hg). Usually bilateral	Blurring of vision, frequent change of glasses. Occasional headaches, often ascribed by patient to "nervous tension" or "sinus problems"	*Topical:* Pilocarpine, timolol maleate, epinephrine, dipivefrin, demecarium bromide *Systemic:* Carbonic anhydrase inhibitors *Surgery:* Subscleral filtering procedure if medication fails
Optic nerve head obscured during attack; may be normal. May show cupping after several attacks. Typical glaucomatous field defects may develop	40 to 70 mm Hg or even higher. Usually unilateral	Severe head & eye ache, blurred vision, halos around lights, general malaise, nausea, sometimes vomiting (GI symptoms may be misleading, delaying proper diagnosis)	*Topical:* Pilocarpine, timolol maleate *Systemic:* Osmotic agents, carbonic anhydrase inhibitors *Surgery:* Peripheral iridectomy when eye is quiet
Usually no cupping. *No visual field loss!*	May be 50 mm Hg or higher. Usually unilateral	Blurred vision, halos around lights, headache. Nausea rare	*Topical:* Corticosteroid drops *Systemic:* Carbonic anhydrase inhibitors *Surgery: Strictly contraindicated*
As for acute angle-closure glaucoma	Up to 70 or higher during attack. Between attacks normal. Usually unilateral	Severe headaches during attacks, blurred vision, halos around lights. Nausea rare.	*Surgery:* Iridectomy; filtering surgery if > 1/2 of iridocorneal angle is permanently closed
Usually hard to evaluate. Later atrophic and may show cupping	Markedly elevated (50 to 70 mm Hg). Usually bilateral	Not assessable	*Surgery:* goniotomy, goniopuncture, trabeculotomy
Initially may appear normal; if condition persists, may be cupped or atrophic. Glaucomatous field defect may develop	May be 50 mm Hg or higher. Usually unilateral	Blurred vision, halos, headache. Nausea rare	*Topical:* Anti-inflammatory management *Systemic:* Anti-inflammatory management, carbonic anhydrase inhibitors
Initially no cupping; if not treated, cupping may develop. Glaucomatous field defect develops	May be 50 mm Hg or higher. Frequently unilateral	Blurred vision and halos initially rare; headaches may be present. Blurred vision common in later stages	*Stop corticosteroids* *Topical:* Pilocarpine 1 to 4%, timolol maleate 0.25 or 0.5%, demecarium bromide 0.125 or 0.25%. *Systemic:* Carbonic anhydrase inhibitors

Treatment

Oral glycerin 1 to 2 gm/kg, mixed with an equal amount of water (cooled and preferably flavored with lemon), will often abort acute attacks, and is excellent initial therapy to reduce elevated intraocular pressure rapidly. Oral carbonic anhydrase inhibitors (e.g., acetazolamide 500 mg), if given immediately, will generally abort an attack. If not, acetazolamide 500 mg IV and frequent instillation of miotics (e.g., pilocarpine 4% q 15 min) for 1 to 2 h are indicated. Once the tension is normal, an oral carbonic anhydrase inhibitor q 6 h can be continued for several doses, together with miotics. If the initial therapy does not reduce the tension, 20% mannitol 500 ml by slow IV drip can be given (unless otherwise contraindicated), to be followed by miotics and a carbonic anhydrase inhibitor. Surgery, peripheral iridectomy or laser iridotomy, prevents further attacks and is often performed prophylactically on the unaffected fellow eye as well, if the angle appears to be narrow by gonioscopy.

Glaucomatocyclic crisis responds to systemic and topical corticosteroids and carbonic anhydrase inhibitors such as dichlorphenamide or acetazolamide; *surgery is strictly contraindicated.*

CHRONIC ANGLE-CLOSURE GLAUCOMA

A disorder characterized by recurrent attacks—usually unilateral, of increased intraocular pressure, pain, and impaired vision—similar to those of acute angle-closure glaucoma but less severe. The causes are similar, but the anterior angle is obstructed gradually, not suddenly. Factors that promote dilation of the pupil may be precipitating causes. The fellow eye frequently becomes involved later. A provocative test for this condition is the **darkroom test**—exposing the patient (who must be awake) to 60 min of darkness with the head bent forward in a prone position (best performed leaning on a Mayo table), then promptly measuring the intraocular pressure.

Treatment
One or two drops of pilocarpine 1 or 2% instilled 3 to 6 times/day is the treatment of choice for temporary management. Timolol maleate 1 drop 0.25 or 0.5% solution used 1 or 2 times/day can be *added*, to aid temporary management; it should not be used without pilocarpine because timolol maleate does not contract the pupil and therefore does not promote the removal of the iris from the iridocorneal angle. Oral glycerin or mannitol by IV drip (see ACUTE ANGLE-CLOSURE GLAUCOMA, above) is useful in aborting attacks. Carbonic anhydrase inhibitors are used only during attacks in narrow-angle glaucoma, and are **contraindicated** in long-term therapy. Early peripheral iridectomy or laser iridotomy usually prevents further attacks. Permanent damage to the iridocorneal angle may necessitate management of the elevated intraocular pressure, even after successful iridectomy or laser iridotomy.

CONGENITAL GLAUCOMA (See Vol. II, Ch. 25)

SECONDARY GLAUCOMA

Glaucoma secondary to an intraocular disorder, usually anterior uveitis.

Etiology and Pathogenesis
This is caused by any interference with the flow of aqueous humor from the posterior chamber through the pupil into the anterior chamber to the canal of Schlemm. Inflammatory disease of the anterior segment may prevent aqueous escape by causing complete posterior synechia and iris bombé, and may plug the drainage channel with exudates. Other common causes are intraocular tumors, enlarged cataracts, central retinal vein occlusion, trauma to the eye, operative procedures, and intraocular hemorrhage.

Treatment
Secondary glaucoma is best treated by an ophthalmologist. The underlying cause, usually uveitis, must be treated. Intensive therapy and probably mydriasis are indicated. Treatment is begun with systemic corticosteroids, and the effect of a mild mydriatic (such as 5% homatropine, 1% cyclopentolate, or 10% phenylephrine) is tested in the office; 1% atropine b.i.d. or t.i.d. is given if the mydriasis is successful. If this fails, use of pilocarpine and/or timolol maleate should be considered. A carbonic anhydrase inhibitor or oral glycerin as for acute angle-closure glaucoma may be useful temporarily during the acute phase. Surgical intervention is indicated in iris bombé, tumor, and swollen cataract.

ABSOLUTE GLAUCOMA

The last stage of any form of uncontrolled glaucoma. The eye is blind from progressive atrophy of the optic nerve head. The pupil usually is widely dilated and fixed, the iris atrophied, and the disc deeply excavated. Pain is no longer prominent but may recur. The eyeball subsequently degenerates.

---

184. OPTIC NERVE; VISUAL PATHWAYS

PAPILLEDEMA
(Choked Disk)

Swelling of the optic nerve head due to increased intracranial pressure. It is usually bilateral and occurs with brain tumor or abscess, cerebral trauma or hemorrhage, meningitis, arachnoidal adhesions, pseudotumor cerebri, cavernous sinus thrombosis, severe hypertensive or renal disease, and pulmonary emphysema.

Vision is not affected initially, but the blind spot is enlarged. The degree of disk elevation is determined by comparing the highest plus lens necessary to bring the most elevated portion of the disk into sharp focus with that used to see an unaffected portion of the retina clearly. Engorged and tortuous retinal veins, a hyperemic disk, and retinal hemorrhages about the disk may be observed. The absence of changes in the arterioles and a normal blood pressure help to differentiate the papilledema of brain tumor from that of hypertension. If the intracranial pressure is not reduced, secondary optic atrophy and loss of vision eventually occur.

PAPILLITIS

(Optic Neuritis)

Inflammation of that portion of the optic nerve visible ophthalmoscopically. It occurs with foci of inflammation in and about the optic nerve, as part of demyelinating conditions following a viral illness or with multiple sclerosis, as a result of infarction of a part or all of the optic nerve head in temporal arteritis or other occlusive disease of the ciliary vessels, from tumorous metastasis to the optic nerve head, from certain chemicals (e.g., lead, ethanol), after bee stings, during meningitis, and from syphilis. It is usually unilateral, though this depends on the etiology. In many cases the etiology remains obscure despite thorough evaluation.

Vision loss, varying from a small central scotoma to complete blindness and frequently maximal within 1 or 2 days, is the only symptom. Ophthalmoscopy discloses hyperemia and edema of the disk with fine vitreous opacities in the early stages, and more noticeable changes in advanced cases. The retina becomes edematous around the nerve head and its vessels engorged; a few exudates and hemorrhages may be present. The condition can last for months.

A particularly important cause of papillitis in patients over age 60 is **cranial giant cell arteritis (temporal arteritis)** (see also TEMPORAL ARTERITIS in Ch. 28). It may present with papillitis in one eye associated with malaise and an elevated ESR. It can rapidly spread to the other eye and result in bilateral blindness. The diagnosis is confirmed by temporal artery biopsy.

With spontaneous remission or successful removal of the cause early in the course, vision is usually restored; otherwise, postneuritic optic atrophy develops, with varying degrees of vision loss depending on the etiology. **Treatment** with corticosteroids, either systemic (e.g., prednisone 60 mg/day orally) or retrobulbar (e.g., methylprednisolone acetate 20 mg), may be helpful. Treatment of cranial giant cell arteritis with systemic corticosteroids is highly effective; see also in Ch. 28.

RETROBULBAR NEURITIS

Inflammation of the orbital portion of the optic nerve, usually unilateral. Multiple sclerosis is responsible for many of the cases; some of the remainder are due to the same factors that cause papillitis, but idiopathic cases are even more common with retrobulbar neuritis than with papillitis. Rapid loss of vision and pain on moving the eye are the principal symptoms. In contrast to papillitis, the fundus usually appears normal, though some mild disk hyperemia is seen occasionally. Spontaneous remission, with normal vision restored, often occurs in 2 to 8 wk. In some cases a central scotoma and pallor of the temporal portion of the disk may remain. Relapses are frequent, especially in multiple sclerosis. Each relapse increases the residual visual damage and temporal pallor; optic atrophy and permanent total visual loss may result. **Treatment** is the same as for optic neuritis.

TOXIC AMBLYOPIA

A reduction in visual acuity believed to be due to a toxic reaction in the orbital portion of the optic nerve. Toxic amblyopia overlaps with retrobulbar neuritis. It is usually bilateral and usually seen in patients who use excessive alcohol or tobacco. In the former case, malnutrition may be the true underlying etiology. Cases of true tobacco amblyopia are rare. Lead, methanol, chloramphenicol, digitalis, and many other chemicals have also been implicated.

An initially small central or pericentral scotoma slowly enlarges and progressively interferes with vision. It may become absolute and lead to blindness. Abnormalities are not usually seen, but later in the course a temporal disk pallor may develop.

Treatment

Vision may improve if the cause is removed immediately, unless the optic nerve has atrophied. Chelation is indicated in lead poisoning.

OPTIC ATROPHY

Atrophy of the optic nerve, commonly divided into primary and secondary. In **primary optic atrophy,** the disk is white or grayish with sharp edges and a saucer-shaped excavation. The lamina cribrosa is clearly visible and the retina is usually normal. In **secondary optic atrophy,** the disk is dirty white with irregular, indistinct margins and is covered by glial tissue that conceals the lamina cribrosa. Evidence of previous inflammation (such as sheathed vessels) may be seen in the retina.

Visual loss is directly proportional to the degree of nerve atrophy. Total blindness with a pupil that is unreactive to direct light can be seen.

Nothing can be done to restore vision once the optic nerve has atrophied. Therapy, rarely of value, must be directed at the underlying factors causing damage to the nerve.

HIGHER VISUAL PATHWAY LESIONS

The site of damage along the optic pathway determines the nature of visual field changes (see Fig. 184–1). Optic nerve lesions result in visual disturbances restricted to the affected eye. Lesions about the chiasm usually affect vision bilaterally. Lesions above or below the chiasm (e.g., a pituitary tumor) destroy nerve fibers supplying the inner (nasal) half of both retinas with consequent defects in the temporal visual fields **(bitemporal hemianopia).** Lesions in the optic tract, optic radiations, or cerebral cortex produce **homonymous hemianopia,** with loss of function in the right or left halves of both visual fields opposite to the side affected. This, the most common type of hemianopia, is usually caused by a brain tumor or CVA.

Treatment is that of the primary lesion.

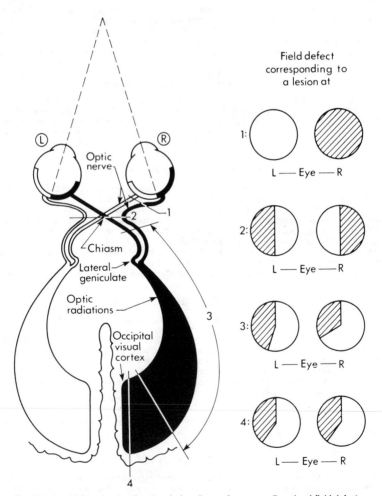

FIG. 184–1.   Higher visual pathways—lesion sites and corresponding visual field defects.

185. CONTACT LENSES

Hard corneal contact lenses are thin, saucer-shaped disks made of polymethyl methacrylate (a hard plastic) that float on the tear layer overlying the cornea. They are 7 to 10 mm in diameter and cover part of the cornea. **Soft hydrophilic contact lenses** are about 13 to 15 mm in diameter and cover the entire cornea. Made of poly-2-hydroxyethyl methacrylate (**HEMA**) and other soft plastics, they mold to the eye. **Flexible nonhydrophilic lenses** (e.g., made of silicone) are being investigated; **cellulose acetate butyrate (CAB) polymer lenses** are available. Both promise increased O_2 transmission to the wearer's cornea.

Contact lenses often provide better visual acuity and peripheral vision than do eyeglasses and are prescribed to correct refractive errors (e.g., nearsightedness and farsightedness, astigmatism, aniso-metropia, aniseikonia, and aphakia after cataract removal) and for keratoconus. Either soft or hard lenses may be prescribed. Toric hard and soft contact lenses (similar to cylindrical lenses in spectacles) are used to correct astigmatism.

Soft contact lenses are prescribed, by an ophthalmologist only, for treatment of bullous keratopathy and other corneal disorders ("bandage lenses"). These lenses are also well-tolerated occluders in children when occlusion therapy is needed (e.g., for amblyopia). Prophylactic antibiotic eyedrops (e.g., 0.5% chloramphenicol ophthalmic solution 1 drop b.i.d. or t.i.d.) may be advisable with a bandage-type soft contact lens. The soft lens as a vehicle for delivering topical medications to the eyes is being studied, but is not very promising. Prolonged wearing of contact lenses, especially for use in aphakia after cataract surgery, is practical and results appear promising.

Hard contact lenses require an adaptation period of as long as a week for complete wearing comfort; during this time the wearer gradually increases the daily number of hours the lenses are worn. Wearers usually experience temporary blurring of vision ("spectacle blur"), which should not exceed 2 h, when wearing eyeglasses after removing their contacts.

No pain should be present at any time; pain is a sign of an ill-fitting contact lens.

Hard contact lenses may occasionally cause superficial corneal abrasions accompanied by severe pain, photophobia, and anxiety if they fit poorly, are worn in a harmful (e.g., oxygen-poor, smoky, windy) environment, or are improperly inserted or removed, or if small foreign particles (e.g., soot, dust) are trapped between the contact lens and the cornea. Discomfort may also occur after removing the lenses, especially after prolonged use ("overwearing syndrome"). Spontaneous healing may occur in a day or so if the lenses are not worn, or treatment may be required—dilation of the pupil with a mydriatic to prevent posterior synechiae of the iris, topical antibiotic eye ointments, a firm eye patch, bed rest, and sedation if necessary. Recovery usually is rapid and complete, with no vision impairment. An ophthalmologist should be consulted before the lenses are worn again.

Because of their size, soft lenses are easier for elderly persons to handle. Since soft contact lenses mold to the eye, they are not apt to eject spontaneously (as hard lenses may) and foreign bodies are less likely to lodge underneath them. Wearing comfort usually is immediate and little or no adaptation period is necessary. Soft lenses apparently do not damage the eye even when the eye is closed and may thus be better for patients who may become unconscious (e.g., epileptics, diabetics). On the other hand, soft lenses are brittle when dry and break easily. Moreover, hard lenses are simpler and less time-consuming to care for than are soft lenses, which require special care and handling.

Because soft lenses are hydrophilic, conventional solutions for hard contact lenses should not be used with soft lenses. Most therapeutic eyedrops can be used in conjunction with soft lenses, though originally there was fear of concentrating the preservative of the eyedrops in the soft lens.

The manufacturer's instructions for hygiene and handling of either type of lens must be strictly observed by the user. Persons susceptible to eye infections, those with a hand tremor or arthritis that interferes with lens insertion or removal, and those who are insufficiently motivated to tolerate the temporary discomfort that may occur while adapting to lenses are unlikely to wear either type of lens successfully. Lenses should not be worn if the eyes are inflamed or infected, during sleep, or when swimming.

Toric soft contact lenses for correction of astigmatic refractive errors are available and are very satisfactory in many cases.

§17. DERMATOLOGIC DISORDERS

186. DIAGNOSIS OF SKIN DISEASES

Many skin diseases can be diagnosed by physical examination alone if one is familiar with the primary and secondary lesions and their arrangement and usual distribution. Except for obviously circumscribed diseases, such as a plantar wart, the patient should undress and be examined completely, since he may not notice or report lesions on clothed areas of the body. The oral mucosa, anogenital area, scalp, and nails also will frequently provide clues to the diagnosis. A good light—preferably daylight—is essential. The history may be invaluable in assessing the physical findings.

PRINCIPAL TYPES OF LESIONS

Primary Lesions

These, the earliest changes to appear, are the most important to recognize and, if necessary, to biopsy.

Macule: *A flat, discolored spot of varied size ($<$ 10 mm) and shape.* **Patch:** *A similar spot $>$ 10 mm.* Examples of macules are freckles, flat moles, tattoos, port-wine marks, and the rashes of rickettsial infections, rubella, and rubeola.

Papule: *A solid, elevated lesion usually $<$ 10 mm in diameter.* **Plaque:** *A plateau-like lesion $>$ 10 mm in diameter or a group of confluent papules.* Many cutaneous diseases begin with papules—warts, psoriasis, syphilis, lichen planus, drug eruptions, pigmented moles, seborrheic and actinic keratoses, some phases of acne, epithliomas.

Nodule: *A palpable, solid lesion, $>$ 5 or 10 mm in diameter, that may or may not be elevated.* Examples are keratinous cysts, small lipomas, fibromas, some types of lymphoma, erythema nodosum, and a variety of neoplasms. Larger nodules (20 mm or greater) are classified as **tumors**, benign or malignant.

Vesicle: *A circumscribed, elevated lesion $<$ 5 mm in diameter containing serous fluid.* **Bulla (blister):** *A vesicle $>$ 5 mm in diameter.* Vesicles or bullae are commonly caused by primary irritants, allergic contact dermatitis, physical trauma, sunburn, insect bites, or viral infections (herpes simplex, varicella, herpes zoster); other causes include drug eruptions, pemphigus, dermatitis herpetiformis, erythema multiforme, epidermolysis bullosa, and pemphigoid.

Pustule: *A superficial, elevated lesion containing pus.* Pustules may result from infection or a seropurulent evolution of vesicles or bullae. Possibilities include impetigo, acne, furuncles, carbuncles, certain deep fungus infections, acne, hidradenitis suppurativa, kerion, pustular miliaria, and pustular psoriasis of the palms and soles.

Wheal: *A transient, elevated lesion caused by local edema.* Wheals are a common allergic reaction; e.g., from drug eruptions, insect stings or bites, or sensitivity to cold, heat, pressure, or sunlight.

Telangiectasia: *Dilation of superficial blood vessels.* Telangiectasias may be seen in rosacea or certain systemic diseases (ataxia telangiectasia, scleroderma) and may result from long-term therapy with topical fluorinated corticosteroids, but most are of unknown etiology.

Secondary Lesions

These result either from the natural evolution of primary lesions (e.g., a vesicle bursts, leaving an eroded area) or from the patient's manipulation of the primary lesion (e.g., scratching a vesicle, leaving an eroded or ulcerated area).

Scales: *Heaped-up particles of horny epithelium* (may be a primary or secondary change). The most common scaling rashes are psoriasis, seborrheic dermatitis, superficial fungus infections, tinea versicolor, pityriasis rosea, and chronic dermatitis of any type.

Crust (scab): *Dried serum, blood, or pus.* Crusting is encountered in a wide variety of inflammatory and infectious diseases.

Erosion: *Loss of part or all of the epidermis.* Erosion is often seen in herpes-group virus infections and in pemphigus.

Ulcer: *Loss of epidermis and at least part of the dermis.* When ulcers result from physical trauma or acute bacterial infection, the etiology usually is apparent. Less obvious causes include chronic bacterial and fungus infections, self-inflicted ulcers, various peripheral vascular diseases and neuropathies, systemic scleroderma, and neoplastic tumors.

Excoriation: *A linear or hollowed-out crusted area, caused by scratching, rubbing, or picking.*

Lichenification: *Thickening of the skin with accentuation of the skin markings.* Atopic dermatitis and lichen simplex chronicus (localized scratch dermatitis) are typically associated with lichenification.

Atrophy: *Thinning and wrinkling of the skin resembling cigarette paper.* Atrophy is seen in the aged, and in discoid LE with long-term use of topical fluorinated corticosteroids.

Scar: *The result of healing after destruction of some of the dermis.* Scars, like ulcers, may have easily recognized origins. Others are evolutionary changes, as in discoid LE.

ARRANGEMENT OF LESIONS

The lesions of certain skin diseases form distinctive patterns. The **grouping** of tense vesicles in herpes simplex and zoster, and their linear configuration in the latter, point to the diagnosis. **Annularity** (a tendency to form rings) is typical in granuloma annulare, erythema multiforme, dermatophyte infections, and secondary syphilis. **Linearity** of lesions is sometimes seen with epidermal nevi, linear scleroderma, and contact dermatitis. Lesions in psoriasis, lichen planus, and flat warts may mimic the shape of trauma to the skin **(the Koebner phenomenon, isomorphic reaction).**

DISTRIBUTION OF LESIONS

Much can be learned from the distribution of the lesions. Occasionally, however, a disease does not follow its common pattern of distribution. Psoriasis, for example, appears most commonly on the extensor surfaces, but may appear on flexor surfaces or even on the tip of the penis or on the palms. Some common patterns of skin involvement are as follows:

Acne: Face, neck, chest, upper back. In "tropical acne" the entire trunk may be involved.

Atopic dermatitis: Characteristically involves the antecubital and popliteal spaces, face, neck, and hands. In infants its distribution is not characteristic.

Erythema multiforme: Primarily on the palms, soles, and mucous membranes, but may be widespread.

Erythema nodosum: The lower legs, principally on the pretibial surfaces.

Lichen planus: Oral mucosa, flexor surface of wrists, trunk, genitalia. Lesions may be widespread.

Chronic discoid LE: Principally on the face, scalp, ears, neck.

Photosensitivity reactions: Areas exposed to natural or artificial light; e.g., the V of the neck, the arms below the sleeves, and the face (especially the cheeks and nose). This characteristic distribution frequently is not recognized and may be confused with contact dermatitis.

Pityriasis rosea: Trunk and proximal extremities in most cases, with the long axis of oval lesions running parallel to the lines of cleavage. Occasionally pityriasis rosea may affect only the extremities and spare the trunk.

Psoriasis: Elbows, knees, scalp, back, anogenital region, nails.

SPECIAL DIAGNOSTIC METHODS

Biopsy is essential for diagnosing any obscure dermatosis, particularly a chronic one, and is imperative if there is any suggestion of neoplasm. A fully developed typical lesion should usually be chosen for biopsy, but early lesions are best in vesicular, bullous, or pustular eruptions. The simplest biopsy procedure is to insert a sharp circular punch, 3 mm or more in diameter, well through the dermis, and snip off the base of the plug. An adequate biopsy of some relatively friable lesions (e.g., seborrheic keratoses) may be obtained with a sharp curet. For a larger tissue sample, and for deep dermal or subcutaneous lesions, a wedge is removed and the incision sutured. For most small tumors, excision allows microscopic diagnosis and cure with one procedure. All excised nevi must be studied histologically. A deep part of the biopsy specimen should be cultured when a mycobacterial or a deep fungal infection is suspected.

Examination of scrapings for fungi: In any suspected superficial fungal infection, the organisms can be demonstrated by microscopic examination of scales that have been taken from the lesion, covered with 10% potassium hydroxide, and warmed gently; hairs from a lesion must be examined in tinea capitis. In dermatophyte infections, only hyphae are seen, while in tinea versicolor and candidal infections both yeast and hyphae are seen; the distinction may be important in selecting specific chemotherapy.

Bacterial and fungal cultures: In acute bacterial infections of the skin, culture and antibacterial sensitivity testing are advisable, although treatment should be started promptly. Adequate sampling is essential. With frankly pustular lesions, a swab sample is sufficient; the swab should be placed immediately in broth culture and not allowed to dry out. In chronic infections (e.g., tuberculosis or deep fungi), where the flora may be mixed and relatively sparse, more ample specimens (including even deep biopsy specimens) must be obtained and special culture media may be needed. Culture of superficial fungal infections will occasionally be positive when the scraping is negative.

Wood's light examination: When the skin is viewed in a darkened room under ultraviolet light filtered through Wood's glass ("black light"), tinea versicolor may fluoresce golden and erythrasma orange-red; scalp hairs in tinea capitis caused by *Microsporum canis* and *M. audouini* are a light bright green. The earliest clue to a *Pseudomonas* infection, especially in burns, may be a green fluorescence under a Wood's light. The depigmentation of vitiligo can be differentiated from hypo-pigmented lesions by its ivory-white color on Wood's light examination.

Cytologic examination: The **Tzanck test** is rapid and reliable in the diagnosis of vesicular erup-tions. A smear of cellular material scraped from the base of a vesicle and stained with Wright's or Giemsa stain shows multinucleated giant cells in herpes simplex, herpes zoster, and varicella, but not in vaccinia and smallpox. Pemphigus can be diagnosed by finding typical acantholytic cells.

Immunofluorescent (IF) tests: Fluorescent microscopy (see TYPE II HYPERSENSITIVITY REACTIONS in Ch. 18) is an important aid in diagnosing and managing certain skin diseases. The indirect IF test demonstrates that the serum of a patient with pemphigus or bullous pemphigoid contains specific antibodies that bind to different areas of the epithelium. In pemphigus, the antibody titer may corre-late with the severity of the disease. In the direct IF test, biopsied skin of patients with pemphigus, pemphigoid, dermatitis herpetiformis, herpes gestationis, SLE, and discoid LE shows specific, diag-nostic patterns.

Electron microscopy: If a viral etiology is suspected, a glass-slide smear of vesicle fluid or crusted tissue may be sent to an electron microscopy unit for identification of the virus.

Other special diagnostic methods include patch tests used for allergic contact dermatitis (see TYPE IV HYPERSENSITIVITY REACTIONS in Ch. 18) and darkfield examination for syphilis (see Ch. 162).

187. GENERAL PRINCIPLES OF DERMATOLOGIC THERAPY

Many substances are applied for topical treatment, including absorbents, anti-infectives, anti-in-flammatory agents, astringents (drying agents that precipitate protein and shrink and contract the skin), cleansing agents, emollients (skin softeners), and keratolytics (agents that soften, loosen, and facilitate exfoliation of the squamous cells of the epidermis). These locally acting agents are used to (1) cleanse, debride, and protect the skin; (2) destroy causative agents (bacteria, fungi, or protozoa); (3) relieve symptoms such as pruritus, burning, and pain; and (4) reduce inflammation and promote healing.

The **vehicle** (base or carrier) for topical medication must be selected carefully, since it may alter the effectiveness of the active ingredient. Allergic and irritating reactions (e.g., contact dermatitis) may be caused by ingredients of the vehicle as well as by the active agent.

Ointments are oleaginous and contain little if any water; they feel greasy, but are generally well tolerated. They are best used to lubricate, especially if applied over hydrated skin; they protect lesions with thick crusts, lichenification, or heaped-up scales, and may be less irritating than a cream on some eroded or open lesions such as stasis ulcers.

Creams, semisolid emulsions of oil in water or water in oil, are the mainstay of dermatologic therapy. They are easy to apply and "vanish" when rubbed into the skin.

Lotions originally were suspensions or dispersions of finely powdered material (e.g., calamine) in a water or alcohol base; however, most modern "lotions" (e.g., some corticosteroid lotions) are really oily emulsions. Convenient to apply, lotions cool and dry acute inflammatory and exudative lesions. The powder suspensions, however, may be irritating if they dry the skin too much. Lotions usually must be shaken before use.

Solutions, homogenous mixtures of 2 or more substances, are convenient to apply, especially in the scalp. Like lotions, solutions are drying. The most commonly used solvents are ethyl alcohol, propylene glycol, and polyethylene glycol.

CLEANSING AGENTS AND PROTECTANTS

The principal **cleansing agents** are detergents and solvents. Soap is the most popular detergent, but synthetic detergents are also used. "Baby type" shampoos are usually well tolerated not only in the eyes but also in cleaning wounds and abrasions and are useful in psoriasis, eczema, and other forms of dermatitis for removal of crusts and scales. Badly irritated, weeping, or oozing lesions, however, should be cleaned only with water.

Various ingredients often are added to detergents and other dermatologic preparations to en-hance or add certain properties. For antidandruff action, dipyrithione or selenium sulfide may be added to a shampoo. Lauryl sulfoacetate, polyethanolamine alkyl sulfate, and sodium lauryl sulfate (anionic wetting agents commonly used in skin cleansing preparations) are often mixed with various medicaments to treat dandruff, psoriasis, and other skin disorders, but these agents may be irritating.

Water is the principal solvent used for cleansing. Plain **tap-water** soaks, baths, or compresses (made from gauze or old sheets) used intermittently for 48 to 72 h will generally soothe acute weeping or oozing lesions and dry them enough so that active medications can be applied. Wet dressings containing aluminum acetate, magnesium sulfate, etc., are seldom better than plain tap water. Ethyl alcohol is the most commonly used organic solvent for topical use.

Topical **protectants** cover and protect the skin against a deleterious influence. **Powders** are often used as protectants in intertriginous areas; i.e., between the toes and in the intergluteal cleft, axillas, groin, and inframammary areas. Powders dry macerated skin and reduce friction by absorbing moisture, thereby providing comfort. However, they tend to "ball up" and can be irritating when they become moist. Powders may be incorporated into protective creams, lotions, and ointments. Collodion and other films are **mechanical protectants** that provide a flexible or semirigid continuous film or coating over the skin. Zinc gelatin (Unna's boot) protects the skin by forming an occlusive dressing. **Sunscreens,** preparations that screen the skin from ultraviolet light, are also protectants (see Ch. 214).

ERADICATION OF CAUSATIVE AGENTS AND RELIEF OF SYMPTOMS

The **eradication of specific agents** causing skin infections is discussed in the appropriate chapters in §17. In general, topical antibiotics are ineffective and in many instances are contraindicated. However, topical fungicides, scabicides, and pediculicides are commonly used in skin disorders, as are systemic antibiotics.

The **relief of symptoms** such as pruritus and pain is discussed elsewhere in this volume. In addition to analgesics for relief of pain, camphor 0.5 to 3% or menthol 0.1 to 0.2% may be used singly or together in topical creams or ointments. Local anesthetics such as lidocaine and dibucaine are generally not used on the skin because they are ineffective; they are sometimes useful on mucosal surfaces.

TOPICAL ANTI-INFLAMMATORY AGENTS

Corticosteroids, the most effective topical agents, are remarkably devoid of major side effects. Itchy and inflammatory dermatoses usually respond favorably to properly used corticosteroids. However, they may worsen a pilosebaceous condition such as acne or rosacea. Topical corticosteroids and other skin preparations are usually made up as creams, lotions, ointments, or solutions, and less commonly as aerosols and tapes.

TABLE 187-1 lists many of the topical corticosteroid preparations currently available. Since hydrocortisone 1%, a nonfluorinated preparation, does not induce facial telangiectasia, perioral dermatitis, atrophy, or striae, it may be preferable to a synthetic corticosteroid for treating facial dermatoses. Although some preparations are available in higher or lower concentrations, a full-strength preparation should usually be prescribed first. The preparations should be applied sparingly t.i.d. For maximum effectiveness, creams should be rubbed in gently until they vanish. The corticosteroid may be diluted with a bland base if large areas of skin are involved.

A useful method for delivering a high concentration of corticosteroid to a chronic lesion or to one resistant to topical corticosteroids is direct **intralesional injection** of a corticosteroid suspension. The major problem with intralesional corticosteroids is dermal atrophy, which is usually reversible. In black skin, hypopigmentation may follow injection. Several corticosteroid suspensions for intralesional injection are listed in TABLE 187-1. These suspensions are usually diluted 2 to 4 times with sterile saline containing a preservative to minimize risk of local atrophy and hypopigmentation. The more insoluble preparations are more persistent and long-acting.

Absorption and effectiveness of topical corticosteroids are increased by covering the treated area with a nonporous occlusive dressing. This **occlusive therapy** is used in such conditions as psoriasis, atopic dermatitis, LE, and chronic hand dermatitis. Usually, a polyethylene film (e.g., a common plastic household wrap) is applied overnight over a cream or ointment preparation, since these tend to be less irritating than lotions for occlusive therapy. A plastic tape impregnated with flurandrenolide is especially convenient for treating isolated or recalcitrant lesions. Miliaria, atrophic striae, and bacterial infections may follow occlusive therapy; children and, less often, adults, may suffer some pituitary and cortisol suppression after prolonged occlusive treatment of large areas.

The use of topical antibiotics, alone or in combination with topical corticosteroids, is seldom warranted, except in the treatment of acne (see Vol. II, Ch. 27). The combinations are no more effective than a corticosteroid alone, and allergic contact dermatitis from topical antibiotics, especially neomycin, is increasingly being encountered.

TABLE 187–1. REPRESENTATIVE TOPICAL CORTICOSTEROID PREPARATIONS

Hydrocortisone Preparations*	
Creams	0.125%–2.5%
Ointments	0.5%–2.5%
Lotions	0.125%–2.5%
Aerosol	0.5%, 1%

Synthetic Corticosteroid Preparations†			
	Lowest Strength	*Low Strength*	*Full Strength*	*High Strength*
Creams	Dexamethasone 0.1% Prednisolone 0.5%	Hydrocortisone valerate 0.2% Fluocinolone acetonide 0.01% Betamethasone valerate 0.01% Flurandrenolide 0.025% Fluorometholone 0.025% Triamcinolone acetonide 0.025% Flumethasone pivalate 0.03% Betamethasone 0.2%	Halcinonide 0.025% Betamethasone benzoate 0.025% Betamethasone valerate 0.1% Desonide 0.05% Fluocinolone acetonide 0.025% Amcinonide 0.1% Flurandrenolide 0.05% Triamcinolone acetonide 0.1%	Fluocinolone acetonide 0.2% Fluocinonide 0.05% Halcinonide 0.1% Triamcinolone acetonide 0.5% Betamethasone dipropionate 0.05% Desoximetasone 0.25% Diflorasone diacetate 0.05%
Ointments	Methylprednisolone acetate 0.25%	Triamcinolone acetonide 0.025% Flurandrenolide 0.025% Methylprednisolone acetate 1.0%	Triamcinolone acetonide 0.1% Betamethasone valerate 0.1% Betamethasone benzoate 0.025% Halcinonide 0.025% Desonide 0.05% Flurandrenolide 0.05% Fluocinolone acetonide 0.025%	Triamcinolone acetonide 0.5% Betamethasone diprorionate 0.05% Halcinonide 0.1% Diflorasone diacetate 0.05% Fluocinonide 0.05%
Lotions		Triamcinolone acetonide 0.025%	Betamethasone benzoate 0.025% Betamethasone valerate 0.1% Flurandrenolide 0.05% Triamcinolone acetonide 0.1%	Betamethasone diprorionate 0.05%
Gels‡	Dexamethasone 0.1%		Betamethasone benzoate 0.025% Triamcinolone acetonide 0.1%	Fluocinonide 0.05%
Solutions		Fluocinolone acetonide 0.01%		Halcinonide 0.1%
Medicated Adhesive Tape				Flurandrenolide 4 µg/sq cm (7.5 cm wide roll × 60 cm/nm)
Aerosols	Dexamethasone 0.01%		Betamethasone diprorionate 0.1% Betamethasone valerate 0.15% Triamcinolone acetonide 0.2%	

(Continued)

TABLE 187–1. REPRESENTATIVE TOPICAL CORTICOSTEROID
PREPARATIONS (*Cont'd*)
Corticosteroid Suspensions for Intralesional Injection

Suspension	Potency (Concentration)—mg/ml
Triamcinolone acetonide	10, 40
Triamcinolone diacetate	25, 40
Triamcinolone hexacetonide	5, 20
Betamethasone sodium phosphate	4
Betamethasone acetate + betamethasone sodium phosphate	6 (3 mg/ml each of sodium phosphate and acetone esters)

* More than 30 companies now provide generic- or brand-labeled hydrocortisone creams, ointments, and lotions.
† Preparations within each group are therapeutically equivalent.
‡ Approximately equivalent to full-strength creams.

188. PRURITUS

(Itching)

A sensation that the patient instinctively attempts to relieve by scratching.

Etiology, Symptoms, and Signs

Itching may accompany a primary skin disease or may be a symptom of systemic disease—sometimes the only symptom.

Skin diseases in which itching is most severe include scabies, pediculosis, insect bites, urticaria, atopic dermatitis, contact dermatitis, lichen planus, miliaria, and dermatitis herpetiformis. Dry skin (especially in the elderly) often is a cause of severe generalized itching.

Systemic conditions in which there is a clear association with generalized itching include obstructive biliary disease, uremia (frequently associated with hyperparathyroidism), lymphomas, leukemias, and polycythemia rubra vera. During the latter months of pregnancy, itching may occur unaccompanied by primary skin lesions. Many drugs (especially barbiturates and salicylanilides) can cause pruritus. Other diseases believed to cause generalized itching, even though an association has not been definitely proved, include hyperthyroidism, diabetes mellitus, and internal cancers of many types. One should always be cautious before attributing a psychogenic etiology to the generalized pruritus, although this is a common problem.

Persistent scratching may produce redness, urticarial papules, excoriated papules, fissures, and elongated crusts along scratch lines. Lichenification and pigmentation may also result from prolonged scratching and rubbing. Frequently, however, the patient who complains of severe generalized itching has no signs of scratching or rubbing the skin.

Treatment

First and foremost, the cause of generalized pruritus should be sought and corrected. If no skin disease is readily apparent, an underlying systemic disorder or drug-related cause should be sought.

If feasible, all medications should be stopped or chemically unrelated drugs substituted. Irritating clothing, such as woolens, should be avoided. Bathing should be minimized, as it may aggravate generalized itching, whatever the cause. Emollients, such as white petrolatum or hydrogenated vegetable oil (e.g., a cooking oil) containing 0.125 to 0.25% menthol, may be soothing. Proprietary anesthetics should be avoided. Topical corticosteroids seldom alleviate generalized itching, but may be useful in essential pruritus of the elderly.

If a drug has been adequately ruled out as the cause of the itching, one may prescribe a tranquilizer, either a "minor" one such as hydroxyzine or, for more severe cases, a "major" one such as chlorpromazine (see TRANQUILIZERS in Ch. 247). Antihistamines, if at all helpful, may be so mainly because of their sedative effect.

189. DERMATITIS

(Eczema)

Superficial inflammation of the skin, characterized by vesicles (when acute), redness, edema, oozing, crusting, scaling, and usually itching. Scratching or rubbing may lead to lichenification.

The terms *dermatitis* and *eczema* are used synonymously in this chapter. There is no general agreement among authorities as to the distinction between them. The term *eczematous dermatitis* is often used to mean a vesicular dermatitis, and some authorities still restrict the term *eczema* to chronic vesicular dermatitides.

For diagnostic purposes, the dermatitides are divided into those with exogenous causes and those with presumably endogenous causes (see TABLE 189-1, Classification of Dermatitides). Many conditions (e.g., hand dermatitis, exfoliative dermatitis) may be either exogenous or endogenous. Dermatitis may also accompany various immune deficiency diseases (e.g., Wiskott-Aldrich syndrome, X-linked agammaglobulinemia), inborn errors of metabolism (e.g., phenylketonuria, ahistidinemia), or nutritional deficiency diseases (e.g., pellagra).

CONTACT DERMATITIS

An acute or chronic inflammation, often sharply demarcated, produced by substances in contact with the skin.

Etiology

Contact dermatitis may be caused by a primary chemical irritant or may be a Type IV delayed hypersensitivity reaction (see Ch. 18).

Direct irritants may damage normal skin or irritate an existing dermatitis. Weak or marginal irritants, such as soap, acetone, or even water, may take several days of exposure to cause clinically recognizable changes. Strong irritants, such as acids, alkalis, or phenol, cause observable changes within a few minutes.

Allergic contact dermatitis is due to delayed hypersensitivity and requires a latent period ranging from 5 or 6 days (in the case of strong sensitizers such as poison ivy) to years between the time of first exposure and the reexposure that precipitates the dermatitis. Patients often find it difficult to believe that they have become allergic to substances they have used for years or to medications used to treat their dermatitis, but the **ingredients in topical medications** constitute a major cause of allergic contact dermatitis: antibiotics (penicillin, sulfonamides, neomycin), antihistamines (diphenhydramine, promethazine), anesthetics (benzocaine), antiseptics (thimerosal, hexachlorophene), and stabilizers (ethylenediamine and derivatives). Other commonly implicated substances include **plants** (poison ivy, oak, and sumac; ragweed, primrose); many potential sensitizers used in the manufacture of **shoes** and **clothing** (tanning agents in shoes; free formaldehyde in durable-press finishes; rubber accelerators and antioxidants in gloves, shoes, underpants, bras, and other wearing apparel); **metal compounds** (nickel, chromates, mercury); *p*-phenylenediamine and other **dyes;** and **cosmetics** (depilatories, nail polish, deodorants). **Industrial agents** capable of producing occupational dermatoses are almost innumerable.

Photoallergic and **phototoxic contact dermatitis** require exposure to light following topical application of certain chemicals. They are manifested as an exaggerated response to sunlight (polymorphous light eruptions—see in Ch. 214). Agents commonly responsible for photoallergic contact dermatitis include aftershave lotions, sunscreening agents, and topical sulfonamides. Phototoxic contact dermatitis is commonly caused by certain perfumes, coal tar, psoralens, and cutting oils. Photoallergic and phototoxic contact dermatitis must be differentiated from photosensitivity reactions to systemically administered drugs.

TABLE 189-1. CLASSIFICATION OF DERMATITIDES

Endogenous	*Contact or Exogenous*
Atopic	Direct irritant
Seborrheic	Non–light-dependent
Nummular	Phototoxic
Chronic dermatitis of hands and feet	
Exfoliative	Allergic
Stasis	Non–light-dependent
Localized scratch dermatitis	Photoallergic
Pruritus ani or vulvae	
Drug eruptions	

Symptoms and Signs

Contact dermatitis ranges from transient redness to severe swelling with bulla formation; itching and vesiculation are common. Any part of the skin that comes in contact with a sensitizing or irritating substance may be involved. Thus, dermatitis on exposed skin surfaces may be due to an airborne substance (e.g., ragweed pollen, insecticide spray). Characteristically, the dermatitis at first is sharply limited to the site of contact; later it may spread to other areas.

The course varies. If the cause is removed, simple erythema disappears within a few days and blisters dry up. Vesicles and bullae may rupture, ooze, and crust. As the inflammation subsides, scaling and some temporary thickening of the skin occur. Continuing exposure to the causative agent or complications such as irritation from or allergy to a topical medication, excoriation, or infection may perpetuate the dermatitis.

Diagnosis

Since contact dermatitis may resemble other types of dermatitis, an allergen or irritant should be suspected as the cause or aggravating factor in any puzzling dermatitis. Characteristic skin changes and a history of exposure facilitate the diagnosis, but identifying the responsible agent may require exhaustive questioning and extensive patch testing. The patient's occupation, hobbies, household duties, vacations, wearing apparel, topical medications, cosmetics, and spouse's activities must all be considered. Knowing the characteristics of topical allergens or irritants, including the typical distribution of lesions, is helpful. The site of the initial lesion is often an important clue to the cause.

Patch testing (see TYPE IV HYPERSENSITIVITY REACTIONS in Ch. 18) with a standard group of contact allergens may be helpful if questioning is fruitless. A specialist should select the test concentrations (particularly for industrial agents or cosmetics). Patch testing is sometimes withheld during the acute phase of the dermatitis because the allergen may worsen the eruption in a very sensitive patient. A positive patch test reaction does not necessarily identify the agent causing the contact dermatitis. There must be a history of exposure to the test agent in the areas where the dermatitis originally occurred before a definite diagnosis can be made. Moreover, a negative patch test does not rule out the diagnosis of contact dermatitis: it may only mean that the offending agent was not included in the tests.

Treatment

Treatment may be ineffective or the dermatitis may promptly recur unless the offending agent is removed. Patients with photoallergic or phototoxic contact dermatitis should avoid exposure to light as well. In the acute phase of dermatitis, such as that caused by poison ivy, gauze or thin cloths dipped in water and applied to the lesions are soothing and cooling; they should be applied for 30 min, 4 to 6 times/day. Blisters may be drained, but the tops should not be removed. An oral corticosteroid (e.g., prednisone 40 to 60 mg/day) should be given for 12 to 16 days in severe or extensive cases or even in limited cases when there is severe facial inflammation. The prednisone dose can be decreased by 10 to 20 mg every 3 to 4 days. Topical corticosteroids are not helpful in the blistering phase, but once the dermatitis is less acute, a topical corticosteroid cream or, if the dermatitis is very dry, an ointment (see TOPICAL ANTI-INFLAMMATORY AGENTS in Ch. 187) should be rubbed in gently t.i.d. Antihistamines (except for their sedative effect) and desensitization are ineffective in contact dermatitis.

ATOPIC DERMATITIS

A chronic, itching, superficial inflammation of the skin, usually occurring in individuals with a personal or family history of allergic disorders (e.g., hay fever, asthma).

Etiology

The cause is unknown. Frequently, numerous inhalants and foods will produce wheal-and-flare reactions on scratch or intradermal tests, but these reactions are usually nonspecific and do not determine a cause for the dermatitis. Patients with atopic dermatitis usually have high serum levels of reaginic (IgE) antibodies and peripheral eosinophilia, but the etiologic significance of these findings is unknown.

Symptoms, Signs, and Course

Atopic dermatitis may begin in the first few months of life, with red, weeping, crusted lesions on the face, scalp, and extremities. In older children or adults, it may take a more localized chronic form. The course is unpredictable. Although the dermatitis usually subsides by age 3 or 4 yr, exacerbations and remissions frequently recur during childhood, adolescence, or adulthood.

Itching is a constant feature. The consequent scratching and rubbing lead to an itch-scratch-rash-itch cycle. In older children and adults, atopic dermatitis typically appears as erythema and lichenification in the antecubital and popliteal fossae and on the eyelids, neck, and wrists. The dermatitis may become generalized. Secondary bacterial infections and regional lymphadenitis are common. Frequent use of medications, proprietary or prescribed, exposes the atopic patient to many topical allergens, and contact dermatitis may aggravate and complicate the atopic dermatitis, as may the generally dry skin that is common in these patients. Intolerance to primary irritants is common, and emotional stress, environmental temperature or humidity changes, bacterial skin infections, and wool garments commonly cause exacerbations.

Complications

Patients with longstanding atopic dermatitis may develop cataracts while in their 20s or 30s. Herpes simplex or vaccinia may induce a grave febrile illness **(Kaposi's varicelliform eruption)** in atopic patients. Therefore, the patient with atopic dermatitis must not be vaccinated against smallpox or be exposed during the active phase to herpes simplex or to recently vaccinated persons.

Diagnosis

Diagnosis is entirely clinical and is based on the distribution of lesions, the long duration, and, often, a family history of atopic allergy. Because atopic dermatitis is often hard to differentiate from seborrheic dermatitis in infancy or from primary irritant dermatitis at any age, the patient should be seen several times before a definitive diagnosis is made. The physician must be careful not to attribute all subsequent skin problems to an atopic diathesis.

Treatment

The following general measures are advisable:

1. Patients should avoid as many offending agents as possible and should be advised against using complex topical medications.

2. Corticosteroid creams or ointments applied t.i.d. are the most effective medications. Because they are expensive, supplemental use of white petrolatum, hydrogenated vegetable oil (as for cooking), or hydrophilic petrolatum and water may be advisable. These emollients are applied between applications of the corticosteroid and help to hydrate the skin, an important objective in treatment. Prolonged, widespread use of high potency corticosteroid creams or ointments should be avoided in infants, as adrenal suppression (reversible) may ensue.

3. Bathing should be minimized and use of soap on the area of dermatitis avoided, since soap and water may be drying and irritating. A nonlipid cleanser can be substituted for soap. Bath oils help to lubricate the skin, and the above-mentioned corticosteroid or emollient ointments should be applied after a bath, preferably before the skin is dried, to enhance their emollient effects.

4. For children, an antihistamine (e.g., diphenhydramine elixir 25 to 50 mg) at bedtime may be a useful sedative when itching is worst.

5. Fingernails should be kept short to minimize excoriations and secondary infections.

6. For secondary infections, oral erythromycin 250 mg q.i.d. for adults and 125 mg q.i.d. for children is advised.

7. If the dermatitis resists home treatment, hospitalization, with its closer psychologic and dermatologic attention and the change in environment, often accelerates improvement.

8. Oral corticosteroids should be considered a last resort. Stunting of growth, osteoporosis, and the other side effects of prolonged systemic corticosteroids are serious hazards when atopic patients take the drug for years, and rebound exacerbations on stopping therapy are frequent. Alternate-day use of corticosteroids may be helpful (e.g., for adults, prednisone 40 to 60 mg every other morning). The initial dose should be continued for several weeks, then slowly decreased while the patient is encouraged to use topical medications.

SEBORRHEIC DERMATITIS

An inflammatory scaling disease of the scalp, face, and, occasionally, other areas of the body. Despite the name, the composition and flow of sebum are normal.

Symptoms and Signs

Onset in adults is gradual, and the dermatitis usually is apparent only as dry or greasy diffuse scaling of the scalp **(dandruff)** with variable itching. In severe disease, yellow-red, scaling papules appear along the hairline, behind the ears, in the external auditory canals, on the eyebrows, on the bridge of the nose, in the nasolabial folds, and over the sternum. Marginal blepharitis with dry yellow crusts and conjunctival irritation may be present. Seborrheic dermatitis does not cause hair loss.

Infants within the first month of life may develop seborrheic dermatitis, with a thick, yellow, crusted scalp lesion **("cradle cap")**, fissuring and yellow scaling behind the ears, and red facial papules. Older children may develop thick, tenacious, asbestos-like, scaly plaques in the scalp that may measure 1 to 2 cm in diameter.

Genetic and climatic factors seem to affect the incidence and severity of the disease; it is usually worse in winter. The prognosis is better than in atopic dermatitis. Very rarely, in infants or adults, the condition may become generalized.

Treatment

This depends on the location and severity of the seborrheic dermatitis. A zinc pyrithione, selenium sulfide, sulfur and salicylic acid, or tar shampoo should be used every other day until the dandruff is controlled and twice/wk thereafter. A corticosteroid lotion (e.g., 0.01% fluocinolone acetonide solution or 0.025% triamcinolone acetonide lotion) should be rubbed into the scalp or other hairy areas b.i.d. until scaling and redness are controlled. Hydrocortisone 1% cream rubbed in b.i.d. or t.i.d. will rapidly improve seborrheic dermatitis of the postauricular areas, nasolabial folds, eyelid margins, and bridge of the nose; the cream is then used once daily if needed. Hydrocortisone cream is best for facial seborrheic dermatitis, as the fluorinated corticosteroids may produce such side effects as telangiectasia, atrophy, and perioral dermatitis. For infantile seborrheic eczema, a mild baby shampoo is used daily and a corticosteroid cream is rubbed in b.i.d. For the thick asbestos-like lesions seen in the scalps of young children, 10% salicylic acid in mineral oil or a corticosteroid gel is applied at bedtime to affected areas and rubbed in with a toothbrush. The scalp is shampooed daily until the thick scale is gone.

NUMMULAR DERMATITIS

Chronic dermatitis characterized by inflamed, coin-shaped, vesicular, crusted, scaling, and usually pruritic lesions.

The etiology of nummular dermatitis is unknown. It is seen most commonly in middle-aged patients under emotional stress and is frequently associated with dry skin, especially during the winter, and most often on the legs. Exacerbations and remissions may occur.

Symptoms and Signs

The discoid lesions start as pruritic patches of confluent vesicles and papules that later ooze serum and then form crusts. The lesions are widespread; they are frequently more prominent on the extensor aspects of the extremities and on the buttocks, but they also appear on the trunk.

Treatment

No treatment is uniformly effective. Oral antibiotics may be given on an empiric basis, since many types of bacteria can be cultured and the therapy has been found to be effective in decreasing the severity of the lesions. Oral cloxacillin or erythromycin 250 mg q.i.d. and tap-water compresses are helpful when there is much weeping and pus. Less infected lesions may also improve with tetracycline 250 mg orally q.i.d. After the lesions have dried, a corticosteroid cream or ointment should be rubbed in t.i.d. and occlusion with a corticosteroid cream under polyethylene film or with flurandrenolide-impregnated tape should be applied at bedtime. Occasionally oral corticosteroids are required; a reasonable starting dose is 40 mg of prednisone given every other day to lessen side effects. Long-term systemic corticosteroid therapy should be avoided.

CHRONIC DERMATITIS OF HANDS AND FEET

The hands and feet are frequent sites of inflammatory eruptions—the hands because they are subjected to mechanical and chemical trauma; the feet because of the warm, moist conditions in shoes. The eruption commonly becomes chronic and can be crippling at home or at work.

The following primary dermatoses may involve the hands and feet:

1. **Contact dermatitis** (see above) is common. Many allergens or irritants—caustics, strong soaps, detergents, organic solvents, vacuum cleaner dust, topical medications—may cause or perpetuate the dermatitis. In any dermatitis of the feet, every effort should be made to obtain patch-test evidence of sensitivity to a component of shoes, since this sensitivity limits the choice of footwear.

2. **"Housewives' eczema,"** a hand dermatitis frequently seen in housewives, has many causes. It is undoubtedly worsened by washing dishes, clothes, and babies, since repeated exposure to even mild detergents and water or prolonged sweating under rubber gloves may irritate dermatitic skin or may even cause a marginal irritant dermatitis.

3. **Pompholyx** is a chronic condition characterized by deep-seated itchy vesicles on the palms, sides of the fingers, and soles. Scaling, redness, and oozing often follow the vesiculation. The condition is also known as **dyshidrosis**—a misnomer, since sweating may be decreased, normal, or excessive. Though no cause is known in most cases, a primary cause, such as a fungus or a contact allergen, should always be sought.

4. **Psoriasis** localized to the hands presents on the dorsum as the typical thick, silvery, scaling papules or plaques, but palmar lesions are not always characteristic. Though pitted grooves in the nails often indicate psoriasis, they can occur with any dermatitis of the fingers.

5. **Recalcitrant pustular eruptions of the palms and soles** are characteristically crops of deep-seated sterile pustules of unknown etiology that resist treatment. They may be associated with psoriasis elsewhere.

6. **Fungal infection** of the feet is common; of the hands, uncommon. Patients with a hand dermatitis should be examined for a fungal infection of the feet, since the latter can produce a nonspecific dermatitis on the hands (**dermatophytid;** see Ch. 191).

Treatment

Treatment should be directed to removing the cause wherever possible. The following general principles are useful if no specific cause is found: (1) A topical corticosteroid cream or ointment applied t.i.d. may decrease the itching, but clearing the dermatitis may require overnight occlusive therapy with polyethylene gloves (or nonpermeable plastic bags on the feet), sealed at the wrists or ankles with cellophane tape, after a 4th application of the cream. (2) Oral cloxacillin or erythromycin, 250 mg q.i.d., should be given if there is any evidence of secondary infection. (3) Wet chores should be limited to short periods, and white cotton gloves should be worn under rubber gloves. (4) A 14-day course of oral prednisone is needed occasionally, starting with 40 mg/day and slowly decreasing the dose while the patient is taught and encouraged to follow the above routines in order to decrease the exacerbation that may ensue when the oral corticosteroid is stopped. (5) If the dermatitis is longstanding and disabling or if benefit from oral corticosteroids is not lasting, 10 to 14 days of hospitalization may be helpful. This removes the patient from his environment, provides intensive therapy, and gives an opportunity for detailed patch testing, cultures, and other diagnostic studies.

GENERALIZED EXFOLIATIVE DERMATITIS

A severe, widespread erythema and scaling of the skin.

Etiology

No cause can be determined in most cases. In some patients, the disorder is secondary to certain dermatitides (e.g., atopic, psoriatic, pityriasis rubra pilaris, contact); or it may be induced by a systemic drug (e.g., penicillin, sulfonamides, isoniazid, phenytoin, or barbiturates) or an irritating topical agent. Exfoliative dermatitis may also be associated with mycosis fungoides or lymphoma.

Symptoms and Signs

The onset may be insidious or rapid. The entire skin surface becomes red, scaly, thickened, and, occasionally, crusted. Itching may be severe or absent. The characteristic appearance of any primary dermatitis is usually lost. Localized areas of normal skin may be seen when the exfoliative dermatitis is caused by psoriasis, mycosis fungoides, or pityriasis rubra pilaris. Generalized superficial lymphadenopathy is frequently present, and biopsy usually shows benign lymphadenitis.

The patient's temperature may be elevated, or he may feel cold from excessive heat loss, because of the increased blood flow to the skin and exfoliation. These may also cause weight loss, hypoproteinemia, iron deficiency, or even (in patients with borderline cardiac compensation) high-output congestive heart failure.

Diagnosis and Treatment

The disease may be life-threatening, and every attempt must be made to determine the cause. A history or signs of a primary dermatitis may be helpful. Biopsy is usually not helpful, but pemphigus foliaceus or mycosis fungoides may be diagnosed by skin biopsy, or lymphoma by a lymph node biopsy. Sézary syndrome may be diagnosed by a blood smear.

Hospitalization is often necessary. Because drug eruptions and contact dermatitis cannot be ruled out by history alone, all possible medications, systemic and topical, should be stopped. Essential systemic medicines should, if possible, be changed to chemically dissimilar ones. Petrolatum applied after tap-water baths will give temporary relief. Subsequent local treatment is the same as for contact dermatitis (see above).

Oral corticosteroids should be used only when topical measures are unsuccessful. Prednisone 40 to 60 mg is given every day; then, after about 10 days, every other day. Usually the dose can be further decreased, but prednisone will be required for long periods if an underlying cause is not found and eliminated.

STASIS DERMATITIS

Persistent inflammation of the skin of the lower legs with a tendency toward brown pigmentation, commonly associated with venous incompetency. (See also in VENOUS DISEASES in Ch. 28.)

Symptoms and Signs

The eruption is usually localized to the ankle, where erythema, mild scaling, and a brown discoloration are seen. Edema and varicose veins are common but by no means always present. Because of the relative lack of symptoms, the condition is often neglected. The usual consequences are increasing edema, secondary bacterial infection, and eventually ulceration.

Treatment

Both topical therapy and measures to increase venous return and prevent tissue edema are necessary. Topical therapy depends on the stage of the process. For acute dermatitis, tap-water compresses should be applied, continuously at first and then intermittently. The compress should be allowed to dry partially so that the crust will be removed with it. When the dermatitis becomes less acute, a corticosteroid cream or ointment should be applied t.i.d. or incorporated into zinc oxide paste. Ulcerative lesions are best treated with compresses and petrolatum or zinc oxide paste. Recent studies have suggested the efficacy of 10 to 20% benzoyl peroxide, but this therapy is still experimental. Elevation of the leg above heart level is important. Oral antibiotics are useful when cellulitis is present; topical antibiotics are useless and often cause contact dermatitis.

In selected instances, ulcers may be healed on an ambulatory basis with an **Unna's paste boot** (zinc gelatin) or the less messy **zinc gelatin bandage**, both available commercially. If the Unna's paste boot is used, it is important to prevent wrinkles in the bandage (particularly over the tibia and foot), to place the gauze layers evenly and smoothly, and to have uniform snugness throughout. A well-mixed paste, thoroughly introduced into the bandage, should be used. After the ulcer has been cleansed and edema of the lower leg has diminished following 1 or 2 days of bed rest, the boot is applied directly over the ulcer. At first it may be necessary to change the boot every 3 or 4 days, but, as edema recedes and the ulcer heals, once/wk is sufficient. Following healing, ambulation should always be with elastic support.

Complex or multiple topical medications or nonprescription remedies should not be used, since the skin in stasis dermatitis is vulnerable to direct irritants and to potentially sensitizing topical agents (antibiotics, anesthetics, and vehicles of topical medications, particularly lanolin or wool alcohols).

LOCALIZED SCRATCH DERMATITIS
(Localized Neurodermatitis)

A chronic, superficial, pruritic inflammation of the skin, characterized by dry, scaling, well-demarcated, hyperpigmented, lichenified plaques of oval, irregular, or angular shape.

Etiology, Symptoms, and Signs
The disease has a strong psychogenic component. Allergy appears to play no part. Women are affected more often than men, with onset usually between ages 20 and 50. An area of skin begins to itch recurrently, as a result of prior irritation or without apparent reason. The principal site is the occipital region, but arms or legs, especially ankles, are frequently involved. Vigorous scratching gives transient relief, but the itching recurs. Stress and tension increase the pruritus, and scratching may become an unconscious habit. The usual course is chronic.

A fully developed plaque has an outer zone of brownish discrete papules and a central zone of confluent papules covered with scales.

Pruritus ani and **pruritus vulvae** are often instances of circumscribed scratch dermatitis. The involved skin may only be red, moist, and hyperpigmented, or may even appear normal.

Diagnosis
Diagnosis is by exclusion. Generalized itching without apparent skin lesions may occur in patients with a variety of systemic disorders (see Ch. 188). Most anal and vulvar pruritus is idiopathic, but may be due to pinworms, trichomoniasis, hemorrhoids, local discharges or fissures, candidiasis, warts, contact dermatitis, or occasionally psoriasis. Unusual but important causes of anal or vulvar dermatitis are extramammary Paget's disease, Bowen's disease, and lichen sclerosis et atrophicus.

Treatment
It is important for the patient to realize that scratching and rubbing produce the skin changes. The pruritus may be controlled with medication; topical corticosteroids are the most effective. A cream may be rubbed in, but surgical tape impregnated with flurandrenolide (applied in the morning and replaced in the evening) may be best, since it simultaneously prevents scratching. Small areas may be locally infiltrated with a long-acting corticosteroid such as triamcinolone acetonide 2.5 mg/ml (achieved by diluting with saline), 0.3 ml/sq cm of lesion; this can be repeated every 3 to 4 wk.

Pruritus ani or vulvae is best treated with a hydrocortisone cream t.i.d. Zinc oxide paste can be applied over the cream for protection; it may be removed with mineral oil. Patients should be cautioned not to rub hard with toilet paper after a bowel movement. Pinworms should be eradicated and warts treated. Hemorrhoids or hypertrophic "tags" should be removed and discharges or fissures corrected surgically if the course is chronic, but this will not always cure the pruritus ani because the itching is frequently psychogenic.

---

190. BACTERIAL INFECTIONS OF THE SKIN

The specific bacterial cause of a skin infection should be identified (see Bacterial and Fungal Cultures in Ch. 186). Knowledge of the normal skin flora helps in interpreting culture reports, since large numbers of bacteria, including micrococci, diphtheroids, and *Corynebacterium acnes*, normally inhabit the skin.

Infection may be the primary cause of a skin lesion or may be superimposed on another skin disease. Primary infections such as impetigo and erysipelas almost always respond promptly to *systemic* antibiotics, but secondary infections may clear more slowly. *Topical* antibiotics are ineffective in most bacterial skin infections and may cause allergic contact dermatitis. Recurrent infections should alert the physician to a possible underlying systemic disorder (e.g., diabetes mellitus).

IMPETIGO; ECTHYMA
(See Vol. II, Ch. 24)

TOXIC EPIDERMAL NECROLYSIS
(Scalded Skin Syndrome; Dermatitis Exfoliativa; Ritter-Lyell Syndrome)

(See also under NEONATAL INFECTIONS in Vol. II, Ch. 21)

A life-threatening skin disease in which the epithelium of the skin, and sometimes the mucosa, peels off in sheets, leaving widespread denuded areas. In infants it is usually due to a staphylococcal infection, but in adults it most often represents a drug reaction.

Etiology, Symptoms, Signs, and Diagnosis
Diagnosis is based on the clinical manifestations and laboratory demonstration of staphylococci.

Infant form: An exotoxin of Group II coagulase-positive penicillin-resistant staphylococci, usually phage type 71, causes this disease. Staphylococci can usually be recovered from the patient's skin and nasopharynx. The disease may occur in epidemics in nurseries or sporadically in children or adults. It starts with a superficial crusted lesion, frequently around the nose or ear, and progresses within 24 h to bright red areas around the primary lesion. Widespread redness, tenderness, and desquamation of the skin develop within 36 to 48 h. The loosened epidermis peels off, often in large sheets, when touched. Blisters of various sizes may exist along with the erosions. Patients may be very ill, with fever, severe malaise, and anorexia, but they usually recover when treated with vigorous systemic antistaphylococcal antibiotics.

Adult form: Large, flaccid blisters that are readily broken may be the first sign of the disease, or the blisters may extend from the blisters of erythema multiforme bullosum. Large sheets of skin may be removed with slight trauma. The full-blown disease usually appears in days. In adults the disease has a grave prognosis.

Treatment

Infant form: Because the disease may progress rapidly, treatment must be started as soon as the clinical diagnosis has been made and specimens for culture have been taken. Treatment should not await culture reports. In early stages, oral cloxacillin 125 mg q.i.d. may be given, but in severe cases methicillin 25 mg/kg IV or IM should be given q 6 h until improvement is noted; oral cloxacillin 25 mg/kg q.i.d. should then be given for at least 10 days. The patient should be watched closely. Fluid and electrolyte balance may need correction; hospitalization and isolation may be required. Topical therapy must be minimized, and the patient should be handled as little as possible. Healing is usually rapid (5 to 7 days) after treatment is started.

Adult form: Fatalities are due to sepsis and to electrolyte and fluid imbalance. Patients should be managed as in severe burns, but debridement should be minimal. Hospitalization with isolation to minimize exogenous infection is urgent. Their value has not been proved, but systemic corticosteroids have been used to try to stop an "allergic" drug reaction. In many cases, corticosteroids seem to enhance gram-negative or other sepsis without improving the skin. Septicemia, often with pulmonary infections, must be recognized and treated promptly.

ERYSIPELAS

A superficial cellulitis caused by Group A β-hemolytic streptococci. The face (often bilaterally), an arm, or a leg is most often involved. The lesion is well demarcated, shiny, red, edematous, and tender; vesicles and bullae often develop. Patches of peripheral redness and regional lymphadenopathy are seen occasionally; high fever, chills, and malaise are common. Erysipelas may be recurrent and may result in chronic lymphedema. A nidus of infection may be an interdigital fungal infection of the foot.

Diagnosis from the characteristic appearance is usually easy. The causative organism is difficult to culture from the lesion, but it may occasionally be cultured from the blood. Erysipelas of the face must be differentiated from herpes zoster; of the arm or hand, from the rare erysipeloid (see in BACTERIAL DISEASES CAUSED BY GRAM-POSITIVE BACILLI in Ch. 8). Contact dermatitis and angioneurotic edema may be mistaken for erysipelas.

Treatment

Penicillin V or erythromycin, 250 mg orally q.i.d., is curative and should be given for at least 2 wk. In acute cases, penicillin G 1.2 million u. IV q 6 h will give a rapid response and should be replaced by oral therapy after 36 to 48 h. Local discomfort may be relieved by cold packs; aspirin 600 mg, with codeine 30 mg if required, may be given orally for pain.

FOLLICULITIS; FURUNCLES; CARBUNCLES

Folliculitis: *A superficial or deep bacterial infection and irritation of the hair follicles.* It is usually caused by *Staphylococcus aureus.* The acute lesion consists of a superficial pustule or inflammatory nodule surrounding the hair. The condition may follow or accompany other pyodermas. Infected hairs are easily removed, but new papules tend to develop. Folliculitis may become chronic where the hair follicles are deep in the skin, as in the bearded area **(sycosis barbae).** Stiff hairs in the bearded area may emerge from the follicle, curve, and reenter the skin, producing a chronic low-grade irritation without significant infection **(pseudofolliculitis barbae;** see Ch. 194. Tinea barbae may be confused with bacterial folliculitis.

Furuncles (boils): *Acute, tender, perifollicular inflammatory nodules resulting from infection by staphylococci.* They occur most frequently on the neck, breasts, face, and buttocks, but are most painful when they occur in skin that is closely attached to underlying structures (e.g., on the nose, ear, or fingers). The initial nodule becomes a pustule 5 to 30 mm in diameter, with central necrosis, which discharges a core of necrotic tissue and sanguineous purulent exudate. The condition may be recurrent and troublesome **(furunculosis),** and often occurs in healthy young individuals.

Carbuncles: *A cluster of furuncles with spread of infection subcutaneously, resulting in deep suppuration, often extensive local sloughing, slow healing, and a large scar.* Carbuncles develop more slowly than single furuncles and may be accompanied by fever and prostration. They occur most frequently in males and most commonly on the nape of the neck. Diabetes mellitus, debilitating diseases, and old age are predisposing factors, though carbuncles do occur in otherwise healthy persons.

Treatment

The treatment of acute folliculitis is similar to that of impetigo. Prompt treatment may prevent development of a chronic infection.

A single furuncle is treated with intermittent moist heat to allow the lesion to point and drain spontaneously, since extensive incision may spread the infection. A furuncle in the nose or central facial area should be treated with systemic antibiotics, the selection depending on the results of culture and sensitivity tests.

Multiple furuncles and carbuncles require culture and sensitivity studies. Usually a penicillinase-resistant penicillin is required, such as cloxacillin 250 mg orally q.i.d., or, for penicillin-allergic patients, erythromycin in the same dosage. For recurrent boils, antibiotic therapy for 2 to 3 mo may be advisable. Clusters of cases are increasing—emphasizing the importance of finding and treating family and friends who may be sources of reinfection for the patients. Immunization with staphylococcal vaccines is ineffective. Extensive necrosis may require debridement, but antibiotics have eliminated the need for mutilating surgery.

HIDRADENITIS SUPPURATIVA

An inflammation of the apocrine glands resulting in obstruction and rupture of the ducts with painful local inflammation. Most lesions occur in the axilla or groin, but they may also be found around the nipples or anus. The lesions may be confused with furuncles but tend to be more persistent and are diagnosed primarily by their location and clinical course. Pain, fluctuation, discharge, and sinus tract formation are characteristic. In chronic cases, coalescence of inflamed nodules may cause palpable cordlike bands in the axilla. The condition may become extensive and disabling; if the pubic and genital areas are severely involved, walking may be difficult.

Treatment

Susceptible patients should avoid antiperspirants or other irritants. Early simple cases are treated with rest, moist heat, and prolonged systemic antibiotic therapy as for furunculosis. Surgical excision and plastic repair of the affected areas may be necessary if the disease persists.

CHRONIC GRANULOMATOUS DISEASE

(See in Vol. II, Ch. 25)

PARONYCHIAL INFECTIONS

Acute or chronic inflammation of the periungual tissues.

In acute paronychia, the causative organisms—usually micrococci, *Pseudomonas*, or *Proteus*, but sometimes *Candida* (see Ch. 223)—enter through a break in the epidermis resulting from a hangnail, trauma (e.g., from manicuring), or chronic irritation (e.g., from excessive exposure to water and detergents). The infection may follow the nail margin ("run-around"), or may extend beneath the nail and suppurate. Rarely, the infection penetrates more deeply into the finger; necrosis of the tendons and further extension of the infection along the tendon sheaths may result. Eventually the chronically infected nail becomes distorted.

Treatment

An acute infection is treated with hot compresses or soaks and, if bacterial, with an appropriate systemic antibiotic. The accumulated debris is painful and should be drained. A purulent pocket should be opened cautiously with the point of a scalpel. Infection extending along the tendon sheaths requires prompt surgical incision and drainage.

In chronic recurrent inflammation, it is important to keep the hands dry. The subungual debris should be cultured. If *Candida* is not present on several cultures, cutting back the nail to the point of its detachment from the underlying skin and applying dilute tincture of iodine, 2 drops b.i.d., will help to keep the subungual and paronychial areas dry and free of infection. If *Candida* is present, miconazole lotion should be applied t.i.d. to the paronychial and subungual areas after the nail is cut back. As the GI tract is a likely source of contamination with *Candida*, oral nystatin 500,000 u. q.i.d. may also be advisable. Women should be examined for an accompanying candidal vaginitis, which should also be treated. Grossly distorted nail plates may have to be removed.

ERYTHRASMA

A superficial skin infection caused by Corynebacterium minutissimum, *found most commonly in adults.* The incidence is higher in the tropics.

Erythrasma resembles a chronic fungus infection or intertrigo. In the toe webs, scaling, fissuring, and slight maceration occur, usually confined to the 3rd and 4th interspaces. In the genitocrural region, principally where the thighs contact the scrotum, patches are irregular and pink, later becoming brown with a fine scale. Erythrasma may widely involve the axillas, trunk, and perineum, particularly in obese middle-aged women or in patients with diabetes mellitus.

Differentiation from ringworm is essential. Diagnosis is established readily with a Wood's light, under which erythrasma shows a characteristic coral-red fluorescence.

Prompt clearing follows oral erythromycin or tetracycline 250 mg q.i.d. for 14 days, but recurrences 6 to 12 mo later are usual.

ERYSIPELOID

(See in Bacterial Diseases Caused by Gram-Positive Bacilli in Ch. 8)

191. SUPERFICIAL FUNGAL INFECTIONS

DERMATOPHYTE INFECTIONS
(Ringworm)

Superficial infections caused by dermatophytes—fungi that invade only "dead" tissues of the skin or its appendages (stratum corneum, nails, hair). Microsporum, Trichophyton, *and* Epidermophyton *are the genera most commonly involved.* Fomites are probably not responsible for transmission of infection. Some dermatophytes produce only mild or no inflammation; in such cases, the organism may persist indefinitely, causing intermittent remissions and exacerbations of a gradually extending lesion with a scaling, slightly raised border. In other cases an acute infection may occur, typically causing a sudden vesicular and bullous disease of the feet; or an inflamed boggy lesion of the scalp **(kerion)** may occur, which is due to a strong immunologic reaction to the fungus and is usually followed by remission or cure.

Clinical Types and Diagnosis

Since clinical differentiation of the related dermatophytes is difficult, these infections are conveniently discussed according to the sites involved. Diagnosis is confirmed by demonstration of the pathogenic fungus in scrapings of lesions, either by direct microscopic examination or by culture (see also Special Diagnostic Methods in Ch. 186).

Tinea corporis (ringworm of the body) is usually caused by a *Trichophyton.* It is characterized by papulosquamous annular lesions with raised borders; they expand peripherally and tend to clear centrally. Differential diagnosis includes pityriasis rosea, drug eruptions, nummular dermatitis, erythema multiforme, tinea versicolor, erythrasma, psoriasis, and secondary syphilis.

Tinea pedis (ringworm of the feet, athlete's foot) is particularly common. *Trichophyton mentagrophytes* infections begin in the 3rd and 4th interdigital spaces and later involve the plantar surface of the arch. The lesions are often macerated and have scaling borders; they may be vesicular. Acute flare-ups, with many vesicles and bullae, are common during warm weather. Infected toenails become thickened and distorted. *T. rubrum* produces scaling and thickening of the soles, often extending just beyond the plantar surface in a "moccasin" distribution. Inflammation or vesiculation may be slight or severe. Tinea pedis may be confused with maceration (from hyperhidrosis and occlusive footgear), with contact dermatitis (from sensitivity to various materials in shoes, particularly adhesive cement), with eczema, or with psoriasis.

Tinea unguium (ringworm of the nails), a form of onychomycosis, is usually caused by a *Trichophyton* species. Toenail involvement is common in longstanding tinea pedis; infections of the fingernails are less common. The nails become thickened and lusterless, and debris accumulates under the free edge. The nail plate becomes separated, and the nail may be destroyed. Differentiating a *Trichophyton* infection from *Candida* infection and psoriasis is particularly important because chemotherapy is specific and prolonged treatment is required.

Tinea capitis (ringworm of the scalp) mainly affects children. It is contagious and may become epidemic. Infections are usually produced by *Microsporum audouini, M. canis,* or *Trichophyton tonsurans. M. audouini* lesions are small, scaly, semi-bald grayish patches with broken, lusterless hairs. Infection may be limited to a small area or extend and coalesce until the entire scalp is involved, sometimes with ringed patches extending beyond the scalp margin. *M. canis* and *M. gypseum* usually cause a more inflammatory reaction, with shedding of the infected hairs. A raised, inflamed, boggy granuloma **(kerion)** may also occur; it is followed shortly by healing. Diagnosis of a *Microsporum* infection is facilitated by examining the scalp under a Wood's light; infected hairs may fluoresce a light bright green. The organism is an ectothrix, producing spores that form a sheath around the hair which can be seen on microscopy. Culture of the fungus is also important in establishing the diagnosis.

T. tonsurans infection of the scalp is more subtle in onset and characteristics. Inflammation is low-grade and persistent; the lesions are not annular or sharply marginated; and the hairs do not fluoresce under Wood's light. Affected areas of the scalp show characteristic black dots resulting from broken hairs. The fungus, an endothrix, produces chains of arthrospores within the hair that can be seen microscopically. *T. tonsurans* infection has become the common cause in recent years; other *Trichophyton* species, such as *T. violaceum*, are common in other parts of the world.

Tinea cruris (jock itch) may be caused by various organisms. Typically, a ringed lesion extends from the crural fold over the adjacent upper inner thigh. Both sides may be affected. Scratch dermatitis and lichenification are often seen. Lesions may be complicated by maceration, miliaria, secondary bacterial or candidal infection, and reactions to treatment. Recurrence is common, since fungi may persist indefinitely on the skin or may repeatedly infect susceptible individuals. Flare-ups occur more often during the summer. Tight clothing or obesity tends to favor growth of the organisms. The infection may be confused with contact dermatitis, psoriasis, erythrasma, or candidiasis. The scrotum is often acutely inflamed in candidal intertrigo, whereas in dermatophyte infections scrotal involvement is usually absent or slight.

Tinea barbae, a mycotic infection of the beard area, is rare. Infections in this area are more commonly bacterial (see FOLLICULITIS in Ch. 190), but may be fungal, especially in agricultural workers. The causative agent is established by microbiologic study.

Dermatophytids or "id" eruptions are fungus-free skin lesions that occur elsewhere on the body during an acute vesicular or inflammatory ringworm infection; they are thought to result from hypersensitivity to the fungus. Vesicular dermatitis of the hands is most commonly due to some other cause (see CHRONIC DERMATITIS OF HANDS AND FEET in Ch. 189).

Treatment

Griseofulvin is effective in treating tinea capitis, corporis pedis, unguium (onychomycosis) caused by *Trichophyton rubrum, T. schoenleini, T. mentagrophytes, T. sulfureum, T. verrucosum, T. interdigitalis, Epidermophyton floccosum, Microsporum audouini, M. canis,* or *M. gypseum*; but it is worthless in candidiasis or tinea versicolor and deep-seated mycoses (e.g., histoplasmosis, coccidioidomycosis). The adult dosage is microsize griseofulvin 250 mg orally b.i.d. to q.i.d. and the drug is best given with a high-fat meal. The micronized form is better absorbed than the nonmicronized form. Some infections, especially those involving the nails, may require > 4 mo of therapy. The drug occasionally causes GI distress, skin rashes, or leukopenia. Angioedema has been reported. Headaches, vertigo, and, rarely, transient hearing reduction may occur. Cross-sensitivity with penicillin is possible, but has not been a significant problem. **Miconazole** 2% cream and **clotrimazole** 1% cream and lotion are very effective topical medications for the treatment of certain types of dermatophyte infections of the skin (but not tinea capitis or onychomycosis). **Ketoconazole,** a new imidazole derivative that has not yet been fully evaluated and is an investigational agent in the USA, appears to be an effective broad-spectrum agent for systemic therapy of dermatomycoses (see also General Therapeutic Principles in Ch. 9).

Tinea corporis: For small to moderately sized lesions, 2% miconazole cream or 1% clotrimazole cream or lotion should be rubbed in b.i.d. until at least 7 to 10 days after lesions disappear. For extensive or resistant tinea corporis, the most effective therapy is griseofulvin. Tinea corporis usually responds readily to specific antifungal medication, but may be extensive and resistant to treatment in persons with debilitating systemic diseases.

Tinea pedis: Griseofulvin is the most effective treatment for mycologically proven tinea pedis, and should be started even though it may have little immediate effect on the acute inflammatory infection. It is useful in chronic infections and in preventing acute exacerbations, but cure may require therapy for many months and is especially difficult if the toenails are involved. Recurrence is frequent and some patients require prolonged medication to prevent disability.

Good foot hygiene is essential. Interdigital spaces must be dried after bathing, macerated skin rubbed away, and a bland, drying dusting powder applied. Light permeable footwear is recommended, especially during warm weather; many patients benefit from going barefoot. During acute vesicular flare-ups, bullae may be drained at the margin, but the keratinous tops should not be removed. Tap-water soaks b.i.d. are drying.

Whitfield's tincture (3% salicylic acid and 6% benzoic acid in 70% alcohol solution) or any of the topical medications used for tinea corporis may be useful in the subacute or chronic phases. Cure with topical treatment is difficult but control may be obtained with long-term therapy.

Tinea cruris: Topical therapy with 2% miconazole cream or 1% clotrimazole cream, as in tinea corporis, is often effective. In some cases, griseofulvin orally for 3 to 4 wk may be needed.

Tinea unguium may respond to griseofulvin if treatment is continued until the nail has regrown completely and all infected material has been cast away. For fingernails, this may require 6 to 12 mo. Treatment of toenails should be discouraged, since 1 to 2 yr may be required, recurrence is usual, and complete cure is unlikely.

Tinea capitis: Children with *Trichophyton* infection should be given microsize griseofulvin 125 to 250 mg orally b.i.d. with meals or milk for at least 4 wk or until all signs of infection are gone. A *single* large dose of 3 gm of griseofulvin given with a meal, ice cream, or milk frequently cures tinea capitis due to a *Microsporum* species, but results of treatment must be assessed in 3 to 4 wk, and if infection persists, daily treatment should be given.

Until the tinea capitis is cured, 1% miconazole or 1% clotrimazole cream should be applied to the affected child's scalp to prevent spread to other children.

Tinea barbae: Griseofulvin is the best treatment. A short course of prednisone should be given in addition if the lesions are severely inflamed, starting with 40 mg/day orally (for adults) and tapering the dose over a 2-wk period.

YEAST INFECTIONS

CANDIDIASIS (Candidosis; Moniliasis)

Candidiasis is usually limited to the skin and mucous membranes; uncommonly, the infection may become systemic and cause life-threatening visceral lesions. Systemic candidiasis (candidosis) is discussed in Ch. 9.

Etiology

Candida albicans is a ubiquitous, usually saprophytic, yeast that can become pathogenic if the organisms proliferate because of a favorable environment and if the host's defenses are weakened. The interrelation of these factors and the mechanisms that increase susceptibility to infection are discussed in Ch. 6. Specifically, the intertriginous and mucocutaneous areas, where heat and maceration provide a fertile environment, are the sites most susceptible to candidiasis; and systemic antibacterial, corticosteroid, or antimetabolic therapy, pregnancy, obesity, diabetes mellitus or other endocrinopathies, debilitating diseases, blood dyscrasias, and immunologic defects increase susceptibility to candidiasis.

Symptoms and Signs

Symptoms vary with the site of the infection. **Intertriginous infections,** the most common, appear as well-demarcated, erythematous, sometimes itchy, exudative patches of varying size and shape. The lesions are usually rimmed with small, red-based pustules and occur in the axillas, inframammary areas, umbilicus, groin and gluteal folds (e.g., diaper rash), between the toes, and on the finger-webs. **Perianal candidiasis** produces white macerative pruritus ani.

Vulvovaginitis is relatively common, especially in pregnancy or diabetes mellitus, and appears as a white or yellow discharge with inflammation of the vaginal wall and vulva. **Infection of the glans penis** is less common but may be seen in men whose sexual partners have candidal vulvovaginitis and in men with diabetes mellitus.

Oral candidiasis (thrush) appears as creamy white patches of exudate that can be scraped off an inflamed tongue or buccal mucosa (see also Ch. 208). **Perlèche** appears at the corners of the mouth and is characterized by inflammation with erosion and fissures.

Candidal paronychia begins as a painful red swelling around the nail that later develops pus. **Subungual infections** are characterized by distal separation of one or several fingernails **(onycholysis)** with white or yellow discoloration of the subungual area.

Defects in cell-mediated immune responses (which, in children, are sometimes genetic) may lead to **chronic mucocutaneous candidiasis (candida granuloma)** (see also in Vol. II, Ch. 25), which is characterized by red, pustular, crusted and thickened lesions, especially on the nose and forehead. In patients with an immune deficiency, other, more typical, candidal lesions or systemic candidiasis is also seen.

Diagnosis

Candida can be demonstrated by finding both yeast and hyphae in gram-stained specimens or in potassium hydroxide mounts of scrapings from a lesion. Because *Candida* is a commensal of man, the culture of a species from the skin, mouth, vagina, urine, sputum, or stool should be interpreted cautiously. To confirm the diagnosis, a characteristic clinical lesion, exclusion of other causes, and, at times, histologic evidence of tissue invasion are needed.

Treatment

Topical nystatin, clotrimazole, and miconazole are all effective against skin and vaginal infections (for genital infections, see also GENITAL CANDIDIASIS in Vol. II, Ch. 5). A vehicle appropriate to the site of infection must be chosen and frequency of administration should be t.i.d. or q.i.d. When antiinflammatory and antipruritic actions are desired, equal amounts of the antifungal cream and a corticosteroid cream can be mixed. Recalcitrant or recurrent cases, especially of oral or anogenital candidiasis, benefit from nystatin oral suspension or tablets, 500,000 u. q.i.d. When one sexual partner has recurrent candidiasis, both partners should be given topical and oral nystatin. For candidal diaper rash, the skin should be kept dry by changing diapers frequently and by generously applying talcum powder containing nystatin; in severe cases, rubber pants and plastic disposable diaper coverings should be avoided. Oral or IM iron has been effective for chronic mucocutaneous candidiasis in some patients with the genetic form of immune deficiency disease. Treatment of paronychial infections is discussed in Ch. 190.

TINEA VERSICOLOR

An infection characterized by multiple, usually asymptomatic, patches of lesions varying in color from white to brown, and caused by Pityrosporon orbiculare (*formerly* Malassezia furfur). It is common in young adults. Tan, brown, or white, very slightly scaling lesions, which tend to coalesce, are seen on the chest, neck, and abdomen and occasionally on the face. The scaling may not be apparent unless the lesion is scratched. The patient may notice the condition only in the summer because the lesions do not tan; instead they appear as variously sized white "sun spots." Itching is rare and usually occurs only when the patient gets overheated. The condition is diagnosed from the clinical appearance and by finding groups of yeast and short plump hyphae on microscopic examination of scrapings from the lesions. The extent of involvement can be determined by the golden fluorescence or pigment changes under a Wood's light. Culture of the organism is difficult.

Treatment

Selenium sulfide in shampoo form (CAUTION: *Keep out of reach of children*) is applied undiluted to all involved areas for 3 or 4 days at bedtime and washed off in the morning; the scrotum should be avoided. If irritation occurs, the selenium sulfide should be washed off after 20 to 60 min or treatment should be stopped for a few days. If irritation is too severe, 25% sodium thiosulfite solution or 2% micropulverized sulfur and 2% salicylic acid in a shampoo base may be applied at bedtime for 2 wk. The lesions may not become repigmented for several months, and the disease may recur in 6 to 12 mo.

---

192. PARASITIC INFECTIONS OF THE SKIN

SCABIES

(The Itch)

A transmissible parasitic skin infection, characterized by superficial burrows, intense pruritus, and secondary infection.

Etiology and Incidence

Scabies is caused by the itch mite *Sarcoptes scabiei.* The impregnated female mite tunnels into the stratum corneum and deposits her eggs along the burrow. The larvae hatch within a few days and congregate around the hair follicles. Lesions are thought to result from hypersensitivity to the parasites.

Scabies is transmitted readily, often through an entire household, by skin-to-skin contact with an infected individual. It is often acquired venereally. It is not spread by clothing or bedding.

Symptoms, Signs, and Diagnosis

Pruritus is marked and is most intense when the patient is in bed. The characteristic initial lesions are the burrows, seen as fine wavy dark lines a few millimeters to 1 cm long with a minute papule at the open end. The inflammatory lesions occur predominantly on the finger-webs, the flexor surface of the wrists, about the elbows and axillary folds, about the areola of the breasts in females and on the genitals in males, along the belt-line, and on the lower buttocks. The face is not involved in adults but may be in infants.

Burrows may be difficult to find, particularly when the disease has persisted for several weeks, because they are soon obscured by scratching or by secondary lesions (e.g., urticaria, scratch dermatitis, eczema, or superimposed bacterial infection). Diagnosis can be confirmed by demonstrating the parasite in scrapings taken from a burrow, mixed with any clear solution (e.g., mineral oil, potassium hydroxide, or even water), and examined microscopically.

Treatment

Treatment is curative and may serve as a "therapeutic test" in doubtful cases. The patient should bathe and then apply 1% gamma benzene hexachloride, 25% benzyl benzoate cream or lotion, or 10% crotamiton over the entire skin surface from the neck down, making certain (with the help of an assistant, if needed) that no areas are missed. For infants < 2 yr, 5 or 10% sulfur ointment is preferred because of a potential neurotoxicity from absorption of gamma benzene hexachloride. The bath and application should be repeated the next morning but not again, because persistent inflammation and itching may be due to scratching, contact dermatitis, or secondary infection rather than to the mite, and further applications may cause irritant dermatitis. Contacts, both adults and children, must be examined for scabies, with prompt treatment as needed.

Retreatment is rarely needed, unless infection is reacquired. A 0.1% fluorinated corticosteroid ointment (see Ch. 187) may be used 2 to 4 times/day for persistent itching, which may take 1 to 2 wk

to subside. Concomitant bacterial infections may require systemic antibiotics but often clear spontaneously when the scabies is cured.

PEDICULOSIS

Infestation by lice may involve the **head** (by *Pediculus humanus capitis*), the **body** (*P. humanus corporis*), or the **genital area** (*Phthirus pubis*). The head louse and pubic (crab) louse live directly on the host; the body louse, in the undergarments. Infestation is widespread where overcrowding or inadequate facilities for personal hygiene or clean clothing exist. The body louse is an important vector of the organisms that cause epidemic typhus, trench fever, and relapsing fever.

Symptoms, Signs, and Diagnosis

Pediculosis capitis is transmitted by personal contact and by such objects as combs and hats. It is common among school children, without regard to social status. Infestation is localized predominantly on the scalp, though it sometimes involves the eyebrows, eyelashes, and beard. Itching is severe, and excoriation of the scalp, sometimes with secondary bacterial infection, may be seen. Moderate discrete posterior cervical adenopathy is frequent. In children, a generalized, nonspecific dermatitis is occasionally caused by lice infesting only the scalp. Diagnosis is simple if infestation is considered and the scalp is inspected, preferably with a lens. Small, ovoid, greyish-white nits (ova) are seen fixed to the hair shafts, sometimes in great numbers; unlike scales, they cannot be dislodged. The nits mature in 3 to 14 days. Lice may be found, less frequently than the nits, around the occiput and behind the ears.

Pediculosis corporis is uncommon under good hygienic conditions. Nits may be found on the body hairs, but both parasites and ova are easily found in underclothing, since the body louse primarily inhabits the seams of clothing worn next to the skin. Itching is invariable. Lesions are especially common on the shoulders, buttocks, and abdomen. Inspection may show small red puncta due to bites, usually associated with linear scratch marks, urticaria, or superficial bacterial infection. Furunculosis is an occasional complication.

Pediculosis pubis is usually transmitted venereally. The crab louse ordinarily infests the anogenital hairs but may involve other areas, especially in hairy individuals. In all itching dermatoses of the anogenital region, careful inspection for the parasites should be made; they may be few in number. The lice are large but not easily seen without a diligent search; they resemble the small crusts of scratch dermatitis. The ova are commonly attached to the skin at the base of the hairs. A sign of infestation is a scattering of minute dark brown specks (louse excreta) on undergarments where they come in contact with the anogenital region. Excoriation and secondary dermatitis, the latter often from self-medication, may develop early. Sometimes the lice may be seen as small bluish spots on the skin, ordinarily on the trunk.

Treatment and Prevention

Cure is rapid with 1% gamma benzene hexachloride, applied once/day for 2 days in shampoo, cream, or lotion form or as a combination of shampoo followed by the cream or lotion. Application may be repeated in 10 days to destroy any nits that survived, but prolonged application of parasiticides should be **avoided,** particularly in males, because persistent genital dermatitis may result. Infestation of the eyelids and eyelashes may be more difficult to manage; the parasites usually must be removed with forceps. Sources of infestation, such as combs, hats, clothing, or bedding, should be appropriately decontaminated by boiling, thorough laundering and steam pressing, or dry cleaning. Recurrence is common.

CREEPING ERUPTION

(Cutaneous Larva Migrans)

This disease is caused chiefly by *Ancylostoma braziliense*, the hookworm of the dog or cat. The ova of the parasites are deposited on the ground in dog or cat feces. The larva persists in warm moist ground or sand and penetrates unprotected skin where it contacts the soil. The feet, legs, buttocks, or back are most commonly involved. The haphazard progress of the parasite as it burrows in the epidermis produces a winding, threadlike trail of inflammation. Itching is marked, and scratch dermatitis and bacterial infection with a bizarre pattern are common.

Treatment

Studies indicate that applying the oral 10% suspension of thiabendazole topically to all affected areas q.i.d. for 7 to 10 days is promptly effective.

193. VIRAL INFECTIONS OF THE SKIN

Herpes simplex and herpes zoster, though they may be considered viral skin infections, are discussed elsewhere in Vols. I and II.

WARTS
(Verrucae)

Common, contagious, benign epithelial tumors caused by papovaviruses. Viral warts may appear at any age, but are most frequent in older children and uncommon in the aged. Their appearance and size depend on their location and on the degree of irritation and trauma to which they are subjected. The course may be erratic. Infection may persist as single or multiple lesions, and lesions may develop by autoinoculation. Complete regression after several months is usual with or without treatment, but warts may persist for years and may recur at the same or different sites. The role of immunologic factors in spontaneous disappearance is unclear.

Common warts (verrucae vulgaris) are sharply demarcated, rough-surfaced, round or irregular, firm, light gray, yellow, brown, or grayish-black tumors 2 to 10 mm in diameter. They appear most frequently on sites subject to trauma (e.g., fingers, elbows, knees, face, scalp) but may spread elsewhere. **Periungual warts** are common warts occurring around the nail plate.

Plantar warts are common warts on the sole of the foot; they are flattened by pressure and surrounded by cornified epithelium. They may be exquisitely tender and can be distinguished from corns and calluses by their tendency to pinpoint bleeding when the surface is pared away. **Mosaic warts** are plaques of myriad small, closely set plantar warts.

Filiform warts are long, narrow, small growths usually seen on the eyelids, face, neck, or lips. **Flat warts** are smooth, flat, yellow-brown lesions and occur more commonly in children and young adults, most often on the face and along scratch marks through autoinoculation. **Warts of unusual shape**— e.g., pedunculated, or resembling a cauliflower—are most frequent on the head and neck, especially on the scalp and bearded region.

Moist or "venereal" warts (condylomata acuminata) are discussed in Vol. II, Ch. 5.

Treatment

No treatment is entirely satisfactory. The virus apparently remains after treatment, and recurrence rates may be as high as 30 to 35%. Destructive procedures, such as full-thickness surgical excision, may cause lasting or painful scars or tissue damage, are usually inappropriate, and should be avoided. X-ray therapy *should not be used.* If a painful procedure is selected, the patient should lie down during treatment to avoid fainting.

For **common warts,** the most satisfactory (though painful) treatment is freezing with liquid nitrogen or solid CO_2. The duration of application depends on the equipment and the amount of pressure applied. The blister that follows in 2 to 3 days may be punctured, but its top should not be removed. Healing occurs in 3 to 4 wk. Electrodesiccation and curettage is satisfactory for solitary or few lesions. After lidocaine is given for local anesthesia, the electric needle is put into the top of the wart and kept in place until the tissues begin to bubble slightly. The wart can then be curetted off easily. Healing follows in about 4 wk.

Less painful and often satisfactory alternatives are available. Cantharidin 0.7% in acetone and collodion may be effective if applied over the entire lesion plus a minute (1-mm) area of adjacent normal-appearing skin and if nonporous adhesive tape is applied after the cantharidin has dried. The tape is removed in 6 h, or earlier if pain becomes severe. A blister forms, and the area heals in 3 to 4 wk. A caustic such as 30% trichloroacetic acid may be applied to the top of the wart (avoiding normal tissue). A 40% salicylic acid plaster can be cut to size and kept in place with adhesive tape; every 2 to 3 days the resulting macerated tissue should be pared and a new plaster applied. In young patients, suggestion accompanied by an impressive manipulation—e.g., shining a Wood's light on the wart after painting it with a fluorescent dye, or warming it with a heat lamp—may be successful.

Periungual warts are often very resistant to treatment because it is difficult to expose the entire lesion. As much of the nail as possible should be cut away and the wart then frozen or treated with cantharidin as described above. Trichloroacetic acid 30% can also be used. **Filiform warts** are best treated by cutting off the lesions at the base.

Plantar warts must be treated with care to avoid lasting, painful scars. The warts should be pared until bleeding or pain occurs. A 40% salicylic acid plaster should then be applied, covered with adhesive tape, and kept in place for 1 wk. The patient should repeat the weekly paring and application of a new plaster at home. Alternatively, 50% trichloroacetic acid can be applied to the pared wart before covering it with 40% salicylic acid plaster and adhesive tape. The area may be extremely painful for 2 to 3 days. The plaster is kept in place for 1 wk if pain is not too severe, and the debris is then removed. Home treatment with salicylic acid plasters and paring should follow. Freezing with liquid nitrogen may be painful enough to prevent walking for 2 to 3 days but often is effective. Electrodesiccation may be used—but with caution, to avoid scarring. If the plantar wart is on a weight-bearing area, a metatarsal bar or foam pad may relieve pressure, aid treatment, and prevent recurrence.

The best treatment for **mosaic warts** is paring and application of salicylic acid plasters as described above.

Light electrodesiccation is useful when **flat warts** are few; however, since the lesions are usually numerous and are superficial, any one of several light peeling agents is preferred. Tretinoin (vitamin

A acid; retinoic acid) 0.05% can be applied nightly until peeling starts or too much irritation occurs; or liquid nitrogen, 30% trichloroacetic acid, or CO_2 snow can be rolled lightly on the affected area to produce mild peeling.

MOLLUSCUM CONTAGIOSUM

A poxvirus infection characterized by skin-colored, smooth, waxy, umbilicated papules 2 to 10 mm in diameter. A "giant" single molluscum may grow 2 or 3 times as large.

Transmission is by direct contact, often venereal. Its contagiousness to others varies. The papules may appear anywhere on the skin and often occur as numerous small papules in the genital and pubic area. The lesions are usually asymptomatic, unless secondarily infected, and may be discovered only when the patient is examined for another sexually transmitted disease. They can be diagnosed easily by the characteristic central umbilication or dell, filled with a semisolid white material that, if expressed and Giemsa-stained, shows many large cells containing inclusion bodies. Inclusion bodies alone may be seen. The disease can spread by autoinoculation, but after months may disappear spontaneously. Areas of eczematous dermatitis may surround several mollusca, especially in young children; the cause of the dermatitis is not known.

Treatment, to be successful, requires destroying each lesion by freezing, curettage, electrocautery, or cantharidin (as for common warts, above), or by removing the central core of the papule with a needle or a comedo extractor.

---

194. DISORDERS OF HAIR FOLLICLES AND SEBACEOUS GLANDS

ACNE

(See Vol. II, Ch. 27)

ROSACEA

A chronic inflammatory disorder, usually beginning in middle age or later, and characterized by telangiectasia, erythema, papules, and pustules appearing especially in the central areas of the face. Tissue hypertrophy, particularly of the nose **(rhinophyma),** may result. Occasionally rosacea occurs on the extremities.

The cause is unknown, but the disease is most common in persons with a fair complexion. Diet probably plays no role in the pathogenesis. Rosacea may resemble acne, but comedones are never present; differential diagnosis also includes drug eruptions (particularly from iodides and bromides), granulomas of the skin, and cutaneous LE.

Treatment

Broad-spectrum oral antibiotics are the only regularly effective treatment. Their mode of action in this disease is unknown. Tetracycline is preferred because side effects with long-term use are few. A starting dose of 250 mg q.i.d. (between meals) should be reduced once a beneficial response is achieved. Often only 250 mg/day or every other day will control the disease. Topical corticosteroids are ineffective; the fluorinated corticosteroids aggravate rosacea and are contraindicated. Rhinophyma may require surgical correction.

PERIORAL DERMATITIS

A red papular eruption of unknown etiology occurring around the mouth and on the chin. The condition occurs predominantly in women aged 20 to 60. It may superficially resemble acne or rosacea. A zone of normal skin lies between the lesions and the vermilion border of the mouth.

Tetracycline 250 mg q.i.d. (between meals) is the most effective **treatment.** The dose should be reduced gradually after I mo to the smallest amount that controls the disease. Topical therapy should be discouraged; as in acne and rosacea, fluorinated corticosteroids worsen the disorder.

HYPERTRICHOSIS

(Hirsutism)

Excessive hair growth in areas usually not hairy. A familial or racial tendency is common. An endocrine disorder may be implicated in women and children—most frequently, adrenal virilism, basophilic adenoma of the pituitary, masculinizing ovarian tumors, and the Stein-Leventhal syndrome. Hirsutism is seen frequently at menopause and with systemic androgenic steroid or corticosteroid therapy, and may occur in porphyria cutanea tarda.

Treatment

Any underlying disorder should be treated. The only safe permanent local treatment is the destruction of individual hair follicles by electrolysis, a tedious process. Widely used temporary measures include plucking, shaving, and use of epilating wax. Chemical depilatories are acceptable if the directions are followed, but may irritate the skin. A hair bleach may mask the condition if the hair is fine.

ALOPECIA

(Baldness)

Partial or complete loss of hair. It may result from genetic factors, aging, or local or systemic disease. (Seborrheic dermatitis and psoriasis, the two dermatoses that affect the scalp most commonly, do not produce alopecia.) **Nonscarring (noncicatricial) alopecia** occurs without prior scarring or gross atrophic changes; **scarring (cicatricial) alopecia** follows scar tissue formation resulting from inflammation and tissue destruction.

Nonscarring Alopecia

Male-pattern baldness is extremely common. It is familial and requires the presence of androgens, but other etiologic factors are unknown. The hair loss begins in the lateral frontal areas or over the vertex. If onset is in the mid-teens, subsequent baldness is commonly extensive. **Female-pattern alopecia** is not infrequent in women. It is confined ordinarily to thinning of the hair in the frontal and the parietal regions; complete baldness in any area is rare.

Toxic alopecia is usually temporary and may follow, by as long as 3 to 4 mo, a severe, often febrile, illness (e.g., scarlet fever). It may also be seen in myxedema, hypopituitarism, or early syphilis, following pregnancy, and with some drugs—particularly cytotoxic agents, thallium compounds, and overdoses of vitamin A.

In **alopecia areata**, sudden hair loss in circumscribed areas occurs in individuals who have no obvious skin disorder or systemic disease. Any hairy area may be involved, the scalp and beard most frequently. Rarely, all the body hair may be lost **(alopecia universalis)**. The prognosis is poor if alopecia is extensive or begins in childhood, but alopecia first appearing in adult life and confined to a few areas is often reversed in a few months, though recurrences may occur. Serum antibodies to thyroglobulin, parietal cells, adrenal cells, and thyroid may be present.

Hair pulling (trichotillomania) is a neurotic habit that usually appears in children; it may remain undiagnosed for a long time. The hairs may be broken off or pulled out. Some stubby regrowth may be visible, but the condition is often hard to differentiate from alopecia areata.

Scarring Alopecia

If hair loss is due to atrophy or scarring, no regrowth can be expected. In injuries (e.g., burns, physical trauma, x-ray atrophy), the cause of the scarring will usually be apparent; if it is not obvious, it should be sought. Cutaneous LE, chronic deep bacterial or fungal infections; deep factitial ulcers; granulomas such as sarcoidosis, syphilitic gummas, or tuberculosis; or inflamed tinea capitis (kerion or favus) may produce scarring alopecia. Certain slow-growing tumors may gradually extend in the scalp with resultant scarring.

Examination should include the entire skin surface and mucous membranes, because related lesions will often be found. Biopsy should be done at an area of active inflammatory change, usually at the border of a bald patch. Cultures for bacteria and fungi may be indicated.

Diagnosis

Microscopic examination of plucked hair may differentiate some forms of nonscarring alopecia. Normally 80 to 90% of hairs are in a growing (anagen) phase; the rest are in a resting (telogen) phase. *All* of the hair (approximately 40 to 60 hairs) should be plucked, using a strong instrument, from a defined area of the scalp and an anagen/telogen count performed. Anagen hairs have sheaths attached to their roots, whereas telogen hairs have no sheaths and have tiny bulbs at their roots. Postpartum and post-illness alopecias are characterized by an increased percentage of telogen hairs, whereas alopecias due to thallium or antimitotic drugs are characterized by a normal percentage of telogen hairs. The anagen hair in the latter conditions may break easily because the hair shaft narrows. Alopecia areata is characterized by hairs that look like exclamation points. Biopsy of the scalp may differentiate various forms of scarring alopecias. Either histologic or immunofluorescent examination may delineate LE, lichen planopilaris (lichen planus of the scalp), and scleroderma. Metastatic lesions, which may also produce localized scarring alopecia, are diagnosed by biopsy.

Treatment

No therapy is known for idiopathic male-pattern baldness, though transplants from hairy to bald areas are effective. In alopecia areata, systemic corticosteroids usually produce regrowth of hair, but the necessarily long-term therapy entails risks that are unjustifiable for cosmetic defects. Triamcinolone acetonide suspension has been injected intradermally but is of little value, as the disorder may recur. Experimental induction of a mild allergic contact dermatitis has shown some benefit.

In scarring alopecia, treatment is directed at eliminating the cause.

PSEUDOFOLLICULITIS BARBAE

Pseudofolliculitis of the beard (**ingrown hairs**) is seen almost exclusively in black men. The stiff hair tips penetrate the skin before leaving the follicle, or else leave the follicle, curve, and reenter nearby skin, provoking small pustules that are more a foreign-body reaction than an infection. The only consistently effective **treatment** is to have the patient grow a beard. A thioglycolate depilatory may be used every 2 to 3 days but is often irritating. Application of tretinoin (vitamin A acid; retinoic acid) 0.05% liquid or cream daily or every other day may be effective in mild or moderate cases; it is initially irritating and should be used every other day at first, then daily.

KERATINOUS CYST

(Wen; Sebaceous Cyst; Steatoma)

A slow-growing benign cystic tumor of the skin containing follicular, keratinous, and sebaceous material and frequently found on the scalp, ears, face, back, or scrotum. On palpation, the cystic mass is firm, globular, movable, and nontender; it seldom causes discomfort unless infected. Puncture of the cyst produces characteristic cheesy, often fetid, contents formed of epithelial debris and greasy material; soft keratin often predominates, and at times calcium deposits may be found. Secondary bacterial infection with abscess formation occurs. A **milium** is a minute superficial keratinous cyst, usually found on the face or scrotum.

Treatment

For milia, expression of the contents through a tiny stab incision is curative. For larger lesions, a small incision is made and the contents are evacuated; then the cyst wall is removed through the incision with a curette or hemostat. Surgical excision is also effective. Infected cysts can be incised and drained; a gauze drain is inserted and gradually removed over 7 to 10 days. Any large cyst may recur after treatment if the cyst wall is not completely removed.

---

195. SCALING PAPULAR DISEASES

PSORIASIS

A common chronic and recurrent disease characterized by dry, well-circumscribed, silvery, scaling papules and plaques of various sizes.

Psoriasis varies in severity from 1 or 2 lesions to a widespread dermatosis with disabling arthritis or exfoliation. The cause is unknown, but the thick scaling is probably due to increased epidermal cell proliferation. About 2 to 4% of the white population, and far fewer blacks, are affected. Onset is usually between ages 10 and 40, but no age is exempt. A family history of psoriasis is common and usually reflects an autosomal dominant inheritance. General health is not affected, except for the psychologic stigma of an unsightly skin disease, unless severe arthritis or intractable exfoliation develops.

Symptoms and Signs

Onset is usually gradual. The typical course is one of chronic remissions and recurrences (or occasionally acute exacerbations) that vary in frequency and duration. Factors precipitating psoriatic eruptions include local trauma (which causes the **Koebner phenomenon,** with lesions appearing at the trauma site) and, occasionally, severe sunburn, irritation, topical medications, chloroquine antimalarial therapy, and withdrawal of systemic corticosteroids. Some patients (especially children) may have explosive psoriatic eruptions after an acute URI.

Psoriasis characteristically involves the scalp (including the postauricular regions), the extensor surface of the extremities (particularly at elbows and knees), the back, and the buttocks. The nails, eyebrows, axillas, umbilicus, or anogenital region may also be affected. Occasionally the disease is generalized.

The lesions are sharply demarcated, usually nonpruritic, erythematous papules or plaques covered with overlapping, silvery or slightly opalescent, shiny scales. The lesions heal without scarring, and hair growth is not altered. Papules sometimes extend and coalesce, producing large plaques in bizarre annular and gyrate patterns. Nail involvement may resemble a fungal infection, with stippling, pitting, fraying or separation of the distal margin, thickening, discoloration, and debris under the nail plate.

Psoriatic arthritis (see in Ch. 103) often closely resembles RA and may be equally crippling, but the patient's serum contains no rheumatoid factor. In **exfoliative psoriatic dermatitis,** which may be intractable and may lead to general debility, the entire skin is red and covered with fine scales; typical psoriatic lesions may be obscured at first. **Pustular psoriasis** is characterized by sterile pustules that may be localized to the palms and soles or may be generalized; typical psoriatic lesions are not always present.

Diagnosis

Diagnosis by inspection is rarely difficult. In psoriasis of the scalp, the well-defined, dry, heaped-up, and scaly lesions are usually not hard to distinguish from the diffuse, greasy, yellowish scaling of seborrheic dermatitis. However, psoriasis may be confused with seborrheic dermatitis, squamous cell carcinoma in situ (when on the trunk), secondary syphilis, fungal infections, cutaneous LE, eczema, lichen planus, or localized scratch dermatitis.

Biopsy findings may be typical, but many other skin diseases may have psoriasiform histologic features that make them difficult to distinguish.

Prognosis and Treatment

The prognosis depends on the extent and severity of the initial involvement and the age of onset. Acute attacks usually clear up, but complete permanent remission is rare. No therapeutic method assures a cure.

The simplest forms of treatment—lubricants, keratolytics, and topical corticosteroids—should be tried first because the number of effective remedies is limited. Exposure to sunlight is recommended, though occasionally sunburn may induce exacerbations. Systemic antimetabolites should be used only in severe skin or joint involvement. Systemic corticosteroids should not be used because of the predictable side effects, including severe exacerbations, that may occur during treatment or after therapy has been stopped.

Lubricating creams, hydrogenated vegetable (cooking) oils, or white petrolatum are applied—alone or with added corticosteroids, salicylic acid, crude coal tar, or anthralin (dithranol)—b.i.d. while the skin is still damp after bathing. Alternatively, crude coal tar ointment or cream may be applied at night and washed off in the morning, followed by exposure to natural or artificial (280 to 320 nm) ultraviolet light in slowly increasing increments sufficient to produce mild erythema.

Anthralin can be effective as an ointment (2%) applied carefully to the lesions under a malocclusive dressing at bedtime; it should be removed in the morning with mineral oil. Anthralin may be irritating and should not be used in intertriginous areas. Anthralin stains sheets and clothing as well as the skin.

Topical corticosteroids may be used as an alternative or adjunct to anthralin or coal tar treatment. As an adjunct they are used b.i.d. or t.i.d. during the day and anthralin or coal tar is used at bedtime. Corticosteroids are most effective when used under occlusive polyethylene coverings or incorporated in adhesive tape. This may be done overnight and a corticosteroid cream rubbed in without occlusion b.i.d. or t.i.d. during the day. The initial choice of concentration usually depends on the extent of involvement. As the lesions improve, the corticosteroid should be applied less frequently or in lower concentration in order to prevent local side effects (atrophy, telangiectasias). Triamcinolone acetonide 0.1% (or equivalent—see Ch. 187) is most effective, but can be expensive; 1 oz (30 gm) of cream is usually needed to cover the entire body. The commercial preparation may be diluted in an appropriate vehicle: ointment in petrolatum, or cream in a vanishing cream base; commercial preparations of lower strength are also available. If potent fluorinated topical corticosteroids are applied to large areas of the body, especially under occlusion, systemic effects can be observed and psoriasis may be aggravated, as with systemic corticosteroids. For small, localized lesions, flurandrenolide-impregnated tape left on overnight and changed in the morning is effective. Relapse after topical corticosteroids is often faster than with other agents.

Thick scalp plaques may be difficult to treat. A preparation containing an oily solution of < 1% phenol and sodium chloride, or 5% salicylic acid in mineral oil, may be rubbed in at bedtime with a toothbrush and washed out the next morning with a detergent shampoo. A shower cap can be worn in bed to enhance penetration and to avoid messiness. Tar-containing shampoos are often used, but must be left on the scalp a half hour or more before rinsing. Topical corticosteroid lotions or gels are applied during the day.

Resistant skin or scalp patches may respond to local superficial injection of triamcinolone acetonide suspension diluted with saline to 2.5 mg/ml, the amount depending on the size of the lesion. Injections should not be repeated more often than every 3 wk, and may cause local atrophy.

Methotrexate taken orally is the most effective treatment in severe disabling psoriasis that is unresponsive to topical agents or psoralens and high intensity ultraviolet A **(PUVA)** therapy (see below), especially severe psoriatic arthritis or widespread pustular or exfoliative psoriasis. Methotrexate seems to act by interfering with the rapid proliferation of epidermal cells. Because the potential toxicity requires careful monitoring of hematologic, renal, and hepatic function and because dosage regimens vary, *methotrexate therapy should be undertaken only by physicians experienced in its use for psoriasis.*

PUVA, a new treatment for extensive psoriasis, is under study. Oral methoxsalen (average dose 40 mg) is followed, at a specific interval, by exposure of the skin to long-wave ultraviolet light (330 to 360 nm). The dosage of both the methoxsalen and the ultraviolet exposure must be tailored to each patient. Although the treatment is clean and may produce remissions for several months, repeated treatments with intensive light may cause skin cancer (especially in those with either prior skin cancer or prior x-ray treatment). Adverse effects on eyes and blood are being sought. Treatment in the USA is available under an investigational new drug application of the FDA.

PITYRIASIS ROSEA

A self-limited, mild, inflammatory skin disease characterized by scaly lesions, possibly due to an unidentified infectious agent. It may occur at any age but is seen most frequently in young adults. In temperate climates, incidence is highest during spring and autumn.

Symptoms and Signs

A "herald" or "mother" patch, found most commonly on the trunk, usually precedes the generalized eruption by 5 to 10 days. It is slightly erythematous, rose- or fawn-colored, and circinate or oval, has a scaly, slightly raised border, and resembles a superficial ringworm infection. Many similar lesions 0.5 to 2 cm in diameter follow the herald patch, sometimes continuing to appear for weeks. They usually appear on the trunk. On the back, the long axes of the lesions parallel the lines of cleavage, typically radiating from the spinal column in a "Christmas tree" pattern. In blacks the eruption may be primarily papular, with little scaling.

At times, lesions principally affect the arms, with relative sparing of the trunk. The face is involved occasionally. Rarely, lesions become generalized, sometimes giving a scarlatiniform appearance. Systemic symptoms are usually absent, but slight malaise and headache occur rarely, and itching is sometimes troublesome. Spontaneous remission within 4 or 5 wk is usual, though the eruption may persist for 2 mo or longer. Recurrences are rare.

Differential Diagnosis

Pityriasis rosea must be differentiated from tinea corporis, tinea versicolor, drug eruptions, psoriasis, and, most importantly, secondary syphilis. A serologic test for syphilis should be done routinely.

Treatment

There is no specific treatment, and usually no treatment is needed. The patient should be reassured that the lesions will clear. Artificial or natural sunlight may hasten involution. Inflamed, itching lesions may be relieved by 0.25% menthol in a vanishing cream base. Prednisone—10 mg orally q.i.d. until the itching subsides, then decreased over a 14-day period—should be used only when itching is severe.

LICHEN PLANUS

A recurrent, pruritic, inflammatory eruption characterized by small discrete angular papules that may coalesce into rough scaly patches, often accompanied by oral lesions. Children are rarely affected.

Etiology

The cause is unknown. Some drugs (e.g., arsenic, bismuth, gold) or exposure to certain color-photography developers may cause an eruption indistinguishable from lichen planus. Quinacrine taken for long periods may produce hypertrophic lichen planus of the lower legs as well as other dermatologic and systemic disturbances.

Symptoms and Signs

Onset may be abrupt or gradual. The initial attack persists for weeks or months, and intermittent recurrences may be noted for years.

The primary papules are 2 to 4 mm in diameter, with angular borders, a violaceous color, and a distinct sheen in cross-lighting. Rarely, bullae may develop. Moderate to severe, often refractory, itching may be present. The lesions are usually distributed symmetrically, most commonly on the flexor surfaces of the wrists and on the legs, trunk, glans penis, and oral and vaginal mucosa. Lesions are occasionally generalized, but the face is rarely involved. Particularly on the lower legs, the lesions may become large, scaly, and verrucous **(hypertrophic lichen planus).** During the acute phase, new papules may appear along a site of minor skin injury such as a superficial scratch (the Koebner phenomenon). Hyperpigmentation (and sometimes atrophy) may develop as lesions persist. Rarely, a patchy scarring alopecia of the scalp appears.

The oral mucosa is involved in about 50% of patients, often before cutaneous lesions develop. The cheek mucosa, tongue margins, and mucosa in edentulous areas show asymptomatic ill-defined, bluish-white linear lesions that may be reticulated at first and increase in size in an angular configuration. An erosive form may occur, in which the patient complains of shallow, often painful, recurrent oral ulcerations. Chronic exacerbations and remissions are common.

Diagnosis

Lichen planus is histologically distinctive. Persistent oral or vaginal lichen planus, with thickening and coalescence of the lesions, may sometimes be difficult to differentiate clinically from leukoplakia. Though always indicated, biopsy may not yield specific findings in old lesions.

Widespread erosive oral lesions must be differentiated from those of candidiasis, leukoplakia, carcinoma, aphthous ulcers, herpetic stomatitis, and erythema multiforme. The peripheries of the lesions should be examined for short dendritic extensions and characteristic delicate bluish-white lacy lesions.

Treatment

Asymptomatic lichen planus does not require treatment. If a drug or chemical is suspected as the cause, its use should be discontinued. An antihistamine (e.g., diphenhydramine 50 mg or chlorpheniramine 4 mg orally q.i.d.) may decrease moderate itching through a sedative effect. Localized pruritic or hypertrophic areas may be treated with triamcinolone acetonide suspension diluted with saline to 2.5 to 5 mg/ml and superficially injected into the lesion, using enough to elevate the lesion slightly (not to be repeated more often than every 3 wk); or with occlusive corticosteroid therapy (e.g., triamcinolone acetonide 0.1% cream or equivalent under polyethylene wrapping at bedtime, or flurandrenolide-impregnated tape). Tretinoin 0.1% solution can also be beneficial in treating lichen planus on glabrous skin. It should be applied with a cotton-tipped applicator at night, followed by t.i.d. application of a full-strength corticosteroid cream (see Ch. 187). For erosive oral lesions, viscous lidocaine mouthwashes before meals and triamcinolone acetonide in emollient dental paste, applied 5 to 6 times/day, should be tried.

Erosive oral lesions and widespread severely pruritic skin lesions often require a systemic corticosteroid; e.g., oral prednisone 40 to 60 mg every morning initially, with the dose decreased by about one third each week. Unfortunately, itching may return after systemic prednisone has been stopped; in this case, a systemic corticosteroid in continued low dosage given every other morning may be tried.

196. INFLAMMATORY REACTIONS OF THE SKIN

DRUG ERUPTIONS

(Dermatitis Medicamentosa)

An eruption of the skin or mucous membranes following oral or parenteral administration of a drug. (See also DRUG HYPERSENSITIVITY in Ch. 19 and ADVERSE DRUG REACTIONS in Ch. 242.)

Etiology

Many drug eruptions are due to allergic mechanisms: specific antibodies to the drug or specifically sensitized lymphocytes may develop during a sensitization period that may be as short as 4 or 5 days after initial drug exposure. A later exposure to the drug results in an eruption, which may appear within minutes or not for hours or days. Other reactions are caused by accumulation of a drug (e.g., pigmentation from silver), the pharmacologic action of a drug (e.g., striae or acne from systemic corticosteroids; purpura from excessive anticoagulation), or interaction with genetic factors (e.g., porphyria cutanea tarda from estrogens, which induce an enzyme involved in porphyrin metabolism).

Symptoms and Signs

Drug eruptions vary in severity from a mild rash to toxic epidermal necrolysis. Onset may be sudden (e.g., urticaria or anaphylaxis after penicillin), or it may be delayed for hours or days (morbilliform or maculopapular eruptions following penicillin or sulfonamides), or even years (exfoliation or pigmentation from arsenic). The lesions may be localized (fixed drug eruptions, oral ulcerations, or dermatitis in light-exposed areas), but many are generalized.

Some drugs produce characteristic eruptions, but reactions may imitate features of practically any dermatosis. The most frequently seen patterns with some typical causative agents are listed below. The drugs added most recently are most likely to be the cause, but drugs that have been taken for long periods must also be suspected.

Urticaria (penicillin, aspirin, tartrazine [the dye FD&C yellow No. 5]) is easily recognized by the typical well-defined edematous wheals.

Morbilliform or maculopapular eruptions (almost any drug, especially barbiturates, sulfonamides, and antibiotics) range in appearance from measles-like to an eruption resembling pityriasis rosea.

Mucocutaneous eruptions (penicillin; barbiturates; sulfonamides, including derivatives used in hypertension and diabetes mellitus) vary from a few small oral vesicles or urticaria-like skin lesions to painful oral ulcerations with widespread bullous skin lesions (see ERYTHEMA MULTIFORME and the Stevens-Johnson syndrome, below).

Acneiform eruptions (corticosteroids, iodides, bromides) resemble acne but lack comedones and usually begin suddenly.

Toxic epidermal necrolysis (barbiturates, hydantoins, penicillin, sulfonamides) is characterized by large areas of loosened, easily detached epidermis that give the skin a scalded appearance. It is often fatal. A similar condition in children is caused by a specific staphylococcal infection (scalded skin syndrome; see in Ch. 190).

Exfoliative dermatitis (penicillin, sulfonamides) is characterized by redness, scaling, and thickening of the entire skin surface; it, too, may be fatal (see in Ch. 189).

Photosensitivity eruptions (phenothiazines, tetracyclines, sulfonamides, chlorothiazide, artificial sweeteners) appear as areas of dermatitis or gray-blue hyperpigmentation (phenothiazines) on skin exposed to the sun.

Fixed drug eruptions (phenolphthalein, tetracycline) are well-circumscribed, frequently isolated, dusky red or purple lesions on the skin or mucous membranes that reappear at the same sites each time the drug is taken.

Lichenoid or lichen planus-like eruptions (antimalarials, gold, chlorpromazine) are angular papules that coalesce into scaly patches (see LICHEN PLANUS in Ch. 195).

Purpuric eruptions (chlorthiazide, carbromal, meprobamate, anticoagulants, apronalide) are nonblanching purple macules that vary in size but are usually tiny. They are most common on the lower extremities but may occur anywhere.

Erythema nodosum (sulfonamides, oral contraceptives, iodides, bromides) is described in this chapter, below.

Diagnosis and Treatment

Identification of the causative agent is essential. A detailed history is often required, with persistent inquiry about *all* medications, including nonprescription drugs used for sleep, pain, colds, constipation, and headache. It is important to remember that some drug eruptions continue for weeks or months after the drug is stopped, and that minute amounts of some drugs may produce a reaction.

Most drug reactions resolve when the offending drug is stopped and require no further therapy. Often, and especially in hospitalized patients who take many drugs, all but life-sustaining medicines must be discontinued, and each reinstituted in order of importance at weekly intervals. A physician well versed in the incidence and types of drug eruptions can frequently withhold the most likely offender and continue the other drugs. When medicines are necessary to the patient's health, chemically unrelated compounds should be substituted when possible.

No laboratory tests are yet available to aid diagnosis, although lymphocyte transformation and penicillin skin tests are under study. Sensitivity can be confirmed only by readministration of the drug, which may be hazardous.

A lubricant (e.g., white petrolatum) may be used for a dry, itching maculopapular eruption. A topical fluorinated corticosteroid ointment (see Ch. 187) should also be applied in one small area q.i.d. and, if effective, applied to the entire eruption. Disabling acute urticaria may require aqueous epinephrine (1:1000) 0.2 ml s.c. or IM. Rarely, soluble hydrocortisone 200 mg IV may be needed. In serious drug reactions, such as severe erythema multiforme or the Stevens-Johnson syndrome, oral or parenteral corticosteroids may be given. A starting dose equivalent to prednisone 60 mg/day or more is continued or increased until a response is seen; the dose is then decreased slowly over 2 to 3 wk. However, some cases of erythema multiforme and other drug eruptions do not respond to systemic corticosteroids.

ERYTHEMA MULTIFORME

(Erythema Multiforme Exudativum or Bullosum)

An inflammatory eruption characterized by symmetric erythematous, edematous, or bullous lesions of the skin or mucous membranes.

Etiology

No cause can be found in > 50% of cases. In the remainder, drugs and x-ray therapy are usually implicated in adults and infectious causes in children and young adults, including herpes simplex (probably the most commonly found etiologic agent), coxsackie- and echoviruses, *Mycoplasma pneumoniae*, psittacosis, and histoplasmosis. Vaccinia, BCG, and poliomyelitis vaccines have also induced erythema multiforme. Almost any drug can cause erythema multiforme; penicillin, sulfonamides, and barbiturates are the most common causes. The mechanism by which infectious agents or drugs cause the condition is unknown, but it apparently is a hypersensitivity reaction.

Symptoms, Signs, and Diagnosis

Onset is usually sudden, with erythematous macules or papules, or wheals, vesicles, and sometimes bullae, appearing mainly on the distal portion of the extremities and on the face; hemorrhagic lesions of the lips and oral mucosa can also occur (see under ORAL ERYTHEMA MULTIFORME in Ch. 208). The skin lesions (target or iris lesions) are symmetric in distribution and often annular, with concentric rings and a central purpura—a grayish discoloration of the epidermis—or vesicle. Itching is variable. Systemic symptoms vary; malaise, arthralgia, and fever are frequent. Attacks that last 2 to 4 wk and recur in the fall and spring for several years are sometimes seen.

The **Stevens-Johnson syndrome** is a severe form of erythema multiforme characterized by bullae on the oral mucosa, pharynx, anogenital region, and conjunctiva. Typical erythema multiforme lesions may or may not be present elsewhere on the skin. The patient may be unable to eat or close his mouth properly and drools continually. The eyes may become very painful, and conjunctivitis with swelling and pus may make it impossible for the patient to open them. The conjunctival lesions may leave residual corneal scarring. The condition is occasionally fatal.

The skin lesions of erythema multiforme must be distinguished from bullous pemphigoid and dermatitis herpetiformis; the oral lesions, from allergic stomatitis, pemphigus, and herpetic stomatitis.

Treatment

When a cause can be found, it should be treated, eliminated, or avoided. Local treatment depends on the type of lesion. Simple erythema often needs no treatment. Vesicles and bullous or erosive lesions can be treated with intermittent tap-water compresses. Cheilitis and stomatitis of erythema multiforme may require special care (see ORAL ERYTHEMA MULTIFORME in Ch. 208). Systemic corticosteroids (see DRUG ERUPTIONS, above, and Treatment, in ORAL ERYTHEMA MULTIFORME in Ch. 208) have often been used in severe erythema multiforme, sometimes with apparent benefit. Other patients, especially those with severe mouth and throat lesions, seem to succumb more readily to fatal respiratory infections if treated with systemic corticosteroids. Intensive systemic antibiotics, fluids, and electrolytes may be life-saving in patients with extensive mucous membrane lesions.

ERYTHEMA NODOSUM

An inflammatory disease of the skin and subcutaneous tissue characterized by tender red nodules, predominantly in the pretibial region but occasionally involving the arms or other areas.

The nodules gradually change from pink to bluish to brown, resembling a bruise. Fever and arthralgia are frequent, hilar adenopathy less frequent. The condition is most common in young adults and may recur for months or years.

Erythema nodosum in children is most commonly caused by URIs, especially from streptococci; in adults, streptococcal infections and sarcoidosis are the most common causes. Less common causes (except in locales where the underlying disease is endemic) include leprosy, coccidioidomycosis, histoplasmosis, primary tuberculosis, psittacosis, lymphogranuloma venereum, and ulcerative colitis. The condition can also be a reaction to drugs (sulfonamides, iodides, bromides, oral contraceptives). A prolonged search for systemic infection or causative drug may be required, and in many cases no cause can be determined. An elevated erythrocyte sedimentation rate is the most common laboratory finding.

Treatment
Bed rest is essential for relief of painful nodules. Appropriate antibiotic therapy—e.g., long-term (at least 1 yr) penicillin, if an underlying streptococcal infection is suspected—is beneficial. If symptoms are severe and there is no evidence of underlying infection or drug etiology, aspirin may be helpful, although the lesions often recur. Systemic corticosteroids reduce the lesions but may mask an underlying systemic disease.

GRANULOMA ANNULARE

A benign, chronic dermatosis characterized by papules or nodules that spread peripherally to form a ring with normal or slightly depressed skin in the center. The lesions are yellowish or the color of the surrounding skin. One or more lesions may be present. They are usually asymptomatic and are usually present on the feet, legs, hands, or fingers. The condition may be seen in children or adults. It is not associated with systemic diseases, except that among adults with many lesions there is a statistically increased incidence of diabetes mellitus. Spontaneous resolution is common. In addition to reassurance and explanation of the benign nature of the disease, high-strength topical corticosteroids under occlusion every night or intralesional corticosteroids (see Ch. 187) may hasten the involution of the disease.

---

197. BULLOUS DISEASES

PEMPHIGUS

An uncommon, potentially fatal skin disorder of uncertain etiology characterized by intraepidermal bullae on apparently healthy skin and mucous membranes.

Etiology and Incidence
Pemphigus usually occurs in middle-aged or older persons and is rare in children. It is probably an autoimmune phenomenon, since the serum and skin of patients in the active stage contain readily demonstrable IgG antibodies that bind at the site of epidermal damage. Puzzling foci of high incidence of pemphigus occur in South America, especially Brazil.

Symptoms and Signs
Tense or flaccid bullae of varying sizes are the primary lesions. They frequently occur first in the mouth, where they soon rupture and remain as chronic, often painful, erosions for variable periods of time before the skin is affected. On the skin, the bullae characteristically arise from normal-appearing skin and leave a raw, denuded, and, later, crusted area when they rupture. The extent of both skin and mucosal involvement varies (e.g., lesions may occur in the oropharynx and upper esophagus). Itching is usually absent.

In some varieties of pemphigus, bullae may not be prominent and the process may resemble exfoliative dermatitis with or without tiny vesicles. The lesions may be localized to the face and suggest a combination of seborrheic dermatitis and cutaneous LE.

Diagnosis

Pemphigus should be suspected in any bullous disorder or chronic mucosal ulceration. It must be differentiated from all other chronic ulcerative oral lesions and from other bullous dermatoses such as bullous pemphigoid, benign mucosal pemphigoid, drug eruptions, toxic epidermal necrolysis, erythema multiforme, dermatitis herpetiformis, and bullous contact dermatitis. In pemphigus the epidermis is easily detached from the underlying skin **(Nikolsky's sign)** and biopsy usually shows typical suprabasal epidermal cell separation. A Tzanck test (see SPECIAL DIAGNOSTIC METHODS in Ch. 186) is frequently diagnostic when one does a Wright's or Giemsa stain on a smear of cells obtained by scraping the base of a lesion. The acantholytic cells typically seen in pemphigus are large, with centrally placed nuclei and condensed dark-blue-staining cytoplasmic membranes. Direct immuno-fluorescence (IF) tests of perilesional skin or mucous membranes invariably show IgG on the epidermal or epithelial cell surfaces. Indirect IF tests usually show pemphigus antibodies in the patient's serum, even when the lesions are localized in the mouth. The antibody titer may correlate with the severity of the disease.

Treatment

Hospitalization and large doses of corticosteroids are indicated because the condition is potentially fatal if inadequately treated. The aim of treatment, both immediate and subsequent, is to stop the eruption of new lesions. The initial dosage is determined by the extent of the disease; prednisone 40 to 80 mg orally b.i.d. (or equivalent) should be doubled if new lesions continue to appear after 1 wk. Skin infections should be treated with the appropriate systemic antibiotics. Generous use of talc on patient and sheets may aid in preventing oozing skin from adhering to the sheets. Silver sulfadiazine cream can be used on erosions to prevent secondary infection.

Corticosteroid dosage may be decreased gradually when no new lesions have appeared for 7 to 10 days, with the total daily dose given every morning at first, then every other morning. The maintenance dose should be as low as possible. It may be possible to discontinue maintenance therapy if no new lesions appear during a trial period without treatment. Methotrexate, cyclophosphamide, azathioprine, and IM gold have each been used successfully, either alone or with corticosteroids, to avoid the undesirable effects of long-term use of corticosteroids, but these drugs carry their own serious risks.

BULLOUS PEMPHIGOID

A chronic, benign bullous eruption seen chiefly in the elderly. It is considered an autoimmune disease because antibodies directed against the basement membrane zone of the epidermis (the site of histologic damage) are found routinely in the serum and skin.

Symptoms and Signs

The characteristic tense bullae develop on normal-appearing or reddened skin and are sometimes accompanied by annular, dusky red, edematous lesions with or without tiny vesicles on the periphery of the lesions. Occasionally, rapidly healing oral lesions are seen. There are usually no other symptoms. As in many of the other bullous diseases, subepidermal blisters may be found on biopsy.

Diagnosis

The disease must be differentiated from pemphigus, erythema multiforme, drug eruptions, benign mucosal pemphigoid, and dermatitis herpetiformis. Finding serum antibodies to the basement membrane zone on an indirect IF test is diagnostic. Antibodies or complement, or both, are bound to the basement membrane zone of perilesional skin.

Treatment

The eruption usually improves with prednisone 40 to 60 mg orally every morning. The dose can be tapered slowly to a maintenance level after several weeks. Occasional new lesions in the elderly should be disregarded (rather than increasing the prednisone dosage, as in pemphigus) because of the burden of side effects. In trials, the corticosteroid dosage has been reduced by giving methotrexate adjunctively.

DERMATITIS HERPETIFORMIS

A chronic eruption characterized by clusters of intensely pruritic vesicles, papules, and urticaria-like lesions.

This disease occurs mainly in patients 15 to 60 yr old. Several immunologic abnormalities have been demonstrated, including IgA deposits in almost all normal-appearing and perilesional skin. Asymptomatic gluten-sensitive enteropathy is found in 75 to 90% of patients and in many of their relatives.

Symptoms, Signs, and Diagnosis

Onset is usually gradual. Tiny vesicles, papules, and urticaria-like lesions appear, usually distributed symmetrically on extensor aspects (elbows, knees, sacrum, buttocks, occiput). Vesicles and papules are not uncommon on the face and neck. Itching and burning are severe, and scratching often obscures the lesions.

The typical histopathologic picture is seen only in early lesions and is characterized by microvesicle formation in the dermal papillary tips, which are infiltrated with neutrophils. Direct IF tests for IgA deposition in the dermal papillary tips or at the dermal-epidermal junction in normal-appearing and perilesional skin are almost always positive and provide an important diagnostic aid.

Treatment

Dapsone 50 mg orally t.i.d. or q.i.d. usually relieves symptoms within 1 or 2 days and improves the rash; a dramatic relief in itching is seen in 1 to 3 days. Up to 100 mg q.i.d. can be given if there is no improvement. Most patients can be maintained eventually on 50 to 150 mg/day. Sulfapyridine may be used as an alternative; initial dosage is 2 to 4 gm/day orally and maintenance dosage is 1 to 2 gm/day. Strict adherence to a gluten-free diet for prolonged periods is somewhat effective in controlling the skin disease. Such diet control either obviates or reduces the patient's requirement for drug therapy.

Patients receiving dapsone or sulfapyridine should have a CBC weekly for 4 wk, then every 2 to 3 wk for 12 to 18 wk, and every 8 to 10 wk thereafter, since hematologic changes are the most common side effects.

---

198.   DISORDERS OF CORNIFICATION

ICHTHYOSIS

(Dry Skin; Xeroderma)

Skin texture is genetically determined, and several ichthyotic skin diseases are inherited. Ichthyosis is a symptom in several rare hereditary syndromes and occurs in several systemic disorders.

1. **Xeroderma,** the mildest form, is neither congenital nor associated with systemic abnormalities. It usually occurs on the lower legs of middle-aged or older patients, most often in cold weather and in patients who bathe frequently. There may be mild to moderate itching and an associated dermatitis due to detergents or other irritants.

2. The **inherited ichthyoses,** all characterized by excessive accumulation of scale on the skin surface, are classified according to clinical, genetic, and histologic criteria (see TABLE 198–1).

3. Ichthyosis is a characteristic of **Refsum's syndrome** (a hereditary ataxia with polyneuritic changes and deafness), and of **Sjögren-Larsson syndrome** (hereditary mental deficiency and spastic paralysis); both syndromes are autosomal recessive.

4. Asymptomatic ichthyosis occurs in some systemic diseases (e.g., leprosy, hypothyroidism, lymphoma) and may be an early manifestation. The dry scaling may be fine and localized to the trunk and legs, or it may be thick and widespread. In sarcoidosis, a thick scaling may appear on the legs and biopsy usually shows the typical granulomas. In other systemic diseases, biopsy of ichthyotic skin is not diagnostic.

Treatment

In any ichthyosis, an emollient—preferably plain petrolatum—should be applied b.i.d. and especially after bathing, while the skin is still moist. An agent particularly effective in removing the scale in ichthyosis vulgaris, lamellar ichthyosis, and sex-linked ichthyosis contains 6% salicylic acid in a gel composed of propylene glycol, ethyl alcohol, hydroxypropylene cellulose, and water. It should be applied after hydration of the skin, b.i.d. plus at bedtime, and should be covered overnight with an occlusive dressing. In children, it should be applied only b.i.d. and should not be occluded. After the scaling has decreased, only occasional application is required. Also useful are 50% propylene glycol in water, hydrophilic petrolatum and water (in equal parts), or cold cream. In lamellar ichthyosis, 0.1% tretinoin (vitamin A acid; retinoic acid) cream is effective.

Soaps should be used only in intertriginous areas. Hexachlorophene products should not be used because absorption and toxicity are increased.

Patients with epidermolytic hyperkeratosis (bullous ichthyosis) may need long-term penicillin (benzathine penicillin G 1.2 million u. IM every 2 to 3 wk) or oral erythromycin, for as long as the thick intertriginous scaling is present, to prevent formation of pyogenic pustules. Lubrication may slightly improve ichthyosis due to an underlying systemic disease, but remarkable improvement follows if the primary disease can be corrected. The most effective therapies for most of the ichthyoses are the synthetic retinoids, given orally. These are not available commercially in the USA, but are available under testing protocols in many medical centers.

TABLE 198–1. CLINICAL AND GENETIC FEATURES OF SOME OF THE INHERITED ICHTHYOSES

Disorder	Inheritance Pattern	Age at Onset	Type of Scale	Distribution	Associated Clinical Findings	Histology
Ichthyosis vulgaris	Autosomal dominant	Childhood	Fine	Usually back and extensor surfaces; spares flexors; usually many markings on palms and soles	Atopy; keratosis pilaris	May be diagnostic
X-linked ichthyosis	X-linked	Birth or infancy	Large, dark (may be fine)	Prominent on neck and trunk; normal palms and soles	Corneal opacities	May be diagnostic
Lamellar ichthyosis (nonbullous congenital ichthyosiform erythroderma; "collodion baby")	Autosomal recessive	Birth	Large, coarse	Most of body; thick palms and soles	Ectropion	Diagnostic
Epidermolytic hyperkeratosis (bullous congenital ichthyosiform erythroderma)	Autosomal dominant	Birth	Thick, warty	Most of body; especially warty in flexural creases	Blisters	Diagnostic

KERATOSIS PILARIS

A common disorder of keratinization in which the orifices of the hair follicles are filled with horny plugs. Multiple small pointed keratotic papules appear mainly on the lateral aspects of the upper arms, thighs, and buttocks. They are most prominent in cold weather. The cause is unknown, the problem is chiefly cosmetic, and **treatment** is usually unnecessary, but hydrophilic petrolatum and water (in equal parts), cold cream, or petrolatum may be beneficial and, with 3% salicylic acid added, may help to flatten the lesions. The 6% salicylic acid gel described above for the treatment of ichthyosis, applied as for that disorder, may be very effective.

CALLUS; CORN

(Tyloma; Heloma)

Callus: *A superficial circumscribed area of hyperkeratosis at a site of repeated trauma.* **Corn:** *A painful conical hyperkeratosis, found principally over toe joints and between the toes.*

Calluses and corns are caused by pressure or friction, usually over a bony prominence. **Calluses** are usually found on the hands or feet but may occur elsewhere, especially in a person whose occupation entails repeated trauma to a particular area (e.g., the mandible and clavicle in a violinist). **Corns** are pea-sized or slightly larger and occur on the feet. "Hard" corns occur over prominent protuberances, especially on the toes; "soft" corns occur between the toes. Corns may ache spontaneously or be tender on pressure.

Diagnosis

Calluses may be differentiated from plantar warts by trimming away the horny skin. A wart will appear sharply circumscribed, sometimes with soft macerated tissue or with central black dots resulting from thrombosed capillaries, and paring it will cause pinpoint bleeding. A callus shows only heaped-up keratin, and skin markings are preserved. A corn, when pared, shows a sharply outlined translucent core that interrupts the normal papillary line.

Treatment

Prophylaxis is important. Completely eliminating undue pressure on the affected site may not be practicable, but pressure should be reduced and redistributed when possible. For foot lesions, soft, well-fitting shoes are important, and pads or rings of suitable shapes and sizes, moleskin or foam-rubber protective bandages, arch inserts, or metatarsal plates or bars may help to redistribute the pressure.

The hyperkeratotic tissue may be removed with keratolytic agents such as 20% salicylic acid in collodion or 40% salicylic acid plasters (taking care to avoid applying the agent to normal skin), or with a nail file or emery board. Salicylic acid plasters can be used on calluses anywhere.

Patients with a tendency to calluses and corns need the regular services of a podiatrist, and those with impaired peripheral circulation, especially if associated with diabetes mellitus, require special care (see under ATHEROSCLEROTIC ARTERIAL DISEASE in Ch. 28).

199.   DECUBITUS ULCER

(Bedsore; Pressure Sore; Trophic Ulcer)

Ischemic necrosis and ulceration of tissues overlying a bony prominence that has been subjected to prolonged pressure against an external object (e.g., bed, wheelchair, cast, splint). It is seen most frequently in patients who have diminished or absent sensation, or are debilitated, emaciated, paralyzed (e.g., from spinal cord injuries or degenerative neurologic diseases), or otherwise long bedridden. Tissues over the sacrum, ischia, greater trochanters, external malleoli, and heels are especially susceptible but other sites may be involved, depending on the patient's position. Decubitus ulcers can affect not only superficial tissues, but also muscle and bone.

Etiology

Both intrinsic and extrinsic factors precipitate decubitus ulcers. **Intrinsic factors** include loss of pain and pressure sensations that ordinarily prompt the patient to shift position and relieve the pressure, and the thinness of fat and muscle padding between bony weight-bearing prominences and the skin. Disuse atrophy, malnutrition, anemia, and infection play contributory roles. In a paralyzed extremity, loss of vasomotor control leads to a lowering of tone in the vascular bed and a lowered circulatory rate. Spasticity, especially in patients with spinal cord injuries, can place a shearing force on the blood vessels to further compromise circulation.

The most important of the **extrinsic factors** is pressure. Its force and duration directly determine the extent of the ulcer. Pressure severe enough to impair local circulation can occur within hours in an immobilized patient, causing local tissue anoxia that progresses, if unrelieved, to necrosis of the skin and subcutaneous tissues. The pressure is due to infrequent shifting of the patient's position; friction and irritation from ill-adjusted supports or wrinkled bedding or clothing may be contributory. Moisture, which leads to tissue maceration, predisposes to decubitus. It may result from perspiration or from urinary or fecal incontinence.

Symptoms, Signs, and Course

The stages of decubitus ulcer formation correspond to tissue layers. The **1st stage** consists of skin redness that disappears on pressure; the skin and underlying tissues are still soft. The **2nd stage** shows redness, edema, and induration, at times with epidermal blistering or desquamation. In the **3rd stage**, the skin becomes necrotic, with exposure of fat. In the **4th stage**, necrosis extends through the skin and fat to muscle; further fat and muscle necrosis characterize the **5th stage.** In the **6th stage**, bone destruction begins, with periostitis and osteitis, progressing finally to osteomyelitis, with the possibility of septic arthritis, pathologic fracture, and septicemia.

Prophylaxis

The best treatment for pressure sores is prevention. *Pressure on sensitive areas must be relieved.* Unless a full-flotation bed (water bed) is used, providing even distribution of the patient's weight through hydrostatic buoyancy, the bedridden patient's position must be changed at least q 2 h until tolerance for longer periods can be demonstrated (by the absence of redness). Air-filled alternating-pressure mattresses, sponge-rubber mattresses, and silicone gel or water mattresses decrease pressure on sensitive areas but do not negate the need for position changes q 2 h. An operative turning (Stryker) frame facilitates turning patients with cord injuries. Protective padding (e.g., sheepskin or a synthetic equivalent) at bony prominences should be used under braces or plaster casts, and at potential pressure sites a window should be cut out of the cast. A wheelchair patient must be able to shift his position every 10 to 15 min even if he is using a pressure-relieving pillow.

Skin inspection is important. Pressure points should be checked for erythema or trauma at least once/day in an adequate light. Able patients, mobile or immobile, and their families must be taught a routine of daily visual inspection and palpation of sites for potential ulcer formation. Exquisite skin care for neurologically damaged parts is necessary to prevent maceration and secondary infection. Lying on a sheepskin helps to keep the patient's skin in good condition and minimize decubiti. Protective padding, pillows, or a sheepskin can be used to keep body surfaces separated.

Maintaining **cleanliness and dryness** helps to prevent maceration. Bedclothes should be changed frequently, using sheets that are soft, clean, and free from wrinkles and particulate matter. Essential hygienic measures include sponging the skin in hot weather and thorough drying after baths.

Oversedation should be avoided and **activity** encouraged. Physiotherapy, when practicable, may be carried out by means of passive and active exercises. Hydrotherapy is also valuable.

Treatment

A well-balanced diet, high in protein, is important. Blood transfusions may be needed for anemia.

Threatened decubitus (lst and 2nd stages) requires energetic use of all the above prophylactic measures to prevent tissue necrosis. The area should be kept exposed, free from pressure, and dry. Stimulating the circulation by gentle massage can accelerate healing. The major problem in treating decubitus ulcer is that the ulcer is like an iceberg, a small visible surface with an extensive unknown base, and there is no good method of determining the extent of tissue damage. Ulcers that have not advanced beyond the 3rd stage may heal spontaneously if the pressure is removed and the area is small.

Fourth stage ulcers require debridement; some may also require surgery. When the ulcers are filled with pus and necrotic debris, application of hydrophilic beads of dextranomer may hasten debridement without surgery. Conservative debridement of necrotic tissue with forceps and scissors should be instituted. Some debridement may be done by cleansing the wound with 1.5% hydrogen peroxide. Enzymatic digestive agents may be useful—e.g., trypsin, applied as dry powder or in frequently changed wet dressings (5000 u./ml). Wet dressings of water will assist in debriding. The granulation that follows removal of necrotic tissue may be satisfactory cover for small areas. A recently described treatment for disabling ulcers is application of petrolatum to the rim of the ulcer followed by 20% benzoyl peroxide lotion (not available in USA) to the ulcer. The solution is applied to a cloth that has first been moistened with saline. The cloth is saturated with the lotion, applied to the ulcer, and covered with polyethylene film.

More advanced ulcers require surgical treatment. Surgical debridement and closure is required for fat and muscle involvement. Affected bone tissue requires surgical removal; disarticulation of a joint may be needed. A sliding full-thickness skin flap graft is the closure of choice, especially over large bony prominences such as the trochanters, ischia, and sacrum, since scar tissue cannot develop the tolerance to pressure that is needed.

For spreading cellulitis, penicillin G, a penicillinase-resistant penicillin, or erythromycin is necessary.

200. PIGMENTARY DISORDERS

HYPOPIGMENTATION

A congenital or acquired decrease in melanin production.

Albinism: *A rare autosomal recessive inherited disorder in which melanocytes are present but do not form melanin.* The hair is white, the skin pale, and the eyes pink; nystagmus and errors of refraction are common. Albinos sunburn easily and frequently develop skin cancers. They should avoid sunlight, use sunglasses, and apply a sunscreen such as 5% aminobenzoic acid alcoholic solution on uncovered skin.

Vitiligo: *An acquired absence of melanocytes, causing hypopigmented areas, usually sharply demarcated and often symmetric, and varying from 1 or 2 spots to near universality.* The hair in vitiliginous areas is usually white, and the lesions are white under a Wood's light. Lesions are prone to sunburn. The cause is unknown, although vitiligo is sometimes familial or may follow unusual physical trauma, especially of the head. The association of vitiligo with Addison's disease, diabetes mellitus, pernicious anemia, and thyroid dysfunction, as well as a high incidence of serum antibodies to thyroglobulin, adrenal cells, and parietal cells, has led to a postulated immunologic and neuro-chemical basis. Antibodies to melanin have been demonstrated only in some patients with associated multiple endocrinopathies. **Treatment** is for the cosmetic disfigurement. Small lesions may be camouflaged with cosmetic creams. Para-aminobenzoic acid **(PABA)** 5% solution or gel gives protection against sunburn. Oral and topical psoralens have been used, but the treatment is protracted and the results vary.

Postinflammatory hypopigmentation follows healing of certain inflammatory disorders (especially bullous dermatoses), burns, and skin infections, and appears in scars and atrophic skin. The skin may not be ivory white as in vitiligo, and spontaneous repigmentation may eventually occur.

HYPERPIGMENTATION

Hyperpigmentation due to deposition of melanin may be a manifestation of hormonal changes as in Addison's disease, pregnancy, or use of anovulatory pills. Darkening may also result from increased melanogenesis, as is seen in hemochromatosis, or from silver deposits, as are seen in argyria.

Melasma (chloasma), dark brown, sharply marginated, roughly symmetric patches of pigmentation on the face (usually on the forehead, temples, and malar prominences) occurs mainly during pregnancy **(melasma gravidarum, the "mask of pregnancy")** and in women taking anovulatory hormones. It may, rarely, occur idiopathically in dark-skinned men. Exposure to sunlight accentuates the pigmentation. In women, the darkening fades somewhat after childbirth, on cessation of the hormone, and with time. **Treatment** with 2 or 4% hydroquinone in a nongreasy, white or opaque base applied b.i.d. may decrease the pigmentation. Hydroquinone should be tested behind one ear for a week before it is used on the face, since it may cause dermatitis or may lighten the skin too much. Sequential use of topical 0.1% tretinoin will enhance the effect of hydroquinone. The patient should use a sunscreen over the hyperpigmented areas when outdoors and should avoid excessive exposure to the sun.

201. DISORDERS OF SWEATING

MILIARIA

(Prickly Heat)

An acute inflammatory pruritic eruption due to retained extravasated sweat. Because of duct obstruction and inflammation, sweat fails to reach the surface, is trapped in the epidermis or dermis, and causes irritation (prickling) and, frequently, severe itching. The characteristic minute lesions are vesicular if obstruction is superficial **(miliaria crystallina)** or red if inflammation is deeper **(miliaria rubra).** Miliaria is usually seen in warm humid weather, but it may occur in cool weather if the patient is overdressed. Treatment is symptomatic and prophylactic, and includes cooling and drying the involved areas and avoiding conditions that may induce sweating. Air conditioning is ideal. Corticosteroid lotions, sometimes with 0.25% menthol added, are often used, but any topical treatment is less effective than changing the environment and the clothing.

HYPERHIDROSIS

Excessive perspiration due to overactivity of the sweat glands. It may be general or confined to the palms, soles, axillas, inframammary regions, or groin. The skin in affected areas is often pink or bluish white. In severe cases, the skin, especially on the feet, may be macerated, fissured, and scaling. The exudate may be malodorous **(bromhidrosis);** the fetid odor is caused by decomposition of the sweat and cellular debris by bacteria and yeasts.

Increased hydration of the skin may be a contributing factor in various skin diseases (fungal or pyogenic infections; contact dermatitis). Generalized hyperhidrosis frequently accompanies fever. An endocrine dysfunction (e.g., hyperthyroidism) or, occasionally, a CNS disorder may also cause generalized sweating. The cause of localized hyperhidrosis is unknown; it usually occurs in otherwise normal individuals. Excessive sweating of the palms and soles may be psychogenic.

Treatment

For generalized hyperhidrosis, the underlying systemic disease must be treated. The hyperhidrosis may be refractory. Side effects make parasympatholytic agents impractical, and sympathectomy may have only a temporary effect.

For localized hyperhidrosis, aluminum chloride or axillary antiperspirants containing an aluminum chlorhydroxy complex are useful. Glutaraldehyde 2% solution may be effective in treating the palms and soles, but it stains the skin yellow and may cause allergic contact dermatitis. Methenamine 5% alcoholic solution (available in some countries) is also effective, and 5% tannic acid in talc may be effective on the feet. A 20% solution of aluminum chloride hexahydrate in absolute ethyl alcohol, applied at night to the dried axilla and covered tightly with a thin polyethylene film, may also be effective. In the morning, the polyethylene film is removed and the area is washed free of salt. Two applications usually protect the area for 1 wk.

Bromhidrosis often responds readily to treatment. Scrupulous cleanliness is essential. Daily bathing and application of an aluminum chlorhydroxy complex preparation is usually adequate. Shaving the axillary hair is important. Extreme axillary hyperhidrosis, especially when accompanied by bromhidrosis, may be relieved by excising the concentrated group of glands in the axillary vault.

---

202. BENIGN TUMORS

WARTS

(See in Ch. 193)

KERATINOUS (SEBACEOUS) CYSTS

(See in Ch. 194)

MOLES

(Pigmented, Nevocytic, or Nevus-Cell Nevi)

Circumscribed pigmented macules, papules, or nodules composed of clusters of melanocytes or nevus cells.

Moles may be small or large; flesh-colored, yellow-brown, or black; flat or raised; smooth, hairy, or warty; and broad-based or pedunculated. Practically every human has a few moles. Most appear in childhood or adolescence. During adolescence and pregnancy, more moles may appear and existing ones may enlarge and darken.

Only about 20 to 30% of malignant melanomas arise from melanocytes in moles; the rest arise from melanocytes in normal skin. The very rare malignant melanomas of childhood arise from large, pigmented moles that are present at birth. Halo nevi usually resolve spontaneously but very rarely are premalignant.

Classification

A **lentigo** is a flat, uniformly pigmented, brown to black spot that is due to an increased number of melanocytes at the epidermodermal junction. Lentigines are darker, sparser, and more scattered than freckles, and do not darken or multiply with sun exposure.

Junctional nevi are usually flat but may be slightly elevated. Light brown to nearly black and from 1 mm to 1 cm in size, they result from clustering of melanocytes at the epidermodermal junction. Moles on the palms, soles, and genitalia are usually junctional.

Compound nevi are usually dark and may be slightly or considerably elevated. Nests of melanocytes occur at the epidermodermal junction and within the dermis.

Intradermal nevi are elevated, flesh-colored to black, and may be smooth, hairy, or warty. Both melanocytes and nevus cells are found, almost entirely confined to the dermis.

Halo nevi are pigmented moles, usually compound or intradermal nevi, surrounded by a ring of depigmented skin.

Treatment

Since moles are extremely common and melanomas uncommon, it is not justifiable to remove moles prophylactically. However, a mole should be excised and examined histologically if it enlarges suddenly, becomes darker or shows spotty color changes, begins to bleed, ulcerates, or becomes inflamed, painful, or pruritic. If the mole is too large for simple excision, it should be biopsied. Extensive surgery—e.g., wide primary excision—is inappropriate before an accurate microscopic diagnosis, since many lesions are misdiagnosed clinically as melanomas. Simple excision or biopsy does not increase the likelihood of metastasis should the lesion prove malignant, and it avoids unnecessary destructive procedures for benign lesions.

Moles can be removed for cosmetic purposes without fear of subsequent malignant changes, but all moles removed should be examined histologically. A hairy mole should be excised completely to prevent hair regrowth.

SKIN TAGS

(Acrochordons)

Common soft, small, flesh-colored or hyperpigmented pedunculated lesions, usually multiple and occurring mainly on the neck, axilla, and groin. They are usually asymptomatic but may become irritated. **Treatment** by freezing with liquid nitrogen or cutting with a scalpel or scissors may be performed if the tags are irritating or for cosmetic reasons.

ANGIOMAS

(Hemangioma; Vascular Nevus; Lymphangioma)

Localized vascular lesions of the skin and subcutaneous tissues, rarely of the CNS, that result from hyperplasia of blood or lymph vessels.

Angiomas are usually either congenital or appear shortly after birth and occur in about a third of newborn infants. Most disappear spontaneously **(immature hemangiomas)**, but some persist and create cosmetic problems. Complications may follow overtreatment, post-traumatic ulceration, or localized tissue hypertrophy from a persistent angioma of the CNS (see ARTERIOVENOUS MALFORMATIONS under VASCULAR DISORDERS in Ch. 129), the face, or an extremity.

Classification and Treatment

Congenital hemangiomas may be classified as follows:

1. Nevus flammeus (portwine stain) is a flat, pink, red, or purplish lesion present at birth and due to vascular ectasia. These lesions are very commonly present in the nuchal area. Nevus flammeus of the trigeminal area may be a component of the **Sturge-Weber syndrome** (leptomeningeal angiomatosis with intracranial calcification). A nevus flammeus usually will not fade, though splotchy small red macular lesions in the area above the nose and on the eyelids may disappear in a few months. No effective **treatment** is known, but a nevus flammeus can usually be hidden with an opaque cosmetic cream prepared by a cosmetician to match the patient's skin color. Argon lasers are being tried, but the long-term results are unknown.

2. Capillary hemangioma (strawberry mark) is a raised, bright red lesion that develops shortly after birth and consists of proliferations of endothelial cells. It tends to enlarge slowly during the first several months of life and usually involutes spontaneously within 2 to 5 yr. Regression is usually complete, but at times a brownish pigmentation and scarring or wrinkling of the skin remains. Since spontaneous regression is the usual course, **treatment** is not indicated, except when a lesion on or near the eye or a body orifice (e.g., urethra, anus) might interfere with function. When treatment is required, prednisone 10 mg orally b.i.d. or t.i.d. should be given for at least 2 wk. If resolution starts, the prednisone should be decreased slowly; if not, it should be stopped. Surgical excision, electrocoagulation, injection of sclerosing solutions, or application of dry ice is used, but often leaves more scarring than would spontaneous resolution.

3. Cavernous hemangioma is a raised red or purplish lesion composed of large vascular spaces. The blood vessels are often mature, in which case the lesion may contain numerous arteriovenous shunts and vascular malformations. Cavernous hemangiomas rarely involute spontaneously. Partial involution may follow ulceration, trauma, or hemorrhage. **Treatment** must suit the type of lesion. Occasionally in children prednisone (as for a capillary hemangioma) may induce spontaneous resolution. Surgical excision and grafting may be considered. Small surface nodules may be excised individually or destroyed by electrocoagulation.

Spider angioma (vascular spider) is a bright red, faintly pulsatile lesion consisting of a central arteriole with slender branches that extend outward like spider legs. Compression of the central vessel temporarily obliterates the lesion. Vascular spiders are not congenital. Single or small numbers of these lesions may be seen in children or adults and are unrelated to internal disease. Most patients with hepatic cirrhosis also develop many vascular spiders that may become quite prominent.

Many women develop lesions during pregnancy or while taking oral contraceptives. As they are asymptomatic and usually resolve spontaneously about 6 to 9 mo postpartum or after discontinuing oral contraceptives, treatment is not usually required. If the lesions do not resolve spontaneously or **treatment** is required for cosmetic purposes, the central arteriole can be destroyed with fine needle electrodesiccation.

Lymphangiomas are elevated lesions composed of dilated and cystic lymphatic vessels, usually yellowish tan but occasionally reddish if small blood vessels are intermingled. Puncture of the lesion yields a colorless fluid. **Treatment** consists of deep excision.

PYOGENIC GRANULOMA

(Granuloma Telangiectaticum)

A bright red, brown, or blue-black vascular nodule composed of proliferating capillaries in an edematous stroma. The term "pyogenic granuloma" is a misnomer because the lesion is neither of bacterial origin nor a true granuloma, but, rather, granulation tissue. The lesion develops rapidly, often at the site of recent injury, and probably represents a vascular and fibrous response to injury. It must be differentiated from a melanoma or other malignant tumor, which it often resembles. There is no sex or age predilection. The overlying epidermis is thin, and the lesion tends to be friable, bleeds easily, and does not blanch on pressure. The base may be pedunculated and surrounded by a collarette of epidermis. During pregnancy, pyogenic granulomas may become large and exuberant—e.g., gingival pregnancy tumors **(telangiectatic epulis).** Pyogenic granulomas sometimes involute spontaneously; if not, a biopsy should be done. **Treatment** consists of removal by excision or electrodesiccation. The lesions may recur.

SEBORRHEIC KERATOSES

(Seborrheic Warts; Senile Warts)

Pigmented superficial epithelial lesions that are usually warty but may occur as smooth papules. The cause is unknown. They occur commonly in middle-aged or older patients and most often on the trunk or temples, though in blacks, especially women, they frequently occur on the malar part of the face **(dermatosis papulosa nigra).** Seborrheic keratoses vary in size and grow slowly. Round or oval and flesh-colored, brown, or black, they usually appear "stuck on" and may have a waxy, scaling, or crusted surface. They are not premalignant, and need no **treatment** unless they are irritated, itchy, or cosmetically bothersome. Curettage with or without electrodesiccation after local injection of lidocaine 1%, or freezing with liquid nitrogen or CO_2 snow, removes the lesions with little or no scarring.

DERMATOFIBROMA

(Fibrous Histiocytoma)

A firm, red to brown, small papule or nodule composed of fibroblastic tissue and usually found on the lower legs. Dermatofibromas are seen often and are usually solitary and asymptomatic, but may be multiple and may or may not itch. Their cause is unknown. **Treatment,** by excision under local anesthesia, is unnecessary unless there are symptoms—irritation, erosion, sudden enlargement, or other change in surface characteristics.

KERATOACANTHOMA

A round, firm, usually flesh-colored lesion with a characteristic central crater containing keratinous material. Onset is rapid, and within 1 or 2 mo the lesion reaches its full size, which may exceed 10 cm. Common sites are the face, forearm, and dorsum of the hand. Spontaneous involution usually starts within a few months, but may result in scarring. This lesion is sometimes difficult to differentiate clinically and histologically from squamous cell carcinoma. Unless the diagnosis is certain and the patient can be observed frequently, the lesion should be surgically excised and examined histologically.

KELOID

A smooth overgrowth of fibroblastic tissue that arises in an area of injury or, occasionally, spontaneously. Keloids are shiny, smooth, often dome-shaped, and slightly pink. They tend to appear on the upper back and chest and on the deltoid area, and may be seen as a consequence of severe acne in these sites. Keloids are more frequent in blacks. **Treatment** with a corticosteroid (e.g., triamcinolone acetonide 40 mg/ml, in amounts up to 20 mg/lesion) injected into the base of the lesion monthly via a Luer-Lok syringe or by jet injection may flatten the keloid but is often ineffective. Excision followed by intralesional injection of the wound with a corticosteroid can also be tried.

203. MALIGNANT TUMORS

Skin cancers of epidermal origin (basal cell and squamous cell carcinoma) are among the most common malignancies of man, and are usually curable. Most of these tumors arise in sun-exposed areas of skin. The incidence is highest in outdoor workers (farmers, sailors, fishermen, etc.), sportsmen, and sunbathers, and is related to the amount of melanin pigment in the skin; light-skinned persons are most susceptible. Such tumors may also develop years after x-ray or radium burns or arsenic ingestion.

Less common malignancies include malignant melanoma, mycosis fungoides, Paget's disease of the nipple, and Kaposi's hemorrhagic sarcoma.

BASAL CELL CARCINOMA
(Rodent Ulcer)

Basal cell carcinomas may appear as small, shiny, firm nodules; ulcerated, crusted lesions; flat, scar-like indurated plaques; or lesions difficult to differentiate from psoriasis or localized dermatitis. Most commonly the carcinoma begins as a small shiny papule, enlarges slowly, and, after a few months, shows a shiny, pearly border with telangiectasias, and a central dell or ulcer. Recurrent crusting or bleeding is not unusual, and the lesion continues to enlarge slowly. Basal cell carcinomas rarely metastasize, but may cause trouble and, rarely, death by invading or impinging on underlying vital structures or orifices (eyes, ears, mouth, bone, dura mater).

Treatment should be by a specialist after the mandatory biopsy and histologic examination. The clinical appearance, size, site, and histologic findings determine choice of treatment—electrodesiccation and curettage, surgical excision, or x-ray therapy. Recurrences (about 5%) are treated with Moh's chemosurgery (microscopically controlled excision after chemical fixation of the tissue) or surgical excision. The recurrence rate with topical fluorouracil is unacceptably high.

SQUAMOUS CELL CARCINOMA

Squamous cell carcinomas arise from the malpighian cells of the epithelium. Most appear on sun-exposed areas, but they may occur anywhere on the body. A squamous cell carcinoma may develop in normal tissue or in a preexisting actinic keratosis or patch of leukoplakia. The tumor begins as a red papule or plaque with a scaly or crusted surface. It may then become nodular, sometimes with a warty surface. In some, the bulk of the lesion may lie below the level of the surrounding skin. Eventually it ulcerates and invades the underlying tissue. About ⅓ of lingual or mucosal lesions have metastasized before they are diagnosed.

A biopsy is essential. **Treatment** is as for basal cell carcinoma; lesions > 2 cm are surgically excised or irradiated. Squamous cell carcinoma on the lip or other mucocutaneous junction should be excised; at times it is difficult to cure, but in general the prognosis for small lesions removed early and adequately is excellent.

Bowen's disease (intraepidermal squamous cell carcinoma) is a superficial squamous cell carcinoma in situ. The lesion is solitary or multiple and resembles a localized patch of psoriasis, dermatitis, or dermatophyte infection. It is red-brown and scaly or crusted, with little induration. **Treatment** is as for basal cell carcinoma. Topical therapy with fluorouracil is rarely curative except for penile lesions.

MALIGNANT MELANOMA
(Melanoma)

A malignant tumor of melanocyte origin. Malignant melanomas arise in areas of the skin, mucous membranes, eye, and CNS where pigment cells occur. They appear in different sizes, shapes, and shades of color (most commonly pigmented), and have a variable propensity for invasion and metastasis. Thus, malignant melanoma may be a highly malignant tumor that spreads so rapidly it is fatal within months of its recognition, while in some forms the 5-yr cure rate is nearly 100%. Early clinical suspicion and an adequate biopsy for histologic determination of the level of invasion are important for effective management and an optimum prognosis.

Most malignant melanomas arise from melanocytes in normal skin; fewer than ⅓ develop from pigmented moles. Danger signals that suggest malignant transformation of pigmented nevi include changes in size; color, especially spread of pigmentation to surrounding normal skin and red, white, and blue colors; surface characteristics; consistency; shape; or surrounding skin, especially with signs of inflammation. Although melanomas are commoner in pregnant than in nonpregnant women, pregnancy does not increase the likelihood that a mole will become a melanoma, nor does it have a deleterious effect on survival. A therapeutic abortion will not induce a remission. Metastasis to the fetus is rare. Malignant melanomas are very rare in children, but can arise from congenitally present large pigmented moles.

Types, Symptoms, and Signs

Three major clinical types of melanoma have been described.

1. Lentigo-maligna melanoma arises from lentigo maligna (Hutchinson's freckle), which appears on the face or other sun-exposed areas in elderly patients as an asymptomatic large (2 to 6 cm), flat, tan or brown macule with darker brown or black spots scattered irregularly on its surface. In lentigo maligna (malignant melanoma-in-situ), both the normal and malignant melanocytes are confined to the epidermis, whereas in lentigo-malignant melanoma, the malignant melanocytes invade the dermis. After 10 yr or more, about ⅓ of lentigo melignas develop a progressive malignant focus with cells invading the dermis.

2. Superficial spreading melanoma accounts for ⅔ of all melanomas. It is initially much smaller than the lentigo-maligna melanoma, is usually asymptomatic, and occurs most commonly on the legs in women and on the torso in men. Consultation is sought because the patient notes enlargement or irregular coloration of the lesion. It usually appears as a plaque with raised, indurated edges, and often shows red, white, and blue spots or small, sometimes protuberant, blue-black nodules. Small indentations may be noted on the surface. Histologically the lesion is characterized by atypical melanocytes invading the dermis and epidermis. The overall mortality rate is 30%.

3. Nodular melanoma comprises 10 to 15% of all melanomas. It may occur anywhere on the body and is seen in patients in their 20s to 60s. It also is asymptomatic, unless it ulcerates. Consultation is usually sought because dark, protuberant papules or a plaque rapidly enlarges, often with little radial growth. Colors vary from pearl to gray to black. Occasionally, a nodular melanoma contains little if any pigment.

Differential Diagnosis

Many lesions colored by melanin pigment or blood can be mistaken for malignant melanomas. Pigmented basal cell carcinoma, seborrheic keratosis, blue nevus, dermatofibroma, all types of moles, hematomas (especially on the hands or feet), venous lakes, pyogenic granulomas, and warts are among the most common lesions confused with melanomas. If doubt exists, an excisional biopsy (or, if impossible because of the size or site of the lesion, incisional biopsy) should be performed. The biopsy should include the full depth of the dermis and extend slightly beyond the edges of the lesion. This enables the pathologist, by doing step sections, to determine the type and deepest thickness of the melanoma. Definitive radical surgery should not be performed before obtaining a histologic diagnosis.

Diagnostic Criteria

Guidelines for selecting those pigmented lesions that need to be excised or biopsied include recent enlargement, darkening, bleeding, or ulceration. These features, however, usually indicate that the melanoma has already invaded the skin deeply. Earlier diagnosis is possible if biopsies can be obtained from lesions having (1) variegated colors—e.g., brown or black with shades of red, white, or blue, (2) irregular elevations that are either visible or palpable, and (3) irregular borders with angular indentations or notches.

Histologic grading: Therapy and prognosis largely depend on recently described histologic criteria that define the level of invasion of malignant melanocytes (see TABLE 203–1) and the actual thickness of the neoplasm, measured histologically. Adequate biopsy specimens are necessary for histologic grading— biopsy should be excisional for small lesions and incisional for larger lesions. Melanomas arising in the CNS and subungual melanomas are not classifiable by these systems.

The degree of lymphocytic infiltration, which represents the patient's immunologic defense system, often correlates well with the level of invasion. Lymphocytic infiltration is maximal in Level II lesions; it decreases with deeper levels of tumor cell invasion, so that little lymphocytic infiltration is seen in Level V tumors.

Prognosis and Treatment

The clinical type of tumor is less important to the survival rate than the depth of invasion or thickness of the tumor at the time of diagnosis. Thus, for example, as indicated in TABLE 203–1, melanomas that have not extended beyond Level II are rarely fatal. No metastases or recurrences have been found with tumors < 0.76 mm thick.

Metastasis of malignant melanoma occurs via both lymphatics and blood vessels. Local metastasis results in the formation of satellite papules or nodules that may or may not be pigmented. Direct metastasis to skin or internal organs may occur, and occasionally metastatic nodules are discovered before the primary lesion is identified. Melanomas arising from mucous membranes have a poor prognosis even though they seem quite limited when first discovered.

Treatment of malignant melanoma is not yet standardized, but appropriate treatment is becoming more rational as new data on grading of lesions accumulates. **Lentigo-maligna melanoma** and its premalignant precursor, lentigo maligna, are usually treated with wide local excision and, if necessary, with skin grafting. This procedure gives a 90 to 100% 5-yr cure rate. Intensive x-ray therapy is far less effective. **Nodular** or **spreading melanomas** limited to Level II have rarely metastasized to lymph nodes and are usually cured by wide local excision extending down to the fascia. Elective lymph node dissection is usually not recommended for Level II lesions.

TABLE 203-1. MALIGNANT MELANOMA—INVASION AND PROGNOSIS

Level of Invasion of Tumor (After Clark)	Approx. Depth of Invasion (mm)	Metastases Found at Elective Lymph Node Dissection	5-Yr Cure Rate	
			Nodes Involved	Nodes Not Involved
I. Entirely within epidermis	< 0.6	0	—	100%
II. Invades papillary dermis with few cells to reticular dermis	0.6	4%	95%	95%
III. Fills papillary dermis and accumulates along interface between papillary and reticular dermis	1.7	7%	60%	90%
IV. Invades reticular dermis	3.3	25%	25%	80%
V. Invades subcutis	7.0	70%	0–15%	0–15%

Tumors thicker than 1.5 mm are considered Levels III and IV melanomas, which have a higher overall mortality rate. When these melanomas occur on an extremity or at a site where drainage is to only one group of nodes, extensive lymph node dissection and lymphadenectomy are indicated after wide local excision of the primary lesion. These two groups clearly benefit from node removal. In Level V melanomas, lymphadenectomy is usually performed, although the outlook is quite poor in any case. Patients with Levels III, IV, and V melanoma may benefit from consultation with experts in newer forms of therapy. For example, chemotherapy with dacarbazine (DTIC) is being used in varying schedules for patients with lymph node involvement. BCG vaccine may increase the patient's immunologic resistance and is being tried experimentally, injected both into accessible lesions and into the uninvolved arm.

PAGET'S DISEASE OF THE NIPPLE

A rare type of carcinoma that appears as a unilateral dermatitis of the nipple and represents extension to the epidermis of an underlying mammary duct carcinoma. The redness, oozing, and crusting closely resemble dermatitis, but the physician should suspect carcinoma because the lesion is unilateral. Biopsy of the nipple shows typical histologic changes. Paget's disease also occurs at other sites, most often in the groin or perianal area. An underlying carcinoma should be sought in all cases. **Treatment** is determined by the surgeon; mastectomy is usual for lesions of the nipple.

MYCOSIS FUNGOIDES
(See in Ch. 98)

KAPOSI'S HEMORRHAGIC SARCOMA (KS)
(Multiple Idiopathic Hemorrhagic Sarcoma)

A neoplasm characterized by vascular skin tumors that may appear in an **indolent form** *or a disseminated macular or aggressive* **lymphoadenopathic form.** The rare indolent form occurs mainly in elderly men of Mediterranean ancestry. The aggressive form, endemic in equatorial Africa, occurs in children and young men and comprises nearly 10% of all malignancies in Zaire and Uganda. Recently, the aggressive form has assumed epidemic proportions in people <45 yr (predominantly male homosexuals) in the USA in association with an acquired immunodeficiency syndrome (AIDS) of unknown etiology. **Clinical Manifestations:** In older men, KS generally appears first in the skin of the toes or legs as purple or dark brown plaques or nodules, which may fungate or infiltrate deeper tissues with lymphedema; disseminated lymph node and visceral involvement may follow in 5 to 10%. Survival in the indolent form is many years. In the epidemic form, asymptomatic cellular immunodeficiency may be the initial stage. Patients become anergic, with lymphopenia and T cell and natural killer cell depletion, while immunoglobulin levels are normal or elevated. Ratios of helper/suppressor T cells are reduced and absolute counts of helper cells tend to be low in most patients. A prodromal wasting syndrome may develop consisting of fever, night sweats, chills, diarrhea, fatigue, and weight loss of >10% body wt. These patients are prone to disseminated KS with involvement of lymph nodes and viscera and also to opportunistic infections similar to those seen in immunosuppressed cancer or transplant patients. **Treatment:** Electrocoagulation or radiotherapy (electron-beam or x-ray) is used for localized lesions or to reduce crippling lymphedema. In disseminated KS, attempts to restore cellular immunity and antimicrobial therapy are used, but 60% of the patients die, most often from infections.

204. DENTISTRY IN MEDICINE

MEDICAL–DENTAL CONSULTATION

A dentist should consult a physician whenever he suspects systemic disease, to evaluate a person's ability to withstand general anesthesia or extensive oral surgery, or because of an emergency occurring in a dental office. A physician should consult a dentist on behalf of children with abnormal growth manifested by peculiar facies, delayed eruption, gross malformation or malalignment of teeth, or for patients with cleft lip or palate, jaw fractures, oral neoplasms, or a newly discovered lump in the neck. Physicians should be familiar with dental procedures and the amount of trauma and risk involved to patients with systemic disease. A dentist who will search for oral cancer and will refuse to extract teeth unless valid dental reasons exist is a consultant to be prized.

Dental consultation is indicated for obscure facial pain, unexplained swelling or cellulitis of the neck that might have originated in an infected tooth, or for infection of the parapharyngeal space that might have followed an abscess of a lower posterior tooth.

Obscure causes of face, head, and neck pain include malocclusion, poorly fitting dental prostheses, disease of the temporomandibular joints, unilateral mastication, spasm of the muscles of mastication, and occult cavities in the jawbones. Referred pain may make diagnosis difficult. For example, pain referred to the ear may arise from an inflammation of the gingival flap about a partly erupted mandibular 3rd molar or from the back of the tongue in glossopharyngeal neuralgia. Paresthesias of the lower lip may follow damage to the inferior alveolar nerve during extraction of a mandibular molar, but may also be a rare sign of an oral neoplasm compressing that nerve. Conversely, percussion tenderness in several maxillary teeth may indicate nasal or antral disease adjacent to the root tips. Clarification of the cause of face, head, and neck symptoms often necessitates the pooled knowledge of both physician and dentist.

At times, the oral surgeon treats a patient who has no primary dental disorder. He may be requested to treat resistant obesity by wiring the jaws. The surgical correction of retrognathia associated with obstructive ventilatory sleep disorders, characterized by collapse of the tongue into the pharynx and myocardial infarction during sleep, is being evaluated as a possible therapy if a nocturnal nasotracheal tube does not work and tracheotomy is unacceptable.

When patients require oral surgery, their preoperative medical workup and postoperative care warrant the same respect accorded to procedures of comparable scope and severity elsewhere in the body. Oral surgical procedures include simple extractions, removal of impacted teeth, which are completely or partially embedded within the jaws, and alveoloplasty, which is remodeling of the alveolar ridge of the jaw so that a denture can be retained better. This may necessitate cartilage grafts to augment the size of the ridge or vestibuloplasty (resection of mucous membrane attachments to increase depth in the mucobuccal fold to aid denture retention). Jaw fractures and correction of protruding mandibles (prognathism) or retruded or small jaws (micrognathism) and segmental alveolar osteotomy for severe malocclusion are other procedures. In the latter, a portion of alveolar bone and its contained teeth is excised and repositioned (orthognathic surgery) to improve occlusion that could not be achieved by traditional orthodontic methods. Excision of soft tissues, bone cysts, and neoplasms is an important part of maxillofacial surgery. Surgical procedures are also done on the temporomandibular joint to remedy arthritis, developmental anomalies, or the results of trauma.

DENTAL CARE OF PATIENTS WITH SYSTEMIC DISORDERS

Dental care is occasionally hazardous. Its risks can be minimized by (1) doing elective dental procedures when the medical patient is best able to withstand the inherent trauma and (2) encouraging healthy individuals to practice oral hygiene so that, should systemic disease develop, massive dental treatment in a belated attempt to remedy prolonged neglect is unnecessary and will not delay medical therapy or cause additional complications.

Routine oral surgery or periodontal treatment puts medical patients at risk when normal inflammation required for healing is inhibited by such drugs as corticosteroids, immunosuppressive agents used in organ transplantation, and cytotoxic drugs given for cancer. Hemorrhage, delayed healing, local infection, and even septicemia may occur. Dental care should be carried out before using such systemic drugs. Otherwise, definitive treatment may not be possible.

Filling a tooth is almost always a bloodless procedure. Exceptions occur: (1) In a tooth with deep decay that has entered the pulp or has almost done so, complete removal of decayed tooth structure, which is mandatory to prevent recurrent caries, will be followed by minimal bleeding from the pulp that is easy to control by pressure. (2) In preparing a cavity to treat interproximal caries (on the surface next to an adjacent tooth), minimal gingival lacerations may occur from instrumentation. Cavity preparation involving the occlusal surface of a tooth that is not deeply decayed should be completely bloodless. Therefore, people with **bleeding disorders** should have teeth filled to avoid subsequent extractions.

Suspected **bleeding or coagulation disorders** should be assessed prior to oral surgery. In patients with acute forms of **leukemia, thrombocytopenia,** or **hepatitis,** extractions should be delayed until the condition improves or stabilizes. Prolonged bleeding following extraction or periodontal procedures may occur in patients with **polycythemia vera** or **macroglobulinemia,** disorders of platelet number and function, and severe **liver disease** with diminished vitamin K-associated plasma coagulation factors or increased fibrinolytic activity. In coagulation disorders, extractions and regional block anesthesia often require pretreatment with the appropriate coagulation factor and perhaps aminocaproic acid immediately before, during, and after the oral surgical procedure.

In **leukemia,** oral hygiene is vital because periodontal disease favors the occurrence of gingival bleeding and probably local tissue infiltration. Infection often follows extraction in disorders with granulocytopenia.

Cardiovascular patients may be adversely affected by dental procedures. Tooth extraction, scaling (removal of calculus), or other periodontal procedures are followed by bacteremia. Patients with congenital or rheumatic heart disease or a prosthetic cardiac valve are predisposed to bacterial endocarditis and should receive antibiotics before and after such dental procedures. It is particularly important for them, as for patients with coagulation disorders, that teeth be filled to avoid extractions; preventive oral hygiene minimizes tooth decay and gingivitis. Following a myocardial infarction, dental procedures should be delayed for 3 mo, if possible.

Epinephrine, used as a vasoconstrictor to potentiate the duration of local anesthetics, may cause arrhythmias or exacerbate hypertension as the exogenous hormone adds to the anxiety or fear-induced endogenous level; cardiac ischemia may result. Sedation or tranquilization is advantageous in fearful cardiovascular patients and facilitates treatment. Electrical equipment such as a cautery, a pulp tester, and even the dental handpiece (drill) can interfere with pacemakers. Such patients and their dentists should be forewarned so that appropriate measures may be taken. Dosage of a long-term anticoagulant may need a temporary reduction (prothrombin time to about 1½ times the control value) to avoid undue postextraction bleeding. The horizontal position of a dental chair may be intolerable to patients with congestive heart failure, and those on antihypertensive drugs may develop orthostatic hypotension on arising. Individuals with pulmonary or cardiac disease who require inhalation anesthesia should be treated in a hospital environment.

Bacteremia follows tooth extraction, particularly of abscessed or periodontally involved teeth. This may result in endocarditis, mediastinitis, thrombophlebitis of the jugular veins, pneumonia, empyema, meningitis, encephalitis, and cavernous sinus thrombophlebitis. Infectious material, such as fragments of teeth or fillings or pus from periodontal infection, may be aspirated and may cause a lung abscess. Such rare complications are sufficient reason for physicians to encourage oral hygiene to minimize periodontal disease and decay.

Chemotherapy for neoplasms includes drugs (e.g., doxorubicin, 5-fluorouracil, bleomycin, dactinomycin, and methotrexate) that cause stomatitis; the severity is often related to the degree of periodontal disease present. Before instituting such drugs, it is advisable to remove calculus (tartar) and improve the health of periodontal tissue to minimize gingival hemorrhage, tissue sloughing, oral pain, and consequent poor food intake. Subsequent proper use of the toothbrush and dental floss will minimize the likelihood of stomatitis.

Prior to radiotherapy of the oral region, patients should have required oral surgery, periodontal treatment, restoration of salvageable teeth, and fluoride treatment (to minimize caries following xerostomia secondary to irradiation and destruction of the salivary glands). Dental work should be completed and healing permitted before radiotherapy begins. *Extraction of teeth from previously irradiated tissues is commonly followed by* **osteoradionecrosis** *of the jaws, a catastrophic complication.* It is thus best to avoid extraction, if possible, by using dental restorations, dental splints, or endodontic treatment (root canal). Careful lifelong attention to oral hygiene is necessary to avoid oral or periodontal surgery. Frequent fluoride applications are also indicated for an indefinite period following radiotherapy. Tissue breakdown and persistent ulceration is likely beneath a partial or a complete denture because of scarring and inelasticity of irradiated tissue. The prostheses should be checked and adjusted whenever discomfort is noted.

Extraction of a tooth adjacent to a carcinoma of the gingiva, palate, or antrum favors invasion of the alveolus (tooth socket) by the neoplasm. Extraction should be done only in the course of definitive treatment.

Subcutaneous and mediastinal emphysema may rarely follow the use of a high-speed air turbine dental drill or compressed air during a root-canal procedure, or to section a tooth or the alveolar bone during an extraction, as the air is forced into the alveolus of the bone and then dissects along fascial planes. The acute onset of jaw and cervical swelling with characteristic crepitus on palpation of the swollen skin is diagnostic.

In **endocrine disorders** tooth extraction is never routine. Dental treatment should usually be postponed until the systemic disease is well controlled. For example, tachycardia may occur in hyperthyroid individuals, accompanying the anxiety often present in dental patients. **Diabetics** are prone to periodontal disease and following periodontal surgery or extractions may require adjustment of insulin dosage and parenteral fluids or diet during the time when food intake is limited due to postoperative pain. Poorly controlled diabetics, often dehydrated, also have a decreased salivary flow that contributes to caries. To avoid undue interference with food intake, extensive restorative dentistry should not be done in one visit. Patients with **adrenocortical insufficiency** may require supplemental corticosteroids during the stress of major dental procedures. Individuals who have **Cushing's syndrome** or are receiving corticosteroids for a systemic disease may have delayed wound healing and increased capillary fragility.

An **allergic** individual might, despite previous interrogation, receive an offending antibiotic, local anesthetic, or other medication given in conjunction with dental treatment.

In **Bell's palsy** the natural cleansing action of the lip and cheek on the tooth surfaces of the involved side is lost; unilateral decay will increase without scrupulous oral hygiene and repeated fluoride treatments.

People with **convulsive disorders** should have fixed (not removable) small dental appliances, to prevent swallowing or aspirating them and causing airways obstruction or possibly esophagitis or enteritis due to the foreign body. Tracheoesophageal or enterocolonic fistulas may develop subsequently.

Hepatitis B virus rarely may be transmitted by dentists with antigenemia who are carriers of the disease to patients via open lesions on the dentist's fingers into the alveolus of an extracted tooth or into the patient's mouth and therefore the GI tract. The hazard is diminished if dentists with digital lesions, particularly with a history of hepatitis, wear rubber gloves. Unfortunately, autoclaving is not the usual means of sterilizing dental instruments, so the use of dental instruments or the probably rarely done reuse of hypodermic needles may infect a subsequent patient. If a patient with viral hepatitis visits a dentist during the incubation period, additional individuals may be placed at risk.

DENTAL RESTORATIONS AND APPLIANCES

Fillings are inserted after removal of decay. A temporary filling is kept in place for weeks in the hope that the tooth will retain its vitality and deposit secondary dentin to seal a pulp exposure. Silicate is a type of porcelain cement used to fill cavities in anterior teeth because of its resemblance to enamel. Recently, plastic resins have been used for the same purpose. Stronger materials are required for the occlusal surfaces of posterior teeth that bear the brunt of mastication. The commonest ones used are amalgam and gold inlay which can be identified by their color. A less common, small filling is gold foil.

If decay is extensive, placing several fillings in one tooth might undermine its structure. To avoid fracture of the natural crown, the dentist removes the decay and fills the sites with cement. He grinds and tapers the outer surfaces so that an artificial **crown**, usually of gold, may be placed. A porcelain jacket crown is used on anterior teeth for its natural appearance. During laryngoscopy, care must be exercised not to dislodge any fixed artificial crowns present on the anterior teeth.

When teeth are missing, a bridge or partial denture can be made. A **bridge** is usually smaller than a partial denture, but it is possible to make 1 or 2 bridges to cover an entire maxillary or mandibular dental arch. Stress in a bridge is largely borne by abutment teeth (usually on either side of the missing tooth or teeth). Abutment teeth have crowns cemented to them; thus, the bridge is a fixed appliance that is not easily removable. False teeth are soldered to the crowns and to each other. A **partial denture** is typically a removable applicance with clasps that snap over the abutment teeth, and the denture may be removed for cleaning. Part of the load of occlusion is borne by the soft tissues underlying artificial teeth, which often are on both sides of the jaw. This appliance is often used when there are no more natural teeth beyond the tooth or teeth to be replaced.

Complete dentures are removable appliances that help a patient chew solid foods and improve his speech and appearance, but they cannot achieve the efficiency or tactile sensations of natural dentition.

All **removable dental appliances** are generally removed before throat surgery, general anesthesia, or convulsive shock therapy to avoid loss, breakage, aspiration, or swallowing during the procedure. They should be stored in water to prevent dimensional changes that may occur with drying. However, some anesthesiologists believe that an appliance aids the passage of an airway tube, keeps the face in a more normal shape so the mask fits better, does not interfere with laryngoscopy, and prevents natural teeth from injuring the opposing gingiva of a completely edentulous jaw.

205. TEETH AND DENTAL STRUCTURES

NORMAL OCCLUSION

In normal occlusion, the teeth are on a gradual curve whose convexity points inferiorly from side to side and from front to back. The maxillary anterior teeth overlie the mandibular anterior teeth. The outer (buccal) cusps of the maxillary posteriors are external to the corresponding cusps of the mandibular posterior teeth. Since the outer parts of all the maxillary teeth are superficial to the mandibular teeth, the lips and cheeks are displaced from between the teeth so they are not bitten. Furthermore, the lingual (inner) surfaces of the lower teeth are nearer each other than are those of the upper teeth, confining the tongue and minimizing the likelihood of its being bitten as the teeth occlude. All the teeth should contact each other, so that the powerful masticatory forces (which may be > 100 lb in the molar region) will be distributed evenly. If these forces are applied to only a few teeth, the latter are likely to loosen.

MALOCCLUSION

A deviation from the normal contact of the maxillary and mandibular teeth.

The commonest **classification** identifies 3 major forms of malocclusion. **Class I:** The upper and lower molars occlude normally, but the anterior teeth are crowded or malpositioned. **Class II:** The maxillary dental arch is anterior to the mandibular arch, so that the lower jaw is retruded and the facial profile is convex. **Class III:** The maxillary arch is posterior to the mandibular arch and is usually small; the mandible appears protruded and the facial profile is concave. Each class has overlapping subdivisions: malocclusion and normal occlusion represent ranges, not fixed points.

Etiology

Malocclusions are commonly due to associated defects: teeth so large that the jaw cannot accommodate them all; supernumerary, malformed, or missing teeth; delayed eruption of permanent teeth; ankylosis of the mandible; cleft lip or palate; rarely, a genetic disease such as cleidocranial dysostosis or Hurler's syndrome. The most frequent cause of acquired malocclusion is early loss of teeth from caries or periodontal disease with shifting of adjacent teeth unless a bridge or partial denture is made. Less frequently, it is from habits like thumb- and finger-sucking or tongue-thrusting. Iatrogenic malocclusions can occur from improper dental restorations, improper fixation of jaw fractures, or a Milwaukee orthopedic back brace, which places constant pressure on the mandible.

Diagnosis and Treatment

Malocclusions are corrected primarily for oral health reasons, although the patient often needs help for cosmetic or psychologic reasons. Because early interceptive **orthodontics** usually eliminates the need for more expensive and difficult technics at a later date, a child should have a dental consultation as soon as malocclusion is suspected. The evaluation includes x-rays of the skull, facial bones, and teeth, and study casts of the teeth. Malocclusion following facial trauma may suggest a jaw fracture.

Therapy increases resistance to dental decay, anterior tooth edge fracture, and periodontal disease, and it improves speaking and mastication. Occlusion can be improved by selective grinding where teeth or restorations contact prematurely, aligning teeth properly, or inserting crowns or onlays to build up those teeth below the plane of occlusion. A constant mild force applied to the teeth (generally by means of braces) moves them through alveolar bone without too rapid resorption of either teeth or bone. Some patients require extraction of 1 or 2 permanent teeth to obtain enough space for a stable alignment. When the final relationship has been achieved, the patient wears a plastic retainer at night until the teeth stabilize in new positions. Surgical correction of skeletal abnormalities contributing to malocclusion is becoming more common, as is adult orthodontics.

206.   APPROACH TO THE DENTAL PATIENT

RELEVANT ASPECTS OF THE HISTORY

Details of dental visits may alert the physician to a particular dental problem or, if infrequent, to a lack of attention to dental care. **Inability to chew food well** suggests insufficient teeth for proper mastication, poorly fitting dental appliances, loose or painful teeth, or disorders affecting the temporomandibular joint (TMJ) or the muscles of mastication. **Slight, occasional bleeding** following brushing suggests bristle damage or mild gingivitis. However, **frequent, spontaneous, or profuse bleeding** may indicate severe gingivitis or a blood dyscrasia. A history of a **single, mild infection** after oral surgery does not necessarily have systemic implications, but with **recurring oral and other infections**, agranulocytosis, neutropenia, leukemia, immunoglobulin defects, and disorders of leukocyte function must be considered. **Root canal treatment,** a common dental procedure when decay has reached the pulp or for devitalization after trauma, occasionally is associated with osteitis at the tip of the root. **Sores, lumps, or pain** may originate from both teeth and soft tissues. **Medication history** will reveal incompatibilites and duplications.

PHYSICAL EXAMINATION OF THE ORAL REGION

The cardinal principles of physical examination—inspection, palpation, percussion, and auscultation, as well as olfaction and ordinary listening—are as applicable in the oral region as elsewhere.

The Face

The face and mouth are inspected for marked asymmetry, lesions, or disproportions. An **unusual facial appearance** characterizes many head and neck syndromes of genetic or developmental origin; often it occurs with atypical positioning or malformations of the pinnae or an unusual skull shape, with or without dental abnormalities. An underweight patient may lack teeth or have severe periodontal disease, caries, or poorly fitting dental appliances that interfere with chewing. Not all involuntary weight loss indicates systemic disease in such individuals.

Slight facial asymmetry is universal. It may be due to preferential chewing on one side causing unilateral enlargement of the masticatory muscles, differences in the contour of the dental arches, angulation of the teeth on one side compared to the other, or to combinations of these. However, **marked facial asymmetry** occurs in individuals with lipodystrophy, hemiatrophy, hemihypertrophy of the face, or congenital absence of the condyle of the mandible. Awareness of the psychologic trauma of facial malformation should lead to referral for possible facial and plastic surgical procedures.

The **contour** of the cheeks depends to a large extent on the posterior teeth. **Swellings** of the face may be cutaneous (e.g., neurofibromas or sebaceous cysts) or arise from deeper tissues. If one or both cheeks appear swollen, the distension may be in the skin, in the parotid glands (which may be enlarged in mumps, Sjögren's syndrome, or by a tumor), or inside the mouth. An excessively thick denture flange gives the wearer a puffy appearance that disappears on removing the denture and can be remedied by a dentist's grinding down its outer thickness. An abscessed tooth may cause soft-tissue swelling as pus drains from the tooth and toward the outer surface of the face or neck. Endodontic (root canal) treatment or extraction promotes drainage and mitigates against further spread of infection. Salivary gland and lymph node enlargement is evident on inspection of the preauricular and submandibular regions.

Fistulas may represent malformations of the embryologic branchial pouches or draining sinuses from abscessed teeth. An abscessed lower molar may drain below the angle of the mandible, eventually leaving a depressed scar.

Breath Odor (see also HALITOSIS, REAL AND IMAGINED in Ch. 51)

If a patient reeks from mouthwash, a physician should wonder why he is self-conscious about his breath. Is it only recent ingestion of alcohol, onions, garlic, use of tobacco, or for another reason? Extensive dental caries, periodontal disease, or tonsillitis causes a fetid odor often accompanied by complaints of a bad taste. Rhinitis, ozena, or sinusitis also causes halitosis. There are **systemic causes** of bad breath: in liver failure, a mousy odor is present; in uremia, it smells uriniferous; and in a lung abscess or bronchiectasis, a putrid odor is present. In diabetic ketosis, acetone is present in the expired air.

Lips

The **movement** of the lips betrays emotion as the patient speaks; in scleroderma or Parkinson's disease, the lips are rigid. With a facial nerve paralysis (Bell's palsy), marked asymmetry occurs when the patient talks or smiles. The **vermilion border** (between the mucosa of the lips and the skin of the face) is the site of recurrent infections (cold sores) and carcinoma. **Generalized thickening** of the lips occurs in myxedema, cretinism, and acromegaly. **Localized swellings** may indicate a lymphangioma or hemangioma, the latter causing a purplish discoloration as well. Besides cosmetics to camouflage the deformity, more definitive treatment is available (see Ch. 202). In the absence of anterior teeth, the lips become shorter and more concave. They are attached to the jaws by prominent midline and smaller lateral frena. Other abnormalities are discussed in Chs. 207 and 212.

Temporomandibular Joint

As the patient opens his mouth, one notes any **deviation of the jaw** that indicates abnormality of the 5th cranial nerve or weakness of jaw muscles. Congenital malformation or absence of the TMJ can cause similar signs, and characteristic abnormalities will appear on x-ray. When the patient opens his mouth, 3 fingers should fit comfortably between his upper and lower incisors (40 to 50 mm). If less space exists **(trismus)**, he may have scleroderma, parotitis, malformation or arthritis of the TMJ, a peritonsillar abscess, or pericoronitis (infection of the gingiva about a partially erupted 3rd molar). Tetanus or a depressed fracture of the zygomatic arch impinging on the coronoid process of the mandible can also impair opening the mouth. An unusually wide opening may indicate a subluxation of the mandible.

By placing his little fingers deeply into the patient's auditory canals, the physician can test the range and smoothness of mandibular condylar motion as the mouth opens and closes.

For complaints of ear or facial pain on chewing, the examiner can use a stethoscope in front of each ear as the patient opens and closes his mouth. A grating noise or crepitus suggests arthritis (e.g., osteoarthritic or post-traumatic) affecting the TMJ.

Teeth (see also Vol. II, Ch. 24)

To record observations, one horizontal and one vertical line, with the symbols in TABLES 206–1 and 206–2 will indicate teeth in a useful shorthand representation. The horizontal line represents the space between the jaws and the vertical line denotes the midline of the face. Teeth are also identified by the letters A to T for the deciduous and numbers 1 to 32 for the permanent teeth, beginning with the last maxillary right molar and extending to the left across the maxilla and then to the right across the mandible to the last mandibular right molar.

TABLE 206–1. RELATIONSHIP BETWEEN DECIDUOUS AND PERMANENT TEETH*

20 Deciduous		32 Permanent	
Symbol	**Name**	**Symbol**	**Name**
A	Central incisor	1	Central incisor
B	Lateral incisor	2	Lateral incisor
C	Canine (cuspid)	3	Canine (cuspid)
D	1st molar	4	1st premolar (bicuspid)
E	2nd molar	5	2nd premolar (bicuspid)
		6	1st molar
		7	2nd molar
		8	3rd molar

* Each quadrant (left or right half of each jaw) contains the teeth listed.

Oral hygiene reflects the patient's general attitude toward himself or his physical, psychologic, or economic ability to care for himself. Are teeth decayed or missing? Teeth that are painful when tapped with a tongue depressor suggest extensive dental caries or periodontal disease. Severe periodontal disease causes most instances of visible mobility of teeth, but rarely, erosion of the alveolar bone by an underlying tumor (e.g., ameloblastoma) will loosen them. A deeply carious tooth may have an infected or necrotic pulp. A dentist can test the patient's reaction of pain to a weak electrical stimulus to determine whether a tooth is alive. A tooth with decay involving the pulp is a potential source of infection into surrounding alveolar bone. **Calculus (tartar),** if present, is deposited particularly near the orifices of the salivary ducts on the buccal surfaces of the maxillary molars and the lingual surfaces of the mandibular anterior teeth.

The commonest motor abnormality of the oral region is probably not Bell's palsy (see Ch. 130) but **bruxism,** which is the clenching or grinding of teeth that erodes and eventually diminishes the height of the dental crowns. Such attrition is common with advancing years; in youth, it often indicates bruxism. The teeth may also become loose. Although the patient may be oblivious of his habit, other family members are aware. The treatment requires that the patient consciously try to overcome the habit, perhaps with the help of sedatives or tranquilizers and abstinence from alcohol. The latter substance often aggravates bruxism. A dentist can make a splint to be worn over the teeth to prevent the grinding movements.

Maxillary incisor **fractures** are common in children with neurologic disorders who fall often. Malocclusion can result in one front tooth's contacting its opponent at an angle so that a corner of an incisor may be chipped.

Defects in tooth form: Once formed, teeth are never remodeled by systemic influences, only by local ones. Thus, they may be compared to stable geologic formations. A careful examination may give evidence of developmental disorders or endocrinopathies. Changes in the contour of the incisors and 1st molars are characteristic of **congenital syphilis.** The incisors show a constriction at the incisal third that produces a pegged or screwdriver shape, and a characteristic notch in the central portion of the incisal edge. The 1st molar is dwarfed, with constriction of the occlusal surface and roughening and hypoplasia of the enamel. With hereditary opalescent dentin (**dentinogenesis imper-**

TABLE 206–2. SHORTHAND REPRESENTATION OF TEETH

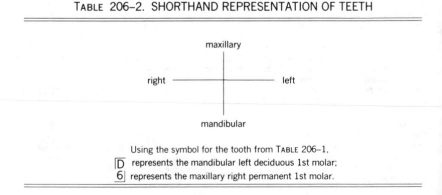

Using the symbol for the tooth from TABLE 206–1,
|D   represents the mandibular left deciduous 1st molar;
6| represents the maxillary right permanent 1st molar.

fecta), an autosomal dominant trait, the dentin is abnormally formed and teeth are a dull bluish-brown. Such teeth cannot withstand occlusal stresses and rapidly become worn. "Peg" lateral incisors are congenitally narrow but are unassociated with systemic disease.

Defects in enamel or tooth color: A dead tooth appears gray. A darkening of the teeth and enamel hypoplasia follow **chronic administration of tetracyclines** during the second half of pregnancy or during tooth development in the child; the affected teeth, rather than fluorescing white in ultraviolet light, have a colored fluorescence, characteristic of the type of tetracycline given. A dark band may be visible after only several weeks of therapy. Abnormal calcium metabolism associated with **rickets** results in enamel hypoplasia. A rough irregular band appears around each tooth. The location of the band indicates the area being calcified at the time of abnormal calcification, and thus provides an estimate of the age when the disease occurred and its duration. Such teeth are not unduly susceptible to dental caries. A **high fever** during odontogenesis can also interfere with enamel formation, and a narrow zone of chalky pitted enamel is visible after the tooth erupts. **Amelogenesis imperfecta,** an autosomal dominant hereditary disease, causes severe enamel hypoplasia. Children who drink water containing $>$ 1 ppm of fluoride during the period of tooth development are likely to develop mottling of the enamel **(fluorosis).** The enamel changes can range, depending on the amount of fluoride ingested, from irregular whitish opaque areas to severe brown discoloration of the entire crown, with a roughened surface. Such teeth have a high resistance to dental caries. In congenital porphyria, teeth fluoresce a reddish color due to deposition of pigment in the dentin. Periapical x-rays show that hypopituitary dwarfs have small dental roots and people with gigantism have large roots. In acromegaly, one sees not only enlargement of the jaws but also hypercementosis of the roots.

The occlusion of the teeth can be examined by retracting the cheek with a tongue depressor as the patient bites. If dental appliances do not replace missing teeth, the adjacent teeth migrate to fill the void and thé opposing teeth extrude from their sockets, thus resulting in abnormalities of occlusion (see also NORMAL OCCLUSION and MALOCCLUSION in Ch. 205).

The patient should be asked to remove dentures so that the underlying soft tissues may be seen. The likelihood of dropping or distorting a dental appliance is greater if the physician attempts to remove it.

Oral Mucosa

With a finger cot for protection against infectious lesions, the physician palpates bimanually (with one finger inside and one outside) to delimit lesions. Most people have yellowish pinhead-size macules in the buccal mucosa. These are harmless **ectopic sebaceous glands** (Fordyce granules). Many persons have a thin white line on the buccal mucosa along the occlusal plane. It represents surface keratinization due to accidental, repeated cheek biting over the years.

The **color** of soft tissues can reflect anemia, polycythemia, cyanosis, or jaundice. One looks for generalized inflammation (stomatitis) as well as localized areas of inflammation, ulceration, petechiae, or thickening. Darkly pigmented areas may indicate a racial characteristic, Addison's disease, or, very rarely, melanoma.

Dryness of the mouth may be from dehydration, mouth breathing, or use of diuretics, or may reflect salivary gland dysfunction or disease (see Ch. 207). The orifices of the parotid ducts open in the cheek beside the maxillary molars. The sublingual and submandibular salivary gland ducts open on the floor of the mouth behind the lower incisors. In case of pain or swelling in those regions, if saliva does not emanate from the appropriate duct, it may be obstructed by a calculus.

The distribution of keratinized and nonkeratinized oral mucosa can be significant. Keratinized epithelium is on the facial aspect of the lips, the dorsum of the tongue, around the teeth, and on the hard palate. It is less likely to be damaged by hard food particles than nonkeratinized mucosa that is mobile, as in the cheek, sides of the tongue, soft palate, and floor of the mouth. Keratinized mucosa in these areas is pathologic and a definite diagnosis must be made (see Ch. 212).

Gingiva

The gum should be firm, nicely contoured about, and adapted to the crowns of the teeth. Pink, stippled tissue should fill the entire interdental space. Keratinized gingiva is present near the crowns. More distant gingiva is nonkeratinized, highly vascular, and continuous with the buccal mucosa. A tongue depressor should express no blood or pus from the gingiva. At the gingival margin, a dark line suggests exposure to lead or a heavy metal. Gingivitis is common.

The Palate (see Ch. 207)

Behind the central incisors are the rugae, little ridges. These are normal. A person with a cleft palate has a very nasal voice. Normal vocal resonance and articulation involve the anterior teeth, lips, tongue, and palate, as well as the lungs and vocal cords.

Tongue and Floor of the Mouth

As the patient touches the tip of his tongue to his palate, one can examine the floor of the mouth and the under surface of the tongue where cancer often starts. The tongue, having a wide range of movement, should be able to twist its tip around the sides of the molar teeth. Normal tongue movement indicates good hypoglossal nerve function but neuromuscular weakness may prevent its holding a midline position or moving rapidly. For a neurologic evaluation of taste, it is possible to use 0.1 M solutions of NaCl, HCl, sucrose, and urea. The tongue may be **enlarged** in myxedema, amyloidosis, acromegaly, or if a rhabdomyoma is present. In edentulous individuals without complete dentures, the tongue tends to broaden.

The **papillae** may be normal or atrophied. The tongue is smooth and pale in pernicious anemia or smooth and fiery red in deficiencies of niacin or riboflavin (see GLOSSITIS in Ch. 207). Oral cancer often occurs on the lateral surface of the tongue (see NEOPLASMS in Ch. 212).

207. COMMON DISORDERS OF THE LIPS AND MOUTH

Most diseases affecting the mucous membrane can occur anywhere in the oral mucosa, but they will be mentioned under the most frequent sites. Also see PHYSICAL EXAMINATION OF THE ORAL REGION in Ch. 206, and Ch. 212.

LIPS

An acute swelling of the lip may be **angioedema** (see URTICARIA; ANGIOEDEMA in Ch. 19). Brownish-black melanin pigmentation spots in association with GI polyposis occur in the **Peutz-Jeghers syndrome**. **Exfoliative cheilitis** is a chronic desquamation of the superficial mucosal cells. If it persists despite removal of very hot or irritating foods, alcoholic beverages, changes of lipstick or dentifrices, triamcinolone acetonide ointment should be tried. A **chancre** has a serosanguineous crust (see SYPHILIS in Ch. 162).

Mucocele (mucous retention cyst), most commonly found on the lower lip, is due to trauma severing the excretory ducts of the accessory salivary glands permitting the mucin-containing saliva to escape into the tissues. A soft nodule forms. If the nodule is superficial, the overlying epithelium is thinned and it assumes a visibly bluish tinge. Treatment is excision.

Tiny painful vesicles characterize two common disorders—herpes labialis ("**cold sore**") is found on the vermilion border while recurrent aphthous ulcers ("**canker sores**") occur on the inner aspects of the lips. For a more detailed consideration see RECURRENT APHTHOUS STOMATITIS and ORAL HERPETIC MANIFESTATIONS in Ch. 208.

Cheilosis (angular cheilitis) is characterized by fissuring and dry scaling of the skin and vermilion surface of the lips and angles of the mouth. The condition is associated with deficiency of some of the B vitamins, particularly riboflavin and pyridoxine, and frequently accompanies other clinical signs of avitaminosis. One must also consider herpetic involvement, the split papule of syphilis, and the pseudocheilosis or wrinkling at the corners of the mouth that accompanies the loss of vertical dimension of the face which reflects the distance between the jaws (particularly in edentulous patients). The treatment is to insert dentures that separate the jaws and diminish the wrinkling. Persistent lesions should be cultured to rule out a mycotic infection, particularly candidiasis **(Perlèche)**. Mixed infections respond best to a preparation of a combination of antifungal, antibacterial, and anti-inflammatory agents. Treatment with high doses of vitamin B complex is beneficial if there is a deficiency.

GINGIVA

VINCENT'S INFECTION (Trench Mouth; Necrotizing Ulcerative Gingivitis; Fusospirochetosis)

A noncontagious infection, associated with a fusiform bacillus and a spirochete, that begins on the interdental papillae and can affect the marginal and attached gingiva by direct extension. Lack of oral hygiene, physical or emotional stress, nutritional deficiencies, blood dyscrasias, debilitating diseases, insufficient rest, and heavy smoking predispose to this disease, which is seen most frequently in young adults.

Symptoms and Signs

Onset, usually abrupt, may be accompanied by malaise. Without a secondary infection, there is usually no fever. The chief symptoms are acutely painful bleeding gums, salivation, and fetid breath. The ulcerations, usually limited to the marginal gingivae and interdental papillae, have a characteristic punched-out appearance, are covered by a grayish membrane, and bleed on slight pressure or irritation. Swallowing and talking may be painful. Regional lymphadenopathy is often present. Lesions on the buccal mucosa are rare but may appear as diffuse ulcerations covered with an easily removed pseudomembrane. Rarely, lesions may occur on the tonsils, pharynx, bronchi, rectum, or vagina.

Diagnosis

The punched-out appearance of the interdental papillae, the interdental grayish membrane, spontaneous bleeding, and pain are pathognomonic. The presence of overwhelming numbers of fusospirochetal forms in stained smears from the lesions confirms the diagnosis. Early differentiation from diphtheria or agranulocytosis is essential when tonsillar or pharyngeal tissues are involved. The differential diagnosis must consider streptococcal or staphylococcal pharyngitis and primary herpetic stomatitis.

Treatment

Gentle local debridement, oral hygiene, adequate nutrition, high fluid intake, and rest are essential. Using a soft brush and irrigating under low pressure or rinsing the mouth with warm normal saline or 1.5% peroxide solution may be helpful for the first few days. Analgesics may be required during the first 24 h after initial debridement. The patient should avoid irritation (e.g., from smoking or from hot or spicy foods). Marked improvement usually occurs within 24 h, and then debridement can be completed. Although the acute stage responds quickly to antibiotic therapy (e.g., penicillin G or V, erythromycin, or a tetracycline, 250 mg q 6 h), antibiotics are seldom necessary and should be avoided unless high fever is present. Poor tissue topography, often produced during the acute phase, may need surgical correction to reduce the possibility of recurrence.

BUCCAL MUCOSA

(See also Ch. 208 and PHYSICAL EXAMINATION OF ORAL REGION in Ch. 206)

Mucosal lesions may cause dentures to hurt or fit poorly. **Koplik's spots** are tiny, grayish-white macules with red margins occurring during the late prodromal and early eruptive stages of measles. **Aspirin burn** is a painful white area of coagulated tissue caused by the local caustic action of aspirin placed against the mucosa in the attempt to relieve a toothache. Wiping off the white film reveals a reddened area. **Irritation "fibroma,"** composed of fibrous tissue, is not a true neoplasm because its growth is limited. It is usually present opposite the occlusal plane where the patient chronically bites or sucks his cheek. Treatment is excision and breaking the habit or reducing the cusps of offending teeth. **Hereditary hemorrhagic telangiectasia** (see in Ch. 95) is characterized by localized dilated blood vessels in the oral cavity, nasal mucosa, and elsewhere. Should bleeding occur, local pressure and the application of absorbable gelatin sponge ordinarily suffice. If not, a cautery may be used. **Lichen planus** often occurs with cutaneous lesions (see Ch. 195). The mucosa is characteristically net-like and hardened, with papules or erosive areas. Violet atrophic or white hyperkeratotic variations may appear on the dorsum of the tongue. **Bullae** of short duration are present in a variety of mucocutaneous disorders (e.g., pemphigus and erythema multiforme), including the severe Stevens-Johnson syndrome. Behçet's syndrome has oral as well as ocular and genital mucosal ulcers. Herpangina, characterized by vesicles in the posterior part of the mouth, and hand-foot-mouth disease with small ulcerated vesicles are both due to different coxsackieviruses (see under Enteroviral Diseases in Vol. II, Ch. 24).

TONGUE

Infants may have **mucocutaneous lymph node syndrome (Kawasaki disease**—see in Vol. II, Ch. 24) in which there is a bright red tongue and face, edema of the extremities, and thrombocytosis. **Ankyloglossia** (tongue-tie) may be diagnosed if the tip of the tongue cannot contact the alveolar ridge or the tips of the teeth or sweep from one corner of the mouth to the other. To increase mobility of the tongue, the lingual frenum may need cutting. Untreated tongue-tie may affect speech and interfere with mastication and passive cleansing of the teeth. A **burning sensation** is often seen postmenopausally in association with poor keratinization, or may be a symptom of diabetic neuropathy; both require treatment of the underlying endocrine disorder.

GLOSSITIS

An acute or chronic inflammation of the tongue.

Etiology

Glossitis may be either a primary disease or a symptom of disease elsewhere. The many and varied causes include the following:

Local: Infectious agents commonly found in the mouth; mechanical trauma (jagged teeth, ill-fitting dentures, oral habits, repeated biting during convulsive seizures); primary irritants (excessive use of alcohol, tobacco, hot foods, spices); or sensitization (by toothpaste, mouthwashes, breath fresheners, candy dyes, and, rarely, plastic dentures or restorative materials).

Systemic: Avitaminosis (particularly of the B group, as in pellagra), anemia (pernicious anemia, iron deficiency anemia), certain generalized skin diseases (lichen planus, erythema multiforme, aphthous lesions, Behçet's syndrome, pemphigus vulgaris, syphilis).

Symptoms, Signs, and Diagnosis

Clinical manifestations vary widely without strong correlation between the appearance of lesions and the severity of symptoms. Reddened tip and edges of the tongue may indicate incipient pellagra, pernicious anemia, irritation from excessive smoking, or a tooth with a rough surface. In later stages of pellagra, the entire tongue is fiery red, swollen, and often ulcerated. In iron deficiency and particularly in pernicious anemia, the tongue is pale and smooth. Painful ulcers may indicate primary herpetic or aphthous lesions, pulmonary tuberculosis with positive sputum, streptococcal infection, erythema multiforme, or pemphigus vulgaris. Whitish patches suggest candidiasis, the mucous patch of syphilis, lichen planus, leukoplakia, or mouth breathing. Denuded smooth areas, if not painful, may indicate **geographic tongue** (benign migratory glossitis), or if moderately painful, anemia or pellagra; if they are very distressing and persistent, they may be the lesions of **Moeller's glossitis** (slick, glossy, or glazed tongue). **Median rhomboid glossitis,** a developmental lesion, consists of a rhomboid-shaped smooth, reddish, nodular area on the dorsal surface of the back portion of the middle third of the tongue. **Hairy tongue,** due to a profuse overgrowth of the filiform papillae, is usually asymptomatic and often follows antibiotic therapy, fever, excessive use of O_2-liberating mouthwashes, or a reduction in salivary flow. Brown papillae are usually from tobacco staining or the overgrowth of chromogenic bacteria. Treatment is to rectify the underlying cause and brush the tongue with a toothbrush.

Severe acute glossitis occasionally results from local infection, burns, or trauma. It may develop rapidly, producing marked tenderness or pain with swelling sufficient to cause protrusion of the tongue and the danger of airway obstruction and suffocation. Mastication, swallowing, and speaking are painful and sometimes impossible. Cervical and sublingual adenitis with evidence of systemic toxicity may be present. Immediate treatment with steroids may be indicated to reduce the edema.

Patients may complain of a painful burning tongue **(glossodynia** and **glossopyrosis)** without obvious clinical evidence of inflammation. Many patients are postmenopausal. Incipient candidiasis, anemias, diabetes mellitus, latent nutritional deficiencies, or malignancies should be excluded.

Each case of glossitis deserves study since the tongue often mirrors disease. History may disclose an irritant, contact allergen, sensitizing drug, deficient diet, or other symptoms of disease. Other mucosal surfaces and the skin should be inspected for evidence of pellagra, erythema multiforme, syphilis, or lichen planus. Studies for an anemia, mild diabetes mellitus, sprue, and syphilis should be performed.

Prognosis

When the cause can be determined and corrected, response is usually prompt, but may be delayed in nonspecific or chronic involvement. The patient should be reassured that persistent lesions such as median rhomboid glossitis and geographic tongue are innocuous. Aphthous ulcers, erythema multiforme, and hairy tongue often recur periodically. Solitary ulcerations that do not respond to treatment after 1 wk should be biopsied.

Treatment

General: Specific causative disorders are treated as indicated. Irritants and sensitizing agents are to be *avoided.* A bland or liquid diet, preferably cooled, is given. Meticulous oral hygiene is imperative.

Local: Oral infections call for specific therapy (see Ch. 208). The pain of large lesions that interfere with eating may be relieved temporarily by rinsing with an obtundent mouthwash before each meal; topical anesthetics (lidocaine 5% ointment or 10% spray; benzocaine 2% ointment; dyclonine 0.5% liquid) applied to discrete lesions also give relief and encourage eating. Occasionally, systemic analgesics (aspirin or acetaminophen 650 mg q 4 h) are required. Topical application of triamcinolone acetonide in emollient dental paste to specific lesions except those of viral etiology t.i.d. or q.i.d. will relieve symptoms and may promote healing.

The patient with symptoms of painful burning but presenting a clinically normal tongue requires special management. Tests for vitamin B_{12} deficiency should be conducted, especially after menopause. For therapy of B_{12} deficiency, see Ch. 92. After systemic causes (anemia, diabetes mellitus) have been ruled out, an emotional basis may be presumed. Reassurance (especially regarding neoplasm) and encouragement are important.

FLOOR OF THE MOUTH

This area may be the site of a **cellulitis** following extraction of, or root canal treatment on, an abscessed mandibular tooth. If the latter procedure was done, the tooth should be extracted to promote drainage. If this proves insufficient, soft tissue incisions may prevent the infection from extending along the pharynx and into the mediastinum. An extensive sublingual infection, termed **Ludwig's angina,** is very hard to palpation (see Submandibular Space Infection in Ch. 4).

An **epidermoid cyst** is an inclusion cyst in the floor of the mouth (usually in the midline) or the mucobuccal fold, which is the junction of the buccal mucosa and the alveolar mucosa. The midline of the floor of the mouth is the most common location for a **dermoid cyst,** which has a doughy feel. All cysts should be excised and carefully examined for evidence of malignancy.

SALIVARY GLANDS

Painless swelling of the parotid glands is often noted in hepatic cirrhosis, in sarcoidosis, in mumps, following abdominal surgery, or associated with neoplasms or infections. The common factors may be dehydration and inattention to oral hygiene. The latter promotes the growth of large numbers of bacteria which, in the absence of sufficient salivary flow, ascend from the mouth into the duct of a gland. Another cause of a painful salivary gland is **sialolithiasis** (salivary duct stone). The submandibular glands are most commonly affected. Pain and swelling associated with eating are characteristic. **Saliva** promotes retention of artificial dentures because of its mucin content. Thus, conditions characterized by diminished saliva flow often adversely affect the ease with which dentures may be worn. Calcium phosphate stones tend to form because of the high pH and viscosity of the submandibular gland saliva which has a high mucin content. Stones are removed by manipulation or excision.

Autoimmune sialosis is the Mikulicz-Sjögren syndrome, a unilateral or bilateral enlargement of the parotid and/or submandibular glands, and often the lacrimal glands. Occasionally painful, it is associated with xerostomia (dry mouth) due to impaired saliva formation that is most common in older women. (See SJÖGREN'S SYNDROME in Ch. 103.)

THE PALATE

The anterior portion of the hard palate is the site of the incisive papilla adjacent to the central incisors. Behind it are the rugae, firm ridges that keep food from slipping as the tongue crushes the food against them.

Torus palatinus is a common benign overgrowth of bone (osteoma) in the midline of the hard palate where the maxillae fuse. No treatment except reassurance is required unless a dentist wishes to cover the hard palate completely with a denture. If so, surgery is required.

A hole in the palate may be a **congenital cleft** involving either or both the hard and soft palates. Clefts of the palate or lip occur once in 700 to 800 births. The cleft may vary from involvement of the soft palate only to a complete cleft of the soft and hard palates, the alveolar process of the maxilla, and the lip. The infant should be referred to a cleft palate team (pediatrician, orthodontist, speech pathologist, plastic surgeon, and psychologist). There are several etiologies of **perforating lesions** other than the congenital cleft; these include salivary gland tumors, the gumma of tertiary syphilis, carcinoma of the palate, and rarely, TB.

In infectious mononucleosis, **petechiae** may occur at the junction of the hard and soft palate. In neutropenia or agranulocytosis, there may be **ulcerations** with little inflammation. Clumps of asymptomatic red **papules** are seen in inflammatory hyperplasia of the palate (pseudopapillomatosis). A denture may irritate such lesions.

The palate may be the site of **Wegener's granulomatosis** (lethal midline granuloma; see also Ch. 104) in which there is destruction of bone with sequestration. A very **high palatal vault** is seen in Marfan's syndrome. Punctate areas of inflammation about the ducts of the numerous minor salivary glands of the palate are common, especially in pipe smokers. The boneless soft palate should rise symmetrically when the patient says "ah." The uvula at the far end of the soft palate's midline varies greatly in length among individuals.

208. STOMATITIS

An inflammation of the mouth, occurring as a primary disease or as a symptom of systemic disease. A fetid breath odor and blood-tinged saliva may accompany any ulcerative lesions of the oral mucosa. Stomatitis is not a disease; it is a syndrome with many possible causes and can present with certain variations that can be described as distinctive entities.

Etiology

Stomatitis may be caused by infection, trauma, dryness, irritants and toxic agents, or hypersensitivity. Infectious agents include streptococci, gonococci, fusospirochetes, *Candida albicans, Corynebacterium diphtheriae, Treponema pallidum, Mycobacterium tuberculosis,* and the viruses of herpes simplex, coxsackie, measles, and infectious mononucleosis. Stomatitis may also result from avitaminosis, particularly lack of the B vitamins or vitamin C (as in pellagra, sprue, pernicious anemia, or scurvy); or from iron deficiency anemia with dysphagia **(Plummer-Vinson syndrome)**, agranulocytosis, or leukemia. Lichen planus, erythema multiforme, SLE, Behçet's syndrome, and pemphigus vulgaris frequently present buccal mucosa signs. Mechanical trauma from cheek biting, mouth breathing, jagged teeth, ill-fitting dentures, or nursing bottles with a hard or too-long nipple may produce characteristic lesions. Xerostomia resulting from drugs, the aging process, or radiation therapy predisposes the mouth to sensitivity and infection. Generalized stomatitis may follow excessive use of alcohol, tobacco, hot foods, or spices; or sensitization to toothpaste, mouthwash, candy dyes, lipstick, and, rarely, acrylic dentures. Phenytoin, iodides, bismuth, mercury, barbiturates, lead, and many other drugs may produce stomatitis. Chemical stomatitis of occupational origin may be due to dyes, heavy metals, acid fumes, or metal or mineral dust. The latter 3 may also cause abrasion of the hard tissues. Mercury causes marked salivation. Some causes are unknown.

Symptoms and Signs

Clinical signs vary widely according to the type of stomatitis present. **Allergic stomatitis** is characterized by an intense, shiny erythema with slight swelling. Itching, dryness, or burning, often present, may be due to sensitivity to foods or to lipstick.

Vincent's infection (necrotizing ulcerative gingivitis—see GINGIVA in Ch. 207) causes ulceronecrotic lesions of the interdental papillae that may extend to the marginal gingivae or produce painful ulcers of the mucous membranes.

Thrush (candidiasis), caused by *C. albicans*, is characterized by white, slightly raised patches resembling milk curds which, when removed, expose a hyperemic area that may bleed slightly. The infection usually begins on the tongue and buccal mucosa and may spread to the palate, gums, tonsils, pharynx, larynx, GI tract, respiratory system, and skin. The mouth usually appears dry. It is common in infants, the debilitated, individuals on long-term antibiotic therapy, and with xerostomia (see SYSTEMIC CANDIDOSIS in Ch. 9).

Pseudomembranous (or **membranous**) stomatitis, an inflammatory reaction that produces a membrane-like exudate, may be caused by chemical irritants (e.g., gold, iodides) as well as bacteria (streptococci, staphylococci, gonococci, *C. diphtheriae*). Fever, lymphadenopathy, and malaise may occur or the infection may be localized.

Mucosal lesions accompanying systemic disease include the mucous patches of syphilis; the strawberry, then raspberry, tongue of scarlet fever; Koplik's spots of measles; the ulcers of erythema multiforme; and the smooth, fiery red tongue and painful mouth of pellagra. Hemorrhagic lesions may occur in scurvy and disorders of platelet number and function. Unprovoked bleeding, decreased salivation, and an ammonia odor accompany uremic stomatitis.

The **mucocutaneous lymph node syndrome (Kawasaki disease)** affects children, causing erythema of the lips and oral mucosa. See MUCOCUTANEOUS LYMPH NODE SYNDROME in Vol. II, Ch. 24.

Acrodynia occurs in children and is characterized by oral ulcerations, profuse salivation, and bruxism (see Bruxism in PHYSICAL EXAMINATION OF THE ORAL REGION in Ch. 206) with loss of teeth. It is caused by a mercurial toxicity reaction.

Diagnosis

Establishing the etiology may be difficult. The history may disclose a systemic disease, a dietary deficiency, or contact with irritants or allergens. Physical examination is obligatory, since it may reveal lesions of other mucous membranes, as in erythema multiforme, candidiasis, or syphilis; lesions of the skin, as in pellagra, pemphigus, lichen planus, or SLE; signs of pulmonary TB, sprue, anemia, or another contributory disease; or a general decrease in exocrine secretions.

Direct smears and cultures from the lesions may disclose a pathogen. Any diphtheria-like membrane should be so examined *promptly*. Vincent's infection usually limits itself to the gingival tissue, differentiating it from primary herpetic gingivostomatitis. Darkfield examination of scrapings from the lesions and STS is indicated in an attempt to rule out syphilis before penicillin is given. In thrush, a history of recent antibiotic therapy is common. To identify *C. albicans*, scrapings from suspect lesions should be cultured and examined microscopically in 10% potassium hydroxide hanging drop preparations or methylene blue stained smears. Blood count, bone marrow examination, gastric analysis, or other laboratory procedures may be indicated.

A solitary, undiagnosed oral lesion of $>$ 1 wk duration which does not respond to treatment must be considered malignant until biopsy proves otherwise.

Treatment

Underlying systemic disorders should be treated specifically. Oral hygiene is always necessary. Thrush usually responds to nystatin oral suspension 100,000 u. as an oral rinse q.i.d. for 10 days; nystatin vaginal tablets, 100,000 u., used as oral lozenges q.i.d. are effective in persistent overgrowths; streptococcal, staphylococcal, and gonococcal infections, to systemic penicillin (see under ANTIBIOTICS in ANTIMICROBIAL CHEMOTHERAPY in Ch. 246). Large, painful ulcers that prevent eating may be relieved temporarily by rinsing the mouth with 2% lidocaine viscous, 15 ml (1 tbsp) before each meal and q 3 h as needed for relief. A mouthwash of ½ tsp sodium bicarbonate in 250 ml (8 oz) warm water q.i.d. is soothing and cleansing. Rinsing after each meal with elixir of dexamethasone 0.5 mg/5 ml (1 tsp) relieves discomfort and promotes healing of nonviral oral lesions.

RECURRENT APHTHOUS STOMATITIS

Acute painful ulcers on the movable oral mucosa, occurring singly or in groups ("canker sores"). Minor ulcers, the most common form, are 3 to 5 mm in diameter and heal without scarring; major ulcers, 7 to 15 mm in diameter, heal with scarring. Recurrent attacks are common, with 2 or 3 ulcers during each attack; however, 10 to 15 ulcers are common in some individuals. Women are affected more often than men.

Etiologically, a precise cause is unknown, but several factors point toward a localized immune reaction. Deficiencies of iron, vitamin B_{12}, and folic acid increase susceptibility. Stress is usually the predominant precipitating factor.

Symptoms and Signs

A vesicular stage is seldom observed. Beginning as a shallow, ovoid erosion with a slightly raised, yellowish border surrounded by a narrow, crimson, hyperemic zone, the ulcer is covered within 5 to 7 days with a yellowish opaque material composed of coagulated tissue fluids, oral bacteria, and WBCs. The acutely painful phase lasts 3 or 4 days; symptoms then diminish until the lesion heals spontaneously, usually without scarring, in 7 to 10 days. Malaise, fever, and lymphadenopathy may accompany severe attacks. Recurrent attacks vary from one lesion 2 to 3 times/yr to an uninter-rupted succession of multiple lesions.

Diagnosis

The mucosal lesion looks distinctive enough to differentiate aphthous stomatitis from primary or recurrent herpetic oral lesions (which may appear concurrently) and from the lesions of erythema multiforme, oral pemphigus, or benign mucosal pemphigoid. Aphthae rarely appear on the immovable mucosa (hard palate, attached gingiva), the prime areas for recurrent intraoral herpetic ulcers. The history and clinical examination exclude herpangina.

Treatment

A topical anesthetic such as 2% lidocaine viscous, 15 ml (1 tbsp) as an oral rinse q 3 h or before meals, provides short-term relief and facilitates eating. A dental protective paste (Orabase®) applied q.i.d. prevents irritation of the ulcers by the teeth, dental appliances, and oral fluids. An application of triamcinolone acetonide in emollient dental paste reduces discomfort and promotes healing.

For multiple lesions, tetracycline oral suspension (250 mg q.i.d. for 10 days) is held in the mouth for 2 to 5 min before swallowing to coat the ulcers. If started early after onset, symptomatic relief occurs during the first day of treatment and new lesions are aborted. Treatment must be repeated for each new attack. Occasionally this therapy will result in oral candidiasis.

ORAL ERYTHEMA MULTIFORME

(See also ERYTHEMA MULTIFORME in Ch. 196)

Acutely painful stomatitis characterized by diffuse hemorrhagic lesions of the lips and oral mucosa and usually associated with constitutional symptoms. Oral, ocular, genital, and dermal lesions can occur concurrently.

Symptoms, Signs, and Diagnosis

Prodromal symptoms may include rhinitis and sinusitis. Multiple vesicles form in the earliest stage. Typical lesions consist of diffuse hemorrhagic eroded areas throughout the mouth; the lips are commonly bloody and crusted, but the gingivae are rarely involved. Extensive oral, conjunctival, and genital lesions may be present, even without dermal eruption.

The patient may have fever as high as 40 to 40.6 C (104 or 105 F) during the early stages. Severe constitutional symptoms (fever, malaise, arthralgia) usually persist for 4 or 5 days; as they regress, the typical lesions develop. The constitutional symptoms may be similar to those in allergic stomatitis, pemphigus, and herpetic stomatitis, which must be differentiated. The lesions are a deeper red than the mucous patches of secondary syphilis.

Treatment

The acute phase of the oral lesions may be treated with systemic corticosteroids (prednisolone 10 mg orally t.i.d. for 5 days) or elixir of dexamethasone 0.5 mg/5 ml (1 tsp) to rinse with and swallow t.i.d. for 5 days. Without corticosteroids, the lesions may persist from 3 to 8 wk or longer. When intraoral lesions cause difficulty in eating, a liquid diet is helpful. Dehydration may necessitate IV fluid therapy. A warm mouthwash of 10% sodium bicarbonate solution and anesthetic troches, ointments, or solutions (e.g., 2% lidocaine viscous) can be used 5 or 6 times/day. Petrolatum ointment may soothe lip lesions. With treatment, improvement is rapid and lesions usually heal without scarring. Recurrence is not usual.

ORAL HERPETIC MANIFESTATIONS

Acute painful vesicular eruptions of the oral mucosa or vermilion borders, caused by the herpes simplex virus. Primary acute herpetic infection is common in infants and young children, and may occur in teenagers and young adults (see also HERPES SIMPLEX in Ch. 12). A history of prior contact with an adult having a herpes simplex eruption is frequent.

In childhood, the initial viral infection usually goes unrecognized unless the stomatitis causes feeding difficulties. After infection, antibody titer remains high throughout life and limits future response to the virus to an occasional recurrent lesion intraorally on the hard palate, or extraorally on the vermilion border, often extending to the skin surfaces of the lips. The latter are often called **fever blisters** or **cold sores**. Mild trauma such as that associated with dental treatment, abrasion of the vermilion border, sunburn, food allergy, onset of menstruation, or any disease that produces a fever or an increased metabolic rate may precipitate lesions.

Symptoms and Signs

In **primary acute herpetic gingivostomatitis,** multiple shallow ulcers of varying size occur throughout the mouth. The oral ulcerations are preceded by inflamed gingivae resembling acute necrotizing ulcerative gingivitis and a 2- to 3-day prodromal period of malaise, fever, and cervical lymphadenopathy. During the first 4 or 5 days, pain may be severe enough to discourage a child from eating and drinking. Although the disease is usually self-limited and symptoms subside in 7 to 10 days, extensive systemic involvement and fatal viremia have occurred in infants and occasionally in older children.

In **recurrent herpes labialis,** patients usually experience a sensation of fullness, burning, and itching before the typical vesicle develops on slightly elevated, erythematous tissue at or near the junction of the vermilion and skin. The greatest extension of the lesion is usually toward the skin. Vesicular lesions may exist for hours before the vesicle breaks leading to formation of yellowish, crusted lesions. Underlying tissues are not indurated, though varying degrees of edema may be present. Lesions seldom last > 10 days.

Recurrent intraoral herpetic palatal and gingival lesions begin with multiple small vesicles that rupture quickly and unite to form large, superficial ulcerations with irregular margins. A large zone of erythema usually surrounds the ulcers.

Diagnosis

Primary acute herpetic stomatitis must be differentiated from drug eruptions and erythema multiforme, and, more rarely in adults, from pemphigus. Allergic forms of stomatitis can usually be suspected from the history. In both erythema multiforme and pemphigus, accompanying skin lesions are common. **Erythema multiforme** (see Ch. 196) may be discerned by more marked constitutional symptoms and widespread hemorrhagic lesions. In **pemphigus** (see also Ch. 197), constitutional symptoms of several weeks' duration are usual, and the patient often recalls a prior episode of large painless bullae without accompanying prodromal symptoms.

Diagnosis of the solitary lesion of **herpes labialis** usually presents no difficulty because of its characteristic appearance and location.

Treatment

In **primary herpetic stomatitis,** a topical analgesic relieves temporary pain; 2% lidocaine viscous, 5 ml (1 tsp) as an oral rinse q 3 h, or diphenhydramine elixir, 5 ml (1 tsp) as an oral rinse q 2 h are used as needed. A sodium bicarbonate mouthwash of 2.5 ml (0.5 tsp) in 250 ml (8 oz) warm water q.i.d. soothes and cleanses. Since children tend to decrease fluid intake, they must be watched for dehydration. Supportive therapy consists of increasing fluids and giving diet supplements. Systemic antibiotics may be used to guard against secondary infection.

Recurrent herpetic labialis (lip lesions) can be reduced in frequency by using a sunscreen containing amino benzoic acid during periods of sun exposure. All proposed treatment is more effective if started in the prodromal stage, i.e., at the first symptoms of local change in sensations.

Topically, antiviral agents such as vidarabine or idoxuridine will discourage spreading and act as a lubricant. Experimentally, 2-deoxy-D glucose shows some promise.

Systemic treatment is directed toward improving the body's resistance to the action of the virus. A combination of equal parts of ascorbic acid and citrus bioflavonoids tablets 400 mg t.i.d. for 3 days may abort or greatly reduce the clinical course of the lesions. Lysine tablets 500 mg t.i.d. for 3 days tend to be effective in reducing the discomfort and duration of the lesions.

Desiccating agents such as alcohol, ether, and chloroform are thought to fractionate the virus thereby inviting resistant and mutagenic strains. Corticosteroids can cause spreading of the virus, especially on mucosal tissue.

There is no cure for herpes simplex.

---

209.   DENTAL CARIES AND ITS COMPLICATIONS

TOOTH DECAY

A gradual pathologic disintegration and dissolution of tooth enamel and dentin, with eventual involvement of the pulp. Except for the common cold, this is the most prevalent human disorder.

Etiology

The interaction of 3 factors results in dental caries: a susceptible tooth surface, the proper microflora, and a suitable substrate for the microflora. Although several oral acidogenic microorganisms can initiate the carious lesion, laboratory and clinical evidence points to *Streptococcus mutans* as the primary pathogen. Some microorganisms also contribute through synthesis of extracellular polysaccharides that adhere to the tooth surface. Mono- and disaccharide sugars serve as the principal substrates for the microbial enzyme systems that produce organic acid (primarily lactic acid) and for extracellular polysaccharide synthesis. Besides providing a source of fermentable carbohydrate for conversion to acid, these gummy extracellular polysaccharides increase the bulk of dental plaque and favor bacterial proliferation. **Dental plaque**—a combination of these polysaccharides, bacteria, and salivary glycoproteins—serves as a localized site of acid production and impedes buffering and remineralization by saliva.

Dietary carbohydrates play a significant role. The types of carbohydrates and their frequency of ingestion are more important than the amounts consumed. Frequent between-meal snacks, especially of sucrose-containing foods, enhance the carious process; sticky foods that linger are potentially more harmful than nonsticky foods.

Pathogenesis

Dental caries begins on the external crown or exposed root surface of the tooth. Bacterial plaque, not food debris, causes caries. Plaque is not flushed away by the action of oral musculature or saliva. The role of saliva in preventing caries is in its buffering capacity and remineralization effect. Acid action first demineralizes enamel with its high inorganic content; proteolysis of its organic matrix follows. When the carious process reaches the dentin or begins on the root surface, the tooth becomes sensitive to temperature or osmotic changes engendered by foods or by touch. Caries spreads rapidly because of the lower mineral content of dentin and cementum. As demineralization and necrosis of the dentin progress, microorganisms may invade the dentinal tubules. The microbial products preceding the organisms in the dentinal tubules may cause inflammation of the dental pulp before destruction of the surrounding dentin is clinically evident.

Symptoms and Signs

The patient is often unaware of the presence of caries until the lesion is well advanced. Common early symptoms are sensitivity to heat and cold and discomfort after eating sugar-containing foods. A darkened area between anterior teeth or cavitation when the carious process has progressed sufficiently may be noticed. Caries is clinically diagnosed by the dentist when softened enamel or dentin is detected with a sharp instrument. On x-ray, caries appears as a radiolucent area, as do most resin filling materials and bases under metallic restorations. Consequently, x-ray diagnosis must be coupled with a visual examination.

Prophylaxis

Teeth are less susceptible to caries if optimum amounts of fluoride (approximately 1 mg/day) are ingested while the teeth are developing. Fluoride combines with some of the apatite crystals in the tooth structure to form the less soluble fluorapatite. Maximum benefit accrues when water containing 1 ppm of fluoride is consumed from birth until the permanent dentition completes eruption (age 11 to 13.) There is no clinical proof that ingesting fluoridated water or fluoride supplements during pregnancy will significantly protect a child's deciduous teeth and permanent lst molars, although these calcify in utero.

Ingestion of excessive fluoride before eruption, while the enamel is forming, may cause permanent mottling of the enamel (see Teeth in Ch. 206). Once erupted, teeth cannot develop mottling when exposed to fluoride. During pregnancy, the placenta acts as a barrier against marked increases in fluoride concentration and thus protects the calcifying fetal teeth against mottling.

If the water supply contains less than the optimum amount of fluoride for the local mean maximum air temperature (as prescribed by the Public Health Service Drinking Water Standards), children should take daily supplements during their tooth-forming years, by using bottled fluoridated water for drinking and cooking, or by taking a sodium fluoride tablet or a fluoride-containing vitamin supplement.

Application of fluoride compounds to erupted teeth enhances the benefit from systemic fluorides in both children and adults; it is not a substitute since the modes of action differ. Periodic applications should be supplemented by daily use of a fluoride-containing dentifrice. Daily use of a mouthrinse containing low fluoride concentrations is also effective for children as prophylaxis against caries.

Food particles and dental plaque should be removed from all accessible tooth surfaces at least once daily. Mechanical removal is the only effective method currently available. Proper use of a soft-bristled toothbrush removes plaque adequately from all areas except interproximal tooth surfaces and deep pits and fissures of the enamel. Interproximal surfaces, highly susceptible to dental caries, should be cleaned daily with dental floss or tape. Plaque-disclosing tablets or liquids composed of food coloring may be used to check the efficacy of plaque removal. Sealing of enamel pits and fissures with a BIS-GMA-type resin is highly effective in preventing caries and is performed increasingly by dentists. The sealed teeth should be checked annually and the sealant replaced when lost.

Treatment

Although caries may be arrested, destroyed tooth structure cannot regenerate. Removal of all affected tooth structure and proper replacement with a restorative material is the best treatment. For details of filling teeth, see DENTAL RESTORATIONS AND APPLIANCES in Ch. 204.

PULPITIS

Inflammation of the dental pulp (containing vascular, connective, and nervous tissue) and of the adjacent periodontal tissues, resulting in **toothache.**

Etiology and Pathology

Pulpitis may result from thermal, chemical, traumatic, or bacterial irritation. Inflammation and infection secondary to caries is the most frequent cause. Since hard dentinal walls surround the pulp, an inflammatory reaction usually results in necrosis. The inflammation extends through the apex of the tooth and involves the periapical tissues (connective tissue of the periodontal membrane and bone).

Diagnosis

In acute suppurative pulpitis, a sharp, throbbing, shooting pain may be intermittent; it is less intense in pulpitis secondary to mechanical debridement of a cavity. Intense pain may be difficult to localize. It may be referred to the opposite mandible or maxilla or to areas supplied by common branches of the 5th nerve. X-rays, pulp testers, percussion, thermal tests, and palpation are aids in diagnosis.

Treatment

In early pulpitis, cleansing of the cavity to remove food debris and the application of clove oil often provide an effective anodyne. Packing the cavity with zinc oxide-eugenol cement (clove oil mixed with zinc oxide powder to form a thick paste) usually affords longer relief and prevents food debris from accumulating. Infected pulpal tissue should be removed and root canal therapy instituted, or the tooth should be extracted.

PERIAPICAL ABSCESS

(Dentoalveolar Abscess)

An acute or chronic suppurative process of the periapical region.

Etiology and Pathogenesis

The abscess is secondary to an infection of the dental pulp usually due to caries. However, it may occur after trauma to the teeth or from periapical localization of organisms, usually α-hemolytic streptococci or staphylococci.

Symptoms and Signs

Pain is gnawing and continuous. The involved tooth is painful when percussed, and often the teeth cannot close without added discomfort. Hot or cold foods may increase the pain. If treatment is delayed, the infection may spread through adjacent tissues, causing **cellulitis**, varying degrees of facial edema, and fever. The infection may extend into osseous tissues or into the soft tissues of the floor of the mouth. Local swelling and **gingival fistulas** may develop opposite the apex of the tooth, especially with deciduous teeth. Drainage into the mouth causes a bitter taste. **Abscesses** from lower molars may drain at the angle of the jaw.

A *chronic* periapical abscess usually presents few clinical signs since it is essentially a circumscribed area of mild infection that spreads slowly. In time, the infection may become granulomatous. As the granuloma enlarges, the lesion may progress to an epithelium-lined cavity and a **periapical cyst** results. Persistent periapical cysts and granulomas may become infected. All are radiolucent on x-ray examination.

Treatment

Extraction or root canal therapy is usually indicated. If high fever persists, antibiotics (e.g., penicillin G or V 250 to 500 mg q 6 h, or erythromycin 250 mg q 6 h, or a tetracycline 250 mg q 6 h) should be given. Hot saline mouth rinses may encourage pointing. If the swelling becomes fluctuant, it should be drained, usually by intraoral incision. An analgesic (e.g., aspirin or acetaminophen 650 mg alone or with codeine 30 to 60 mg orally q 3 to 4 h) is usually needed. Bed rest, a soft diet, and forced fluids may be necessary.

---

210.   PERIODONTAL DISEASE

(Pyorrhea)

Inflammation or degeneration of tissues that surround and support the teeth: gingiva, alveolar bone, periodontal ligament, and cementum. Periodontal disease most commonly begins as gingivitis and progresses to periodontitis. If the severity of the disease is disproportionate to the amount of plaque and calculus, **systemic disease** may be present; however, in widespread periodontal disease, local factors are also present. For example, diabetes mellitus, scurvy, leukemia and other disorders of leukocyte number or function, hyperparathyroidism, and osteoporosis aggravate local factors.

GINGIVITIS

Inflammation of the gingivae, characterized by swelling, redness, change of normal contours, and bleeding. Swelling deepens the crevice between the gingiva and the teeth, forming gingival pockets. Gingivitis may be acute, chronic, or recurrent.

Etiology

The greatest single cause is poor hygiene, characterized by bacterial plaque (microbial colonies growing in carbohydrate residues tenaciously attached to the tooth surfaces). Other local factors such as malocclusion, dental calculus (calcified plaque, called tartar), food impaction, faulty dental restorations, and mouth breathing play important secondary roles.

Gingivitis is commonly noted at puberty and during pregnancy, presumably due to endocrine factors. Gingivitis may be the first sign of a systemic disorder with lowered tissue resistance, e.g., hypovitaminosis, leukopenic disorders, allergic reaction, endocrine disturbance (e.g., diabetes mellitus), or a debilitating disease. Prolonged ingestion of phenytoin may cause enlargement of the gingiva; the use of birth control pills may increase inflammatory changes; heavy metals (e.g., lead and bismuth) may also cause gingivitis. Correction of gingivitis would prevent most periodontal disease.

Symptoms, Signs, and Diagnosis

Simple gingivitis: The outstanding signs are a band of red, inflamed gum tissue surrounding the necks of teeth, edematous swelling of the interdental papillae, and bleeding on minimal injury. Pain is usually absent. The inflammation, usually acute in onset, may subside or persist.

Gingivitis of diabetes mellitus: Uncontrolled diabetics have an exaggerated response to gingival irritants; secondary infections and acute gingival abscesses are common.

Gingivitis of pregnancy: A mild inflammation of the gingiva may develop in pregnancy; hyperplasia, especially of the interdental papillae, is likely to occur. Pedunculated gingival growths **(pregnancy tumors)** often arise from the papillae in the first trimester, may persist throughout pregnancy, and may or may not subside after delivery. It tends to recur if excised before term and may or may not regress following delivery. A similar lesion, **pyogenic granuloma,** is a soft, reddish mass in the interdental gingiva that develops rapidly and then remains static. Treatment is excision. A similar gingivitis may accompany dysmenorrhea.

Desquamative gingivitis is characterized by deep red, painful, easily bleeding gingival tissue. Vesicles may precede the stage of desquamation. It often occurs during menopause. The gingivae are soft due to the absence of cornified cells that would resist masticatory trauma. Sequential administration of estrogens and progestins is often beneficial. A similar gingival lesion may be associated with bullous pemphigoid or benign mucosal pemphigoid (see Ch. 197).

Gingivitis in leukemia: Engorged, edematous, painful, enlarged, livid gums that bleed readily suggest leukemia. They result from reduced tissue resistance, the presence of leukemic infiltrates in the periodontal tissues, and characteristic bleeding abnormalities. The gingiva may become secondarily infected with fusospirochetal organisms, resulting in necrotizing ulcerative gingivitis (see GINGIVA in Ch. 207).

Phenytoin gingivitis: Prolonged intake of phenytoin may cause fibrotic gingival hyperplasia. The interdental papillae enlarge initially. The process may progress until the gums are entirely involved and the teeth are partially obscured. The hyperplastic tissue is firm and less prone to bleed than in other forms of gingivitis. Excision may afford temporary benefit.

Gingivitis in hypovitaminosis: The gingiva in **scurvy** is inflamed, hyperplastic, engorged with blood, and bleeds easily. It may appear as "bags of blood." Petechial and ecchymotic areas may be on the gums and elsewhere in the mouth. Destruction of periosteum and periodontal tissue, resulting in loosened teeth, is common. Gum changes are not seen in edentulous patients. In **pellagra,** the gingiva is inflamed, bleeds easily, and is subject to secondary infection. The lips are reddened and cracked, the mouth feels scalded, the tongue is smooth and bright red, and tongue and mucosa may show ulcerations.

Pericoronitis: Recurrent episodes of acute inflammation of the gingival flap overlying a partially erupted tooth are common—this occurs most often around the 3rd molar and extraction may be considered after the acute process subsides. The gingival flap disappears when the tooth is fully erupted. Treatment is local aqueous irrigation. Antibiotics may be required if the infection is severe.

Gingival abscess (parulis) develops from a periapical abscess at the tip of the root of a nonvital tooth. Pus escapes from a sinus that opens on the mucosal surface. A periodontal abscess may drain similarly.

Prophylaxis

Daily removal of plaque with dental floss and a toothbrush, and routine cleaning by a dentist every 4 to 6 mo are essential preventive procedures, especially when systemic conditions predispose to gingivitis.

Treatment

The treatment is to control or correct both plaque and local and systemic factors. Some cases require extensive treatment such as scaling, selective grinding of teeth to eliminate traumatic occlusion, and replacement of overhanging fillings and poorly contoured restorations. Otherwise food trapped against the gingiva may become impacted into the gingival margin. Excision of excess gingiva is required in specific situations as noted above.

OTHER GINGIVAL DISORDERS

Enlargement of the gingivae occurs frequently during puberty, particularly where local irritation exists, as with malocclusion or calculus. **Idiopathic fibromatosis** is characterized by diffuse enlargement of the gingivae, either smooth or nodular (see also Phenytoin Gingivitis, above). Removal of the hypertrophied tissue is often done.

Gingival **fibromas** often occur near sites of chronic irritation. A **giant cell epulis,** which looks similar, may arise from the periodontal ligament. If the tissue contains such cells, blood chemistry should be investigated for the possibility of hyperparathyroidism.

Denture sore mouth is chronic inflammation due to frictional trauma of the mucosa under a poorly fitting denture. Treatment is replacement with a proper fit. Frequently this condition is accompanied by an oral candidiasis which requires concomitant treatment with nystatin.

In thrombocytopenic purpura or disorders of platelet function, gingival petechiae and **hemorrhage** may occur. Localization is predominantly at sites of periodontal disease.

PERIODONTITIS

Progression of gingivitis to the point that loss of supporting bone has begun. It is the primary cause of tooth loss in adults.

Etiology

Periodontitis results from the same local and systemic factors that cause gingivitis. The rate of osseous resorption is influenced by the duration and severity of these factors as well as by the resistance and repair potential of the patient. Faulty occlusion that results in an excessive functional load on the teeth may contribute to the progress of the disease.

Symptoms, Signs, and Diagnosis

The early symptoms and signs of periodontitis are similar to those of gingivitis. The gingival pockets between the gingivae and the teeth deepen, calculus deposits often enlarge, the gums lose their attachment to the teeth, and bone loss begins. The pockets collect debris and allow microbes to proliferate, thus promoting the disease. Destruction of the supporting osseous tissue in varying degree is the earliest evidence seen on x-ray. Loosening of teeth and possible recession of the gums follow progressive bone loss; tooth migration is common in later stages. Pain is usually absent unless an acute infection (e.g., abscess formation in one or more periodontal pockets) is superimposed on the chronic process.

Treatment (see also GINGIVITIS, above)

Systemic disorders require correction. Astringent agents, mouthwashes, and antibiotics are of little value in long-term treatment. Dental referral is indicated to correct or eliminate local irritative factors and instruct in home care to limit further destruction. If abnormal gum shape and pockets go uncorrected, surgery will be required. Advanced periodontitis with deep pocket formation and mobility of the teeth is likely to require extensive periodontal surgery. Selective grinding of tooth surfaces to eliminate traumatic occlusion, and splinting of loose teeth may be necessary. Extractions are often imperative in advanced disease.

PERIODONTOSIS

An uncommon widespread degeneration of the periodontal tissues with loss of alveolar bone so that teeth may be lost at an early age. It differs from periodontitis in its lack of associated inflammation and pus formation. While its cause and treatment are unknown, improving the occlusion and splinting the teeth may be of value. Periodontal surgery may stabilize the condition.

---

211. TEMPOROMANDIBULAR JOINT (TMJ) DISORDERS

The TMJ is susceptible to common congenital and developmental anomalies, fractures, dislocations, ankylosis, arthritis, and neoplastic diseases. Nonarticular disorders that affect the area and can mimic true TMJ disease and the muscular disorder known as **myofascial pain-dysfunction (MPD) syndrome** (see below), which may secondarily involve the TMJ, must be considered in differential diagnosis. **Examination of the TMJ** is described in Ch. 206.

CONGENITAL AND DEVELOPMENTAL ANOMALIES

Agenesis: Congenital absence of the condyloid process results in severe facial deformity. The coronoid process, the ramus, and parts of the mandibular body may also be absent. Abnormalities of the external, middle, and inner ear, the temporal bone, and the facial nerve are often associated. Without the condyle, the mandible deviates to the affected side, and the unaffected side is elongated and flattened. Mandibular skewing results in severe malocclusion. X-rays of the mandible and TMJ show the degree of agenesis and distinguish this condition from others which affect the growing condyle and produce similar facial deformities, but which are not associated with severe structural loss.

Treatment: Jaw reconstruction by autogenous bone grafting should be initiated as soon as possible to limit progression of the facial deformity. Mentoplasty and onlay grafts of bone, cartilage, or soft tissue are also frequently used to improve facial symmetry. Orthodontic treatment helps correct malocclusion.

Condylar hypoplasia may be developmental in origin but usually results from local injury due to trauma, infection, or irradiation during the growth period. Hypoplasia produces facial deformity characterized on the affected side by a short mandibular body, fullness of the face, and deviation of the chin. On the unaffected side, the body of the mandible is elongated and the face appears flat. Malocclusion results from the mandibular deviation. Diagnosis is based on a history of progressive facial asymmetry during the growth period, x-ray evidence of condylar deformity and antegonial notching, and, frequently, a history of trauma. **Treatment** by surgical shortening of the normal side of the mandible or lengthening of the affected side is usually functionally and esthetically corrective. Presurgical orthodontic therapy helps to achieve an optimal result.

Condylar hyperplasia is a disorder of unknown etiology characterized by persistent or accelerated growth at a time when growth should be diminishing or ended. Slowly progressive unilateral enlargement of the mandible causes cross-bite malocclusion, facial asymmetry, and shifting of the midpoint of the chin to the unaffected side. The patient may appear prognathic. The lower border of the mandible is often convex on the affected side. On x-ray, the TMJ may appear normal or the condyle may be symmetrically enlarged and the mandibular neck elongated. The condition is self-limiting. Since chondroma and osteochondroma may produce similar symptoms and signs, they must be ruled out. These grow more rapidly and usually cause asymmetric condylar enlargement.

Treatment: Condylectomy is recommended during the period of active growth, as determined by serial cephalometric x-rays and bone scan. If growth has already stopped, orthodontics and surgical mandibular repositioning are indicated. If the height of the mandibular body is greatly increased, facial symmetry can be further improved by reduction of the inferior border.

TRAUMA AND DISLOCATION

(See Ch. 213)

ANKYLOSIS

Ankylosis of the TMJ is most often a sequel to trauma or infection, though it may accompany RA or be congenital. Chronic, painless limitation of movement occurs. When associated with condylar growth arrest or tissue loss, facial asymmetry is usual (see **condylar hypoplasia,** above). True (intra-articular) ankylosis must be distinguished from false (extra-articular) ankylosis. The latter may be caused by such things as enlargement of the coronoid process, depressed fracture of the zygomatic arch, or scarring from surgery or irradiation. In most cases of true ankylosis, x-rays of the TMJ show loss of normal bony architecture.

Treatment: Forced opening of the jaws is generally ineffective because of bony fusion. Condylectomy can be used if the ankylosis is intra-articular. An ostectomy in the ramus may be needed if the coronoid process and zygomatic arch are also involved. Prolonged use of jaw-opening exercises is essential to maintain the surgical correction.

ARTHRITIS

(See also Ch. 103)

Most forms of arthritis can involve the TMJ; the most common ones are infectious, traumatic, rheumatoid, and degenerative (osteoarthritis).

Infectious arthritis may be part of a generalized systemic disease, may arise from direct extension of adjacent infection, or may result from localization of blood-borne organisms from a distant infection. Inflammation and limitation of jaw movement are present. Early x-rays are negative but bone destruction becomes evident later. Local signs of inflammation, associated with evidence of a systemic disease or an adjacent infection, suggest the diagnosis. In suppurative arthritis, joint aspiration may confirm the diagnosis and identify the causative organism.

Treatment includes antibiotics, proper hydration, control of pain, and restriction of motion. Suppurative infections should be aspirated or incised. Once the infection is controlled, jaw-opening exercises are important to prevent scarring and limitation of function.

Traumatic arthritis may be caused by acute injury or excessive opening—e.g., during yawning, tooth extraction, or endotracheal intubation. Pain, tenderness, and limitation of motion occur. X-rays are negative except for occasional widening of the joint space due to intra-articular edema or hemorrhage. The diagnosis includes a history of trauma and x-rays negative for fracture. **Treatment** includes analgesics, heat application, a soft diet, and restriction of jaw movement.

In **RA**, the TMJ is involved in > 50% of cases, in both adults and children. Pain, swelling, and limited movement are the most common findings. In children, destruction of the condyle results in growth disturbance and facial deformity. Ankylosis may follow in all patients. X-rays of the TMJ are usually negative in early stages, but bone destruction is seen later; it may result in an anterior open-bite deformity. TMJ inflammation in association with polyarthritis suggests the diagnosis. Confirmation depends upon positive laboratory findings.

Treatment is similar to that for RA of other joints. In the acute stage, anti-inflammatory drugs are given and jaw function should be limited. When symptoms subside, mild jaw exercises help prevent excessive loss of motion. Surgical correction is necessary if ankylosis develops, but should not be undertaken until the condition is quiescent.

Primary degenerative arthritis (osteoarthritis) may involve the TMJ as well as other joints. Relatively asymptomatic, patients complain only occasionally of stiffness, crepitation, or mild pain. Joint involvement is generally bilateral. X-rays may show flattening and lipping of the condyle. **Treatment** is symptomatic.

Secondary degenerative arthritis usually occurs in persons aged 30 to 50, usually after trauma or persistent MPD syndrome (see below). It is characterized by limitation of opening and unilateral pain on motion, joint tenderness, and crepitation. When associated with MPD syndrome, the symptoms intermittently become more severe and some muscles of mastication are tender. X-rays generally show condylar flattening, lipping, spurring, or erosion. The unilateral joint involvement helps to distinguish secondary from primary degenerative arthritis. **Treatment** is conservative, as for MPD syndrome, though arthroplasty or high condylectomy may be necessary. Intra-articular injection of corticosteroids or of 2% lidocaine may bring symptomatic relief but may harm the joint if repeated often.

NONARTICULAR CONDITIONS MIMICKING TEMPOROMANDIBULAR JOINT DISORDERS

Conditions unrelated to the TMJ that can produce preauricular pain, limitation of jaw movement, or a combination of both include pulpitis, pericoronitis, otitis, parotitis, trigeminal neuralgia, atypical (vascular) neuralgia, temporal arteritis, nasopharyngeal carcinoma, myositis and myositis ossificans, tetanus, scleroderma, depressed fracture of the zygomatic arch, and osteochondroma of the coronoid process. Pain due to these, unlike intrinsic TMJ disorders, is usually not exacerbated by finger pressure on the TMJ as the patient opens his mouth.

MYOFASCIAL PAIN-DYSFUNCTION (MPD) SYNDROME

The most common disorder involving the TMJ area, MPD syndrome occurs in women more frequently than in men. Most cases are psychophysiologic in origin and result from tension-relieving jaw-clenching or -grinding habits, or a centrally generated increase in masticatory muscle tonus in response to stress. The ensuing muscle fatigue in turn induces spasm of the masticatory muscles, the immediate cause of MPD. Poorly aligned teeth or ill-fitting dentures occasionally contribute to the condition. Secondary degenerative arthritis may involve the joint in the late stages.

Diagnosis is based on clinical findings. Characteristically, the patient complains of unilateral, dull, aching preauricular pain that radiates to the temporal region, the angle of the jaw, and the occiput; tenderness in one or more of the muscles of mastication; jaw limitation; and occasional "clicking" or "popping" sounds in the joint. Joint pain on awakening may indicate bruxism during sleep. X-rays are usually normal although secondary degenerative changes are seen occasionally in very late stages. Degenerative arthritis, which causes similar symptoms, must be excluded. Primary degenerative arthritis is usually bilateral. Both primary and secondary degenerative arthritis produce x-ray changes in the joint, and secondary degenerative arthritis causes tenderness of the TMJ on lateral or intrameatal palpation; these findings help to distinguish the arthritides from MPD syndrome.

Treatment includes a soft, non-chewy diet; limited use of the jaw; hot, moist applications or diathermy; diazepam 2 to 5 mg q.i.d. (the last dose taken at bedtime) as a muscle relaxant and tranquilizer; analgesics (e.g., aspirin 650 mg q.i.d.) for pain; and use of a biteplate. Clenching or grinding the teeth should be avoided. Possible causative life stresses should be discussed with the patient. Psychologic counseling may be helpful in persistent cases.

212.   PRENEOPLASTIC AND NEOPLASTIC LESIONS

ORAL LEUKOPLAKIA

A potentially precancerous lesion appearing as an adherent white patch or plaque on the oral mucosa that cannot be characterized clinically or histologically as any other specific disease.

Etiology

Many factors, local or systemic, act independently or in combination to result in leukoplakia. Most frequently implicated are tobacco, including its chemical constituents and combustion end-products; alcohol, because of irritation to the mucosa; chronic irritation from causes such as cheek biting (e.g., due to malocclusion), ill-fitting dentures, sharp, broken, or worn-down teeth, or spicy foods; syphilis, especially among patients who have had syphilitic glossitis; vitamin deficiency, especially of A or B; other factors, e.g., hormonal changes and *Candida albicans* have been implicated but the data are inconclusive.

Symptoms and Signs

Leukoplakia is more common in men between ages 40 and 70. Although it occurs anywhere in the mouth, the buccal and alveolar mucosa, palate, floor of the mouth, and tongue are sites of predilection. Lesions vary from small, well-localized white patches to diffuse areas involving much of the oral mucosa, and from a smooth, flat or slightly elevated, translucent white plaque to a thick, fissured, papillomatous lesion that is firm to palpation. The lesions of leukoplakia may be gray or yellowish-white, and excessive tobacco use may cause a brownish-yellow color. The lingual papillae are usually absent if lesions involve the dorsum of the tongue. White patches interspersed with areas of erythema ("speckled leukoplakia" or "erythroplakia") are potentially more serious than other types (see NEOPLASMS, below).

Leukoplakia may become epidermoid carcinoma in some cases. The frequency of serious pathologic alteration varies according to anatomic site. Those in the floor of the mouth have the highest incidence of epithelial alteration. The patient may feel a firmness of the involved tissues, or be asymptomatic until ulceration, fissuring, or malignant degeneration has developed. Pain usually announces an advanced lesion.

Diagnosis

Leukoplakia is suggested by the appearance of lesions, as described above and confirmed by biopsy. *Since potentially dangerous lesions look like innocuous ones, all leukoplakic lesions should be biopsied (by excision when possible).*

Treatment

Any recognizable irritation should be eliminated. Thus, faulty restorations and prosthetic devices should be corrected or removed. Chemical irritants, including tobacco in any form and hot, highly seasoned foods, should be eliminated. Small localized lesions should be totally excised or cauterized. Larger lesions may be removed by a series of operations. Every patient with leukoplakia should be reexamined at 3- to 6-mo intervals regardless of treatment and any lesions found should be biopsied.

NEOPLASMS

Any ulcer of the oral mucosa that does not improve after 1 wk of treatment should be considered malignant until proved otherwise. A neoplasm should be suspected when no local cause is found for a hypertrophic lesion in or around the mouth, particularly when associated with a burning sensation. The primary site may involve the gingiva, palate, tongue, mucosa of the lip and cheek, or floor of the mouth. Early stages of tumors in these areas are seldom symptomatic or painful. When gingiva bleed spontaneously, the patient should be evaluated for a blood dyscrasia.

The most common malignancies of the oral cavity are epidermoid carcinoma of the lip, cheek, and tongue; lymphoepithelioma; melanoma; and myelocytic and lymphocytic leukemias. Benign lesions that may be confused with oral cancer include irritation, fibroma, papilloma, granuloma (including pregnancy tumor), the glossitis of avitaminosis, geographic tongue, median rhomboid glossitis, hemangioma and lymphangioma, fibrous hypertrophy of the gingiva, melanosis, myoblastoma, retention cysts (including ranula), xanthomatosis, torus palatinus, submandibular duct calculus, hypertrophy of the foliate papillae, radiculodental cysts, and ameloblastoma. Syphilis, benign ulcer, tuberculosis, leukoplakia, and dental abscess should also be considered. Exfoliative cytology is useful in screening, but biopsy is essential to establish the diagnosis.

NEOPLASMS OF SPECIFIC TISSUES

Lips and Gingiva

Smoker's patch is a firm, brownish, keratotic plaque on the vermilion border of the lower lip, most common in smokers who hold a cigarette or pipe in one location. *Only a biopsy can rule out squamous cell carcinoma.* Cessation of smoking and careful observation are recommended even if it is not malignant. **Actinic cheilosis** occurs in adults, especially redheads with fair skin, who spend much time out of doors. The lips are dry with many erosive areas. A person with this *precancerous* lesion should be seen every 3 to 6 mo, avoid prolonged exposure to sunlight, wear a broad-brimmed hat or cap, and use an antiactinic cream. **Squamous cell carcinoma** usually appears on the vermilion border of the lower lip as a nonhealing ulcer with a convex, indurated margin, or less commonly, as a keratotic patch. It may be fixed to the underlying tissues. If treated early, prognosis is excellent. In **leukemia**, the gingival tissue may be infiltrated and prone to bleed.

Tongue and Floor of the Mouth

Leukoplakia (see above) is commonly a white keratotic patch. Even more likely to become carcinomatous is the **"speckled" type of leukoplakia** or **erythroplakia** in which small white patches form on an erythematous base. This type often appears on the ventral surface of the tongue and the floor of the mouth. Biopsy is mandatory. It is usually carcinoma in situ or frankly invasive. **Squamous cell carcinoma** often arises in chronic glossitis or in an area of leukoplakia. A deep ulcer with smooth, indurated, rolled margins and fixed to deeper tissues is characteristic. It is most common in heavy users of both alcohol and tobacco. Syphilis is a predisposing factor. **Rhabdomyoma** of the tongue causes a palpable interior mass. It is much rarer than squamous cell carcinoma which arises in the mucosa.

Cheek
Irritation of the mucosa is commonly seen in the mucobuccal fold, where chewing tobacco or snuff may be habitually retained. This may progress to leukoplakia or erythroplakia and squamous cell carcinoma.

Palate
Accessory salivary gland tumor is usually a mixed tumor with both epithelial and mesenchymal components, an adenoid cystic carcinoma, or a mucoepidermoid carcinoma. Typically, it appears as a firm, smooth, painless mass lateral to the midline. Any such swelling that is not bony hard should be considered a salivary gland tumor until a biopsy proves otherwise. A **fullness of the palate** can represent extension of a malignant tumor of the lining of the nose or the antrum rather than a primary lesion of the palate. The soft palate may become immobile if a cancer is in the nasopharynx.

Jaws
If not initially detected on x-ray, jaw tumors are diagnosed clinically because their growth causes **swelling** of the face, palate, or alveolar process (the area of the jaw surrounding the teeth). They cause bone tenderness and severe pain originating in the involved bone. **Ameloblastoma** is the most common odontogenic neoplasm. It most frequently arises in the posterior mandible and is slowly invasive, but rarely metastatic. On x-ray, it typically appears as a multiloculated or soap-bubble radiolucency. **Odontomas** are tumors of the dental follicle or the dental tissues that usually appear in the mandibles of young people; several types include fibrous odontomas and cementomas. An absent molar tooth suggests a composite odontoma. **Other neoplasms** include osteogenic sarcoma, giant cell tumor, Ewing's tumor, multiple myeloma, and metastatic tumors.

Salivary Glands
The two main types of tumors are the **mixed tumor** (pleomorphic adenoma), 60% of which occur in the parotid glands, and **mucoepidermoid carcinoma.** These tumors occur not only in major salivary glands but also in accessory salivary glands located in the palate and the buccal mucosa (see above). Slowly developing swellings may be painless: the patient complains of a change in appearance, but because of dense fascia surrounding it, acute swelling of the parotid gland is painful. A parotid tumor causes facial paralysis if it compresses or infiltrates the facial nerve, which may also be inadvertently damaged during surgery to remove the tumor. Tumors of the submandibular salivary glands are often painful because of close association with the lingual branch of the trigeminal nerve.

---

213.   DENTAL EMERGENCIES

Emergency dental treatment by a physician is sometimes required when dentists are unavailable, but dental consultation is desirable as soon as possible.

TOOTHACHE AND INFECTION

Pain localized to a particular tooth and provoked by sweets or cold is usually caused by **caries** that do not yet involve the dental pulp (nerve). Because this type of pain is usually fleeting, the patient should avoid provoking stimuli, use mild analgesics, and seek prompt treatment.

Localized pain that is usually intensified by heat most commonly denotes caries that has reached the dental pulp (see PULPITIS in Ch. 209). Associated **periapical inflammation,** often present, may be diagnosed by tenderness to percussion. (If all maxillary posterior teeth on one side are sensitive to percussion, maxillary sinusitis should be suspected.) Initial treatment with an analgesic (e.g., acetaminophen 325 mg with codeine 30 mg orally q 4 h) and an antibiotic (e.g., erythromycin or penicillin V 250 mg q 6 h) is indicated until dental therapy can be initiated.

Periapical infection, often accompanied by swelling of contiguous soft tissues, will usually develop from untreated pulpitis. Emergency treatment consists of analgesics and antibiotics, as described above in periapical inflammation. A **periapical abscess** that has spread beyond the alveolar bone causing swelling and fluctuation in adjacent soft tissue requires incision and drainage; antibiotics alone are inadequate. An intraoral incision is usually appropriate, but a percutaneous incision may be necessary for dependent drainage. (See also PERIAPICAL ABSCESS in Ch. 209.) **Erupting or impacted molar teeth,** particularly 3rd molars, can be painful and may cause adjacent soft tissue inflammation that can progress to serious infection; erythromycin or penicillin V 250 mg orally q.i.d. should be started. **Less common causes of acute perioral swelling** include periodontal abscess, infected cysts, antritis, allergy, salivary gland obstruction or infection, peritonsillar infection, or skin infection.

POSTEXTRACTION PROBLEMS

Swelling is normal after intraoral surgical procedures and is proportional to the degree of manipulation and trauma. If it does not begin to subside by the 3rd postoperative day, infection should be suspected and an antibiotic (e.g., erythromycin or penicillin V 250 mg orally q.i.d.) should be started.

Postoperative pain, usually moderate, can be controlled with acetaminophen or aspirin 325 mg with codeine 30 mg orally q 4 h.

Postextraction alveolitis (dry socket) is usually peculiar to the removal of a mandibular 3rd molar. Typically, the pain begins on the 2nd or 3rd postoperative day, is referred to the ear, and lasts from a few days to many weeks. Alveolitis is best treated with topical analgesic medication: 1/4-in. gauze saturated in eugenol and/or guaiacol, placed in the socket and changed daily, usually reduces the need for prolonged systemic analgesics. Infection is uncommon. However, rarely, **osteomyelitis** may be confused with alveolitis, but osteomyelitis is characterized by fever, local swelling, and later x-ray changes. If osteomyelitis is suspected, antibiotics should be instituted and the patient referred for definitive care.

Postextraction bleeding usually oozes from small vessels. After removing any superfluous clot with gauze, a pressure dressing (cotton wrapped in gauze, or a tea bag) is applied directly and continuously to the extraction site for 20 to 30 min. This is repeated 2 or 3 times. If the bleeding continues, the site may be anesthetized with 2% lidocaine with 1:100,000 epinephrine by nerve block or infiltration as appropriate, and the socket area sutured under tension, allowing space between the sutures for packing if necessary. Local hemostatic agents such as oxidized cellulose or topical thrombin on a gelatin sponge or microfibrillar collagen may be placed in the socket. If these measures fail, a systemic cause should be sought. Rarely, blood loss may require transfusion.

FRACTURED AND AVULSED TEETH

If a small portion of a crown is fractured and the dental pulp is not exposed, analgesic medication (e.g., aspirin 650 mg q 4 h) and a topical covering with zinc-eugenol or similar cement are appropriate. If the pulp is exposed or the tooth is mobile, erythromycin or penicillin V 250 mg q 6 h should also be given.

Permanent retention of a completely avulsed tooth is possible *if it is immediately replaced into the socket without washing and with minimal handling.* The long-term prognosis is very poor (retention for a few months to a few years) if there is a delay of even a few minutes in replacement or if the tooth is washed or handled excessively. Root resorption invariably occurs after delayed replacement. Thus, patients should be instructed to replace the avulsed tooth immediately and seek professional care to stabilize it. If this is not possible, the tooth should be kept moist in saline, or in the patient's mouth, and then replaced and stabilized as indicated.

Partially avulsed teeth should be repositioned, immobilized, and stabilized. With any partially or completely avulsed tooth, antibiotic therapy should be prescribed for several days.

FRACTURES OF THE JAW AND CONTIGUOUS STRUCTURES

Fractures of the jaws and contiguous structures are diagnosed primarily by physical examination and x-ray. Fracture should be suspected if there is malocclusion, mobility of the maxillae, discrepancy in the smooth contour of the orbital rims, diplopia, infraorbital anesthesia, tenderness to palpation (particularly over the condyle or condylar neck of the mandible), and restriction or deviation when the mouth is open. A facial fracture is an emergency if there is airway obstruction, uncontrollable hemorrhage, or trauma to the eye or CNS. Routine x-rays usually confirm the diagnosis for fractures of the mandible, but may not for midface fractures. *Fracture of a cervical vertebra should be considered when a blow has been sufficient to fracture facial bones.* An oral surgeon should be consulted for a fractured jaw because unrecognized malocclusions may otherwise result.

Treatment: Manually holding the mandible in a protruded position or inserting an orotracheal or oropharyngeal airway may be necessary temporarily to maintain an airway (see Ch. 31). If there is hemorrhage into the oropharynx, an orotracheal airway should be placed or the patient positioned to allow the oropharynx to drain dependently. Until definitive care is available, the jaws usually can be temporarily stabilized and hemorrhage minimized by use of a Barton bandage. If a jaw fracture can be treated within the first few hours after injury, closure of lip lacerations is best delayed until the fracture has been reduced.

Fractures through a tooth socket are compound fractures, usually requiring antibiotic prophylaxis (e.g., with penicillin V or erythromycin 250 to 500 mg orally in liquid form q 6 h).

Fractures of the mandibular condyle are usually characterized by preauricular pain, swelling, and limitation of opening. With a unilateral fracture, the jaw deviates to the affected side on attempted opening. Bilateral fracture can produce an anteriorly opened bite. Posterior-anterior and Towne's views of the mandible usually show the fracture on x-ray. **Treatment** is usually closed reduction and intermaxillary fixation, though severely displaced, bilaterally fractured condyles may require open reduction and fixation. Jaw opening exercises are used to reestablish normal function after fixation is discontinued.

DISLOCATED MANDIBLE

A dislocated mandible will be fixed in a markedly open position with only the most posterior teeth contacting. If the midline is deviated, the dislocation is unilateral rather than bilateral. Injecting a local anesthetic agent (e.g., 1% lidocaine 2 to 5 ml) in the joint area and in the area of insertion of the lateral pterygoid muscle may allow the mandible to reduce spontaneously.

Alternatively, or in addition, manual reduction may be necessary. Premedication with diazepam (5 mg IV) and a narcotic (e.g., meperidine 50 mg IV or IM) is desirable. With the patient well below the operator, and his head stabilized to obtain leverage, the operator's thumbs are placed on the external oblique line of the mandible (lateral to the 3rd molar area) and the fingers are placed under the tip of the chin. A rotary motion is used with the thumbs pressing inferiorly and anteriorly and the fingers pressing superiorly until the mandible is reseated.

The jaw should be stabilized with a Barton bandage to maintain the mandible in the reduced position. The patient should restrict opening his mouth for about 6 wk. If this is not the first such dislocation, an oral-maxillofacial surgeon should be consulted.

214. REACTIONS TO SUNLIGHT

The skin responds to excessive sunlight with an acute reaction (sunburn); a chronic reaction that may lead to skin cancer after many years; or an unusual photosensitivity that may be due to the ingestion or application of certain drugs or chemicals, may be indicative of systemic disease, or may be idiopathic.

Etiology and Predisposing Factors

Solar radiation that reaches the earth's surface ranges in wavelength from 2900 to 18,500 angstroms (Å), or 290 to 1850 nm. The character and amount of such radiation varies greatly with the seasons and with changing atmospheric conditions. Sunburn-producing rays—those below 3200 Å (320 nm)—are filtered out completely by ordinary window glass and to a great extent by smoke and smog; most are filtered out during the winter months in northern temperate zones, especially in urban areas. Large amounts of sunburn-producing rays may pass through light clouds or fog, and many persons unwittingly sustain severe reactions under such conditions. Snow, sand, and water enhance exposure by reflecting the rays.

Following exposure to sunlight, the epidermis thickens and the melanocytes produce melanin at an increased rate, providing some natural protection against further exposure. Persons differ greatly in their reactivity to sunlight. Uneven melanin deposition occurs in many fairhaired individuals and results in freckling. Pigmentation does not occur in the skin of albinos because of a defect in melanin metabolism, nor in areas of vitiligo because of the absence of melanocytes. Blondes and redheads are especially susceptible and should avoid overexposure. Blacks and other nonwhites are not immune to the effects of the sun and can become sunburned with prolonged exposure.

ACUTE SUNBURN

Ordinary sunburn results from overexposure of the skin to ultraviolet rays of about 3000 Å (300 nm). **Symptoms and signs** appear in 1 to 24 h and, except in severe reactions, pass their peak in 72 h. Skin changes range from mild erythema with subsequent evanescent scaling, to pain, swelling, skin tenderness, and blisters from more prolonged exposure. Sunburn affecting the lower legs, particularly the pretibial surfaces, is especially uncomfortable and often slow to heal. Constitutional symptoms (fever, chills, weakness, shock), similar to a thermal burn, may appear if a large portion of the body surface is affected; these may be due to heatstroke or heat exhaustion (see Ch. 216).

Secondary infection and miliaria-like eruptions are the most common late complications. Following exfoliation, the skin may be hypervulnerable to sunlight for one to several weeks.

Prophylaxis

Simple precautions will prevent most cases of severe sunburn. Initial summer exposure to bright midday sun should not be $>$ 30 min, even in persons with dark brunette skin. In temperate zones, exposure is less hazardous before 10:00 AM and after 4:00 PM because sunburn-producing wavelengths are usually filtered out. In winter, the greatest danger of sunburn (and snow blindness) comes during foggy days on fresh snow and is increased at high altitude.

Formulations of 5% aminobenzoic acid (p-aminobenzoic acid; **PABA**) in ethyl alcohol or in a gel are very effective in preventing sunburn. They take about 30 min to bind strongly to the skin, and therefore should be applied about 30 to 60 min before sun exposure so that perspiration or swimming will not wash them away. PABA esters are only slightly less effective. PABA may stain clothing and, rarely, causes allergic contact dermatitis. Those who cannot tolerate PABA or its esters may use a benzophenone sunscreen. Opaque formulations containing zinc oxide or titanium dioxide are physical **sunscreens** and prevent radiation from reaching the skin. They are unacceptable cosmetically to many people but may be very useful on the nose or lips. Newer, highly effective, nonopaque lotions containing both a PABA ester and benzophenone are now available. Sunscreens are now rated by SPF (sun protection factor) numbers: 15 is the most protective and 1 the least.

Treatment

Further exposure should be *avoided* until the acute reaction has subsided. Topical corticosteroids are no more effective than cold tap-water compresses in relieving symptoms. Sensitizing preparations, especially ointments or lotions containing local anesthetics such as benzocaine, should be *avoided.*

Early treatment of extensive and severe sunburn with a systemic corticosteroid (e.g., prednisone 10 mg orally q.i.d. for 4 to 6 days for adults or teenagers) will decrease the discomfort considerably. (For treatment of heatstroke and heat exhaustion, see Ch. 216.)

CHRONIC EFFECTS OF SUNLIGHT

Chronic exposure to sunlight ages the skin. Wrinkling and elastosis (yellow discoloration with small yellow nodules) and pigment alterations are the most common troubling consequences of long-term exposure, especially for women. The atrophic effects in some persons may resemble those seen after x-ray therapy. Precancerous keratotic lesions **(actinic keratoses)** are a frequent, disturbing consequence of many years' overexposure. Blondes and redheads are particularly susceptible; blacks are rarely affected. The keratoses are usually hard, and gray to dark in color. They should be differentiated from *seborrheic* keratoses, which occur on covered as well as uncovered areas of the body and are not premalignant.

The incidence of squamous and basal cell carcinoma of the skin in fair, white-skinned persons is directly related to the amount of yearly sunlight in the area. Such lesions are especially common in sportsmen, farmers, ranchers, sailors, and sunworshipers. Malignant melanomas may also increase in incidence with increasing sun exposure.

Treatment

If there are only a few lesions, cryotherapy, e.g., freezing with liquid nitrogen, is the most rapid and satisfactory treatment.

Actinic keratoses usually respond dramatically to small amounts of 5-fluorouracil **(5-FU),** applied to the affected area nightly. For face lesions, 1% 5-FU in propylene glycol is best; elsewhere (e.g., on the arm), 2 or 5% 5-FU cream can be used; if no response is seen, 0.1% tretinoin solution should be applied a few hours before the 2 or 5% 5-FU application. Treatment is continued for at least 2 wk or until a brisk reaction with redness, scaling, and slight burning is seen, often including patches with no previously detected gross changes. If the reaction is too brisk, application should be suspended for 2 or 3 days. Topical 5-FU therapy is remarkably free of significant adverse effects.

PHOTOSENSITIVITY REACTIONS

In addition to the acute and chronic effects of sunlight, a variety of unusual reactions may occur after only a few minutes' exposure: e.g., areas of erythema or frank dermatitis; urticarial and erythema multiforme-like lesions; bullae; and chronic, thickened, scaling patches.

Numerous factors (many unknown) may contribute to increased photosensitivity: (1) SLE or cutaneous LE—unless the cause is obvious, every patient with pronounced photosensitivity should be studied for these conditions; (2) herpes simplex—sunlight commonly precipitates "cold sores"; (3) ingestion of a variety of drugs (e.g., sulfonamides, tetracyclines, thiazides, griseofulvin), though sensitivity appears in only a small percentage of patients taking such compounds; (4) external application of or contact with various substances (see also Ch. 189), including toilet waters and perfumes, sulfonamides, coal tar, soaps containing halogenated salicylanilides, and certain plants (e.g., meadow grass, parsley); (5) xeroderma pigmentosum and certain porphyrias are less common but serious diseases also associated with photosensitivity.

Polymorphous light eruptions are unusual reactions to light that are not associated with systemic disease or drugs, as far as can be determined. Eruptions may be papular or plaque-like, dermatitic, urticarial, or erythema multiforme-like, and appear on sun-exposed areas. Direct immunofluorescence of lesions and of normal-appearing skin is negative. Diagnosis is by exclusion or by reproduction of the lesions with artificial or natural sunlight when the patient is not using any medication (systemic *or* topical).

Prophylaxis and Treatment

Avoidance of sunlight is important, and the patient should wear protective clothing (e.g., hats and long-sleeved shirts) when outdoors on sunny days. Sunscreening preparations (see ACUTE SUNBURN, above) may be helpful. Other treatment is directed to the underlying cause, where possible. Polymorphous eruptions manifested as papules, plaques, or dermatitis may respond to topical corticosteroids. In patients with polymorphous photosensitivity or cutaneous LE, prolonged administration of hydroxychloroquine 200 to 400 mg/day orally often reduces or completely suppresses photosensitivity and may be tried if treatment is required and sunscreens are not effective. Potential eye toxicity should be watched for by an ophthalmologist.

215. BURNS

Tissue injury caused by thermal, electrical, or chemical agents. The extent of injury varies with the etiology and its duration and intensity. Tissues in direct contact with heat (e.g., the skin and sometimes the mucosa of the respiratory and GI tracts) are damaged most quickly, but the systemic effects of severe burns generally pose a greater threat to life than do local effects.

Pathology and Pathophysiology

Local effects: All burns denature protein, resulting in cell injury or death. The first local effect of a burn is dilation of capillaries and small vessels, with increased capillary permeability. The resultant plasma loss under the epidermis produces edema. Later, the cellular injury can be seen histologically as swollen or pyknotic nuclei with cytoplasmic coagulation; collagen fibrils lose their definition.

In spontaneous healing, dead tissue sloughs off as new epithelium begins to cover the injured area. In **superficial burns,** regeneration occurs rapidly from uninjured epidermal elements, hair follicles, and sweat glands; little scarring results unless infection occurs. With **deep burns** (destruction of the epidermis and much of the dermis), reepithelialization starts from the edges of the wound or from the scattered remains of integument. The process is slow, and excessive granulation tissue forms before being covered by epithelium. Such wounds generally contract and develop into disfiguring or disabling scars unless treated promptly by skin grafting.

In **electrical burns,** injury results from the generation of heat up to 5000 C. Since most of the resistance to electric current is at the point of skin contact with the conductor, electrical burns usually involve the skin and subjacent tissues and may be of almost any size and depth. Progressive necrosis and sloughing are usually greater than the original lesion would indicate. **Chemical burns** may be due to strong acids and alkalies, phenols, cresols, mustard gas, or phosphorus. All produce necrosis that may extend slowly for several hours. **Inhalation (respiratory tract) injury** accompanying thermal burns is due to inhalation of the incomplete products of combustion, which are potent chemical irritants to the respiratory mucosa. Only steam inhalation causes actual thermal damage to the respiratory tract.

Systemic effects: These may quickly endanger life. **Primary (neurogenic) shock** causes sudden collapse from generalized vasodilation, presumably as a reflex reaction to pain, fright, or anxiety; it is rarely fatal. The more serious **secondary shock** results from hypovolemia; it develops insidiously, or rapidly if the burn is extensive. Increased capillary permeability resulting from damage to vessel walls allows large amounts of fluid (approximately 4 ml/kg body wt/% burned BSA in the first 24 h) to exude into the wound area from the burned surface. This fluid, lost at the expense of the plasma, consists of water, plasma crystalloids, and about 2/3 of the plasma protein.

Bacterial invasion occurs whenever the epidermis is broken. Dead tissue, warmth, and moisture provide ideal conditions for bacterial growth. Streptococci and staphylococci usually predominate shortly after a burn, and gram-negative bacteria after 5 to 7 days, but mixed flora are always found.

Electrical injury, particularly from alternating current, may cause immediate respiratory paralysis, ventricular fibrillation, or both (see Ch. 219).

Symptoms and Signs

Burns are usually classified by the degree of tissue damage. In **first-degree burns,** damage is limited to the outer layer of the epidermis, with erythema, increased warmth, tenderness, and pain. Edema, but not vesiculation, usually occurs. In **second-degree burns,** damage extends through the epidermis and involves the dermis, but not sufficiently to interfere with rapid regeneration of epithelium. Vesicles, blebs, or bullae form. In **third-degree (full-thickness) burns,** both the epidermis and dermis are destroyed. Because nerve endings are destroyed, severe pain is unusual after the acute initial pain. The surface may be charred, coagulated, or white and lifeless (as from scalds), and is sometimes insensitive to pinprick. Vesiculation is often absent. The degree of damage varies in different areas of the burn, and it is often difficult to distinguish second- from third-degree burns until areas of third-degree depth demarcate.

The physician must immediately estimate the degree and extent of the burn. A rapid, reasonably accurate, and easily remembered guide is the "**Rule of 9**": head and neck, 9% of BSA; each hand and arm (including deltoid), 9%; each foot and leg as far up as the inferior gluteal fold, 18%; anterior and posterior trunk including buttocks, 18% each; perineum, 1%. For a somewhat more accurate estimate the **Lund and Browder body surface chart** (see Fig. 215–1) is often used, especially for children.

In adults with burns of > 15% of BSA or small children with burns of > 10% of BSA, shock should always be anticipated. **Incipient shock** is suggested by restlessness, thirst, and an increase in pulse rate or a fall in BP when the patient is moved from the recumbent to the sitting position. The symptoms of **advanced shock** include: low BP, weak thready pulse, cold clammy extremities, pale face with beads of cold perspiration and an anxious expression, increased respiration, restlessness, confusion, and oliguria.

Inhalation injury is serious and should be diagnosed promptly. A history of being burned in a closed space, singed nasal hairs, hyperemia of the nasal and pharyngeal mucosa, cough, hoarseness, expectoration of blood or carbon particles, and wheezing (bronchospasm) are early signs of inhalation injury. Laryngeal or pulmonary edema usually develops rapidly. Obstruction, wheezing, sloughing of the mucosa, and pulmonary edema are also signs of **pulmonary thermal injury,** as from steam inhalation.

Treatment

Therapy for all burns includes relief of pain, strict asepsis and wound care, prevention or relief of shock, control of infection, correction of attendant anemia, and maintenance of nutrition. *Treatment of shock* (see below) *takes precedence over local therapy.* In **electrical injury,** the burn must be ignored temporarily if circulatory or respiratory failure occurs, and cardiopulmonary resuscitation is imperative (see CARDIAC ARREST AND CARDIOPULMONARY RESUSCITATION in Ch. 25). Treatment is otherwise the same as for thermal burns of similar extent and depth.

Initial local treatment of **chemical burns** depends on the causative agent. Contaminated clothing must be removed. **Acid and alkali burns** should be washed immediately with large quantities of water and the chemicals neutralized with an appropriate agent (e.g., dilute sodium bicarbonate solution for acid burns, vinegar or dilute acetic acid for alkali burns). **Phenols or cresols** should be neutralized and removed with ethyl alcohol or castor oil. **Phosphorus burns** should be immersed immediately in water to avoid contact with air. Phosphorus particles are removed gently under water and the wound is washed with 1% copper sulfate solution to coat any residual particles with a protective film of copper phosphide; these fluoresce and can be readily removed in a darkened room. Following initial treatment, chemical burns should be treated as thermal burns of comparable size and extent.

1. **General measures:** Pain can usually be relieved by codeine 30 to 60 mg orally or s.c. and aspirin 650 mg orally q 4 to 6 h. Some patients may require morphine 8 to 10 mg s.c. or meperidine 50 to 100 mg orally or IM q 4 to 6 h. **Hypoxia** or mania due to hypoxia requires O_2 therapy.

A **tetanus toxoid booster**, 0.5 to 1 ml s.c. or IM, may be given to patients immunized within 4 to 5 yr; otherwise, tetanus immune globulin (human) 250 u. IM should be given (and repeated every 6 wk as necessary), and concomitant active immunization should be started.

Systemic antibiotics are ineffective as prophylaxis and are given only if needed for concomitant injuries, preexisting disease, or infected burns as determined by cultures and sensitivity studies.

The need for **bed rest** depends on the severity of the injury. The patient's **diet** should be moderately high in calories and high in protein and vitamins. Large amounts of vitamin C (up to 200 mg/day) and vitamin B complex should be given routinely to every burn patient. With burns of > 30% BSA, a diet of 1800 to 2200 kcal/m² is required with a calorie-nitrogen ratio of 150/1.

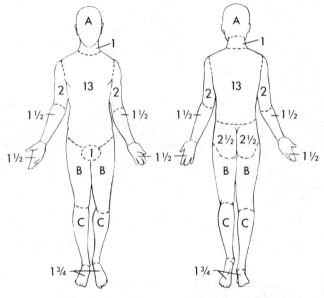

ANTERIOR   POSTERIOR

Relative percentage of areas affected by growth

	Age in years					
	0	1	5	10	15	Adult
A—1/2 of head	9 1/2	8 1/2	6 1/2	5 1/2	4 1/2	3 1/2
B—1/2 of 1 thigh	2 3/4	3 1/4	4	4 1/4	4 1/2	4 3/4
C—1/2 of lower leg	2 1/2	2 1/2	2 3/4	3	3 1/4	3 1/2

FIG. 215–1. **Lund and Browder chart for estimating extent of burns.** (Redrawn from *The Treatment of Burns* by C. P. Artz and J. A. Moncrief, ed. 2. Copyright 1969 by W. B. Saunders Company. Used with permission of W. B. Saunders Company.

2. First- and second-degree burns involving < **10% of BSA (small children) or** < **15% (adults):** The burned areas should be gently cleaned with soap and water and rinsed thoroughly with saline. All dirt, grease, and broken epidermis should be removed; intact epidermis, though burned, should be left in place because healing will progress more effectively beneath it. Unbroken blebs should be evacuated and the overlying epidermis allowed to cover the wound in a flat sheet.

Either open (exposure) or closed treatment is acceptable. **Open treatment** is especially suitable for burns of the hands and extremities because it allows continued mobilization of the joints, which is crucial in preventing joint stiffness and contractures. It is also best for burns of the face, neck, and perineum. In open treatment, the wounds are allowed to dry; this may be hastened by use of a lamp (e.g., a 100-watt bulb in a goose-neck lamp).

In **closed treatment**, sterile, fine-mesh, absorbent gauze is applied first, and is covered by a bulky pressure dressing composed of additional layers of sterile, absorbent gauze, topped by abdominal pads, and all finally enclosed by a firmly applied bandage that provides even compression over the burned area. *Care must be taken to avoid a multiple tourniquet effect.* Burned extremities are often more comfortable if immobilized and elevated; pressure dressings provide good splinting. Ambulatory patients with burns of the arm or hand may find a sling helpful. Pressure dressings on burns uncomplicated by infection may be left in place until the burn has healed (usually in 2 wk), except that the burned area is usually inspected for signs of infection at 5 to 7 days. If the wound is dry and a hard crust has formed, the dressing immediately adjacent to the burn is usually left intact.

Infected burns should be treated q 12 h with a topical antibacterial agent, such as 0.5% silver nitrate solution, mafenide or gentamicin ointment, or 1% silver sulfadiazine cream. Cytotoxins such as tannic acid, picric acid, butamben picrate, or gentian violet or other dyes should *not* be applied, nor should systemic antibiotics be given unless needed for another indication (e.g., pneumonia).

3. Third-degree burns (and deep second-degree burns except on face and hands) involving < **15% of BSA (adults) or** < **10% (children):** Shock is not usually a problem. Treatment is identical with that outlined previously, though burns of more than a few square centimeters require skin grafting to avoid slow healing and disfiguring scars. In small areas of obvious third-degree depth, grafting can be done within a few days of the injury by excision of the burned area, followed by application of split-thickness grafts. Less clearly defined areas should first be dressed, then inspected after 3 to 5 days, by which time second-degree areas can be clearly distinguished from areas of full-thickness skin destruction. The full-thickness areas can then be cleaned, excised, and grafted immediately or after healthy granulation tissue has formed.

4. Third-degree and extensive second-degree burns involving > **15% of BSA (adults) or** > **10% (children):** While the general principles described here apply to all patients, specific requirements for children are discussed separately below.

Shock should be anticipated; its treatment takes precedence over treatment of the burn. Calculation of **IV fluid requirements** during the first 48 h is based on body weight and the amount of BSA burned. Any recognized formula may be used to determine the type, rate, and amount of fluid to be given, but formulas are merely guides and therapy must be modified according to the patient's response. In calculations, patients with burns of > 50% BSA should be considered as having a 50% burn.

Precise clinical and laboratory monitoring of the patient is necessary so that formulas may be altered as needed. An indwelling catheter should be inserted immediately and urinary output measured hourly in all severely burned or anuric patients. A suitable vein should be cannulated at once in all patients for determination of Hb, Hct, blood type, and cross-match. Hb is determined q 3 to 4 h for the first 72 h, and therapy is regulated so that the Hb does not rise above 16 or fall below 11 gm/100 ml. Hct should be maintained at about 40%. Urine volume should be maintained at 50 to 100 ml/h. **Insufficient therapy** can be recognized by a decline in urine volume, an increase in hemoconcentration, and symptoms of shock. **Too rapid IV therapy** may overload the circulation, resulting in pulmonary edema and congestive failure, and should be prevented by monitoring the pulse, respiration, BP, and neck vein distention or the central venous pressure. The lung bases should be auscultated frequently for rales.

During the first 24 h, the patient should receive electrolyte solution to expand plasma volume and increase cardiac output. Colloid is no more effective and is reserved for the second 24-h period postburn. Ringer's lactate solution is the preferred electrolyte solution, since it approximates the ionic concentration of plasma. Isotonic saline can be given if necessary, but hypernatremia and hyperchloremia must be avoided. The Ringer's lactate solution, 4.5 ml/kg body wt/1% of BSA burned, is given IV at a rate sufficient to maintain the urinary output at 50 to 100 ml/h, usually 4 ml/kg/h. At this rate, about ½ the calculated 24-h fluid requirement will be given in the first 8 h.

Progressive and severe **anemia** develops rapidly in patients with extensive infected burns and should be treated vigorously with whole blood transfusions.

If shock is not profound and the likelihood of vomiting is not acute, an oral electrolyte solution (⅓ tsp table salt and ⅓ tsp baking soda in 1 L flavored, sweetened water) can be given. Patients with burns of < 20% of BSA can generally tolerate oral fluids well. Those with burns of 20 to 30% of BSA can be sustained by this route alone if they are not vomiting and can be kept recumbent (since orthostatic hypotension is likely to occur). In those with burns of > 30% of BSA, immediate resuscitation cannot be accomplished with oral fluids alone and IV therapy is required. All burn patients should also be offered electrolyte-free fluids orally, such as sweetened tea or fruit juices.

Patients with preexisting cardiovascular-renal disease present a special problem. Fluid, electrolyte, and colloid administration should be limited to amounts sufficient to produce minimal adequate urinary output (25 ml/h) and the patient watched for signs of circulatory overload. If possible, all fluid except colloids should be given orally or by gavage.

In the second 24 h, the patient is given glucose and water, and no electrolyte solution is given. If this does not maintain the urinary output at 50 to 100 ml/h, colloid (as plasma or plasma protein fraction) is given to expand plasma volume. Urinary output then usually increases and can be readily maintained with glucose and water alone.

By the third day, the patient is usually able to tolerate a high-protein, moderately high-caloric, high-vitamin oral diet containing adequate minerals. Hb, serum electrolytes, and serum proteins should be checked frequently and maintained at as near optimal levels as possible by appropriate therapy.

For children, guidelines for the initial 24 h of therapy include IV fluid maintenance therapy plus plasma in amounts equivalent to 0.5 ml/kg body wt/1% BSA burned and Ringer's lactate equivalent to 1.5 ml/kg body wt/1% BSA. Generally, 1/2 of this quantity is given within the first 8 h following the time of the burn (not the time after reaching the hospital) and 1/4 in each of the ensuing 8-h periods. If shock is not imminent, not over 20 ml/kg body wt of fluid should be given in any 45-min interval. If the burn area exceeds 50% of the body surface, fluid requirements should be computed as if only 50% of the body had been burned. In the second 24-h interval, maintenance fluids plus 50% of the first day's colloid and electrolyte are given.

The rate of IV fluid administration should be adjusted so that (1) urine output averages 1 to 1.5 ml/kg body wt/hr (a urine of high sp gr may indicate either fluid deficit or the onset of inappropriate antidiuretic hormone release), (2) Hb is maintained between 11 and 16 gm/100 ml, (3) vital signs and central venous pressure remain stable, (4) BUN, creatinine, and electrolyte levels remain normal, and (5) cardiopulmonary function is maintained. Children are best given nothing by mouth until their condition has stabilized and bowel function appears adequate. Blood should be given only when the Hb falls below 8 to 9 gm/100 ml.

Burn treatment: Extensive third-degree burns are best treated by the open method and topical antimicrobial therapy. After the burned area is cleaned and debrided, the patient is placed on surgically clean sheets with a cradle over the bed. The room temperature should be about 30 to 32 C (86 to 89.5 F). The burned areas are covered b.i.d. with either 0.5% silver nitrate solution, mafenide, or gentamicin ointment, or 1% silver sulfadiazine cream. Silver nitrate is applied as a saturated 1/2-inch-thick gauze dressing laid directly on the wound and held in place with a light dressing or light cotton blanket. Mafenide, gentamicin, or silver sulfadiazine cream is applied without a dressing, though a single layer of gauze may occasionally be used to hold the cream in place. Occlusive dressings must *not* be used. The wounds are debrided daily. As the necrotic tissue is removed and clean underlying tissue forms, a biologic dressing of homograft or heterograft skin can be applied to prepare the wound for autografting (see SKIN TRANSPLANTATION in Ch. 20).

Following topical applications of silver nitrate, patients may develop excessive Na losses, hypokalemia, hypochloremia, alkalosis, and methemoglobinuria. Mafenide acetate cream applied topically as an antibacterial inhibits carbonic anhydrase activity and may produce compensated metabolic acidosis and, occasionally, proximal renal tubular acidosis.

5. Inhalation injury: Pulmonary edema may develop rapidly in the immediate postburn period or 48 to 72 h later. When present, fluid and colloid therapy should be limited to a volume consistent with a minimal adequate urinary output of 25 ml/h. The respiratory tract must be kept clear by gentle suctioning. O_2 therapy and mechanical ventilators may be necessary. Tracheostomy is indicated if upper airways obstruction occurs. Bronchospasm is common and a bronchodilator (e.g., aminophylline 250 mg IV slowly or isoproterenol aerosol mist) may be helpful.

6. Disaster: Warfare or other disaster may require treating large numbers of burn victims. Minimal early therapy for all but those with minor burns consists of oral electrolyte fluids (1/3 tsp table salt and 1/3 tsp baking soda in 1 qt water, flavored and sweetened if feasible). If it can be retained, one to two 8-oz glasses/h should be given. The demand for parenteral colloid may vastly exceed the supply and it should be reserved for those most likely to benefit from it. Open treatment of burned areas without dressings usually is a logistic necessity. Tetanus toxoid booster immunization should be given (see 1 above, under Treatment). Morphine 10 to 15 mg IV should be given to those in great pain and despair.

216. HEAT DISORDERS

HEAT STROKE AND HEAT EXHAUSTION

Mild to grave reactions to high temperature due to inadequate or inappropriate responses of heat-regulating mechanisms.

Etiology

Prolonged exposure to high ambient temperatures may lead either to excessive fluid loss and hypovolemic shock (heat exhaustion) or to failure of heat loss mechanisms and dangerous hyperpyrexia (heat stroke). Dehydration, excessive sweating, vomiting, diarrhea, age, and debility predispose to either; high humidity, strenuous exertion, poor ventilation, and heavy clothing contribute. Though stemming from the same cause, these 2 reactions to heat are sharply different (see TABLE 216–1).

Prophylaxis

Common sense is the best preventive; strenuous exertion in a very hot environment, inadequately ventilated space, or heavy, insulating clothing should be avoided; loss of fluid and electrolytes (often imperceptible in very hot, very dry air) should be replaced by continuous oral fluids slightly salty to taste (i.e., near isotonic). Sometimes exertion in a hot environment cannot be avoided; every effort should then be made to replace lost fluid and salt and to keep the skin temperature cool by evaporation. Salt tablets occasionally cause gastric distress and are less desirable than lightly salted beverages and foods.

HEAT STROKE (Sunstroke; Hyperpyrexia; Thermic Fever; Siriasis)

Symptoms and Signs

An abrupt onset is sometimes preceded by prodromal headache, vertigo, and fatigue. Absence or cessation of sweating is a key sign, as is a hot, flushed, dry skin. The pulse rate increases rapidly and may reach 160 to 180; respirations usually increase, but BP is seldom affected. Disorientation may briefly precede unconsciousness or convulsions. The temperature climbs rapidly to 40 or 41 C (105 or 106 F) and the patient feels as if burning up. Circulatory collapse may precede death; after hours of extreme hyperpyrexia, survivors may have permanent brain damage.

Diagnosis and Prognosis

Hot, dry, flushed skin, high body temperature, and rapid pulse in a person exposed to a hot environment are usually enough to distinguish heat stroke from food, chemical, or drug poisoning. Heat stroke is a *serious emergency* and unless promptly and energetically treated, results in convulsions and death or permanent brain damage. Core temperature of 41 C (106 F) is a grave prognostic sign; temperature a degree higher is often fatal. Old age, debility, or alcoholism worsen the prognosis.

Treatment

Heroic measures should be instituted immediately. If distant from a hospital, the patient should be wrapped in wet bedding or clothing, immersed in a lake or stream, or even cooled with snow or ice while waiting for transportation. WARNING: *The temperature should be taken every 10 min and not allowed to fall below 38.5 C (101 F) to avoid converting hyperpyrexia to hypothermia.* Once in hospi-

TABLE 216–1. DIFFERENTIATION BETWEEN HEAT STROKE AND HEAT EXHAUSTION

	Heat Stroke	Heat Exhaustion
Cause	Inadequate or failure of heat loss	Excessive fluid loss—hypovolemic shock
Warnings	Headache, weakness, sudden loss of consciousness	Gradual weakness, nausea, anxiety, excess sweating, syncope
Appearance and Signs	Hot, red, dry skin; little sweating; hard rapid pulse; very high temperature	Pale, grayish, clammy skin; weak, slow pulse; low BP; faintness
Management	Emergency cooling by wrapping or immersion in cold water or ice; immediate hospitalization	As for simple syncope: head down; replace lost salt and water (usually orally, rarely IV)

tal, more exact control measures are instituted and the core temperature is monitored continuously to avoid hypothermia. Stimulants and sedatives including morphine are avoided; diazepam or a barbiturate may be given IV if convulsions are not otherwise controllable. Electrolyte determinations should guide IV therapy. Bed rest is desirable for a few days after severe heat stroke, and temperature lability may be expected for some time.

HEAT EXHAUSTION (Heat Prostration, Collapse, or Syncope)

Symptoms and Signs

Due to excessive fluid loss, this disorder gives adequate warning by increasing fatigue, weakness, anxiety, and drenching sweats, leading to circulatory collapse with slow thready pulse, low or imperceptible BP, cold, pale, clammy skin, and disordered mentation followed by a shock-like unconsciousness. Temperature is *below* normal and the picture is that of simple syncope.

Diagnosis and Prognosis

Heat exhaustion causing vasomotor collapse is more difficult to differentiate than heat stroke from insulin shock, poisoning, hemorrhage, or traumatic shock. Usually the history of heat exposure, failure of hydration, absence of other apparent cause, and response to treatment are sufficient for diagnosis. The condition is usually transient and the prognosis is good unless circulatory failure is prolonged.

Treatment

Heat exhaustion requires restoration of normal blood volume and assurance of adequate brain perfusion. The patient should be placed flat or with head down. Small amounts of cool, slightly salty fluids should be given orally every few minutes to restore normovolemia. Isotonic saline IV, cardiac stimulants, or plasma volume expanders (albumin, dextran) are seldom needed, and should be given cautiously to avoid overloading an embarrassed circulatory system.

HEAT CRAMPS

Severe cramps of striated muscle resulting from excessive sweating due to exertion and/or high ambient temperatures.

Etiology

Heat cramps are due to excessive loss of sodium chloride by profuse sweating during strenuous activity at high atmospheric temperatures ($>$ 38 C [100 F]). It is common in manual laborers (e.g., engine room personnel, steel workers, and miners), in mountaineers or skiers overdressed against the cold, and in those not acclimatized to hot, dry climates where excessive sweating is almost undetected because of rapid evaporation.

Symptoms and Signs

Onset is often abrupt, with muscles of the extremities affected first. Severe pain and carpopedal spasm may incapacitate the hands and feet. Often episodic, the cramping makes the muscles feel like hard knots. When the cramps affect only the abdominal muscles, the pain may simulate an acute abdomen. Vital signs are usually normal. The skin may be either hot and dry or clammy and cool, depending on the humidity.

Prophylaxis and Treatment

In most instances, heat cramp is prevented and also rapidly relieved by drinking fluids or eating foods containing sodium chloride. If the patient cannot take food or drink orally, IV saline may be necessary. Sodium chloride tablets are often used for prophylaxis, but can cause stomach irritation, and overdose may lead to edema. Awareness of the problem is usually sufficient to prevent it.

---

217. COLD INJURY

(Frostnip; Frostbite; Accidental Hypothermia; Exposure; Immersion or Trench Foot; Chilblains;
Pernio)

Injury of the extremities by cold, with secondary structural and functional disturbances of the smaller surface blood vessels, the nerves, and the skin; or generalized lowering of body temperature.

Etiology

Exposure to damp cold (temperatures around freezing) causes immersion or trench foot, chilblains, and frostnip. Exposure to dry cold (temperatures well below freezing) more often causes frostbite and exposure (accidental hypothermia). The risk and extent of cold injury are increased by heat loss by conduction (wet clothing, contact with metals), convection (windchill), and radiation (dependent on the temperature gradient between body and surroundings). Vulnerability to cold injury is also increased when circulation is impaired by cardiovascular disease, drunkenness, impaired consciousness, exhaustion, hunger, or very young or old age (see also ACCIDENTAL HYPOTHERMIA in Ch. 232).

Pathology

Ice crystals may form in or between cells; capillaries may thrombose due to sludging of RBCs; neurovascular impulses may cause shunting of blood, thus sacrificing the injured area to ensure survival of the whole; or, most likely, combinations of all the above occur. Cold injuries range from mild to severe. Most dry-cold injury is superficial; the gangrenous area is often less than a few mm thick and consists of a hard black carapace over healthier tissue. Deeper damp-cold injury causes more physiologic aberrations (e.g., edema, blotchy cyanosis, increased sweating, and paresthesias) than it does tissue loss. The pathophysiology of the long-term sequelae that may follow cold injury is unknown.

Diagnosis

Frostnip (superficial damp-cold injury) leaves firm, white, cold areas on the face, ears, or extremities. Peeling or blistering (as from mild or severe sunburn) may occur in 24 to 72 h and there may occasionally be mild long-term cold sensitivity. In **other damp-cold injury** (e.g., **immersion or trench foot, chilblains**), the feet or hands are pale, edematous, numb, and clammy; the tissue is often macerated; and there are usually prolonged symptoms (e.g., increased sweating and cold susceptibility, hyperesthesia, and edema) due to neurovascular instability. In **frostbite**, the injured area is cold, hard, white, and anesthetic, and becomes blotchy-red, swollen, and painful on rewarming. Depending on the extent of injury, symptoms may subside with few residua, or gangrene may ensue. **Exposure** (hypothermia) may result in lethargy, mental confusion, hallucinations, partial or total loss of consciousness, slowed or arrested respiration, and slowed, irregular, and ultimately arrested heartbeat. The victim's rectal temperature may be as low as 27 C (80 F). It is important to differentiate possible coexisting disorders (e.g., CVA, cardiac disease, diabetic coma, insulin shock, drunkenness) from the cold injury and to treat both concurrently.

Prophylaxis

Preventive measures, though obvious, are often ignored. Warm, multilayered clothing with good hand and foot protection (avoiding constricting wrist bands and tight socks and shoes) should be worn. Warm headgear is particularly important since much heat is lost through the unprotected head. Fatigue, hunger, young or old age, circulatory illness, fear, alcohol, windchill, and hypoxia increase the risk of cold injury.

Treatment

The old methods of slow rewarming or rubbing with or without snow are *contraindicated*. The best treatment for **frostnip** is by rapid local rewarming with the unaffected hands or with a warm object. **Frostbite** is also treated by rapid rewarming. The best method, if available, is a warm bath. Hot drinks to warm the whole body from within, heating pads, or hot water bottles are also effective. The temperatures used for rewarming should be 38 to 43 C (100 to 110 F). Since the affected tissues are anesthetic and therefore susceptible to burns, **the temperature must not exceed 43 C (110 F)**, whatever method of rewarming is used. Snuggling next to a warm companion or rewarming the hands or feet against the abdomen or axilla may be effective in the field. If water is used for rewarming, it should be followed by careful drying of the skin so as to avoid injury. Frozen feet must *not* be thawed or warmed if the victim must walk for any considerable distance to care.

Immediate in-hospital treatment should include low molecular weight dextran (20 ml/kg q 24 h) infusion, and reserpine (2 mg q 6 h IV) to decrease sludging and improve microcirculation. Damaged tissue should be carefully cleaned using sterile technics and protected with sterile drapes but left open to air circulation. Blisters should not be broken. A tetanus booster should be given and infection prevented by antibiotics (tetracycline or ampicillin 250 mg q 6 h).

Pain may be relieved by morphine if necessary (up to 15 mg IM q 3 h, being careful not to depress respiration in an unconscious patient or when at high altitudes), though aspirin (650 mg q 3 h) is usually sufficient and may, through inhibition of platelet aggregation, decrease capillary sludging and thrombosis. The patient's nutrition and morale require special attention. Surgery should be delayed. The adage "Freeze in January, operate in July" is sound. Most severe cold injury is more superficial than it seems; even severe gangrene causes less tissue loss than at first appears inevitable. As the area of tissue damage becomes more sharply demarcated over weeks or months, it should be kept sterile and observed for signs of infection; debridement should be *avoided*. Whirlpool baths (t.i.d. with water containing disinfectant) are often helpful but may increase risk of infection.

Severe exposure (hypothermia) is a major emergency. The victim is found semiconscious or unconscious, often some distance from shelter. *At the scene*, if cardiac arrest has occurred, cardiopulmonary resuscitation is the first priority (see CARDIAC ARREST AND CARDIOPULMONARY RESUSCITATION in Ch. 25), but it may be difficult to restore sinus rhythm if core temperature is below 29 C (85 F). The cold heart is usually slow, weak, and highly vulnerable to ventricular fibrillation **(VF)**. Therefore, vigorous efforts to improve the airway and ventilation should be avoided; jarring, sudden motions, or other stress should be minimized. Many authorities believe it preferable to have a slow, regular heart rhythm, even with impaired respiratory exchange, rather than risk precipitating VF. Since unconscious or semiconscious victims cannot generate sufficient heat to rewarm themselves, they must be rewarmed externally. However, if rewarming is too rapid, further heat may be lost because of peripheral vasodilation. The victim should be taken to a hospital immediately; but if this is delayed, rewarming can be started at the scene by immersing the victim's hands and forearms in water maintained at 45 to 48 C (113 to 118 F) and controlled by a thermometer. The water should feel uncomfortably but bearably hot to the rescuer's elbow. If conscious, the victim may be given hot drinks. Although alcohol has been considered to be contraindicated, some recent research indicates that it does not decrease core temperature by peripheral vasodilation as previously believed and that its euphoric effect may be beneficial.

The optimal method of *in-hospital* rewarming is controversial. Some persons advocate whole-body immersion in hot water maintained at 45 to 48 C (113 to 118 F). Others believe that nothing will succeed if the victim's rectal temperature continues to fall after rescue, and that whole-body immersion may actually tip the scales against recovery. Once rectal temperature begins to rise, the patient's metabolic status should be monitored q 3 h. Acidosis should be anticipated and corrected, and O_2 should be given to sustain Pa_{O_2} at above normal levels. IV fluids are given through a central venous catheter that is also used to measure central venous pressure. Core temperature may be raised by gastric lavage with warm D/W; peritoneal dialysis or hemodialysis has also been recommended. It is prudent, though debated, to give antibiotics. A tetanus booster is often recommended, though its necessity is unclear. Massive IV doses of corticosteroids are often recommended, especially for severe, stubborn shock. Vasodilators and anticoagulants are now rarely used, though the latter may be indicated if thromboembolic disease (not uncommon in cold injury) is suspected. A high-caloric diet with supplemental vitamins is desirable during recovery.

---

218.   RADIATION REACTIONS AND INJURIES

The harmful effects—acute, delayed, or chronic—produced in body tissues by exposure to ionizing radiations.

Etiology

Harmful sources of ionizing radiation once were limited primarily to high-energy x-rays used for diagnosis and therapy, and to radium and related radioactive materials. Present sources of potential radiation injury include nuclear reactors, cyclotrons, linear accelerators, alternating gradient synchrotrons, and sealed cobalt and cesium sources for cancer therapy. Numerous artificial radioactive materials have been produced for use in medicine and industry by neutron activation in reactors.

The accidental escape of large amounts of radiation from reactors has occurred several times. Most of these events occurred in the early developmental phase of research reactors and were due to control failure or major breaches of safety regulations. Radiation exposure from such accidents during the first 30 yr up to 1975 resulted in $>$ 30 serious exposures with 7 deaths. The possibility of further mishaps, although remote, has increased because of the use of fissionable fuel for commercial power reactors. Nuclear power generators must meet stringent federal standards that limit effluent radioactivity to extremely low levels. Although background radioactivity in the earth and in its atmosphere increased after the years of atmospheric nuclear weapons testing, it appears to have stabilized at present levels. Ionizing radiation—whether in the form of x-rays, neutrons, protons, α or β particles, or γ-rays—acts either directly or by secondary reactions to produce ionization in tissues. Interaction with water and other protoplasmic constituents causes biochemical lesions that initiate a series of histologic changes and physiologic symptoms and signs that vary with the dose of radiation and the time after exposure. In addition to the early somatic effects of large doses (clinically observable within days), changes in the DNA of rapidly proliferating cells may become manifest as a disease or as a genetic effect in offspring many years later.

Total dose and dose rate determine somatic or genetic effects. The units of measurement commonly used in determining radiation exposure or dose are the roentgen, the rad, and the rem. The **roentgen (R)** is a measure of quantity of x or γ ionizing radiation in air. The **radiation absorbed dose (rad)** is the amount of energy absorbed in any tissue or substance from exposure and applies to all types of radiation. The R and the rad are nearly equivalent for practical purposes. The **rem** is used in describing the observation that some types of radiation, such as neutrons, may produce more biological effect for an equivalent amount of absorbed energy; thus the rem is equal to the rad times a constant called the "quality factor." For x and γ radiation, the rem is equal to the rad. The rad and the rem are currently being replaced in the scientific nomenclature by 2 units that are comparable with the International System of Units, namely, the **gray (Gy)**, equal to 100 rads, and the **Sievert (Sv)**, equal to 100 rem.

The **dose rate** is the radiation dose/unit of time. From the very low dose rates of unavoidable background radiation (about 0.1 rad/yr), where no effect can be detected, the probability of measurable effects increases as the dose rate and/or total dose increases. An observable effect becomes quite certain after a single dose of several hundred rads, but may require higher doses if given at a low dose rate, or intermittently. As a rule, large doses are of concern because of their immediate somatic effects, while low doses are of concern because of the potential for possible late somatic and long-term genetic effects. The effects of radiation exposure on an individual are cumulative.

The **body area** exposed is also an important factor. The entire human body can probably absorb up to 200 rads without fatality; however, as the whole-body dose approaches 450 rads the death rate will approximate 50% (i.e., LD50), and a total wholebody dose of > 600 rads received in a very short time will almost certainly be fatal. By contrast, many thousands of rads delivered over a long period of time (e.g., for cancer treatment) can be tolerated by the body when small volumes of tissue are irradiated. **Distribution of the dose** within the body is also important. For example, protection of bowel or bone marrow by appropriate shielding will permit survival of the exposed individual from what would be an otherwise fatal whole-body dose.

Pathophysiology

Tissues vary in response to immediate radiation injury according to the following descending order of sensitivity: (1) lymphoid cells, (2) gonads, (3) proliferating cells of the bone marrow, (4) epithelial cells of the bowel, (5) epidermis, (6) hepatic cells, (7) epithelium of the lung alveoli and biliary passages, (8) kidney epithelial cells, (9) endothelial cells (pleura and peritoneum), (10) nerve cells, (11) bone cells, (12) muscle and connective tissue. Generally, the more rapid the turnover of the cell, the greater the radiation sensitivity.

If the absorbed dose of radiation is sufficiently high, death of any living cell (as judged by pathologic criteria of necrosis) will occur. Large but sublethal doses of radiation may produce disturbances in cell proliferation: (a) the rate of mitosis is decreased and (b) DNA synthesis is impaired in 2 ways—first, the rate of synthesis is slowed; second, cells may continue DNA synthesis and become polypoid. These and other ill-defined effects of radiation are reasonably certain to occur after significant tissue doses in categories 1 to 4, above, are received.

Diminished production of new cells in tissues that normally undergo continual renewal (e.g., enteric mucosa, marrow, gonads) results in progressive hypoplasia, atrophy, and eventually fibrosis, depending on the dose. Some cells, injured but still capable of mitosis, may be so damaged that they will pass through 1 or 2 generative cycles, producing abnormal progeny such as giant metamyelocytes and hypersegmented neutrophils before they die.

Symptoms and Signs

The disruption of cell renewal systems and direct injury of other tissues produce clearly defined clinical syndromes:

1. Acute radiation syndromes: The syndromes, depending on dose, dose rate, area of the body, and time after exposure, can be divided into cerebral, GI, and hematopoietic categories.

The **cerebral syndrome** is produced by extremely high total body doses of radiation (> 3000 rads), is always fatal, and consists of 3 phases: a prodromal period of nausea and vomiting; then listlessness and drowsiness ranging from apathy to prostration (possibly due to nonbacterial inflammatory foci in the brain or the effects of radiation-induced toxic products); and, finally, a more generalized component characterized by tremors, convulsions, ataxia, and death within a few hours.

The **gastrointestinal syndrome** (400 or more rads) occurs when the total body dose of radiation is smaller but still high. It is characterized by intractable nausea, vomiting, and diarrhea that lead to severe dehydration, diminished plasma volume, vascular collapse, and death. The GI syndrome results from the initial "toxemia" due to necrosis of tissue and is perpetuated by progressive atrophy of the GI mucosa. Ultimately, the intestinal villi are denuded, with massive loss of plasma into the intestine. Regeneration of intestinal epithelial cells may be possible after large doses of radiation; massive plasma replacement and antibiotics during the first 4 to 6 days will keep patients alive until the epithelium regenerates. However, even if the patient does survive, the respite is temporary, since hematopoietic failure will ensue, commencing within 2 or 3 wk.

The **hematopoietic syndrome** (200 to 1000 rads), characterized by anorexia, apathy, nausea, and vomiting, may be maximal within 6 to 12 h. Symptoms then subside, so that within 24 to 36 h after exposure the subject is asymptomatic. During this period of relative well-being, lymph nodes, spleen, and bone marrow begin to atrophy, leading to pancytopenia. This atrophy is the result of 2 distinct processes—direct killing of radiosensitive cells and inhibition of new cell production. In the peripheral blood, lymphopenia commences immediately, becoming maximal within 24 to 36 h. Neutropenia develops more slowly. Thrombocytopenia may be prominent within 3 or 4 wk.

Increased susceptibility to infection develops due to (1) a dose-dependent decrease in circulating granulocytes and lymphocytes, (2) a dose-dependent impairment of antibody production, (3) impairment of granulocyte migration and phagocytosis, (4) decreased ability of the reticuloendothelial system to kill phagocytized bacteria, (5) diminished resistance to diffusion in subcutaneous tissues, and (6) hemorrhagic areas of the skin and bowel that encourage entrance and growth of bacteria. Susceptibility to infection by both saprophytic and pathogenic organisms is present. Hemorrhage is mainly due to the thrombocytopenia.

With acute total body radiation doses of > 600 rads, hematopoietic or GI malfunction will be fatal; with doses < 600 rads, the probability of survival is inversely related to the total dose.

2. Acute "radiation sickness" following therapeutic irradiation (particularly of the abdomen) is characterized by nausea, vomiting, diarrhea, anorexia, headache, malaise, and tachycardia of varying severity. The discomfort subsides within a few hours or days; its cause is not understood.

3. Delayed effects: (a) *Intermediate effects*: Prolonged or repeated exposure to low dose rates from internally deposited or external sources of radiation may produce amenorrhea, decreased fertility in both sexes, decreased libido only in the female, anemia, leukopenia, thrombocytopenia, and cataracts. More severe or highly localized exposure causes loss of hair, skin atrophy and ulceration, keratosis, and telangiectasia, and ultimately may cause squamous cell carcinomas. Osteosarcomas may appear years after ingestion of radioactive bone-seeking nuclides such as radium salts.

Serious injury to exposed organs may occur occasionally after extensive radiotherapy for cancer. Renal functional changes include a decrease in renal plasma flow, GFR, and tubular function. Clinical manifestations may occur acutely after extremely high doses (after a latent period of 6 mo to 1 yr) and may include proteinuria, renal insufficiency of varying degree, anemia, and hypertension. When cumulative kidney exposure is > 2000 rads in less than 5 wk, radiation fibrosis and oliguric renal failure will occur in about 37% of cases. The remainder will develop variable changes over a prolonged time. Large accumulated doses to muscles may result in painful myopathy with atrophy and calcification. Very rarely, these changes may be followed by a neoplastic change, usually a sarcoma. Radiation pneumonitis and subsequent pulmonary fibrosis may be severe when lung metastases are irradiated, and can be fatal after a cumulative dose of > 3000 rads if treatment is not spread over a sufficient period. Radiation pericarditis and myocarditis have been produced by extensive mediastinal radiotherapy. Catastrophic myelopathy may develop after a segment of the spinal cord has received cumulative doses > 4000 rads. Following vigorous therapy of abdominal lymph nodes for seminoma, lymphoma, or ovarian carcinoma, chronic ulceration, fibrosis, and perforation of the bowel may develop. Skin erythema and skin ulceration were observed fairly often during the era of orthovoltage x-ray therapy, but the high-energy photons produced by cobalt units or accelerators penetrate deeply into tissues and have virtually eliminated these complications.

(b) *Late somatic and genetic effects*: Radiation alters the "information system" of proliferating somatic and germ cells. With somatic cells this may be manifested ultimately as somatic disease—e.g., cancer (leukemia, thyroid, skin, bone) or cataracts—or, as suggested in animal models, by nonspecific shortening of life. Leukemia from substantial radiation in humans has been observed. It is asserted, but not proved, that there is no "threshold" dose for leukemia, and that the incidence increases with dose. Thyroid carcinoma has been observed 20 to 30 yr after x-ray treatment for adenoid and tonsillar hypertrophy, and x-ray treatment for nonmalignant conditions is now considered inappropriate except in highly unusual situations.

With germ cell exposure, the number of mutations is increased. If mutations are perpetuated by procreation, in the course of generations we can extrapolate from animal studies that they will be expressed as an increasing number of genetic defectives. Although this has not been observed in man as a direct result of germ cell irradiation, the possibility presents a serious medical, ethical, and philosophic problem with respect to unborn generations. It imposes a moral obligation to limit radiation exposure to that which is absolutely necessary for valid diagnostic or therapeutic purposes, and to strictly control occupational exposure. The potential harm, however, should be kept in perspective. Some investigators suggest that no measurable effects will occur below a certain threshold while others insist that any radiation is potentially harmful. The long-term probability of a measurable genetic or somatic effect appearing in a given individual is about 10^{-4}/rad.

Diagnosis and Prognosis

When a person is receiving therapeutic radiation or has been exposed during a radiation accident, the etiology is obvious. However, prognosis depends on the dose and its distribution within the body. Extensive review of the accident and serial hematologic and bone marrow studies to gauge the severity of marrow injury are necessary to accurately determine the prognosis.

When the cerebral or GI syndromes are present after an accident, the diagnosis is simple but the prognosis grave. Death occurs with the cerebral syndrome within a few hours to a few days; with GI symptoms within 3 to 10 days; and with hematopoietic symptoms in 8 to 50 days. In the last syndrome, death may occur from a supervening infection in 2 to 4 wk or from massive hemorrhage between weeks 3 and 6.

In **chronic** cases, where external exposure is either unknown, overlooked, or low-level, a diagnosis may be difficult or impossible. A search for possible occupational exposure is required. In institutions licensed by federal or state governments, records of exposure to radiation are maintained. Serial chromosome studies can be performed to watch for types and frequency of chromosomal abnormalities that are likely to occur after significant radiation exposure, but such abnormalities may have preexisted or been induced by nonradiation causes. Periodic examination for early cataracts is appropriate in situations leading to chronic radiation exposure of the eye, especially to neutrons.

Cases of alleged exposure to radiation are difficult to evaluate since emotional or psychologic factors tend to predominate. Unless the individual has received a documented external or internal dose, exact diagnosis is probably impossible. Normal hematologic values and absence of objective clinical illness would permit reassurance of the patient and others concerned.

Prophylaxis

Many drugs and chemicals are known to increase the survival rate in animals if given prior to irradiation; e.g., sulfhydryl compounds. However, none are of practical value in man. The only certain way to avoid fatal or serious overexposure is the rigorous enforcement of protective measures and adherence to the maximum permissible dose (MPD) levels. These values are listed in *Basic Radiation*

Protection Criteria, NCRP Report No. 39, published by the National Council on Radiation Protection and Measurements (P.O. Box 30175, Washington, D. C. 20014).

Treatment

Contamination of the skin by radioactive materials should be immediately removed by copious water irrigation and special chelating solutions containing EDTA when available (Radiac Wash®). Small puncture wounds must be treated vigorously to remove contamination. Irrigation and debridement are indicated until the wound is free of radioactivity. Ingested material should be removed promptly by induced vomiting or lavage if exposure is recent. If radioiodine is inhaled or ingested in large quantities, the patient should be given Lugol's solution or saturated solution of potassium iodide to block thyroid uptake for days to weeks, and diuresis should be promoted. Monitoring of exposed patients is mandatory, using hand-type rate-meter probes or sophisticated whole-body counting. Urine should be analyzed for non–gamma-emitting radionuclides if exposure to these agents is suspected. Radon breath analysis can be done in cases of suspected radium ingestion.

For the **acute cerebral syndrome,** treatment is palliative, since this syndrome is uniformly fatal, and is directed toward combating shock and anoxia, relieving pain and anxiety, and sedation for control of convulsions.

Symptoms of **radiation sickness due to therapeutic irradiation of the abdomen** can be controlled in part by an antiemetic (e.g., prochlorperazine 5 to 10 mg orally or IM q.i.d.) and may be prevented by administering the drug beforehand. Attention to nutrition and fluid balance through close cooperation between radiotherapist and referring physician is mandatory. Most difficulties can be avoided or minimized by careful planning of the overall management (e.g., dose, time interval between treatments, supportive therapy).

If the **gastrointestinal syndrome** develops after external whole-body irradiation, the type and degree of therapy will be dictated by the severity of the symptoms. After modest exposure, antiemetics and sedation may suffice. If oral feeding can be started, a bland diet is tolerated best. Fluid, electrolytes, and plasma, by appropriate routes, may be required in huge volumes. The amount and type will be dictated by blood chemical studies (especially electrolytes and proteins), blood pressure, pulse, fluid exchange, and skin turgor.

Management of the **hematopoietic syndrome,** with its obvious potentially lethal factors of infection, hemorrhage, and anemia, is similar to therapy of marrow hypoplasia and pancytopenia from any cause. Antibiotics, fresh blood, and platelet transfusions are the main therapeutic aids. Rigid asepsis during all skin-puncturing procedures is mandatory as is strict isolation to prevent exposure to pathogens.

Concurrent antineoplastic chemotherapy or use of other marrow-suppressing drugs, unless strongly indicated because of some preexisting clinical condition or sudden complication, should be *avoided* because of the potential for further suppression of blood-forming elements in bone marrow.

Bone marrow transplants have proved helpful in genetically identical animals. If a dose > 200 rads is suspected, tissue typing and search for a compatible bone marrow should be made. If an identical twin is available, a marrow transplant will increase the probability of survival. If granulocytes and platelets continue to decrease at a constant rate and fall to < 500 and 20,000/cu mm, respectively, homotransplantation of marrow should be considered, though the likelihood of success is small and the transplant may be followed by a potentially fatal immunologic graft-vs.-host reaction.

In dealing with **late somatic effects due to serious chronic exposure,** removal of the patient from the radiation source is the first step. With radium, thorium, or radiostrontium deposition in the body, prompt administration of oral and parenteral chelating agents (EDTA) will increase the excretion rate. However, in the late stages these agents are useless. Radiation ulcers and cancers require surgical removal and plastic repair. Radiation-induced leukemia is treated like any similar spontaneous leukemia. Anemia is corrected by whole-blood transfusion. Thrombocytopenic bleeding may be reduced by platelet transfusions. However, these measures are of only temporary value since the probability is slight that an extensively damaged bone marrow will regenerate. No effective treatment for sterility, or for ovarian and testicular dysfunction, except for hormonal supplementation, has been devised.

---

219. ELECTRIC SHOCK

Injury resulting from the passage of an electric current through the body. Electric shock may be caused by contact with lightning, high-voltage transmission lines, low-voltage lines in the home and industry, etc. The modern hospital, with its many electric devices, appliances, and instruments, is also a potential source of electric shock, particularly where equipment is attached directly to the patient's body.

Pathogenesis

Factors that determine the form and severity of injury (which may range from a small minor burn to death) include (1) the type and magnitude of current, (2) the resistance of the body at the point of contact, (3) the current pathway, and (4) the duration of current flow.

In general, **direct current (DC)**, which has zero frequency (although it may be intermittent or pulsating), is less dangerous than **alternating current (AC)**, which is the type of current generally used in the USA. The effects of AC on the body depend to a great extent on the frequency—low-frequency currents, 50 to 60 Hz (cycles/second), usually being more dangerous than high-frequency currents. Both types may affect the body by either altering physiologic functions (involuntary muscular contractions and seizures, ventricular fibrillation, respiratory arrest due to CNS injury or muscle paralysis, etc.) or producing thermal, electrochemical, or other damage (burns, necrosis of muscle and other tissue, hemolysis, coagulation, dehydration, vertebral and other skeletal fractures, muscle and tendon avulsion, etc.). Electric shock often causes a combination of these effects.

The **threshold of perception** for DC entering the hand is about 5 milliamperes (mA); for AC, 60 Hz, about 1 mA. The maximum current that can cause contraction of the flexor musculature of the arm but still permit the subject to release his hand from the current source is termed the "**let-go**" **current.** For DC this value is about 75 mA; for AC, about 15 mA. A low-voltage (110 to 220 volts) 60-Hz AC traveling through an intact skin and a transthoracic pathway for a fraction of a second can induce **ventricular fibrillation** at currents as low as 60 to 100 mA; about 300 to 500 mA of DC are required. If the current has a direct pathway to the heart (e.g., via a cardiac catheter or pacemaker electrodes), much smaller currents (< 1 mA, AC or DC) can produce fibrillation.

Body resistance (measured in ohms) is concentrated primarily in the skin, and varies directly with the skin's condition. Dry, well-keratinized, intact skin may have a resistance of several hundred thousand ohms, whereas the resistance of moist, thin skin is about 500 ohms. If the skin is punctured (e.g., from a cut or abrasion, or by a needle), or if current is applied to moist mucous membranes (e.g., mouth, rectum, vagina), the resistance may be as low as 200 to 300 ohms.

The **pathway of current** through the body can be crucial in determining human injury. Conduction from arm to arm or between an arm and a foot at ground potential is much more dangerous than contact between a leg and ground since the current may traverse the heart.

The **duration of current flow** through the body is another major factor. While the heart is vulnerable to small currents at relatively low voltages (see ventricular fibrillation, above), the effects of prolonged electric contact with the body are twofold: (1) sweating increases, reducing the skin resistance and increasing the current flow; and (2) heat is produced, which causes severe burns, coagulation of protein, and necrosis of tissues.

Symptoms and Signs

The effects and clinical manifestations of electrical injuries depend on the factors discussed above. Electricity can startle a person and cause him to fall down or to drop objects. It may cause severe, spastic stimulation and contraction of the muscles, followed by excitation, hyperventilation, loss of reflex control, and unconsciousness. Both respiratory paralysis (apnea) and ventricular fibrillation may occur. Sharply demarcated electrical burns may be present on the skin and extend well into the subjacent tissues (see also Ch. 215).

Treatment

Treatment consists of (1) separating the patient from the current source, and (2) reestablishing vital functions immediately.

Breaking contact between the victim and the current source can be done either by **shutting off the current** or by **removing the person from contact with it.** The best method is to cut off the source if it can be done rapidly (e.g., throwing a circuit breaker or switch, disconnecting the device from its electrical outlet, or cutting the wires, using insulated tools such as an axe with a wooden handle); otherwise, the victim must be removed from the source. The rescuer should first ensure that he himself is well insulated from ground, and then should use an insulating material (e.g., cloth, dry wood, rubber, leather belt) to pull the person free.

Immediately after separating the victim from the source, **a rapid examination for vital functions should be performed** (e.g., radial, brachial, or carotid pulses; respiratory function; level of consciousness). If no pulses are palpable, external cardiac massage should be administered until pulses return, or until the patient is pronounced dead. If spontaneous respiration is not observed, mouth-to-mouth resuscitation should be instituted until it does return, or until a more adequate means of maintaining ventilatory assistance is provided. Heart-lung resuscitation technics are detailed in CARDIAC ARREST AND CARDIOPULMONARY RESUSCITATION, in Ch. 25.

Once vital functions have been reestablished, the full nature and extent of the injury must be evaluated (see Pathogenesis, above) and treated.

Prevention

Prevention of electrical injuries entails proper design and installation of all electric devices, whether in the home, office, hospital, or industry. Education and compliance are essential. Any electric device that touches or may be touched by the body and has life-threatening potential should be properly grounded and incorporated in circuits containing fail-safe equipment. **Ground-fault cir-**

cuit breakers, which trip at current leakage to ground levels of as low as 5 mA, are excellent safety devices and are commercially available.

---

220. MOTION SICKNESS

A disorder caused by repetitive angular and linear acceleration and deceleration and characterized primarily by nausea and vomiting. Sea-, air-, car-, train-, and swing-sickness are specific forms. Prevention is easier than treatment.

Etiology

Excessive stimulation of the vestibular apparatus by motion is the primary cause. There is great individual variation in susceptibility. The pathways of the afferent impulses from the labyrinth to the vomiting center in the medulla are undefined, but motion sickness only occurs when the 8th nerve and cerebellar vestibular tracts are intact. Visual stimuli (e.g., a moving horizon), poor ventilation (fumes, smoke, and carbon monoxide), and emotional factors (e.g., fear, anxiety) commonly act in concert with motion to precipitate an attack.

Symptoms and Signs

Cyclic nausea and vomiting are characteristic. They may be preceded by yawning, hyperventilation, salivation, pallor, profuse cold sweating, and somnolence. Aerophagia, dizziness, headache, general discomfort, and fatigue may also occur. Once nausea and vomiting develop, the patient is weak and unable to concentrate. With prolonged exposure to motion, individuals may adapt and gradually return to well-being. However, symptoms may be reinitiated by more severe motion or by recurrence of motion after a short respite.

Prolonged motion sickness with vomiting may lead to arterial hypotension, dehydration, inanition, and depression. Motion sickness can be a serious complication in patients who are already ill.

Prophylaxis and Treatment

Susceptible individuals should minimize exposure by positioning themselves where there is the least motion (e.g., amidships or, in airplanes, over the wings). A supine or semirecumbent position with the head braced is best. Reading should be avoided. Keeping the axis of vision at an angle of 45° above the horizon will reduce the susceptibility of the labyrinthine receptors to stimulation. Avoiding visual fixation on waves or other moving objects is helpful to some. A well-ventilated cabin is important and going out on deck for a breath of fresh air is helpful. Alcoholic or dietary excesses before or during travel are contraindicated. Small amounts of fluids and simple food should be taken frequently during extended periods of exposure; if the exposure is short, as in air travel, food and fluids should be avoided.

Prophylactic drugs should be given before nausea and vomiting occur. One hour before departure, susceptible individuals may be given diphenhydramine, meclizine, or cyclizine 50 mg orally; promethazine 25 mg or diazepam 5 to 10 mg orally; or scopolamine HBr 0.6 mg orally to minimize the vagal mediated GI symptoms. If emotional factors are significant, phenobarbital 15 to 30 mg may be given orally 1 h prior to departure. Sedation with pentobarbital 100 mg orally to induce light sleep may be helpful if alertness is not required. However, sedation should be mild enough to allow mental clarity when the passenger arrives at the destination. All dosages should be appropriately modified for prolonged exposure. Once vomiting begins, medication must be given rectally or parenterally to be effective. With prolonged vomiting IV fluids and electrolytes may be required for replacement and maintenance.

---

221. MEDICAL ASPECTS OF AIR TRAVEL

Commercial aviation safely and comfortably transports hundreds of millions of passengers each year, but imposes a variety of potential medical stresses for which the physician may be consulted. Although most people can fly as passengers safely, planning and precautions are necessary for some patients; however, absolute prohibitions on flying exist for very few conditions. **General aviation,** a rapidly growing area for business and recreational flying, also presents a number of potential health hazards.

The FAA requires periodic medical examination by specially designated physicians, but the vast majority of the nearly 1 million pilots licensed in the USA receive their medical care from private practitioners. Of the more than 4000 accidents that occur each year in general aviation, the vast majority occur in recreational aircraft, and are often related to the injudicious use of alcohol or drugs. The physician may provide counseling to his pilot patient in these areas, as well as cautioning about side effects of medications (e.g., antihistamines) and providing for current tetanus immunization. Commercial pilots are rigorously screened and accidents due either to their illness or to substance abuse are extremely rare.

Aircraft of all types represent a growing **environmental health hazard** in terms of urban noise and air pollution, occasional large scale disasters, and toxic contamination in agricultural areas. Physicians in urban areas should be aware that for patients living near large airports, continuous high level noise and air pollution has been shown to aggravate a wide variety of medical conditions. Local disaster facilities near airports should be prepared to provide initial management of major trauma and burns of air crash survivors. Physicians in agricultural communities should know the toxic manifestations of the chemicals used in crop dusting that may accidentally contaminate farm workers or nearby populated areas (see Ch. 258).

Air Travel Stresses

Major problems imposed on the air traveler relate to (1) changes in barometric pressure, (2) decrease in O_2 tension, (3) turbulence, (4) circadian dysrhythmia, and (5) psychologic stress.

1. Changes in barometric pressure: All modern jet aircraft, including supersonic, maintain cabin pressure equivalent to 5000 to 8000 ft. At that altitude free air in body cavities tends to expand by about 25% and may aggravate certain medical problems. Upper respiratory inflammation or allergy may obstruct eustachian tubes or sinus ostia, resulting in **barotitis media** (see Ch. 166) or **barosinusitis** (see Ch. 168). Frequent yawning or closed-nose swallowing during descent, decongestant nasal sprays, and antihistamines before or during the flight often prevent or relieve these conditions. Children are particularly susceptible to barotitis media and should be given oral fluids or feedings during descent to encourage swallowing (chewing gum or hard candy is more effective than eating). Facial pain of dental origin may occur with change in air pressure. Air travel is *contraindicated* in the following: procedures involving air injection (e.g., pneumoencephalography) until air is absorbed; in patients with pneumothorax or potential for its development (e.g., large pulmonary blebs or cavities); and where air or gas is trapped and even modest expansion may cause pain or stress tissue (e.g., incarcerated bowel or recent [< 10 days] laparotomy). Patients with a colostomy should wear a large bag and expect frequent filling. The occasional accidental loss of cabin pressure and the fact that some airplanes in service are unpressurized must be kept in mind.

2. Decreased O_2 tension: Cabin pressure at a 7500-ft altitude-equivalent results in a Pa_{O_2} of about 70 mm, which is well tolerated by healthy travelers. Problems may arise, however, in a number of conditions, including moderate or severe **pulmonary disease** (e.g., asthma, emphysema, cystic fibrosis, etc.), **congestive heart failure, anemia** with a Hb < 8.5 gm/dl, severe **angina pectoris, sickle-cell disease** (but not trait, see Ch. 92), and some **congenital heart diseases.** Patients with these conditions can usually fly safely with continuous O_2, available from most airlines if arranged for in advance (all commercial aircraft carry O_2 for use during an in-flight emergency). Patients recovering from **myocardial infarction** may fly when stable, often within 10 to 14 days. Ankle edema is common on long flights and should not be confused with an increase in congestive heart failure. **Hypertension** is influenced only by psychologic stress of flight which may be controlled by the use of a mild pre-flight tranquilizer. Smoking can aggravate mild hypoxia and should be avoided. In general, anyone able to walk 100 yd or climb one flight of stairs and whose disease is stable should tolerate normal cabin conditions without additional O_2.

3. Turbulence may cause air sickness (see Ch. 220) or injury and can occur at any time. Passengers should keep their seat belts fastened at all times while seated.

4. Circadian dysrhythmia: Rapid travel across multiple time zones creates many biologic and psychologic stresses; after long trips, travelers should plan on 24- to 48-h rest upon arrival and avoid major commitments or decisions during this adjustment period. A gradual shift in sleeping and eating patterns before departure may partly alleviate the problem. During flight, dehydration may develop because of very low cabin humidity, but can be avoided by adequate intake of fluids and avoidance of alcohol. Some therapeutic regimens require alteration to compensate for circadian dysrhythm, e.g., diabetics using long-acting insulin may need to change to regular insulin until they have accommodated to the destination time, available food, and activity. Digitalis, steroids, anticonvulsants, peptic ulcer, and other medication schedules may require adjustment based on elapsed rather than local time.

5. Psychologic stress: Fear of flying and claustrophia are psychologic and not influenced by logic or reason; hypnosis and behavioral modification psychotherapy have reduced the fear of flying for some. Fearful passengers may benefit from mild sedation before and during flight. Hyperventilation may provoke unconsciousness, tetany-like convulsions, or simulate cardiovascular disease; physician-passengers may be asked to volunteer Good Samaritan services in such inflight situations. Mentally ill patients with violent or unpredictable tendencies must be accompanied by an attendant and appropriately sedated.

Other Considerations

(1) **Thrombophlebitis** is a possibility for anyone sitting for long periods, especially during pregnancy and for patients with venous disease; frequent (q 1 to 2 h) walks around the cabin and isomet-

ric exercises should be practiced. **(2) Wired jaw:** Maxillofacial injury immobilized by fixed wires, unless fitted with a special quick-release device, is a *contraindication* to air travel since air sickness may result in aspiration of vomitus. **(3) Pacemakers:** Newer models are effectively shielded from interference from security devices; older units may be affected. The metal content of pacemakers, however, may trigger a security alarm; a physician's letter should be carried to avoid security difficulties. **(4) Communicable disease:** Patients with any communicable disease posing a threat to others in a crowded aircraft are not acceptable as passengers. International immunization requirements change frequently; current information may be obtained from local or state health departments. **(5) Contact lens** wearers should instill artificial tears frequently to avoid corneal irritation resulting from low cabin humidity. **(6) Medications and records:** The experienced traveler carries on his person essential medications sufficient to assure continued therapy in the event of lost baggage, theft in hotels, delayed arrival, or local unavailability. Patients who must carry narcotics should have a verifying letter from the physician to avoid possible security complications. A summary of a patient's medical record (including ECG) may be invaluable should a patient become ill away from home. Patients subject to disabling illness (e.g., epilepsy) or who are at high risk should wear a medical identification bracelet or necklace (e.g., as provided by Medic-Alert Foundation, Turlock, CA 95380). **(7) Uncomplicated pregnancy** through the 8th mo is acceptable; high-risk patients must be individually evaluated if travel is planned. Acceptance during the 9th mo usually requires a physician's written approval dated within 72 h of departure and indicating delivery date. Seat belts should be worn across the thighs. Thrombophlebitis is a specific risk when sitting for long periods (see above). **(8) Children:** Infants under 7 days of age are not accepted for travel. For children with chronic disease (e.g., congenital heart disease, chronic lung disease, anemia), the same precautions apply as for adults. **(9) Elderly and the handicapped:** There is no upper age limit and airlines make all reasonable efforts to accommodate patients with handicaps. Wheel chair and litter patients can often be accommodated on commercial aircraft; otherwise, air ambulance service will be required if travel is necessary. Some airlines will accept patients requiring special equipment (IV fluids, respirators, etc.) provided appropriate personnel accompany the patient and arrangements have been made in advance.

Further advice regarding air travel may be obtained from the medical department of major airlines or from the FAA Regional Flight Surgeon. Special arrangements (e.g., O_2, wheelchair, etc.) can be made through regular reservations clerks, but at least 72 h advance notice is usually required.

Foreign travel may involve significant difficulties in case of illness. Millions travel abroad yearly; about 1 in 30 requires emergency care. Many insurance plans, including Medicare, are not valid in foreign countries; overseas hospitals often require a substantial cash deposit regardless of insurance. Special insurance programs, including some that will arrange for emergency evacuation (e.g., NEAR, 1900 N. MacArthur, Oklahoma City, OK 73127) are available. Directories listing English-speaking physicians in foreign countries are available from several organizations (e.g., InterMedic, 777 Third Avenue, New York, NY 10017); U.S. Consulates may also assist in obtaining emergency medical services. The book *Traveling Healthy,* by Hillman and Hillman, Penguin Books, 1980, contains valuable information for persons traveling abroad, including those with special health needs (e.g., hemodialysis, anticoagulation, cancer chemotherapy, etc.).

---

222.   NEAR-DROWNING

Asphyxiation due to submersion.

Pathophysiology

Near-drowning victims, because of aspiration or laryngospasm, usually sustain significant hypoxemia, with the consequent danger of respiratory failure and hypercapnea. Acute reflex laryngospasm may occur and result in asphyxia without aspiration of water. Aspiration of fluid and particulate matter may cause chemical pneumonitis, damaging cells lining the alveoli, and may impair alveolar secretion of surfactant, resulting in patchy atelectasis. Surfactant, a lipoprotein, normally lowers the surface tension at the alveolar capillary membrane and prevents alveolar collapse.

The perfusion of nonaerated, atelectatic areas of the lungs leads to intrapulmonary shunting of blood and aggravates hypoxemia. The more fluid aspirated, the greater the surfactant loss, atelectasis, and hypoxemia. With aspiration of large quantities of water, the patient may develop sizable areas of atelectasis and, later, stiff noncompliant lungs and respiratory failure (see Ch. 33). The hypoxemia and tissue hypoxia in near-drowning patients often result in pulmonary edema and even cerebral edema.

The mammalian diving reflex in cold water allows survival after long periods of submersion. The **diving reflex,** first identified in seagoing mammals, slows the heartbeat and constricts the peripheral arteries, shunting oxygenated blood away from the extremities and the gut to the heart and brain. In cold water the O_2 needs of the tissues are reduced, extending the possible time of survival.

Respiratory insufficiency is more critical than changes in electrolytes and blood volume, which vary in magnitude depending on the type and volume of aspirated fluid. Sea water may cause a mild elevation of Na and Cl, but the levels are rarely life-threatening. By contrast, aspirating large quantities of fresh water can cause a sudden increase in blood volume, profound electrolyte imbalance, and hemolysis. Victims may succumb to the effects of these changes, asphyxia, and, possibly, ventricular fibrillation, at the scene of the tragedy. Cardiac arrest, usually preceded by fibrillation, causes many of the deaths attributed to drowning.

One of the commonest complications of near-drowning is the late development of pulmonary edema. On x-ray this may simulate atelectasis and the 2 conditions may coexist. However, current belief is that the pulmonary edema which follows near-drowning is a direct result of hypoxemia and analogous to pulmonary edema of high altitude.

Prevention

Eating and drinking shortly before swimming should be avoided. Children require proper supervision at beaches and near pools or ponds. All swimmers should be accompanied by an experienced swimmer and swim only in areas where a lifeguard is present; these precautions are essential for those with a history of seizures. Nonswimmers and small children should wear flotation jackets when in boats or playing near bodies of water. Children should be taught to swim as early as possible, and adults and children over 12 should be familiar with the basics of resuscitation.

Treatment

The key factors for surviving submersion without permanent injury appear to be the duration of submersion, the water temperature, the age of the individual (the diving reflex is more active in children), and the speed of resuscitation efforts. Survival depends more on the prompt correction of hypoxemia and acidosis (ventilatory insufficiency) than correction of electrolyte imbalance, the goal being to prevent pulmonary edema due to hypoxia and cerebral edema also secondary to hypoxia.

If the near-drowning takes place in very cold water, the victim *may be hypothermic*. There is sharp controversy about the management of hypothermia; some experts argue strongly that no jarring, sudden movements, or manipulation should be done on a hypothermic patient whose heart is beating, however slowly. Others feel the danger of initiating ventricular fibrillation by a sudden blow is exaggerated. However, in cases of near-drowning, hypothermia should be strongly suspected, even though the water may not seem extremely cold. Rectal or core temperature should be taken as soon as practical.

Emergency mouth-to-mouth resuscitation should begin immediately if the victim is apneic—in the water, if necessary. If heart beat and carotid pulse cannot be detected, closed chest cardiac massage (see CARDIAC ARREST AND CARDIOPULMONARY RESUSCITATION in Ch. 25) is initiated as soon as artificial ventilation is started. Mechanical ventilators, which supply higher inspired O_2 concentrations, should be used if available. Electrical defibrillation may be necessary.

Time should not be wasted in attempts to drain water from the lungs in a fresh-water victim, because the hypotonic fluid passes rapidly into the circulation. Sea water, being hypertonic, draws plasma into the lung, and the Trendelenburg position may help to promote drainage.

Hospitalization is mandatory for all victims. Resuscitation should continue during transport, regardless of the patient's condition. Consciousness is not synonymous with recovery, since *delayed death from hypoxia can occur*. A key goal is to prevent both pulmonary edema and cerebral edema secondary to hypoxia.

Initial emphasis in the hospital should be on intensive pulmonary care to achieve adequate arterial blood-gas and acid-base levels. Required measures range from simple O_2 administration for a spontaneously breathing patient to continuous ventilatory support of an apneic patient by tracheal intubation with a cuffed tube connected to a mechanical ventilator. Sodium bicarbonate IV is usually indicated, since metabolic acidosis almost invariably accompanies the hypoxia. Further bicarbonate administration and ventilatory support, and proper inspired O_2 concentrations are determined by monitoring blood gases. In all cases, high supplemental levels of O_2 inhalation must be continued until the arterial blood-gas studies indicate that lesser O_2 concentrations are adequate. Consciousness usually returns when arterial oxygenation and pH improve.

Frequent manual hyperinflation of the lungs is indicated to re-expand atelectatic alveoli. Isoproterenol by inhalation or IV injection helps to reduce bronchospasm. Since near-drowning with fluid aspiration is a form of aspiration pneumonitis, corticosteroids and antibiotics may be considered depending on the individual case.

Fluid and electrolyte solutions are required to correct significant electrolyte imbalance. A large quantity of fluid may be extravasated into the lungs, producing a reduced blood volume that may be reflected by lowered central venous pressure; infusion of volume expanders may be indicated. Fluid restriction is usually not advisable, since the pulmonary and cerebral edema caused by hypoxia are related to direct pulmonary epithelial damage or osmotic gradients rather than to circulatory overload as in congestive failure. RBC replacement to increase the O_2-carrying capacity of the blood, and forced diuresis to facilitate excretion of the free plasma Hb may be necessary if there is significant hemolysis.

The patient who develops acute respiratory distress syndrome requires mechanical ventilation (see Ch. 33). Pulmonary care may be necessary for hours or days, depending on the arterial blood-gas and pH analyses. Permanent brain damage from hypoxemia and tissue hypoxia may be a residual problem in some cases.

223. MEDICAL ASPECTS OF DIVING AND WORKING IN COMPRESSED AIR

Medical problems caused by **increased environmental pressure** have long been recognized in deep-sea divers and tunnel and caisson workers. They are now commonly seen in divers using **scuba (self-contained underwater breathing apparatus** such as the Aqua-Lung®) for sport, scientific study, or commerce (e.g., in offshore oil development). The high-pressure environment of hyperbaric chambers, used for medical and scientific applications, can also cause similar problems.

PRESSURE CONSIDERATIONS

Pressure is commonly measured in pounds per square inch **(psi)** or in mm Hg. In diving, pressure is often expressed in units of depth (e.g., feet or meters of water) or in atmospheres **(atm)**. One atm is the average barometric pressure at sea level (14.7 psi or 760 mm Hg). With descent into water, the ambient pressure increases rapidly. Every 33 ft of descent in sea water adds 1 atm to the pressure encountered at depth. The total (absolute) pressure exerted upon a submerged object is the pressure of the water plus the atmospheric pressure. Therefore, at 33 ft below the water surface, the total pressure is 2 atmospheres absolute **(atm abs,** or **ata)**; at 66 ft, 3 atm abs, and so on.

Effects of Increased Pressure

Exposure of the body to increased pressure can cause a variety of medical problems as shown in the following examples.

1. Local differences in pressure: As external pressure on the body increases, the pressure of gas in the lungs and airways usually increases correspondingly. If the eustachian tubes can be opened normally (e.g., by yawning or swallowing), pressure in the middle ear can be kept equal to the increasing external pressure. If structural abnormalities, allergic or vasomotor rhinitis, or an URI prevent such equalization, the excess external pressure is exerted directly on the eardrum and the blood vessels in the middle ear. The mucosal blood vessels may dilate, leak, and rupture, causing bleeding into the middle ear space. If the edema fluid and extravasated blood do not occupy enough volume to equalize the pressure, the eardrum may rupture. Middle ear infections from this **barotitis media** (see also Ch. 166) are a likely consequence. In like manner **barotrauma** may also occur in the paranasal sinuses or lungs. A similar pressure differential in any rigid or semirigid airspace attached to the body (e.g., face masks, diving suits) can cause discomfort and local hemorrhage and tissue damage. Ear plugs must not be used in diving.

2. Compression and expansion of gas: As Boyle's law indicates, the volume of a given mass of gas varies inversely with its absolute pressure. For example, 1 L of gas at the surface (1 atm abs) is compressed to $\frac{1}{2}$ L at 33 ft of depth (2 atm abs). The equalization of pressure in body airspaces on descent reflects such changes, and compression of lung gas limits the safe depth of a "breath-hold" dive, in which scuba is not used.

Gas compression involves the middle ear in 2 types of **vertigo.** (1) If the tympanic membrane ruptures when a diver is bareheaded in cold water, the effect is like that of the caloric test (see in Ch. 164), producing severe and potentially disastrous vertigo. (2) Unequalized pressure differences in the middle ear may affect the inner ear via the round window, causing **alternobaric vertigo,** a possible cause of the dysequilibrium sometimes experienced by divers on starting ascent. **Perilymph fistula** is an uncommon but serious cause of vertigo, and one that requires prompt intervention.

Increased gas density due to compression at depth has several consequences. When a given mass of a gas is compressed, the total number of molecules remains constant, and the number of molecules/unit volume increases in accordance with Boyle's law. Since a scuba diver breathes with about the same tidal volume and number of breaths/min for a given work rate at depth as he does at the surface, the number of gas molecules inspired/min increases markedly at depth. Not only does the duration of the diver's air supply decrease proportionately, but breathing can become difficult because of the respiratory limitations of the scuba and of the diver's own airways. This can considerably accentuate overexertion, which, with respiratory exhaustion and general fatigue, can be a serious diving problem even under ideal conditions.

More serious medical problems can arise with the expansion of pulmonary gas on ascent. If a diver inspires compressed gas at depth and fails to exhale freely on ascent, the expanding gas may then overinflate the lungs, possibly causing pneumothorax, mediastinal and subcutaneous emphysema, and air (gas) embolism. **Gas embolism** (see Table 223–1 and the discussion below) is an extreme emergency and is probably second only to drowning as a cause of death among divers.

TABLE 223-1. CONDITIONS REQUIRING RECOMPRESSION

	Decompression Sickness	Gas Embolism
Signs and symptoms	**Extremely variable.** Three main types (singly or in combination): 1. **"Bends"**—pain, most often in a joint (about 90% of cases) 2. **Neurologic** involvement of almost any type or degree (about 10%) 3. **"Chokes"**—respiratory distress followed by circulatory collapse (rare—extreme emergency)	Usual: **unconsciousness,** frequently with convulsion (Mediastinal and subcutaneous emphysema may also be present) **Assume that any unconscious diver has air embolism and treat promptly**
Onset and immediate course	Gradual or sudden onset during decompression or as long as 24 h after one or more* dives or hyperbaric exposures beyond 2 atm abs (Also possible in exposure to low pressure at altitude) *Repetitive dives are a particular source of trouble	Sudden onset during or very shortly after . . . 1. Ascent, even from very shallow depth 2. Decompression from any increased pressure 3. Any accident or procedure that could permit gas to enter circulation
Proximate cause	Usual: Diving or hyperbaric exposure beyond no-decompression limits and without proper decompression stops Occasional: 1. Pressure exposure within no-decompression limits or with proper decompression 2. Low-pressure exposure as in loss of cabin pressure in aircraft at altitude	Usual: Breath holding or airway obstruction during ascent from dive or decompression from hyperbaric exposure Other: Entry of free gas into cardiovascular system in open heart surgery or other medical/surgical procedure
Mechanism	Excess dissolved gas forms bubbles in blood or tissues upon reduction of pressure Bubbles then produce local circulatory obstruction or mechanical effects	Usual: Overinflation of lungs causes entry of free gas into pulmonary circulation Resulting arterial gas-embolization usually involves the brain Other: Pulmonary, cardiac, or systemic circulatory obstruction by free gas from any source

3. Partial pressure effects: The partial pressure of a gas is proportional to the number of molecules of that gas present in a given volume of gas. If, for example, the volume of a gas mixture is halved by compression, the number of gas molecules/unit volume doubles, and the partial pressure of each gas in the mixture also doubles. The physiologic effects of gases are related to their partial pressure and are thus subject to modification by changes in depth.

O_2 displays toxic effects as its partial pressure increases. Pulmonary damage can occur with extended exposure to O_2 above approximately 0.5 atm P_{O_2} (equivalent to 50% O_2 at surface or 25% O_2 at 33 ft). Beyond about 2 atm P_{O_2} (100% O_2 at 33 ft or 50% O_2 at 99 ft), convulsive O_2 toxicity can occur.

Increased partial pressure of N_2 results in **nitrogen narcosis,** a condition resembling alcohol intoxication. In divers breathing air, this becomes noticeable at 100 ft or less and is incapacitating at about 10 atm abs (300 ft), where the effect resembles breathing 30% nitrous oxide at sea level. Helium lacks this anesthetic property and is therefore used as an inert gas diluent in deep diving.

Partial pressures of O_2 and CO_2 in alveolar gas are also modified by depth and are especially important in breath-hold swimming and diving (when breathing apparatus is not used). A swimmer who hyperventilates in order to increase his underwater swimming capability will blow off CO_2 without much effect on his O_2 stores. He may become **unconscious from hypoxia** before his P_{CO_2} rises enough to warn him that he must surface and resume breathing. Making a breath-hold dive to a significant depth will temporarily elevate the alveolar P_{O_2}, but both P_{O_2} and P_{CO_2} will then drop precipitously as the external pressure decreases on ascent. A diver who has "pushed his limits" under such circumstances may lose consciousness without warning before he reaches the surface. This phenomenon is probably responsible for many unexplained drownings among spearfishermen and others who frequently do breath-hold diving. It is sometimes called **shallow-water blackout,** but that term is more correctly applied to mishaps due to high P_{CO_2} levels in rebreathing types of scuba. Hypoxia is also a potential problem in rebreathing units.

CO_2 retention results from inadequate pulmonary ventilation during exertion in some divers and may occasionally be responsible for loss or impairment of consciousness at depth. Unusually low air-use rates and severe post-dive headaches may be indicative of the retention tendency.

Increased partial pressures also dissolve unusual amounts of gas directly into the blood and tissues. If later the pressure is reduced too rapidly gas bubbles may form with various consequences (see TABLE 223–1 and DECOMPRESSION SICKNESS, below).

4. Pressure per se: Neuromuscular abnormalities known as the "high-pressure neurologic syndrome" are observed in deep diving beginning at about 600 ft on descent. The phenomenon bears no evident relationship to partial pressures or to gas compression and is attributed to hydrostatic pressure alone. Such effects have no recognized medical importance at shallower depths.

5. Complicating factors include environmental elements such as poor visibility, currents requiring excessive effort, and cold. **Hypothermia** can develop very rapidly in water, and early effects may include crucial loss of dexterity and judgment. Cold water can trigger fatal cardiac arrhythmias in susceptible individuals. **Hypoglycemia** may be a serious hazard, especially with alcoholic indulgence and inadequate food intake. **Drugs,** including medications as well as drugs of abuse, may have unanticipated effects at depth.

CONDITIONS REQUIRING RECOMPRESSION

GAS EMBOLISM (Air Embolism)

A disorder resulting from overinflation of the lungs due to expanding pulmonary gas during reduction of surrounding pressure (e.g., ascent from diving), generally characterized by abrupt loss of consciousness with or without other CNS manifestations, and attributed to cerebral gas emboli originating in the lungs. (See TABLE 223–1.)

Etiology

The victim of gas embolism is most commonly a diver who held his breath during ascent from a dive (as shallow as 6 ft, possibly less) in which he was using breathing apparatus or had some other source of inspired gas at depth. Compressed gas inspired beneath the surface expands on ascent and, if not allowed to escape freely, overinflates the lungs. Overinflation and accompanying elevation of intra-alveolar pressure result in escape of gas from the alveoli into the pulmonary blood vessels. Embolization of cerebral arteries usually results, and prompt loss of consciousness is almost inevitable.

Symptoms, Signs, and Diagnosis

Whatever the source of bubble emboli, gas embolism is an extreme emergency requiring prompt and adequate recompression. Any diver who loses consciousness during or very shortly after ascent must be assumed to have gas embolism and should be recompressed as promptly as possible.

Overinflation of the lungs may produce mediastinal and subcutaneous emphysema, alone or with gas embolism. Pneumothorax is a much less frequent consequence. Not infrequently, convulsions or other cerebral manifestations accompany loss of consciousness in gas embolism.

DECOMPRESSION SICKNESS (Caisson Disease; The Bends)

A disorder resulting from reduction of the surrounding pressure (as in ascent from a dive, exit from a caisson or hyperbaric chamber, or ascent to altitude), attributed to formation of gas bubbles in tissues or blood vessels, and characterized most commonly by pain, less frequently by neurologic symptoms, and rarely by pulmonary complications. The pathophysiologic and clinical differences between decompression sickness and gas embolism are summarized in TABLE 223–1.

Pathophysiology

A diver or compressed-air worker breathing air under increased pressure takes up increased quantities of O_2 and N_2 in solution in the blood and tissues. O_2 is utilized continuously, but N_2 (or any other "inert" gas present) leaves the body only via the reverse of its entry through the lungs and circulation. Gradients of partial pressure govern uptake and elimination of the gas, but the degree of supersaturation (excess of tissue gas pressure over ambient pressure) is crucial in determining whether symptomatic bubbles will form during or after ascent. The consequences of bubble formation from dissolved gas are known as **decompression sickness, caisson disease,** or "the bends" (see TABLE 223–1). Although "the bends" strictly refers to painful symptoms, it is often used as a synonym for decompression sickness.

Consequential bubble formation can usually be avoided by (1) restricting the uptake of gas, as by limiting the depth and duration of dives to a range that does not require decompression stops on ascent ("**no-decompression limits**"; see TABLE 223–2), or (2) using a standard air **decompression table** (available in the *US Navy Diving Manual*, obtainable from the Superintendent of Documents, US

Government Printing Office, Washington, D.C. 20402) to provide a pattern of ascent that allows excess inert gas to escape harmlessly. Breathing O_2 accelerates the exit of inert gas by increasing the "outward partial pressure gradient" without lowering the ambient pressure. Decompression sickness rarely occurs after dives within the limits given in TABLE 223–2, but the diver's account of depth and duration is often unreliable. **Repetitive dives** are a major source of difficulty, since some excess of inert gas remains in the body after any dive and increases with each subsequent dive. Repetitive dives occurring less than 12 h apart must be handled according to special tables as provided in the *US Navy Diving Manual.*

US Navy decompression tables have not been tested for adequacy in females or older divers. Dives conducted at **altitude** and **flying after diving** require special procedures or precautions.

Symptoms and Signs

Local pain (**"the bends"**) is the most common manifestation of decompression sickness. It is most often localized in the knee, elbow, shoulder, or hip, and is commonly described as being deep and "like something boring into bone." At first, pain may be mild or intermittent, but it is apt to increase steadily and may become very severe. Local tenderness or inflammation is uncommon and the pain may not be exacerbated by motion.

Neurologic manifestations are less common and may occur alone or with pain. They are extremely variable, ranging from mild paresthesias to major cerebral symptoms. Spinal cord involvement is a particular hazard.

"Chokes" are rare in occurrence but grave in significance. The condition is thought to represent massive bubble embolization of the pulmonary vascular tree. If not promptly treated, "chokes" can lead to circulatory collapse and death. Substernal discomfort and coughing on deep inspiration or inhalation of tobacco smoke must be viewed as premonitory symptoms. "Chokes" and other serious manifestations appearing at **altitude** are not necessarily remedied by a return to ground level and may require immediate chamber recompression.

Other manifestations of decompression sickness include itching, rash, and severe fatigue. These are seldom treated by recompression, but they may be forerunners of more consequential problems. Cutaneous edema, a rare manifestation, may require recompression if it progresses. Mottling ("marbling") of the skin, though relatively uncommon, may precede or accompany symptoms that require recompression. **Abdominal pain** may be a manifestation of local bubble formation that demands treatment in its own right. Especially in the form of girdle pain, it is important as a signal of spinal cord involvement.

Late manifestations of decompression sickness may occur. **Aseptic bone necrosis** (dysbaric osteonecrosis) is more common in compressed-air workers than in divers, but divers are by no means immune. Bone necrosis is presumed to be a consequence of bone infarction by bubbles, as in delayed or inadequate treatment of clinical "bends." Juxta-articular bone lesions are most common at the hip and shoulder and can cause great damage to the joint, with chronic pain and severe permanent disability. Bone necrosis is a particularly insidious hazard because it becomes symptomatic or is detected on x-ray only months or years after the responsible insult.

TABLE 223–2. NO-DECOMPRESSION LIMITS

(Single dives not requiring decompression stops on ascent)

Depth	Time[1]
30 ft	(no limit)
35	310 min
40	200
50	100
60	60
70	50
80	40
90	30
100	25
110	20
120	15
130–140	10
150–190	5

Notes:
1. Times include time of descent as well as time actually at depth.
2. *Important:* If one "no-decompression" dive was followed by others within a 12-h period, the subsequent dives probably required stops on ascent (see *Repetitive dives* in text).
3. Diver's recollection of depth and time is commonly inaccurate.

Adapted from *The New Science of Skin and Scuba Diving.* Copyright 1980 by the Council for National Cooperation in Aquatics. Used with permission.

Permanent neurologic defects are almost always an obvious result of failure to relieve original manifestations. Post-decompression **paraplegia,** for example, is frequently attributable to delayed or inappropriate treatment of spinal cord involvement. In some instances, the initial damage may be too severe to remedy, even with prompt and careful treatment.

RECOMPRESSION TREATMENT

General Principles

Recompression is the crucial treatment in both decompression sickness and gas embolism. Its objective is to compress bubbles to asymptomatic size, to put their gaseous content back into solution, and to restore adequate oxygenation to affected tissues. Despite the differences between the 2 conditions (outlined in Table 223–1, above), decisions concerning treatment are governed much more by presenting symptoms and response than by differential diagnosis.

Guidelines for the selection and use of appropriate US Navy treatment tables may be found in the *US Navy Diving Manual.* These tables should yield good therapeutic results in most cases of decompression sickness that follow ordinary diving with air as the breathing medium. Dives involving unusual gas mixtures or extraordinary depths or durations may require special therapeutic procedures.

In determining whether or not chamber recompression is needed, thorough examination and detailed history-taking are less vital than having a strong suspicion that a condition requiring recompression exists. Sometimes, a definite diagnosis cannot be made without a "test of pressure." Failure to provide prompt and appropriate treatment of decompression sickness or gas embolism entails unacceptable risk of serious and lasting injury (see late manifestations, above). Unnecessary recompression entails far less risk than does prescribing palliative measures in the hope that symptoms or signs of decompression sickness will subside without recompression.

When a physician recommends recompression but cannot be sure that the patient will seek and receive appropriate treatment in an adequate chamber, it is prudent to obtain signed and witnessed acknowledgment of the recommendation. Medical installations and rescue and police units in popular diving areas should know the *location* of the nearest hyperbaric chamber, the *means of reaching it* most rapidly, and the most appropriate source of *consultation* by telephone. A national diving accident network is coordinated by the Duke University Medical Center, Durham, N.C. (919–684–8111).

Recompression in the water should not be attempted. O_2 should be administered during transport of the patient to a chamber. Marked saving of time justifies transport by air, but exposure to the reduced pressure of altitude must be kept to a minimum. In suspected gas embolism, the patient should be kept supine.

Medical adjuncts to recompression: Although recompression alone suffices in most cases, a patient may also need resuscitation, first aid, or other medical or surgical treatment. Both recompression and other measures usually can be accomplished simultaneously. If not, recompression takes precedence over any therapy that can be postponed without risk to life; other priorities are usually clear.

Adequate fluid intake is extremely important. Intake and output should be measured and recorded together with vital signs. The possibility of bladder paralysis and need for catheterization should be kept in mind.

Corticosteroids (e.g., dexamethasone sodium phosphate 20 to 40 mg IV, then 4 mg IM q 6 h) may be useful, especially when spinal cord edema is suspected. Effective means of reducing brain swelling are indicated when cerebral manifestations are present, especially if these do not respond promptly to recompression.

Sedatives and narcotics may obscure symptoms and produce respiratory insufficiency. They should be avoided before and during recompression or given in smallest effective dosage, with careful attention to respiratory status. Aspirin (0.5 to 1.0 gm) is administered early in some centers.

EVALUATION OF FITNESS FOR DIVING

Increasingly often, physicians are asked to judge the fitness of candidates for diving and similar activity. Uniform standards do not yet exist, but certain basic principles are widely accepted.

Diving can involve unusually heavy **exertion** even for an individual who intends to avoid arduous underwater activities. The diver should be free of significant cardiac or pulmonary disease and should have normal or superior exercise capacity. Gross **obesity** is commonly associated not only with poor exercise tolerance but also with increased susceptibility to decompression sickness. Rigid **age limits** are unrealistic, but older candidates deserve special scrutiny from the standpoint of cardiorespiratory fitness. Family history and coronary risk factors need to be considered. Certain arrhythmias contraindicate diving even in younger individuals.

All body airspaces must be able to **equalize pressure** uneventfully. Pulmonary conditions that involve air trapping may cause gas embolism on ascent; absolute *contraindications* to diving include lung cysts, active asthma, and a history of spontaneous pneumothorax. Failure of equalization in the middle ear spaces and paranasal sinuses can have serious consequences. Chronic nasal congestion, perforated eardrum, and certain otologic surgical procedures are *contraindications*. Diving should be avoided during respiratory infections and episodes of vasomotor or allergic rhinitis.

Any **impairment of consciousness or judgment**, even if momentary, can lead to a fatal mishap underwater. Epileptic seizures or syncopal attacks, diabetes, and alcoholism or drug abuse are not compatible with diving. Medications that cause drowsiness or lessened alertness are undesirable in diving and may potentiate nitrogen narcosis. **Lack of emotional stability** is perilous for the diver and his companions; it may be suspected from inappropriate motivation, a history of impulsive behavior, or accident-proneness.

Pregnancy presents unknown hazards, especially from the standpoint of possible decompression injury to the fetus.

Evaluation of **commercial divers** and others at unusual risk warrants special procedures including pulmonary function testing, stress electrocardiography, audiometry, and bone x-rays.

Individuals who are inclined to dive despite medical advice to the contrary should be clearly informed of the potential risks involved, and the physician's disapproval should be made a matter of record.

Adequate training is absolutely essential for safety in diving, and the physician should emphasize its importance. Courses sanctioned by national organizations are widely available.

224.   HIGH-ALTITUDE ILLNESS

(Acute Mountain Sickness [AMS]; High-Altitude Pulmonary Edema [HAPE]; Hypoxia; Soroche; Puna; Mareo)

Hypoxic syndromes due to rapid exposure to O_2 lack.

Etiology and Pathophysiology

Barometric pressure decreases as altitude increases, but the percentage of O_2 in the atmosphere remains constant. Therefore, the partial pressure of O_2 in air decreases with altitude and at 18,000 ft (5500 m) is about 1/2 that at sea level. Persons ascending to high altitudes faster than adaptation can accommodate often develop symptoms and signs of hypoxic stress. Illnesses and injuries that cause hypoxia at sea level can also produce similar symptoms. Although rest does not prevent altitude illness, strenuous exertion increases the risk. Persons who have had one attack appear somewhat more vulnerable to another under similar conditions, but there is wide variation between individuals and in the same person on different occasions. Infants, children, and women in the premenstrual phase are especially susceptible. Residents of altitudes above 10,000 ft (3000 m) may be more vulnerable on reascent after a brief stay at low altitude, although this is controversial. Very rapid ascent (unpressurized aircraft, balloons, decompression chambers) or only a brief stay (few hours) at an elevated altitude may produce adverse effects but rarely causes typical high-altitude illness.

Hypoxia stimulates ventilation, which increases tissue oxygenation but also produces respiratory alkalosis. This begins to be compensated within 24 to 72 h by loss of HCO_3 in urine. It is hypothesized that hypoxia impairs the O_2-dependent ATP "sodium pump," resulting in the accumulation of Na and water within and movement of K out of cells, leading to disturbed fluid and electrolyte distribution. Increased ADH secretion may be precipitated by hypoxia in some individuals.

No specific pathology has been demonstrated in acute mountain sickness. Asymptomatic interstitial edema, which recedes in mild cases, precedes frank alveolar edema, which sometimes occurs in the usual hilar butterfly distribution, but more often in asymmetrical, sometimes unilateral, patches. Cerebral edema may occur; papilledema is present in severe cases. Platelet and fibrin microemboli are found in lungs and brain. The heart is normal and passive congestion is not noted. Petechial hemorrhages, splinter hemorrhages beneath the fingernails, and hemorrhages involving different layers of the retina are common at elevations above 16,000 ft (5000 m), but their specific pathogenesis is unknown. Endocrine glands, liver, and kidneys appear normal, but reversible derangements of function are common.

Symptoms, Signs, and Diagnosis

Altitude illness must be distinguished from motion sickness with which it is sometimes confused. Different hypoxic syndromes often overlap and can be considered parts of a spectrum of pathophysiology. However, they may appear as discrete conditions and it is helpful to describe them as separate illnesses. **Acute mountain sickness (AMS)** can begin at about 6500 ft (2000 m) and is manifested by headache, weakness, nausea, vomiting, sleep disturbances, dyspnea, and forceful, rapid heartbeat. Unless dehydration is severe or hyperventilation excessive, AMS, though unpleasant, is rarely serious and improves within 1 or 2 days. Laboratory studies are nonspecific and rarely helpful.

High-altitude pulmonary edema (HAPE) develops within 24 to 72 h after rapid ascent above 10,000 ft (3000 m), and is characterized by increasing dyspnea, cough productive of white, pink, or occasionally bloody sputum, low-grade fever, and tachycardia. Cyanosis and dyspnea may be severe, and widespread rales are often audible even without a stethoscope. The symptoms may be mistaken for pneumonia. Chest x-rays show Kerley lines and all degrees of pulmonary edema. Atrial pressure is normal while pulmonary artery pressure is elevated. Headache, coma, and death (sometimes within a few hours of onset) are characteristic of severe HAPE.

High-altitude cerebral edema (HACE) is less common but more dangerous. In HACE headache is usually severe, the gait is ataxic, clumsy hand movements and diplopia are seen, and auditory and visual hallucinations are common. Papilledema is not necessary for diagnosis. HACE must be distinguished from other causes of coma (e.g., infection, vascular accident, or ketoacidosis) by history of rapid ascent, absence of significant fever or paralysis, and normal blood and spinal fluid studies where feasible. Coma and death may develop rapidly.

Retinal hemorrhages are asymptomatic unless the macula is involved and occur alone or in combination with other forms of altitude illness. They are absorbed without sequelae, though in rare instances a scotoma may persist. Retinal hemorrhages may be found on ophthalmoscopy and must be differentiated from those due to hypertension, diabetes, or uremia.

Prophylaxis

Although physical fitness improves the ability to work with less O_2 consumption, it does not protect against altitude illness. The best prevention is to allow time for acclimatization by ascending no faster than 800 to 1000 ft (250 to 300 m)/day above 8000 ft (2500 m) with occasional rest days above 13,000 ft (4000 m). Complete rest appears to make some people worse, but strenuous exertion should be avoided. Because of individual variation, mountaineers should be advised to climb at rates which leave them relatively symptom-free, to stop if symptoms progress, and to descend immediately if symptoms become severe.

Acetazolamide 250 mg orally b.i.d. for 1 or 2 days before and during the climb is helpful. It inhibits carbonic anhydrase, permitting better O_2 transport with less respiratory alkalosis, and improves oxygenation during sleep by decreasing or eliminating periodic breathing. Breathing low flow O_2 during the night minimizes the increase in hypoxia due to periodic breathing during sleep. Progesterone, ammonium chloride, cytochrome, and respiratory stimulants have been advocated, but side effects generally outweigh benefits. Drinking more water than usual seems to help. Antacids to prevent exercise acidosis have been advocated, but their value is unproven.

Acclimatization is a gradual process consisting of a series of integrated physiologic changes that tend to restore the partial pressure of O_2 in tissues toward normal. Full acclimatization above 13,000 ft (4000 m) may take years to achieve and cannot be expedited with medications. Short-term acclimatization has enabled individuals to perform astonishing feats as high as 29,000 ft (8800 m), but during long stays above 20,000 ft (6000 m), deterioration outstrips acclimatization. The dominant features of acclimatization include moderate hyperventilation and slightly increased cardiac output, followed by polycythemia, increased myoglobin, increased tissue capillarity, and decreased blood alkaline reserve. Excessive polycythemia may lead to thrombophlebitis; consequently, polycythemia is considered by some to be an adverse response to hypoxia.

Treatment

AMS rarely requires any treatment beyond fluid replacement, decreased activity, and occasionally descent. **HAPE** is treated by halting the ascent and decreasing activity; *if symptoms worsen, immediate descent is essential.* Breathing O_2 relieves HAPE only in early stages and is less effective as the condition progresses, because of the interference with O_2 diffusion caused by progressive interstitial and alveolar edema. Although morphine is effective, respiratory depression may outweigh its benefits. Since cardiac function is normal, digitalis is of no value. Furosemide (20 to 40 mg orally q 2 h or 20 mg slowly IV) is often effective. (Caution: *Too brisk a diuresis may cause hypovolemic shock, changing a mildly ill individual into a litter case*) Waiting to observe the effects of medication should not delay descent in severe cases, because going down 1000 to 1600 ft (300 to 500 m) often causes dramatic improvement. Placing the victim in a pressurized bag or chamber, though effective, is of limited value because symptoms return when the victim is removed. **HACE** responds slowly to steroids (dexamethasone or betamethasone 4 to 8 mg IV q 4 h). Other measures to reduce intracranial pressure have not been assessed in altitude illness. O_2 only relieves headache temporarily. Diuresis is less effective and recovery after descent is slower than in HAPE. Retinal hemorrhages require no treatment and alone are not major reasons for descent. They are resorbed during stay at altitude; few leave permanent scars.

Chronic mountain sickness (Monge's disease), an uncommon complication of high-altitude living, is characterized by excessive polycythemia, dyspnea, thromboses, and cardiac failure; it is relieved by moving to a low altitude, and temporarily by phlebotomy. The syndrome is similar to **alveolar hypoventilation (pickwickian disease).**

§20. SPECIAL SUBJECTS

225. COMPUTERIZED TRANSVERSE TOMOGRAPHY
(Computerized Tomography [CT]; Computerized Transverse Axial Tomography [CTT];
Computerized Axial Tomography [CAT]; Computer-Assisted Transaxial Tomography; EMI Scan)

Computerized tomography **(CT)** combines the technologies of radiology, computer processing, and cathode ray tube **(CRT)** display. The result is an image of the transverse section of the body part studied, which looks much like an anatomic section. It is a computer reconstruction of the area, utilizing the computer's ability to calculate small differences in the attenuation of various tissues swept by a tightly collimated radiographic beam. These attenuation coefficients may be separable even though minimal, as in the difference between soft tissue and water, which ordinarily cannot be seen with conventional radiography. Considerable clinical experience has been gained with computerized tomography of the brain and experience is rapidly increasing with applications to the rest of the body.

CT is a noninvasive procedure without significant risk, morbidity, or discomfort. It provides clear radiographic definition of structures that are not visible by other technics, thus permitting earlier diagnosis and treatment, more effective and efficient follow-up studies of postoperative complications, monitoring of the evolution of a lesion, and evaluation of treatment.

CT is relatively expensive compared to other imaging modalities, but this expense is mitigated by the possible elimination of procedures, such as angiography, which require hospitalization. Although early scanners required a moderate dose of radiation, recent units have reduced the required levels significantly.

Principles of Operation
Common to all scanners is a narrow beam or beams of x-ray emitted from a standard heavy-duty x-ray tube and recorded by one or more scintillation crystals which travel parallel to the x-ray beam. Utilizing various motions and technics, including single beam, fan beam, multiangular transverse motion, and circular motion, the beam sweeps across the area of the body to be imaged and multiple measurements of the transmitted radiation are recorded. These recordings, as electronic impulses, are converted into digital form and entered into the computer where x-ray absorption (attenuation) coefficients of the thousands of readings (picture points) are calculated. Usually each picture point or **pixel** approximates 1 mm in its x and y diameters and about 1 cm in its thickness or z diameter. Using the absorption coefficient of water as a baseline, the computer converts the absorption coefficients of the readings into brightness or density ratios on a CRT, which may be photographed. Alternatively, the absorption coefficients of the various pixels can be displayed digitally on a hardcopy printout. Because of the narrow pencil-beam phenomenon achieved by tight collimation and minimal scatter of the transmitted x-ray beam, CT can detect and portray radiographic density differences as low as $\pm$ 0.5%. In comparison, the sensitivity of standard radiography usually ranges between $\pm$ 4 to 5%. Consequently, CT generates an anatomic portrayal of a transverse section of the brain or other part of the body that allows clear depiction of the relationships of the structures in the "slice."

Clinical Applications
Brain: CT can depict various intracranial abnormalities, some of which might otherwise require clarification by invasive procedures or even surgical exploration. In brain studies, 8 slices about 1.3 cm thick are usually generated and portrayed at an angle of about 20° cephalad from the orbital-meatal line. Due to the angulation, the entire posterior fossa can be evaluated. Other views, including coronal, can be obtained either directly or by computer reconstruction from the axial slices. One can clearly identify the CSF-filled ventricular system and evaluate its normalcy or displacement. Additionally, various lesions can be identified from their disruption of normal anatomic relationships or from their alterations in densities compared to that of normal brain tissue. Increased densities are usually caused by blood-filled structures, blood being denser than normal tissues. Lower densities are usually due to an increase in the water content of the brain tissue (edema), which shows up as a marked lucency. Space-occupying brain lesions (e.g., tumor, hematoma, cyst, cerebral infarct, hemorrhagic change, calcification, metastatic disease, and hydrocephalus) are all generally identifiable by CT.

CT has revolutionized pediatric neurology, and CT studies of the ventricular system have rendered air or positive contrast encephalography obsolete. The characterization of various types of congenital and developmental brain anomalies has been aided markedly by this technic.

In children and adults, intracranial tumors have been diagnosed with about 98 to 99% accuracy. The baseline scan often shows the effects of a tumor; i.e., a midline shift, edema, or both. The evaluation of many brain lesions may be aided by the IV injection of iodinated contrast material (e.g., meglumine iothalamate, meglumine diatrizoate). The circulating iodine shows the vascularity of the brain tumor and, as some of the iodine leaks through the damaged blood-brain barrier, enhances visualization of the solid portion of the tumor. Thus, the extent and size of the main portion of the mass may be defined.

Acute hemorrhages, such as subdural and epidural hematomas, are well delineated because blood density is quite high compared to normal brain tissue. They may also be identified by analysis of their effects on the brain. In time, the blood density diminishes and, when significant absorption has occurred, hematomas become lucent. During the transition from density to lucency, the clot may be isodense with the brain, making identification difficult. However, IV contrast injection may show membranes associated with subdural hematomas and help in their localization.

Cerebral infarction may be indiscernible if the lesion is small or does not cause much edema. However, if the lesion is large and the edema extensive, shifts of the brain structures and the lucency due to edema are often apparent. Hemorrhagic infarcts in particular can be definitively localized and characterized. Old infarcts, because of loss of brain tissue and replacement with fluid, become markedly lucent. The shrinkage of the brain on the side of the infarct, loss of the cortical pattern, and dilation of the ventricle into this area may also characterize encephalomalacia. Brainstem and cerebellar infarctions may be difficult to identify unless they are quite large.

Aneurysms of the circle of Willis, if larger than about 1 cm, are usually demonstrable by CT. Arteriovenous (A-V) malformations may show a slight increase in density due to their circulating blood, and focal speckled increases in density may be due to calcification, but sometimes these lesions are impossible to demonstrate. A-V malformations and small aneurysms may be better visualized after the injection of contrast material. CT cannot replace angiography when the precise delineation of vascular abnormalities (such as aneurysms) or the site of vascular obstruction is required before surgery.

False-negative and false-positive errors are possible with CT, as with any other diagnostic procedure; however, CT corroboration by postmortem brain sections made in the plane of the scan has resulted in nearly identical findings as to the location and extent of primary intracranial tumors, obstructive hydrocephalus, intracerebral hemorrhage, ischemic and hemorrhagic infarctions, thermal burn encephalopathies, and other lesions. In one large study, CT, with a diagnostic error of significantly under 5%, was second only to cerebral pneumoencephalography in accurately diagnosing and evaluating a variety of intracranial disorders. CT is considerably more useful in evaluating brain lesions than is radionuclide scanning, heretofore the primary noninvasive technic. **CT of the spine** can demonstrate herniated discs and certain other conditions such as syringomyelia.

Abdomen, General Principles: With the development of scanners that can now scan in 5 seconds or less, motion (which degrades images) is no longer a serious technical limitation. Millisecond scanners, designed to evaluate cardiac function, are being developed.

The usefulness of CT in the abdomen, as in the brain, lies in its ability to define organ contours and to display contrast differences. Organs such as the liver, spleen, and kidneys are displayed as homogeneous-appearing soft tissue densities. Alterations in soft tissue composition, such as replacement by tumor, abscess, or cyst, appear as areas of differing densities on the scan. Cysts will appear at water density, tumors will usually appear at a soft tissue density less than that of the parent organ, while abscesses will show up at densities somewhere in between the two. The definition and contour of organ boundaries is used in the evaluation of the retroperitoneal organs, mainly the adrenals, pancreas, and lymph nodes. In evaluating the retroperitoneum, there must be sufficient retroperitoneal fat to separate one organ from the other. Without adequate fat, organ boundaries are not readily separable, hindering diagnostic evaluations.

Liver: Intrahepatic space-occupying lesions can be detected in much the same fashion as with radionuclide scanning. However, since CT scanning displays tissue densities, a more precise characterization of space-occupying lesions can be made. Tumors, cysts, and abscesses all have a respective range of attenuation coefficients, which may overlap, but usually are separate enough to allow characterization. Dilation of the intrahepatic biliary ducts can be demonstrated, and appear as branching, tubular, low attenuation areas dispersed throughout the liver. By following the dilation of the intra- and extrahepatic ductal system to its most proximal point, the etiology of the obstruction can usually be identified.

Pancreas: Pancreatic abnormalities are usually identified by alterations in the normal contour of the organ. Small pancreatic lesions that do not affect organ morphology cannot be defined, because there is no difference between their attenuation coefficients and normal pancreas. Larger pancreatic neoplasms are identified by their bulk and irregular margins. Pancreatic pseudocysts are identified as low attenuation areas within the pancreas. Pancreatitis usually results in diffuse enlargement of the gland.

Kidneys: Space-occupying lesions of the kidneys are easily characterized as to cyst or tumor. If a tumor is identified, CT can also give other important information such as local spread of tumor beyond the capsule or invasion of adjacent retroperitoneal structures. Inferior vena caval spread of hypernephroma can, at times, be identified.

Adrenal glands: Adrenal adenomas as small as 1 cm in diameter can be visualized when the patient has adequate retroperitoneal fat. Pheochromocytomas and adrenal carcinomas can also be identified in most cases. Adrenal hyperplasia can be identified as enlargement of an otherwise normal appearing adrenal gland.

Retroperitoneum: Enlargement of retroperitoneal lymph nodes, whether due to infection or tumor, can be identified. The reproducibility of CT scanning of the retroperitoneum makes this method ideal for following patients with known retroperitoneal lymphadenopathy.

Pelvis: With 2 exceptions, CT of the pelvis does not offer any appreciable advantage over ultrasound examination. Once a tumor of the pelvic organs has been identified by other clinical or radiographic means, its extent can be more easily defined by CT than by any other means, including ultrasound. Staging of bladder carcinoma by CT has also proven to be extremely useful. The bladder is scanned after the installation of a small amount of gas to allow determination of bladder wall thickness. Thus, it is possible to determine whether a mucosal lesion has grown through the wall or has spread to adjacent structures such as the seminal vesicles or adjacent pelvic lymph nodes.

Chest: CT demonstrates mediastinal and hilar lymphadenopathy and small intrapulmonary metastases, which may go undetected on routine studies, with a high degree of accuracy. Aortic aneurysms can be easily demonstrated. Currently, scanners are being developed that will allow evaluation of the cardiac chambers and pulmonary vessels.

CT-guided biopsy: The ability of CT to define lesions as small as 1 cm in diameter makes percutaneous aspiration biopsy an easily performed procedure. After a lesion has been identified, the aspirating needle is inserted through the skin to the mass. The precise location of the tip of the needle can then be verified by CT. With this method, it is possible to biopsy safely masses of the pancreas, adrenal glands, lymph nodes, and pelvis.

---

226. DIAGNOSTIC ULTRASONOGRAPHY

The use of ultrasonic pulse-echo imaging technics to detect tissue density differences within the body and thus display pathologic processes that are not adequately seen by other diagnostic procedures.

The development of radar and sonar (and of the flaw detector for materials testing) during World War II made possible the use of ultrasound for medical diagnostic purposes. Ultrasonic pulse-echo technics have been refined and can accurately present anatomic images of tissue and fluid interfaces within the body, providing valuable diagnostic information on many internal disorders. Evidence indicates that the power levels used for routine diagnostic studies with ultrasound cause no adverse effects, even in pregnancy. These power levels average < 10 mW/sq cm, a value at least 100 times less than that used in physical medicine (1 to 4 W/sq cm) for many years in the treatment of arthritis.

The diagnostic applications of ultrasound and CT scanning (see above) now comprise a very significant proportion of the radiology department space, equipment, budget, personnel, and general diagnostic load. Ultrasonography and CT are usually considered as a single diagnostic unit and while they may provide some similar information, each plays a special role. Ultrasonography has special capabilities, including the display of motion, simplicity of examination (no prior preparation is required), greater sensitivity than x-rays to soft tissue density differences, and elimination of the hazards associated with radiation and contrast dyes. It is particularly effective in determining depth and in guiding needle probes for diagnostic taps for renal cysts, ascites, aminocentesis, pericardial fluid, or pleural fluid.

The use of the Doppler effect and the ability to display pulsating structures as wave motion is an advantage in locating large blood vessels within a tumor mass prior to surgery. Real-time equipment can be easily moved to the bedside, a special advantage in emergencies and in trauma to the spleen, aorta, liver, or kidney. Phased array systems can demonstrate motion (e.g., cardiac or fetal) up to 40 frames/second and can automatically provide successive tissue sections as close as 2 mm apart.

In obstetrics, because it does not involve x-radiation, ultrasonography is the diagnostic method of choice. In many places almost all of the women have an ultrasonic evaluation at least once during pregnancy. It is invaluable in guiding the needle for amniocentesis and fetal transfusion. Ultrasound also has special diagnostic applications in ophthalmology and provides the only approach presently available to evaluate the retina and choroid in patients with opacity of the cornea. Diagnostic applications for the heart using ultrasonography as the initial screening procedure may eliminate the need for more hazardous tests such as arteriograms or cardiac catheterization. Many obstetricians, cardiologists, and ophthalmologists have units in their office. Furthermore, many radiologists use mobile units, especially in the West, to service small hospitals in their areas.

Principles of Operation and Clinical Applications

In standard ultrasonic diagnostic equipment, a transducer (usually a crystal of barium titanate), designed to oscillate between 1 and 15 MHz, is pulsed at a rate between 300 and 1000 times/second, producing bursts of ultrasonic energy that are directed into the tissue as a collimated or focused beam. When the ultrasound strikes a tissue or fluid interface of different density, sonic echoes are reflected back to the transducer face, converted into electrical impulses, amplified, and displayed on an oscilloscope as pips or dots.

Three standard modes of presentation of the echo data are currently used diagnostically. **(1) A-mode presentation:** The returned echoes are displayed as pips on a time base. Precise measurements can be made between the transducer face and each tissue interface returning echoes. This display is no longer used extensively but was used frequently in echoencephalography and for measurement of the biparietal diameter of the fetal head. **(2) Time-motion:** By using an intensity modulation display, the echo information appears on the oscilloscope as a dot whose intensity is roughly proportional to the magnitude of the returned echoes. When an echo-producing structure has motion, the echo information can be displayed in a wave form by proper synchronization of the oscilloscope sweep frequency. This type of display is used for echocardiography to show valvular motion, ventricular wall motion, etc. **(3) Compound B-scan:** When a dot is displayed for each echo-reflecting tissue interface at the rate of $>$ 300 times/second, movement of the transducer across the skin surface causes the dots to coalesce and form an echo anatomic outline of structures beneath the skin. This type of cross-sectional display is used for diagnostic studies of the liver, kidney, pancreas, spleen, bladder, and pregnant abdomen.

The **Doppler principle** was used first in pregnancy for detecting the fetal heart and in evaluating peripheral vascular disease. When a continuous or pulsed beam of ultrasonic energy passes through a column of flowing blood or other moving fluid to a receiving transducer, the frequency shift of the detected sound will vary with the rate and direction of flow. Thus, the slower flow through the umbilical vein can easily be differentiated from rapid flow through a maternal artery. A technic has been developed using pulsed Doppler and ultrasonic echo visualization of vessel size to calculate blood flow with $\pm$ 10% accuracy in carotid artery, umbilical vein, and other superficial vessels. The technic should soon be applicable to deeper vessels such as the renal artery, and will have many other diagnostic applications.

The Doppler technic is also used for serial measurements of BP (e.g., every 2 min), fetal heart monitoring, measuring BP in areas like the ankle, detecting large vessel occlusion, and bubble detection in dialysis and cardiac bypass systems.

Only those echoes reflected at right angles to the face of the transducer are registered by the oscilloscope while echo information reflected at an angle often does not impinge on the transducer face. Therefore, positioning of the body so that the interface of an organ, such as the kidney, is perpendicular to the transducer face is extremely important in obtaining maximum echo information. A tumor not visualized in one body position may become apparent when examined in another body position.

Several major ultrasonic equipment developments have expanded the current uses of diagnostic ultrasonography. The first is the capability of displaying echoes of 6 to 20 different magnitudes simultaneously on the same screen, either as different shades of gray or by color coding. This display (called gray-scale) accentuates visualization of such structures as the bile duct, Wirsung duct, portal vein, superior mesenteric artery, and gallbladder. This has significantly improved the localization and visualization of pancreatic lesions. In obstetrics, the gray-scale technic can more accurately outline the placenta, measure its thickness, and detect alterations in homogeneity.

A second development is the incorporation of computers, both digital and analog. These have smoothed out and presented a more recognizable image. A synchronized scanning system developed in Australia uses eight 2-in. transducers, each recording successively to provide a complete picture of the abdomen in approximately 2 seconds. The patient lies on a plastic sheet stretched over a water-filled tank. Advantages include improved definition provided by the water path system and a mechanical standardized scanning that eliminates operator variability.

Real-time scanning employs a multiple transducer array interphased successively to display motion of the heart, the fetus, and the larger blood vessels without use of contrast media at up to 40 frames/second. In linear arrays the transducers operate successively, whereas in phased arrays they operate in a planned pattern.

Finally, there are new phased transducer systems which automatically provide a series of pictures at 2 mm intervals. This has been of particular value in breast scanning or in tumor differentiation in a single organ. One system employs 3 transducers mounted on a wheel and by using 2 such wheels achieves a compound picture rapidly and with improved detail.

Since the real time scanner can be easily moved to the patient's bedside, ultrasound has proved invaluable as a screening procedure in emergencies.

Tissue characterization is a new concept for an imaging technic. Since ultrasound is a pressure wave, in contrast to the electromagnetic wave used in other types of image processing, it behaves differently in transmission through tissue. Measurement of specific parameters, such as velocity of sound transmission, spectral frequency absorption, attenuation, and echo reflection characteristics, may make it possible to establish a specific measurement pattern for each tumor or other pathologic process. Investigators are currently measuring attenuation and velocity of sound in the same sections of breast tissue and displaying the echo information on a single screen. An acoustic microscope has been constructed and is commercially available. It should help in establishing the ultrasonic pattern of various pathologic processes.

Echoencephalography (see Ch. 117)

Echocardiography (see Ultrasound in Ch. 23)

Peripheral Arteries (see Ch. 28)

Lung

Air rapidly attenuates ultrasound. Whenever there is consolidation or fluid, then ultrasound is readily transmitted through the lesion area demonstrated by x-ray. In complex pulmonary lesions, ultrasound may contribute important diagnostic information and should be tried when other studies are inconclusive.

The use of ultrasound for detecting pulmonary embolism has not had wide application in the USA, but has been used more extensively in England. Anatomic changes in the lung (manifested as echo changes) can occur within 1 h after emboli production. The skillful use of ultrasound can be helpful in determining the causes of acute chest pain.

Thyroid

Ultrasonic studies of a thyroid nodule can differentiate between a fluid-filled cyst and a tumor. A cyst is smoothly outlined, remains sonolucent (echo-free) when receiver sensitivity is increased, and the far border is accentuated, while a tumor usually has an irregular border, fills in with echoes when sensitivity is increased, and may have shadowing at its distal edge. Use of a short-focused transducer and higher frequencies may improve the display of thyroid detail. Demonstration of the anatomic relations of the mass to the jugular vein and carotid artery may also be of use whenever surgery is planned.

Internal Hemorrhagic Conditions

In patients with hemophilia or other causes of internal bleeding, ultrasonography can often be helpful in locating the site of hemorrhage, the extent of the hemorrhage, and the presence of internal echoes, suggesting organization of the clot. Serial examinations often show when hemorrhage has stopped after therapy.

Abdomen

Ultrasound is particularly effective in demonstrating the presence of ascitic fluid, in determining whether the fluid is free or loculated, and in precisely localizing the best site for diagnostic paracentesis. In a series of > 100 patients with ascites, in whom abdominal palpation was difficult, ultrasound demonstrated unsuspected intra-abdominal pathology in > 40%. Some authorities believe that paracentesis should not be done until the presence and location of suspected fluid is checked with ultrasound.

When echoes are not attenuated by gas in the bowel, intra-abdominal vessels can be identified and their function assessed. These include the portal vein and its major branches, the superior mesenteric artery and vein, the splenic vein, the hepatic vein, the renal arteries and veins, and the inferior mesenteric vein.

One of the most important new diagnostic applications of ultrasound has been the display of biliary and pancreatic ducts. While they can be seen in the normal subject under ideal conditions, in the patient with biliary obstruction they can be readily demonstrated and the presence of obstruction verified. In the jaundiced patient ultrasonography should be the first imaging technic ordered. Because blood vessels and secretory ducts vary greatly in size and course, it may be necessary to scan in several different planes to differentiate between ducts or blood vessels.

Pancreas and Gallbladder

Through the identification of blood vessel positions, one can localize the pancreatic area anatomically quite precisely and in > 80% of diagnostic problems specifically identify changes in the echo pattern suggestive of a specific pathology. More than 90% of pseudocysts can be identified correctly and usually any errors are in the identification of the source of the cyst, since mesenteric, splenic, renal, and hepatic cysts may be mistaken for pseudocyst of the pancreas. Tumors can be either echogenic or sonolucent, which means there is no specific recognizable echo pattern for pancreatic tumors. On the other hand, the ultrasonic echo pattern combined with other medical data usually leads to the correct diagnosis. Ultrasonic visualization of tumors as small as 1 to 2 cm have been reported. In acute pancreatitis there will often be increased sonolucence in the pancreas. Patients with suspected chronic pancreatitis may have increased intrapancreatic echoes, but there is no consistency in the echo pattern for chronic pancreatitis.

The gallbladder is readily visualized. In the longitudinal plane it appears as a pear-shaped sonolucent area that disappears when emptying is stimulated. Presence of echoes within the gallbladder associated with a sonic shadow beyond is the characteristic echo pattern for gallstones. In many patients, ultrasonography now precedes oral cholecystography.

Recent studies utilized filling of the stomach with fluid (methylcellulose 1% or orange juice) as a sonic window to look at the pancreas. Fluid in the stomach has often resulted in good sonic delineation of the duodenum. In thinner patients, it has been possible to demonstrate the inner surface of the stomach and to pick up lesions of the stomach wall. Further development of this technic may improve visualization of the pancreas and provide the ultrasonic capability for picking up gastric lesions.

Liver and Spleen

Both organs appear as low echo areas on the gray-scale echogram and changes in size and position can be readily estimated. By integrating the cross-sectional area of ultrasonic serial scans taken at 1-cm intervals, the total splenic volume can be determined. These calculated volumes range within about ± 12% when compared with displacement volume measurements of surgically removed spleens. Measurement of splenic size can be important in obese patients where palpation is difficult and for monitoring splenic size during chemotherapy. Of diagnostic importance is the anteriorly placed spleen that is often palpable but not enlarged. The ratio of the maximal cross-sectional area of the liver and the area of the corresponding abdominal cross section provide a rapid semiquantitative assessment of liver size.

Hepatic lesions (cyst, tumor, abscess, or cirrhosis) often have a distinctive echo pattern. Radioisotope studies demonstrate functional uptake by the liver cells, whereas ultrasound demonstrates density differences. Various types of liver tumors may differ in their echo patterns, which makes interpretation of present day records more difficult, but in the future may well prove useful in predicting the type of liver tumor present. (See also Ch. 65.)

Kidney and Bladder (see in Ch. 144)

Retroperitoneal Pathology

Ultrasonography and CT scanning have proved to be the most effective imaging methods for demonstrating retroperitoneal and intrapelvic pathology. When intestinal gas does not attenuate the sound, retroperitoneal lymphadenopathy and tumor can be demonstrated easily. In radiation therapy both CT and ultrasound have been used in evaluating therapeutic effectiveness by showing changes in lymph node size.

Aorta and Vena Cava

These structures are well visualized by ultrasound and the echo information provides primary diagnosis of lesions. Additionally, they serve as landmarks for identifying other anatomic structures within the abdomen. In patients with aortic aneurysm, ultrasound or CT has been the diagnostic method of choice, since either can differentiate between blood lumen and associated clot within the aneurysm. Ultrasound also displays constriction or generalized dilation of these vessels, hemorrhage surrounding them, and displacement by contiguous lesions.

Tumor

Ultrasonography has proved very promising for early tumor detection and evaluation. At present there are at least 5 different ultrasonic echo patterns associated with tumors. These include (1) a dense echo nest, (2) a cystic appearance due to surface reflection from the tumor, (3) an irregular sonolucent area indicating better sound transmission in tumor, (4) lack of echoes beyond tumor due to attenuation of sound, and (5) ultrasonic pattern of a cyst due to hemorrhage or necrosis within the tumor. Development of new technics may make tissue characterization of the tumor more accurate. This has already been done for the eye.

When a tumor can be outlined accurately using ultrasonics, the planning of radiation fields and thus radiation therapy can be more efficient. Furthermore, ultrasonography can identify anatomic structures adjacent to the tumor, such as the kidney or bladder, so that they can be protected from radiation injury. It can also determine the effectiveness of radiation or chemotherapy by monitoring changes in tumor size. In planning radiotherapy, rapid advances indicate that ultrasound or CT will be used routinely during radiation therapy.

Breast

Ultrasonography has developed as an imaging technic effective for evaluation of breast tumor and palpable masses. As a mass screening technic for detection of early breast tumors and especially for detection of nonpalpable tumors, ultrasonography is not yet practical. There are many problems associated with ultrasonic visualization of the breast, especially those relating to changes in breast tissue characteristics throughout a woman's life and also to the variations between breasts even in the same woman. Another difficulty is holding the breast in a fixed position for scanning without compression. The recent use of water path screening and multiple sections (every 2 mm) should help overcome the positioning problem. However, recent scans suggest that better evaluations can be obtained with ultrasonography than with other imaging technics.

Gynecology

Ultrasonography is used to detect pelvic, uterine, and ovarian lesions. The full-bladder technic of examination not only improves visualization of the uterus and other structures posterior to the bladder, but through contour changes assists in locating a pelvic lesion anatomically. Ultrasonography is the method of choice in locating IUDs and in determining if they are still within the uterine cavity.

Ophthalmology

Because of the limited area of examination, even the early transducers provided good visualization of the eye. Thus, use of ultrasound in ophthalmology started early using both A and B mode technics. Definition in the orbit is improved by the use of higher frequencies (7 to 10 MHz). Ultrasonography has been useful in locating metallic and nonmetallic foreign bodies and in demonstrating intraocular tumor, hemangioma, hemorrhage, retinal detachment, and many intraorbital lesions. In the presence of opacities of the cornea, diagnostic ultrasonography is the only method for detecting retinal or choroidal lesions. Ultrasonic measurements are used for refraction prior to implantation of plastic lenses.

The recent development of a hand-held B scanner has simplified ultrasonic examination of the eye and made it possible to do such studies in the ophthalmologist's office. By using a biologic standard, an accuracy of > 90% in differentiating between melanoma and metastatic carcinoma of the orbit has been claimed. This is the most successful application of ultrasonic tissue characterization at present.

---

227. DIAGNOSTIC USE OF RADIOISOTOPES

The medical use of radionuclides (radioactive isotopes) anticipated at the beginning of the atomic era in the late 1940s has become a routine part of practice and serves many areas and specialties faced with diagnostic problems. Appropriate facilities or access to the services of nuclear medicine is required for hospital accreditation by the Joint Commission on Hospital Accreditation. In 1972 the American Board of Nuclear Medicine was created to certify physicians, thus formally establishing a significant presence in the field of medicine.

Radiopharmaceuticals and the Radiotracer Concept

The most useful property of a radionuclide is its emission of electromagnetic radiation in the form of γ-rays, which are readily detectable with modern instrumentation. Each radioactive isotope decays at a unique rate (half-life) and has a characteristic spectrum of γ-ray energies. These 2 properties permit its identification. Many radionuclides emit β rays in addition to or instead of γ-rays that may be useful for in vitro analysis such as radioimmunoassay or competitive binding analysis of serum. However, β emission that occurs in association with γ emission is usually undesirable, since it results in a higher total radiation dose when administered internally.

Exceedingly small amounts of radiation produced by a fraction of a μg (tracer dose) of radionuclide can be detected, thus eliminating the potential for chemical or physical toxicity and any pharmacologic considerations. For example, a tracer dose of radioactive iodine may be given safely to a patient with a known iodine sensitivity. Nuclear medical procedures provide clinical information with a much lower dose of radiation than alternative radiographic technics. They have an excellent safety record and it is accepted practice to use them in children when indicated. While most radiopharmaceuticals are used as tracers for diagnosis, a small number are used as radiation sources for therapy.

Radioactive isotopes may be used as simple salts of an element (sodium radioiodide), or they may be chemically bound to another molecule to produce a "labeled" compound. In either instance, these substances are physiologically and biochemically identical to the stable or nonradioactive form. For example, radioiodine (^{131}I) behaves in the body in a manner similar to nonradioactive or stable iodine (^{127}I). If radioiodine is attached to a molecule such as albumin, the molecule continues to behave as albumin, but its fate and location in the body may be "traced" by external detection of the γ-rays from the radioiodine. These tracers may be administered by parenteral, oral, or intracavitary routes.

Radiation Detectors

Equipment capable of detecting the emitted radiation of radioisotopes usually includes some form of scintillation detector, a device which contains (1) a special crystal that absorbs ionizing radiation and converts it into light flashes or scintillations and (2) a mechanism for counting these scintillations or converting them into an image. Several types of scintillation detectors are used currently. The stationary probe type is used in thyroid uptake, kidney function, and red cell survival studies. The rectilinear scanner is a mechanized version of the probe-type detector using a special focused collimator. It moves a scintillation detector back and forth across the patient in a series of parallel lines, detecting radioactivity on a point-by-point basis, while a photorecorder connected to the moving detector mechanically and electronically creates an image. The rectilinear scanner has now been largely replaced by camera imaging devices and is used with decreasing frequency, but remains very useful in a few specific test situations.

The scintillation camera is a more sophisticated stationary imaging device that combines the advantages of the stationary probe and the scanner and is widely used for virtually all imaging procedures. Changing levels of radioactivity throughout a large area can be monitored rapidly, providing both image and count rate information thus allowing the study of dynamic processes.

Computers are now routinely used with camera imaging devices. These permit storage of data for later playback in many modes. Quantitation of data is possible since the computer enables the operator to review localized portions of the camera image as a regional image, integrated count rate, or time-activity histogram. Computer technology has also made possible the cardiovascular technics discussed below and is being used with increasing application in other organs.

The Meaning of Dose

The term "dose" in nuclear medicine is used in 2 senses. The given dose of a radiopharmaceutical used for diagnosis is measured in microcuries (μCi) or millicuries (mCi), which are units of measurement of the quantity of radioactivity. The radiation dose, on the other hand, refers to the amount of radiation energy absorbed by tissue. It is commonly expressed as the rad (radiation absorbed dose) and is discussed in more detail in Ch. 218. Calculation of the rad requires a complex computation involving the given dose of radioactivity; the type, energies, and half-life of the radioactive emissions;

the density and volume of organs exposed to the radiation; and the biologic half-life of the isotope within those organs. Though difficult to calculate with high precision, the radiation dose from most radioisotope diagnostic procedures generally is less than or comparable to that obtained from conventional x-ray procedures.

RADIONUCLIDE IMAGING METHODS

Radionuclide incorporation into an organ depends upon particular physiologic or biochemical properties of that organ and the specific radiocompound used. Imaging procedures in nuclear medicine have less spatial resolution of structures than radiographs but more physiologic significance. In some instances, there is no comparable practical x-ray procedure for visualizing the organ of interest; e.g., the thyroid. In others, the x-ray findings and radionuclide imaging findings are complementary. Additional information from the history, clinical examination, x-rays, and other laboratory data contribute to the reliability and applicability of the scan information.

Thyroid

The concentration of radioiodine or pertechnetate in the thyroid depends on the presence of functioning tissue and adequate thyroid-stimulating hormone (TSH). Any zone of absent or diminished uptake of radioactivity usually indicates abnormal hypofunctional tissue, which may be caused by a cyst, hemorrhage, inflammation, or neoplasm. Focal zones of increased radioactivity indicate hyperfunctional tissue such as may be found in occasionally adenomatous changes, or more frequently, in hyperactive pre-toxic or frankly toxic nodules. Goiter is characterized by an enlarged gland. When the concentration of uptake is diffusely increased, toxic diffuse goiter (Graves' disease) probably is present, while irregular uptake is associated with Plummer's disease.

A solitary palpable thyroid nodule requires differentiation between a benign cyst or adenoma and a malignancy. The absence of radioactivity in the nodule ("cold nodule") signifies an increased probability of neoplasm, whereas normal or increased radioactivity in the nodule ("hot nodule") is strong evidence against neoplasm. Ultrasonography may demonstrate the presence of a cyst, helping greatly in the differential diagnosis, but definitive diagnosis of a cold nodule requires either direct needle biopsy (currently the procedure of choice) or open neck exploration. If metastasis from thyroid carcinoma (papillary-follicular) has occurred, the lesion usually does not concentrate radioiodine in the presence of an intact thyroid gland. Only after complete surgical removal and radioiodine ablation of the original thyroid remnants will metastatic lesions in the neck, lungs, or bone become visible by scanning. Radioiodine does not concentrate in undifferentiated carcinomas and has no practical application in these disorders.

In patients over age 40, there is a greater incidence of benign multinodular goiter related to focal areas of degeneration or inflammation interspersed with islands of intact normal tissue. These islands usually have undergone various degrees of hypertrophy in response to endogenous thyroid requirements. Considerable difficulty may be encountered in differentiating these cases from the uncommon case of advanced multifocal carcinoma.

Patients with solitary or multiple hyperfunctional ("hot") nodules may have typical clinical findings of thyrotoxicosis (toxic nodular goiter). The administration of TSH may stimulate nonvisualized zones of suppressed normal tissue. This finding and failure to reduce the radioiodine uptake in the active nodules with triiodothyronine suppression confirm the autonomous nature of these nodules. Since the incidence of neoplasm in such nodules is negligible, diagnosis is important in the choice of therapy.

Liver

Evaluation of primary or secondary hepatic disease is enhanced by liver scanning. When combined with data from serologic tests, liver scan data may indicate the best additional diagnostic or therapeutic measures. Technetium Tc 99m sulfur colloid given IV is trapped rapidly by the Kupffer cells (reticuloendothelial) of the liver. The normal scan shows a typical triangular organ with a homogeneous distribution of activity. A variety of pathologic processes change the size, shape, or the patterns of distribution of activity that raise or lower the probability of particular diagnoses. Liver scanning is most useful when specific diagnostic questions are posed as a result of the history and physical findings.

Liver scanning may help evaluate the relationship of a palpable abdominal mass to the liver. The presence of a palpable liver is not pathologic per se, but often is an anatomic displacement due to a flattened diaphragm or an unusual shape. A mass in the right lower quadrant may be Reidel's lobe or a large dependent gallbladder attached to the liver. The liver may not be palpable with tense ascites, in which case the scan will show the liver's size and shape and the presence of possible intrahepatic masses.

The liver scan is rarely normal when jaundice due to intrahepatic causes, especially a focal neoplasm, is present. Intrahepatic biliary tract obstruction is accompanied by diffuse hepatomegaly, sometimes with some overall anatomic distortion. Extrahepatic obstruction often results in dilation of the large intrahepatic bile ducts and a displacement of tissue visible as a "Y" defect in the porta hepatis.

The finding of solitary or multiple, discrete, focal defects suggests metastatic neoplasms, but artifacts do occur. Serial scans showing progressive change are highly suggestive of neoplasm. Liver scans fail to show these discrete changes in about 15 to 20% of cases with proved metastases, probably because of diffuse involvement with small lesions below the limits of resolution. At times, the changes in the liver scan may be confused with other lesions, notably those resulting from scarring or healing after injury due to drugs or alcohol. Negative findings must be viewed with caution, but a positive scan can lead to more precise biopsy. Percutaneous needle biopsy alone may miss as many as 32% of liver metastases. The combination of liver scan and needle biopsy will detect more hepatic neoplasms than either method alone.

In chronic liver disease, widespread necrosis, scarring, or nodular regeneration causes distortion of liver anatomy with left lobe enlargement and irregularity of radionuclide distribution. Many hepato-toxins and malnutrition will produce diffuse, nonspecific, mild to moderate liver enlargement and varying degrees of decreased uptake of labeled colloid on the scans. These changes regress when the conditions are reversed. Diffuse hepatomegaly is also seen in infiltrative disorders such as amy-loidosis, sarcoidosis, xanthomatosis, leukemia, and lymphoma.

The liver scan is a useful noninvasive means of detecting a bacterial or amebic liver abscess. In an acutely ill, febrile patient with right upper quadrant pain or tenderness, an elevated right hemidia-phragm, and a typical liver scan defect, an intrahepatic abscess is the most likely diagnosis. A right subphrenic abscess, often the consequence of abdominal surgery, trauma, or a perforated viscus, can be demonstrated by a zone of absent radioactivity between the lung and liver. The liver-lung scan, however, is generally undependable. The exact relationship between the value of liver scan-ning with radioisotopes and computerized tomography (CT) of the liver has not yet been defined. It does not appear at present that CT will replace the radioisotope liver scan.

Biliary Scanning Agents

The introduction of iminodiacetic acid derivatives (HIDA) labeled with 99mTc has made possible a new generation of liver scan. HIDA and related compounds achieve high biliary concentrations and are used to image the gallbladder and bile ducts. They are of great diagnostic accuracy in the detection of acute cholecystitis characterized by nonvisualization of the gallbladder. Differential di-agnosis of obscure cases of abdominal pain is facilitated by this procedure. Bile duct obstruction can be demonstrated by failure of the radioactivity to enter the bowel. The exact role of these agents in liver disease is not yet clear, but their use in the differential diagnosis of acute cholecystitis appears secure.

Spleen

The spleen scan is a reliable noninvasive method of determining if the spleen is normal and can help to differentiate left upper quadrant masses. Splenic views usually are taken routinely in the course of liver scanning. Reticuloendothelial cells in the spleen will trap technetium Tc 99m sulfur colloid in a manner similar to the liver. In normal individuals, the apparent concentration of activity in liver and spleen are about equal. Marked reduction in spleen uptake compared to liver uptake indi-cates either splenic arterial obstruction or pathologic infiltration. Increases in relative spleen uptake occur usually with decreases in hepatic portal blood flow accompanying parenchymal liver disease, but may result from increased blood flow in patients with acute splenitis. Primary neoplasms of the spleen are unusual, but splenic involvement in the presence of leukemia, lymphoma, or melanoma is not. Patients with Hodgkin's disease generally have diffuse splenic enlargement. In some lympho-mas, nodular or focal changes are present, but this is most frequent in reticulum cell sarcoma involving the spleen. A major use of splenic scanning, especially in children, is after abdominal trauma when splenic rupture or subcapsular hematoma is suspected. Focal scan defects in the spleen are uncommon and are mostly due to infarcts or small abscesses; they may suggest injury.

Pancreas

Detection of abnormalities in the exocrine portion of the pancreas depends on incorporation of selenomethionine Se 75 in the enzyme protein of acinar cells. An active, functional, anatomically intact pancreas will take up sufficient radio-labeled amino acid to produce usable images. A normal study usually excludes pancreatic disease. A diffuse decrease in radionuclide uptake may occur with any process that impedes the normal secretory sequences that lead to stimulation of pancreatic enzyme formation and secretion into the bowel. Vagotomy, antral cancer, acute peptic ulcer, starva-tion, advanced ascites, carcinomatosis, the use of anticholinergic drugs, and gastroenterostomy are the most common of such processes. Focal lesions of the pancreas are strong evidence of neoplasm or chronic inflammation, but the two cannot be distinguished by scan alone. This procedure pres-ents great difficulties in interpretation and has only very limited usefulness.

Lung

Lung perfusion scans are performed after IV injection of 20- to 50-μ particles of biodegradable albumin labeled with 99mTc. These particles traverse the right heart and are distributed to the right and left lungs through the pulmonary arteries, ultimately lodging in the small precapillary arterioles. Nearly 100% of the particles remain in the lung, except when right-to-left shunting is present either at the cardiac or pulmonic level. The regional distribution of these particles is directly proportional to regional pulmonary arteriolar blood flow. This distribution is relatively homogeneous in normal per-sons, but visible activity is greater at the base and gradually diminishes up to the apex, reflecting gravitational effects on perfusion when the patient is injected in the sitting position. The distribution of particles depends on the position of the patient and pulmonary blood flow distribution at the time of injection. Any alteration of the normal pattern in relation to a standard injection procedure represents pathologic regional perfusion and may result from vascular obstruction, displacement of lung by fluid, masses in the chest, or any condition causing left atrial hypertension or pulmonary hypertension.

The lung perfusion scan is a valuable noninvasive method of detecting **acute pulmonary embolism**, especially when x-rays are normal. A normal lung scan excludes life-threatening pulmonary embolism with an accuracy of over 98%. Conversely, single or multiple wedge-shaped marginal scan defects, especially in a segmental distribution, are highly suggestive evidence of vascular obstruction or of another process leading to regional vascular shunting. In most cases the patterns are so typical as to be unmistakable to an experienced observer, characteristically revealing "cold" or nonradioactive areas of the lung. Sometimes, however, acute or chronic airway obstruction (emphysema) may produce a confusing pattern due to extensive focal perfusion abnormalities. Often this can be recognized by poorly defined, mid-zonal areas of decreased radionuclide distribution. In many cases, superimposed small emboli cannot be excluded by a single study. Serial scans over a 3- to 6-day period often resolve the issue. Progressive resolution of lesions favors a diagnosis of emboli, while a static picture favors chronic preexisting changes. Edema and alveolar secretions caused by lung infection will produce perfusion defects related to hypoxia and secondary regional arterial shunting. Characteristic x-ray changes of pneumonia and positive microbiologic studies help differentiate pneumonia from embolism.

In cases where differentiation between pulmonary embolism and chronic obstructive lung disease is difficult, the ^{133}Xe lung **ventilation scan** is useful. The radioactive gas is inhaled and distributes with the respiratory air. In pulmonary embolism the radioxenon scan is usually normal, exhibiting ventilation/perfusion mismatches. Areas of parenchymal disease usually show abnormalities of both perfusion and ventilation, and will demonstrate delayed ventilation and trapping of radioactive gas.

Any process leading to increased left atrial pressure, such as congestive heart failure, mitral valve disease, or veno-occlusive disease, will produce reversal of the normal preponderance of radioactivity at the base of the lung and can be detected even before x-ray or clinical changes of heart failure appear. The apical/basilar distribution of radioactivity in the pulmonary perfusion scan has been shown to be proportional to left atrial pressure.

Cardiovascular System

The transit of an IV bolus of Tc 99m sodium pertechnetate through the right and left sides of the heart can be recorded on rapid sequential views with the scintillation camera and stored in a computer for later analysis. Obstruction of the superior vena cava by tumor; mass lesions in the right heart, such as myxomas, neoplasms, valve lesions, fibrous bands, and thrombi; and pulmonary arterial obstruction or post-stenotic dilation can be demonstrated. On return to the left heart, the bolus may show enlargement of both left chambers and changes in the appearance of the left ventricular wall due to aneurysm and dyskinetic segments following myocardial infarction. A left-to-right shunt at the atrial level results in delayed pulmonary transit reflected as a prolonged activity washout over the lungs. Right-to-left shunts are readily discernible by observing early appearance of activity over the left heart or aorta. Aneurysmal dilations of the aortic arch and of the descending and abdominal aorta are demonstrable in rapid sequential views. The bolus technic may be used to evaluate any mediastinal mass to determine its vascularity or connection with major vessels and is the technic for first-pass studies discussed below.

Pericardial effusion suspected from clinical or x-ray findings may be confirmed by a rapid sequential bolus study by detecting a space between right atrial heart blood pool and the medial border of the right lung blood pool, but this is a less sensitive method than detection with diagnostic ultrasound. The scan method is sufficiently accurate to detect most hemodynamically significant effusions (200 ml or more). Smaller amounts may be significant in some cases if fluid accumulates suddenly. Ultrasonic examination is less valuable in loculated effusions in postoperative heart surgery patients or when left pleural effusion is present.

Cardiac Function

The most impressive development in clinical nuclear medicine in the past 5 yr is in cardiovascular nuclear medicine. There are now several distinct categories of cardiac procedures.

"Cold spot" imaging employs radiothallium which behaves as an analog of potassium. Its distribution in the heart is proportional to coronary blood flow. After IV injection, thallium is concentrated in the left ventricle especially. A patient who has had a myocardial infarction, either recent or old, shows a decreased or absent area of uptake. The test is particularly useful in the differential diagnosis of angina pectoris. Patients with suspected coronary artery disease are subject to maximum-tolerated stress levels and thallium is injected. If a significant coronary stenosis is present, there will be a reduction in myocardial perfusion showing up as a "cold spot" in that area. After the patient rests, the thallium redistributes throughout the myocardium. The filling in of a "cold spot" with radioactivity confirms that the lesion is due to ischemia and not to an old infarct that would not fill in. The thallium scan is most useful in patients who are carefully screened and when other procedures have not produced definite results.

"Hot spot" imaging, unlike thallium, depends on selective uptake of an agent in an abnormal area of myocardium. The most commonly used agent is ^{99m}Tc pyrophosphate, but technetium-labeled glucoheptonate, tetracycline, and other agents have been used also. In patients with a myocardial infarction 24 to 48 h old, these agents are concentrated in the abnormal area. Although thought to be related to microscopic Ca deposition, the mechanism of the uptake is not clear. Low-grade uptake is nonspecific, while intense focal uptake usually is seen in infarction. The value of these agents is limited by delay before a positive result and by the wide variety of conditions that can cause uptake, including cardiomyopathy, trauma, pericarditis, and many others. However, they are useful in clarifying difficult diagnostic situations and in evaluating possible reinfarction or extension.

To evaluate cardiac function, a variety of technics are available. Ejection fraction can be measured by either a first-pass or a gated technic. In the first-pass method, a bolus of ^{99m}Tc is recorded as it passes through the left ventricle. The data are then played back by computer to provide quantitative as well as qualitative analysis. Alternatively, a gated technic may be used in which a series of usually 120 or more cardiac cycles are summated through ECG gating. A compound confined to the bloodstream is required for the gated method; ^{99m}Tc labeled albumin or ^{99m}Tc labeled RBCs are used. RBC labeling is quite simply accomplished by giving an IV injection of Sn pyrophosphate followed 15 min later by a ^{99m}Tc pertechnetate injection, which results in labeling of the tin-coated erythrocytes.

The ejection fraction is the stroke volume of the heart divided by the end-diastolic volume. It is used generally in reference to the left ventricle. In isotonic exercises normal subjects increase the inotropic force of the heart, raising the ejection fraction significantly, while patients with heart disease will tend to dilate the heart moving along Starling's curve with a resultant fall in ejection fraction. The normal range is about 50 to 70% with a significant change being about 3 to 5 ejection fraction units, depending on the laboratory and the exact method. Ejection fraction measurements provide an accurate, sensitive measure of myocardial function.

It also is possible to play back the cardiac images so that the observer can see the change in distribution of radioactivity as the heart contracts. Abnormal areas show up as decreased wall movement (hypokinesia), absent movement (akinesia) or paradoxical movement (dyskinesia). Dyskinesia suggests ventricular aneurysm. Wall motion studies have been reported to be a very sensitive method of detecting coronary artery disease, especially when used in conjunction with exercise testing.

Urogenital

Several radiopharmaceuticals (such as ^{99m}Tc-labeled glucoheptanate, dimercaptosuccinate, and ^{131}I-labeled iodohippurate) concentrate in the renal parenchyma. Any focal parenchymal lesion (e.g., tumor, abscess, cyst, or infarction) will produce a focal defect visible in static scans in which the radiotechnetium agents are most useful. Ultrasound is the procedure of choice for differentiating most renal masses noninvasively, but lesions within the renal parenchyma, irregular renal shapes, and hypertrophied columns of Bertini may be best diagnosed by nuclear methods. Renal masses seen on urography can be evaluated by confirming a pathologic change or by demonstrating an intact parenchyma free of disease. Additional data on renal vascular integrity are obtained by rapid sequential views of a ^{99m}Tc pertechnetate or ^{99m}Tc-DTPA bolus entering the kidneys from the aorta (renal perfusion study). With this procedure, cysts appear as unperfused areas and hypernephroma is highly perfused. Renal arterial obstruction or focal avascular sites in the renal parenchyma may be observed with the flow study. Patients with hypertension from surgically curable unilateral renal disease are infrequent, but a combination of radionuclide studies may be used to screen patients for this entity with an accuracy equal to that of urography.

DTPA labeled with ^{99m}Tc is excreted at about 5% less than the GFR. It can be used in most situations and results in a relatively low radiation dose, so it is especially suited for repetitive studies and studies in children. It does not provide the same image resolution as the compounds mentioned above and is not concentrated like orthoiodohippurate in kidneys with poor renal function (see below).

Another approach to renal functional evaluation can be achieved wih iodohippurate sodium I 131. The intrarenal transit and distribution of this agent reflects renal plasma flow and secretory activity of the renal tubules. Sequential scans taken every 3 min following injection show the uptake, concentration, and transit of the radiolabeled compound from the cortical area of the nephron, through the medulla, into the pelvocaliceal system, and down the ureter. Obstruction due to any lesion may be demonstrated with great sensitivity. Focal retention of radioactivity within kidney parenchyma signals the possible presence of caliceal obstruction, such as is caused by neoplasm, stone, or infection. Similarly, ureteral stenosis or chronic bladder neck obstruction may occasionally show ureteral dilation and trapping of activity above the obstruction. If the radioiodine or ^{99m}Tc-DTPA data are computerized, curves may be generated from various portions of the kidney. These curves facilitate qualitative comparison of individual and segmental renal function. They are of great help in evaluating urinary tract obstruction.

Renal failure: An advantage of iodohippurate sodium I 131 in renal imaging is its ability to scan the kidney at very low levels of renal function, permitting evaluation of size and location in acute renal failure. Failure to image the kidneys with iodohippurate sodium I 131 in a patient with renal insufficiency is a grave prognostic sign.

Ureteral reflux usually is demonstrated by x-ray contrast cystourethrography. However, this method has certain disadvantages, especially the high gonadal radiation exposure in children. Such repetitive studies of this type can be avoided by using sodium pertechnetate Tc 99m cystourethrography, which is highly sensitive and satisfactory for long-term follow-up of previously diagnosed patients. It is equally useful for detecting early cases of ureteral urinary reflux.

Sodium pertechnetate Tc 99m is of value in the early differential diagnosis of sudden testicular pain. Torsion of the testicle appears as an unperfused area, while epididymitis is usually detected by relative hyperperfusion.

Adrenal Gland

Synthesis of ^{131}I labeled 19-iodocholesterol permits semiquantitative imaging of the adrenal gland. Absent unilateral uptake suggests destruction of gland tissue by neoplasm, infection, infarction, or suppression. Small aldosteronomas may be detected by a refined technic that distinguishes normal tissue from the tumor. Bilateral hyperplasia is reflected by an increased uptake of the radiopharmaceutical. Adrenal suppressibility can be determined by prescan treatment with corticosteroids. The procedure has achieved greatest use in localizing adrenal adenomas and in differentiating adenoma from bilateral hyperplasia. Medullary tumors such as pheochromocytoma may occasionally be detected as defects. Unfortunately, the radiation dose with this procedure is high and the relative roles of CT scanning and nuclear scanning have not been defined.

Bone and Joint

Focal injury to bone from any cause leads to new bone formation in that site. The associated biochemical changes result in an increased concentration and turnover of Ca and PO_4 compounds. ^{99m}Tc-labeled pyrophosphate, dimethylphosphate, and a variety of lesser-used analogs are agents of choice for bone scanning. Total-body bone scanning is a proven adjunct to cancer management. Well-defined abnormal sites of labeled phosphate in the skeleton are highly suggestive of metastatic cancer, especially when primary breast or prostate carcinoma is present. These areas are detectable on scans long before they can be seen by x-rays but, in some instances, highly lytic lesions seen on x-ray may not show phosphate uptake until treatment begins and healing or reactive bone formation occurs. Certain types of lesions, such as Hodgkin's tumor in bone and myeloma, may appear as a negative or "skip" area, while diffuse metastatic disease as seen in prostate carcinoma may cause increased uptake in virtually the entire skeleton.

Acute osteomyelitis is usually ruled out by a negative bone scan. Occasionally, osteomyelitis may show up as decreased uptake on a phosphate scan. In such cases, a ^{67}Ga scan usually reveals the diagnosis. Septic joint, osteomyelitis, and cellulitis usually can be differentiated. Bone infarction in sickle cell crisis cannot always be distinguished from osteomyelitis by scan alone, since both may be positive. However, the time course of the 2 diseases differs; early on, infarction is almost always "cold," while infection is "hot." Rib fractures, even when unsuspected clinically, may be found on a scan in an aged patient with osteoporosis.

Metabolic bone disease such as Paget's disease is readily detected by bone scans even in its earliest stages. The true extent of skeletal involvement cannot be ascertained without a total-body bone scan.

Arthritis or inflammatory synovial changes result in an increased concentration of labeled phosphate in the joint capsule. This appears as a "hot" joint, often with obliteration of the joint space; while this appearance is nonspecific, the degree of injury is readily apparent. One of the earliest confirmatory signs of rheumatoid arthritis is a positive scan over an asymptomatic joint in a patient with at least one other positive symptomatic joint. The scan appearance reflects activity of the disease and may return to normal in cases treated early.

Total Body Scanning

Gallium citrate Ga 67 has been shown to localize in certain types of soft tissue cancers, especially lymphomas, reticulum cell sarcomas, osteosarcomas, melanomas, and squamous cell or oat cell carcinoma of the lung, with a concentration several times that in normal tissue. Other tumor types, mainly well-differentiated adenocarcinomas of the gastrointestinal tract, take up ^{67}Ga less predictably and to a lesser degree. These scans are not particularly helpful for initial diagnosis of cancer but are useful in staging and in ascertaining the extent of the disease as well as in management and follow-up. Positive studies typical of neoplastic spread are characterized by increased ^{67}Ga concentrations in nodal areas, the mediastinum, the retroperitoneum, or bone. Occasionally, neoplasm can be confirmed in liver (mainly hepatoma) and spleen (melanoma). Metastases to the liver from most primary cancers are variable in their uptake of ^{67}Ga, depending on the mass of normal liver relative to tumor mass. ^{67}Ga uptake is not specific for neoplasm, since it also concentrates in sites of active occult infection.

In FUO, the usual search may fail to find a site of localized infection. ^{67}Ga scans have detected a number of such occult infections of practically every variety and are also valuable in searching for an abscess. Patients with sarcoid have increased uptake of gallium in mediastinal nodes. The finding of hilar nodes on gallium scan and increased plasma concentration of converting enzyme is diagnostic of sarcoid.

Central Nervous System (see Ch. 117)

Transplantation

Nuclear medical procedures have been used in liver, lung, pancreas, and kidney transplantation. Their greatest use is in providing a very sensitive method for detection of renal transplant rejection that is visually characterized by decreased perfusion, decreased function, and some urine production. Acute tubular necrosis in transplantation is characterized by minimal perfusion reduction, better uptake of iodohippurate than rejection, and virtually no urine production. Kidney transplants may also concentrate ^{99m}Tc sulfur colloid during rejection.

Emission Tomography

Although not yet beyond the research stage, emission tomography is an exciting development in nuclear medicine. It combines the tomographic capabilities of CT scanning with the physiologic advantages of tracer technics. It is possible with emission tomography to image those areas of the brain associated with specific functions, such as the uptake of deoxyglucose in the occipital area as a light is flashed before the eye. This development will have profound impact on the future practice of nuclear medicine.

228. GASTROINTESTINAL AND GENITOURINARY PROCEDURES

GASTRIC AND INTESTINAL INTUBATION

The **stomach** may be intubated to relieve nausea, vomiting, and gastric dilation (e.g., in pyloric obstruction, in ileus, after surgery, or during mechanically assisted respiration), to obtain gastric contents for analysis, to feed unconscious or debilitated patients, and to remove ingested noncorrosive poisons.

Gastric intubation via a nasal **Levin tube** is usually performed with the patient sitting up. The Levin tube may be stiffened in ice, as well as lubricated, before insertion into the nose. Entry into the pharynx induces a reflex cough. Having the patient swallow continuously and breathe deeply while the tube is *slowly* advanced will assist passage into the esophagus and stomach. Violent coughing with flow of air through the tube during respiration indicates that the tube is in the trachea. Aspiration of gastric juice verifies entry into the stomach. Tube position may be determined by instilling 20 to 30 ml air in the stomach and listening for the rush of air with a stethoscope.

For **gastric feeding,** once the tube's position has been verified in the stomach, about 100 to 300 ml of formula (see ELEMENTAL OR DEFINED FORMULA DIETS in Ch. 76), warmed to about 37.8 C (100 F), is instilled *slowly* into the tube via a funnel, 50-ml catheter-tip syringe, or gavage container. The patient's head must be elevated to prevent aspiration. (In **drip gavage,** the bottle of fluid is suspended from a stand and the drip regulated by a clamp.) Care is taken to prevent air from entering the tube and stomach. After the feeding, about 50 ml of water is given to rinse the tube, which is then clamped and taped in place with its end covered by sterile gauze or a commercial plug to prevent leaking. If tube feedings are required for an extended period of time, a 10 or 12 French pediatric feeding tube will prevent esophageal irritation. Before a tube is removed, it is tightly clamped to prevent leakage of fluid into the trachea.

A large tube passed via the mouth is used for **gastric lavage** to remove ingested noncorrosive poisons (see GENERAL PRINCIPLES OF TREATMENT in Ch. 258). Small volumes of the appropriate fluid (5% sodium bicarbonate solution, tap water, physiologic saline, antidotes, etc.) are repeatedly instilled and removed. In unconscious patients, lavage should be preceded by endotracheal intubation to prevent aspiration.

Intestinal intubation is performed to aspirate intestinal contents, relieve dilation associated with intestinal obstruction, or decompress the bowel postoperatively. A long, double-lumen **Miller-Abbott tube** with balloon is usually used. The balloon, when inflated, fills the gut lumen and the tube is moved along by peristalsis. A single-lumen long intestinal tube, passed in a similar manner, is sometimes used. There is less control of the balloon, but the effective diameter of the tube for suction is greater.

The Miller-Abbott tube, as with a Levin tube, is passed through the nose into the stomach. The balloon is then inflated and the tube withdrawn until it catches at the cardia. The patient is turned on his right side, still in a half-sitting position, the air is withdrawn, and 2 ml of mercury are instilled into the balloon. The gastric contents are aspirated and the tube advanced slowly to the antrum. Progress of the tube should be followed by fluoroscopy or x-ray at frequent intervals. The tube will usually pass into the duodenum by peristalsis if the patient remains on his right side for 2 or 3 h. Once in the duodenum, the balloon is reinflated and its inlet lumen clamped.

Long intestinal tubes should be irrigated with saline at hourly intervals. Continuous aspiration may be provided by attaching the passed tube to low-pressure suction with suitable trap bottles to collect the aspirate.

The tube is removed slowly by withdrawing 12 to 18 in. every 30 to 60 min. Intussusception or an intestinal injury may result if the tube is removed more rapidly.

CARE OF FISTULAS AND STOMAS

INTESTINAL FISTULAS

Intestinal fistulas present problems in maintaining fluid and electrolyte balance as well as in the care of the surrounding skin. The higher the intestinal origin of the fistula, the greater the metabolic disturbance produced. A duodenal fistula causes the greatest disturbance and may bring about rapid deterioration of the patient's condition because of excessive loss of fluids, electrolytes, and unabsorbed food; moreover, the pancreatic enzymes severely irritate the skin. With high fistulas, fluid and electrolyte replacement becomes a major problem and central venous alimentation is practically mandatory. A sigmoid colostomy, by contrast, produces little disturbance.

Skin irritation due to a fistula may be reduced by daily application of (1) karaya gum powder, (2) 10% aluminum powder in equal parts of lanolin and zinc oxide ointment, or (3) a commercially available skin protectant. A paste of boiled Maalox® is effective in neutralizing acid secretions. All are more effective when applied to dry intact skin before maceration or ulceration develops.

Removal of wound secretions, particularly those containing proteolytic enzymes, requires continuous suction. A wide glass, plastic, or rubber tube is first inserted in the wound; a rubber catheter is placed inside the tube and attached to a source of suction. A combination of this maneuver and use of protective skin coatings is usually effective in protecting the skin.

COLOSTOMY CARE

The patient with a permanent colostomy should be assured that convenient management is possible; explanations and demonstration of procedures greatly help the patient to adjust. Discussions with and guidance from others who have successfully adapted to a colostomy can be especially helpful; many cities have organized "ostomy clubs" whose members provide such services. "Stoma" therapists are available in some communities to assist with the selection and proper use of devices.

Management of a colostomy should begin as soon as GI function commences. Relative constipation is achieved by limiting the fresh fruits and vegetables in the diet, after which irrigations are begun (usually daily). Colostomy irrigation is usually performed with tap water, using a catheter and special collecting devices. The catheter should be inserted no more than 1 in. into the stoma before the water is allowed to flow. The catheter can then be safely advanced 4 to 6 in. into the colon *with the water running*. Commercially available collecting devices are accompanied by literature explaining their use. Peristomal skin irritation may be treated as for fistulas (see above).

Complete training may take several months. When this has been accomplished, the diet can be liberalized and only a small dressing will be required over the opening. The patient is assured that no bowel movement will occur until the next irrigation.

ILEOSTOMY CARE

Because a salt deficiency often occurs immediately after an ileostomy, continuous efforts must be made to prevent or correct fluid or electrolyte imbalance (see Ch. 81) or nutritional deficiency, and to maintain healthy peristomal skin (see INTESTINAL FISTULAS, above). Special appliances are available to handle the copious discharge that is always present. A projecting segment of ileum, which has been everted and protrudes 1 to 3 cm, is desirable for the application of necessary special fittings.

BLADDER CARE

URINARY CATHETERIZATION

Catheterization may be necessary to obtain a urine specimen, to relieve urinary retention, to check for residual urine, or to monitor kidney function. Every bladder treatment is directed toward preventing infection and maintaining urinary tract integrity. Urinary catheterizations have precipitated infections within 24 h and 95% of patients with long-term indwelling catheters have an infection which cannot be eradicated while the catheter remains in place. Urinary catheterizations should be considered in the light of alternatives. A male patient, whenever possible, should be allowed to assume the standing position for voiding to stimulate the normal reflex mechanism. External collecting devices (e.g., condoms) can be used for the incontinent male patient, but not for overflow incontinence due to obstruction or flaccid bladder.

Catheterizations in hospital must be carried out aseptically with a small catheter to prevent trauma and compromised urethral circulation, both sources of infection. The catheter should be well lubricated. Force should never be used to insert a catheter if resistance is felt. A retention catheter, such as the Foley catheter with an inflatable balloon that keeps the catheter in place, is used to monitor kidney output and prevent urinary retention during shock of trauma, after burns, and following certain pelvic surgery. A chronically distended bladder is emptied in stages (beginning with 500 ml, then 100 ml every hour) to prevent hemorrhage and other complications. Because the indwelling retention catheter serves as an entrance for organisms to the entire urinary tract, it should be used only when intermittent catheterization is not feasible. When the retention catheter is used, it should be changed when it does not drain freely. The urethral meatus should be cleaned t.i.d. with soap and water and an antibiotic ointment (e.g., neomycin) applied. For long-term drainage, the male patient should have the catheter and penis taped upward on the abdomen to eliminate the urethral penal-scrotal junction curve, which is prone to external fistula formation. A closed sterile drainage system with a valve to prevent reflux must be used and changed daily or more often if contamination occurs.

For patients who form kidney stones and require an indwelling catheter, daily Renacidin® (which dissolves and prevents formation of calcifications) instillations can be used to maintain catheter patency. The catheter and bladder may require irrigations when mucus and infection are present. Sterile 0.9% sodium chloride solution is the usual irrigant, which is instilled in 30- to 60-ml amounts by a sterile syringe. Irrigations are continued until the returns are clear and all irrigant returned. The catheter must be removed if it cannot be irrigated.

A patient should have a 2.5 to 3.0 L fluid intake daily to flush the urinary tract if a catheter is used for an extended time. The prophylactic use of antibiotics is controversial since relatively innocuous organisms are often replaced by virulent pathogens. Maintaining a low urine pH with ascorbic acid or potassium acid phosphate along with sulfisoxazole allows for therapeutic use of antibiotics when infection occurs. The urine must be monitored daily for pH and at least once a week for organisms.

BLADDER TRAINING

When voluntary bladder control is lost, conditioning may avoid the need for catheterizations, although a flaccid bladder can never be conditioned. Bladder training should be initiated as soon as kidney function is normal. The patient is catheterized on a schedule whereby the bladder volume is no more than 500 ml. The normal filling and complete emptying of the bladder stimulates an earlier return of the normal reflex emptying of the bladder as well as eliminating residual urine that may serve as a media for organisms. A q 6 h schedule of catheterizations is desirable and is achieved by limiting the fluid intake to 1.5 L/day. This schedule can be tapered to q 8 h when the patient begins to void spontaneously, when the patient voids 300 to 400 ml consistently, or when there is residual urine of 200 to 300 ml or less (by catheterization immediately after voiding), and q 3 to 4 days when the residual falls to $\leq$ 100 to 150 ml. After a good voiding pattern has been established, the patient can liberalize his fluid intake, and can be assisted in voiding in the normal upright position. The paraplegic patient may learn certain trigger points to initiate voiding, such as stroking the inner aspect of the thigh, tapping the abdomen over the bladder (percussion technic), or tugging on the pubic hair. This program is practical for women only if they have the ability to use a toilet independently. Otherwise, an indwelling catheter may be the method of choice. Patients with flaccid bladders may continue intermittent catheterizations indefinitely or use the indwelling catheter.

A clean catheterization procedure has been found satisfactory for some in long-term management of the flaccid bladder, especially those with spina bifida or low spinal cord injuries. The patient uses a sterile catheter (well lubricated) for each catheterization, preps himself with soap and water, and uses good hand washing technic (see also Treatment under NEUROGENIC BLADDER in Ch. 156).

---

229.   AIDS FOR THE DISABLED PATIENT

The family that must provide long-term home care for a bedridden or partially disabled patient requires guidance in routine nursing care as well as instruction in more complicated procedures. Personnel from the Visiting Nurse Association or the local Board of Health can provide invaluable instruction and assistance.

The **ambulatory, partially disabled patient** and his family should learn together, at the beginning of treatment, the new methods of ambulation, the needed safety measures, and any ongoing treatments. The patient should optimally be able to direct and be responsible for any measures that he cannot manage for himself. Family members should be helped to acquire a proficiency that makes them relatively secure and they should feel free to ask questions.

Equipment

A **wheelchair** must have brakes and be chosen with consideration of the patient's disability, size, weight, and activity, in order that a stable sitting position without contractures is maintained. **Crutches** are measured and adjusted with the patient standing against a wall or supported by a chair. In use, the top bar should be 2 in. below the anterior axillary fold and the tips 6 to 8 in. ahead of and to each side of the toes, so that the crutches and legs form a supporting tripod. The patient's weight is borne on the hand pieces, which should be adjusted to allow a 15° angle at the elbow.

A **cane** should provide 25° of elbow flexion. To walk correctly with a cane, the patient stands in a normal walking position with the cane held on the side opposite to his bad leg. With his weight on the cane and the bad leg, he moves his good leg forward. Then he puts his weight on his good leg and moves the cane and the bad leg forward. An alternative method is to place the cane a step ahead of his feet, move his bad leg forward, shift his weight to the cane and his bad leg, and then move his good leg forward.

Building Modifications

Stairs should be 10 in. deep, a maximum of 7 in. high, preferably snub nose, and have at least one **railing,** which should be 32 in. high and extend 18 in. beyond the top and bottom steps. **Wheelchair access** requires 32-in. doorways; a space 60 × 60 in. for turns; and **ramps** with a nonskid surface, a grade of 1 in./ft (8.33%), and railings 48 in. apart, 32 in. high, and extending 1 ft beyond the ramp at top and bottom. A small wheelchair elevator is useful for outside accessibility when space prohibits a ramp. An elevator may be installed along the inside stairway.

Toilet bars should be 1½ in. in diameter, 33 in. above and parallel to the floor, and 1½ in. from the wall. Bars that can be attached to the toilet are commercially available. An elevated toilet seat may aid in wheelchair transfers. Two **tub grab bars** are needed: one parallel to the tub and 4 in. above the tub surface, and the other vertical to the tub starting 9 in. from the tub surface. Both should be 1½ in. from the wall. **Shower grab bars** should reach from the floor to head height (minimally knees to head) and be 1½ in. from the wall. A number of tub seats or shower seats are available, including shower chairs. Roll-in shower chairs are available, and "telephone" shower head allows greater independence for the severely disabled.

Kitchen requirements include counters 26¼ in. (or 26½ in.) from the floor or waist high; a stove with controls at the front, an oven at chair-arm height; and a sink that is open below and with the pipes flush to the wall to allow a chair to roll under.

230.   LABORATORY MEDICINE

Improved instrumentation and automation have permitted mass production of various tests and increased the availability of biochemical screening at economical rates with improved quality control. Organ test panels are being used to detect abnormalities or to determine the state of health. Several technics, including multiple enzyme analyses, isoenzyme separations, and radioimmunoassays (replacing bioassay methods) providing more specific information, have contributed to increased laboratory utilization.

The nature of the equipment (such as physical size, cost), the specialized operating skills required, and the need for significant quality control have made it less possible to utilize these technics in a small office. Only relatively simple tests can and should be performed in the office, and these should be considered on an individual basis. Many large laboratories provide either pickup or mail service of specimens on a regional basis.

Since the same laboratory test may be done by different technics, it is necessary to know the normal ranges for each specific method and laboratory. The units may differ, thereby giving divergent values. It is also important to know that the usually reported normal range encompasses the 95% confidence level ($\pm$ 2 standard deviations from the mean). This means that 1:20 values may fall outside of the normal range but still be normal for the individual from whom the specimen was drawn.

Standard methods of specimen collection, storage, and preparation are extremely important in assuring reliable results. Such factors as being certain that the appropriate anticoagulant is added, that hemolysis does not take place, and that serum is separated from clot without delay are among the important considerations.

Many substances interfere with laboratory determinations. These should be known and considered in the interpretation of results. Where significant, these will be noted in the descriptions of some of the individual tests that follow.

PRINCIPLES OF MEASUREMENTS

A number of basic physical and chemical principles are used to produce measurable effects that relate to the substance of interest in the specific determination reported. A listing and brief discussion of each are included.

1. Atomic absorption spectrophotometry depends upon the ability of an element in its gaseous, atomic state to absorb light of specific wavelengths emitted from a source derived from that element. A quantitative relationship exists between the amount of light absorbed and the amount of the element in the specimen, which is placed in a flame or other volatizing mechanism to produce an excited atomic state. This technic is valuable for the measurement of trace amounts of many elements in biologic fluids. Calcium, magnesium, copper, lead, nickel, zinc, mercury, cadmium, and lithium, among others, can be measured by this method.

2. Chromatography involves the *separation* of very closely related substances by a packed column, liquid column, paper, gas, thin layer, or gel permeation. A stationary and a motile phase or countercurrent phases are required to accentuate the differences in mobility, which are dependent upon molecular size, polarity, adsorption, entrapment, or ion-exchange. It is a physical process.

Many substances, such as hormones and their degradation products, drugs used therapeutically or abused, enzymes, and carrier proteins, may be separated by chromatographic technics and then identified by chemical methods.

3. Colorimetry (absorption spectrophotometry) is the most commonly used final step in quantitative determinations made in the clinical laboratory. It provides adequate specificity and sensitivity, ease of use, and ready availability at low cost, and is readily adaptable to automation.

A wavelength that is optimal for the substance to be measured is selected and a measurement is made on both a prepared standard (containing a known concentration of the material) and the unknown. An equation may then be used to calculate the concentration of the unknown. This equation relates the proportion of light absorption of the unknown and known to the concentrations of the substance in both specimens.

This principle is used in autoanalyzers, kinetic enzyme analyses, and end-point analyses, as well as in a wide variety of manual procedures.

4. Electroanalytical chemistry deals with measurements of the interactions of electricity with liquid or dissolved substances in specimens. **Potentiometry** requires 2 electrodes. One is the standard or reference electrode and the other is the working or indicator electrode. A difference in potential (voltage) develops across the 2 electrodes when they are placed in a solution of the unknown; this difference is directly related to the activity of the measured ion.

This principle applies in the measurement of pH, where a glass electrode is used generally in combination with a calomel reference electrode. Ion-specific electrodes have been developed to determine ions directly. Sodium, potassium, calcium, and other substances may be measured in this way. As the technology advances, new electrodes will become available. Electrodes for the measurement of blood gases are available and widely used.

Coulometry involves the generation of a reagent at the surface of an electrode that reacts with the substance to be measured. When all of the substance in the sample has reacted with the electrode-generated reagent, a small excess of free reagent limits the current, indicating the end-point. An example of this is the titration of chloride with silver ion (electrogravimetric analysis).

Anodic stripping voltammetry involves the use of a metal-exchange reagent that releases bound metals such as lead from macromolecular binding sites. A composite mercury/graphite electrode provides this sensitive technic for trace metal analysis.

5. Electrophoresis is the movement of suspended particles under the influence of an electric field. The direction, distance, and rate of travel of the particles depend upon the strength of the field, the polarity, the pH of the medium through which migration takes place, and the nature of the particle (size, shape, physicochemical makeup). Separation of the components of a mixture takes place because of differences in migration rates. After separation, the constituents are treated in such a way as to permit densitometric readings of the bands that form. Serum proteins, lipoproteins, isoenzymes, Hb, haptoglobins, and abnormal proteins may be separated and identified by this technic.

6. Flame photometry is used to quantitate cations that produce characteristic colors when fed into a flame. These colors are due to *ions* as opposed to the excited but nonionized *atoms* in atomic absorption technics. Applications in the clinical laboratory include the measurement of sodium, potassium, and lithium.

7. Fluorometry measures those substances that fluoresce in ultraviolet light or that produce fluorescence upon excitation with intense radiant energy. Characteristic wavelengths may be selected for certain substances measured by this method, and instruments that resemble spectrophotometers are designed that are unaffected by incident light. Substances in the μg to ng/ml quantities may be detected. There are several factors that interfere with these measurements both negatively and positively. This method measures triglycerides, catecholamines, urinary estrogens, and other substances.

A fluorescent tag is also used to identify certain antigen-antibody complexes.

8. Immunodiffusion is used in detecting and quantitating substances for which an antibody is available. The antibody is added to a gel and the body fluid specimen is placed in a well and given time to diffuse. A precipitin ring forms around the well. The diameter of the ring is proportional to the quantity of antigen in the sample. This process is sometimes modified, to speed it up, by applying an electric current to the system, and is then called **immunoelectrodiffusion. Immunoelectrophoresis** is also available to detect and identify abnormal proteins.

Practical application of these technics lies in detecting abnormal immunoglobulins and components of complement and other proteins, such as macroglobulins, ceruloplasmin, transferrin, antitrypsins, and hepatitis-associated antigen, in the globulin fraction that is often associated with specific diseases.

9. Isotope technics in the clinical laboratory are employed mainly in vitro, as opposed to scanning of parts of the patient's body after administration of radioisotopes. In the laboratory, isotopes are measured by their characteristic production of photons, usually in a crystal of sodium iodide, when their β-particles or γ-rays are absorbed and scintillations are produced in the crystal. Liquid scintillation counters substitute a dissolved organic compound for the crystal. This system is useful when the emitting particle from the isotope is of low energy, such as a β-particle. An example of the liquid system is naphthalene or anthracene dissolved in toluene.

10. Mass spectrometry is a technic which uses the mass of compounds to identify and quantitate them. The principle involves ionizing the substance and separating the resulting molecular and fragment ions by means of electric and magnetic fields. Quantitative determinations can be made by measuring the magnitude of ion currents at different mass settings. Ionization is essential since uncharged particles do not separate rapidly according to mass. This technic has been used to identify peptides, steroid hormones, catecholamines, bile acids, vitamins, drugs, and other substances. Its usefulness is limited in the clinical laboratory because of its complexity and low volume capability.

11. Protein binding is a property that is utilized in the measurement of certain substances that are bound to serum protein when it is precipitated. Competition for these binding sites between an isotopically labeled compound and the radioinert compound permits an estimate of the amount present in the serum. Quantities as small as a ng/ml may be measured by this technic. Serum thyroxine (T_4), cortisol, folate, and vitamin B_{12} levels may be measured using this technic.

12. Radioimmunoassay (RIA) integrates radiochemical technics with immunologic technics, affording a high level of sensitivity and specificity. These assays provide the ability to measure physiologic substances in ng or pg/ml concentrations. The principles involve the reaction between antigen and antibody. High affinity and high specificity are required of the antibody. The label must be an isotope that is easily measured, such as ^{125}I, tritium, ^{14}C, or ^{57}Co. The actual test procedures differ in detail although the RIA principle is the same for all. A wide variety of substances may be measured in this fashion, including hormones, proteins, vitamins, drugs, and other compounds that are either antigenic alone or may be made so by adding them as a hapten to an antigenic substance.

13. Enzyme immunoassay (EIA) refers to methods in which enzyme-labeled antigens, antibodies, or haptens produce a measurable reaction with their respective immune counterparts. Homogeneous assays depend upon the conjugation of the enzyme to a hapten without hindering enzyme activity. Enzyme activity is inhibited by binding of hapten-specific antibody to the label. Free hapten in samples competes for antibody thereby making enzyme activity proportional to the concentration of free hapten. The "EMIT" assay of the SYVA Co. is based on this principle and is used to measure a number of drugs.

Heterogeneous assays involve solid-phase immunoassay in which an enzyme tag to an antiglobulin produces a color change on contact with a specific substrate. An example of this is the enzyme-linked immunosorbent assay (ELISA). This method is most used in serology associated with infectious disease, especially in virology.

14. Turbidimetry is the measurement of transmitted light through a suspension. It has the advantage of permitting quantitation without separation from solution. Measurements can be made with any spectrophotometer or against a series of visual, comparative standards. This method has been used to test for protein in urine or spinal fluid, using sulfosalicylic acid; for thymol turbidity determinations of plasma proteins, indicative of liver disorders; and for quantitation of bacteria, lipase, and immunoprecipitates such as antigen-antibody complexes.

15. Nephelometry differs from turbidimetry in that the light is measured at right angles to the incident beam. It permits greater sensitivity at lower concentrations of particulate suspended matter. This method also lacks specificity unless one can be certain that the turbidity is the result of a single substance. It has been used in the analysis of fibrinogen, thrombin, triglycerides, antigen-antibody complexes, and other substances.

16. Osmometry utilizes the relationship that exists between the number of particles in a solution and their collective effect upon the depression of the freezing point of that solution. Serum and urine are usually measured in such conditions as diabetes insipidus and hyperosmolar coma, and to assess the level of hydration.

17. Ultracentrifugation takes place when a specimen is spun at 25,000 rpm or more. Macromolecules migrate through the solvent. This technic is used in determining the sedimentation and diffusion coefficients of biopolymers and synthetic macromolecules, in examining the purity of macromolecules, and in identifying biologic materials. It has been useful in separating lipoproteins and has applicability in the confirmation of Type III hyperlipidemia and in separation of various protein fractions such as the macroglobulin rheumatoid factor.

CLINICAL CHEMISTRY

Some of the more frequently used clinical chemistry tests are described elsewhere in this volume and in Vol. II under the disease(s) with which they are associated. A table of normal laboratory values listed in alphabetical order is located at the end of this chapter.

CLINICAL HEMATOLOGY

Blood Specimen Collection

Blood is preferably collected by venipuncture, though fingertip puncture with a sterile lancet may sometimes suffice. The tests to be performed determine which anticoagulant, if any, should be in the collection tubes. Vacuum tubes which have double-ended needles for ease in specimen collecting and which contain suitable amounts of the appropriate anticoagulants for most routine hematologic procedures are available. However, most commercially available vacuum tubes are nonsterile and backflow of blood from the filled tube to the vein may occur, permitting the entry of bacteria. Several maneuvers may help to avoid such infections: (1) It is essential to remove the tourniquet well before blood flow into the tube has stopped and, preferably, before the tube stopper is completely punctured. (2) Moving the patient's arm during sampling should be avoided; even a few centimeters' elevation after the tube draw is complete may lower venous pressure sufficiently to produce backflow. (3) No pressure should be exerted on the stopper end of the tube. Whenever possible, sterile tubes or needle and tube arrangements that have a check valve in the system should be used.

EDTA (ethylenediaminetetraacetic acid) is the preferred anticoagulant when blood counts are desired since morphology is less distorted and platelets are better preserved. It can be added to clean test tubes, or vacuum tubes containing EDTA may be obtained commercially. Slides should be prepared within 3 to 4 h after the blood has been drawn, or within 1 to 2 h for platelet counts.

When small quantities of blood are required or venipuncture is not feasible, the finger, earlobe, or, in infants, the plantar surface of the heel is punctured quickly with a sterile disposable lancet, piercing deeply enough to ensure spontaneous flow of blood. Undue pressure which might cause dilution of the blood with tissue fluids should be avoided while collecting the specimen.

Bleeding Time (see Laboratory Tests in Ch. 95)

Bone Marrow

Bone marrow aspiration is not difficult and should be done early in suspected hematologic diseases. About 1 ml of marrow is withdrawn by aspiration from the marrow space of the sternum, iliac crest, or dorsal spine of a lumbar vertebra. A few drops are smeared directly on slides and the rest is placed in a tube with either heparin or EDTA. If larger volumes of marrow are withdrawn, there usually is dilution with peripheral blood, making interpretation difficult. The anticoagulated marrow may be spun in a centrifuge to separate the plasma from RBC and myeloid-erythroid layers. Additional smears of the concentrated myeloid-erythroid layer help in interpretation. The smears are stained with Wright's stain and then examined under the microscope. Thicker smears are made for iron stores and stained with Prussian blue.

Bone marrow examination is helpful in anemia, other cytopenias, unexplained leukocytosis, thrombocytosis, or when leukemia or myelophthisis is suspected, since it permits evaluation of the site of blood production and an assessment of iron stores.

Clot Retraction and Observation (see Laboratory Tests in Ch. 95)

Complete Blood Count (CBC)

The CBC, along with the urinalysis, is a basic "screening" test in all patients. The CBC usually includes determination of Hb, Hct, WBC count, WBC differential count, an estimation of platelet number, and a description of the blood smear, including RBC morphology. An RBC count is frequently included, especially when calculation of RBC indices is desired. Anemia, erythrocytosis, inflammation, leukemia, bone marrow failure, and adverse drug reactions may be detected.

Examination of the blood smear can aid in detecting certain abnormalities (e.g., thrombocytopenia, malarial parasites, significant rouleau formation, and the presence of nucleated RBCs or immature granulocytes) which may occur despite normal counts. It is important in evaluating RBC morphology and abnormal WBCs.

Blood counts are normally made by diluting a measured volume of blood with an appropriate diluent or lysing agent and counting in a chamber under the microscope. Hb can be measured colorimetrically after treatment with dilute hydrochloric acid or with Drabkin's reagent, which will permit colorimetric or spectrophotometric comparison with standards of hematin or cyanmethemoglobin, respectively. The Hct is measured by centrifuging a volume of blood and determining the percentage of RBCs. From a knowledge of the RBC count, Hb, and Hct, one may calculate **RBC indices**, namely **MCV** (mean corpuscular volume), **MCH** (mean corpuscular hemoglobin), and **MCHC** (mean corpuscular hemoglobin concentration). These indices may be useful in helping to establish the character of anemia.

All of the CBC values except the WBC differential count, but including the RBC indices, can be measured very quickly on venous blood by automated equipment. The WBC differential count is made by spreading a small drop of blood on a glass slide and staining with Wright's stain. The smear is examined by oil immersion microscopy and a count kept of each type of leukocyte identified. A minimum of 100 cells are counted and the various types are reported as a percentage. Automated equipment is available to do differential counts by computerized pattern recognition. The number of platelets is estimated.

Normal values for the total leukocyte (WBC) count range between 4,300 and 10,800 cu mm; normal values for the various cell types (**differential leukocyte count**) are: segmented neutrophils (SEGS) 34 to 75%, band neutrophils (BANDS) 0 to 8%, lymphocytes (LYMPHS) 12 to 50%, monocytes (MONOS) 3 to 15%, eosinophils (EOS) 0 to 5%, and basophils (BASOS) 0 to 3%.

The RBCs are studied for the presence of anisocytosis, poikilocytosis, hypochromia, stippling, and other abnormalities. Occasionally the RBC indices may be anticipated from such an inspection. The cells should be studied in an area of the smear where they just touch one another.

Erythrocyte Sedimentation Rate (ESR)

Venous blood, collected in anticoagulant, is added to a Wintrobe Hct tube to the 10-cm mark and placed in a vertical position. The distance the RBCs fall in 1 h is the ESR. Alternatively, a Westergren tube is filled to the 200-mm mark and read at the end of 1 h. A modified Westergren method in which blood is diluted with saline (4 parts blood to 1 part saline) provides greater reproducibility.

This is a nonspecific screening test and may be elevated in infection, inflammatory disease, and malignancy. An elevated ESR frequently signifies an increase in fibrinogen and γ-globulin. The test is useful in the follow-up evaluation of rheumatoid arthritis and acute rheumatic fever, and may help to distinguish between serious disease and functional symptoms when other findings are unremarkable.

Fibrin/Fibrinogen Degradation Products (see Laboratory Tests in Ch. 95)

Haptoglobin

Haptoglobin is an α_2-globulin with a specific affinity for Hb. It is ordinarily reduced in the presence of hemolysis. The determination may be useful in distinguishing Hb from myoglobin. While many methods for measuring haptoglobin are available, immunodiffusion is the simplest.

Iron and Iron-Binding Capacity (see Laboratory Evaluation on p. 706)

Lupus Erythematosus (LE) Cell Preparation

LE cells when treated with Wright's stain appear as amorphous inclusions about the size of a lymphocyte nucleus, lavender in color, with the lobes of the neutrophil nucleus displaced to the cell margin. This nonspecific test is positive in SLE and is also often positive during therapy with certain drugs, including hydralazine and procainamide. Determination of antinuclear antibodies has become the preferred test for the diagnosis of SLE since the technic and interpretation of the "LE prep" are so variable. (See also SLE in Ch. 104.)

Partial Thromboplastin Time and Prothrombin Time (see Laboratory Tests in Ch. 95)

Platelet Aggregation

The ability of platelets to aggregate and stick together may be measured; it provides a useful tool for elucidating some coagulation defects.

Platelet Count

A direct platelet count is useful in evaluating purpura and other bleeding disorders and is indicated when platelets appear to be decreased on blood smear. Periodic platelet counts are helpful in following the course of leukemia, aplastic anemia, and other conditions associated with bone marrow failure.

Diluting fluid is prepared by dissolving 1 gm ammonium oxalate in 100 ml distilled water. Venous blood is drawn to the 0.5 mark of a white cell pipet (with tubing) and diluting fluid is added to the 11 mark. The pipet is shaken for 3 min. The first 5 drops are discarded and a counting chamber is filled. The counting chamber is placed in a Petri dish containing moist filter paper, is covered, and is left to stand for 15 min to permit settling. The platelets are then counted as if doing an RBC count, using the high-power objective or phase microscope. The number of platelets counted multiplied by 1000 equals the total number of platelets/cu mm. Automated platelet counters are available and are used widely. Normal values range between 200,000 and 400,000/cu mm.

RBC Fragility (Osmotic Fragility)

A series of 12 small test tubes containing sodium chloride (NaCl) solutions varying from 0.28 to 0.5% in 0.02% increments is prepared. A drop of the patient's blood is placed in each of these tubes and the blood of a normal control is added to another series of tubes. The percent of NaCl at which hemolysis begins and the first tube showing complete hemolysis are noted. Normal blood begins to hemolyze at 0.44% NaCl or less. The process is usually complete at about 0.32% NaCl. Normal values may vary by ± 0.04%. If many spherocytes are present, as in familial hemolytic jaundice, hemolysis will appear at higher concentrations. If the predominating cell is abnormally thin, as in thalassemia major, hemolysis will appear first at lower concentrations and in some cases may never be complete.

RBC Indices

These are helpful in identifying iron deficiency and macrocytic anemias (see in Complete Blood Count, above).

Reticulocyte Count (see Laboratory Evaluation on p. 706)

IMMUNOHEMATOLOGY
(See in Ch. 93)

MICROBIOLOGY
(See Ch. 2)

NORMAL LABORATORY VALUES

Normal laboratory values are listed alphabetically in TABLE 230–1. They reflect methods used at The Massachusetts General Hospital and published in The New England Journal of Medicine.

Note that SI units are given in addition to the conventional units. The SI units are SYSTÈME INTERNATIONAL units that have been used uniformly in the European literature for several years. The benefits consist in scientific standardization in reporting and the use of molar concentration units of SI which are more meaningful as they represent relative combining power of chemical species.

TABLE 230–1. NORMAL LABORATORY VALUES IN THE MASSACHUSETTS GENERAL HOSPITAL*
BLOOD, PLASMA, OR SERUM VALUES

| Determination | Reference Range | | Minimal ml Required | Note |
	Conventional	SI		
Acetoacetate plus acetone	0.3–2.0 mg/100 ml	3–20 mg/L	2-S	
Aldolase	1.3–8.2 mu./ml	12–75 nmol·s⁻¹/L	2-S	Use fresh, unhemolyzed serum
Alpha amino nitrogen	3.0–5.5 mg/100 ml	2.1–3.9 mmol/L	5-P	Collect with heparin
Ammonia	80–110 µg/100 ml	47–65 µmol/L	2-B	Collect in heparinized tube; deliver *immediately* packed in ice
Amylase	4–25 u./ml	4–25 arb. u.	3-S	
Ascorbic acid	0.4–1.5 mg/100 ml	23–85 µmol/L	7-B	Collect in heparin tube before any food is given
Barbiturate	0 Coma level: phenobarbital, approx. 10 mg/100 ml; most other drugs, 1–3 mg/100 ml	0 µmol/L	5-S	
Bilirubin (van den Bergh test)	One min: 0.4 mg/100 ml	up to 7 µmol/L	3-S	
	Direct: 0.4 mg/100 ml. Total: 1.0 mg/100 ml Indirect is total minus direct	up to 17 µmol/L		
Blood volume	8.5–9.0% of body wt	80–85 ml/kg		
Bromide	0 Toxic level: 17 mEq/L	0 mmol/L	3-S	
BSP	Less than 5% retention	<0.05 L	3-S	Inject IV 5 mg of dye/kg; draw blood 45 min later

* Abbreviations used: SI, Système International d'Unités; P, plasma; B, blood; S, serum.
Modified from *The New England Journal of Medicine*, Vol. 302, pp. 37–48, January 3, 1980. Used with permission of the *Journal* and The Massachusetts General Hospital.

TABLE 230–1.   NORMAL LABORATORY VALUES IN THE MASSACHUSETTS GENERAL HOSPITAL   *(Cont'd)*
BLOOD, PLASMA, OR SERUM VALUES   *(Cont'd)*

| Determination | Reference Range | | Minimal ml Required | Note |
	Conventional	SI		
Calcium	8.5–10.5 mg/100 ml (slightly higher in children)	2.1–2.6 mmol/L	3-S	BSP dye interferes
CO₂ content	24–30 mEq/L; 20–26 mEq/L in infants (as bicarbonate)	24–30 mmol/L	3-S	Draw without stasis under oil or fill tube to top
CO	Symptoms with >20% saturation	0 (L)	5-B	Fill tube to top; tightly stopper; use anticoagulant
Carotenoids	0.8–4.0 µg/ml	1.5–7.4 µmol/L	3-S	Vitamin A may be done on same specimen
Ceruloplasmin	27–37 mg/100 ml	1.8–2.5 µmol/L	2-S	
Chloride	100–106 mEq/L	100–106 mmol/L	1-S	
Cholinesterase (pseudo-cholinesterase)	0.5 pH u. or more/h 0.7 pH u. or more/h for packed cells	0.5 or more arb. u.	1-S 1-S	
Copper	Total: 100–200 µg/100 ml	16–31 µmol/L	3-S	
CPK	Female: 5–35 mu./ml Male: 5–55 mu./ml	0.08–0.58 µmol·s⁻¹/L	3-S	Immediately separate & freeze serum
Creatinine	0.6–1.5 mg/100 ml	60–130 µmol/L	1-S	
Ethanol	0.3–0.4%, marked intoxication; 0.4–0.5% alcoholic stupor; 0.5% or over, alcoholic coma	65–87 mmol/L 87–109 mmol/L >109 mmol/L	2-B	Collect in oxalate & refrigerate
Glucose	Fasting: 70–110 mg/100 ml	3.9–5.6 mmol/L	2-F	Collect with EDTA-fluoride mixture
Glutethimide	0 mg/100 ml	0 µmol/L	5-S	
Iron	50–150 µg/100 ml (higher in males)	9.0–26.9 µmol/L	5-S	Shows diurnal variation higher in AM
Iron-binding capacity	250–410 µg/100 ml	44.8–73.4 µmol/L	5-S	

Lactic acid	0.6–1.8 mEq/L	0.6–1.8 mmol/L	2-B	Collect with oxalate fluoride mixture; deliver immediately packed in ice
Lactic dehydrogenase	60–120 u./ml	1.00–2.00 μmol·s^{-1}/L	2-S	Unsuitable if hemolyzed
Lead	50 μg/100 ml or less	up to 2.4 μmol/L	2-B	Collect with oxalate fluoride mixture
Lipase	2u./ml or less	up to 2 arb. u.	3-S	
Lipids				
Cholesterol	120–220 mg/100 ml	3.10–5.69 mmol/L	2-S	Fasting
Cholesterol esters	60–75% of cholesterol		2-S	Fasting
Phospholipids	9–16 mg/100 ml as lipid phosphorus	2.9–5.2 mmol/L	5-S	Fasting
Total fatty acids	190–420 mg/100 ml	1.9–4.2 gm/L	10-S	Fasting
Total lipids	450–1000 mg/100 ml	4.5–10.0 gm/L	5-S	Fasting
Triglycerides	40–150 mg/100 ml	0.4–1.5 gm/L	2-S	Fasting
Lipoprotein electrophoresis (LEP)			2-S	Fasting; do not freeze serum
Lithium	Toxic level 2 mEq/L	2 mmol/L	1-S	
Magnesium	1.5–2.0 mEq/L	0.8–1.3 mmol/L	1-S	
Methanol	0		5-B	May be fatal as low as 115 mg/100 ml; collect in oxalate
5'-Nucleotidase	0.3–3.2 Bodansky u.	30–290 nmol·s^{-1}/L	1-S	
Osmolality	285–295 mOsm/kg water	285–295 mmol/kg	5-S	
Oxygen saturation (arterial)	96–100%	0.96–1.001	3-B	Deliver in sealed heparinized syringe packed in ice
P_{CO_2}	35–45 mm Hg	4.7–6.0 kPa	2-B	Collect and deliver in sealed heparinized syringe
pH	7.35–7.45	same	2-B	Collect without stasis in sealed heparinized syringe; deliver packed in ice
P_{O_2}	75–100 mm Hg (dependent on age) while breathing room air / Above 500 mm Hg while on 100% O_2	10.0–13.3 kPa	2-B	

TABLE 230-1. NORMAL LABORATORY VALUES IN THE MASSACHUSETTS GENERAL HOSPITAL *(Cont'd)*
BLOOD, PLASMA, OR SERUM VALUES *(Cont'd)*

| Determination | Reference Range | | Minimal ml Required | Note |
	Conventional	SI		
Phenylalanine	0–2 mg/100 ml	0–120 μmol/L	0.4·S	
Phenytoin	Therapeutic level, 5–20 μg/ml	19.8–79.5 μmol/L	3·S	
Phosphatase (acid)	Male–Total: 0.13–0.63 Sigma u./ml Female–Total: 0.01–0.56 Sigma u./ml Prostatic: 0–0.7 Fishman-Lerner u./100 ml	36–175 nmol · s⁻¹/L 2.8–156 nmol · s⁻¹/L	1·S	Must always be drawn just before analysis or stored as frozen serum; avoid hemolysis
Phosphatase (alkaline)	13–39 IU/L; infants and adolescents up to 104 IU/L	0.22–0.65 μmol · s⁻¹/L up to 1.26 μmol · s⁻¹/L	1·S	BSP dye interferes For Bodansky u. multiply IU/L by 0.15 up to 90 u.: 0.13 to 256 u.
Phosphorus (inorganic)	3.0–4.5 mg/100 ml (infants in 1st year up to 6.0 mg/100 ml)	1.0–1.5 mmol/L	2·S	Obtain blood in fasting state; serum must be separated promptly from cells
Potassium	3.5–5.0 mEq/L	3.5–5.0 mmol/L	2·S	Serum must be separated promptly from cells (within 1 h)
Primidone	Therapeutic level 4–12 μg/ml	18–55 μmol/L	3·S	
Protein: Total	6.0–8.4 gm/100 ml	60–84 gm/L	1·S	Patient should be fasting; avoid BSP dye
Albumin	3.5–5.0 gm/100 ml	35–50 gm/L	1·S	
Globulin	2.3–3.5 gm/100 ml	23–35 gm/L		Globulin equals total protein minus albumin
Electrophoresis	% of total protein		1·S	Quantitation by densitometry
Albumin	52–68	0.52–0.68 L		
Globulin:				
α₁	4.2–7.2	0.042–0.072 L		
α₂	6.8–12	0.068–0.12 L		
β	9.3–15	0.093–0.15 L		
γ	13–23	0.13–0.23 L		

Test	Conventional Value	SI Value	Code	Notes
Pyruvic acid	0–0.11 mEq/L	0–0.11 mmol/L	2·B	Collect with oxalate fluoride; deliver *immediately* packed in ice
Quinidine	Therapeutic level: 1.5–3 µg/ml; Toxic level: 5–6 µg/ml	4.6–9.2 µmol/L; 15.4–18.5 µmol/L	1·S	
Salicylate:	0	0	5·P	Collect in heparin or EDTA
Therapeutic	20–25 mg/100 ml; 25–30 mg/100 ml to age 10 yr 3 h post dose	1.4–1.8 mmol/L; 1.8–2.2 mmol/L		
Toxic	Over 30 mg/100 ml; Over 20 mg/100 ml after age 60	over 2.2 mmol/L; over 1.4 mmol/L		
Sodium	135–145 mEq/L	135–145 mmol/L	2·S	
Sulfate	2.9–3.5 mg/100 ml	0.3–0.36 µmol/L	3·S	Avoid hemolysis
Sulfonamide	0 mg/100 ml; Therapeutic: 5–15 mg/100 ml	0 mmol/L	2·S,B	Value given as unconjugated unless total is requested
Thymol				
Flocculation	Up to 1+ in 24 h	up to 1 + arb. u.	1·S	Checked with phosphate buffer of higher molarity to rule out false-positive reaction
Turbidity	0–4 u.	0–4 arb. u.		
Transaminase				
(AST or SGOT)	10–40 u./ml	$0.08\text{–}0.32\ \mu\text{mol} \cdot \text{s}^{-1}/\text{L}$	1·S	
(ALT or SGPT)	6.0–36 u./ml	$0.05\text{–}0.29\ \mu\text{mol} \cdot \text{s}^{-1}/\text{L}$		
BUN	8–25 mg/100 ml; urea = BUN × 2.14	2.9–8.9 mmol/L	1·S,B	Use oxalate as anticoagulant
Uric acid	3.0–7.0 mg/100 ml	0.18–0.42 mmol/L	1·S	Serum must be separated from cells at once & refrigerated
Vitamin A	0.15–0.6 µg/ml	0.5–2.1 µmol/L	3·S	
Vitamin A tolerance test	Rise to twice fasting level in 3 to 5 h	Rise to twice fasting level in 3 to 5 h	3·S	Samples taken fasting & at intervals up to 8 h after test dose

TABLE 230–1. NORMAL LABORATORY VALUES IN THE MASSACHUSETTS GENERAL HOSPITAL *(Cont'd)*
URINE VALUES

Determination	Reference Range Conventional	Reference Range SI	Minimal Quantity Required	Note
Acetone plus acetoacetate (quantitative)	0	0 mg/L	2 ml	Keep cold
α amino nitrogen	64–199 mg/day; not > 1.5% of total nitrogen	4.6–14.2 mmol/day	24-h specimen	Preserve with thymol; refrigerate
Amylase	24–76 u./ml	24–76 arb. u.		
Calcium	150 mg/day or less	3.8 or less mmol/day	24-h specimen	Collect in special bottle with 10 ml of concentrated HCl
Catecholamines Epinephrine Norepinephrine	<20 μg/day <100 μg/day	<55 nmol/day <590 nmol/day	24-h specimen	Collect with 12 ml of concentrated HCl (pH should be 2.0–3.0)
Chorionic gonadotropin	0	0 arb. u.	First morning voiding	Sp gr should be at least 1.015
Copper	0–100 μg/day	0–1.6 μmol/day	24-h specimen	
Coproporphyrin	50–250 μg/day; Children <80 lb 0–75 μg/day	80–380 nmol/day 0–115 nmol/day	24-h specimen	Collect with 5 gm of sodium carbonate
Creatine	<100 mg/day or <6% of creatinine. In pregnancy, up to 12%. In children <1 yr, may equal creatinine; in older children, up to 30% of creatinine	<0.75 mmol/day	24-h specimen	Order serum creatinine also
Creatinine	15–25 mg/kg/day	0.13–0.22 mmol · kg^{-1}/day	24-h specimen	
Creatinine clearance	150–180 L/day (104–125 ml/min)/1.73 m² of BSA	1.7–2.1 ml/sec	24-h specimen	Order serum creatinine also
Cystine or cystine	0	0	10 ml	Qualitative

Determination	Normal Values (conventional)	Normal Values (SI)	Specimen	Notes
Follicle-stimulating hormone:		same	24-h specimen	Radioimmunoassay
Follicular phase	5–20 IU/day			
Mid-cycle	15–60 IU/day			
Luteal phase	5–15 IU/day			
Menopausal	50–100 IU/day			
Men	5–25 IU/day			
Hemoglobin & myoglobin	0		Freshly voided sample	Chemical examination with benzidine
Homogentisic acid	0		Freshly voided specimen or 24-h specimen kept cold	Must be refrigerated if not determined at once. Test also measures gentisic acid & may be positive in patients on high doses of salicylates
5-Hydroxyindole acetic acid	2–9 mg/day (women lower than men)	10–45 μmol/day	24-h specimen	Collect in special bottle with 10 ml of concentrated HCl
Lead	0.08 μg/ml or 120 μg or less/day	0.39 μmol/L or less	24-h specimen	
PSP	At least 25% excreted by 15 min; 40% by 30 min; 60% by 120 min	0.25 L	Total ouput of urine collected 15, 30, & 120 min after injection	Inject 1 ml (6 mg) IV; BSP interferes
Phenylpyruvic acid	0	0	Freshly voided specimen unless quantitation needed	
Phosphorus (inorganic)	Varies with intake; average 1 gm/day	32 mmol/day	24-h specimen	Collect in special bottle with 10 ml of concentrated HCl
Porphobilinogen	0	0	10 ml	Use freshly voided urine
Protein:				
Quantitative	<150 mg/24 h	<0.15 gm/day	24-h specimen	
Electrophoresis	(See Blood Protein, above)			

TABLE 230–1. NORMAL LABORATORY VALUES IN THE MASSACHUSETTS GENERAL HOSPITAL *(Cont'd)*
URINE VALUES *(Cont'd)*

Determination	Reference Range				Minimal Quantity Required	Note
	Conventional		SI			
	Male	Female				
Steroids:						
17-Ketosteroids (per day)	Age		$\mu mol/day$	$\mu mol/day$	24-h specimen	Not valid if patient is receiving meprobamate
	1–4 mg	1–4 mg	3–14	3–14		
	10 6–21	4–16	21–73	14–56		
	20 8–26	4–14	28–90	14–49		
	30 5–18	3–9	17–62	10–31		
	50 2–10	1–7	7–35	3–24		
	70					
17-Hydroxy-steroids	3–8 mg/day (women lower than men)		8–22 $\mu mol/day$ as hydrocortisone		24-h specimen	Keep cold: chlorpromazine & related drugs interfere with assay
Sugar:						
Quantitative glucose	0		0 mmol/L		24-h or other timed specimen	Collect with toluene; refrigerate
Identification of reducing substances					50 ml	Use freshly voided urine; no preservatives
Fructose	0		0 mmol/L		50 ml	Use freshly voided urine; also quantitate total reducing substances
Pentose	0		0 mmol/L		50 ml	Use freshly voided urine
Titratable acidity	20–40 mEq/day		20–40 mmol/day		24-h specimen	Collect with toluene; refrigerate
Urobilinogen	Up to 1.0 Ehrlich u.		to 1.0 arb. u.		2-h specimen (1–3 PM)	
Uroporphyrin	0		0 nmol/day		See Coproporphyrin	
Vanillylmandelic acid (VMA)	Up to 9 mg/24 h		up to 45 $\mu mol/day$		24-h specimen	Collect as for catecholamines

SPECIAL ENDOCRINE TESTS

Determination	Reference Range		Minimal ml Required	Note
	Conventional	SI		
Steroid hormones				
Aldosterone	Excretion: 5–19 µg/24 h	14–53 mmol/day	5/day	Keep specimen cold
	Supine: 48 ± 29 pg/ml	133 ± 80 pmol/L	3-S,P	Fasting, at rest, 210 mEq Na diet
	Upright: (2 h) 65 ± 23 pg/ml	180 ± 64 pmol/L		Upright, 2 h, 210 mEq Na diet
	Supine: 107 ± 45 pg/ml	279 ± 125 pmol/L		Fasting, at rest, 110 mEq Na diet
	Upright: (2 h) 239 ± 123 pg/ml	663 ± 341 pmol/L		Upright, 2 h, 110 mEq Na diet
	Supine: 175 ± 75 pg/ml	485 ± 208 pmol/L		Fasting, at rest, 10 mEq Na diet
	Upright: (2 h) 532 ± 228 pg/ml	1476 ± 632 pmol/L		Upright, 2 h, 10 mEq Na diet
Cortisol	8 AM: 5–25 µg/100 ml	0.14–0.69 µmol/L	1-P	Fasting
	8 PM: < 10µg/100 ml	0–0.28 µmol/L	1-P	At rest
	4 h ACTH test: 30–45 µg/100 ml	0.83–1.24 µmol/L	1-P	20 u. ACTH IV/4 h
	Overnight suppression test: < 5 µg/100 ml	<0.14 nmol/L	1-P	8 AM sample after dexamethasone midnight
	Excretion: 20–70 µg/24 h	55–193 nmol/day	2-day	Keep specimen cold
11-Deoxycortisol	Responsive: >7.5 µg/100 ml	>0.22 µmol/L	1-P	8 AM sample preceded by metyrapone 4.5 gm orally/24 h or by single 2.5-gm dose orally at midnight
Testosterone	Adult male: 300–1100 ng/100 ml	10.4–38.1 nmol/L	2-P	AM sample
	Adolescent male: >100 ng/100 ml	>3.5 nmol/L		
	Female: 25–90 ng/100 ml	0.87–3.12 nmol/L		
Unbound testosterone	Adult male: 3.06–24 ng/100 ml	106–832 pmol/L	2-P	AM sample
	Adult female: 0.09–1.28 ng/100 ml	3.1–44.4 pmol/L		
Polypeptide hormones				
ACTH	15–70 pg/ml	3.3–15.4 pmol/L	5-P	Place specimen on ice and send promptly to laboratory
Calcitonin	Undetectable; >100 pg/ml in medullary carcinoma	0 >29.3 pmol/L	5-P	Test done only on known or suspected cases of medullary carcinoma of the thyroid

TABLE 230–1. NORMAL LABORATORY VALUES IN THE MASSACHUSETTS GENERAL HOSPITAL (Cont'd)
SPECIAL ENDOCRINE TESTS (Cont'd)

Determination	Reference Range Conventional	Reference Range SI	Minimal ml Required	Note
Polypeptide hormones (Cont'd)				
Growth hormone	<5 ng/ml	<233 pmol/L	1-S	Fasting, at rest
	Children: >10 ng/ml	>465 pmol/L		After exercise
	Male: <5 ng/ml	<233 pmol/L		
	Female: Up to 30 ng/ml	0–1395 pmol/L		After glucose load
	Male: <5 ng/ml	<233 pmol/L		
	Female: <10 ng/ml	0–465 pmol/L		
Insulin	6–26 μu./ml	43–187 pmol/L	1-S	Fasting
	<20 μu./ml	<144 pmol/L		During hypoglycemia
	Up to 150 μu./ml	0–1078 pmol/L		After glucose load
Luteinizing hormone	Male: 6–18 mu./ml	6–18 u./L	2-S,P	Pre- or post-ovulatory
	Female, 5–22 mu./ml	5–22 u./L		Mid-cycle peak
Parathyroid hormone	30–250 mu./ml	30–250 u./L	5-P	Keep blood on ice, or plasma must be
	<10μl equiv/ml	<10 ml equiv/L		frozen if it is to be sent any distance; AM sample
Prolactin	2–15 ng/ml	0.08–6.0 nmol/L	2-S	
Renin activity	Supine: 1.1 ± 0.8 ng/ml/h	0.9 ± 0.6 (nmol/L)h	4-P	EDTA tubes, on ice; normal diet
	Upright: 1.9 ± 1.7 ng/ml/h	1.5 ± 1.3 (nmol/L)h		
	Supine: 2.7 ± 1.8 ng/ml/h	2.1 ± 1.4 (nmol/L)h		Low Na diet
	Upright: 6.6 ± 2.5 ng/ml/h	5.1 ± 1.9 (nmol/L)h		
	Diuretics: 10.0 ± 3.7 ng/ml/h	7.7 ± 2.9 (nmol/L)h		Low Na diet
Thyroid hormones				
Thyroid-stimulating hormone (TSH)	0.5–3.5 μu./ml	0.5–3.5 mu./L	2-S	
Thyroxine-binding globulin capacity	15–25 μg T₄/100 ml	193–322 nmol/L	2-S	
Total tri-iodothyronine by radioimmuno-assay (T₃)	70–190 ng/100 ml	1.08–2.92 nmol/L	2-S	

Determination	Reference Range		Minimal ml Required	Note
	Conventional	SI		
Total thyroxine by radioimmunoassay (T₄)	4–12 µg/100 ml	52–154 nmol/L	1-S	
T₃ resin uptake	25–35%	0.25–0.35	2-S	
Free thyroxine index (FT₄I)	1–4 ng/100 ml	12.8–51.2 pmol/L	2-S	

HEMATOLOGIC VALUES

Determination	Reference Range		Minimal ml Required	Note
	Conventional	SI		
Coagulation factors				
Factor I (fibrinogen)	0.15–0.35 gm/100 ml	4.0–10.0 µmol/L	4.5-P	Collect in vacuum tube containing sodium citrate
Factor II (prothrombin)	60–140% of control	0.60–1.40	4.5-P	Collect in plastic tubes with 3.8% sodium citrate
Factor V (accelerator globulin)	60–140% of control	0.60–1.40	4.5-P	Collect as for factor II
Factor VII-X (proconvertin-Stuart)	70–130% of control	0.70–1.30	4.5-P	Collect as for factor II
Factor X (Stuart factor)	70–130% of control	0.70–1.30	4.5-P	Collect as for factor II
Factor VIII (antihemophilic globulin)	50–200% of control	0.50–2.0	4.5-P	Collect as for factor II
Factor IX (plasma thromboplastic cofactor)	60–140% of control	0.60–1.40	4.5-P	Collect as for factor II
Factor XI (plasma thromboplastic antecedent)	60–140% of control	0.60–1.40	4.5-P	Collect as for factor II
Factor XII (Hageman factor)	60–140% of control	0.60–1.40	4.5-P	Collect as for factor II

TABLE 230-1.   NORMAL LABORATORY VALUES IN THE MASSACHUSETTS GENERAL HOSPITAL *(Cont'd)*
HEMATOLOGIC VALUES *(Cont'd)*

Determination	Reference Range		Minimal ml Required	Note
	Conventional	SI		
Coagulation screening tests				
Bleeding time	3–9 min	180–540 sec		
Prothrombin time	<2-sec deviation from control	<2-sec deviation from control	4.5-P	Collect in vacuum tube containing 3.8% sodium citrate
Partial thromboplastin time (activated)	25–37 sec	25–37 sec	4.5-P	Collect in vacuum tube containing 3.8% sodium citrate
Whole-blood clot lysis	No clot lysis in 24 h	0/day	2.0 whole blood	Collect in sterile tube & incubate at 37 C
Fibrinolytic studies				
Euglobin lysis	No lysis in 2 h	0 (in 2 h)	4.5-P	Collect as for factor II
Fibrinogen split products	Negative reaction at >1:4 dilution	0 (at >1:4 dilution)	4.5-S	Collect in special tube containing thrombin & aminocaproic acid
Thrombin time	Control ± 5 sec	Control ± 5 sec	4.5-P	Collect as for factor II
"Complete" blood count			1-B	Use EDTA as anticoagulant; the 7 listed tests are performed automatically on the Coulter Counter Model S, which directly determines cell counts, Hb (as the cyanmethemoglobin derivative), & MCV, computes Hct, MCH, & MCHC
Hematocrit	Male: 45–52% Female: 37–48%	Male: 0.42–0.52 Female: 0.37–0.48		
Hemoglobin	Male: 13–18 gm/100 ml Female: 12–16 gm/100 ml	Male: 8.1–11.2 mmol/L Female: 7.4–9.9 mmol/L		
Leukocyte count	4300–10,800/cu mm	$4.3–10.8 \times 10^9$/L		
Erythrocyte count	4.2–5.9 million/cu mm	$4.2–5.9 \times 10^{12}$/L		
MCV	80–94 cu microns	80–94 fl (femtoliter)		
MCH	27–32 pg	1.7–2.0 fmol		
MCHC	32–36%	19–22.8 mmol/L		
ESR	Male: 1–13 mm/h Female: 1–20 mm/h	Male: 1–13 mm/h Female: 1–20 mm/h	5-B	Use EDTA as anticoagulant

Test				Special handling
Erythrocyte enzymes				
Glucose-6-phosphate dehydrogenase	5-15 u./gm	5-15 u./gm Hb	9-B	Use special anticoagulant (ACD solution)
Pyruvate kinase (serum)	13-17 u./gm	13-17 u./gm Hb	8-B	Use special anticoagulant (ACD solution)
Ferritin (serum)				
Iron deficiency	0-20 µg/L	0-20 ng/ml		
Iron excess	>400 µg/L	>400 ng/L		
Folic acid				
Normal	>4.3 mmol/L	>1.9 ng/ml	1-S	
Borderline	2.3-4.3 mmol/L	1.0-1.9 ng/ml	1-S	
Haptoglobin	1.0-3.0 gm/L	100-300 mg/100 ml	1-S	
Hemoglobin studies				
Electrophoresis for abnormal Hb			5-B	Collect with anticoagulant
Electrophoresis for A_2 Hb	0.015-0.035	1.5-3.5%	5-B	Use oxalate as anticoagulant
Fetal Hb	<0.02	<2%	5-B	Collect with anticoagulant
Met. & sulf-Hb	0	0	5-B	Use heparin as anticoagulant
Serum Hb	1.2-1.9 µmol/L	2-3 mg/100 ml	2-S	
Thermolabile Hb	0	0	1-B	Any anticoagulant
Lupus anticoagulant	0	0	4.5-P	Collect as for factor II
LE cell preparation				
Hargraves Method	0	0	5-B	Use heparin as anticoagulant
Barnes Method	0	0	5-B	Use defibrinated blood
Leukocyte alkaline phosphatase:				
Quantitative method	15-40 mg/h	15-40 mg of phosphorus liberated/h/10^{10} cells	20-Isolated blood leukocytes	Special handling of blood necessary
Qualitative method	33-188 u., 30-160 u.	Males: 33-188 u. Females (off contraceptive pill): 30-160 u.	Smear-B	
Muramidase	3-7 mg/L, 0-2 mg/L	Serum, 3-7 µg/ml Urine, 0-2 µg/ml	1-S, 1-U	

TABLE 230–1. NORMAL LABORATORY VALUES IN THE MASSACHUSETTS GENERAL HOSPITAL *(Cont'd)*
HEMATOLOGIC VALUES *(Cont'd)*

Determination	Reference Range		Minimal ml Required	Note
	Conventional	*SI*		
Osmotic fragility of erythrocytes	Increased if hemolysis occurs in >0.5% NaCl; decreased if hemolysis is incomplete in 0.3% saline		5-B	Use heparin as anticoagulant
Peroxide hemolysis	<10%	<0.10	6-B	Use EDTA as anticoagulant
Platelet count	150,000–350,000/cu mm	150–350 × 10⁹/L	0.5-B	Use EDTA as anticoagulant. Counts are performed on Clay Adams Ultraflow. Low counts are confirmed by hand counting
Platelet function tests				
Clot retraction	50–100%/2 h	0.50–1.00/2h	4.5-P	Collect as for factor II
Platelet aggregation	Full response to ADP, epinephrine, & collagen	1.0	18-P	Collect as for factor II
Platelet factor 3	33–57 sec	33–57 sec	4.5-P	Collect as for factor II
Reticulocyte count	0.5–1.5% red cells	0.005–.015	0.1-B	
Vitamin B₁₂	90–280 pg/ml (borderline: 70–90)	66–207 pmol/L (borderline: 52–66)	12-S	

CEREBROSPINAL FLUID VALUES

Determination	Reference Range		Minimal ml Required	Note
	Conventional	SI		
Bilirubin	0	0 μmol/L	2	
Cell count	0–5 mononuclear cells		0.5	
Chloride	120–130 mEq/L		0.5	20 mEq/L higher than serum chloride
Colloidal gold	0000000000–0001222111	same	0.1	
Albumin	Mean: 29.5 mg/100 ml ± 2 SD:11–48 mg/100 ml	0.295 gm/L ± 2 SD:0.11–0.48 ml	2.5	
IgG	Mean: 4.3 mg/100 ml ± 2 SD:0–8.6 mg/100 ml	0.043 gm/L ± 2 SD:0–0.086		
Glucose	50–75 mg/100 ml	2.8–4.2 mmol/L	0.5	30–50% less than blood glucose
Pressure (initial)	70–180 mm of water	70–180 arb. u.		
Protein:				
Lumbar	15–45 mg/100 ml	0.15–0.45 gm/L	1	
Cisternal	15–25 mg/100 ml	0.15–0.25 gm/L	1	
Ventricular	5–15 mg/100 ml	0.05–0.15 gm/L	1	

MISCELLANEOUS VALUES

Determination	Reference Range		Minimal ml Required	Note
	Conventional	SI		
Ascorbic acid load test	0.2–2.0 mg/h in control sample	0.3–3.2 nmol/sec	Urine–approx. 1½-h sample	Administer ascorbic acid 500 mg orally
	24–49 mg/h after loading	38–77 nmol/sec	Urine–2 timed samples of about 2 h each	

TABLE 230-1. NORMAL LABORATORY VALUES IN THE MASSACHUSETTS GENERAL HOSPITAL *(Cont'd)*
MISCELLANEOUS VALUES *(Cont'd)*

Determination	Reference Range		Minimal ml Required	Note
	Conventional	SI		
Autoantibodies				
Thyroid colloid & microsomal antigens	Absent		2-S	Low titers in some elderly normal women
Stomach parietal cells	Absent		2-S	
Smooth muscle	Absent		2-S	
Kidney mitochondria	Absent		2-S	
Rabbit renal collecting ducts	Absent		2-S	
Cytoplasm of ova, theca cells, testicular interstitial cells	Absent		2-S	
Skeletal muscle	Absent		2-S	
Adrenal gland	Absent		2-S	
Carcinoembryonic antigen (CEA)	0–2.5 ng/ml, 97% healthy nonsmokers	0–2.5 µg/L 97% healthy nonsmokers	20-P	Must be sent on ice
Chylous fluid				Use fresh specimen
Cryoprecipitable proteins	0	0 arb. u.	10-S 5-P 10-P	Collect & transport at 37 C
Digitoxin	17 ± 6 ng/ml	22 ± 7.8 nmol/L	1-S	Medication with digitoxin or digitalis
Digoxin	1.2 ± 0.4 ng/ml	1.54 ± 0.5 nmol/L	1-S	Medication with digoxin 0.25 mg/day
	1.5 ± 0.4 ng/ml	1.92 ± 0.5 nmol/L	1-S	Medication with digoxin 0.5 mg/day

Test			Amount	Comments
Duodenal drainage				pH should be in proper range with minimal amount of gastric juice
pH	5.5–7.5	5.5–7.5	1	
Amylase	>1200 u./total sample	>1.2 arb. u	1	
Trypsin	From 35 to 160% "normal"	0.35–1.60	1	
Viscosity	3 min or less	180 sec or less	4	Run ice cold in 34-sec viscosimeter
Gastric analysis				
Basal:				
Females 2.0 ± 1.8 mEq/h		0.6 ± 0.5		
Males 3.0 ± 2.0 mEq/h		0.8 ± 0.6 μmol/sec		
Maximal: (after betazole or pentagastrin)				
Females 16 ± 5 mEq/h		4.4 ± 1.4 μmol/sec		
Males 23 ± 5 mEq/h		6.4 ± 1.4 μmol/sec		
Gastrin-I	0–200 pg/ml	0–95 pmol/L	4-P	Heparinized sample
Immunologic tests				
α-Fetoglobulin	Abnormal if present		5-clotted blood	
α 1-Antitrypsin	200–400 mg/100 ml	2.0–4.0 gm/L	10-B	Send to laboratory promptly
Antinuclear antibodies	Positive if detected with serum diluted 1:10		10-clotted blood	
Anti-DNA antibodies	<15 u./ml		10-B	
Bence-Jones protein	Abnormal if present		100 U.	
Complement, total hemolytic	150–250 u./ml		10-B	Must be sent on ice
C3	Range 55–120 mg/100 ml	0.55–1.2 gm/L	10-B	
C4	Range 20–50 mg/100 ml	0.2–0.5 gm/L	10-B	
Immunoglobulins				
IgG	1140 mg/100 ml Range 540–1663	11.4 gm/L 5.5–16.6 gm/L		
IgA	214 mg/100 ml Range 66–344	2.14 gm/L 0.66–3.44 gm/L		
IgM	168 mg/100 ml Range 39–290	1.68 gm/L 0.39–2.9 gm/L		

TABLE 230-1. NORMAL LABORATORY VALUES IN THE MASSACHUSETTS GENERAL HOSPITAL *(Cont'd)*

MISCELLANEOUS VALUES *(Cont'd)*

Determination	Reference Range		Minimal ml Required	Note
	Conventional	SI		
Iontophoresis	Children: 0–40 mEq Na/L Adults: 0–60 mEq Na/L	0–40 mmol/L 0–60 mmol/L		Value given in terms of sodium
Propranolol (includes bioactive 4-OH metabolite)	100–300 ng/ml	386–1158 nmol/L	1-S	Obtain blood sample 4 h after last dose of beta blocking agent
Serum viscosity	1.4–1.8		10-B	Expressed as the relative viscosity of serum compared to water
Stool fat	<5 gm in 24 h or <4% of measured fat intake in 3-day period	<5 gm/day	24-h or 3-day specimen, preferably with markers	
Stool nitrogen	<2 gm/day or 10% of urinary nitrogen	<2 gm/day	24-h or 3-day specimen	
Synovial fluid				
Glucose	Not <20 mg/100 ml lower than simultaneously drawn blood sugar	see blood glucose mmol/L	1 ml of fresh fluid	Collect with oxalate-fluoride mixture
Mucin	Type 1 or 2	1–2 arb. u.	1 ml of fresh fluid	Grades as Type 1–tight clump Type 2–soft clump Type 3–soft clump that breaks up Type 4–cloudy, no clump
D-Xylose absorption	5–8 gm/5 h in urine 40 mg/100 ml in blood after 2 h	33–53 mmol 2.7 mmol/L	5-U 5-B	Administer 25 gm of D-xylose orally

231. BIOSTATISTICS FOR CLINICIANS

FUNDAMENTAL SCIENTIFIC PROCESSES

For a nonstatistical reader, the statistical tactics reported in medical literature may create a sense of insecurity. The reader may feel intimidated by the magisterial numbers of the descriptive statistics, confused by the mathematical intricacies of the associative indexes, or oppressed by the probabilistic theories of the inferential P values and confidence intervals. Abandoning hope of understanding or critically evaluating the results, the reader may assume that the work must be satisfactory, since it was published in a respectable journal after approval by a suitable expert.

This reliance on experts and on literary prestige has not always been justified, since prominent experts (as well as prominent journals) have sometimes been strikingly wrong. For example, statistical data were once used to support expert opinions that cholera was caused by low atmospheric pressure. After a long, careful statistical investigation, a prominent governmental commission concluded that pellagra was an infectious disease.

To avoid being misled either by arcane statistics or by mistaken experts, readers may therefore want to rely on their own critical capacities of evaluation. In trying to make use of these capacities, the reader should focus not on the secondary statistical activities, but on the primary scientific processes that underlie all the statistical data. These fundamental processes consist of observation and comparison, and no mathematical training is needed for their critical evaluation.

The observational processes provide the sources of the raw data. Their evaluation depends on answers to the following questions: Where did the data come from? How do we know that the stated information is correct? What has been left out? The processes of comparison provide the various analytic contrasts created by the investigator. Their evaluation depends on answers to the following questions: Are the comparisons fair? What sort of bias or unrecognized distortion may have occurred to favor one group against another? These evaluations of reliability in data and of validity in comparison require only clinical wisdom and common sense.

Observational Processes and Sources of Data

The trustworthiness of raw data depends on their accuracy, reproducibility (or consistency), and relevance to the problem under consideration.

The idea of demonstrating accuracy and reproducibility is well established for the dimensional data of laboratory tests, which are usually performed with standard procedures and can be checked through quality control inspections. This type of quality control is seldom available or employed, however, when the data are obtained from patients' responses to an oral or written set of questions. Thus, no investigative efforts may have been made to verify information about a patient's age, eating patterns, alcohol consumption, daily exercise, or maintenance of prescribed medication. Responses to such questions might be verified by repeating the questions on another occasion, by questioning relatives, or by such external procedures as checking birth certificates and doctors' office records. Unfortunately, however, the data of large statistical compilations, particularly in epidemiologic surveys, are usually obtained by a single interrogation that is seldom repeated or confirmed.

The verification process becomes even more difficult when the raw data come from value judgments or clinical conclusions. On what basis was a diagnosis established for atherosclerosis or ulcerative colitis? How consistent were the observers who decided on the histologic type of a cancer or on the interpretation of a roentgenographic silhouette? How was the cause of death determined and uniquely ascribed to a single disease? What criteria were used to conclude that improvement had occurred after treatment or that an unwanted event was an adverse reaction to a particular drug? The standards used for all of these decisions may differ remarkably from one occasion to another, or from one physician to the next.

To provide consistency in the published data, an investigator should establish criteria that denote the elements, rules, and tactics for all such clinical decisions and judgments. If such criteria are lacking, a reader may begin to doubt whether the same basic "facts" would be found by another investigator.

The problems caused by the absence of satisfactory criteria can be particularly well illustrated with studies of so-called adverse drug reactions. To prove the benefits of a drug, investigators are usually required to perform prospective research in the form of controlled, randomized, double-blind trials. By contrast, no such rules have been required for allegations of a drug's toxicity. The study can be retrospective; the treatment need not be randomly assigned; no control drug need be used; the control group can be chosen capriciously; and an adverse drug reaction can be diagnosed not only without double-blind methods, but even without effort to standardize the way multiple observers made their ad hoc diagnoses.

Scientific problems become embellished in the registries used for collecting data on adverse drug reactions. Collected information is stored in computers and subjected to diverse statistical analyses, even though no criteria may have been established to validate the accuracy of reported reactions, or to demonstrate that other clinicians, observing the same events, would reach the same diagnostic conclusion. As a result of this scientific double standard, if a clinician says that something bad happened after use of a drug, the report may be accepted into the registry and immortalized by the computer as an adverse drug reaction. But if a clinician says that something good happened, the report may be dismissed as testimonial evidence.

In addition to being trustworthy, data should also be relevant. Is the entity that is measured really germane to the question being asked? The blood level of penicillin seems clearly germane to a study of treatment for infections, but do general mortality rates for myocardial infarction really indicate the incidence of the infarctions? Is a change in survival time an adequate index of palliative therapy for patients with advanced cancer? Is infant mortality rate a suitable measurement of a nation's health care? Is an individual doctor's professional skill really assessed by the average length of time that his patients remain in the hospital? The issue of relevance is particularly important because of the "substitution game" that commonly occurs in modern statistical data. The information that the investigator really wanted to get was unavailable, unobtainable, or regarded as unreliable. Consequently, in search of hard, objective, dimensional data, the investigator substituted one form of information for another.

The statistics derived from these displaced data may often be valuable and helpful. In many other instances, however, the results are fallacious or misleading.

Acts of Cause–Effect Comparison

The most frequent comparisons that appear in clinical biostatistical literature involve cause–effect relationships. The most commonly investigated causative agents are either an etiologic factor suspected of leading to a disease or a therapeutic regimen believed to produce a favorable (or unfavorable) outcome in treatment of a disease. In the reasoning used for the comparisons, the results observed in people who received the principal maneuver of etiology or therapy are contrasted with the results observed in a control group of people who received either no maneuver or some other maneuver. The fairness of such a comparison can be distorted by bias that produces inequality in one or more of 4 components of the comparative procedure. The groups under comparison may have had different baseline susceptibilities to the outcome event; the maneuvers may have been performed with differences in proficiency; the outcome events may have been detected in an unequal manner; and the members of the groups counted at the end may have migrated in unequal proportions from the starting groups. These 4 biases can be illustrated as follows:

Susceptibility bias: As an example of different baseline susceptibilities in people receiving the compared maneuvers X and Y, a group of operable patients with cancer are more likely to have high survival rates than an inoperable group, even if no operation is performed. Because of this bias, the results of a surgically treated operable group cannot be compared fairly against the results of alternative treatment for an inoperable group.

This type of susceptibility bias, which arises from decisions made when patients are selected for treatment, can usually be removed in therapeutic trials if the treatment is assigned by a randomization mechanism. Since randomization is not used in surveys of causes of disease or in surveys of therapeutic agents, susceptibility bias must always be carefully contemplated as a source of distortion in such studies. Perhaps the most commonly omitted potential sources of bias in etiologic research are the roles of constitutional and psychic factors in predisposing to development of disease. In studies of therapeutic agents, the most commonly neglected potential sources of bias are the indication for use of the agent, the clinical severity of the ailment under investigation, and the comorbidity of associated diseases.

Performance bias: In contrast to people assigned to Agent Y, the people assigned to Agent X may not have taken it faithfully, may have received it in an unsatisfactory way, or may have received additional agents (or co-interventions) that could affect their outcome. As an example of the first of these problems, which refers to inequalities in *compliance*, two oral regimens may have equal pharmacologic efficacy when maintained faithfully, but one may seem less active simply because its taste or inconvenience makes people unwilling to take it faithfully. The second problem refers to an unequal proficiency in administration of the compared agents. This type of problem would occur if the merits of two different surgical operations were being compared, with the first operation having been performed by a highly-skilled surgeon and the other by an inexperienced intern. The third problem, which refers to inequalities in the associated interventions, can be illustrated in a comparison of two antibiotic regimens intended to prevent streptococcal infections and recurrences of rheumatic fever. If the patients assigned to prophylactic regimen X have also received substantially more additional antibiotic therapy than the patients assigned to prophylactic regimen Y, the subsequent comparisons of prophylactic efficacy for X vs. Y are unfair.

Detection bias: The problem of detection bias arises from inequalities in the intensity of diagnostic surveillance or in the diagnostic criteria used to detect the outcome of either treatment or exposure to a suspected etiologic agent. A simple example of this problem is the availability of roentgenographic and cytologic procedures for diagnosing cancer. The occurrence rate of certain cancers may rise or fall according to the technologic availability, dissemination, and usage of these procedures. Consequently, the cancer rates found in one era or geographic region may differ from those found in another, not because the true incidence has changed, but because of differences in diagnostic technology.

The problem becomes particularly striking when certain agents are compared as causes of disease. Thus, does thrombophlebitis really occur more often in women receiving oral contraceptive agents than in those using diaphragms, or does the use of oral agents invoke the greater diagnostic surveillance that makes thrombophlebitis more likely to be detected? Does reserpine usage predispose to breast cancer or is an otherwise undetected breast cancer more likely to be found in women who receive frequent medical examinations in the course of therapy for hypertension? Problems of detection bias, often overlooked in contemporary epidemiologic research, constitute major hazards for the validity of the comparisons performed in many cause–effect studies.

Migration bias: In many studies of etiology or therapeutic agents, a long period of time may intervene between initiation of the alleged causal agent and the development of subsequent effects. During this time, various members of the original groups may depart from observation. Departures may be due to death, geographic migration, or choice of other sources of medical care. If these migrations (or drop-outs) occur unequally in the principal groups under comparison, the subsequent analyses may be greatly distorted. Distortions are particularly likely to happen if the comparisons take place long after the original groups were assembled.

For example, suppose Groups A and B both have a 4-yr death rate of 30% after their exposures to Agents A and B, but that the 2-yr death rates are respectively 5% and 25%. In other words, of 100 people starting in Group A, 5 will be dead at 2 yr and 25 more will die in the next 2 yr, whereas in Group B, 25 of the 100 members die in the first 2 yr and 5 in the next 2 yr. Now suppose that we do not assemble Groups A and B at the time that they were first exposed to Agents A and B. Instead, we assemble them 2 yr later. Group A will contain 95 members, of whom 25 (or 26%) will die in the next 2 yr. Group B will contain 75 members of whom 5 (or 6%) will die in the next 2 yr. The death-rate difference of 26% vs. 6% in the next 2 yr will be statistically significant and will make Group A seem much worse off than Group B. In fact, however, Group A fared substantially better than Group B at 2 yr, and the mortality results in the 2 groups were identical at 4 yr.

Another type of migration problem, sometimes known as Berkson's bias, occurs if patients with condition X are much more likely to be referred to a hospital than patients with condition Y. Erroneous results will then be noted at that hospital for the concurrence of conditions X and Y.

These and several other kinds of problems in migration bias create hazards in epidemiologic studies of risk factors when a cross-sectional population is followed prospectively, and in retrospective hospital-based ("case-control") studies of causes of disease or adverse drug reactions.

Design of Cause–Effect Studies

To establish a cause–effect relationship, the preferred model in most forms of scientific research is an experimental investigation in which the results that occur after the causal agent is imposed upon a susceptible group are compared against the results noted with a comparative agent, or "control." This model can readily be used, in laboratory settings, for animals or inanimate systems, but the model cannot easily be applied for cause–effect studies of the impact of etiologic or therapeutic agents in human beings. Accordingly, several alternative research structures have been developed and used to make cause–effect decisions in clinical science.

Experimental trials: The randomized controlled clinical trial is an experimental procedure, which is the preferred method (when feasible) for demonstrating causal efficacy. Many of the biases cited in the previous section can be prevented or reduced because the design of such a trial customarily includes the use of a concurrent control group, randomized assignment of treatment, and double-blind methods (when possible) for detecting outcome events. Because of complex logistics and other features to be cited later, however, such trials cannot be applied to all types of therapy, and because of ethical constraints, the trials cannot be used to study agents strongly suspected of having noxious effects.

Observational cohort studies: An observational cohort (or "longitudinal") study is concerned with the follow-up of groups of persons exposed or not exposed to the therapeutic or etiologic agent whose efficacy is under evaluation. The basic design is similar to that of an experimental trial, but the agents are assigned by selective judgment (of either the recipient or the physician), not by randomization; the compared groups may have received different co-interventions beyond the agents under study; and the methods of detecting outcome events may not have been similar. An observational cohort study may be performed prospectively (or "prolectively") with deliberate advance planning for collecting the research data; or the data may be obtained retrospectively (or "retrolectively") from medical records or other available sources of information. In some cohort studies, the control group is not concurrent, and is collected in an "historical" manner, based on results found during a previous calendar period.

Because of the cited nonexperimental features, observational cohort studies contain the potential for bias in susceptibility, performance, and detection. With careful methods of defining and following the population under analysis, migration bias can usually be minimized.

Case-control studies: When the outcome event has a very low rate of occurrence or does not appear until long after exposure to the etiologic or therapeutic agent, the longitudinal approach—in either an experimental trial or observational cohort study—becomes unfeasible because too many people would need to be studied for too protracted a period of time. Accordingly, a "retrospective" case-control study may become the best practical way of investigating certain cause–effect relationships.

In a case-control study, the customary scientific direction of observations is reversed. The investigator begins at the end, rather than at the beginning, of the causal pathway. The cases consist of a group of people, who are chosen because they have already developed the outcome event under consideration. The *controls* are a comparative group, chosen from people who have not developed the outcome event. The two groups are then examined to determine (and contrast) their antecedent rates of exposure to the suspected etiologic or therapeutic agent. Such studies can potentially contain all of the biases that may arise in observational cohort research, but also can be distorted by diverse aspects of migration bias, particularly since the "control" group is chosen according to arbitrary standards.

Associative trend studies: In this form of research, no specific groups of people are actually assembled and studied. Instead, the investigator assembles general calendrical or geographic data showing how the occurrence rates of a particular condition may have changed with calendar time or geographic region. The trends are then associated with data showing the prevalence of usage of the suspected agent during the same calendar periods or in the same geographic regions. An association (or lack of association) in these two sets of data may then be used to support (or refute) the idea of a causal relationship.

The results noted in this type of study may be distorted by all of the four main types of bias noted earlier, as well as by the investigator's capacity for self-delusion in choosing and evaluating the plausibility of an association.

Illustration of the four approaches: To illustrate the four types of approach, suppose we suspected that regular tea-drinking produces gallstones. In an *experimental trial,* we would randomly assign a large group of healthy adults, without gallstones, to drink or not drink tea regularly for the next 20 yr. At the end of that time we would compare the incidence of gallstones in the two groups. In an *observational cohort study,* we would find a group of tea-drinkers and a group of non–tea-drinkers, eliminate the members of either group who already have gallstones, and follow the remaining people in the two groups for the next 20 yr. The incidence of gallstones would then be compared in the two groups.

In a *case-control study,* we would find a group of people with gallstones and assemble a control group without gallstones. After interrogating the members of the two groups about their antecedent patterns of beverage intake, we would compare the rates of previous exposure to tea-drinking in the two groups. In the *associative trend approach,* we might assemble national data about the general occurrence rate of gallstones in 12 different countries. We would also assemble data about the consumption of tea in those 12 countries. We would then draw a graph and do statistical tests associating national tea intake with gallstone occurrence rates.

Conclusion

Some of the most crucial distinctions of collected statistics in scientific research, particularly those distinctions that may lead to erroneous data or unfair comparisons, can become readily evident to a reader who contemplates the basic principles of both science and clinical medicine, rather than the intricate strategies of the mathematical procedures. Statistical quantification and statistical analysis can make (and have made) invaluable contributions to clinical science. The ultimate value of the contributions depends, however, on the basic quality of data and comparisons made during the statistical activities. To assess and create that basic quality, the prerequisite principles are those of clinical science, not mathematics.

INTRODUCTION TO STATISTICS

The word "statistics" is applied to at least 2 distinctly different activities: descriptive statistics and inferential statistics.

Descriptive statistics consists of individual items of data or specific expressions to summarize the contents, contrasts, or associations of groups of data. Items of data can describe single observations, such as a serum cholesterol of 250 mg/dl; single enumerations, such as a frequency count of 27 women; or a collection of such observations and counts. The summary expressions for a group of data may indicate a mean or proportion for the collected results; and 2 means or 2 proportions can be contrasted with comparative expressions, such as an increment or ratio. The procedures used for the summaries and contrasts of descriptive statistics usually require no knowledge of mathematics beyond elementary arithmetic. A separate branch of descriptive statistics produces indexes of association, derived from distinctively mathematical technics that provide the correlation indexes, regression coefficients, and other numerical expressions used to indicate associations or interrelations of data.

Inferential statistics, which depends on mathematical theories of probability and concepts about random variation, provides the procedures that are used to estimate the characteristics of a parent population from the results found in a sample; and to draw conclusions about the role of chance in numerical contrasts of data from two or more groups. These probabilistic procedures produce the confidence intervals, P values, and tests of "statistical significance" that are encountered so often in modern medical literature.

Although usually regarded as the special domain of statisticians, the associative and inferential procedures cannot be applied until the fundamental data have been obtained and descriptively summarized. Consequently, a reader who is familiar with the phenomena under observation and with the basic structure of the research can often arrive at cogent statistical judgments, despite a lack of mathematical knowledge. By evaluating the structure, quality, and pertinence of the basic descriptive data and by noting whether the data were suitably acquired and expressed, a mathematically unsophisticated reader who understands the primary scientific issues of the research may be able to avoid struggling with the secondary mathematical strategies. If the basic data and design of the research are too poor to be worthy of associative and inferential statistical analyses, the results of those analyses can often be ignored.

The rest of the discussion here is divided into 3 principal parts: the arithmetical structures of descriptive statistics; the mathematical tactics of associative statistics; and the basic ideas of inferential statistics. All 3 types of statistical activity, however, depend on the underlying fundamental scientific processes.

DESCRIPTIVE STATISTICS

Items that are called *data* consist of expressions that are the "values" of variables. Before any data become summarized, contrasted, or associated, they must first be suitably expressed.

TYPES OF VARIABLES

The name "variable" is applied to a single class of data that can take on different values in a scale of available categories. A variable is called dimensional, ordinal, existential, or nominal according to the interrelationship of the categories in the scale.

A **dimensional** (which is also called **continuous** or **interval**) **variable** contains a scale of ranked categories with measurably equal intervals between each pair of adjacent categories. *Age* and *temperature* are examples of dimensional variables having the respective categories of *1, 2, 3, . . . 98, 99, . . .* yr and *. . . 36.9, 37.0, 37.1, 37.2, . . .* C. For a particular person, these categories might have the values of *57* yr for age and *37.1 C* for temperature.

An **ordinal variable** contains ranked categories that are established arbitrarily without measurably equal intervals between them. *Severity of dyspnea* is an ordinal variable expressed in such categorical values as *none, mild, moderate,* and *extreme*. *Briskness of reflexes* is another ordinal variable, with categories of *0, 1+, 2+, 3+,* and *4+*.

Existential variables are a subdivision of ordinal variables, in which the existence of an entity, such as chest pain or a particular disease, is expressed in a dichotomous scale of categories, such as *yes* and *no*, or *present* and *absent*. Such a scale can be expanded into the overtly ordinal categories of *definitely yes, probably yes, uncertain whether yes or no, probably no,* and *definitely no*.

A **nominal variable** is expressed in categories that have no ranks. *Gender* is a nominal variable with categories *female* and *male*. Other examples of nominal variables are occupation, religion, birthplace, and social security number. A particular person might have the values of *male* in **gender**, *physician* in **occupation**, and *California* in **birthplace**.

Composite variables are constructed by combining elements from two or more other variables. The wind–chill factor and temperature–humidity index are composite variables encountered in daily life. The scale of categories for a composite variable can be dimensional, ordinal, existential, or nominal according to the expressions that emerge from the type of procedure used for forming the categories. Examples of composite medical variables are the following: **ponderal index**, which is the dimensional result of dividing weight by the cube root of height; **Apgar score**, which has the ordinal ranks *0, 1, 2, . . ., 9, 10* formed by adding arbitrary numerical values for the presence or absence of five different clinical manifestations in a newborn infant; and **diagnosis of rheumatic fever**, which is expressed as *yes* or *no*, based on fulfillment of a series of specifications in the individual variables that constitute the eligibility requirements of the modified Jones diagnostic criteria.

SUMMARIES OF A COLLECTION

Although any value of any variable for a particular person can be regarded as a statistical item of data, the main concepts of descriptive statistics become applied when a series of values have been collected. For a single variable, such as **BP**, the collection can comprise the individual values noted for each member of a group of people, or a series of values determined at different times for the same person. Thus, a collection might include the values of cholesterol for a group of people with a particular disease; or the values noted at a series of weekly measurements of an individual person's cholesterol.

Frequency Counts

The simplest way of summarizing a collection of data for a single variable is to note the total number of members in the group, and to list the counted frequency of occurrences of each value of the variable. These direct frequency counts are especially useful for nominal or ordinal variables that have a small number of categories. Thus, we might note that a group of 87 people contains, for the variable **gender**, 52-*women* and 35-*men;* and for the variable **severity of dyspnea**, 36-*none*, 28-*mild*, 15-*moderate*, and 8-*extreme*.

For dimensional variables that contain a large number of categories, the categorical values are sometimes consolidated into an ordinal array for citing frequencies. Thus, in the group of people just cited, we might count 2 persons with age $\leq$ 10; 5 with age 11 to 20; 11 persons at age 21 to 30; and so on. Categories can also be consolidated for nondimensional variables. In baseball statistics, for example, the variable **result of time at bat** contains such categories as *single, double, triple,* and *home run.* For many enumerations of frequency in a player's batting performance, however, these four categories are consolidated into a single category called *hit.*

Relative Frequencies

After the frequencies at each value have been counted, the relative frequencies can be calculated as a proportion (or percentage) of the total. Thus, the 87 people mentioned in the previous section can be listed as containing 52/87 women, which is a proportion of 0.60. Proportions are often multiplied by 100 and expressed as percentages. The percentages in the cited group for the variable **severity of dyspnea** would be 41%, *none;* 32%, *mild;* 17%, *moderate;* and 9%, *extreme.*

The listing of relative frequencies is particularly helpful for comparing different collections of data, since the use of proportions (or percentages) helps "standardize" the results for groups of different total size. Relative frequencies are also often used for graphic portraits of a distribution, as described in the next section.

Distribution Curves

A common method of demonstrating the collection of data for a particular variable is to show, at each value of the variable, the associated frequency count or proportionate relative frequency. These pairs of data can be converted into graphic form by placing the values of the variable on the abscissa (x-axis) and the associated frequency result on the ordinate (y-axis).

For the graphs, ordinal and dimensional variables are arrayed according to the rank of their values; and the adjacent heights of the frequency columns form a **histogram.** Alternatively, the associated frequency at each value can be shown on a graph as a point and the points can be connected with lines to form a structure called a **frequency polygon.** For the multiple points of dimensional data, the frequency polygon may resemble a curved line. Since the values of nominal variables cannot be arranged in rank order, the associated frequencies can be shown as a group of vertical columns that form a **bar graph.**

The varied shapes of these graphic portraits denote the **distribution** of the variable. For ordinary descriptive purposes, the distribution curve serves merely to illustrate the scope of the collected data. For certain statistical maneuvers, however, the collected data are regarded as a sample taken from a larger population, having its own characteristic distribution curve.

The best known of these statistical distributions has a "cocked-hat" or "bell-shaped" form that is called a **normal** or **Gaussian curve.** One major characteristic of the Gaussian curve is its centripetal symmetry around a single apex, occurring at the central value of the curve. If the apex of a distribution is displaced substantially to the right or left of the center, the distribution is called **skewed.**

A particularly important statistical feature of a distribution curve is the interpretation given to the arrangement of relative frequencies. For each demarcated category along the abscissa of the curve, the associated relative frequency can be regarded as the likelihood or probability of obtaining that value if any single member of the category were randomly selected from the distribution. The area that lies under the curve beyond a selected dimensional or ordinal value will represent the probability (or P value) of obtaining a more extreme value if some other member of the distribution were chosen at random. Since the sum of the relative frequencies is 1, the total area of probability that lies under the curve is also 1.

Central Tendency

The frequency counts, relative frequencies, and shape of a distribution curve give a general description of a collection of data, but do not summarize it. One type of summary item is a single result, often called the **index of central tendency,** that denotes a center or focal point of the collected data. Its choice will depend on the type of variable and the purpose of the selection.

For nominal variables, which cannot be ranked, no central tendency can be cited. For a variable that has only two categories, only one choice of central tendency is possible. It is the **mode,** which is *the particular value that has the highest relative frequency.* In the group of 52 women and 35 men mentioned earlier, the mode is the value, *woman.*

A mode can also be determined for ordinal variables, but because the ordinal values are ranked, an alternative point of central focus can be selected. It is called the **median**—*the value that occurs midway in the ordered ranks of the distribution.* In the group of 87 people whose values were cited earlier for severity of dyspnea, the median value will be the 44th ranked value, counted from either end of the distribution. Since 36 people were in the *none* category, the 44th ranked person will occur in the *mild* group. Accordingly, the median value for this distribution is *mild.* The modal value would be *none.*

A mode and a median can be determined for dimensional data, but since these data have equal intervals between adjacent categories, the array of values can also be averaged. In the customary procedure, each of the observed values in the distribution is added and their sum is divided by the total number of observations. The result is called the **mean** (or **arithmetic mean**). In the standard statistical symbols that are regularly used to show this process, the symbol X is used both as a name for the variable and as a representative of any one of the values of the variable. The symbol X_i is used to represent a specified value in the group. (The symbol x_i is often used to represent the deviations of an individual value, X_i, from the mean of the data. To simplify the typography, however, most authors follow a different convention, using x for the variable itself and x_i for the individual values. The latter convention is employed in this chapter.)

The symbol Σ is used to indicate the process of summation, so that Σx_i or, more simply, Σx, denotes that all the observed values of the variable x are to be added. With $\bar{x}$ representing the arithmetic mean, and n representing the number of observations, the calculation of a mean is then symbolized as

$$\bar{x} = \frac{\Sigma x}{n}$$

or, expressed on a single line, as $\bar{x} = \Sigma x / n$.

The choice of whether to use the mode, median, or mean as the best index of central tendency is often a matter of judgment. The mode is seldom used in medical science, although it is important in marketing research and it is the only expression that can be used to cite a central tendency in nominal data. The mean, which is the traditional and most commonly used index, has the advantage of being mathematically "tractable"; i.e., it is readily amenable to the concepts and manipulations used in statistical formulas. The main disadvantages of the mean are that it may sometimes be impossible, unrealistic, or unrepresentative. A mean value cannot be rationally determined for nominal, existential, or ordinal data, and it is unrealistic when calculated for integer dimensions that may yield such peculiar results as a "mean of 2.3 children per family." The mean may be unrepresentative if its value is greatly affected by isolated items in certain extreme (or "**outlier**") values in the distribution.

An example of the latter problem occurs in a distribution of the survival times for 10 patients with advanced cancer, listed as: 1, 1, 2, 2, 3, 3, 3, 3, 4, and 12 mo. The mean value of survival time for this group is 3.4 mo. If the last-cited patient had survived 40 mo rather than 12 mo, however, the mean value would be 6.2 mo. The mean is also sometimes incalculable. Thus, if the last patient has not yet died, the mean survival of this group cannot be determined. By contrast, the median value for the group would be 3 mo, regardless of the survival duration of the last patient.

For this reason, many investigators prefer to use the median as a general index of central tendency. In certain instances, such as bacterial counts or antibody titers, where the data are expressed in powers of a number, such as 10^2, 10^3, etc., the most appropriate index may be a **geometric mean**, obtained by taking the nth root of the product of the n items of data.

Dispersion

A second salient characteristic of a collection of dimensional data is its dispersion or spread around the point of central tendency. Consider two distributions of 10 values: 11, 11, 11, 12, 12, 12, 12, 13, 13, 13; and 1, 5, 8, 10, 12, 12, 14, 16, 19, 23. Each of these distributions has a mean, median, and mode of 12; yet the first distribution is much more compact than the second.

The simplest way of denoting the spread of a distribution is to cite its **range**, which is simply the distance from the highest value to the lowest. In the two distributions just cited, the respective ranges are 2 (= 13 to 11) and 22 (= 23 to 1). The main disadvantage of using the range to denote spread is that this measurement, like the mean, can be profoundly altered by extreme outlier values. Thus, the 10 values that form the distribution 1, 11, 11, 12, 12, 12, 12, 13, 13, 23 also have a mean, median, and mode of 12 and a range of 22; but this distribution differs substantially from the immediately preceding one that had those same summary characteristics.

The traditional statistical method of indicating spread of a distribution is the **standard deviation**. This is calculated in several steps. The first involves finding the deviation from the mean for each value in the collecton of data. The individual deviations are squared (to avoid negative values) and the squared deviations are added together. The result, which is the sum of squared deviations around the mean, is often symbolized as $S_{xx} = \Sigma(x - \bar{x})^2$. The two subscripts indicate that the deviations for x are calculated around the mean of the x values. For another variable, y, the corresponding notation would be $S_{yy} = \Sigma(y - \bar{y})^2$.

An average value, called the **variance**, is then calculated for S_{xx} by dividing it by a suitably chosen number. If the data come from a complete population and are being used descriptively, S_{xx} is divided by n to form the variance. If the data are regarded as a sample of a population and are used inferentially, S_{xx} is divided by n − 1. The square root of the variance is the **standard deviation**. Thus, for inferential purposes, the standard deviation is $s = \sqrt{[\Sigma(x - \bar{x})^2]/(n - 1)}$.

In addition to certain mathematical virtues, the standard deviation has the advantage of providing a single value that can summarize the dispersion of a distribution. For the three distributions that were noted earlier, the respective standard deviations (calculated with n − 1) are 0.82, 6.50, and 5.23 respectively. The differences in these three standard deviations indicate the relative compactness (or "density") of the distribution. This distinction can be determined by calculating a **coefficient of variation**, which is simply the ratio, $s/\bar{x}$. The smaller this coefficient, the less is the relative spread of the distribution around the mean.

Another advantage of the standard deviation is that it can be used to denote the inner range of a Gaussian distribution: about 65% of all the frequency data lie in a zone that symmetrically spans one standard deviation on either side of the mean (expressed as $\pm$ s), and 95% of the data lie in the symmetric zone that spans almost two standard deviations ($\bar{x} \pm 1.96s$) around the mean.

When applied to a distribution of data that is not Gaussian, the standard deviation can produce odd or unrealistic results. Consider the following set of values for fasting blood sugar in 10 people: 85, 87, 88, 95, 97, 100, 110, 150, 170, 500. The mean value for this group is 148.2 and the standard deviation is 126.9. If we take 1.96 standard deviations on either side of this mean, the 95% inner range would be expected to lie from –100.5 to 396.9. The lower value of this range is obviously unrealistic.

To avoid some of these problems of the range and standard deviation, the **percentile technic** has become increasingly used for showing the dispersion of a distribution. When the array of observations is arranged in rank order from the lowest to highest, the particular value that occurs at each 100th of these ranks is a percentile. For example, if the collection of data contains 199 values, the 20th ranked value is at the 1st decile, the 40th ranked value is at the 1st quintile, and so on. The 100th ranked value would be the 50th percentile, which is the median. To obtain the 95% inner range of the distribution, we would cite the values that correspond to the 2.5 and 97.5 percentile ranks.

The percentile method, which is now the standard procedure for indexing the distribution of heights and weights of normal growing children, is not as mathematically easy to work with as a standard deviation, but offers the major descriptive advantage of being applicable to any form of dimensional data, regardless of distributional characteristics. The standard deviation, calculated with $n - 1$, is particularly valuable for its role in the inferential statistics discussed later.

COMPOUND QUOTIENTS

A quotient is formed by dividing one number, called the numerator, by another called the denominator. Three such statistical quotients have already been discussed: the proportions or percentages that represent relative frequencies; the calculation of a mean as $\Sigma x/n$; and the calculation of a variance as $S_{xx}/(n - 1)$. Each of these quotients was simple in that the numerator and denominator were obtained from the same set of data for a single variable. Many other statistical expressions, however, are obtained as compound quotients, representing frequency counts from two or more different variables. These compound quotients are often called **rates** or **ratios**.

An example of a compound quotient is the entity called an **annual mortality rate**. The denominator of this rate consists of the number of people determined, by census count, to be the population of a defined geographic region during a particular year. The numerator consists of the number of people in that region who, according to death certificate enumerations, died during that year. The proportion that emerges in the calculation is often multiplied by 1000 or by 100,000 to yield a number cited as an annual mortality rate per 1000 or per 100,000. Because of migration of people in and out of the geographic region and because of the logistic difficulties in maintaining surveillance over a large human population, a single counting process cannot simultaneously indicate the number of people who were alive and dead in that region. Accordingly, the mortality rate becomes a compound quotient via numerator and denominator data that come from two different sources: census counts and death certificate counts.

In epidemiologic data, a **prevalence rate** refers to *the frequency with which an event exists at a particular time in a particular group*. An **incidence rate** refers to *the frequency with which new occurrences of an event are noted as the group is observed during a defined period*. For example, if we examine a group of 2000 school children and find that 50 of them have positive throat cultures for streptococcal infection, the prevalence rate is 25/1000. If we continue to examine the 2000 children during the next year and find that 80 of them develop new infections in that interval, the incidence rate is 40/1000 for that year.

In addition to these usages, the term "rate" is commonly applied to quotients that are really simple proportions or percentages, in which the numerator group is actually a subset of the denominator. Thus, in a **case fatality rate**, the denominator consists of the number of people known to have a particular disease at a certain point in time; and the numerator consists of the number of those people who died at a later date. An alternative expression, with living rather than dead people counted in the numerator, is called a **survival rate**.

EXPRESSION OF COMPARATIVE CONTRASTS

Three kinds of statistical expressions—increments, ratios, and proportional increments—are used to achieve a single index that can be used for decisions about the **quantitative significance** of a contrast of results in two groups. For example, suppose that in a well-designed, properly conducted clinical trial, the rate of success is 50% with Treatment A and 33% with Treatment B. Expressed as an increment, the difference can be reported as Treatment A being 17% higher than B, or B 17% lower than A. Expressed as a ratio, success occurred 1.52 times ($= 50\%/33\%$) as frequently with A as with B, or .67 times ($= 33\%/50\%$) as frequently with B as with A. Expressed as a proportional increment, Treatment A was 52% [$= (50\% - 33\%)/(33\%)$] relatively more successful than B; or B was 34% [$= (33\% - 50\%)/(50\%)$] relatively less successful than A.

Since all six of these expressions (+17%, –17%, 1.52, .67, 52%, and 34%) are available to describe a single comparison, at least two different acts of judgment are required for decisions of quantitative significance. The first is to choose the particular expression(s) in which the comparison will be cited. The second is to decide the magnitude(s) that will be regarded as "significant." For this decision to be as sensible as possible, *both* the increment *and* the ratio (or proportionate increment) will be examined concomitantly. For example, one treatment may seem substantially better than another if the ratio of success is 3.5 times higher, but if the actual rates of success for the two treatments are 7% and 2%, the increment of 5% may make the ratio seem less impressive. Nevertheless, if "success" is measured by survival rather than by improvement of headache, an increment as small as 5% may again seem impressive. Consequently, decisions about quantitative significance usually involve an appraisal of both the increment and the ratio.

A ratio index is commonly used in epidemiology to contrast the risk of disease in people exposed or nonexposed to a suspected etiologic agent. Thus, if we know the attack rate of infectious hepatitis in people who eat raw clams and the corresponding attack rate in those who do not eat them, the 2 rates can be divided to form a "risk ratio" for infectious hepatitis in raw-clam eaters.

INDEXES OF ASSOCIATION

An association can be determined for two (or more) variables whenever their points of data can be linked together. The item of linkage can be a particular person, a particular time period, or a pair of measurements for the same entity. Thus, we can relate hematocrit and cholesterol values for each of a group of people; the sale of backgammon sets and the number of crimes committed during each of a group of years; the values of weight for each of a group of people before and after a reduction diet; or the measurements of triglyceride as performed on the same group of specimens in two different laboratories or on two occasions in the same laboratory.

In one type of mathematical model for expressing association, we assume that the two variables are *dependent*, i.e., that the value of one is affected by the value of the other. Since this assumption is purely mathematical, it may or may not be correct in reality. Thus, we can mathematically determine the dependence of either Hct on cholesterol or cholesterol on Hct; but in biological reality neither one of these variables may be affected by the other. In a different mathematical technic, we determine the correlation of two variables as an expression of their *interdependency*. Do the values of one variable tend to rise or fall as the other variable's values rise and fall? The mathematical answer to this question does not require that the variables actually be related—they can be as unrelated perhaps as crime and backgammon sets.

For doing either the dependent or interdependent calculations, we make use of an entity called **covariance.** Just as variance for an individual variable was derived from the squared products of the deviation from the mean (so that $S_{xx} = \Sigma[x - \bar{x}]^2$ and $S_{yy} = \Sigma[y - \bar{y}]^2$), the covariance of two variables is derived from the cross products of the individual deviations. Thus, the covariance of two variables, x and y, is determined from $S_{xy} = \Sigma(x - \bar{x})(y - \bar{y})$.

The Regression Coefficient

If x and y are dimensional variables, their dependent relationship is commonly expressed as the equation for a straight line, $y = a + bx$, where x is assumed to be the independent variable upon whose values y depends. This equation is called the *regression* of y upon x. The a and b values for the equation are usually calculated from the data by a mathematical procedure that makes use of the method of least squares for fitting a straight line to a series of points. With this procedure, b, the slope of the line, is determined as $b = S_{xy}/S_{xx}$. It is often called the **regression coefficient.** It indicates the amount of change that takes place in variable y with a unit of change in variable x. Thus, if b = –2.5, a rise of 2 units in x would be accompanied by a fall of 5 units in y. The value of a, which is the y-intercept of the line when x = 0, is calculated as $\bar{y} - b\bar{x}$. The line can be drawn by connecting the point $(0, \bar{y} - b\bar{x})$ to the point $(\bar{x}, \bar{y})$.

If y is believed to depend on only one variable, x, the foregoing relationships are called **simple regression.** When y is believed to depend upon more than one independent variable—such as x_1, x_2, x_3, etc.—the dependency equation describes a linear "surface" in multidimensional space. The expression is $y = b_0 + b_1x_1 + b_2x_2 + b_3x_3 + \ldots$, and the procedure is called **multiple linear regression.**

The Correlation Coefficient

The interdependent linear relationship of two variables x and y is expressed with a correlation coefficient, r, which is calculated as $S_{xy}/\sqrt{(S_{xx})(S_{yy})}$. The absolute value of r will range between 0 and 1. When r is close to 1, the correlation is high. When r is near 0, the two variables have little or no correlation. When r is negative, the variables have an inverse correlation, so that one of the variables tends to rise as the other falls.

Advantages and Problems

The main advantages of correlation and regression coefficients are that they provide single values that summarize the linear relationships of two (or more) variables. Because the regression coefficients are calculated with mathematical models that fit a straight line (or its multidimensional equivalent) to the data, the results will not be appropriate if the data do not actually have a linear relationship or if the relationship becomes nonlinear beyond the points contained in the data. A separate limitation, when multiple variables are used, is that the customary linear model deals with each variable as making a separate additive contribution, ignoring the synergistic or antagonistic effects (which statisticians call "interactions") that can occur when certain features (such as old age and major co-morbidity) are concurrent. The problem can be avoided if the multiple regression equation is expanded to contain special "interaction terms," but such terms are seldom included in the calculations.

Another potential difficulty is that regression coefficients are dependent on the units in which the data are expressed. Thus, the regression coefficient for age expressed in months will be 12 times higher than the corresponding value for age in years. For this reason, the relative "importance" of different variables in a multiple regression equation cannot be determined unless their regression coefficients have been expressed in a "standardized" manner that makes provision for differences in dimensional units.

A different problem in regression occurs when the dependent variable, y, is existentially expressed as present or absent (in values of *1* or *0*). In this situation, the coefficients of a regression equation may sometimes provide peculiar results for the data of an individual person, because the predicted value of y that emerges from the equation may exceed *1* or be < 0. To avoid this problem the data are often "transformed" with a tactic called **logistic regression**, which contains the values of y to lie between the limits of 0 and 1. The equation is expressed as $y = 1/(1 + e^{-A})$, where $A = b_0 + b_1x_1 + b_2x_2 + b_3x_3 + \ldots$

Three important precautions should be observed in using the correlation coefficient. The first is that the coefficient indicates linear association rather than agreement between two variables. Consequently, correlation coefficients are not the best way to express the results when quality control is tested for laboratory procedures or for observer variability. A second precaution is that the closeness of fit in a correlation is expressed better with r^2 than with r. Thus, when the correlation coefficient is 0.4, the linear model used in the correlation has achieved a proportional reduction in variance of only 0.16. Finally, when a correlation coefficient is associated with a P value (as described later), the likelihood of obtaining "statistical significance" depends mainly on the size of the sample. Thus, if the number of observations is sufficiently large, a correlation coefficient as unimpressive as .01 can become "statistically significant" at $P < .05$.

Other Expressions of Association

The coefficients of regression and correlation are calculated as described if the data are dimensional. If the data are not dimensional, other expressions and mathematical models are employed. The names of some of these expressions are cited here for the sake of indicating their existence. Their application is described in appropriate textbooks. For calculating correlations in nondimensional data, the available procedures include *Spearman's rho*, *Kendall's tau*, and such coefficients as *phi*. When the dependent variable is expressed in nominal, non-ranked categories, its relationship to multiple independent variables is determined with discriminant function analysis, rather than with the standard multiple regression model.

Indexes of Agreement

The described indexes of association denote the *trend* of a relationship between 2 variables, but do not indicate effectively the *agreement* between variables. Thus, if laboratory A gets triglyceride results that are exactly twice as high as those of laboratory B, the correlation between the 2 sets of results will be perfect, but the agreement will be terrible. Furthermore, 2 observers may appear to have an excellent score for agreement, even though much of the concordance arises by chance because of an inadequate scope of the challenge group. Thus, in examining 200 healthy college students, 2 ophthalmologists may agree that 195 students have normal retinas, and that 2 have abnormal retinas. Because a disagreement of normal–abnormal occurs in only 3 of the 200 students, the 98.5% of agreement may make the ophthalmologists seem extraordinarily consistent in their diagnoses. Nevertheless, it can be shown that, in these circumstances, an agreement of 96.5% would have occurred by chance alone.

A desirable index of agreement will therefore measure actual concordance, rather than mere trend, in the 2 variables, and will make provision for agreement that might have occurred by chance. Indexes that perform these roles are Kappa (for dichotomous data), weighted Kappa (for ordinal data), and the intraclass correlation coefficient (for dimensional data). Their values range from $+1$, for perfect agreement; to -1, for total disagreement. A value of 0 indicates that agreement is no better than what might have occurred by chance.

INFERENTIAL STATISTICS

Mathematical theories of probability are used in two major forms of statistical inference: parametric estimations and stochastic contrasts. In **parametric estimation**, *the value of a parameter in a parent population is inferred from the result found in a sample of that population.* In a **stochastic contrast**, *the numerical results in two (or more) groups are compared for their "statistical significance," testing whether the observed differences are likely to have occurred by chance alone.* (Statisticians usually employ the term **hypothesis testing** for this type of contrast, but since a scientific **hypothesis** contains many more ideas than the numerical equivalence examined in statistical hypothesis testing, the term **stochastic contrast** provides a clearer label for the statistical activity.)

PARAMETRIC ESTIMATIONS

The simplest illustration of parametric estimation is a political poll. If a properly performed survey of 200 voters shows 106 favoring party A, 86 favoring party B, and 8 undecided, we estimate that the larger electorate will also be distributed in the ratio of 53% for A, 43% for B, and 4% undecided.

Since the polled sample is supposed to indicate what is happening in the parent population, we may want to know the reliability of the estimate. Can party A really count on 53% of the vote? The answer to this question requires recourse to the **theory of probability,** which allows the calculation of a confidence interval around the mean or the percentage value found in the sample.

For this purpose, we first calculate the **standard error** of the sample mean or proportion. For the mean of a randomly selected sample, the standard error is calculated as $s/\sqrt{n}$, with $s = \sqrt{S_{xx}/(n-1)}$ for this inferential usage. For a proportion, p, the standard error is calculated as $\sqrt{p(1-p)/n}$. Thus, for the proportion of 0.53 found in the poll of 200 people, the standard error is $\sqrt{(0.53)(0.47)/200} = 0.035$, or 3.5%. To determine the size of the **confidence interval,** the standard error is multiplied by a factor derived from considerations of probability. For a 95% confidence interval, this factor is 1.96 (which is commonly listed as 2). The result of the multiplication is then (essentially) added to and subtracted from the proportion or mean to form the confidence interval.

Thus, for the cited value of 53%, the confidence interval is $53\% \pm (1.96)(3.5\%) = 46.1\%$ to 59.9%. The actual meaning of a 95% confidence interval here is that if random samples of 200 people were repeatedly drawn from the parent population, 95% of the intervals calculated in this manner would include the value of the true populational mean. We can thus be 95% confident that the parametric mean is included in the interval between 46.1 and 59.9%. Consequently, since the true populational parameter may be below 50%, Party A cannot be fully assured of victory. On the other hand, if the proportion of 0.53 had been found in a poll of 1500 rather than 200 people, the standard error of the proportion would be 1.3% and the 95% confidence interval would run from 50.5% to 55.5%. With this result in the larger sample, Party A could feel more "confident" of victory.

For a confidence interval to be applied appropriately, the sample under study should have been obtained by a **randomization procedure.** In a simple random sampling, every member of the parent population has the same chance (or probability) of being selected for the sample. *The selection procedure cannot be performed in a casual (haphazardly "at random") manner and requires the specific use of a formal randomization mechanism, which is commonly obtained from tables of random numbers.*

Although randomization is usually employed to assign the therapeutic agents tested in clinical trials, the basic population studied in the trials is obtained from the patients conveniently available to the investigator. In fact, random samples have not been used for any of the existing studies of etiology or therapy that appear in contemporary medical literature, despite the extensive application of random sampling in political science and marketing surveys.

Consequently, two principal sources of error must be considered whenever a sampling procedure is used to estimate a populational parameter. The first source is sometimes called **sampling** or **stochastic error.** It arises, as a purely quantitative problem, from the fact that small samples can never be as reliable as large ones. *As sample size increases, sampling error is reduced.* This quantitative type of sampling error can be calculated, however, only if the sample is chosen randomly. The second type of error, sometimes called **non-sampling** or **selection error,** arises from the bias or distortion that can occur if the sample is not chosen randomly. Thus, whenever the person who selects a sample can make deliberate choices, rather than using a random mechanism for the choices, the opportunity exists for overt or subtle forms of bias to enter the selections. Since random samples are used so seldom in clinical medicine and epidemiology, the main errors to beware are those that arise from distortion during the selection process.

If the sampling mechanism allows distortion, increasing the size of the sample will simply increase the distortion, which may be difficult or impossible to remove. (If the source of the problem is suitably recognized and if adequate data are available, appropriate adjustments can be attempted.) The classical example of a distorted sampling occurred in the Literary Digest's presidential poll of 1936. The magazine assembled a sample of 2,000,000 people by random selection of names from telephone books throughout the USA. When the sampled people indicated an overwhelming preference for Landon rather than Roosevelt, the magazine (in view of the huge sample size) confidently predicted that Roosevelt would be defeated in a landslide. After the election produced a landslide that went in the opposite direction, the magazine went into an eclipse that led to its demise. The "post-mortem" examination revealed that the original sampling technic was erroneous. Although people's names were randomly selected from telephone directories, the directories were a poor place to begin. In 1936, a depression year, people who could afford to have telephones were particularly likely to be Republicans, voting for Landon.

STOCHASTIC CONTRASTS (Hypothesis Testing)

The principles applied to the results of a single group for estimating a parametric mean can be extended to allow a stochastic contrast of the results of 2 groups. The process involves the construction of a hypothetical sample, composed of the differences found in the means of 2 samples repeatedly drawn from their own hypothetical parent populations. Under the **null hypothesis,** these 2 parent populations are assumed to have equal means (and perhaps equal variances). With this assumption, the observed difference in the 2 means becomes regarded as a single sample randomly drawn from a parent population whose mean is zero and whose variance is estimated from the results noted (and perhaps "pooled") in the 2 observed samples. A test statistic, such as t or Z, is calculated as the ratio between the observed difference in means and the standard error of their difference, which is the square root of the estimated variance. With tables that show the sampling distribution of the test statistic, a P value can be associated with each calculated ratio of t or Z.

Because of the many mathematical ideas that are involved in this "hypothesis testing" procedure, the strategies of a stochastic contrast are seldom clearly understood by nonstatistical readers. The strategy can be explained more simply and understood more easily when the procedure is performed with a nonparametric **"random permutation"** test, which is described as follows: In a clinical trial of therapy, suppose the rate of successful results is found to be 33% with treatment A and 50% with treatment B. The increment of 17 percentage points (or the ratio of 1.52) in favor of treatment B would probably be regarded as quantitatively significant. Before concluding that treatment B was superior to A, however, we would want to examine the numerical sources of the 33% and 50% values. Our possible enthusiasm for treatment B would vanish if we discovered that treatment A was given to only 3 patients and treatment B to 2, so that the compared data were actually 1/3 vs. 1/2. With numbers this small, the distinction could easily arise simply by chance. On the other hand, if the compared numbers were much larger, such as 100/300 vs. 150/300, the success rates would still be 33% and 50%, but the results would be much more convincing.

The role of statistical **"tests of significance"** is to establish the numerical magnitudes that allow a substantively significant difference to be regarded as statistically (or stochastically) significant. The basic reasoning can be illustrated in reference to the 5 people in the preceding paragraph who were treated with agents A and B.

Suppose those people are distributed as follows:

PERSON	RESULT	TREATMENT
u	success	A
v	failure	A
w	failure	A
x	success	B
y	failure	B

Under the null hypothesis, we assume that treatments A and B are essentially identical. If so, the 5 observed people would have had exactly the same outcomes regardless of whether they received A or B. Let us now contemplate all possible ways in which those 5 people might have been allocated in a group of 3 to A and 2 to B. (In Table 231–1, below, the two successful people, u and x, are shown in **italics**). Of the 10 possible arrangements, the difference in percentage points for the outcomes of B and A would have been –67% on 3 occasions, 17% on 6 occasions, and 100% on 1 occasion. If any of these 10 possible arrangements were chosen at random, the probability would be 0.7 (= 0.6 + 0.1) of getting a difference of 17% or higher in favor of B. The probability of getting a difference of at least 17% in either direction—in favor of either B or A—would be 1, since each of the 10 arrangements produces such a difference.

Regardless of whether we consider the two-sided (or "two-tailed") arrangement or the one-sided arrangement, the observed difference of 17% could have happened quite readily in the 5 people under comparison even if treatments A and B are identical. The high likelihood of obtaining the observed difference by chance alone would make us conclude that the observed difference was not "statistically significant."

TABLE 231–1. POSSIBLE ARRANGEMENTS AND RESULTS

Assignment to A	Assignment to B	Results	Differences (B–A)
u, v, w	*x*, y	1/3 vs. 1/2	17%
u, v, *x*	w, y	2/3 vs. 0/2	–67%
u, v, y	w, *x*	1/3 vs. 1/2	17%
u, w, *x*	v, y	2/3 vs. 0/2	–67%
u, w, y	v, *x*	1/3 vs. 1/2	17%
u, *x*, y	v, w	2/3 vs. 0/2	–67%
v, w, *x*	*u*, y	1/3 vs. 1/2	17%
v, w, y	*u*, *x*	0/3 vs. 2/2	100%
v, *x*, y	*u*, w	1/3 vs. 1/2	17%
w, *x*, y	*u*, v	1/3 vs. 1/2	17%

Determination of a P Value

The reasoning in the procedure that has just been described is the basis for most statistical "tests of significance." The logic follows the same general pattern used to prove theorems in grade school geometry. We begin by making an assumption that is contrary to the thing we want to establish. If the consequences of the assumption lead to an obvious absurdity or impossibility, we reject the assumption. In the statistical use of this reasoning, the process is slightly modified. We reject the assumption, not if it leads to an impossibility (which would have a P value of 0), but to a sufficiently remote possibility. The strategy of the statistical procedure follows a distinctive sequence of steps:

1. We have observed a difference, d_o, in the results of 2 groups, A and B. Because the difference is *quantitatively* or *clinically* significant, we want to be sure that it did not occur merely as an event of random chance.

2. To explore this issue, we begin with an assumption, called the **null hypothesis,** that the causal or therapeutic agents given to groups A and B have essentially similar effects.

3. If these agents are similar, the people who received them would have had the same results, regardless of whether they happened to be in Group A or Group B.

4. With this assumption, we can contemplate all the ways in which the entire original group might have been divided into two groups, each having the same number of members as A and B.

5. For each of these possible arrangements of members in the two groups, we note the results that would have been found for each group, together with the associated difference.

6. We then tabulate the list of arrangements, results, and differences in a manner analogous to that of TABLE 231–1.

7. From this tabulation of the frequencies and relative frequencies for each of the possible differences, we can note the relative frequency of occurrence for a difference as large or larger than d_o. This relative frequency, called a P value, tells us the likelihood of such a difference if any one of the 2-group arrangements had occurred at random. (The procedure does not require the actual construction of a table like 231–1. Certain mathematical formulas can be used to obtain the P value more directly and rapidly.)

Associated with this determination of a P value are two acts of judgment. One of these is to draw a conclusion from the P value. The other judgment, which actually precedes all the cited activity, is to choose the mathematical model to be used for the calculations.

Interpretation of a P Value

At what level of chance are we willing to conclude that an impressive result was not likely to occur purely by chance? For example, the random chance of getting 5 consecutive heads in 5 tosses of a fair coin is $(1/2)^5$, which is $1/32$ or 0.03. If this event occurred, would it make us decide that the coin is unfair? The chance of getting a royal flush if someone randomly selects 5 cards from a fair deck of 52 cards is 0.0000015 (about 1.5 in a million). If this event should occur, would we conclude that the deck was improperly stacked?

Perhaps the best answer to these questions is that we might not want to draw a conclusion on the basis of a single occurrence of the extraordinary event. We would want to make additional observations of the presumably random phenomenon. If the extraordinary event happened repeatedly, we would then decide that something was amiss.

Unfortunately, however, the strategy of waiting for further observations cannot be used in the usual circumstances of statistical evaluation. In most medical studies, the investigator will not be able to repeat the proceedings. What is available is the observed collection of data and the P value that was determined for it in the statistical test procedure. This single P value, derived from the single collection of data from a single research project, is the available evidence. On the basis of this evidence, a decision must be made.

The generally accepted method of making the decision is to select a certain critical boundary value, which separates the **rejection zone** of "remote possibility" from the **concession zone** of nonremote possibility. The symbol α, which refers to the demarcated region, indicates the probability of the observed event's falling into the rejection zone. If the P value that emerges from the statistical test is at or below α, the observed event will be regarded as too uncommon to be ascribed to random chance. Accordingly, the null hypothesis (that agents A and B are similar) will be rejected; and the difference in groups A and B will be regarded as statistically (or stochastically) significant at the calculated level of P. If the P value exceeds α, the null hypothesis is conceded; and the observed event is not regarded as statistically significant.

The value usually chosen for α is 0.05 (or 1 in 20). Since 95% of the data of a Gaussian distribution are encompassed by an interval that extends 1.96 standard deviations on both sides of the mean, the 5% of data that are not included in this interval are regarded as the uncommon, unusual, or extraordinary members of the distribution. With this standard, P values of 0.05 or below are proclaimed to be "statistically significant."

The standards of these decisions are entirely arbitrary. For greater confidence, α may be decreased to levels of 0.025, 0.01, or 0.001, and in some circumstances, the decisive level of α may be set higher than .05. *The nomenclature that juxtaposes the words "statistically" and "significant" is also arbitrary.* The substantive significance of the observed statistics depends on the clinical importance of the events and on the quantitative magnitude of d_o, not on the calculation of P. Another noteworthy point is that rejection of the null hypothesis implies that the observed difference did not occur by random chance, but there still exists a P probability that chance alone was responsible.

Finally, the statistical decision refers only to the numerical role of random chance. *The decision provides no information about the nonrandom phenomena caused by distortions, bias, and other sources of error in the design of the research and collection of data.* For example, despite the statistical confidence produced by the large sample size of the Literary Digest 1936 presidential poll, the results were egregiously incorrect.

False-Positive and False-Negative Decisions

Tests of "statistical significance" are analogous to diagnostic marker tests, since the results may lead to false-positive and false-negative decisions. In the most common type of stochastic contrast, the observed difference is the positive result under scrutiny, and the α level indicates the risk of reaching a false-positive conclusion if the two treatments are not really different. When the P value exceeds α, however, the null hypothesis must be conceded, rather than accepted; and the investigator concludes that the observed difference is not statistically significant, rather than insignificant.

The reason for this distinction is that acceptance of the null hypothesis is associated with a risk of a false-negative decision; i.e., the situation in which the treatments are really different but the difference has not been substantiated. Since β is the probability of incorrectly accepting the null hypothesis, the false-negative conclusion is often called β **error** or **Type II error.** (The false-positive conclusion is called α **error** or **Type I error.**) If a value of Δ is selected as the size of the notable difference between treatments, two different probability values can be calculated for any stochastic contrast. The first is the customary P value for the likelihood of a false-positive decision if the two treatments are actually similar. The second is a P value for the likelihood of a false-negative decision if the two treatments actually differ by the amount, Δ. The second P value (or a selected level of β) is customarily subtracted from 1, and the result is called the *power* of the stochastic test. These two different strategies, together with selected levels of α, β, and Δ, are commonly used to calculate the necessary sample size for a clinical trial.

Mathematical Models

For the mathematical strategy illustrated here, the P value was determined directly from the relative frequencies noted among all possible arrangements (or permutations) of the observed data. These combinatorial arrangements can be formed and readily appraised with the aid of a computer, but the performance of the calculations was often a formidable event in the era before computers. For this and other reasons, alternative statistical procedures have been the preferred mathematical models for determining P values in an indirect manner more amenable to simple calculations. Although the alternative procedures have now become traditional in testing statistical significance, their current eminence may be altered as the increasing availability and decreased cost of computers allows a more direct determination of P values.

In most of the alternative mathematical models, the observed groups are regarded as random samples from a larger parent population. The sampling process yields characteristic, theoretical distributions, for whose shapes the names of Gauss, Poisson, and Bernouilli are often used as eponyms. With assumptions about the shapes of these theoretical distributions, the populational parameters are estimated from the means, standard deviations, or proportions found in the observed samples.

For stochastic contrasts, certain **test statistics,** such as t- or **chi-square,** are calculated from the observed data. Under the null hypothesis, each test statistic has its own characteristic distribution, so that a P value can be mathematically associated with the calculated value of the test statistic.

For the chi-square procedure, the test statistic is calculated by first noting the difference between each observed value and the corresponding value that would be expected under the null hypothesis. This difference is squared and divided by the expected value. The sum of each of these results is X^2, a test statistic that is interpreted as having the sampling characteristics of a chi-square (χ^2) distribution. For the appropriate "degrees of freedom," a P value can be associated with each value of X^2.

For example, suppose the 33 and 50% success rates with treatments A and B arose from the corresponding numerical proportions 25/76 and 39/78. The tabulation would have the form

	SUCCESS	FAILURE	TOTAL
TREATMENT A	25	51	76
TREATMENT B	39	39	78
TOTAL	64	90	154

Under the null hypothesis, the expected success rate would be $64/154 = .416$ and the failure rate would be $90/154 = .584$ for each treatment. The expected numbers in the interior of the table would then be

	SUCCESS	FAILURE	TOTAL
TREATMENT A	31.6	44.4	76
TREATMENT B	32.4	45.6	78
TOTAL	64	90	154

The value of X^2 would be calculated as $(25 - 31.6)^2/31.6 + (51 - 44.4)^2/44.4 + (39 - 32.4)^2/32.4 + (39 - 45.6)^2/45.6 = 4.66$.

In this type of "fourfold" or "2×2" table, there is one "degree of freedom." At one degree of freedom, the P value is $< .05$ whenever X^2 exceeds 3.84. The observed difference is therefore statistically significant.

The calculation of X^2 can be substantially simplified by the use of computational formulas. For a fourfold table containing the elements a, b, c, d, and a grand total N, the $X^2 = (ad - bc)^2 N/[(a+b)(c+d)(a+c)(b+d)]$. Thus in the foregoing table, $X^2 = [(25 \times 39) - (51 \times 39)]^2 \times 154/[(76)(78)(64)(90)] = 4.64$. The minor difference in the 2 methods of computing X^2 is due to the "rounding" performed in calculating the expected values.

The interpretation of P values does not depend on the mathematical models used for the test. The most direct type of model is the permutation (or randomization) procedure described earlier, which uses all possible arrangements of the observed data, without resort to theoretical distributions and parameters. Procedures that depend on distributions and parameters, such as the t and chi-square tests, have been traditionally popular because they are easy to calculate and also because, especially when sample sizes are large, their results are essentially similar to those noted with the permutation tests. The growing popularity of nonparametric tests probably arises because they require no assumptions about the parameters or distributional shape of a parent population. Nonparametric tests can be performed directly with the observed values of the data, or more often, with permutations of the ranks (rather than actual values) of the observed numbers.

Types of Tests

The choice of a stochastic test depends on many features, including the type of data, number of groups, and relationship under study. *In a contrast of results for two groups*, the usual procedures are the t test for dimensional data and the chi-square test for existential or nominal data. (The chi-square procedure is replaced by a permutation test—the Fisher exact probability test—when the numbers are small.) A nonparametric test, such as the Mann-Whitney U test, is used for the ranks of ordinal data.

When the two groups have been "matched," so that a single set of differences can be contemplated, the corresponding respective procedures are the paired t-test, the McNemar chi-square test, and the Wilcoxon signed–ranks test. When more than two groups are being contrasted simultaneously, the chi-square test is still applicable for existential or nominal data, but the F test of the analysis of variance is used for dimensional data. For ordinal data, several nonparametric procedures can be used, including the Kruskal-Wallis and Friedman tests.

For an index of association, such as a regression or correlation coefficient, the populational parameter for the index is assumed to have a value of 0 under the null hypothesis. The observed value of the index is then contrasted against 0, using a t test or some other suitable procedure.

Conclusion

The activities of biostatistics can be divided into at least 3 different types of reasoning. One type involves the evaluation of quantitative importance for the observed magnitudes of the indexes used to describe summaries, contrasts, and associations of collected data. The second type involves the use of probabilities and inferences to estimate parameters and to perform "tests of significance" (or stochastic contrasts) for comparisons of data. The third type involves an appraisal of the scientific design, structure, and quality of data in the research. Although the second activity requires many intensively mathematical procedures, relatively little mathematics is needed for evaluating quantitative magnitudes, and no mathematics is needed for the fundamental scientific appraisals. Even when puzzled or confused by the inferential statistics, a clinical reader who concentrates on the indexes and architecture of the research can often arrive at effective evaluations of its scientific merit.

232. GERIATRIC MEDICINE

Gerontologic investigation includes distinguishing normal aging from disease effects. Most age-related biologic changes appear to show physiologic functioning at a peak before age 30 with subsequent gradual linear decline. Some changes have no practical implications for daily activity but can become critical in periods of great stress. Thus, disease rather than normal aging appears to be the prime decompensating factor in old age. Declines with age include renal blood flow and creatinine clearance, cardiac output, glucose tolerance, vital capacity of the lung, lean body mass, and cellular immunity. But liver function and total lung capacity remain the same across the age spectrum, and secretion of ADH in response to osmolar stimuli actually increases with age. Studies on aging are hampered by the fact that, as people age, healthy subjects are harder to find. Cross-sectional studies, which compare individuals of different ages, are relatively easy to do, but may be less useful than longitudinal studies in which long-term monitoring compares the same persons to their younger selves. Such studies are difficult because of the long duration and subject drop-out.

Geriatrics is an interdisciplinary approach to manage sickness and disability in the aged population, particularly dealing with those degenerative and immunosenescent diseases that are more prevalent with age. Caring for an elderly person with multiple interacting diseases—and often difficult socioeconomic circumstances—demands the highest expression of the diagnostic, analytic, and synthetic and interpersonal skills of the physician. The last is of major significance, for often it is the physician's familiarity with patient behavior, history, satisfaction, fears, and aspirations that underlies early recognition of disease and the preparation and acceptance of suitable interventions. These often involve lifestyle adjustments. The value of knowing the patient through a thorough life history and mental performance test cannot be emphasized enough. Studies indicate that first signs of physical illness, often reversible, are mental or emotional, tending to confirm the stereotype of "senility" and thereby deterring proper diagnosis and treatment if casually accepted.

DEMOGRAPHY AND HEALTH CARE DELIVERY

Maximum human life span (about 100 yr, but with an estimated potential of reaching 110 to 120 yr) has not changed, but many more people are surviving to the oldest ages. The old-old population is chiefly female, because women outlive men. Although they are an increasingly healthy and active group, many problems emerge, especially after age 75. Burdens of multiple diseases are complicated by social disadvantage, emotional vulnerability, and poverty (as individuals outlive their resources and supportive age peers). One hundred years ago, 2% of Americans were over age 65. At the turn of the century, 4% were over age 65. Currently, $> 11\%$ of our citizens (25 million) are over age 65, and there is a net daily gain of > 1000 people into the ranks of elders. A full picture suggests that more recent cohorts of elderly persons are reaching age 65 in better health than their predecessors. Old age in its conventional but erroneous image as severe debilitation after age 65 may actually apply far more aptly to the post-75 population.

Today a 65-yr-old man has a 13-yr life expectancy; if he lives to 75, he has 9 more years ahead of him. A 65-yr-old woman will live 18 yr on the average, and at age 75 she can expect to live 12 more years. It is estimated that in 2030, when the peak of the post-World War II baby boom will reach age 65, there will be 50 million Americans (1:5) over age 65. The "over 85s" are expected to experience the highest percentage increase of all. Women live about 8 yr longer than men, probably the result of genetic, biologic, and environmental factors. Survival differences are likely to narrow as women begin to suffer the effects of accelerated smoking habits and mobility into traditionally male job markets; morbidity figures already show the effects of cumulative heavy smoking.

Caring for increasing numbers of old and infirm citizens makes extraordinary demands on traditional systems of health care delivery; the strains increase disproportionately, since the elderly, having more illness and complicating psychosocial sequelae, use more medical and socially supportive services. Though $< 11\%$ of our population, they occupy $> 33\%$ of our acute hospital beds, buy 25% of all prescription drugs, and spend 30% of our 160 billion dollar health budget ($> 50\%$ of the 40 billion dollar federal health budget). Nursing home care cost 18 billion dollars in 1978 and rose 25% the following year with few beds added. As early as 1972, annual nursing home costs began to exceed acute hospital costs. Of the 1.2 million nursing home beds in America, 1 million are occupied by people over age 65, but $< 5\%$ of Americans over age 65 live in nursing homes or other institutions.

Other ways of looking at the same data give a different perspective. Among the "over 65s," 20% will spend time in a nursing home before death, and of those surviving beyond 80, nearly 50% will die in a nursing home. Nursing home beds in America outnumber acute hospital beds, but twice as many immobilized elderly live in the community as in nursing homes, and 25% of the community-dwelling elderly have no living relatives. A segment of our "over 65" population can be identified as being institutionalized or at high risk for future institutionalization (especially in the absence of community services). These approximately 6 million older Americans consume a disproportionate share of health resources. Special attention to their needs and their function within our health care system could add quality and years to their lives while restraining cost increases.

Several instructive studies, done in the early 1950s in Scotland, examined the response of older people to illness; they illustrate *qualitatively* different demands on traditional health care delivery systems. Each patient had a doctor responsible for continuing outpatient care, the doctor's office was conveniently located, and care was free to the patient. Although this system appeared adequate, startling numbers of people were identified with multiple medical problems that were *unknown to the responsible physician*. The problems unearthed by screening with history, physical examination, laboratory tests, and a questionnaire given in the home were not esoteric. Common treatable conditions, such as B_{12} or iron deficiency anemia, congestive heart failure, GI bleeding, uncontrolled diabetes mellitus, active TB, foot disease interfering with mobility, oral disorders interfering with eating, correctable hearing and vision defects, and a high incidence of depression often go undiagnosed in the elderly for several reasons.

(1) Elderly patients tend to conceal legitimate complaints pointing to serious treatable diseases. Elderly people, with others in their society, believe that old age is a time of sickness and disability, and not feeling well is a natural part of aging. The prevalence of depression, combined with the cumulative losses of old age and the discomfort of illness, reduces interest in regaining health. Impaired cognition impedes the patient's complaining and reduces the physician's diagnostic

searching. Today's old people grew up when hospitals were places for dying, discouraging them from seeking care now.

(2) **The phenomenon of multiple disorders** in the elderly means that numerous problems are likely to complicate and interfere with diagnosing and treating the presenting illness. An average of 6 diseases was found in each of several thousand people studied, and the primary physician was unaware of ½ of the disorders. Disease in one organ system puts stresses on another weakened system which begins an irreversible concatenation of deteriorations, passing multiple points of no return, leading to infirmity, dependence, and, if uninterrupted, death. Active case-finding surveillance mechanisms for the aging must be added to our current passive health care system. Alert intervention at an early stage may prevent compounding and improve the quality of life through relatively minor maneuvers.

(3) **Disorders often present atypically** (see below for further discussion).

(4) **"Predeath,"** *a period of dependency due to immobility, incontinence, or impaired cognition* (frequently in combination) that precedes nearly ¾ of deaths in old age is another illness phenomenon common in the elderly. This period, usually spent in the hospital and in nursing homes, is strongly age-related and approaches 3 mo in the group > 85 yr old. The cost, in human suffering and in money, is substantial. Immobility, incontinence, and cognitive impairment are clarions of serious underlying disease that demand prompt evaluation and specific treatment to avoid prolonged dependency.

BASIC PRINCIPLES IN CARING FOR THE ELDERLY

Predictable hazards for aged hospitalized patients include (1) nighttime confusion or "sundowning," (2) falls, (3) fractures with no identifiable trauma, (4) sudden appearance of decubiti, (5) fecal impaction and urinary retention, (6) falling victim to diagnostic and therapeutic endeavors, (7) prolonged convalescence, and (8) loss of the home while the patient is hospitalized. There is special need to identify multiple concomitant pathologic processes. Treating one disorder without considering simultaneous associated ones may accelerate decline rather than result in improvement. Common conditions coexist in the elderly (e.g., congestive heart failure, chronic renal failure, angina pectoris, osteoporosis, osteoarthritis, frail gait, chronic constipation, urinary precipitancy, venous and arterial insufficiency in the legs, diabetes mellitus, chronic pain, sleep disturbance, depression, cognitive impairment, and multiple drug regimens with poor compliance). When an average of 6 or more problems coincide in one elderly patient, bed rest, surgery, drugs, and other treatments may be disastrous if not scrupulously monitored and well integrated.

Disorders in old age can be divided into 2 broad groups—those seen commonly *only* in the elderly and those which, though occurring also in other age groups, present *unusual features* or present *without usual features* in the elderly.

DISORDERS COMMON ONLY IN THE ELDERLY

Diseases usually restricted to the elderly are diabetic hyperosmolar nonketotic coma; stroke; polymyalgia rheumatica—giant cell arteritis; metabolic bone disease, including osteoporosis and osteoarthritis; hip fracture and its rehabilitation; causes of the dementia syndrome; causes of falls; prostatic carcinoma; gammopathies, including multiple myeloma, chronic lymphatic leukemia, angioimmunoblastic lymphadenopathy with dysproteinemia (lymphoma); TB (especially miliary); herpes zoster; basal cell carcinoma; and parkinsonism. Separate discussions elsewhere in this volume are listed in the index.

NORMAL PRESSURE HYDROCEPHALUS (NPH)

Cerebral ventricular dilation with normal lumbar CSF pressure, presenting with a characteristic clinical syndrome of dementia, dyspraxia of gait, and urinary incontinence. Etiology may be attributed to recent surface inflammation of the brain, usually from subarachnoid hemorrhage or diffuse meningitis, presumed to result in scarring of the arachnoid villi over the brain convexities where CSF absorption usually occurs. Supporting data are meager, however, and many elderly NPH patients have no history of predisposing disease.

Clinical Manifestations

The syndrome consists of dementia, incontinence, and a distinctive dyspraxia of gait (resembling ignorance of walking coordination), associated with ventricular dilation and normal CSF pressure. There is neither motor weakness nor staggering, but rather what has been described as the "slipping clutch" phenomenon. NPH has also been described in association with various psychiatric manifestations that are not distinctive, and it should be considered in the differential diagnosis of any new psychiatric illness in old age.

Treatment

Shunting CSF from the dilated ventricles sometimes results in clinical improvement. No radiographic or pressure measurements in patients with the syndrome predict the clinical outcome of shunting, but the longer the disease has been present, the less likely shunting will be curative.

ACCIDENTAL HYPOTHERMIA (AH; Hypothermia)

Unexpected fall of body temperature to < 35 C (95 F). The sudden appearance of low body temperature in the elderly as a common winter event was noted 20 yr ago. The afflicted are at high risk for a potentially fatal clinical syndrome mimicking stroke or metabolic derangement. No American studies have been done, but British investigations speculate that between 100 and 20,000 elderly people die each year in Great Britain from AH. The wide range of estimates can be explained by the lack of definitive pathologic evidence of hypothermia death. Stated simply, most dead people are cold; therefore, death cannot confidently be attributed to AH postmortem. Temperatures of elderly patients entering hospitals in Britain during winter months were accurately recorded using a low-reading thermometer, disclosing that > 3.5% of patients over age 65 had body temperatures below 35 C. Lack of central heating or indoor plumbing was not a risk factor for these patients. If these data can be extrapolated, nearly 50,000 elderly Americans may be entering hospitals each winter with occult hypothermia.

Etiology and Pathogenesis

Elderly people with borderline low temperatures have age-related autonomic defects producing low peripheral resting blood flow, a nonconstrictor vasomotor response to cold, and easily provoked orthostatic hypotension. These defects are unmasked by phenothiazines, especially chlorpromazine, and correlate with hypothermia risk.

The provocative cold stress is not prolonged exposure to severe cold conditions; rather, these aged patients may become hypothermic while in their mildly cool homes (as warm as 18.3 C [65 F]), though most episodes are initiated by temperatures < 18.3 C. Besides inadequate environmental heating in the winter, contributory factors include diminished perception of cold and poor heat conservation mechanisms. AH takes many hours to several days to develop. Body temperature, once falling below 35 C, continues to fall slowly and insidiously, terminating in death if the environment is unaltered. The mortality rate is about 50% and increases in the presence of complicating disease.

Phenothiazine treatment, congestive heart failure, hypothyroidism, hypopituitarism, uremia, Addison's disease, starvation, ketoacidosis, pulmonary infection, sepsis, brain injury, any sort of immobilizing illness predispose to hypothermia.

Symptoms and Signs

As body temperature drops, the patient proceeds from fatigue, weakness, incoordination, apathy, and drowsiness to an acute confusional state that, when body temperature falls below 32.2 C (90 F), progresses to stupor and coma. Hallucinations, combativeness, and resistance to aid may be seen. While hands and feet of many people are cold to the touch in winter, these patients have cold abdomens as well. Shivering and pallor are strikingly absent, respirations are shallow and infrequent, slow pulse and low BP with a host of atrial and ventricular arrhythmias are common, and the face may be puffy and pink. The ECG may show a characteristic J wave early—a small positive deflection following the QRS complex in the left ventricular leads—which is found in no other condition. Unfortunately, it appears in slightly < 50% of hypothermic patients. More commonly, the ECG shows baseline oscillation produced by a fine rapid muscle tremor that is often mistaken for electrical interference or voluntary motion. This fine trembling is usually not apparent grossly but probably is the elderly hypothermic patient's physiologic equivalent of shivering. Neurologic signs of tremor, ataxia, pathologic and depressed reflexes, coma, seizures, and a marked increase in muscle tone resembling acute parkinsonism may all occur. If temperature fall is uninterrupted, death usually occurs between 23.9 C (75 F) and 29.4 C (85 F) from cardiac standstill or ventricular fibrillation.

General metabolic effects of hypoxia and tissue necrosis are the rule, though if the patient survives, low temperature may delay the onset of many complications. The commonest complications are pancreatitis, pulmonary edema, pneumonia, metabolic acidosis, renal failure, and gangrene of the extremities.

Diagnosis

Knowledge of the disorder and a low-reading thermometer are required. The standard clinical thermometer reads from 34.4 C (94 F) to 42.2 C (108 F) and is rarely shaken down below 35.6 C (96 F). A low-reading thermometer, registering 28.9 C (84 F) to 42.2 C (108 F), is available from standard hospital supply companies. Reorientation of health personnel to body temperature is needed, since the usual custom is to verify only normal or elevated temperatures; elderly patients at risk for AH must be evaluated considering low body temperature.

Treatment

Slow spontaneous rewarming, which allows body temperature to return to normal gradually (not faster than 0.6 C [1 F]/h) by conserving heat still being produced by the hypothermic patient, is recommended. *More rapid rewarming has often resulted in irreversible hypotension.* Heat conservation is achieved with blankets or more sophisticated insulating materials in a warm room. Careful monitoring and anticipation of common complications are essential to successful treatment.

URINARY INCONTINENCE

The involuntary loss of urine while awake or asleep. It is a malodorous social stigma, commonly concealed by its embarrassed victim with a mountain of absorbent pads. The prevalence ranges from 5 to 15% of people over age 65 at home, as high as 50% of elderly in the hospital, and is even higher in chronic institutional beds. As much as 25% of nursing time in geriatric hospitals is consumed dealing with incontinence. Incontinent patients require a 200% increase in alloted nursing time to deal with bedpans and urinals, and nearly 600% more time to be bathed satisfactorily, compared with the nursing required by continent peers.

The causes of urinary incontinence may be temporary or fixed. Specific types and their management are discussed in Ch. 157.

DISORDERS WITH UNUSUAL PRESENTATIONS IN THE ELDERLY

The characteristic complex of symptoms or signs of any disorder frequently is absent in old age; the expected findings are often replaced with one or more nonspecific problems, such as refusal to eat or drink, falling, incontinence, dizziness, acute confusion, worsening dementia, weight loss, and failure to thrive. Depression is probably the most common disease in the "over 65" population. Organic psychoses, other affective disorders, paranoid states, hypochondriasis, and suicide become more common with age; all may present atypically.

Diseases that are especially likely to be diagnostic enigmas in the elderly are drug intoxication, alcoholism, myxedema, myocardial infarction, pulmonary embolism, pneumonia, malignant disease (especially colon, lung, and breast), surgical abdomen, and thyrotoxicosis. Thyrotoxicosis is discussed illustratively below.

OCCULT THYROTOXICOSIS

Apathetic and masked thyrotoxicosis are 2 variant syndromes of hyperthyroidism lacking the readily recognizable constellation of typical symptoms and signs (see Ch. 86). Although > 50% of thyrotoxic patients are 40 to 60 yr of age, 15% are over age 65. Occult hyperthyroidism is found in 1 to 2% of newly hospitalized patients over age 65 in Great Britain. These elderly thyrotoxics show no goiter 40% of the time and no eye signs or tachycardia in > 50%. The constellation of diffuse goiter, eye signs, and thyroid bruit occurs in only 20% of older thyrotoxic patients. One explanation of the paucity of classic findings in the elderly is that their diminished physiologic reserve is depleted quickly by hypermetabolic stress. T_3 toxicosis is uncommon in the elderly.

Symptoms and Signs

Masked hyperthyroidism is the more common of the 2 syndromes. The usual features of multisystem involvement in thyrotoxicosis are absent, and symptoms and signs referrable to a single organ system, most often the heart, dominate the clinical picture. Congestive heart failure poorly responsive to digitalis, atrial fibrillation with slow ventricular response, other fixed or paroxysmal arrhythmias, cardiomegaly, and palpitations are common. GI involvement can include constipation, weight loss with anorexia, and hepatomegaly. Psychiatric manifestations include confusion, psychomotor retardation, chronic depression, and apparent "senile" dementia. Increased bone calcium turnover is reflected in elevated serum calcium, bone pain, osteoporosis, and frequent fracture.

Apathetic hyperthyroidism, the less common occult presentation of thyrotoxicosis in the elderly, occurs in 10 to 15% of aged thyrotoxics. Apathy and inactivity replace the usual hyperkinesis and dominate the clinical picture even though there may be associated cardiac or other organ system findings. These patients look extremely old and wizened, but with treatment rapidly lose wrinkling and become more youthful-looking. They have been described as having a "characteristic senile appearance" of mild chronic illness, but when afflicted with an acute illness or stress, they "quietly and peacefully sink into coma and die an absolutely relaxed death without activation."

Laboratory values are generally the same for older and younger adults, but T_3 levels decline 10 to 20% in euthyroid elderly (see Ch. 86). **Treatment** is usually effective with radioactive iodine, but up to 50% of the patients need temporary prior and subsequent pharmacologic thyroid suppression.

PHARMACOTHERAPEUTICS

Elderly patients, in or out of the hospital, are at twice the risk for an adverse drug reaction compared with younger patients. These adverse reactions are likely to be more serious and extend hospitalization longer than for a younger patient. Old people at home take nearly 3 times as many drugs as the general population and women take twice as many as men. (The average older person fills 13 prescriptions annually and spends 20% of personal funds on drugs.) When the prevalence of intellectual and visual impairment in the elderly is juxtaposed to the similar size, shape, and color of many medicines, errors in administration seem likely. More than 50% of elderly patients do not take their drugs as prescribed and about 25% make errors likely to result in drug-induced illness.

Elderly patients are more susceptible to side effects and toxic effects of most drugs, and they often bear the brunt of reflexive prescribing for uninvestigated symptoms. Multiple phenomena make old people more vulnerable to adverse drug reactions. Although body composition and drug distribution, metabolism, excretion, and response have special features in the elderly, most clinical trials and pharmacologic studies are performed in young people. Drug treatment standards developed in the young and applied to the old are predictably hazardous.

Physiologic data demand that extreme care be used in selecting drugs and doses used to treat old people. When a drug is indicated for the treatment of a specific disease, it should not be withheld because of a patient's age, but extra thoughtfulness is required in prescribing for and supervising the elderly.

Drug absorption can be influenced by numerous changes in the aging GI tract. Decline of gastric acid secretion, decreased mesenteric blood flow, shrinkage of total surface area of the gut, and decline of active transport mechanisms tend to decrease absorption and result in a lower serum level of an orally administered drug. Decreasing motility, largely due to higher pH of gastric contents, makes absorption more complete and thus elevates serum levels. The net effect of these factors is small, so that blood levels for most drugs in the elderly are not predictably influenced by differences in absorption. The predictable decline in cardiac index of 0.8%/yr from age 20 to 90 slows drug transport to and from sites of action.

Body composition changes occurring with age collaborate to make blood levels of drugs higher after standard doses. Weight declines, but body fat doubles in men and increases by 50% in women. Lean body mass relative to total weight and total body water both decline, resulting in more drug/wt of metabolically active tissue, and generally a smaller volume of distribution with standard doses of drug. Serum albumin falls, so that the many drugs which bind substantially to protein circulate less bound and are more active. These changes in body composition add up to make toxic accumulation of drugs more likely in the elderly.

Metabolism, largely by liver enzymes, accounts for inactivation of many drugs. The scanty available data suggest a decline in the vigor of some hepatic enzyme systems, but currently there are insufficient data to make any general statements about drug inactivation with age. Smoking and alcohol consumption have more influence on hepatic metabolism of drugs than does aging.

Changes in kidney function are major factors responsible for elevated blood levels of drugs in the elderly. Renal blood flow falls about 1%/yr between ages 30 and 80, resulting in a 50% decrease in the elderly. Diminished renal blood flow is reflected by a similar 40 to 50% fall in GFR, urea, and creatinine clearance. However, serum creatinine, the commonly used measure of renal function, rises little or not at all, largely because of decreased muscle mass and creatinine production in the elderly. Similarly, BUN rises far less than expected because of diminished protein intake in old age. Therefore, creatinine clearance is the only reliable indicator of drug-clearing capacity of the aging kidney. It is generally predictable by an age-creatinine clearance nomogram.

Neuronal dropout in the aging brain reduces reserve capacity and makes cognitive decline a particularly high-risk early event when elderly patients accumulate high blood levels of many drugs. Tissue sensitivity to some drugs increases, producing greater effects using standard doses.

233.   OFFICE CLINICAL RECORDS

The primary purpose of the office medical record is to document appropriate patient care, whether related to a single illness or to long-term care. The record aids the physician's recall, enhances communications among physicians and others involved in the patient's care, and provides documentation for research and legal protection.

COMMON PROBLEMS IN RECORD KEEPING

Lack of organization: Information that is filed haphazardly impedes retrieval and follow-up care. Pages should be organized according to content, numbered sequentially, and labeled with the patient's name and/or chart number.

Omission of vital information: When findings are written in the physician's shorthand or omitted, reconstruction of what the patient said or what the physician observed may be impossible at a later date. Inability to document good care may leave a physician vulnerable to suit.

Lack of adequate problem identification: A probable diagnosis or "clinical impression" without supporting data is often stated immediately as the basis for further workup and treatment. This may lead to inappropriate tests or therapy based upon an unsubstantiated hypothesis. The scientific approach states the problem at the current level of resolution, whether this be a symptom, a physical finding, a laboratory abnormality, or a diagnosis. The diagnostic plan can then spell out data to be gathered as the next step in reaching the diagnosis.

Inability to recall vital data: Particularly in group practices, but even in busy solo practices, a physician may diagnose or treat a patient's presenting complaint without regard for other problems unless they are easily identifiable in the record. For example, the question "When was your last period?" is embarrassing if the patient has had a hysterectomy. The failing can be more serious, as when an adverse drug reaction occurs that could have been anticipated. Summary lists of problems, including past surgery and medications, can reduce such pitfalls.

Poor communications: Many records can be read or interpreted only by the physician who wrote them. This hampers patient care by colleagues, by consultants, or by the office staff. It also complicates transfer of information to insurance companies or other agencies when the patient seeks reimbursement or services. Commonly, problems include illegible handwriting, lack of structure in the record, lack of documentation for diagnosis or therapy, or simply "too many pieces of paper" in the chart. For clear communications, the essentials of a record include an adequate data base, a problem list, a medication list, and dictated or clearly written progress notes that document the findings, assessment, and plans for each patient visit. Each note should be signed or initialed by the physician or allied health person making the entry.

Fragmented, ineffective patient care: A medical record in itself cannot ensure good patient care, but lack of a well-organized medical record can deprive the patient of care that carries over from one visit to another. The mobility of people and the degree of specialization in medicine require that every record be an organized repository of information that does not rely upon the memory of an individual physician.

TYPES OF RECORD SYSTEMS

The source-oriented record: Physicians have traditionally arranged records by the source of the information; i.e., x-ray reports, lab reports, consultants' reports, and physicians' progress notes. Within each section, information is arranged in chronologic order, with the most recent entry usually on the face sheet. A source-oriented record includes the results of one or more complete history and physical examinations, hospital discharge summaries, flow sheets and the like, each of which must be reviewed for a complete picture of any particular disorder. Each progress note usually contains a record of the history and physical findings on the visit of that date, often a diagnosis or clinical impression, and further diagnostic tests to be ordered and drug or diet prescribed. Sometimes laboratory, x-ray, or ECG findings are included in the progress note as well as in the appropriate source section.

The chief advantages of the source-oriented record are that it is commonly used and understood and is relatively easy to maintain. However, support is frequently lacking for action taken. Those unfamiliar with the patient find that substantial time is needed to review the patient's problems or to trace the history of a particular problem.

The problem-oriented medical record (POMR): As its name implies, this format differs from the source-oriented record by being arranged according to each of the patient's problems. Creation of a POMR starts with the development of a comprehensive data base drawn from a complete history and physical examination, supplemented by diagnostic tests appropriate to the patient's age, sex, and condition. From this data base, an initial problem list is drawn up, with each physical, emotional, or environmental problem titled, numbered, and dated (see Fig. 233–1). Each problem should be listed at the level of definition justified by the information at hand and by the physician's level of understanding. Problems may be a symptom, a physiologic abnormality, an unusual laboratory finding, a demographic problem ("lives alone"), or an emotional problem. In some cases, separate lists are maintained of acute and chronic problems. As a symptom is resolved into a diagnosis, or as an acute problem becomes chronic, this resolution is noted through a correction to the problem list. Next, an initial management plan evolves for each problem, either diagnostic (which may include lab tests, x-

Name *Heckler, Ruth*			ALLERGIES/SENSITIVITIES				
Number *3241*		Blood Type: **A**	*Codeine, Sulfa*				
Prob. No.	Date	PROBLEM DESCRIPTION	Date Resolved	Index	Prob. No.	Date	PROBLEM DESCRIPTION
1	*10/76*	*Hypertension - essential*		✓			
2	*10/76*	*Diabetes mellitus (mild) FEM*		✓			
~~*3*~~	~~*1/79*~~	~~*Early retinopathy — FEM—*~~	*See below*				
4	*4/79*	*Atherosclerosis, with*					
		cerebrovascular insuffic. FEM					
5	*4/81*	*Hearing loss, bilateral FEM*					
6	*1/81*	*BP medicine noncompliance*	*2/83*				
3	*1/81*	*Bilateral Grade II*					
		retinopathy FEM					

FIG. 233–1. **Example from a problem-oriented medical record.** From medical record formats, © Miller Communications, Inc. Reproduced by permission.

ray, or consultation) or therapeutic (which may include drugs, diet, or patient education). A "resolved" problem, such as an uncomplicated appendectomy, requires no management plan. The ongoing record is maintained in progress notes organized according to the "**SOAP**" structure: date, number and title of the problem, followed by **S**ubjective findings (chief complaint and present history); **O**bjective findings (physical and lab data); **A**ssessment, the documented resolution of the findings; and **P**lan for further diagnostic or therapeutic action, including when the patient is to return (see FIG. 233–2). If a patient presents with more than one problem, separate SOAP notes are entered for each problem reviewed. All laboratory, x-ray, ECG, consultants' reports, and other pieces of information are integrated into the progress note, so as to document fully the diagnosis and therapy. The source data from the laboratory, radiologist, or consultant are usually filed separately for reference. A summary list of medications and diets, keyed to the problems, is included adjacent to the problem list.

There are many **advantages** of the POMR: it helps to define the patient's problems; it formulates logical and orderly plans of care; it evaluates specific problems in the context of all problems; and it summarizes care according to the problem list, so that another physician or paraprofessional can monitor the patient's progress toward the resolution of the problems. The **disadvantages** include time-consuming rearrangement of data according to problems, difficult separation of interrelated problems; and highly structured format, which makes POMR more suited for teaching residents than for delivery of patient care in a busy office practice.

The modified problem/source record: In this combined approach, the data base may be obtained either at one time from the comprehensive history and physical examination or in the course of several visits, each time recording data on a standardized history and physical examination form. After completion of each segment of the data base, new problems can be identified and recorded. Only chronic problems need be titled and numbered, except for any acute problem likely to become chronic (e.g., otitis media in children, urinary tract infection in women). Each progress note should indicate the number and title of each problem being evaluated, but data may be entered under one set of SOAP headings rather than under separate sets for each problem. In most cases, brief notations of findings clearly substantiate the assessment, even if 2 or more problems are active. Similarly, the relationship between most diagnostic or treatment plans and the appropriate problem are obvious. Where necessary, data may be keyed to the appropriate problem; e.g., "Prob. 3, consultation arranged" (see FIG. 233–3). The data base flow sheets, lab, x-ray, and consultant reports are organized behind the progress notes and may be cross-referenced without repeating the full findings in the progress note; a one-line reference keyed to the problem should always be made for each such finding. If the patient has multiple chronic diseases, a flow sheet should be maintained on top of the progress notes as an aid to guide the review of interrelated data.

PROGRESS NOTES

Patient Name _BerKow, Robert_ _____ Number _1379_____ Page _3___

Date/Problems (No. and Description)	FINDINGS (Subjective and Objective)	PLANS
5/12/85	S: Follow-up asthma. Symptoms diminishing.	
	O: Ears, nose, and throat clear	
# 1	chest clear	CONT: Ephedrine sulfate, theophyllin
Asthma	A: Resolving Asthma	hydroxyzine HCl 4ml q 4 to 6 h
# 2	S: Using flurandrenolide on skin	
Eczema	O: Still scaling, but improved	RETURN ~ 2 wk
	A: Resolving eczema	
# 3	O: Testes not palpable	Refer to pediatric surgeon, Dr. K.
Undescended Testes	A: Undescended Testes	Humber (see letter)
		F.E. Manson

FIG. 233–2. **Example of notes organized according to "SOAP" structure.** From medical record formats, © Miller Communications, Inc. Reproduced by permission.

PROGRESS NOTES

Patient Name _Ferguson, Doris_ _____ Number __3042__ Page __8__

Date/Problems (No. and Description)	FINDINGS (Subjective and Objective)	PLANS
1/19/83	S: Here for 3mo BP check; chief	1. Restart hydrochlorothiazide
#1. Hypertension	complaint of blurred vision - this is	50 mg b.i.d.
	bilateral and without a pattern	Counseling regarding care of
	as to time.	hypertension given as well as
#3. Retinopathy	Denies chest pain, shortness of	#18 Patient Aid on subject;
	breath or related symptoms.	main points personally stressed.
#6. Compliance	Not taking hydrochlorothiazide for	2. Schedule fasting blood sugar
	past 2mo. "Tired of taking medication	and 2h postprandial blood sugar.
	and felt good!"	Also patient to recheck urine
	O: BP $\frac{190}{105}$ Right and left arms. Wt 109	q.i.d. x 2 wk.
	Fundoscopic now reveals bilateral	3. Consultation arranged with
	Grade II retinopathy-? diabetic component!	Dr. Aniter for
	Rest of physical exam unchanged.	ophthalmologic evaluation.
	A: Poor compliance! -? of diabetic state	4. Return in 2 wk.
	Needs evaluation of vision and fundi.	
	? etiology of blurred vision - from	
	#1, #2, or #3. FEM	

FIG. 233-3. **Example of a problem/source record.** From medical record formats, © Miller Communications, Inc. Reproduced by permission.

INFORMATION RETRIEVAL

Color coding: Office clinical records should be kept in color-coded manila folders and carefully filed by name or number. Medical record jackets should be marked with the year of the last visit so that inactive records can be pulled every 2 to 3 yr and stored for the years indicated in each state's statute of limitations.

Problem indexing: An index card file arranged by problem, and listing each patient with chart number and telephone number, should be maintained in order to recall patients when appropriate (e.g., for Pap smears, flu shots, a drug recall, a new method of therapy) as well as for practice analysis.

234. READY REFERENCE GUIDES

CALCULATION OF DOSAGES FOR INFANTS AND CHILDREN

Drug dosages for children can be calculated by using Young's, Cowling's, or Clark's rules. To use **Young's rule,** the child's age should be divided by the age plus 12; the result is the fraction of the adult dose recommended for the child. For example, a child aged 3 yr will require $\frac{3}{3 + 12} = 1/5$ of the adult dose.) **Cowling's rule** divides the age at the next birthday by 24. (Thus, for a child aged 5 yr, the dose is 6/24 or 1/4 of the adult dose.) **Clark's rule** divides the weight (in lb) by 150 to give the appropriate fraction of the adult dose. (Thus, for a 50-lb child, the dose is $\frac{50}{150}$ or 1/3 of the adult dose.)

Body surface area (BSA) can also be used to calculate pediatric drug dosages or fluid and electrolyte requirements. A nomogram for estimating the BSA is given in Fig. 22–1 in Vol. II, Ch. 22. The dosage is determined as follows:

$$\frac{\text{BSA (sq m)}}{1.7} \times \text{Adult Dose} = \text{Approximate Dose}$$

It should be emphasized that these calculations give only approximate values, that individual requirements vary widely, and that young children may be unduly susceptible to certain drugs (e.g., opiates) or relatively insusceptible to others (e.g., belladonna). Individual drug characteristics and idiosyncrasies make it prudent to review the manufacturer's instructions on the drug package insert.

WEIGHTS, MEASURES, AND EQUIVALENTS

TABLE 234–1. METRIC SYSTEM

Weight:

1 kilogram (kg)	=	1000 grams (10^3 Gm)
1 gram (Gm, gm)	=	1000 milligrams (10^3 mg)
1 milligram (mg)	=	1000 micrograms (10^{-3} Gm)
1 microgram (μg, mcg)	=	1000 millimicrograms (10^{-6} Gm)
	=	1000 nanograms (ng) (10^{-6} Gm)
1 millimicrogram (mμg)	=	1000 micromicrograms (μμg) (10^{-9} Gm)
	=	1000 picograms (pg) (10^{-9} Gm)

Volume:

1 liter (L)	=	1000 milliliters (ml)
	=	1000 cubic centimeters (cc)

TABLE 234–2. EQUIVALENTS
(all approximate)

Liquid:

Metric		Apothecaries'
30 ml	=	1 fluid ounce
250 ml	=	8+ fluid ounces
500 ml	=	1+ pint
1000 ml	=	1+ quart
(1 liter)		

Weight:

65	mg =	1	grain (gr)
28.35	gm =	1	ounce (oz)
1	kg =	2.2	pounds (lb)

Linear:

1	millimeter (mm)	=	0.04 inch (in.)
1	centimeter (cm)	=	0.4 inch
2.5	centimeters	=	1 inch
1	meter (m)	=	39.37 inches

TABLE 234–3. HOUSEHOLD MEASURES
(with approximate equivalents)

1 teaspoon (tsp)	=	4 ml		
1 teaspoon, medical	=	5 ml		
1 dessert spoon	=	8 ml		
1 tablespoon (tbsp)	=	15 ml	=	1/2 fluid ounce
1 teacup	=	120 ml	=	4 fluid ounces

TABLE 234–4. ATOMIC WEIGHTS (APPROXIMATE)
OF SOME COMMON ELEMENTS

Hydrogen (H)	=	1	Magnesium (Mg) = 24
Carbon (C)	=	12	Phosphorus (P) = 31
Nitrogen (N)	=	14	Chlorine (Cl) = 35.5
Oxygen (O)	=	16	Potassium (K) = 39
Sodium (Na)	=	23	Calcium (Ca) = 40

MILLIGRAM-MILLIEQUIVALENT CONVERSIONS

The unit of measure of electrolytes is the milliequivalent (mEq), which expresses the chemical activity, or combining power, of a substance relative to the activity of 1 mg of hydrogen. Thus, 1 mEq is represented by 1 mg of hydrogen, 23 mg of sodium, 39 mg of potassium, 20 mg of calcium, and 35 mg of chlorine. Conversion equations are as follows:

$$mEq/L = \frac{(mg/L) \times Valence}{Formula\ Wt}$$

$$mg/L = \frac{(mEq/L) \times Formula\ Wt}{Valence}$$

(NOTE: Formula Wt = Atomic or Molecular Wt)

Milliosmol

The mEq is roughly equivalent to the milliosmol (mOsm), the unit of measure of osmolality or tonicity. Normally, the body fluid compartments each contain about 280 mOsm of solute/L.

TABLE 234–5. CENTIGRADE–FAHRENHEIT EQUIVALENTS

Centigrade°	Fahrenheit°	Centigrade°	Fahrenheit°
Freezing (water at sea level):		Pasteurization (holding), 30 min at:	
0	32	61.6	143.0
Clinical range:		Pasteurization (flash), 15 sec at:	
36.0	96.8	71.1	160.0
36.5	97.7	Boiling (water at sea level):	
37.0	98.6	100.0	212.0
37.5	99.5		
38.0	100.4		
38.5	101.3	Conversion	
39.0	102.2	To convert degrees F to degrees C, subtract 32, then multiply by 5/9 or 0.555	
39.5	103.1		
40.0	104.0		
40.5	104.9	To convert degrees C to degrees F, multiply by 9/5 or 1.8, then add 32	
41.0	105.8		
41.5	106.7		
42.0	107.6		

§21. CLINICAL PHARMACOLOGY

235. DRUG ABSORPTION AND BIOAVAILABILITY

Absorption: *The process of drug movement from the site of application toward the systemic circulation.*

Bioavailability: *The rate at which and the extent to which the active moiety (drug or metabolite) enters the general circulation, thereby permitting access to the site of action.*

Drug product: *The actual dosage form of a drug, consisting of the drug itself plus other inert ingredients formulated into a usable medicine; e.g., as a tablet, capsule, or solution.*

In the present context, absorption describes drug movement, while bioavailability refers to a specific net result. Whereas the physicochemical properties of a drug govern its absorptive potential, the properties of the dosage form, or both, can be major determinants of its bioavailability. Hence, the concept of equivalence among drug products is important in clinical decisions. However, there is often confusion about different types of equivalence. **Chemical equivalence** refers to *preparations that contain the same compound in two or more dosage forms and meet present official standards.* **Bioequivalence** refers to *chemical equivalents that, when administered to the same individual in the same dosage regimen, result in equivalent concentrations of drug in blood and tissues.* **Therapeutic equivalence** refers to *two drugs that, when administered to the same individual in the same dosage regimen, provide essentially the same therapeutic effect, even though they may not be chemically equivalent.*

Bioavailability depends upon a number of factors, some of which relate to how a drug product is designed and manufactured and others which relate to its physicochemical properties. Therefore, preparations which are chemically equivalent may not be bioequivalent, but bioequivalence suggests therapeutic equivalence.

Sometimes therapeutic equivalence may be achieved despite differences in bioavailability. For example, the margin between an effective concentration of penicillin and its toxic level is so great that the prescribed dosage usually achieves a blood concentration far above the minimum effective level. Moderate blood concentration differences due to bioavailability differences in penicillin products might therefore not affect therapeutic effect or safety. In contrast, bioavailability differences would be important for a drug with a relatively narrow range between therapeutic and toxic drug levels. These matters will be discussed below and in the ensuing chapters.

DRUG ABSORPTION

Drug products are formulated for administration by a variety of routes, including oral, buccal, sublingual, rectal, parenteral, topical, and inhalation. The physicochemical properties of drugs, their formulations, and the routes of administration are important in absorption. A prerequisite to absorption of any drug is that it be able to enter into a solution. The active ingredients in solid drug products (e.g., a tablet) must undergo disintegration, deaggregation, and dissolution before the drug can be absorbed.

Except when a drug is given IV, it must traverse several semipermeable cell membranes before it reaches the general circulation. These membranes act as biologic barriers that selectively permit the passage of certain solutes or drug molecules and are remarkably similar in chemical composition and spatial arrangement throughout the body. Cell membranes are composed primarily of a bimolecular lipid matrix, containing mostly cholesterol and phospholipids, in which are embedded globular protein macromolecules of random size and composition. The membrane proteins may be involved in transport processes and may also function as receptors for cellular regulatory mechanisms. Membrane lipid confers both hydrophilic and hydrophobic properties, providing stability to the membrane and determining its permeability characteristics. Compounds are transported across this biologic barrier by passive diffusion, facilitated diffusion, active transport, and pinocytosis.

Passive diffusion: *Transport across the cell membrane in which the driving force for movement is the concentration gradient of the solute.* Most drug molecules are transported across a membrane by simple diffusion from a high concentration area (e.g., GI fluids) to a low concentration area (e.g., blood) without expenditure of energy by the biologic system. Diffusion rate is directly proportional to this gradient and depends upon lipid solubility, degree of ionization, molecular size, and the area of the absorptive surface. Since the drug is transported away by the systemic circulation and distributed into a large volume, the concentration of drug in the blood is initially low compared to that at the site of administration, and the large concentration gradient serves as the driving force for absorption. However, since the cell membrane is lipoid in nature, drugs that are highly lipid-soluble diffuse more rapidly than drugs that are relatively lipid-insoluble. Small molecules tend to penetrate membranes more rapidly than do large molecules.

Most drugs exist as weak organic acids or bases in both undissociated and dissociated form in an aqueous environment. The undissociated or nonionized fraction is usually lipid-soluble and diffuses readily across the cell membrane. The dissociated or ionized form cannot penetrate the cell membrane easily because of its low lipid solubility. The importance of lipid solubility in transport can be illustrated by the absorption of three barbiturates as shown in TABLE 235-1. At pH 1, all are essentially nonionized, yet absorption rates vary because of their different lipid solubilities. The charged groups on the protein surfaces of the cell membrane may also impede passage of the ionized fraction. Thus, the combination of low lipid solubility and greater electrical resistance make penetration of the ionized form so slow that the penetration rate may be attributed mainly to the undissociated fraction.

The distribution of a weak electrolyte across a membrane will be determined by its pK and the pH gradient. If a pH gradient exists, the extent of ionization of a weak electrolyte on the two sides of a membrane will differ—for a weak acid, the higher the pH, the lower the ratio of nonionized to ionized fractions. Consider the partitioning of a weak acid (e.g., pK_a 4.4) between plasma and gastric juice. In plasma (pH 7.4) the ratio of nonionized to ionized forms is 1:1000; in gastric juice (pH 1.4) the ratio is reversed, i.e., 1000:1. When the weak acid is given orally, a large concentration gradient is established between the stomach and the plasma, a condition favorable to diffusion through the gastric mucosa. At equilibrium, the concentration of nonionized drug will be equal in the stomach and in the plasma because it is the only moiety that can penetrate membranes. However, the concentration of ionized fraction in the plasma will be approximately 1000 times greater than that in the gastric lumen. For a weak base with a pK_a of 4.4, the situation is reversed. Thus, weakly acidic drugs (e.g., aspirin) are more readily absorbed from an acid medium (gastric lumen) than weak bases (e.g., quinidine). However, regardless of pH, most drug absorption occurs in the small intestine because of its large surface area.

Facilitated diffusion: For certain molecules driven across the cell membrane by the concentration gradient, the rate of penetration is greater than would be expected on the basis of their low lipid solubility (e.g., glucose). It is postulated that a "carrier component" combines reversibly with the substrate molecule at the cell membrane exterior and that the carrier-substrate complex diffuses rapidly across the membrane with release of the substrate at the interior surface. This carrier-mediated diffusion process is characterized by **selectivity** and **saturability**. The carrier mechanism accepts for transport only those substrates having a relatively specific molecular configuration and the process is further determined by the availability of carrier. No expenditure of energy is required by this process; substrate is not transported against a concentration gradient.

Active transport: In addition to the same selectivity and saturability described for facilitated diffusion, active transport *requires energy expenditure by the cell, and substrates may be accumulated intracellularly against a concentration gradient.* Active transport processes appear to be limited to agents with close structural similarities to normal body constituents. These agents are usually absorbed from specific sites in the small intestine. Active transport processes have been identified for various ions, vitamins, sugars, and amino acids.

Pinocytosis refers to *the engulfing of particles or fluid by a cell.* The cell membrane invaginates, encloses the particle or solute, and then fuses again, forming a vesicle which later buds off within the interior of the cell. This mechanism also requires the expenditure of energy. Pinocytosis probably plays a minor role in drug transport.

Absorption of Oral Solutions

The GI mucosa acts as a semipermeable barrier. Oral solutions may be absorbed along the entire alimentary canal and must pass through various fluids and tissues and survive encounters with several enzyme systems. The epithelial lining, its organization, and physiologic factors affecting acid secretion, stomach emptying, intestinal transit, and bile and mucus flow can affect drug absorption and bioavailability. Thus some segments favor the absorption process. The **oral mucosa** has a thin

TABLE 235-1. INFLUENCE OF LIPID SOLUBILITY
ON RATE OF ABSORPTION

Barbiturate	pK_a	Partition Coefficient $CHCl_3/H_2O$	% Absorbed from Stomach in 1 h at pH 1
Barbital	7.8	1	4
Secobarbital	7.8	52	30
Thiopental	7.6	580	46

Modified from L. S. Schanker et al: "Absorption of Drugs from the Stomach; I. The Rat," *Journal of Pharmacology and Experimental Therapeutics* Vol. 120, pp. 528–539, 1957. Copyright 1957 by The Williams and Wilkins Co., Baltimore. Used with permission of The Williams and Wilkins Co. and the author.

epithelium and a rich vascularity that favors drug absorption, but solutions are in contact too briefly for any appreciable absorption.

The **stomach** has a rich blood supply and a large epithelial surface, but the rate at which the stomach empties determines the length of time a substance remains in the stomach and is influenced by many factors. For some drugs, physiologic processes that delay gastric emptying increase the degradation of the drug in the stomach and profoundly decrease systemic absorption. Penicillin G is an example of a drug that is acid-labile. The acidic environment of the stomach favors the absorption of weak acids which are largely in the lipid-soluble, nonionized form. Under normal conditions, absorption from the stomach is highly variable and minor compared to absorption from the small intestine.

The **small intestine** presents the largest GI surface area for absorption; however, its environment varies. In the duodenum the pH is 4 to 5, but the intraluminal pH becomes progressively more alkaline farther along the alimentary canal (e.g., the pH of the lower ileum is about 8). The GI flora may inactivate certain drugs, reducing their absorption and bioavailability. Compared to passage through the stomach, drug transit through the small intestine is usually slow, but other factors, including blood flow, metabolism in the intestinal wall, and permeability characteristics, influence the passage of intact drug across the intestinal mucosa. Decreased blood flow (e.g., in shock) may lower the concentration gradient across the intestinal mucosa and decrease absorption by passive diffusion. (Decreased peripheral blood flow also alters drug distribution and metabolism.)

Certain physiologic factors or disease states can influence bioavailability after the drug has penetrated the intestinal wall but before it has reached the systemic circulation. Certain drugs (e.g., salicylamide) are well absorbed but are extensively metabolized by enzymes in the gut wall during absorption. The rate of hepatic clearance may be so high for some drugs (e.g., propranolol) that only a fraction absorbed from the intestine reaches the systemic circulation. Individual variations in age, sex, activity, genetic phenotype, stress, disease (e.g., achlorhydria, malabsorption syndromes), and previous GI surgery can alter or impair drug bioavailability.

In contrast to the small intestine, the **large intestine** has no villi and its main function is not one of absorption. Nevertheless, molecules that escape absorption in the small intestine may be absorbed, albeit less efficiently, in the colon.

Absorption of Solid Dosage Forms

Most drugs administered orally are in the form of tablets or capsules, primarily for convenience, economy, stability, and patient acceptance. They must disintegrate and dissolve before absorption can occur. **Disintegration** greatly increases the surface area of the drug, brings it into contact with the gastrointestinal fluids, and promotes dissolution. Disintegrants and other excipients (e.g., diluents, lubricants, surfactants, binders, and dispersants) are often added in the manufacturing process to facilitate these processes. Factors capable of causing variable or retarded disintegration of solid drug products include excessive pressure applied during the tableting procedure and special coatings applied to protect the tablet from the digestive processes of the gut. Hydrophobic lubricants (e.g., magnesium stearate) may bind to the active drug and reduce its bioavailablility. Surfactants may influence the wettability, solubility, and dispersibility of the active drug and thereby alter its dissolution rate.

The **dissolution rate** determines the availability of the drug for absorption. When slower than the absorption rate, dissolution will be the rate-limiting step. It can be altered by manipulating the drug or the dosage formulation. Some factors that may alter the dissolution rate are salt form, particle size, crystal form, and hydrates. For example, the Na salts of weak acids (e.g., barbiturates and salicylates) dissolve faster than their corresponding free acids regardless of the pH of the medium. Reduction of particle size is a frequent approach to increasing the surface area of a drug and is an effective method of increasing the rate and extent of GI absorption of a drug which is rate-limited by slow dissolution. Certain drugs exhibit polymorphism, existing in amorphous or various crystalline forms. Chloramphenicol palmitate exists as two polymorphs, A and B, but only the latter has sufficient dissolution, absorption, and bioavailability to be of clinical value. A hydrate is formed when one or more water molecules associate with a drug molecule in crystal formation. The solubility of such a solvate may be markedly different from the nonsolvate form of a drug. For example, anhydrous ampicillin has a greater rate of dissolution and in vivo absorption than its corresponding trihydrate.

Absorption from Parenteral Sites

Direct placement of a drug into the bloodstream (usually IV) ensures bioavailability of all the drug administered. However, administration by a route that requires penetration through one or more biologic membranes to reach the bloodstream precludes a guarantee that all of the drug will eventually be absorbed. IM or subcutaneous injection of drugs bypasses the skin barrier, but the drug must penetrate into the capillaries. The rate of entry into capillaries is usually determined for lipid-soluble drugs by their oil/water partition coefficients and for lipid-insoluble drugs by their molecular size. The rate of capillary blood flow is also a major factor in the rate of absorption.

Absorption may be delayed or erratic when salts of poorly soluble acids and bases are injected IM. For example, the parenteral form of phenytoin is the Na salt, which has a pH of about 12. When it is injected IM, tissue fluids act as buffers and the pH decreases, causing a shift in the equilibrium between the ionized and free acid form of the drug, forming more of the poorly soluble free acid which precipitates and is absorbed very slowly.

Absorption via the lymphatic system contributes little to the total absorption of small molecules because the flow of lymph is slow compared to that of blood. However, lymphatic absorption may be significant in the case of larger molecules (e.g., insulin).

Prolonged-Release Dosage Forms

Prolonged- (sustained-) release dosage forms are designed to reduce the frequency of dosing and to maintain more uniform plasma drug concentrations, thus providing a more uniform pharmacologic effect. Additionally, greater patient convenience may improve compliance with the therapeutic regimen. Ideally, suitable drugs for such dosage forms are those that require frequent dosing because of a short biologic half-life and a short duration of effect. Drugs with a narrow therapeutic index (e.g., anticoagulants) are not suitable because of the larger doses required and variable absorption may lead to poor control of therapy or unwanted side effects.

Oral prolonged-release dosage forms are usually designed to maintain therapeutic concentrations of drug for up to 12 h. They generally release a normal therapeutic dose of drug initially, and subsequently release sustaining amounts more slowly. Reduction of the absorption rate can be achieved in various ways: by coating the drug particles with wax or related water-insoluble material, by embedding the drug in a matrix from which it is released slowly during transit through the GI tract, or by complexing the drug with ion-exchange resins.

Many nonintravenous parenteral preparations have been formulated to provide sustained blood levels. In some cases, insoluble salts (e.g., fluphenazine enanthate) injected IM may provide activity for several weeks or a month. For other drugs, suspensions or solutions in nonaqueous vehicles are formulated; e.g., insulin may be injected in crystalline suspensions for prolonged action. Amorphous insulin, with a high surface area for dissolution, has an intermediate onset and duration. The procaine salt of penicillin is poorly soluble and slowly absorbed when injected IM. Its duration of action can be further prolonged by suspending the procaine penicillin in an oil containing aluminum stearate. The oil prevents contact of the salt with an aqueous medium, thereby retarding dissolution, and the aluminum stearate further delays dissolution by increasing the viscosity of the preparation.

BIOAVAILABILITY OF DRUGS

The concept of bioavailability relates to the efficiency of the dosage formulation as an extravascular drug delivery system and permits comparison of drug products for relative availability or bioequivalence. Bioavailability is determined either by measuring the concentration of drug in body fluids or by the magnitude of the pharmacologic or therapeutic response produced in humans. For most drugs, determining the blood level at predetermined times after a single dose is the easiest and, generally, the most quantitative method.

Qualitative analysis of the serum concentration-time curve allows assessment of bioavailability, which usually involves three parameters: the maximum (or peak) serum drug concentration, the time of occurrence of maximum serum drug concentration, and the area under the serum concentration-time curve (FIG. 235–1). The serum drug concentration increases with the rate and extent of absorption; the peak is reached when the rate of drug removal equals the rate of absorption.

Slow or incomplete absorption may result in capricious absorption, since more factors affect bioavailability in this situation than when drugs are rapidly and completely absorbed. Variations in bioavailability are more consequential for drugs with a narrow therapeutic index (e.g., digoxin and dicumarol) than for drugs with a wide therapeutic margin (e.g., many antibiotics). Formulation-modi-

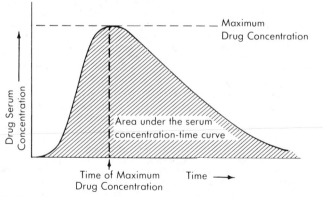

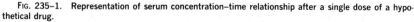

FIG. 235–1.   Representation of serum concentration–time relationship after a single dose of a hypothetical drug.

fied and physiologically-modified factors influencing bioavailability are described under Drug Absorption, above.

Bioavailability determinations based on maximum serum concentration alone can be misleading, since drug removal begins immediately upon entry into the bloodstream. The peak serum concentration time is related to the absorption rate and is the most widely used index of this parameter, but absorption is not complete when the serum concentration has peaked, except in the case of an IV bolus.

The **area under the concentration curve (AUC)** is the most important measurement of bioavailability based on serum concentration determinations. It is directly proportional to the total amount of unchanged drug in the blood. To describe the serum concentration curve accurately it is necessary to sample blood at frequent intervals; the extent of absorption is determined by taking samples for a sufficient time. Drug products may be considered bioequivalent if their serum level curves are essentially superimposable. Two drug products which have similar AUC's but different shapes of serum level-time profiles are equivalent in *extent* of availability but are absorbed at different *rates*.

Multiple dosing also permits evaluation of bioavailability, and this procedure has several advantages. In some cases, it more closely represents the usual clinical situation (e.g., use of most antibiotics). Higher serum levels are usually achieved than following a single dose and less sensitive analytical methods are required for determining the drug concentration. After 5 to 10 consecutive doses of a drug are administered at an equal dosing interval, the blood concentration should reach an approximate steady state, provided the dosing interval is about equal to the elimination half-life of the drug. The completeness of absorption can be analyzed by measuring the AUC during one dosing interval after reaching the steady-state.

For drugs that are primarily excreted unchanged in the urine, bioavailability may be estimated by measuring the total amount of drug excreted. Ideally, urine collection should be made over a period of 5 to 10 elimination half-lives for complete recovery of the drug and to evaluate the extent of absorption. Comprehensive bioavailability studies utilize both serum and urinary excretion data.

236. DRUG DISTRIBUTION

After a drug enters the general circulation, it distributes throughout the body and partitions in various tissues. Distribution through various fluid compartments and tissues is generally unequal and is affected by the extent of protein binding, regional variations in pH, and the permeability of various membranes.

The rate of entry of a drug into a tissue depends upon the rate of blood flow to the tissue, the tissue mass, and the partition characteristics of the drug between blood and tissue. Richly vascular areas achieve equilibrium more rapidly than poorly perfused areas, if the drug readily crosses the vascular membrane barriers. After **distribution equilibrium** is attained, the concentrations of drug in tissues and extracellular fluids reflect changes in the plasma concentration. Metabolism and excretion occur simultaneously with distribution, making the process dynamic and complex. The means for measuring the rate and extent of drug distribution are described in Ch. 237, while factors affecting drug distribution are discussed below.

Magnitude of Distribution

If one assumes that the body acts as a single fluid compartment, the amount of fluid into which a drug appears to be distributed is called the **apparent volume of distribution** (see Ch. 237). Every drug is distributed in the body in a characteristic manner. It is useful and customary to describe the extent of distribution in terms of the water content of compartments that are anatomically and functionally distinct. For instance, a drug whose volume of distribution is approximately 3 L can be conceptualized as being contained almost completely within the plasma water. A volume of distribution of 12 L corresponds to that of extravascular interstitial fluid plus plasma water, and about 40 L is equal to the total water content of the body. To assume that a drug is contained within a particular compartment is an oversimplification; however, it does allow some valid generalizations about the extent of drug distribution. *The greater the volume of distribution of a drug, the smaller the fraction likely to reach the receptor site to produce the desired pharmacologic effect.*

Most drugs have a volume of distribution of < 500 L/70 kg; some typical values are shown in Table 236–1. Many acids (e.g., warfarin and salicylates) are highly protein bound and too water soluble to enter the cellular water, and thus have a low volume of distribution. Many bases (e.g., amphetamine and meperidine) are avidly taken up by the tissues and thus have a very large volume of distribution, which can be larger than the volume of the entire body. This paradox is the result of the mathematical method for calculating the "apparent" volume of distribution.

TABLE 236–1. SOME EXAMPLES OF THE VOLUME OF DISTRIBUTION

Drug	Liters/70 kg
Warfarin	8
Acetylsalicylic acid	10
Gentamicin	18
Theophylline	35
Phenytoin	45
Acetaminophen	66
Lidocaine	77
Procainamide	133
Quinidine	189
Propranolol	273
Amitriptyline	581

Protein Binding

Drugs are transported in the bloodstream partly in solution (as free drug) and partly bound to various blood components (e.g., plasma protein). The major determinant of the ratio of bound to free drug is the reversible interaction between a drug molecule and a molecule of protein, an interaction governed by the Law of Mass Action. Although many plasma proteins can interact with drugs, albumin is the most important and can interact with anions or cations. The extent to which a drug binds with an albumin molecule depends upon the molecular structure of the drug. Acidic drugs are generally bound more extensively than basic drugs. TABLE 236–2 gives some values for drug binding to serum albumin.

The α- and β-lipoproteins of the plasma are an important group of proteins with a high binding affinity, but a relatively low binding capacity, for many endogenous (e.g., corticosteroids) and foreign compounds. Plasma γ-globulins do not interact significantly with drugs except where they occur as specific antibodies to protein hormones (e.g., insulin). Such antibodies may lessen the hormone's therapeutic effects.

Since only unbound drug is available for passive diffusion to the extravascular or tissue sites where pharmacologic effects occur, plasma protein binding influences the distribution and pharmacologic activity of drugs. As free drug leaves the circulation, the remaining protein-drug complex begins to dissociate, releasing more free drug for diffusion. Some highly protein-bound drugs (e.g., diazoxide) may be confined largely to the plasma compartment, serving as depots and releasing more drug as it is removed from the circulation by metabolism and excretion. As the dose of a drug increases, the available protein-binding sites decrease, and the relative amount of free drug increases. If the dose exceeds protein-binding capacity, the addition of more drug will increase only the free drug concentration. In practice, saturation of protein-binding sites by drugs with high association constants (e.g., sulfonamides) occurs only when such drugs are given in large (i.e., gm) doses.

TABLE 236–2. SOME VALUES OF DRUG BINDING IN HUMAN SERUM

Drug	Percent Bound
Warfarin	99
Diazepam	99
Furosemide	96
Dicloxacillin	94
Propranolol	93
Tolbutamide	93
Sulfisoxazole*	88–92
Phenytoin	89
Quinidine**	71
Lidocaine	50
Digoxin	25

 * Function of drug blood level, see text.
 ** Significant binding to serum protein other than albumin.

Generally, only unbound drug is available for metabolism; however, some highly bound drugs (e.g., propranolol) are rapidly metabolized. Only free drug is available for glomerular filtration, but active processes such as secretion by the renal tubules and carrier-mediated transport across other cell membranes are not restricted to free drug.

Sequestration (Storage)

Various tissues can act as reservoirs for drugs; e.g., tetracycline may be stored in bone, chlorinated insecticides in fat, and the antimalarial chloroquine in the eye or liver. These stored drugs are in equilibrium with the drug in the plasma and are released into the plasma as the drug is eliminated from the body, but their rate of release is usually too slow to produce pharmacologic effects. Consequently, this type of storage represents a site of loss (and possible local toxicity) rather than a depot for continued drug action. Chloroquine, for example, binds to nucleic acids of the cell nucleus and its concentration in the liver may reach 200 to 700 times the plasma concentration. When chloroquine is used to treat malaria, this sequestration site must be saturated before plasma levels adequate for systemic antimalarial therapy can be attained.

Passage of Drugs into the Central Nervous System

Drugs enter the CNS by 2 routes: the capillary circulation and the CSF. Although the brain receives a large proportion of the cardiac output (about $1/6$), rapid distribution of drugs to brain tissue is restricted. While some lipid-soluble drugs (e.g., thiopental) do enter and exert their pharmacologic effects very rapidly, many drugs, particularly the more water-soluble agents, enter the brain very slowly. The endothelial cells of the brain capillaries, which appear to be more tightly joined to one another than are those of other capillary beds, contribute to the slow diffusion of water-soluble substances. Another important barrier to water-soluble substances is the close approximation of the glial connective tissue cells (astrocytes) to the basement membrane of the capillary endothelium. The capillary endothelium and the astrocytic sheath together are referred to as the **blood-brain barrier.** They confer permeability characteristics on the brain different from those of other tissues and constitute a relative obstacle to drug penetration.

Drugs may enter the ventricular CSF directly via the choroid plexus, gaining access to brain tissue by passive diffusion from the CSF. The choroid plexus is also a site of active tranport of organic acids (e.g., penicillin) from CSF to blood.

The major factors that determine the rate of drug penetration into the CSF include the extent of protein binding, the ionization state, and especially the lipid/water partition coefficient of the compound. The penetration rate into the brain is slow for highly protein-bound drugs, and for the ionized form of weak acids and bases is so slow as to be virtually nonexistent. Differences in pH between the plasma and brain compartments may appreciably influence the distribution ratio of drugs between the compartments through an ion-trapping effect. Under normal conditions there is a small pH difference between plasma (pH 7.4) and CSF (pH 7.3), which particularly affects weak electrolytes with pK's near these pH values. Lipid-soluble substances diffuse across brain capillaries and capillary barriers elsewhere at similar rates.

---

237. PHARMACOKINETICS AND DRUG ADMINISTRATION

Pharmacokinetics is the study of the time course of a drug and its metabolites in the body following drug administration.

Drugs are administered to achieve a therapeutic objective, which requires the attainment and maintenance of a pharmacologic response. To accomplish this, an appropriate concentration of drug is required at the site of action. What is appropriate and the dosage needed depends upon the patient's clinical state, the severity of the condition being treated, the presence of other drugs and concurrent disease, and other factors.

The pharmacologic response observed relative to the concentration at the active site depends upon the **pharmacodynamics** of the drug, while the attainment and maintenance of the appropriate concentration depends upon the **pharmacokinetics** of the drug. The former is concerned with how a drug acts on the body; the latter, which is emphasized in this chapter, deals with how the body acts on a drug.

Because of individual differences, successful therapy requires planning drug administration according to each patient's needs. Traditionally, this has been accomplished by empirically adjusting dosage until the therapeutic objective is met. This method is frequently inadequate because of delays or because of undue toxicity. An alternative approach is to initiate drug administration according to the expected absorption and disposition (distribution and elimination) of the drug in a patient and to adjust dosage by monitoring the plasma drug concentration, a reflector of drug at the active site, in addition to drug effects. This approach requires knowledge of the drug's pharmacokinetics as a function of age and weight, and of the presence of renal, hepatic, cardiovascular, or other disease.

To identify and quantitate the variables in pharmacokinetics, isolation of the input and disposition processes is helpful. Absorption, distribution, and elimination and the factors affecting them are described in Chs. 235, 236, and 238. The quantitative aspects of these processes and the application of pharmacokinetic principles to drug administration are discussed in this chapter.

BASIC PHARMACOKINETIC PARAMETERS

The pharmacokinetic behavior of most drugs may be summarized by 10 parameters that relate variables to each other (see TABLE 237-1). The parameters are constants, although their values may differ from patient to patient and in the same patient under different conditions.

Bioavailability and Absorption Rate Constant

The extent of drug absorption into the general circulation is expressed by the **bioavailability**, the fraction of a dose reaching the plasma site of measurement. The rapidity of absorption is often expressed by the **absorption rate constant**, provided absorption follows Relationship 2 in TABLE 237-1. Changes in these two parameters influence the maximum (or peak) concentration, the time at which the maximum concentration occurs, and the area under the concentration-time curve after a single oral dose. In chronic drug therapy bioavailability is the more important measurement because it relates to the average level obtained, whereas only the degree of fluctuation is related to the absorption rate constant.

Volume of Distribution and Unbound Fraction

The **apparent volume of distribution** and the **fraction unbound** in plasma are the two most widely-used parameters for drug distribution. The volume of distribution is useful because it allows estimation of the dose required to achieve a given concentration and, conversely, the concentration

TABLE 237-1. BASIC PHARMACOKINETIC PARAMETERS AND THEIR DEFINING RELATIONSHIPS

Relationship			Parameter		
Absorption					
1.	Rate of Absorption	=	**Absorption Rate Constant**	×	Amount Remaining to be Absorbed
2.	Amount Absorbed	=	**Bioavailability**	×	Dose
Distribution					
3.	Amount in Body	=	**Volume of Distribution**	×	Plasma Drug Concentration
4.	Unbound Drug Concentration in Plasma	=	**Fraction Unbound**	×	Plasma Drug Concentration
Elimination					
5.	Rate of Renal Excretion	=	**Renal Clearance**	×	Plasma Drug Concentration
6.	Rate of Metabolism	=	**Metabolic Clearance**	×	Plasma Drug Concentration
7.	Rate of Elimination	=	**Clearance**	×	Plasma Drug Concentration
8.	Rate of Renal Excretion	=	**Fraction Excreted Unchanged**	×	Rate of Elimination
9.	Rate of Elimination	=	**Elimination* Rate Constant**	×	Amount in Body

* Another conceptually useful parameter is biologic half-life. Its relationship to the elimination rate constant is: Half-life = 0.693/Elimination Rate Constant.

achieved on administering a given dose. The unbound fraction is useful because it relates the measured total concentration to the unbound concentration, which is presumably more closely associated with drug effects. It is a particularly useful parameter when plasma protein binding is altered, e.g., in hypoalbuminemia, renal disease, hepatic disease, and displacement interactions.

Clearance, Renal Clearance, and Fraction Excreted Unchanged

The rate at which a drug is eliminated from the body is proportional to the plasma concentration, Relationship 7, Table 237-1; the parameter relating the two is clearance. The parameters relating rate of renal excretion of unchanged drug and rate of metabolism to the plasma concentration are **renal clearance**, Relationship 5, and **metabolic clearance**, Relationship 6, respectively. Because the rate of elimination is the sum of the rates of renal excretion and extrarenal elimination, usually metabolism, it follows that

$$\text{Total clearance} = \text{Renal clearance} + \text{Extrarenal (metabolic) clearance}$$

The ratio of the rate of renal excretion to the rate of total elimination, also the ratio of renal clearance to (total) clearance, is the **fraction excreted unchanged,** Relationship 8. This parameter is useful in assessing the potential effect of renal and hepatic diseases on drug elimination.

The rate of extraction of a drug from the blood in an eliminating organ, such as the liver, cannot exceed the rate of its presentation to the organ. Thus, clearance has a limiting value. When high extraction exists, elimination is limited by drug delivery and hence by blood flow to the organ. Furthermore, when the eliminating organ is the liver and a drug is given orally, a portion of the dose administered is lost on its requisite passage through the liver to the general circulation. This is called the **first-pass effect**; it applies to metabolism in the gut wall as well as in the liver. Thus, whenever a drug is highly extracted (high clearance) in either of these locations, the bioavailability is low, sometimes precluding oral administration or resulting in an oral dose much larger than the equivalent parenteral dose. A large first-pass effect is shown by a number of drugs, such as morphine, meperidine, propranolol, alprenolol, lidocaine, nitroglycerin, hydralazine, and isoproterenol.

Elimination Rate Constant and Half-life

The **elimination rate constant** relates the rate of elimination to the amount of drug in the body. As the rate of elimination equals clearance times plasma drug concentration (Relationship 7, Table 237-1) and the amount of drug in the body equals volume of distribution times plasma drug concentration (Relationship 3), it is apparent from Relationship 9 that

$$\text{Elimination rate constant} = \frac{\text{Clearance}}{\text{Volume of distribution}}$$

Expressed in these terms, the elimination rate constant is a function of how a drug is cleared from the blood by the eliminating organs and how the drug distributes throughout the body.

Half-life (biologic) is a convenient parameter. It is the time required for the plasma drug concentration or the amount in the body to decrease by 50%. For most drugs, the half-life remains constant regardless of how much drug is in the body. It is related to the elimination rate constant by

$$\text{Half-life} = \frac{0.693}{\text{Elimination rate constant}}$$

VARIABILITY IN PARAMETER VALUES

Many of the variables affecting pharmacokinetic parameters have been recognized and can be taken into account to adjust drug administration to an individual patient's needs, although even after dosage adjustment there is usually often sufficient variability remaining to require careful monitoring of drug response and, in many cases, of plasma drug concentration.

Age and Weight

For some drugs, changes in pharmacokinetics with age and weight are well-established. In children (6 mo to 20 yr), renal function appears to correlate best with body surface area. Thus, for drugs primarily eliminated unchanged by renal excretion, clearance varies with age according to the change in surface area. In persons over age 20, renal function decreases about 1%/yr. Taking these changes into account permits adjusting dosage with age for these drugs. Body surface area also has been found to correlate with metabolic clearance in children, although exceptions are common. For neonates and young infants, both renal and hepatic functions are not fully developed and no generalization, except for the occurrence of rapid change, can be made.

Disease

Renal function impairment causes several pharmacokinetic changes. The renal clearance of most drugs appears to vary directly with creatinine clearance, regardless of the renal disease present. The change in the (total) clearance is dependent upon the contribution of the kidneys to the total elimination. Thus, (total) clearance is expected to be proportional to the renal function (creatinine clearance) for drugs solely excreted unchanged and not to change at all for drugs eliminated by metabolism.

Sometimes the volume of distribution changes in renal failure. For digoxin, a decreased volume of distribution is observed because of decreased tissue binding. For phenytoin, salicylic acid, and many other drugs, the volume of distribution increases because of decreased binding to plasma proteins.

In physiologic stress, e.g., myocardial infarction, surgery, ulcerative colitis, Crohn's disease, etc., the concentration of the acute phase protein, α_1-acid glycoprotein, is increased. Consequently, the binding of several basic drugs, such as propranolol, quinidine, and disopyramide, to this protein is increased. The volume of distribution of these drugs is decreased accordingly.

Hepatic disease produces changes in metabolic clearance, but good correlates or predictors of the changes are unavailable. Dramatically reduced drug metabolism has been associated with hepatic cirrhosis. Reduced plasma protein binding is also often observed in this disease because of lowered plasma albumin. Acute hepatitis, with elevated serum enzymes, is usually not associated with altered drug metabolism. Congestive heart failure, pneumonia, hyperthyroidism, and many other diseases also alter the pharmacokinetics of drugs.

Drug Interactions

Drug interactions also cause variability in the values of pharmacokinetic parameters and, therefore, in drug response. Interactions are known that affect each of the parameters in TABLE 237–1. Most of these interactions are graded, and the extent of the interaction depends upon the concentration of both of the interacting drugs. For these reasons, predicting and adjusting drug administration in these situations are difficult. The prevention and management of drug interactions is discussed in DRUG INTERACTIONS in Ch. 241.

Dose and Time Dependence

In some instances, the values of the pharmacokinetic parameters change with the dose administered, with the concentration in plasma, or with time; e.g., a decreased bioavailability of griseofulvin as the dose is increased, a disproportionate increase in the steady-state phenytoin concentration on increasing its dosing rate, and a decrease in carbamazepine concentration during its chronic administration. The decreased bioavailability of griseofulvin is due to the drug's low solubility in the GI tract. Phenytoin shows a concentration (dose) dependency because the metabolizing enzymes have a limited capacity to eliminate the drug, and the usual rate of administration approaches the maximum rate of metabolism. Carbamazepine shows time dependence because it induces its own metabolism.

Although relatively uncommon, these dose and time dependencies introduce variability into the kinetics and response to several drugs. Other causes of dose- and time-dependent kinetics are saturable plasma protein and tissue binding (phenylbutazone), saturable secretion in the kidney (high dose penicillin therapy), and saturable metabolism during the first pass through the liver (propranolol).

DRUG ADMINISTRATION

Pharmacokinetic parameter values are obtained experimentally. When these values are known, the kinetics of a drug can be predicted. The kinetic consequences of administering a drug as a single IV dose, by constant-rate infusion, as an oral dose, and in multiple doses are described below using the drug aminophylline as an example. The metabolism of this drug shows concentration dependence in some individuals, especially children; however, for illustrative purposes, consider a 70 kg individual (Patient A) whose metabolism is concentration independent. The patient's parameter values are bioavailability, 1.0; absorption rate constant, 1.0 h^{-1}; volume of distribution, 0.5 L/kg; clearance, 43 ml/kg/h; and half-life, 8 h.

Single Intravenous Bolus

The expected time course of theophylline in plasma following the IV administration of a 300-mg bolus dose of aminophylline (85% theophylline) to Patient A is shown in FIG. 269–1 with both linear and semilogarithmic plots. The predicted initial plasma concentration is 7.29 mg/L (Dose [mg]/Volume of distribution [L]). The subsequent decline is estimated from the half-life; q 8 h the concentration decreases by a factor of 2.

The discrepancy between the observed (solid line) and the predicted (dashed line) concentration-time profiles is explained by the time required to distribute drug throughout the body. This is often called the **distribution phase** and explains why bolus doses of many drugs, including aminophylline, must be administered by infusion over a period of 5 to 10 min or more.

Constant Rate Intravenous Infusion

The expected plasma concentration of theophylline on IV infusion of aminophylline to Patient A at a constant rate of 42.5 mg/h is shown in Curve A of FIG. 237–2.

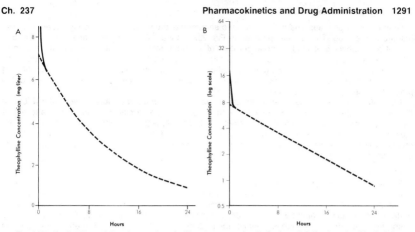

FIG. 237–1.   Decline of the plasma theophylline concentration in Patient A following the IV administration of a single 300-mg dose of aminophylline. Shown on linear (A) and semilogarithmic (B) plots. Key: observation (——); prediction from parameter values given (– – – – –).

Plateau concentration: The plasma concentration of theophylline and the amount of drug in the body rise until the rate of elimination equals the rate of infusion. The plasma concentration and amount of drug in the body are then at steady state—having reached a plateau level. From Relationships 7 and 9, TABLE 237–1, it follows that

$$\text{Rate of infusion} = \text{Clearance} \times \text{Plateau plasma drug concentration}$$

and

$$\text{Rate of infusion} = \text{Elimination rate constant} \times \text{Plateau amount of drug in body}$$

Thus, the plateau plasma concentration is controlled only by the clearance value and the rate of infusion; the plateau amount of drug in the body is determined only by the elimination rate constant and the rate of infusion.

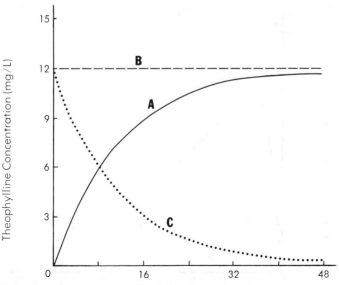

FIG. 237–2.   Time course of the plasma theophylline concentration following the constant-rate IV infusion of 42.5 mg/h of aminophylline without (——, Curve A) and with (– – – –, Curve B) the administration of an IV loading dose of 500 mg of aminophylline to Patient A. Curve C (····) shows drug remaining from the loading dose.

Time to reach plateau: The time required to accumulate theophylline in the body depends on the half-life of the drug. This is demonstrated in Fig. 237–2 by the administration of a bolus dose (500 mg) of aminophylline to attain a concentration of 12 mg/L followed immediately by an infusion of 42.5 mg/h to maintain the level, Curve B of Fig. 237–2. Drug from the bolus dose disappears as shown in Curve C, with 1/2 remaining at one half-life, 1/4 at 2 half-lives, and so on. The amount of drug in the body from the infusion, therefore, increases (Curve A) so that 1/2 of the plateau amount is present at one half-life, 3/4 at 2 half-lives, etc.

If the infusion were stopped at 48 h, the postinfusion curve would resemble Curve C, but would be displaced in time. The important principle is that the time frame for both accumulation and disappearance of drug is determined by the half-life. In Patient A, without a loading dose, aminophylline must be infused for at least 24 h (3 to 4 half-lives in the patient) for the concentration to approach the plateau value. Measuring a plasma concentration after this time would then provide an accurate estimate of theophylline clearance.

Single Oral Dose

The predicted concentration of theophylline in this patient after administering a 300-mg dose of aminophylline is shown in Fig. 237-3. Several points are pertinent: (1) The time course is different from that of an IV bolus (Fig. 237-1), because time is required to absorb the drug; however, the area under the curve is the same because this drug is virtually totally bioavailable. (2) The more rapid the absorption, the closer the curve is to that of the IV dose. (3) At the peak concentration, absorption is not over; here, the rate of absorption is simply equal to the rate of elimination.

Multiple Dosing, Drug Accumulation, and Dosage Regimens

On repetitively administering 300 mg of aminophylline orally q 6 h to Patient A, the theophylline concentration increases as shown in Curve A of Fig. 237-4. As with IV infusion, the average concentration at plateau depends upon the clearance, and the time required to accumulate the drug is a function of the half-life. Here, however, the levels fluctuate because of intermittent dosing. The kinetic consequence of an altered clearance of theophylline is demonstrated by Curves B and C. Curve B is the time course of plasma theophylline concentration in Patient B, who has congestive heart failure and whose clearance is only 21.5 ml/kg/h (about half that of Patient A). On administering 300 mg of aminophylline q 6 h to Patient B, the drug accumulates to levels about double those of Patient A. Furthermore, the time to reach the plateau levels is twice as long, a result of a 16-h half-life in Patient B.

Plasma concentrations of 10 to 20 mg/L are usually associated with optimal theophylline therapy. Above 20 mg/L the probability of toxicity increases. Thus, Patient B is at risk of developing toxicity (nausea, vomiting, CNS stimulation, seizures) that could have been averted, with prior knowledge of

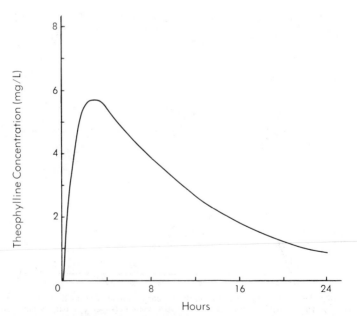

Fig. 237–3.   Time course of the plasma theophylline concentration following the oral administration of a single 300–mg dose of aminophylline to Patient A.

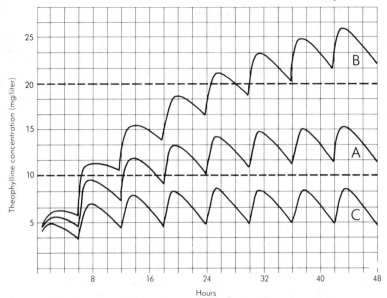

FIG. 237–4. **Accumulation of theophylline on orally administering 300 mg of aminophylline every 6 h.**
Curve A: in Patient A. Curve B: in Patient B, whose clearance is ½ that of Patient A. Curve C: in Patient C,
whose clearance is twice that of Patient A. The dashed lines are the usual therapeutic limits and represent
the *therapeutic window.*

decreased metabolism in congestive heart failure, by decreasing the dosage. The slow metabolism
also might have been detected by plasma concentration monitoring.

The requirement of Patient B for theophylline would probably be met with 200 mg aminophylline q
8 h (25 mg/h). However, because of the long half-life and the slow accumulation in this individual,
rapid attainment of a therapeutic concentration (and response) cannot be achieved without administering a loading dose. The loading dose of aminophylline required (volume of distribution × desired
concentration) is about 500 mg:

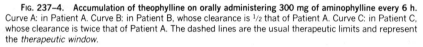

$$\left(35\ L \times \frac{12\ mg}{L} \times \frac{100\ mg\ aminophylline}{85\ mg\ theophylline}\right)$$

Curve C of FIG. 237–4 shows the time course of theophylline in a young, otherwise healthy, asthmatic adult (a heavy smoker). The clearance in this patient is 86 ml/kg/h and the half-life is 4 h.
Administration of 300 mg aminophylline q 6 h (50 mg/h) would probably be ineffective. The need for
more drug could have been anticipated. Measurement of a plasma concentration, just before the
next dose, would support this need. However, administration of aminophylline to this patient would
be difficult because of the short half-life, high clearance, and large dosage requirements (100 mg/h).
This is an example of a patient for whom the use of prolonged-release type of dosage form may be
indicated. Because absorption is more or less sustained, 600 mg q 6 h is reasonable, since widely
fluctuating levels would be avoided.

In summary, pharmacokinetic principles can be helpful in initiating and monitoring drug therapy
and in making adjustments to provide the optimum dosage requirements for each patient. The most
useful pharmacokinetic parameters are bioavailability, clearance, volume of distribution, half-life,
and fraction excreted unchanged.

238. DRUG ELIMINATION

The sum of the processes of loss of drug from the body. Removal of active drugs from the body
depends on **metabolism** and **excretion.** Although these are separate and distinct processes, their
functions in eliminating drugs are similar.

METABOLISM
(Biotransformation)

The process of chemical alteration of drugs in the body. The liver is the principal site of drug metabolism. Metabolites are sometimes pharmacologically active (see TABLE 238–1). When the substance administered is inactive and an active metabolite is produced, the administered drug form is called a **prodrug.** Metabolic reactions may be classified as nonsynthetic and synthetic.

In **nonsynthetic reactions,** the drug is chemically altered by either (1) oxidation, (2) reduction, (3) hydrolysis, or (4) a combination of these processes. These reactions usually represent only the first stage of biotransformation; metabolic products formed may subsequently undergo a synthetic reaction prior to elimination. Unlike the conjugated products of synthetic reactions, the metabolites of nonsynthetic processes may be pharmacologically active. Most oxidation and reduction reactions are catalyzed by the microsomal enzyme systems in the endoplasmic reticulum of the liver. The hydrolysis reactions and a few oxidative and reductive reactions are mediated by nonmicrosomal enzyme systems.

Examples of drugs metabolized by nonsynthetic reactions include amphetamine, chlorpromazine, imipramine, meprobamate, phenacetin, phenobarbital, phenytoin, procainamide, quinidine, and warfarin.

In **synthetic reactions** (or **conjugations**) the parent drug, or intermediate formed by nonsynthetic reactions, combines with an endogenous substrate, such as an amino acid or glucuronic acid, to yield an addition or conjugation product. Metabolites formed from synthetic reactions are biologically inactive and, because they are more polar, are more readily excreted by the kidney (in urine) and the liver (in bile) than those derived from nonsynthetic reactions.

The most important synthetic reactions are: (1) **Glucuronidation,** the most common synthetic reaction, is the only one that takes place in the liver microsomal enzyme system. Glucuronides are eliminated in the urine and are also secreted in the bile. Examples of drugs metabolized this way are salicylic acid, morphine, meprobamate, and chloramphenicol. (2) **Amino acid conjugation** with glutamine and glycine produces conjugates that are readily excreted in the urine but are not secreted into bile. (3) **Acetylation** is the primary metabolic pathway for sulfonamides. Other drugs that are acetyl-

TABLE 238–1. EXAMPLES OF DRUGS FORMING THERAPEUTICALLY IMPORTANT METABOLITES

Drug	Metabolite
Acetohexamide	Hydroxyhexamide
Acetylsalicylic acid*	Salicylic acid
Amitriptyline	Nortriptyline
Chloral hydrate*	Trichloroethanol
Chlordiazepoxide	Desmethylchlordiazepoxide
Codeine	Morphine
Diazepam	Desmethyldiazepam
Flurazepam	Desethylflurazepam
Glutethimide	4-Hydroxyglutethimide
Imipramine	Desipramine
Lidocaine	Desethyllidocaine
Meperidine	Normeperidine
Phenacetin*	Acetaminophen
Phenylbutazone	Oxyphenbutazone
Prednisone*	Prednisolone
Primidone*	Phenobarbital
Procainamide	N-Acetylprocainamide
Propranolol	4-Hydroxypropranolol

* Prodrugs. Metabolites are primarily responsible for their therapeutic effects.

ated include isoniazid and aminosalicylic acid. (4) **Sulfate conjugation:** Phenolic acid and alcoholic groups may be conjugated with sulfate derived from sulfur-containing amino acids such as cysteine to form sulfate esters, which are readily excreted in the urine. (5) **Methylation** is a major metabolic pathway for inactivation of some catecholamines. Other compounds that are methylated are niacinamide and thiouracil.

Effects of age on drug metabolism: Neonates have incompletely developed liver microsomal enzyme systems and, consequently, have difficulty with the metabolism of many drugs, such as hexobarbital, phenacetin, amphetamine, and chlorpromazine. The experience with chloramphenicol in neonates highlights the serious consequences that may occur because of slower conversion to the glucuronide. Equivalent mg/kg doses of chloramphenicol that are well tolerated by older subjects can result in serious toxicity in neonates **(the gray baby syndrome)** and are associated with prolonged and elevated blood levels of chloramphenicol. Elderly patients often show a reduced ability to metabolize drugs. The reduction varies depending on the drug and is not as severe as that in neonates. (See PHARMACOTHERAPEUTICS in Ch. 232)

Individual variation in the rate of drug metabolism (see also Ch. 241) makes it difficult to predict an individual's clinical response to a given dose of a drug. Some patients may metabolize a drug so rapidly that therapeutically effective blood and tissue levels are not achieved; in others, metabolism may be so slow that toxic effects result with usual doses. For example, phenytoin blood levels vary from 2.5 to > 40 mg/L in different persons given the same dose. Some of this variability is due to differences in the amount of the key enzyme, cytochrome P_{450}, available in the liver, and to differences in the affinity of the enzyme for the drug. Genetic factors play a major role in determining these differences. Concurrent disease states, particularly chronic liver disease, drug interactions, especially those involving induction or inhibition of metabolism, and other factors also contribute.

EXCRETION

The process by which a drug or metabolite is eliminated unchanged from the body. The kidney is the major organ of excretion and is responsible for eliminating water-soluble substances. The biliary system also excretes certain drugs and metabolites. Although drugs may also be eliminated via other pathways (e.g., intestine, saliva, sweat, breast milk, and lungs), the overall contribution of these routes is generally small. An exception is the excretion of volatile anesthetics, whose major route of elimination is via the lung.

RENAL EXCRETION OF DRUGS

Glomerular filtration and tubular reabsorption: About 1/5 of the plasma reaching the glomerulus is filtered through pores in the glomerular endothelium; the remainder passes along the efferent arterioles to the renal tubules. Drugs bound to plasma proteins are not filtered; only unbound drug appears in the filtrate. The principles that govern renal tubular reabsorption of drugs are those of any transmembrane passage (see DRUG ABSORPTION in Ch. 235). Polar compounds and ions are unable to diffuse back into the circulation and are excreted unless a specific transport mechanism for their reabsorption exists, as there is, for example, for glucose, ascorbic acid, and the B vitamins.

Effects of pH on the reabsorption and excretion of drugs: Although the glomerular filtrate which enters the proximal tubule has the same pH as plasma, the pH of voided urine varies from 4.5 to 8.0, and this may markedly affect the rate of drug excretion. Since the nonionized forms of nonpolar weak bases and weak acids tend to be reabsorbed readily from the tubular urine, acidification of the urine increases the reabsorption (i.e., decreases the elimination) of weak acids and decreases the reabsorption of weak bases (excreted more rapidly). The opposite is true for alkalinization of the urine.

These principles may be applied in some cases of overdosage to enhance the elimination of weakly basic or acidic drugs. With the weak acids phenobarbital or aspirin, for example, alkalinization of the urine increases their excretion. Conversely, urinary acidification may accelerate the urinary elimination of certain bases, such as methamphetamine. The overall extent to which changes in urinary pH alter the rate of drug elimination depends upon the contribution of the renal route to total drug elimination.

Tubular secretion: Mechanisms for active tubular secretion exist in the proximal tubule and are important in the elimination of many drugs; e.g., penicillin, mecamylamine, and salicylic acid. This process is energy-dependent and may be blocked by metabolic inhibitors. The secretory transport capacity can be saturated at high concentrations and each substance has its own characteristic maximum secretion rate, termed **tubular maximum (Tm).** Anions and cations are handled by separate transport mechanisms. Normally, the anion secretory system eliminates metabolites that have been conjugated with glycine, sulfate, or glucuronic acid. The various anionic compounds compete with one another for secretion. This tendency can be used therapeutically; e.g., probenecid blocks the normally rapid tubular secretion of penicillin and thus produces higher plasma penicillin concentrations for a longer period of time. Organic cations also compete with each other but not with anions.

BILIARY EXCRETION OF DRUGS

Drugs and their metabolites that are excreted in the bile must be transported across the biliary epithelium against a concentration gradient, requiring an active secretory process. This transport mechanism may become saturated by high plasma concentrations of a drug (transport maximum), and substances with similar physicochemical properties may compete for excretion via the same mechanism. This secretory process is utilized in the sulfobromophthalein (**BSP**) test (see Ch. 65). BSP, which is actively secreted by liver cells into the bile, is measured in the blood to assess liver function. Impaired liver function decreases the rate of biliary excretion of BSP, and higher levels consequently persist in blood. Elevated blood levels of BSP can also be found in a patient receiving a drug that competes for the same transport system (e.g., rifampin).

Biliary elimination is enhanced by (1) a mol wt over 300 (smaller molecules are generally secreted only in negligible amounts); (2) the presence of both polar and lipophilic groups; and (3) conjugation, particularly with glucuronic acid. Biliary excretion is only occasionally a major route of drug elimination.

ENTEROHEPATIC CYCLE

When a drug undergoes biliary secretion and reabsorption from the intestine, it completes an **enterohepatic cycle.** Drug conjugates that are secreted into and hydrolyzed in the GI tract, where the drug is reabsorbed, also undergo enterohepatic cycling. Biliary excretion is a route of elimination from the body only when the enterohepatic cycling is incomplete, i.e., when all the secreted drug is not reabsorbed.

---

239. PLASMA CONCENTRATION MONITORING

Once a therapeutic objective is defined and a drug and dosage regimen are chosen for a patient, drug therapy is conventionally managed by monitoring the incidence and intensity of both therapeutic and undesirable effects. Although preferable, the use of a direct measure of the therapeutic effect is not always possible. For a number of drugs alternative endpoints are used, e.g., prothrombin time for oral anticoagulants, Rosette Inhibition Test for immunosuppressive agents, blood or urine glucose for hypoglycemic drugs, and serum uric acid for uricosurics. Signs of toxicity are also used, e.g., tinnitus and nystagmus in therapy with salicylate and phenytoin, respectively. Because minor toxicities do not always occur before more severe toxicities and because of the inherent undesirability of toxic reactions, this procedure clearly has limitations. An alternative procedure is **plasma concentration monitoring.**

MONITORING DRUG IN PLASMA

Plasma concentration monitoring can provide additional information to guide and assess drug therapy. A plasma drug concentration may be useful in the initiation as well as in the maintenance of drug therapy. The basic idea is to achieve and maintain a target concentration or range of concentrations. Such monitoring is of value, for example, in reducing toxicity when the probability and severity of toxicity are closely related to the plasma concentration. A plasma concentration then serves as an intermediate therapeutic endpoint to help prevent toxicity. A strategy for drug administration may be entirely developed based on the plasma drug concentration, but this approach must be placed in perspective with all methods of monitoring.

Plasma concentration monitoring is useful when certain criteria, some related to the drug and others to the situation of its use, are satisfied. A few of the criteria are absolutely necessary; others are only relatively important. However, most of them must be met for the strategy to be effective.

Criteria Related to the Drug

Direct effect-concentration relationship: The intensity and probability of therapeutic or toxic effects must quantitatively correlate with the plasma level.

Nature of the therapeutic regimen: The objective of the regimen must be to attain and maintain a therapeutic effect. This usually requires maintenance of plasma concentration within a limited range. Drugs for which only acute or intermittent effects are desired are therefore excluded. Tolerance also diminishes the potential for applying the method.

Lack of other dosing guides: When readily assessed therapeutic endpoints are lacking, plasma concentration monitoring becomes particularly attractive. For example, this situation occurs in antiepileptic therapy for which the therapeutic endpoint is the absence of seizures.

Low therapeutic index: The probability of a therapeutic problem is greater for a drug with a narrow range between those concentrations giving the desired response and those producing toxicity, e.g., a drug with a low margin of safety or a low therapeutic index.

Current state of information: Prior knowledge of the therapeutic concentrations and the pharmacokinetic parameters of a drug is essential for plasma concentration monitoring to be effective. Furthermore, knowledge of the conditions in which these concentrations and parameters are likely to be altered is also important. However, this requirement is relative, in that by monitoring the concentration, adjustments in dosage can be made.

Analytical procedure: A sensitive, accurate, and specific assay for the drug must be available. Furthermore, the results of the assay must be available within a reasonable period of time so that a prudent therapeutic decision can be made. The half-life of the drug is an index of this "turn-around" time, as it is the time frame of accumulation on multiple dosing and of disappearance on discontinuing the drug.

Variability in pharmacokinetics: Interindividual differences and, in certain conditions, intraindividual differences in the pharmacokinetics of drugs are the principal reasons for monitoring plasma concentrations. Those drugs with poor and erratic absorption and those which are primarily metabolized, in contrast to those mostly excreted unchanged, are often candidates for monitoring. The larger the variability in the absorption and disposition of the drug, the greater is the need for monitoring it.

TABLE 239–1 lists drugs for which plasma level monitoring is now commonly used as well as the respective plasma concentrations usually associated with optimal therapy—**the therapeutic window** (see below).

Criteria Related to the Situation

There are drugs for which plasma level monitoring is not *routinely* suggested, but for which it might be helpful in certain situations.

Anticipation of a therapeutic problem: When there is a high probability of encountering a therapeutic failure because of the patient's clinical status, a plasma concentration measurement can be helpful. For a patient with GI disease or with a gastric resection, a drug with potentially poor availability may be a candidate for monitoring. Similarly, the presence of renal, hepatic, thyroid, or cardiovascular disease may also suggest monitoring. For drugs that are primarily excreted unchanged, the presence of renal disease requires special attention, particularly if renal function is severely impaired or variable with time.

The concurrent administration of several drugs, especially those known to interact pharmacokinetically, is also a situation in which plasma monitoring should be more seriously considered (see DRUG INTERACTIONS in Ch. 241). Finally, plasma concentration monitoring may be useful where noncompliance is likely to occur (see Ch. 243).

Presence of a therapeutic problem: Plasma concentration monitoring may also be helpful when a therapeutic problem arises. The lack of a response at usual or even higher dosages or a toxic reaction at customary or lower dosages represent typical situations. Appropriately planned plasma levels may help explain whether noncompliance, poor availability, altered metabolism, or an unusual pharmacodynamic resistance or sensitivity to the drug is the cause of the problem.

TABLE 239–2 lists additional drugs for which situations may arise in which monitoring may be useful. This list is illustrative, not exhaustive. As more clinical pharmacokinetic information becomes available the status of these drugs and those in TABLE 239–1 will undoubtedly change.

TABLE 239–1. COMMONLY MONITORED DRUGS AND THEIR THERAPEUTIC PLASMA CONCENTRATIONS

Drug	Plasma Concentration Usually Associated with Optimal Therapy (mg/L)
Digitoxin	0.01–0.03*
Digoxin	0.0006–0.002*
Phenobarbital †	10–30
Phenytoin	7–20
Procainamide ‡	4–8
Quinidine	2–5
Theophylline	10–20

* Often expressed in units of ng/ml: digitoxin, 10–30 ng/ml; digoxin, 0.6–2.0 ng/ml.
† When used as an anticonvulsant.
‡ Concentration of active metabolite, N-acetylprocainamide, should also be monitored.

TABLE 239–2. SITUATIONS AND ADDITIONAL DRUGS FOR WHICH PLASMA
CONCENTRATION MONITORING MAY BE USEFUL*

Drug	Plasma Concentration Usually Associated with Optimal Therapy (mg/L) †	Situation(s) Suggesting Monitoring of Drug Concentration
Amikacin	12–25 (1 h after last dose)	Patient with impaired or changing renal function
Ethosuximide	25–75	Question of compliance or when coadministered with other anticonvulsants & source of toxicity is desired
Gentamicin	4–12 (1 h after last dose)	Patient with impaired or changing renal function
Kanamycin	12–25 (1 h after last dose)	Patient with impaired or changing renal function
Lidocaine	1.4–6.0	Patient with chronic hepatic disease or when infusion of drug is prolonged
Lithium	0.7–2.0 (mEq/L)	Patient with partially impaired renal function or on a low sodium diet
Methotrexate		In high dose therapy, concentration is used as a measure of potential toxicity & of a requirement for citrovorum factor rescue
Nortriptyline	0.05–0.15 (50–150 ng/ml)	Inadequate patient response. Plasma concentrations above 0.15 are less effective
Propranolol	0.02–0.2 (20–200 ng/ml)	Question of compliance or low availability. Patient with chronic hepatitis
Primidone ‡	8–12	Question of compliance. Also when coadministered with other anticonvulsants & source of toxicity is desired
Salicylates §	100–300 (10–30 mg/100 ml)	Patient with impaired hearing or patient on high-dose antacid therapy that increases urine pH
Tobramycin	4–12 (1 h after last dose)	Patient with impaired or changing renal function

* Selected examples of situations are given.

† For each drug the therapeutic window is defined in terms of the concentration at the time of sampling. Usually a trough concentration is measured. When concentration units other than mg/L are commonly used, they are so noted.

‡ Metabolized to phenobarbital. The concentration of phenobarbital should also be monitored.

§ Metabolism and protein binding are dose dependent. Serum albumin must be considered in the interpretation of a salicylate concentration. Therapeutic window refers to the anti-inflammatory use of the drug.

Complicating Factors

The use of plasma concentration monitoring for some drugs is limited by a number of complicating factors. One of the major limitations is the occurrence of active metabolites. The antiarrhythmic agent, procainamide, for example, forms an active acetylated metabolite, N-acetylprocainamide, by a hepatic enzyme that shows genetic differences. Procainamide is partially excreted unchanged, while the metabolite is almost entirely handled by the kidneys. Thus, in patients who are rapid acetylators and who have compromised renal function, the correlation between response and procainamide concentration is expected to differ from that observed in patients who are slow acetylators and have normal renal function. The concentration of both the drug and its metabolite should be monitored.

Another complicating factor is delay in the response to a given drug concentration. The effects of digoxin on the heart exemplify a delay caused by the time required to distribute the drug to the active site. For this reason, digoxin concentrations should not be measured within 6 h of a dose, even after IV administration, as the plasma concentration within this time does not reflect the concentration at the active site. An observed response that is an indirect measurement of the actual drug effect may be another cause of delay. The measurement of serum uric acid concentrations following the administration of a uricosuric agent and the determination of the one-stage prothrombin time following use of an oral anticoagulant are examples.

THE THERAPEUTIC WINDOW

The therapeutic window is the range of plasma concentrations with the greatest probability of therapeutic success. However, values of the typical population may be inappropriate for an individual patient. Higher than usual values may be appropriate if the condition is severe and the converse if the condition is mild. Individual exceptions are not uncommon.

For drugs that are bound to plasma proteins and in situations in which an alteration in binding is anticipated, the total concentration (bound + unbound) must be adjusted to give the desired unbound concentration. Conditions which reduce binding to albumin (a protein to which many acidic drugs bind) include end-stage renal disease, cirrhosis, hypoalbuminemia, severe burns, and pregnancy. Binding to α_1-acid glycoprotein and lipoproteins (proteins to which many basic drugs bind) has been observed to be increased during stress and decreased in chronic hepatic disease. In these situations, adjustment of the therapeutic window is accomplished by estimating the fraction unbound in plasma in the patient and comparing it to the usual fraction unbound. Thus,

$$\text{Adjusted concentration} = \frac{\text{Usual fraction unbound}}{\text{Anticipated fraction unbound}} \times \text{Usual concentration}$$

For example, the fraction unbound for phenytoin is increased from 0.1 to about 0.25 in severe renal disease. Therefore, the usual therapeutic window, 7 to 20 mg/L, becomes 3 to 8 mg/L after adjustment.

EVALUATION OF A MEASURED CONCENTRATION

In contrast to usual clinical laboratory tests, the interpretation of plasma drug concentrations requires the application of pharmacokinetic principles. The subsequent presentation is a brief discussion of this application.

Collection of Data

To use plasma concentrations effectively, the history of drug administration, the clinical status of the patient, and a firm knowledge of the clinical pharmacokinetics of the drug are required. TABLE 239-3 lists information that must be collected. The drug administration history, including the doses and times of dosing, and the time of sampling are mandatory, as are the age and weight of the patient.

The need for other information (e.g., renal, hepatic, and cardiovascular functions; serum proteins; active metabolites; assay methods) varies with the drug and the situation. This information must be known by the individual who evaluates the concentration. An ability to estimate renal function from a serum creatinine is also important (see Ch. 144).

Interpretation of Data

After collecting the information needed, including the present and previous, if any, plasma concentrations, two approaches may be taken. One is to compare the observed value with that predicted from known information. This approach is helpful in identifying problems such as noncompliance, low or high availability, or unusually slow or rapid elimination. The other approach is to determine the pharmacokinetic parameters of the drug in the individual. The results of this latter type of analy-

TABLE 239-3. DATA COLLECTION

History of Drug Administration
Drug, dosage, dosage forms, routes of administration, times of administration, compliance, inpatient or outpatient

Time of Sampling (Relative to Dose)

Present and Previous (If Any) Plasma Drug Concentrations

Clinical Status of Patient
Weight, age, sex, condition being treated, concurrent disease states (especially cardiovascular, hepatic, and renal diseases)

Laboratory Data
Renal function (serum creatinine, creatinine clearance, blood urea nitrogen)
Hepatic function (prothrombin time, serum albumin, serum bilirubin, hepatic enzymes in blood)
Protein binding (plasma proteins and albumin)

Concurrent Drug Therapy
Drug interactions
Assay interferences

Active Metabolites

Assay Method (Accuracy, Sensitivity, and Specificity)

Usual Pharmacokinetic Parameters Associated with Type of Patient in Question
Availability, absorption rate constant, volume of distribution, unbound fraction in plasma, renal clearance, hepatic clearance

sis are particularly useful in determining an individual patient's dosage requirements. Whether the measured value is a good estimate of the minimum, average, or maximum concentration at steady state on a fixed-dose, fixed-dosing interval regimen, or a nonsteady-state value obtained shortly after starting the drug or following an unequal dosage schedule, must be immediately established from the dosing history and the time of sampling.

Steady state: A value which represents an estimate of the average steady-state concentration on a fixed-dose, fixed-dosing interval regimen is most readily handled. For a concentration to approximate such a value, a plasma sample must be obtained after dosing for at least 3 half-lives (in the patient). Furthermore, the fluctuation of the concentration within a dosing interval must be small, especially if the sample is obtained just before the next dose. This condition is essentially satisfied if the dosing interval is < 1 half-life. For example, this occurs for the daily administration of digoxin (half-life of 2 days or more). The observed concentration can then be evaluated by comparing it with the expected concentration.

The predicted average concentration, C_{av}, is a function of the expected values of availability, F, and clearance, Cl, and the rate of administration, (D/τ, dose/dosing interval), that is,

$$C_{av} \text{ (expected)} = \frac{F}{Cl} \text{ (expected)} \cdot \frac{D}{\tau} \tag{1}$$

If the ratio of concentrations, observed to predicted, is > 1, either the input is greater or the elimination is slower than expected, or both. The converse is true for a ratio < 1. Thus, a set of explanations is consistent with either observation.

Causes of either an altered input or an altered elimination are summarized in TABLE 239–4. Perhaps the most common cause is the difference between how the patient takes the drug and how he is supposed to or is believed to take it—a compliance problem. Availability is a factor that only needs to be considered for drugs whose availability is low or variable or for situations in which malabsorption is suspected. Renal and hepatic clearances may explain altered elimination depending on the major route of drug elimination. Plasma protein binding is a concern for highly bound drugs because of the dependence of clearance upon it.

Fluctuation: The dosage regimens of many drugs are such that there is considerable fluctuation in the plasma concentration. The dosing interval may be comparable to or greater than the half-life, or the regimen may be similar to a 9–1–5–9 regimen in which the drug is taken q 4 h for 4 doses and then a 12-h interval intervenes. In either case, if there is much fluctuation it must be considered.

For drugs in which the regimen involves considerable fluctuation, the preferred time of sampling is usually just before the next dose. The concentration, C, expected at the end of a fixed dosing interval, τ, following the administration of a fixed dose, D, under steady-state conditions, is

$$C = \frac{F \cdot D \cdot e^{-\frac{Cl}{V} \cdot \tau}}{V \left(1 - e^{-\frac{Cl}{V} \cdot \tau}\right)} \tag{2}$$

where Cl is total clearance, V is the apparent volume of distribution, and F is the availability. Again, the observed concentration may be compared to the value predicted from the expected values of the parameters.

A maximum concentration, that is, from a sample obtained soon after an IV dose or at the peak time after an oral dose, is often unreliable. Either absorption or distribution, or both, may take time to be essentially complete; they also often vary with time and between patients.

When absorption and distribution are rapid, e.g., after the IM administration of the aminoglycosides, measurement of plasma concentration soon after the dose and close to the peak has been found to be useful. Under these conditions, the peak concentration can be estimated from

$$C_{peak} = \frac{F \cdot D}{V \left[1 - e^{-\frac{Cl}{V} \cdot \tau}\right]} \tag{3}$$

or from the relationship

$$C_{peak} = C + F \cdot D/V \tag{4}$$

where $F \cdot D/V$ is the increment of change in the concentration on adding $F \cdot D$ to the body.

TABLE 239-4. CAUSES OF AN UNEXPECTED STEADY-STATE PLASMA CONCENTRATION

Factor Involved	Concentration Ratio >1*	Comment	Concentration Ratio <1	Comment
Compliance	Noncompliance—taking more than directed	Probably less frequently a cause than taking less than directed	Noncompliance—taking less than directed	A very frequent problem
Availability	Higher than usual	Only an explanation if availability is usually low	Lower than usual	A more frequent problem for drugs that are usually poorly absorbed
Renal Clearance	Lower than usual	A valid explanation for drugs whose major route of elimination is renal excretion. May be altered pH, inhibition of secretion, or simply decreased renal function	Greater than usual	Not a frequent explanation. May occur because of altered urine pH or flow. The renal route must usually be or become the major route of elimination
Hepatic Clearance	Lower than usual	An explanation for drugs whose major route of elimination is metabolism or biliary secretion. May be competitive inhibition by another drug, decreased blood flow, hepatic disease, or genetic in origin	Greater than usual	An explanation if hepatic elimination is or becomes the major route of elimination. May be enzyme induction, or activation, or genetic in origin
Plasma Protein Binding	Greater than usual	Not usually an explanation	Less than usual	May be a result of displacement, hypoalbuminemia, hepatic and/or renal disease

* Observed concentration divided by expected concentration

Nonsteady state: A plasma sample may be obtained at a time when the drug has not fully accumulated or following an erratic pattern of previous doses and dosing intervals. Steady-state principles cannot be applied in these circumstances; however, other methods may be used here.

Estimation of Parameter Values

For adjusting dosage in an individual patient, the most useful procedure is to estimate the value of clearance and sometimes the values of the volume of distribution and half-life from the monitored concentration(s). Clearance is the most valuable parameter because it is needed to predict the dosage required to achieve a given concentration and the converse.

From a steady-state value: When a concentration is a good estimate of an average steady-state concentration, availability is not variable, compliance is assured, and the patient is on a fixed-dose fixed-interval dosage regimen, clearance is readily estimated from

$$Cl = \frac{F \cdot D/\tau}{C_{av}} \tag{5}$$

a rearrangement of equation 1. For example, if a digoxin concentration of 1.2 µg/L were obtained on chronically administering 0.125 mg IV (F = 1.0) per day to a patient, the clearance would be 104 L/day. From equation 1, then, a concentration of 1.4 µg/L, a value near the middle of the usual therapeutic window, would be expected on orally (F = 0.6) administering 0.25 mg/day.

Clearance may be calculated from the relationship:

$$Cl = \frac{V}{\tau} \cdot \ln\left[\frac{F \cdot D}{V \cdot C} + 1\right] \tag{6}$$

when a trough concentration is obtained under steady-state conditions, large fluctuations are anticipated (dosing interval $\gg$ half-life), and the drug is given IV or absorption is rapid. As an example, consider gentamicin, a drug whose concentrations fluctuate extensively because the usual half-life and dosing interval are 2 and 8 h, respectively. If a steady-state trough gentamicin concentration of 3 mg/L were obtained in a 70-kg patient on an IV regimen of 80 mg q 8 h, the clearance would be 2.0 L/h (F = 1, V = 0.25 L/kg). One's confidence in the estimate depends on several factors, including variability in the values of V and F, assay errors, and the assumptions above.

The dosage required to achieve a given average concentration can then be computed from the clearance and availability estimates as follows:

$$D/\tau = \frac{Cl}{F} \cdot C_{av} \tag{7}$$

In the example of digoxin above, the daily oral dose required to achieve a concentration of 1.4 µg/L is 0.25 mg. For gentamicin, the 12-h IV dose required to maintain an average concentration of 3 mg/L, from equation 5, is then 72 mg. The peak, equations 3 or 4, and trough, equation 2, are then 5.5 and 1.4 mg/L, respectively.

From a nonsteady-state value: Clearance may also be estimated from a nonsteady-state concentration. As an example, consider the interpretations that would be given to theophylline concentrations obtained in 3 different 70-kg patients 12 h after starting an IV infusion of 42.5 mg/h (aminophylline, 50 mg/h). Clearance is highly variable for theophylline, whereas the volume of distribution is relatively constant (0.5 L/kg). On infusing the drug in patients A, B, and C who have clearances of 20, 40, and 80 ml/h/kg respectively, the plasma concentrations rise as shown in Fig. 239–1. The plasma concentration in patient A reaches toxic levels, but it takes > 24 h of infusion. The concentration in patient B approaches a steady-state value within the therapeutic window. The values for patient C remain subtherapeutic.

For a plasma sample obtained 12 h after starting an infusion, the concentration in patient C is close to a steady-state value and clearance is reasonably estimated using the steady-state approach. The concentrations in patients A and B are not near the steady-state, but the levels do provide some information. The concentration expected at this point in time may be calculated from the values of clearance, Cl, and volume, V, using the relationship

$$C = \frac{R}{Cl} \cdot \left(1 - e^{-\frac{Cl}{V}t}\right) \tag{8}$$

where R is the rate of infusion and t is the duration of the infusion. The steady-state concentration is R/Cl.

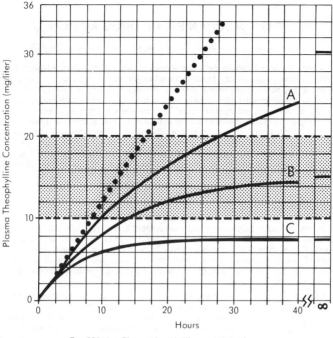

FIG. 239-1. Plasma theophylline concentration.

The observed concentration in patient B is identical to that calculated, indicating that a steady-state concentration of about 15 mg/L will be approached. For patient A, however, the observed value of 12 mg/L is above that expected at this time. A steady-state concentration in the potentially toxic range is possible, but one has little confidence in estimating what the value will be. The reason for the lack of confidence is seen by the dotted line in FIG. 239-1. This line represents the increase in the plasma concentration in a patient who is totally unable to eliminate the drug. The concentration at 12 h in patient A, about 12 mg/L, is close to that, 15 mg/L, which would be observed if no elimination occurs and, as a consequence of analytical and other sources of error, the only valid conclusions to be drawn are that the patient may approach potentially toxic levels and that a subsequent sample should be obtained.

Concentration Dependent Kinetics

For a drug, like phenytoin, whose clearance is concentration dependent, the principles above cannot be applied. Yet, because of its kinetic behavior, monitoring is particularly useful. Michaelis-Menten enzyme kinetic concepts apply here, but they are beyond the scope of this chapter.

FREQUENCY OF MONITORING

How frequently the concentration should be monitored depends on the drug, the confidence one has in estimates from previous measurements, and the presumed change in those factors which influence drug response. For example, digoxin may need to be monitored only occasionally in patients with congestive heart failure whose state of health and drug therapy remain stable, but if their health deteriorates or drugs known to interact with digoxin, e.g., quinidine, are added, more frequent monitoring is indicated. For theophylline, daily or even more frequent monitoring may be required for a patient in an intensive care unit, especially if congestive heart failure, pulmonary edema, or severe constrictive airway disease is present. These conditions alter theophylline metabolism; consequently, dosage requirements are likely to vary.

In summary, plasma concentration monitoring can aid in the management of drug therapy. It permits a more facile and rapid estimation of dosage requirements than by observing drug effects alone. For some drugs it is routinely useful; for others it can be helpful in certain situations.

240.   MECHANISM OF DRUG ACTION

Receptors are specialized cellular or tissue elements with which a drug interacts to produce its characteristic pharmacologic effects. Much work is being devoted to the isolation of actual receptor molecules and it may soon be possible to discuss receptors in terms of their specific structural and physicochemical characteristics. Structurally, receptors appear to be macromolecules such as proteins, enzymes, lipoproteins, and nucleic acids. The formation of a complex between a drug and the receptor is thought to trigger a series of events that alter biologic systems and lead to a pharmacologic effect. Thus, this concept is linked to considerations of the molecular basis of drug action.

Receptors are studied and defined in terms of a known quantity (the drug) and an unknown quantity (the steps between the receptor-drug interaction and observable effects). These effects may be as diverse as inhibition of an enzyme, release of a neurotransmitter, or interference with reabsorption in the renal tubule. However, the effect may be separated both in time and nature from the drug-receptor interaction, which initiates a series of events that only eventually results in the observed response. A drug reacts with a specific receptor but may have multiple effects based upon the organ in which the receptor is located.

The pharmacologic actions of certain drugs apparently are *not* mediated by receptor interaction. For example, neutralization of gastric acid by an antacid is a direct chemical reaction between an acid and a base. Hyperosmotic diuresis is an example of drug action based on the physical properties of solutes. Chelation of heavy metals by some drugs is also not a classic receptor-drug interaction. The lack of reactivity of certain volatile general anesthetics and their varied chemical structures suggest that this action is not mediated by formation of a specific complex with endogenous macromolecules or receptors.

Several theories of drug-receptor interaction have been proposed, but most experimental observations are best explained by a combination of current hypotheses. The Law of Mass Action and the reversibility of drug-receptor interaction served as the basis for the receptor occupation theories, which postulate that the magnitude of the drug-induced effect is proportional to the concentration of the drug-receptor complex. Inherent in this theory are the concepts of **affinity** (the propensity of a drug to bind with a given receptor) and **intrinsic activity** or **efficacy** (the biologic effectiveness per unit of drug-receptor complex). A plot of the drug effect (in terms of **percent of maximum response**) vs. the logarithm of the dose results in a typical sigmoid curve (FIG. 240–1). The increase in response depicted by Curve A represents a graded, continuous process whose magnitude is directly proportional to the combination with, or occupancy of, receptors by the drug molecules.

Curves A and B in FIG. 240–1 illustrate the principles of intrinsic activity and maximal response, which are also called **potency** and **ceiling effect** in clinical terminology. Examination of the log dose-effect relationships for various doses of Drug A and Drug B reveals that more Drug B than Drug A is needed to confer the same degree of pain relief. Thus, Drug A has greater biologic activity per unit

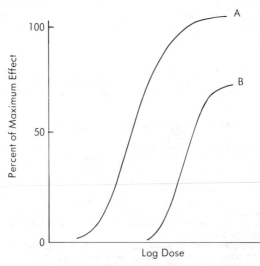

FIG. 240–1.   Log dose–effect curves for morphine (A) and codeine (B).

weight and is more potent than Drug B. In addition, no matter how much Drug B is given, there is a point beyond which no further effect will occur. This is also true of Drug A, but the plateau occurs at a much greater degree of effect. Thus, Drug A is not only more potent than Drug B but it also has a higher maximum or ceiling of activity.

Dose-effect curves and the concepts of affinity and intrinsic activity are useful in defining the interaction of 2 drugs acting on the same receptors. **Such interactions** include competitive antagonism, noncompetitive antagonism, potentiation, and partial agonist (i.e., dual agonist-antagonist) activity.

In some cases, the chemical structure or steric configuration of 2 different drugs is sufficiently similar that both molecules possess an affinity for the same receptor sites. **Agonists** are drugs whose interaction with a receptor serves as the stimulus for a biologic response; such drugs possess both receptor affinity and intrinsic activity (efficacy). Drugs that interact with a receptor but do not initiate the sequence of events leading to an effect are referred to as **antagonists;** such drugs have affinity but lack intrinsic activity. When both agonist and **competitive antagonist** are present in the same biologic system, they compete for the same receptor sites, and a larger dose of the agonist is required to induce the biologic effect at every response level. The dose-effect curve is shifted to the right but is parallel to the curve obtained with the agonist alone (FIG. 240–2). For example, naloxone (N-allyl noroxymorphone), which is structurally similar to morphine, has little or no morphine-like activity, but blocks the expected effects when given before or after morphine. More morphine is needed to overcome the competition, resulting in the characteristic shift to the right of the dose-response curve.

One explanation for the phenomenon of competitive antagonism relates to the **stereospecificity** of the drug-receptor interaction. In some instances, only one of several stereoisomers of the same drug exhibits full agonist activity. Others may be partial agonists or even antagonists. The d and l isomers of epinephrine are structurally identical except for the spatial arrangement of the substitutions on one carbon atom, a seemingly minor difference that results in profound biologic differences. The spatial arrangement may affect the ease with which the drug can approach the crucial area of the receptor or perhaps the binding of the molecule to areas adjacent to the specific receptor site.

Drugs are also **selective,** reacting only with **specific** receptors; selectivity and specificity are hallmarks of the receptor theory of drug action.

The term **noncompetitive antagonism** is used to explain the effect of the antagonist preventing the agonist from having any action at a particular receptor site. In some cases, a noncompetitive antagonist may form a covalent bond with the same receptor with which the corresponding agonist interacts. Noncompetitive antagonist effects may occur at distant sites which prevent the result of the receptor-agonist interaction. The efficacy of one drug is reduced as the concentration of the 2nd drug increases. Affinity of the agonist for the receptor remains unchanged. Instead of a parallel shift in the dose-response curves as with competitive antagonism, in noncompetitive antagonism the curves start at the same point but shift to the right and have a depressed maximum effect (see FIG. 240–3).

Two agonists that react with the same receptor, when administered together, may produce an additive or supra-additive effect at low concentrations, although the maximum attainable response is no greater than that elicited by the more active member of the drug pair (FIG. 240–4). The term **potentiation** describes the effect obtained by a drug combination that is greater than the algebraic sum of the effects of each component. However, the term is also used to describe the ability of one drug to increase the action of another by interfering with its inactivation or elimination.

Certain structural analogs of agonist molecules may exhibit a complex mixture of both agonist and antagonist activities; such dual-acting drugs are referred to as **partial agonists** (FIG. 240–5). Recep-

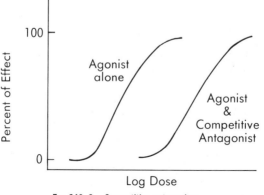

FIG. 240–2.   Competitive antagonism.

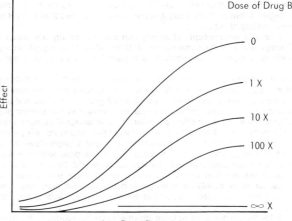

Fig. 240-3.   Theoretical log dose–response curves for noncompetitive interaction between drug A and drug B.

tor activation is usually predominant at low concentrations, whereas receptor blockade is dominant at higher concentrations. Dichloroisoproterenol is a typical partial agonist; at low doses it produces adrenergic β-receptor-mediated effects similar to those of isoproterenol; at higher doses it acts similar to propranolol, blocking interaction of isoproterenol at β-receptor sites.

A variety of physicochemical forces attract the drug to the receptor site, bind it to the receptor, and trigger the characteristic response. Ionic forces (those between oppositely charged atoms) seem most important in the approach of a drug molecule to the receptor site. These are gross forces, however, and may not be as critical as hydrogen bonding and Van der Waals forces in properly aligning and stabilizing the drug-receptor complex. Covalent binding of drugs to receptors usually results in stable long-lasting complexes; such is the case with nitrogen mustard alkylating agents used in chemotherapy of neoplastic diseases.

Tolerance is defined as *either a power or an ability to resist or endure and includes the concept of lack of injury, relative impunity from undesired drug action, or of not being affected in any manner by a drug or poison.* Current medical usage looks at the practical aspects of tolerance—the need to increase the size of subsequent drug doses in order to achieve the same effect obtained previously. Tolerance may be present as a constitutional attribute or it may be acquired. One may exhibit tolerance to continuous or to very large doses of active drug or poison. The complex causes for this phenomenon include preexisting genetic, physiologic, or pathophysiologic factors, such as reduction in drug concentration at its site of action resulting from changes in the number or functional capacity of receptors, changes in cellular responsiveness to drug effects, stimulation or creation of alternative biochemical or metabolic pathways which act to contravine drug effects, and changes in

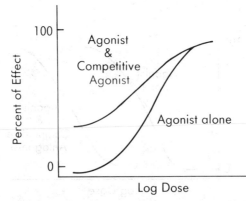

Fig. 240-4.   **Potentiation.** Both agonist and competitive agonist react with the same receptor.

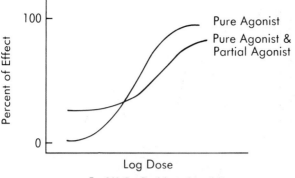

FIG. 240–5. Partial agonist activity.

behavior or psychology which decrease response to a drug. Tolerance may be gradual, requiring many doses and a long period of time (weeks or months) to develop, or acute, requiring a few doses and a short period of time (seconds or minutes). Rapidly developing tolerance to repeated doses of the same drug is termed **tachyphylaxis.** One example of tachyphylaxis involves displacement and depletion of neurotransmitter by repeated doses of an indirect-acting adrenergic agent. Each dose has less effect because it releases less transmitter, since the pool of available transmitter has not been replenished.

241. MODIFICATION OF DRUG RESPONSE

PHARMACOGENETICS

Pharmacogenetics deals with *genetic factors responsible for variations in drug response among individuals.* The original definition was limited to genetic disorders initially revealed by the administration of a drug. Now, the scope includes all of the applications of formal genetic analysis to pharmacology and therapeutics (e.g., therapy of genetic disorders). This discussion, however, is limited to conditions covered by the original definition. Many unexpected and peculiar adverse reactions occurring in a small percentage of individuals exposed to a drug, commonly referred to as "**idiosyncrasies,**" can be explained as genetically determined abnormal reactivity to a drug.

Just as normal ranges exist for physiologic parameters, a random population of individuals given the same dosage of a drug usually will show a quantitative range of responses. This variation is due to both environmental and hereditary factors and in most instances follows a unimodal normal distribution pattern. Occasionally, however, drug responses follow a more complex distribution pattern and there may be two or more recognizable populations (bimodal distribution, FIG. 241-1). There may be a large population showing a normal range and a smaller population (or populations) behaving differently, or the populations may be of equivalent size. These differences are usually due to single inherited factors.

Genetic factors can affect drug response in two ways: by altering drug metabolism, or by modifying the individual's response to the drug. It is important to differentiate between these two interactions. Individuals who manifest *quantitative* abnormalities in the absorption, distribution, biotransformation, or excretion of a specific drug may be given that drug if suitable dosage adjustments are made and the blood or urinary levels of the drug are monitored. However, persons who respond abnormally to a drug, despite dosage adjustments, should generally not be given that drug.

Alteration of the Drug by the Individual

This refers to genetic differences in the absorption, metabolism (biotransformation), transport, and excretion of drugs. For example, persons with plasma **pseudocholinesterase deficiency** (frequency, about 1:2500) have a decreased ability to inactivate succinylcholine (a depolarizing skeletal muscle relaxant), resulting in prolonged paralysis of the respiratory muscles when conventional dosages are used. Prolonged apnea may occur, requiring extended artificial ventilation.

About 50% of the population of the USA have a **defect in isoniazid acetylase** in the liver that results in slow inactivation of isoniazid and other drugs metabolized by the same enzyme system (e.g., hydralazine, sulfamethazine, phenelzine). Slow acetylators tend to be more susceptible to adverse effects, e.g., peripheral neuritis with isoniazid and hydralazine-induced lupus erythematosus, when given conventional dosages of these drugs. Rare genetic biotransformation defects include **deficient**

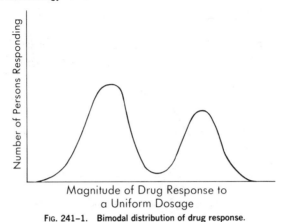

Magnitude of Drug Response to
a Uniform Dosage

Fig. 241-1.   Bimodal distribution of drug response.

parahydroxylation of phenytoin, and certain varieties of **phenacetin-induced methemoglobinemia.** In all the above conditions, the therapeutic dosage of the drug should be reduced or the dosage interval increased.

Normally, chemicals introduced into the body are metabolically detoxified, mainly in the liver. However, in the case of some drugs and chemical agents the metabolites are more toxic (e.g., acetaminophen, methanol, glutethimide, and organophosphorus insecticides), a process that may be referred to as **metabolic toxification.** Agents that have an inducing effect on hepatic enzymes (see DRUG INTERACTIONS below) may lead to increased production of such metabolites. This is clinically relevant, for example, when a patient taking acetaminophen also consumes alcohol or phenobarbital. Inhibiting agents that block the appropriate metabolic pathway may be used to advantage in treatment, e.g., giving N-acetylcysteine for acetaminophen overdose or ethanol for methanol overdose.

Alteration of the Individual's Response to the Drug

Persons with **glucose-6-phosphate dehydrogenase (G6PD) deficiency** may develop hemolytic anemia when given oxidant drugs such as antimalarials, sulfonamides, and certain analgesics. As G6PD is a key enzyme in RBC reduction reactions and these reactions appear to be essential for maintenance of cellular integrity, a deficiency of this enzyme results in an exaggerated sensitivity to the hemolytic effect of certain oxidant drugs. The condition is inherited as a sex-linked recessive trait. Many varieties of drug-induced hemolytic anemia have been described, but the two most important are the African and Mediterranean types. In the former (occurring in about 10% of U.S. blacks), the deficiency is manifested only in the older RBCs, the younger cells being normal. The G6PD levels in these persons are usually 8 to 20% of normal. In the Mediterranean type, levels are lower and the deficiency involves the entire RBC population. (See also ANEMIA DUE TO EXCESSIVE RED CELL DESTRUCTION in Ch. 92.)

Malignant hyperthermia occurs in 1:20,000 surgical procedures involving muscle relaxants and general inhalation anesthetics (most often succinylcholine and halothane). Muscular rigidity is often the first sign of the disorder; other symptoms include tachycardia, arrhythmias, rapidly rising temperature, acidosis, and shock. This rapidly progressive reaction, which is inherited as an autosomal dominant trait, is often fatal (70% in untreated cases); *therapy should be initiated immediately.* All anesthetic agents should be discontinued at once and dantrolene administered by rapid IV push, starting with 1 mg/kg and continuing until symptoms begin to subside, or up to a total dose of 10 mg/kg. Corrective therapy should also include management of metabolic acidosis and core and surface cooling. Susceptible family members can be identified by elevated CPK levels and muscle biopsy for histochemistry, electronmicroscopy, and in vitro exposure to halothane. If a susceptible person needs an operation, it should be done under local anesthesia or neuroleptic analgesia.

Approximately 5% of the U.S. population respond abnormally to **corticosteroids** by marked increases in intraocular pressure; glaucoma may develop. The condition is inherited as an autosomal recessive trait.

Genetic **warfarin resistance** is inherited as an autosomal dominant trait. The exact mechanism is unclear, but it probably operates at a receptor or enzymatic level in the liver. Genetic **warfarin sensitivity** also occurs.

In patients with certain types of **porphyria** (see ANOMALIES IN PIGMENT METABOLISM in Ch. 82), acute attacks can be precipitated by barbiturates and other drugs (e.g., sulfonamides, aminopyrine, phenylbutazone). The mechanism involves induction of the enzyme δ-aminolevulinic acid synthetase (ALA synthetase), which results in increased porphyrin production.

INDIVIDUAL VARIATION DUE TO ENVIRONMENTAL FACTORS

Apart from the genetically determined differences in drug response mentioned above, individuals may differ widely in their response to drugs because of environmental factors. Both internal and external environmental factors can cause marked variation in drug response, even within the same individual. For example, diurnal and circadian variations, changes in temperature, diet, disease states, menstruation, various drugs, and changes in posture may influence response to a particular drug, mainly by altering its pharmacokinetics (e.g., decreased renal function in elderly patients on conventional dosages of digitalis may lead to retention and an increased incidence of toxicity), but also by altering the response of the body to the drug (e.g., hypokalemia, hypomagnesemia, or hypercalcemia may potentiate certain effects of digitalis).

DRUG INTERACTIONS

Alteration of the effects of one drug by the prior or concurrent administration of another. The usual result is an increase or decrease of the effects of one of the drugs. Desired interactions are usually considered in the context of combination therapy (e.g., in the treatment of hypertension, asthma, certain infections, and malignancy), in which two or more drugs are used to increase therapeutic effects and/or reduce toxicity. Unwanted interactions can cause adverse drug reactions (ADRs) or produce therapeutic failure.

Relatively few of the known or suggested drug interactions have been sufficiently analyzed to determine their clinical significance, and the possibility of problems developing must be viewed in perspective. If an interaction appears likely, therapeutic alternatives should be considered; however, a patient should not be deprived of needed therapy because of the possibility of an interaction. Drug interactions are either pharmacodynamic or pharmacokinetic. **Pharmacodynamic interactions** include the concurrent administration of drugs having the same (or opposing) pharmacologic actions and alteration of the sensitivity or the responsiveness of the tissues to one drug by another. Many of these interactions can be predicted from a knowledge of the pharmacology of each drug. By monitoring the patient clinically, deviations from the expected effect can often be quickly detected and the dosage adjusted accordingly. Although the majority of drug interactions are of the pharmacodynamic type, most of the literature deals with the pharmacokinetic type.

Pharmacokinetic interactions are more complicated and difficult to predict because the interacting drugs have unrelated actions and the interactions are mainly due to the processes of absorption, distribution, metabolism, and excretion, which change the amount and duration of a drug's availability at receptor sites. The *type* of response expected from the component drugs is *not* changed, only the *magnitude* and *duration*. Thus, a pharmacokinetic interaction is confined to an altered effect of one of the participating drugs and is predictable from a knowledge of what the individual drugs can do. Such interactions may be detected by the usual patient-monitoring procedures. A change in blood drug levels usually occurs and useful information may be obtained by measuring these levels.

PHARMACODYNAMIC INTERACTIONS

Drugs With Opposing Pharmacologic Effects

Interactions resulting from the use of two drugs with opposing pharmacologic effects should be among the easiest to detect. However, there may be factors that preclude early identification of such an antagonism. For example, an ophthalmologist may prescribe a cholinergic drug (e.g., pilocarpine) for a patient who is also taking an anticholinergic preparation (e.g., propantheline) prescribed by his family physician for a GI condition.

Drugs With Similar Pharmacologic Effects

An example of this type of interaction is the increased CNS-depressant effect that often occurs when persons taking sedatives or tranquilizers consume alcoholic beverages. Many individuals risk this combination and experience no difficulty, but it can be lethal.

An excessive anticholinergic effect can develop with the concurrent use of drugs that all produce such effects, for example, an antipsychotic agent (e.g., chlorpromazine), an antiparkinson drug (e.g., trihexyphenidyl), and a tricylic antidepressant (e.g., amitriptyline). In some individuals, particularly geriatric patients, this response may result in an atropine-like delirium that could be mistakenly interpreted as a worsening of the psychiatric symptoms. Distinguishing between the symptoms of the condition being treated and the effects of the drugs being employed as therapy may be difficult, but is essential.

Interactions Involving the Adrenergic System

The enzyme monoamine oxidase (MAO) metabolizes catecholamines such as norepinephrine. Increased levels of norepinephrine accumulate within the adrenergic neurons when MAO is inhibited. Any drug that releases greater than usual amounts of norepinephrine can bring about exaggerated responses, including severe headache, hypertension (possibly a hypertensive crisis), and cardiac arrhythmias. Such an interaction may occur between MAO inhibitors (e.g., isocarboxazid, phenelzine, tranylcypromine, and pargyline) and indirectly-acting sympathomimetic amines. Although most sympathomimetic amines (e.g., amphetamine) are available only by prescription, others (e.g., ephedrine, phenylephrine, and phenylpropanolamine), known to interact with MAO inhibitors, are present in many popular nonprescription cold and allergy remedies. Patients taking MAO inhibitors should *avoid* using such products.

Serious reactions (hypertensive crises) have occurred in patients being treated with MAO inhibitors following the ingestion of certain foods and beverages having a high tyramine content, including certain cheeses, beer and wines, chocolate, and pickled herring. Tyramine is metabolized by MAO, normally found in the intestinal wall and the liver; this enzyme protects against the pressor actions of amines in foods. When the enzyme is inhibited, unmetabolized tyramine can accumulate, releasing norepinephrine from the adrenergic neurons.

The antineoplastic drug procarbazine and the anti-infective drug furazolidone (or probably its metabolite) can also inhibit MAO and the same warnings apply to these drugs as to other MAO inhibitors. With furazolidone, however, the enzyme inhibition usually does not occur within the first 5 days of therapy and the course of treatment is often completed within that time.

The antihypertensive agent guanethidine is transported to its site of action within adrenergic neurons by a system that is also responsible for the uptake of norepinephrine and several indirectly-acting sympathomimetic amines such as ephedrine and the amphetamines. Concentration of guanethidine in these neurons is necessary for its hypotensive effect. Tricyclic antidepressants can inhibit the uptake of guanethidine into the neuron terminal, thereby preventing its concentration at these sites and antagonizing the hypotensive effect. The effect of guanethidine is also antagonized by amphetamine, ephedrine, methylphenidate, chlorpromazine, and other antipsychotic agents.

Alteration of Electrolyte Levels (see Ch. 255)

PHARMACOKINETIC INTERACTIONS

Alteration of Gastrointestinal Absorption

Interactions that involve a change in the absorption of a drug from the GI tract are of variable importance. Overall absorption of the drug may be reduced and its therapeutic activity compromised, or absorption may be delayed though the same amount of drug is eventually absorbed. A delay in drug absorption is undesirable when a rapid effect is needed to relieve acute symptoms, such as pain, or when the effects of a drug may be unduly prolonged (e.g., the patient may have excessive residual sedation in the morning).

Alteration of pH: Since many drugs are weak acids or weak bases, the pH of the GI contents can influence absorption. Since the nonionized (more lipid-soluble) form of a drug is more readily absorbed than the ionized form, acidic drugs are usually more readily absorbed from the upper regions of the GI tract, where they are primarily in a nonionized form. By raising the pH of the GI contents, antacids may delay the absorption of pentobarbital, an acidic substance, and decrease, or delay, its hypnotic effect.

Complexation and adsorption: Tetracycline derivatives can combine with metal ions (e.g., calcium, magnesium, aluminum, and iron) in the GI tract to form poorly absorbed complexes. Thus, certain dietary items (e.g., milk) or drugs (e.g., antacids, products containing magnesium, aluminum, and calcium salts, or iron preparations) can significantly decrease the amount of tetracycline absorbed. Absorption of two tetracyclines, doxycycline and minocycline, is apparently not markedly influenced by the simultaneous ingestion of food or milk; one of these agents might thus be preferred when gastric irritation occurs or appears likely. Aluminum-containing antacids will, however, decrease the absorption of these tetracyclines; it is likely that the increase in pH of the GI contents also contributes to the reduction of absorption of the tetracyclines.

Complexation can be expected with cholestyramine and colestipol. In addition to binding with and preventing reabsorption of bile acids, these agents can bind with drugs in the GI tract, having the greatest affinity for acidic drugs. They can interfere with the absorption of thyroid hormone, warfarin, and other drugs. Therefore, to minimize the possibility of an interaction, the interval between the administration of cholestyramine or colestipol and another drug should be as long as possible (preferably, at least 4 h).

The absorption of digoxin may be significantly reduced by the simultaneous use of kaolin-pectin mixtures or antacids. Physical adsorption of digoxin to these agents represents the most likely explanation for the occurrence of the interaction, although other mechanisms also may be involved.

Alteration of motility: By increasing GI motility, a cathartic may hasten the passage of drugs through the GI tract, resulting in decreased absorption, particularly of drugs that require prolonged contact with the absorbing surface and those that are absorbed only at a particular site along the GI tract. Similar problems can occur with enteric-coated and sustained-release formulations.

By decreasing GI motility, anticholinergics may either reduce absorption by retarding dissolution and slowing gastric emptying, or increase absorption by keeping a drug for a longer period of time in the area of optimal absorption.

Alteration of Distribution

Displacement of drugs from protein-binding sites: This type of interaction may occur when two drugs capable of protein-binding are given concurrently, especially when they are capable of binding to the same sites on the protein molecule **(competitive displacement)**. Since there are a limited number of plasma or tissue protein-binding sites, drugs can displace one another. Although the protein-bound fraction of a drug is not pharmacologically active, an equilibrium exists between the bound and unbound fractions. As the unbound or free drug is metabolized and excreted, the bound drug is gradually released to maintain the equilibrium and pharmacologic response. The risk of interactions from protein displacement is significant primarily with drugs that are highly protein-bound ($>$ 90%) and have a small apparent volume of distribution, and during the first few days of concurrent therapy.

Both phenylbutazone and warfarin are extensively bound to plasma proteins, especially albumin, though phenylbutazone has a greater affinity for the binding sites. When the two are taken concurrently, fewer binding sites are available for warfarin, the amount of free drug is increased, and the activity of the free anticoagulant and the risk of hemorrhage are increased.

Chloral hydrate also may potentiate warfarin response. Trichloroacetic acid, a highly protein-bound major metabolite of chloral hydrate, can displace warfarin from protein binding sites and thus increase the anticoagulant response. However, the clinical importance of this phenomenon is limited.

Alteration of Metabolism

Stimulation of metabolism: Many drug interactions result from the ability of one drug to stimulate the metabolism of another by increasing the activity of hepatic microsomal enzymes involved in their metabolism **(enzyme induction).** In this manner, phenobarbital increases the rate of metabolism of coumarin anticoagulants such as warfarin, resulting in a *decreased* anticoagulant response. The dose of the anticoagulant must be increased to compensate for this effect, though this is potentially dangerous if the patient discontinues the phenobarbital without appropriately reducing the anticoagulant dose. The use of alternative sedatives (e.g., the benzodiazepines) eliminates this risk. Phenobarbital also accelerates the metabolism of other drugs, such as digitalis and steroid hormones. Enzyme induction is also caused by other barbiturates and by various therapeutic agents (e.g., glutethimide) and chemicals (e.g., insecticides).

Studies have associated disturbed calcium metabolism and osteomalacia with the use of anticonvulsants such as phenobarbital and phenytoin. The reduced serum calcium levels are due to vitamin D deficiency, resulting from enzyme induction by the anticonvulsants. The possibility of deficiency developing is greatest when the patient's dietary intake of vitamin D is borderline.

Pyridoxine can antagonize the activity of the antiparkinson drug levodopa by accelerating the conversion of the levodopa to its active metabolite, dopamine, in the peripheral tissues. In contrast to levodopa, dopamine cannot cross the blood-brain barrier, where it is required for the antiparkinson effect. In patients receiving both levodopa and carbidopa (a decarboxylase inhibitor), the addition of pyridoxine does not reduce the action of levodopa.

Recent studies show that the efficacy of certain drugs (e.g., chlorpromazine, diazepam, propoxyphene, and theophylline) may be decreased in individuals who smoke heavily. This is due to increased hepatic enzyme activity resulting from the action of polycyclic hydrocarbons found in cigarette smoke.

Inhibition of metabolism: One drug may inhibit the metabolism of another, causing its prolonged and intensified activity. For example, disulfiram, used in the treatment of alcoholism, inhibits the activity of aldehyde dehydrogenase, thus inhibiting the oxidation of acetaldehyde, an oxidation product of alcohol. This results in the accumulation of excessive acetaldehyde and causes the characteristic disulfiram effect (see under Treatment in DEPENDENCE ON ALCOHOL in Ch. 136). Disulfiram exhibits several other inhibitory actions that can result in drug interactions. It has been reported to enhance the activity of warfarin, phenytoin, and isoniazid, presumably by inhibiting their metabolism.

Allopurinol reduces the production of uric acid by inhibiting the enzyme xanthine oxidase. However, xanthine oxidase is involved in the metabolism of such potentially toxic drugs as mercaptopurine and azathioprine; when the enzyme is inhibited, the effect of these two agents can be markedly increased. Therefore, when allopurinol is given concurrently, a *reduction* to about one third to one fourth the usual dose of mercaptopurine or azathioprine is advised. Thioguanine, which is closely related chemically and pharmacologically to mercaptopurine and azathioprine, is apparently not influenced by allopurinol.

Alteration of Urinary Excretion

Alteration of urinary pH: Urinary pH influences the ionization of weak acids and bases and thus affects their reabsorption and excretion. A drug in its nonionized form more readily diffuses from the glomerular filtrate into the blood. More of an acidic drug is in the nonionized form in an acid urine than in an alkaline urine, where it primarily exists as an ionized salt. Thus, more of an acidic drug (e.g., a salicylate) diffuses back into the blood from an acid urine, resulting in a prolonged and perhaps intensified activity. Opposite effects are seen for a basic drug like dextroamphetamine. When the urinary pH was maintained at about 5 in one investigation, 54.5% of a dose of dextroamphetamine was excreted within 16 h, compared to a 2.9% excretion when the pH value was maintained at about 8.

Interference with urinary excretion: Probenecid can increase the serum levels and prolong the activity of penicillin derivatives, primarily by blocking their tubular excretion. Such combinations have been used to therapeutic and economic advantage. For example, probenecid improves the effectiveness of penicillin and its analogs when used in single-dose regimens in the treatment of gonorrhea.

PRINCIPLES OF MANAGEMENT

The following general points concerning drug interactions warrant emphasis:

1. The drugs for which interactions are most significant clinically are those with potent effects, low safety margins, and a steep dose-response curve; e.g., warfarin, digoxin, cytotoxics, hypotensives, and hypoglycemic agents.

2. It may be difficult to distinguish a drug interaction from other pathophysiologic factors affecting the response to therapy.

3. Not all patients develop reactions, even when it is known that interactions may occur. Individual factors, such as dose and metabolism, determine whether the phenomenon occurs.

4. When the effects of drugs are being closely monitored, an interaction usually requires a change of dosage or therapy (physician response) and does not result in significant problems for the patient.

5. *In the displacement-from-protein-binding types of interaction, one fact is often overlooked.* Any displacement alters the relationship between total and unbound drug and thus complicates the clinical interpretation of total drug levels in the blood. Total plasma concentrations of highly bound and displaceable drugs do not have the same meaning in the presence of displacing drugs as in their absence. Awareness of this becomes more important as blood levels are increasingly used to aid in the therapeutic control of patients on a variety of drugs. It would be desirable, and in some cases it may be necessary, to use ultrafiltrates of plasma samples rather than whole plasma for determinations of drug concentrations.

To minimize the incidence and clinical consequences of drug interactions, the prescriber should (1) know the patient's total drug intake, including all agents prescribed by others and those that are purchased without a prescription; (2) prescribe as few drugs in as low doses for as short a time as needed to achieve a desired effect and avoid unnecessary combinations; (3) know the effects, both wanted and unwanted, of all the drugs used (since the spectrum of drug interactions is usually contained within these effects) and know the slope of dose-response curves (i.e., the drug should be one for which the dosage range permits a considerable margin of error); (4) observe and monitor the patient for the drugs' effects, particularly after any alteration in therapy (some interactions, e.g., metabolic effects depending on enzyme induction may take a week or more to appear); and (5) consider drug interactions as possible causes of any unanticipated troubles. If unexpected clinical responses do occur, blood levels of drugs being taken should be measured, if possible; the literature or someone with specific knowledge of drug interactions should be consulted; and, most importantly, the dose of the drug should be altered until the desired effect is obtained. If this fails, the drug should be changed to one that will not interact with the other being taken.

---

242. DRUG TOXICITY

PRECLINICAL AND CLINICAL EVALUATION OF TOXICITY

Before a drug is approved for general clinical use by the FDA, preclinical and clinical data showing substantial evidence of safety and efficacy are required by law. Drug studies proceed through various phases.

Preclinical Investigation (Animal Studies)

Current guidelines issued by the FDA specify a stepwise increase in the duration of the animal toxicity testing required before certain levels of human exposure are allowed. For most drugs, initial human administration (Phase I clinical studies, see below) can be started after 2- to 4-wk studies in 2 animal species; Phase II clinical studies require the completion of 90-day studies in 2 animal species; and before the manufacturer submits an application for marketing of his product, he must have completed 1-yr dog, 18-mo mouse, and 2-yr rat studies. Certain classes of drugs (e.g., oral contraceptives) have different requirements.

Once data have been derived from these studies, it is possible to plot drug effects, both therapeutic and toxic, against the log dosage. This provides dose-response curves for wanted and unwanted effects, and the relationship between these gives an indication of the safety margin. The **therapeutic index** refers to the dose ratio between toxic and therapeutic effects (see FIG. 242–1). The therapeutic index in animals can be expressed as the ratio LD50/ED50, where LD50 is the dose lethal to 50% of a population and the ED50 is the dose therapeutically effective in 50% of a comparable population. Therefore, the greater the therapeutic index, the greater the safety margin for a particular drug. This concept becomes less important in clinical situations dealing with individuals, where the concern is usually related to nonlethal events and the smallest dose that will be associated with a serious toxic reaction. The concept is more complex to apply in clinical practice because of the multiplicity of toxic effects, each of which may have its own dose-response curve, and because the toxic and therapeutic curves may not be parallel.

Clinical Investigation (Human Studies)

Clinical studies of new drugs are conducted in 3 phases. The widespread general use of the drug (and postmarketing surveillance of drug use) can be regarded as a 4th phase.

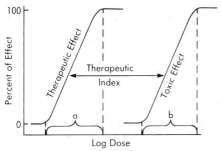

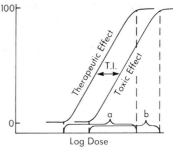

FIG. 242-1. Therapeutic index.

Drug A: Large therapeutic index with no overlap between therapeutic (a) and toxic (b) dose range; thus, a wide safety margin.

Drug B: Small therapeutic index with overlap between therapeutic (a) and toxic (b) dose range; thus, a small safety margin.

Phase 1 represents the first administration of a new drug to man. As in all human experimentation, informed consent is a prerequisite. Phase 1 studies can be performed only after certain legal requirements have been met, such as submitting the results of animal studies, information about product composition and manufacture, the intended clinical study protocol, approval from the local Institutional Review Board (IRB), and information about the training and experience of the investigators to the FDA, whose permission is required to initiate the study. These investigational drug studies are performed under a permit from the FDA known as an investigational new drug exemption permit **(IND)**. A small number of closely monitored subjects, mainly healthy volunteers, are usually involved. Initially, each receives a single dose of the drug to determine a safe dose range and assess pharmacokinetic data.

Phase 2 can begin after satisfactory preliminary evidence regarding safety has been obtained. It involves the carefully supervised administration of the drug to patients for treatment of, or prophylaxis against, the disease or symptoms for which the drug is intended, usually in randomized clinical trials. This is also often the first opportunity to observe the effect of long-term administration of the drug in humans.

Phase 3 begins after the initial phases have provided reasonable evidence of safety and efficacy. It consists of more widespread clinical trials that may move from the realm of full-time investigators to practicing physicians. Phase 3 extends up to the time of release of the drug for general use.

Phase 4 is the naturalistic phase of study and, though often not recognized as a phase of clinical investigation, is a most important one from a clinical standpoint. Increasingly, this phase is being formalized with specific protocols for post-marketing surveillance. Feedback is obtained from the use of a drug that is past the legally required investigational phase. Because the drug may be given to large numbers of people, new therapeutic effects may be discovered, rare or long-term side effects may be spotted, and drug-drug or drug-disease interactions may be discovered. An example is the fortuitous observation that the antiviral drug amantadine also improves extrapyramidal symptoms in parkinsonian patients.

ADVERSE DRUG REACTIONS

Adverse drug reactions (ADRs) embody *a wide variety of toxic drug reactions, dose- or non-dose-related, that occur in therapeutic situations.* The term usually excludes nontherapeutic overdosage due, for example, to accidental exposure or attempted suicide, and also usually excludes situations where the drug fails to have its intended effect (i.e., excludes lack of efficacy).

Assessing the incidence and consequences of ADRs is extremely difficult. Cause-effect relationships are often difficult or impossible to prove. The ultimate proof, which may be unobtainable in cases of severe reactions, depends on disappearance of the effect on withdrawal of the suspected drug (although some severe reactions are irreversible) and reappearance on rechallenge. It is also difficult to select a control population in a clinical setting to differentiate drug-related symptoms and signs from those that are non-drug-related; thus, there is a wide variation in the methods used to collect data on ADRs. Some studies rely on reactions reported voluntarily by physicians; others involve selected patient groups (such as medical inpatients); information from patients may be collected by direct questioning or by patients volunteering information.

There is also a potential for both under- and overestimating the incidence of ADRs. Perhaps 1 to 3% of admissions to hospital *medical* services are due to drug reactions (excluding deliberate overdose or drug abuse). This figure is reduced considerably when all services in a hospital are considered, since drug reactions contribute insignificantly to admissions on some services; e.g., surgical admissions. Among patients hospitalized on a general medical service the incidence of mild to severe side effects may be as high as 10%. These data are difficult to interpret in terms of cause-effect relationships, mortality, morbidity, and cost. The incidence of drug-related deaths is unknown, but probably only a few deaths in medical units are drug-related, and these are often in patients with serious diseases that warrant such risks.

The incidence and severity of drug toxicity can also be influenced by such patient variables as age, sex, disease, genetic factors, geographic factors, and by such drug-related factors as type of drug, route of administration, duration of therapy, dosage, and bioavailability. The extent to which misprescribing and patient compliance errors also contribute to the incidence of ADRs is not clear.

The most commonly reported causes of drug-related deaths are (1) **gastrointestinal hemorrhage and peptic ulceration** (corticosteroids, aspirin, other anti-inflammatory drugs, anticoagulants); (2) **other hemorrhages** (anticoagulants, cytostatic agents); (3) **aplastic anemia** (chloramphenicol, phenylbutazone, gold salts, cytostatic agents); (4) **hepatic damage** (chlorpromazine, isoniazid); (5) **renal failure** (analgesics); (6) **infection** (corticosteroids, cytostatic drugs); and (7) **anaphylaxis** (penicillin, antisera). Allergy is an important factor in nonfatal drug reactions, but is less important as a cause of death.

Dose-Related, Predictable Drug Reactions

Although individuals vary considerably in their responsiveness to a particular drug effect, most drug toxicity is related to the amount of drug taken; the nature of the toxic manifestations is determined by the properties of the drug molecule. Previous contact with the drug is not necessary for the development of toxic reactions. Dose-related reactions can occur as side effects or overdosage toxicity.

Side effects are *unwanted, predictable pharmacologic effects that occur within therapeutic dose ranges.* These effects may be wanted under certain circumstances. For example, antihistamines given for hay fever may cause drowsiness as a side effect, but drowsiness may be a wanted effect when an antihistamine is given as a mild hypnotic. Other examples of predictable dose-related side effects are dyspepsia and tinnitus that occur with high doses of aspirin.

Overdosage toxicity is *the predictable toxic effect that occurs with dosages in excess of the therapeutic range for a particular patient.* It overlaps with side-effect toxicity to some extent, especially in drugs with a small therapeutic index. The higher the dose, the more severe the effect (e.g., hemorrhage with oral anticoagulants or convulsions due to local anesthetic agents). A number of drugs may be ototoxic (see Ch. 167).

Non-Dose-Related, Unpredictable Effects

Drug allergy: Allergic reactions depend on altered reactivity of the patient as a result of prior contact with a drug that functions as an antigen or allergen. Allergic reactions are not related to dose level; the symptoms and signs which develop are determined by antigen-antibody interactions and are largely independent of the pharmacologic properties of the drug molecule. In a strict sense, allergic reactions are not completely unpredictable because a careful clinical history and appropriate skin tests may enable some definition of a population at risk. This subject is discussed in greater detail under Drug Hypersensitivity in Ch. 19 (see also Drug Eruptions in Ch. 196).

Idiosyncrasy is an imprecise term which has been used as a catch-all classification for unexpected and peculiar adverse reactions occurring in a small percentage of individuals exposed to a drug. Idiosyncratic reactions are not related to a drug's known pharmacologic effects and are not obviously allergic in nature. The aplastic anemia occurring with chloramphenicol might be considered as an example. Idiosyncrasy has been recently defined by some as *a genetically determined abnormal reactivity to a drug,* but not all idiosyncratic reactions have a pharmacogenetic cause. The term "idiosyncrasy" may become obsolete as specific mechanisms of adverse drug reactions become elucidated (see Pharmacogenetics in Ch. 241). For example, hemolysis occurring in individuals taking certain drugs (e.g., antimalarials) can no longer be considered idiosyncratic, because a genetic predisposition (G6PD deficiency) can be detected in the laboratory and hemolysis is therefore predictable and dose-related.

Management and Prevention

Prevention requires a familiarity with the drug used and an awareness of the potential reactions to it, since ADRs can often be recognized before serious effects develop.

If a reaction occurs, the type and any precipitating factors (e.g., digitalis toxicity occurring from hypokalemia due to concurrent diuretic therapy) must be determined if possible. With dose-related side effects, dose modification or attention to precipitating factors may suffice; increasing the rate of drug elimination is rarely necessary. With non-dose-related side effects, the drug should usually be withdrawn and re-exposure avoided.

CARCINOGENESIS

A carcinogen is a *chemical or physical agent that has the potential of producing neoplasia.* Carcinogens have several important characteristics: (1) Effects are usually dose-dependent, additive, and irreversible. A single dose of a carcinogen can be equivalent in effect to the same total dosage incurred gradually over a long period. (2) There is usually a latent period (equivalent to at least 30 cell divisions in in vitro systems) following exposure before malignant change develops. In humans, carcinogenesis may take years; e.g., some victims of the Hiroshima bomb developed leukemia 15 yr after exposure, and an association has been found between women who took diethylstilbestrol during pregnancy and some of their daughters who developed vaginal carcinoma 15 to 20 yr later. (3) Although certain carcinogens have similarities in chemical structure, it is impossible to predict all carcinogenicity on this basis. (4) There are marked species, strain, and sex differences in susceptibility to carcinogens. (5) Many carcinogens require metabolic activation to produce the carcinogenically active form. This makes in vitro testing methods for carcinogenicity problematical and accounts for some of the species differences.

Malignancies may be produced with many therapeutic agents if the species, route of administration, and dosage are appropriate. It is important not only to determine whether a drug is carcinogenic in experimental situations, but also to evaluate the clinical significance of the carcinogenic potential. Determining which drugs have a high potential for carcinogenesis is a major problem. Animal screening tests may reveal tumor development in certain species that would not occur in humans; conversely, certain tumors may occur in humans which would not be detected in laboratory animals. The detection of a low incidence of carcinogenesis is another problem. For example, if a carcinogen induces neoplasia in 1% of experimental animals at a specific dosage, 300 animals must be tested to be sure of seeing even one tumor at 95% confidence limits.

Because of the latent period, restricted dosages, and the small numbers of experimental subjects, carcinogenic potential not evident in animal tests is unlikely to be manifested in clinical trials prior to marketing of the drug. Once a drug is marketed, it is usually administered to large numbers of patients, often on a long-term basis, making this the most likely time for detection of carcinogenic associations. Controlled clinical studies of this nature are difficult, if not impossible, to conduct, and associations usually become apparent through clusters of cases or "epidemics" of neoplasia discovered at a later date.

Therapeutically, all drugs with a high carcinogenic potential should be avoided if possible and benefit-risk assessments should be made in all instances. For example, though alkylating chemotherapeutic agents are potent carcinogens in a variety of animals, it would be illogical to withhold them from a patient with a potentially lethal disease. (The situation is analogous to exposure to x-rays, which also have carcinogenic potential.)

There are actually very few drugs in use for which there is good evidence of carcinogenesis in humans. Oral contraceptives appear rarely to cause hepatic adenomas, which are benign in terms of their own growth, but they are extremely vascular and can cause fatal hemorrhage. An association between reserpine and carcinoma of the breast has been claimed by some workers on the basis of case-control studies, but has not been confirmed by others in cohort studies. There is convincing evidence that some nondrug chemicals are carcinogens. This evidence includes the associations between aflatoxin and hepatoma, vinyl chloride and liver hemangiosarcoma, coal tars and skin cancer, cigarette smoke and lung carcinoma, and aniline dyes and bladder tumors.

BENEFIT-TO-RISK RATIO

In every therapeutic endeavor, risks must be weighed against benefits for each particular clinical situation and patient. Drug therapy is justified only if the possible benefits outweigh the possible risks after considering the qualitative and quantitative impact of the use of a drug and the likely outcome if drug therapy is withheld. This decision depends on adequate clinical knowledge of the patient, knowledge of the disease and its natural history, and knowledge of the drugs pertinent to the specific situation.

Although the term "benefit-to-risk ratio" is convenient and often used, for individual patients numerical predictions of benefit or risk do not exist, and the mathematical division (to obtain a ratio) is never performed. The term is used to describe informed clinical judgment.

Patient factors: Age, sex, presence or capability of pregnancy, occupation, social circumstances, genetic traits, etc., may change the magnitude of risks and benefits by influencing the course and severity of the disease or the response to medication. Examples include the poor prognosis of very young or old patients with pneumonia that requires aggressive therapy, the sensitivity of the fetus to drugs which may be relatively safe for a nonpregnant woman, and industrial exposure to organophosphates or genetic cholinesterase deficiency resulting in increased sensitivity to depolarizing muscle relaxants. A 60-yr-old patient with atherosclerosis, a poor cerebral blood flow, and a blood pressure of 200/120 requires different therapy than would an otherwise healthy young patient with the same blood pressure.

Disease factors such as the course, duration, mortality, and morbidity influence risks and benefits of treatment. It makes little sense to treat a self-limiting disease causing little debility, such as herpes labialis with a potent systemic drug such as cytarabine, whereas such therapy may be justified in herpetic encephalitis, which is otherwise usually fatal.

Drug factors include the frequency, severity, and predictability of adverse reactions, the relationship of such reactions to dosage, the means by which they can be prevented or treated, and the availability of alternative drugs or therapies. For example, penicillin anaphylaxis is rare, but it is potentially fatal and may sometimes be avoided by taking an adequate history and doing appropriate skin tests. If anaphylaxis occurs when one is prepared for it, successful treatment is possible. Penicillin, therefore, should not ordinarily be withheld in streptococcal pharyngitis for fear of anaphylaxis. On the other hand, aplastic anemia due to chloramphenicol is also fatal and relatively rare, but it is unpredictable and often irreversible. Therefore, although chloramphenicol is also effective against streptococcal pharyngitis, safer alternatives exist, and its use is not justified. However, for a serious disease such as *Haemophilus influenzae* meningitis, few alternative drugs exist and chloramphenicol therapy may be justified.

A drug's efficacy should also be known, including the predictability of a favorable response, whether the effect is symptomatic or curative, the relationship to dosage, and the duration of the beneficial effect. Acute myeloid leukemia in children responds to aggressive combination chemotherapy and is justified. However, use of aggressive chemotherapy is debatable in such malignancies as gastric carcinoma, where the response to chemotherapy is poor and therapy may increase morbidity.

Judicious use of drug combinations may increase benefits and reduce risks; e.g., the use of adrenergic blocking agents with a thiazide diuretic and potassium supplements in the treatment of hypertension.

---

243.   PATIENT COMPLIANCE

The degree to which patients adhere to a treatment plan.

Even the most thorough and well-designed therapeutic regimen will fail without patient compliance. Depending on the variable studied and the strictness of definition, from 15% to 95% of patients studied have been found to be noncompliant. Overall, probably a third to a half of patients make some error with their medications—incorrect dose, errors in timing, adding unprescribed medications, or not taking medication. Capricious or irregular dosing exposes a patient to the risks of medication without concomitant therapeutic benefit. While most patients occasionally default or make errors, some never stray and others continually fail to comply.

It is difficult to identify patients who do not take their medications as prescribed. The same patient may act differently depending on the treatment, disease, adverse effects, or other factors in his life. In dealing with noncompliance, *the prescriber must discuss it with the patient and ascertain why the patient is not following the prescribed treatment.* The cause for noncompliance may be remediable with such a discussion, or the therapeutic regimen may need to be modified.

Patient factors in noncompliance: Age, sex, race, and educational level are not predictors of compliance. "Forgetfulness" is the most frequently cited reason, but it is not really an explanation. It may be a rationalization to cover unconscious or partly conscious concerns about the patient's health status, his diagnosis, and the taking of medication. Commonly, there is fear of adverse effects, of addiction, of the disease state that treatment implies, and of loss of independence. For example, patients with hypertension have an asymptomatic disease and must cope with medical advice from physicians, public health advertisements, and well-intentioned friends regarding their risks of stroke, heart attack, and renal disease. Many deal with the resultant anxiety by attempts at denial of illness, a prominent sign of which is neglecting to take medication. Medications may be stopped because symptoms and signs decrease or disappear. Although medications comprise < 10% of total personal health expenditures, some patients decrease the dose or the duration of treatment to save money. Rarely, a patient may not fill the prescription at all for financial or other reasons.

Medication factors in noncompliance: Complex regimens with frequent dosing or many medications increase errors in dosage times, scheduling with meals, etc. If preparations look alike, patients may confuse medications and inadvertently repeat or omit doses. Other factors include adverse effects (real or imagined), unpleasant tastes or smells, and precautions imposed by therapeutic regimens (no alcohol or cheese, etc.).

Disease factors in noncompliance: Certain types of illness, such as chronic diseases with day-to-day fluctuation in symptoms (or without symptoms), seem to be important in predisposing to compliance problems. When prophylactic medication is prescribed or when the medication causes more symptoms than the disease under therapy (e.g., hypertension), noncompliance or defaulting is more likely.

The physician's role in improving patient compliance: Making a correct diagnosis and designing a simple, effective therapeutic regimen starts the therapeutic process. Good communication between the physician and the patient is essential. Directions must be clear, precise, and tailored to the vagaries and necessities of the patient's life and the disease process. Inappropriate termination of the therapeutic regimen may be prevented if the physician explains the delay associated with the onset of apparent benefit characteristic of some drugs, e.g., antidepressants. Inquiring about adherence to the regimen and the reasons for any problems may help to correct noncompliance and is necessary, since patients often do not volunteer such information. The belief that education promotes rational choices and improves compliance is not supported by hard evidence. Dealing specifically with patient factors that underlie noncompliance is far more effective. Trust—in the personal physician, in the prescribed therapy, or perhaps in medical science in general—appears most crucial to patient compliance. Explaining the purpose of the components in the regimen and the beneficial and adverse effects of a medication, as well as its shape, color, and dosage schedule, are educational, but, more important, they may help create a relationship of trust.

The pharmacist's and nurse's role in improving compliance: Nurses or pharmacists may detect compliance problems. Information that patients do not discuss with physicians may be transmitted to less threatening figures and can be relayed to the physician; e.g., by the pharmacist who notes that the patient cannot pay for a full prescription or does not obtain refills. Illogical or incorrect prescriptions may be noted and corrected by consulting the prescriber. Nurses and pharmacists may instruct patients on their medications, especially prior to discharge from the hospital. By reviewing the physical characteristics of medications, directions, side effects, drug interactions, precautions, specific patient concerns, and the necessity for each medication with the patient, they can uncover misunderstandings and fears and can enhance the patient's knowledge. Some institutions have experimented with programs of patient self-medication under modified supervision with promising results.

The role of the pharmaceutical industry and pharmacologists in improving compliance: The pharmaceutical industry and pharmacologists can help by discovering effective medications with few adverse effects and convenient dosage schedules. Making medications taste better and varying the shape and color of tablets also help. Better sustained-release and rational combination products may help improve compliance by reducing the number of doses needed per day and the number of medications ingested. Pharmacologists contribute by studying the ways in which medications can be administered to take advantage of their pharmacokinetic properties with the goal of reducing missed doses and errors. For example, many psychotropic drugs have long half-lives and can be given once a day in a large dose (e.g., at bedtime) instead of in 3 or 4 smaller doses throughout the day. Better definition of the patients who will respond to a medication and of those at risk for adverse effects should help the physician to assess pharmacologic response, maximize benefit, and design an optimum dosage schedule of the logical agent.

Misuse of medication, such as taking outdated prescription drugs or those prescribed for other apparently similar illnesses, also forms part of a broadened definition of compliance to therapy. Following the spirit but not the sense of prescription directions is another type of noncompliance. Examples include inappropriate ingestion of certain medications with food, and taking medications with interacting over-the-counter preparations.

Patients may not take medications for valid and important reasons. In fact, "intelligent non-compliance" (where the patient discontinues or decreases the dose of medication based on a correct interpretation of the clinical situation) may decrease adverse effects and improve the therapeutic outcome. Too often, however, the therapist does not know of these efficacious maneuvers. If the patient can act as a therapeutic monitor, noting benefit and detriment and communicating these observations to the physician, both will benefit. The physician can better adjust therapy, exploring the dose-effect relationship or discontinuing unneeded drugs. Patients are more likely to have a satisfactory outcome through adherence to the *cooperatively* designed program. Finally, physicians can gain valuable knowledge about responses to medication and the course of a disease which may be valuable in treating other patients. Such cooperative compliance demands patient and physician education about therapeutic monitoring and involves time, money, and sharing responsibility. Nevertheless, it would seem beneficial to expend the time and effort to achieve cooperative compliance.

244. PRESCRIPTION WRITING

Prescriptions measure physicians' therapeutic knowledge. Fewer than 1% of prescriptions are now compounded by pharmacists, a trend that has provided more efficacious and more uniform drug products but that has led in part to decreased skill in prescription writing. A high degree of misinterpretation and noncompliance with prescription directions exists and desultory prescription directions contribute to these problems. Instruction in prescription writing is often cursory, with little corrective feedback for poor practices. The patient rarely complains about poorly communicated directions, and the pharmacist commonly asks only minimal polite questions to determine the essential information needed to complete the prescription.

The General Format of the Prescription

The prescription should follow a definite pattern (see Fig. 244-1). It should be written legibly and should contain the patient's name, address, age, and the date of prescription (Federal law *requires* that the patient's full name and address be included on prescriptions for narcotics) (1). The drug name is written out and the dosage clearly specified (2 and 3). (There are few instances in which the name of the drug should not be included on the label.) The number of units and the dosage form (tablets, capsules, etc.) are also stated exactly (4). The label directions transmitted to the pharmacist should be clear, preferably without abbreviations or jargon (5). An exact number of refills is specified (6) and the prescriber's signature and degree are written clearly (7).

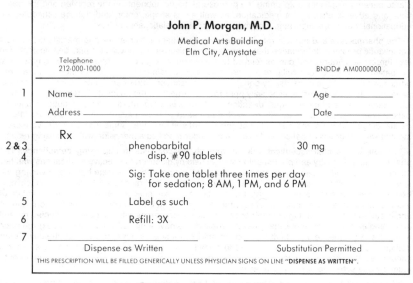

FIG. 244-1. Sample prescription.

COMMON PROBLEMS AND ERRORS

Identification Data

The patient's address is seldom written out by prescribers and is often sought for identification by the pharmacist. Dating the prescription helps the pharmacist to detect outdated ones. The patient's age helps the pharmacist to identify variations in dosage and other factors. An alternative is to add the word "infant," "child," or "adult" after the patient's name.

Drug Name

Drugs may be prescribed by their official generic names, which are those included in the current edition of the *United States Pharmacopeia* (**USP**); by their nonofficial generic names, which are those assigned by the *United States Adopted Names* (**USAN**) *Council*, many of which are cited in *AMA Drug Evaluations*; by their nonproprietary names, which, in the case of recently marketed drugs, may not yet be cited in official or nonofficial compendia; or by the manufacturer's proprietary (trade or brand) names.

In some states, using the manufacturer's proprietary name mandates that only that specific drug product may be used in filling the prescription. Recently, however, most states have declared that, *unless* the physician specifies no substitution, the pharmacist can dispense a chemically identical product. The physician may signal his wishes by signing in a designated place on the blank. In some states the physician must add in writing, "Do not substitute" or a similar statement. When a drug product is marketed by more than one manufacturer, using a nonproprietary or generic name or not signing on the "dispense as written" line leaves the choice of product to the pharmacist. The majority of prescriptions written in the USA still bear a proprietary name, but changes in state laws are altering this.

Many educators and government officials recommend using non-branded drugs whenever possible, to reduce costs to the patient, but this practice does not guarantee savings for the patient. Another unresolved issue is that of bioavailability (see Ch. 235). The fact that 2 different manufacturers' drug products may be identical, according to labeled composition, is no assurance of equivalent bioavailability of the active ingredient(s) and, hence, of therapeutic performance.

Abbreviations of drug names should be avoided; the use of chemical notations ($FeSO_4$, KCl) is often confusing. "Chlor" may mean both chloral and chlorate. The failure to specify a particular salt of a drug can be important. Morphine virtually always means morphine sulfate, but with a prescription for erythromycin the patient can receive the estolate, the ethylsuccinate, the stearate, or the base. Many other types of synonyms may be confusing. The prescriber who wishes to obtain phenoxymethyl penicillin may write phenoxymethyl penicillin, potassium phenoxymethyl penicillin, Penicillin VK. Pen VK (all nonproprietary terms), or Pen-Vee K (a brand name) and receive the same drug.

If a brand name is used, it should be carefully and fully written because many are similar and confusing. A hastily scribbled Ornade might be read as Orinase or even Ananase. The specific brand name is necessary when prescribing a precompounded combination product.

Dosage

Prescriptions should be written in metric units. For tablets and capsules the terms "gram" and "milligram" should be used and preferably should be written out. The term "μg," although occasionally useful, should not be used because of its confusing similarity to the larger measure (mg); "mcg" is acceptable. Those who have forgotten the quantities indicated by a minim or a scruple or a grain nevertheless still use the measure ounce, but ml should be used as a fluid measure. If one knows that 5 ml of the liquid contain the unit dose, the number of doses desired can be calculated and the exact quantity should be written on the prescription.

The number of units dispensed is determined in various ways. One may order a small supply because this will remind the patient to return for follow-up or because a large supply of drug may be dangerous in terms of suicidal or accidental poisoning. Dispensing large quantities may lead to significant wasting of drug. However, when a patient requires a drug long-term, a large quantity may be more economical.

Labeling and Directions

Abbreviations and fashionable jargon, whether in English or in Latin, should be avoided. Gtt., p.c., q.d., t.i.d., and p.r.n. may be confusing even when written clearly. Label directions to the pharmacist written so that they may be transcribed directly without translation or literary transmogrification help to avoid errors or confusion. Complete, precisely stated sentences are preferred. If the medication must be taken 3 or 4 times daily, the times should be specified on the prescription, since patients are often confused by directions such as "every 6 hours." However, if it is important to take a particular drug at a 6-hour interval, that should be emphasized and explained to the patient. If a drug can be taken safely and effectively once daily, it is important to discard traditional divided doses because patients will often comply better with once/day dosage. If the drug is affected by food, the relationship must be made explicit to the patient.

All directions should be explicit and should begin with the verb; e.g., *take* 3 capsules, *place* in rectum, *apply* to rash, *instill* in affected ear. There are prescriptions—the "as needed" or "p.r.n." prescriptions—in which the patient assumes responsibility for the treatment within certain limits set by the prescriber. For example, the directions may say to take 2 tablets every 4 to 6 hours as needed for pain. Generally, the patient is given a time interval that he should not compress and a medication volume that he should not expand. An "as needed" prescription should name the symptom that the patient monitors; e.g., pain, nausea, tremulousness, itching, sleeplessness.

The frequently used phrase "as directed" is undesirable (even with oral contraceptives) unless printed or written directions are also given to the patient.

For liquids, prescribers have relied for years on household measures despite the non-uniformity of teaspoons, tablespoons, droppers, and wine glasses. In cases where precise dosage is required, the medication should be dispensed with an appropriate measuring device and instructions on proper use. Compulsive adherence to the rules should not interfere with common sense; in many cases it suffices to remember that a teaspoon equals about 5 ml, a tablespoon equals about 15 ml, and there are about 20 drops to 1 ml.

Refills

According to the Durham-Humphrey Act (1952), a prescription cannot be refilled unless expressly authorized by the prescriber. In many cases, the prescriber may specify the number of times a prescription may be refilled by a pharmacist. Centrally-acting drugs (e.g., narcotics, barbiturates, amphetamines) regulated by the Federal Controlled Substances Act (1970) are assigned to one of five "schedules" (I through V). Schedule I drugs are experimental agents with no approved clinical utility. Prescriptions for Schedule II drugs are not refillable; Schedule III and IV drugs may be refilled up to 5 times within 6 mo of the initial issuance, if authorized by the prescriber. Schedule V drugs are not subject to any restrictions that do not also apply to nonscheduled prescription drugs. Refills at the pharmacist's discretion may occasionally be justified.

---

245. PLACEBOS

Inactive substances used in controlled studies for comparison with presumed active drugs or prescribed with the intent to relieve symptoms or meet a patient's demands. A placebo may be any type of therapeutic maneuver, including surgical and psychologic technics or medication in any form (e.g., oral, parenteral, topical), but this discussion is limited to drug formulations.

The term placebo harks back to the 116th Psalm in the Hebrew Bible. Through a number of translating errors, the Vulgate Latin version came to contain the word "placebo" (I shall please). Over the centuries, the term placebo was applied to the Vespers for the Dead, derisively to servile flatterers and toadies, and to laments sung at funerals by professional mourners.

In 1785, the word placebo appeared in a medical dictionary for the first time as "a commonplace method or medicine." Two editions later, the placebo had become a "make-believe medicine," allegedly inert and harmless. We now know that administration of placebos may have profound effects, both good and bad.

The Binary Nature of Placebo Effects

The medical literature is replete with reports on the power of the placebo to help patients with anxiety, tension, melancholia, schizophrenia, pain of all sorts, headaches, cough, insomnia, seasickness, chronic bronchitis, the common cold, arthritis, peptic ulcer, hypertension, nausea, and senile dementia, among others. But the placebo is not only able to help; it has also been associated with "side effects." These have included nausea, headache, dizziness, sleepiness, insomnia, fatigue, depression, numbness, hallucinations, itching, vomiting, tremor, tachycardia, diarrhea, pallor, rashes, hives, ataxia, and edema, to name only a partial list.

This remarkable list of *subjective and objective* changes, both desirable and unwanted, becomes more understandable and is put into perspective once one recognizes that there are 2 components of the placebo response. One is the anticipation (usually optimistic) of effects because of the expectations associated with medication. One can call this "suggestibility," "faith," "hope," or whatever.

The 2nd component, however, is at times even more important—spontaneous change. If a placebo has been taken before spontaneous improvement, it may be given credit, just as a placebo may be blamed if someone spontaneously develops a headache or a rash after taking an inert capsule or tablet.

The "Placebo Reactor"

Studies to determine whether or not certain personality characteristics correlate with responses to placebos have disagreed extravagantly with one another. This is not surprising, since some investigators have called a "placebo reactor" one who gets benefit from placebos, and others have used the term for people who report side effects after placebos. It seems unlikely that the same personality traits would predispose to such different types of responses.

It is probably more correct to talk about a spectrum of "placebo reactivity" than about placebo reactors, since virtually anyone is suggestible under some circumstances. However, some people seem more prone to influence than others. We can only speculate, but these differences at times may relate to the recipient's personality; e.g., dependent personalities, who tend to want to please their physicians, may be more likely to report beneficial effects, and histrionic personalities may be more likely to note some sort of effect, good or bad. Probably the most important factors are those that relate to specific attitudes toward the illness, medications, and physician. For example, when a patient with acute pain has a favorable attitude toward medicines and is given the placebo by a concerned and confident physician, a better response may occur than when a patient has moderate pain, views drugs as dangerous chemicals, and is given the placebo by a gruff physician who appears uncertain.

Placebo addicts: At least 2 patients have been reported who were addicted to placebos. One consumed 10,000 placebos in 1 yr. The other showed many of the characteristics of a true drug addict: a tendency to increase the dose; inability to stop the "medicine" without psychiatric help; a compulsive desire to take the tablets; and an abstinence syndrome when deprived of the tablets.

Use in Research

Difficulty in sorting out the 2 components of the placebo response does not detract from the utility of the placebo as a standard in clinical trials, where it serves in much the same way as a "blank" serves the chemist to assay "background noise" that must be subtracted from the overall treatment effect. Whatever the relative importance of suggestibility and spontaneous change, the drug must perform better than placebo to justify its being marketed. For regulatory purposes, attention is paid only to positive ("good" therapeutic) responses. In some studies, e.g., comparison with a new drug to relieve angina pectoris, relief with placebo commonly exceeds 50%, presenting quite a challenge to demonstrate effectiveness with an active agent.

Use in Therapy

There is a placebo element in every therapeutic maneuver; therefore, the effects of a drug will vary from patient to patient and doctor to doctor, depending on placebo reactivity. People with a "positive" orientation to drugs, doctors, nurses, hospitals, etc. are more likely to respond favorably to placebos than are people with a "negative" orientation. The latter may deny benefit or complain of untoward effects. Thus, as with any other prescribed agent, giving a placebo has potential benefits and risks that must be evaluated. A positive placebo effect is more likely when both patient and doctor believe that therapeutic benefit will result from a drug. Thus, an active agent with no pharmacologic effect on the process being treated (e.g., vitamin B_{12} in a patient with arthritis) may provide a favorable response, or a mildly active agent may have an enhanced effect (e.g., aspirin in a patient with metastatic bone pain).

With deliberate placebo use (which is extraordinarily rare in clinical practice, as opposed to research trials), in addition to the adverse effects described above, there are several major **hazards:** (1) Since the doctor is deceiving the patient, there may be an adverse alteration in the doctor-patient relationship. At the very least, the doctor must be more guarded, lest his deception be discovered. Should it be discovered, the patient will lose face, feel betrayed, and his confidence in the physician will be impaired. (2) The doctor may misinterpret the patient's response; particularly pernicious is the unwarranted conclusion that a positive response means that the patient's symptoms are psychogenic or neurotically exaggerated. (3) Where other doctors or nurses are involved in the deception (as in a group practice or hospital setting), the potential for adversely modifying the attitudes and behaviors of any or all of the others toward the patient and the potential for discovery are greatly increased. Considering the availability of a host of drugs that have at least the potential to alleviate most of the complaints seen in practice and the danger of destroying a patient-doctor relationship with placebo use, placebos qua placebos are rarely indicated.

Today, doctors may prescribe vitamin "tonics" or B_{12} injections that are often tantamount to placebos, but they rarely prescribe lactose tablets or "sterile hypos." However, such practice is appropriate as a risk-to-benefit calculation in certain circumstances. For example, most young physicians pick up patients from another who has left practice. Often, a doctor acquires patients who have taken B_{12} or other vitamins as a "tonic" with great faith and perceived benefit for many years; denied their "medicine," such patients often feel ill and can become seriously upset. Based on cultural or psychologic sets, some patients genuinely seem to require and obtain benefit from either an unrequired medication or a particular dosage form (e.g., by injection when an oral agent should suffice). Denying them may result in their turning to unscrupulous charlatans and sometimes hazardous practices. In dealing with incurable chronic or malignant disease, placebos may also offer needed hope.

246. ANTI-INFECTIVE DRUGS

TOPICAL ANTISEPTICS

Agents that can kill or inhibit the growth of microorganisms when applied to living tissues without significant harm to the tissues.

Antiseptics are widely used but their efficacy and hazards are poorly understood. An ideal antiseptic should possess high germicidal activity, a broad spectrum of effectiveness, and a wide margin of safety. It should act promptly, even in the presence of exudate or necrotic tissue, and should have prolonged therapeutic effectiveness. Its surface tension should be low, for easy and effective topical application, and it should be painless, stable, odorless, and nonstaining. Since no such product exists, therapeutic selection must be based on the most important characteristic required for each case. Several typical antiseptics are discussed here under broad chemical categories.

Phenols: A 1 to 2% solution of phenol (carbolic acid) is effective against nonsporulating bacteria and fungi, but clinical usefulness is limited due to systemic toxicity manifested by CNS stimulation with muscle tremors and seizures, possibly followed by CNS depression, respiratory failure, and death. Several phenol derivatives are more effective and less toxic than phenol. **Hexylresorcinol** is a useful agent when applied in a 1:1000 dilution; its low surface tension allows effective penetration and spreading, but it may produce skin irritation.

Hexachlorophene, a chlorinated bis-phenol, is a highly effective bacteriostatic agent in concentrations of 2 to 5% against both gram-positive and gram-negative organisms. Although often used in combination with soaps, maximum effectiveness is only achieved with regular use when a deposit of hexachlorophene forms on the skin. This deposit exerts a prolonged bacteriostatic effect but is readily removed by soap. *Hexachlorophene should not be applied to denuded skin,* since excessive absorption results in systemic toxicity manifested by vomiting, abdominal cramps, diarrhea, disorientation, and seizures. Routine bathing of newborn infants with hexachlorophene soaps or solutions greatly reduces the incidence of staphylococcal infections, but CNS toxicity with cerebral degeneration has been reported, especially in premature and low-birth-weight infants. For this reason, *routine infant bathing with hexachlorophene preparations should be restricted* to nurseries having a serious risk of staphylococcal infections. It is wise to avoid bathing low-birth-weight and premature infants with such products.

Chlorhexidine is an effective antiseptic against gram-positive and gram-negative bacteria when used as a 4% sudsing scrub or 1.0% aqueous solution, and is most effective as a 0.5% solution in 70% isopropyl alcohol. Antibacterial activity is cumulative with regular use and persists for > 6 h on gloved hands. Local skin reactions are unusual, but *avoid contact with the eyes and ears.* Chlorhexidine may cause hearing loss if it reaches the middle ear and should *not* be used as a skin antiseptic before ear surgery. It is effective in combination with silver sulfadiazine to control infection in burn wounds.

Alcohols: Ethyl alcohol (50 to 70% solution) and isopropyl alcohol (70 to 90% solution) are both effective antiseptics. Isopropyl alcohol is less volatile and has slightly greater antiseptic activity. Neither alcohol is suitable for sterilization, since they are not sporocidal. Alcohols are not used to disinfect wounds, since they form a coagulum with protein under which bacteria can thrive.

Halogens: Iodine, an old and potent antiseptic, is highly effective, low in cost, and has low tissue toxicity. In a 1:20,000 solution, it is bactericidal after 1 min and sporocidal after 15 min. Iodine solutions are also fungicidal, amebicidal, and weakly virucidal. Iodine preparations are available as tincture of iodine, containing 2% iodine and 2.4% sodium iodide in 50% alcohol, and as iodine solution, containing 2% iodine and 2.4% sodium iodide in water. Despite the efficacy of iodine preparations, clinical applications have been limited by the disadvantages of skin staining, tissue irritation, pain, and occasional hypersensitivity reactions manifested by fever and generalized skin eruptions.

Iodophors are complexes of iodine, usually with a surface active agent. Following application, free iodine is slowly released for germicidal activity. Iodophors are somewhat less effective than the aqueous and alcoholic iodine solutions, but may be less irritating and less toxic. Iodophor compounds such as povidone-iodine are available in aerosol spray, ointment, shampoo, skin cleanser, solution, and vaginal douche preparations containing 0.5% to 1% available iodine.

Acids: Boric acid is weakly bacteriostatic and nonirritating to devitalized tissues and delicate eye structures. However, it is readily absorbed if applied to large or denuded skin areas and can cause severe systemic toxicity with GI disturbances, hypothermia, rash, renal impairment, vascular collapse, shock, and death, particularly in infants and children. *Clinical use of boric acid should be limited to the ophthalmic preparations.*

Oxidizing agents: Hydrogen peroxide as a 3% solution is a weak and very unstable antiseptic, but is useful for cleansing wounds. The brief antibacterial activity is due to the release of O_2, which also aids in the mechanical removal of material from wound cavities.

Aldehydes: Formaldehyde (0.5% solution) is germicidal after 6 to 12 h, but is too irritating for clinical use. **Methenamine,** a condensation product of formaldehyde and ammonia, is rapidly excreted in the urine, where under acid conditions it decomposes to ammonia and formaldehyde. The formaldehyde then acts as a urinary antiseptic. The usual adult dosage of methenamine is 1 gm orally q.i.d., and the urine pH must be maintained at 5.5 or less. Since some ammonia is released following oral administration, *methenamine should not be used in patients with hepatic insufficiency.*

Heavy metals: Mercury compounds exert antibacterial action by reversible binding to sulfhydryl enzymes in microorganisms. However, they are highly toxic to tissues, they penetrate poorly, and their activity can be blocked by extraneous proteins. Therefore, these preparations are not recommended.

Silver nitrate solution in a 1:1000 dilution rapidly destroys most microorganisms. Silver nitrate as a 0.5% solution has been used extensively in the treatment of burns for reducing the incidence of infections and promoting eschar formation. Prolonged use may result in argyria, and bacterial reduction of silver nitrate to nitrite in the burn may cause methemoglobinemia. One to 2 drops of 1% silver nitrate ophthalmic solution is commonly used as prophylaxis for gonorrheal ophthalmia neonatorum, but may cause a chemical conjunctivitis, especially following repeated applications (see NEONATAL CONJUNCTIVITIS in Vol. II, Ch. 21).

Cerium nitrate is effective against many bacteria and fungi when used for the treatment of burns. The combination of 0.05 M cerium nitrate with silver sulfadiazine cream suppresses both grampositive and gram-negative bacteria better than either drug alone without increasing toxicity. Bacterial reduction of cerium nitrate to nitrite in the burn may cause methemoglobinemia. Local tissue irritation may occur.

Surface-active agents: Many anionic and cationic surfactants possess antiseptic properties. Most anionics are effective against gram-positive bacteria, while the cationics are effective against grampositive and gram-negative bacteria as well as some fungi and viruses. Anionic and cationic surfactants inactivate each other, so cationic surface active agents cannot be used with ordinary soaps, which are anionic detergents. The mechanism of antimicrobial activity is not known but may be related to alterations in bacterial cell membrane permeability. The clinically useful cationic surfactants are the quaternary ammonium compounds such as **benzalkonium chloride, cetylpyridinium chloride,** and **benzethonium chloride.** They possess rapid onset of antiseptic action, good tissue penetration, and low systemic toxicity; the disadvantages are inactivation by soaps and formation of a film on the skin with a weakly antiseptic inner surface under which some bacteria may survive and grow, despite a highly bactericidal outer surface. Aqueous solutions of these antiseptics may become contaminated with resistant gram-negative bacteria and serve as a source of nosocomial infections.

Furans: Nitrofurazone is bactericidal against many gram-positive and gram-negative organisms in dilutions up to 1:75,000. It is clinically useful as a topical antiseptic on surgical wounds and superficial skin lesions, including burns, ulcers, and abrasions, but systemic toxicity may result from absorption from large wound areas. It is available as a 0.2% solution, cream, and ointment. Rash, pruritus, and, rarely, exfoliative dermatitis have been reported with this agent.

Miscellaneous agents: Mafenide acetate is a useful topical sulfonamide, available as an 8.5 to 10% cream, for applying to burns to prevent bacterial infection. It provides effective *prophylaxis* against both gram-positive and gram-negative organisms, especially *Pseudomonas aeruginosa*, but should not be used to treat established *Pseudomonas* infections. Unlike other sulfonamides, it is effective in the presence of pus and has a low incidence of hypersensitization. A disadvantage is severe pain on application or removal. Systemic absorption inhibits carbonic anhydrase activity in the renal tubule and may cause hyperchloremic acidosis. Mafenide hydrochloride is also available as a 5% solution.

Silver sulfadiazine is a topical antiseptic effective against many bacteria and fungi, but some gram-negative organisms are resistant. It is clinically useful for burn treatment, where it both prevents and eradicates *Pseudomonas* infections, and is painless on application and removal. However, systemic absorption may result in the same toxicity as seen with any systemic sulfonamide.

ANTIMICROBIAL CHEMOTHERAPY

Antibacterial, antirickettsial, and antifungal agents are derived either from bacteria and molds (the *antibiotics*, though some can be synthesized) or from total chemical synthesis. Antibiotics that are sufficiently nontoxic to the host are used as chemotherapeutic agents. They act through interference with the organism's (1) cell wall synthesis, (2) cell membrane synthesis or permeability, and (3) molecular mechanisms of replication, information transfer, and protein synthesis.

SELECTION OF A CHEMOTHERAPEUTIC AGENT

An ever-increasing number of antimicrobial drugs is available for treating infections. A working knowledge of the common pathogenic microorganisms is essential for best results. Although etiology can often be inferred from the onset and clinical features of a disease, culture studies and antibiotic sensitivity tests are frequently desirable and are essential for the proper treatment of most serious infections. Experienced laboratory help must be available. It may be necessary to begin treatment in critically ill patients before culture and sensitivity studies indicating a specific drug are completed. In such cases, it is advisable to give maximum doses of the likeliest agent from the outset, but culture specimens should always be taken before therapy is begun.

In vitro sensitivity of organisms is difficult to interpret unless test methods are standardized. In vitro sensitivity of an organism to any antimicrobial may *not* be a true index of the drug's clinical effectiveness, since efficacy depends in part on the concentration of the drug in body fluids, host defense mechanisms, the presence of inhibiting substances in body fluids, and the extent to which the drug is protein-bound. Generally, however, agents active in vitro are therapeutically effective.

The choice of drug is not automatic even when the etiology of infection and the sensitivity of the causative organism are known. The nature and gravity of the illness, the toxicity of the drug, the patient's history of hypersensitivity or other serious reaction, and the cost of the drug must also be considered.

Antimicrobial agents in combination are superior to a single agent in some instances. In brucellosis and tuberculosis, the combination of streptomycin and one or more other agents enhances therapeutic activity. Penicillin and streptomycin are more effective in Group D streptococcal (enterococcal) infections than is penicillin alone.

Administration: Parenteral administration, preferably IV, is usually mandatory in severe infection; oral preparations are often used for maintenance once the infection is under control. Therapy should be continued until there is objective evidence that active systemic infection has been absent for several days (e.g., absence of fever, of leukocytosis, and of abnormal laboratory findings).

Administration of antimicrobials to patients with impaired kidney function must be carefully supervised, since many antimicrobials are excreted mainly in the urine. Such patients run the risk of having drug concentrations in blood and tissue rise to toxic levels because of renal insufficiency. They may tolerate the usual doses for the first 24 h, but subsequent doses must be reduced or the intervals between doses prolonged. Dosages must be carefully supervised in infants (see NEONATAL INFECTIONS in Vol. II, Ch. 21) and the aged for the same reason.

COMPLICATIONS OF CHEMOTHERAPY

Undesirable effects may follow the use of any chemotherapeutic agent and can involve most organ systems. These adverse effects may be due to direct toxicity or to hypersensitivity. Reactions do not always require cessation of treatment, especially if the offending drug is the only effective one available, but the severity and type of reactions, their expected course, and the possibility of influencing them by proper management must be weighed against the gravity of the infection.

Cutaneous reactions are mostly due to hypersensitivity and may occur with any drug. Morbilliform and other eruptions, purpura, erythema multiforme, erythema nodosum, and exfoliative dermatitis may occur. Contact dermatitis may develop in persons handling antibiotics, especially streptomycin and penicillin. **Other manifestations of hypersensitivity** include fever; angioedema; serum sickness, possibly with subsequent polyarteritis or SLE; and, rarely, anaphylactic shock (mainly with penicillin). **Oral reactions** occur most commonly with the broad-spectrum antibiotics and include dryness, burning, soreness, and itching of the mouth and tongue; stomatitis; acute glossitis; cheilosis; and black or brown coating of the tongue. **GI reactions,** also most common with the broad-spectrum antibiotics, include nausea; vomiting; diarrhea; *Staphylococcus aureus* enteritis; membranous colitis; oral, pharyngeal, rectal, and perianal *Candida* infection; liver damage (from tetracyclines IV in doses > 1.5

gm/day), jaundice, and hepatitis; and steatorrhea. **Urinary tract complications** include hematuria (semisynthetic penicillins and sulfonamides); crystalluria, acute tubular necrosis, and obstruction to urine flow (sulfonamides); proteinuria and cylindruria (streptomycin in acid urine); and nephrotoxicity (cephaloridine, polymyxin, neomycin, gentamicin, kanamycin, and vancomycin). **Neurologic reactions** include peripheral neuritis (broad-spectrum antibiotics and nitrofurantoin), paresthesias (streptomycin, kanamycin, polymyxin, vancomycin), 8th nerve damage (streptomycin, dihydrostreptomycin, neomycin, vancomycin, kanamycin, gentamicin, tobramycin, and amikacin), encephalitis (some sulfonamides and penicillin), encephalopathy from excessive intrathecal doses, psychosis or convulsions (cycloserine), and respiratory paralysis (polymyxin, kanamycin, colistin). **Hematologic complications** include hemolytic anemia (sulfonamides, the nitrofurans, nalidixic acid), eosinophilia (sensitization to any of the antibiotics), aplastic anemia (chloramphenicol), thrombocytopenia, and leukopenia.

Organisms may develop **resistance** to any antimicrobial agent. The resistance may appear rapidly or after long or repeated courses of therapy. For this reason, infections must be controlled as rapidly as possible by promptly (1) identifying the causative organism, (2) determining its in vitro sensitivity, and (3) providing effective in vivo concentrations of the drug. Initially inadequate doses promote the development of resistance, and even greatly increased doses may later fail to control the infection.

For a discussion of superimposed infections by resistant organisms, see Ch. 6.

MISUSES OF CHEMOTHERAPY

Antimicrobial agents are often used needlessly, or used improperly with poor clinical results. The most frequent misuse is probably in the treatment of FUO. Fever is not necessarily due to infection. Without strong evidence of microbial invasion, chemotherapy should be delayed, if possible, until clinical and laboratory studies confirm the presence of an infection and guide the choice of an appropriate agent.

Other common misuses and errors include (1) choice of an ineffective antibiotic, (2) inadequate or excessive doses, (3) use in such insusceptible infections as uncomplicated viral disease, (4) improper route of administration, (5) continued use after bacterial resistance has developed, (6) continued use in the presence of a serious toxic or allergic reaction, (7) failure to alter chemotherapy when superimposed infections with resistant organisms occur, (8) use of improper combinations of chemotherapeutic agents, and (9) reliance on chemotherapy or prophylaxis to the exclusion of surgical intervention (e.g., drainage of localized infection).

ANTIBIOTICS

THE PENICILLINS

Penicillin G	Amoxicillin	Dicloxacillin
Penicillin V	Methicillin	Nafcillin
Ampicillin	Oxacillin	Carbenicillin
Hetacillin	Cloxacillin	Ticarcillin

The penicillins are a large group of bactericidal antibiotics having the **6-aminopenicillanic acid (6-APA)** nucleus in common. Naturally occurring penicillins, the most important of which is benzyl penicillin (penicillin G), are produced by several mold species. All the other penicillins in common use are semisynthetic, obtained by substituting various side chains on the 6-APA nucleus.

Penicillins affect only actively multiplying bacteria. Their antibacterial action seems to reside in their ability to inhibit metabolic functions vital to bacterial cell wall synthesis. The precise mechanism is unknown.

Penicillin absorption from the GI tract is incomplete and takes place mainly from the duodenum, much less so from the stomach and large intestine. To ensure maximum absorption, all oral penicillins should ideally be taken on an empty stomach, at least 1/2 h before or 2 h after meals. Penicillins are distributed rapidly to most body fluids and tissues after IV or IM injection, more slowly after oral administration. Concentrations are low in normal joint, ocular, pericardial, and pleural fluids, and somewhat higher in peritoneal fluid. However, with active inflammation the penicillins penetrate well into most body fluids and spaces. Penetration into the CSF also varies, but the levels are often therapeutic when the meninges are inflamed. High concentrations are found in the liver, bile, lungs, intestine, and skin.

Penicillins are reversibly bound to plasma protein; activity occurs when the complex dissociates. A highly bound penicillin may be therapeutically comparable to one less strongly bound if it is inherently more potent (has a lower minimum inhibitory concentration) against a specific organism.

Penicillin is largely excreted unchanged. Little work has been done on identifying penicillin metabolites, probably because most are virtually nontoxic. However, penicilloic acid, a metabolite of benzylpenicillin, appears to be an important intermediate in the formation of certain antigenic determinants in vivo and may be an important factor in allergic reactions. Benzylpenicilloyl-polylysine is available as a skin test for determining sensitivity to penicillin. (See also in Ch. 19.)

Excretion of penicillins occurs, with varying rapidity, mainly by a renal tubular mechanism and to a lesser degree via the bile. Parenteral penicillin G is so rapidly absorbed and excreted that repository preparations have been formulated; these slowly release the antibiotic from the injection site, thereby producing a lower, but more prolonged, blood concentration. The penicillinase-resistant penicillins differ significantly in their degree of oral absorption and serum binding, and in their rate of urinary excretion.

Indications: The penicillins are the antibiotics of choice in infections caused by pneumococci, meningococci, aerobic and anaerobic streptococci, gonococci, and non-penicillinase-producing staphylococci; and in the treatment of syphilis, actinomycosis, anthrax, Vincent's angina, and yaws. They are useful in ratbite fever and infections due to *Listeria*, *Corynebacterium*, and *Clostridium* organisms. Specific information on indications and dosages is given in the discussions of individual agents.

The penicillins are qualitatively similar in their antimicrobial spectrum, but differ significantly in their degree of effectiveness against specific species and strains of bacteria. Although each of the semisynthetic penicillins has advantages, penicillin G remains the preferred agent for the majority of penicillin-susceptible infections. Other penicillins, whether acid-or penicillinase-resistant or both, frequently are not as active as penicillin G against susceptible organisms, including non-penicillinase-producing staphylococci. In addition, the many available forms of penicillin G provide high, intermediate, or low levels of serum activity for various lengths of time, as necessary. Penicillins that are penicillinase-resistant or that have a broader gram-negative spectrum should be reserved for infections in which penicillin G is not indicated.

Administration: Injectable penicillin is recommended for severely ill patients and when nausea and vomiting are present; aqueous parenteral penicillin is used in severe infections when a rapid, high penicillin serum level is needed. Oral penicillin is not adequate in these instances, but it is used for maintenance therapy once the infection is under control, and is also given for mild or moderate infections. Topical use is discouraged because of the high risk of sensitization.

Side effects: True toxic reactions seldom occur with the penicillins. They are potent sensitizers, however, and allergic reactions are not uncommon. Previous hypersensitivity to any penicillin is generally a *contraindication* to their use, and they must be used cautiously in individuals with a history of any allergy. An untoward effect is not always repeated on future exposures to penicillin. Patients with mild reactions are sometimes given penicillin at a later date, after appropriate skin tests (see DRUG HYPERSENSITIVITY in Ch. 19, and TYPE I REACTIONS in Ch. 18), without serious effects. A patient who suffers a serious reaction or who survives an anaphylactic reaction *should not be given penicillin again* except with special precautions in unusual circumstances when no substitute can be found.

Hypersensitivity responses include (1) skin rashes (urticaria; erythematous, macular, papular, morbilliform, scarlatiniform, or purpuric rashes; bullous eruptions; angioedema; exfoliative dermatitis) appearing 7 to 10 days after therapy begins, and, rarely, persisting or recurring for weeks after therapy is stopped; (2) serum sickness; and, rarely, (3) anaphylactic shock with sudden death after oral or parenteral administration.

Some allergic responses are mild and disappear even if penicillin is continued, or subside quickly if it is stopped. Mild reactions may be managed with an oral antihistamine. More severe reactions may require corticosteroids and epinephrine. Specific treatment for urticaria is given in Ch. 19; for exfoliative dermatitis, in Ch. 189; for serum sickness, in DRUG HYPERSENSITIVITY in Ch. 19; and for anaphylactic shock, in ATOPIC DISEASES in Ch. 19.

CNS toxicity may occur with high penicillin doses if renal function is reduced, if the blood-brain barrier is altered by cardiopulmonary bypass, or with excessive intrathecal doses.

Other reactions include pain at the site of IM injection, thrombophlebitis when the same site is used repeatedly for IV injection, and GI disturbances with oral preparations. Black tongue may occur, more often with oral preparations, and is due to irritation of the glossal surface and keratinization of the superficial layers. Superinfection by nonsusceptible bacteria or fungi may occur as with other antibiotics. There is some evidence that superinfections may be more frequent with the newer penicillins than with penicillin G. This may be related to the higher dosage of the new agents and also to their use in more debilitated patients.

General-Purpose Penicillins

The antibacterial spectrum of penicillins G and V is quite similar. Penicillin G is highly effective in vitro against many, but not all, species of gram-positive and -negative cocci. Some gram-negative bacilli are susceptible to very large parenteral doses of penicillin G, but most gram-negative organisms, except *Hemophilus influenzae*, gonococci, and meningococci, are beyond the range of clinically practicable doses. Clinical use of penicillin V is primarily for infections due to susceptible gram-positive organisms; it should *not* be used to treat gonorrhea. The spectrum of ampicillin is similar to that of penicillin G, but it is more active against several species of gram-negative bacteria. All of these compounds are inactivated by penicillinase and are *contraindicated* for infections caused by organisms elaborating that enzyme.

Penicillin G (benzyl penicillin) is highly effective in acute and chronic gonorrhea; infections due to meningococci, pneumococci, and β-hemolytic and anaerobic streptococci; most cases of SBE; fusospirochetal diseases; anthrax; streptobacillosis; actinomycosis; and all stages of syphilis. Although many nosocomial staphylococcal infections are penicillin G-resistant, many staphylococci are penicillin-sensitive. Penicillin G may be used to prevent streptococcal pharyngitis, recurrent rheumatic fever, acute gonococcal urethritis, and SBE (after surgical procedures such as dental extractions). Penicillin G is marketed in many forms, the most important of which are discussed here.

Penicillin G, potassium or sodium may be given IM or IV. When infection is severe or the organism is relatively resistant, IM doses of 1 to 3 million u. may be given q 3 h; higher doses may be given IV. Severe infections, such as enterococcal endocarditis, may rarely require as much as 100 million u./day. In most susceptible mild or moderate infections 300,000 to 600,000 u. given b.i.d. or t.i.d. are as effective as a dosage schedule aimed at maintaining a relatively constant blood level. Injection intrathecally, intracisternally, or into pleural or joint spaces is rarely necessary.

Repository forms of penicillin G are given IM, the slow absorption from IM depots providing prolonged therapeutic blood levels. The **aqueous suspension of procaine penicillin G** is probably used most extensively; blood levels may be detectable for as long as 12 to 48 h. Doses of 600,000 u. given b.i.d. suffice for most penicillin-susceptible infections. Many physicians advocate a concomitant initial large dose of penicillin G potassium for prompt high penicillin blood levels, but it is unclear whether this is necessary. A single IM injection of 600,000 u. of **benzathine penicillin G** produces detectable blood levels for 1 wk or longer. A dose of 1,200,000 u. IM once/mo is used in preventing recurrent rheumatic fever. Because penicillin suspended in oily preparations may cause fatty abscesses, the other repository forms are usually preferred.

Oral penicillin G is used in mild to moderate infections such as scarlet fever and streptococcal pharyngitis; it is *not* recommended for severe infections because it is incompletely absorbed. The usual oral dose is 200,000 to 400,000 u. q 6 h for 10 days.

Penicillin V (phenoxymethyl penicillin) is given orally only. It is acid-resistant and better absorbed than oral penicillin G. Like the latter, it is indicated in mild to moderate infections due to streptococci, pneumococci, and susceptible staphylococci. For most infections, the usual oral dose is 200,000 to 400,000 u. (125 to 250 mg) q 4 to 8 h.

Ampicillin (α-aminobenzyl penicillin) is primarily indicated for certain gram-negative infections and for enterococcal infections. It is ineffective against *Klebsiella*, *Enterobacter*, and *Pseudomonas* species. It is effective in urinary tract infections due to *Escherichia coli* and *Proteus mirabilis*, and in meningitis due to susceptible *H. influenzae*, pneumococci, and meningococci. Ampicillin compares favorably with the tetracyclines in bronchitis caused by *H. influenzae*. Cholangitis and cholecystitis due to susceptible organisms may respond since biliary levels of the drug are high. It effectively controls some chronic typhoid carriers, but its role in acute typhoid fever has not been established; it has been successfully used in typhoid fever associated with chloramphenicol-resistant strains. It appears to be effective in shigellosis and salmonellosis, although antimicrobials are usually not needed in uncomplicated *Salmonella* gastroenteritis.

Ampicillin may be given orally, IM, or IV; oral absorption is variable, and absorption may be decreased when it is given with food. Peak blood levels are attained about 2 h after oral or IM administration; significant activity lasts for several hours. By any route, the usual dose is 250 to 500 mg q 4 to 6 h.

Skin rashes, particularly delayed responses, occur more often with ampicillin than with other penicillins, but the reported incidence varies greatly. The incidence is high in *Salmonella* infections, in patients with impaired renal function, and in conditions often associated with a rash (typhoid, paratyphoid, and glandular fevers). Patients with infectious mononucleosis and lymphatic leukemia are especially prone to react to ampicillin with a characteristic skin eruption. Most ampicillin rashes are probably not allergic in origin.

Hetacillin is a prodrug which, following absorption, is hydrolyzed to ampicillin. The antimicrobial spectrum and clinical indications are therefore similar to orally given ampicillin. It does not seem to possess any advantage over ampicillin.

Amoxicillin (*p*-hydroxy α-aminobenzyl penicillin) is almost identical to ampicillin except that it is absorbed better in the GI tract. It is less active than ampicillin against *Shigella*.

Penicillinase-Resistant Penicillins

Methicillin, oxacillin, cloxacillin, dicloxacillin, and nafcillin are primarily indicated for infections due to penicillinase-producing staphylococci. Methicillin-resistant strains are almost always resistant to the other 4 agents.

Methicillin (dimethoxyphenyl penicillin) is highly effective in severe infections caused by penicillinase-producing staphylococci. Most strains of *S. aureus* are sensitive to concentrations of 1.6 to 6.2 μg/ml. Methicillin is ineffective against enterococci and gram-negative bacilli.

Methicillin is not absorbed when taken orally and is rapidly excreted after parenteral injection. Blood concentrations for the first 2 h after a 1-gm IM dose are about 4 times the minimal inhibitory level, but little or no drug remains at the end of 4 h. Thus, in severe infections, the interval between injections should not exceed 3 to 4 h. Probenecid elevates and prolongs the blood levels, but is rarely necessary.

The usual dosage for adults is 6 to 8 gm/day IM, in divided doses q 4 to 6 h; for children, 100 mg/kg/day IM in divided doses q 6 h. Solutions of methicillin are unstable, but the drug is stable for 4 to 6 h in such IV solutions as isotonic saline or D/W. Continuous IV drip may produce inadequate blood levels because of the rapid renal excretion; it is preferable to divide the total daily dose into equal amounts and give each as a freshly prepared IV solution over 30 min.

Reversible bone marrow suppression and nephritis are rare but potentially serious complications. Interstitial nephritis appears to occur more frequently during therapy with methicillin than with other penicillins.

Oxacillin, cloxacillin, and dicloxacillin (isoxazolyl penicillins) are acid-stable and well absorbed, although absorption of oxacillin varies. **Nafcillin** (ethoxynaphthamido penicillin) is not as well absorbed orally as are the isoxazolyls. With equivalent oral doses, the plasma concentrations and duration of action of the three isoxazolyls, in the above order, are in the ratio of 1:2:4. The plasma concentration is also higher with dicloxacillin than with nafcillin. Methicillin-resistant strains of *S. aureus* are cross-resistant to these agents. Oxacillin is more active against pneumococci and streptococci than is methicillin, but is also more highly protein-bound.

Oxacillin and nafcillin are usually given orally, but are initially given parenterally in seriously ill patients; the usual adult dose is 0.5 to 1.5 gm q 4 to 6 h. Cloxacillin and dicloxacillin are given orally only; the usual adult dose is 250 to 500 mg q 6 h. Dosages for children are 50 mg/kg/day of oxacillin, cloxacillin, or nafcillin, or 25 mg/kg/day of dicloxacillin, usually given as 4 equally divided doses q 6 h.

Other Penicillins

Carbenicillin (carboxybenzyl penicillin) is indicated for infections due to *Pseudomonas*, indole-positive strains of *Proteus* species, and strains of *E. coli* that are resistant to other antibiotics. It is not well absorbed orally and must be given parenterally. **Carbenicillin indanyl sodium** can be given orally but is recommended only for urinary tract infections.

Carbenicillin is excreted relatively slowly, but because the minimal inhibitory concentration is high even for susceptible organisms, large parenteral doses are needed to yield adequate serum levels of antibiotic. Dosages, with the quantity depending on the site and severity of the infection, are as follows: systemic *Pseudomonas* infections—adults, 24 to 40 gm IV; children, 400 to 500 mg/kg/day IV. Urinary tract *Pseudomonas* infections—adults, 200 mg/kg/day; children, 50 to 200 mg/kg/day; IM or IV. Infections due to other organisms—adults, 4 to 15 gm/day; children, 50 to 250 mg/kg/day; IM or IV. The usual adult dosage for carbenicillin indanyl sodium is 1 to 2 tablets q.i.d. orally. Each tablet contains the equivalent of 382 mg of carbenicillin. The oral ester of carbenicillin is reserved for treatment of urinary tract infections only.

Ticarcillin is more active in vitro against *Pseudomonas aeruginosa* than is carbenicillin. Since less of the drug is necessary for systemic infection, the patient may benefit from receiving a lower concentration of sodium. This may be beneficial in patients with uremia or congestive heart failure.

THE CEPHALOSPORINS

Cephalothin	Cephapirin	Cefadroxil
Cephaloridine	Cephradine	Cefaclor
Cefazolin	Cefamandole	Cephaloglycin
	Cefoxitin	Cephalexin

As with the penicillins, molecular manipulation has been applied to the cephalosporins, and these drugs have been developed at so rapid a pace that it is difficult to predict the potential usefulness of a new agent before another appears on the scene. Cephalosporin C is the parent substance from which were derived the first cephalosporins to find clinical use. Although cephalosporin C had a broad spectrum of action, including relative insensitivity to penicillinase, not much could be done clinically until the discovery of a method for the large scale production of 7-aminocephalosporanic acid.

Indications: As a group of compounds, cephalosporins often are used as prophylactic drugs, without clear-cut indications that they are clinically effective or necessary. Although they have a broad spectrum of activity, they are the *primary* drugs of choice against few bacterial species. In most instances, they are employed before the specific etiologic organism is known and, in addition, are often alternatives for patients hypersensitive to penicillin. Such use, however, is not without risk, since severe reactions occasionally have followed their administration to penicillin-sensitive patients. The cephalosporins have been used extensively because of their broad spectrum of activity against many gram-positive cocci (except enterococcus) and against numerous gram-negative rods (except *Pseudomonas*). Prior to the availability of cefamandole and cefoxitin, except for the greater potential nephrotoxicity of cephaloridine, differences among them were primarily related to variations in antibacterial activity and clinical pharmacology. However, cefamandole and cefoxitin are active against certain gram-negative organisms that are resistant to other cephalosporins. Cefoxitin and cefamandole, by virtue of their apparent resistance to degradation by cephalosporinase, extend the antibacterial spectrum of the cephalosporins. Cefoxitin, while resembling cephalothin, is actually a member of the cephamycin group of antibiotics. Although cefoxitin and, to a lesser degree, cefamandole are less active in vitro against *S. aureus* than some of the other cephalosporins, cefoxitin appears active against indole-positive *Proteus* spp. as well as against strains of *Bacteroides fragilis* and some strains of *Serratia*. In contrast to cefoxitin, the primary in vitro advantage of cefamandole appears to be its activity against some strains of *Enterobacter*. Cefamandole is also more active than other cephalosporins against *H. influenzae*, including ampicillin-resistant strains. However, there are insufficient clinical data to justify the use of cefamandole in the treatment of meningitis.

Side effects: In general, potential side effects are similar to those listed under the penicillins. Pain at the site of IM injection and thrombophlebitis following IV use are observed in various degrees with most of the cephalosporins. Although cephaloridine appears to be the least painful cephalosporin following IM injection, it is potentially the most nephrotoxic of the group. Some studies suggest that cephapirin is well tolerated by the parenteral route, whereas others report intolerance similar to that observed with cephalothin.

Administration and Dosage

Cephalothin is given IM or IV. The adult dosage ranges from 0.5 to 2 gm given q 4 to 6 h depending upon the severity of infection. It rarely is necessary to exceed 12 gm/day.

Cephaloridine is given IM or IV. The adult dosage is 0.5 to 1 gm q 6 to 8 h and should not exceed 4 gm/day because of possible renal tubular injury. *It should be avoided in patients with azotemia.*

Cefazolin is given IM or IV. The usual adult dosage in patients with moderate or severe infection is 0.5 to 1 gm q 6 to 8 h. In pneumococcal pneumonia and other infections of mild severity, 0.5 gm q 8 h is adequate treatment. Serum concentrations of cefazolin after comparable doses given IM are about twice those reached with cephaloridine and 4 times those achieved with cephalothin. Cefazolin enters the CSF very poorly, and is contraindicated in CNS infections.

Cephapirin possesses attributes almost identical to those of cephalothin. In fact, in many hospitals they are considered interchangeable. The dosage is the same as for cephalothin.

Cephradine is the only cephalosporin presently available as an oral and a parenteral formulation. The parenteral drug offers no advantage over cephalothin or cephapirin and is prescribed in the same dosage. However, unlike cephalothin or cephapirin, cephradine accumulates in serum when renal function is severely impaired. The oral formulation is very similar in activity and pharmacology to cephalexin. The usual dosage of cephradine is 250 to 500 mg orally q 6 h.

Cefamandole is prescribed IM or IV in usual adult dosage of 0.5 to 1 gm q 4 to 8 h. Peak serum concentrations are about 1½ times higher than those observed with comparable amounts of cephalothin. Unlike cephalothin, cefamandole is excreted unchanged into the urine and modifications of the dose are necessary in the presence of renal failure.

Cefoxitin is given IM or IV. The usual adult dosage range is 1 to 2 gm q 6 to 8 h. For IM use, cefoxitin may be diluted with 0.5% lidocaine to minimize discomfort. Cefoxitin has been shown by in vitro tests to have activity against certain strains of *Enterobacteriaceae* found resistant when tested with the cephalosporin class disc. For this reason, the cefoxitin disc should not be used for testing susceptibility to cephalosporins, and cephalosporin discs should not be used for testing susceptibility to cefoxitin.

Dilution methods, preferably the agar plate dilution procedure, are most accurate for susceptibility testing of obligate anaerobes. A bacterial isolate may be considered susceptible if the MIC value for cefoxitin is not more than 16 μg/ml. Organisms are considered resistant if the MIC is > 32 μg/ml.

Cefadroxil is prescribed orally in an initial dose of 1 gm followed by 0.5 gm q 12 to 36 h, depending on creatinine clearance.

Cefaclor is prescribed orally in a dose of 0.25 to 0.5 gm q 8 h. It is more active against some organisms in vitro than are other cephalosporins.

Cephaloglycin is prescribed only orally and its use has been restricted to urinary tract infections. However, since cephradine, cefadroxil, and cephalexin are better absorbed, cephaloglycin has been outmoded and superseded.

Cephalexin is prescribed orally in a dose of 250 to 500 mg q 6 h.

The Aminoglycosides

Streptomycin	Kanamycin	Gentamicin
Neomycin	Amikacin	Tobramycin

The aminoglycosides differ widely in clinical indications although they are chemically related and are qualitatively similar in absorption, distribution, excretion, antibacterial activity, and toxicity. All are poorly absorbed from the GI tract; most of an oral dose is excreted in the feces. Streptomycin, kanamycin, and gentamicin are well absorbed after injection and are primarily excreted by the kidney; neomycin is too toxic to be given parenterally.

The aminoglycosides can cause serious renal injury and severe irreversible 8th nerve damage with impaired hearing, vestibular dysfunction, or both. Eighth nerve damage is generally dose-related, though it has sometimes followed the use of small doses, and occurs most often when renal impairment reduces excretion and results in drug accumulation. The risk of ototoxicity is increased when a potent diuretic such as ethacrynic acid is used concurrently. Elderly patients are most susceptible to ototoxic effects. Audiometric tests should be performed at least twice/wk in patients receiving the drugs for > 7 days. However, deafness or vestibular damage may not appear until several days after the drug is stopped and may progress to complete loss of hearing. Because of the ototoxicity, the aminoglycosides should not be used parenterally for minor infections, or for severe infections that can be treated with safer antimicrobials. Renal injury is related to dosage and duration of therapy, and is usually reversible if the drug is discontinued at the first signs of toxicity. Oto- and nephrotoxicity are most severe with neomycin.

Streptomycin is chiefly effective against gram-negative and acid-fast bacteria. Its use in most infections has been largely superseded by kanamycin, gentamicin, tobramycin, and amikacin. **Dihydrostreptomycin**, a closely related modification, can produce irreversible deafness from cochlear 8th nerve damage and *should not be used.*

For the treatment of tuberculosis, streptomycin is effective when combined with other chemotherapeutic agents. It is also effective in granuloma inguinale, plague, tularemia, chancroid, and glanders. It may be given with tetracycline in brucellosis and Klebsiella pneumonia (Friedlander's pneumonia), and with penicillin in enterococcal infections, particularly endocarditis.

The drug is usually given IM, though it is well tolerated subcutaneously. Oral administration is ineffective in systemic infections. The optimum dosage for most infections is 1 to 2 gm/day, given in 500-mg doses. In tuberculosis, 1 gm is usually given daily or 2 or 3 times/wk. Following IM administration, streptomycin passes into the peritoneal, pericardial, pleural, and intraocular fluids, and into the bile (in the absence of hepatic or biliary damage); it also enters the amniotic fluid and the fetal circulation. It does not diffuse into thick-walled abscesses or empyema cavities, and passage into the CSF is variable. Since 60 to 80% of the drug is excreted in the urine within 24 h, relatively small doses give therapeutically effective urinary levels. Alkalinization of the urine increases the activity and effectiveness of aminoglycosides, including streptomycin, for urinary tract infections. Renal impairment causes low concentrations in the urine and high blood levels. Intrathecal injection has been abandoned. Intrapleural and intraperitoneal administration at the time of surgery is inadvisable, since streptomycin and other aminoglycosides have a neuromuscular blocking action, and respiratory arrest may result. Topical use of streptomycin is to be avoided because of the high incidence of sensitization.

Toxic reactions are more apt to develop with impaired renal function or with large doses given over prolonged periods. Disturbances of the 8th cranial nerve (vestibular portion) occur in about 20 to 25% of patients receiving 1 gm/day over prolonged periods. Increasing the dosage increases the possibility of damage. Damage to the 8th nerve is manifested by vertigo, tinnitus, loss of equilibrium, and, less frequently, hearing loss. Vestibular function may recover slowly after cessation of streptomycin, though damage can be permanent; auditory changes are irreversible. Mild reactions such as skin eruptions, eosinophilia, arthralgia, malaise, fever, and proteinuria may occur; some of these respond to antihistamines or desensitization. Dermatitis may develop in susceptible individuals handling streptomycin without rubber gloves.

Neomycin is bactericidal in vitro against a number of gram-negative organisms and staphylococci. Though the in vitro effectiveness is impressive, its clinical usefulness is limited by toxicity, and, with the availability of kanamycin, amikacin, tobramycin, and gentamicin, neomycin is no longer used for systemic infections. Apnea or severe hypotension due to neuromuscular blockade may follow intraperitoneal use of large amounts (usually 2 gm or more) during abdominal surgery, particularly during deep anesthesia and when other neuromuscular blocking agents are being used. Treatment consists of neostigmine, artificial respiration, and levarterenol.

Applied topically, the drug is well tolerated but may produce sensitization. Oral neomycin, because it is negligibly absorbed, rarely causes systemic toxic effects and is used for pre- and postoperative bowel sterilization and to suppress nitrogen-forming bacteria in patients with hepatic cirrhosis. However, deafness has resulted from prolonged oral therapy, and large oral doses (12 gm/day) can produce a malabsorption syndrome.

Kanamycin is active against gram-negative bacteria such as *E. coli, Enterobacter aerogenes,* and *Proteus* and *Salmonella* species, and against many staphylococci and the tubercle bacillus. Like other aminoglycosides, it is ineffective against streptococci, pneumococci, and all anaerobes, including *Clostridium* and *Bacteroides* species.

Kanamycin is useful in the initial treatment of sepsis thought due to gram-negative bacteria. In many instances, however, it has been superseded by gentamicin, which, in addition to encompassing the spectrum of kanamycin, is also active against *Pseudomonas.* The recommended dose of kanamycin for systemic infections is 15 mg/kg/day IM in divided doses q 8 to 12 h (not over 1.5 gm/day). Peak blood levels appear 1 to 2 h after injection; half-life is about 4 h. CSF levels are low. Excretion is mainly through the kidneys. Since it is poorly absorbed and has a minimal risk of toxicity, kanamycin, 50 mg/kg/day in divided doses, is given orally to reduce intestinal bacteria, either for preoperative bowel sterilization or in patients with hepatic cirrhosis. Smaller oral and parenteral doses should be given to patients with renal insufficiency.

Skin eruptions may follow parenteral use. More important, toxic reactions include 8th nerve damage, affecting primarily hearing rather than vestibular function, and renal irritation. The incidence of these reactions is related to the total dosage. The risk of ototoxicity can be reduced by decreasing the daily dose in patients with renal dysfunction and by restricting therapy to 5 to 7 days. Most patients receiving kanamycin develop cylindruria; many show proteinuria and other evidence of renal damage. Respiratory arrest has followed parenteral administration in patients with decreased renal function and has occurred with intraperitoneal administration during abdominal surgery.

Amikacin is a kanamycin derivative that is also active against *Pseudomonas* organisms. It is a semi-synthetic derivative of kanamycin that is available for parenteral treatment of infections caused by susceptible strains of gram-negative bacteria, and is not a substrate for many of the enzymes (resistant transfer factors) which inactivate other aminoglycoside antibiotics such as kanamycin, gentamicin, and tobramycin. Some bacterial strains possessing amikacin-inactivating enzymes, however, have been isolated, and nonenzymatic mechanisms can confer resistance to amikacin, as they do to other aminoglycosides. Most gram-negative strains resistant to amikacin are generally, although not invariably, resistant to kanamycin, gentamicin, and tobramycin.

The daily dosage of amikacin is the same as for kanamycin. Patients with impaired renal function need serum levels monitored and should be given smaller doses at longer intervals, after the recommended initial dose. One theoretical advantage of amikacin appears to be its relative stability in the presence of high concentrations of carbenicillin when compared to the lability of gentamicin or tobramycin in the presence of carbenicillin. There is some controversy as to policies for use of the various aminoglycosides that are currently available. Some feel that amikacin should not be used unless there is a high proportion of resistance to gentamicin and tobramycin in a given hospital.

Gentamicin is bactericidal against many strains of *S. aureus*, *E. coli*, *Klebsiella*, *Enterobacter*, *Serratia*, *Proteus*, and *Pseudomonas aeruginosa*. Many gentamicin-sensitive organisms are resistant to other antimicrobials, including other aminoglycosides. This is probably because gentamicin is less susceptible to inactivation by resistance transfer factor. The drug is used primarily for serious infections (e.g., pneumonia, urinary tract infections, septicemia) caused by gram-negative organisms resistant to the more commonly used antibiotics, especially *Pseudomonas* species.

Gentamicin is not absorbed from the GI tract. The usual dosage for adults and children is 3 mg/kg/day IM in divided doses q 8 h. Some cases of sepsis may require up to 5 mg/kg/day. Peak blood levels appear 30 to 90 min after an IM dose and effective levels persist for 6 to 8 h. Since gentamicin is almost completely excreted by the kidney, patients with impaired renal function should be given smaller doses at longer intervals after the recommended initial dose.

Like other aminoglycosides, gentamicin may cause 8th nerve injury, mainly vestibular, particularly if renal function is impaired or if dosage is high or prolonged. Dizziness may be the earliest sign of ototoxicity and should prompt discontinuance of the drug. The ototoxic effects are usually reversed when the drug is stopped, but permanent damage has occurred. Gentamicin is occasionally nephrotoxic, but apparently less frequently and less severely so than are kanamycin, neomycin, and the polymyxins. The topical preparation is well tolerated.

Tobramycin is administered similarly to gentamicin and its sole advantage appears to be its enhanced activity in vitro against *Pseudomonas aeruginosa*. Conversely, tobramycin appears to be less active in vitro against members of the Klebsiella-Enterobacter-Serratia group of organisms. Whereas tobramycin has not been used as extensively as gentamicin, there are some animal data to suggest that this agent is less nephrotoxic.

THE TETRACYCLINES

Oxytetracycline	Demeclocycline	Doxycycline
Tetracycline	Methacycline	Minocycline

These drugs are closely related broad-spectrum antibiotics, similar in antibacterial spectrum and toxicity. They are effective against many α-hemolytic streptococci, nonhemolytic streptococci, gram-negative rods, rickettsias, spirochetes, *E. histolytica*, *Mycoplasma*, and *Chlamydia*. Although tetracycline-resistant strains of pneumococci are increasing, they account for under 5% of isolates from pneumonia patients. Infections due to Group A β-hemolytic streptococci should not be treated with a tetracycline, since as many as 25% may be resistant when tested in vitro. Serious staphylococcal disease is also not a primary indication for any of the tetracyclines. Bacterial resistance to one tetracycline is generally accompanied by cross-resistance to the others.

Among the diseases amenable to tetracycline treatment are Rocky Mountain spotted fever, rickettsialpox, typhus (epidemic, murine, and scrub), Q fever, most pneumococcal pneumonia, brucellosis, some *H. influenzae* infections, urinary tract infections due to some gram-negative bacteria, meningococcemia, gonococcemia, lymphogranuloma venereum, psittacosis, and amebiasis.

Potential toxicity must be considered before using these drugs. GI side effects, especially diarrhea, are common. Tetracyclines may be dangerous in patients with renal dysfunction and may produce an abrupt rise in BUN, most probably from increased nitrogen breakdown, resulting in azotemia. Evidence suggests that some of the newer preparations (e.g., doxycycline) may be safer in azotemic patients. Outdated or deteriorated preparations may cause reversible renal tubular dysfunction indistinguishable from the Fanconi syndrome. Tetracyclines are active chelating agents (see DRUG INTERACTIONS in Ch. 241) and readily attach to calcium complexes in bones and teeth, often resulting in discolored teeth when given during pregnancy or childhood while dental calcification is occurring.

Tetracyclines, therefore, should be avoided after the first trimester of pregnancy, and from birth up to age 8. Because of a possible photosensitivity reaction, patients taking a tetracycline should avoid direct exposure to natural or artificial sunlight. Oral iron preparations and aluminum-, calcium-, or magnesium-containing antacids impair the absorption of oral tetracyclines and should not be taken concomitantly.

Oxytetracycline serum levels are antibacterial 1 h after oral administration and persist for as long as 24 h. The serum concentration is the same whether the agent is given in the fasting or nonfasting state. The usual oral dose given q 6 h is 1 to 2 gm/day for adults and 25 to 50 mg/kg for children. Since IM injection can be painful, other routes are preferred. Injection should be reserved for severe illnesses or when oral administration is impossible.

Tetracycline is closely related to oxytetracycline. It penetrates the blood-brain barrier with relative ease. For oral treatment, 1 to 2 gm/day for adults and 25 to 40 mg/kg/day for children, given in 2 to 4 divided doses, are usually adequate. IV use should be reserved for patients unable to take oral medication. The average adult IV dose is 500 mg q 12 h; this may be increased to a maximum of 500 mg q 6 h. For children, dosage is 10 to 20 mg/kg/day in 2 divided doses. The drug is relatively stable in solution, maintaining its activity at 37 C (98.6 F) for at least 7 days.

Demeclocycline (demethylchlortetracycline) has a slower renal clearance rate than other tetracyclines. The usual adult dosage is 600 mg/day orally in 2 to 4 divided doses; the dosage for children is reduced proportionately. Photosensitivity appears to be more frequent with demeclocycline than with other tetracyclines.

Methacycline is qualitatively similar to the other tetracyclines. The usual oral dose is 600 mg/day for adults and 7.5 to 15 mg/kg/day for children in 2 to 4 divided doses.

Doxycycline, a synthetic derivative of methacycline, is almost completely absorbed from the GI tract. It may be given IV when oral therapy is not indicated. The usual adult dosage is 200 mg on the first day and 100 mg/day thereafter in 1 or 2 divided doses; the dosage for children is 5 mg/kg on the first day and 2.5 mg/kg/day thereafter in 1 or 2 divided doses. Doxycycline, unlike other tetracyclines, can be used without special concern in patients with renal failure.

Minocycline has antibacterial activity comparable to other tetracyclines; it appears to be more effective than other tetracyclines in the meningococcal carrier state. A single 200-mg dose produces high blood serum concentrations in 1 h, and the serum half-life ranges from 11 to 17 h. The usual oral dosage is 200 mg initially, followed by 100 mg q 12 h. A limitation of minocycline is that dizziness, nausea, and lightheadedness occur frequently.

THE MACROLIDES

Erythromycin   Troleandomycin

Erythromycin: Gram-positive organisms, including pneumococci, Group A hemolytic streptococci, and many *S. aureus* strains, are highly sensitive to erythromycin. Strains of some gram-negative bacteria (such as *Neisseria*, *Hemophilus*, and *Brucella*) are inhibited, but to a lesser degree than some gram-positive organisms. The antibiotic is active against various rickettsias and *E. histolytica*, appears to be effective against the lymphogranuloma venereum organism, and is very effective against *Mycoplasma pneumoniae*. Coliform organisms, *Proteus*, and *Ps. aeruginosa* are all resistant. In clinical practice, use of erythromycin should be restricted to infections due to gram-positive bacteria in patients allergic to penicillin. Erythromycin appears to be effective in treating **Legionnaire's disease.**

Erythromycin is usually given orally, as the parent compound, the stearate, or the estolate. Dosage for adults is 0.25 to 1.0 gm q 6 h, and for children, 30 to 50 mg/kg/day, the larger quantities for infections that do not respond quickly. The maximal blood level roughly correlates with the dose. Erythromycin ethylsuccinate may be given orally (400 mg q 6 h for adults; 30 to 50 mg/kg/day for children). Erythromycin is given IV as the gluceptate or lactobionate in severe infections; dosage is 15 to 20 mg/kg/day (up to 4 gm/day).

Side effects include fever, skin eruptions, GI distress, pain on IM injection, and thrombophlebitis on IV injection. Erythromycin *estolate* may cause jaundice, which usually appears after 1 or 2 wk of therapy or after several courses of the drug; rarely, it may appear after only a few days of treatment. Eosinophilia may occur and liver function tests are frequently abnormal. Symptoms subside promptly when the drug is stopped. Erythromycin *base* and erythromycin *stearate* have not been associated with hepatotoxicity.

Troleandomycin (triacetyloleandomycin) is a chemical derivative of oleandomycin for oral use only. It is not affected by food or gastric acidity. Antibacterial activity closely resembles that of erythromycin. While most staphylococci demonstrate cross-resistance between these two drugs, some remain sensitive to troleandomycin. The usual adult dose is 250 to 500 mg orally q.i.d. for not > 10 days.

Toxic effects include skin reactions, GI upsets, and rare episodes of anaphylaxis. Patients receiving troleandomycin for > 10 days often show liver function changes. As with erythromycin, esterification appears to confer hepatotoxicity not found in the parent drug. Liver function returns to normal if the drug is discontinued promptly. Because of the high incidence of such reactions, troleando-mycin is *not recommended for routine or prolonged use.*

THE POLYPEPTIDES

Polymyxin B   Colistin   Bacitracin

Polymyxin B is principally effective against gram-negative bacteria, especially *Ps. aeruginosa*, though its use in *Pseudomonas* infection has been largely superseded by gentamicin and carbenicil-lin. Most strains of *Proteus* are resistant.

Following parenteral injection, the drug disappears rapidly from the blood. It does not appear in the CSF and cannot be detected in the bowel or urine in biologically active form. The drug may be given IM at 8-h intervals, the total daily dose being 1.5 to 2.5 mg/kg (15,000 to 25,000 u./kg), not to exceed 200 mg/day.

Parenteral polymyxin B may be nephrotoxic, with effects usually appearing about the fourth or fifth day of treatment. This danger is not pronounced when the recommended dosage is not exceeded. There may be proteinuria, oliguria, or nitrogen retention. Parenteral use may also result in neurologic disturbances (dizziness; weakness; facial, and sometimes extremity, paresthesias), usually not seri-ous enough to stop the drug. However, respiratory paralysis is a potential complication. Small quan-tities of the drug may be given intrathecally in severe meningeal infection, but this route should be avoided if possible.

Polymyxin B is not absorbed from the bowel, from which it eliminates sensitive organisms; 75 to 100 mg q.i.d. may be given orally for enteritis due to such gram-negative bacteria as *Shigella*.

Colistin (polymyxin E) is mainly effective against gram-negative bacteria. Similar to polymyxin B in its structure and range of activity, it is particularly effective in *Ps. aeruginosa* infections, though like polymyxin B, this use has been superseded to a large extent by gentamicin and carbenicillin. It is used in oral and otic products as colistin sulfate, and IM, IV, and intrathecally as sodium colistimeth-ate. If formulated with dibucaine it *cannot* be given intrathecally. Oral use is limited to enteric infec-tions, since it is not absorbed orally. Dosage for adults is: oral, 5 to 15 mg/kg/day in 3 divided doses; IM and IV, 2.5 to 5 mg/kg/day in 2 to 4 divided doses. In side effects, analogous salts of colistin and polymyxin B are identical.

Bacitracin has a range of activity similar to that of penicillin. It inhibits the growth of streptococci, staphylococci, gonococci, meningococci, clostridia, *Treponema pallidum*, and *E. histolytica*. The effect of bacitracin is not altered by serum, pus, or necrotic tissue.

Since bacitracin is not absorbed from the GI tract, oral administration is ineffective; because baci-tracin is nephrotoxic, it is rarely used parenterally. However, topical ointments are available for ophthalmic and dermal use. Bacitracin may be dissolved in saline to a concentration of 500 u./ml for topical use.

MISCELLANEOUS ANTIBIOTICS

Chloramphenicol   Rifampin   Vancomycin
Lincomycin   Cycloserine   Spectinomycin
Clindamycin

Chloramphenicol inhibits the growth of a wide range of gram-positive and -negative bacteria and rickettsia. It is the drug of choice in typhoid fever and is effective in *H. influenzae* meningitis, typhus, Rocky Mountain spotted fever, lymphogranuloma venereum, psittacosis, and *Salmonella* and *Shi-gella* infections. In addition, it is active against most anaerobic organisms, including *Bacteroides* spp.

Chloramphenicol is effective when given orally; therapeutic blood levels appear 30 min after inges-tion. It can also be given IV, but IM absorption is erratic. The dose, oral or IV, is 50 to 75 mg/kg/day in divided doses q 6 h. The serum level of chloramphenicol (normal effective range is 5 to 20 μg/ml) should be monitored closely and the dosage adjusted accordingly.

Chloramphenicol may produce bone marrow depression with neutropenia, agranulocytosis, or, in the most severe cases, aplastic anemia. It is impossible to protect against this rare but potentially fatal complication even with monitoring of the blood count. *For this reason, chloramphenicol should not be used unless clearly indicated for severe infection; it should not be used in trivial infections or for prophylaxis.* A distinct advantage of chloramphenicol is its penetration into the CNS. For this reason it is the drug of choice for brain abscess of unknown etiology. Prolonged use of large doses may cause a reversible maturation arrest of the RBC precursors, indicated by a sudden drop in the reticulocyte count and an abrupt rise in the serum iron level. Newborns receiving over 25 mg/kg/day have developed the **gray baby syndrome,** a state of cardiovascular collapse with abdominal disten-tion, lethargy, respiratory distress, and gray cyanosis which is fatal if the drug is continued. It results from excessive blood concentrations of chloramphenicol due to a deficient glucuronic-acid conju-gating mechanism plus diminished renal function, both of which are normal in the newborn, espe-cially if premature. In adults, impaired hepatic or renal function may reduce the ability to metabolize and excrete the drug, and dosage may have to be adjusted accordingly.

Lincomycin is effective against most gram-positive organisms, including staphylococci, streptococci, and pneumococci, as well as most anaerobes. Most enterococci and *Neisseria* species, and some erythromycin-resistant staphylococci, are resistant. Lincomycin may be given orally or parenterally. It appears to penetrate well into bone and CNS. The usual oral dosage for adults is 500 mg t.i.d. or q.i.d.; for children, 30 to 60 mg/kg/day in 3 or 4 divided doses. The usual IM dosage for adults is 600 mg q 12 to 24 h; for children, 10 mg/kg q 12 to 24 h. In serious infections, the drug may be given IV as an infusion. Severe diarrhea, sometimes with blood and mucus, is the main side effect. Hypersensitivity and reversible blood dyscrasias have also been reported.

Clindamycin, an analog of lincomycin, is useful in anaerobic infections, including those produced by *Bacteroides* spp. It is better absorbed orally and produces fewer GI side effects than the parent compound, but, unlike lincomycin, it does *not* penetrate well into CNS and bone. The usual oral adult dosage is 150 to 300 mg q 6 h; for children, 8 to 16 mg/kg/day divided into 3 or 4 doses. Side effects are primarily GI. This antibiotic may produce serious pseudomembranous colitis more frequently than originally thought. It should not be used for ordinary infections. The clindamycin-associated colitis appears to be the result of an enterotoxin produced by strains of clostridia.

Rifampin, a derivative of rifamycin, is effective in vitro against a variety of gram-positive and -negative organisms. However, its use in these infections is limited by the rapid emergence of resistant strains. Rifampin is absorbed from the GI tract and excreted mainly in the bile. It is used, in combination with at least one other antituberculous drug, in the treatment of pulmonary tuberculosis (see TUBERCULOSIS in Ch. 8). It may be useful alone for the eradication of *Neisseria meningitidis* in asymptomatic carriers during outbreaks. The oral dosage is 600 mg once/day for adults and 10 to 20 mg/kg/day for children (maximum 600 mg/day). Side effects include liver dysfunction; anticoagulant antagonism; red-orange staining of urine, feces, saliva, and tears; hypersensitivity phenomena; GI reactions; and, infrequently, neurologic disturbances.

Cycloserine has antibacterial activity of wide range but of relatively low degree, inhibiting many gram-positive and -negative organisms in vitro. Clinically, it has been useful in tuberculosis resistant to other agents. Because of the hazard of neurotoxicity, cycloserine should be used with caution and only when other drugs have been ineffective. The dosage is 500 mg to 1 gm/day in 2 to 4 equal oral doses.

Vancomycin is active against β-hemolytic streptococci, staphylococci, *Streptococcus faecalis, Streptococcus pneumoniae, Neisseria gonorrhoeae, Corynebacterium diphtheriae,* and *Clostridium tetani,* and ineffective against gram-negative rods. Staphylococci develop slight or no resistance to vancomycin. Although highly effective against resistant staphylococci, it has largely been replaced by newer drugs that are less toxic and easier to give. However, it still remains a useful drug in methicillin-resistant staphylococcal infections and in penicillin-allergic patients with staphylococcal infections or enterococcal endocarditis.

Vancomycin is not absorbed from the GI tract and must be given IV. The usual dosage is 250 to 500 mg q 6 h for 2 to 4 wk. The 500-mg dose is given in staphylococcal bacteremia; 1 gm/day is used in endocarditis or meningitis.

Pain and thrombophlebitis at the injection site are common. Skin eruptions, usually morbilliform, result from sensitization. Auditory impairment may occur, especially with prolonged therapy or high dosage. Many patients receiving the drug develop cylindruria and proteinuria, and facial paresthesias are common. Rarely, azotemia and decreased PSP excretion may appear when large doses are given for 2 wk or more.

Spectinomycin is active in vitro against most strains of *N. gonorrhoeae* and is used when susceptible strains cause acute gonorrheal urethritis and proctitis in the male and acute gonorrheal cervicitis and proctitis in the female. It is not used in treating syphilis. No cross-resistance of *N. gonorrhoeae* between spectinomycin and penicillin has been shown in vitro. The drug is rapidly absorbed after IM injection; excretion is largely renal. The drug is given as a single 2-gm IM dose. Adverse reactions include soreness at the injection site, urticaria, nausea, fever, and, after multiple doses, a decrease in Hb, Hct, and creatinine clearance, and an elevation of alkaline phosphatase, BUN, and SGPT. These untoward effects are uncommon.

SULFONAMIDES

The sulfonamides are synthetic antimicrobial agents with a wide antibacterial spectrum encompassing most gram-positive and many gram-negative organisms. Especially among the latter, however, many strains of an individual species may be resistant. The sulfonamides are bacteriostatic, not bactericidal. They inhibit growth and multiplication of bacteria by interfering with bacterial uptake of aminobenzoic acid. They also depress the activity of some fungi and protozoa. Bacterial sensitivity is the same for the various sulfonamides, and cross-resistance is absolute.

Most sulfonamides are absorbed rapidly and well by mouth, the small intestine being the major site of absorption, although 90% of succinylsulfathiazole and phthalylsulfathiazole is excreted unchanged in the feces. Parenteral administration is difficult, since the soluble sulfonamide salts are highly alkaline and irritating to the tissues.

The sulfonamides are widely distributed throughout all tissues, a clinically important point. High levels are achieved in pleural, peritoneal, synovial, and ocular fluids. CSF levels are effective in meningeal infections. Sulfonamides are loosely and reversibly bound in varying degrees to serum albumin. Since the bound sulfonamide is inactive and nondiffusible, the degree of binding can affect antibacterial effectiveness, distribution, and excretion rate. The antibacterial action of sulfonamides is also inhibited by pus.

The sulfonamides are metabolized mainly by the liver to acetylated forms and glucuronides, both therapeutically inactive. Excretion is primarily by glomerular filtration with minimal tubular secretion or reabsorption.

Precautions: The relative insolubility of most sulfonamides, especially their acetylated metabolites, may cause them to precipitate in the renal tubules. The more soluble analogs should be chosen for systemic therapy, and the patient must be well hydrated. To avoid crystalluria and renal damage, fluid intake should be sufficient to produce a urinary output of 1200 to 1500 ml/day. If therapy is to be prolonged, blood counts and urinalyses should be performed initially and at 2-wk intervals. Since sulfonamides easily pass the placenta and enter the fetus in concentrations sufficient to produce antibacterial and toxic effects, they should not be given to pregnant women at term. In addition, they should not be used in neonates, especially premature infants, since sulfonamide competes with bilirubin for serum albumin binding. Increased levels of free bilirubin result, possibly causing kernicterus in the infant.

Side effects of the sulfonamides include (1) GI reactions, such as nausea, vomiting, and diarrhea; (2) hypersensitivity reactions, such as rashes, the Stevens-Johnson syndrome (see ERYTHEMA MULTIFORME in Ch. 196), serum sickness, anaphylaxis, and angioedema; (3) crystalluria, oliguria, and anuria; (4) hematologic reactions, such as methemoglobinemia, agranulocytosis, thrombocytopenia, kernicterus in the newborn, and hemolytic anemia in patients with G6PD deficiency; and (5) neurologic effects, such as peripheral neuritis, insomnia, and headache. Other side effects include hypothyroidism, potentiation of sulfonylureas with consequent hypoglycemia; and potentiation of coumarin anticoagulants. The incidence of side effects is different for the various sulfonamides, but cross-sensitivity is common.

Indications: Sulfonamides are used mostly in urinary tract infections, particularly acute uncomplicated infections. Chancroid and lymphogranuloma venereum may be treated with sulfonamides until syphilis has been ruled out, at which time therapy is changed. Sulfonamides are given orally for antistreptococcal prophylaxis in patients with a history of rheumatic fever. Sulfonamides are often effective in nocardiosis. Nonabsorbable sulfonamides have been used for pre- and postoperative bowel sterilization and to treat bacillary dysentery. Since the antibacterial activity of the various analogs is similar, the choice in any given infection rests primarily on the pharmacologic properties or formulation desired.

CLASSES OF SULFONAMIDES

The sulfonamides can be classified according to duration of action or use. The specific drugs mentioned below are representative examples.

Short-Acting Sulfonamides

These are rapidly absorbed and excreted and are the preferred sulfonamides for the treatment of systemic and urinary tract infections.

Sulfadiazine has relatively high antibacterial activity. The initial adult dose, 2 to 4 gm orally, is followed by 500 mg to 1 gm q 4 to 6 h. The dose in children is 35 to 50 mg/kg orally initially, then 13 to 20 mg/kg q 4 h. Sulfadiazine sodium is given IV as a 5% solution, 100 mg/kg IV initially, then 30 to 50 mg/kg IV q 6 to 8 h. Parenteral therapy is used only if oral administration is impossible.

Sulfisoxazole is used in GU infections. The dosage is the same as for sulfadiazine.

Sulfachlorpyridazine and **sulfamethizole** are used in GU infections, and are given orally. For sulfachlorpyridazine, the initial adult dose is 2 to 4 gm, followed by 2 to 4 gm/day divided in 3 to 6 doses; For sulfamethizole, the adult dose is 500 mg 5 or 6 times/day.

Sulfonamide mixtures are combinations of 2 or 3 short-acting sulfonamides. They provide therapeutic sulfonamide levels with a reduced risk of crystalluria and renal damage (though not a lesser risk of other reactions). Trisulfapyrimidines are such a triple sulfonamide mixture, combining equal parts of sulfadiazine, sulfamerazine, and sulfamethazine. The oral dosage is 4 gm initially, then 1 gm 4 to 6 times/day.

Intermediate-Acting Sulfonamides

These are rapidly absorbed but more slowly excreted, and doses need to be given only once or twice daily. They are most commonly used for rheumatic fever prophylaxis or in GU infections.

Sulfamethoxazole is similar to sulfisoxazole except for its slower excretion rate. The usual oral adult dosage is 1 gm initially, then 2 gm q 12 h.

Sulfaethidole is a short-acting oral sulfonamide prepared in a sustained-released formulation. Adult dosage is 4 gm initially, then 2 gm q 12 h. For children, the dosage is 60 mg/kg initially, then 30 mg/kg q 12 h.

Long-Acting Sulfonamides

These are excreted very slowly (serum half-life is 30 to 40 h) and need to be given only once daily. *Because of serious side effects (e.g., Stevens-Johnson syndrome), their use is seldom justified.* **Sulfamethoxypyridazine** is given orally, 1 gm initially, then 500 mg/day. It is given as a weekly oral dose of 30 mg/kg for prophylaxis after rheumatic fever. **Sulfameter** is similar to the other long-acting oral sulfonamides. The dose is 1500 mg orally initially, then 500 mg/day.

Poorly Absorbed Sulfonamides

These are used specifically for their effect on intestinal flora. They are given for pre- and postoperative bowel sterilization, although the value of such therapy is disputed, and for bacillary dysentery, although soluble sulfonamides are more effective and antibiotics are superior to sulfonamides. Side effects seldom occur.

Phthalylsulfathiazole dosage is 50 to 100 mg/kg/day (not over 8 gm/day) in 6 equal oral doses q 4 h. **Succinylsulfathiazole** dosage is 250 mg/kg/day orally in 6 equal doses q 4 h.

Sulfamethoxazole-trimethoprim is a combination of 2 agents that inhibit different steps in folic acid synthesis by bacteria. Sulfamethoxazole is a competitive inhibitor of para-aminobenzoic acid and trimethoprim, a diaminopyrimadine, inhibits dihydrofolate reductase. The 2 drugs are synergistic in vitro against many species of bacteria. The combination has been approved in the USA for treatment of recurrent urinary tract infection caused by susceptible *Enterobacteriaceae*, i.e., *E. coli*, *Klebsiella*, *Enterobacter*, and *Proteus* spp. Isolates of *Pseudomonas* and enterococci are generally resistant. Other indications are Shigellosis, otitis media caused by susceptible isolates, and treatment of *Pneumocystis carinii* infection.

The combination is available as an oral preparation containing 80 mg of trimethoprim and 400 mg of sulfamethoxazole. In addition, there is a double strength formulation containing 160 mg trimethoprim and 800 mg of sulfamethoxazole. The usual adult dosage for urinary tract infection is 160 mg trimethoprim and 800 mg sulfamethoxazole q 12 h for 10 to 14 days. An identical daily dosage is used for 5 days in the treatment of Shigellosis. The recommended dose for children with urinary tract infection or otitis media is 8 mg/kg trimethoprim and 40 mg/kg sulfamethoxazole per 24 h, given in 2 divided doses q 12 h for 10 days. The same daily dosage is used for 5 days in the treatment of Shigellosis in children. Dosage of the drug has to be reduced in the presence of renal failure. Side effects are identical to those reported with sulfonamide therapy.

OTHER SYNTHETIC ANTIMICROBIALS

Nitrofurantoin is active in vitro against some strains of *S. aureus*, enterococci, and most gram-negative organisms. For practical purposes, at levels achieved in the urine, it is effective primarily against *E. coli*. It is used in urinary tract infections at oral doses of 50 to 100 mg q.i.d. in adults and 5 to 7 mg/kg/day in 4 divided doses in children. The macrocrystal form is better tolerated orally. The drug may be given IM or IV when oral therapy is impossible; dosage for patients weighing over 55 kg (120 lb) is 180 mg b.i.d., and for those under 55 kg it is 3 mg/kg b.i.d.

Nitrofurantoin may cause hemolytic anemia in neonates because of their immature enzyme systems (glutathione instability), and is contraindicated in infants < 1 mo old. Hemolytic anemia is also a risk in patients with G6PD deficiency. Peripheral neuropathy, hypersensitivity, and GI side effects also occur.

Furazolidone, another nitrofuran, is indicated for GI infections. Its spectrum of effectiveness covers the majority of GI pathogens, including *E. coli*, staphylococci, *Salmonella*, *Shigella*, *Proteus*, *Aerobacter aerogenes*, *Vibrio cholerae*, and *Giardia lamblia*. The recommended oral doses are 100 mg q.i.d. in adults, and 25 to 50 mg q.i.d. in children over 5 yr of age. Monoamine oxidase inhibitors, tyramine-containing foods, and indirectly acting sympathomimetics are contraindicated in patients receiving furazolidone. The drug may produce a disulfiram-like reaction, and alcohol should be avoided during or within 4 days of furazolidone therapy. Other side effects resemble those of nitrofurantoin. Furazolidone is contraindicated in children < 1 mo old.

Nalidixic acid is orally absorbed and active against gram-negative organisms, except *Pseudomonas* species. Doses are given orally, 1 gm q.i.d. for adults and up to 55 mg/kg/day in 4 doses for children. Side effects include hemolytic anemia, photosensitivity reactions, GI and visual disturbances, and toxic psychoses. The drug is of limited usefulness, since gram-negative organisms often develop resistance during therapy. **Oxolinic acid** is similar in activity to nalidixic acid but dosage is 750 mg b.i.d. orally.

Isoniazid (INH) and **ethambutol (EMB),** are discussed under Tuberculosis in Ch. 8.

ANTIVIRAL DRUGS

Difficulties with antiviral chemotherapy arise because of the obligatory dependence of viruses on host cell metabolism for replication and because few virus-specific enzyme systems are as yet vulnerable to chemotherapeutic intervention. Agents that block viral replication also block normal host cell processes, and the limits between effective and toxic doses are very narrow. There are numerous complications for the clinically useful antiviral agents, including a wide variety of side effects and a relatively low therapeutic index. Patients receiving antiviral agents must be monitored carefully. Further, some resistant virus strains have developed in patients receiving initially effective therapy.

Chemotherapeutic intervention could occur at the time of viral particle attachment to host cell membranes or of uncoating of viral nucleic acids, by blocking transcription in some deoxyribo-viruses and riboviruses that require a virus-specific DNA-dependent RNA polymerase, by blocking translation at the level of viral messenger RNA (which must be different from mammalian host cell messenger RNA, since the interferon-induced translation inhibitory protein can recognize the difference), and by blocking specific virus-coded enzymes produced in the host cells that are essential for viral replication but not for normal host cell metabolism.

Amantadine is primarily used for influenza *prophylaxis* and appears to act at the early stage of virus-host interaction, blocking either virus penetration into the host cells or uncoating. Given orally, 90% of the drug may be recovered unchanged in the urine; about 50% of a single dose is recovered in 20 h. Amantadine is partially protective against influenza A_2 infection and is recommended for prophylactic treatment of high-risk patients during A_2 epidemics. Prophylaxis is immediate. Antibody formation following influenza infection apparently is not blocked. In addition, evidence suggests that when the drug is given as *treatment* the clinical course of illness may be shortened. Side effects include CNS reactions (e.g., nervousness, insomnia, dizziness, lightheadedness, slurred speech, ataxia, inability to concentrate, hallucinations, and depression); skin rashes; and anorexia, nausea, and constipation. Side effects usually develop within 48 h after starting amantadine and often resolve during continued use. Amantadine has anticholinergic activity and may intensify peripheral and central adverse effects of other anticholinergic drugs administered concomitantly. The usual prophylactic dose is 100 mg orally b.i.d. for the duration of the epidemic. For children aged 1 to 9 yr, the daily dose is 4 to 8 mg/kg in 2 or 3 divided doses, to a maximum of 150 mg/day.

Methisazone (not available in the USA) is effective for smallpox prophylaxis in susceptible individuals exposed to active smallpox infection, but it does not supersede vaccination as the primary modality for preventing the disease. It is also effective in treating the complications of vaccination: (1) eczema vaccinatum; (2) vaccinia gangrenosa, an otherwise fatal complication that may develop in immune-deficient persons; and (3) ectopic vaccinia, which may result from either autoinoculation or heteroinoculation and may develop in a dangerous site such as the face or eyes.

Methisazone must be given orally. Peak blood levels are attained in 4 to 7 h; there is no detectable drug in the blood after 10 to 12 h. For smallpox prophylaxis, the usual adult dose is either 1.5 gm orally b.i.d. for 4 days, or 3 gm orally for 2 doses 12 h apart. For vaccinia gangrenosa and eczema vaccinatum, the recommended regimen is 200 mg/kg orally initially, followed by 50 mg/kg orally q 6 h for 8 doses. The main side effects are nausea, vomiting, and alcohol intolerance.

Idoxuridine (IDU) apparently acts by being phosphorylated and incorporated into newly synthesized DNA, irreversibly replacing thymidine and producing an abnormal and essentially nonfunctional DNA molecule. The drug acts on both viral and host cell DNA and is *highly toxic to host cells*. Clinical use of IDU has been limited to topical therapy because of its high systemic toxicity. An ophthalmic preparation has been used to treat herpes simplex keratoconjunctivitis, but is less effective for recurrent herpes keratitis, probably because of the development of drug-resistant virus strains. Two such topical ophthalmic preparations are available: a 0.1% aqueous solution and a 0.5% ointment. The solution is given hourly as 1 drop instilled conjunctivally during waking hours and q 2 h at night. The ointment is given 5 times/day (q 4 h), the last dose given before the patient retires. Ophthalmic IDU may cause irritation, pain, pruritus, and inflammation or edema of the eyelids; rare allergic reactions and photophobia have also been reported.

Vidarabine (adenine arabinoside, Ara-A) interferes with viral DNA synthesis and is effective in the treatment of herpes simplex virus infections. Ophthalmic preparations of vidarabine are effective for acute keratoconjunctivitis and recurrent superficial keratitis caused by herpes simplex virus types 1 and 2. Vidarabine appears less susceptible to the development of drug resistant viral strains than idoxuridine, and IDU resistant infections often respond to vidarabine treatment. A 3% ophthalmic ointment is available and is given 5 times/day (q 3 h). Treatment should be continued for several days after complete healing to prevent recurrent infection. Ophthalmic vidarabine may cause tearing, irritation, pain, photophobia and superficial punctate keratitis.

In recent clinical trials, systemic vidarabine for herpes encephalitis has reduced mortality from 70% to 28%. It is most effective when therapy is initiated early, and little benefit ensues when therapy is started after the patient is comatose. Systemic vidarabine is given as an intravenous infusion of 15 mg/kg/day over 12 hours for 10 days. Side effects include nausea, vomiting, tremor and phlebitis at the infusion site. Bone marrow toxicity and hepatotoxicity may occur with high doses.

Trifluridine (trifluorothymidine), a thymidine analog, interferes with DNA synthesis and is effective in treating acute herpes keratitis caused by herpes simplex virus types 1 and 2. Trifluridine is as effective as vidarabine and may be effective in patients who have not responded to idoxuridine or vidarabine. A 1% ophthalmic solution is available, and 1 drop should be instilled into the affected eye q 2 h while the patient is awake. The maximum recommended dose is 9 drops/day until the corneal ulcer is re-epithelialized, then 5 drops/day (1 drop q 4 h) for 7 days. If there is no improvement in 7 days, another agent should be considered.

Side effects include burning or stinging in the eye and palpebral edema; less frequently, punctate keratopathy and hypersensitivity reactions may develop.

Levamisole is an immunotropic drug that has been used experimentally, but its exact mechanism of action in viral illness is not understood. In clinical trials levamisole has been effective for treatment of herpes progenitalis. Pain was dramatically relieved with levamisole therapy in acute genital herpes but recurrent genital herpes responded only when both partners were treated simultaneously. The recommended dosage for acute infection is 50 mg levamisole orally t.i.d. for 4 days with a 2nd course of treatment after 10 to 14 days. Recurrent genital herpes requires 50 mg levamisole orally 3 times/day for 2 consecutive days each week for 4 to 8 wk.

Prophylactic use of levamisole in children with a history of frequent wintertime viral respiratory infections decreased the number of viral URIs and the duration and severity of the illnesses. The levamisole dosage was 1.25 mg/kg orally twice a day for 2 consecutive days each week during the winter months. This use of levamisole is investigational and does not represent an FDA-approved clinical indication. Side effects with levamisole are uncommon and may include nervousness, nausea, vomiting, diarrhea, dysosmia, metallic taste and skin rash.

Interferon is a natural cellular product formed in response to viral or other foreign nucleic acids. It is detectable as early as 2 h after infection. It is released from infected host cells and induces production of translation inhibitory protein **(TIP)** in other host cells. TIP binds to cellular ribosomes and selectively blocks translation of viral RNA, stopping viral replication without disturbing host messenger RNA translation and permitting normal host cell function. Interferon is not virus-specific and may be active against many viruses; it is species specific, however, and can be used only in the same species as initially produced it. Recent work with recombinant DNA technics may allow production of human interferon from bacterial cells.

---

247. DRUGS ACTING ON THE CENTRAL NERVOUS SYSTEM

GENERAL CENTRAL NERVOUS SYSTEM DEPRESSANTS

Drugs that depress the central nervous system **(CNS)** make up the most widely employed group of pharmacologic agents. General (nonselective) CNS depressants include the anesthetic gases, alcohol, barbiturates, and many of the sedative-hypnotics, including antianxiety agents. All depress brain function by decreasing the activity of both the sensory and motor areas of the brain. The action of these drugs is dose-dependent and progresses from sedation through somnolence, hypnosis, anesthesia, coma, and death, usually from respiratory failure. Other CNS depressants are more selective and act on specific brain centers. These drugs include certain analgesics (narcotic and non-narcotic), anticonvulsants, antipsychotics, antiparkinsonian agents, antipyretics, and antitussives.

SEDATIVES AND HYPNOTICS

Sedatives are drugs that calm and relax a patient without necessarily producing sleep. **Hypnotics** are drugs that induce sleep. However, terms such as sedative, hypnotic, antianxiety agent, minor tranquilizer, and anxiolytics are ambiguous and often used interchangeably; there is no clear distinction among them. Often a single drug is useful in more than one therapeutic category, depending on the dosage (for a discussion of nonhypnotic use of these drugs see under Tranquilizers below).

The ideal hypnotic, even in large doses, should induce sleep or improve its quality without producing profound depression; drug effects should dissipate rapidly upon awaking. However, none of the available hypnotics are ideal and all involve some risk of overdose, habituation, tolerance, and addiction, as well as withdrawal symptoms that include temporary recurrence of sleeplessness. In the treatment of insomnia, short-term (2 to 4 wk) use of hypnotics is preferred; it should not be assumed that chronic use is required. Ambulatory patients given sedative-hypnotics should be warned to avoid activities requiring mental alertness, judgment, and physical coordination (e.g., driving a vehicle or operating machinery). Hypnotic drugs should be used with special caution in patients with severe pulmonary insufficiency. For clinical discussion of insomnia see Ch. 121; for potential problems of hypnotic drug use see Chs. 136 and 141.

Adverse effects: Drowsiness, lethargy, and hangover are observed commonly after excessive intake of sedative-hypnotics. Rarely, skin eruptions (e.g., urticaria, angioneurotic edema, and bullous erythema multiforme) and GI disturbances (e.g., nausea and vomiting) may be seen. With any sedative, the elderly may exhibit restlessness, excitement, or exacerbations of symptoms of organic brain disorders. Barbiturates are contraindicated in patients with porphyria, since they may provoke an acute episode.

Many patients take higher doses of hypnotics than they admit, and slurring of speech, incoordination, tremulousness, and nystagmus should arouse suspicion of overdosage. Serum levels of many drugs can be determined in the laboratory.

Sedative-hypnotics are additive in effect with other CNS depressants (e.g., alcohol, antianxiety agents, opiates, antihistamines, phenothiazines, and antidepressants). Doses should be reduced when these drugs are given concurrently. Barbiturates, chloral hydrate, chloral betaine, and gluteth-imide can interact with coumarin anticoagulants (see DRUG INTERACTIONS in Ch. 241).

Commonly Used Hypnotic Drugs

TABLE 247–1 lists a number of drugs and their average dosages known to be effective in the short-term treatment of insomnia. A hypnotic should be selected with attention to the cause of the sleep problem and the pattern of the sleep disorder. The choice of drug should be based on physician and patient preference and past experience. Barbiturates and chloral hydrate, although they have many of the same disadvantages, are effective and cheaper than the newer agents. Flurazepam has mini-mal suicidal risk, minimally alters REM sleep, and does not cause REM rebound.

The **barbiturates** are the hypnotics to which all others are compared; their adverse effects and the dangers of overdosage and chronic use are well known. Tolerance, habituation, and drug depen-dence may develop with barbiturates. They also induce hepatic drug-metabolizing enzymes that can adversely interact with other drugs, such as coumarin anticoagulants. The different barbiturates act similarly, but dosage, onset, and duration of sedation may differ.

In chronic insomnia or inverted sleep pattern due to long-term use of barbiturates, habituation to the drug may outlast the initial reason for taking it. Attempts by the patient to discontinue the drug may lead to withdrawal symptoms, reinforcing his belief that he needs it. Often a patient can be gradually weaned from the drug. If he strongly resists withdrawal, it may be worthwhile to change to a different drug.

Flurazepam and nitrazepam, benzodiazepine derivatives, can have a marked hypnotic effect and may be used instead of barbiturates in insomnia. Doses of 15 to 30 mg of flurazepam or 5 to 10 mg of nitrazepam (not available in the USA) suffice in most cases; smaller doses may be used for the elderly. These compounds have much less addiction potential than other hypnotics, and overdoses rarely are fatal. The dosage that induces serious respiratory and vital center depression is consider-ably greater with benzodiazepines than with barbiturates and most other nonbarbiturate sedative-hypnotics. Flurazepam has gained great popularity for this reason. It is reasonable to select it or other benzodiazepines as the agent of choice for many patients with insomnia. However, these drugs (like the others) may increase the effects of alcohol, and serious CNS depression may result if they are taken together. Flurazepam is converted to a slowly active metabolite; nightly or alternate-night use may result in drowsiness or ataxia during the day. After several days of use, impairment of visual-motor coordination may be greater than that resulting from the use of a short-acting barbiturate.

Chloral hydrate is a relatively weak hypnotic, particularly suited for elderly patients. The usual oral dose is 0.5 to 1 gm; if necessary, an additional 0.5 gm may be given after 1 h. It is available in capsules and in solutions that have a pungent, unpleasant taste. Chloral hydrate is similar to the barbiturates in its potential for tolerance, addiction, and induction of hepatic drug-metabolizing en-zymes.

Ethchlorvynol acts rapidly, is a somewhat less effective hypnotic than chloral hydrate, and does not stimulate hepatic enzyme activity. The recommended oral dose is 0.5 gm, although 1 gm fre-quently is given.

Glutethimide and **methyprylon** are related hypnotics. They have a fairly long duration of action and, like barbiturates, can produce tolerance and addiction. The usual oral hypnotic doses are glutethimide 500 mg and methyprylon 200 to 400 mg. *Overdosage with glutethimide is particularly dangerous because the toxic dose is not much larger than the hypnotic dose.* Perhaps because the

TABLE 247–1. COMMONLY USED HYPNOTICS

Drug	Range of Single Hypnotic Dose (mg)
Barbiturates	
Amobarbital	100–200
Butabarbital	100–200
Pentobarbital	100–200
Phenobarbital	100–300
Secobarbital	100–200
Nonbarbiturates	
Chloral hydrate	500–2000
Ethchlorvynol	500–1000
Ethinamate	500–1000
Flurazepam	15–45
Glutethimide	500–1000
Methaqualone	150–300
Methyprylon	200–400
Triclofos sodium	750–1500

drug is recycled through the GI tract, blood levels fluctuate and produce cyclic changes in the depth of coma. If hemodialysis is used to counteract an overdose of glutethimide, a non-polar solvent used as the dialysate may enhance removal of the drug from the bloodstream.

Methaqualone is used as a hypnotic in oral doses of 150 to 300 mg. It has been subject to significant abuse; coma caused by large doses may be accompanied by seizures.

NARCOTICS AND NARCOTIC ANTAGONISTS

If possible, the underlying cause of the pain should be sought and removed. Therapeutic goals vary with the pain's etiology, nature, and expected duration, and with the location of treatment (home or hospital). A reasonable goal is to decrease pain to a level that allows the patient to eat, sleep, and convalesce with minimal disturbance. The dosage should be modified after assessing the patient's response, since each patient is his own bioassay system.

Drugs that exert their effect peripherally at the locus of pain (e.g., local anesthetics, certain anti-inflammatory analgesics) usually relieve pain without disrupting the patient's ability to function. In contrast, sedation resulting from centrally acting drugs, which alter the patient's perception of pain, may decrease his ability to function and limit him to bedrest. Patients with severe pain can often tolerate higher analgesic doses without untoward CNS depression; but such resistance disappears once the pain has been controlled. The patient's respiratory function and ability to clear secretions must be maintained.

Narcotic analgesics are often underused, resulting in needless suffering. The required dose is often underestimated and the duration of action overestimated. Physician and nurse's concern over creating narcotic addiction is often excessive. Fewer than 1% of hospitalized patients given large doses of narcotics for 10 days or longer develop true addiction. Adequate pain relief produced early during therapy may decrease the total amount of medication needed and increase the patient's comfort. This may be accomplished in the hospital by giving the drug **at the request of the patient** but no more often than q 1 h for the first two doses. After that, it should be given no more often than q 3 h. The patient should be asked q 4 h if medication is needed. It is frequently helpful to analyze the 24 h pattern of a patient's pain. An increased or supplemental dose of analgesic at a particular time (e.g., prior to a bath or procedure) may lessen discomfort dramatically and diminish the overall need for pain medication.

Opiate effects apparently are mediated via specific receptors in the CNS and gut. Endogenous opioids (enkephalins, endorphins) are the primary ligands for these receptors, but these have not yet become clinically useful materials. Strong, opiate-like analgesics acting at these sites with fewer undesirable effects may be developed, and ways of increasing the body's own stores of or sensitivity to endogenous analgesic peptides are being sought. Specific reviews of the rapidly expanding knowledge in this field are recommended for a more complete analysis of opioid action.

Morphine, an opium alkaloid, is the prototype of the narcotic analgesics. It provides analgesia at a dose (about 10 mg IM) that does not result in severe alterations in consciousness. Although its exact mechanism and locus of action are not known, morphine affects both the initial perception of pain and the emotional response to it. Pain relief is usually not complete, but the level of distress or suffering is markedly decreased. Patients with severe pain rarely obtain pleasant, euphoric sensations after morphine administration, but may become drowsy and relaxed, partly because of decreased distress. Paradoxically, in people without pain morphine frequently produces unpleasant psychologic sensations (dysphoria). Many chemical variations of the morphine molecule have been developed to increase potency and oral effectiveness and to reduce undesired side effects, but the desired and undesired effects are intertwined. Though the possibility of psychologic and physical dependence is a major constraint on the clinical use of morphine and related narcotic analgesics, true addiction rarely occurs.

Morphine is not very effective when taken orally. It is rapidly transformed by the liver and other tissues to inactive metabolites and excreted in the urine. Morphine sulfate is the most commonly used water-soluble salt, and a reasonable starting dose for a 70 kg patient is 8 to 10 mg IM or s.c. If administered IV (2 to 10 mg), it must be given slowly (over 4 to 5 min) to prevent serious hypotension. Epidural and intrathecal morphine administration are currently under study and may provide long-lasting effective pain relief with very low doses. Pain relief generally begins within 15 to 20 min (sooner after IV administration) and lasts 3 to 4 h. Higher doses provide greater analgesic effect and longer duration of action. The ceiling of morphine's analgesic effect is very high and, in large doses, it may be used as a surgical anesthetic. However, adverse effects limit the maximum tolerated dose.

The dose-related adverse effects of morphine include CNS depression, with decreased respiratory responsiveness to CO_2, decreased cough reflex, nausea, and vomiting. Morphine also produces miosis and stimulates release of ADH from the hypothalamus. Peripheral smooth muscle effects decrease propulsive movements in the GI tract, causing constipation (a useful effect in the treatment of diarrhea by opiates). The venules (capacitance vessels) dilate following morphine administration, and hypotension may occur in hypovolemic patients or those who suddenly assume an upright position. Depression of central vasomotor centers and histamine release may be involved in causing hypotension. The hypotensive effect of opiates is intensified by concomitant administration of phenothiazines.

Morphine and other narcotics should be used with great caution (if at all) in patients with chronic obstructive pulmonary disease. Since morphine increases CSF pressure, patients with suspected CNS disease should probably not receive opiates. In patients with liver disease, smaller starting doses and careful titration are advisable. Patients with markedly decreased renal function may have unusually prolonged CNS depressant effects from opiates, so that repeated doses of narcotic antagonists (perhaps for several days following the last opiate dose) may be needed to reverse respiratory depression in anuric patients. Neonates, especially premature babies, lack adequate metabolic pathways to eliminate morphine and other opiates and are unusually sensitive to them.

The development of tolerance to morphine varies from one physiologic system to another; e.g., the pupillary and GI effects of morphine exhibit little tolerance. However, during chronic therapy it may become necessary to increase the dose to achieve the same degree of pain relief, since the duration of action shortens and the peak analgesic effect decreases. CNS stimulants such as amphetamines potentiate the analgesic effect of morphine.

Codeine, also derived from opium, has analgesic activity when given orally, and 65 mg is equivalent to about 600 mg of aspirin. However, since codeine acts centrally, it complements aspirin, acetaminophen, and other peripherally acting analgesics. It is also useful in treating cough and diarrhea and has little abuse potential. Unwanted effects of codeine are similar to those of other opiates (respiratory depression, nausea, vomiting, and constipation).

Meperidine is a synthetic narcotic analgesic. Between 75 and 100 mg parenterally is equivalent to 10 mg of morphine sulfate, but its duration of action (about 3 h) is shorter than that of morphine. The adverse effects of these drugs are similar, but meperidine has less smooth muscle effect and seems to have less depressant effect on the newborn, probably because it less readily crosses the placental barrier. Meperidine has a relatively high abuse potential. Serious hypotension may occur when meperidine is given to a patient on monoamine oxidase inhibitors. It is not useful for cough or diarrhea.

Methadone is a synthetic drug with excellent analgesic activity when given orally. The usual dose for pain relief is 5 to 10 mg orally q 6 to 8 h. Methadone is used extensively in the USA for short-term treatment of heroin withdrawal (detoxification), for long-term maintenance therapy of narcotic addiction, and for analgesia in cancer patients. These uses are made possible by methadone's long duration of action, oral effectiveness, ability at high dosage to block heroin-induced euphoria, and less prominent sedation. Adverse effects of methadone resemble those of morphine and are reversible by narcotic antagonists. It is easily differentiated from morphine by a urine test. Some narcotic addicts legally receiving methadone regularly, function better socially than when taking heroin, although controversy surrounds such maintenance therapy.

Combinations: Opiate analgesia may be potentiated by a CNS stimulant such as amphetamine or cocaine. A liquid analgesic-stimulant-alcohol combination has been successfully used in cancer hospitals and may be useful in other selected patients with pain. A flavored combination of methadone, amphetamine (or cocaine), and alcohol may diminish the sedative effect of the narcotic, potentiate its analgesic effect, and delay the appearance of opiate tolerance.

Phenothiazines (e.g., chlorpromazine), while having little direct analgesic activity, are useful as analgesic adjuvants because they potentiate narcotic analgesia and decrease associated nausea and vomiting. However, hypotension may also be potentiated with such concomitant use. In some clinical syndromes (e.g., postherpetic neuralgia and atypical facial pain), combinations of a phenothiazine and a tricyclic antidepressant are often effective.

Other analgesics: Methotrimeprazine, a phenothiazine analgesic, has many important differences from the narcotic analgesics. It does not induce tolerance or psychologic or physical dependence and thus has no abuse or addiction potential. In analgesic activity, 15 to 20 mg of methotrimeprazine given IM is equivalent to about 10 mg of morphine. This drug should not be given IV or s.c. Therapeutic doses do not produce respiratory depression, pupillary changes, or constipation, but orthostatic hypotension and sedation are common adverse effects.

Narcotic antagonists: The N-allyl analogs of morphine and levorphanol (**nalorphine** and **levallorphan,** respectively) diminish or abolish the narcotic effects of opiates and methadone and precipitate an acute withdrawal syndrome in physically dependent addicts, but they have partial agonist activity and elicit narcotic effects when given alone. CNS depression can be exacerbated if these antagonists are given to patients with respiratory depression caused by nonnarcotic drugs such as barbiturates or other sedative-hypnotics. **Nalorphine** is an effective analgesic, but its use is limited by a significant incidence of hallucinations. The medications discussed in this section, with the exception of **naloxone** (see below), are perhaps best termed partial agonists rather than narcotic antagonists.

Pentazocine, a weak narcotic antagonist with considerable analgesic activity, is less subject to abuse than pure narcotic agonists. However, it has some abuse potential, especially if given parenterally. The analgesic activity of 40 to 50 mg of pentazocine IM is comparable to 10 mg of morphine. The drug may also be given orally. Pentazocine can cause unpleasant hallucinations. If given to someone dependent on narcotics, it can precipitate withdrawal symptoms. Pentazocine overdosage is reversible by **naloxone,** but not by other narcotic antagonists.

Newer partial-agonist–narcotic–antagonist analgesics include **butorphanol, nalbuphine,** and **buprenorphine.** Each is derived from a different narcotic class. They have different ratios of antagonist to agonist properties and are all effective analgesics. Only buprenorphine is currently available in an orally administered form. The abuse potential of these drugs, while less than morphine or meperidine, has not yet been established.

Naloxone is virtually free of the undesirable effects of the other narcotic antagonists. It is almost a pure narcotic antagonist without significant agonist action. It does not cause respiratory depression nor psychotomimetic effects when given alone, and it can reverse the effects of pentazocine, propoxyphene, and all other narcotic analgesics. Onset of action is extremely rapid (within minutes) when given IV and slightly less rapid when given IM. However, the duration of antagonism is frequently not as long as the duration of narcotic-induced respiratory depression, so that clinical vigilance and repeated doses of naloxone may be necessary. A common starting dose is 0.4 mg IV every 2 to 3 min as needed.

TRANQUILIZERS

ANTIANXIETY AGENTS (Anxiolytics; "Minor" Tranquilizers; Sedatives)

Using drugs to relieve anxiety is common, although their precise efficacy is uncertain. Their utility is affected by patient and physician acceptance, placebo effect, and the episodic nature of most anxiety (see ANXIETY NEUROSES in Ch. 138).

The benzodiazepines (e.g., chlordiazepoxide, diazepam) have largely supplanted other antianxiety drugs, including the barbiturates, meprobamate, and the diphenylmethane antihistamines, such as diphenhydramine and hydroxyzine. The phenothiazines (e.g., thioridazine) are occasionally used as antianxiety agents; however, the clinically effective dosage of these agents is generally accompanied by limiting side effects including restlessness, dizziness, oversedation, and atropine-like effects, making them generally unacceptable to ambulatory patients without marked anxiety. The degree of CNS depression that most of these compounds produce is dose-dependent and can be severe with overdosage. The larger dose preparations used mainly as tranquilizers or hypnotics retain their position as the most common agents of drug suicide attempts (see Ch. 141).

Clinical Principles

Since most antianxiety drugs have a long biologic half-life, the traditional t.i.d. or q.i.d. dosage is unnecessary. The benzodiazepines (particularly diazepam) may persist in the serum for over 24 h after a single dose. Since many patients with anxiety complain of insomnia, the largest portion of the dosage may be given at bedtime, thus promoting sleep and providing some tranquilizing effect the next day. Smaller doses can be taken during the day as needed.

There is wide variation in dosage requirements. The dose may be increased to above conventional levels in those patients who are disabled by significant anxiety. Because a patient has had drug therapy once, there is no reason to assume that it will always be needed. Some may need treatment only once or intermittently. Counseling and supportive maneuvers are always indicated and may preclude the need for constant drug therapy.

Choice of an Antianxiety Drug

The choice of agent depends on an evaluation of its potential toxicity, because the antianxiety effects of the above drugs are nonspecific. The benzodiazepines, particularly chlordiazepoxide and diazepam, have important advantages and are often the drugs of choice. Phenobarbital is inexpensive and effective, but unwanted sedation is common. Meprobamate is occasionally a useful drug and costs less than the benzodiazepines, but is generally regarded as less effective. Both meprobamate and the barbiturates have abuse potential including tolerance, physical dependence, and a withdrawal syndrome. This danger, particularly with phenobarbital, is overrated, but remains an important consideration for many physicians who fear that exposing an anxious patient to small doses of a drug may lead to larger doses and drug abuse. The benzodiazepines have less abuse potential and a minimal hazard of CNS depression and death following overdose. TABLE 247–2 lists the commonly used drugs and their average dosage ranges. Recently, β-adrenergic blockers such as propranolol have been used to decrease some manifestations of anxiety (e.g., tremor, palpitations). They block anxiety-induced increases in heart rate, decrease tremor, and also appear to have a central anxiolytic effect. They may be used alone or in combination with other anxiolytic drugs *as an investigational procedure.*

Barbiturates: (See SEDATIVES AND HYPNOTICS, above)

Meprobamate is rapidly absorbed from the GI tract, metabolized by the liver, and excreted by the kidneys. The usual adult dose for anxiety is 400 mg orally t.i.d. Beneficial effects appear within a few days. The drug is relatively safe at normal doses. Drowsiness is the most common side effect. Other adverse effects include allergic reactions, nausea and vomiting, hypotension, muscular weakness, and, rarely, blood dyscrasias. Tolerance and dependence may occur and chronic intoxication with confusion and ataxia has been seen. In patients receiving high doses (> 3 gm/day) for long periods, abrupt cessation of therapy produces a withdrawal syndrome that can present as convulsions or as a state resembling delirium tremens.

TABLE 247–2. COMMONLY USED ANTIANXIETY AGENTS

Drug	Daily Dose Range (mg) Often Divided into 2–4 Daily Doses
Barbiturates	
Phenobarbital	30–100
Butabarbital	25–120
Benzodiazepines	
Clorazepate	15–60
Chlordiazepoxide	15–300
Diazepam	5–60
Oxazepam	10–120
Prazepam	20–60
Lorazepam	2–6
Other antianxiety agents	
Chlormezanone	200–800
Hydroxyzine	100–400
Meprobamate	800–2400
Tybamate	750–3000

Benzodiazepines, particularly diazepam and chlordiazepoxide, are the most widely used antianxiety drugs. They are highly effective in nonpsychotic anxiety, but offer no benefits for thought disorder of schizophrenics; in some they may exacerbate it. In affective disorders these drugs have no mood elevating or antidepressant effect, but reduce anxiety in anxious depressed patients. Their use in endogenous depression can increase suicidal tendency. Benzodiazepines are useful in treating acute and chronic alcoholism, and are effective as anticonvulsants and as muscle relaxants. They are often helpful in patients with emotionally induced clinical exacerbation of pathologic conditions such as allergies, dermatologic lesions, GI and cardiovascular abnormalities. With therapeutic doses, these drugs are not likely to cause any significant cardiovascular or respiratory depression, but they do potentiate the effects of alcohol and the barbiturates. Ethanol significantly enhances diazepam absorption and, possibly, oral absorption of other benzodiazepines. Derivatives such as flurazepam can be effectively used as hypnotics (see SEDATIVES AND HYPNOTICS, above).

The **mechanism of action** of benzodiazepines as antianxiety agents is not well established. Diazepam is rapidly absorbed after oral administration reaching peak plasma concentrations in 1 h; chlordiazepoxide is slowly absorbed, reaching peak plasma concentrations in several hours. The plasma half-life of diazepam is 20 to 50 h; of chlordiazepoxide, 7 to 28 h. The benzodiazepines are highly protein bound, especially in plasma and in tissues of the GI tract and brain. Diazepam distributes rapidly to the adipose tissues after administration, explaining the initial rapid plasma decline in a few hours, followed by a slow decline and, in about 6 h, a resurgence of blood levels that is associated with another phase of drowsiness. Certain benzodiazepines are metabolized into active and inactive metabolites. Chlordiazepoxide, chlorazepate, diazepam, and prazepam are metabolized to active metabolites that concentrate in the brain; they stay longer than the parent compound. Because of long plasma half-life and the presence of active metabolites, significant body accumulation can occur on repeated administration of these 4 benzodiazepines. In contrast, oxazepam and lorazepam are eliminated by the kidney without formation of active intermediate metabolic products.

Clinical toxicity of benzodiazepines is low; skin rash, nausea, headache, impairment of sexual function, vertigo and lightheadedness occasionally occur. Side effects such as drowsiness and ataxia may be extensions of the pharmacologic effects. Paradoxical responses like increased anxiety, psychosis, and sudden suicidal impulses have been reported.

Tolerance does occur and habituation is common, particularly with high doses. Because of the long half-life of diazepam and its conversions to active metabolites, withdrawal symptoms may appear weeks after discontinuation of the drug.

The use of chlordiazepoxide in the elderly has been associated with oversedation and ataxia, thus dosage should be limited to the smallest effective amount.

The use of antianxiety drugs (benzodiazepines, meprobamate, etc.) is not advised in pregnancy, especially during the first trimester, because of increased risk of congenital abnormalities, notably cleft lip and palate (0.2 to 0.4% incidence). However, they are sometimes used during labor and delivery for the relief of anxiety and emotional tension and to potentiate analgesia. Perinatal use can sedate the newborn.

Excretion of benzodiazepines and their metabolites is mainly by the kidney and a small portion by hepatobiliary excretion and the feces. Differences in the clinical performances of the various benzodiazepines appear to be due more to their pharmacokinetics than to inherent neuropharmacologic effects. Changes in the pharmacokinetics of benzodiazepines by factors such as liver disease, renal failure, age (elderly), sex, and concomitant drug administration can enhance toxicity. Individual drugs and their average adult daily **dosages** for anxiety are given in TABLE 247-2. Requirements vary widely and the dose must be tailored to the individual; larger doses may be used with caution in patients with severe anxiety and in alcoholism.

ANTIPSYCHOTIC DRUGS (Neuroleptics; "Major" Tranquilizers)

Over the past 35 yr psychotropic drugs have produced major changes in the management of psychiatric illness. Fewer patients need hospital care; family physicians offer more effective treatment in the office; and psychiatrists are consulted more selectively for diagnosis and treatment of difficult cases. As with many physical disorders, the realistic objective of psychiatric treatment may not be complete remission, but rather the restoration of an adequate level of basic functions necessary for a satisfying and productive life. When this goal is attained, medication must not be discontinued abruptly. Maintenance therapy may be necessary. In schizophrenia, the more florid the symptoms and the more acute the onset, the more likely is a good response. Little change can be expected in chronic schizophrenics. The 3 major classes of antipsychotic drugs are the phenothiazines, the butyrophenones, and the thioxanthenes. (See TABLE 247-3.)

Antipsychotic drugs do not cure schizophrenic patients. Regardless of which neuroleptic is prescribed, patients usually achieve maximal benefit in the first 3 to 6 mo of treatment. This initial improvement can be sustained with maintenance therapy in most patients. Some clinicians have proposed as a rule of thumb that after the first episode a schizophrenic patient should be maintained on medication for at least 1 yr, and after the second episode, for at least 2 yr; in the event of further relapse, the patient should be kept on drug therapy indefinitely. Early cessation of therapy has led to relapse in 25% of patients within 4 wk, in 50% within 8 wk, and in 75% within 12 wk.

Paranoid schizophrenics do better on neuroleptics than do nonparanoid schizophrenics. Haloperidol (a butyrophenone) is preferred over the phenothiazines in nonparanoid patients. Among the phenothiazines, the more sedative ones such as chlorpromazine or thioridazine are preferable for agitated patients. Less sedative drugs such as trifluoperazine and perphenazine are best for patients with symptoms of withdrawal and retardation. The notion that different antipsychotic drugs affect target symptoms selectively does not have convincing experimental support. Individual response to each phenothiazine varies, and may reflect pharmacokinetic differences more than inherent pharmacologic differences among the drugs.

TABLE 247-3. COMMONLY USED ANTIPSYCHOTIC DRUGS

Drug	Daily Oral Dose Range (mg)
Phenothiazines, aliphatic	
Chlorpromazine	50–2000
Promazine	50–600
Triflupromazine	25–150
Phenothiazines, piperidine	
Mesoridazine	50–400
Piperacetazine	20–160
Thioridazine	20–300
Phenothiazines, piperazine	
Acetophenazine	40–80
Butaperazine	15–60
Carphenazine	25–100
Fluphenazine	1–8*
Perphenazine	4–32
Prochlorperazine	25–150
Trifluoperazine	1–20
Butyrophenones	
Haloperidol	2–30
Thioxanthenes	
Chlorprothixene	30–400
Thiothixene	6–60
Dihydroindolone	
Molindone	20–200
Dibenzoxazepine	
Loxapine	60–250

* Oral fluphenazine is currently being used in much larger doses: 15 mg to the extremely high dose of 1200 mg after careful titration of doses in chronic schizophrenic patients.

Often the choice of an antipsychotic drug depends on avoiding side effects detrimental to a particular patient. Haloperidol and the piperazine phenothiazines are preferred where sedation is undesirable and there is risk of CVS symptoms, e.g., arrhythmias and hypotension. Haloperidol is preferred for patients with suspected liver abnormalities. If there is a risk of developing extrapyramidal symptoms (e.g., in the aged, or in those with neurologic problems), thioridazine is the drug of choice. *Avoid* thioridazine in patients with heart disease and with ejaculation problems. Children and young adults are susceptible to extrapyramidal side effects; therefore, haloperidol and piperazine phenothiazines should be *avoided*. Chlorpromazine appears to be safest to use in children and young adults when doses are properly titrated.

PHENOTHIAZINES

The clinically important subgroups of phenothiazines are the **aliphatics** (the most widely known is **chlorpromazine [CPZ]**); the **piperazines** (e.g., fluphenazine, trifluoperazine, perphenazine); and the **piperidines** (e.g., thioridazine). The pharmacologic properties of the various phenothiazines are qualitatively similar, but the relative potency and toxicity depend on the chemical structure.

Clinically, the aliphatics are the least potent drugs. Piperidines have intermediate potency, and piperazines are generally the most potent. Thioridazine (a piperidine derivative), for example, causes less hypotension and fewer extrapyramidal side effects than CPZ (an aliphatic derivative), although it has a greater tendency to produce pigmentary retinopathy and ECG changes in high dosage. In contrast, the piperazine derivatives (fluphenazine, trifluoperazine, perphenazine, etc.) produce less drowsiness, hypotension, and tachycardia, but more extrapyramidal reactions than CPZ.

Plasma levels of CPZ vary widely in different patients with a given dose, due to differences in absorption, distribution, metabolism, and excretion of the drug. After absorption, CPZ is rapidly distributed and bound by most tissues, resulting in a high tissue/plasma concentration. There is extensive hepatic and extrahepatic metabolism of CPZ with more than 150 potential metabolites, some of which are pharmacologically active. The plasma half-life of CPZ is about 9 to 12 h and it takes 7 to 10 days of oral intake to achieve a steady state. CPZ and its metabolites are excreted in both urine and feces, where they can be detected in trace amounts for 6 to 18 mo after cessation of treatment. Psychotic patients with plasma levels < 50 ng/ml generally show no improvement. Those with 50 to 300 ng/ml show clinical improvement, and when plasma levels reach 700 to 1000 ng/ml, toxicity often appears (e.g., convulsions or extrapyramidal symptoms). The optimum therapeutic plasma concentration in children is lower than that of adults (40 to 80 ng/ml). Unfortunately, plasma levels do not usually correlate with dosage, but are affected by such factors as (1) dosage form; (2) age (children are rapid metabolizers and, despite moderate doses of 3 to 10 mg/kg of CPZ, they achieve low plasma CPZ concentrations); and (3) duration of neuroleptic therapy (institutionalized patients on long-term therapy achieve very low plasma levels—17 to 50% of values seen in patients on short-term therapy—despite moderately high [600 to 1000 mg/day] CPZ doses).

Clinical Effects

The phenothiazines are effective in acute and chronic schizophrenia and do not produce drug dependence. They have a marked effect on thought disturbances associated with paranoid ideation, delusions, anxiety, and agitation. CPZ, the prototype phenothiazine, produces psychomotor slowing, emotional quieting, and an affective indifference that is described as a neuroleptic action. CPZ also produces considerable drowsiness and hypotension, to which tolerance develops quite rapidly, and has a central antiemetic and hypothermic effect. Endocrine effects include suppression of ovulation, induction of lactation, increased release of ADH, and inhibition of oxytocin release. CPZ also has antihistaminic, anticholinergic, and muscle relaxant activity. Important biochemical effects are blockade of catecholamines (norepinephrine and dopamine), of serotonin uptake in the brain, and inhibition of dopamine-sensitive adenylate cyclase activity in the limbic system.

In acute psychosis, a starting dose of 300 to 400 mg/day of CPZ is increased rapidly to as much as 1000 to 2000 mg/day in 1 or 2 wk. Thereafter it is lowered to a maintenance dose of 300 to 400 mg/day, depending on the clinical picture. Young adults in their 20s should be given relatively lower doses in a therapeutic trial of not less than 3 to 6 wk. Single daily maintenance doses can be tried in order to improve patient compliance.

Adverse effects include drowsiness, sedation, hypotension, extrapyramidal symptoms (e.g., akathisia, dystonia, tremors, and rigidity), reduction of convulsive seizure threshold, ocular and skin pigmentation, photosensitization, tardive dyskinesia, hepatotoxicity, and blood dyscrasias. Phenothiazines may produce abnormalities in myocardial repolarization and phenothiazine-induced arrhythmias are common.

The phenothiazines may cause drug-induced dyskinesia with vigorous chorea and athetosis, muscular facial spasms, and torticollis. This appears to be an idiosyncratic phenomenon that is not dose-related. Treatment of severe reactions with diphenhydramine 50 mg IV or benztropine 2 mg IM is usually effective. Small oral doses of benztropine, biperiden, trihexyphenidyl, or diphenhydramine usually suffice for mild reactions.

High doses of phenothiazines given over a long time may cause an oral-facial dyskinesia (**tardive dyskinesia**), particularly in older patients and in those with brain injury, that does not disappear when the drug is discontinued and that resists standard treatments for movement disorders. Anticholinergics can exacerbate tardive dyskinesia. The incidence has increased with the common and prolonged use of phenothiazines. Reintroduction or increase in dosage of piperazine phenothiazines or haloperidol may aggravate or, paradoxically, may suppress the dyskinesia. Reserpine 0.1 to 1.0 mg/day or clonazepam 1 to 3 mg/day is sometimes helpful. Deanol acetamidobenzoate and choline chloride, precursors for acetylcholine, are also sometimes helpful. Lithium, tricyclic antidepressants, and baclofen have also been useful in some patients.

Skin and eye complications, drowsiness, and hypotension appear to be dose-related. Extrapyramidal symptoms (e.g., persistent dyskinesia) and hepatotoxicity are influenced by other factors such as age, sex, duration of drug administration, and individual hypersensitivity. Older women on long-term therapy have a higher incidence of tardive dyskinesia than men. Hepatotoxicity and blood dyscrasias appear to be hypersensitivity reactions.

Interaction of CPZ with other drugs includes the following: (1) CPZ potentiates the action of CNS depressants, e.g., alcohol, narcotics, hypnotics, and sedatives; (2) CPZ plasma levels are lowered by trihexyphenidyl and possibly by other anticholinergics; (3) CPZ absorption is impaired by insoluble antacids; (4) CPZ potentiates the hypotensive effect of antihypertensives; (5) the use of L-dopa in phenothiazine-induced parkinsonism in psychiatric patients aggravates schizophrenia and does not control the extrapyramidal symptoms; and (6) lithium lowers plasma CPZ levels.

Long-acting parenteral preparations of fluphenazine decanoate or enanthate may be used to manage problems of compliance, absorption, and erratic plasma levels, particularly in patients on long-term therapy. These dosage forms are given IM or s.c. (25 to 50 mg) every 1 to 3 wk and are usually well tolerated. Side effects generally consist of minor autonomic disturbances, infrequent hypotension, and dermatologic disorders. Drowsiness and lethargy may occur in some individuals after the initial injection, but are generally mild and abate spontaneously within 1 wk; when pronounced, they can be counteracted by methylphenidate 10 to 20 mg orally once or twice daily for a few days. Extrapyramidal symptoms occur within 4 to 5 days of treatment, in contrast to the greater delay often seen after oral neuroleptics. With oral treatment, 90% of dyskinesias, parkinsonism, and akathisias occur in 4 to 5, 72, and 73 days, respectively. With parenteral fluphenazine, dyskinesia may occur in some patients in 12 to 24 h, akathisia in 1 to 4 days, and parkinsonism in 2 to 5 days post-injection. Symptoms of parkinsonism are well controlled by anticholinergic antiparkinsonian agents such as benztropine mesylate. Akathisia responds to the same drugs and also to small doses of barbiturates or antihistamines. Dystonic reactions are readily relieved by diazepam IV or benztropine mesylate 1 to 2 mg IM. Convulsions, jaundice, agranulocytosis, and major skin and eye changes are rare complications of therapy. Interaction of fluphenazine decanoate with other drugs appears to be of minor significance.

BUTYROPHENONES

Haloperidol and droperidol are the only butyrophenones available in the USA at present; however, droperidol is used primarily as an adjunct to anesthesia rather than as a neuroleptic. Haloperidol blocks dopamine receptors in the CNS. It is effective against aggressive behavior in disturbed children, organic psychosis, alcoholic delirium, and assaultive behavior. It is also useful in managing confused, negativistic geriatric patients, senile psychosis, mania and paranoid reactions, and other behavior disorders of the elderly. Neurologic disorders such as Gilles de la Tourette's syndrome, Huntington's chorea, spasmodic torticollis, hemiballismus and hyperkinesia of organic origin, and intractable hiccups are also benefited by haloperidol. It is a potent antiemetic. Compared with the phenothiazines, it causes less hypotension, anticholinergic effects, cardiac complications, and sedation. The risk of drug-induced liver disease with haloperidol appears minimal.

Haloperidol induces more extrapyramidal side effects than phenothiazines; these effects may be minimized by using low doses. The drug-induced extrapyramidal effects are also dependent on age, sex, and physical condition. Young patients (children and adolescents) are most likely to develop dystonic reactions, middle-aged patients usually develop akathisia, and elderly individuals tend more to develop parkinsonism.

Overdosage of haloperidol usually involves an exaggeration of the pharmacologic effects and adverse reactions. Gastric lavage or induction of emesis should be followed by administration of activated charcoal. Treatment is primarily supportive. Haloperidol should be used in pregnancy only if the benefits clearly justify a potential risk to the fetus.

The usual initial dosage of haloperidol is 1 to 2 mg/day orally, increasing by 0.5 to 1 mg every 3 days until remission is achieved. For maintenance, dosage is reduced to the smallest effective amount. Haloperidol is readily absorbed orally. Peak plasma concentration occurs 2 to 6 h after ingestion and may plateau for as long as 72 h; plasma levels may be detectable for weeks. In acute cases, haloperidol 2 to 5 mg IM may be given.

Haloperidol potentiates the effect of CNS depressants and anticoagulants. It diminishes the effect of L-dopa. It can diminish dyskinesia but aggravates parkinsonism in patients on L-dopa therapy. Since prolonged neuroleptic treatment is associated with development of tardive dyskinesias, haloperidol is not recommended for the treatment of tardive dyskinesias or L-dopa dyskinesias.

THIOXANTHENES

Of the 4 thioxanthenes marketed in various countries, only **chlorprothixene** and **thiothixene** are available in the USA for clinical use. The thioxanthenes resemble the phenothiazines in chemical structure, absorption, metabolism, excretion, and clinical effects. Chlorprothixene and thiothixene have been used in the treatment of schizophrenia and depression. The average oral daily adult dosage is 75 to 200 mg for chlorprothixene and 10 to 30 mg for thiothixene; however, individual patient requirements vary.

Like other neuroleptics, the thioxanthenes interfere with conditioned reflex activity without affecting unconditioned reflex activity. They increase limbic system activity and inhibit proprioceptive arousal reactions. Psychoactive thioxanthenes share some of the properties of tricyclic antidepressants. Thiothixene is comparable to chlorpromazine in therapeutic impact and is particularly effective against affective symptoms. It is especially useful for patients who are socially withdrawn, and is also effective in the management of psychotic depression, tension-agitation, and anxiety.

Fever, fatigue, and drowsiness are the most frequent adverse effects. The sensitivity to sunlight seen with phenothiazines is usually not observed. The relative frequency of adverse effects with thiothixene is lower than with the corresponding phenothiazine analogs. The lower incidence of extrapyramidal effects in long-term maintenance therapy is especially advantageous. Thiothixene has fewer adverse effects on the myocardium than does thioridazine.

OTHER ANTIPSYCHOTIC DRUGS

Reserpine, a rauwolfia alkaloid, was used as an antipsychotic drug in the past. However, its present use in psychiatry is almost obsolete because other neuroleptics are more effective.

Loxapine, a tricyclic dibenzoxazepine derivative, is chemically distinct from thioxanthenes, butyrophenones, and phenothiazines. Its pharmacologic and toxicologic properties are similar to those of the phenothiazines. Therapeutic efficacy is comparable with that of other neuroleptics in schizophrenia. Side effects include involuntary movements, hypotension, and somnolence. Oral doses range from 60 to 100 mg/day, although some patients may require up to 250 mg/day.

Molindone, a dihydroindolone derivative, is structurally different from the phenothiazines, butyrophenones, and thioxanthenes, but it is pharmacologically similar to the phenothiazines. The daily oral dose range is 20 to 200 mg.

ANTIDEPRESSANTS

Depression has several subcategories based upon clearness of precipitating events, the age of the subject, and other clinical aspects (see Chs. 138 and 139 for a more complete discussion of depression and additional discussion of clinical use of antidepressants). Many patients with psychomotor retardation experience significant anxiety, and antianxiety agents are useful in their treatment. In addition to their sedative effect some phenothiazine compounds (e.g., thioridazine, mesoridazine) may have an antidepressant effect. The most popular tricyclic antidepressants also have sedative effects and this fact has been exploited in the treatment of mixed anxiety-depression.

Most drugs used in depression and most psychostimulants have catecholamine-like activity or they incrementally alter catecholamine concentration or activity in the CNS, hence the elaboration of a catecholamine hypothesis of depression. Patients with depression (particularly those with recurrent episodes) may have a functional decrease in the activity or concentration of CNS catecholamines, but this supposition lacks proof.

Many episodes of depression are mild and self-limiting and need no drug therapy. When drugs are used the choice is generally made from among (1) tricyclic antidepressants, (2) monoamine oxidase inhibitors, or (3) amphetamine-like drugs. Currently the tricyclic antidepressants (often in combination with an antianxiety drug) are preferred.

TRICYCLIC ANTIDEPRESSANTS

These compounds differ slightly in chemical structure from the phenothiazines, which are also "tricyclic" compounds. Imipramine was developed in a search for an antipsychotic drug similar to chlorpromazine, which it closely resembles structurally. Amitriptyline and doxepin are the most sedative tricyclics. Desipramine is an active metabolite of imipramine, and nortriptyline is the corresponding active metabolite of amitriptyline.

The similarity of tricyclics to phenothiazines is important in cataloging their effects. Most tricyclic antidepressants have some sedative effect. Both types of agent possess anticholinergic activity, although that of the antidepressants is more pronounced. Both tricyclics and phenothiazines are active at the neural synapse, but here the functional effects diverge. While phenothiazines largely block the central dopamine receptors (thereby impairing functional dopaminergic neurotransmission), the tricyclic antidepressants interfere with the reuptake of norepinephrine into presynaptic adrenergic neurons, presumably facilitating adrenergic neural transmission, an important mechanism in the psychic effects. Tricyclic antidepressants also inhibit serotonin reuptake and may block central histamine H_2-receptors; the contribution of these pharmacologic effects to their antidepressant action remains unresolved.

The antidepressant effects of tricyclic compounds are often slow to appear. A 2- to 4-wk trial is necessary in most cases; some of their success may be due to spontaneous improvement in the patient. In patients who are anxious or agitated, a phenothiazine may be used in combination with a tricyclic antidepressant.

The dosages of currently available tricyclic antidepressants are listed in TABLE 247–4. Therapy is usually started with imipramine or amitriptyline 25 mg t.i.d. or q.i.d. Although the dosage may be increased until the desired response is obtained, few patients need as much as 300 mg/day. Additional doses may be added at nighttime. A single nighttime dose during maintenance is often adequate and some manufacturers have developed dosage formulations designed for bedtime use. Plasma levels of tricyclic antidepressants vary greatly in individuals on the same dose.

Clinical manifestations may recur if the drug is stopped prematurely; therefore, therapy should be continued for some time after symptoms have disappeared, and the dose should then be reduced gradually. If symptoms recur, the dose should be increased to the original level immediately and, thereafter, may be reduced on a trial basis but not precipitously.

Side Effects

Because of their anticholinergic activity, tricyclics can cause dry mouth, blurring of vision, urinary hesitation, and constipation; therefore, they should be used with caution in patients with glaucoma or prostatic hypertrophy, or in parkinsonian patients taking anticholinergic agents. These drugs should also be used cautiously in patients with cardiac arrhythmias, angina pectoris, and congestive heart failure, since they can produce arrhythmias, sinus tachycardia, and prolongation of the conduction time.

Dizziness, vertigo, tachycardia, and postural hypotension may occur early in treatment. Weakness, fatigue, lethargy, and drowsiness are common initially but usually disappear after a few weeks. Transient episodes of peripheral, glottal, and orbital edema have been reported. Headache is a fairly common complaint. Hyperreflexia and tremors are seen. The seizure threshold is reduced. Mania or hypomania may follow relief of depression in some patients and can usually be controlled by adding a phenothiazine to the regimen. Giving both a tricyclic and a phenothiazine from the outset may be useful if the patient's history includes such episodes.

In the treatment of tricyclic-induced adverse effects, physostigmine salicylate (1 to 3 mg IV) is a useful drug, having beneficial effects against arrhythmias and CNS manifestations of toxicity. The dosage of physostigmine may need to be repeated because the drug is rapidly metabolized. Propranolol has been effective in cases of protracted arrhythmia.

MONOAMINE OXIDASE (MAO) INHIBITORS

The MAO inhibitors were discovered to be "psychic energizers" when some antitubercular compounds that had MAO-inhibiting qualities were noted to elevate the mood of tuberculous patients. They have been widely used to treat depression, but occasional serious interactions with a variety of foods and drugs have reduced their popularity. They are currently used in depressed patients who do not respond to tricyclic antidepressants. TABLE 247–4 lists some common MAO inhibitors and their daily dosages.

MAO is an important enzyme in the degradation process of catecholamines and indolethylamines. If the enzyme is inhibited, catecholamines and serotonin increase in concentration. The increase in CNS catecholamine concentration is assumed to cause psychostimulation.

MAO inhibitors can cause severe hypertensive reactions accompanied by hypertensive encephalopathy and cerebrovascular accidents. The mechanism is now well understood. Patients on MAO inhibitor therapy suffer from adrenergic crises when they consume sympathomimetic drugs or dietary catecholamine precursors. The commonly available nasal decongestants often contain sympathomimetic drugs such as phenylephrine or phenylpropanolamine. Certain foods and beverages

TABLE 247–4. COMMONLY USED ANTIDEPRESSANTS

Drug	Daily Oral Dose (mg) Often Divided into 3 or 4 Doses
Tricyclic Antidepressants	
Amitriptyline	75–300
Desipramine	50–200
Doxepin	50–300
Imipramine	75–300
Nortriptyline	20–100
Protriptyline	15–60
Trimipramine	75–300
Monoamine Oxidase Inhibitors	
Isocarboxazid	10–30
Phenelzine	7.5–45
Tranylcypromine	20–60

(particularly aged cheeses and Chianti wines) contain tyramine. Hypertensive reactions may also ensue when patients on MAO inhibitors are treated with such catecholamine depletors as reserpine, guanethidine, or bretylium because these agents act initially to cause a release of catecholamines. Therefore, MAO inhibitors should be used with special care regarding food and drug intake.

MAO inhibitors have a paradoxical hypotensive effect that is poorly understood, and one (pargyline) is used to treat hypertension. Other side effects that may be encountered include CNS stimulation, insomnia, headache, palpitations, nausea, dysuria, and constipation.

AMPHETAMINE AND RELATED DRUGS

Amphetamine and related psychostimulant drugs (methylphenidate, phenmetrazine) have been used in depression. They are less effective than the tricyclic antidepressants or the MAO inhibitors in serious depressions and, unlike the other antidepressants, are subject to abuse; rebound depression may follow withdrawal. (See GENERAL CENTRAL NERVOUS SYSTEM STIMULANTS AND ANOREXIANTS, below.)

LITHIUM (See under Treatment in Ch. 139)

GENERAL CENTRAL NERVOUS SYSTEM STIMULANTS AND ANOREXIANTS

CNS stimulants are widely used to increase alertness, inhibit fatigue, suppress the appetite, manage certain children with minimal brain dysfunction or hyperkinesis, and treat narcolepsy. Many of these drugs are related to amphetamine and share the phenethylamine structure. Their activity as psychostimulants is primarily due to an ability to act indirectly by displacing endogenous catecholamines from storage sites in neural tissues, but may also be partly related to direct catecholamine-like adrenergic receptor activation in the CNS. They are widely used in clinical medicine but there has been criticism of their use to induce brief mood elevation or to suppress fatigue and a fear that inappropriate prescribing may have contributed to abuse (see also Ch. 136). Such use is often questioned, even though the use of tranquilizers to combat anxiety and tension has gained general acceptance.

The failure of most obese patients to lose weight satisfactorily by attempting to decrease food intake alone has led to widespread use of anorectic agents. Though these drugs may be of value in beginning a weight reduction program, their long-term utility has been seriously questioned. Amphetamine and related compounds such as diethylpropion, phentermine, and phenmetrazine are most effective for the first 3 to 6 wk. The suggestion that they might be useful intermittently over a long period to aid in weight control has not been documented by controlled clinical trials. The dosage usually is divided and given before meals, but some agents have a long duration of action and may be given less frequently. Most anorexiants may disturb sleep if given late in the day.

Amphetamine is the prototype CNS stimulant. There are a variety of amphetamine salts and mixtures in various formulations. It produces mood elevation with increased wakefulness, alertness, concentration, and physical performance. Systolic and diastolic blood pressures are raised, the respiratory center is stimulated, and appetite is suppressed through a central effect. It is rapidly absorbed from the GI tract, reaches high concentrations in the CNS, and is excreted by the kidneys. Its prolonged duration of action relates to its resistance to metabolic degradation by enzymes that metabolize catecholamines. Amphetamine and related compounds, when taken repeatedly, induce tolerance to some degree, but this is partially dependent on dosage.

Insomnia, dizziness, excessive sweating, tremors, and euphoria may occur and feelings of depression and fatigue often accompany withdrawal. Anxiety and panic states are seen, particularly at the high dosage levels associated with amphetamine abuse. Lethal overdose is uncommon because of the large difference between an effective and fatal dose and because tolerance has often occurred. Symptoms of **chronic abuse** include insomnia, weight loss, irritability, and restlessness. A syndrome resembling paranoid schizophrenia may appear; patients display marked anxiety, paranoid delusions, and visual and auditory hallucinations. These dramatic effects are most often seen with IV use of methamphetamine. Patients should be hospitalized for treatment of amphetamine addiction. A severe stereotyped withdrawal syndrome is not usually present. For a detailed discussion of amphetamine withdrawal and its management, see Ch. 136.

Methylphenidate is a mild CNS stimulant with effects similar to that of amphetamine. It is used to treat hyperkinesis in children (see LEARNING DISORDERS in Vol. II, Ch. 24) and for narcolepsy (see Ch. 121).

Mazindol and **fenfluramine**, newer anorexiants, vary from amphetamine, and thus far appear to have minimal abuse potential. Mazindol resembles the tricyclic antidepressants in chemical structure, has a slightly dysphoric effect, and has anticholinergic actions that may be unpleasant. Fenfluramine, although a phenethylamine, has sedation as its principal side effect and may be given late in the day without disturbing sleep. However, its use has been limited by this sedative effect and its tendency to cause melancholia. It should be *avoided* in patients with a history of mental depression.

ANTIEMETICS

Drugs that prevent or relieve nausea and vomiting. Nausea and vomiting may be symptoms of disease processes or responses to stimuli such as drugs, radiation, or motion. The underlying cause should be sought and corrected if possible, as the etiology suggests which antiemetic is optimal for symptomatic treatment.

TABLE 247–5. SOME ANTIEMETIC DRUGS

Agent	Usual Adult Dosage (mg)	Route of Administration	Frequency
Phenothiazines			
Chlorpromazine	10–25	oral	q 4–6 h
	50–100	rectal	q 6–8 h
	25	IM	q 3–4 h
Perphenazine	8–16	oral	daily in divided doses
	5	IM or IV	only as necessary
Prochlorperazine	5–10	oral	t.i.d. or q.i.d.
	25	rectal	b.i.d.
	5–10	IM	q 3–4 h
Promethazine	10–25	oral	b.i.d.
	10–25	rectal	b.i.d.
	12.5–25	IM or IV	q 4–6 h
Thiethylperazine	10	oral	once daily to t.i.d.
	10	rectal	once daily to t.i.d.
	10	IM	once daily to t.i.d.
Triflupromazine	20–30	oral	daily
	5–15	IM	q 4 h
	1–3	IV	daily
Antihistamines			
Cyclizine	50	oral	q.i.d.
	50	IM	q 4–6 h
Dimenhydrinate	50	oral	q 4 h
	100	rectal	b.i.d.
	50	IM or IV	q 4 h
Diphenhydramine	50	oral	t.i.d. or q.i.d.
	10–50	IM or IV	q 3–4 h
Meclizine	25–100	oral	once daily
Hydroxyzine	25–100	oral	t.i.d. or q.i.d.
Buclizine	50	oral	b.i.d.
Anticholinergics			
Scopolamine	0.3–1.0	oral	prior to travel
Sedatives			
Phenobarbital	30–60	oral	b.i.d. or t.i.d.
Miscellaneous			
Benzquinamide	50	IM	q 3–4 h
	25	IV	1st dose only
Diphenidol	25–50	oral	q 4 h
	20–40	IM	q 4 h
	20	IV	1st & 2nd doses only
Trimethobenzamide	250	oral	t.i.d. or q.i.d.
	200	rectal	t.i.d. or q.i.d.
	200	IM	t.i.d. or q.i.d.

Stimulation of the vomiting center in the medulla can arise in the chemoreceptor trigger zone **(CTZ)**, cerebral cortex, or vestibular apparatus, or can be relayed directly from peripheral areas (e.g., gastric mucosa). Though the mechanism of action of the antiemetics is not well understood, they appear to act on the CTZ, cerebral cortex, vestibular apparatus, or vomiting center.

Some nausea and vomiting is mild, self-limited (e.g., usually that occurring during the first trimester of pregnancy), and does not require drug therapy. Drugs should be avoided if possible during the first 3 mo of pregnancy, but certain antihistamines may be tried if drug therapy is absolutely necessary. In other settings, untreated vomiting may delay or interrupt wound healing after surgery or may cause fluid and electrolyte loss perpetuating the symptoms of nausea and vomiting. Persistent vomiting precludes oral administration.

Most of the drugs mentioned in this chapter (See also TABLE 247-5) are discussed in more detail elsewhere in this volume; the primary focus here is on their antiemetic effect.

Phenothiazines

The phenothiazines are the most effective antiemetics. They appear to act by selective depression of the CTZ and are useful in treating nausea and vomiting that is postoperative, radiation- or drug-induced, or associated with gastroenteritis, pregnancy, carcinoma, or uremia. Except for promethazine, they are not useful in treating motion sickness. Since most phenothiazines (except thioridazine and mesoridazine) appear to be equally effective, if given in sufficient dosage, the choice of drug may depend upon consideration of side effects (see PHENOTHIAZINES under ANTIPSYCHOTIC DRUGS, above).

The butyrophenone derivatives, haloperidol and **droperidol,** have antiemetic activity. Only droperidol is approved for use in nausea and vomiting of surgical and diagnostic procedures. However, preliminary, uncontrolled studies suggest IV droperidol may be useful for the intractable nausea and vomiting associated with cancer therapy.

Antihistamines

These appear to act on the neural pathways originating in the labyrinth. Certain antihistamines (e.g., diphenhydramine, buclizine, cyclizine, meclizine) are effective in treating motion sickness and the vertigo of Ménière's disease. They are useful, but less effective, in treating postoperative nausea and vomiting and that associated with pregnancy.

Buclizine and meclizine have been demonstrated to be teratogenic in preclinical studies and are contraindicated during pregnancy; cyclizine, although not contraindicated, should be used with caution in pregnancy; the dose and duration of treatment should be kept to a minimum. (See also PRENATAL CARE in Vol. II, Ch. 13.)

Anticholinergics

Scopolamine is more effective than antihistamines for preventing motion sickness, but its clinical use is limited by a short duration of action and by side effects, including blurred vision, dry mouth, drowsiness, fatigue, and the possibility of increased intraocular pressure in patients with glaucoma.

Sedatives

Barbiturates and other nonspecific CNS depressants possess weak antiemetic properties.

Miscellaneous Agents

Benzquinamide appears to be as effective an antiemetic as the phenothiazines. The drug increases cardiac output and BP and may be useful in patients with CNS depression (e.g., postoperative patients and those treated with sedatives or analgesics). Drowsiness is the most common side effect; shivering and chills, and reactions similar to phenothiazines have also been reported.

Diphenidol acts upon the aural vestibular apparatus. It is useful in treating nausea and vomiting associated with malignancy, radiation sickness, anesthetics and antineoplastics, and is also effective in treating the vertigo of motion sickness and Ménière's disease. Diphenidol should be used only after safer agents have failed. Therapy should be closely supervised and discontinued if auditory or visual hallucinations, disorientation, or confusion occur. Drowsiness, dizziness, and dryness of the mouth may also occur.

Metoclopramide inhibits the CTZ; it also has unique actions in the upper GI tract. It raises pressure at the lower esophageal sphincter, increases both the frequency and amplitude of gastric contractions, and speeds the rate of transit through the small bowel. It benefits patients who are likely to vomit because of gastric retention or cancer chemotherapy. Side effects are uncommon, although lassitude, drowsiness and occasional extrapyramidal reactions may be seen.

Trimethobenzamide is useful for preventing postanesthetic nausea and for treating the vomiting of pregnancy. The incidence of side effects is low, though drowsiness, diarrhea, extrapyramidal reactions, hypersensitivity reactions, and pain at the injection site may occur.

248. AUTONOMIC DRUGS

To provide a basis for understanding the action of autonomic drugs and their effective use in clinical practice, fundamental anatomic and physiologic aspects of the autonomic nervous system are described first, following which the clinically relevant aspects are reviewed, along with a discussion of specific agents.

PHYSIOLOGY OF THE AUTONOMIC NERVOUS SYSTEM

The autonomic nervous system consists of neurons, ganglia, and plexuses that innervate and regulate the heart, blood vessels, visceral smooth muscles, and many exocrine glands. Mediation of autonomic responses usually involves a reflex arc containing afferent, CNS, and efferent components.

Autonomic Nervous System Reflex Arc

The afferent fibers from visceral structures (visceral afferents) are the first link in the reflex arcs of the autonomic nervous system. The sensory receptors distributed throughout the body, including pressor or baroreceptors, chemoreceptors, and smooth muscle stretch receptors, activate visceral afferents. The visceral afferents mediate visceral sensation and vasomotor, respiratory, and viscerosomatic stimuli and carry them into the cerebrospinal axis via the vagus, pelvic, splanchnic, and other autonomic nerves. The cell bodies of visceral afferents lie in the dorsal root ganglia of the spinal nerves and in the corresponding sensory ganglia of certain cranial nerves.

Most autonomic reflexes are mediated through the CNS. The visceral afferents that enter the spinal cord send branches up the cord before synapsing with the cell bodies of the preganglionic efferent fibers and completing the reflex arc. The visceral afferents of cranial nerves terminate in the brainstem, where branches synapse with cell bodies of the preganglionic efferent parasympathetic fibers. Extensive central ramifications of the autonomic nervous system exist in the brain; various groups of cells located in the medulla are concerned with integration and control of specific autonomic functions (the cardioaccelerator and inhibitory centers, the vasomotor center, the respiratory center, etc.). Descending fibers from these centers synapse with cell bodies of the preganglionic efferent fibers in the medulla and spinal cord. All spinal and lower brainstem autonomic centers are controlled and coordinated by the hypothalamus, which has extensive connections with the cerebral cortex and pituitary gland. Through these connections autonomic nervous system activity is coordinated with somatic neural and endocrine activity.

There are 2 divisions of the peripheral efferent autonomic nervous system, the **parasympathetic** and the **sympathetic**. FIG. 248-1 diagrams the way these 2 systems innervate the various tissues, and TABLE 248-1 summarizes the major effects of stimulation of the 2 divisions. In general, sympathetic stimulation produces responses which prepare the body for emergency (increased cardiac output, increased BP, mydriasis, bronchodilation, etc.), while irrelevant activities are suppressed (decreased tone and motility of the GI tract, relaxation of smooth muscles of the GU tract with contraction of the sphincter, etc.)— the "fight, fright, flight syndrome." Parasympathetic stimulation, in general, prepares the body for more sedentary activities; most responses are opposite to those evoked by the sympathetic system.

Neurohumoral Transmission

Transmission of nerve impulses at ganglion synapses and in neuroeffector junctions occurs through **neurotransmitters** (chemical mediators), which are shown in FIG. 248-2. **Acetylcholine** is the neurotransmitter at the nerve endings of all preganglionic autonomic nerves including the adrenal medulla, all postganglionic parasympathetic nerves, the postganglionic sympathetic nerves to sweat glands and vasodilatory blood vessels of the skeletal muscle, and all skeletal neuromuscular junctions. The actions of acetylcholine and substances acting like it at postganglionic cholinergic nerve endings (parasympathetic nerves and cholinergic sympathetic nerves) and the blood vessels are described as **muscarinic** because they resemble those of muscarine. Actions of these agents at autonomic ganglia, the adrenal medulla, and skeletal neuromuscular junctions are described as **nicotinic** because they resemble those of nicotine. **Norepinephrine** is the neurotransmitter at all postganglionic sympathetic nerve endings except those supplying the sweat glands and vasodilatory blood vessels of the skeletal muscle. Other neurotransmitters may exist in the peripheral autonomic system, but none has been firmly established.

The major steps in the process of neurohumoral transmission (FIG. 248-3) are as follows: (1) The nerve impulse (action potential) is conducted along the prejunctional neuron. (2) This impulse depolarizes the prejunctional membrane facing the postjunctional surface and (3) Ca ions enter the prejunctional axoplasm and facilitate release of the excitatory or inhibiting chemical transmitter (as the case may be) from storage (synaptic) vesicles into the junctional space. (4) The neurotransmitter diffuses across the junctional space and combines with receptors at the postjunctional membrane

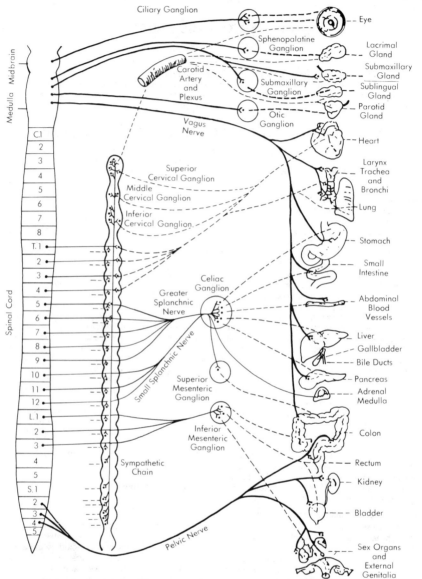

FIG. 248-1. **Diagram of the efferent autonomic pathways.** Preganglionic neurons are shown as solid lines, postganglionic neurons as broken lines. The heavy lines are parasympathetic fibers; the light lines are sympathetic. (From W.B. Youmans, *Fundamentals of Human Physiology,* ed. 2, 1962, Used with permission. Year Book Medical Publishers, Inc.)

surface, resulting in permeability changes to small ions (Na, K) and depolarization (in case of an excitatory transmitter) or hyperpolarization (in case of an inhibitory transmitter) of the membrane. (5) The effector response then occurs (contraction or relaxation of muscle, or glandular secretion, or continuation of impulse conduction in a postganglionic nerve). (6) Termination of neurotransmitter activity occurs in several ways; the most common are degradation by enzymes (e.g., acetylcholinesterase hydrolyzes acetylcholine) and reuptake of the neurotransmitter by the prejunctional axon.

TABLE 248-1. RESPONSES OF EFFECTOR ORGANS TO AUTONOMIC NERVE IMPULSES

Effector Organs	Adrenergic Impulses		Cholinergic Impulses
	Receptor Type	Responses*	Responses*
Eye			
Radial muscle, iris	α	Contraction (mydriasis) + +	———
Sphincter muscle, iris		———	Contraction (miosis) + + +
Ciliary muscle	β	Relaxation for far vision +	Contraction for near vision + + +
Heart			
S-A node	β_1	Increase in heart rate + +	Decrease in heart rate; vagal arrest + + +
Atria	β_1	Increase in contractility and conduction velocity + +	Decrease in contractility, and (usually) increase in conduction velocity + +
A-V node	β_1	Increase in automaticity and conduction velocity + +	Decrease in conduction velocity; A-V block + + +
His-Purkinje system	β_1	Increase in automaticity and conduction velocity + + +	Little effect
Ventricles	β_1	Increase in contractility, conduction velocity, automaticity, and rate of idioventricular pacemakers + + +	Slight decrease in contractility claimed by some
Arterioles			
Coronary	α, β_2	Constriction +; dilatation ‡ + +	Dilatation ±
Skin and mucosa	α	Constriction + + +	Dilatation ‡
Skeletal muscle	α, β_2	Constriction + +; dilatation ‡§ + +	Dilatation ** +
Cerebral	α	Constriction (slight)	Dilatation ‡
Pulmonary	α, β_2	Constriction +; dilatation ‡	Dilatation ‡
Abdominal viscera; renal	α, β_2	Constriction + + +; dilatation § +	———
Salivary glands	α	Constriction + + +	Dilatation + +
Veins (systemic)	α, β_2	Constriction + +; dilatation + +	———
Lung			
Bronchial muscle	β_2	Relaxation +	Contraction + +
Bronchial glands	?	Inhibition (?)	Stimulation + + +
Stomach			
Motility and tone	α_2, β_2	Decrease (usually) †† +	Increase + + +
Sphincters	α	Contraction (usually) +	Relaxation (usually) +
Secretion		Inhibition (?)	Stimulation + + +
Intestine			
Motility and tone	α_2, β_2	Decrease †† +	Increase + + +
Sphincters	α	Contraction (usually) +	Relaxation (usually) +
Secretion		Inhibition (?)	Stimulation + +
Gallbladder and ducts		Relaxation +	Contraction +
Kidney	β_2	Renin secretion + +	———
Urinary bladder			
Detrusor	β	Relaxation (usually) +	Contraction + + +
Trigone and sphincter	α	Contraction + +	Relaxation + +

(Continued)

TABLE 248–1. RESPONSES OF EFFECTOR ORGANS TO AUTONOMIC NERVE IMPULSES *(Cont'd)*

Effector Organs	Receptor Type	Adrenergic Impulses Responses*	Cholinergic Impulses Responses*
Ureter Motility and tone	α	Increase (usually)	Increase (?)
Uterus	α,β_2	Pregnant, contraction (α); nonpregnant: relaxation (β)	Variables §§
Sex organs, male	α	Ejaculation + + +	Erection + + +
Skin Pilomotor muscles Sweat glands	α α	Contraction + + Localized secretion *** +	——— Generalized secretion + + +
Spleen capsule	α,β_2	Contraction + + +; relaxation +	———
Adrenal medulla		———	Secretion of epinephrine and norepinephrine
Liver	α,β_2	Glycogenolysis, gluconeogenesis †††	Glycogen synthesis +
Pancreas Acini Islets (β cells)	α α β_2	Decreased secretion + Decreased secretion + + + Increased secretion +	Secretion + + ——— ———
Fat cells	α,β_1	Lipolysis ††† + + +	———
Salivary glands	α β	Potassium and water secretion + Amylase secretion +	Potassium and water secretion + + +
Lacrimal glands		———	Secretion + + +
Nasopharyngeal glands		———	Secretion + +
Pineal gland	β	Melatonin synthesis	———

* Responses are designated 1+ to 3+ to provide an approximate indication of the importance of adrenergic and cholinergic nerve activity in the control of the various organs and functions listed.

† Dilatation predominates *in situ* due to metabolic autoregulatory phenomena.

‡ Cholinergic vasodilatation at these sites is of questionable physiological significance.

§ Over the usual concentration range of physiologically released, circulating epinephrine, β-receptor response (vasodilatation) predominates in blood vessels of skeletal muscle and liver; α-receptor response (vasoconstriction), in blood vessels of other abdominal viscera. The renal and mesenteric vessels also contain specific dopaminergic receptors, activation of which causes dilatation, but their physiological significance has not been established (*see* review by Goldberg *et al.*, 1978).

** Sympathetic cholinergic system causes vasodilatation in skeletal muscle, but this is not involved in most physiological responses.

†† It has been proposed that adrenergic fibers terminate at inhibitory β receptors on smooth muscle fibers, and at inhibitory α receptors on parasympathetic cholinergic (excitatory) ganglion cells of Auerbach's plexus.

§§ Depends on stage of menstrual cycle, amount of circulating estrogen and progesterone, and other factors.

*** Palms of hands and some other sites ("adrenergic sweating").

††† There is significant variation among species in the type of receptor that mediates certain metabolic responses.

Adapted from "Drugs Acting at Synaptic and Neuroeffector Junctional Sites," pp. 60, 61, in GOODMAN AND GILMAN'S THE PHARMACOLOGICAL BASIS OF THERAPEUTICS, ed. 6, 1980, edited by A. G. Gilman, L. S. Goodman, and A. Gilman. Copyright © 1980 by Macmillan Publishing Co., Inc. Used with permission.

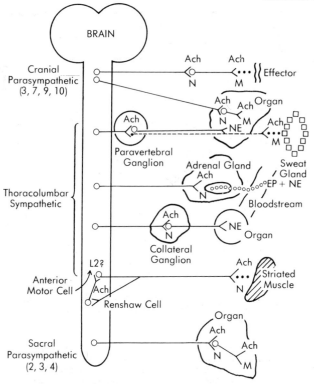

Fɪɢ. 248–2. Diagrammatic summary of transmitter location in the autonomic nervous system. Transmitters at each location: Ach, acetylcholines; NE, norepinephrine; EP, epinephrine. Receptors at each location: N, nicotinic; M, muscarinic. (From O. Carrier, Jr.: PHARMACOLOGY OF THE PERIPHERAL AUTONOMIC NERVOUS SYSTEM. Copyright ©1972 by Year Book Medical Publishers, Inc., Chicago. Used with permission.)

Synthesis, Storage, Release, and Destruction of Neurotransmitters

Acetylcholine: After being synthesized from choline and acetyl coenzyme A by the enzyme choline acetylase in the cell body of the neuron, acetylcholine migrates down the axon to the prejunctional area and is stored in synaptic vesicles. A nerve impulse causes a synchronous breakdown of many vesicles, and fixed packages or quanta of acetylcholine are released into the junctional gap to effect transmission. Action is terminated by the destruction of acetylcholine brought about by acetylcholinesterase (present in nervous tissue and striated muscle), which hydrolyzes the molecule into choline and acetic acid. There are also pseudocholinesterases in plasma, intestine, skin, and many other tissues, which can destroy choline esters, and their action may be important in terminating the effects of therapeutically administered choline esters (e.g., succinylcholine).

Catecholamines: The most important of these are norepinephrine, epinephrine, and dopamine. **Norepinephrine** is the neurotransmitter in most sympathetic postganglionic nerve terminals. **Epinephrine** is released from the adrenal medulla by sympathetic stimulation and is thought to act as a neurotransmitter in some areas in the brain. **Dopamine,** a precursor of norepinephrine and epinephrine, may function as a neurotransmitter in certain areas of the brain (e.g., basal ganglia) and in certain peripheral vascular beds.

These catecholamines are enzymatically synthesized from the amino acid tyrosine by a series of steps: tyrosine → dihydroxyphenylalanine (dopa) → dopamine → norepinephrine → epinephrine. In the sympathetic nerves, norepinephrine is synthesized mainly in the varicosities of the nerve terminal and stored in synaptic vesicles. In the adrenal medulla, where part of norepinephrine is converted to epinephrine, the catecholamines are stored in chromaffin granules, and released by a process termed exocytosis. The action of norepinephrine released from the sympathetic neuron is terminated mainly by reuptake by the prejunctional axon; this norepinephrine can be used again for neurotransmitter function. The same mechanism also takes up epinephrine and dopamine. The action may also be terminated by enzymatic inactivation. Catecholamine-O-methyltransferase (**COMT**—present in the effector cells and in the liver) and monoamine oxidase (**MAO**—present in effector cells, liver, and

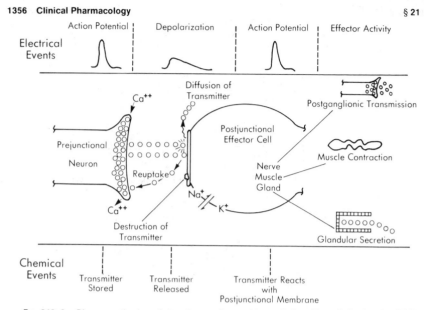

Fig. 248–3. Diagrammatic view of steps in neurohumoral transmission. (From O. Carrier, Jr.: PHAR-MACOLOGY OF THE PERIPHERAL AUTONOMIC NERVOUS SYSTEM. Copyright ©1972 by Year Book Medical Publishers, Inc., Chicago. Used with permission.

also in the prejunctional axon, where it can inactivate any excess norepinephrine that may leak out of storage vesicles) are important enzymes in catecholamine degradation. Catecholamines released from the adrenal medulla are inactivated in the liver primarily by COMT and MAO. The main metabolites of norepinephrine and epinephrine in the body are 3-methoxy-4-hydroxymandelic acid (generally, but incorrectly, called vanillylmandelic acid—**VMA**), normetanephrine, and metanephrine. The main biotransformation product of dopamine is homovanillic acid.

NEUROTRANSMITTERS IN THE CENTRAL NERVOUS SYSTEM

The enormous structural and functional complexity of the CNS has posed many problems in the identification of central neurotransmitters. The following monoamines and amino acids have been strongly implicated as neurotransmitters in the CNS.

Acetylcholine is nonhomogeneously distributed in the CNS and is probably a synaptic transmitter agent in many regions. The spinal **Renshaw cell** is the best example of a central cholinoceptive neuron. Other sites where acetylcholine has been implicated as a transmitter include the basal ganglia, cerebral cortex, and hippocampus. In most regions of the CNS the effects of acetylcholine appear to be generated by interaction with a mixture of nicotinic and muscarinic receptors. In the Renshaw cell, the receptor appears to be of the nicotinic type.

Catecholamines that have been strongly implicated as central neurotransmitters include dopamine, norepinephrine, and epinephrine. The neuronal systems that utilize the 3 catecholamines seem to be distinct from one another. **Dopamine** has been implicated as an inhibitory neurotransmitter in the caudate nucleus and the putamen, playing an important role in integration of movement. The main lesion in Parkinson's disease is thought to be in this region, where severe depletion of dopamine allows the activity of cholinergic neurons to predominate, causing the parkinsonian symptoms. Dopamine has also been implicated in other CNS activities (e.g., inhibition of prolactin release). **Dopamine receptor agonists** (notably bromocriptine) have been found useful in a number of clinical situations; their beneficial effect is presumably through stimulation of dopamine receptors normally activated by dopamine in the body. Thus in some cases of hyperprolactinemia with galactorrhea and amenorrhea, bromocriptine has been successfully used. Similarly, dopamine agonists have been shown to have beneficial effects in parkinsonism. The use of bromocriptine in treatment of acromegaly is paradoxical. It is known that dopamine facilitates the release of growth hormone and in normal individuals bromocriptine and L-dopa both have been shown to increase growth hormone release; how or why bromocriptine causes decreased growth hormone release in acromegalic patients is unclear.

Most **norepinephrine**-containing neurons in the brain arise either in the locus ceruleus of the pons or in neurons of the lateral tegmental portion of the reticular formation. From these neurons, multiple branched axons innervate specific target cells in the cortical, sub-cortical, and spinomedullary areas. The effect of norepinephrine in most brain areas seems to be inhibitory. Norepinephrine has been implicated with other biogenic amines in a wide variety of centrally mediated physiologic functions including sleep and arousal, affect, memory, learning, and most of the essential homeostatic mechanisms (e.g., regulation of temperature, BP, and food and fluid intake).

Epinephrine-containing neurons have been found in the medullary reticular formation making connections with a few pontine and diencephalic neurons. The physiologic properties of these neurons are not well understood, but their effects are probably inhibitory.

The **amino acids, γ-aminobutyrate (GABA)** and **glycine** have been strongly implicated as neurotransmitters in the CNS. Evidence suggests that GABA mediates the inhibitory actions of local interneurons in many brain regions including cerebellar cortex, olfactory bulb, hippocampus, and cerebral cortex. GABA may also mediate presynaptic inhibition within the spinal cord. Glycine has been strongly implicated by neurochemical and electrophysiologic evidence to be an inhibitory neurotransmitter between spinal interneurons and motor neurons.

Other biogenic amines (e.g., 5-hydroxytryptamine, histamine) and amino acids (glutamate, aspartate) have been hypothesized to be neurotransmitters in the brain. Evidence in their support is still preliminary and incomplete.

Recently, many endogenous **neuropeptides** with striking effects on the activity of neural systems have been discovered. These include the **enkephalins** and **endorphins, luteinizing hormone-releasing hormone (LHRH), somatostatin, substance P,** and **thyrotropin-releasing hormone (TRH).** Until now, none of these has been clearly shown to meet all the rigorous criteria required to be definitely identified as a neurotransmitter. The role of these peptides in central and peripheral neural functions is not yet well defined. However, it seems likely that many of them will prove of importance in both physiologic and pathologic states.

CHOLINERGIC DRUGS
(Parasympathomimetics)

Drugs that act at sites in the body where acetylcholine is the neurotransmitter of the nerve impulse. In addition, these drugs, like acetylcholine, act directly on peripheral blood vessels (which lack parasympathetic innervation), resulting in vasodilation. They produce parasympathetic stimulation (see TABLE 248–1), and stimulate autonomic ganglia (the ganglionic effects are overshadowed by peripheral parasympathetic effects) and the neuromuscular junction, causing muscle fasciculation in small doses and persistent depolarization or neuromuscular block in large doses. The effect of cholinergics on the CNS is variable and depends on the extent to which they enter the CNS; they usually result in stimulation followed by depression. Not all the effects are seen with all the drugs in the group, the effects vary with dosage, and there is little organ or regional selectivity in their effects. Side effects caused by most of these drugs are parasympathomimetic effects produced at sites other than those desired. Cholinergics are **contraindicated** in asthma, coronary insufficiency, and peptic ulcer. They may be grouped into 2 categories: choline esters and cholinergic alkaloids.

Choline Esters

Choline esters act wherever acetylcholine acts. **Bethanechol,** the most clinically useful drug in this group, is a long-acting muscarinic drug, resistant to hydrolysis by cholinesterases. It acts chiefly on the urinary bladder and the bowel and is useful in urinary retention and for increasing bowel motility. The usual oral dose is 5 to 20 mg t.i.d. It may be given s.c. 2.5 mg q 15 to 30 min until there is a response or prohibitive side effects occur; e.g., sweating, salivation, intestinal pain, cramps, diarrhea, flushing, hypotension, and difficulty in breathing. Atropine can alleviate these side effects. **Methacholine** has predominantly cardiovascular effects; it is occasionally used in doses of 10 to 30 mg s.c. to stop supraventricular tachycardia. **Carbachol** mainly affects the bladder and bowel. It is sometimes used topically in the eyes as a miotic (1.5% solution or ointment b.i.d. or t.i.d.). **Acetylcholine** (1% solution) is used in cataract extractions and certain other ophthalmic surgery when it is necessary to produce miosis rapidly.

Cholinergic Alkaloids

Cholinergic alkaloids act mainly on end-organs affected by acetylcholine. **Pilocarpine,** the most clinically useful drug of this group, exhibits predominantly muscarinic effects. Its chief use is in ophthalmology as a miotic (0.5 to 10% solution; 1 to 2 drops several times/day as required). It is a potent stimulator of sweat glands and salivary glands and is occasionally used as a sialagogue. **Muscarine** itself has no therapeutic uses. It can be poisonous when ingested, causing symptoms of excess parasympathetic stimulation (see NONBACTERIAL FOOD POISONING in Ch. 55).

Anticholinesterases

These are drugs capable of inactivating the enzymes that terminate the action of acetylcholine and other choline esters in the body; they act as parasympathomimetics by allowing acetylcholine and its effects to persist. They potentiate the action of all cholinergics. *Atropine antagonizes only the muscarinic effects of anticholinesterases.*

Anticholinesterases are classified as reversible or irreversible, according to the duration of the blocking effect. This depends on how fast the body can disrupt the anticholinesterase drug-enzyme complex (inhibitor-enzyme complex). The blocking effect usually lasts from a few minutes to several hours with the reversible anticholinesterases and days or weeks with the irreversible ones. The reversible anticholinesterases are primarily used as miotics in ophthalmology and in treating myasthenia gravis and anticholinergic drug poisoning.

Reversible anticholinesterases: 1. Physostigmine, an alkaloid found in the West African plant *Physostigma venenosum,* is well absorbed from the GI tract and readily enters the CNS. It produces generalized anticholinesterase effects when given systemically. Physostigmine salicylate is the drug of choice for treating anticholinergic drug poisoning (e.g., atropine, scopolamine, tricyclic antidepressants) because it antagonizes both central and peripheral effects. It is given slowly IV in doses of 1 to 4 mg (not to exceed 1 mg/min) and may be repeated as needed. More commonly, it is used topically as a miotic in ophthalmology, in which its duration of action is about 6 to 12 h. One or two drops of the 0.25% solution can be used several times/day as required; the 0.25% ointment is usually applied at bedtime.

2. Neostigmine, a synthetic anticholinesterase, is structurally similar to acetylcholine and hence has a direct stimulatory effect of its own in addition to its acetylcholine potentiating effect. It is poorly absorbed from the GI tract and penetrates poorly into the CNS. Its main use is in myasthenia gravis (usual dosage: 15 to 375 mg/day orally in 4 to 8 divided doses; 0.25 to 1 mg s.c. or IM t.i.d. or q.i.d.). It is also used to combat poisoning with anticholinergics (0.5 mg q 2 to 3 h), to terminate paroxysmal atrial tachycardia (0.5 to 2 mg s.c.), and as an antidote to overdosage with the competitive type of neuromuscular blocking agents (e.g., *d*-tubocurarine).

3. Pyridostigmine is similar to neostigmine, with a slower onset and longer duration of action. The usual dose range is 360 mg to 1.5 gm/day orally in 4 to 6 divided doses for the treatment of myasthenia gravis.

4. Ambenonium is also similar to neostigmine but is more potent, with a longer duration of action and possibly fewer side effects. The usual dosage in treatment of myasthenia gravis is 20 mg orally q 4 to 6 h.

5. Demecarium consists of 2 neostigmine molecules joined together. It is a long-acting anticholinesterase chiefly used in ophthalmology (0.125 to 0.25% solution), and as a long-acting miotic (effect of a single dose lasts up to 5 days) in the treatment of glaucoma.

6. Edrophonium has a short duration of action (less than 5 min) and is used mainly in testing for myasthenia gravis and for differentiating between myasthenic and cholinergic crisis. **For the diagnostic test,** a syringe is loaded with 10 mg of edrophonium; 2 mg is given IV and if no reaction occurs within 30 seconds, the rest is injected. In myasthenics there is a sudden, though short-lasting, improvement in muscle function. When the test is performed to differentiate between myasthenic and cholinergic crisis, the effect on muscle function and general condition indicates the diagnosis: a myasthenic crisis improves and a cholinergic crisis worsens. Dangerous respiratory depression can occur and *facilities to maintain respiration and atropine (as an antidote) must be available during the test.* Edrophonium is also often used to terminate paroxysmal atrial tachycardia (10 mg by slow IV push, repeated if necessary after 15 min).

Irreversible anticholinesterases: These compounds are therapeutically useful only as long-acting miotics in treating certain types of glaucoma. (1) Isoflurophate ¼ in. of ointment (0.025%) is applied in each eye daily at bedtime. The drug may be absorbed and cause systemic effects. (2) Echothiophate iodide solutions (0.06, 0.125, and 0.25%) may be prepared from the marketed powder. (3) Many organophosphorous insecticides (parathion, malathion, tetraethyl pyrophosphate, etc.) are irreversible anticholinesterases without therapeutic use. They are medically important because humans are sometimes accidentally poisoned with them (see under Parathion in TABLE 258–4 in Ch. 258).

ANTICHOLINERGIC DRUGS
(Parasympatholytics)

Anticholinergics primarily oppose the actions of acetylcholine at postganglionic cholinergic nerve endings. They also block direct acetylcholine action on blood vessels and in the CNS; the muscarinic actions of other cholinergic drugs are also opposed. In high doses most of these drugs also block the autonomic ganglia; none block the neuromuscular junction.

Since most organs receive both sympathetic and parasympathetic nerves and these tend to oppose each other, parasympathetic blockade in most organs results in sympathetic dominance and sympathomimetic effects (see FIG. 248–1 and TABLE 248–1). Thus, in therapeutic doses, anticholinergics produce mydriasis, cycloplegia, tachycardia, and enhanced conduction in the bundle of His. All exocrine secretions, except milk, decrease (dry mouth is the most prominent effect), gastric secretion decreases (with no change in pH), smooth muscles of the bronchi relax, and the tone and motility of the GI tract and urinary bladder decrease. All of these effects may not be seen with all of the drugs in this group. CNS effects vary with individual drugs and depend upon the extent to which the drugs enter the CNS.

Poisoning with these drugs presents with peripheral and CNS signs (excitement or depression); variations depend on drug and dosage. The drugs are **contraindicated or should be used with caution** in narrow angle glaucoma, cardiac failure, achalasia, pyloric obstruction, paralytic ileus, bladder neck obstruction, and prostatic hypertrophy. The common drugs in this group are described below. Atropine or scopolamine are usually the anticholinergic drugs of choice. Other drugs may offer some advantage in special circumstances; e.g., homatropine, tropicamide, and cyclopentolate may be advantageous for topical application to produce mydriasis and cycloplegia because of their short duration of action.

Atropine (*dl*-hyoscyamine), a plant alkaloid, is the prototype drug of the group, and when used systemically in adequate doses it provides all of the effects described above for the group as a whole. In most cases it produces an initial transitory central vagal *stimulant* action before the blocking effect is manifested.

The CNS is stimulated by atropine; restlessness, mental excitement, mania, delirium, and hallucinations occur with large doses. Large doses also cause hyperpyrexia because of a combination of central and peripheral effects (decreased sweating).

Atropine is well absorbed when given orally and is rapidly eliminated from the body. About equal amounts of unchanged atropine and inactive metabolites are excreted in the urine; excretion is nearly complete in 24 h. Usually, 3 or 4 doses/day are needed to sustain pharmacologic effects, but cycloplegia and mydriasis may persist for days after a single dose, especially if given topically. The usual dose range of atropine sulfate is 0.4 to 3 mg/day orally or parenterally (s.c., IM, or IV). Above 3 mg, mental status and behavior usually change. The dose and route depend on the condition being treated. For chronic use in peptic ulcer, the maximum *tolerated* daily dose is usually given orally in 3 or 4 divided doses. Its use in the treatment of sinus bradycardia and incomplete atrioventricular block is described under CARDIAC ARRHYTHMIAS in Ch. 25. In ophthalmology it is used topically as a mydriatic and cycloplegic drug (1% solution, 0.5 and 1% ointment for cycloplegia, 1 drop t.i.d. for 3 days prior to examination and 1 drop on day of examination; for iritis, solution or ointment b.i.d. or t.i.d.). Atropine can also be given orally as tincture of belladonna (0.03% solution, 0.3 to 3 ml daily) or belladonna extract (15 to 60 mg daily).

Poisoning with atropine is best treated with physostigmine salicylate (see above), which antagonizes atropine effects both in the CNS and in the periphery.

Scopolamine (hyoscine) differs from atropine chiefly in being a CNS depressant instead of a stimulant. It is used mainly in obstetrics (where its sedative and amnesic properties are useful), as an antiemetic, and to prevent motion sickness. The usual dose is 0.3 to 3 mg. Many hypnotics sold without a prescription contain scopolamine in combination with a mildly sedative antihistamine; the hypnotic efficacy of these preparations is minimal.

Other atropine-like compounds: Homatropine has a shorter duration of action than atropine and is used mainly for its ocular effects; it may not be effective in children. For mydriasis and complete cycloplegia, repeated instillations of a 2% solution q 15 min for 1 to 2 h may be needed. **Benztropine** is a potent antimuscarinic drug often used in parkinsonism (2 to 12 mg/day orally in divided doses).

Tertiary amines with atropine-like properties are less specific and weaker antimuscarinic drugs than atropine and the others mentioned. They have less ganglion blocking activity and lack the ocular and certain other side effects of atropine-like drugs. This group includes dicyclomine, methixene, oxyphencyclimine, and others. In general they are useful when spasmolytic action is desired, as in the treatment of GI disorders associated with hypermotility or spasm.

Quaternary ammonium compounds with atropine-like properties: This group includes propantheline, methantheline, glycopyrrolate, methscopolamine, methylatropine, oxyphenonium, diphemanil, isopropamide, and others. Because of their net positive charge, these drugs do not readily enter the CNS and thus offer an advantage over atropine and scopolamine. For the same reason, however, their absorption from the GI tract is poor. Anticholinergic effects are most marked at the parasympathetic nerve endings; action is not selective. These drugs are used to treat peptic ulcer and GI hypermotility.

Other drugs with anticholinergic properties: Important groups of drugs in this category are (1) ethanolamine antihistamines (diphenhydramine, orphenadrine), (2) piperazine antihistamines (cyclizine, meclizine), and (3) phenothiazines (ethopropazine, promethazine). They are mainly used to treat Parkinson's disease and nausea and vomiting due to vestibular disturbances (as in Ménière's disease and motion sickness). Tropicamide and cyclopentolate are 2 synthetic compounds with anticholinergic properties that are often used topically as mydriatics and cycloplegics in ophthalmology.

ADRENERGIC DRUGS

(Sympathomimetics)

Drugs that mimic the effects of stimulation of the sympathetic division of the autonomic nervous system (see TABLE 248–1). Many synthetic and naturally occurring drugs belong to this category, which can be broadly classified into 3 groups: (1) **direct-acting drugs** (e.g., epinephrine, norepinephrine, isoproterenol, and phenylephrine), which produce their effect primarily by direct stimulation of the adrenergic receptor; (2) **indirect-acting drugs** (e.g., tyramine), which act by releasing norepinephrine from its storage site in the adrenergic nerve endings; and (3) **drugs acting by both mechanisms** (e.g., ephedrine, dopamine, metaraminol, and mephentermine).

   Sympathetic nerve stimulation produces effects of at least 2 different types, mediated by 2 different adrenergic receptors, α and β. TABLE 248–1 lists the major organ systems and the adrenergic receptor type associated with each. The standard α stimulants (α agonists) are phenylephrine and methoxamine, although both produce some β effects as well. The relative potency for α stimulation among the 3 important catecholamines is epinephrine $>$ norepinephrine $>$ isoproterenol. Alpha effects appear mainly as vasoconstriction (chiefly in skin and viscera) and mydriasis. All the α effects are antagonized by the nonselective α-blocking drugs (phentolamine, dihydroergocryptine, etc.). Activation of β receptors produces cardiac stimulation, peripheral inhibition in the form of vasodilation (chiefly in skeletal muscles), and bronchial and uterine relaxation. The standard β agonist is isoproterenol. The relative potency for β stimulation among the 3 important catecholamines is isoproterenol $>$ epinephrine $>$ norepinephrine. All β effects are antagonized by the β-blocking agents (propranolol, nadolol, etc.). Some adrenergic effects do not clearly fall into the α or β group (e.g., some metabolic effects).

   Recently, the development of more selective agonists and antagonists that act at adrenergic receptors has resulted in the subclassification of both β- and α-adrenergic receptors. β-Adrenergic receptors have been subclassified into β_1 and β_2. β_1-Adrenergic receptors predominate in the heart and adipose tissue while β_2 receptors are present primarily in smooth muscles of the bronchus, uterus, GI tract, blood vessels, and gland cells. Different tissues may possess β_1 and β_2 receptors in varying proportions. At β_1 receptors, isoproterenol is more potent than epinephrine, which is equipotent with norepinephrine. In contrast, at β_2 receptors, isoproterenol is equal to or more potent than epinephrine, which is much more potent than norepinephrine. These differences in β_1 and β_2 receptors presumably reflect structural dissimilarities in the receptors. Drugs, both agonists and antagonists, with greater potency at one or the other subtype of β receptor have been developed. Thus for example, while propranolol has equal potency at β_1 and β_2 receptors, the β-blocker metoprolol is approximately 10 times more potent at β_1 receptors than at β_2 receptors. Similarly, agonists such as salbutamol and terbutaline are much more potent at β_2 receptors than at β_1 receptors, in contrast to isoproterenol, which is equipotent at β_1 and β_2 receptors. The availability of selective β agonists and antagonists is of distinct advantage in some special situations (e.g., in treatment of bronchial asthma, selective β agonists have the distinct advantage of having much less cardiac side effects in comparison to nonselective β agonists).

   Subclassification of α-adrenergic receptors into α_1 and α_2 receptors has been made more recently. The α_1-adrenergic receptors are the classic postsynaptic α receptors, such as those that mediate the effects of α agonists in constricting smooth muscle cells. The α_2 receptors are classically found at presynaptic sites on the nerve ending itself and they mediate the presynaptic feedback inhibition of neural release of norepinephrine and, perhaps, acetylcholine. The α_2 receptors are also found in locations other than presynaptic, as for example, on human platelets, where they mediate the effects of epinephrine in causing platelet aggregation. These α_1 and α_2 adrenergic receptors can be distinguished because of differences in affinities for various selective α-adrenergic agonists and antagonists. Among agonists, methoxamine and phenylephrine are considered α_1 selective, clonidine α_2 selective, and epinephrine and norepinephrine relatively nonselective. Among antagonists, prazosin and phenoxybenzamine are considered α_1 selective, yohimbine (a plant alkaloid) α_2 selective, and phentolamine and dihydroergocryptine nonselective. The therapeutic advantage (if any) of selective α agonists and antagonists over the nonselective agents is currently being investigated.

   Use of high-affinity-radiolabeled agonist or antagonist binding technics has recently provided new information on the regulation of the adrenergic receptors. It has become apparent that the number and function of the adrenergic receptors can be modified by a number of factors that can be broadly classified as homologous and heterologous. **Homologous regulation** is regulation of the receptors by ligands (hormones or agonists) that normally interact with those receptors. The most common type of homologous regulation of the adrenergic receptors involves the endogenous catecholamines. The regulation is usually time and concentration dependent and takes the form of an inverse relationship between the ambient concentration of the catecholamines and the receptor number. Thus, elevated concentration of catecholamines "down-regulate" and lowered concentrations "up-regulate" the adrenergic receptor number. In contrast to homologous regulation, **heterologous regulation** refers to regulation of receptors by ligands that do not normally interact with the receptor under consideration. Thus, in the case of adrenergic receptors in some tissues, other hormones besides the catecholamines have been found to regulate the receptor number. For example, animal studies have shown that in the heart, salivary glands, and some other tissues, hyperthyroidism results in an increase in β-adrenergic receptor number. Similarly, estrogen and progesterone have been shown to regulate the α-adrenergic receptor number in the uterus. The hormone or drug-related changes in adrenergic receptor number often are associated with corresponding changes in tissue responsiveness to catecholamines; thus, increased receptor number is often associated with supersensitivity and decreased number with decreased responsiveness. Many phenomena such as tachyphylaxis and supersensitivity observed with adrenergic agents may be explicable on the basis of this knowledge about the regulation of the adrenergic receptors.

   The molecular mechanisms by which the adrenergic effects are mediated is beginning to be understood, especially in reference to the β effects. In most, if not all cases, the key compound involved in mediation of β-adrenergic effects seems to be cAMP. The β agonist causes intracellular accumulation of cAMP by activating (via β receptors) a membrane-bound enzyme, adenylate cyclase, which catalyzes the conversion of ATP to cAMP. This in turn activates protein kinases that phosphorylate specific substrates, which then lead to the characteristic β-adrenergic effects. The mechanisms seem qualitatively similar for both β_1 and β_2 subtypes. Much less is known about details of α-adrenergic activation. In some cases changes in Ca flux may be involved. The α_2 receptors are often coupled (in an inhibitory manner) to adenylate cyclase. Thus, effects produced through their stimulation may be mediated through inhibition of adenylate cyclase and the consequent decrease in intracellular cAMP.

Adverse effects of sympathomimetic agents are usually predictable from their known pharmacologic effects, are usually due to a lack of selective action, and are in the form of sympathomimetic effects occurring at sites other than the one at which the effect is desired (e.g., tachycardia when bronchodilation is desired). Tissue necrosis due to intense vasoconstriction at the injection site can occur if there is leakage during IV infusions. Excess cardiac stimulation (possibly leading to ventricular arrhythmia and death) may occur with excessive or too rapid administration of the drugs, especially by the parenteral route. Dangerous synergistic effects (especially on the heart) can occur when 2 or more of these agents are used concurrently (e.g., isoproterenol by inhalation and epinephrine parenterally). *Sympathomimetics should be used with extreme caution in patients with heart disease, hypertension, cerebral ischemia, and hyperthyroidism.*

Individual Sympathomimetic Agents

Norepinephrine (levarterenol): The chief therapeutic use of norepinephrine is to raise BP. However, since it reduces blood flow to the kidney and brain, its use in shock may be harmful (see SHOCK in Ch. 24). Gangrene of the extremities and necrotic ulceration of large areas around the infusion vein can occur with prolonged IV use; the risk can be minimized by using large veins and a rapid flow of solution for the shortest time possible. If extravasation is detected, the α-blocking agent phentolamine (5 to 10 mg in 10 ml saline) should be infiltrated into the site, within 12 h, to prevent tissue necrosis. Norepinephrine infusions should be stopped gradually because their sudden cessation may be followed by a catastrophic fall in BP. Norepinephrine is ineffective orally.

Epinephrine affects all α and β subtypes; it is ineffective orally. Its use in treating bronchial asthma and anaphylactic shock is discussed in Chs. 34 and 19, respectively. In Stokes-Adams syndrome, 3 ml of 1:1000 aqueous epinephrine are diluted in 300 ml of 5% D/W; the rate of administration is adjusted according to adequacy of the heart rate. Epinephrine (1:80,000 or less concentrated) is often used with local anesthetics to prolong their effect. Overdose with epinephrine should be treated with both an α blocker (usually phentolamine) and a β blocker (e.g., propranolol).

Isoproterenol primarily affects the β receptors, being equipotent at β_1 and β_2 receptors. It is poorly absorbed from the intestine, although sometimes a large dose in sustained-release form is used for prolonged effect; given sublingually, it is quite effective. For its use in bronchial asthma, see Ch. 34. In Stokes-Adams syndrome it is used as an IV infusion (see under INFRANODAL A-V BLOCK in CARDIAC ARRHYTHMIAS in Ch. 25).

Dopamine, a precursor of norepinephrine in the body, has unique effects that make it especially useful in the treatment of shock due to various causes (myocardial infarction, trauma, endotoxic septicemia). Its use has also been advocated in some cases of chronic refractory congestive heart failure, hepatorenal syndrome, and acute renal failure. Although relative dopamine deficiency in the basal ganglia is felt to be the primary defect in parkinsonism, IV dopamine is ineffective in this condition, since it does not cross the blood-brain barrier.

Dopamine has effects both on β receptors (primary β_1 receptors) and α receptors (the predominantly observable effects are on the postjunctional α_1 receptors). In addition it stimulates specific dopamine receptors (present in renal, mesenteric, coronary, and intracerebral arterial beds) causing vasodilation. The specific dopamine effects are not antagonized by α or β blockers. Haloperidol and other butyrophenones, phenothiazines, and morphine have been shown to be capable of antagonizing these effects. Some of the effects of administered dopamine are due to release of norepinephrine from its storage sites in sympathetic nerve endings. In general, when dopamine is administered in relatively low doses, the predominant effects are due to β_1 receptor and dopamine receptor stimulation. In higher doses the α_1 effects predominate.

The hemodynamic effects of dopamine in humans depend on the dose and the patient. In normal subjects, with infusion rates in the range of 1 to 10 μg/kg/min, there is increased cardiac contractility and cardiac output. Heart rate is unchanged and the mean arterial BP is unchanged or slightly decreased. Myocardial O_2 consumption is unchanged. Total peripheral resistance is decreased with skeletal muscle vasoconstriction and renal and mesenteric vasodilation. Renal blood flow, GFR, urine flow, and Na excretion are enhanced. With higher doses of dopamine, there is increased BP, systolic rising more than diastolic. The effect on the heart rate is variable with the direct cardioaccelerator action of the drug being antagonized by the reflex bradycardic effects mediated through the vagus. With very high doses there is usually a decrease in heart rate.

Dopamine is ineffective orally and has to be administered as an IV infusion. For most uses, the appropriate dilution is 200 mg of dopamine in 250 or 500 ml of 5% D/W, 5% D/S, or 0.9% saline. Dopamine is inactivated in alkaline solution. In patients with shock, infusion rates ranging from 2 to 5 μg/kg/min are suitable for initiating therapy. The infusion rate should be gradually increased until the desired hemodynamic and renal effects are obtained. Most patients respond to infusion rates below 20 μg/kg/min though rates up to 50 μg/kg/min have been used. If hypotension persists even with high doses of dopamine, alternative therapy with a more potent vasoconstrictor such as levarterenol should be considered. (See also SHOCK in Ch. 24.)

In **chronic refractory congestive heart failure** unresponsive to digitalis and diuretics, dopamine may be useful. The initial infusion rate should be 0.5 to 1 μg/kg/min. The dose should be increased gradually until urine flow increases or diastolic BP or heart rate starts to rise. If the latter events occur, the infusion rate should be decreased to prevent an increase in myocardial O_2 consumption. Most patients respond to doses of 1 to 3 μg/kg/min.

Adverse effects reported with dopamine include ventricular arrhythmias, tachycardia, angina pectoris, nausea, and vomiting.

Dobutamine is a synthetic catecholamine that chemically resembles dopamine but has a slightly different spectrum of hemodynamic effects. It is a direct-acting agent with primary effect on β_1 receptors and only slight effects on β_2 and α receptors. It does not stimulate the specific dopamine receptors and has only minimal indirect effects through release of endogenous norepinephrine. Dobutamine is relatively more effective in enhancing the contractile force of the heart than in increasing heart rate. The reason for this relative selectivity is not clear, but it may be related to a less pronounced effect of the drug on the sinoatrial node than on ventricular contractile tissue. Dobutamine appears to have advantages over other catecholamines for the improvement of myocardial function in heart failure. Since the effects of dobutamine on heart rate and systolic pressure are minimal in comparison to other catecholamines, the O_2 demands of the myocardium are increased less. The drug is particularly useful in patients who have undergone procedures involving cardiopulmonary bypass.

Dobutamine is not effective orally. Its plasma half-life is approximately 2 min and thus it must be administered by continuous IV infusion. The starting dose is 1 to 2 μg/kg/min and the dosage is increased until maximum hemodynamic improvement is achieved. Usual effective dose range is 2.5 to 10 μg/kg/min. Possible *adverse effects* are similar to those reported with other IV administered sympathomimetic amines. It has been reported that dobutamine causes a lower incidence of arrhythmias than isoproterenol or dopamine.

Ephedrine has α and β effects similar to epinephrine but differs from it in being effective orally, having a slower onset and longer duration of action, and a greater stimulant effect on the CNS, producing alertness, anxiety, insomnia, and tremor. The peripheral actions of ephedrine are partly due to direct effects and partly to release of endogenous norepinephrine. Tachyphylaxis is seen when repeated doses are administered parenterally within a brief time interval, probably because of discharge and depletion of norepinephrine stores. **Pseudoephedrine,** an isomer of ephedrine, has similar actions but is less potent and is less stimulating to the CNS and BP. The use of ephedrine in the treatment of bronchial asthma is discussed in Ch. 34. Ephedrine is sometimes used parenterally (15 to 50 mg s.c. or IM) for treating heart block. It is used as a nasal vasoconstrictor in 1 or 3% solution (2 to 3 drops b.i.d. or t.i.d.). In some patients with myasthenia, ephedrine 25 mg orally t.i.d. or q.i.d., in addition to the anticholinesterases, provides further benefit, possibly by enhancing neuromuscular junction transmission.

Metaproterenol, salbutamol, isoetharine, and **terbutaline** are predominantly β_2-adrenoceptor stimulants with special usefulness in the treatment of bronchial asthma (see Ch. 34).

Adrenergics with Predominant α Activity

Metaraminol is a direct α stimulator, although some of its effect is due to norepinephrine release from sympathetic nerve endings. It is less potent than norepinephrine but has a more prolonged action and lacks CNS stimulant effects. Like norepinephrine, it reduces blood flow to the kidney and brain; thus, its use in hypotensive states must be carefully considered. It is available as a 10 mg/ml solution; dosage is 5 to 10 mg IM or, after suitable dilution, 25 to 100 mg in 500 ml of 5% D/W by IV infusion.

Phenylephrine is predominantly a direct α_1 stimulator, although some effect is indirect through norepinephrine release. The most prominent effects of parenteral administration are an increase in BP and a reflex bradycardia. It is used topically as a nasal decongestant (see Ch. 256), as a mydriatic (2.5 and 10% solution, 1 to 2 drops instilled), as a vasoconstrictor in conjunction with local anesthetics, in the relief of paroxysmal atrial tachycardia (0.5 to 1 mg IV over 2 to 3 min), and sometimes in hypotensive states (0.5 to 1 mg IV over 2 to 3 min, or 5 to 10 mg IM or s.c.).

Methoxamine is predominantly a direct α_1 stimulator and increases BP. It is less useful than other agents in hypotensive states. Its effects last for 60 to 90 min. Reflex bradycardia is usually prominent and this effect is sometimes used to relieve attacks of paroxysmal atrial tachycardia. It is given IM 10 to 20 mg or IV 5 to 10 mg, *slowly*. Methoxamine is also used as a nasal decongestant (0.5% solution, 2 to 3 drops t.i.d. or q.i.d.).

Amphetamines: See GENERAL CENTRAL NERVOUS SYSTEM STIMULANTS AND ANOREXIANTS in Ch. 247.

Mephentermine has both α and β stimulant activity. It acts both directly and by release of endogenous norepinephrine. It does not offer any advantage over other pressor drugs and is not as potent;

however, it sometimes is used in hypotensive states (2 to 10 mg IM, or slow IV infusion of 10 to 30 mg in 1000 ml 5% D/S).

ADRENERGIC BLOCKING DRUGS

(Sympatholytics)

Drugs capable of antagonizing the effects of sympathetic stimulation or of sympathomimetic agents. Alpha and beta effects, mediated through different adrenergic receptors, are blocked by α- and β-adrenergic blocking drugs, respectively.

α-Adrenergic Blocking Drugs

The α-adrenergic blockers as a class have few clinical applications, but prazosin, a new agent, appears to have great value in treating heart failure. Their main effect is to produce peripheral vasodilation by antagonizing the sympathetic tone normally present in the peripheral vasculature. A brief discussion of the important drugs in this group follows.

Prazosin (see discussions on pp. 278 and 1369)

Tolazoline has a moderate α-blocking effect and a direct relaxant effect on the smooth muscle of the arteriolar wall. Theoretically, this makes it well suited for use in peripheral vascular disease, but, in practice, tolazoline increases skin blood flow more than muscle blood flow. Untoward effects include palpitations and aggravation of angina (due to stimulation of the heart), diarrhea, orthostatic hypotension, and cutis anserina ("gooseflesh"). It may also activate dormant peptic ulcers because of a histamine-like effect on gastric secretion. The usual dosage is 25 to 100 mg orally q.i.d. for the treatment of Raynaud's disease, postfrostbite syndrome, arteriosclerosis obliterans, and thromboangiitis obliterans; results generally are not dramatic. For use in sudden arterial thrombosis or embolism, 25 to 75 mg is given intra-arterially or IV.

Phenoxybenzamine is a powerful α-adrenergic blocker relatively specific for α_1 receptors. Its effects may last for 3 or 4 days and are not easily reversed with sympathomimetic agents, therefore *dosage must be increased gradually.* Phenoxybenzamine is used for the same disorders as tolazoline. Untoward effects include nasal congestion, hypotension, headache, tachycardia, indigestion, and nausea. The usual dosage is 10 to 20 mg orally b.i.d. to q.i.d.

Phentolamine is a short-acting nonselective α blocker with effects similar to tolazoline and is used principally in the diagnosis and control of hypertension due to pheochromocytoma. It may also be used as an α-antagonist in sympathomimetic overdosage, to control hypertensive crises due to monoamine oxidase inhibitor-adrenergic amine interactions, and to prevent tissue sloughing in norepinephrine extravasation. It is erratically absorbed when taken orally. The usual dosage is 5 to 30 mg IV or IM.

Ergot alkaloids with α-adrenergic blocking effects: A mixture of 3 semisynthetic alkaloids of ergot—dihydroergocryptine, dihydroergocristine, and dihydroergocornine as the mesylates—is marketed for symptoms attributed to cerebral arteriosclerosis (e.g., depression, anxiety, confusion, unsociability) in the elderly. There are reports of increased cerebral blood flow without reduction in BP and of subjective improvement in patients suffering from cerebral ischemia. It is given sublingually or orally 0.5 to 3 mg/day in divided doses. Nasal stuffiness, malaise, nausea, vomiting, and headache may be seen as side effects.

β-Adrenergic Blocking Agents (β Blockers)

The β-adrenergic blockers vary in the magnitude of their effects, depending on the prevalent sympathetic tone at the time of their administration. Cardiovascular effects are the most prominent and consist of reduced heart rate, contractility, and stroke volume, with a consequent decrease in cardiac output and myocardial O_2 consumption. The resting BP is usually little affected by a single dose, but long-term administration generally lowers BP. Other effects of β blockade depend on sympathetic tone. At rest they are slight, but during exercise the β effects of epinephrine and norepinephrine are blocked. Activation of the renin-angiotensin-aldosterone pathway is decreased by propranolol through an inhibitory effect on renin secretion, possibly through interference with specific renal β-adrenergic receptors.

The β blockers are potentially useful in any condition in which sympathetic activity can be detrimental to the patient. These may be cardiac (angina pectoris, arrhythmias, hypertension, or hemodynamic problems consequent to abnormalities such as idiopathic hypertrophic subaortic stenosis, mitral stenosis, and tetralogy of Fallot), endocrine (thyrotoxicosis, pheochromocytoma), or CNS (anxiety states) conditions. The large functional reserve of the heart permits the use of β blockers in many noncardiac conditions despite their depressant effect on the heart. In many conditions in which β blockers are useful, it is not clear what effects are due to β-adrenergic blockade and what effects are due to other inherent properties of these drugs.

The classification of β blockers is based on 2 pharmacologic properties besides β-receptor blockade: intrinsic sympathomimetic activity (ISA) and membrane-stabilization (local anesthetic) activity. It has been suggested that ISA may reduce the degree of cardiodepression and thus a β blocker with

ISA may have fewer side effects than one without ISA. There is no definite evidence to suggest that membrane-stabilizing property in a β blocker is of any clinical importance. Current classification of β blockers is as follows:

Group 1 drugs (e.g., oxprenolol and alprenolol) have ISA and local anesthetic activity.
Group 2 drugs (e.g., propranolol) have local anesthetic activity but no ISA activity.
Group 3 drugs (e.g., pindolol) have β-blocking activity and ISA but no local anesthetic activity.
Group 4 drugs (e.g., nadolol, timolol, sotalol) have only β-blocking activity.
Group 5 drugs selectively block β receptors in specific tissues and thus are likely to have fewer unwanted effects. Metoprolol and atenolol, for example, selectively block β receptors in the heart while sparing β receptors in the bronchi and blood vessels, a potential advantage in treating cardiac conditions with coexisting obstructive pulmonary disease.

Among the β blockers, most of the clinical experience in the USA is with propranolol. It is discussed in detail below. Metoprolol, nadolol, atenolol, pindolol, and timolol are other β blockers available for use in the USA for treatment of cardiovascular disorders. Timolol has also been approved as an ophthalmic preparation for the treatment of chronic wide-angle glaucoma. In Europe other β blockers are available.

Adverse effects with the use of β blockers are low in frequency (approximately 5%), if patients with heart failure, asthma, and heart block are excluded. Patient acceptance is generally excellent. The most common complaint is fatigue and lethargy. Other untoward effects include hypotension, bowel disturbances, nightmares, depression, insomnia, skin rashes, thrombocytopenia, and alopecia. Some patients complain of cold extremities and Raynaud's phenomenon may be exacerbated. Bradycardia both at rest and during exercise is to be expected with these drugs, and depends on the vagal tone. In general, most patients tolerate heart rates as low as 50/min well. If symptomatic bradycardia occurs, the drug should be withdrawn or the dosage reduced. Insulin hypoglycemia may be prolonged, since sympathetic glycogenolysis, which occurs as a homeostatic response, is a β effect. Diabetics using β-adrenergic blockers may be unaware of hypoglycemia because the symptoms due to sympathetic discharge (such as palpitations) are suppressed. CAUTION: *These agents should be used cautiously (if at all) in patients with congestive heart failure, asthma, and heart block.*

The **pharmacokinetics** of propranolol are of some interest and importance. When given orally, it is well absorbed from the intestine, producing peak concentrations in 1 to 2 h. The plasma half-life is short (3.5 to 6 h). It is rapidly metabolized in the liver. The active metabolite, 4-hydroxypropranolol, is formed to a significant extent only after oral administration. A substantial variation in hepatic hydroxylation of the drug has been noted in different individuals; thus the plasma concentrations of parent drug and metabolite vary widely (about 20-fold) between individuals after the same oral dose. By the IV route, effects appear sooner but persist for a correspondingly shorter time. In most patients, propranolol plasma levels of 50 to 100 ng/ml produce a high degree of peripheral β blockade, alleviation of angina pectoris, antiarrhythmic activity, and diminished plasma renin activity. Effective blood levels are generally attained with oral doses of 80 to 320 mg/day and should be carefully individualized. The usual oral starting dose is 10 to 20 mg t.i.d. or q.i.d. before meals and at bedtime. Increments should be gradual until optimal response is obtained. Specific therapy is discussed below.

There are potential problems associated with the abrupt withdrawal of propranolol in patients with coronary artery disease. Rapid withdrawal of the drug may precipitate arrhythmias, angina, or even myocardial infarction, especially in patients receiving high doses. If possible, doses should be gradually reduced over a 2-wk period. There may be increased risks associated with surgery in patients on propranolol, and a 24- to 48-h period off the drug prior to surgery is recommended. In patients on high doses of the drug who require emergency surgery, excessive β blockade may be counteracted with atropine, glucagon, or isoproterenol.

Arrhythmias: Propranolol is useful in treating supraventricular and ventricular arrhythmias. It is the drug of choice in arrhythmias due to pheochromocytoma, but must be used only subsequent to administration of an α blocker to avoid a precipitous increase in BP. Propranolol is also useful in atrial fibrillation (to slow ventricular response), paroxysmal supraventricular tachycardias, digitalis-induced arrhythmias, and arrhythmias associated with mitral valve prolapse. For life-threatening arrhythmias, 0.5 to 3 mg of propranolol is given IV *cautiously under careful monitoring* at a rate not to exceed 1 mg/min to avoid lowering BP and causing cardiac standstill. If necessary a second dose may be given after 2 min. Thereafter, additional propranolol should not be given for at least 4 h.

Idiopathic hypertrophic subaortic stenosis: Propranolol can be used in this condition both as an aid to diagnosis and in treatment. The dosage ranges from 40 to 320 mg/day.

Angina pectoris: Propranolol reduces the number of attacks, increases exercise tolerance, and reduces the need for nitroglycerin. The starting dosage of 10 to 20 mg t.i.d. or q.i.d. is gradually increased every 3 to 7 days until an optimum response is obtained. Optimum dosage may range from 40 to 480 mg/day. Nitrates neutralize the undesired effects (prolongation of ejection time, dilation of the ventricle) of propranolol and the 2 drugs constitute a rational combination in angina.

Hypertension: Use of propranolol in hypertension is discussed in Ch. 24.

Pheochromocytoma: Patients with hypertension due to pheochromocytoma are often treated medically to stabilize them for later surgery. Propranolol in combination with an α-blocking agent is often used. The α blocker must be administered prior to or concomitantly with the β blocker, otherwise the BP may rise precipitously due to the β blockade of the skeletal blood vessel vasodilatory effect of epinephrine (which is the predominant circulating catecholamine in this condition), leaving the constrictor effect in the rest of the body unopposed. For details see PHEOCHROMOCYTOMA in Ch. 88.

Migraine prevention: Propranolol is sometimes useful as a prophylactic for migraine. The initial dosage is 80 mg/day in divided doses; the effective dosage range is 80 to 240 mg/day. Propranolol is not indicated for treating the acute migraine attack.

Miscellaneous uses: In the USA, the FDA-approved indications for propranolol are those discussed above. Clinical studies have suggested an even broader range of therapeutic uses. These are briefly outlined below.

Thyrotoxicosis: Propranolol is useful as an adjunct in the treatment of thyrotoxicosis and thyroid storm. The effectiveness is possibly related to its blocking the peripheral conversion of T_4 into T_3. The drug can be used orally or intravenously depending on the urgency of the condition being treated.

Anxiety states: Propranolol has been reported to be useful in anxious patients with predominantly somatic complaints including palpitations, shakiness, tremor, breathlessness, and hyperventilation.

Schizophrenia: In certain chronic schizophrenic patients, propranolol addition to standard neuroleptics has been reported to be useful.

Tremors: Several studies have demonstrated that propranolol is useful in the treatment of action tremors.

Alcohol withdrawal: Propranolol has been used successfully to manage patients undergoing acute alcohol withdrawal.

Myocardial infarction: In clinical trials conducted outside the USA, timolol has been shown to be effective in significantly reducing the rate of reinfarction and mortality in patients during at least the 2 yr after an acute myocardial infarction. (See MYOCARDIAL INFARCTION in Ch. 25.)

Metoprolol is a selective β_1-receptor blocking agent recently marketed in the USA. Currently it is approved for use only for the treatment of hypertension. Studies conducted mostly outside the USA have shown that metoprolol has the same general range of clinical usefulness as propranolol. The advantage of metoprolol over propranolol is its selectivity for β_1 receptors (in the heart) over the β_2 receptors (bronchial and vascular smooth muscle), even though the selectivity is not absolute. Thus it can be used with caution in patients with bronchospastic diseases. The suggested initial dosage for treatment of hypertension is 50 mg b.i.d. The dose can be increased at weekly intervals until optimum response is obtained. The usual maintenance dosage is 100 to 450 mg/day. Potential adverse effects are similar to those described for propranolol above.

Nadolol is a nonselective β blocker but, unlike propranolol, it has little or no local anesthetic or membrane-stabilizing activity. Nadolol is not metabolized to any appreciable degree prior to renal elimination; it has a long half-life (20 to 24 h) and thus may be administered once daily. Currently, nadolol is approved for the treatment of hypertension (40 mg/day initially; maintenance dose, 80 to 320 mg) and angina pectoris (same initial dose as in hypertension; maintenance: 80 to 240 mg/day).

GANGLIONIC BLOCKING DRUGS

The ganglionic blockers have limited therapeutic use because they are not selective and have many untoward effects due to blocking of both sympathetic and parasympathetic ganglia. The effect of ganglionic blockade can be predicted from knowing which division of the autonomic nervous system (sympathetic or parasympathetic) exercises dominant control in an organ, since blockade tends to produce an *opposite* effect. In the heart, eye, GI tract, urinary bladder, and salivary glands, the parasympathetic system dominates, and ganglionic blockade results in tachycardia, mydriasis and cycloplegia, reduced tone and motility (constipation), urinary retention, and dry mouth, respectively. In the arterioles, veins, and sweat glands, where sympathetic tone is dominant, ganglionic blockade results in vasodilation and hypotension, peripheral pooling (decreased venous return and cardiac output), and skin dryness, respectively.

The only current use of ganglionic blockers is in the treatment of severe hypertension and hypertensive crisis. Even here they are being replaced by newer potent agents, such as **nitroprusside** and **diazoxide.** The ganglionic blockers currently in use are discussed below.

Trimethaphan is given as an IV drip for control of high BP. Usually, a 1 mg/ml solution of the drug is added to 5% D/W and the rate of flow is regulated as needed (usual range: 1 to 10 mg/min). Oral therapy with other agents should be started as soon as possible because tachyphylaxis to trimethaphan develops rapidly.

Mecamylamine is used in moderately severe to severe essential hypertension and in uncomplicated cases of malignant hypertension. The dosage ranges from 2.5 to 60 or more mg/day orally. It should not be given to patients with azotemia, since a neurologic syndrome characterized by severe tremor and incoordination usually occurs.

VASODILATORS

A wide variety of drugs with different modes of action (most do *not* act via the autonomic nervous system), but with the common property of being able to dilate blood vessels in one or more regions of the body, come under the broad category of "vasodilator drugs." Based on therapeutic rather than pharmacologic considerations, they can be classified into 3 groups—peripheral, coronary, and antihypertensive vasodilators.

PERIPHERAL VASODILATORS

Inadequacies of cutaneous, skeletal muscle, and cerebral blood flows are the conditions most commonly treated with this group of drugs. In general, results are unsatisfactory. The drugs are more useful in arteriospastic conditions than in those due to organic occlusive disorders, where reconstructive arterial surgery or regional sympathetic denervation may produce better results.

Peripheral vasodilators act either directly to relax the smooth muscle of the arterioles or indirectly by antagonizing sympathetic effects. It is important to titrate the dose of these drugs in each individual, starting with the lowest effective dose and increasing slowly and in increments not exceeding the starting dose until the desired response is attained or unacceptable side effects occur.

Selective Sympathetic Inhibiting Agents

Reserpine 1 mg/day orally is used in Raynaud's disease or in secondary Raynaud's phenomenon and is usually effective in > 50% of cases. Single injections of 0.5 to 1 mg intra-arterially into the brachial artery may provide relief for 1 wk to several months. Side effects include lassitude, drowsiness, depression (sometimes suicidal), postural hypotension, nasal congestion, and activation of peptic ulcer.

α-Adrenergic blocking agents are discussed above under ADRENERGIC BLOCKING DRUGS.

β-Adrenergic stimulating agents, most importantly **nylidrin** and **isoxsuprine,** dilate the blood vessels supplying the skeletal muscles and stimulate the heart to increase cardiac output. Nylidrin may also increase cerebral blood flow. Relaxation of smooth muscle in other organs occurs to a small extent. Disturbing side effects occurring occasionally include nervousness, trembling, weakness, dizziness, palpitation, nausea, and vomiting. The drugs are especially indicated in treatment of intermittent claudication caused by chronic occlusive arterial disease. The usual dosages are nylidrin 6 to 24 mg orally q.i.d. and isoxsuprine 5 to 10 mg orally q.i.d.

Drugs Acting Directly on Arteriolar Smooth Muscle

Cyclandelate is useful in almost all the peripheral vascular disorders. Untoward effects are flushing, tingling, dizziness, sweating, nausea, and headache. The usual dose range is 100 to 300 mg q.i.d.

Papaverine 30 to 60 mg intra-arterially or IV is of use only in conditions of sudden arterial occlusion (thrombosis or embolism). Untoward effects include hypotension and respiratory depression. Oral papaverine for peripheral vasodilation is probably not effective.

Ethyl alcohol in doses of 30 to 60 ml orally q.i.d. is of some use in chronic arterial occlusive disease. Possible untoward effects include intoxication, GI irritation, and exacerbation of peptic ulcer.

CORONARY VASODILATORS

Nitrates: See ANTIHYPERTENSIVE VASODILATORS, below, and ANGINA PECTORIS in Ch. 25.

Dipyridamole, although more potent than nitrates in increasing coronary blood flow and decreasing coronary vascular resistance, is much less effective in treating angina pectoris. This may be due to the fact that unlike nitrates, dipyridamole does not reduce myocardial O_2 requirement. Dipyridamole also lacks the ability to dilate collateral vessels (in contrast to nitrates), an effect possibly important in nitrates producing beneficial effects in angina. The suggested dose of dipyridamole is 25 to 50 mg b.i.d. to t.i.d., at least 1 h before meals. Occasional side effects include nausea, vomiting, diarrhea, headache, and vertigo.

Recent studies have shown dipyridamole to have an inhibitory effect on platelet aggregation. The use of dipyridamole and aspirin together in prevention of myocardial infarction and thromboembolic disorders is being investigated.

Calcium "antagonists" (or **"blockers"**) are a group of drugs that appear to work by modifying (generally preventing or slowing) calcium flow into muscle cells, an essential step for activating contraction of cardiac and arterial muscle. Different agents vary in their primary sites of activity and effects, but they are becoming important therapeutic agents in angina pectoris and a variety of other cardiovascular disorders (e.g., heart failure, hypertension, hypertrophic cardiomyopathy, supraventricular tachycardias). When coronary artery spasm is prominent, as in variant (Prinzmetal's) angina, drugs such as **nifedipine** and **verapamil** are becoming primary agents. They are also effective in many patients with angina of effort, generally being used after treatment with nitrates and β-blockers.

ANTIHYPERTENSIVE VASODILATORS

Vasodilators in this group reduce BP via a relaxing action on arterial smooth muscles. BP is reduced, both in the upright and recumbent positions. Because of the decreased peripheral resistance caused by these drugs, there is a tendency for reflex tachycardia (through the baroreceptors) and increased cardiac output; this reflex effect varies with each drug and depends upon whether the drug has additional effects in the form of increasing venous capacitance and/or direct depressant effect on the heart, both of which would tend to negate the reflex effects. All the drugs in this group tend to cause Na and water retention, expansion of plasma and extracellular fluid volumes, weight gain and edema formation. These effects are probably mediated through the renin-angiotensin-aldosterone system and tend to oppose the antihypertensive effect. If the plasma and extracellular fluid volume expansion are prevented by the concomitant administration of an appropriately potent diuretic, tolerance to the antihypertensive effects of these drugs does not develop. In general, a combination of these drugs with β blockers such as propranolol markedly potentiates the antihypertensive effects; this potentiation is greater for those drugs that have a significant reflex component causing increased cardiac output (e.g., hydralazine).

Sodium nitroprusside is an extremely potent and short-acting vasodilator that directly relaxes vascular smooth muscle *in both the arteries and veins,* thus reducing both the preload and afterload on the heart. In a subject with a normal or nearly normal left ventricle, venous pooling caused by the drug has a more profound effect on cardiac output than a concomitant reduction of impedance (afterload); thus cardiac output falls. In contrast, when left ventricular function is severely impaired, the heart is operating on a flat Frank-Starling curve and the impedance is high. The peripheral pooling and the arterial-dilating effects of nitroprusside together cause a fall in the abnormally elevated end-diastolic pressure and a sharp increase in cardiac output. Heart rate generally increases moderately when nitroprusside reduces BP in normal or hypertensive subjects. In heart failure, however, nitroprusside usually produces a slight or no decrease in heart rate. In normal or hypertensive states, the overall effect on the BP is a significant fall due to substantially reduced peripheral resistance and slightly reduced cardiac output. In contrast, in low output states (such as in the acute phase of myocardial infarction) the decrease in peripheral resistance and the resultant tendency for a fall in BP is mostly offset by the augmented cardiac output (within limits) and the overall effect is no change or a minimal fall in BP. *Thus, sodium nitroprusside can produce varying hemodynamic effects, depending on the prevailing state of the left ventricle and the peripheral resistance;* this fact explains the apparent paradox of its use in hypertensive crisis on one hand and cardiogenic shock on the other.

Sodium nitroprusside, in doses producing hypotension, also decreases pulmonary and renal vascular resistance. In the usual clinical doses, nitroprusside does not affect other smooth musculature in the body.

The effects of nitroprusside infused IV are apparent in minutes. The fall in arterial pressure is dose dependent. The effects of nitroprusside in the body are transient (effects are lost within a few minutes of the stoppage of infusion) due to its rapid conversion to thiocyanate.

The acute **toxicity of nitroprusside** is secondary to excessive vasodilation and hypotension. Symptoms include nausea, vomiting, sweating, restlessness, headache, palpitation, and substernal distress; they disappear promptly when the infusion is stopped or the rate reduced. With prolonged use, the toxicity is due to thiocyanate accumulation, and its principal manifestations are fatigue, nausea, and anorexia followed by disorientation, psychotic behavior, and muscle spasms. There is a rare possibility of temporary hypothyroidism from the effect of the thiocyanate ion. Symptoms of thiocyanate toxicity begin to appear at plasma levels of 5 to 10 mg/100 ml. Fatalities have been reported at levels of 20 mg/100 ml. The drug should be discontinued if thiocyanate levels reach 10 to 12 mg/100 ml. Thiocyanate is removed almost exclusively by the kidney with a half-life of approximately 1 wk in the presence of normal renal function. Rapid reduction of thiocyanate plasma levels is possible by peritoneal dialysis.

Sodium nitroprusside is supplied as a 50-mg lyophilized powder. It should be dissolved in D5W (250 or 500 ml) and administered as an IV drip. Usual initial infusion rate is between 0.5 to 1.5 μg/kg/min. Dosage must be carefully titrated, with frequent monitoring of BP. Even after the appropriate infusion rate has been reached, frequent follow-up monitoring of BP and other vital signs is indicated, since, in an occasional patient, the drug response may change with time. Nitroprusside decomposes in light. Thus the IV bottle (and the translucent plastic tubing) should be covered with an opaque wrapper. Solutions $>$ 4 h old should be discarded. Specific clinical uses for sodium nitroprusside include the following:

Hypertensive crisis: Nitroprusside is very effective in this setting. A dose of 1 to 3 μg/kg/min usually produces a prompt drop in pressure. The suggested maximum dose is 10 μg/kg/min.

Dissecting aneurysm: Nitroprusside is one of the drugs of choice in reduction of BP in acute dissecting aortic aneurysms. In this condition a reduction in cardiac impulse is felt to be at least as important as reduction in overall BP. Nitroprusside does not have a myocardial depressant effect and thus it should be combined with propranolol (or possibly reserpine or guanethidine) when being used to treat dissecting aneurysms.

Acute myocardial infarction: Nitroprusside improves cardiac pump function in patients with left ventricular failure during the acute phase of myocardial infarction. The dose required to reduce aortic impedance varies from 15 to 400 μg/min (usual dose is about 50 μg/min). If normalization or near normalization of left ventricular filling pressure (pulmonary artery wedge pressure) cannot be obtained without reduction of arterial pressure to dangerously low levels, then combination therapy with an inotropic agent such as dopamine or dobutamine may produce the desired effect.

Acute pulmonary edema: Sodium nitroprusside may be the agent of choice in the treatment of acute pulmonary edema, since it reduces pulmonary and ventricular pressures and increases cardiac output. IV infusion should be started at about 20 μg/min with increments at 5-min intervals until the pulmonary congestion subsides or arterial pressure falls to hypotensive levels. A diuresis usually ensues with the treatment and can be enhanced by concomitant administration of furosemide.

Acute therapy of refractory chronic congestive heart failure: In chronic congestive heart failure that has progressed to a stage of refractoriness to digitalis and diuresis, therapy with sodium nitroprusside may dramatically improve left ventricular performance and promote a diuresis. Dosage is similar to that used in treating acute myocardial infarction discussed above. In some cases, parenteral vasodilator therapy must be continued for days or even weeks. Following effective use of nitroprusside, patients may become responsive to previously ineffective diuretics. In some cases combining nitroprusside with inotropic agents such as dopamine or dobutamine may increase the effectiveness of therapy.

Miscellaneous: Use of nitroprusside in the treatment of ergot poisoning and for producing controlled hypotension during surgical procedures to reduce bleeding has been reported.

Diazoxide is a very potent and unique antihypertensive agent that acts through direct relaxation of *arteriolar* smooth muscle. It has very little effect on the venous capacitance vessels and no direct effect on cardiac function. Thus reflex increases in heart rate, stroke volume, and cardiac output accompany the hypotensive action of diazoxide. Because of this, blood flow is generally well maintained or increased in all circulatory beds after diazoxide administration (the reflex effects may be detrimental in patients with limited coronary or cardiac reserve). Retention of Na and water with diazoxide is more marked than with other drugs in this group because of its direct tubular antinatriuretic action (even though it is chemically related to thiazides, it has no natriuretic or chloruretic effect).

Proper clinical use of diazoxide requires awareness of some pharmacokinetic and clinical aspects of the drug. After IV injection of diazoxide into hypertensive patients, arterial pressure falls within 1 min and reaches its lowest level within 2 to 5 min. Reduction of pressure below normotensive levels is rare and the magnitude of the antihypertensive effect increases with the level of the pretreatment BP. Both intensity and duration of the hypotensive action also increase with the rate of IV injection. To be most effective the full dose (usual IV dose is 300 mg or 5 mg/kg) should be injected within 10 to 30 sec. This time dependence has been attributed to the fact that diazoxide is 90% bound to plasma protein and the concentration reaching the vascular smooth muscle is inadequate if time is allowed for equilibration with the binding proteins. Slow IV infusion and repeated oral dosing of diazoxide can both produce a gradual sustained fall in arterial pressure, but these modes of administration are rarely used clinically in the management of hypertension and IV bolus administration is the method of choice. During the 10 to 20 min following the initial hypotensive effect of the IV bolus injection of diazoxide, a part of the fall in arterial pressure is reversed, presumably due to cardiovascular reflex responses. Thereafter, the BP increases very gradually, reaching pretreatment levels within 3 to 15 h. If the hypotensive response to the first dose is unsatisfactory, a second dose may be given after 30 min (preferably at a more rapid rate). The subsequent dosage schedule is individualized according to response.

Recent studies have shown that minibolus administration of diazoxide (doses of 1 to 3 mg/kg repeated at intervals of 5 to 15 min) is as effective as the administration of 300 mg in a single dose in reducing BP while offering improved safety and control.

After each dose of diazoxide, patients should remain recumbent and should be closely monitored for 30 min. Subsequent constant supervision is unnecessary, since maximum hypotensive effect of the drug has already occurred within this early period and the return to pretreatment levels is always gradual. On the rare occasion when the BP falls below normal levels with the bolus injection, the hypotension will respond to the usual pressor agents. The oral preparation is not marketed in the USA.

Diazoxide should always be administered with a diuretic (preferably a potent loop diuretic such as furosemide or ethacrynic acid) to prevent Na retention. The diuretic is administered 30 to 60 min before each diazoxide injection after the first. As with other agents in this group, the antihypertensive effect of diazoxide is increased by β-blockers such as propranolol. Thus, in patients recently treated with propranolol (or guanethidine or reserpine), a smaller than usual dose of diazoxide should be used to prevent excessive hypotension. Patients with impaired renal function generally require the usual dosage of diazoxide even though the drug is primarily eliminated by the kidneys.

The most important clinical use for diazoxide is the treatment of **hypertensive emergencies.** Its effect is apparent in minutes. In comparison to other agents such as nitroprusside and trimethaphan, which are used in similar situations, diazoxide has the distinct advantage of not requiring constant patient monitoring, and the possible disadvantage that minute-to-minute adjustments are not possible. Diazoxide should not be used in hypertension with dissecting aortic aneurysms because its reflex cardiac stimulatory effect is undesirable. Diazoxide is also best avoided in hypertension associated with subarachnoid, subdural, intracerebral, and post-operative bleeding.

The **major side effects of diazoxide** (besides the occasional excessive hypotension and salt and water retention discussed above) are hyperuricemia and hyperglycemia. These do not present major problems in short-term therapy, but preclude the use of the drug for the long-term management of hypertension. The hyperglycemic effect (which is primarily due to antagonism of insulin secretion), while being a serious obstacle to the chronic use of the drug for treating hypertension, has proven of use in medical treatment of insulinomas (hypertrichosis has been a side effect with such chronic usage). Atrial and ventricular arrhythmias, palpitation, angina, headache, and flushing occur in occasional patients after diazoxide administration; these usually respond well to treatment with propranolol. When diazoxide is used for treatment of hypertensive crises of eclampsia, it may arrest labor because of its uterine relaxant effect; the uterine contractions can be reestablished with oxytocin. Diazoxide solution is very alkaline, and extravasation can cause severe local pain and cellulitis; thus, diazoxide should be injected into an established IV line.

Hydralazine is an antihypertensive which has been in use for many years. It exerts its hypotensive effect by direct relaxation of *arteriolar* smooth muscle. It has no direct actions on the heart and minimal effect on venous capacitance vessels. Thus its administration results in reflex increase in heart rate and cardiac output which greatly offset the hypotensive effect of the arteriolar dilation. As a single agent in the treatment of hypertension, hydralazine is not very potent. In recent years, the role of hydralazine in antihypertensive therapy has greatly expanded with the appreciation of the fact that when it is combined with propranolol or other β-blockers (which will block its reflex cardiac stimulatory effects), its antihypertensive potency is markedly increased. Like other drugs of this group, hyalazine causes salt and water retention and thus a diuretic should be administered concomitantly.

The most appropriate hypertensive patient for treatment with hydralazine is one whose arterial pressure remains elevated despite therapy with a diuretic and a β-blocker such as propranolol. The diuretic-propranolol-hydralazine regimen is effective in most patients with moderate to severe hypertension. When used orally, hydralazine should be started in small doses (25 mg b.i.d.) after the patient has been receiving a diuretic and β-blocker for 2 to 3 wk. Dosage should be gradually increased, depending upon response. A dose of 200 to 300 mg/day is usually well tolerated and can be reached in 10 to 14 days. Greater reduction of BP can be achieved with higher daily doses up to 800 mg/day, but such doses carry an unacceptable risk of side effects. Traditionally, hydralazine has been given q.i.d., but recent observations suggest that the same daily dose can be administered b.i.d. to give equally effective BP control and improve patient compliance.

Hydralazine can be used IM or IV for treatment of hypertensive emergencies; however, it is not as potent or effective for this purpose as other available drugs (diazoxide, sodium nitroprusside, trimethaphan). The usual dose is about 20 mg and the onset of action is in 15 to 30 min.

The **adverse effects** that appear within the first day or two of hydralazine treatment are usually more annoying than serious and include headaches, palpitation, tachycardia, flushing, unpleasant taste, nausea, vomiting, anxiety and transient depression. More serious early adverse effects (usually requiring withdrawal of drug) may be in the form of exacerbation of coronary insufficiency, chills, fever, and toxic psychosis. The incidence of early side effects is very much less in patients who are already on propranolol or other such agent. Chronic administration of hydralazine can lead to an acute rheumatoid state with generalized aching and stiffness. This may progress to a systemic lupus erythematosus-like illness complete with positive antinuclear antibodies and LE cell phenomenon. This incidence of "**hydralazine lupus syndrome**" increases with dosage and duration of exposure and is higher in slow than in fast acetylators (acetylation in the liver is a major pathway of biotransformation of hydralazine). The syndrome rarely develops when the daily dose is $<$ 300 mg and is almost always entirely reversible when hydralazine is stopped. Several other adverse effects of hydralazine such as drug fever, skin eruptions, and peripheral neuropathy also appear to be dose related; the peripheral neuropathy can be corrected by giving pyridoxine.

Recently, the use of hydralazine in the treatment of chronic congestive heart failure has been reported. Its usefulness in this situation is related to its vasodilator effect (afterload reduction). This mode of therapy is still investigational.

Prazosin is a relatively new antihypertensive vasodilator which reduces peripheral resistance in part by direct action on the arterioles, but primarily by selective blockage of postjunctional α_1-adrenergic receptors. Unlike nonselective α-adrenergic blockers (such as phentolamine), prazosin usually does not incite a reflex increase in cardiac rate and output. This may be related to its relative lack of effect on prejunctional α_2 receptors that allow the released norepinephrine to exert negative feedback control on its own release. Like other vasodilators, it does tend to cause Na and water retention and thus a diuretic should be used concomitantly.

Prazosin is useful in the treatment of hypertension of mild to moderate severity. The initial starting dose is 1 mg orally t.i.d. The dose can be gradually increased depending on response. The maximum suggested dose is 20 mg/day in 2 or 3 divided doses.

Adverse effects reported with prazosin include syncope with sudden loss of consciousness. These syncopal episodes have usually occurred 30 to 90 min after the initial administration of the drug and are believed to be due to excessive postural hypotension. Syncope is rare when the starting dose is 1 mg. Other occasional side effects include dizziness, faintness, headache, nervousness, drowsiness, and depression.

Recently, the use of prazosin in treatment of chronic congestive heart failure has been suggested. Its usefulness in this situation may be related to its effect of reducing the pre- and afterload on the heart (see also p. 278).

Minoxidil is a potent *oral* vasodilator. It is indicated only for treatment of patients with severe symptomatic or organ-damaging hypertension refractory to other drug therapy, and is particularly useful as an alternative to bilateral nephrectomy in patients with end-stage renal failure. Like hydralazine it causes reflex tachycardia and increased cardiac output as well as fluid retention. Thus it should be used with a β-blocker and a diuretic (usually a loop diuretic such as furosemide or ethacrynic acid when renal failure is present). The initial dose is 5 mg/day, increased to 40 mg/day in divided doses; some patients may require as much as 100 mg/day. Minoxidil causes facial hirsutism, and its prolonged use has been associated with an unusual hemorrhagic degenerative lesion in the right atrium of dogs and humans, the exact significance of which is unknown.

---

249. NONNARCOTIC ANALGESICS; ANTIPYRETICS; NONSTEROIDAL ANTI-INFLAMMATORY DRUGS

MILD ANALGESICS

Analgesics for relief of mild to moderate pain described in this chapter include antipyretic/anti-inflammatory types (salicylates); para-aminophenol derivatives (acetaminophen); anthranilic acid derivatives (mefenamic acid); and those related to potent narcotics (propoxyphene).

Acetylsalicylic acid (aspirin, ASA): Though salicylates are not identical, ASA can serve as a prototype for discussion of this group. Unlike narcotic analgesics, which act on the CNS, salicylates act, at least partially, at the peripheral or local level—the site of origin of the pain—and do not (in therapeutic dosage) alter consciousness or mood. ASA is often combined with a centrally acting analgesic. The exact mechanism of action of ASA is unknown. Its ability to decrease the synthesis of prostaglandins and lipoperoxidases may explain its anti-inflammatory actions. ASA also decreases fever, a usually desired but not always beneficial effect, perhaps by the same mechanism.

ASA 650 mg is an effective analgesic, equal to about 32 mg of codeine, 65 mg of propoxyphene, or 50 mg of oral pentazocine. Peak analgesic effects develop at about 45 min; duration of analgesia is generally 3 to 4 h. ASA is most useful in mild to moderate pain arising from injury or inflammation in structures such as the skin, teeth, or musculoskeletal system. ASA is rapidly absorbed from the gut and is hydrolyzed to free salicylate by nonspecific esterases shortly after entering the bloodstream. At higher doses, elimination of ASA follows zero-order kinetics; its metabolism is a capacity-limited process at higher doses; i.e., there is a limit to the amount of drug that can be metabolized in any time period. Hence the elimination half-life and serum concentration of active drug may rise out of proportion to dose increases if the processes for metabolizing salicylate are saturated. Excretion of unchanged ASA may be promoted by alkalinization of the urine. This causes a larger percentage of the filtered drug to become ionized, and decreases its ability to diffuse passively from the glomerular filtrate across the tubular cells back into the blood.

ASA also possesses uricosuric properties which are dose-dependent. Low doses compete with uric acid in the renal tubular organic acid secretory system and may decrease urate excretion. However, larger doses compete for the more important, higher capacity renal tubular organic acid reabsorptive system, resulting in uricosuria and lower serum urate levels.

Dose-related and reversible **adverse effects** of aspirin include tinnitus and decreased hearing acuity, which may foretell more serious toxicity. Hyperventilation, resulting in respiratory alkalosis, may be followed by metabolic acidosis as a result of ASA overdose in children (see ACCIDENTS AND POISONINGS in Vol. II, Ch. 24). In adults, overdose usually results in respiratory alkalosis. Interference with the clotting mechanism occurs at doses lower than those causing acid-base disturbances: ASA decreases platelet aggregation by blocking the synthesis of prostaglandin A_2 (thromboxane) and release of ADP, mediators of the second phase of platelet aggregation. This may be a serious problem in neonates or patients who have coagulation disorders, are taking anticoagulants, are undergoing surgery, or are receiving blood transfusions. Decreased platelet aggregation may be helpful in avoiding strokes and preventing recurrent myocardial infarctions. At higher doses, ASA interferes with prothrombin production or function, resulting in potentiation of the effects of oral anticoagulants. Aplastic anemia and thrombocytopenia are rare but serious adverse effects.

Direct GI irritation and subsequent GI blood loss can be caused by particles of ASA adhering to the mucosa, apparently a dose-related phenomena. However, serious hemorrhage and peptic ulceration are idiosyncratic and may occur at normally tolerated doses in susceptible patients. Various buffered preparations have been used in an attempt to decrease GI intolerance to ASA. Excessive buffer such as sodium bicarbonate may lead to systemic and urinary alkalosis, with increased excretion of active drug. Delayed- or sustained-release formulations may cause less GI upset, but absorption may be variable. Various salts (aluminum, calcium, magnesium, choline, and sodium) and other salicylates have been used in efforts to decrease toxicity, prolong effect, or increase efficacy; none is as efficacious as ASA.

A small number of patients are hypersensitive to ASA and small doses may cause skin rashes and asthmatic-type anaphylactic reactions. The incidence is greater among those with asthma, hay fever, or nasal polyps. Salicylates other than ASA rarely cause these effects.

Acetaminophen, a metabolic product of both phenacetin and acetanilid, is the major para-amino-phenol derivative in common use today. It is an effective analgesic and antipyretic, but lacks anti-inflammatory action and does not inhibit prostaglandin synthesis. The mechanism of its analgesic activity is unknown. In similar doses, it is therapeutically equivalent to aspirin in analgesic potency and duration of action; however, unlike aspirin it does not cause GI or bleeding disorders. There is no cross-sensitivity between aspirin and acetaminophen.

Acetaminophen is rapidly absorbed following oral administration. It is conjugated in the liver with glucuronide and sulfate; both the conjugates and some of the parent drug ($<$ 10%) are then excreted in the urine. In overdose, acetaminophen can cause hepatic necrosis through failure to inactivate a toxic metabolite. Administration of a sulfur containing amino acid such as acetylcysteine within 12 h of overdosing may decrease the extent and severity of this reaction (see Ch. 70). Some patients (particularly those who are poorly nourished or alcoholics) on chronic acetaminophen therapy may also develop hepatic damage of a less dramatic type.

Acetaminophen (650 mg) is a useful drug for the relief of mild to moderate pain, especially in patients who are aspirin-sensitive, whose hemostatic system is impaired or under stress (e.g., postpartum or after surgery), or who have gout. Acetaminophen is convenient for pediatric use because it can be formulated as a liquid. Following ingestion of large single doses, the acute toxicity of acetaminophen may be greater than that of aspirin, but it has fewer nuisance side effects. Combinations of centrally active agents (propoxyphene, codeine) and acetaminophen are effective.

Mefenamic acid, an anthranilic acid derivative, is a newer antipyretic, anti-inflammatory drug. Clinical evidence of its analgesic efficacy is limited. The initial dose is 500 mg, followed by 250 mg q 6 h as needed. Unwanted effects are generally mild and infrequent, but may include GI distress, diarrhea, dizziness, vertigo, skin rash, and, rarely, blood dyscrasias. Short courses of less than I wk are recommended to avoid serious adverse effects.

Propoxyphene is related chemically to methadone and other narcotics, but has less addiction liability. Propoxyphene 65 to 130 mg has central-type analgesic activity, but does not cause significant respiratory depression, GI upset, or clotting difficulties. It is clinically useful alone or in combination with aspirin or acetaminophen. The drug's toxicity resembles that of narcotic analgesics. Sedation, nausea, and dizziness may occur. CNS depression caused by overdosage may be reversed by naloxone, a narcotic antagonist. True physical dependence is rare with propoxyphene. Narcotic restrictions are not presently necessary with propoxyphene, but deaths have occurred with overdosage and it should be prescribed with discretion. Its hazards are increased if the drug is combined with alcohol or other CNS depressants.

In analgesic activity, 100 mg of propoxyphene napsylate is equivalent to 65 mg of propoxyphene hydrochloride. Because of its physical characteristics, it is possible to make suspension and tablet formulations of the napsylate salt, allowing more flexibility in dosage and administration. Propoxyphene napsylate may be useful in "detoxifying" narcotic addicts.

NONSTEROIDAL ANTI-INFLAMMATORY DRUGS

Anti-inflammatory drugs are a heterogeneous group of medications useful in the symptomatic treatment of undesired tissue inflammation. Only the nonsteroidal agents are discussed in this chapter, some of which appear to be most useful as analgesics. Generally, anti-inflammatory drugs are organic acids which are highly bound to plasma proteins. In vitro, several of these drugs have been shown to uncouple oxidative phosphorylation and stabilize lysosomal membranes. These effects and the inhibition of synthesis of prostaglandins, also shown in vitro for some agents (e.g., ASA, indomethacin), may be related to their clinical effects. Anti-inflammatory drugs are useful adjuncts in the treatment of rheumatoid arthritis, acute gout, ankylosing spondylitis, and osteoarthritis. Each "inflammatory disorder" may respond differently and only some aspects of inflammation (such as cellular infiltration) may respond to any given drug. Although the symptoms of a disease such as rheumatoid arthritis may be ameliorated by anti-inflammatory drugs, tissue destruction may continue unabated. A single drug is often sufficient, but occasionally two agents that affect different aspects of inflammation may be more effective. Drugs work best in chronic conditions if given continuously rather than according to the presence of pain or other symptoms. Sudden cessation of therapy may result in a flare-up of disease activity. Anti-inflammatory agents may irritate the GI tract and predispose to peptic ulceration.

Indomethacin, an indole derivative, also has analgesic, antipyretic, and anti-inflammatory actions, but because of its potential toxicity is not recommended as a simple analgesic. It is indicated primarily for rheumatoid arthritis and related diseases. (See also Ch. 103.)

Propionic acid derivatives: The newer nonsteroidal anti-inflammatory agents such as ibuprofen, fenoprofen, ketoprofen, naproxen, and others are also useful as analgesics. Sodium naproxen has been shown to be effective for dysmenorrhea. The other agents of this class can also be useful for that indication, as well as for mild to moderate pain from athletic injuries, skin, bone, and teeth disorders, and postoperative pain. Propionic acid derivatives can help relieve pain in cancer patients as well, particularly the pain arising from bony metastasis.

Zomepirac, a new drug that is related chemically to indomethacin and tolmetin, has some nonsteroidal anti-inflammatory properties. It seems most useful as an analgesic (100 mg of oral zomepirac was shown to be as effective as 8 to 16 mg of IM morphine), and may also have additional central (but nonnarcotic) analgesic action. Zomepirac is administered orally 50 mg initially q 4 to 6 h with a maximum of 100 mg orally q 4 to 6 h. Zomepirac is well tolerated; adverse effects include GI reactions (nausea, heartburn, abdominal pain) and occasional CNS effects (drowsiness, dizziness, insomnia). *Anaphylactoid reactions and deaths have occurred.* Careful dose adjustment in patients with decreased renal function is necessary because the drug is primarily eliminated by the kidneys.

Nefopam (available in some countries) has a chemical structure unrelated to other nonnarcotic analgesics. It is useful in mild to moderate pain. Nefopam has a different adverse-effect profile and thus may be tolerated by some patients who suffer adverse effects from other analgesics.

Diflunisal, a difluorophenyl derivative of salicylic acid, has analgesic and anti-inflammatory properties. It appears to be useful for treatment of mild to moderate pain as well as for rheumatoid and osteoarthritis. It is long-acting and can generally be given orally every 12 h.

Anti-inflammatory drugs, including salicylates, gold compounds, D-penicillamine, hydroxychloroquine, indomethacin, phenylbutazone, propionic acid derivatives, and several newer agents are also discussed in Ch. 103.

250. CANCER CHEMOTHERAPY

Cancer chemotherapy has been under intensive development during the past 25 yr, resulting in cures of certain types of disseminated, previously fatal cancer. Most cures occur in uncommon tumors, but they provide leads for applying theory to the control of common ones. Overt metastatic cancer should no longer be considered irrevocably fatal. In 15 of the more than 100 forms of clinical cancer (TABLE 250–1) the use of effective drugs results in normal life expectancy for many patients.

TABLE 250–1. PERCENTAGES OF DISSEMINATED CANCERS CURABLE
WITH CHEMOTHERAPY

Type of Cancer	Percentage of Patients Reaching Normal Life Expectancy	
	Estimated % Prior to Chemotherapy	Estimated % with Chemotherapy
Wilms' tumor	30	90
Choriocarcinoma	20	80
Rhabdomyosarcoma	10	60
Advanced Hodgkin's disease	5	58*
Ewing's sarcoma	10	55
Burkitt's lymphoma	5	55
Retinoblastoma	20	55
Acute lymphoblastic leukemia	0	50
Mycosis fungoides	5	50*
Osteosarcoma	20	50*
Diffuse histiocytic lymphoma	0	42
Metastatic embryonal testicular carcinoma	0	32–70*
Acute myelocytic leukemia	0	20*
Ovarian cancer	0	20*
Nodular mixed lymphoma	0	20*

* Longer observation required to be certain of this percentage.

PRINCIPLES OF THERAPY

Understanding cancer chemotherapy rests on the knowledge that antitumor drugs are more effi-cient in killing tumor cells during DNA synthesis and active division; that is, they are more active against cycling than against noncycling cells. Some tumors are cured by drugs because the majority of their cells, at any given moment, are making DNA and dividing (i.e., have a large **growth fraction)**. When drug reaches the tumor, the great majority of the cells in these phases of the cell cycle die. When the tumor is young, most of its cells are making DNA; as it ages, the growth fraction decreases, growth is slowed, and drug sensitivity is reduced. The curable tumors are usually discovered while young and 30 to 100% of their cells are in the growth fraction.

Nonresponsive tumors are usually diagnosed when they are old and have low growth fractions; they require combining systemic chemotherapy with surgery and radiation, which are effective means of removing the old portions of the tumor. Chemotherapy should kill the 2 categories of tumor cells often left behind following local removal—the microscopic nests of cells in the tissue planes adjacent to the primary tumor left outside the surgical margin, and clinically inapparent distant me-tastases. Both categories of cells are in the infancy of their growth cycle and are highly susceptible to drugs given after surgery. Unfortunately, active specific drugs are not available for all types of tumor cells. Old, large tumors are more likely to contain drug-resistant cells because the large num-ber of cell divisions is accompanied by the development of drug-resistant mutants, especially if the cells have been exposed to chemotherapeutic agents.

Normal tissues that have a high percentage of cells synthesizing DNA, such as the hair roots, hematopoietic tissues, and the various GI epithelia from mouth to rectum, are also destroyed by chemotherapy. However, sufficient differences in the post-drug repopulation rates between normal and tumor cells make it possible to give a short course of drug followed by a rest period, permitting the normal cells to regrow before the next course. For some drugs, specific organ toxicities can be avoided if the total dose is kept below a certain threshold.

The strategy of cancer chemotherapy is based upon the therapeutic situations that the physician faces. These fall into 3 categories: (1) curative attempts when overt metastatic disease is present; (2) curative attempts in the absence of manifest metastatic disease, but when the prognosis following local removal is poor; and (3) palliative use of drugs (i.e., to reduce symptoms and to gain prolonged survival when cure is not possible).

Only 2 large growth fraction tumors, Burkitt's lymphoma and choriocarcinoma, have a large enough drug-susceptible fraction of cells to permit cure by a single agent when demonstrable metas-tases are present. **Burkitt's lymphoma** (occurring most commonly in African children) appears in the jaw, rapidly spreads to many areas of the body, and eventually invades the CNS. Virtually 100% of its cells are in active mitosis, so that size doubles q 24 h and death occurs in 2 to 3 mo. Because practically all cells in Burkitt's lymphoma are in cycle, it can be cured by a single dose of cyclophos-phamide in a substantial percentage of patients. Most failures underscore an important concept in cancer chemotherapy, the existence of **"pharmacologic sanctuaries,"** such as metastases in the CNS where highly active drugs cannot reach tumor cells because of the blood-brain barrier. A similar situation exists in acute lymphocytic leukemia, and a successful therapeutic solution is discussed below.

Choriocarcinoma originates in the trophoblastic elements of the placenta and also has rapid growth and similar cell population kinetics. The cure rate was 20% with surgery and radiation therapy (now largely abandoned). With chemotherapy, over 75% of these patients are curable by several courses of either dactinomycin or methotrexate. Four to 5 days of drug therapy is followed by a rest period (usually about 2 to 3 wk) to allow repopulation of granulocytes, platelets, and oro-gastrointes-tinal epithelia. The tumor elaborates chorionic gonadotropin, which appears in the blood and urine and can be used as a marker for the continued presence of cancer. Drug treatment is repeated until gonadotropin has returned permanently to normal values (emphasizing the value of using biochemi-cal or immunologic products of tumors to guide the intensity and duration of therapy).

Certain tumors with intermediate growth fractions (between 10 and 40%) are curable by drugs, albeit not by single agents. Those cells not active in DNA synthesis will switch into active synthesis after a course of a drug has killed the dividing cells. The tumor growth is slowed, but a single drug will not eradicate all cells because the reservoir repopulates the tumor soon after the course is completed. **Combinations of drugs** have greater killing capacity than single drugs because several drugs with different modes of action and toxicities can increase tumor-killing capacity without adding toxicity.

In addition to killing cells during DNA synthesis or during physical mitosis, most drugs have a variable secondary killing capacity for cells in other stages of the cell cycle, designated G_1, G_2. A combination may eradicate cells in these stages of the cell cycle, but it must be given more inten-sively and for relatively long durations. For example, in **acute lymphocytic leukemia**, single drugs or drugs given sequentially cure fewer than 1% of patients, but a combination of 4 drugs given inten-sively for 3 yr or more in a regimen spanning several phases increases the cure rate to 25%. In the **remission induction phase**, vincristine and prednisone rapidly produce complete remission in about 90% of patients. However, **remission maintenance** requires other drugs, most commonly methotrex-ate and 6-mercaptopurine. Other drugs are often added and many variations on this regimen have been developed. Recently the use of cytarabine, thioguanine, and doxorubicin have resulted in 5-yr apparent cures of **acute myelocytic leukemia.**

Failures are often due to CNS relapse (pharmacologic sanctuary). Prophylactic x-irradiation of the brain and intrathecal methotrexate may prevent CNS relapse and increase the cure rate to over 50%. Similar strategies with different drug combinations are effective in Hodgkin's disease Stages III and IV, diffuse histiocytic and nodular mixed lymphomas, ovarian cancers, and embryonal testicular cancers.

A different therapeutic problem is present when a primary tumor is apparently completely resectable (or controllable by x-irradiation), yet the prognosis for life is poor. For example, in breast cancer with lymph node metastases the cure rate is only 10% even though all axillary nodes are removed, because microscopic nests of cells are left in the tumor bed or in metastatic sites. This circumstance most often occurs in the common slow-growing, or small growth fraction, tumors (e.g., bronchogenic or colon cancer) but also is seen in the rare, large growth fraction tumors, and the latter have provided the clue to cure. For example, in Wilms' tumor, surgery, x-irradiation, or both give at best a 40% cure rate. When dactinomycin or vincristine is added after operation and irradiation, the cure rate is more than 90%. This approach, called **combined modality treatment,** has improved the cure rate in Ewing's sarcoma, rhabdomyosarcoma, retinoblastoma, mycosis fungoides, and osteosarcoma.

A remaining problem is late discovery of the primary tumor, especially with the common carcinomas that are slow-growing. However, the multi-modal approach appears to offer hope. In one study of women with breast cancer and axillary nodal involvement who had radical mastectomy, the use of melphalan beginning postoperatively and continuing for 18 mo sharply reduced the expected metastatic and local relapses after 3 yr of observation. A combination of cyclophosphamide, methotrexate, and 5-fluorouracil used as adjuvants after mastectomy has significantly increased the survival rate after a 4-yr observation period. In both studies, these effects occurred in premenopausal but not in postmenopausal women.

Palliation is of value when cure is impossible but when the tumor can be partially destroyed by drugs, resulting in reduced symptoms and sometimes prolonged life. Also, the drug or drug combination should be able to produce regression in at least 20% of patients with a particular tumor. Intensive palliative chemotherapy leading to severe side effects cannot often be justified. **Contraindications** include recent extensive surgery, malnutrition, intestinal obstruction, reduced bone marrow reserve due to extensive x-irradiation, infection or bleeding, and renal or hepatic insufficiency.

ANTITUMOR DRUGS

Traditionally, antitumor drugs are divided into alkylating agents, antimetabolites, antibiotics, alkaloids and other natural products, hormones, and miscellaneous compounds, thus grouping drugs of similar structure and mechanism of action.

Alkylating Agents

These drugs, developed from wartime research on mustard gases, alkylate (affix an alkyl group to) a biologically important cellular constituent, modifying its properties. With cancer cells, these agents alkylate DNA, causing cross-linking between the 7-nitrogen atom of guanine in each of the double strands, interfering with the separation of strands, and preventing mitosis. Most of these drugs are absorbed after oral administration, but a few require IV use. Their active moieties disappear rapidly from the blood, usually in 2 to 15 min. They distribute to all tissues *except the CNS.* All are toxic to the bone marrow, cause immunodepression, and are carcinogenic and mutagenic. Some of the agents have additional side effects.

Mechlorethamine (mustine, HN_2), the original agent, has largely been supplanted by newer congeners. It is (like mustard gas) a strong vesicant, cannot be taken by mouth, and is usually injected into the tubing of a running infusion and repeated at monthly intervals. The maximum effect on granulocytes, lymphocytes, and reticulocytes is at 10 days; recovery is complete at 21 to 28 days. Nausea and vomiting occur within minutes to an hour after injection in most patients, and prophylactic sedation and administration of antiemetics is advisable. The principal use of mechlorethamine is in combination chemotherapy of Hodgkin's disease and the non-Hodgkin's lymphomas. It has activity in a wide variety of cancers, but has been replaced by alkylating agents that are easier to give.

Cyclophosphamide depresses platelets less, has a broad spectrum of activity, and is the most widely used alkylating agent. It is the only alkylating agent that is not active in vitro, and must be enzymatically oxidized by liver microsomes to active metabolites. Phenobarbital accelerates and proadifen slows the rate of active metabolite production. Cyclophosphamide may be given orally, even though absorption is incomplete, but often is used IV for maximum effectiveness. This alkylating agent usually causes alopecia. Sterility and testicular atrophy, ovarian fibrosis, and amenorrhea occur, and the drug is teratogenic. Hemorrhagic cystitis occurs unless fluids are forced during administration. Large doses cause myocardial necrosis.

Chlorambucil has a greater effect on lymphocytes than on other formed elements and is chiefly used in chronic lymphocytic leukemia, usually orally in daily doses. It is also used in combination for testicular cancer and sometimes for lymphomas.

Busulfan has its greatest effect on granulocytes and is used in chronic myelocytic leukemia. It is given orally daily, titrating dose to the granulocyte count. Overdosage can lead to severe irreversible granulocytopenia, and generally the drug should be halved when the WBC count is 30,000 to 40,000 and discontinued when the count is 20,000. Side effects include skin pigmentation, ovarian suppression leading to amenorrhea, and, rarely, pulmonary fibrosis. Prolonged administration can be associated with a syndrome that mimics adrenal insufficiency.

Dibromomannitol, a good substitute for busulfan in chronic myelocytic leukemia, is also given by mouth daily. It is of pharmacologic interest because it crosses the blood-brain barrier.

Melphalan (phenylalanine mustard, LPAM) is effective in multiple myeloma and is widely used as an adjuvant to surgery for breast cancer. It is given orally in monthly or 6-wk courses and can be given IV.

Carmustine (BCNU) and **lomustine (CCNU)** are nitrosureas with a broad spectrum of activity. They are alkylating agents, but also inhibit DNA repair by isocyanate formation. They have 2 other distinguishing features: (1) Toxicity to the bone marrow does not reach its maximum until 6 to 8 wk after administration, which places certain limitations on the dose schedule. (2) They are highly lipid-soluble and easily transported across the blood-brain barrier, making them drugs of choice in tumors involving the CNS (e.g., glioblastoma multiforme). BCNU is given only IV as a 15-min infusion in a single dose. CCNU can only be given orally.

Streptozocin, discovered as a natural product, is a nitrosurea without bone marrow depressant toxicity. It has specific effectiveness in islet cell tumors of the pancreas and in disseminated carcinoid.

Triethylenemelamine (TEM), an early alkylating agent, was used when combined with radiation therapy for retinoblastoma. It has largely been replaced by cyclophosphamide.

Thiotepa, another early drug, has effects quite similar to those of mechlorethamine. In bladder cancer, for which it is now largely used, thiotepa is instilled in the bladder once weekly for 4 wk.

Mitomycin C is another natural product whose mechanism of action is through alkylation. It has some effectiveness in GI cancer. Recent studies have shown greater effectiveness and less toxicity when given in large doses intermittently.

Antimetabolites

Antimetabolites inhibit a metabolic pathway essential for the viability or reproduction of a cancer cell; e.g., through inhibition of folate, purine, pyrimidine, and pyrimidine nucleoside pathways required for DNA synthesis. No metabolic pathway unique for cancer cells has been found, yet antimetabolites can be used to kill tumor cells without killing the host. The differences that permit selective toxicity are probably in the growth fractions of the tumor and bone marrow cells rather than in metabolic pathways. The antimetabolites have a much narrower spectrum of use than the other classes of anticancer drugs.

Methotrexate acts as an antifolate, by binding almost irreversibly to the enzyme dihydrofolate reductase and preventing the formation of the coenzyme tetrahydrofolate, essential for DNA synthesis and for replication of animal cells. In spite of its impressive potential toxicities, physicians have learned to use methotrexate safely and to the great benefit of patients with choriocarcinoma, the acute leukemias, osteosarcoma, head and neck cancer, and breast cancer. Methotrexate is readily absorbed from the GI tract and distributed to the liver and kidneys, but it is virtually excluded from the CNS. It is not significantly metabolized and biliary excretion is < 5%; excretion is mainly through the kidney by both glomerular filtration and active tubular transport. *The recommended therapeutic dosages depend on normal renal function, and in the presence of diminished clearance, toxic plasma concentrations may result from full dosage.* Concomitant salicylates inhibit tubular secretion of methotrexate. Vincristine increases the cellular uptake of methotrexate and this effect has been utilized in the treatment of osteosarcoma. Methotrexate can be given by any route, including the intrathecal. Toxicity is a function of the *duration* of administration, and a prolonged 24-h infusion is far more toxic than a push injection of the same amount. Dosages are 2.5 to 10 mg/day, but much larger doses (up to 1 gm) in 24 h can be given IV when **"leucovorin rescue"** is used. Leucovorin supplies the cells with tetrahydrofolate, and when started after the methotrexate and continued for 72 h, it diminishes the toxicity to the host without abolishing the antitumor effect. Toxicity to the bone marrow follows the same time pattern as for mechlorethamine. In addition, methotrexate is toxic to the oro-gastrointestinal epithelium, and 2 to 7 days after administration one often sees oral reddening and ulceration, nausea, and vomiting. Diarrhea, dysphagia, and GI bleeding may result as more serious side effects. Skin rashes and alopecia occasionally are seen. With very large doses, hepatic damage or renal damage progressing to uremia may occur. Prolonged usage (2 to 5 yr), as for psoriasis, is associated with liver damage with a cirrhosis-like syndrome. Leukoencephalopathy sometimes occurs when intrathecal methotrexate is used in repeated doses together with whole brain irradiation.

6-Mercaptopurine (6MP) and **6-thioguanine (6TG)** are antagonists to purines which are essential constituents of DNA. Their usefulness is limited to the acute leukemias and chronic myelocytic leukemia; 6MP is effective in choriocarcinoma but is rarely so used in the USA. It is first converted to the ribonucleotide and interferes with a number of metabolic pathways, most importantly with the first step in purine biosynthesis. Absorption is incomplete after oral administration. There is rapid metabolic degradation of 6MP by xanthine oxidase; therefore, dosage must be reduced if a patient is concomitantly receiving allopurinol, a xanthine oxidase inhibitor. Toxicity consists of bone marrow depression and oro-gastrointestinal damage similar to that seen with methotrexate.

6TG differs from 6MP because it is actually incorporated into the DNA of normal and cancer cells. Its sole use is the treatment of acute myelocytic leukemia in combination with cytarabine. 6TG can be given orally or IV; its pharmacology and toxicity are similar to those of 6MP.

Cytarabine (ARA-C, arabinosylcytosine) is a pyrimidine nucleoside antagonist. Its major use is in acute myelocytic leukemia and, when combined with thioguanine, it gives the highest percentage of complete remission so far observed. ARA-C must be converted into the nucleotide to be active and as such inhibits the incorporation of thymidine triphosphate into DNA. It must be given IV and can safely be used intrathecally. In the body it is rapidly deaminated by a kinase to an inert moiety, arabinosyl uridine, which is excreted in the urine. Because of this rapid degradation, ARA-C must be given by continuous infusion. It is a marked bone marrow depressant, causes lesions of oro-gastro-intestinal epithelia, and occasionally gives rise to hepatic and renal toxicity.

5-Fluorouracil (5FU), a pyrimidine antagonist, is the most active drug available for colorectal cancer and has modest activity in pancreatic and other GI tumors. 5FU has also been effectively used intra-arterially for treatment of hepatic metastases from colorectal cancer but has considerable toxicity. It is active in metastatic breast cancer and is used in some of the drug combinations. 5FU is effective against actinic keratoses when applied locally and is also used when there are a number of basal cell or squamous cell cancers of the skin not readily treated by surgery or irradiation. Local reaction in the involved skin can be severe. 5FU must be phosphorylated to the nucleotide to be active, and as such inhibits thymidylate synthetase, a key enzyme in the biosynthesis of DNA. While some 5FU is absorbed after oral administration, it should be used IV. The half-life of 5FU in the blood is 15 to 30 min. It is rapidly catabolized, many products appear in the urine, and many of the carbon residues are disposed of via respiratory CO_2. It crosses the blood-brain barrier but, when given intrathecally or into a carotid artery, it forms fluorocitrate, a metabolite that causes cerebellar ataxia. 5FU is given on an intermittent schedule, either a 4- to 5-day course at about 3- to 6-wk intervals or once weekly after an initial course. It can cause devastating bone marrow and GI toxicity, but these effects can be obviated by intermittent schedules and careful monitoring. Alopecia, skin rashes, or cerebellar dysfunction are noted occasionally.

Dacarbazine (DTIC) is an analog of AIC (5-aminoimidazole-4-carboxamide) which is used by tumor cells in DNA synthesis. DTIC has been shown to inhibit DNA synthesis, probably through this pathway. It is the most active drug in malignant melanoma and is also used in combination therapy of several soft tissue sarcomas. DTIC is used IV and has a half-life of 30 min. It is metabolized and its products appear in the urine. Toxicity includes bone marrow depression, GI erosions, marked vomiting, and occasionally an influenza-like syndrome.

Antibiotics

A number of natural antibiotics have antitumor activities. Some are complex alkylating agents; the remainder are rather large molecules that bind to DNA.

Dactinomycin (actinomycin D) is the most active of a series of cyclic pentapeptides derived from a streptomycete. It is used in choriocarcinoma and Wilms' tumor, and in combination for testicular cancer, Ewing's sarcoma, and soft tissue sarcomas. Dactinomycin interferes with DNA function by intercalation; i.e., the drug is inserted between base pairs across the helix. Absorption is variable. The dosage schedule consists of 5-day courses at monthly intervals. The drug is always given IV into a running infusion to avoid local irritation. It disappears rapidly from the blood and is not metabolized, and most of the excretion is through the biliary tract, with only small amounts in the urine. It is distributed in good concentration to most organs, but does not reach the CNS. Toxicity includes bone marrow depression, oro-gastrointestinal ulceration, nausea and vomiting, and alopecia. A specific side effect is a severe skin reaction wherever there has been previous (or concomitant) radiation.

Doxorubicin (adriamycin) and **daunorubicin** (daunomycin, rubidomycin) are close analogs obtained from cultures of streptomyces. Doxorubicin is the more important of the two drugs, daunorubicin being used largely in the acute leukemias. Doxorubicin has the broadest spectrum of any antitumor drug, and is especially useful in the sarcomas and acute myelocytic leukemia. In addition, it has major activity in cancers of the breast, bladder, and prostate, and in the lymphomas; and there is evidence of minor activity in a number of other cancers. Doxorubicin and daunorubicin both intercalate with DNA, with resulting uncoiling of the helix and inhibition of both RNA and DNA polymerases. They are chemically irritating and should be given as part of a running IV infusion. Both drugs disappear rapidly from the blood, being excreted mainly in the bile. For this reason the risk of toxicity from usual doses increases if hepatic disease is present. Both accumulate in tissues, especially in cardiac muscle. Toxicity includes bone marrow depression, alopecia, and oro-gastrointestinal reactions. They also can cause cardiac failure, often severe and irreversible. Apparently the drugs accumulate in cardiac muscle and cause severe cardiac damage if a certain total dosage is exceeded. Because of this limitation, the drugs cannot be given for more than 6 to 8 mo, which severely limits their use for maintenance.

Bleomycin is the name given to a group of peptides with antitumor activity. They cause strand scission and fragmentation of DNA. The clinical preparation is a mixture of bleomycin A_2, A_21, B_1, B_2, B_3, B_4, etc., with A_2 being the predominant moiety. Bleomycin is active in lymphomas and testicular cancer and provides the basis of new combinations, especially because it lacks marrow toxicity and immune suppression. It has modest activity in a variety of squamous cell cancers. Bleomycin is not absorbed orally, but can be given IV, IM, or s.c. It is a mixture, and hence little is known of its pharmacokinetics. It is rapidly inactivated by all tissues except the skin and lung, where its specific toxicities lie. Bleomycin causes erythema, pain, and hypertrophic changes in the skin in areas where there is a lot of keratin, and ulceration of these areas and pigmentation of the nails may occur. Pulmonary fibrosis, which is sometimes fatal, occurs in 5 to 15% of patients who receive more than 100 mg/m². Bleomycin is usually not given to patients over age 50 or with pulmonary disease. The maximum total dose is usually limited to 300 mg/m².

Mithramycin has limited usefulness in embryonal testicular cancer. It binds to DNA but is even more inhibitory to RNA. It is given as a running infusion. Little is known of its pharmacology but it does cross the blood-brain barrier. Bone marrow toxicity is marked. Mithramycin also causes bleeding by depressing the coagulation factors manufactured by the liver, and it inhibits the activity of osteocytes, depressing serum levels of Ca and P. It has some use in controlling hypercalcemia and Paget's disease of bone.

Alkaloids

Vincristine and **vinblastine** are alkaloids obtained from the plant *Vinca rosea*. Vincristine is included in the highly effective combinations for acute lymphocytic leukemia, the lymphomas, breast cancer, sarcomas, and the various childhood neoplasms. Vinblastine has similar capacities in lymphomas, choriocarcinoma, testicular cancer, and breast cancer but not in acute lymphocytic leukemia. It is less popular in combination regimens because of its more marked myelosuppression. Both drugs arrest cells in metaphase—as does colchicine—and have subtle effects on nucleic acid synthesis. The antimitotic action of the vinca alkaloids is due apparently to specific binding to the protein tubulin, a vital component of cellular microtubules. They are not dependably absorbed after oral administration and are given IV. Their pharmacology is poorly understood, but apparently little of these alkaloids appears in the urine, with moderate amounts being excreted in bile. Metabolic degradation is extensive. Considerable vinblastine is absorbed on blood platelets. Both drugs cause alopecia and bone marrow depression, but leukopenia is less marked for vincristine. Oro-gastrointestinal reactions are not seen, but both drugs have reversible neuromuscular toxicity (which is more marked for vincristine) leading to severe constipation, paresthesias, loss of reflexes, and weakness of extremities.

Miscellaneous Compounds

Procarbazine, a hydrazine derivative, is important in the treatment of Hodgkin's disease, but is markedly carcinogenic, producing leukemia in monkeys. It is a component of the "MOPP" combination, which is so effective in Hodgkin's disease, and has modest effects in mesothelioma. It must be converted to an azo derivative in vivo to become active against tumor cells by interfering with DNA by alkylation and perhaps by aberrant transmethylation. Procarbazine is absorbed in the GI tract and crosses the blood-brain barrier, has a plasma half-life of 10 min, is distributed to liver and kidney, and is extensively metabolized. The kidneys excrete about 70%, but 10 to 20% appears in respiratory CO_2. The drug is usually given by mouth, but can be given IV. In addition to nausea, vomiting, and bone marrow depression, there are neurologic effects—somnolence, confusion, and cerebellar ataxia—related to the drug's ability to enter the CNS. Procarbazine is a weak monoamine oxidase inhibitor and is therefore subject to the same precautions regarding concomitant use of other drugs and foods (see PHARMACODYNAMIC INTERACTIONS in Ch. 241).

Hydroxyurea interferes with DNA synthesis by inhibiting ribonucleoside diphosphate reductase and has modest effects in melanoma; it is sometimes used to enhance radiation. The drug is usually given by mouth but can be given IV, is extensively metabolized to urea, and crosses the blood-brain barrier. Its main toxicity is bone marrow depression. It is useful in rapidly but transiently lowering the high WBC counts of chronic myelocytic leukemia in the blastic phase. It has some effect in melanoma.

Asparaginase, an enzyme obtained from *Escherichia coli* and a few other bacteria, is used only for inducing remission in acute lymphatic leukemia. It hydrolyzes and deprives tumors of extracellular sources of the supposedly nonessential amino acid asparagine, causing cell death. Marrow depression is not seen, nor does it affect GI mucosa or hair follicles, but asparaginase produces many other serious toxicities in man, especially upon those organs that synthesize large amounts of proteins, such as the liver and pancreas. The liver toxicity is moderate, but an occasional patient can develop fulminating pancreatitis. There are occasional CNS manifestations and, because it is a protein given IV, some patients (about 5%) develop allergic reactions, and sometimes anaphylactic shock.

The 2 groups of hormones of most importance in cancer chemotherapy are the corticosteroids and the antiestrogens. **Prednisone** is the analog usually used and is an essential and valuable component of curative combination chemotherapy in acute lymphocytic leukemia, Hodgkin's disease and other lymphomas, and breast cancer. It, or dexamethasone, is valuable in the management of metastatic and primary brain cancer, in part due to rapid control of cerebral edema. **Tamoxifen** is an antiestrogen which is the drug of choice in treating estrogen-dependent breast cancer. Estrogen dependence can in large measure be determined by the estrogen receptor assay, which should be done as a baseline in all patients who have breast cancer tissue removed. When the assay is positive, 70% of these women will be responsive to hormonal therapy; when it is negative, less than 10% will respond and thus the indication is for chemotherapy rather than hormonal manipulation. While tamoxifen is not curative, it does give extensive palliation lasting 6 to 9 mo in metastatic breast cancer. Common side effects are pruritus vulvae, hot flashes, and vaginal bleeding. Fluid retention usually does not occur unless the dosage exceeds 40 mg per day.

Mitotane (ortho, para'-DDD) is related to DDT, has specific toxicity for the cells of the adrenal cortex, and is useful in the management of adrenal cortical carcinoma. Long-term survival has been noted in patients with metastatic involvement. It is given in large doses by mouth and has a variety of side effects, including anorexia, nausea, vomiting, and diarrhea. Lethargy and somnolence occur in some patients; less common effects include skin rashes, bone marrow depression, and liver damage.

Cisplatin, a new but widely used drug, is *cis*-platinum-diammine-dichloride **(CPDD)**. Its mechanism of action is unknown but it probably functions as an alkylating agent. In combination with other active drugs it has provided a major advance in the treatment of testicular cancer. It is also active in cancers of the head and neck area, bladder and ovary. In addition to severe nausea and vomiting and hematologic depression, its specific side effects are renal damage and ototoxicity. These can be in large part avoided by premedication hydration and the use of diuretics.

---

251.   CORTICOTROPIN (ACTH) AND CORTICOSTEROIDS

While the adrenal corticosteroids are essential for life, they do not *initiate* cellular and enzymatic activity; they *permit* many biochemical reactions to proceed at optimal rates. Except as specific replacement therapy in adrenocortical insufficiency or for suppression of adrenal overactivity, clinical use of corticosteroids and their synthetic analogs depends on their anti-inflammatory, antiallergic, and lympholytic properties.

Endogenous ACTH and corticosteroids are not produced and do not function in isolation; they operate as an integral component of the hypothalamic-pituitary-adrenal system. This system is important in maintaining homeostasis under resting conditions and in response to many stimuli and stresses. The corticosteroids affect all organs and tissues. They aid in keeping the internal environment constant through their actions on the metabolism of water and electrolytes, carbohydrate, fat, and protein. The pituitary rapidly augments its release of ACTH into the circulation in response to environmental stress; the increased ACTH stimulates the adrenal cortex to secrete more hydrocortisone (cortisol). The mechanisms of interaction of the hypothalamic-pituitary-adrenal system and their clinical significance are detailed in Chs. 84, 85, and 88.

CORTICOTROPIN (ACTH)

ACTH maintains the weight of the adrenal and stimulates its secretion of corticosteroid hormones. Excess ACTH, endogenous or administered, induces adrenal hypertrophy and provokes increased adrenocortical secretion of hydrocortisone. The increase in hydrocortisone and dehydroepiandrosterone **(DHEA)** production is reflected by sharp increases in urinary excretion of 17-hydroxycorticosteroids and 17-ketosteroids. The plasma hydrocortisone level rises in minutes in response to ACTH, which also has some influence on aldosterone production, causing only small and transient increases in adrenal secretion of aldosterone.

ACTH given IV has a short plasma half-life. Repository, long-acting preparations such as ACTH in a gelatin vehicle or in combination with zinc are used for IM injection. Lyophilized preparations are partially inactivated in muscle. Though ACTH is distributed throughout the body after injection, its therapeutic effects are due to stimulation of hydrocortisone overproduction by the adrenal. The clinically desirable effects of ACTH can be achieved with corticosteroids, which are generally preferred to ACTH because they can be given orally. Some believe ACTH to be more effective in selected situations (e.g., to avoid adrenal suppression, and, possibly, to lessen growth retardation in children), but this has been questioned (see PRINCIPLES FOR USING CORTICOSTEROIDS, below).

THE CORTICOSTEROIDS

Chemistry and Classification

Over 50 corticosteroids have been isolated from the adrenal glands of animals and humans, but few have biologic importance. They are classified according to their biologic activities: (1) **glucocorticoids** (e.g., hydrocortisone, cortisone, corticosterone) affect mainly carbohydrate and protein metabolism; (2) **mineralocorticoids** (chiefly aldosterone, but also desoxycorticosterone) regulate electrolyte and water metabolism; and (3) **androgens** (e.g., DHEA, androstenedione, testosterone, 11β-hydroxyandrostenedione) are anabolic and cause masculinization.

The **synthetic analogs of hydrocortisone (cortisol)** possess no significant properties that hydrocortisone lacks; they differ chiefly in relative mineralocorticoid vs. anti-inflammatory potencies (see TABLE 251-1). The other chief difference is the long half-life of many of these synthetic analogs, which contributes significantly to their increased potency. The lesser potency of **cortisone** (80%)

compared to **hydrocortisone** correlates well with the observation that about 80% of cortisone is converted in vivo to hydrocortisone, the active hormone at the tissue level. **Desoxycorticosterone acetate,** which lacks the anti-inflammatory activity of hydrocortisone, is a potent mineralocorticoid. However, since it must be given parenterally, it has been supplanted in the treatment of Addison's disease by **fludrocortisone** (the most potent mineralocorticoid), which can be given orally. The addition of a fluorine atom to the hydrocortisone molecule enhances anti-inflammatory potency. However, the much greater augmentation of mineralocorticoid activity precludes the use of this compound as a systemic anti-inflammatory agent.

Dehydrogenation at the 1 and 2 positions of the hydrocortisone and cortisone molecules yields **prednisolone** and **prednisone,** respectively, which possess more potent anti-inflammatory properties but have less sodium and water-retaining effect. The addition of a 16α-hydroxyl, a l6α-methyl, and a 16β-methyl group to the 9α-fluoro substituent **(fludrocortisone)** forms **triamcinolone, dexamethasone,** and **betamethasone,** respectively, and reduces the sodium-retaining properties of the parent compound. All 3 compounds evoke little or no sodium retention in effective anti-inflammatory doses. The reason for the differences in relative potencies of these compounds is not known. Most synthetic corticosteroids disappear from the blood more slowly and are less firmly bound to serum protein than hydrocortisone.

Absorption, Metabolism, and Excretion

Hydrocortisone is readily and quickly absorbed from the gut, even in malabsorption syndromes or after total or partial gastrectomy. High corticosteroid blood levels are reached within 1 h and persist (though falling) for 6 to 8 h. Sustained action requires administration at 4- to 8-h intervals. The **oral route** is preferred for long-term therapy. Onset of action is rapid, but, for acute allergic emergencies (e.g., status asthmaticus, angioedema), epinephrine acts faster.

The therapeutic effects of glucocorticoids are achieved most rapidly by the **IV route.** Hydrocortisone sodium succinate exemplifies a water-soluble preparation that can be dissolved in a small volume of sterile water and given as a rapid IV injection over a 2-min period. The ester hydrolyzes quickly in the blood, yielding free hydrocortisone; the level remains elevated for 4 h. An effect (e.g., on blood pressure after adrenalectomy) may appear in minutes. This agent can also be given as a prolonged infusion in 5% D/W or saline (500 to 1000 ml over 4 to 12 h).

The **IM route** is probably the least satisfactory method of giving corticosteroids because absorption is slow and variable. However, the sustained action of IM hydrocortisone makes it suitable for adrenal suppression when continuous adequate blood levels are essential. Hydrocortisone sodium succinate and similar esters can also be given IM, but are absorbed and metabolized more rapidly, thus requiring several injections daily for sustained effect.

Glucocorticoids can also be absorbed **through the skin and from joint spaces,** only rarely producing adverse systemic effects.

Hydrocortisone enters all body tissues and compartments, including the CSF, and is eliminated from the body within 24 to 48 h. The major metabolic site is the liver, where the steroid undergoes degradation, yielding compounds readily excreted in the urine. Minute amounts of corticosteroid are also excreted unchanged. Metabolism of hydrocortisone is delayed in patients with hepatic cirrhosis, hypothyroidism, and severe renal insufficiency.

Pharmacologic Actions and Undesirable Effects

Qualitatively, the pharmacologic actions of hydrocortisone and of the synthetic glucocorticoids are identical; quantitatively, they differ in their respective effects on various tissue and organ functions. See TABLE 251–1 for the relative biologic potencies of various corticosteroids.

Carbohydrate metabolism: Administration of hydrocortisone repletes liver glycogen and raises blood glucose in adrenalectomized animals and humans, largely through enhancement of gluconeogenesis from protein. Hydrocortisone also impedes peripheral utilization of glucose. While glucose intolerance occurs in many patients with spontaneous Cushing's syndrome, clinical diabetes mellitus is not common in corticosteroid-treated patients. When glucosuria occurs, latent or subclinical diabetes mellitus must be ruled out. "Steroid diabetes" is characterized by insulin resistance and, usually, the absence of ketosis and acidosis. A family history of diabetes mellitus demands extra vigilance when glucocorticoids are given.

Protein metabolism: Large doses of hydrocortisone invoke increased amino acid production from protein, negative nitrogen balance, and, after prolonged administration, depletion of body protein, as in the severe muscle wasting and osteoporosis of both spontaneous and corticosteroid-induced Cushing's syndrome.

Fat metabolism: Hydrocortisone is antiketogenic as a result of increased availability of carbohydrate. High doses cause redistribution of fat, with depletion in the extremities and increased deposition in the face and the cervicodorsal, interscapular, and abdominal regions.

Electrolyte and water metabolism: Mineralocorticoids and, to a lesser extent, glucocorticoids produce Na and water retention. *Absence* of these hormones (as in Addison's disease) results in renal Na wasting, with concomitant loss of water, hemoconcentration, hyponatremia, hypovolemia, and, ultimately, vascular collapse, hypotension, and shock. In addition to renal loss of Na and water, electrolyte and water shifts to and from the intracellular compartment occur; hyperkalemia is a feature of addisonian crisis. Hydrocortisone acts with aldosterone to maintain electrolyte balance.

TABLE 251-1. RELATIVE BIOLOGIC POTENCIES OF COMMONLY USED CORTICOSTEROIDS

Corticosteroid	Relative Potency* (mEq)	
	Glucocorticoid (Anti-inflammatory)	Mineralocorticoid (Sodium-retaining)
Hydrocortisone (Cortisol)	1	1
Cortisone	0.8	0.8
Desoxycorticosterone	0	30–50
Fludrocortisone	10	125
Prednisone	4–5	0.8
Prednisolone	4–5	0.8
Methylprednisolone	5–6	0.5
Triamcinolone	4–5	Minimal
Dexamethasone	30	Minimal
Betamethasone	30	Minimal

* Hydrocortisone expressed as unity. Potencies vary considerably depending upon whether determination is at 4, 12, or 24 h following administration. The above rough approximations are taken chiefly from bioassays and do not necessarily apply to individual patients.

Glucocorticoids (but not mineralocorticoids) also help maintain the capacity to excrete a water load. This effect is due to enhancement of renal plasma flow and increased GFR.

High dosages of hydrocortisone may produce Na and water retention with hypervolemia, edema, and, especially in elderly patients, congestive heart failure. Hypokalemic alkalosis occurs and can be treated with K salts.

Effects on the endocrine system: In addition to its diabetogenic effect, hydrocortisone causes adrenocortical atrophy by suppressing endogenous pituitary ACTH secretion. Such atrophy is accompanied by failure to secrete increased amounts of corticosteroid in response to an acute illness or other environmental stress; the ensuing adrenocortical insufficiency may be of clinical import (as in too hasty withdrawal) and occasionally is fatal.

Hydrocortisone may induce mild hirsutism in women. Disturbances in menstrual function are not likely to occur unless very high serum corticosteroid levels follow prolonged administration.

Effects on connective tissue: Glucocorticoids induce many chemical changes in ground substance and alter the response of connective tissue to injury. They inhibit inflammatory reactions, which explains their usefulness in suppressing manifestations of the collagen diseases but also accounts for their deleterious effect on wound healing. Suppression of the inflammatory reaction in patients receiving large doses may be so complete as to mask the clinical symptoms and signs of major diseases (e.g., perforation of a peptic ulcer or spread of infection).

The anti-inflammatory actions of glucocorticoids are only suppressive. Thus, their withdrawal is generally followed by recrudescence of the disease.

Effects on hypersensitivity reactions: The antiallergic action of hydrocortisone on bronchial asthma may be due to interference with the mechanism by which tissue injury results from an antigen-antibody reaction. Suppression of prostaglandin production may also be important.

Effects on the musculoskeletal system: Hydrocortisone in physiologic quantities appears to be essential for muscular contraction. In large doses it evokes muscle weakness and atrophy due to inhibition of protein synthesis; K depletion may also play a role. Corticosteroids may induce myopathies characterized by loss of muscle substance and focal myositis.

Osteoporosis, which may accompany corticosteroid therapy, results from a decrease in the protein matrix of bone and an increased calcium removal. Hydrocortisone impedes growth in children, partially through its inhibition of protein synthesis. Daily doses of prednisone (or equivalent) of more than 4 mg/sq m of BSA retard skeletal maturation. Catch-up growth after treatment is stopped is slow and variable.

Effects on the hemopoietic system: Large doses of hydrocortisone induce peripheral lympholysis and slower lymphocyte production; the polymorphonuclear leukocytes are relatively increased and may be markedly increased shortly after administration is started. Leukemoid reactions rarely occur. Leukocytosis is uncommon in spontaneous Cushing's syndrome. This lympholytic property is exploited in the treatment of acute lymphoblastic leukemia, particularly in children.

Effects on the GI system: Gastric or duodenal ulcer may follow administration of hydrocortisone, especially in patients with RA. Corticosteroids combat the malabsorption of fat in sprue and in Whipple's disease through an unknown mechanism. Rarely, pancreatitis occurs during corticosteroid therapy.

Effects on the cardiovascular system: Hypervolemia, edema, and congestive heart failure occasionally follow administration of high doses of hydrocortisone. Hypertension is rarely produced.

Effects on the skin: Administration of excessive amounts of hydrocortisone is associated with thinning of the subcutaneous tissue and splitting of elastic fibers, with red or purple striae and ecchymoses. The acne and hirsutism of induced hypercorticism are due to androgenic breakdown products.

Effects on the CNS: Hydrocortisone increases brain excitability; seizures may result, especially in children and in those with established convulsive disorders. The abnormal EEG of Addison's disease usually becomes normal after a small dose of replacement hydrocortisone is taken.

Emotional disturbances including psychoses may be seen in patients with Addison's disease or Cushing's syndrome. It cannot be predicted from the patient's underlying personality whether psychologic changes will occur in patients who receive large doses of glucocorticoids. Changes in affect vary from euphoria to depression. Agitation and insomnia are not uncommon. Psychotic reactions with delusions and hallucinations may occur. Pseudotumor cerebri is a rare untoward event. Serious psychiatric symptoms are directly, though roughly, correlated with higher dosage.

Corticosteroids, especially when applied topically, raise intraocular pressure. The increase is greater in patients with glaucoma.

PRINCIPLES FOR USING CORTICOSTEROIDS

Corticosteroids are used to treat disorders of adrenal hypo- and hyperfunction (see Ch. 88). The pharmacologic properties of corticosteroids also make them valuable in many other disorders (e.g., RA, SLE, bronchial asthma, hypersensitivity diseases). Specific details of corticosteroid use in these conditions are discussed in their appropriate chapters. Topical corticosteroid preparations are discussed in Ch. 187. General principles of corticosteroid use are described here.

1. Possible benefits should be weighed against risks of undesirable effects.

2. Patients should be evaluated with regard to a history of (a) peptic ulcer; (b) emotional instability; (c) personal or family diabetes mellitus (blood sugar should be determined 2 h after a meal); or (d) tuberculosis. A chest x-ray and tuberculin skin test should be ordered routinely for all patients. If the latter is positive, isoniazid should be given concomitantly with corticosteroids.

3. The synthetic analogs are generally preferable to hydrocortisone or cortisone because of their lower sodium-retaining effects.

4. The lowest effective dose should be prescribed for the shortest possible time; moderation of symptoms with minimal untoward effects is preferable to complete palliation with major complications.

5. Committing a patient to long-term corticosteroid therapy should be considered only after other therapeutic measures have failed.

6. Corticosteroids may be given orally (except for acute emergencies or in infants) in divided doses, 1 to 4 times/day.

7. All dosages should be individualized. The effective dose varies with different diseases, with different phases of the same disease, and from patient to patient.

8. The dosage should be kept flexible, being raised or lowered according to the activity of the disease or the development of undesirable effects.

9. In stable treatment programs, use of the *alternate-day (intermittent) dosage schedule* should be considered; e.g., prednisone 40 mg orally on alternate days instead of 20 mg/day. Usually, results are satisfactory with this regimen and the undesirable effects are fewer and less severe.

10. If an acute infection, trauma, or surgery occurs during treatment, the dosage should be *increased* and given parenterally if necessary; e.g., hydrocortisone sodium succinate 300 mg IV on the day of surgery, 200 mg on the 1st postoperative day, and 100 mg on the 2nd postoperative day, after which the previous prednisone doses are resumed. ACTH should not be used in these circumstances, since the adrenal response to ACTH is suppressed and the desired increases in endogenous hydrocortisone are not achieved.

11. Patients who have received cortisone 50 mg or more/day (or equivalent amounts of other corticosteroids) for periods of more than 1 to 2 mo should be considered to have some degree of pituitary-adrenal suppression for at least I yr after corticosteroid withdrawal.

12. Corticosteroids should be withdrawn gradually.

Contraindications

Active, healed, or questionably healed TB was once considered an absolute contraindication to corticosteroid use. However, corticosteroids, combined with antituberculous therapy, may be lifesaving in overwhelming tuberculous infections and are essential in TB patients who develop adrenal insufficiency.

Ocular herpes simplex is an **absolute contraindication** to corticosteroid therapy. **Relative contraindications** are acute or chronic infections (especially chickenpox), pregnancy, diabetes mellitus, hypertension, peptic ulcer, osteoporosis, recent intestinal anastomoses, diverticulitis, psychotic tendencies, renal insufficiency, and diminished cardiac reserve or congestive heart failure other than that due to active rheumatic carditis. With any of these conditions, the advantages of corticosteroid therapy must be carefully weighed against the possibility of deleterious results.

Generally, corticosteroids should not be given if prophylactic immunization is imminent because of the possible interference with immune response. However, if the continued administration of corticosteroids is mandatory, as in adrenal insufficiency or SLE, concurrent immunization should be carried out as indicated.

No injection of these drugs should be made into an infected area.

Management During Long-Term Treatment

Precautions to be taken prior to corticosteroid therapy are as outlined above. During treatment, close attention should be given to the appearance of undesirable effects: weight gain, edema, hypertension, signs of intercurrent infection, glucosuria, hyperglycemia, or psychiatric abnormalities. If back pain occurs, x-rays of the spine should be taken for possible osteoporosis or compression fractures. If pathologic fractures occur but the patient's condition requires continuation of corticosteroid therapy, additional Ca and protein are indicated with or without anabolic steroids. Abdominal pain or GI bleeding, major or minor, demands upper GI x-ray study to detect peptic ulcer. Peptic ulceration or severe mental disturbance requires stopping corticosteroids. With acute abdominal crisis (e.g., perforated ulcer), increased corticosteroid dosage is needed during the acute phase or during surgery for its treatment; then the corticosteroid should be gradually withdrawn.

Dietary salt restriction is usually not needed at the outset, and need not be stringent with synthetic glucocorticoids. Body weight should be watched and, if edema develops, diuretics should be given or corticosteroid dosage reduced, or both. Hypokalemic alkalosis can be prevented or corrected with potassium chloride. Disturbances in carbohydrate metabolism may be controlled by dietary readjustment or by proper doses of insulin.

Infections occurring during therapy may be controlled by antibiotics, which should not be given prophylactically, but for emergent infections. If the infecting organisms are not readily treatable by available antibiotics (as in candidiasis), corticosteroids should be discontinued gradually.

Withdrawal of ACTH and Corticosteroids

Treatment with ACTH produces adrenal hypertrophy, but at the same time it suppresses secretion of endogenous ACTH because of the pituitary-suppressive effect of the induced hypercortisolemia. Cessation of ACTH therapy removes the stimulus to adrenocortical secretion, resulting in a temporary state of relative adrenal insufficiency.

Administration of corticosteroids causes atrophy of the adrenal cortex and decreased production of endogenous hormones. Abrupt withdrawal of exogenous corticosteroids produces a hypoadrenal state. Therefore, drug dosage should be decreased gradually when therapy is being discontinued. Adrenal stimulation with exogenous ACTH is not helpful. Adrenal function is usually restored within a few weeks, but relative adrenal insufficiency may occasionally persist for as long as 1 yr or more.

Patients with adrenal or pituitary suppression or both cannot tolerate stress (e.g., surgery, trauma, infection). They must be prepared for surgery by increasing the amount of exogenous corticosteroid before, during, and after the stressful situation. For emergency surgery, an IV solution of hydrocortisone (or one of the synthetic corticosteroids) should be used until oral absorption is possible. After the stress has abated, corticosteroids should be continued in gradually decreasing doses to previous maintenance levels.

A small increase in corticosteroid dosage is advisable for minor surgical procedures, slight injuries, or mild infections. Stressed patients should be watched for fall in BP, weakness, circulatory collapse and shock, or other evidence of adrenal insufficiency.

TESTS OF ADRENOCORTICAL FUNCTION

The best methods of assessing adrenocortical function, in addition to direct measurement of plasma ACTH, plasma corticosteroids, and urinary corticosteroids, are those which depend on the response of plasma or urinary corticosteroid levels to stimulation with ACTH or metyrapone, or suppression by exogenous corticosteroids. These are more specific and safer than the provocative tests. (For further discussion of tests, see Chs. 85 and 88.)

252. PROSTAGLANDINS

Prostaglandins **(PGs)** are a group of cyclic fatty acids that possess diverse and potent biologic activities affecting cell function in every organ system. Originally isolated as lipid-soluble extracts from sheep and human prostates, they are found in most mammalian tissues. The parent compound, prostanoic acid, contains a 20-carbon chain with a cyclopentane ring. Variations in the number and position of the double bonds and hydroxyl groups determine the physiologic activities of the different PGs. The important substitutions are on the cyclopentane ring.

PGA_1 primarily affects the cardiovascular-renal system. PGE_1 has hypotensive and other actions. $PGF_{1\alpha}$ has diverse and potent physiologic effects on many organ systems but, unlike PGA_1 and PGE_1, does not lower BP. Although differences exist between PG_1s and PG_2s, in general they are physiologically similar. PGE_3 and $PGF_{3\alpha}$ have also been isolated and described but are found in much lower concentrations and in far fewer tissues than the PG_1 or PG_2 compounds. Recently PGD_2, PGI_2 (prostacyclin), thromboxane A_2, and the leukotrienes have been shown to be major end products of prostaglandin synthesis.

PGs are synthesized ubiquitously in the body from unsaturated fatty acid precursors with high rates of production by the seminal vesicles and renal medulla. These precursors initially are converted to the cyclic endoperoxides PGG_2 and PGH_2 by PG cyclo-oxygenase, and then to various PGs and thromboxanes. PG synthesis is inhibited by aspirin, indomethacin, and other nonsteroidal anti-inflammatory agents. Metabolism takes place mostly in the lungs, renal cortex, and liver. Metabolites are excreted in the urine.

BIOLOGIC ACTIONS

REPRODUCTIVE SYSTEM

PGE and PGF (but not PGAs) induce luteolysis, decrease progesterone secretion, stimulate the gravid uterus to contract at all stages of pregnancy, and act at the hypothalamic-pituitary level as mediators of luteinizing hormone releasing factor (LRF) on luteinizing hormone (LH) secretion.

Effects on the Ovulatory Cycle

It is thought that during the secretory phase of the ovulatory cycle progressively larger amounts of estradiol produced by the maturing follicle increase uterine $PGF_{2\alpha}$ (uterine luteolysin), resulting in luteolysis and decreased progesterone secretion. In the human, $PGF_{2\alpha}$ is probably secreted by the oviduct and delivered directly to the ovary. $PGF_{2\alpha}$ reduces luteal blood flow and inhibits progesterone synthesis; this effect may be mediated through the hypothalamic-pituitary axis, so that $PGF_{2\alpha}$ increases pituitary cAMP. Hypothalamic extracts increase LH release through stimulation of cAMP; prostaglandin antagonists inhibit this stimulation.

Effects on the Uterus

Endogenous $PGF_{2\alpha}$ is present in amniotic fluid, and its plasma concentration rises steadily during pregnancy, reaching high levels immediately prior to delivery. This results in decreased progesterone, an increased uterine sensitivity to oxytocin, and the onset of labor. PGEs and PGFs are useful as 2nd-trimester abortifacients and as oxytocics. In 1st-trimester abortion, they have no advantage over suction curettage. For induction of labor at term, PGs offer little clinical advantage over oxytocin.

CARDIOVASCULAR-RENAL SYSTEMS

PGs have major effects on the cardiovascular-renal system. The isolation and identification of PGA_2 (originally called medullin) and PGE_2 from the rabbit renal medulla was the first direct evidence that the kidney possessed potent vasodilating compounds and, thus, an important antihypertensive function. These PGs, as well as the more recently discovered PGD_2 and PGI_2, also have other important effects on renal blood flow, Na and water excretion, and renin release.

Renal Blood Flow and Sodium and Water Excretion

Administration of PGA, PGE, PGD, PGG, PGH, and PGI all increase renal blood flow and natriuresis. The pronatriuretic action of PGs may be due to nonspecific renovasodilation such as is observed with any renovasodilator (e.g., acetylcholine, bradykinin, etc.). Similarly, the PG precursor arachidonic acid produces a rise in deep cortical and inner medullary flow accompanied by Na and water loss; these actions are inhibited by indomethacin. Loop diuretics (e.g., ethacrynic acid and furosemide) also increase renal blood flow, natriuresis, and urinary PGE excretion, suggesting that they act through PG release.

PGs probably do not directly maintain resting blood flow, but act to oppose renal vasoconstriction due to angiotensin, norepinephrine, sympathetic nervous stimulation, and renal artery occlusion by providing an offsetting vasodilatory action. This is important in diseases such as lupus nephritis, where renal blood flow becomes partially dependent on PG synthesis and release. Administration of indomethacin to such patients results in a marked deterioration of renal function. Thus, such compounds should be administered cautiously in patients with compromised renal blood flow, particularly those in renal failure.

Suppositions regarding the interaction of PGs with the renal handling of Na are controversial. Recent studies have shown a rise in plasma PGA and urinary PGE during volume depletion induced by low Na intake, diuretics, or hemodialysis. The apparent antinatriuretic response of PGs to volume depletion may be due to renin release and increased aldosterone secretion and Na retention.

PGEs may attenuate vasopressin-stimulated adenyl cyclase and the accompanying increase in water movement. Aspirin, indomethacin, or meclofenamate can increase vasopressin-stimulated water reabsorption and maximal urinary osmolality. Thus PGE_2, which is normally secreted by the collecting duct cells, may be a physiologic antagonist of vasopressin acting at the site of vasopressin-induced water movement in the collecting duct cell.

Renin Release and Blood Pressure Regulation

Arachidonic acid, PGA_1, PGA_2, PGE_1, PGE_2, and PGI_2 all stimulate renin production. PG synthesis inhibition results in marked renin reduction and partial inhibition of the natriuretic and antihypertensive effects of loop diuretics, which suggests that volume depletion leads to a reduction in renal blood flow that triggers PG release leading to an increase in renin, angiotensin II, and aldosterone. Theoretically, volume depletion such as that resulting from a low Na intake or diuretic therapy should not lower BP as is clinically observed, since there is a marked activation of the renin-angiotensin-aldosterone axis under these conditions. Possibly the rise in plasma, renal, or local vascular PGs offsets the vasoconstricting effects of angiotensin II, thus lowering BP. The fact that indomethacin and aspirin increase BP in normotensives and hypertensives when plasma renin activity is markedly decreased supports this contention and suggests that inhibition of the vasodepressor PG system allows pressor mechanisms such as the renin-angiotensin system to act unopposed, even at lower plasma concentrations. Clinically, this has important connotations in **Bartter's syndrome** (see Ch. 153) where hyperreninemia, hyperaldosteronism, and hypokalemic alkalosis have been shown to be associated with increased plasma and urinary levels of PG, all of the above being reversed by PG synthesis inhibition with aspirin or indomethacin.

In summary, the evidence supports an antihypertensive function for renal and systemic PGs by antagonizing the vasopressor activity of the renin-angiotensin or the adrenergic nervous systems.

Effects in Hypertensive Humans

The first PG given to a hypertensive human was PGA_2. When given IV, the total calculated peripheral resistance fell as the result of direct peripheral arteriolar vasodilation and a fall in BP associated with a reflex baroreceptor-mediated increase in cardiac output. Subsequently, PGA_1 was shown to have the same mechanism of action as PGA_2. However, following infusion of PGA_1, the BP did not fall immediately; rather, there was an initial increase in renal blood flow and in Na, K, and water excretion. Later, when the BP fell to normotensive levels, there was a return to control levels in renal blood flow and in Na, K, and water excretion. Thus, normotension induced by PGAs is associated with normal renal blood flow and normal Na and water excretion, in contrast to antihypertensive agents that compromise renal blood flow. The initial natriuresis and diuresis are associated with about a 10% fall in plasma volume, which is in part responsible for the hypotensive action of PGA. Thus, PGA_1 and PGA_2 appear to act as "ideal" antihypertensives, reversing many of the known abnormalities in patients with essential hypertension. They favorably influence total peripheral resistance, renal resistance, cardiac output, baroreceptor activity, plasma volume, and Na and water balance.

GASTROINTESTINAL SYSTEM

Effect on Smooth Muscle

PGE and PGF contract longitudinal smooth muscle in both the small and large intestine. By contrast, PGEs inhibit contraction of circular smooth muscle, whereas PGFs increase circular muscle peristalsis. Since PGE and PGF are normally present and released by various stimuli in the GI tract, intestinal peristalsis may be mediated partially by PGs. In patients with medullary carcinoma of the thyroid, PGs are released in large amounts into the bloodstream, with an associated watery diarrhea. However, there is little other clinical evidence to delineate their role in peristalsis.

Gastric Secretion and Intestinal Absorption

Administration of PGE_1, PGE_2, and PGA_1 and their 16,16-dimethyl analogs inhibits gastric HCl secretion stimulated by histamine, pentagastrin, or food ingestion. In addition, experimental ulcer production in animals (produced by pyloric ligation, stress, or steroids) is prevented by administration of PGEs and PGAs either orally, IV, or by inserting them into the jejunum. The hyperchlorhydric and ulcerogenic effects of aspirin and indomethacin are probably the result of inhibition of synthesis of antichlorhydric and antiulcerogenic PG.

Both PGE_1 and cholera toxin produce a rise in mucosal adenyl cyclase and cAMP that is capable of inhibiting intestinal Na and water transport. Diarrhea due to cholera toxin may be mediated by increased cAMP and inhibition of luminal Na and water transport resulting from increased intestinal PG release.

The most likely clinical GI use of PGEs and PGAs will be in the treatment of gastric hyperacidity and peptic ulceration. However, advantages over existing drugs and effectiveness in long-term therapy must be demonstrated.

RESPIRATORY SYSTEM

PGE_1 and PGE_2 relax human bronchiolar smooth muscle and increase pulmonary blood flow; $PGF_{2\alpha}$ and leukotrienes C and D contract bronchiolar smooth muscle and inhibit the bronchodilating effect of isoproterenol. This suggests that pulmonary synthesis and release of PGE may be clinically significant in increasing pulmonary blood flow in response to hypoxia. Furthermore, some bronchial asthma may be caused by a reduced PGE to PGF ratio, leading to bronchial vasoconstriction. PGE produces bronchial dilation by different mechanisms than isoproterenol, since PGE is devoid of β-adrenergic stimulation. Theoretically, PGEs could be very useful in the treatment of asthma, since they are metabolized by the lung and would not have the cardiovascular side effects associated with β-adrenergic stimulants.

THE INFLAMMATORY RESPONSE

At high concentrations PGs are considered anti-inflammatory because they ameliorate experimental adjuvant arthritis in animals. However, at low concentrations, PGEs, PGD_2, and PGG_2 elicit all the typical signs of the inflammatory response. Furthermore, increased amounts of PGs are present in local areas of inflammation. PG synthetase activity is inhibited by nonsteroidal anti-inflammatory agents, and many of their actions, (as well as their side effects) have been attributed to this inhibition of PG synthesis.

PGs may play an important role during systemic, as well as local, inflammatory reactions. Pyrogen-induced fever, which has been associated with an increased $PGF_{2\alpha}$ content in the third ventricle, can be reduced by prior administration of a PG synthetase inhibitor such as indomethacin or aspirin. The analgesic effect of aspirin in headache may also be mediated by inhibition of PG synthesis, since PGE produces severe headaches in man.

In rheumatoid arthritis, large amounts of PGs in the synovium may contribute to inflammation and to periarticular bone demineralization from their Ca resorptive actions.

IMMUNE RESPONSE

PGEs and PGAs, in contrast to the PGFs, have marked effects on the immune response. PGEs are capable of inhibiting antigen-induced histamine release from Ig-antibody-sensitized basophils and lung tissue; they are much more potent than catecholamines in this respect. Furthermore, catecholamine inhibition of histamine release can be blocked by propranolol, whereas no such inhibition occurs with PGE_1. Delayed hypersensitivity reactions are also inhibited. Lastly, phytohemagglutinin-induced lymphocyte transformation, as measured by protein DNA and RNA synthesis, is not only inhibited by cAMP but also by PGA and PGE, with a concomitant return of cell morphology toward normal.

In general, PGEs and PGAs inhibit both T and B cell activity, possibly in the former instance by inhibition of lymphokines. Since PGE is released by activated macrophages, a homeostatic feedback action of PGE inhibition of lymphocyte activation is believed to exist. However, it is premature to speculate on the clinical usefulness of PGs in various immune responses.

METABOLIC AND ENDOCRINE EFFECTS

Many of the actions of the PGEs and PGFs can be explained on the basis of their ability to stimulate or inhibit the production of cAMP, an intracellular hormonal mediator. Tropic hormones such as LH, TSH, and ACTH interact with cell membrane receptors, leading to increased PG synthetase activity and PG production. The increased levels of PG in turn stimulate the enzyme adenylate-cyclase to convert ATP to cAMP where a biological action would be exerted. However, the same PG may accelerate production of cAMP within the target cell in one tissue and *inhibit* the activation of adenylatecyclase in another tissue. This puzzling and unexplained nonspecificity of PG interaction with cAMP does not occur with other hormone mediators. Specificity must relate to factors other than biochemical interactions between PGs and cAMP.

PGE_1 inhibits the lipolytic effects of ACTH, epinephrine, and glucagon, which act primarily by increasing adenylatecyclase activity and intracellular cAMP. In vitro, the antilipolytic effect of PGE_1 is associated with a decrease in cAMP, suggesting that it inhibits adenylatecyclase. Studies in humans, however, have shown both lipolytic and antilipolytic effects.

In carbohydrate metabolism, PGEs inhibit both basal and glucose-stimulated insulin release. Since PG synthesis inhibition with salicylates markedly improves the acute insulin response to glucose in diabetics, an excessive stimulation of pancreatic PG production has been postulated to be a contributing factor to impaired insulin release and carbohydrate intolerance in these patients.

PGs stimulate thyroid, adrenal, and pituitary hormonogenesis. Thyroid hormone production is increased by PGE_1, apparently a TSH-like action with stimulation of adenylatecyclase and cAMP. In the adrenal gland, PGE_2 accelerates corticosterone and aldosterone production, the former in association with a rise in cAMP. PGs also act on pituitary hormone secretion, releasing growth hormone, prolactin, ACTH, and LH.

HEMATOLOGIC EFFECTS

PGE_1 is a potent inhibitor of platelet aggregation, while PGE_2 stimulates platelet aggregation. Both actions are mediated through cAMP, with PGE_1 causing a rise in cAMP and PGE_2 a fall in cAMP during the corresponding changes in platelet adherence. Although platelets normally contain PGE_2, which is released during clotting, the major compounds now believed to be involved in the clotting process are the recently discovered PGI_2 **(prostacyclin)** and thromboxane A_2 **(TXA_2)**. PGI_2 is synthesized ubiquitously in blood vessel walls from arachidonate derived either from the vessel wall or from the platelet. It is the most potent of all inhibitors of platelet aggregation and has vascular dilatory properties as well. Conversely, TXA_2, a potent platelet aggregator and vasoconstrictor, is synthesized primarily by the platelet.

Following endothelial damage, platelets adhere to the subendothelial connective tissue releasing catecholamines, serotonin, ADP, and TXA_2, which promote platelet aggregation through a decrease in platelet cAMP formation. TXA$_2$ is thought to be the main compound in this platelet aggregating process; it has a very short half-life and breaks down into the stable thromboxane B$_2$ (TXB$_2$). Conversely, once an interaction between the platelet and the vessel wall takes place, PGG$_2$ is converted to PGI$_2$ (prostacyclin), which tends to promote vasodilation and inhibition of TXA$_2$-induced platelet aggregation by stimulation of cAMP (FIG. 252–1). Whether or not physiologic or pathologic clot formation ensues appears to depend on the relative amount of PGI$_2$ versus TXA$_2$ production. The net effect appears to be on the anticlotting activity, since inhibition of TXA$_2$ synthesis occurs during the entire platelet lifetime and its effects on vascular PGI$_2$ synthesis is shorter lasting. This may be one of the main mechanisms involved in the beneficial effects of aspirin on thrombotic processes. The status of PGI$_2$ and TXA$_2$ in this process have important implications for the control of deep venous thrombosis, myocardial infarction, stroke and hypertension, and are receiving widespread attention.

CALCIUM AND BONE METABOLISM

PGE$_1$ and PGE$_2$, in contrast to the other PGs and thromboxanes, are potent stimulators of bone resorption in vitro, acting by increasing cAMP synergistically with parathyroid hormone. Excess PGE has been demonstrated in hypercalcemic animals with experimental tumors. In such animals, indomethacin markedly reduces hypercalcemia caused by the tumor secreting PGE$_2$. In humans, the hypercalcemia of some solid tumors has been shown to be associated with low parathyroid hormone secretion and excessive plasma PGE, with both the high PGE levels and hypercalcemia being reversed by indomethacin. In contrast, hematologic tumors, hyperparathyroidism, and breast tumors are not associated with PG-induced hypercalcemia.

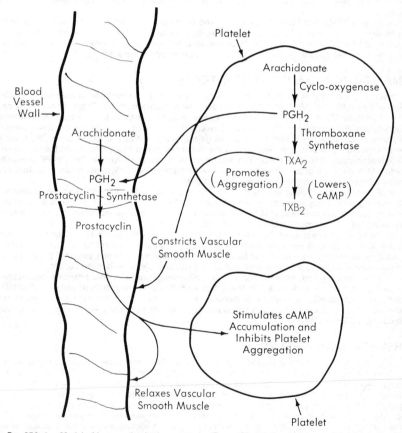

FIG. 252–1. **Model of human platelet homeostasis.** (From "Modulation of human platelet function by prostacyclin and thromboxane A$_2$," pp. 83–88, by R. R. Gorman, in *Federation Proceedings* Vol. 38, No. 1, January 1979. Used with permission of the Federation of American Societies for Experimental Biology, and the author.)

NERVOUS SYSTEM

Central

In animals, PGE_1 has sedative, tranquilizing, and anticonvulsant actions. Further, PGEs antagonize norepinephrine inhibition of Purkinje cell discharge, leading to the theory that PGs may function as CNS neuromodulators.

Peripheral

PGE_1, PGE_2, and PGI_2 reversibly inhibit norepinephrine in the peripheral nervous system with consequent inhibition of synaptic transmission. Presumably, a feedback mechanism exists whereby sympathetic stimulation leads to an increase in PGE_2 formation, thus reducing the amount of norepinephrine released.

OCULAR EFFECTS

In animals, PGE_1, PGE_2, and $PGF_{2\alpha}$ produce miosis; thus light-adapted miosis may be mediated in large part by local PG synthesis and release in the iris. This action is inhibited by norepinephrine. In rabbits, PGEs cause an increase in intraocular pressure, but this effect has not been duplicated in other animals. Nevertheless, PG antagonists may be found clinically useful in certain forms of wide-angle glaucoma.

POTENTIAL THERAPEUTIC APPLICATIONS

TABLE 252-1 summarizes the potential therapeutic applications of the PGs. A major problem regarding the clinical use of PGs is finding an appropriate delivery system, particularly for the PGEs and PGFs. Since these compounds are metabolized during circulation through the lungs and appear to function as local hormones, their use would be limited if given orally or parenterally. However, PGA and PGI compounds, which are not degraded in the lungs, conceivably could be given as oral systemic antihypertensive agents.

In general, unique delivery systems that can provide local delivery are required for clinical use; e.g., the intrauterine administration of PGE or PGF for abortion. Aerosol delivery of a PGE preparation may be feasible in bronchial asthma, and oral administration of PGA or PGE may have value for inhibition of HCl secretion.

TABLE 252-1. POTENTIAL THERAPEUTIC APPLICATIONS OF THE PROSTAGLANDINS

Hypertension	Patent ductus arteriosus
Congestive heart failure	Hypercalcemia of malignancy
Induction of labor	Periodontal inflammation
Infertility	Cholera and certain diarrheal states
Coronary and deep thrombosis	Burns
Peptic ulceration	Lupus erythematosis
Gastric hyperacidity	Glaucoma
Bronchial asthma	Nasal congestion

Modified from "The Prostaglandins," by J. B. Lee, in *Textbook of Endocrinology*, ed. 8, edited by R. H. Williams. Copyright 1974 by W. B. Saunders Company. Used with permission of W. B. Saunders Company and the author.

253. ANTIHISTAMINES

Many antihistamines, in addition to blocking the effects of histamine, have other useful therapeutic effects. Pharmacologic differences among them are most apparent in their sedative, antiemetic, and other CNS effects, and in their anticholinergic, antiserotonin, and local anesthetic properties.

Histamine

Histamine is widely distributed in mammalian tissue. In man the highest concentrations are in skin, lungs, and stomach. Histamine is present mainly in the intracellular granules of mast cells, but there is also an important extra-mast-cell pool in the gastric mucosa, with smaller amounts in the brain, heart, and other organs. The release of histamine from the mast-cell storage granules can be triggered by physical tissue disruption, various chemicals (including tissue irritants, surface active agents, and polymers), and most prominently by antigen-antibody interactions.

The specific homeostatic function of histamine remains unclear. Its actions in man are exerted primarily on the cardiovascular system, extravascular smooth muscle, and exocrine glands, and they appear to be mediated by 2 distinct histamine receptors, termed H_1 and H_2.

Histamine H_1 Receptor Effects

Cardiovascular system: Histamine is a potent arteriolar and capillary dilator that can cause extensive peripheral pooling of blood and hypotension. It also increases capillary permeability by distortion of the endothelial lining of the postcapillary venules, with widening of the gap between endothelial cells and exposure of basement membrane surfaces. This accelerates loss of plasma and plasma proteins from the vascular space and, combined with arteriolar and capillary dilation, can produce circulatory shock. Histamine also dilates cerebral vessels, which may be a factor in histamine headache.

The "**triple response**" is mediated by local *intracutaneous* histamine release, causing (1) local erythema from capillary dilation, (2) wheal due to local edema from increased capillary permeability, and (3) flare from a neuronal reflex mechanism producing a surrounding area of arteriolar vasodilation. **Other smooth muscle:** In man, histamine may cause severe bronchoconstriction in susceptible individuals. Histamine also stimulates GI motility. **Exocrine glands:** Histamine increases salivary and bronchial gland secretions. **Sensory nerve endings:** Local instillation of histamine may produce intense itching.

Histamine H_2 Receptor Effects

Cardiovascular system: Histamine increases heart rate, contractility, and coronary blood flow, and the H_2 receptor plays some role in the histamine vasodilator and depressor response. Administration of either a histamine H_1 or H_2 receptor blocker alone has little effect on histamine-induced vasodepression, but H_1 and H_2 receptor antagonists together can reverse the hypotension, suggesting that both types are involved in the cardiovascular response to histamine.

Exocrine glands: Histamine is a potent stimulator of gastric acid secretion. **Leukocytes:** H_2 receptor stimulation inhibits histamine release from sensitized basophils and mast cells (negative feedback system).

HISTAMINE H_1 RECEPTOR ANTAGONISTS

The conventional antihistamines, now termed histamine H_1 receptor antagonists, possess a substituted ethylamine side-chain (similar to that of histamine) linked to one or more cyclic groups. The similarity between the ethylamine moiety of histamine and the substituted ethylamine structure of the H_1 receptor antagonists suggests that this molecular configuration is important in receptor interactions. Histamine H_1 receptor antagonists appear to act by competitive inhibition; they do not significantly alter histamine production, release, or metabolism.

The H_1 blocker antihistamines are generally well absorbed from the GI tract following oral or rectal administration. Onset of action usually occurs within 15 to 30 min, with peak effects attained in 1 h; duration of action is generally 3 to 6 h, but some of these drugs act considerably longer.

Antihistaminic effects of H_1 receptor antagonists are noted only in the presence of increased histamine activity. They block the effects of histamine on GI tract smooth muscle, but in man the allergic reaction of the bronchial smooth muscle is not dependent primarily on histamine release and does not respond effectively to antihistamines. Histamine H_1 receptor antagonists effectively block histamine-induced increased capillary permeability and sensory nerve stimulation, thus inhibiting the wheal, flare, and pruritus responses. However, these agents are only partially effective in reversing histamine-induced vasodilation and hypotension.

Clinically useful effects other than histamine antagonism are discussed below.

Therapeutic Indications

Antihistamines are useful for treating the symptoms of allergies, including seasonal hay fever, allergic rhinitis, and conjunctivitis. They are mildly effective in perennial vasomotor rhinitis. Acute and chronic urticaria and certain allergic dermatoses respond well, and pruritus may be alleviated. They are also useful for treating minor transfusion incompatibility reactions and systemic reactions to IV x-ray contrast media. The H_1 blockers have no role, however, in the treatment of bronchial asthma or systemic anaphylaxis. They provide little benefit in the therapy of the common cold, but because of their anticholinergic effects (see below) they may control rhinorrhea.

TABLE 253–1 summarizes the dose, route, and frequency of administration of some commonly available histamine H_1 receptor antagonists. These agents are all effective H_1 receptor blockers; their pharmacologic differences are primarily in the type and intensity of their other effects.

Other Clinically Useful Effects

CNS depression is prominent with many H_1 receptor antagonists, and they have been used as sedatives, tranquilizers, and hypnotics. Most have some anticholinergic properties that may account centrally for modest antiparkinsonian activity and peripherally for symptomatic relief of rhinorrhea in URIs. Several of the H_1 blockers are potent local anesthetics and are often applied to the skin in the form of creams and lotions to reduce itching. However, topical application of antihistamines incurs considerable risk of drug sensitization. Some antihistamines have a quinidine-like effect on myocardial conduction and have had limited use as antiarrhythmics.

TABLE 253-1. DOSAGE, ADMINISTRATION, AND PREPARATIONS OF SOME HISTAMINE H_1 RECEPTOR ANTAGONISTS

Agent	Usual Adult Dosage	Route of Administration	Frequency	Available Preparations
I. Alkylamines				
Brompheniramine maleate	4–8 mg	Oral	t.i.d. or q.i.d.	4-mg tablets 2 mg/5 ml elixir 8- and 12-mg tablets (timed-release)
	5–20 mg	IM or IV	q 6–12 h	10 mg/ml
Chlorpheniramine maleate	2–4 mg	Oral	q 6–8 h	2-mg tablets 4-mg tablets 2 mg/5 ml syrup 8- and 12-mg tablets (timed-release)
	5–20 mg	IV, IM, or s.c.		10 mg/ml injection 100 mg/ml injection
Dexchlorpheniramine maleate	2 mg	Oral	t.i.d. or q.i.d.	2-mg tablets 2 mg/5 ml syrup 4- and 6-mg tablets (extended-release)
Dimethindene maleate	2.5 mg	Oral	once daily or b.i.d.	2.5-mg tablets (extended-release)
Triprolidine HCl	2.5 mg	Oral	b.i.d. or t.i.d.	2.5-mg tablets 1.25 mg/5 ml syrup
II. Ethanolamines				
Carbinoxamine maleate	4–8 mg	Oral	t.i.d. or q.i.d.	4-mg tablets 4 mg/5 ml elixir 8- and 12-mg tablets (timed-release)
Dimenhydrinate	50–100 mg	Oral	q 4 h	50-mg tablets 12.5 mg/4 ml liquid
	100 mg	Rectal	b.i.d.	100-mg suppositories
	50 mg	IM or IV	q 4 h	50 mg/ml injection
Diphenhydramine HCl	25–50 mg	Oral	t.i.d. or q.i.d.	25-mg capsules 50-mg capsules 12.5 mg/ml syrup 12.5 mg/5 ml elixir
	10–50 mg	IV or deep IM	q 3–4 h	10 mg/ml injection 50 mg/ml injection
Diphenylpyraline HCl	2 mg	Oral	q 4 h	2-mg tablets 5-mg capsules (sustained-action)
Doxylamine succinate	12.5–25 mg	Oral	q 4–6 h	12.5- and 25-mg tablets 6.25 mg/5 ml syrup
III. Ethylenediamines				
Tripelennamine citrate	25–50 mg	Oral	q 4–6 h	37.5 mg/5 ml elixir
Tripelennamine HCl	25–50 mg	Oral	q 4–6 h	25-mg tablets 50-mg tablets 50- and 100-mg tablets (timed-release)

(Continued)

TABLE 253-1. DOSAGE, ADMINISTRATION, AND PREPARATIONS OF SOME HISTAMINE H₁ RECEPTOR ANTAGONISTS *(Cont'd)*

Agent	Usual Adult Dosage	Route of Administration	Frequency	Available Preparations
IV. Piperazines				
Cyclizine HCl	50 mg	Oral	q 4–6 h	50-mg tablets
	50 mg	IM	q 4–6 h	50 mg/ml injection
Hydroxyzine HCl	25–100 mg	Oral	t.i.d. or q.i.d.	10-mg tablets
				25-mg tablets
				50-mg tablets
				100-mg tablets
				10 mg/5 ml syrup
	25–100 mg	IM	q 4–6 h	25 mg/ml injection
				50 mg/ml injection
Meclizine HCl	25–50 mg	Oral	once daily	12.5-mg tablets
				25-mg tablets
V. Phenothiazines				
Methdilazine HCl	4 mg	Chewable	q 6–12 h	8-mg tablets
	8 mg	Oral	b.i.d. or q.i.d.	4 mg/5 ml syrup
Promethazine HCl	12.5–25 mg	Oral	b.i.d.	12.5-mg tablets
				25-mg tablets
				50-mg tablets
				6.25 mg/5 ml syrup
				25 mg/5 ml syrup
	12.5–25 mg	Rectal	q 2 h prn	12.5-mg suppositories
			q 6 h	25-mg suppositories
				50-mg suppositories
	12.5–25 mg	IV or IM	q 6 h	25 mg/ml injection
		IM only	q 6 h	50 mg/ml injection
Trimeprazine tartrate	2.5 mg	Oral	q.i.d.	2.5-mg tablets
				2.5-mg/5 ml syrup
				5-mg capsules (timed-release)
VI. Other				
Cyproheptadine HCl	4 mg not to exceed 0.5 mg/kg/day	Oral	t.i.d. or q.i.d.	4-mg tablets
				2 mg/5 ml syrup

The alkylamines have relatively little sedative effect and are useful as H₁ antihistamines for daytime use. The ethanolamines are significant CNS depressants and are useful as sedatives and hypnotics, although they are less potent and dependable than the barbiturates and other central depressants. The ethanolamines also have marked anticholinergic properties. The ethylenediamines produce less CNS depression but more GI side effects than the ethanolamines.

Diphenhydramine, an ethanolamine derivative, and dimenhydrinate, its chlorotheophyllinate salt, the phenothiazine congener promethazine, and the piperazines, cyclizine and meclizine, are all used to prevent or treat motion sickness and relieve the nausea and vertigo associated with labyrinthitis. Cyclizine, hydroxyzine, and meclizine have been implicated as teratogens in animals, and probably should not be given during pregnancy. The phenothiazine group of H₁ receptor antagonists, notably promethazine, are useful as tranquilizers and are effective in controlling the nausea associated with radiotherapy and certain antineoplastic drugs; for this latter use they are less effective than prochlorperazine and chlorpromazine.

Side Effects and Toxicity

Undesirable effects of the H₁ antihistamines include anorexia, nausea, vomiting, constipation, diarrhea, epigastric distress, decreased alertness, impaired ability to concentrate, muscular weakness, and drowsiness. Topical administration can produce dermatitis and urticaria. Blood dyscrasias, such as leukopenia, agranulocytosis, thrombocytopenia, and hemolytic anemia, occur relatively rarely. The manifestations of overdosage are dominated by anticholinergic effects, including dry mouth, palpitations, chest tightness, urinary retention, visual disturbances, convulsions, hallucinations, and, later, by respiratory depression, fever, hypotension, and mydriasis. The common side effects of several histamine H₁ receptor antagonists are summarized in TABLE 253-2.

TABLE 253–2. COMMON SIDE EFFECTS OF HISTAMINE H_1 RECEPTOR ANTAGONISTS

Agent	Peripheral Atropine Effects	Sedation	Stimulation	Antiemetic	Antitremor	Local Anesthetic	GI Effects	Other
Pyrilamine (mepyramine)	+	+	+	0	0	++	++	
Antazoline	+	+	+	−	−	++	−	Antiarrhythmic
Diphenhydramine	+++	+++	+	++	++	+	0	
Chlorpheniramine	++	+	+	−	−	−	−	
Triprolidine	+	+	+	−	−	−	−	Photosensitization
Cyclizine	+	+	+	+++	−	−	+	
Meclizine	+	+	+	+++	−	−	+	
Promethazine	+++	+++	+	++	+	+++	+	Photosensitization
Cyproheptadine	++	++	+	−	−	++	−	Serotonin antagonism

Key: +++ = well-marked effect; ++ = moderate effect; + = effect present; 0 = no effect; − = insufficient information.
Modified from "Today's Drugs," Jan. 24, 1970, pp. 217–219. Used with permission of the *British Medical Journal.*

HISTAMINE H₂ RECEPTOR ANTAGONISTS

CIMETIDINE

In contrast to the H_1 receptor antagonists, which possess a side-chain similar to the ethylamine moiety of histamine, the H_2 receptor blocking agent, cimetidine, incorporates a longer and more complex side-chain but retains the imidazole ring structure of histamine. This suggests that the imidazole ring is necessary for interaction of both histamine and cimetidine with the H_2 receptor site.

Cimetidine is a competitive inhibitor of histamine at H_2 receptors. In the stomach it blocks gastric acid secretion stimulated by histamine, gastrin, parasympathetic activity, and food, and diminishes both basal and nocturnal gastric acid secretion. Pepsin secretion, gastric juice volume, and intrinsic factor secretion are also reduced. In the gall bladder, H_2 blockers potentiate cholecystokinin-induced contraction. Cimetidine augments delayed hypersensitivity responses in the immune system.

Cimetidine is well absorbed from the GI tract after oral administration. Onset of action begins within 30 min after an oral dose, and peak effects are attained in 1 to 2 h. IV administration produces a more rapid onset of activity. Duration of action is generally 4 to 6 h with either route. Cimetidine is largely eliminated unmetabolized from the body mainly by renal excretion, but several hepatic metabolites have been identified after oral doses. In renal failure the dosage should be reduced to prevent drug accumulation (see TABLE 253–3). Hemodialysis removes cimetidine, and patients on dialysis may need an extra dose at the end of the procedure.

Therapeutic Indications

The principal indication for cimetidine is treatment of peptic ulcer disease. Cimetidine 300 mg orally q.i.d. (with meals and at bedtime) relieves pain and promotes ulcer healing. This regimen should be continued until the ulcer heals, and then be followed by maintenance therapy using 400 to 800 mg daily for 6 mo. Maintenance therapy can be given as a single 400-mg dose at bedtime. Cessation of therapy is often associated with recurrence of ulcers, and perforation of duodenal ulcers has occurred when cimetidine was stopped abruptly. Patients should be cautioned that ulcers may recur weeks or months after discontinuing therapy.

Cimetidine has also been used to treat gastric ulcers, but clinical trials have given conflicting results and the role of cimetidine in gastric ulcer therapy is unclear.

Cimetidine is useful in the symptomatic treatment of patients with **Zollinger-Ellison syndrome.** Incapacitating pain, diarrhea, and peptic ulcers are often controlled with cimetidine, using oral doses of up to 2400 mg daily; surgery can often be avoided. Treatment should be continued as long as necessary for symptomatic relief; however, cimetidine has no effect on tumor progression.

Prophylactic cimetidine administration reduces gastric mucosal damage and GI bleeding associated with aspirin use, and decreases the risk of upper GI hemorrhage after renal transplantation. Cimetidine is also a useful adjunct to oral pancreatic enzyme replacement in patients with pancreatic insufficiency. It reduces acid-peptic degradation of the ingested enzymes.

Severe metabolic alkalosis may develop after prolonged nasogastric suction, especially in patients with gastric hypersecretion. Cimetidine reduces both gastric juice volume and acid output, thus effectively decreasing acid loss and allowing correction of the metabolic alkalosis.

Side Effects and Toxicity

Cimetidine is generally well tolerated. A mild increase in serum creatinine and serum transaminases often occurs without apparent clinical significance. Diarrhea, rash, drug fever, and myalgias have been reported, and mental confusion with agitation may develop, especially in elderly patients with impaired renal function. Cimetidine increases plasma prolactin levels, and gynecomastia and, rarely, galactorrhea may ensue. Other rare side-effects include ileus in patients with extensive burns, sinus bradycardia, hypotension after rapid IV injection, and hyperglycemia. Reversible bone-marrow suppression with granulocytopenia, thrombocytopenia, and anemia has occurred. Potentiation of warfarin-type anticoagulants may occur with concomitant administration of cimetidine.

TABLE 253–3. RECOMMENDED CIMETIDINE DOSAGE BASED ON
RENAL FUNCTION

Creatinine Clearance	Approximate Half-life	Recommended Dose Interval (300 mg dose)
Normal	2 h	q 6 h
50–90 ml/min	2 ½ h	q 6 h
20–35 ml/min	3 h	q 8 h
< 10 ml/min	4 h	q 12 h

254. ANTICOAGULANTS

Agents used to prevent or counteract pathologic intravascular clotting consist of anticoagulants (notably heparin and vitamin K antagonists), thrombolytic agents, and drugs that impair platelet function.

Indications
Anticoagulants, especially heparin, are useful in treating acute deep (and extensive superficial) venous thrombosis, pulmonary embolism, acute arterial embolization of the extremities, and disseminated intravascular coagulation. Given prophylactically, they prevent (1) recurrent embolism secondary to intracardiac thrombi in patients with rheumatic and arteriosclerotic heart disease and recurrent venous thromboses in thrombophilic individuals and (2) thromboembolic complications of surgery or delivery in selected surgical or obstetric patients. Anticoagulants reduce formation of atrial thrombi in patients with atrial fibrillation, and heparin reduces the incidence of thromboembolic complications from mural thromboses in patients with myocardial infarction, but vitamin K antagonists do not. Heparin is also used to prevent thromboembolic complications in patients undergoing organ transplantation, open-heart surgery with extracorporeal circulation, and hemodialysis. Anticoagulation has less value in cerebrovascular disease and in transient ischemic attacks.

Thrombolytic agents decrease the period of morbidity in patients with venous and pulmonary embolism and are most useful in arterial embolism. They have no established value in cerebral thrombosis and myocardial infarction.

Drugs that impair platelet function are valuable in preventing emboli from prosthetic heart valves and in preventing myocardial infarction and strokes in patients with cerebral vascular disease.

Contraindications
Anticoagulants should not be given to patients with a hemorrhagic diathesis (unless it is due to disseminated intravascular coagulation; see Ch. 95), hypertension, suspected current hemorrhage (excluding hemoptysis due to pulmonary embolism or mitral stenosis), or dissecting aneurysms. The possible benefit of anticoagulants must be weighed against the risk of hemorrhage in patients with a history of GI bleeding; in those with severe hepatic disease, SBE, thoracic or abdominal aneurysms, or pericarditis complicating acute myocardial infarction; and in those anticipating surgery (especially of the lung, prostate, spinal cord, or brain). Vitamin K antagonists should *not* be given to pregnant women; rather, heparin (which does not pass the placental barrier) may be given.

HEPARIN

Pharmacology and Action
Several steps in blood coagulation are mediated by serine proteases. These enzymes can be inhibited by a serine protease inhibitor, antithrombin III. The affinity of this inhibitor for serum proteases is markedly increased by heparin; thus heparin inhibits several steps in blood coagulation. In high concentration, heparin also inhibits platelet aggregation.

Laboratory Control
The Lee-White clotting time and the activated partial thromboplastin time **(PTT)** are the usual tests for monitoring heparin therapy. Significant inhibition of the coagulation process with minimal risk of bleeding is achieved when the Lee-White clotting time is 20 to 30 min (about 2 to 3 times the normal control) or when PTT times are 1½ to 2 times the normal control. The PTT method is now most commonly used because of its convenience.

Administration and Dosage (see also in Ch. 37)
Heparin should be prescribed in USP units rather than in milligrams, since different preparations vary in potency. (NOTE: There are claims that the USP heparin unit is 10 to 15% more potent than the IU used in all Canadian and European studies.) The preparation of choice is aqueous sodium heparin given IV (intermittently or continuously) or s.c. The repository form is not recommended because absorption is irregular and hematomas may form at the site of injection.

Low-dose heparin is indicated for prophylaxis in high-risk surgical patients. It is not suitable for prophylaxis in maximal challenges, such as after hip replacement. The dosage is 5,000 u. s.c. (deep intrafat) injection 2 h before surgery and 5000 u. q 8 to 12 h thereafter for 7 days or until the patient is fully ambulatory, whichever is longer.

Medium-dose heparin is indicated for patients with active phlebitis and with pulmonary emboli and, in the lower dosage ranges, for prophylaxis in patients with hip replacements. The dosage is 20,000 to 60,000 u./day, usually given by continuous IV infusion, although it may be given by intermittent IV push q 6 to 8 h and monitored by PTT as described above.

Large-dose heparin is indicated in patients with massive pulmonary embolism, in a dosage of 60,000 to 120,000 u./day given by continuous infusion. Dosages should be decreased to medium-dose range after 24 h.

Adverse Reactions

Hemorrhage is the chief complication of therapy with any anticoagulant. Toxic reactions are unusual, but hypersensitivity reactions (e.g., fever, skin rashes, rhinitis, bronchial asthma, chest pain, hypertension) may appear, as well as thrombocytopenia. Transient alopecia 3 to 4 mo after administration has been reported. Osteoporosis and spontaneous fractures may occur in patients taking heparin for 6 mo or longer.

Management of Complications

Minor bleeding manifestations (ecchymoses at the site of injections, microscopic hematuria, bleeding from gums) or a prolongation of clotting times to > 60 min can usually be controlled by withholding the next scheduled dose of heparin and reducing subsequent doses. If major bleeding occurs, protamine, a protein that combines with heparin to form an inactive complex, should be used to neutralize the anticoagulant effect of heparin. One ampul containing 50 mg/5 ml diluted with isotonic saline 20 ml and injected IV over a 5-min period (CAUTION: *Rapid injection may cause hypotension, dyspnea, and bradycardia*) neutralizes about 5000 u. of heparin and usually suffices to counteract overheparinization. The therapeutic effect of protamine may be checked by testing the clotting time 5 min after the injection. Higher doses are usually needed for post–open-heart surgery with extracorporeal circulation. Blood transfusions may be required to cover major blood losses but do not reduce the anticoagulant effect of overheparinization.

VITAMIN K ANTAGONISTS

The coumarin and the indandione derivatives are the 2 major groups. Dicumarol and warfarin, coumarin derivatives, are the safest and most commonly used preparations.

Pharmacology and Action

These drugs are given orally and act as competitive inhibitors of vitamin K, suppressing the synthesis of the 4 vitamin-K-dependent factors in the liver: prothrombin (Factor II); Factor VII; Factor IX (PTC [plasma thromboplastin component], Christmas factor); and Factor X (Stuart-Prower factor). They do so by blocking the carboxylation of glutamic acid residues of protein precursor clotting factors. Gamma-carboxyl glutamic acid is necessary for the activity of the vitamin-K-dependent clotting factors. In the absence of vitamin K, the descarboxy precursor proteins are inactive. Even when the synthesis of the vitamin-K-dependent factors is markedly inhibited, these factors do not reach therapeutically depressed levels for a few days. Their approximate biologic half-lives are: Factor VII, 5 to 6 h; Factor IX, 20 to 24 h; Factor X, 40 h; prothrombin, 60 h.

Laboratory Control

Prothrombin time is the test used in controlling dosage of vitamin K antagonists.

Preparations and Administration

Coumarin derivatives: Dicumarol has slow onset of effect (48 to 96 h) and prolonged action (elimination half-time, 1 to 4 days depending on dose); it is well suited for long-term anticoagulation. *Dosage* on the first day is 300 mg; 2nd day, 200 mg; 3rd and following days, usually 37.5 to 100 mg, depending on daily prothrombin time.

Warfarin has intermediate to prolonged action (elimination half-time, 50 h), is easy to control, and is suited for both long- and short-term anticoagulation. The *dosage* on the first day is 30 to 40 mg; 2nd day, 10 to 20 mg; thereafter, depending on daily prothrombin time, 2 to 25 mg, but usually in the 5- to 10-mg range.

Phenprocoumon: Slow onset (48 to 72 h); persistent action (5 to 8 days). *Dosage*: First day, 21 to 24 mg; 2nd day, 9 mg; maintenance dose, 0.75 to 6 mg, depending on prothrombin time.

Indandione derivatives: Anisindione has slow onset of effect and long action. *Dosage* on the first day is 300 mg; 2nd day, 200 mg; 3rd day, 100 mg; and maintenance dosage, 25 to 250 mg/day, depending on prothrombin time.

Phenindione has short to intermediate action. *Dosage* on the first day is 200 mg (given in 2 divided doses); the maintenance dosage is 25 to 150 mg/day (in divided doses), depending on prothrombin time.

Potentiators and Antagonists (see also Ch. 240)

The action of coumarin and indandione derivatives may be potentiated by various drugs and factors, including broad-spectrum antibiotics (which suppress intestinal flora that produce vitamin K); phenylbutazone, chloral hydrate, salicylates, quinine, and quinidine, which displace coumarin from its bound form, making more available to the liver; and any form of hepatocellular damage. The therapeutic response to coumarins may be decreased significantly by simultaneous use of barbiturates, haloperidol, glutethimide, griseofulvin, or antihistamines, agents that enhance hepatic microsomal enzyme activities, thereby increasing catabolism of the anticoagulant.

Side Effects and Toxicity

Except for hemorrhages, side effects with the coumarin derivatives are rare and consist of rashes, nausea, vomiting, and diarrhea. A more serious effect is a toxic vasculitis leading to hemorrhagic infarction and necrosis of the skin and subcutis. The indandione derivatives are more toxic than the coumarin derivatives. Agranulocytosis, thrombocytopenia, hepatitis, nephropathy, and exfoliative dermatitis have been reported after their use.

Management of Complications

Minor bleeding episodes (e.g., microhematuria, ecchymoses, bleeding from the gums) are common and do not demand discontinuation of therapy. Major bleeding occurs in about 3 to 5% of patients receiving long-term anticoagulant treatment. If the prothrombin activity is > 10%, the bleeding is often due to some underlying organic pathologic change (duodenal ulcer, kidney disease, carcinoma of the GI tract); hence, a thorough diagnostic study should be performed.

If the prothrombin activity is excessively reduced (< l0%) but there is **no bleeding**, omission of 1 dose of the short-acting or 2 doses of the long-acting anticoagulants, daily monitoring of the prothrombin time, and a slight reduction in the subsequent doses are often the only corrective actions required.

Mild bleeding with or without excessive reduction of the prothrombin activity can usually be controlled by phytonadione (vitamin K_1) 5 to 10 mg orally. An excessively depressed prothrombin activity will rise to a safe level in 8 to 12 h.

Moderately severe bleeding should be treated with phytonadione 10 to 20 mg IM. The prothrombin time should be tested b.i.d.; if necessary, a 2nd dose of phytonadione should be given 24 to 48 h after the 1st (the biologic half-life of phytonadione is less than the half-life of long-acting vitamin K antagonists).

For life-threatening bleeding, the preferred therapy is Factor IX complex, human, a concentrate of the vitamin-K-dependent clotting factors (prothrombin and Factors VII, IX, and X). The contents of 1 bottle (500 u.) dissolved in saline 20 ml contains the clotting factor activity equivalent to 500 ml of normal human plasma; 1500 u. (60 ml) are given by IV infusion over a 15- to 30-min period. In addition, phytonadione 20 mg is given IM or IV (*slowly*). Massive blood losses are best replaced with whole blood. Fresh blood is not necessary because the coagulation factors that are depressed in these conditions are present in nearly normal amounts in stored blood. If the patient has been massively overdosed with a long-acting vitamin K antagonist, a 2nd dose of phytonadione may be needed after 24 to 48 h, depending on the prothrombin time activity.

Surgery: If minor or major elective surgery or tooth extraction must be performed in a patient receiving coumarin or indandione anticoagulants, the drug should be discontinued until the prothrombin time has risen to about 35 to 40%, when surgery can be performed without a significantly increased risk of bleeding. Phytonadione administration should be **avoided** because of the increased risk of thromboembolic complications after abrupt termination of anticoagulation. Anticoagulant therapy should be reinstated after surgery. For major emergency surgery, treatment should be administered as described for life-threatening bleeding, above.

Combination Therapy with Heparin and Vitamin K Antagonists

Heparin and vitamin K antagonists in full doses may be given simultaneously for the first 2 to 3 days. Immediate anticoagulation is achieved with heparin, and usually the vitamin-K-dependent factors are sufficiently depressed after 3 days of therapy with warfarin or dicumarol so that heparin may then be discontinued. This procedure is used for patients with acute deep thrombophlebitis *without* pulmonary embolism for whom a lengthy hospitalization is not anticipated. Alternatively, heparin may be given for the first 7 to 14 days or until the patient becomes ambulatory and then vitamin-K-dependent inhibitors are added. Prothrombin times and PTT's should be performed simultaneously on the 3rd day of combined therapy at least 4 h after the last heparin injection. If the prothrombin time is < 30% in the presence of a PTT of < 40 seconds, heparin can be discontinued (note that high concentrations of heparin also inhibit prothrombin activity; if the PTT is > 40 seconds, the assays should be repeated about 4 h later).

Termination of Therapy

When therapy is to be terminated, the dosage should be reduced gradually over several weeks because a rebound phenomenon with increased frequency of thromboembolic complications is thought by some to follow sudden discontinuation of vitamin K antagonists after long-term administration.

THROMBOLYTIC THERAPY

Streptokinase and urokinase have been extensively studied but are not widely used, in part because of the need for specialized laboratory control; nonetheless, both agents are available commercially. The major uses are in massive pulmonary embolism and in peripheral arterial embolism. Allergic reactions may occur with streptokinase.

AGENTS THAT IMPAIR PLATELET FUNCTION

These agents act in general by inhibiting the synthesis of a parent prostaglandin from its precursor, arachidonic acid. This parent molecule can be converted to many other prostaglandins, including thromboxane A_2, a potent platelet aggregator (see under HEMATOLOGIC EFFECTS in Ch. 252). Agents that impair platelet function should be avoided in patients who are on anticoagulant therapy as noted above or who have a bleeding tendency of any kind. Therapeutic dosage ranges have not been firmly established, but aspirin 1.2 gm/day, sulfinpyrazone 600 mg/day, or dipyridamole 300 mg/day is commonly used. When used in combinations, dosages of each of these agents may be decreased. However, 300 mg/day of aspirin alone may be adequate.

255.   DIURETICS

Drugs that promote urine formation by increasing the GFR or by decreasing reabsorption in the renal tubules.

Diuretics are commonly used to prevent or eliminate edema; they improve function of vital organs and relieve symptomatic distress. Edema is always secondary to an underlying disorder and, except when due to obstruction of veins or lymphatics, represents an attempt by the body to restore its intravascular volume. Thus, its treatment should always be accompanied by other measures.

Diuretics are also used in nonedematous states such as hypertension, hypercalcemia, idiopathic hypercalciuria, and nephrogenic diabetes insipidus. This chapter emphasizes the pharmacology of diuretics and their clinical application; uses in specific disorders are discussed elsewhere in this volume.

General Guidelines

Since the success of a diuretic program is affected by the amount of Na in the diet, Na restriction usually accompanies use of a diuretic. In mild edema, such as may occur in chronic congestive heart failure, a "no-added salt" diet (about 2 to 4 gm [87 to 174 mEq] Na) will generally suffice; when Na retention is severe, a 1 gm (43 mEq) Na diet (the minimum most patients can manage at home) may be required. In the hospital, reduction of dietary Na to 500 mg (22 mEq) daily may occasionally be necessary in severe edema or poorly responsive patients.

Potent diuretics profoundly reduce ECF (and therefore intravascular) volume. Thus diuresis that is too rapid can produce **hypovolemia,** with orthostatic hypotension, tachycardia, azotemia, and impaired cardiac and CNS function.

Hypokalemia is probably the most common adverse effect of diuretics. Nearly all diuretics in effective doses, except those noted below to be K-sparing, inhibit Na and water reabsorption in the nephron at a point proximal to the site in the distal tubule where K is secreted. Thus they increase the load of Na and water delivered to the distal tubule where K secretion partly depends upon Na delivery. In some edematous patients, elevated aldosterone levels also augment K secretion. Serum K must be closely monitored when initiating diuresis, and supplemental K should be given to patients with low or low-normal values. Alternatively, a K-sparing diuretic may be used.

The combination of hypovolemia and hypokalemia frequently results in metabolic alkalosis. Since most potent diuretics produce urine in which Cl is the predominant anion with little or no HCO_3, the HCO_3 concentration in ECF is increased and that of Cl depressed. Hypokalemia also enhances renal HCO_3 reabsorption. The **hypokalemic-hypochloremic metabolic alkalosis** that results is not an indication that the diuretic should be discontinued, because the alkalosis and K deficit can be treated (or

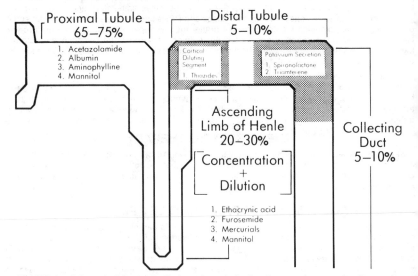

FIG. 255–1. **Schematic diagram of a single nephron,** indicating the normal ranges of sodium reabsorption (expressed as percent of filtered load) for each segment and the major site of action for various diuretics.

prevented) with potassium chloride. The more palatable K salts (e.g., potassium bicarbonate, potassium citrate, potassium gluconate, or potassium acetate) deliver an alkali equivalent and thus will not correct the metabolic alkalosis. *Enteric-coated K preparations cause small-bowel ulcerations and should be avoided.*

Except in an emergency, therapy is begun with a single diuretic. Intermittent administration (once or twice/wk) is often sufficient to control fluid accumulation safely during the early stages of illness. As the disease state progresses, the dosage and frequency usually have to be increased. Since the principal sites of action within the nephron have been localized, appropriate drug combinations with additive effects can then be selected for patients who become refractory to a single-drug program.

In the following discussion, individual diuretics are classified by primary site of action within the nephron, as schematically diagrammed in Fig. 255-1. Table 255-1 summarizes the effect of the most important diuretics on urinary excretion of Na, K, Cl, HCO_3, and PO_4 ions.

DISTAL TUBULAR DIURETICS

Thiazide and Related Sulfonamide Diuretics

The thiazides are sulfonamide derivatives and include bendroflumethiazide, benzthiazide, chlorothiazide, cyclothiazide, hydrochlorothiazide, hydroflumethiazide, methyclothiazide, polythiazide, and trichlormethiazide. They were the first potent oral diuretics. Certain general statements apply to all thiazides and related sulfonamides such as chlorthalidone, quinethazone, and metolazone. The potency of thiazides varies widely between patients because of such factors as previous treatment and differing mechanisms of fluid retention. The thiazides all have a similar site of action, are equipotent when given in maximal doses, and, except for minor differences in onset and duration of action, are interchangeable.

These agents inhibit renal tubular reabsorption of Na, increasing urinary excretion of both Na and water. They also increase the urinary excretion of Cl and K ions. The thiazides probably have some action throughout the nephron, but their greatest effect appears to be in the distal tubule, at the cortical diluting site. Some carbonic anhydrase inhibitory activity occurs, but this effect is minimal at usual clinical doses; thiazides have little diuretic action in the proximal tubule.

Since the thiazides have a low incidence of side effects and are well tolerated orally, they are generally used before other diuretics. They are effective in edema associated with heart failure, renal and liver disease, pregnancy, the premenstrual syndrome, and edema caused by corticosteroids. Perhaps their most important use is in hypertension, either alone or in combination with other drugs. Thiazides decrease Ca excretion in hypercalciuric patients during chronic administration and also paradoxically reduce the polyuria of nephrogenic and central diabetes insipidus.

Thiazides are rapidly absorbed from the GI tract. The usual initial dose is 50 mg of hydrochlorothiazide orally once or twice daily. The maximum effective dose is 200 mg/day. Diuretic effects usually begin within 1 h. Peak action occurs at 3 to 6 h, and most of the drug is excreted during this interval. Thiazides differ mainly in duration of effect, which allows choice of a particular derivative. For example, trichlormethiazide may act for 24 h, and chlorthalidone for up to 72 h.

Hypovolemia and **hypokalemic metabolic alkalosis** are common with prolonged use of thiazides. Weakness, postural hypotension, and azotemia may result. Azotemia is a manifestation of decreased GFR, secondary to progressive ECF depletion, and is an indication for withholding all diuretics pending further evaluation. Serum K levels must be monitored; they may drop to 2 to 3 mEq/L, and occasionally ECG signs of K deficiency appear. A suitable K preparation (e.g., potassium chloride 40 to 80 mEq/day orally) should be given concurrently with the thiazide if dietary K intake is not adequate, especially during treatment of corticosteroid-induced edema, since steroids also increase K loss. K supplementation may not be needed if low doses, an intermittent dosage schedule, or combi-

TABLE 255-1. URINARY EFFECTS OF DIURETICS

Drug	Maximal Excretion of Sodium (% of Filtered Load)	K^+	Cl^-	HCO_3^-	PO_4^-
Acetazolamide	5	↑	↔ or ↑	↑	↑
Thiazides	8	↑	↑	↔	↔
Mercurials	20	↔ or ↓	↑	↔	↔
Ethacrynic acid	25	↑	↑	↔	↔
Furosemide	25	↑	↑	↔ or ↑	↔ or ↑
Spironolactone	2	↓	↔	↔ or ↑	↔
Triamterene	2	↓	↔	↔ or ↑	↔
Amiloride	2	↓	↔	↔ or ↑	↔

Key: ↑ = increased urinary excretion of ion; ↓ = decreased urinary excretion of ion; ↔ = no change in urinary excretion of ion.

nation therapy with spironolactone or triamterene is used. It is usually unnecessary when thiazides are used for the treatment of hypertension.

Hyperuricemia is a common side effect of the thiazides that is shared with furosemide and ethacrynic acid (see below) and is due to impaired renal excretion of urate, but acute attacks of gout are rare. If thiazides must be used in the presence of severe hyperuricemia, allopurinol will nearly always reduce the serum level by blocking uric acid production.

An infrequent but worrisome side effect of the thiazides is the precipitation or worsening of **hyponatremia.** Since they block one of the Na reabsorptive sites responsible for urinary dilution, thiazides may interfere with water excretion. ECF depletion may induce the neurohypophysis to secrete antidiuretic hormone. Severe hyponatremia by these mechanisms is uncommon and can be corrected by discontinuing the drug or by water restriction.

Thiazides may also **impair glucose tolerance,** which is rarely of consequence in nondiabetic patients, but hyperglycemia in overt or prediabetic patients may be aggravated. This diabetogenic effect can occur with most diuretics.

Hypersensitivity phenomena are unusual, but include thrombocytopenic purpura, leukopenia, photosensitivity, and necrotizing vasculitis. **Other side effects** of thiazides include nausea, vomiting, and rashes. Serious toxicity resulting in exfoliative dermatitis, agranulocytosis, jaundice, acute pancreatitis, or glomerulonephritis is rare.

Metolazone, a nonthiazide sulfonamide diuretic, acts mainly at the cortical diluting segment, similar to the thiazides. The usual daily dose of 5 to 20 mg orally is rapidly absorbed from the GI tract. Natriuresis is comparable to that produced by the thiazides and begins about 1 h after ingestion, with a peak action at 2 h. However, because of enterohepatic recirculation of the drug, natriuretic effects persist for up to 24 h, allowing administration once a day. Another potential advantage of metolazone over thiazides is its effectiveness even with moderate degrees of renal insufficiency. In certain patients who appear refractory to "loop" diuretics, the addition of metolazone may produce a marked natriuresis.

POTASSIUM-SPARING DISTAL TUBULAR DIURETICS

Spironolactone competitively inhibits aldosterone at the distal tubule where Na is reabsorbed and reciprocal K and H ion secretion occurs. It does not affect electrolyte excretion in adrenalectomized animals, but in the presence of aldosterone, spironolactone can increase Na and HCO_3 excretion and decrease K excretion. Spironolactone may be absorbed poorly and promotes Na and water excretion slowly. Its immediate effect is much weaker than that of the mercurials, "loop" diuretics, or the thiazides. Used alone, even in states of severe hyperaldosteronism, it is a relatively weak natriuretic agent, since Na reabsorption proximal to the distal tubule is enhanced. Nevertheless, it is useful as an effective adjunct to K-losing diuretics, particularly when K depletion may cause cardiac arrhythmias (e.g., in patients receiving digitalis).

Because of its different mode of action, spironolactone is useful in resistant cases to potentiate other agents and is most effective in edematous states associated with excessive aldosterone production, such as cirrhosis and the nephrotic syndrome. In congestive heart failure, results are less striking, possibly because hemodynamic factors are more important than hormonal factors in sustaining the edema.

The usual daily dose of spironolactone is 100 mg orally in divided doses, but as much as 400 mg/day may be required, particularly in patients with severe secondary hyperaldosteronism. The usual dose in children is 3.3 mg/kg body wt. Duration of action is 4 to 6 h. It is well tolerated and free of serious toxicity.

Hyperkalemia, the most significant adverse effect, is most likely to occur in uremic patients or those receiving supplemental K. **Metabolic acidosis** and hyperkalemia may occur, particularly in diabetics and patients with a decreased GFR. *Such patients should be treated with extreme caution. They should rarely, if ever, be given spironolactone combined with potassium chloride therapy.* GI irritation has been reported. **Other side effects** are probably related to the drug's structural similarity to progesterone and include painful gynecomastia, hirsutism, and impotence. Spironolactone has been shown to be a tumorigen in chronic toxicity studies in rats; its use should be restricted to conditions in which the benefits justify the potential risks.

Triamterene and **amiloride** are mild natriuretics that decrease K excretion. They apparently act in the distal tubule and retard K loss during thiazide therapy. Their effect is similar to that of spironolactone, but they do not require aldosterone for their action, which can be demonstrated in patients with adrenal insufficiency. The combined effect of either of these drugs and spironolactone may be additive. They can be used interchangeably with spironolactone and may be preferred when the diagnosis of hyperaldosteronism is uncertain.

The usual oral dose of triamterene is 100 to 300 mg/day in divided dosage. It is readily absorbed from the GI tract. Action begins within 2 to 4 h and generally tapers off within 7 to 9 h. However, the maximum therapeutic effect may not appear for several days.

Amiloride is readily absorbed from the GI tract. Action begins within 2 h and lasts for about 24 h. The usual dose is 5 to 10 mg once daily.

Adverse reactions of triamterene and amiloride are uncommon and relatively mild but include nausea, vomiting, leg cramps, and light-headedness. BUN may be reversibly increased and they may at times cause mild H ion retention and **hyperchloremic acidosis**. As with spironolactone, **hyperkalemia** is the major danger, especially in azotemic patients. *Triamterene or amiloride can be dangerous when given concomitantly with K supplementation or in the presence of hyperkalemia.*

DIURETICS THAT ACT PRIMARILY IN THE LOOP OF HENLE

Furosemide and Ethacrynic Acid

Furosemide and ethacrynic acid are the most potent diuretics currently in use (about 5 times as potent as the thiazides). At maximal effectiveness, they can cause as much as 25% of filtered Na to be excreted. Both induce K and H ion depletion, and both interfere with urinary dilution and concentration. They are useful in patients refractory to other diuretics, particularly in chronic renal failure, the nephrotic syndrome, cirrhosis of the liver with ascites, and congestive heart failure. They are effective adjuncts in acute pulmonary edema and hypertensive crisis because IV administration produces a rapid diuresis and a transient reduction in peripheral vascular resistance. Either drug should be given initially in low doses with stepwise increments if necessary. Intermittent dosage regimens allow for correction of electrolyte derangements.

Furosemide, in usual doses, acts primarily in the ascending limb of the loop of Henle by inhibiting active Cl transport. It also has minor activity in the proximal tubule, possibly because it is a weak carbonic anhydrase inhibitor (like acetazolamide, it is a sulfonamide derivative). Normally, the proximal action is not important to natriuresis, but it may be responsible for significant increases in HCO_3 and PO_4 excretion. The urine resulting from a furosemide diuresis has a high Na and Cl content.

Furosemide is rapidly absorbed from the GI tract and is given orally in doses of 40 to 120 mg up to t.i.d. Diuresis usually begins within 30 min, reaches a peak in 1 to 2 h, and is usually complete within 6 to 8 h. About $2/3$ of the dose is excreted in the urine within 24 h; the remainder is excreted in the feces. In congestive heart failure refractory to thiazides, furosemide 40 mg orally once or twice daily is usually adequate. In acute pulmonary edema it should be given as an IV bolus of 20 to 40 mg in 5 to 15 min. Diuresis usually begins within 5 min, reaches a peak in 30 to 60 min, and ends within 3 to 4 h. This dose may be repeated once or twice until other measures to improve cardiac function have taken effect. In refractory edema, up to 240 to 320 mg/day may be needed, along with other diuretics such as thiazides, metolazone, or those that spare K. When large total IV or oral doses are needed, 1 or 2 daily doses are more effective than several smaller divided ones.

Aside from excessive diuresis and hypokalemia, toxicity is rare, but includes GI distress, skin rashes, thrombocytopenia, neutropenia, and paresthesias. Marked kaliuresis is also common, particularly in states of secondary hyperaldosteronism.

Ethacrynic acid is chemically dissimilar to furosemide, but its effects are remarkably similar, and the drugs can be used almost interchangeably. Most of the indications and precautions for furosemide apply. Ethacrynic acid is not a carbonic anhydrase inhibitor and therefore has limited action in the proximal tubule. It acts primarily in the ascending limb by inhibition of Cl transport, and is readily absorbed from the GI tract. It is given in doses of 25 to 100 mg (50 mg is equivalent to 40 mg of furosemide). Diuresis begins 1 to 2 h after oral and within 30 min of IV administration. The response usually lasts 6 to 8 h. Excretion is $2/3$ renal and $1/3$ hepatic.

Side effects of ethacrynic acid usually relate to excessive diuresis or kaliuresis. Less frequent side effects include gastric distress, vomiting, and diarrhea, particularly with long-term administration. GI bleeding has been reported. Large IV doses of ethacrynic acid, particularly in patients with renal insufficiency, can produce transient or permanent bilateral nerve deafness. This adverse effect is rare with furosemide.

Mercurials

The organic mercurial diuretics include mercaptomerin sodium, merethoxylline procaine, and mersalyl with theophylline. They are potent diuretics, but must be given parenterally, and are contraindicated in the presence of renal disease. Therefore, they are seldom used.

However, mercurials are unique among the potent diuretics in being relatively non-kaliuretic. For any degree of natriuresis they cause less kaliuresis than ethacrynic acid or furosemide, and acute administration may produce no kaliuresis; hence, mercurials are used occasionally in cirrhotic patients who have low K intake, or in patients with heart failure in whom acute K loss might precipitate digitalis toxicity.

DIURETICS ACTING IN THE PROXIMAL TUBULE

Carbonic Anhydrase Inhibitors

The enzyme carbonic anhydrase catalyzes the formation of carbonic acid and then of H^+ and HCO_3^- in the renal tubule; its inhibitors decrease the rate of carbonic acid formation and hence H^+ production. Renal tubular secretion of H^+ and reabsorption of HCO_3^- and Na^+ are thereby inhibited. Urinary output is increased because of larger excretion of solutes. **Acetazolamide** is a potent inhibitor of carbonic anhydrase and also inhibits proximal NaCl reabsorption. Other carbonic anhydrase inhibitors include dichlorphenamide, methazolamide, and ethoxzolamide; they are primarily used in treating glaucoma and are not used as diuretics.

Although not usually useful alone, the carbonic anhydrase inhibitors may be combined with more distally acting diuretics, particularly in situations where proximal reabsorption is enhanced. The proximal inhibition produced by acetazolamide delivers more Na to distal sites where the second diuretic can act. Acetazolamide may be used to correct metabolic alkalosis or to potentiate or restore the effectiveness of mercurial diuretics, and it is helpful in glaucoma by decreasing the rate of aqueous humor secretion and reducing intraocular tension.

The usual dose of acetazolamide is 250 to 500 mg orally or IV daily or b.i.d. This dosage may be used effectively on alternate days in some patients. Acetazolamide produces marked kaliuresis, because of increased delivery of Na to distal K secretory sites, and because distal K secretion is enhanced by alterations in intracellular pH produced by the drug. With repeated dosage hypokalemic metabolic acidosis occurs as a result of urinary excretion of potassium bicarbonate, but this effect is self-limiting, since acidosis prevents acetazolamide from producing its usual renal effects. Because of this loss of effectiveness after 2 or 3 days, carbonic anhydrase inhibitors should be given only when an interrupted dosage regimen is feasible. Serious toxicity is infrequent, although large doses may cause drowsiness and paresthesias. Hypersensitivity is rare, with occasional reports of skin rash, fever, and leukopenia.

Aminophylline

Caffeine, theobromine, and theophylline are the major xanthine derivatives, but only the soluble derivative of theophylline, aminophylline, is currently used as a diuretic. Because it is much weaker than other diuretics and it tends to produce nausea and vomiting when given orally, it is used only as an adjunct to other diuretics in refractory edema.

Aminophylline produces renal vasodilation and stimulates cardiac function, thus increasing renal plasma flow and GFR. It may also directly inhibit Na reabsorption in the proximal tubule. Na and Cl excretion are increased, but renal acidification and K excretion are not significantly affected. Delivery of filtrate from the proximal tubule to sites where more distally-acting diuretics exert their major effect is increased. Acid-base disturbances have little effect on the diuretic response. It is given in a dose of 250 to 500 mg IV *slowly* over 20 min to prevent hypotension and peripheral circulatory collapse; children may receive 3 to 4 mg/kg body wt. Peak action occurs after about 30 min but is short-lived (within 2 h). Aminophylline should be given so that this peak coincides with that of the second drug. Reported reactions include dizziness, faintness, nausea and vomiting, palpitations, syncope, and sudden death; all are apparently due to an excessive rate of infusion.

Albumin Human, Concentrated

In nephrotic or cirrhotic patients with hypovolemia due to hypoalbuminemia, diuresis may sometimes be begun only by acutely expanding the intravascular volume. The osmotic effect of concentrated human serum albumin given IV expands the intravascular volume, thus increasing GFR and decreasing Na reabsorption in the proximal tubule. Albumin is most effective when used in conjunction with a diuretic acting in the loop of Henle. After pretreatment with a loop diuretic, 25 or 50 gm of albumin should be infused IV over 30 to 60 min. The dose may have to be repeated every 1 to 2 days, since the albumin is usually retained only transiently in the circulation. Albumin is expensive and should be used only for refractory edema that is life-threatening or that severely limits activity.

Osmotic Diuretics

Mannitol: Any nonreabsorbable solute in the proximal tubule or loop of Henle impairs Na and water reabsorption and thus increases the tubular fluid delivered to the distal nephron. As much as 5 to 10% of the filtered Na may be excreted during osmotic diuresis with IV mannitol. Mannitol is nontoxic, is not metabolized, and is excreted principally by glomerular filtration. Its most important natriuretic action occurs in the ascending limb of the loop of Henle. It is rarely used in the treatment of edema. Mannitol is specifically recommended for enhancing drug excretion (e.g., salicylates and barbiturates) after poisoning, for reducing elevated CSF pressure, and for preventing oliguric renal failure during cardiopulmonary bypass operations.

Mannitol is given as 1 to 2 IV boluses of 12.5 gm administered in 15 to 30 min. To promote diuresis as an adjunct in drug intoxication, 100 to 200 gm may be given over 24 to 48 h. Serious adverse reactions are infrequent if that dose is not exceeded. *Extreme caution must be used in patients with cardiac disease because of the rapid expansion of vascular volume.* The patient must be constantly monitored for signs of circulatory decompensation. *Mannitol should not be used in patients with pulmonary vascular congestion.* Because osmotic diuretics cause more water than Na to be lost, prolonged use may result in water depletion and hypernatremia. Fluid and electrolyte balance should be monitored.

A special use of mannitol is in the reversal of acute oliguria and anuria secondary to hypovolemia and/or hypotension, in which it may prevent or modify the progression to acute renal failure. The mechanism of action is uncertain. If adequate ECF volume expansion does not restore urine flow, 25 gm of mannitol IV should be given cautiously. If urine flow is increased, up to 100 gm/24 h may be given in divided doses to maintain urine flow at approximately 100 ml/h. If the first 1 or 2 doses do not initiate diuresis within 2 h, no additional mannitol should be given since its primary route of excretion is renal.

256. RESPIRATORY DRUGS

NASAL DECONGESTANTS

Nasal decongestants provide symptomatic relief in many respiratory conditions, including allergic rhinitis, hay fever, acute coryza, and sinusitis.

Sympathomimetic Amines as Nasal Decongestants

The most important group of nasal decongestants are the sympathomimetic amines with α-adrenergic receptor stimulating actions; they cause vasoconstriction of the nasal mucosal blood vessels and thereby lessen secretions and edema (see also in ADRENERGIC DRUGS in Ch. 248). Phenylephrine and the longer acting congeners (imidazoline derivatives) are the most useful and are usually applied topically, although oral administration may be preferred if prolonged therapy is indicated.

Topical preparations are available as nasal drops, sprays, or inhalers containing the volatile bases of certain decongestants. Sprays and inhaled vapors reach a greater area of the mucous membrane. Adverse reactions, associated particularly with repeated application of nasal decongestants, include rebound congestion after the effect has worn off, allergic reactions, and **rhinitis medicamentosa,** *a condition of chronic edema of the nasal mucosa caused by over-use of topical nasal decongestants*; it occurs when the drugs are used more frequently than q 3 h and for longer than 3 wk, and is treated by stopping the medication. Individual drugs in the group may have other adverse reactions. For example, systemic absorption of sympathomimetic amines may cause generalized vasoconstriction and tachycardia that may be undesirable in patients with hypertension, heart disease, hyperthyroidism, diabetes, and advanced arteriosclerotic conditions. Systemic absorption of naphazoline and tetrahydrozoline can cause CNS depression and coma in children, especially infants. Sympathomimetic nasal decongestants are contraindicated in patients on monoamine oxidase inhibitor or tricyclic antidepressant therapy.

The common drugs in this group include the following: (1) Phenylephrine (0.125, 0.25, and 0.5% solution), 2 to 3 drops or 2 to 4 sprays q 4 h. (2) Naphazoline (0.05% solution), 3 to 4 drops or 2 to 3 sprays t.i.d. or q.i.d. CAUTION: *Avoid use in children; can cause CNS depression.* (3) Oxymetazoline (0.05% solution), 2 to 4 drops or 2 to 3 sprays b.i.d. *Use with caution in children.* (4) Xylometazoline (0.05 and 0.1% solution), 2 to 3 drops or 1 to 2 sprays t.i.d. or q.i.d. *Use with caution in children.* (5) Ephedrine (1 and 3% solution), 2 to 3 drops b.i.d. or t.i.d. (6) Propylhexedrine (inhaler), two inhalations in each nostril as needed. (7) Other available topical decongestants include epinephrine (0.1%), methylhexaneamine (inhaler), tetrahydrozoline (0.1%), and tuaminoheptane (inhaler and 1% solution).

Oral use: Sympathomimetic agents that are useful as oral decongestants include phenylpropanolamine (25 mg q 3 to 4 h), ephedrine (25 to 50 mg q 3 to 4 h), pseudoephedrine (30 to 60 mg q 3 to 4 h) and phenylephrine (10 mg t.i.d.). Systemic side effects due to sympathomimetic activity occur more frequently by this route, but rhinitis medicamentosa is avoided.

Other Nasal Decongestants

Other drugs are often used in combination with the sympathomimetic amines; e.g., antihistamines when an allergy is involved (e.g., acute allergic rhinitis). They can be administered topically or orally. Intranasal topical corticosteroids (usually dexamethasone) are useful in certain conditions; e.g., vasomotor rhinitis. Dexamethasone is available as a metered spray; the usual dose range is 1 to 2 sprays in each nostril 2 to 3 times/day (each metered spray delivers 0.084 mg of dexamethasone). Systemic absorption is low but may sometimes cause side effects (e.g., adrenal suppression).

COUGH REMEDIES

Cough is a protective reflex (FIG. 256–1) which can serve to expel secretions, exudates, transudates, or extraneous materials from the respiratory tract (see also in COUGH in Ch. 29). When cough is serving a productive function, it should not be suppressed except under special circumstances (e.g., when it is exhausting the patient or preventing rest and sleep). Useless cough should either be suppressed or made productive. Any symptomatic treatment of cough should be accompanied by measures aimed at diagnosis and treatment of the underlying cause.

An **antitussive agent** *inhibits or suppresses the act of coughing by acting on either the central or peripheral components of the cough reflex.*

Centrally Acting Antitussive Agents

These agents suppress the cough reflex by depressing the medullary cough center or associated higher centers. The most commonly used drugs in this group are codeine and dextromethorphan.

Codeine: Codeine has antitussive, analgesic, and slight sedative effects and is especially useful in relieving painful cough. It also exerts a drying action on the respiratory mucosa which may be useful (e.g., in bronchorrhea) or deleterious (e.g., when bronchial secretions are already viscous). The

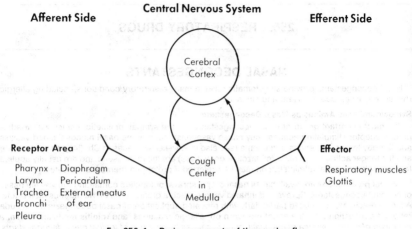

FIG. 256–1. Basic components of the cough reflex.

average adult dose is 8 to 15 mg orally q 3 or 4 h as required, but single doses as high as 60 mg may be necessary. The usual dose for children is 5 to 15 mg daily in divided doses. Codeine in these doses has minimal respiratory depressant effects. Nausea, vomiting, and constipation can occur, as well as tolerance and physical dependence, but abuse potential is low.

Dextromethorphan, a congener of the narcotic analgesic levorphanol, possesses no significant analgesic or sedative properties, does not depress respiration in usual doses, and is nonaddicting. No evidence of tolerance has been found during long-term use. The average dose for adults is 15 to 30 mg 1 to 4 times/day, given as a tablet or syrup; for children 1 mg/kg daily is given in divided doses. Extremely high doses may depress respiration.

Other agents in this group include benzonatate, chlophedianol, levopropoxyphene, and noscapine in the non-narcotic group; and hydrocodone, hydromorphone, methadone, and morphine in the narcotic group.

Peripherally Acting Antitussive Agents

These agents may act on either the afferent or the efferent side of the cough reflex. On the afferent side, they may reduce the input of stimuli by acting as a mild analgesic or anesthetic on the respiratory mucosa, by modifying the output and viscosity of the respiratory tract fluid, or by relaxing the smooth muscle of the bronchi in the presence of bronchospasm. On the efferent side, they may render secretions more easily removable, thereby increasing the efficiency of the cough mechanism. Peripherally acting agents are grouped as follows.

Demulcents are useful against cough arising above the larynx. They act by forming a protective coating over the irritated pharyngeal mucosa. They are usually given as syrups or lozenges and include acacia, licorice, glycerin, honey, and wild cherry syrups.

Local anesthetics such as benzocaine, cyclaine, and tetracaine are used to inhibit the cough reflex under special circumstances; e.g., before bronchoscopy or bronchography. Benzonatate (50 to 100 mg orally t.i.d.), a congener of tetracaine, is a local anesthetic; its antitussive effect may be due to a combination of local anesthesia, depression of pulmonary stretch receptors, and nonspecific central depression.

Humidifying aerosols and steam inhalations exert an antitussive effect by demulcent action and by decreasing the viscosity of bronchial secretions. Inhalation of water as an aerosol or steam, with or without medicaments (sodium chloride, compound benzoin tincture, eucalyptol), is the most common method of humidification. The efficacy of the added medicaments has not been clearly proven.

Expectorants produce their antitussive effect by decreasing the viscosity of bronchial secretions, thus facilitating their removal, and by increasing the amount of respiratory tract fluid, which exerts a demulcent action on the mucosal lining. Most expectorants produce increased secretions through reflex irritation of the bronchial mucosa. Some, like the iodides, also act directly on the bronchial secretory cells and are excreted into the respiratory tract.

The use of expectorants in clinical practice is highly controversial. There are no objective experimental data showing that any of the available expectorants decrease sputum viscosity or ease expectoration. This may be partly due to the fact that the available technology is inadequate for obtaining such evidence. Thus the use and choice of expectorants is often based on tradition and the widespread clinical impression that they are effective in at least some circumstances.

Adequate hydration is the single most important measure that can be taken to encourage expectoration. If this is unsuccessful, additional use of an expectorant may produce the desired result.

Iodides have been used as expectorants for many years for liquefying tenacious bronchial secretions in conditions such as later stages of bronchitis, bronchiectasis, and asthma.

Saturated solution of potassium iodide is the least expensive and the most common iodide preparation used. The initial dose is 0.5 ml orally q.i.d., after meals and at bedtime, and is increased gradually to 1 to 4 ml q.i.d. It is usually given with milk to conceal its unpleasant taste. To be effective, iodides must be taken in doses approaching intolerance. Their usefulness is limited by low patient acceptance due to their unpleasant taste and also by the common occurrence of side effects in the form of acneiform skin eruptions, coryza, erythema of face and chest, and painful swelling of the salivary glands. The side effects are reversible and subside when the medication is stopped. **Iodinated glycerin** is better tolerated than potassium iodide solution but is probably less effective. The usual oral dose is 60 mg (tablets) or 5 ml of elixir q.i.d.; *avoid in patients sensitive to iodide.*

Syrup of ipecac, 0.5 ml orally q.i.d. (NOTE: This is much less than the emetic dose), can be used as an antitussive in patients sensitive to iodides. Some studies have reported that it is useful in relieving spasm of the larynx in children with croup and often clears up thick, tenacious mucus from the bronchi.

Guaifenesin (100 to 200 mg orally q 2 to 4 h) is the most commonly used expectorant in the OTC cough remedies. It has no serious adverse effects. However, there is no clear evidence for its efficacy.

Many of the other traditional expectorants, such as ammonium chloride, terpin hydrate, creosote, and squill, are ingredients in numerous OTC cough remedies. Their efficacy is doubtful and they are probably of little value in the doses contained in most cough preparations.

Mucolytics: Chemical mucolytic agents such as **acetylcysteine** have free sulfhydryl groups that open mucoprotein disulfide bonds, thus reducing the viscosity of mucus. As a rule, their usefulness is restricted to a few special instances such as liquefying thick, tenacious mucopurulent secretions in conditions like chronic bronchitis and cystic fibrosis. Acetylcysteine is given as a 10 to 20% solution by nebulization or instillation. In some cases, airway obstruction may be aggravated by these agents. If this occurs, treatment with the mucolytic may be preceded by inhalation of a nebulized sympathomimetic bronchodilator.

Proteolytic enzymes such as pancreatic dornase are useful only where grossly purulent sputum is a major problem. They seem to offer no advantage over chemical mucolytic agents. Local irritation of the buccal and pharyngeal mucosa and allergic reactions are common after repeated doses.

Antihistamines serve little or no purpose in the treatment of cough. Their drying action on the respiratory mucosa may be helpful in the early congestive phase of acute coryza, but may be deleterious especially to patients with a nonproductive cough resulting from retained viscous secretions.

Decongestants such as phenylephrine are *not* useful in relieving cough.

Bronchodilators such as ephedrine and theophylline may be useful if cough is complicated by bronchospasm. Atropine is *undesirable* because it thickens bronchial secretions.

Drug Combinations in the Treatment of Cough

Many prescription and nonprescription cough remedies are mixtures containing two or more drugs, usually in a syrup. Typically, they may include a centrally acting antitussive, an antihistamine, an expectorant, and a decongestant. Bronchodilators and antipyretics are also often present. These mixtures are aimed at treatment of symptoms of an acute URI, which, in addition to cough, produces nasal congestion, painful throat, headache, etc. They should not be used for management of cough alone. Some combinations of antitussive drugs are rational (e.g., combination of a centrally acting antitussive such as dextromethorphan with a peripherally acting demulcent syrup for cough originating above the larynx). However, the components of some drug mixtures have opposing effects on respiratory tract secretions (e.g., expectorants and antihistamines). Many combination cough remedies contain suboptimal or ineffective concentrations of potentially useful ingredients.

Choice of Drug Therapy in Cough

As a rule, when cough alone is a major problem, it is better to use full dosage of a single drug aimed at a specific component of the cough reflex. The following are some general principles and recommendations: (1) For simple suppression of useless cough, dextromethorphan is preferred, but codeine also is useful. The more potent narcotic antitussives should be reserved for patients in whom analgesic and sedative effects are required. (2) To increase bronchial secretion and liquefy viscous bronchial fluid, adequate hydration (water or steam inhalation) is used; saturated solution of potassium iodide or syrup of ipecac orally may be tried if hydration by itself is unsuccessful. (3) To relieve cough originating in the pharyngeal region, demulcent syrups or lozenges, combined if necessary with dextromethorphan, are used. (4) For bronchoconstriction complicating cough, bronchodilators, possibly combined with expectorants, are advised.

ASTHMA PREPARATIONS

(See BRONCHIAL ASTHMA in Ch. 34)

257. SOME TRADE NAMES OF GENERIC (NONPROPRIETARY) DRUGS

Most prescription drugs placed on the market are given trade names (also called proprietary, brand, or specialty names) to distinguish them as being produced and marketed exclusively by a particular manufacturer. In the USA these names are usually registered as trademarks with the Patent Office and confer upon the registrant certain legal rights with respect to their use. A trade name may be registered as representing a product containing a single active ingredient (with or without additives) or one containing 2 or more active ingredients.

A drug marketed by several companies may have several trade names. Drugs manufactured in one country and marketed in many countries may have different trade names in each country.

Throughout this book we have used nonproprietary or "generic" names whenever possible. However, since trade names are found in many publications and are used extensively in clinical medicine, as a convenience to our readers, we have included a list of most of the drugs mentioned throughout this volume and Vol. II, in alphabetic order, followed by many of their trade names (see TABLE 257–1 below).

With few exceptions, we have limited the trade names in this list to those marketed in the USA. This list is by no means all-inclusive and no effort has been made to list every trade name in current use for each drug. A few are investigational and may subsequently be released as approved new drugs. The inclusion of a drug in this list does not indicate approval or disapproval of its use in any category, neither does it imply efficacy nor safety of its action.

Finally, the reader must keep in mind that many drugs are marketed almost exclusively by their official nonproprietary name and that the inclusion of a trade name in this list does not indicate its endorsement by this book nor its preference as the product of choice.

Constant changes in information resulting from new research and clinical experience, reasonable differences in opinion among authorities, and the unique aspects of individual clinical situations require that the physican exercise his own best judgments in the choice and use of a drug. In particular, the physician is advised to check the product information included in each package of drug that he plans to administer or prescribe, especially if the drug is one that is unfamiliar or is used only infrequently, or is one in which the effective therapeutic levels are close to the toxic levels.

TABLE 257–1. SOME TRADE NAMES OF COMMONLY USED GENERIC DRUGS

Generic Name	Trade Name(s)	Generic Name	Trade Name(s)
Acetaminophen	DATRIL, TYLENOL	Beclomethasone	BECLOVENT, VANCERIL
Acetazolamide	DIAMOX	Dipropionate	
Acetohexamide	DYMELOR	Bendroflumethiazide	NATURETIN
Acetophenazine	TINDAL	Benzalkonium Cl	ZEPHIRAN
Acetylcysteine	MUCOMYST	Benzene	See Lidane
ACTH	See Corticotropin	Hexachloride,	
Allopurinol	ZYLOPRIM	Gamma	
Albuterol	PROVENTIL, VENTOLIN	Benzonatate	TESSALON
Amantadine	SYMMETREL	Benzquinamide	EMETE-CON
Ambenonium	MYTELASE	Benzthiazide	AQUATAG, EXNA
Amikacin	AMIKIN	Benztropine	COGENTIN
Aminocaproic Acid	AMICAR	Mesylate	
Aminophylline	AMINODUR, SOMOPHYLLIN	Benzylpenicilloyl-polylysine	PRE-PEN
Amitriptyline	ELAVIL, ENDEP	Beta-Carotene	SOLATENE
Amoxicillin	LAROTID	Betamethasone	CELESTONE
Amphotericin B	FUNGIZONE	Betamethasone	BENISONE
Ampicillin	AMCILL, OMNIPEN, POLYCILLIN, PRINCIPEN	Benzoate	
		Betamethasone	VALISONE
		Valerate	
Anisotropine	VALPIN	Bethanechol Cl	DUVOID, URECHOLINE
Anthralin	ANTHRA-DERM	Bisacodyl	DULCOLAX
Asparaginase	ELSPAR	Bleomycin	BLENOXANE
Azathioprine	IMURAN	Busulfan	MYLERAN
Baclofen	LIORESAL	Bromocriptine	PARLODEL

TABLE 257–1. SOME TRADE NAMES OF COMMONLY USED
GENERIC DRUGS *(Cont'd)*

Generic Name	Trade Name(s)	Generic Name	Trade Name(s)
Brompheniramine	DIMETANE	Cortisol	CORTEF,
Butaperazine	REPOISE		HYDROCORTONE,
Butorphanol	STADOL		SOLU-CORTEF
Calcifediol	CALDEROL	Cosyntropin	CORTROSYN
Calcitonin-Salmon	CALCIMAR	Co-Trimoxazole, see	
Calcitriol	ROCALTROL	Trimethoprim-	
Calusterone	METHOSARB	Sulfamethoxazole	
Capreomycin	CAPASTAT	Cromolyn Sodium	INTAL
Captopril	CAPOTEN	Cyclacillin	CYCLAPEN
Carbamazepine	TEGRETOL	Cyclandelate	CYCLOSPASMOL
Carbenicillin	GEOPEN, PYOPEN	Cyclizine	MAREZINE
Carbenicillin Indanyl	GEOCILLIN	Cyclobenzaprine	FLEXERIL
Sodium		Cyclopentolate	CYCLOGYL
Carbidopa	LODOSYN	Cyclophosphamide	CYTOXAN
Carbidopa-Levodopa	SINEMET	Cyproheptadine	PERIACTIN
Carbinoxamine	CLISTIN	Cytarabine	CYTOSAR-U
Carboprost	PROSTIN/15M	Dacarbazine	DTIC-DOME
Tromethamine		Dactinomycin	COSMEGEN
Carisoprodol	SOMA	Danazol	DANOCRINE
Carmustine	BiCNU	Danthron	MODANE
Carphenazine	PROKETAZINE	Dantrolene	DANTRIUM
Cefaclor	CECLOR	Dapsone	AVLOSULFON
Cefadroxil	DURICEF	Daunorubicin	CERUBIDINE
Cefamandole	MANDOL	Deanol	DEANER
Cefazolin	ANCEF, KEFZOL	Deferoxamine	DESFERAL
Cefoxitin	MEFOXIN	Demeclocycline	DECLOMYCIN
Cephalexin	KEFLEX	Desipramine	NORPRAMIN,
Cephalothin	KEFLIN		PERTOFRANE
Cephapirin	CEFADYL	Dexamethasone	DECADRON, HEXADROL
Cephradine	ANSPOR, VELOSEF	Dexchlor-	POLARAMINE
Chloral Hydrate	NOCTEC, SOMNOS	pheniramine	
Chlorazepate	TRANXENE	Dextromethorphan	ROMILAR, SYMPTOM 1
Dipotassium		Diazepam	VALIUM
Chlorazepate	AZENE	Diazoxide, IV	HYPERSTAT
Monopotassium		Diazoxide, Oral	PROGLYCEM
Chlorambucil	LEUKERAN	Dicloxacillin	DYNAPEN
Chloramphenicol	CHLOROMYCETIN	Dicyclomine	BENTYL
Chlordiazepoxide	LIBRIUM	Diethylpropion	TENUATE
Chlorhexidine	HIBICLENS, HIBITANE	Digitoxin	CRYSTODIGIN,
Chlormezanone	TRANCOPAL		PURODIGIN
Chlorotrianisene	TACE	Digoxin	LANOXIN
Chlorothiazide	DIURIL	Dihydrotachysterol	HYTAKEROL
Chlorphedianol	ULO	Dimercaprol	BAL
Chlorpheniramine	CHLOR-TRIMETON;	Dinoprostone	PROSTIN E2
	TELDRIN	Diphenhydramine	BENADRYL
Chlorpromazine	THORAZINE	Diphenidol	VONTROL
Chlorpropamide	DIABINESE	Diphenoxylate with	LOMOTIL
Chlorprothixene	TARACTAN	Atropine	
Chlorthalidone	HYGROTON	Dipyridamole	PERSANTINE
Cholestyramine	QUESTRAN	Disulfiram	ANTABUSE
Cimetidine	TAGAMET	Dobutamine	DOBUTREX
Cisplatin	PLATINOL	Docusate Sodium	COLACE
Clindamycin	CLEOCIN	Dopamine	INTROPIN
Clofibrate	ATROMID-S	Doxepin	ADAPIN, SINEQUAN
Clomiphene	CLOMID	Doxorubicin	ADRIAMYCIN
Clonazepam	CLONOPIN	Doxycycline	VIBRAMYCIN
Clonidine	CATAPRES	Doxylamine	DECAPRYN
Clotrimazole	LOTRIMIN, MYCELEX	Droperidol	INAPSINE
Cloxacillin	TEGOPEN	Echothiophate Iodide	ECHODIDE;
Colestipol	COLESTID		PHOSPHOLINE IODIDE
Corticotropin (ACTH)	ACTHAR		

TABLE 257–1. SOME TRADE NAMES OF COMMONLY USED
GENERIC DRUGS *(Cont'd)*

Generic Name	Trade Name(s)	Generic Name	Trade Name(s)
Edetate Disodium (EDTA)	SODIUM VERSENATE	Isoniazid	INH, NYDRAZID
Edrophonium	TENSILON	Isopropamide Iodide	DARBID
Ergocalciferol	CALCIFEROL, DRISDOL	Isoproterenol	ISUPREL
Erythromycin	E-MYCIN, ERYTHROCIN, ILOSONE	Isosorbide Dinitrate	ISORDIL, SORBITRATE
		Isoxsuprine	VASODILAN
Ethacrynic Acid	EDECRIN	Kanamycin	KANTREX
Ethambutol	MYAMBUTOL	Lactulose	CEPHULAC, CHRONULAC
Ethoheptazine	ZACTANE	Levallorphan	LORFAN
Ethosuximide	ZARONTIN	Levarterenol	
Etidronate Disodium	DIDRONEL	Bitartrate, see	
Factor IX Complex (Human)	KONYNE, PROPLEX	Norepinephrine bitartrate	
		Levodopa	DOPAR, LARODOPA
Fenfluramine	PONDIMIN	Levopropoxyphene	NOVRAD
Fenoprofen	NALFON	Levothyroxine (T₄)	SYNTHROID
Fentanyl	SUBLIMAZE	Lidocaine	XYLOCAINE
Flucytosine	ANCOBON	Lincomycin	LINCOCIN
Fludrocortisone	FLORINEF	Lindane	KWELL
Flumethasone Pivalate	LOCORTEN	Liothyronine (T₃)	CYTOMEL
		Liotrix	EUTHROID, THYROLAR
Fluocinolone Acetonide	FLUONID, SYNALAR	Lithium Carbonate	LITHANE, LITHONATE
		Lomustine	CeeNU
Fluocinonide	LIDEX	Loperamide	IMODIUM
Fluoxymesterone	HALOTESTIN	Lorazepam	ATIVAN
Fluphenazine	PERMITIL, PROLIXIN	Loxapine	LOXITANE
Flurandrenolide	CORDRAN	Lypressin	DIAPID
Flurazepam	DALMANE	Mafenide	SULFAMYLON
Furazolidone	FUROXONE	Magaldrate	RIOPAN
Furosemide	LASIX	Maprotiline	LUDIOMIL
Gentamicin	GARAMYCIN	Mazindol	SANOREX
Glutethimide	DORIDEN	Mebendazole	VERMOX
Gold Sodium Thiomalate	MYOCHRYSINE	Mecamylamine	INVERSINE
		Mechlorethamine	MUSTARGEN
Griseofulvin	GRIFULVIN, GRISACTIN, FULVICIN P/G, FULVICIN U/F	Meclizine	ANTIVERT, BONINE
		Meclofenamate	MECLOMEN
		Medroxy- progesterone	PROVERA
Guaifenesin	HYTUSS, ROBITUSSIN		
Guanethidine	ISMELIN	Mefenamic Acid	PONSTEL
Haloperidol	HALDOL	Megestrol Acetate	MEGACE
Haloprogin	HALOTEX	Melphalan	ALKERAN
Hydralazine	APRESOLINE	Menadiol	SYNKAYVITE
Hydrochlorothiazide	ESIDRIX, HydroDIURIL, ORETIC	Menotropins	PERGONAL
		Meperidine	DEMEROL
Hydrocortisone	See Cortisol	Mephenytoin	MESANTOIN
Hydromorphone	DILAUDID	Mephobarbital	MEBARAL
Hydroquinone	ELDOPAQUE, ELDOQUIN	Meprobamate	EQUANIL, MILTOWN
Hydroxychloroquine	PLAQUENIL	Mercaptopurine	PURINETHOL
Hydroxy- progesterone Caproate	DELALUTIN	Mesoridazine	SERENTIL
		Metaproterenol	ALUPENT, METAPREL
		Metaraminol	ARAMINE
Hydroxyurea	HYDREA	Metaxalone	SKELAXIN
Hydroxyzine	ATARAX, VISTARIL	Methadone	DOLOPHINE
Ibuprofen	MOTRIN	Methamphetamine	DESOXYN
Idoxuridine	DENDRID, STOXIL	Methandrostenolone	DIANABOL
Imipramine	PRESAMINE, TOFRANIL	Methaqualone	QUAALUDE, SOPOR
Indomethacin	INDOCIN	Methdilazine	TACARYL
Iodochlor- hydroxyquin	VIOFORM	Methanamine Hippurate	HIPREX
Iron Dextran	IMFERON	Methenamine Mandelate	MANDELAMINE
Isoetharine	BRONKOSOL		
Isoflurophate	FLOROPRYL	Methicillin	STAPHCILLIN

TABLE 257–1. SOME TRADE NAMES OF COMMONLY USED
GENERIC DRUGS *(Cont'd)*

Generic Name	Trade Name(s)	Generic Name	Trade Name(s)
Methimazole	TAPAZOLE	Paramethadione	PARADIONE
Methocarbamol	ROBAXIN	Paramethasone	HALDRONE
Methohexital	BREVITAL	Pargyline	EUTONYL
Methoxsalen	OXSORALEN	Parmomycin	HUMATIN
Methotrimeprazine	LEVOPROME	Penicillamine	CUPRIMINE
Methsuximide	CELONTIN	Penicillin G	BICILLIN, PERMAPEN
Methyldopa	ALDOMET	Benzathine	
Methylphenidate	RITALIN	Penicillin G	PENTIDS
Methylprednisolone	MEDROL	Potassium	
Methyltestosterone	ORETON METHYL	Pencillin G Procaine	DURACILLIN A.S.,
Methyprylon	NOLUDAR		DURACILLIN,
Methysergide	SANSERT		CRYSTICILLIN A.S.,
Metoclopramide	REGLAN		WYCILLIN
Metolazone	DIULO, ZAROXOLYN	Penicillin V	PEN·VEE, V-CILLIN
Metoprolol	LOPRESSOR	Penicilloyl-polylysine,	
Metronidazole	FLAGYL	see	
Metyrapone	METOPIRONE	Benzylpenicilloyl·	
Miconazole	MICATIN, MONISTAT	polylysine	
Minocycline	MINOCIN	Pentaerythritol	PERITRATE
Minoxidil	LONITEN	Tetranitrate	
Mithramycin	MITHRACIN	Pentazocine	TALWIN
Mitomycin	MUTAMYCIN	Pentobarbital	NEMBUTAL
Mitotane	LYSODREN	Pentylenetetrazol	METRAZOL
Molindone	LIDONE, MOBAN	Perphenazine	TRILAFON
Nadolol	CORGARD	Phenacemide	PHENURONE
Nafcillin	UNIPEN	Phenazopyridine	PYRIDIUM
Nalbuphine	NUBAIN	Phenelzine	NARDIL
Nalidixic Acid	NegGRAM	Phenmetrazine	PRELUDIN
Naloxone	NARCAN	Phenobarbital	LUMINAL
Nandrolone	DURABOLIN	Phenoxybenzamine	DIBENZYLINE
Naphazoline	PRIVINE	Phensuximide	MILONTIN
Naproxen	NAPROSYN	Phentermine	IONAMIN
Neostigmine	PROSTIGMIN	Phentolamine	REGITINE
Nitrofurantoin	FURADANTIN,	Phenylbutazone	AZOLID, BUTAZOLIDIN
	IVADANTIN,	Phenylephrine	NEO-SYNEPHRINE
	MACRODANTIN	Phenyl-	DEXATRIM, PROPADRINE
Nitrofurazone	FURACIN	propanolamine	
Nitroprusside	NIPRIDE	Phenytoin	DILANTIN
Norepinephrine	LEVOPHED	Physostigmine	ANTILIRIUM
Bitartrate		Phytonadione	AquaMEPHYTON,
Nortriptyline	AVENTYL		MEPHYTON
Noscapine	TUSSCAPINE	Piperacetazine	QUIDE
Nylidrin	ARLIDIN	Piperazine	ANTEPAR
Nystatin	MYCOSTATIN, NILSTAT	Pipobroman	VERCYTE
Orphenadrine Citrate	NORFLEX	Polythiazide	RENESE
Orphenadrine HCl	DISIPAL	Pralidoxime	PROTOPAM
Oxacillin	BACTOCILL,	Prazepam	CENTRAX
	PROSTAPHLIN	Prazosin	MINIPRESS
Oxandrolone	ANAVAR	Prednisolone	DELTA-CORTEF,
Oxazepam	SERAX		HYDELTRASOL
Oxolinic Acid	UTIBID	Prednisone	DELTASONE,
Oxybutynin	DITROPAN		METICORTEN
Oxymetazoline	AFRIN, DURATION	Primidone	MYSOLINE
Oxymetholone	ADROYD, ANADROL	Probenecid	BENEMID
Oxyphenbutazone	OXALID, TANDEARIL	Probucol	LORELCO
Oxytetracycline	TERRAMYCIN	Procainamide	PRONESTYL
Oxytocin	PITOCIN, SYNTOCINON	Procaine	NOVOCAIN
Pancreatin	ELZYME, VIOKASE	Procarbazine	MATULANE
Pancrelipase	COTAZYM, ILOZYME	Prochlorperazine	COMPAZINE
Pancuronium	PAVULON	Procyclidine	KEMADRIN
Papaverine	CERESPAN, PAVABID	Progesterone	PROGELAN

TABLE 257–1. SOME TRADE NAMES OF COMMONLY USED
GENERIC DRUGS *(Cont'd)*

Generic Name	Trade Name(s)	Generic Name	Trade Name(s)
Promazine	SPARINE	Theophylline	ELIXOPHYLLIN,
Promethazine	PHENERGAN		SUSTAIRE, THEO-DUR,
Propantheline	PRO-BANTHINE		THEOPHYL
Proparacaine	OPHTHETIC, OPHTHAINE	Thiabendazole	MINTEZOL
Propiomazine	LARGON	Thiethylperazine	TORECAN
Propoxyphene	DARVON, DOLENE	Thioridazine	MELLARIL
Propranolol	INDERAL	Thiothixene	NAVANE
Propylhexedrine	BENZEDREX	Thiphenamil	TROCINATE
Protriptyline	VIVACTIL	Thyroglobulin	PROLOID
Pseudoephedrine	SUDAFED	Thyrotropin	THYTROPAR
Pyrantel Pamoate	ANTIMINTH	Ticarcillin	TICAR
Pyridostigmine	MESTINON	Timolol	TIMOPTIC
Pyrimethamine	DARAPRIM	Tobramycin	NEBCIN
Pyrvinium Pamoate	POVAN	Tolazamide	TOLINASE
Quinacrine	ATABRINE	Tolazoline	PRISCOLINE
Quinethazone	HYDROMOX	Tolbutamide	ORINASE
Quinidine	CARDIOQUIN,	Tolmetin	TOLECTIN
	QUINAGLUTE,	Tolnaftate	TINACTIN
	QUINIDEX, QUINORA	Tranylcypromine	PARNATE
Reserpine	RAU-SED, SERPASIL	Tretinoin	RETIN-A
Rifampin	RIFADIN, RIMACTANE	Triacetin	ENZACTIN
Secobarbital	SECONAL	Triamcinolone	ARISTOCORT,
Selenium Sulfide	SELSUN		KENACORT, KENALOG
Semustine	Methyl-CCNU	Triamterene	DYRENIUM
Silver Sulfadiazine	SILVADENE	Trichlormethiazide	NAQUA
Simethicone	MYLICON, SILAIN	Triclofos	TRICLOS
Spectinomycin	TROBICIN	Trifluridine	VIROPTIC
Spironolactone	ALDACTONE	Trifluoperazine	STELAZINE
Stanozolol	WINSTROL	Triflupromazine	VESPRIN
Streptokinase	KABIKINASE, STREPTASE	Trihexyphenidyl	ARTANE, TREMIN
Streptokinase-	VARIDASE	Trimeprazine	TEMARIL
Streptodornase		Trimethadione	TRIDIONE
Streptozocin	ZANOSAR	Trimethaphan	ARFONAD
Sulfacytine	RENOQUID	Trimethobenzamide	TIGAN
Sulfamethizole	THIOSULFIL	Trimethoprim	PROLOPRIM, TRIMPEX
Sulfamethoxazole	GANTANOL	Trimethoprim-	BACTRIM, SEPTRA
Sulfasalazine	AZULFIDINE	Sulfamethoxazole	
Sulfinpyrazone	ANTURANE	Trimipramine	SURMONTIL
Sulfisoxazole	GANTRISIN	Tripelennamine	PBZ
Sulfoxone	DIASONE	Triprolidine	ACTIDIL
Sulindac	CLINORIL	Tromethamine	THAM
Tamoxifen	NOLVADEX	Tropicamide	MYDRIACYL
Terbutaline	BRETHINE, BRICANYL	Tybamate	TYBATRAN
Testolactone	TESLAC	Urokinase	ABBOKINASE,
Testosterone	ORETON		BREOKINASE
Testosterone	DEPO-TESTOSTERONE	Valproic Acid	DEPAKENE
Cypionate		Vancomycin	VANCOCIN
Testosterone	DELATESTRYL	Vasopressin	PITRESSIN
Enanthate		Vidarabine	VIRA-A
Tetanus Immune	HU-TET, HYPER-TET	Vinblastine	VELBAN
Globulin (Human)		Vincristine	ONCOVIN
Tetracycline	ACHROMYCIN V,	Warfarin	COUMADIN, PANWARFIN
	TETRACYN, TETREX	Xylometazoline	OTRIVIN
Tetrahydrozoline	TYZINE	Zomepirac	ZOMAX

258. POISONING

(See also ACCIDENTS AND POISONINGS in Vol. II, Ch. 24)

Some general principles of diagnosing and treating poisoning will be discussed first. Highlights of symptoms and treatment for individual chemicals and drugs, or groups of substances will follow in alphabetic order.

Poisoning due to bacterial or other toxins in food is discussed in Ch. 55. Venomous bites and stings are dealt with in Ch. 259. Alcoholism and drug dependence are discussed in §12. Drug reactions are discussed in Chs. 19, 196, and 242.

GENERAL PRINCIPLES OF TREATMENT

Diagnosis

Worldwide, $>$ 4 million natural and synthetic chemicals have been identified; fortunately, fewer than 3000 cause more than 95% of accidental and deliberate poisonings. The identification of a poison and an accurate assessment of its potential toxicity are critical to a physician's successful management of poisoning. In their absence, one must rely on simple general supportive treatment unless a specific "toxidrome" (toxicologic symptom complex) is pinpointed. Increasingly, physicians are depending upon local or regional "Poison Centers" for technical information.

Poisoning should be considered in the differential diagnosis of any unexplained symptoms or signs, especially in children $<$ 5 yr. Similarly, for the young adult, any disparity between expected history and clinical findings should suggest poisoning. Often the type and speed of onset of the total clinical picture will confirm or refute a suspicion of poisoning. Occasionally, the absence of a specific finding will be of as much import as its presence. Any pertinent history should be secured and the person and premises inspected for traces of drugs, alcohol, etc., particularly for the unconscious patient.

Ingredients, first aid measures, and antidotes often are printed on product containers, but may be inaccurate or out of date. Information about household and industrial chemicals can be obtained through poison centers in all parts of the USA and Europe. Consultation with the centers is encouraged. The nearest center is often listed under Emergency Numbers in the local telephone directory, or is available from the operator.

Immediate Care

1. Determine adequacy of cardiac and respiratory function and begin resuscitation if needed (see CARDIAC ARREST AND CARDIOPULMONARY RESUSCITATION in Ch. 25).

2. Determine quickly what has happened. Identify the substance ingested, its route of entry into the body, and its toxicity potential. *Save any containers and appropriate specimens of the product or of emetic returns.* Determine the need for medical care, recognizing that many substances (see TABLE 258–1) need no further treatment. At all times, recall that overtreatment per se may be a hazard.

3. Unless contraindicated, immediately dilute and remove the toxic substance from the body. A person who has ingested a toxic substance may also have spilled it on the skin and may be inhaling fumes as well.

Ingested poison: Emesis will usually remove more of the toxic substance than will gastric lavage. Immediately induce vomiting with ipecac syrup 15 to 30 ml (1 to 2 tbsp) for children and adults; follow with water or soft drinks (orally; 15 ml/kg for infants; 1 qt [1 L] for adults), and keep the patient actively moving if possible. The dose of ipecac may be repeated in 15 min if necessary. If ipecac is not available, give soapy water, anionic or non-anionic detergent (handwashing liquid detergent) plus water, and induce vomiting by inserting a finger or blunt instrument into the patient's throat. Avoid being bitten. Place a child in the head-down position. Save a portion of the vomitus for analysis. (CAUTION: *Do not induce vomiting if the patient is comatose, is having convulsions [or is likely to], or has ingested petroleum distillates or corrosive substances. Emesis of petroleum distillates is hardly ever indicated unless some other compound has been dissolved in the distillates that requires evacuation [e.g., parathion]*)

When **gastric lavage** is carried out (*do not use lavage if the patient is convulsing or if the ingested substance is corrosive*), use the largest tube appropriate for the patient. For comatose or sedated patients $>$ 2 yr of age, use a cuffed endotracheal tube to prevent aspiration. For those $<$ 2, no cuff is needed on the endotracheal tube because of the snug fit. Have the patient in a head-low position.

TABLE 258-1. GENERALLY NONTOXIC SUBSTANCES*

Ball-point inks (amt. in 1 pen)	Lipstick
Barium sulfate	Magnesium silicate (antacid)
Bathtub toys (floating)	Matches
Blackboard chalk (calcium carbonate)	Methylcellulose
Candles (insect-repellent type may be toxic)	Modeling clay
Carbowax (polyethylene glycol)	Paraffin, chlorinated
Carboxymethylcellulose (dehydrating material packed with drugs, film, etc.)	Pencil lead (graphite)
	Pepper, black (except inhaled in mass)
Castor oil	Petrolatum
Cetyl alcohol	Polyethylene glycols
Crayons (children's: marked A.P., C.P., or C.S. 130–46)	Polyethylene glycol stearate
	Polysorbate (Tweens®)
Detergents, anionic and nonionic	Putty
Dichloral (herbicide)	Red oil (turkey-red oil, sulfated castor oil)
Dry cell battery	Silica (silicon dioxide)
Glycerol	Spermaceti
Glyceryl monostearate	Stearic acid
Graphite	Sweetening agents
Gums (acacia, agar, ghatti, etc.)	Talc
Hormones	Tallow
Kaolin	Thermometer fluid or mercury
Lanolin	Titanium oxide
Lauric acid	Triacetin (glyceryl triacetate)
Linoleic acid	Vitamins, multiple without iron
Linseed oil (not boiled)	

* Substances listed here may, however, be present in combination with phenol, petroleum distillate vehicles, or other toxic chemicals. Since manufactured products may be changed in their composition, this table is intended only as a guide, and prudence requires that a poison center be consulted for up-to-date information.

For adults, physiologic (0.9%) sodium chloride solution or tap water may be used; for children, 0.45% sodium chloride solution is recommended. Introduce lavage fluids in 20- to 30-ml aliquots and remove the stomach contents by siphon or syringe after each instillation. Continue the rinsing procedure until the washings return free of the toxin. After the return is clear, instill a specific antidote if one is available; otherwise instill a slurry of activated charcoal (see below).

The use of **cathartics** remains controversial; some evidence suggests that they may actually enhance absorption rather than promote excretion. If a cathartic is used, it is best limited to sodium sulfate 30 gm dissolved in 250 ml water, with proportionally reduced amounts for children.

When taken internally, **activated charcoal** with its molecular configuration and large surface area adsorbs significant amounts of many poisons, precluding their absorption from the gut. The earlier the charcoal is used, the more effective it is. From 5 to 10 times the amount of charcoal as that of the poison suspected of being ingested should be used. For children < 5 yr the usual dose is 25 gm; for older children and adults, 50 to 100 gm. Charcoal is administered as a slurry (20 to 200 gm in water), preferably by stomach tube; it should be administered before or after syrup of ipecac has been given.

Specific antidotes: While not large in numbers, specific antidotes are remarkably effective—e.g., naloxone in opiate overdoses, atropine in organo-phosphate encounters, physostigmine for tricyclic antidepressants, methylene blue for methemoglobinemia, N-acetylcysteine for acetaminophen. A poison center should be contacted to determine if new specific antidotes have been developed, particularly for new drugs.

Inhaled poison: The patient should be removed from the contaminated environment, his respiration supported, and other personnel protected from contamination.

Skin and eye contamination: Contaminated clothing (including shoes and socks) should be removed. The skin should be thoroughly washed and the eyes flushed out with water (see also Chs. 174 and 215). Helpers should be protected from contamination.

CNS stimulation by the poison may require sedation. Usually, diazepam or a barbiturate is used. In pure amphetamine poisoning, chlorpromazine is the drug of choice. To terminate convulsions, diazepam (5 to 10 mg for adults; 0.1 to 0.2 mg/kg for children) is given slowly IV; phenobarbital (100 to 200 mg for adults and 4 to 7 mg/kg for children) may be used IV or IM to either terminate or prevent the recurrence of a convulsion. Refractory seizures very rarely require general anesthesia; the above measures usually are satisfactory to control the hypoxic and cardiovascular consequences of convulsions.

Continuing Care

Symptomatic and supportive treatment depends on symptoms and signs and on anticipation of the clinical course, based upon identification of the poison. Continuation of the appropriate measures already begun and attempts to enhance the excretion of poison already absorbed are basic considerations. Stimulants are unlikely to be effective and are generally *contraindicated*. **Severe CNS depression** requires support of the circulation and ventilation (see Ch. 32). Endotracheal intubation and, rarely, tracheostomy may be necessary. In suspected or known narcotic poisoning, naloxone should be used (see NARCOTIC ANTAGONISTS in Ch. 247).

Cerebral edema is common in poisonings due to sedatives, carbon monoxide, lead, and other CNS depressants. A 20% mannitol solution (5 to 10 ml/kg) is given slowly IV over a 30- to 60-min period. Corticosteroids are also used (dexamethasone 1 mg/sq m of BSA q 6 h by IV drip). The use of intracranial monitoring with hyperventilation to alter the degree of cerebral edema enjoys widespread favor. The use of "barbiturate coma" in cerebral edema associated with hypoxic episodes has been advocated, but the practice must be considered experimental.

Renal failure may occur in poisoning, and dialysis may be required. Elimination of poisons sometimes can be hastened either by augmenting normal excretory pathways or by using artificial means such as dialysis, depending upon the nature of the poisoning, the availability of the facilities, and the condition of the patient. Flushing out the poison by simply increasing urine volume is rarely helpful. Alkalinization or acidification of the urine can occasionally be helpful (e.g., in acute salicylate ingestions, giving 2 to 3 mEq/kg of sodium bicarbonate IV will augment excretion significantly). In general, weak acids are captured in alkalinized urine and weak bases in acidified urine.

Over the past decade, **hemo-** and **peritoneal dialysis** have been augmented by the development of "**lipid dialysis**," aimed at removal of lipid-soluble substances from the blood, and **hemoperfusion,** to provide an even more rapid and efficient clearance of toxic substances from the blood. However, these technics are of no value if the involved substance has a large "apparent volume of distribution"—i.e., if it is stored in fatty tissue or extensively bound to tissue protein. In select circumstances these technics may be effective, but in many instances their yield is negligible. Thus, while digoxin is rapidly cleared from the blood via hemoperfusion, such a small amount (3 to 5%) of the total body digoxin is present in the blood that hemoperfusion is ineffective. Tricyclic antidepressants are also largely confined to other than the vascular compartment, and the use of hemoperfusion for overdoses is likewise not warranted. TABLE 258-2 lists some representative toxic substances that are dialyzable (see also DIALYSIS, and HEMOPERFUSION in Ch. 146).

Chelating agents are useful in treating poisoning by many metals and other toxic substances. The most commonly used agents, the toxic substances that they effectively chelate, and the usual doses required are given in TABLE 258-3.

Prevention

Widespread, voluntary, and now mandatory use of child-resistant containers (safety caps) has produced a dramatic decline in aspirin poisoning. Labeling of household products and prescription items, use of drug imprints on solid medication forms, improved monitoring of toxic exposures within industry and throughout the environment, widespread public and professional education programs such as that built around the **Mr. Yuk Program**® of the National Poison Center Network, and intense community-wide efforts to make syrup of ipecac available in each home and to make each home aware of the nearest poison center's phone number are examples of successfully implemented and effective activities aimed at preventing poisoning.

TABLE 258-2. SOME DIALYZABLE TOXIC SUBSTANCES*

Alcohols	Chlorates	Methaqualone
Aminoglycoside antibiotics	Chlordiazepoxide	Methyprylon
Amphetamines	Chromic acid	Monoamine oxidase inhibitors
Aniline	Diphenhydramine	Paraldehyde
Barbiturates	Ethchlorvynol	Penicillins
γ-Benzene hexachloride	Ethinamate	Phenytoin (diphenylhydantoin)
(lindane)	Ethylene glycol	Potassium
Boric acid	Glutethimide	Salicylates
Bromides and other halides	Isoniazid	Sodium
Calcium	Lithium	Tetracycline
Camphor	Meprobamate	Theophylline
Cephaloridine	Metals (arsenic, copper, iron,	Thiocyanates
Chloral hydrate	lead, magnesium, strontium,	
Chloramphenicol	zinc)	

* It should be emphasized that only in unusual circumstances is dialysis or hemoperfusion actually clinically useful.

TABLE 258–3. CHELATION THERAPY

Calcium disodium edetate (calcium disodium edathamil; CaNa$_2$-EDTA)
Toxic substances:

Cadmium	Lead	Tungsten
Chromium	Manganese	Uranium
Cobalt	Nickel	Vanadium
Copper*	Radium	Zinc
Copper salts	Selenium	Zinc salts

Dosage: Dilute to 3% (or less) for IV use
Give 25 to 35 mg/kg IV slowly (over 1 h) q 12 h for 5 to 7 days
Interrupt for 7 days, then repeat

Dimercaprol (BAL)
Toxic substances:

Antimony	Chromic acid*	Nickel
Arsenic	Chromium trioxide*	Tungsten
Bichromates*	Copper salts	Zinc salts
Bismuth	Gold	
Chromates*	Mercury	

Dosage: Use 10% BAL in oil; give IM only
1st day: 3 to 4 mg/kg q 4 h
2nd day: 2 mg/kg q 4 h
3rd day: 3 mg/kg q 6 h
Then 3 mg/kg q 12 h every 10 days until recovery

Penicillamine
Toxic substances:

Bichromates	Chromium trioxide	Mercury*
Cadmium	Cobalt	Nickel
Chromates	Copper salts	Zinc salts
Chromic acid	Lead	

Dosage: 15 to 20 mg/kg orally b.i.d.

NOTE: Neither iron nor thallium salts are chelated effectively by the above agents, but each has its own chelating agent (see Iron and Thallium salts in TABLE 258–4, below).

* Chelator of choice.

SPECIFIC POISONS

TABLE 258–4. SPECIFIC POISONS: SYMPTOMS AND TREATMENT

Poison	Symptoms	Treatment
Acetaminophen	Early: Often asymptomatic; mild nausea, vomiting, diaphoresis, pallor; beginning signs of hepatotoxicity; oliguria Later (at 24–48 h): Nausea & protracted vomiting, right upper quadrant pain, jaundice, coagulation defects, hypoglycemia, encephalopathy, hepatic failure; renal failure, myocardiopathy may occur	Emesis; gastric lavage. Monitor plasma drug levels for prognosis; if > 160–200 μg/ml at 4 h, hepatic necrosis may occur; if plasma level >300 μg/ml at 4 h, hepatic damage is almost certain. If given before 18 h, oral N-acetylcysteine (Mucomyst®) 140 mg/kg to start and 70 mg/kg q 4 h for 4 to 18 doses has been effective in preventing significant hepatotoxicity.
Acetanilid Aniline (indelible) inks Aniline oils Chloroaniline Phenacetin (acetophenetidin)	Cyanosis due to formation of methemoglobin & sulfhemoglobin; dyspnea; weakness; vertigo; anginal pain; rashes & urticaria; vomiting; delirium; depression; respiratory & circulatory failure	(1) Inhalation: Give O$_2$; support respiration. Blood transfusion. For severe cyanosis, methylene blue 1–2 mg/kg IV (2) Skin: Remove clothing & wash area with copious soap & water; then as in (1) (3) Ingestion: Give ipecac emetic; if this fails, gastric lavage; then as in (1)

TABLE 258-4. SPECIFIC POISONS: SYMPTOMS AND TREATMENT *(Cont'd)*

Poison	Symptoms	Treatment
Acetic acid: see Acids and alkalis		
Acetone Nail polish remover Ketones Model airplane glues, cements	Inhalation: Bronchial irritation, pulmonary congestion & edema, decreased respirations, dyspnea, drunkenness, stupor, ketosis Ingestion: As above except direct pulmonary effect	Remove from source; evacuate stomach; support respirations; give O_2 & fluids; correct metabolic acidosis
Acetophenetidin: see Acetanilid		
Acetylene gas: see Carbon monoxide		
Acetylsalicylic acid: see ASPIRIN AND OTHER SALICYLATE POISONING in Vol. II, Ch. 24		
Acids & alkalis (see also specific acids & alkalis by name in alphabetic order and INGESTION OF CAUSTICS in Vol. II, Ch. 24)		
Acids Acetic Hydrochloric Nitric Phosphoric Sulfuric (some drain or toilet bowl cleaners, some dishwasher detergents) Alkalis Ammonia water (ammonium hydroxide) Potassium hydroxide (potash) Sodium hydroxide (caustic soda, lye) Carbonates of the above Detergent powders Some drain or toilet bowl cleaners; some dishwasher detergents	Corrosive burns from inhalation, skin contact, eye contact, & ingestion; local pain. In general, alkali is more damaging to the GI tract	Skin or eye: Flush with water for 15 min Ingestion: Dilute with water or milk; *do not stimulate vomiting;* consider gastric lavage if large amounts of alkali granules have been consumed Hospitalize; give opiates for pain; treat shock if present; endoscopy is recommended; tracheostomy may be needed; for verified esophageal burns, give antibiotics and dexamethasone 1 mg/sq m BSA q 6 h or equivalent for 2–3 wk
Airplane glues, cements (model-building): see Acetone, Benzene, Petroleum distillates		
Alcohol, ethyl (ethanol) Brandy, whiskey, & other liquors	Emotional lability, impaired coordination, flushing, nausea & vomiting, stupor to coma, respiratory depression	Emesis; gastric lavage; support respirations; IV glucose to prevent hypoglycemia; dialysis if blood levels > 300–350 mg/100 ml; generous fluid administration as serum alcohol increases serum osmolarity
Alcohol, isopropyl Rubbing alcohol	Dizziness, incoordination, stupor to coma, gastroenteritis, hypotension; *no* retinal injury	Emesis; gastric lavage; IV glucose; correct dehydration & electrolyte changes; dialysis
Alcohol, methyl (Methanol, wood alcohol) Paint solvent Varnish Antifreeze Solid canned fuel	Very toxic: 60–250 ml (2–8 oz) fatal in adults; 8–10 ml (2 tsp) in children. Latency period 12–18 h; headache, weakness, leg cramps, vertigo, convulsions, dimness of vision, decreased respiration	Combat acidosis with IV sodium bicarbonate; give 10% ethanol/5% dextrose solution IV; initially, a loading dose of 0.7 gm/kg of ethanol to impede methanol metabolism is infused over 1 h followed by 0.1 to 0.2 gm/kg hourly to maintain a blood ethanol level of 100 mg/ml; *hemodialysis*

TABLE 258–4. SPECIFIC POISONS: SYMPTOMS AND TREATMENT *(Cont'd)*

Poison	Symptoms	Treatment
Aldrin: see DDT		
Alkalis: see Acids & alkalis		
Aminophylline	Wakefulness, restlessness, anorexia, vomiting, dehydration, convulsions; with hypersensitivity, immediate vasomotor collapse may occur	If ingested use emetic; if by rectal suppository, use enema. Stop medication; obtain theophylline blood level; phenobarbital for convulsions; give parenteral fluids; maintain blood pressure; if serum level > 50–100 mg/100 ml, consider dialysis
Amitriptyline: see Tricyclic antidepressants		
Ammonia gas	Irritation of eyes & respiratory tract; cough, choking; abdominal pain	Flush eyes with tap water for 15 min. *No gastric lavage or emetic.* If severe, positive pressure O$_2$ to prevent pulmonary edema; support respiration
Ammonia water: see Acids & alkalis		
Ammoniated mercury: see Mercury		
Ammonium carbonate: see Acids & alkalis		
Ammonium fluoride: see Fluorides		
Ammonium hydroxide: see Acids & alkalis		
Amobarbital: see Barbiturates		

Amphetamines
  Amphetamine sulfate, phosphate
  Dextroamphetamine
  Methamphetamine
  Phenmetrazine
	Increased activity, exhilaration, talkativeness, insomnia, irritability, exaggerated reflexes, anorexia, dry mouth, arrhythmia, anginal chest pain, heart block, psychotic-like states	Emesis or lavage effective long after ingestion because of recycling via gastric mucosa
		Sedate with chlorpromazine 0.5–1 mg/kg IM or orally q 30 min as needed; reduce external stimuli; hypothermia; combat cerebral edema; peritoneal dialysis (NOTE: For amphetamine/barbiturate combination use ¹/₂ chlorpromazine dose)

Amyl nitrite: see Nitrites		
Aniline: see Acetanilid		
Ant poison: see DDT (chlordane); Thallium salts		
Antifreeze: see Alcohol, methyl; Ethylene glycol		
Antihistamines	Excitation or depression, drowsiness, nervousness, disorientation, hallucinations, tachycardia, arrhythmias, hyperpyrexia, delirium, convulsions	Ipecac emesis, gastric lavage; support respiration and blood pressure; control seizures; physostigmine salicylate 0.5–2.0 mg IM or IV (slowly)
Antimony: see Arsenic & antimony		

Antineoplastic agents
  Methotrexate
  Mercaptopurine
  Vincristine
	Effects on hematopoetic system; nausea; vomiting	Emesis > lavage; supportive care; "folinic acid rescue"

TABLE 258-4. SPECIFIC POISONS: SYMPTOMS AND TREATMENT *(Cont'd)*

Poison	Symptoms	Treatment

Arsenic & antimony
  Antimony compounds
    Stibophen
    Tartar emetic
  Arsenic
    Donovan's solution
    Fowler's solution
    Herbicides
    Paris green
    Pesticides
	Throat constriction, dysphagia; burning GI pain, vomiting, diarrhea; dehydration; pulmonary edema; renal failure; liver failure	Emesis; gastric lavage, then a demulcent; chelation with penicillamine; BAL if patient cannot take oral medication; hydration; treat shock, pain; saline cathartic (sodium sulfate 15–30 gm in water)

Arsine gas	Acute hemolytic anemia	Transfusions; diuresis
Asphalt: see Petroleum distillates		
Aspirin: see ASPIRIN AND OTHER SALICYLATE POISONING in Vol. II, Ch. 24		
Atropine: see Belladonna		
Automobile exhaust: see Carbon monoxide		

Barbiturates
  Amobarbital
  Pentobarbital
  Phenobarbital
  Secobarbital
	Headache, confusion, ptosis, excitement, delirium, loss of corneal reflex, respiratory failure, coma	Empty stomach up to 24 h after ingestion. If immediately after, use ipecac emetic; if sedated, use lavage with cuffed endotracheal tube. Give saline cathartic (sodium sulfate 15–30 gm); good nursing care; support respirations, give O_2; correct any dehydration. Rarely hemodialysis or peritoneal lavage, especially for long-acting barbiturates

Barium compounds
  (soluble)
  Rodenticides
  Depilatories
  Fireworks
  Barium acetate
        carbonate
        chloride
        hydroxide
        nitrate
        sulfide
	Vomiting, abdominal pain, diarrhea, tremors, convulsions, hypertension, cardiac arrest	To precipitate barium in stomach, give 60 gm sodium or magnesium sulfate orally. Then emesis or gastric lavage. 10% Sodium sulfate 10 ml slowly IV; repeat q 15 min until symptoms subside. Control convulsions with diazepam; atropine 0.5–1 mg for colic; sublingual nitroglycerin 1/100–1/50 for hypertension; O_2 for dyspnea & cyanosis; quinidine 0.1–0.3 gm to prevent ventricular fibrillation; correct hypokalemia

Belladonna
  Atropine
  Hyoscyamine
  Hyoscyamus
  Scopolamine
    (Hyoscine)
  Stramonium
	Dry skin and mucous membranes; pupils dilated; flushing, hyperpyrexia; tachycardia, restlessness; coma; respiratory failure; convulsions	Emesis; support respiration; give fluids to augment excretion. May need to catheterize bladder. Physostigmine salicylate 0.5–2.0 mg IM or IV (slowly) may reverse peripheral and central effects

Benzene
  Benzol
  Hydrocarbons
  Toluene
  Toluol
  Xylene
  Model airplane glue
	Dizziness, weakness, headache, euphoria, nausea, vomiting, ventricular arrhythmia, paralysis, convulsions; with chronic poisoning, aplastic anemia	If sizeable ingestion (> 0.5–1 ml/kg), emesis or cautious gastric lavage. Give O_2; support respiration; monitor ECG—ventricular fibrillation can occur. Control seizures with diazepam. Blood transfusion for severe anemia. *Do not give epinephrine*

TABLE 258–4. SPECIFIC POISONS: SYMPTOMS AND TREATMENT *(Cont'd)*

Poison	Symptoms	Treatment
γ-Benzene hexachloride BHC Hexachlorocyclo- hexane Lindane	Irritability, CNS excitation, muscle spasms, atonia, clonic & tonic convulsions, respiratory failure, pulmonary edema	Emesis immediately after ingestion; gastric lavage; saline cathartic (sodium sulfate 15–30 gm). Diazepam for convulsions. Avoid all oils—they promote absorption. Charcoal hemoperfusion p.r.n.
Benzin, benzine: see Petroleum distillates		
Benzodiazepines Dalmane® Librium® Valium®	Sedation to coma, particularly if accompanied by alcohol	Emesis; lavage; supportive care
Benzol: see Benzene		
BHC: see γ-Benzene hexachloride		
Bichloride of mercury: see Mercury		
Bichromates: see Chromic acid		
Bishydroxycoumarin: see Warfarin		
Bismuth compounds	Poorly absorbed. Ulcerative stomatitis, anorexia, headache, rash, renal tubular damage	Ipecac emesis; gastric lavage; respiratory support; BAL (see TABLE 258–3, Chelation Therapy)
Bitter almond oil: see Cyanides		
Bitter almond oil, artificial: see Nitrobenzene		
Bleach, chlorine: see Hypochlorites		
Borates Boric acid	Nausea, vomiting, diarrhea, hemorrhagic gastroenteritis, weakness, lethargy, CNS depression, convulsion, "boiled lobster" skin rash, shock	Ipecac emesis; gastric lavage; remove from skin; prevent or treat electrolyte changes & shock; control convulsions. Dialysis for severe poisoning
Boric acid: see Borates		
Brandy: see Alcohol, ethyl		
Bromates: see Chlorates		
Bromides	Nausea, vomiting, rash (may be acneiform), slurred speech, ataxia, confusion, psychotic behavior, coma, paralysis	Ipecac emesis, gastric lavage for acute ingestion; stop use as medication; promote mild diuresis by hydration & sodium chloride IV; ethacrynic acid is specifically useful. Hemodialysis if severe
Bromine: see Chlorine		
Bulan: see DDT		
Cadmium Solder	Severe gastric cramps, vomiting, diarrhea; dry throat, cough, dyspnea; headache; shock, coma; brown urine, renal failure	Ipecac emesis; gastric lavage with milk or albumin; saline catharsis; respiratory support; hydration; IPPB for pulmonary edema. Give calcium disodium edetate (see TABLE 258–3, Chelation Therapy); *not BAL*
Caffeine	Tachycardia, extrasystoles, convulsions, restlessness, excitement, urinary frequency, tinnitus, nausea, vomiting, tremors	Ipecac emesis; gastric lavage; diazepam; consider dialysis

TABLE 258-4. SPECIFIC POISONS: SYMPTOMS AND TREATMENT *(Cont'd)*

Poison	Symptoms	Treatment
Calomel: see Mercury		
Camphor Camphorated oils	Camphor odor on breath, headache; confusion, delirium, hallucinations, convulsions, coma	Ipecac emesis; gastric lavage. Prevent & treat convulsions with diazepam; support respiration. Lipid dialysis is being explored
Canned fuel, solid: see Alcohol, methyl		

Cantharides
  Spanish fly
  Cantharidin
	Skin and mucous membranes irritated, vesicles; nausea, vomiting, bloody diarrhea; burning pain in back and urethra; respiratory depression; convulsions, coma; abortion, menorrhagia	Avoid all oils; ipecac emesis; support respiration; treat convulsions; maintain fluid balance

Cantharidin: see Cantharides		
Carbolic acid: see Phenols		
Carbon bisulfide: see Carbon disulfide		
Carbon dioxide	Dyspnea, weakness, tinnitus, palpitations	Respiratory support; O_2
Carbon disulfide Carbon bisulfide	Garlic-breath odor, irritability, weakness, manic depression, narcosis, delirium, mydriasis, blindness, parkinsonism, convulsions, coma, paralysis, respiratory failure	Wash skin; emesis; gastric lavage; O_2; diazepam sedation; support respiration & circulation

Carbon monoxide
  Acetylene gas
  Automobile exhaust
  Carbonyl iron
  Coal gas
  Furnace gas
  Illuminating gas
  Marsh gas
	Toxicity varies with length of exposure, conc. inhaled, resp. & circ. rates. Symptoms vary with % carboxyhemoglobin in blood. Headache, vertigo, dyspnea, confusion, dilated pupils, convulsions, coma	100% O_2 by mask; respiratory support if needed; absolute bed rest (minimum 48 h); watch for cardiac problems & for nerve or brain injury (may appear up to 3 wk). *Do not use stimulants.* Hyperbaric O_2 is being used

Carbon tetrachloride
  Cleaning fluids
    (nonflammable)
	Nausea, vomiting, abdominal pain, headache, confusion, visual disturbances, CNS depression, ventricular fibrillation, renal injury, hepatic injury	Wash from skin; emesis or gastric lavage; give O_2; support respiration; monitor renal & hepatic function & treat appropriately. *Avoid alcohol, epinephrine, ephedrine*

Carbonates (ammonium, potassium, sodium): see Acids & alkalis		
Caustic soda: see Acids & alkalis		
Chloral amide: see Chloral hydrate		
Chloral hydrate Chloral amide	Drowsiness, confusion, shock, coma; respiratory depression; renal injury, hepatic injury	Ipecac emesis; gastric lavage; saline enema if rectal instillation; respiratory support

Chlorates
  Bromates
  Nitrates
  Permanent wave
    neutralizers
	Vomiting, nausea, diarrhea, cyanosis (methemoglobin), toxic nephritis, shock, convulsions, CNS depression, coma, jaundice	Ipecac emesis; gastric lavage; early renal or peritoneal dialysis; transfusion for severe cyanosis; *do not use methylene blue.* Treat shock; O_2

Chlordane: see DDT		
Chlorinated lime: see Chlorine		

TABLE 258-4. SPECIFIC POISONS: SYMPTOMS AND TREATMENT *(Cont'd)*

Poison	Symptoms	Treatment

Chlorine (see also Hypochlorites)
  Bromine
  Chlorinated lime
  Chlorine water
	Inhalation: Severe respiratory & ocular irritation, glottal spasm, cough, choking, vomiting; pulmonary edema; cyanosis
	Ingestion: Irritation, corrosion of mouth & GI tract, possible ulceration or perforation; abdominal pain, tachycardia, prostration, circulatory collapse
		Inhalation: O$_2$; respiratory support; watch for & treat pulmonary edema
		Ingestion: Ipecac emesis; gastric lavage; treat shock

Chloroaniline: see Acetanilid		

Chloroform
  Ether
  Nitrous oxide
  Trichloromethane
	Drowsiness, coma; with nitrous oxide, delirium	Inhalation: Respiratory, cardiac, and circulatory support
		Ingestion: Ipecac emesis; gastric lavage; observe for renal and hepatic damage

Chlorophenothane: see DDT		
Chlorothion: see Parathion		
Chlorpromazine: see Phenothiazine		
Chromates: see Chromic acid		

Chromic Acid
  Chromates
  Chromium trioxide
  Bichromates
	Corrosive due to oxidation. Ulcer and perforated nasal septum; severe gastroenteritis; shock, vertigo, coma; nephritis	Milk or water to dilute; BAL (or penicillamine) for severe symptoms; fluids & electrolytes, with caution, to support renal function

Chromium: see TABLE 258-3, Chelation Therapy		
Chromium trioxide: see Chromic acid		
Clonidine	Sedation; periodic apnea; hypotension	Emesis; lavage; supportive care; tolazoline IV and dopamine drip
Coal gas: see Carbon monoxide		
Cobalt: see TABLE 258-3, Chelation Therapy		
Cobaltous chloride: see Nitrogen oxides		
Cocaine	Stimulation, then depression; nausea & vomiting; loss of self-control, anxiety, hallucinations; sweating; respiratory difficulty progressing to failure; cyanosis; circulatory failure; convulsions	Emetic early; gastric lavage; if needed, propranolol 10-15 mg orally or 0.1 mg IV, diazepam for excitation; O$_2$, respiratory & circulatory support
Codeine: see Narcotics		
Copper: see TABLE 258-3, Chelation Therapy		

Copper salts
  Zinc salts
  Cupric sulfate, acetate, subacetate
  Cuprous chloride, oxide
	Emesis; burning sensation, metallic taste, diarrhea; pain; shock; jaundice; anuria; convulsions	Emesis; gastric lavage; penicillamine or BAL (see TABLE 258-3, Chelation Therapy); electrolyte & fluid balance; respiratory support; monitor GI tract; treat shock, control convulsions; monitor for hepatic & renal failure

Corrosive sublimate: see Mercury		
Creosote; cresols: see Phenols		

TABLE 258–4. SPECIFIC POISONS: SYMPTOMS AND TREATMENT (Cont'd)

Poison	Symptoms	Treatment

Cyanides
  Bitter almond oil
  Wild cherry syrup
  Hydrocyanic acid
  Nitroprusside
  Potassium cyanide
  Prussic acid
  Sodium cyanide
	Tachycardia, headache, drowsiness, hypotension, coma, convulsions, death; plasma bright red; *very rapidly lethal* (1–15 min)	*Speed essential.* Remove from source of inhalation; immediate emesis or lavage, amyl nitrite inhalation, 0.2 ml (1 capsule) 30 sec of each min, 100% O_2, support respiration; 10 ml 3% sodium nitrite 2.5–5 ml/min IV (in child: 10 mg/kg) then 50 ml 25% sodium thiosulfate 2.5–5 ml/min IV; repeat the above if symptoms recur. Lilly kit

DDD: see DDT		

DDT(chloro-
    phenothane)
  Chlorinated organic
    insecticides
  Aldrin
  Bulan
  Chlordane
  DDD
  Dieldrin
  Dilan
  Endrin
  Heptachlor
  Methoxychlor
  Prolan
  Toxaphene
	Vomiting (early or delayed); paresthesias, malaise; coarse tremors, convulsions; pulmonary edema, ventricular fibrillation, respiratory failure	Emesis; gastric lavage if not convulsing; 15–30 gm sodium sulfate or charcoal left in stomach; diazepam or phenobarbital to prevent & control tremors & convulsions; avoid epinephrine & sudden stimuli; parenteral fluids; monitor for renal & hepatic failure

Deodorizers, household: see Naphthalene, Paradichlorobenzene		
Depilatories: see Barium compounds		
Detergent powders: see Acids & alkalis		
Dextroamphetamine: see Amphetamines		
Diazinon: see Parathion		
Dicumarol: see Warfarin		
Dieldrin: see DDT		
Diethylene glycol: see Ethylene glycol		
Digitalis, digitoxin, digoxin: see CONGESTIVE HEART FAILURE in Ch. 25		
Dilan: see DDT		
Dinitrobenzene: see Nitrobenzene		

Dinitro-o-cresol
  Herbicides
  Pesticides
	Fatigue, thirst, flushing; nausea, vomiting, abdominal pain; hyperpyrexia, tachycardia, loss of consciousness; dyspnea, respiratory arrest. Absorbed through skin	Emesis; gastric lavage with 5% sodium bicarbonate; leave 0.5–1 L (1–2 pt) in stomach; saline catharsis; fluid therapy; O_2; anticipate renal & hepatic toxicity

Diphenoxylate with atropine	Lethargy, nystagmus, pinpoint pupils, tachycardia, coma, respiratory depression (NOTE: toxicity may be delayed up to 12 h)	Ipecac emesis, gastric lavage; activated charcoal; naloxone; admit all children to ICU for observation
Dipterex: see Parathion		
Dishwasher detergents: see Acids & alkalis		
Diuretics, mercurial: see Mercury		
Drain cleaners: see Acids & alkalis		
Endrin: see DDT		

TABLE 258-4. SPECIFIC POISONS: SYMPTOMS AND TREATMENT *(Cont'd)*

Poison	Symptoms	Treatment
Ergot derivatives	Thirst, diarrhea, vomiting, light-headedness, burning feet; convulsions, hypotension, coma, abortion; gangrene of feet; cataract	Ipecac emesis; gastric lavage; short-acting barbiturate for convulsions; amyl nitrite 0.3 ml by inhalation; papaverine 60 mg IV
Eserine: see Physostigmine		
Ethanol: see Alcohol, ethyl		
Ether: see Chloroform		
Ethyl alcohol: see Alcohol, ethyl		
Ethyl biscoumacetate: see Warfarin		
Ethylene glycol Diethylene glycol Permanent antifreeze	Eye contact iridocyclitis: Ingestion: Inebriation but no alcohol odor on breath; nausea, vomiting; carpopedal spasm, lumbar pain; oxalate crystalluria; oliguria progressing to anuria & acute renal failure; respiratory distress, convulsions, coma	Flush eyes Ingestion: Emesis; gastric lavage, support respiration, correct electrolyte imbalance; give ethanol (see Alcohol, methyl); hemodialysis
Explosives: see Barium compounds (fireworks); Nitrogen oxides		
Fava bean (favism): see Nonbacterial Food Poisoning in Ch. 55		
Ferric salts: see Iron		
Ferrous gluconate, ferrous sulfate: see Iron		
Fireworks: see Barium compounds		
Fluorides Ammonium fluoride Hydrofluoric acid Rat poisons Roach poisons Sodium fluoride Soluble fluorides generally	Inhalation: Intense eye, nasal irritation; headache; dyspnea, sense of suffocation, glottal edema, pulmonary edema, bronchitis, pneumonia; mediastinal & subcut. emphysema from bleb rupture Skin & mucosa: Superficial or deep burns Ingestion: Salty or soapy taste; tremors, convulsions, CNS depression; shock; renal failure	Inhalation: O₂, respiratory support; prednisone for chemical pneumonitis (adults 30–80 mg/day in divided doses); manage pulmonary edema Skin: Copious flushing with cold water; debride white tissue; for late pain, inject 10% calcium gluconate locally & apply magnesium oxide paste Ingestion: Ipecac emesis; gastric lavage—leave aluminum hydroxide gel in stomach; IV glucose & saline; 10% calcium gluconate, 10 ml IV (1 ml/kg in child); monitor for cardiac irritability; treat shock & dehydration
Formaldehyde Formalin (Note: May contain methyl alcohol)	Inhalation: Irritation of eyes, nose, respiratory tract; laryngeal spasm & edema; dysphagia; bronchitis, pneumonia Skin: Irritation, coagulation necrosis; dermatitis, hypersensitivity Ingestion: Oral & gastric pain, nausea, vomiting, hematemesis, shock, hematuria, anuria, coma, respiratory failure	Inhalation: Flush eyes with saline; O₂; support respiration Skin: Wash copiously with soap & water Ingestion: Give water or milk to dilute; treat shock, correct acidosis with sodium bicarbonate; support respiration; observe for perforations

TABLE 258-4. SPECIFIC POISONS: SYMPTOMS AND TREATMENT *(Cont'd)*

Poison	Symptoms	Treatment
Fowler's solution: see Arsenic & antimony		
Fuel, canned: see Alcohol, methyl		
Fuel oil: see Petroleum distillates		
Furnace gas: see Carbon monoxide		
Gamma benzene hexachloride: see γ-Benzene hexachloride		

Gas
   Acetylene, automobile exhaust, coal, furnace, illuminating, marsh: see Carbon monoxide
   Ammonia: see Ammonia gas
   Tear: see Chlorine
   Nerve: see Parathion
   Sewer, volatile hydrides: see Hydrogen sulfide		

Gasoline: see Petroleum distillates		
Glues, model airplane: see Acetone, Benzene, Petroleum distillates		
Glutethimide	Drowsiness, areflexia, mydriasis, hypotension, respiratory depression, coma	Ipecac emesis; gastric lavage, activated charcoal; support respiration, maintain fluid & electrolyte balance; hemodialysis may help; treat shock
Gold salts: see TABLE 258-3, Chelation Therapy; see also RHEUMATOID ARTHRITIS in Ch. 103		
Guaiacol: see Phenols		
Halogenated hydrocarbons: see DDT		
Heptachlor: see DDT		
Herbicides: see Arsenic & antimony, Dinitro-*o*-cresol		
Heroin: see Narcotics		
HETP (hexaethyl tetraphosphate): see Parathion		
Hexachlorocyclohexane: see γ-Benzene hexachloride		
Hormones—single acute oral overdose—no toxicity		
Hydrides, volatile: see Hydrogen sulfide		
Hydrocarbons: see Benzene		
Hydrocarbons, halogenated: see DDT		
Hydrochloric acid: see Acids & alkalis		
Hydrocyanic acid: see Cyanides		
Hydrogen chloride, fluoride: see Nitrogen oxides		

Hydrogen sulfide
   Alkali sulfides
   Phosphine
   Sewer gas
   Volatile hydrides
	"Gas eye" (subacute keratoconjunctivitis), lacrimation & burning; cough, dyspnea, pulmonary edema; caustic skin burns, erythema, pain; profuse salivation, nausea, vomiting, diarrhea; confusion, vertigo; sudden collapse & unconsciousness	Give O_2, support respiration; amyl nitrite & sodium nitrite as for cyanide (*no thiosulfate*)

Hyoscine, hyoscyamine, hyoscyamus: see Belladonna		

Hypochlorites
   Bleach, chlorine
   Javelle water
	Usually mild pain & inflammation of oral & GI mucosa; cough, dyspnea, vomiting; skin vesicles	Usual 6% household preparations require little except milk dilution; treat shock; esophagoscope only if concentrated forms have been ingested

Table 258–4. SPECIFIC POISONS: SYMPTOMS AND TREATMENT *(Cont'd)*

Poison	Symptoms	Treatment
Illuminating gas: see Carbon monoxide		
Imipramine: see Tricyclic antidepressants		
Indelible markers: see Acetanilid—usually no problem		
Ink, aniline: see Acetanilid—usually no problem		
Insecticides: see DDT, Paradichlorobenzene, Parathion, Pyrethrum		
Iodine	Burning pain in mouth & esophagus; mucous membranes stained brown; laryngeal edema; vomiting, abdominal pain, diarrhea; shock, nephritis, circulatory collapse	Give milk, starch, or flour orally; gastric lavage; fluid & electrolytes; treat shock; tracheostomy for laryngeal edema
Iodoform Triiodomethane	Dermatitis; vomiting; cerebral depression, excitation; coma; respiratory difficulty	Skin: Wash with sodium bicarbonate or alcohol Ingestion: Emetic or gastric lavage; respiratory support

Iron
  Ferric salts
  Ferrous salts
    Ferrous gluconate
    Ferrous sulfate
  Carbonyl iron: see
    Carbon monoxide
  Vitamins with iron
	Vomiting; upper abdominal pain, pallor, cyanosis, diarrhea, drowsiness, shock; concern if >40–70 mg/kg of elemental iron ingested	Ipecac emesis, gastric lavage with sodium bicarbonate; if serum iron >400 mg/100 ml, give deferoxamine 1–2 gm IM q 3–12 h (urine turns red within 2 h; if no color change, no further dose is needed); for shock, give deferoxamine 1 gm IV (max. rate 15 mg/kg/h); exchange transfusion

Isoniazid	CNS stimulation, seizures, obtundation, and coma	Emesis; lavage; diazepam sedation; pyridoxine 200 mg slowly IV for seizures; NaHCO₃ for acidosis
Isopropyl alcohol: see Alcohol, isopropyl		
Javelle water: see Hypochlorites		
Kerosene: see Petroleum distillates		
Ketones: see Acetone		

Lead
  Lead salts
  Some paints & painted
    surfaces
  Solder
	Acute inhalation: Insomnia, headache, ataxia, mania, convulsions
	Acute ingestion: Thirst, burning abdominal pain, vomiting, diarrhea, CNS symptoms as above
	Lead encephalopathy: see Lead Poisoning in Vol. II, Ch. 24
		See Lead Poisoning in Vol. II, Ch. 24

Lead, tetraethyl	Vapor inhalation, skin absorption, ingestion: CNS symptoms—insomnia, restlessness, ataxia, delusions, mania, convulsions	Supportive treatment; e.g., diazepam, chlorpromazine, fluid & electrolytes
Lime, chlorinated: see Chlorine		
Lindane: see γ-Benzene hexachloride		
Liquor: see Alcohol, ethyl		
Lye: see Acids & alkalis		
Malathion: see Parathion		
Manganese: see Table 258–3, Chelation Therapy		

TABLE 258-4. SPECIFIC POISONS: SYMPTOMS AND TREATMENT *(Cont'd)*

Poison	Symptoms	Treatment
Marsh gas: see Carbon monoxide		
Meperidine: see Narcotics		
Meprobamate: see Barbiturates		
Mercurial diuretics: see Mercury		
Mercuric chloride: see Mercury		
Mercury All mercury compounds Ammoniated mercury Bichloride of mercury Calomel Corrosive sublimate Diuretics Mercuric chloride Mercury vapor Merthiolate	Acute: Severe gastroenteritis, burning mouth pain, salivation, abdominal pain, vomiting; colitis, nephrosis, anuria, uremia. Skin burns from alkyl & phenyl mercurials Chronic: Gingivitis, mental disturbance; neurologic deficits	Gastric lavage, activated charcoal; give penicillamine (or BAL)—see TABLE 258-3, Chelation Therapy; maintain fluid & electrolyte balance; hemodialysis for renal failure, observe for GI perforation Skin: Scrub with soap & water
Merthiolate: see Mercury—usually no problem		
Metals	Symptoms vary with metals; see specific metals	See TABLE 258-3, Chelation Therapy
Methadone: see Narcotics		
Methamphetamine: see Amphetamines		
Methanol: see Alcohol, methyl		
Methoxychlor: see DDT		
Methyl alcohol: see Alcohol, methyl		
Methyl salicylate: see ASPIRIN AND OTHER SALICYLATE POISONING in Vol. II, Ch. 24		
Mineral spirits: see Petroleum distillates		
Model airplane glues, solvents: see Acetone, Benzene, Petroleum Distillates		
Morphine: see Narcotics		
Moth balls, crystals, repellent: see Paradichlorobenzene, Naphthalene		
Mushrooms, Poisonous: see NONBACTERIAL FOOD POISONING in Ch. 55		
Nail polish remover: see Acetone		
Naphtha: see Petroleum distillates		

Naphthalene (see also Paradichlorobenzene)
  Moth balls, crystals,
   repellent cakes
  Deodorizer cakes
	Contact: Dermatitis, corneal
	 ulceration
	Inhalation: Headache, confusion,
	 vomiting, dyspnea
	Ingestion: Abdominal cramps,
	 nausea, vomiting; headache,
	 confusion; dysuria;
	 intravascular hemolysis;
	 convulsions. Hemolytic
	 anemia in persons with G6PD
	 deficiency
		Contact: Remove clothing if formerly
		 stored with naphthalene moth balls;
		 flush skin and eyes
		Ingestion: Ipecac emesis, gastric
		 lavage; blood transfusion for severe
		 hemolysis; alkalize urine for
		 hemoglobinuria; for severe
		 hemolysis, blood transfusions as
		 necessary; control convulsions

Naphthols: see Phenols		

TABLE 258–4. SPECIFIC POISONS: SYMPTOMS AND TREATMENT *(Cont'd)*

Poison	Symptoms	Treatment
Narcotics (see also Chs. 136 and 247) 　Alphaprodine 　Codeine 　Heroin 　Meperidine 　Methadone 　Morphine 　Opium 　Propoxyphene	Pinpoint pupils, drowsiness, shallow respirations, spasticity, respiratory failure	*Do not give emetics.* Gastric lavage, respiratory support. Naloxone 5 μg/kg IV to awaken & improve respiration; if patient does not respond, give 2–20 mg naloxone (dosage must be repeated as many as 10–20 times); fluids IV to support circulation

Neostigmine: see Physostigmine

Nerve gas agents: see Parathion

Nickel: see TABLE 258–3, Chelation Therapy

Nicotine: see Tobacco

Nitrates: see Chlorates

Nitric acid: see Acids & alkalis

Nitrites 　Amyl nitrite 　Butyl nitrite 　Nitroglycerin 　Potassium nitrite 　Sodium nitrite	Methemoglobinemia, cyanosis, anoxia; GI disturbance, vomiting; headache, dizziness, hypotension, respiratory failure, coma	Ipecac emesis, gastric lavage; O_2; for methemoglobinemia, 1% methylene blue 1–2 mg/kg slowly IV; when >40% methemoglobin, transfusion with whole blood
Nitrobenzene 　Artificial bitter 　　almond oil 　Dinitrobenzene	Bitter almond odor (suggests cyanides); drowsiness, headache; vomiting; ataxia, nystagmus; brown urine; convulsive movements; delirium; cyanosis; coma, respiratory arrest	See Acetanilid

Nitrogen oxides (see also Chlorine; Hydrogen sulfide; Sulfur dioxide; and Ch. 40)

(Air contaminants that form atmospheric oxidants. Liberated from missile fuels, explosives, agricultural wastes) 　Cobaltous chloride 　Fluorine 　Hydrogen chloride 　Hydrogen fluoride	Delayed onset of symptoms with nitrogen oxides unless heavy concentration; other irritant gases give warnings—local burning in eye, nasal, pharyngeal mucous membranes. Fatigue, cough, dyspnea, pulmonary edema; later, bronchitis, pneumonia	Absolute bed rest; pure O_2 as soon as symptoms develop; for excessive pulmonary foam: suction, postural drainage, tracheostomy; to prevent pulmonary fibrosis: prednisone 30–80 mg/day has been used

Nitroglycerin: see Nitrites

Nitrous oxide: see Chloroform

Oil of wintergreen: see ASPIRIN AND OTHER SALICYLATE POISONING in Vol. II, Ch. 24

Oils
　Aniline: see Acetanilid
　Fuel, lubricating: see Petroleum distillates

OMPA (octamethyl pyrophosphoramide): see Parathion

Opiates: see Narcotics

Oxalates: see Oxalic acid

Oxalic acid 　Oxalates 　Ethylene glycol	Burning pain in throat, vomiting, intensive pain; hypotension, tetany, shock; glottal & renal damage; oxaluria	Give milk or calcium lactate; careful gastric lavage if at all; 10% calcium gluconate 10–20 ml IV; pain control, saline IV for shock; demulcents by mouth; watch for glottal edema & stricture

TABLE 258-4. SPECIFIC POISONS: SYMPTOMS AND TREATMENT *(Cont'd)*

Poison	Symptoms	Treatment
Paint solvents: see Mineral spirits (under Petroleum distillates) and Turpentine		
Paints: see Lead		

Paradichlorobenzene
  Insecticide
  Moth repellent
  Toilet bowl deodorant
	Abdominal pain, nausea, vomiting, diarrhea, seizures, and tetany	Ipecac emesis, gastric lavage; fluid replacement; diazepam for seizure control

Paraldehyde	Paraldehyde odor on breath, incoherent, pupils contracted, respirations depressed, coma	Ingestion: Ipecac emesis, gastric lavage; support respiration, O_2
Paraquat	Immediate: GI pain and vomiting; within 24 h: respiratory failure	Emesis, fuller's earth plus Na_2SO_4; limit O_2; call poison center or manufacturer

Parathion
  Chlorothion
  Demeton
  Diazinon
  Dipterex (trichlorfon)
  HETP (hexaethyl tetraphosphate)
  Malathion
  Nerve gas agents
  OMPA (octamethyl pyrophosphoramide)
  Systox
  TEPP (tetraethyl pyrophosphate)
	Nausea, vomiting, abdominal cramping, excessive salivation; increased pulmonary secretion, headache, rhinorrhea, blurred vision, miosis; slurred speech, mental confusion; breathing difficulty, frothing at mouth, coma. Absorbed through skin	Remove clothing, flush & wash skin. Empty stomach; atropine: adults 2 mg, children 1–2 mg, IV or IM q 15–60 min, if no signs of atropine toxicity, repeat as needed; pralidoxime chloride (PAM): adults 1–2 gm, children 0.25 gm, IV over 5–10 min, repeat in 12 h if needed; O_2; support respiration; correct dehydration. *Do not use morphine or aminophylline*

Paris green: see Arsenic & antimony		
Pentobarbital: see Barbiturates		
Permanent wave neutralizers (bromates): see Chlorates		
Pesticides: see Arsenic & antimony, Barium compounds, DDT, Dinitro-o-cresol, Fluorides, Paradichlorobenzene, Parathion, Phosphorus, Pyrethrum, Thallium salts, Warfarin		
Petroleum distillates (see also HYDROCARBON POISONING in Vol. II, Ch. 24)		

Asphalt
  Benzine (benzin)
  Fuel oil
  Gasoline
  Kerosene
  Lubricating oils
  Mineral spirits
  Model airplane glue
  Naphtha
  Petroleum ether
  Tar
	Vapor inhalation: Euphoria; burning in chest; headache, nausea, weakness; CNS depression, confusion; dyspnea, tachypnea, rales. Ingestion: Burning throat & stomach, vomiting, diarrhea; pneumonia; late pulmonary changes. Aspiration: Early acute pulmonary changes	Since major problems are consequential to aspiration, as opposed to GI absorption, in most instances no gastric evacuation is warranted; gastric lavage only with rapid-onset depression from large amounts ingested; arterial blood gas levels to monitor care; supportive care for pulmonary edema; O_2, respiratory support

Petroleum ether: see Petroleum distillates		
Phenacetin: see Acetanilid		
Phencyclidine (PCP)	"Spaced-out," unconscious; hypertension	Quiet environment; prolonged gastric lavage; propranolol and diazepam
Phenmetrazine: see Amphetamines		
Phenobarbital: see Barbiturates		

1426 Poisoning; Venomous Bites and Stings

TABLE 258–4. SPECIFIC POISONS: SYMPTOMS AND TREATMENT *(Cont'd)*

Poison	Symptoms	Treatment
Phenols Carbolic acid Creosote Cresols Guaiacol Naphthols	Corrosive. Mucous membrane burns; pallor, weakness, shock; convulsions in children; pulmonary edema; smoky urine; respiratory, cardiac, & circulatory failure	Remove clothing, wash external burns. Lavage with water, activated charcoal. *Do not use alcohol or mineral oil.* Demulcents; pain relief; O_2; support respiration; correct fluid balance; watch for esophageal stricture (rare)
Phenothiazine Chlorpromazine Prochlorperazine Promazine Trifluoperazine (etc.)	Extrapyramidal tract symptoms (ataxia, muscular & carpopedal spasms, torticollis), usually idiosyncratic; overdose results in dry mouth, drowsiness, coma, hypothermia, respiratory collapse. Leukopenia, jaundice, coagulation defect, skin rashes	Ipecac emesis, gastric lavage; diphenhydramine 2–3 mg/kg IV or IM for extrapyramidal symptoms; diazepam for convulsions; warm patient. Avoid levarterenol & epinephrine
Phosphoric acid: see Acids & alkalis		
Phosphorus (Yellow or white) Rat poisons Roach powders (NOTE: Red phosphorus is unabsorbable & nontoxic)	3 Stages of symptoms: 1st—Garlicky taste; garlic odor on breath; local irritation, skin burns, throat burns; nausea, vomiting, diarrhea 2nd—Symptom-free 8 h to several days 3rd—Nausea, vomiting, diarrhea; liver enlargement, jaundice; hemorrhages; renal damage; convulsions, coma Toxicity enhanced by alcohol, fats, digestible oils	Protect patient & attendant from vomitus, gastric washing, feces. If phosphorus is imbedded in skin, keep patient's body submerged in water. Gastric lavage copiously—preferably with potassium permanganate (1:5000) or cupric sulfate (250 mg in 250 ml water); mineral oil 100 ml (to prevent absorption) & repeat in 2 h; combat shock; vit. K_1 IV; transfusion with fresh blood
Physostigmine Eserine Neostigmine (Prostigmin) Pilocarpine Pilocarpus	Dizziness, weakness, vomiting, cramping pain; pupils dilated, then contracted	Atropine sulfate 0.6 to 1 mg s.c. or IV
Pilocarpine, pilocarpus: see Physostigmine		
Potash: see Acids & alkalis		
Potassium bichromate, Potassium chromate: see Chromic acid		
Potassium carbonate: see Acids & alkalis		
Potassium cyanide: see Cyanides		
Potassium hydroxide: see Acids & alkalis		
Potassium nitrate: see Chlorates		
Potassium nitrite: see Nitrites		
Potassium permanganate	Brown discoloration & burns of oral mucosa, glottal edema; hypotension; renal involvement	Gastric lavage, demulcents; maintain fluid balance
Prochlorperazine: see Phenothiazine		
Prolan: see DDT		
Promazine: see Phenothiazine		

TABLE 258-4. SPECIFIC POISONS: SYMPTOMS AND TREATMENT *(Cont'd)*

Poison	Symptoms	Treatment
Propoxyphene: see Narcotics		
Propranolol	Confusion and seizures	Emesis; lavage; supportive care; diazepam sedation
Prostigmin: see Physostigmine		
Prussic acid: see Cyanides		
Pyrethrin: see Pyrethrum		
Pyrethrum Pyrethrin	Allergic response (including anaphylactic reactions, skin sensitivity) in sensitive people. Otherwise low toxicity, unless vehicle is a petroleum distillate (see that entry)	For sizeable ingestion, emesis if patient is alert; otherwise, endotracheal tube & gastric lavage; wash skin well
Radium: see TABLE 258-3, Chelation Therapy		
Rat poison: see Barium compounds, Fluorides, Phosphorus, Thallium salts, Warfarin		
Resorcinol (resorcin)	Vomiting, dizziness, tinnitus; chills, tremor; delirium, convulsions, respiratory depression, coma	Emetic or gastric lavage; support respiration
Roach poison: see Fluorides, Phosphorus, Thallium salts		
Rodenticides (rat poison): see Barium compounds, Fluorides, Phosphorus, Thallium salts, Warfarin		
Rubbing alcohol: see Alcohol, isopropyl		
Salicylates: see ASPIRIN AND OTHER SALICYLATE POISONING in Vol. II, Ch. 24		
Salicylic acid: see ASPIRIN AND OTHER SALICYLATE POISONING in Vol. II, Ch. 24		
Scopolamine: see Belladonna		
Secobarbital: see Barbiturates		
Selenium: see TABLE 258-3, Chelation Therapy		
Sewer gas: see Hydrogen sulfide		

Silver salts
  Silver nitrate
  (NOTE: Chloride, bromide, iodide, & oxide salts are usually benign)
	Stain on lips (white, then black); gastroenteritis, shock, vertigo, convulsions	Gastric lavage with saline soln; control pain; control convulsions with diazepam

Smog: see Sulfur dioxide		
Soda, caustic: see Acids & alkalis		
Sodium carbonate: see Acids & alkalis		
Sodium cyanide: see Cyanides		
Sodium fluoride: see Fluorides		
Sodium hydroxide: see Acids & alkalis		
Sodium nitrite: see Nitrites		
Sodium salicylate: see ASPIRIN AND OTHER SALICYLATE POISONING in Vol. II, Ch. 24		
Solder: see Cadmium; Lead		
Stibophen: see Arsenic & antimony		
Stramonium: see Belladonna		

TABLE 258–4. SPECIFIC POISONS: SYMPTOMS AND TREATMENT *(Cont'd)*

Poison	Symptoms	Treatment
Strychnine	Restlessness, hyperacuity of hearing, vision, etc.; convulsions from minor stimuli, complete muscle relaxation between convulsions; perspiration; respiratory arrest	Isolate & restrict stimulation to prevent convulsions. Activated charcoal orally; control convulsions with IV diazepam, curariform drugs; support respiration; acid diuresis with ammonium chloride or ascorbic acid; gastric lavage *after* convulsions controlled
Sulfur dioxide Smog	Respiratory tract irritation; sneezing, cough, dyspnea, pulmonary edema	Remove from contaminated area, give O_2; positive pressure breathing, respiratory support
Sulfuric acid: see Acids & alkalis		
Syrup of wild cherry: see Cyanides		
Systox: see Parathion		
Tar: see Petroleum distillates		
Tartar emetic: see Arsenic & antimony		
Tear gas: see Chlorine		
TEPP: see Parathion		
Tetraethyl lead: see Lead, tetraethyl		

Thallium salts
  Ant poison
  Rat poison
  Roach poison
	Abdominal pain (colic), vomiting (may be bloody), diarrhea (may be bloody), stomatitis, excessive salivation; tremors, leg pains, paresthesias, polyneuritis, ocular & facial palsy; delirium, convulsions, respiratory failure; loss of hair approx. 3 wk after poisoning	Ipecac emesis, gastric lavage; activated charcoal; potassium chloride 5–25 gm/day orally; treat shock, control convulsions with diazepam; chelation (experimental) with sodium diethyldithiocarbamate 30 mg/kg/day orally or diphenylthiocarbazone 10 mg/kg orally; BAL, EDTA are of no use

Tobacco Nicotine	Excitement, confusion, muscular twitching, weakness, abdominal cramps, clonic convulsions, depression, rapid respirations, palpitations, collapse, coma, CNS paralysis, respiratory failure	Ipecac emesis, gastric lavage; activated charcoal; support respiration, O_2; diazepam for convulsions; wash skin well if contaminated
Toilet bowl cleaners, deodorizers: see Acids & alkalis; Paradichlorobenzene		
Toluene, toluol: see Benzene		
Toxaphene: see DDT		
Trichlorfon: see Parathion		
Trichloromethane: see Chloroform		

T<small>ABLE</small> 258–4. SPECIFIC POISONS: SYMPTOMS AND TREATMENT *(Cont'd)*

Poison	Symptoms	Treatment
Tricyclic antidepressants Amitriptyline Desipramine Doxepin Imipramine Nortriptyline Protriptyline	Anticholinergic effects (e.g., blurred vision, urinary hesitation); CNS effects (e.g., drowsiness, stupor, coma, ataxia, restlessness, agitation, hyperactive reflexes, muscle rigidity, and convulsions); CVS effects (tachycardia and other arrhythmias, bundle branch block, impaired conduction, congestive heart failure). Respiratory depression, hypotension, shock, vomiting, hyperpyrexia, mydriasis, and diaphoresis may also be present	Symptomatic and supportive; emesis, gastric lavage; monitor vital signs and ECG; maintain open airway and adequate fluid intake. Physostigmine salicylate (slowly IV) is reported to reverse both CNS and cardiac manifestations of overdosage—adults: 2 mg with repeat of 1–4 mg p.r.n. at 20- to 60-min intervals; children: 0.5 mg repeated p.r.n. at 5-min intervals to maximum 2 mg; sodium bicarbonate as a bolus IV (0.5–2 mEq/L), repeat periodically to maintain blood pH >7.45, precludes development of arrhythmias

Trifluoperazine: see Phenothiazine

Triiodomethane: see Iodoform

Tungsten: see T<small>ABLE</small> 258–3, Chelation Therapy

Turpentine Paint solvent Varnish	Turpentine odor; burning oral & abdominal pain, coughing, choking, respiratory failure; nephritis	Emesis (alert patient), gastric lavage; support respiration, O_2; control pain; monitor renal function

Vanadium: see T<small>ABLE</small> 258–3, Chelation Therapy

Varnish: see Alcohol, methyl; Turpentine

Vitamins—single acute oral ingestion of isolated or multiple dose form—no toxicity

Warfarin Bishydroxycoumarin Dicumarol Ethyl biscoumacetate Rat poisons	Single ingestion not serious, multiple overdoses result in coagulopathy	For hemorrhagic manifestations, vit. K_1 1 mg/kg IV, 10 mg/min till prothrombin time normal, transfusion with fresh blood if necessary

Wax, floor: see Carbon tetrachloride

Whiskey: see Alcohol, ethyl

Wild cherry syrup: see Cyanides

Wintergreen oil: see A<small>SPIRIN AND</small> O<small>THER</small> S<small>ALICYLATE</small> P<small>OISONING</small> in Vol. II, Ch. 24

Wood alcohol: see Alcohol, methyl

Xylene: see Benzene

Zinc: see T<small>ABLE</small> 258–3, Chelation Therapy

Zinc salts: see Copper salts

259. VENOMOUS BITES AND STINGS

POISONOUS SNAKES

In the USA, about 20 of the 120 species of snakes are venomous. These can be divided into the **pit vipers** (Crotalidae) and the **coral snakes** (Elapidae). TABLE 259-1 lists some medically important snakes of the USA and their usual habitats.

Epidemiology

Although > 45,000 people/yr are bitten by snakes in the USA, just under 7000 cases of snake poisoning are reported. Fewer than 12 fatalities/yr occur, mostly in children, in untreated or under-treated cases, or in members of religious sects who handle venomous serpents. Rattlesnakes account for about 60% of venomous snake bites and for almost all the deaths. Most other venomous snake bites can be attributed to the copperhead, and to a lesser extent the cottonmouth. Coral snakes inflict < 1% of all bites. Imported snakes are found in zoos, schools, snake farms, and amateur and professional collections, and account for about 5 bites/yr.

Chemistry, Pharmacology, and Pathology

Snake venoms are complex mixtures, chiefly proteins, many having enzymatic activity. Although the enzymes contribute to the deleterious effects of the venom, the lethal effects, and some of the more important toxic effects, may be caused by certain of the venom polypeptides, which are gener-

TABLE 259-1. SOME MEDICALLY IMPORTANT

Snakes	Wash., Ore., Id.	Calif., Nev.	Ariz., New Mex.	Texas
PIT VIPERS (Crotalidae)				
Cottonmouths and Copperheads (*Agkistrodon*)				
Cottonmouths (*A. piscivorus*)				X
Copperheads (*A. contortrix*)				X
Rattlesnakes (*Crotalus*)				
Eastern diamondback (*C. adamanteus*)				
Western diamondback (*C. atrox*)		X	X	X
Sidewinder (*C. cerastes*)		X	Ariz.	
Timber (*C. horridus*)				X
Rock (*C. lepidus*)			X	X
Speckled (*C. mitchelli*)		X	Ariz.	
Black-tailed (*C. molossus*)			X	X
Twin-spotted (*C. pricei*)			Ariz.	
Red diamond (*C. ruber*)		Calif.		
Mojave (*C. scutulatus*)		X	X	X
Tiger (*C. tigris*)			Ariz.	
Western (*C. viridis*)				
Prairie (*C.v. viridis*)	Ore., Id.		X	X
Grand Canyon (*C.v. abyssus*)			Ariz.	
Southern Pacific (*C.v. helleri*)		Calif.		
Great Basin (*C.v. lutosus*)	Ore., Id.	X	Ariz.	
Northern Pacific (*C.v. oreganus*)	X	X		
Ridge-nosed (*C. willardi*)			Ariz.	
Massauga and Pigmy (*Sistrusus*)				
Massauga (*S. catenatus*)			X	X
Pigmy rattlesnake (*S. miliarius*)				X
CORAL SNAKES (Elapidae)				
Western coral snake (*Micruroides euryxanthus*)			X	
Eastern coral snake (*Micrurus fulvius*)				X

Certain groups of adjoining states are treated here as units. The symbol X indicates that distribution of the species is widespread within the unit. Restriction of a species to a part of a unit is indicated appropriately.

ally 5 to 100 times more lethal than the crude venom. These polypeptides appear to have specific chemical and physiologic receptor sites.

In addition to the activities of various venom components and their metabolites, envenomation may be complicated by the release of autopharmacologic substances that can make diagnosis and treatment difficult. *Thus, the arbitrary grouping of snake venoms into categories such as "neurotoxins," "hemotoxins," "cardiotoxins" is pharmacologically superficial and can lead to grave errors in clinical judgment.* A so-called neurotoxic venom can produce marked cardiovascular changes or direct hematologic effects. The so-called hemolytic venoms can also produce changes in the nervous system or in vascular dynamics. A patient with snake poisoning may present with perhaps 3 or more toxic reactions.

Rattlesnake and many viper venoms produce local tissue damage, blood cell changes, coagulation defects, blood vessel injury, and changes in vascular resistance. The Hct may fall rapidly, although hemoconcentration may occur during the very early stages. Thrombocytopenia is uncommon. Pulmonary edema is common in severe poisoning, and bleeding may occur in the lungs, peritoneum, kidneys, and heart. These changes are often accompanied by alterations in cardiac and renal function. Renal failure may occur because of a critical deficit in glomerular filtration secondary to hypotension; or because of the effects of hemolysis, hemoglobinuria, myoglobinuria, or all of the above; or because of the direct effects of venom components. Although cardiac dynamics may be disturbed, the early cardiovascular collapse seen in an occasional patient bitten by a rattlesnake is due chiefly to a marked fall in circulating blood volume. This appears to be caused by a loss of blood plasma and protein through the vessel walls, and by blood pooling. Most North American crotalid venoms produce relatively minor changes in neuromuscular transmission, but the venoms of the Mojave rattlesnake and the tropical rattlesnake markedly alter neuromuscular transmission.

SNAKES OF THE UNITED STATES

Mont., Mich., Wis., (W.) Minn., S. Dak., N. Dak., Neb., Iowa, Wyo., Utah, Colo.	Kan., Okla., Ark., Mo.	Tenn., Ky., Ill., Ind., Ohio	N.C., S.C., Ga., Ala., Miss., La.	Fla.	Pa., N.J., Md., Del., Va., W. Va. N.Y., N. Eng.
Neb., Iowa	X	Tenn., Ky., Ill.	X	X	Va.
Neb., Iowa	X	X	X	X	X
			X	X	
	Okla., Ark.				
Utah					
Minn., Wis., Neb., Iowa	X	X	X	X	X
Not Mich., Minn., Wis.	Kan., Okla.				
Utah					
Mich., Wis., Minn., Neb., Iowa, Colo.	X	Ill., Ind., Ohio			N.Y., Pa.
	Okla., Ark., Mo.	Tenn.	X	X	
	Ark.		X	X	

Adapted from U.S. Navy Bureau of Medicine and Surgery: *Poisonous Snakes of the World*, ed. 2, U.S. Govt. Printing Office 1968; and *Snake Venom Poisoning* by F. E. Russell, 1980, J. B. Lippincott.

Most elapid venoms also cause marked changes in neuromuscular transmission, in nerve conduction, and, to a much lesser extent, in the CNS. However, some elapid venoms cause local tissue damage and necrosis, blood changes, and severe renal complications.

Symptoms, Signs, and Diagnosis

Venomous snake bites are medical emergencies, requiring immediate attention and considerable judgment. Before treatment is begun, it is essential to determine whether the snake was venomous and whether envenomation occurred, since a venomous snake may bite and not inject venom (no poisoning develops in about 20 to 30% of crotalid bites and in about 40% of cobra and certain other elapid bites). When no envenomation occurs or the bite is inflicted by a nonvenomous snake, it should be treated as a puncture wound.

Positive diagnosis of snake poisoning requires identification of the snake and evidence of envenomation. Although the identity of the offending snakes can be suggested by the fang marks, *these should never be relied on for positive identification.* "Typical" fang-mark patterns are based on the anatomy of the snake's jaw and laboratory experiments and are infrequently seen under field conditions. Rattlesnake bites may leave one or two fang marks as well as other teeth marks; single fang punctures are very common and are not uncommon in bites by some nonvenomous snakes.

Numerical grading of rattlesnake bites is sometimes described in the literature, but it is more practical to describe cases as minor, moderate, or severe, depending on all the symptoms, signs, and laboratory findings rather than on just 1 or 2, such as swelling and pain. Bites by the Mojave rattlesnake, for example, can give rise to minimal edema, local tissue changes, or pain and therefore be graded as I; the consequence can be administration of insufficient antivenin and a poor, even fatal, outcome.

Pit viper envenomation: The symptoms and signs of crotalid poisoning vary considerably, depending on the species of snake, the amount of venom injected, and other factors. If there is evidence of poisoning soon after a bite, the possible consequences must not be underestimated.

Bites by rattlesnakes, cottonmouths, and copperheads usually cause immediate swelling, edema, and pain. Contrary to popular opinion, severe pain is not a constant finding; in bites by some species, pain is minimal or even absent. Generally, however, some degree of pain immediately follows envenomation, and swelling and edema usually appear within 10 min—they are rarely delayed more than 15 to 20 min. By the time the patient arrives at the doctor's office, a diagnosis of crotalid bite with envenomation can usually be made (or envenomation excluded) on the basis of fang marks, swelling and edema, pain, and, in bites by some species, tingling or numbness periorally or in the fingers or toes, or a metallic or rubbery taste in the mouth.

Untreated, the edema progresses rapidly and may involve the entire extremity within several hours. There may be lymphangitis and enlarged, tender, regional lymph nodes. Skin temperature over the injured part and body temperature are usually elevated, although the patient may complain of chills. Weakness, syncope, sweating, and nausea may be present. Vomiting may occur and the pulse may be rapid and weak. BP often drops and, in severe cases, shock may develop early. Particularly following bites by the Mojave rattlesnake, respiratory distress may be marked, muscle fasciculations, spasms, and weakness are not uncommon, and true paralysis may occur in some cases. The patient may complain of headache, blurred vision, ptosis, and marked thirst.

Ecchymosis is common in most cases of moderate or severe rattlesnake poisoning and usually appears over the bite within 3 to 6 h. It is severe following bites by the eastern and western diamondbacks and the prairie and Pacific rattlesnakes, and less severe following copperhead and Mojave rattlesnake bites. The skin may appear tense and discolored; vesicles often appear in the area of the bite within the first 8 h, often becoming blood-filled. These changes tend to be relatively superficial, since the bites of the North American rattlesnakes tend to be superficial. Necrosis is common around the bite area in untreated cases, and surrounding superficial blood vessels may be thrombosed. Most of the effects produced by the venom reach their peak by the 4th day.

There may be hemorrhage from the gums, hematemesis, melena, and hematuria. Bleeding and clotting times are prolonged, and platelet counts may fall sharply in moderate or severe envenomations. In most cases, a marked rise in the packed cell volume soon occurs, although in moderate or severe cases hemolysis may cause a rapid fall in the Hct.

Coral snake envenomation: The bite is usually associated with little or no pain, which is often transitory. Swelling is either absent or very minor. Paresthesia is often noted around the bitten area, and some weakness of the part becomes evident within several hours. Muscular incoordination may subsequently develop, and the patient may complain of marked weakness and lethargy. There may be increased salivation, difficulties in swallowing and phonation, and visual disturbances. Respiratory distress and failure may ensue. In fatal cases, shock, leading to complete cardiovascular failure, usually precedes death.

Laboratory Tests

In all but trivial cases, a CBC, platelet count, and urinalysis are essential; the following tests should also be obtained: blood typing and cross-matching; bleeding and clotting times; clot retraction, prothrombin, and partial thromboplastin times; ESR; Na, K, Cl, and Ca blood levels; and CO_2 combining power. Serum bilirubin and RBC fragility tests are often useful. An ECG is indicated in all severe cases.

Treatment

Pit viper: If the patient is seen within 10 min of being bitten and is more than 30 min from a hospital, a constriction band should be placed close to the bite or above the first joint proximal to it. The band should be tight enough to occlude lymph flow and superficial venous return, but not tight enough to impede deep venous or arterial flow. The fang marks are cut through, making incisions no longer than 1/4 in. and no deeper than 1/8 in. Incisions should not be made elsewhere. Suction, applied directly over these incisions, is of value only during the first 30 to 60 min following the bite. The affected part should be immobilized at heart level and in a physiologic position. The patient should be kept warm and at rest and should be given reassurance. If the patient is within 30 min of a medical facility, he should be transported there, at rest, without any first aid other than reassurance and immobilization of the affected part.

At the hospital, if antivenin is needed, a skin test for horse serum sensitivity should be performed as described in the antivenin brochure. If the patient is mildly sensitive to horse serum, diphenhydramine IV may be indicated before giving the antivenin. A tourniquet, O_2, epinephrine, and other drugs and equipment for treating anaphylaxis should be available during antivenin administration.

The amount of Antivenin (Crotalidae) Polyvalent (Wyeth) to be given depends on many factors, most important of which is the severity and progression of the symptoms and signs. In minimal rattlesnake venom poisoning, 30 to 50 ml (3 to 5 vials) of antivenin (reconstituted) will usually suffice. Moderate cases may require 50 to 100 ml (5 to 10 vials); severe cases may need 150 ml (15 vials) or more. Water moccasin poisoning usually requires lesser doses; with copperhead bites, antivenin is usually required only for children and the elderly. Reconstituted antivenin should be diluted in sterile isotonic saline or 5% dextrose and given by IV drip in most cases. If necessary to inject IM, give in the buttocks. *Never inject antivenin into a toe or finger.* Measuring the circumference of the extremity at 3 points increasingly proximal to the bite and recording the measurements every 15 to 30 min provides a guide to antivenin dosage. If additional antivenin is needed, it is added to the IV drip and given over 3 to 4 h. Antivenin is probably of less value if not administered within 12 h; after 24 h its use is of questionable value. IV fluids should be kept to a minimum, except when shock or hypovolemia is present.

Antitetanus and broad-spectrum antimicrobial therapy should be given in serious cases. In many cases, either early or late in the poisoning, blood volume decreases and perfusion fails, often with concomitant lysis of RBCs and platelet destruction, necessitating transfusions and parenteral fluids. Plasma or albumin may be used to treat hypovolemia. If there is a decrease in RBC mass, either through lysis or bleeding, packed cells or whole blood should be given. When these complications are accompanied by defects of hemostasis—i.e., abnormal clotting or lysis of cells or clots, or a disturbance of platelet activity—replacement with specific clotting factors, fresh frozen plasma, or platelet transfusions is indicated.

At the first sign of respiratory distress, O_2 should be given and preparations made to provide mechanical support (see Ch. 32). Tracheal intubation or tracheostomy may be indicated, particularly if trismus, laryngeal spasm, or excessive salivation is present. Aspirin or codeine may be used for pain, meperidine or morphine if the pain is severe. Mild sedation with phenobarbital is indicated in all severe bites when respiratory failure is not a problem. Sedation should reduce the amount of analgesic necessary.

The wound should be cleansed and covered with a sterile dressing. The injured part should be immobilized in a position of function. Surgical debridement of blebs, bloody vesicles, or superficial necrosis, if present, should be carried out between the 3rd and 10th day, and may need to be done in stages. The injured part should be soaked in 1:20 Burow's solution t.i.d. for 15 min. O_2 bubbled through the solution around the injured part may be of value. The injured part can be cooled (10 to 15 C) during the first 60 h to reduce pain, but an extremity should never be left in contact with ice for an extended period, since this risks a high incidence of amputation.

Corticosteroids are useless during the acute stages of poisoning and may be contraindicated. Short-term corticosteroid therapy may be useful in an anaphylactic crisis, but corticosteroids are not substitutes for catecholamines in shock caused by envenomation. Continued corticosteroid use is not advised. Local infiltration of small amounts of 0.05 M EDTA in isotonic saline around the bite area may reduce some of the local necrotizing effects of the venom if carried out within 30 min of the bite. The volume of the injection should be kept to a minimum.

Follow-up care is of the utmost importance. Amputations and contractures can be avoided by early corrective measures and exercises. Fasciotomy should be discouraged. It is usually unnecessary and reflects the use of insufficient antivenin during the first 12 h of the poisoning. It may be necessary, however, when there is strong evidence of severe vascular embarrassment. Within 4 days of the injury, a complete evaluation should be made of joint motion, muscle strength, sensation, and girth measurements. Immobilization is then interrupted by frequent periods of gentle exercise, progressing from passive to active. Follow-up care should also include sterile whirlpool treatment, debridement as indicated, daily cleansing of the wound with 3% hydrogen peroxide followed by 15-min soaks in 1:20 Burow's solution, and twice weekly painting of the wound with an aqueous triple dye of brilliant green 1:400, gentian violet 1:400, and acriflavine 1:1000. A 5% scarlet red ointment or polymyxin-bacitracin-neomycin ointment can be applied at bedtime. Daily exposure to continuous flowing O_2 while the part is immobilized in a plastic bag may be of value. The lesion should be covered with a sterile dressing and a loose bandage when the patient is supine, and a reasonably firm bandage when the patient is ambulatory.

Coral snake: The general principles noted above for pit viper envenomation should also be considered in coral snake bites, but incision and suction and other such first aid measures are of little value. Three vials of specific antivenin should be given on admission. The physician should contact a poison control center, zoo, or Wyeth Laboratories for the nearest source of this antivenin. In severe cases, respiratory and cardiac intensive care may be indicated.

Imported species: The local zoo is the first place to call when dealing with a bite by an imported venomous snake. The American Society of Zoological Parks and Gardens maintains a list of available antivenins, as does the Oklahoma City Poison Information Center (1–800–522–4611). Poison control centers in the major cities also maintain some listings for antivenins for exotic species. However, recent federal regulations on the use of foreign-prepared antivenins indicate that it is prudent to contact a local public health officer before giving these antivenins.

POISONOUS LIZARDS

Only 2 lizards, the Gila monster (*Heloderma suspectum*) found in Arizona and Sonora and adjacent areas, and the beaded lizard (*H. horridum*) of Mexico are known to be venomous. Their venom contains one or more salivary kallikreins, similar to those of some snakes, which cause the release of certain enzymes. Hyaluronidase and phospholipase A are also present.

Symptoms and signs following poisoning include localized pain, swelling and edema, ecchymosis, and lymphangitis around the wound. Systemic manifestations may develop in moderate or severe poisonings, including weakness, sweating, thirst, headache, and tinnitus. The findings and clinical course are generally similar to those of a mild to moderate case of western diamondback rattlesnake bite. In severe cases, there may be cardiovascular collapse.

In **treatment,** supportive measures are similar to those recommended above for pit viper envenomation. No specific antiserum is available.

SPIDERS

With the exception of 2 small groups, all spiders are venomous. Fortunately, the fangs of most species are too short or fragile to penetrate the skin. Nevertheless, at least 60 species in the USA have been implicated in bites on humans. Those species which are dangerous include the black widow spider, *Latrodectus mactans*, and related species; the brown or violin spider, *Loxosceles reclusa* (sometimes called the brown recluse), and related species; the jumping spiders, *Phidippus* species; the tarantulas, *Aphonopelma* and *Pamphobeteus* species; the trap-door spider, *Bothriocyrtum* and *Ummidia* species; the so-called banana spiders, *Phoneutria* and *Cupiennius sallei*, *Lycosa* (wolf spider), and *Heteropoda*; the crab spider, *Misumenoides aleatorius*; the running spiders, *Liocranoides* and *Chiracanthium*; the orbweavers, *Neoscona vertebrata*, *Araneus* species, and *Argiope aurantia* (orange argiope); the running or gnaphosid spiders, *Drassodes*; the green lynx spider, *Peucetia viridans*; and the comb-footed or false black widow, *Steatoda grossa*. *Pamphobeteus, Cupiennius,* and *Phoneutria* are not native to the USA, but may be brought into the country on produce or other materials.

The incidence of spider bites in the USA is unknown. In Southern California, about 400/yr are reported to physicians. Fewer than 4 fatalities/yr occur in the USA, usually in children.

Chemistry and Pharmacology

Only a few spider venoms have been studied in any detail. Black widow venom consists chiefly of proteins, a few of which are enzymatic. The lethal fraction appears to be a peptide with a marked effect on neuromuscular transmission. Brown or violin spider venom consists of at least 7 or 8 proteins. Its enzyme activity is greater than that of *Latrodectus* venom, but no fraction of *Loxosceles* venom has been isolated that produces the unusual necrotic lesion characteristic of *Loxosceles* bites. The lesion may be the product of an autopharmacologic response and not of any specific venom component. Tarantula venom contains a number of proteins but has a much lower enzymatic content than does *Loxosceles* venom. At least one protein has a cardiovascular effect, but it is highly unlikely that the bite of one tarantula would produce a deleterious cardiac response in a human.

Symptoms and Signs

Black widow spiders: A *Latrodectus* bite usually gives rise to a sharp pinprick-like pain, followed by a dull, sometimes numbing, pain in the affected extremity and by pain and some muscular rigidity in the abdomen or the shoulders, back, and chest. Associated symptoms may include pain on inspiration, headache, dizziness, ptosis, eyelid edema, skin rash and pruritus, respiratory distress, nausea, vomiting, anxiety, increased perspiration, salivation, weakness, and increased skin temperature over the affected area. Blood and CSF pressures are usually elevated, as is the Hct.

Brown or violin spiders: A *Loxosceles* bite gives rise to little or no immediate pain, but some localized pain develops within an hour or so. The bite area becomes erythematous and skin temperature is elevated. A small bleb forms, surrounded by an ischemic ring which is outlined by an erythematous ring that becomes redder and more tender in time. The lesion has the appearance of a bull's eye and often becomes larger, ruptures, and leaves an ulcer which may increase in size and involve the underlying tissues, including muscle. A black eschar forms, eventually sloughs, and leaves a large tissue defect. Pain may become severe and involve the entire injured area. Systemic symptoms and signs may develop, including nausea and vomiting, malaise, hemolysis, and thrombocytopenia.

Diagnosis

Far more common than spider bites are flea, bedbug, tick, mite, and biting fly bites; these are often mistaken for spider bites. Some arthropod bites may give rise to bullous lesions which rupture and ulcerate, resembling those produced by the violin and certain other spiders. Numerous reports of necrotic or gangrenous arachnidism attributed to *L. reclusa*, particularly in areas where this species is not usually found, are probably caused by spiders other than *Loxosceles*. Therefore, every attempt should be made to capture and identify the offending spider. If help is needed in identification, a county or state health department, poison control center, local zoo, or university department of entomology may be able to assist.

Treatment

Black widow spider: There are no first aid measures of value. An ice cube may be placed over the bite to reduce pain. All patients who are under 16 or over 60 yr, or who have hypertensive heart disease and have symptoms and signs of severe envenomation, should be hospitalized. On admission, 1 ampul of Antivenin *Latrodectus mactans* should be given IV in 10 to 50 ml of saline after the appropriate skin test. One ampul is usually sufficient. Children with severe envenomation may require respiratory assistance. Vital signs should be checked frequently during the first 12 h following the bite.

For muscle pain and spasms, 10 ml of 10% calcium gluconate may be given slowly IV. Several doses at 4-h intervals may be necessary. In adults, a relaxant, particularly methocarbamol, mephenesin, or orphenadrine citrate, given IV, is often effective; diazepam 10 mg t.i.d. has had varying degrees of success. Meperidine 50 to 100 mg, or morphine 6 to 16 mg q 6 h, may be used. Hot baths may afford relief in mild cases.

Brown or Violin Spider: Excision of the bite is recommended in proved cases of envenomation seen within several hours of the bite. Persons bitten by this spider (or by an unidentified species) who develop a skin lesion within the first 12 h that increases in size during the next 12 h should receive a corticosteroid such as dexamethasone 4 mg IM q 6 h during the acute phase, then in decremental doses in accordance with standard practice. If the patient is not seen until 48 h or more after the bite and a well-developed cutaneous lesion is present at the wound site, corticosteroids may be of little value but should be used, barring contraindications.

Ulcerating lesions should be cleansed daily with peroxide; soaked in 1:20 Burow's solution t.i.d. for 10 min; painted 3 times/wk with the aqueous triple dye used for pit viper bites (see above); and debrided as necessary. A 5% scarlet red ointment or polymyxin-bacitracin-neomycin ointment can be applied at bedtime. O_2 applied several times/day to the bite through an improvised face mask or plastic bag is of some value.

BEES, WASPS, HORNETS, ANTS

While it may take over 100 bees to inflict a lethal dose of venom in most adults, one sting can cause a fatal anaphylactic reaction in a hypersensitive person. There are 3 to 4 times more deaths in the USA from bee stings than from snake bites. In the few fatalities that have resulted from multiple bee stings, death has been attributed to acute cardiovascular collapse. The venoms of these insects contain, among other components, peptides and nonenzymatic proteins, such as apamin and melittin or kinins; enzymes, such as phospholipase A and B and hyaluronidase; and amines, such as histamine and 5-hydroxytryptamine.

Treatment

The stingers of many *Hymenoptera* may remain in the skin and should be removed by teasing or scraping rather than pulling. An ice cube placed over the sting will reduce pain; an analgesic–corticosteroid lotion is often useful. Persons with known hypersensitivity to such stings should carry a kit containing an antihistamine and epinephrine when in endemic areas. Desensitization can be carried out using insect whole-body antigens or, preferably, whole-venom antigens. (See also Ch. 19, particularly ATOPIC DISEASES, ANAPHYLAXIS, and URTICARIA.)

OTHER BITING ARTHROPODS

In the USA, a number of biting arthropods possess salivary secretions that can produce various reactions and lesions. Among the more common biting and sometimes bloodsucking arthropods are the ticks and mites; sand, horse, and deer flies; mosquitoes; fleas; lice; bedbugs; kissing bugs; and certain water bugs. The composition of the saliva of these arthropods varies considerably, and the lesion produced by their bites can vary from a small papule to a large ulcerating wound with swelling and acute pain. Dermatitis may also occur. Most serious bites are complicated by sensitivity reactions or infection. In hypersensitive persons, these bites can be fatal.

Treatment

The offending arthropod should be quickly removed. For ticks and some of the bugs, this is best accomplished by direct application of a petroleum product or other irritant to the animal. Care should be taken not to leave the capitulum in the wound, as it may induce chronic inflammation or may migrate into deeper tissues and give rise to a granuloma. The bite should be cleansed and a corticosteroid lotion applied. A piece of ice placed over the wound will usually reduce pain. Serious hypersensitivity reactions should be treated as described in Ch. 19, particularly ATOPIC DISEASES, ANAPHYLAXIS, and URTICARIA.

TICKS AND MITES

Ticks are vectors of many diseases. In addition to the reactions noted above under BITING ARTHROPODS, ticks are also involved in poisonings. In North America, some species of *Dermacentor* and *Amblyomma* cause **tick paralysis**. Symptoms and signs include anorexia, lethargy, muscle weakness, incoordination, nystagmus, and ascending flaccid paralysis. Bulbar or respiratory paralysis may develop. The bite of some *Ornithodorus* ticks ("pajaroello"), found in Mexico and southwestern USA, causes a local vesiculation, pustulation, rupture, ulceration, and eschar, with varying degrees of local swelling and pain.

Mite infestations are quite common and are responsible for "chiggers" (intensely pruritic dermatitis caused by the mite larva, or chigger), various forms of scabies, demodicidosis, and a number of other diseases. The bites produce varying degrees of local tissue reaction, with or without sensitization.

Treatment

Treatment of tick paralysis is symptomatic. O_2 and respiratory assistance may be needed. An antitoxin is presently under study. Pajaroello tick lesions should be cleansed, soaked in 1:20 Burow's solution, debrided, and painted with the aqueous triple dye used for pit viper bites (see above). Corticosteroids are of value in severe reactions. Infections are not uncommon during the ulcer stage but rarely require more than local antiseptic measures.

Mite infestations may be treated as described under SCABIES in Ch. 192.

CENTIPEDES AND MILLIPEDES

Some of the larger centipedes of the genus *Scolopendra* can inflict a painful bite, with some localized swelling and erythema. Lymphangitis and lymphadenitis are not uncommon. Necrosis is rare and infection almost unknown. Symptoms and signs seldom persist for > 48 h. The millipedes do not bite but when handled may discharge a toxic secretion that can cause local skin irritation and, in severe cases, some necrosis. Some non-USA species can spray a highly irritating repugnant secretion that may cause severe conjunctival reactions.

Treatment

An ice cube will control the pain of most centipede bites. Local infiltration of the wound with an anesthetic may be of value. Corticosteroids have been used as anti-inflammatory agents. The toxic secretions of millipedes should be washed from the skin with copious amounts of soap and water. Cleansing with alcohol should be avoided. A corticosteroid lotion or cream should be applied if a skin reaction develops. Eye injuries require immediate irrigation and the application of a corticosteroid-analgesic ointment.

SCORPIONS

The active components and modes of action of scorpion venoms vary considerably with the genus. All North American scorpions except *Centruroides sculpturatus* are relatively harmless, their stings usually causing no more than some localized pain and paresthesia with minimal swelling, some lymphangitis with regional lymph gland swelling, and an increase in skin temperature and tenderness around the wound. Vesicles may form at the injury site and some localized tissue reaction may occur. *C. sculpturatus* is found in Arizona, New Mexico, and the California side of the Colorado River. Its sting causes some immediate pain and subsequent numbness or tingling over the involved part. The injured area is often hypersensitive to touch, pressure, heat, and cold. Weakness of the extremity may occur. Moving the part may be painful and in severe cases there may be paralysis. Respiratory difficulties may develop, particularly in children. The venom can also provoke a hypertensive crisis.

Treatment

The stings of most North American scorpions require no specific treatment. An ice cube over the wound area reduces pain. Antihistamines and corticosteroids are of little value. Persons stung by *C. sculpturatus* should be observed for 24 h; children should be hospitalized. Antivenin may be required, particularly in children. The physician should consult the local poison control center for the nearest location of the antivenin. Oxygen and, in some cases, intensive care respiratory support may be needed. Atropine can be used as an anticholinergic drug. For the rare case of convulsions, IV phenobarbital can be given with caution and drugs for a hypertensive crisis should be available. Opiates and meperidine should be avoided.

MARINE ANIMALS

Stingrays cause about 750 stings/yr along the North American coasts. The venom is contained in one or more spines located on the dorsum of the animal's tail. Injuries usually occur when the unwary victim treads on the fish while wading in the ocean surf, bay, or slough. The pressure provokes the fish to thrust its tail upward and forward, driving the dorsal spine (or spines) into the victim's foot or leg. The integumentary sheath surrounding the spine is ruptured and the venom escapes into the victim's tissues, causing immediate and severe pain. While the pain is often limited to the area of injury, it may spread rapidly, reaching its greatest intensity in < 90 min, and often persists (if untreated), though gradually diminishing, for 6 to 48 h. Syncope, weakness, nausea, and anxiety are common and may be due, in part, to peripheral vasodilation. Lymphangitis, vomiting, diarrhea, sweating, generalized cramps, inguinal or axillary pain, and respiratory distress are sometimes reported. The wound is usually jagged, bleeds freely, and is often contaminated with parts of the integumentary sheath. The edges of the wound are often discolored and some localized tissue destruction may occur. Generally, there is some swelling and edema. Wound infections are rare.

Mollusks include the cones, octopuses, and bivalves. *Conus californicus* is the only dangerous cone found in North American waters. Its sting produces localized pain, swelling, redness, and numbness. The bites of North American octopuses are rarely serious. Paralytic **shellfish poisoning,** caused by eating certain bivalves that have ingested toxic dinoflagellates, is discussed under Non-bacterial Food Poisoning in Ch. 55.

Echinoderms contain several classes known to be venomous. Certain of the **sea urchins** have venom organs (globiferous pedicellariae) which have calcareous jaws capable of penetrating human skin, but injuries from these are rare. Far more common are injuries by sea urchin spines, which can break off in the skin and give rise to local tissue reactions. If not removed they may migrate into deeper tissues, causing a granulomatous nodular lesion, or they may wedge against bone or nerve. Joint and muscle pains may also occur, as well as dermatitis.

Coelenterates include the corals, sea anemones, jellyfishes, and hydroids (the Portuguese man-of-war is a colonial hydroid). Many of these animals contain a highly developed stinging unit (the nematocyst) that is capable of penetrating the skin. These are abundant on the animal's tentacles, and a single tentacle may fire hundreds of nematocysts into the skin following contact. The lesions vary with the type of coelenterate involved. Generally, the initial lesions appear as small papular eruptions in one or several discontinuous lines, at times surrounded by an erythematous zone. The papules develop rapidly and the area becomes red and raised. Pain may be severe and itching is common. The papules may vesiculate and proceed to pustulation and desquamation. Systemic manifestations include weakness, nausea, headache, muscle pain and spasms, lacrimation and nasal discharge, increased perspiration, changes in pulse rate, and chest pain that increases on respiration.

Treatment

Stingrays and most other fish stings: Injuries to an extremity should be irrigated with the salt water at hand. An attempt should be made to remove the integumentary sheath if it can be seen in the wound. The extremity should then be submerged in water as hot as the patient can tolerate without injury, for 30 to 90 min. Sodium chloride or magnesium sulfate may be added to the hot water. The wound should again be examined for remnants of the sheath, debrided, and sutured if necessary, and the appropriate antitetanus agent should be given. The injured extremity should be kept elevated for several days.

If the initial first aid measures were delayed, the injured area may be blocked with procaine. Meperidine is the drug of choice for pain. The primary shock that sometimes immediately follows stingray injuries usually responds to simple supportive measures.

Mollusks: The treatment of *Conus* stings and octopus bites is largely empirical. Local measures appear to be of little value. A tourniquet, local injection of epinephrine, and subsequent use of neostigmine have all been suggested. Severe *Conus* stings may require mechanical ventilation and measures to combat shock.

Echinoderms: Pedicellariae stings are treated by washing the area and applying an analgesic–corticosteroid cream. Sea urchin spines should be quickly removed. Vinegar dissolves most superficial spines, and soaking the wound in vinegar several times/day and covering the area with a wet vinegar compress is usually sufficient; surgery is seldom necessary. If still present after days or weeks have passed, the spine may have migrated into deeper tissues. A bluish discoloration where the spine entered the skin will aid in locating the structure, which may sometimes be seen on x-ray. Removing these spines surgically may be tedious.

Coelenterates: Various remedies for coelenterate stings have been advocated. In some parts of the world, no treatment is advised except the local application of ammonia or vinegar. In the USA, the local application of meat tenderizers (e.g., papain) is now popular. Sodium bicarbonate, boric acid, lemon juice, gasoline, alcohol, and many other agents have also been espoused, and it may be that merely changing the pH of the skin alleviates some of the symptoms. The following procedures are suggested: ocean water (not fresh water) is poured over the injured areas; the tentacles are removed, preferably with instruments or a gloved hand; alcohol is poured over the wounds and then flour, baking powder, or shaving soap (not dry sand, unless none of the others are readily available); the applied material is then scraped from the wounds with a sharp knife or instrument (not a razor) and the areas are washed again with salt water; a topical corticosteroid–analgesic is then applied, preferably by aerosol.

More serious cases require additional therapeutic measures. O_2 or respiratory assistance may be required. Painful muscle spasms may be relieved with 10 ml of 10% calcium gluconate given IV. Meperidine is preferred for pain. IV fluids and epinephrine may be needed in the few cases in which shock develops. An antivenin for the stings of certain Australian species of coelenterates is available.

INDEX

Page numbers followed by *f* indicate Figure; by *t*, Table

F